Introductory Medical-Surgical Nursing

EDITION 10

Barbara K. Timby, RN, BC, BSN, MA
Professor Emeritus
Medical-Surgical Nursing
Glen Oaks Community College
Centreville, Michigan

Nancy E. Smith, MS, RN
Professor and Chair
Department of Nursing
Southern Maine Community College
South Portland, Maine

 Wolters Kluwer | Lippincott Williams & Wilkins
Health
Philadelphia • Baltimore • New York • London
Buenos Aires • Hong Kong • Sydney • Tokyo

Executive Acquisitions Editor: Elizabeth Nieginski
Product Manager, Development Editor: Betsy Gentzler
Director of Nursing Production: Helen Ewan
Art Director, Design: Joan Wendt
Art Director, Illustration: Brett MacNaughton
Art Coordinator: Robert Galindo
Manufacturing Coordinator: Karin Duffield
Production Services: Cadmus Communication

10th Edition

9 8 7 6 5 4

Printed in China.

Library of Congress Cataloging-in-Publication Data

Timby, Barbara Kuhn.
Introductory medical-surgical nursing / Barbara K. Timby, Nancy E. Smith. – 10th ed.
  p. ; cm.
Includes bibliographical references and index.
ISBN 978-1-60547-063-4
1. Nursing. 2. Surgical nursing. I. Smith, Nancy E. (Nancy Ellen). 1949-II. Title.
[DNLM: 1. Nursing Care. 2. Perioperative Nursing. WY 150 T583i 2010]
RT41.S38 2010
610.73–dc22

2009020193

LWW.COM

This edition is dedicated to student nurses who will join the collective body of practicing nurses in making substantial contributions to combat the healthcare crises facing people in the United States and foreign countries.

BKT

For my mother, Jane Miller Wolfe Eddy, who encouraged me in countless ways to be a nurse and nurse educator, and who also taught me that caring and quality matter. I wish she were here to see one more edition.

NES

Contributors

Stephanie C. Butkus, MSN, RN, CPNP
Assistant Professor
Kettering College of Medical Arts
Kettering, Ohio
Drug Therapy Tables

Susan G. Dudek, RD, CDN, BS
Nutrition Instructor
Erie Community College
Williamsville, New York
Nutrition Notes

Debbie Faulk, PHD, RN, CNE
Associate Professor
EARN Coordinator
Auburn Montgomery School of Nursing
Montgomery, Alabama
Gerontologic Considerations

Arlene H. Morris, EDD, RN, CNE
Distinguished Teaching Associate Professor of Nursing
Auburn Montgomery School of Nursing
Montgomery, Alabama
Gerontologic Considerations

Sally S. Roach, MSN, RN, CNE, AHN-BC
Associate Professor
University of Texas at Brownsville
Brownsville, Texas
Pharmacologic Considerations

Reviewers

LaVon Barrett, MSN, RN
Assistant Professor
Coordinator Vocational Nursing
Amarillo College
Amarillo, Texas

Judith Bartels, BSN, RN, PN
Instructor
Butler Technology and Career Development Schools
Hamilton, Ohio

Terry Bichsel, BSN, RN
Practical Nursing Coordinator
Moberly Area Community College
Moberly, Missouri

Michele Blash, MSN, RN
Assistant Professor of Nursing
Hagerstown Community College
Hagerstown, Maryland

Karen Brown, PHD
Associate Dean Kirtland Community
College
Roscommon, Michigan

Victoria J. M. Brown, MSN, RN
Professor of Nursing
Jefferson College
Hillsboro, Missouri

Tamara Campbell, MSN, RN
Nursing Professor
Schoolcraft College
Livonia, Michigan

Carol Carr, MS, RN
Associate Professor
Program Head, Practical Nurse Program
J. Sargeant Reynolds Community College
Richmond, Virginia

Carla Carter
Spencerian College
Louisville, Kentucky

Mary Ann Cosgarea, BSN, BA, RN
Coordinator Portage Lakes Career Center
W Howard Nicol School of Practical
Nursing
Green, Ohio

Linda Crawford
Coastal Georgia Community College
Brunswick, Georgia

Susanne Cubberley, MSN, RN
Nurse Educator

Pinellas County Schools
Largo, Florida

Jennie C. Denker, EDDC, MSN, RN
Program Administrator
Brown Mackie College
Akron, Cincinnati, Findlay, and North Canton, Ohio

Linda Douglas
Nevada Regional Technical Center
Nevada, Missouri

Jennifer Duhon
Assistant Professer of Nursing
Illinois Central College
Peoria, Illinois

Patricia Duick
Retired, Former Director of Nurses
Bucks County Community College
Newtown, Pennsylvania

Patricia Dusek, RN
Assistant Professor
Brazosport College
Lake Jackson, Texas

Linda Elias-Thomas, BSN, RN, LT, NC, USN
Nursing Instructor
The Robert T. White School of Practical
Nursing
Alliance, Ohio

Stephanie Ellis
Practical Nursing Instructor
Moultrie Tech College
Moultrie, Georgia

Marie Fagan, MN, RN
Director
Annenberg School of Nursing
Reseda, California

Freeman BJ, MS, RN
Associate Professor
Ivy Tech Community College
Sellersburg, Indiana

Evelyn A. Grace, MSN, RN
Interim Director, Practical Nursing
Program
Bucks County Community College
Newtown, Pennsylvania

Kimberly Guard, MSN, RN
Nursing Instructor
Ivy Tech Community College – Richmond
Richmond, Indiana

Ericka Guz, BSN, MED, MSN
Associate Professor
Jefferson Community College
Steubenville, Ohio

Teresa Harden
Associate Professor
Ivy Tech State College Columbus
Columbus, Indiana

Elaine C. Hein, MS, RN
Practical Nurse Instructor
Everest College
Merrillville, Indiana

Ardyce Hill, MSN, BSN, RN
Coordinator, Outreach Practical Nursing
Western Wyoming Community College
Evanston, Wyoming

Judith Hince, MS, RN
Associate Professor
Jefferson Community College
Steubenville, Ohio

Kerri Hines, BSN, RN
Vocational Nursing Instructor
San Jacinto College
Houston, Texas

Beulah A. Hofmann, MSN, RN
Nursing Department Chairperson
Ivy Tech Community College Greencastle
Greencastle, Indiana

Jane Irwin, MSN, RN
Coordinator, Practical Nursing
Central Pennsylvania Institute of Science
and Technology
Pleasant Gap, Pennsylvania

Lenetra Jefferson
Delgado Community College
New Orleans, Louisiana

Melissa Jones, BSN, RN
Practical Nurse Coordinator
Waynesville Career Center
Waynesville, Missouri

Mariatu Kargbo, MSN, RN, CFNP
Doctoral Student
Executive Director
Global Health Nurse Training Services
Alexandria, Virginia

Dolores Kaulbach
Dallas Nursing Institute
Dallas, Texas

Francine Kirby, MSN, RN
Coordinator Practical Nursing
McDowell County Career and Technology
  Center
Welch, West Virginia
Associate Professor
Mountain State University
Welch, West Virginia

Donna M. Kuenstler, MSN, RN
Department Chair
Vocational Nursing Program
Sul Ross State University
Alpine, Texas

Karen Kulhanek, BSN, MED, RN
Nursing Instructor
Kellogg Community College
Battle Creek, Michigan

Christina Lamb, BSN, RN
Director of Practical Nursing Education
Bolivar Technical College
Bolivar, Missouri

Lynda Logan, BSN, RN
Assistant Instructor
Ivy Tech Community College
Lafayette, Indiana

Tracy Lohstroh
Nursing Instructor
Shawnee Community College
Ullin, Illinois

Karen Malloy, MSN, RN
Department Chair Allied Health Programs
San Jacinto College Central
Pasadena, Texas

Claire Marshall, BTSN, RN, CMH
Instructor
Vancouver Island University
Nanaimo, British Columbia

Linda Mollino, BSN
Practical Nursing Faculty
Rogue Community College
Medford, Oregon

Robbie L. Murphy, BSN, RN, BC-G
Instructor
San Jacinto College, North Campus
Houston, Texas

Diana L. Mustacchio, BSN, RN
Course Coordinator Level II
Clinical Coordinator
The Robert T. White School of Practical
  Nursing
Alliance, Ohio

Francine P. Pappalardo, MSN, RN
Nursing Program Curriculum Coordinator
Northern Essex Community College
Lawrence, Massachusetts

Sue Parker, MSN, APN, FNP-BC, CNOR
Assistant Professor
University of Arkansas-Fort Smith
Fort Smith, Arkansas

Mary Jane Pignatelli, BSN, ADN
Assistant Professor of Practical Nursing
Berkshire Community College
Pittsfield, Massachusetts

Rosalie M. Poyntz, MPH, EDS, RN
Department Chairperson
Health Science Department
Lindsey Hopkins Technical Educational
  Center
Miami Dade County Public Schools
Miami, Florida

Linda Reader, MED, BSN, RN
Practical Nursing Coordinator
Trumbull Career & Technical Center
Warren, Ohio

Carolyn Reese
Blinn College
Bryan, Texas

Sandra Reider, RN, BA, BSN, MSN
Associate Professor, Practical Nursing
  Program
Reading Area Community College
Reading, Pennsylvania

**Elaine M. Rissel-Muscarella, BSN,
  RN**
PNI Lead Instructor, Jamestown Site
Erie 2 Chautauqua Cattaraugus BOCES
Adult and Community Education
Jamestown, New York

Priscilla Rivera, BS, RN
Faculty, Lead Instructor
Americare Institute
Hanover Park, Illinois

Lyndi Shadbolt, MS, RN
Associate Professor, Nursing
Amarillo College
Amarillo, Texas

Gregory F. Sherrill, RN-AAS
Senior Practical Nursing Instructor
Tennessee Technology Center Crossville
Crossville, Tennessee

Cinda Siekbert, MSN, RN
Nursing Instructor
Great Oaks School of Practical Nursing
Cincinnati, Ohio

**Deborah Simmons-Johnson, MED,
  BSN, RN**
Department Chair Vocational Nursing
  Program
Houston Community College
Houston, Texas

Sherrill Sorensen
Keiser College
Miami Lakes, Florida

Russlyn St. John, MSN, RN
Professor, Practical Nursing Coordinator
St Charles Community College
Cottleville, Missouri

Lisa Streeter, BSN, RN
Instructor
Madison Oneida BOCES
Verona, New York

Lynne A. Sullivan, MS, RN
Director, Practical Nurse Program
Bristol Plymouth Regional Technical
  School
Taunton, Massachusetts

Kay Swartzwelder, MSN, RN
Director of Nursing, Collins Career Center
Director of Health Technology, Ohio Uni-
  versity Southern
Ironton, Ohio

Brigitte Thiele
Coordinator
Kennett Career and Technology Center
Kennett, Missouri

Iona Thomas-Connor, MA, RN, CNE
Associate Professor
LaGuardia Community College
Queens, New York

Sandra Thompson
Licensed Practical Nursing Staff
Mercer County Technical Education Center
Princeton, Wisconsin

Peggy Thweatt, MSN, BSN, RN
Medical Career Institute
Newport News, Virginia

Debra Tymcio
Southern Ohio College Northeast
Akron, Ohio

Alicia L. Warren, MSN, RN
Assistant Professor of Nursing
Washington State Community College
Marietta, Ohio

Christina Wilson, BAN, PHN, RN
Faculty
Anoka Technical College Practical Nursing
  Department
Anoka, Minnesota

Margaret A. Yoder, MS, MHA, RN
Associate Professor Nurse Education
Practical Nursing Program Coordinator
Quinsigamond Community College
Worcester, Massachusetts

Pamela Young, BSN, RN
Lead Instructor, Practical Nursing
Trumbull Career and Technical Center
Warren, Ohio

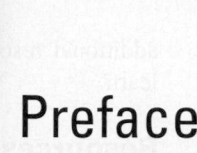

Preface

In today's changing health care environment, nurses continue to face many challenges and opportunities. *Introductory Medical-Surgical Nursing* provides the information that will help nurses meet these challenges and embrace expanding opportunities. The text addresses the common adult disorders that are treated medically and surgically and also covers basic concepts student nurses need to know to care for clients with these disorders. Written at a level appropriate for the practical/vocational nursing student, the text provides comprehensive information about medical-surgical nursing that is easy to understand.

For the 10th edition, the entire text has been reviewed, revised, and updated to reflect current medical and nursing practice. Additionally, one new chapter has been added. Chapter 70, *Caring for Clients with Eating Disorders*, is a new chapter that introduces students to the spectrum of abnormal eating problems ranging from self-starvation to binge eating and compulsive overeating. Other highlights of this edition include improved organization of the table of contents, new and updated features, and hundreds of new illustrations and photos.

ORGANIZATION OF THE TEXT

The 10th edition of *Introductory Medical Surgical Nursing* has been organized to improve readability and clarity. Unit 3, *Foundations of Medical-Surgical Nursing* and Unit 4, *Caring for Clients with Multis-System Disorders*, have been reorganized to provide a broad foundation for conditions that may accompany the care of clients with system-specific disorders in chapters that follow. The chapter entitled *Caring for Clients with Burns* is now included as part of Unit 16, *Caring for Clients with Integumentary Disorders*. The chapter on *Interaction of Body and Mind* has been relocated to Unit 17, *Caring for Clients with Psychobiologic Disorders*.

The 10th edition contains 72 chapters organized into 17 units:

- Unit 1, *Nursing Roles and Responsibilities,* includes foundational chapters covering concepts and trends in healthcare, nursing roles and settings, nursing process, interviewing and physical assessment, legal and ethical issues, and leadership and management.
- Unit 2, *Client Care Concerns,* explores areas in which nurses interact and work with clients to manage their health. Topics include nurse–client relationships, culture, complementary and alternative therapies, and end-of-life care.

- Unit 3, *Foundations of Medical-Surgical Nursing*, includes chapters on frequent and regular topics in medical-surgical nursing care. These include pain, infection, intravenous therapy, perioperative care, and disasters.
- Unit 4, *Caring for Clients with Multisystem Disorders,* includes chapters on fluid, electrolyte, and acid–base imbalances; shock; and cancer.
- Units 5 through 16 present information on disorders according to body systems. Each unit begins with an introductory chapter that includes a general review of anatomy and physiology, a discussion of client assessment, and common diagnostic and laboratory tests that pertain to particular disorders.
- Unit 17, *Caring for Clients with Psychobiologic Disorders,* contains chapters on frequently encountered emotional and behavioral issues: anxiety disorders, mood disorders, eating disorders, chemical dependency, and dementia and thought disorders.

At the end of the text, Appendix A provides a list of useful *Nursing Resources*, Appendix B lists *Commonly Used Abbreviations and Acronyms*, and Appendix C provides a convenient reference for *Laboratory Values*. A *Glossary* provides a quick reference to definitions for Words to Know that appear throughout the text. The text concludes with a comprehensive listing of *References and Suggested Readings*, including general recommendations as well as unit-specific citations, that provides a streamlined guide to current literature about topics discussed in the text. A quick reference to the most current *NANDA-Approved Nursing Diagnoses* is printed on the inside back cover to help students become familiar with the expanding taxonomy of problems that falls within nursing's domain.

FEATURES AND LEARNING TOOLS

The 10th edition includes new and updated features, as well as many features that long-time users of Timby and Smith love:

- *NEW!* **A full-color art program** offers a brilliant design and **more than 300 new full-color photographs and illustrations** to assist visual learners and enhance readers' interest.
- **Words to Know** listed at the beginning of each chapter are set in bold type within the text where they appear with or near their definition. Additional technical terms are italicized throughout the text.

- **Learning Objectives** at the beginning of each chapter help focus the student's reading and identify important information to learn in each chapter.
- **Stop, Think, and Respond Exercises,** appearing within the flow of chapter text, ask students to consider scenarios related to pertinent topics and to respond quickly based on their understanding. The exercises are numbered for quick reference, with answers provided for students and instructors on thePoint at http://thePoint.lww.com/Timby MedSurg10e.
- **Drug Therapy Tables** address the major categories of medications prescribed for common disorders. They include drug categories, examples of generic and trade names, mechanisms of action, common side effects, and nursing considerations. They reinforce the beginning student's knowledge of drug therapy and coordinate pharmacology for students whose nursing curricula integrate this content.
- **Client and Family Teaching** displays found throughout clinical chapters highlight important education points for nurses to communicate to clients and their families.
- **Nursing Guidelines** present essential information nurses need to perform specific nursing skills or to manage care for a client with a particular disorder.
- **Nursing Process** sections accompany major disorders and emphasize the importance of the nursing process. These sections clearly distinguish each step of the process. Interventions describe not only what to do, but why, with rationales provided in italics.
- **Nursing Care Plans** provide detailed examples of nursing-focused management for clients with such diverse issues and problems as Alzheimer's disease, cancer, myocardial infarction, cerebrovascular accident, diabetes mellitus, modified radical mastectomy, and chronic renal failure. More than 30 care plans are included. (See Quick Reference to Nursing Care Plans on p. xxiv.)
- *NEW!* **Nutrition Notes** in new, special displays, present information about diet and nutrition that the nurse should consider when caring for clients with specific conditions.
- **Pharmacologic Considerations** and **Gerontologic Considerations,** written by experts in their fields, demonstrate how nursing care is multidisciplinary. *NEW* to this edition is an integrated format that presents these considerations within the context of relevant chapter discussion.
- **Critical Thinking Exercises** at the end of each chapter facilitate application of chapter material, using clinical situations or rhetorical questions. *NEW* questions have been added so that each chapter includes at least four exercises. Suggested answers are provided on thePoint at http://thePoint.lww.com/Timbymedsurg10e.
- *NEW!* **NCLEX-Style Review Questions** added to the end of each chapter help students apply their knowledge and prepare for multiple choice and alternative item formats on the NCLEX-PN. Answers are provided on thePoint at http://thePoint.lww.com/TimbyMedSurg10E so students can check their learning.

TEACHING–LEARNING PACKAGE

The 10th edition of *Introductory Medical-Surgical Nursing* features a compelling and comprehensive complement of additional resources to help instructors teach and students learn.

Resources for Instructors

Tools to assist you with teaching your course are available upon adoption of this text on thePoint at http://thePoint.lww.com/TimbyMedSurg10e and on the Instructor's Resource DVD:

- The **Test Generator** lets you put together exclusive new tests from a bank containing hundreds of questions to help you in assessing your students' understanding of the material.
- An extensive collection of materials is provided for each book chapter:
  - **Pre-Lecture Quizzes** (and answers) are quick, knowledge-based assessments that allow you to check students' reading.
  - **PowerPoint Presentations** provide an easy way for you to integrate the textbook with your students' classroom experience, either via slide shows or handouts. Multiple-choice and true/false questions are integrated into the presentations to promote class participation and allow you to use i-clicker technology.
  - **Guided Lecture Notes** walk you through the chapters, objective by objective, and provide you with corresponding PowerPoint slide numbers.
  - **Discussion Topics** (and suggested answers) can be used as conversation starters or in online discussion boards.
  - **Assignments** (and suggested answers) include group, written, clinical, and web assignments.
  - **Case Studies** with related questions (and suggested answers) give students an opportunity to apply their knowledge to a client case similar to one they might encounter in practice.
- An **Image Bank** lets you use the photographs and illustrations from this textbook in your PowerPoint slides or as you see fit in your course.
- **Answers to Questions in the Book** (Stop, Think, and Respond Exercises; Critical Thinking Exercises; and NCLEX-Style Review Questions) are provided for each chapter.
- A **sample syllabus** provides guidance for structuring your medical-surgical nursing course.
- **Journal Articles** offer access to current research available in Lippincott Williams & Wilkins journals.

Resources for Students

An exciting set of free resources is available to help students review material and become even more familiar with vital concepts. Students can access all these resources on thePoint at http://thePoint.lww.com/TimbyMedSurg10e using the codes printed in the front of their textbooks. Many of these resources are also available on the CD-ROM bound in this textbook. Resources include the following:

- **NCLEX-Style Review Questions** for each chapter help students review important concepts and practice for NCLEX.
- **End-of-Unit Exercises** offer additional opportunities to review and apply content from each unit of the textbook.

Activities include true/false, fill-in-the-blank, and short answer questions.

- **Concepts in Action Animations** bring physiologic and pathophysiologic concepts to life and enhance student learning. Icons appear throughout the text to direct students to relevant animations.
- **Answers to Questions in the Book** (Stop, Think, and Respond Exercises; Critical Thinking Exercises; and NCLEX-Style Review Questions) are available to allow students to check their knowledge and understanding.
- A **Spanish–English Audio Glossary** provides helpful terms and phrases for communicating with clients who speak Spanish.

- **Journal Articles** offer access to current research available in Lippincott Williams & Wilkins journals.

Student Workbook

The *Workbook to Accompany Introductory Medical-Surgical Nursing, 10th edition,* has been updated to provide an engaging review of important material and is available for purchase. Featuring images from the text, **review exercises, application activities,** and more **NCLEX-style practice questions,** the Workbook complements this textbook and reinforces the information students need to learn. Answers to the Workbook questions are provided for instructors on thePoint and on the Instructor's Resource DVD.

Acknowledgments

The authors wish to thank all those who helped in the preparation of this edition. We remain grateful to the skilled and knowledgeable professionals at Lippincott Williams & Wilkins. Although we never met most of them, we appreciate their expert ability to keep us on track and in turn respond to our many requests and needs as this textbook was in production. We would like to personally thank Elizabeth Nieginski, Executive Acquisitions Editor. Our immense thanks go to Betsy Gentzler, Development Editor and Product Manager, who manages the work of revisions ably and efficiently, providing great guidance and oversight. Betsy has an amazing ability to see the whole picture, which was particularly useful when we were focused on parts. The 10th edition reflects her attention to excellence and quality.

We appreciate the efforts of Laura Scott, Senior Editorial Assistant, for coordinating numerous project details. To Ruth Einstein, Project Manager at Cadmus Communications, we appreciate the work on the final editing and proof process.

We hope that *Introductory Medical-Surgical Nursing,* 10th edition, provides the readers with the practical knowledge and skills to manage the nursing care of clients in today's changing health care environments. We also hope that our contributions provide students with similar joys and rewards that we have experienced in our nursing careers.

Barbara K. Timby, RN, BC, BSN, MA
Nancy E. Smith, MS, RN

Contents

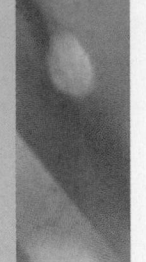

Quick Reference to Nursing Care Plans

UNIT 1
Nursing Roles and Responsibilities

1

Concepts and Trends in Healthcare

Words To Know

capitation
client
clinical pathways
diagnosis-related group (DRG)
disease
early detection
health
healthcare delivery system
healthcare team
health maintenance
health maintenance organization (HMO)
health promotion
holism
illness
illness prevention
integrated delivery system
managed care organization (MCO)
morbidity
mortality
physician hospital organization (PHO)
point-of-service (POS)
preferred provider organization (PPO)
primary care
prospective payment system (PPS)
secondary care
tertiary care
wellness

Learning Objectives

On completion of this chapter, you will be able to:

1. Explain the concepts of health, holism, wellness, illness, disease, and the health-illness continuum.
2. Describe how clients with chronic illness may still be considered healthy.
3. Differentiate health maintenance and health promotion.
4. Identify members of the healthcare team.
5. Describe three levels of care that the healthcare delivery system provides.
6. Describe problems related to access to healthcare.
7. Describe Medicare, Medicaid, and Medigap insurance.
8. Explain how a prospective payment system (PPS) works.
9. Explain how the different types of managed care organizations work.
10. Discuss the difference between capitation and fee-for-service insurance.
11. Discuss the effects of cost-driven changes on healthcare.
12. Discuss methods for monitoring quality of care.
13. Describe national and worldwide healthcare campaigns designed to improve healthcare and healthcare outcomes.
14. Identify trends that influence future healthcare policy.

The roles of nurses in the healthcare delivery system are multiple and complex. Nurses collect data, diagnose human responses to health problems, plan and provide care, and evaluate outcomes of care. They work in various settings, adhering to facility policies and state nurse practice acts. Nurses educate clients, families, and staff; manage resources; and act as advocates for clients. In addition, they participate in disease prevention and health promotion activities for clients, families, and communities.

CONCEPTS RELATED TO HEALTH

Health and Wellness

The constitution of the World Health Organization (WHO) defines **health** as "a state of complete physical, mental, and social well-being and not merely the absence of disease and infirmity" (WHO, www.who.int, 2007). Although this definition of health is useful, it presents health and illness in absolute terms: if a person is not functioning optimally in every way, he or she is not healthy. It also implies that an infirmity negates the possibility of health. Nurses practice from the perspective of holism. **Holism** means viewing a person's health as a balance of body, mind, and spirit. Treating only the body will not necessarily restore optimal health. In addition to physical needs, nurses must also consider clients' psychological, sociocultural, developmental, and spiritual needs.

Wellness describes a state of being. It is a constant and intentional effort to stay healthy and achieve the highest potential for total well-being. It requires life-style choices that assist individuals to strive for and maintain a balance in their physical, occupational/leisure, environmental, intellectual, spiritual, and emotional/social domains. Activities and choices should help individuals to promote good physical self-care, prevent illness and injury, use one's full intellectual potential, express appropriate emotions in response to changes and others' behaviors, manage stress, and maintain positive interpersonal relationships. As with health and illness, one's determination of a state of wellness is highly individual.

Illness and Disease

Theoretically, **illness** refers to a state of being sick. Illness may be viewed as catastrophic (sudden, traumatic), acute, chronic, or terminal. **Disease** refers to a pathologic condition of the body that presents with clinical signs and symptoms and changes in laboratory values. The term *disease* has related terminology and concepts. Table 1-1 provides a list of these terms with brief definitions.

The major difference between illness and disease is that illness is highly individual and personal, whereas disease is something more definitive and measurable. For example, a client with arthritis presents with distinct pathologic changes associated with the disease. A person, however, may or may not be ill with arthritis. The degrees of pain, suffering, and immobility vary with each person.

The Health-Illness Continuum

In contrast to definitions of health and illness, the health-illness continuum considers level of health, which continually changes for each person. The health-illness continuum illustrates this process of change, in which individuals face various states of health and illness, ranging from extremely good health to death (Fig. 1-1). Within this continuum, clients adapt physically, emotionally, and socially, enabling maintenance of comfort, stability, and self-expression. Therefore, clients with chronic illness can achieve a high level of wellness if they can experience a high quality of life within the limits of that illness. For example, physically disabled people are considered healthy if they are physiologically stable and engaged in personal and social activities that they find meaningful.

Health Maintenance and Promotion

Many people now believe they have control over their well-being and are taking more responsibility for their health status. **Health maintenance** refers to protecting one's current level of health by preventing illness or deterioration, such as by complying with medication regimens, being screened for diseases such as breast and colon cancers, or practicing safe sex. **Health promotion** refers to engaging in strategies to enhance health. Such strategies include eating a diet high in grains and complex carbohydrates, exercising regularly, balancing work with leisure activities, and practicing stress-reduction techniques. **Illness prevention** involves identifying risk factors such as a family history of hypertension or diabetes and reducing the effects of risk factors on one's health. In addition, **early detection** uses screening diagnostic tests and procedures to identify a disease process earlier, so that treatment may be initiated earlier and be more effective. Examples include mammography and colonoscopy (Chitty, 2007).

A **client** is an active partner in nursing care. Thus, the person receiving healthcare services no longer plays a passive, ill role but is an active purchaser of healthcare services. The use of the term *client* in this textbook reflects the attitude

TABLE 1-1 Disease-Related Terminology

TERM	DEFINITION
Etiology	The cause of a disease
Incidence	The frequency of a particular disease in a specific population during a specific period
Morbidity	The number of sick persons with a particular disease in a specific population
Mortality	The death rate or the ratio of the number of deaths for a specific population
Pathophysiology	Study of how disease alters normal physiologic processes
Prevalence	The number of cases of a disease in a specific population during a specific period
Primary prevention	Prevention of the development of disease in a susceptible or potentially susceptible population; includes health promotion and immunization
Secondary prevention	Early diagnosis and treatment to shorten duration and severity of an illness, reduce contagion, and limit complications
Sign	Objective manifestation of a disease; can be seen, heard, measured, or felt
Symptom	Subjective manifestation of a disease or illness; what the client relates is happening
Tertiary prevention	Healthcare to limit the degree of disability or promote rehabilitation in chronic, irreversible diseases

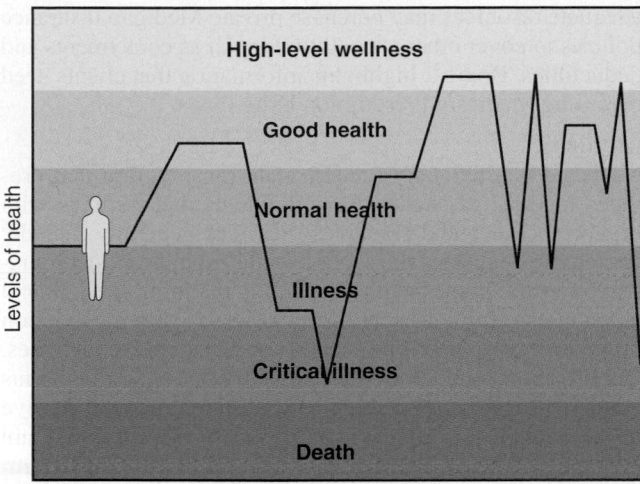

FIGURE 1-1. The health-illness continuum.

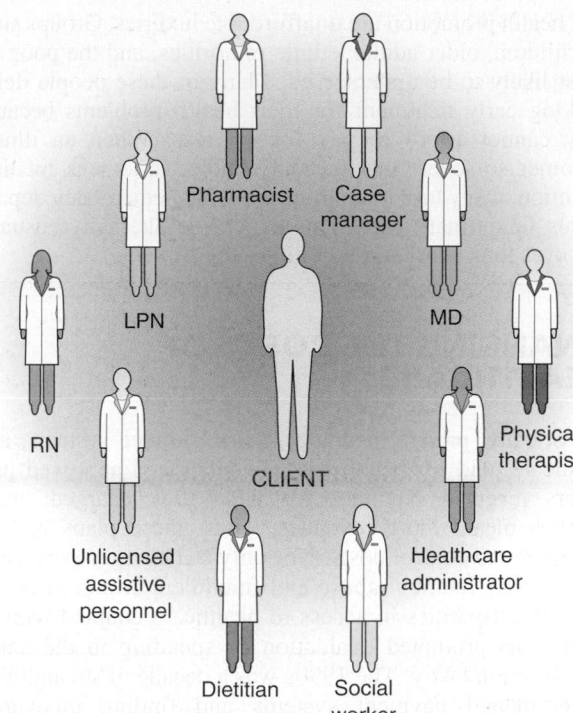

FIGURE 1-2. Members of the healthcare team.

of personal responsibility for health. Clients may or may not be ill, but they take great responsibility for meeting their health maintenance and promotion needs and actively participate in treatment decisions regarding health restoration.

> ▶ *Stop, Think, and Respond Exercise 1-1*
>
> *A homeless client, who collapsed on the street, is brought to the emergency room by the local police for treatment. Without knowing the actual diagnosis, what factors related to health and illness concepts may have contributed to this client's poor health?*

HEALTHCARE

Just as the concept of health has changed in recent decades, so too has the healthcare industry. Rapid advances in science and technology have contributed to the development of highly sophisticated methods for diagnosing and treating disease. At the same time, escalating healthcare costs have created difficult economic conditions, disparity in access to care, and brief lengths of stays in hospitals. The healthcare system has grown to include multiple outpatient, short-term, and long-term care facilities with care given by various providers.

Healthcare Providers

The **healthcare team** consists of specially trained personnel who work together to help clients meet their healthcare needs. The team includes physicians, nurses, psychologists, pharmacists, dietitians, social workers, respiratory and physical therapists, occupational therapists, nursing assistants, technicians, and insurance company staff (Fig. 1-2). All members of this team collaborate on client issues (medical, social, and financial) to achieve the best possible outcomes.

The Healthcare Delivery System

The **healthcare delivery system** refers to the full range of services available to people seeking prevention, identification, treatment, or rehabilitation of health problems. The first resource person or agency that clients contact about a health

need provides **primary care**. This initial contact is often with a family practitioner, internist, or nurse practitioner. **Secondary care** includes referrals to facilities for additional testing such as cardiac catheterization, consultation, and diagnosis. **Tertiary care** is provided in hospitals where specialists and complex technology are available.

In addition to their roles at the settings already mentioned, nurses provide care in a variety of other settings. Skilled nursing care occurs in facilities or units that offer prolonged health maintenance or rehabilitative services, such as long-term care or extended-care facilities. Examples include nursing homes, skilled nursing facilities, rehabilitation centers, and subacute care units. Home care is an important adjunct to inpatient care; visiting nurses and home health aides make earlier discharge to home possible by providing services formerly done in hospitals or long-term care facilities. Hospices and home hospice care are resources for terminally ill clients and their families.

> ▶ *Stop, Think, and Respond Exercise 1-2*
>
> *A client in an acute tertiary care setting is ready for discharge. This client will require follow up for wound care. Discuss two possibilities for how this can be managed.*

Access to Care

As the types of health services expand, the healthcare delivery system becomes more complex, costly, and, in many cases, inaccessible. An estimated 44.8 million U.S. citizens (more than 1 in 7) do not have access to healthcare because of the economic burden it poses (U.S. Census Bureau, 2005). Another estimated 30 million citizens have inadequate healthcare coverage. For many, health maintenance and health promotion are unaffordable luxuries. Groups such as children, older adults, ethnic minorities, and the poor are most likely to be underserved. Many of these people delay seeking early treatment for their health problems because they cannot afford to pay for services. When an illness becomes so severe that the only choice is to seek medical attention, many turn to their local hospital emergency departments for primary care. This expensive alternative usually involves long waits and no follow-up care.

FINANCING THE COSTS OF HEALTHCARE

Historically, private insurance, self-insurance systems, and Medicare paid for healthcare. Hospitals and approved providers received payment for what they charged; more charges meant more revenues. Thus, these plans had no incentives to control costs. Not only did charges escalate at an alarming rate, but abuse and fraudulent billing escalated as well. Disparities in access to healthcare coupled with its high costs prompted evaluation of spending in the entire healthcare industry. The 1990s was a decade of streamlining governmental payment systems and finding innovative approaches from private insurers and corporate health plans.

Government-Funded Healthcare

In 1965, federal legislation created Medicare and Medicaid.

Medicare

Medicare is a federally run program financed primarily through employee payroll taxes. It covers individuals who are 65 years of age or older, permanently disabled workers of any age with specific disabilities, and persons with end-stage renal disease. Medicare has several parts (Medicare and You, 2008):

- Part A—Covers hospital care, skilled care, hospice, and home health services; may require participants to pay $423.00 per month for this coverage if they did not pay Medicare taxes when they were working.
- Part B—Covers physician services, outpatient care, and other selected services not covered under Part A; requires an annual $135.00 deductible and a monthly premium of $96.40, which may be adjusted based on income.
- Part C, Medicare Advantage Plan—Combines Parts A and B and sometimes Part D as well. Private insurance companies approved by Medicare manage these plans and may implement different premiums, copays, coinsurance, or deductibles.
- Part D, Medicare Prescription Drug Coverage—Helps to cover and possibly reduce prescription drug costs and protect against catastrophic drug expenses. Premiums vary depending on the plan manager and a person's income.

Clients on Social Security automatically participate in Part A, whereas the other parts are optional. Although Medicare is primarily for older Americans, it does not cover long-term care and limits coverage for health promotion and illness prevention. The increased costs of Medicare coupled with decreases in benefits make the program prohibitively expensive for many older adults. Those people with adequate resources may purchase private Medigap insurance policies to cover other expenditures such as copayments and deductibles. Box 1-1 highlights information that clients need regarding Medicare Prescription Drug Plans.

Medicaid

Medicaid is a federally funded, state-run program that provides medical assistance for individuals and families with limited incomes and resources. Services generally include: doctor and dentist services; clinic and hospital services; nursing home and home healthcare; family planning services and prenatal care; pediatric care; mental healthcare; prescription drug coverage; and optometrist services and eyeglasses. Qualifications vary from state to state, but typically clients qualify if they: have children and a limited income; receive or are eligible for Supplemental Security Income (SSI); are pregnant women who meet income requirements; have family assets of less than $2,000; or receive adoption assistance or foster care assistance. Older adults who cannot afford Medicare may qualify for Medicaid.

Prospective Payment Systems

In 1983, Medicare implemented a **prospective payment system (PPS)** in an attempt to control costs. A PPS is a method of reimbursement in which healthcare providers receive payment for services based on a predetermined, fixed rate. The payment amount for a particular service is derived from the classification system of that service. One

---

| **BOX 1-1** | **Medicare Prescription Drug Coverage, 2008** |

Who is eligible for a Medicare Prescription Drug Plan (PDP)?
Everyone enrolled in Medicare.

When does a client join?
The client must join when first eligible for Medicare or wait for the enrollment period and pay a late penalty fee. If a client is unable to do this himself or herself, Medicare will enroll that person.

What types of PDP plans are there?
- *Medicare PDP:*
  - Original Medicare Plan
  - Medicare Cost Plan
  - Medicare Private Fee-For-Service (PFFS)
  - Medicare Medical Savings Account (MSA)
- *Medicare Advantage Plan:* A plan for clients with Medicare Parts A, B, and D that includes prescription drug care; sometimes called MA-PDs.

What needs to be considered when selecting a plan?
- Does the plan include the client's prescription drugs?
- What are the costs, such as premiums, deductibles, or co-payments?
- Does the client's preferred pharmacy accept the plan?

Source: Centers for Medicare and Medicaid Services (2008). *Medicare & You.* www.medicare.gov/publications

classification system for inpatient hospital services uses **diagnosis-related groups (DRG)** to group services for clients with similar diagnoses. For example, all clients receiving a hip, knee, or shoulder replacement fall into DRG 209, Total Joint Replacement, and their surgeries are reimbursed at basically the same rate. Other classification systems may be used for other healthcare services. Private insurers may use DRGs or other classification systems for reimbursement.

PPSs are largely responsible for the marked decreases in hospital lengths of stay since the early 1980s. Possible premature discharge of clients and increased responsibility for family members who may be unable to provide adequate care has created much criticism of PPS. These systems have also caused shifts in costs from clients with Medicare to those who have private insurance. Providers charge privately insured clients inflated amounts to make up for losses in Medicare revenues. In response to this cost shifting and other economic forces, insurers have challenged hospital charges aggressively, refused payment when hospital level of care is not provided, and shifted their clients into cost-containment reimbursement systems known as *managed care.*

Managed Care

Managed care organizations (MCOs) are insurers who carefully plan and closely supervise the distribution of healthcare services. Although it is a business venture that emphasizes costs of services and economic use of resources, managed care focuses on prevention as the best way to manage healthcare costs (Box 1-2). The two most common types of managed care systems are health maintenance organizations (HMOs) and preferred provider organizations (PPOs). Two other models—point-of-service (POS) plans and physician hospital organizations (PHOs)—are becoming more prominent.

Health Maintenance Organizations

A **health maintenance organization (HMO)** is a group insurance plan in which participants pay a preset, fixed fee in exchange for healthcare services. The fee is not based on the number of services provided, but rather is projected to the number of participants and expected services. This type of financial management is referred to as **capitation**, which refers to the actual head or person count. Physicians have an incentive to keep costs low because the fee paid to the physicians remains the same regardless of the actual services or frequency of care provided. The financial stability of HMOs is based on their ability to keep their members healthy and out of the hospital through periodic screening, health education, and preventive services. Participant fees cover all medical costs incurred and are paid regardless of whether members require healthcare services. If they do not require much high-cost care, providers make money; if members use many high-cost resources, providers lose money. This method of financing provides the strongest incentives for limiting use of expensive services and focusing healthcare on health maintenance and health promotion.

Health maintenance organizations provide ambulatory, hospitalization, and home care services. Some HMOs have their own facilities; others use community agencies for services. Members of an HMO must receive authorization (referral) for secondary care, such as second opinions from specialists or diagnostic testing. If members obtain unauthorized care, they are responsible for the entire bill. In this way, HMOs serve as gatekeepers for healthcare services.

Preferred Provider Organizations

A **preferred provider organization (PPO)** operates on the principle that competition can control costs. Acting as agents for health insurance companies, PPOs create a community network of providers who are willing to discount their fees for service in exchange for a steady stream of referred customers. Consumers can lower their healthcare costs if they receive care from the preferred providers. If they select providers outside the network, they pay a higher percentage of the costs.

Point-of-Service Plans

Point-of-service (POS) organizations involve a network of providers. Clients select a primary care physician within the group who then serves as the gatekeeper for other healthcare services. Clients can use healthcare providers in or out of the provider group but may pay additional fees, such as a higher deductible or copayment, for providers outside the group, unless the primary physician approves. Benefits for the insurer include discounted services, reduced services, and elimination of unnecessary referrals (Chitty, 2007).

Physician Hospital Organizations

Physician hospital organizations (PHOs) evolved as a result of the financial concerns of hospitals and physician practices. The PHO creates a corporate structure between hospitals and groups of physicians—they contract with a managed care organization to negotiate fees for services for their self-insured employees (Chitty, 2007). The goals are to maintain high quality service and contain costs, while fostering group contracts, collaboration, and capitation.

> ### ▶ *Stop, Think, and Respond Exercise 1-3*
>
> *An older client tells you that he receives Social Security benefits, but is not clear about his Medicare benefits. What information would you provide to this client?*

CHANGES AND TRENDS IN HEALTHCARE

Effects of Cost-Driven Changes

Changes in reimbursement structures and practices have created a shift in economic and decision-making power from hospitals, nurses, and physicians to insurers. Much concern and criticism accompany this shift, as physicians, nurses,

---

> **BOX 1-2 Goals of Managed Care**
>
> - Use healthcare resources efficiently
> - Deliver high-quality care at a reasonable cost
> - Measure, monitor, and manage fiscal and client outcomes
> - Prevent illness through screening and health promotion activities
> - Provide client education to decrease risk of disease
> - Case manage clients with chronic illness to minimize number of hospitalizations

other providers, and consumers find themselves unable to obtain or provide care free from the insurer's economic pressures. As a result of managed care's influence, hospitals have downsized, restructured, or sometimes closed. Consequently, many regions are left with fewer hospitals, higher nurse/client ratios, and higher client acuity levels on general medical–surgical units, skilled nursing facilities, long-term care facilities, and home health settings. Thus, many claim that profits posted by large insurance companies come at the expense of quality care and jobs of healthcare providers. Box 1-3 summarizes some of the economic issues and trends.

Changes in the healthcare industry have also affected employment for healthcare workers. Hospitals employ unlicensed assistive personnel (UAPs) to perform some duties that practical and registered nurses once provided. Many are concerned that the use of UAPs will jeopardize quality of care. In addition, physicians' income decreased in recent years. This trend will most likely continue, partly because of the growth of nurse practitioners and physician assistants. The predicted decreased income may lead to fewer men and women entering the medical profession. Rural areas already suffering with inadequate numbers of physicians will not see an improvement in this situation.

These changes also may affect the client's experience and satisfaction with healthcare. A single episode of illness can involve negotiating for a referral, receiving testing at a site other than the hospital, staying a shorter time in the hospital, transferring to a skilled nursing facility, and obtaining outpatient rehabilitation and home health services. Although much effort is made to coordinate care, particularly by nurse case managers (see Chap. 2), this fragmentation forces clients to repeatedly build therapeutic relationships and may leave them unsure of who is in charge.

Cost-driven changes have had positive effects as well. In an attempt to reduce redundancy of healthcare services and increase economic leverage, hospitals and other healthcare facilities are forming networks known as **integrated delivery systems (IDCs)** (Box 1-4). IDCs provide a full

---

BOX 1-4 | **Integrated Delivery Systems**

Fully integrated healthcare delivery systems will provide:
- Wellness programs
- Preventive care
- Ambulatory care
- Outpatient diagnostic and laboratory services
- Emergency care
- General and tertiary hospital services
- Rehabilitation
- Long-term care
- Assisted-living facilities
- Psychiatric care
- Home healthcare services
- Hospice care
- Outpatient pharmacies

---

range of healthcare services with a goal of achieving highly coordinated and cost-effective care. Mandated shorter hospital stays may result in fewer nosocomial (acquired in the hospital) complications and a quicker return to self-care. Nurses have a greater ability to take an active role in advocating for high-quality, nurse-provided care. Nurses work in new and expanded positions in the healthcare industry (see Chap. 2). There is also increased attention to monitoring quality and best practices in healthcare.

Measures of Quality of Care

Demand for evidence that hospitals and practitioners provide high-quality, cost-effective care comes from insurers, regulatory bodies such as The Joint Commission, and consumers. To meet this demand, hospitals form performance improvement committees. These groups or hospital departments also may be called *quality improvement* or *outcomes management committees*. These committees use standardized indicators to measure healthcare quality.

One example of standardized indicators are the Quality Indicators (QIs) provided by the Agency for Healthcare

---

BOX 1-3 | **Economic Issues and Trends**

From:		To:
Illness/crisis emphasis	→	Preventive emphasis
Acute care	→	Preventive, home care
Hospital/institution-based	→	Non-institution–based (clinic/home)
Fee-for-service (cost-based)	→	Prospective payment and managed care
Physician-directed	→	Diverse decision-makers and managed care
If it helps, use it (regardless of cost)	→	Outcomes measurement and cost-effectiveness
Independent decisions	→	Protocols/guidelines (best practices)
Local perspective	→	Global perspective (protocols/guidelines/practice)
Introduce new technologies	→	Outcomes measurement and cost-effectiveness
Paper records, medical charts	→	Information systems, computer records
Specific, specialist	→	Holistic
Quantity of care	→	Quality of care
Retrospective payment	→	Prospective payment
Fee-for-service	→	Managed care

Adapted from Cherry B., & Jacob, S. R. (2008). *Contemporary nursing issues, trends, and management* (4th ed.). St. Louis, MO, Elsevier Mosby.

Research and Quality (AHRQ). These QIs can be used to measure healthcare quality at the federal, state, and local levels. Although specifically for use by hospitals, similar tools for other healthcare organizations are used or are in process. The AHRQ uses hospital administrative data to highlight potential quality concerns, identify areas that need further study and investigation, and track changes over time. The AHRQ QIs consist of the following four modules (AHRQ, 2008):

- Prevention QIs, which identify hospital admissions that could be avoided through high-quality outpatient care
- Inpatient QIs, which reflect quality of care inside hospitals, including inpatient mortality for medical conditions and surgical procedures
- Patient safety QIs, which also reflect quality of care within hospitals, but focus on potentially avoidable complications and iatrogenic events
- Pediatric QIs, which reflect quality of care inside hospitals and identify potentially avoidable hospitalizations among children

The Joint Commission has also established national patient safety goals (NPSG), which are updated annually. As described by Rafter and Keown (2006), "These goals have helped nurses change how they identify patients, prepare them for surgery, monitor their care, and protect them from preventable adverse events (such as infections or falls)." Some of the goals for 2009 include: improving the accuracy of client identification; improving the safety of using medications; reducing the risk of healthcare–associated infections; reconciling medications across the continuum of care; reducing the risk of client harm resulting from falls, influenza and pneumococcal disease in institutionalized older adults, and from surgical fires; and improving recognition and response to changes in a client's condition (The Joint Commission, 2008).

As concern for cost meets concern for quality, practitioners search for ways to ensure that they accomplish all care, teaching, and preparation before the client discharge date without overusing expensive resources. Stemming from such concerns, protocols (also known as *guidelines* or *standards*) for managing care have been developed. Multidisciplinary teams use **clinical pathways** or care mapping for specific diagnoses or procedures, which standardize important aspects of care such as diagnostic work-ups, nursing care, education, physical therapy, and discharge planning across the estimated length of stay. By analyzing variances from the pathway (unexpected events such as delayed discharge or transfer to a more intensive level of care), clinicians can identify trends that are beneficial or detrimental. The team who develops the pathway can then redesign care to address the identified trend. Clinical pathways often are considered a tool of case management (see Chap. 2). Figure 1-3 is an example of a clinical pathway for a client with pneumonia.

Many other methods exist for determining quality of care. Patient satisfaction surveys, quality-of-life questionnaires, functional assessment tools, number of hospital admissions per year for clients with chronic illnesses, and morbidity (complications) and mortality (deaths) rates are a few important measures assessed when examining quality.

Future Trends and Goals for Healthcare

The healthcare system will continue to respond to changes in the demographics and cultural diversity, as well as technological innovations and the impact of the shortage of nurses. It is predicted that the number of people over the age of 65 years will exceed 20% of the U.S. population by 2030 (U.S. Census Bureau, 2000). In addition, it is predicted that 40% of the population in 2030 will be ethnic minority groups. Concern remains regarding the health of all Americans. Several initiatives are directed at promoting health and monitoring progress toward health goals and prevention of treatable problems, as well as actual treatment of illness without complications.

The United States Department of Health and Human Services (2005) has identified national health goals. *Healthy People 2010* provides an overall action plan to improve the health and quality of life for people living in the United States. The plan describes two broad goals (U.S. Department of Health and Human Services, 2005):

- Increase quality and years of healthy life
- Eliminate health disparities

The Healthy People initiative targets the improvement of health for all. It promotes a systematic approach to health improvement by setting goals, objectives, determinants of health, and general health status. Focus areas include specific concerns, such as diseases (diabetes, arthritis), environmental issues (environmental health, food safety), and social issues (substance abuse, family planning). In addition, the *Healthy People 2010* initiative developed leading health indicators for measuring the overall health of the U.S. population (Box 1-5). These include outcomes for health and disease, preventive health behaviors, indicators of mental health, access to healthcare, and ecologic factors such as injuries and deaths related to firearms. The initiative includes 467 measurable objectives designed to improve Americans' health. Data are provided from healthcare agencies at all levels to the National Center for Health Statistics (NCHS) Progress reports are available quarterly and annually. A final report will be released in 2010, and work is already underway for *Healthy People 2020* (Office of Disease Prevention and Health Prevention, 2008).

Another initiative, called the *100,000 Lives Campaign,* was launched in 2004 by the Institute for Healthcare Improvement (IHI), in an effort to reduce preventable deaths in U.S. hospitals. With the participation of 3100 hospitals, an estimated 122,000 lives were saved within an 18-month time period. The IHI extended this campaign to the *5 Million Lives Campaign*, with a goal of protecting clients from 5 million incidents of harm between December 2006 and December 2008. The primary aim of this effort was to "support the improvement of medical care in the U.S., significantly reducing current levels of morbidity … and mortality" (Institute for Healthcare Improvement, 2008).

As the 21st century progresses, economics, consumer satisfaction, effectiveness of traditional medical care, alternative medicine, disease prevalence, global emergence of drug-resistant organisms, and cultural diversity are forces that influence the direction of worldwide healthcare. The continued effects of infectious diseases on global health, particularly in developing nations, and epidemics of cancer and

EMERGENCY DEPARTMENT CLINICAL PATH: PNEUMONIA Exclusion Criteria: Clients with HIV, neutropenia, severe hypotension, steroid dependency > 20mg/day, those requiring mechanical ventilation, or clients on immunosuppressive or chemotherapy.

	2ND HOUR	3RD HOUR	4TH HOUR
ASSESSMENTS	REASSESSMENT/ASSESSMENT RESPONSE TO TREATMENT	REASSESSMENT/ASSESSMENT RESPONSE TO TREATMENT	REASSESSMENT/ASSESSMENT RESPONSE TO TREATMENT
CONSULTS	IF INDICATED NOTIFY ADMITTING RESIDENT		
LABS, DIAGNOSTICS PROCEDURES	1. AP/LAT CXR RESULTED 2. CBC, SMA7 3. BLOOD CULTURES X2 4. SPUTUM C + S/gmst. Y__N__ 5. ABG IF PULSE OX <92% RA 6. EKG FEMALE >55 MALE >45 OR CLINICALLY INDICATED		
INTERVENTIONS	SAFETY MEASURES AS PER STANDARD		
IV/MEDICATION	1. SALINE LOCK 2. O2 THERAPY AS PER ORDER 3. ANTIBIOTIC AS PER ALGORITHM AFTER BLOOD CULTURE AND ATTEMPT AT SPUTUM CULTURE		

Community Acquired Is the client allergic to PCN?		Institutional Is the client allergic to PCN?	
No Ceftriaxone 1gm q24 •	Yes TMP/SMX 2amps (320mg/1600mg) IV q12 •	No Ticarcillin/Clavulanate 3.1gm q6 •	Yes Ciprofloxacin 400mg IV q12 • and Clindamycin 600mg IV q8 •
CIRCLE MEDICATION: TIME OF ADMINISTRATION		CIRCLE MEDICATION: TIME OF ADMINISTRATION	

TEACHING	1. REASSURE AND INFORM PT/SO RE: TX PLAN AND INTERVENTIONS 2. PROVIDE CLIENT WITH PSYCHOLOGICAL SUPPORT 3. PT/FAMILY CAN VERBALIZE DISCHARGE INSTRUCTIONS? Y__N__ 4. PT/FAMILY RECEIVED WRITTEN DISCHARGE INSTRUCTIONS? Y__N__	1. REASSURE AND INFORM PT/SO RE: TX PLAN AND INTERVENTIONS 2. PROVIDE CLIENT WITH PSYCHOLOGICAL SUPPORT 3. PT/FAMILY CAN VERBALIZE DISCHARGE INSTRUCTIONS? Y__N__ 4. PT/FAMILY RECEIVED WRITTEN DISCHARGE INSTRUCTIONS? Y__N__	1. REASSURE AND INFORM PT/SO RE: TX PLAN AND INTERVENTIONS 2. PROVIDE CLIENT WITH PSYCHOLOGICAL SUPPORT 3. PT/FAMILY CAN VERBALIZE DISCHARGE INSTRUCTIONS? Y__N__ 4. PT/FAMILY RECEIVED WRITTEN DISCHARGE INSTRUCTIONS? Y__N__
D/C PLANNING AND FOLLOW-UP	DISPOSITION: 1. ADMITTED RM#____ 2. TREATED AND REFERRED 3. TX TO OTHER INSTITUTION 4. NOT EXAMINED OR TREATED 5. LEFT AMA 6. DOA/DIED IN ED TIME OF DISCHARGE_____	DISPOSITION: 1. ADMITTED RM#____ 2. TREATED AND REFERRED 3. TX TO OTHER INSTITUTION 4. NOT EXAMINED OR TREATED 5. LEFT AMA 6. DOA/DIED IN ED TIME OF DISCHARGE_____	DISPOSITION: 1. ADMITTED RM#____ 2. TREATED AND REFERRED 3. TX TO OTHER INSTITUTION 4. NOT EXAMINED OR TREATED 5. LEFT AMA 6. DOA/DIED IN ED TIME OF DISCHARGE_____
OUTCOMES	1. CLINICALLY STABLE 2. PULSE OX > 92% (W OR W/O O2) Y__N__ 3. HR 60–135 Y__N__ 4. RR 12–35 Y__N__ 5. SBP >90 Y__N__ 6. RECEIVED FIRST DOSE OF ANTIBIOTICS Y__N__	1. CLINICALLY STABLE 2. PULSE OX > 92% (W OR W/O O2) Y__N__ 3. HR 60–135 Y__N__ 4. RR 12–35 Y__N__ 5. SBP >90 Y__N__ 6. RECEIVED FIRST DOSE OF ANTIBIOTICS Y__N__	1. CLINICALLY STABLE 2. PULSE OX > 92% (W OR W/O O2) Y__N__ 3. HR 60–135 Y__N__ 4. RR 12–35 Y__N__ 5. SBP >90 Y__N__ 6. RECEIVED FIRST DOSE OF ANTIBIOTICS Y__N__

SIGNATURE	TIME	INITIAL	SIGNATURE	TIME	INITIAL

**Shaded Area Represents MD Decision Point

FIGURE 1-3. An emergency department (ED) clinical pathway for pneumonia. This generic clinical pathway covers the first hour of care, which includes the general interventions and baseline diagnostics that lead to a working diagnosis and a specific critical pathway. (ABG = arterial blood gas; AMA = against medical advice; AP/LAT CXR = anterior, posterior, and lateral chest x-rays; CBC = complete blood count; DOA = dead on arrival; EKG = electrocardiogram; HR = heart rate; pulse ox = pulse oximetry; PT/SO = patient/significant other; RR = respiratory rate; SBP = systolic blood pressure; SMA7 = electrolytes, glucose; Sputum C & S/gmst = sputum culture, sensitivity, and Gram stain; Tx = treatment or transfer; W or W/O = with or without.)

other chronic diseases remain likely. The World Health Organization (WHO, 2005) estimates that women and children increasingly lack access to healthcare. Eleven million children younger than 5 years die from largely preventable causes, including 4 million infants who do not survive the first month. One-half million women die annually during pregnancy or childbirth, or shortly after delivering their babies. WHO has established goals in 2005 that address the health of women and children, stressing the need for increased access to healthcare (Box 1-6).

In the midst of these dramatic changes and challenges, nurses must continue to provide safe, high-quality, cost-effective care to individuals, families, and communities. It also is imperative that nurses distinguish and communicate to clients the various choices that the clients may make about their healthcare.

BOX 1-5 Leading Health Indicators

1. Physical activity
2. Overweight and obesity
3. Tobacco use
4. Substance abuse
5. Responsible sexual behavior
6. Mental health
7. Injury and violence
8. Environmental quality
9. Immunization
10. Access to healthcare

U.S. Department of Health and Human Services. (2000). *Healthy people 2010: Understanding and improving health.* (2nd ed.). (On-line.) Available at: http://www.healthypeople.gov, accessed November 27, 2007.

BOX 1-6 Millennium Development Goals

Goal 1: Eradicate extreme poverty and hunger
Goal 2: Achieve universal primary education
Goal 3: Promote gender equality and empower women
Goal 4: Reduce child mortality
Goal 5: Improve maternal health
Goal 6: Combat HIV/AIDS, malaria, and other diseases
Goal 7: Ensure environmental sustainability
Goal 8: Develop a global partnership for development

(Available at: http://millenniumindicators.un.org, accessed November 27, 2007.)

CRITICAL THINKING EXERCISES

1. Interview an older client to explore their understanding of the healthcare coverage, including access to prescription drugs. Compare their knowledge with information available from Medicare & You (www.medicare.gov/publications).
2. Ask the nurse manager on your assigned clinical unit about the quality indicators the unit must provide data on, and what impact they have had on client care.

NCLEX-STYLE REVIEW QUESTIONS

1. A client with chronic illness always tells the nurses that the client feels great. This may be due to this client's ability to:
   1. define health in a positive way
   2. dismiss his chronic illness
   3. engage in meaningful activities
   4. put on a positive demeanor
2. A client is scheduled for a physical examination with a physician. When reviewing the client's new insurance plan, the client recognizes that this type of service falls under:
   1. Acute care
   2. Primary care

3. Secondary care
   4. Tertiary care
3. An LPN is employed at a physician's office that is part of an organization that provides client referrals to this practice. In exchange, the physician's office offers services at a reduced cost. This practice is part of a(n):
   1. HMO—health maintenance organization
   2. PHO—physician-hospital organization
   3. PPO—preferred provider organization
   4. PPS—prospective payment system
4. The nurse is meeting with a group of clients to discuss health promotion activities, in an effort to target poor lifestyle habits. Which of the following activities promote health? Select all that apply.
   1. Engage in activities to manage stress
   2. Exercise for 30 to 40 minutes five times a week
   3. Increase fiber in the diet
   4. Reduce caloric intake
   5. Sleep at least 6 hours a night
5. An LPN is assigned to serve on her unit's quality improvement committee. The nurse manager explains that the primary purpose of this committee is to:
   1. Audit client care based on standard measures
   2. Determine safe nurse-client ratios
   3. Develop systems to improve client care
   4. Establish standards of care

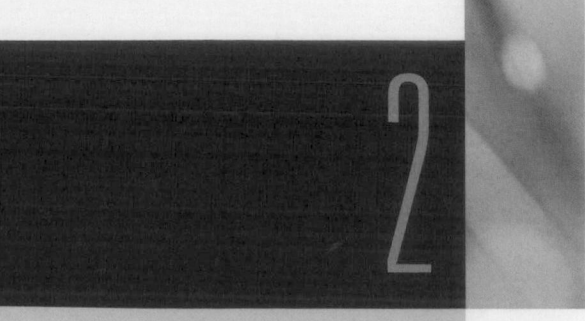

Settings and Models for Nursing Care

2

Learning Objectives

On completion of this chapter, you will be able to:

1. Define nursing.
2. Describe the different roles of the LPN/LVN and RN.
3. List three ways to classify healthcare agencies in which nurses practice.
4. Describe settings in which nurses practice and nurses' roles in each setting.
5. Compare nursing care delivery models.
6. Define case management and explain the nurse case manager's role.

Today's dynamic healthcare environment challenges traditional roles and responsibilities of healthcare providers and institutions. Clients and family members now manage, with the support of visiting nurses, conditions and treatments that were previously relegated to intensive care units. Procedures that formerly required clients to stay in the hospital for at least one week may now be done on a short-stay unit (less than 24 hours). In many instances, insurance companies and case managers dictate choice of services, treatment options, and hospital lengths of stay, which were formerly determined by attending physicians. No matter the setting or circumstances, current healthcare mandates that nurses provide high-quality nursing care wherever needed and function in both traditional and evolving roles.

NURSING CARE

Nursing is concerned with caring for individuals, families, or groups. Nurses not only care for clients when they are ill, but also play a significant role in health education, illness prevention, and promotion. Nurses attend to client needs related to hygiene, activity, diet, the environment, medical treatment, and physical, emotional, and spiritual comfort.

Definitions of Nursing

Arriving at a clear and comprehensive definition of nursing is difficult. Florence Nightingale (1859) described the role of the nurse as putting "the patient in the best condition for nature to act upon him." Virginia Henderson (1966), one of the first nursing theorists, envisioned the nurse's role as helping people (sick or well) to carry out those activities contributing to health, recovery, or a peaceful death that they would do for themselves if they had the necessary strength, will, or knowledge. Her definition also focused on regaining independence.

Since nursing has evolved, the American Nurses Association (ANA) now identifies six essential features of contemporary nursing practice (ANA, 2003):

- Provision of a caring relationship that facilitates health and healing
- Attention to the range of human experiences and responses to health and illness within the physical and social environments
- Integration of objective data with knowledge gained from an appreciation of the client's or group's subjective experience
- Application of scientific knowledge to the processes of diagnosis and treatment through the use of judgment and critical thinking
- Advancement of professional nursing knowledge through scholarly inquiry
- Influence on social and public policy to promote social justice.

Table 2-1 provides other definitions of nursing by selected theorists.

> ▶ **Stop, Think, and Respond Exercise 2-1**
>
> Imogene M. King stated that clients are open systems in constant interaction with their environment. Compare King's definition with Virginia Henderson's. What is different? What is the same?

Nursing Roles

Nurses with different levels of education perform various care activities in diverse settings. The licensed practical or vocational nurse (LPN/LVN) provides care to clients under the direction of a registered nurse (RN) or physician in a structured healthcare setting. LPN/LVNs care for clients with well-defined, common problems that often require a high level of technical competency and expertise. They frequently work in settings in which RN supervision is available but must be sought after the LPN/LVN determines the need to do so. The RN's role is more complex, involving the management and coordination of all the care provided to a group of clients. As healthcare delivery models continue to change, LPN/LVN and RN roles are likely to change as well.

SETTINGS AND TYPES OF NURSING CARE

Nursing care is provided in various settings, with many classifications of healthcare agencies. Healthcare agencies can be classified by length of stay (Table 2-2), ownership (Table 2-3), or type of care.

Although hospitals employ all levels of nurses in outpatient care areas (e.g., dialysis units, clinics, same-day surgery units, related diagnostic departments), inpatient units have been the traditional site for much of the nursing work force. Trends in financing suggest that nursing care will rely less on hospital settings in the future. However, there is a great deal of interest in determining the best, most cost-effective methods and settings for providing care as well as meeting clients' needs. Client needs determine the setting for care.

The following sections discuss the various healthcare agencies according to the type of care.

Acute Care

The term **acuity** refers to the gravity and the degree to which a person's condition changes. Higher acuity refers to clients with severe illness whose condition changes rapidly. Generally,

TABLE 2-1 Definitions of Nursing by Selected Theorists

THEORIST	DEFINITION
Florence Nightingale (1859)	Nurses alter the environment to put the client in the best condition for nature to act.
Virginia Henderson (1966)	Nurses assist clients to carry out those activities that they would perform unaided if they possessed the necessary strength, will, or knowledge.
Ernestine Weidenbach (1964)	Nursing is a helping, nurturing, and caring service delivered sensitively with compassion, skill, and understanding.
Dorothea Orem (1980)	Nursing care is directed at restoring self-care abilities, which are activities that clients initiate on their own behalf in maintaining health, life, and well-being.
Imogene M. King (1981)	Nursing is the care of human beings; individuals and groups are viewed as open systems in continual interaction with the environment.

TABLE 2-2 Healthcare Institutions Classified by Length of Stay

LENGTH OF STAY	DESCRIPTION
In-and-out care	Contact with client is measured in minutes versus hours. Typical examples are office visits, emergency department visits, and therapy sessions.
Short stay	Provides care to clients who suffer from acute conditions or need treatments that require fewer than 24 hours of care and monitoring. Diagnostic tests or minimally invasive surgeries are examples.
Acute care	Traditionally occurs in hospitals where clients stay more than 24 hours but fewer than 30 days. Stays have been shortened since the advent of managed care and DRGs (see Chap. 1).
Long-term care	Provides care to residents for the remainder of their lives; care also includes services to clients with limited recovery needs, functional losses, chronic disease, mental illness, or major rehabilitation, which may range from 30–90 days.

Source: Ellis, J. R., & Hartley, C. L. (2008). *Nursing in today's world: Trends, issues, and management* (9th ed.). Philadelphia: Lippincott Williams & Wilkins.

TABLE 2-3 Healthcare Institutions Classified by Ownership

OWNERSHIP	DESCRIPTION
Government-owned or public facilities	Receive at least some tax support for costs and can be governed by federal, state, or local governments. Examples include veterans' hospitals (federal), mental health facilities (state), and visiting nursing agencies (county).
Proprietary agencies	Often referred to as for-profit agencies. These facilities are owned and operated by corporate groups with investors and stockholders. Prominent examples include Humana Incorporated (full array of healthcare facilities) and Hillhaven Corporation (nursing homes).
Nonprofit agencies	Include facilities owned and operated by nonprofit groups, such as universities or religious organizations. The term *nonprofit* means that any income that exceeds operating and maintenance costs must be used for growth and development of the facility as opposed to distribution to stockholders.

higher client acuity requires a greater need for highly skilled care. Clients with complicated or high-risk surgery, massive trauma, or critical illness will be cared for in an acute care hospital, where a high level of professional, skilled, and technological care is available. RNs are instrumental in caring for these clients.

Long-Term Acute Care

Clients who require long-term wound care or ventilator support, or who have other conditions that are potentially unstable but do not have rapid changes may receive care in a *long-term acute care* facility. The development of these hospitals includes a different method of funding for clients who need "a high intensity of care but whose conditions are not changing rapidly" (Ellis & Hartley, 2008, p. 7). RNs manage clients' care.

Subacute Care

Subacute care refers to care that is more intense than traditional long-term care, but less intense than acute inpatient care (Chitty & Black, 2007). The treatment plan requires frequent assessments and periodic review of clients' progress. Generally, clients are in these facilities for a brief period, up to 30 days. Some subacute units may have a longer length of stay, up to 90 days. RNs coordinate clients' care, and LPN/LVNs provide and oversee care provided by unlicensed assistive personnel (UAP).

Skilled Nursing Care

Skilled nursing care facilities provide skilled nursing and rehabilitative care to people who have the potential to regain function but need skilled observation and nursing care during an acute illness. Clients using these facilities may also require invasive procedures and therapies (e.g., tube feedings, intravenous fluids, and sterile dressing changes). An RN must be in charge of clients' care, although other healthcare providers, particularly LPN/LVNs, participate in their care. Skilled nursing facilities are often referred to as SNFs or "sniffs."

Intermediate Care Facilities

Intermediate care facilities (ICFs) are nursing homes that provide custodial care for people who cannot care for themselves because of mental or physical disabilities. Clients must meet specific criteria related to an inability to meet their own activities of daily living (ADLs). ICFs do not receive

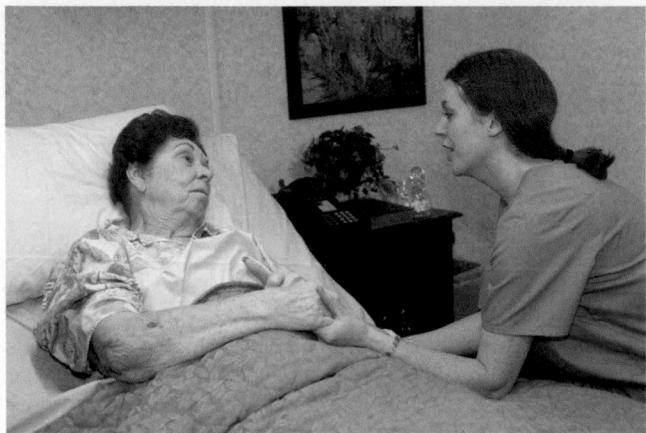

FIGURE 2-1. LPN/LVNs may provide care in intermediate care facilities for clients who cannot care for themselves.

reimbursement from Medicare because they are not considered medical facilities. LPN/LVNs and nursing assistants generally provide care under the supervision of RNs (Fig. 2-1).

Rehabilitation Care

Rehabilitation centers provide physical and occupational therapy to clients and families to help individuals regain as much independence with ADLs as possible. RNs are part of a multidisciplinary team that provides a full range of rehabilitative services.

Hospice Care

Hospices provide care for clients diagnosed with a terminal illness whose life expectancy is fewer than 6 months. Hospices allow terminally ill clients to live as fully as possible while managing pain, discomfort, and other symptoms. Hospice staffs, generally supervised by RNs, are specially trained to help families with the grief process. Medicare covers many of the services provided by hospice care.

Ambulatory Care

Ambulatory care is also referred to as outpatient care. Many settings qualify as outpatient settings: diagnostic centers, such as gastroenterology centers; day surgery centers; and medical treatment centers, such as those for specific therapies or dialysis. Clinics and primary care centers are also considered outpatient settings. Depending on the purpose of the outpatient setting, RNs and LPN/LVNs may or may not play a prominent role.

Home Care

Cost containment measures in the last 20 years have resulted in the expansion of home healthcare services. **Home healthcare** addresses both long-term and short-term health needs and can provide comprehensive services. Home health nurses provide specialized care, such as intravenous infusion of fluids, medications, and chemotherapy; hospice care; postcardiac surgery care; and care to ventilator-dependent clients (Fig. 2-2). RNs manage and coordinate the care clients receive and have a high level of competency in assessment skills, communication, teaching, management, and documentation abilities. The RN encourages clients and family members to develop self-care skills, with support from community resources. Box 2-1 lists other functions of

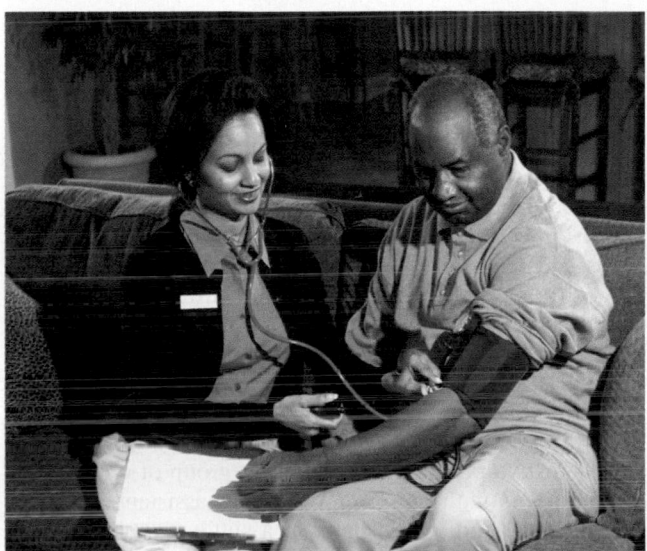

FIGURE 2-2. Home health nurses provide specialized care in the client's home.

BOX 2-1	Functions of the Home Healthcare Nurse

- Plan, coordinate, and provide care in consultation with hospital and physician.
- Teach client and family to perform procedures, monitor symptoms, administer medications, and report to physician.
- Assess client and consult with physician as needed.
- Evaluate the home environment for safety hazards, cleanliness, ability to safely store medication, family support, and adequacy of food supplies.
- Connect client and family with community resources.
- Advocate for the client when additional services are needed.
- Document care and teaching provided.
- Complete forms required for reimbursement.

the home health nurse. Beside nursing, home healthcare agencies provide many other services (Table 2-4).

Community Health Centers

Community health centers and local health departments provide a range of services to the districts, counties, or communities they serve. These agencies receive partial or complete funding from federal, state, and local governments. Community mental health centers are also part of this network. Neighborhood health clinics make healthcare more accessible, and when health facilities are more accessible, people are more likely to seek prompt treatment and reduce the need for acute care.

Alternative Healthcare Settings

In addition to the community-based settings described previously, other facilities and services are available for seniors and adults with physical or mental disabilities. These individuals are relatively healthy and do not need extended care, but may need some assistance with ADLs. The goal of alternative care facilities is to provide the least restrictive living arrangements, while maintaining safety and quality. These facilities include congregate housing, boarding homes, and assisted-living facilities.

Congregate housing provides independent living for seniors or disabled adults who need minimal to no assistance. There are freestanding apartments, private rooms, or both. Often residents must meet certain qualifications and may have subsidized rent based on income. Some congregate housing centers may provide other services such as serving one or more meals per day in a common dining room and offering recreational activities. In general, congregate housing is affordable, but residents may not have any other resources to purchase extra services or goods. They are assured of appropriate housing, but may lack the resources, ability, or opportunity to participate in outside activities.

Boarding homes usually are small homes with individual rooms where residents pay for room and board and minimal nursing services. Residents often share rooms. Boarding homes usually have a common dining area for all meals. Often, boarding homes also oversee employment for disabled adults and provide a stable environment for those who cannot live independently. In this type of setting, residents receive needed supervision but may relinquish some independence and privacy.

Assisted living facilities provide care to residents who require assistance with up to three ADLs. Residents maximize their independence in a setting that maintains their privacy and dignity. These facilities are not regulated as long-term care facilities are, and there is some concern that the quality of care is not at an appropriate level. The Joint Commission is developing a voluntary accreditation process for assisted living facilities to ensure consistency and quality of care. In many instances, this type of living arrangement is very expensive. Residents must provide a large, up-front investment and then a high monthly fee. The facility may or may not provide such services as housekeeping, laundry, transportation, and meals. Residents can, however, maintain a lifestyle more similar to that which they previously

TABLE 2-4 Services Provided by Home Health Agencies

TYPE OF SERVICE	DESCRIPTION
Physical therapy	Therapist assesses the client's mobility after orthopedic surgery, injury, or stroke. He or she assesses the need for assistive devices. Client must meet Medicare requirements to receive physical therapy.
Speech therapy	Therapist provides rehabilitation to clients with speech or swallowing disorders. Client must meet Medicare requirements.
Occupational therapy	Therapist assesses need for assistive devices to aid in activities of daily living and identify issues related to fine motor movements and muscle retraining.
Social services	Social worker meets with client and family to identify difficulties with managing illness at home and provides information about financial assistance and community services.
Home health aides	Aides provide personal care such as bathing and dressing and basic skills such as taking vital signs.
Homemakers	Homemakers clean, do laundry, and shop for groceries.

enjoyed. They also are more able to participate in decisions that affect their future care needs.

MODELS FOR NURSING CARE DELIVERY

Over the years, the delivery of nursing care has been structured in different ways. The structures or models of care used today may vary in different settings depending on client needs and cost of services.

Case Method

Nursing care was historically provided on a **case method** basis, by which one nurse provided all the services that a particular client required. Although the nurse would accompany the client to the hospital if necessary, the nurse provided care in the home and performed many household duties as well. As times changed and care became more complex, this method become impractical, and different models for the hospital-based delivery of nursing care evolved. A modern version of the case method is private duty nursing.

Functional Nursing

Functional nursing, a task-oriented method, evolved during the 1930s. In **functional nursing**, distinct duties are assigned to specific personnel. For example, one nurse takes all the vital signs, someone else makes all the beds, a third nurse does all the dressing changes, and so on. Tasks are divided, and clients see several people during the shift. Although efficient, functional nursing fragments care and is confusing for clients.

Team Nursing

Team nursing emerged in the 1950s, partially in response to the fragmented care of functional nursing and to accommodate staff with varying levels of education and skill. In **team nursing**, teams made up of an RN team leader, other RNs, LPN/LVNs, and nursing assistants provide care to a group of clients. The RN team leader directs the care provided by the RNs, LPN/LVNs, and aides, and works with them in various capacities. Team conferences allow for discussion and care planning.

Total Care

Total care refers to assignments in which a nurse assumes all the care for a small group of clients. This method focuses more on the client as a whole rather than the collection of nursing tasks that need to be accomplished. Total care often is practiced in intensive care units where nurses are assigned one or two clients.

Primary Nursing

In **primary nursing**, an RN assumes 24-hour accountability for the client's care and has total responsibility for the nursing care of assigned clients during his or her shift. Secondary nurses carry out the plan of care in the primary nurse's absence. This approach, initiated in the 1970s, is expensive because it relies entirely on RNs. An advantage, however, is that the client has a caregiver who sees to all of his or her needs and who provides holistic and comprehensive care. Some settings, such as home care, still use this model effectively.

Patient-Focused Care

An updated version of primary care and team nursing called **patient-focused care** uses an RN partnered with one or more assistive personnel to care for a group of clients. The RN may work with an LPN/LVN and an assistant, a respiratory therapist and an assistant, or a similar combination of staff. The licensed and unlicensed assistants are cross-trained to do many functions formerly done by separate departments, such as drawing blood or obtaining electrocardiograms. The RN may have a role in resource management and may be held accountable for outcomes of nursing care such as skin breakdown (negative outcome) or early ambulation (positive outcome).

Case Management

Although it is not a model of primary nursing care, a new role and responsibility for nurses that affects delivery of care is case management. **Case management** maximizes fiscal outcomes without sacrificing quality through careful oversight of a client's healthcare. The person responsible for overseeing the client's care, usually an RN with a bachelor's or master's degree or another highly experienced health professional, is called the *case manager* (Fig. 2-3).

In some specialized settings, a case manager may have a very specific group of clients, such as those with renal failure or diabetes. Insurance companies and hospitals employ case managers. A hospital-based case manager may have a caseload of 15 to 25 clients, depending on the acuity (degree of

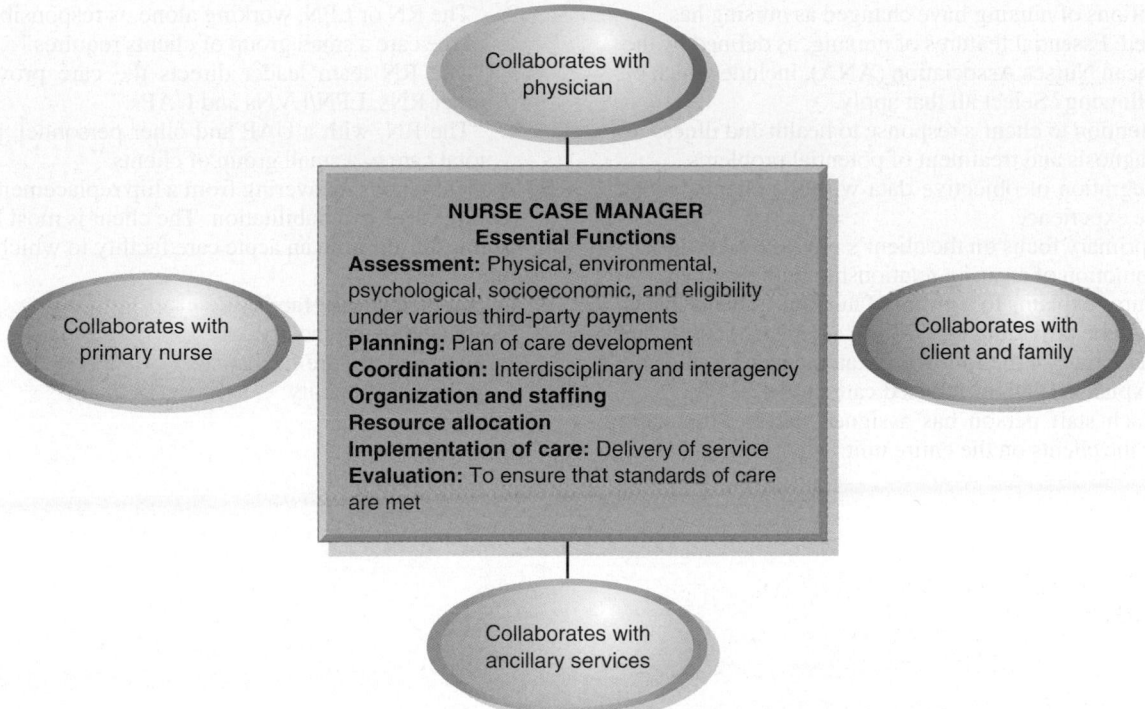

FIGURE 2-3. Functions of the nurse case manager.

illness) of the clients. Not every client is aggressively case managed; those who are sickest, experience complications, or have chronic illnesses that require more intensive case management. The case manager follows clients when they are scheduled for admission until the day of discharge. An insurance-based case manager often maintains contact with the client, especially one with a chronic illness, in the home. Regardless of the employer, case managers plan and coordinate the client's progress through the various phases of care to avoid delays, unnecessary diagnostic testing, and overuse of expensive resources. An important function of case managers is early, thorough discharge planning. Case managers often use tools such as clinical pathways (see Chap. 1), practice guidelines, and standards of care to help them plan and coordinate care. Hospitals and insurance companies may develop their own or rely on published protocols for guidance. (A cautionary note: Experts using published research should develop all protocols.)

▶ **Stop, Think, and Respond Exercise 2-2**

A 70-year-old client was admitted to the hospital with several chronic diagnoses, including diabetes, arthritis, and emphysema. The client tells you that he has a case manager, but he does not understand what that means. How would you explain the case manager's role to this client?

Along with the increase in responsibility, autonomy, and power, nurse case managers have increased accountability for financial and health outcomes of care. Many employers, particularly insurance companies, measure costs of services provided to the case managers' clients as a means of

assessing their effectiveness. One of the complaints about case management, and its parent, managed care, is that the "bottom line" can become more important than quality. For this reason, and because they are in the best position to collect outcome data, case managers often are integral members of hospital-based and insurance-based quality improvement programs.

CRITICAL THINKING EXERCISES

1. How do you think nurses will practice in 2020?
2. What is your definition of nursing?
3. Discuss the pros and cons of case management for both the client and the nurse case manager.

NCLEX-STYLE REVIEW QUESTIONS

1. Which of the following describes the service provided by home health nurses?
   1. 24-hour accountability for the client's care
   2. Care planning in the primary nurse's absence
   3. Total care for a small group of clients
   4. Care adapted for a client's long- and short-term needs
2. Student nurses are reviewing nursing roles. A student is correct to state that nurses care for people when they are ill, but also are involved with which of the following? Select all that apply.
   1. Managing health finances
   2. Preventing illness
   3. Providing spiritual comfort
   4. Teaching clients self-care

3. Definitions of nursing have changed as nursing has evolved. Essential features of nursing, as defined by the American Nurses Association (ANA), include which of the following? Select all that apply.
   1. Attention to client's response to health and illness
   2. Diagnosis and treatment of potential problems
   3. Integration of objective data with the client's subjective experience
   4. A primary focus on the client's physical problems
   5. Promotion of a caring relationship with the client

4. The nurse explains to a group of nursing students that they will be providing care within a patient-focused care model. Which of the following statements by a student best explains a patient-focused care model?
   1. "Each staff person has assigned duties when caring for the clients on the entire unit."
   2. "The RN or LPN, working alone, is responsible for all of the care a small group of clients requires"
   3. "The RN team leader directs the care provided by other RNs, LPN/LVNs and UAPs."
   4. "The RN, with a UAP and other personnel, provides total care to a small group of clients."

5. A client who is recovering from a hip replacement requires further rehabilitation. The client is most likely to be transferred from an acute care facility to which of the following?
   1. ambulatory care facility
   2. assisted living facility
   3. intermediate care facility
   4. skilled care facility

3

The Nursing Process

Words To Know
actual nursing diagnosis
assessment
client database
collaborative problems
concept mapping
critical thinking
documentation
evaluation
expected outcomes
health promotion diagnosis
implementation
interventions
nursing diagnosis
nursing orders
nursing process
planning
risk nursing diagnosis
syndrome diagnosis
wellness nursing diagnosis

Learning Objectives

On completion of this chapter, you will be able to:

1. State the purpose of the nursing process.
2. Describe the five steps of the nursing process.
3. Define assessment.
4. Discuss the parts of a nursing diagnostic statement.
5. Differentiate types of nursing diagnoses.
6. Explain the five levels of human needs as identified by Maslow.
7. Explain how nurses use the hierarchy of needs to establish nursing priorities.
8. Define expected outcomes.
9. Explain the implementation phase of the nursing process and its relationship with documentation.
10. Explain the purpose of evaluation.
11. Give reasons why expected outcomes may not be accomplished.
12. Define critical thinking and its relevance to the nursing process.
13. List characteristics of critical thinkers.
14. Discuss the use of concept mapping as a means to master the nursing process and develop critical thinking skills.

Providing healthcare is a process of problem solving. Clients present with multiple healthcare needs that the caregiver must approach in an organized, systematic manner to provide efficient and effective care. The purpose of the **nursing process** is to provide a systematic method for nurses to plan and implement client care to achieve desired outcomes. The nursing process for making clinical decisions grew from problem-solving techniques and the scientific process. It includes collecting information, identifying problems, developing an outcome-based plan, carrying out the plan, and evaluating the results. Other reasons for learning and using the nursing process include the following:

- The nursing process provides the framework for nursing care in all healthcare settings.
- Most states' nurse practice acts include the nursing process as part of the definition of nursing.
- Nursing educators use the nursing process in the organizational structure of nursing curricula.
- The nursing process forms the basis for the National Council Licensing Examinations (NCLEX) RN and PN.

Learning the nursing process is essential to all nursing practice. The use of computerized and standardized nursing care plans may seem to negate the necessity to learn the nursing process. However, as stated by Alfaro-LeFevre (2006, p. 5), "If you don't understand the purpose of each step, the relationship among the steps, and how each step is accomplished, it's like using a calculator without having learned what it means to add, subtract, multiply, or divide." Nursing students and nurses must be very familiar with all aspects of the nursing process.

STEPS OF THE NURSING PROCESS

The nursing process begins when a client enters the health-care system. It consists of five steps:

1. Assessment
2. Diagnosis (nursing) or analysis
3. Planning
4. Implementation
5. Evaluation

The nurse collects data (assessment), defines problems or needs (diagnosis), establishes outcomes and actions that will help achieve the overall goals (planning), puts the plan into action (implementation), and determines the client's responses to the care provided (evaluation). Figure 3-1 depicts these five steps in a dynamic, circular model, showing that each component not only is separate and distinct, but interrelated and continuous with the others. Table 3-1 compares the roles of the LPN and RN in each step of the nursing process.

Assessment

Assessment is the careful observation and evaluation of a client's health status. During assessment, the nurse collects information to determine abnormal function and risk factors that contribute to health problems, as well as client strengths (Alfaro-LeFevre, 2006). Not only is assessment the first step in the nursing process, it is an important, recurring nursing activity that continues as long as a need for healthcare exists. During assessment, the nurse methodically obtains data about the client's health and illness. Chapter 4 describes the assessment process and data collection in greater detail.

The nurse documents the data in the medical record, which contributes to the client database. The **client database** includes all the information obtained from the medical and nursing history, physical examination (see Chap. 4), and diagnostic studies. Baseline data serve as a comparison for future signs and symptoms, and provide a reference for determining if a client's health is improving. Initial and ongoing assessment is essential to the provision of nursing care.

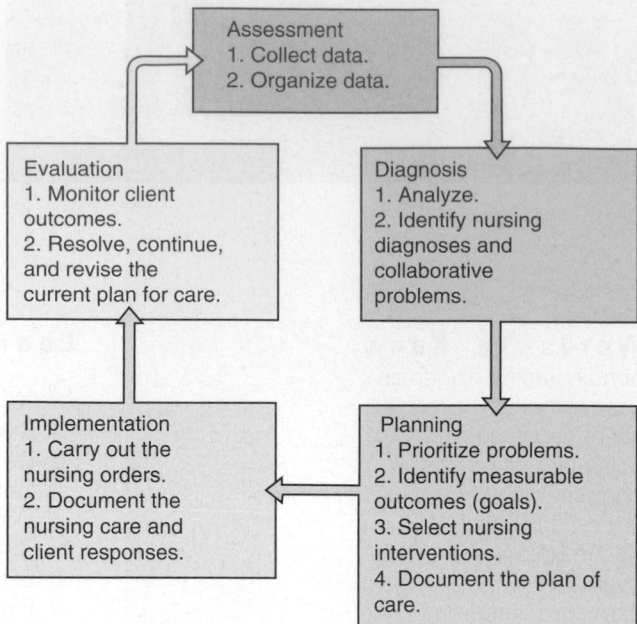

FIGURE 3-1 Steps in the nursing process.

Nursing Diagnosis

During the **nursing diagnosis**, the second phase of the nursing process, the nurse reports or analyzes data to identify and define health problems that independent or physician-prescribed nursing actions can prevent or solve. As in other phases of the nursing process, the nurse's role depends on his or her level of practice. Licensed practical/vocational nurses (LPN/LVNs) report information that suggests actual or potential health problems. Registered nurses (RNs) examine and analyze the client database to formulate nursing diagnoses.

The North American Nursing Diagnosis Association (NANDA) developed the classification system for client problems and nursing diagnoses. NANDA meets every 2 years to review and update the list, the most recent version of which is on the inside cover of this text. Nurses should

TABLE 3-1 Comparison of the Role of the Licensed Practical/Vocational Nurse (LPN/LVN) and Registered Nurse (RN) in the Nursing Process

NURSING PROCESS PHASE	ROLE OF LPN/LVN	ROLE OF RN
Assessment	Gathers data, performs assessment, identifies client's strengths	Gathers more extensive biopsychosocial data, groups and analyzes data, researches additional data needed, identifies client resources
Nursing diagnosis	Does not establish nursing diagnoses, but needs to understand diagnoses written by RN	Draws conclusions, uses judgment, makes diagnosis
Planning	Contributes to development of care plans	Establishes priorities, sets short- and long-term client outcomes, collaborates, and refers
Implementation	Provides basic therapeutic and preventive nursing measures, provides client education, records information	Manages client care (performs and delegates), provides client and family teaching, provides referrals, records and exchanges information with healthcare team
Evaluation	Evaluates effects of care given	Evaluates effectiveness of overall plan, analyzes new data, modifies and redesigns plan, collaborates with health team members

use NANDA-approved nursing diagnoses whenever possible. If a client's problem does not fit into any of the NANDA-approved diagnoses, the nurse can use her or his own terminology. The NANDA-approved diagnoses are very comprehensive, however, and provide student nurses with the appropriate terminology to formulate nursing diagnoses.

Nursing Diagnostic Statements

A diagnostic statement includes one to three parts: (1) the name, or label, of the problem; (2) the cause of the problem; and (3) the signs and symptoms, or data, that indicate the problem. The name or label portion of the statement is linked to the cause with the phrase *related to,* and the data are linked to the name/label and cause by the phrase *as manifested by* or *as evidenced by* (Fig. 3-2). The following is an example of a nursing diagnostic statement:

> *Constipation* (name of the problem) *related to decreased fluid intake, lack of dietary fiber, and lack of exercise* (causes) *as manifested by no bowel movement for the past 3 days, abdominal cramping, and straining to pass stools* (signs and symptoms).

Sometimes the cause is explained in more depth using the term *secondary to,* as in *decreased fluid intake secondary to nausea.* Different types of diagnoses, as outlined below, also have different prefixes or stems.

Types of Nursing Diagnoses

NANDA identifies five types of nursing diagnoses: actual, health promotion, risk, wellness, and syndrome. Some sources also use *possible nursing diagnoses* (discussed below). Nursing diagnoses can refer to an individual client, family, or community. **Actual nursing diagnoses** identify existing problems, such as Constipation or Anxiety. **Health promotion nursing diagnoses** reflect clinical judgment of a client's motivation to increase well-being and enhance health-seeking behaviors (NANDA International, 2007). Health-seeking behaviors would be those made by a client with stable health (but not necessarily wellness) who desires a higher level of health, such as Health-seeking Behavior related to concern about environmental conditions that impact the client's breathing status.

Risk nursing diagnoses identify potential problems and use the stem *risk for,* as in Risk for Impaired Skin Integrity related to inactivity. Risk nursing diagnoses do not include the third part of the statement, the data, because the data are undeveloped or incomplete. The use of *possible nursing diagnoses* (Carpenito-Moyet, 2008) includes the stem *possible* to indicate uncertainty, as in Possible Sexual Dysfunction. Sometimes the cause of a possible diagnosis may be unknown; in such cases, the nurse can omit the second part of the statement as well.

Wellness diagnoses describe a client's transition from one level of wellness to a higher level of wellness. The diagnostic statement begins with the stem *readiness for enhanced* and does not include related factors or supporting data. According to Carpenito-Moyet (2008), "two cues should be present: (1) a desire for increased wellness and (2) effective present status or function" (p. 17). An example of a wellness diagnostic statement is Readiness for Enhanced Family Coping.

Syndrome diagnoses identify a diagnosis associated with a cluster of other diagnoses. NANDA identifies five syndrome diagnoses: Disuse Syndrome, Impaired Environmental Interpretation Syndrome, Post-trauma Syndrome, Rape Trauma Syndrome, and Relocation Stress Syndrome.

Table 3-2 explains the different types of nursing diagnoses and provides examples of diagnostic statements for each type.

Collaborative Problems

Collaborative problems denote complications with a physiologic origin and differ from nursing diagnoses, which address client responses to various circumstances and are managed by nursing interventions (Carpenito-Moyet, 2008). Collaborative problems involve activities of nurses to monitor clients for the purpose of detecting physiologic changes or the onset of physiologic problems. Carpenito-Moyet (2008) explains, "Nurses manage collaborative problems using physician-prescribed interventions and nursing-prescribed interventions to minimize the complications of the events" (p. 24). Collaborative problems begin with the stem *potential complication* (abbreviated PC), as in PC: Pulmonary Embolism. Nurses do not include related factors and supporting data when writing collaborative problem statements.

Planning

The third step of the nursing process is **planning**, which involves several steps: setting priorities, defining expected (desired) outcomes (goals), determining specific nursing interventions, and recording the plan of care. Respecting clients' rights to participate in their healthcare is an important ethical principle. Actively involved clients are more committed to carrying out the plan and achieving the outcomes. Thus, nurses ensure that clients and families participate in care planning as much as possible. Nurses consult with clients about specific activities that are equally effective in achieving the outcomes.

For example, a female client has a nursing diagnosis of Imbalanced Nutrition: Less than Body Requirements related to poor appetite and medication side effects as manifested by an intake of less than 1000 calories per day and weight loss of 3 kg in 10 days. When planning care for this client, the nurse must talk with her about the importance of increased caloric intake and ways to accomplish it, including different types of foods, frequency of meals, and timing of medications. If the nurse simply decides to add certain high-calorie foods to the client's food tray, it is highly possible that the client will reject the foods because she may not like them.

FIGURE 3-2 Nursing diagnostic statement. (From Carpenito-Moyet, L. J. [2008]. Nursing diagnosis: Application to clinical practice [12th ed.]. Philadelphia: Lippincott Williams & Wilkins.)

Problem		Etiology		Symptom
Diagnostic label	*related to*	Contributing factors	*as evidenced by*	Signs and symptoms

TABLE 3-2 Types and Examples of Nursing Diagnoses and Collaborative Problems

TYPE	EXPLANATION	EXAMPLE OF DIAGNOSTIC STATEMENT
Actual diagnosis	A problem that already exists	*Feeding Self-Care Deficit related to right hemiparesis as manifested by inability to grasp utensils* *Impaired Verbal Communication related to hearing deficit as evidenced by inability to hear or read lips*
Health promotion diagnosis	Desire to increase well-being and enhance specific health behaviors	*Health-seeking behavior (specify) related to desire to learn more about healthy practices as demonstrated by lack of knowledge about healthy behaviors.*
Risk diagnosis	A problem that the client is at high risk for developing	*Risk for Disturbed Sleep Pattern related to changed environment (intensive care unit)* *Risk for Impaired Skin Integrity related to prescribed bed rest and decreased sensation and mobility of the lower extremities*
Possible diagnosis	A problem that is suspected but more data are needed before making a decision	*Possible Parental Role Conflict related to impending divorce* *Possible Ineffective Airway Clearance related to excessive mucus*
Wellness diagnosis	No problem exists; the client desires a higher level of wellness	*Readiness for Enhanced Spiritual Well-Being* *Readiness for Enhanced Fluid Balance*
Syndrome diagnosis	Used when the diagnosis is associated with a cluster of other diagnoses	*Disuse Syndrome: Impaired Physical Mobility, Risk for Constipation, Risk for Ineffective Breathing Pattern, Risk for Infection, Risk for Activity Intolerance, Risk for Injury, Risk for Disturbed Thought Processes, Risk for Disturbed Body Image, Risk for Powerlessness, Risk for Impaired Tissue Integrity*
Collaborative problem	A problem that is monitored and managed by the nurse using physician-prescribed and nursing-prescribed interventions	*Potential Complication (PC): Phlebitis* *PC: Pneumothorax*

Establishing Priorities

Some problems require immediate action, whereas others may not have high priority (Lipe & Beasley, 2004). The nurse prioritizes the client's multiple problems by first ranking the diagnoses that are the client's most important, serious, or immediate needs, followed by the remainder in descending order of importance. A framework that nurses frequently use when prioritizing client problems is the hierarchy of human needs developed by Abraham Maslow (1968). Maslow proposed five levels of needs that motivate human behavior and grouped them as follows, according to their significance:

1. Physiologic needs (first level)
2. Safety and security needs (second level)
3. Love and belonging needs (third level)
4. Esteem and self-esteem needs (fourth level)
5. Self-actualization needs (fifth level)

The first-level needs, sometimes called *baseline survival needs,* have the highest priority. These activities, such as eating, breathing, and drinking, sustain life. Maslow believed humans could not or would not seek to fulfill higher-level needs until physiologic needs were satisfied. Thus, nurses must rank any problem that poses a threat to physiologic functioning first. For example, nursing diagnoses such as Ineffective Breathing Pattern and Deficient Fluid Volume demand the nurse's attention more than other diagnoses because these conditions may be life-threatening.

Nursing diagnoses such as Anxiety or Risk for Injury address the second-level needs of safety and security. Parental Role Conflict and Social Isolation are examples of nursing diagnoses that apply to the third level of love and belonging needs. Examples of nursing diagnoses that affect the fourth level of esteem and self-esteem needs are Powerlessness and Ineffective Coping. Delayed Growth and Development and Spiritual Distress are examples of nursing diagnoses that interfere with an individual's ability to achieve fifth-level, self-actualization needs.

Defining Expected Outcomes

Defining **expected outcomes** is an important part of the care planning process. The nurse includes the client and family in establishing outcomes. Outcomes are specific and realistic, so the client can attain them and not become frustrated, and measurable so the nurse can reliably determine to what extent the client is meeting the goals.

The nurse determines client-centered outcomes from the nursing diagnoses, so that the focus is on the treatments and results, as opposed to what the nurse hopes to achieve. For example, a nurse may desire the outcome that the client understands everything the nurse teaches. Instead, the outcome needs to focus on the essential care techniques for the client to master before leaving the healthcare facility. Thus, an appropriate outcome in this scenario would be "Before discharge, the client will demonstrate clean technique when changing the dressing on his left calf wound."

Specifically, outcomes are as follows (Alfaro-LeFevre, 2006):

- Derived from nursing diagnoses
- Documented as measurable goals
- Developed with the client and family and other healthcare providers when possible
- Realistic in relation to the client's present and potential capabilities
- Achievable in relation to the client's available resources
- Written to include
  - Time estimate for achievement
  - Direction for continuity of care

When writing expected outcomes, the nurse should relate them directly to the nursing diagnoses and make them clear and specific. For example, if the nursing diagnosis is "Acute Pain related to left knee replacement surgery, movement, and physical therapy," an expected outcome is that "the client will experience minimal pain throughout hospitalization." Table 3-3 provides examples of client-centered outcomes for each type of nursing diagnosis.

In some settings, it may be necessary to identify short-term outcomes and long-term outcomes. For example, in a rehabilitation center, clients may be involved in therapy for weeks or months. The expected outcomes need to reflect this length of treatment. In this situation, a short-term outcome is "the client will ambulate 20 feet on the first postoperative day," whereas a long-term outcome is "the client will ambulate with a walker by the end of 3 weeks."

Unlike nursing diagnoses that require client-centered outcomes, collaborative problems need nurse-centered outcomes, because the nurse is managing situations that rely on physician and nursing interventions. For example, the outcome for Potential Complication: Increased intracranial pressure would be *The nurse will monitor the client for signs of changes in level of consciousness.*

Determining Specific Interventions

The plan of care identifies **interventions** or actions for achieving the outcomes. Relieving the cause of the problem directs the interventions. If the cause cannot be fixed, such as in permanent injury, then the interventions focus on reducing consequences of the problem.

For example, if a client has the nursing diagnosis of "Impaired Skin Integrity related to the effects of pressure secondary to decreased mobility as manifested by a 2-cm ulcer on the right heel," the nurse needs to identify measures directed at relieving pressure and its effects (decreased circulation). Such interventions would include elevating the heel off the bed to relieve pressure and having the client do ankle-pumping exercises to increase blood flow to the area. If the diagnosis is "Feeding Self-Care Deficit related to right hemiparesis (paralysis affecting one side of the body) secondary to stroke as manifested by inability to grasp utensils," the nurse may provide utensils with large rubber grips to decrease the effects of the problem.

Recording the Plan of Care

Once the RN determines the interventions, he or she writes the interventions in the written plan as nursing orders. **Nursing orders** are specific nursing directions so that all healthcare team members understand exactly what to do for the client (Box 3-1). Different people are likely to interpret a vague nursing order such as "Encourage fluids" differently, resulting in inconsistent care. In such cases, if outcomes are not met, determining whether the nursing measures themselves were ineffective or whether they were carried out ineffectively becomes difficult. A more appropriate nursing order would be "Give the client 100 mL of juice, water, tea, or milk every hour while awake." Interventions in the nursing care plan also must be compatible with the medical orders. For instance, if the physician has prescribed complete bed rest, a nursing order should not call for ambulation.

Many agencies have preprinted or computer-generated care plans that help identify nursing interventions for specific nursing or medical diagnoses. They save time by providing general suggestions for common conditions. The nurse selects appropriate interventions from the list, makes the orders specific for the individual client, and eliminates whatever is unnecessary.

A complete plan of care provides a means to communicate to all shifts of nursing personnel. This communication establishes a basis for continuity of care.

Implementation

As the fourth step of the nursing process, **implementation** means carrying out the written plan of care, performing the interventions, monitoring the client's status, and assessing and reassessing the client before, during, and after treatments. Carrying out the plan involves the client and one or

---

TABLE 3-3 Examples of Expected Outcomes Derived from Nursing Diagnoses

NURSING DIAGNOSIS	EXPECTED OUTCOME
Ineffective Airway Clearance related to excessive secretions secondary to inflammation	The client will demonstrate optimal positioning to facilitate drainage of secretions on day of admission.
Health-seeking Behavior related to desire to increase control of weight maintenance	The client will discuss healthy eating strategies within two sessions of nutrition classes.
Risk for Deficient Fluid Volume related to nausea and vomiting and increased loss of fluids and electrolytes from gastrointestinal tract	The client will maintain fluid balance as evidenced by total intake greater than or equal to 2500 mL, with output equal to intake or differing from intake by no more than 500 mL.
Possible Constipation	The client will have soft bowel movements as evidenced by client report.
Disuse Syndrome: Impaired Physical Mobility related to mechanical immobilization	The client will demonstrate ability to turn with assistance, maintaining restrictions, by second postoperative day.
PC: Congestive Heart Failure	The nurse will monitor the client for shortness of breath, dyspnea on exertion, and orthopnea.

Nursing interventions and orders are:
• Directed at preventing or minimizing the underlying causes of a problem
• Directed at minimizing problems when the cause cannot be changed
• Compatible with medical orders and other therapies
• Compatible with professional and facility standards of care
• Specific and outline what, how, when, how often, and how much
• Safe
• Individualized
• Supported by scientific rationales

more members of the healthcare team. It also may include the client's family and the community. It requires that the nurse not only act but also think before acting. For example, the nurse looks for any changes in the client's condition, reviews the client's responses to changes or care, and determines if changes need to be made in the plan of care.

An important element of implementation is documentation. Accurate and thorough **documentation** in the medical record serves five functions (Alfaro-LeFevre, 2006):

1. Communicates care
2. Shows trends and patterns in client status
3. Creates a legal document
4. Supplies validation for reimbursement
5. Provides a foundation for evaluation, research, and quality improvement

By law, nurses must document all nursing actions, observations, and client responses in a permanent record. This record of nursing actions should be a mirror image of the written plan. Appropriate documentation is essential in maintaining communication among members of the healthcare team and ensuring that nurses monitor the client's progress.

Evaluation

Evaluation, the fifth step of the nursing process, consists of assessment and review of the quality and suitability of care given and the client's responses to that care (Box 3-2). During evaluation, nurses compare the actual outcomes to the expected outcomes. This process enables the nurse to revise the expected outcomes or select alternative plans of action when expected outcomes are not met. The nurse may reach one of several conclusions during evaluation:

Evaluation includes the following components:
• Determining if expected outcomes have been met
• Identifying factors that interfered with achieving expected outcomes
• Deciding whether to continue, modify, or discontinue the plan

• The outcome is achieved, the problem is solved, and the nursing orders are discontinued.
• The outcome is not met, but progress is being made and the plan of care is continued or revised with minor changes.
• The outcome is not achieved, and the plan requires critical re-evaluation and major revision.

A client's lack of progress may result from unrealistic expectations, incorrect diagnosis of the original problem, development of additional problems, ineffective nursing measures, or a premature target date. Once nurses identify the deficiency in the plan, they may implement a revision. See the sample Nursing Care Plan 3-1.

THE NURSING PROCESS AND CRITICAL THINKING

Critical thinking is intentional, contemplative, and outcome-directed thinking. In nursing, critical thinking (Alfaro-LeFevre, 2006):

• Involves purposeful, outcome-directed thinking
• Considers client, family, and community needs
• Is based on principles of nursing process and scientific method
• Requires knowledge, skills, and experience
• Is guided by professional standards and codes of ethics
• Makes judgments based on evidence rather than conjecture
• Involves constant re-evaluation, revision, and striving for improvement
• Requires strategies that maximize human potential (using individual strengths) and compensate for problems

When caring for clients, nurses continually assess their clients' needs and frequently confront situations that require multiple interventions. Developing good critical thinking skills will make nurses more efficient and effective at resolving these situations. This careful, deliberate, outcome-directed thinking has predictable features that nurses can practice and learn. One key feature is the ability to maintain a questioning attitude. "Why is this occurring?," "Do I have all the information I need?," and "What does this mean?" are examples of questions that critical thinkers ask themselves (Alfaro-LeFevre, 2006). Box 3-3 outlines other characteristics of critical thinkers.

The use of the nursing process in nursing combines critical thinking with problem-solving methods. Nurses identify client problems and develop and implement plans of care with a logical, purposeful, and outcome-based method. The nursing process assists nurses to acquire critical thinking and problem-solving skills because it entails scientific problem-solving in a systematic, client-centered, outcome-based way. It also is a dynamic continuous process. Nurses must use specific cognitive and mental activities when thinking critically (Smeltzer & Bare, 2008):

• Ask questions to determine why a situation occurred and if more information is needed.
• Gather relevant information to consider all factors.
• Validate information for accuracy, ensuring that it is not just supposition or opinion—it needs to be factual and based on evidence.

NURSING CARE PLAN 3-1* | Postoperative Abdominal Surgery Care

Assessment
- Check the client's abdominal dressing
- Assess the Hemovac drain
- Check the nasogastric tube
- Assess the Foley catheter
- Review the intravenous (IV) infusion rate

- Assess the patient-controlled analgesia (PCA)
- Evaluate the IV insertion site
- Take the client's vital signs
- Determine the client's ability to ambulate
- Assess the client's level of consciousness
- Assess the client's pain

Nursing Diagnosis: **Risk for Ineffective Airway Clearance** related to depressed respiratory function, pain, and bed rest

Expected Outcomes: Client maintains a patent airway at all times.
Client's breath sounds remain clear.

Interventions	Rationales
Monitor breath sounds at least every 4 hours for 48 hours.	Breath sounds with crackles and wheezes indicate retained secretions.
Instruct client to deep breathe and cough every 2 hours.	Lung expansion prevents atelectasis and keeps secretions cleared.
Turn client at least every 2 hours.	Turning promotes lung expansion and movement of secretions.

Evaluation of Expected Outcomes
- Client's respirations are unlabored and regular.
- Client's bilateral breath sounds are clear.
- Client performs deep breathing and coughing exercises with coaching.
- Client turns every 2 hours with maximum assistance.

Collaborative Problem: **PC:** Wound Infection

Expected Outcome: The nurse will minimize the client's potential for a wound infection.

Interventions	Rationales
Observe incision for signs and symptoms of infection.	Redness, warmth, fever, or swelling indicates a wound infection.
Monitor wound drainage, dressing, and Hemovac drain.	Changes in wound drainage from serosanguinous to purulent indicate a wound infection.
Maintain sterile technique for dressing changes.	Sterile technique reduces potential for development of infection.

Evaluation of Expected Outcomes
- Incision remains free of redness, warmth, and swelling.
- Drainage is decreased and serosanguinous.
- The nurse changes the dressing every 8 hours, with scant serosanguinous drainage on old dressings.

*Sample care plan only. See more complete care plan for postoperative clients in Chapter 15.

- Analyze information to determine what it means—does it form patterns that lead to specific conclusions?
- Use past clinical experience and knowledge to explain what is happening and to anticipate what may occur.
- Acknowledge personal bias and cultural influences.
- Maintain a flexible attitude so that facts guide thinking.
- Consider all possibilities.
- Determine all possible options, considering the advantages and disadvantages of each.
- Make decisions that are creative and show independent decision-making.

Nurses use critical thinking skills in all practice settings. Each client presents with unique and dynamic issues. The nurse considers all factors and interprets the information to focus on the most needed elements and make decisions relevant to the individual client's care. Developing critical thinking skills requires knowledge, practice, and experience. This text presents critical thinking exercises at the end of each chapter, as well as "Stop, Think, and Respond Exercises" in many chapters. These exercises encourage the reader to begin the process of critical analysis and interpretation, as well as providing a foundation for critical decision-making

BOX 3-3 Characteristics of Critical Thinkers

Critical thinkers are:

- Aware of their strengths and capabilities (show confidence)
- Aware of their own limitations (know when to ask for help)
- Open minded (listen to new ideas and other viewpoints)
- Humble (do not have to know everything all the time)
- Creative (look for ways to improve performance)
- Proactive (anticipate problems and prevent them)
- Flexible (can modify priorities and adapt to change)
- Aware that mistakes lead to new knowledge (learn from errors)
- Willing to persevere (accept that answers may not come easily)
- Aware that the world is not ideal (realize that the best solution may not be perfect)
- Logical thinkers (establish facts, determine what is relevant, search for cause and effect, avoid jumping to conclusions)
- Able to weigh advantages and disadvantages before making decisions (foresee probable outcomes)

▶ **Stop, Think, and Respond Exercise 3-1**

A do-not-resuscitate (DNR) order was just added to a terminally ill client's plan of care. Using critical thinking skills, what must the nurse consider when adapting the nursing care plan? What types of nursing diagnoses should the nurse consider adding to the care plan?

CONCEPT MAPPING

One helpful way to master the nursing process and develop thinking skills is to practice concept mapping. **Concept mapping** links important ideas about the care a client requires. It provides a means for students and nurses to consider all of the client's problems as a whole and then develop a plan to treat the problems. Specifically, a concept map presents the client's medical and nursing diagnoses with the relevant clinical data. It provides a means not

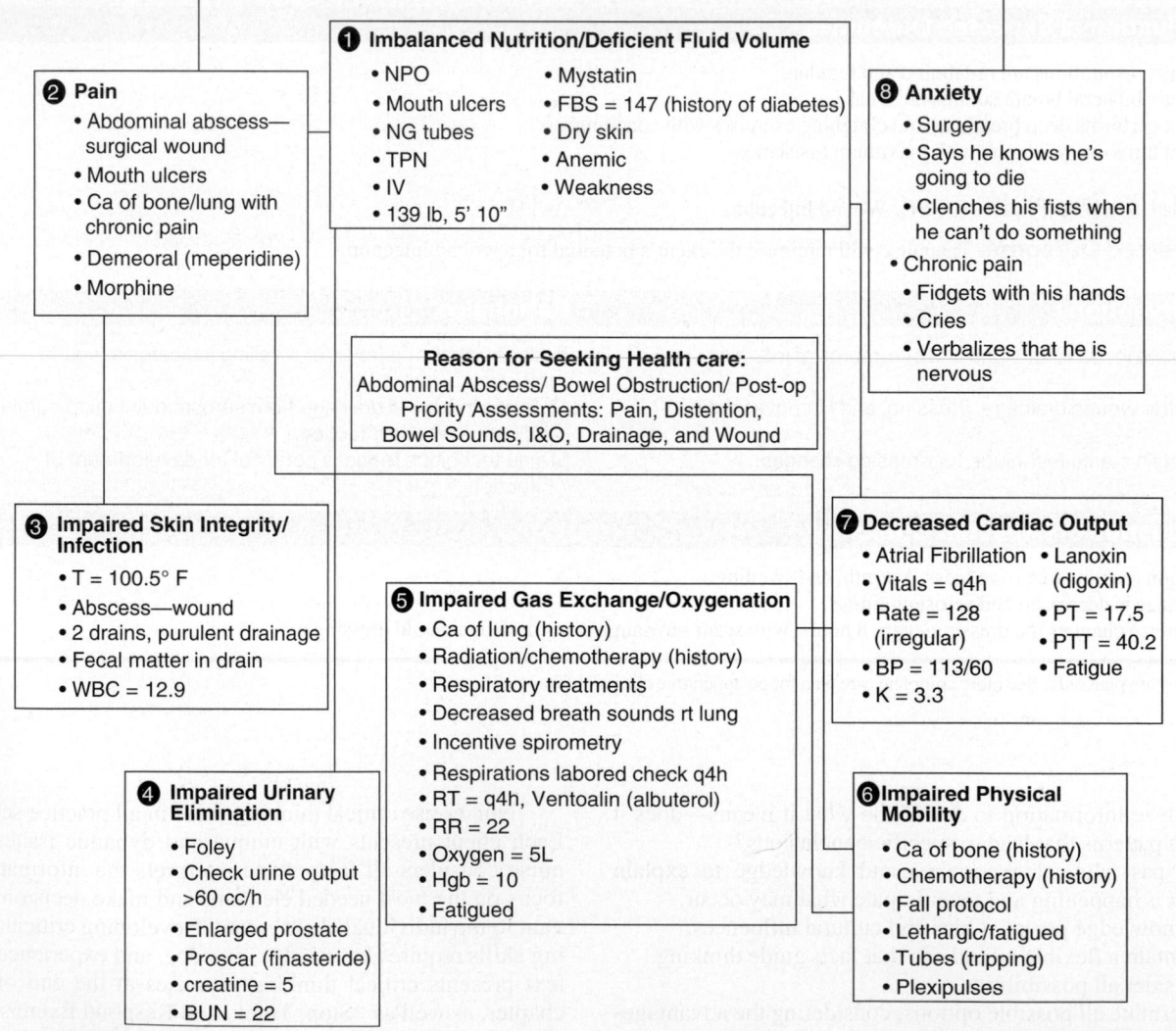

FIGURE 3-3 Relationships between diagnoses. Ca=cancer; BP=blood pressure; BUN=blood urea nitrogen; FBS=fasting blood sugar; Hgb=hemoglobin; I&O=intake and output; IV=intravenous; K=potassium; NG=nasogastric; NPO=nothing by mouth; PT=prothrombin time; PTT=partial thromboplastin time; RR=respiratory rate; RT=respiratory therapy; T=temperature; TPN=total parenteral nutrition; WBCs=white blood cells. (From Schuster, P. M. [2008]. *Concept mapping: A critical-thinking approach to care planning* [2ⁿᵈ ed.]. Philadelphia: F. A. Davis.)

only to assess what is known about the client but also to determine what other information is needed. Schuster (2008) delineates five steps when developing a concept map:

• **Step 1**—*Develop a basic skeleton diagram.* The skeleton evolves from the clinical data that the nurse collects. In the middle of a blank sheet of paper, the nurse writes the reason the client seeks care, usually the medical diagnosis. Around this central diagnosis, the nurse then writes problems or nursing diagnoses that relate to the client's response to the central problem (Fig. 3-3). When mapping the nursing care problems, the nurse generally selects only actual problems based on his or her assessment. At times, however, nurses may include potential problems if the client's health status indicates this possibility.

• **Step 2**—*Analyze and categorize data.* In this step, the nurse places clinical assessment data, client history data, treatments, and medications under the appropriate nursing diagnosis/problem. Refer to Figure 3-3 for examples. The nursing diagnoses flow from why the client sought healthcare and include the clinical evidence, as well as current information of tests and results, treatments, and medications. The client's history also may be included if pertinent. The final part of this step involves prioritizing the most important assessments.

• **Step 3**—*Label and analyze nursing diagnoses relationships.* In this step the nurse determines relationships among nursing diagnoses. In Figure 3-3, note that all the problems are interrelated and provide a means to "see" the client holistically. For that client, pain and nutrition may seem less obviously connected until one considers that the

---

Problem No. 1:   Imbalanced Nutrition, Imbalanced Fluid Volume
Goal: Improve Nutrition
Outcomes: Client's NG, TPN, and JP drains will remain patent, and client's intake of fluids and electrolytes will balance outputs.

STEP 4	STEP 5
Nursing Nutrition/Fluid Interventions	**Client Response (Evaluation)**
1. Assess new lab values	1. No new lab values except shown below
2. Assess I&O	2. Intake 600/ Output 650
3. NPO	3. NPO except ice and medications
4. Mouth care with nystatin mouth wash	4. Liked the taste, said it helped a lot
5. Ice chips	5. Sucked on for sore throat
6. Monitor NG tube, check drainage	6. Nurse checked (skill not yet learned)
7. Monitor TPN	7. Nurse checked (skill not yet learned)
8. Assess FBS	8. 109 at 6 A.M.
9. Assess abdominal pain	9. Grimacing, moaning: "15"
10. Morphine for pain	10. Gave MS at 8:10: "2" at 9:15
11. Bowel sounds	11. Hypoactive
12. Distention	12. None, soft (has NG tube)
13. Skin turgor	13. Poor, dry: Lubricated with bath
14. Drainage, JP	14. Purulent yellow, foul-smelling A– and purulent green E–

Impressions: Nutritional status in balance with intake equal to output, electrolytes stable, tubes remain patent, bowels remain hypoactive

---

Problem No. 2:   Pain
Goal: Control pain
Outcome: Client's pain remains below 3 on a 10-point scale.

STEP 4	STEP 5
Nursing Pain Interventions	**Client Responses (Evaluation)**
1. Assess pain with scale and medicate with Demerol (meperidine) and morphine	1. As above
2. Positioning	2. As above
3. Check noise, lighting	3. Positioned with pillow in bed
4. Guided imagery	4. Decreased light and fell asleep
5. Backrub	5. Visualized a beach
	6. Stated that it hurt to be touched

Impressions: client needs narcotics to control pain and likes the nondrug measures of positioning, noise and light control, and guided imagery

FIGURE 3-4 An example of the planning phase for a client with Imbalanced Nutrition, Imbalanced Fluid Volume, and Pain. (From Schuster, P. M. [2008]. *Concept mapping: A critical-thinking approach to care planning* [2nd ed.]. Philadelphia: F. A. Davis).

client has mouth ulcers and an uncomfortable nasogastric tube, both of which contribute to the client's pain.

- **Step 4**—*Identify goals, outcomes, and interventions.* On a separate page, the nurse writes the client goals, outcomes, and nursing interventions in the numbered order indicated on the concept map for each nursing diagnosis. This corresponds to the planning phase of the nursing process. Figure 3-4 provides an example of this step.
- **Step 5**—*Evaluate client's responses.* In this step, the nurse evaluates, in writing, the client's responses. Refer to Figure 3-4 for some examples. This process provides a thorough foundation for documentation in the client record. Steps 1, 2, and 3 of concept map care planning are used as the basis for documenting assessment data. Step 4, involving outcomes and interventions, is used to guide documentation of nursing interventions. Step 5 guides documentation of client responses and progress toward outcomes.

Concept mapping is dependent on clinical assessment skills and the ability to organize client data. When concept mapping is completely applied, it forms a foundation for individualizing client care while maintaining standards of nursing practice.

CRITICAL THINKING EXERCISES

1. List several reasons why including clients in care planning is important.
2. Explain the importance of the five steps of the nursing process. Give examples of what problems might arise if the nurse skips any steps.
3. Think of a client problem and a personal problem you encountered recently, and refer to the characteristics of critical thinkers to determine which characteristics you demonstrated. Apply the other characteristics to the problems and discuss how the outcomes might have been different.
4. Take the following medical diagnosis (in center of diagram below) and consider associated problems that could be part of a concept map. (Italicized words are possible answers; add additional blank circles as needed.)

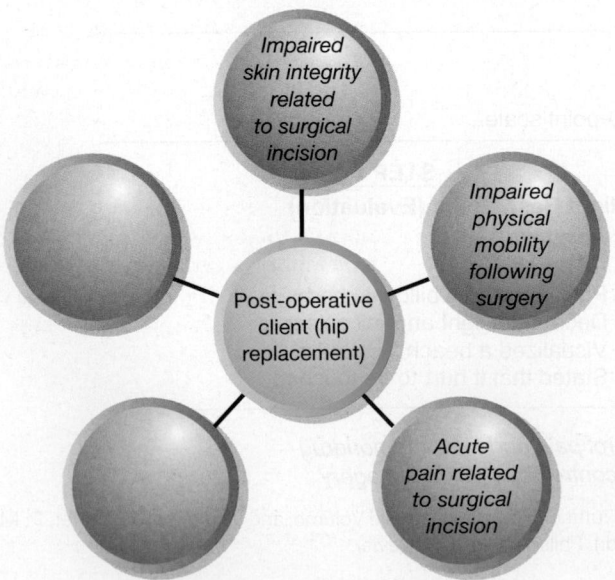

NCLEX-STYLE REVIEW QUESTIONS

1. A nurse stops to assist an adult individual involved in a motor vehicle accident. The victim was not wearing a seat belt and was thrown from the car. Of the following emergency measures, which one should the nurse perform first?
   1. Assess for signs of injuries
   2. Check the victim's breathing
   3. Cover the victim with a blanket
   4. Move the victim to the curb
2. A student nurse is assigned to care for a client who just had bowel surgery. When the nurse enters the client's room, the nurse knows that assessment of the client begins with:
   1. analysis of all collected data
   2. initial interview of the client
   3. collection of baseline data
   4. the initial contact with the client
3. Nursing diagnoses include nursing and collaborative problems. When determining care for a client, the nurse identifies which of the following as a collaborative problem?
   1. Risk for constipation related to inadequate fluid intake
   2. Ineffective health maintenance related to cognitive impairment
   3. Potential complication: Hypoglycemia
   4. Urinary retention related to dysuria
4. Which of the following nurses is thinking critically?
   1. The nurse who is concerned about the dosage of an ordered medication but administers it anyway.
   2. The nurse who makes rounds on her clients in the order of the rooms.
   3. The nurse who places a seriously ill client near the nurses' station.
   4. The nurse who resets an intravenous pump without adequate instruction.
5. "Imbalanced nutrition: Less than body requirements related to loss of appetite, difficulty swallowing, and side effects of chemotherapy" is an example of a(n):
   1. actual nursing diagnosis
   2. risk nursing diagnosis
   3. syndrome nursing diagnosis
   4. wellness nursing diagnosis

4

Interviewing and Physical Assessment

Words To Know

auscultation
chief complaint
closed questions
cultural history
focus assessment
functional assessment
head-to-toe method
inspection
objective data
open-ended questions
palpation
past health history
percussion
physical assessment
psychosocial history
signs
subjective data
symptoms
systems method

Learning Objectives

On completion of this chapter, you will be able to:

1. Explain the purpose of the interview and physical assessment.
2. Define subjective and objective data, symptoms, and signs.
3. Summarize the three phases of the interview process.
4. Explain the components of an interview.
5. Differentiate a systems method of assessment from a head-to-toe method of assessment.
6. Identify four assessment techniques.
7. Describe general assessment measures that all nurses can perform.

Assessment is the process of gathering information about a client's health (see Chap. 3). Through systematic assessment, the nurse identifies the client's:

- Current and past health status.
- Current and past functional status.
- Coping patterns.
- Health beliefs and relevant cultural practices.
- Risks for potential health problems.
- Responses to care.
- Nursing care needs.
- Referral needs.

The nurse first assesses the client when he or she is admitted to the healthcare system. Findings from this comprehensive initial assessment establish a database that gives all team members relevant client information and become a yardstick for measuring effectiveness of care. The initial assessment consists of two parts: the interview and the physical assessment.

During the interview, the nurse gathers subjective data. **Subjective data** are statements the client makes about what he or she feels. When the client tells the nurse about nausea, pain, fear, bloating, or other feelings of discomfort, he or she is providing subjective data. These feelings of discomfort are called **symptoms.**

During the physical assessment, the nurse gathers objective data. **Objective data** are facts obtained through observation, physical examination, and diagnostic testing. When the nurse assesses blood pressure or heart rate or examines results from urinalysis, he or she obtains objective data. When objective data are abnormal, they are called **signs.** Objective data often support the subjective data.

THE INTERVIEW PROCESS

The length of the interview depends on variables such as the severity of the client's condition, level of discomfort, ability to cooperate, age, and mental state. The interview process is divided into three parts: the preinterview period, the interview, and the postinterview period (Box 4-1).

Preinterview Period

The preinterview period determines the direction of the interview process. The nurse begins by establishing rapport with the client and family members and ensuring that the client is comfortable. Putting the client physically and emotionally at ease facilitates the exchange of information and helps to establish a bond between the client and the nurse. When making introductions, the nurse should address the client by his or her surname. A private setting for the interview is essential to eliminate interruptions and maintain the client's confidentiality (Fig. 4-1). The nurse should explain that the information obtained during the interview helps with planning care. He or she should tell the client that all information is kept confidential, although all members of the healthcare team share the data.

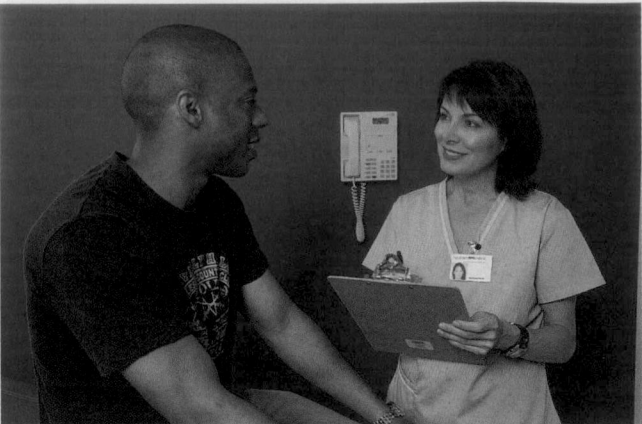

FIGURE 4-1 The nurse provides a relaxed and private atmosphere when conducting an interview.

▶ *Stop, Think, and Respond Exercise 4-1*

Describe approaches you would use in the preinterview period for a client who is hearing or vision impaired.

The Interview

During the interview, the nurse asks the client questions to gather data for the client database. Good communication skills are essential. The nurse should avoid using medical terms. Questions are best phrased as **open-ended questions** that require discussion rather than **closed questions** that require only "yes" or "no" answers. Giving the client ample time to answer each question and maintaining frequent eye contact are important measures.

Many institutions have assessment forms that help ensure the database is complete. If the nurse asks the client to complete the assessment form, he or she should clarify information that the client gives during the interview. Many hospitals are using hand-held or bedside computers to complete the database. Whether entering data on a computer or writing on a form, the nurse should connect with the client in a meaningful way and not focus entirely on the process of data entry.

The interview includes the following components (Box 4-2):

B O X 4 - 1 **Parts of the Interview**

Preinterview Period
Establish rapport
Explain the purpose of the interview

Interview
Collect subjective data
Ask open-ended questions

Postinterview Period
Summarize what transpired during the interview
Thank client and family for their cooperation

- Psychosocial and cultural history
- Chief complaint
- Functional status—self-care ability
- History of the present illness
- Past health history
- Family history
- Review of body systems

It is unnecessary to discuss these topics in a specific pattern in the interview. The examiner can rearrange the order in which topics are discussed, digress from an established format if additional information seems pertinent, or omit areas that are not applicable.

Psychosocial and Cultural History

The **psychosocial history** and **cultural history** include the client's age, occupation, religious affiliation, cultural background, and health beliefs (see Chap. 8), marital status, and home and working environments. Although some of this material is found on the face sheet of the client's chart, specific aspects may need further exploration. If, for example, the client is a factory worker, the examiner would ask if the client works around hazardous chemicals or has had job-related injuries.

Chief Complaint

The **chief complaint** is the current reason the client is seeking care. The primary purpose of the interview is to discover what the client perceives as the health problem that needs treatment. Recording information in the client's own words is best. For example, "I had a terrible pain in the right side of my stomach after I ate. I never had it so bad. The doctor said maybe it's my gallbladder."

Functional Assessment

A **functional assessment** determines how well the client can manage activities of daily living (ADLs). ADLs include self-care activities such as walking moderate distances, bathing, and toileting, and instrumental activities, such as preparing meals, obtaining transportation, and dialing the telephone. This assessment component is particularly important when assessing older adults or physically challenged clients of any age.

BOX 4-2 **Interview Guide**

The interviewer establishes a database by asking the client questions about his or her health.

Psychosocial and Cultural History

Age; gender; marital status; number of children; occupation; highest level of education; religious affiliation; place of residence; country of origin; primary language; military service; date, location, and length of foreign travel or residence

Chief Complaint

Reason for seeking care; type, location, and severity of symptoms

Functional Assessment

Ability to walk, get in and out of bed, bathe, dress, eat, and get to and from the bathroom; ability to drive, take public transportation, get groceries, or prepare meals

History of Present Illness

Chronologic description of the onset, frequency, and duration of current symptoms; attempts and outcomes of self-treatment; what the client thinks caused the problem; how the illness affects the client's life at home, at work, and socially

Past Health History

Childhood diseases, physical injuries, major illnesses, previous medical or psychiatric hospitalizations, surgical procedures, drug history, use of alcohol and tobacco, allergy history

Family History

Health problems among relatives living and deceased; longevity and cause of death among deceased blood relatives

Review of Systems

General. Usual weight, recent weight change, weakness, fatigue, fever

Skin. Rashes, lumps, sores, itching, dryness, color change, changes in hair or nails

Head. Headache, head injury

Eyes. Vision, glasses or contact lenses, last eye examination, pain, redness, excessive tearing, double vision, blurred vision, spots, specks, flashing lights, glaucoma, cataracts

Ears. Hearing, tinnitus, vertigo, earaches, infection, discharge, use of hearing aids

Nose and sinuses. Frequent colds; nasal stuffiness, discharge, or itching; hay fever; nosebleeds; sinus trouble

Mouth and throat. Condition of teeth and gums; bleeding gums; dentures, if any, and how they fit; last dental examination; sore tongue; dry mouth; frequent sore throats; hoarseness

Neck. Lumps; "swollen glands," goiter, pain or stiffness in the neck

Breasts. Lumps, pain or discomfort, nipple discharge, self-examination

Respiratory. Cough; sputum (color, quantity); hemoptysis, wheezing, asthma, bronchitis, emphysema, pneumonia, tuberculosis, pleurisy, last chest x-ray film

Cardiac. Heart trouble, high blood pressure, rheumatic fever, heart murmurs, chest pain or discomfort, palpitations, dyspnea, orthopnea, paroxysmal nocturnal dyspnea, edema, past electrocardiogram or other heart test results

Gastrointestinal. Trouble swallowing, heartburn, appetite, nausea, vomiting, regurgitation, vomiting of blood, indigestion, frequency of bowel movements, color and size of stools, change in bowel habits, rectal bleeding or black tarry stools, hemorrhoids, constipation, diarrhea, abdominal pain, food intolerance, excessive belching or passing of gas, jaundice, liver or gallbladder trouble, hepatitis

Urinary. Frequency of urination, polyuria, nocturia, burning or pain on urination, hematuria, urgency, reduced caliber or force of the urinary stream, hesitancy, dribbling, incontinence, urinary infections, stones

Genital. Male: Hernias, discharge from or sores on the penis, testicular pain or masses, history of sexually transmitted diseases and their treatments, sexual preference, interest, function, satisfaction, and problems. *Female:* Age at menarche; regularity, frequency, and duration of periods; amount of bleeding; bleeding between periods or after intercourse; last menstrual period; dysmenorrhea; premenstrual tension; age at menopause; menopausal symptoms; postmenopausal bleeding. If the client was born before 1971, exposure to diethylstilbestrol from maternal use during pregnancy. Discharge, itching, sores, lumps, sexually transmitted diseases and their treatments. Number of pregnancies, deliveries, or abortions (spontaneous and induced); complications of pregnancy; birth control methods. Sexual preference, interest, function, satisfaction; any problems, including dyspareunia (painful intercourse)

Peripheral vascular. Intermittent claudication, leg cramps, varicose veins, past history of blood clots in the veins

Musculoskeletal. Muscle or joint pains, stiffness, arthritis, gout, backache. If present, describe location and symptoms (e.g., swelling, redness, pain, tenderness, stiffness, weakness, limitation of motion or activity)

Neurologic. Fainting, blackouts, seizures, weakness, paralysis, numbness or loss of sensation, tingling or "pins and needles," tremors or other involuntary movements

Hematologic/immunologic. Anemia, easy bruising or bleeding, past transfusions and any reactions to them, status for human immunodeficiency virus infection, autoimmune disorders

Endocrine. Thyroid trouble, heat or cold intolerance, excessive sweating, diabetes, excessive thirst or hunger, polyuria

Psychobiologic. Nervousness, tension, mood, memory

Adapted from Bickley, L. S., (2006). *Bates' guide to physical examination and history taking* (9th ed.). Philadelphia: Lippincott Williams & Wilkins.

History of Present Illness

The nurse asks the client to describe all present problems, including the onset, frequency, and duration of symptoms. Asking for more detailed information about one body system or problem is called a **focus assessment** because it adds depth to the original data. For example, a client may reveal that he or she has experienced abdominal pain for the past several weeks. The questioning then addresses what causes the pain, how long the pain lasts, what the quality of the pain is, and what makes it better or worse.

Past Health History

The client's **past health history** includes identifying childhood diseases, previous injuries, major illnesses, prior hospitalizations, surgical procedures, and drug history. Obtaining this information is important because it may affect current care. When discussing the client's past medical problems, the nurse should ask the age at which the problem was diagnosed, treatments prescribed, and whether the problem still exists. Information about past surgeries includes types, when each was done, and whether recoveries were uneventful or accompanied by complications.

The nurse identifies any current and past use of prescription and nonprescription drugs or herbal products. He or she asks about the client's use of alcohol and tobacco, because these drugs can create or contribute to other health problems.

The nurse compiles a list of the client's allergies, including sensitivities to drugs, foods, and environmental substances. If the client has a drug allergy, the drug and the client's reaction are described; some clients confuse a drug's side effects with an allergic response. If the client or family cannot remember the name of the drug, the nurse should try to identify it from another source, such as the prescribing physician or past hospital records.

Family History

The family history is important because many disorders are hereditary. The nurse asks if parents, siblings, and grandparents are living or dead. If any blood relatives in the immediate family have died, the nurse documents the causes of their deaths and the ages at which they died. The nurse identifies health problems that affect other living relatives.

Review of Body Systems

The nurse asks general questions about each body system to trigger the client's memory of inadvertently overlooked health problems. For example, when reviewing the gastrointestinal system, the nurse should ask if the client has a history of nausea, vomiting, food intolerance, bowel irregularity, stomach ulcer, changes in the color of stool, and similar questions that suggest a current or past health problem. Asking an exhaustive number of questions for each system may be unnecessary, but the review should include a few questions about each system. If the client affirms that a problem exists, the nurse asks more focused questions until he or she has obtained adequate data about the problem.

Postinterview Period

An effective way of ending the interview is to summarize what occurred and thank the client for cooperating. Asking the client if he or she needs more information provides an opportunity for the client to express concerns and ask questions.

Gerontologic Considerations

- Before interviewing the older client, be certain that assistive sensory devices (e.g., glasses, hearing aids) are in place and functioning.

- Ask the client to describe activities in a usual day. Also ask questions about family and social supports. Use this information as a foundation for other interview questions.

- Allow a friend or family caregiver to remain during the history if the client requests.

- Use silence to allow more time for the client to respond to questions.

- Include questions regarding changes that may affect nutrition such as taste, smell, swallowing, ability to obtain or prepare foods, fit of dentures, fit of clothing, and if meals are eaten alone or with whom.

- Data obtained from the interview may need to be validated with family or significant others involved in the client's care.

THE PHYSICAL ASSESSMENT

The second part of the assessment process is the collection of objective data through a physical assessment. During the **physical assessment**, the nurse examines body structures and observes the client's physical appearance, mood, mental status, behaviors, and ability to interact. Licensed practical/vocational nurses (LPN/LVNs) participate in some of aspects of the physical assessment, but are generally limited by education and experience, as well as scope of practice. Understanding the role of registered nurses, nurse practitioners, and physicians is essential so that the LPN/LVN can provide explanations to the client and assist the other healthcare providers as they assess the client.

The physical assessment is conducted using one of two methods: the systems method or the head-to-toe method. The **systems method** approaches the examination by assessing each body system separately (Box 4-3). The **head-to-toe method** of assessment begins at the top of the body and progresses downward. Sometimes, healthcare providers use parts of both methods.

Assessment Techniques

There are four assessment techniques that the nurse or other healthcare provider performs during a physical assessment: inspection, palpation, percussion, and auscultation (Fig. 4-2).

Inspection

Inspection is the systematic and thorough observation of the client and specific areas of the body (see Fig. 4-2A). The nurse (including the LPN/LVN who learns and practices inspection techniques) uses the senses of vision, smell, and hearing to inspect a client. Inspection includes examining the client for changes in skin color, temperature, or both; observing a wound for signs of healing or infection; or generally noting color, size, location, texture, symmetry, odors, and sounds. The technique of inspection includes the following measures (Weber, 2008):

- Expose the area being inspected while draping the rest of the client
- Look before touching
- Use adequate lighting
- Provide a warm room for examination

Palpation

Palpation is assessing the characteristics of an organ or body part by touching and feeling it with the hands or

BOX 4-3 **Components of the Physical Assessment**

Using inspection, palpation, percussion, and auscultation, the examiner assesses and records findings about the following attributes, body functions, and systems:

General Appraisal

Physical appearance, age, overall physical development, hygiene, grooming, posture, mobility, use of ambulatory devices, weight, height, and vital signs

Skin and Related Structures

Color, moisture, temperature, texture, turgor, skin integrity, rash, edema (swelling caused by the collection of fluid in the tissues), warts, moles, petechiae (hemorrhagic spots on the skin), distribution of body hair, condition and shape of fingernails and toenails

Head

Shape and size of head; texture, color, and distribution of hair

Eyes

External structures of the eyes (upper and lower lids, eyelashes, cornea, conjunctiva, sclera, iris, and pupil), pupil size and reaction to light, eye movement, anterior chambers of the eye, visual acuity

Lips and Mouth

Condition of the teeth and gums, oral cavity and mucous membranes, oral pharynx, tonsils, uvula

Ears

External ear (the earlobe, auricle, and surrounding tissues), tympanic membrane, hearing

Neck

Lymph nodes, thyroid, position of trachea, carotid arteries, neck veins

Thorax and Lungs

Shape of the chest, expansion, axilla (armpits), breathing patterns, respiratory rate and depth, use of accessory muscles, breath sounds

Breasts

Appearance, skin characteristics, nipples, presence of lumps or masses

Cardiovascular System

Radial pulse rate; apical pulse rate; heart sounds; blood pressure measurements in both arms while standing, sitting, and lying down; pedal pulses

Abdomen

Bowel sounds, tenderness, pain, muscle resistance or rigidity, masses, scars, hernia, liver size, spleen, kidneys, abdominal aorta

Rectum

Hemorrhoids, fissures, prostate gland in male clients, stool

Genitalia

Male: penis, scrotum, inguinal lymph nodes. *Female:* external genitalia (labia, clitoris, urethral orifice, and vaginal opening), internal structures (vaginal wall and the cervix), inguinal lymph nodes

Musculoskeletal System

Contour and size of joints, range of motion, muscle size and strength

Neurologic System

Level of consciousness; orientation; intellectual functioning; emotional state; speech patterns; short-term and long-term memory, perception of pain, heat, cold, light touch, and vibration; gait; reflexes; cranial nerves; muscle strength; movement; coordination; tendon reflexes; proprioception (or position awareness)

---

fingertips (see Fig. 4-2*B*). The process of palpation provides information about texture, temperature, moisture, motion, and consistency or firmness of structures (solid vs. fluid). Palpation detects abnormal conditions, such as enlarged organs, tumors, or fluid in a cavity. When palpating, the nurse uses the fingertips to detect pulsations or to differentiate between surfaces, the surface of the palm to sense vibrations, and the back of the hand to determine temperature. Techniques for palpation include using first light then deep palpation and palpating tender areas last (Weber, 2008). The LPN/LVN does some palpation for initial gathering of data, but generally the RN, nurse practitioner, or physician perform this assessment technique. The LPN/LVN assists the client to move or turn so that the examiner can more easily palpate a particular area on the client.

Percussion

Percussion is tapping a portion of the body to determine if there is tenderness or to elicit sounds that vary according to the density of underlying structures (see Fig. 4-2*C*). Table 4-1 provides a description of sounds that may be heard with percussion. The procedure for percussion is as follows:

1. Place the index or middle finger of the nondominant hand firmly on the surface to be percussed. Only the finger should have contact with skin surface. Raise the other fingers and heel of the hand off the surface.
2. Use quick, light, firm strikes with the tip of the middle finger of the dominant hand against the distal end of the nondominant finger. Use wrist motion to make tapping movements—keep forearm stable.
3. Deliver one to three taps, and then move the nondominant finger to another area.

The technique of percussion requires practice and skill and is generally performed by nurse practitioners and physicians. LPN/LVNs assist the client to move or turn so that the examiner may more easily percuss a particular area on the client.

Auscultation

Auscultation means listening with a stethoscope for normal and abnormal sounds generated by organs and structures such as the heart, lungs, intestines, and major arteries (see Fig. 4-2*D*). When performing auscultation, nurses describe normal and abnormal sounds using descriptive terms such as *high-pitched, low-pitched, harsh, blowing, crackling, loud, distant,* and *soft.* They auscultate the lungs, heart, and abdomen.

Depending on the healthcare setting, LPN/LVNs may auscultate breath and bowel sounds, but generally RNs,

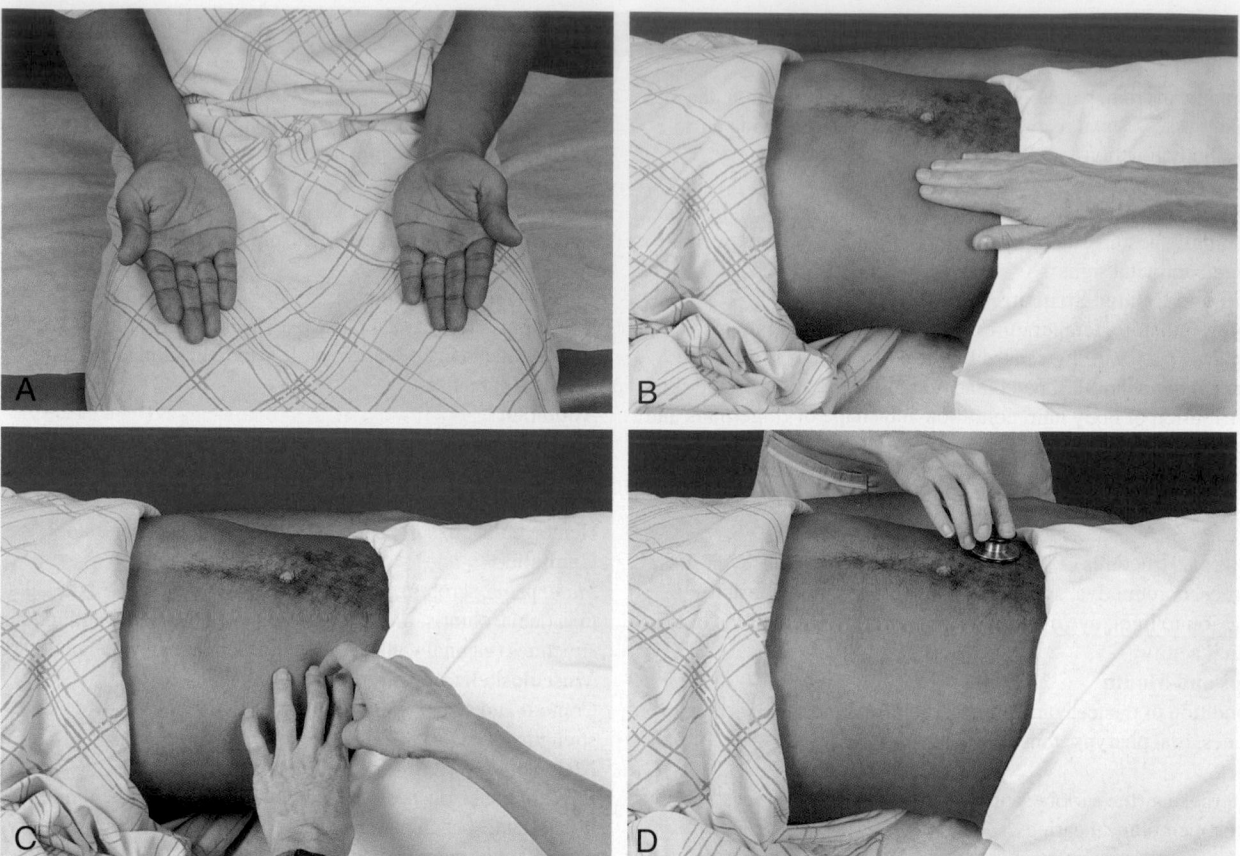

FIGURE 4-2 Assessment techniques: (**A**) inspection, (**B**) palpation, (**C**) percussion, and (**D**) auscultation.

nurse practitioners, and physicians perform this assessment technique. LPN/LVNs assist the client to move or turn so that the examiner is able to auscultate the client more easily.

Performing the Assessment

As stated above, in-depth physical assessment requires practice and skill. Nurse practitioners or physicians perform many components of the physical assessment. The extent of the assessment performed by the LPN/LVN or registered nurse depends on the nurse's skill, the client's condition, and facility practices. In any case, the nurse gives the client an examination gown or drape and maintains the client's privacy. He or she should ensure that there is adequate lighting in the examination area and gather all equipment, such as a penlight, stethoscope, and sphygmomanometer. Another im-

portant nursing measure is to maintain Standard Precautions (see Chap. 12).

Clients often feel anxiety, embarrassment, and fear when undergoing a physical examination. They are concerned about the findings and implications of those findings for their future well-being. Explaining what will happen helps the client prepare for the examination and assists in obtaining the most accurate information. The nurse should avoid showing surprise or concern at any findings to prevent increasing the client's anxiety level.

At the conclusion of the examination, the nurse allows the client to dress privately or help the client dress if needed, help the client get in a comfortable position, and ask if he or she has any questions. Finally, the nurse informs the client and family that data will be shared with the physician.

TABLE 4-1 Percussion Sounds

PERCUSSION SOUNDS	ORIGIN	SOUND	EXAMPLES
Tympany	Enclosed air	Drumlike	Puffed-out cheek, air in bowel
Resonance	Part air and part solid tissue	Hollow	Normal lung
Hyper-resonance	Mostly air	Booming	Lung with emphysema
Dullness	Mostly solid tissue	"Thud" sound	Liver, spleen, heart
Flatness	Very dense tissue	Flat	Muscle, bone

From Weber, J. R. (2001). *Nurses' handbook of health assessment* (4th ed.) Philadelphia: Lippincott Williams & Wilkins, p. 41.

▶ *Stop, Think, and Respond Exercise 4-2*

Refer to Table 3-1 and consider the role of the LPN when a client is having a physical assessment. For each aspect of the physical assessment, list one activity for the LPN.

Gerontologic Considerations

When performing a physical assessment for an older client, keep the following in mind:

- Ask what chronic condition may impact the assessment (e.g., arthritis may limit range of motion of a particular extromity).
- Avoid tiring the client—allow rest periods if needed.
- Keep the older client warm and away from drafts.
- Be aware of privacy issues if the older client's hearing impairments require louder interactions.
- Allow ample time for the client to respond to directions and change position.
- If possible, observe the client performing ADLs. Include an unaided "Get-up-and-go" assessment of the client rising from a seated position and ambulating to assess ability.

CRITICAL THINKING EXERCISES

1. How might you handle a situation in which a client's spouse answers questions asked of the client? Role-play a possible nurse–client scenario.

2. How might room temperature, lighting, lack of privacy, or limited time affect the assessment of a client?

3. A client is admitted with the medical diagnosis of chronic obstructive lung disease. What focus assessment data might be essential?

4. A client admitted to a nursing facility is disoriented and confused. How might the assessment be different for this client?

NCLEX-STYLE REVIEW QUESTIONS

1. A student nurse is learning the process of physical examination. Palpation is most likely to detect which of the following findings?
1. Abnormal body tenderness
2. Abnormal lung sounds
3. Abnormal organ size
4. Abnormal skin color

2. A client recovering from abdominal surgery complains of feeling full and bloated after a clear liquid lunch. What type of assessment should the nurse conduct?
1. Focus assessment
2. Functional assessment
3. Head-to-toe assessment
4. Systems assessment

3. Which of the following documented findings is classified as subjective data? Select all that apply.
1. The UAP reports vital signs of 100°C, 88, 24, and 148/72 mm/Hg.
2. The client states that the pain is worse at night
3. "I have not had a bowel movement for three days."
4. The client voided 120 mL of dark yellow urine.

4. During a systems assessment, the nurse is assessing the client's neurologic status. Which of the following assessment techniques should be included? Select all that apply.
1. Ask the client to count backward from 100.
2. Ask the client what the date and time are.
3. Assess the client's bilateral muscle strength.
4. Inspect the color of the client's sclera.
5. Note any signs of swelling in the extremities.
6. Palpate the contour and size of the joints.

5. A nurse is obtaining information from a client as part of the admission to the medical unit. Which of the following questions/statements are most likely to elicit more information from the client?
1. "Do you have children living at home?"
2. "How many packs of cigarettes do you smoke?"
3. "Tell me why you are being admitted to the hospital."
4. "What do you estimate is your daily beer consumption?"

5

Legal and Ethical Issues

Learning Objectives

On completion of this chapter, you will be able to:

1. Explain the difference between laws and ethics.
2. Categorize sources of U.S. law.
3. Differentiate intentional and unintentional torts.
4. Summarize negligence, malpractice, and liability.
5. Describe measures such as risk management that help limit nurses' liability in malpractice suits.
6. Describe procedures and regulations to protect client information.
7. Discuss informed consent, advance directives, and do-not-resuscitate orders.
8. Explain utilitarianism, deontology, duties, and rights.
9. Summarize the characteristics of ethical values.
10. Define six professional values.
11. Describe factors that affect healthcare ethics.
12. Explain an ethical decision-making model.

A system of laws and ethical beliefs helps to establish and maintain order and harmony within a society. **Laws** are written rules for conduct and actions. They are binding for all citizens and ensure the protection of rights. **Ethics** are moral principles and values that guide the behavior of honorable people. Ethical standards dictate the rightness or wrongness of human behavior. Box 5-1 highlights the differences between laws and ethics.

The healthcare delivery system affects and is affected by societal beliefs, values, and laws. It is accountable to society for maintaining established legal and ethical standards. In turn, legal and ethical situations that healthcare personnel face also may become issues for society. Nurses today require a basic understanding of laws and ethics that may affect their practice. Issues related to competence, safety, optimal care, protecting clients' rights, and practicing according to professional standards of care are of most concern to nurses. This chapter provides an introduction to the legal and ethical dimensions of nursing practice.

LEGAL ISSUES IN NURSING PRACTICE

Federal and state legislation directly affects the healthcare industry. Laws and regulations that affect nursing practice and the safety of clients are essential for nurses to know.

Sources of Law

Laws stem from several sources. Types of law discussed in this section include constitutional, statutory, administrative, common, criminal, and civil law.

Laws
Serve as rules of conduct
Guide actions and interactions within a society
Are regulated by authorized organizations and law officers

Ethics
Deal with right and wrong
Consider beliefs about morals and values
Do not have a formal enforcement system

Constitutional Law

Constitutional law is based on the constitution, which guarantees fundamental freedoms to all people in the United States. This type of law affects nurses in that it protects their basic rights, just as it protects the rights of clients. For example, freedom of speech and the right to privacy are rights that nurses and clients have as citizens of the United States.

Statutory Law

Statutory law is a law that any local, state, or federal legislative body enacts. These laws can significantly affect healthcare providers. For example, the "DRG law" described in Chapter 1 greatly influenced healthcare reimbursement and length of hospital stays.

Another example of statutory law is the nurse practice act in each state. **Nurse practice acts** define nursing practice and set standards for nurses in each state. These legal statutes regulate the practice of nursing to protect the health and safety of citizens. Although each state has its own nurse practice act, they all share common components:

- Define the scope of practice
- Establish requirements for licensure and entry into practice
- Create a board of nursing to oversee nursing practice
- Identify legal titles for nurses, such as *registered nurse* and *licensed practical/vocational nurse*
- Determine what constitutes grounds for disciplinary action

Administrative Law

Statutory law empowers regulatory agencies to create and carry out the laws. These federal and regulatory agencies practice **administrative law**, the rules and regulations that concern the health, welfare, and safety of federal and state citizens. For example, the Occupational Safety and Health Administration (OSHA) is the federal agency that develops the rules and regulations governing workplace safety. State statutory law forms nurse practice acts, but the authority to regulate that act is given to an administrative agency, usually called the state board of nursing.

The primary responsibility of a state **board of nursing** is to protect the public's health and well-being. Other responsibilities include reviewing and approving nursing education programs in the state, forming criteria for granting licensure, overseeing procedures for licensure examinations, issuing or transferring licenses, investigating complaints, and implementing disciplinary procedures.

- Because of the vulnerability of older adults, federal and state governments carefully regulate the treatment provided in licensed healthcare facilities. These regulations address almost every aspect of life in a nursing facility and include sanctions to force compliance.

Common Law

Common law, also known as *judicial law,* is based on earlier court decisions, judgments, and decrees. These earlier decisions set precedents for interpretation of laws. Common law evolved when courts began to present written decisions based on prior court cases. Stated another way, if one court has previously decided on a particular case and another court reviews a similar case, the second court will make the same decision, citing the precedent of the previous case. The court will make new rules if the precedent is outdated.

Criminal Law

Criminal law concerns offenses that violate the public's welfare. A crime is a violation of criminal law. There are two categories of offenses: (1) misdemeanors, which are minor offenses; and (2) felonies, which are serious offenses. Misdemeanors involving healthcare workers are similar to those for all citizens (e.g., driving violations). Examples of felonies involving healthcare workers include falsification of medical records, insurance fraud, and theft of narcotics. If an individual misrepresents himself or herself as a licensed nurse, this person commits the crime of practicing without a license.

Civil Law

Civil law applies to disputes that arise between individual citizens. Civil laws protect each individual's personal freedoms and property rights. Some civil laws include the right to be left alone, freedom from threats of injury, freedom from offensive contact, and freedom from character attacks. The plaintiff is the individual who brings a dispute to the court; the complaint is the formal written dispute and the restitution that the plaintiff seeks. The individual or party against whom the complaint is filed is the defendant. **Liability** means legal responsibility. If a client receives the wrong medication and is harmed as a result, the nurse is liable, or held responsible, for that harm.

Although there are various branches of civil law, tort law is most likely to affect nurses. **Tort law** is the body of law that governs breaches of duty owed by one person to another. A **duty** is an expected action based on moral or legal obligations. A **tort** is an injury that occurred because of another person's intentional or unintentional actions, or failure to act. This injury can be physical, emotional, or financial. If the defendant is found to have breached his or her duty and that breach causes harm, he or she must pay restitution for damages. The types of torts that involve nurses are intentional and unintentional.

Intentional Torts

An **intentional tort** is a deliberate and willful act that infringes on another person's rights or property. Examples of intentional torts include assault, battery, false imprisonment, invasion of privacy, and defamation.

Assault. *Assault* is an act that involves a threat or attempt to do bodily harm. Types of assault include physical intimidation, verbal remarks, or gestures that lead the client to believe that force or injury may be forthcoming. For example, a nurse is frustrated because a client constantly turns on the call light. The nurse threatens to restrain the client's hands if he or she continues this action. This verbal threat constitutes assault.

Battery. *Battery* is actual physical contact with another person without that person's consent. The contact can include touching a person's body, clothing, chair, or bed. A charge of battery can be made even if the contact did not cause physical harm to the individual. To protect healthcare workers from being charged with battery, clients sign a general permission for care and treatment at the time of admission (Fig. 5-1). They also sign a written consent before undergoing special tests, procedures, or surgery. A parent or guardian must provide consent if the client is a minor, mentally retarded, or mentally incompetent. In an emergency, healthcare providers can infer consent, meaning the law assumes that in life-threatening circumstances clients would provide consent.

Nonconsensual physical contact sometimes is justified. When mentally ill or intoxicated clients are endangering their own safety and/or the safety of others, health professionals may use physical force to subdue them. The nurse must clearly document that the situation required the degree of restraint used. Excessive force never is appropriate when less force would have been just as effective. When recording these incidents, the nurse must document the behavior that resulted in the use of force and the client's response when the nurse tried lesser forms of restraint first. Healthcare facilities have specific requirements related to the use of physical and chemical restraints. Nurses need to adhere strictly to agency policies related to restraints.

False Imprisonment. *False imprisonment* occurs when healthcare workers physically or chemically restrain an individual from leaving a healthcare institution. Mentally impaired, confused, or disoriented clients may be restrained if their safety or the safety of others is at risk. This confinement requires restraining orders, court-ordered commitments, or medical orders. A nurse, however, cannot detain a competent client who wishes to leave a hospital or long-term care facility before being discharged by the physician. If a client wishes to leave the facility against medical advice, he or she signs a form (Fig. 5-2) that releases the healthcare facility from responsibility.

The unnecessary or unprescribed application of physical or chemical restraints also creates potential liability for battery and false imprisonment. If the nurse must apply restraints and no current medical order exists, the best legal defense is to show just cause through accurate documentation. Because confined and restrained clients cannot protect themselves or meet their own needs, charting must show that the nurse assessed the client frequently, offered fluids and nourishment, and provided an opportunity for bowel and bladder elimination. It is expected that the restraints will be discontinued when the client no longer poses a threat to self or others.

Invasion of Privacy. The right to privacy means that persons have the right to expect that they and their property will be left alone. Failure to do so is an *invasion of privacy*. Nonmedical torts of this nature generally include trespassing, illegal search and seizure, or wiretapping. Invasion of privacy also applies to releasing private information about a person, regardless of whether or not the information is true.

Examples of invasion of privacy in healthcare include photographing an individual without consent, revealing a client's name in a public report or research paper, and allowing unauthorized persons to observe a client during treatment or care. Health professionals protect a client's privacy by:

* Obtaining a signed release for recognizable photographs for publications or presentations.
* Using initials or code numbers instead of names in written reports or research papers.
* Closing bedside curtains when giving personal care.
* Obtaining a client's permission for a nursing student or other healthcare person to observe treatment.

Defamation. *Defamation* is an act that harms a person's reputation and good name. If a person orally utters a character attack in the presence of others, the action is called *slander*. If the damaging statement is written and read by others, it is called *libel*. Nurses must avoid offering unfounded or exaggerated negative opinions about clients, the expertise of physicians, or other coworkers. Injury occurs because the derogatory remarks may mar a person's public image or keep potential clients from seeking the services of the defamed person. If a client accuses a nurse of defamation of character, the client must prove that there was malice, misuse of privileged information, and spoken or written untruths. Nurses are at risk for defamation of character suits if they make negative comments in public areas (e.g., elevators, cafeterias) or assert opinions regarding a client's character in the medical record.

Unintentional Torts

Unintentional torts involve situations that result in injuries, although the person responsible did not mean to cause any harm. Types of unintentional torts involve negligence and malpractice.

Negligence describes the failure to act as a reasonable person would have acted in a similar situation. If harm results from the action (or failure to act), a person may sue that individual for negligence. For example, a homeowner fails to repair a broken step or warn a visitor to be careful. The visitor falls and suffers an injury. The jury decides if another reasonable, prudent person would have repaired the step and/or warned the visitor to be careful.

The law defines **malpractice** as professional negligence. It refers to harm that results from a licensed person's actions or lack of action. A jury must determine if the responsible person's conduct deviated from the standard expected of others with similar education and experience. Box 5-2 provides a summary of elements that must be demonstrated for malpractice claims.

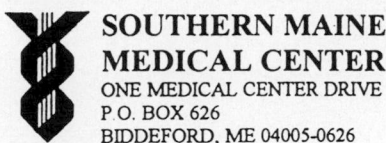

SOUTHERN MAINE
MEDICAL CENTER
ONE MEDICAL CENTER DRIVE
P.O. BOX 626
BIDDEFORD, ME 04005-0626

NOTICE
You are being admitted to SMMC as an inpatient.

CONSENT TO TREAT AND/OR ADMIT
When I sign this form, I agree to let SMMC treat me in the emergency department, or as an outpatient, or to admit and treat me as an inpatient at this hospital.

1. SMMC may examine me and perform tests and treatments to help learn about, and care for, my injury or illness.
2. This could mean emergency care or outpatient services with more visits.
3. It could also mean hospital care with a need for inpatient hospital services.

I know that inpatient hospital treatment may mean medications, tests, and nursing care. I agree to this.

I know I can stop all or part of my treatment at any time.

I know my consent is needed to have me take part in any experiments or research.

I know that medicine and surgery have risks. Some tests and treatments could cause harm even death. In some cases I may be asked to sign a separate consent form. SMMC has not told me that any test or treatment will guarantee a certain result.

I know that many staff doctors are not employed by SMMC, but may use the hospital as a place to care for their patients. Other doctors at SMMC may be in post-graduate training programs. Some other health care workers at SMMC may also not be employees of SMMC.

MEDICAL RECORDS RELEASE
I know that, under Maine law, SMMC may give parts of my medical record to those who pay for health care services, check for insurance claims or do medical reviews. SMMC may also release my medical record to other people who may be responsible for my further care. Only parts of my record that relate to these purposes may be released. Maine law also allows SMMC to share health care information about me with my family and household members, unless I instruct SMMC not to do so.

I know that Maine Worker's Compensation law gives my employer(s) and their agents the right to review my record if I may have an injury or illness covered by that law. I know also, that state and federal laws may provide additional protection against giving out information regarding HIV status, mental health services, or services received from an alcohol or drug abuse treatment program.

I know that Maine law gives me the right to decide whether certain health care information may be disclosed to others. I may tell SMMC if I wish to exercise this right. If I do, one of my choices is to have my name left out of the directory that lists people being cared for at SMMC. Leaving my name out of this directory may prevent SMMC from directing visitors and telephone calls to me.

ASSIGNMENT OF INTEREST AND FINANCIAL AGREEMENT
I know I must pay any charges not covered by insurance. I agree to have the payments of insurance and plan benefits (including Medicare) go directly to SMMC. If the payment is in keeping with the provisions of the insurance policy or plan, this will end the claim on the payor to the extent of the payment. If charges are denied, or are not covered by my insurance or plan, I must pay SMMC for these charges. If my account is referred for collection, I may be responsible for all fees required to collect it (including attorney's fees).

ADVANCE APPROVAL FOR MEDICAL SERVICES
If my insurance or health plan says I need an OK for a test or treatment before it is provided, SMMC will try to help me. SMMC cannot, however, promise to get this OK for me. If some services are denied later by my payor, I must pay the balance of my bill.

MEDICARE
_____ I have received a copy of the *Important Message from Medicare*.
(Initial)

_____   _____
Patient   Date

_____   _____   _____
Legal Representative   Relationship to Patient   Date

INPATIENT

_____
Witness

FIGURE 5-1 Example of a form to obtain consent for treatment.

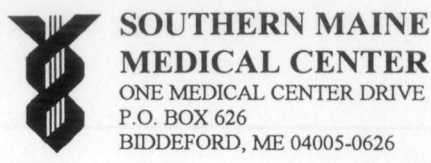

**SOUTHERN MAINE
MEDICAL CENTER**
ONE MEDICAL CENTER DRIVE
P.O. BOX 626
BIDDEFORD, ME 04005-0626

LEAVING HOSPITAL AGAINST MEDICAL ADVICE

I certify that I am leaving the hospital voluntarily, against the advice and recommendation of the attending physician and the hospital. I acknowledge that I have been informed of the following risks and possible medical consequences involved:

_____

_____

_____

I release the attending physician, his associates or assistants, the hospital, and its personnel from any and all responsibility for any ill effects which may result from this action.

_____   _____
Witness   Patient Signature

_____ _____ A.M. / P.M.
Date   Time

* Because the above patient is an unemancipated minor, _____ years of age, or is unable to sign for the following reasons:

_____

_____

the above consent is given on the patient's behalf by:

_____   _____
Witness   Closest Relative or Legal Guardian

_____ _____ A.M. / P.M. _____
Date   Time   Relationship

FIGURE 5-2 Example of a release form for leaving against medical advice.

One determination of a nurse's duty to a client involves standards of practice. **Standards of practice** are guidelines that the nursing profession establishes for clinical decision-making. These standards include standards of care (Box 5-3). These standards evolve as research and evidence change treatments and procedures. Nurses continually have to revise their methods of delivering care as standards change. In addition, "court cases and legislation…clarify the duties nurses owe patients" (LaDuke, 2003).

Unintentional tort law holds healthcare workers to a higher standard than that used in negligence cases. Several factors have contributed to increased malpractice suits against nurses (Croke, 2003):

| BOX 5-2 | Essential Elements of Malpractice |

- Harm to an individual
- Duty of a professional toward an individual
- Breach of duty by the professional
- Breach of duty as the cause of harm

(From Ellis, J. R., & Hartley, C. L. 2008. *Nursing in today's world: Trends, issues and management* [9th ed.]. Philadelphia: Lippincott Williams & Wilkins.)

- Delegation of more tasks to unlicensed assistive personnel
- Early discharge of clients
- Shortage of professional nurses and past downsizing of hospitals
- Technological advances that require greater expertise
- Better-informed consumers
- Expanded legal definitions of liability

Rather than being held accountable for acting as an ordinary, reasonable layperson, the court will determine if a nurse acted in a manner comparable with that of his or her peers. For example, if a client sustains a burn from warm soaks, the nurse who failed to check the water temperature could be found liable because he or she violated professional standards by not checking the temperature of the water before applying the soak to the skin. Published standards, the testimony of expert witnesses, written agency policies and procedures, a bill of rights for patients (Box 5-4), and standardized care plans are examples of documents that establish professional standards of care (Fig. 5-3). These help familiarize the jury with the scope of a nurse's practice.

| BOX 5-3 | Standards of Care |

Standard I. Assessment
The nurse collects client health data.
Standard II. Diagnosis
The nurse analyzes the assessment data in determining diagnoses.
Standard III. Outcome Identification
The nurse identifies expected outcomes individualized to the client.
Standard IV. Planning
The nurse develops a plan of care that prescribes interventions to attain expected outcomes.
Standard V. Implementation
The nurse implements the interventions identified in the plan of care.
Standard VI. Evaluation
The nurse evaluates the client's progress toward attainment of outcomes.

Reprinted with permission from Standards of Clinical Nursing Practice, 2nd ed., 1998. Washington, D.C.: American Nurses Association.

Stop, Think, and Respond Exercise 5-1

An elderly client refuses to take his medication for hypertension. The nurse informs him that if he does not take it, his blood pressure will skyrocket and he will have a stroke that may kill him or leave him severely disabled. The nurse also states that she may need to restrain the client so that he will take his medication as ordered. Is the nurse threatening the client or merely providing important information?

Measures to Limit Liability

Some measures protect nurses and other healthcare workers from litigation (lawsuits) or provide a foundation for legal defense. Good Samaritan laws, statutes of limitations, principles regarding assumption of risk, documentation, risk management, anecdotal records, and liability insurance can limit or reduce a nurse's liability.

Good Samaritan Laws

Many states have enacted **Good Samaritan laws**, which provide legal immunity for rescuers who provide first aid in an emergency to accident victims. The law defines an emergency as one occurring outside a hospital, not in an emergency department.

None of the Good Samaritan laws provides absolute exemption from prosecution in the event of an injury. The law still holds paramedics, emergency medical technicians, physicians, nurses, and other healthcare providers who stop to provide assistance to a higher standard of care because they have training above and beyond that of laypersons. In cases where there has been gross negligence (total disregard for another's safety), individuals may be charged with a criminal offense.

Statute of Limitations

Each state establishes statutes of limitations related to civil laws. A **statute of limitations** is the designated time in which a person can file a lawsuit. The time usually is calculated from when the incident occurred. When the injured party is a minor, however, the statute of limitations sometimes does not commence until the victim reaches adulthood. Once the period expires, an injured party can no longer sue.

Assumption of Risk

If a client is forewarned of a potential hazard to his or her safety and chooses to ignore the warning, the court may hold the client responsible. For example, if the client objects to having the side rails up or lowers the rails independently, the nurse or healthcare facility may not be held fully accountable if an injury occurs. It is essential that the nurse document that he or she warned the client and that the client disregarded the warning. The same recommendation applies when nurses caution clients about ambulating only with assistance.

Documentation

A major component in limiting liability is accurate, thorough documentation. Nurses are held responsible or liable for information that they either include or exclude in reports and documentation. Each healthcare setting requires accurate and complete documentation. The medical record is a legal

---

BOX 5-4 **A Patient's Bill of Rights**

1. The patient has the right to considerate and respectful care.
2. The patient has the right to and is encouraged to obtain from physicians and other direct caregivers relevant, current, and understandable information concerning diagnosis, treatment, and prognosis.
3. The patient has the right to make decisions about the plan of care prior to and during the course of treatment and to refuse a recommended treatment or plan of care to the extent permitted by law and hospital policy and to be informed of the medical consequences of this action.
4. The patient has the right to have an advance directive (such as a living will, healthcare proxy, or durable power of attorney for healthcare) concerning treatment or designating a surrogate decision maker with the expectation that the hospital will honor the intent of that directive to the extent permitted by law and hospital policy.
5. The patient has the right to every consideration of privacy. Case discussion, consultation, examination, and treatment should be conducted so as to protect each patient's privacy.
6. The patient has the right to expect that all communications and records pertaining to his/her care will be treated as confidential by the hospital, except in cases such as suspected abuse and public health hazards when reporting is permitted or required by law.

7. The patient has the right to review the records pertaining to his or her medical care and to have the information explained or interpreted as necessary, except when restricted by law.
8. The patient has the right to expect that, within its capacity and policies, a hospital will make reasonable response to the request of a patient for appropriate and medically indicated care and services. The hospital must provide evaluation, service, and/or referral as indicated by the urgency of the case.
9. The patient has the right to ask and be informed of the existence of business relationships among the hospital, educational institutions, other healthcare providers, or payers that may influence the patient's treatment and care.
10. The patient has the right to consent to or decline to participate in proposed research studies or human experimentation affecting care and treatment or requiring direct patient involvement, and to have those studies fully explained prior to consent.
11. The patient has the right to expect reasonable continuity of care when appropriate and to be informed by physicians and other caregivers of available and realistic patient care options when hospital care is no longer appropriate.
12. The patient has the right to be informed of hospital policies and practices that relate to patient care, treatment, and responsibilities.

American Hospital Association. (1992). Available at: http://www.aha.org/resource/pbillofrights.asp, accessed April 5, 2008.

---

document and is used as evidence in court. Records must be timely, objective, accurate, complete, and legible. The quality of the documentation, including neatness and spelling, can influence a jury's decision. Box 5-5 lists rules for legally safe documentation.

Documentation serves several purposes. It meets client needs by serving as a communication tool for healthcare providers. Client records are essential for agency accreditation

BOX 5-5 **Rules for Legally Safe Documentation**

- Follow agency procedures for written and/or electronic documentation
- Chart promptly
- Write legibly
- Chart objectively, accurately, and concisely
- Use only standard and accepted abbreviations
- Do not leave vacant lines
- Sign every entry
- Keep charting free of criticism or complaints
- Make no mention of an incident report
- Do not destroy or attempt to obliterate documentation
- Record the date of a return visit, cancellation, or missed appointments
- Document all telephone conversations and follow-up instructions

and financial reimbursement from third-party payers. They also protect nurses and other healthcare providers because they verify that such personnel adhered to practice standards (Gialanella, 2004).

Electronic medical records are becoming more common. In many ways they provide methods that improve accuracy, in that they eliminate illegible writing and immediately flag contraindicated medical orders (Sullivan, 2004). Nevertheless, the same rules—confidentiality, accuracy, and timeliness—apply whether a medical record is written or electronic. Sullivan (2004) suggests the following safeguards when using electronic records:

- Do not share access codes or passwords.
- Position the monitor so that passersby cannot view it.
- Do not leave client information on the screen when not using the information.
- If using a hand-held device, do not leave it lying around; transfer information to the electronic record as early as possible.
- When printing medical information, use a printer in a secure area; retrieve the record immediately.
- Dispose of printed records according to agency policy.

The sharing of private information has been problematic for as long as there has been documentation. Because of problems related to unregulated use of healthcare information, the federal government implemented the Health Insurance Portability and Accountability Act (HIPAA) of 1996. The original purposes of this act include ensuring health

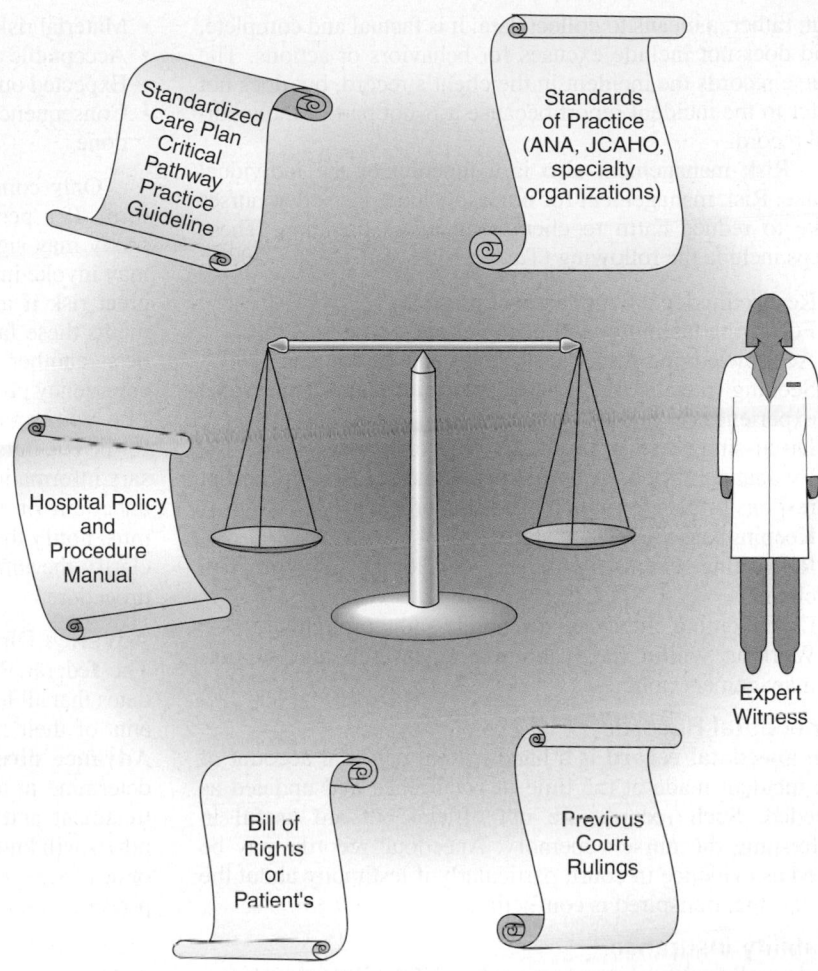

FIGURE 5-3 How the court establishes professional standards of care.

insurance portability for people who change jobs, reducing healthcare fraud and abuse, guaranteeing security and privacy of health information, limiting exclusions for preexisting conditions, improving access to health insurance coverage for small employers, and enforcing standards for health information (Catalano, 2006; Chitty & Black, 2007). In 2000, HIPAA added rules for the exchange of electronic information related to the administration of healthcare. Standardized electronic forms are now required for claims for healthcare services. The following year HIPAA required that clients must consent to the use or disclosure of any information for treatment, payment, or healthcare procedures. In 2003, an amendment referred to as the Privacy Rule was enacted. The regulations have several major client protections, which are outlined in Box 5-6.

Risk Management

Risk management, a concept developed by insurance companies, refers to the process of identifying and then reducing the costs of anticipated losses. Healthcare institutions that employ risk managers now use this term. The risk manager has responsibility for reviewing all the problems that occur at the workplace, identifying common elements, and then developing methods to reduce the risk of their occurrence.

One of the primary tools of risk management is the **incident report**. Healthcare workers complete incident reports when they make or discover errors, or when an event occurs that results in harm. The incident report identifies the nature of the incident (who, what, where, and when), witnesses, what actions were taken at the time, and the client's condition. The incident report is not intended to be a punitive tool

---

B O X 5 - 6 **Major Client Protections Provided by HIPAA**

- Clients may see and obtain copies of their medical records. If they detect errors, they may request correction. Clients may be asked to pay for the copying and mailing costs.
- Healthcare providers must give clients written notice describing their information practices and explaining clients' rights. Clients sign the written notices as confirmation of their agreement to these practices.
- Limits are placed on the length of time records may be retrieved, what information can be shared, and who can be present when information is shared.

From Chitty, K. K. & Black, B. P. (2007). *Professional nursing: Concepts & challenges* (5th ed.). St. Louis, MO: Elsevier Saunders.

but, rather, a means to collect data. It is factual and complete, and does not include excuses for behaviors or actions. The nurse records the incident in the client's record, but does not refer to the incident report because it is not part of the medical record.

Risk management also is a function of the individual nurse. Risk management for nurses includes steps that nurses take to reduce harm to clients and avoid litigation. These steps include the following (Taylor, Lillis, & LeMone, 2008):

- Respecting legal boundaries of practice
- Following institutional procedures and policies
- Acknowledging personal strengths and weaknesses
- Seeking means of growth, education, and supervised experiences
- Discussing issues or problems with colleagues
- Evaluating proposed assignments and refusing to accept responsibilities for which one is not prepared
- Keeping knowledge and skills current
- Respecting client rights and developing rapport with clients
- Documenting client care accurately and thoroughly
- Working within the institution to develop and support management policies

Anecdotal Records

An **anecdotal record** is a handwritten, personal account of an incident made at the time of occurrence and updated as needed. Such records are not official but are useful in refreshing the nurse's memory. Anecdotal records may be used as evidence in court, particularly if testimony about the events that transpired is conflicting.

Liability Insurance

Today, all healthcare professionals need liability or malpractice insurance. Liability insurance provides funds for attorneys' fees and damages awarded in malpractice lawsuits. All healthcare institutions carry liability insurance, and some may insure their employees. Nurses also should carry their own personal malpractice insurance, however, so they have a separate attorney working on their sole behalf. Because the damages sought in malpractice lawsuits are so high, the attorneys hired by healthcare institutions sometimes are more committed to defending the institution rather than the nurse against liability. There also have been instances in which healthcare facilities have countersued negligent nurses for reimbursement of damages.

Other Legal Issues

Some legal issues and regulations affect client care. Two prominent issues are informed consent and advance directives. Another issue involves do-not-resuscitate orders.

Informed Consent

Informed consent is the voluntary permission granted by a client, or the client's assigned *medical proxy* (a person who legally may make medical decisions for a client), for medical staff to perform an invasive procedure or surgery on the client. The physician obtains the informed consent and must inform the client of the following:

- Description of treatment, procedure, or surgery proposed
- Potential benefits

- Material risk involved
- Acceptable alternatives available
- Expected outcome
- Consequences if treatment, procedure, or surgery is not done

Only competent adults may sign the informed consent form. If a person is not competent, a guardian or medical proxy may sign for the client. In an emergency, physicians may invoke implied consent if the client cannot sign but is at great risk if a procedure is not done. The physician documents these facts in the medical record, and, in most facilities, another physician must verify the need for the emergency procedure (Marquis & Huston, 2003).

Nurses may witness the client's signature on the consent form. The nurse must be certain that the client has the necessary information before signing. If it appears that the client is uncertain or lacks the appropriate information, the nurse must notify the physician. Sometimes the nurse just needs to clarify the information and teach the client more about the procedure.

Advance Directives

The federal Patient Self-Determination Act of 1990 mandates that all federally funded healthcare facilities inform clients of their right to have and prepare advance directives. **Advance directives** provide an opportunity for clients to determine in advance their wishes regarding life-sustaining treatment and other medical care, so that their significant others will know what decisions clients desire. The two types of advance directives are the living will and medical durable power of attorney.

Living Will

A **living will** is a document that states a client's wishes regarding healthcare if he or she is terminally ill (Fig. 5-4). It is specific about what the client will accept and not accept for medical treatment if he or she is no longer competent or able to make medical decisions. The living will does not necessarily mean legal consent, but it does indicate the client's wishes (Ellis & Hartley, 2008).

Medical Durable Power of Attorney

A client may designate another person to be the **medical durable power of attorney** or healthcare proxy. This person has the authority to make healthcare decisions for the client if he or she is no longer competent or able to make these decisions. Although durable power of attorney forms are available in office supply stores, it is desirable to consult a lawyer when making these arrangements. The document may simply name the appointed person, or it may also include the client's preferences for end-of-life care.

 Gerontologic Considerations

- The ability to give informed consent is an issue that arises every time an older adult is asked to agree to treatment or to execute an advance directive. Cognitive impairment does not automatically constitute incompetence. Older people with fluctuating cognitive status may retain sufficient ability to make some, if not all, of their healthcare decisions. For example, an older adult may be unable to decide to have a

---

TO MY FAMILY, MY PHYSICIAN, MY CLERGYMAN, MY LAWYER

If the time comes when I can no longer take part in decisions for my own future, let this statement stand as the testament of my wishes:

If there is no reasonable expectation of my recovery from physical or mental disability,

I, _____

request that I be allowed to die and not be kept alive by artificial means or heroic measures. Death is as much a reality as birth, growth, maturity and old age—it is the one certainty. I do not fear death as much as I fear the indignities of deterioration, dependence and hopeless pain. I ask that medication be mercifully administered to me for terminal suffering even if it hastens the moment of death.

This request is made after careful consideration. Although this document is not legally binding, you who care for me will, I hope, feel morally bound to follow its mandate. I recognize that it places a heavy burden of responsibility upon you, and it is with the intention of sharing that responsibility and of mitigating any feelings of guilt that this statement is made.

Signed _____

Date _____

Witnessed by:

_____

_____

FIGURE 5-4 Example of a living will. (From Ellis, J. R., & Hartley, C. L. [2008]. *Nursing in today's world: Trends, issues and management* [9th ed.]. Philadelphia: Lippincott Williams & Wilkins.)

feeding tube but can appoint a daughter or son to make such decisions. Client and family education regarding anticipated disease trajectories may prompt discussion of client desires and designation of a trusted person to serve as the medical durable power of attorney.

Do-Not-Resuscitate Orders

Legally, nurses cannot act on a client's advance directive without a physician's order. *Do-not-resuscitate (DNR) orders* involve a written medical order for end-of-life instructions. If a DNR order is written, the client wishes to have no resuscitative action taken if he or she experiences a cardiac arrest. Often DNR instructions may be part of an advance directive, but when a client is in the hospital or other healthcare facility, there must be a written medical order for a "no code." Each facility should have a policy regarding DNR orders.

▶ *Stop, Think, and Respond Exercise 5-2*

A physician tells the nurse that he informed the client about his lung biopsy scheduled for the following day and that the client just needs to sign the form for the procedure to move forward. The doctor asks the nurse to take the form to the client for his signature. When the nurse asks the client if he understands what the lung biopsy will involve, the client states that after the biopsy the spot on his lung will be gone. Should the nurse allow the client to sign the form at this time or take other action?

ETHICAL ISSUES IN NURSING PRACTICE

Nurses frequently encounter complex situations that require decisions based on determining not what is legally right or wrong, but what is morally good or bad. Ethical issues do not have absolute answers. Conflicts may arise related to the desire to maintain the client's rights and yet uphold professional values and institutional policies.

For example, a mildly confused, order client has liver cancer but is expected to live at least several more months. The client eats and drinks some, but overall her intake is poor. Efforts to help the client drink and eat more have failed. The physician obtains consent from the client's medical durable power of attorney to place a feeding tube in the client. The physician asks the nurse to assist while the tube is placed. The client resists placement, and the nurse must restrain the client's hands to place the feeding tube. Because the client makes frequent attempts to remove the feeding tube, the restraints remain in place, with frequent checks by the nursing staff. In such a situation, knowing the ethically right course of action is difficult. The client receives better nutrition this way but must endure the discomfort of the tube and wrist restraints. What are the benefits and harms of the feeding tube and the wrist restraints? Should the client be forced to accept a treatment that necessitates the use of physical restraints? In the following material, theories of ethical practice and an ethical decision-making model provide essential information to consider situations such as the one just described. Refer to Box 5-7 for definitions of terms related to ethics.

BOX 5-7 Terms Related to Ethics

Ethics: Decisions regarding what is right and wrong; often a system that is used to protect the rights of individuals or groups

Code of ethics: Standards of conduct and values as defined by a profession; forms the basis for ethical decision-making by a profession.

Values: The ideals and beliefs held by an individual or group; usually influenced by family, society, and religion; greatly influence behavior

Morals: An individual's standards of right and wrong; formed in childhood; also influenced by family, society, and religion

Bioethics: Ethical questions surrounding life and death questions and concerns regarding quality of life as it relates to advanced technology

Ethical dilemma: A situation in which an individual must choose between two undesirable alternatives; often involves examining rights and obligations of particular individuals, choice frequently defended

 Gerontologic Considerations

- The aging process and presence of one or more chronic diseases may necessitate older adults' reliance on the healthcare team to a greater extent than they may have in younger years. However, the older adult should always be considered as being central in care decisions, rather than the recipient of care mandated by the healthcare team for the client. Planning with older adults and families to meet unique needs presents meaningful legal and ethical questions.

Theories of Ethics

Ethical theories provide a means to determine if a particular action is good or bad. In nursing ethics, two systems or theories predominate: utilitarianism and deontology.

Utilitarianism

Utilitarianism, also referred to as *teleologic theory,* is an outcome-oriented approach for decision-making. There are two important principles: "the greatest good for the greatest number" and "the end justifies the means." When individuals or groups use utilitarianism to make ethical decisions, they consider the consequences of their actions and make decisions that benefit the greatest number and harm the fewest. Furthermore, an action is not good or bad in and of itself. Instead, the consequences of the action (the end) determine if the action (the means) was good or bad. Utilitarianism compels the individual or group to evaluate consequences. Theorists suggest that:

- Consequences are good if they bring pleasure.
- The primary consideration is the outcome desired by those who are most affected.

Allocation of healthcare dollars provides an example of the use of utilitarianism. If a group is considering funding vaccines for many children or organ transplants for a few, the group will decide to give the money for the vaccines because a greater number will benefit.

Deontology

Another theory of ethics, **deontology**, argues that consequences are not the only important consideration in ethical dilemmas. Deontology states that duty is equally important. Duties are part of our understanding of the situations and relationships in which we find ourselves. We know intuitively that we must keep promises, return borrowed items, or help an injured person (Quinn & Smith, 1987). We have an obligation to perform or avoid some actions, regardless of the consequences, because of our duties to others. For example, the deontologist would say that lying is never acceptable because it disregards one's duty to tell the truth. He or she would believe abortion is unethical because it violates the duty to respect and preserve life (Zerwekh & Claborn, 2006).

Implied in the concept of duties is the idea of rights. **Rights** are freedoms or actions to which individuals have a just moral or legal claim. Another individual is entitled to what we have a duty to provide. For example, a person has a right to have his or her belongings returned or to have promises kept. This concept is particularly important in nursing practice. Nurses have a professional duty to their clients, and those clients have a right to expect that the nurse will perform his or her duties (see Box 5-3).

The deontologic approach considers the rights of each person—a distinct advantage. A second advantage is that the obligation to duty and moral thinking is foremost, and thus the decisions for similar situations are the same. Applying the deontologic method may be difficult, however, when the consequence of the decision can be harmful to an individual. For example, the decision to maintain life for all infants regardless of the outcome may be difficult when the infant is severely deformed and will require many invasive and expensive procedures to survive in a vegetative state.

Factors That Influence Ethical Decision-Making

Selecting a system for ethical decision-making should simplify the process; however, most nurses do not necessarily use one system or another. Other factors influence their decisions, not just knowledge of ethical theory.

Professional Values

Values are the beliefs that individuals find most meaningful. People value many different ideas, and not all ideas are ethical. Ethical values are rules or principles a person uses to make decisions about right and wrong. They share four characteristics (Quinn & Smith, 1987). Ethical values:

- Are consistent
- Take priority over other values
- Concern the treatment of others
- Are well thought out

Professional values are principles intended to support the ethical conduct of the profession. Some of those values do not differ from personal values, whereas some may come from a person's professional education. Several professional values guide the decisions that nurses make: beneficence, nonmaleficence, autonomy, justice, fidelity, and veracity.

Beneficence

Beneficence is the duty to do good for the clients assigned to the nurse's care. This 'good' includes technical competence and a humanistic, holistic approach. Stated another way, a nurse ought to prevent or remove harm, and promote or do good. The nurse has a duty to remove wrist restraints whenever possible (removing a harm) and to help the client regain independence (promoting and doing good). The principle of beneficence directly supports the nurse's role of client advocacy. **Advocacy** is safeguarding clients' rights and supporting their interests. For example, if a client is being discharged before mastering a complicated dressing change, the nurse advocates for an additional day in the hospital or home health visits.

Nonmaleficence

Nonmaleficence is the duty to do no harm to the client. If a nurse fails to check an order for an unusually high dose of insulin and administers it, he or she has violated the principle of nonmaleficence. Sometimes it is difficult to reconcile nonmaleficence with medical care because the choice of treatment may initially cause harm, even though the outcome is potentially good. For example, a client with colon cancer has a resection with a colostomy and endures the pain of surgery. In addition, the client undergoes unpleasant chemotherapy and radiation treatments. Although the client is harmed in many ways, the ultimate goal is for the client to be free of cancer. In these cases, the treatment still is ethically right because the intended effect is good and outweighs the bad effect. If the outcome is likely to be poor despite the treatment, what is ethically right may be difficult to determine.

Autonomy

Autonomy refers to a client's right to self-determination or the freedom to make choices without opposition. Nurses respect the client's right of autonomy even if the client's decision conflicts with the nurse's values. Through their advocacy role, nurses support clients' autonomy.

Justice

Justice is the duty to be fair to all people regardless of age, sex, race, sexual orientation, or other factors. The American Nurses Association Code of Ethics (Box 5-8) has the principle of justice as its first statement. A conflict can occur if healthcare resources are limited or when fairness to one means discrimination to another.

Fidelity

Fidelity is the duty to maintain commitments of professional obligations and responsibilities. Such obligations and responsibilities usually are defined by nurse practice acts.

Veracity

Veracity is the duty to tell the truth. The nurse must provide factual information to the client so that he or she may exercise autonomy. There are potential conflicts if the family or physician withholds information from the client. The issues of beneficence and nonmaleficence can enter into this ethical conflict.

BOX 5-8 **American Nurses Association Code of Ethics for Nurses**

1. The nurse, in all professional relationships, practices with compassion and respect for the inherent dignity, worth, and uniqueness of every individual, unrestricted by considerations of social or economic status, personal attributes, or the nature of health problems.
2. The nurse's primary commitment is to the patient, whether an individual, family, group, or community.
3. The nurse promotes, advocates for, and strives to protect the health, safety, and rights of the patient.
4. The nurse is responsible and accountable for individual nursing practice and determines the appropriate delegation of tasks consistent with the nurse's obligation to provide optimum patient care.
5. The nurse owes the same duties to self as to others, including the responsibility to preserve integrity and safety, to maintain competence, and to continue personal and professional growth.
6. The nurse participates in establishing, maintaining, and improving healthcare environments and conditions of employment conducive to the provision of quality healthcare and consistent with the values of the profession through individual and collective action.
7. The nurse participates in the advancement of the profession through contributions to practice, education, administration, and knowledge development.
8. The nurse collaborates with other health professionals and the public in promoting community, national, and international efforts to meet health needs.
9. The profession of nursing, as represented by associations and their members, is responsible for articulating nursing values, for maintaining the integrity of the profession and its practice, and for shaping social policy.

From American Nurses Association. (2001). *Code for nurses with interpretive statements.* Washington, DC: Author.

Legislative and Judicial Influences

Society's struggles with ethical issues result in legislative and judicial decisions that affect ethical decisions. For example, the issue of declaring death and removing life support has become more difficult with advances in technology. Often there are examples in the news that highlight legislative and judicial involvement with decisions related to removal of life support and termination of tube feedings. Formerly, the loss of cardiac and respiratory function was the deciding factor in determining death. With greater abilities to maintain cardiac and respiratory function, however, society, through laws and judicial decisions, has redefined death. Definitions of death now include brain criteria, including lack of movements or breathing, absence of reflexes, a flat reading on an electroencephalogram, and unresponsiveness. Most states accept such criteria. The ethical issues for many nurses are related to their own beliefs about the dignity of life, harvesting of donor organs from an individual who is brain dead, and supporting the family members who may be asked to make decisions. The legality of brain death has removed some of the uncertainties for nurses regarding ethical issues.

Another topic that creates debate is physician-assisted suicide and euthanasia. Many people fear a prolonged and painful death. This has given rise to a movement for a legally sanctioned, medically assisted, peaceful death as an option for clients of sound mind with terminal illnesses. Nurses are committed to preserving life and also to maintaining quality of life. Nurse practice acts prohibit nurses from assisting clients to die; however, nurses have a unique understanding of their clients' wishes and suffering. Some nurses may face dilemmas in advocating for their clients.

Influence of Technology

Developments in science and technology produce ethical issues that were unheard of even 10 years ago. Some examples include the following:

- Successful impregnation of a woman past menopause—some governments are considering age limitations for such procedures.
- Genetic engineering—such procedures may potentially harm humans, create a "perfect" being, or lead to discrimination.
- Cloning animals, humans, or both—this raises difficult questions about the creation of life and individuality.

These advances, once in the realm of science fiction, now pose serious ethical dilemmas. Nurses definitely will play a key role in the decisions involved with these issues. They also will have particular problems if the need to promote science and progress obscures the nurse's duty to clients.

Healthcare Reform

Cost control, shortened hospital stays, increased client acuity, and interest in alternative healthcare are factors that affect ethical decision-making. The discharge of clients to their homes when they are sicker and more vulnerable is of great concern. Issues related to the allocation of healthcare dollars to those who need it the most or who have the greatest potential to have a positive outcome also are ethically challenging. Nurses will face questions that make them examine their own values as they relate to providing quality care to clients and their families.

Ethical Decision-Making Process

Nurses use a problem-solving method (the nursing process) to provide care to clients. Healthcare providers use a similar problem-solving approach for ethical dilemmas. Nurses can use the following steps when making ethical decisions:

1. Obtain as much information as possible to understand the situation. Identify the problem and describe it. Determine what values are involved and whom the decision will affect. A statement of the dilemma (after considering all the data) helps to define the issue as clearly as possible.
2. List all the possible options for solving the dilemma; this process is referred to as *brainstorming*. Do not determine the consequences at this point.
3. Examine the pros and cons of each option, foreseeing possible consequences from both a utilitarian and a deontologic approach. Consider the effects on the individual.

4. Make the decision and follow through on it.
5. Evaluate the decision in terms of effects and results.

> ▶ *Stop, Think, and Respond Exercise 5-3*
>
> *A kidney becomes available for transplantation. The tissue matches that of an adolescent and a middle-aged client, both of whom need the organ. If you were responsible for deciding which client receives the kidney transplant, how would you decide?*

Ethics Committees

Hospitals and other healthcare institutions often have ethics committees to help resolve ethical dilemmas and make decisions on a case-by-case basis. Ethics committees are composed of individuals with diverse backgrounds. They often include physicians, nurses, clergy, social workers, and community members. Ethics committees establish guidelines and policies before an ethical dilemma develops. They also may be called on to act as an advocate for clients who no longer are mentally capable of making their own decisions. Ethics committees are a valuable resource for reviewing difficult cases and help ensure a careful and unbiased decision.

CRITICAL THINKING EXERCISES

1. A confused client has attempted to get out of bed by climbing over the side rails. What actions would you take to protect yourself from being sued?
2. Consider the case of the client who needed to be restrained to receive tube feedings (presented earlier in this chapter). Discuss the ethical issues involved from the standpoint of values. Assess the situation from a utilitarian and a deontologic viewpoint using the ethical decision-making model. Do you think inserting the feeding tube and using wrist restraints were ethically good decisions?
3. You are caring for a female client who had a hysterectomy two days ago. When you enter the room to administer her medications, the client's husband tells you that he has a history of high blood pressure and would like you to take his blood pressure and tell him if he needs to increase his blood pressure medication. What is your best response?
4. In the following situation, determine if there are the necessary elements that could bring about a claim of malpractice. The LPN is working in a long-term care facility and is responsible for administering medications to 20 residents. One of the clients has a new order for a heart medication that the LPN is familiar with. She thinks it may be a higher dose than usually ordered, but does not have time to look it up and decides to give it, because the physician who ordered it is reliable. Later that day the client's blood pressure and pulse fall, and the client becomes unresponsive. The client is transferred to the hospital and is hospitalized for several days. It is later determined that the medication was transcribed incorrectly, and the client received twice the normal dose. The family is very unhappy and hires a lawyer.

NCLEX-STYLE REVIEW QUESTIONS

1. There are potential conflicts if a client's family members or physician withhold information from the client. Which of the following is an issue that can enter into this ethical conflict?
1. Beneficence
2. Malpractice
3. Negligence
4. Unintentional tort

2. A nurse who witnesses a motor vehicle accident stops to provide emergency assistance to the injured motorists. To reduce the risk for liability, it is most appropriate for the nurse to do which of the following?
1. Avoid giving the accident victim any personal identification.
2. Conceal the fact that he or she is a nurse.
3. Let others at the scene provide direct care.
4. Remain with the accident victim until paramedics arrive.

3. When a client is injured following a seizure, which fact is most important to document on the accident report to reduce the risk for liability?
1. The client's signal cord was within reach

2. The client's vital signs had been stable
3. The client was assigned to a licensed nurse
4. The client was last observed to be reading

4. A friend shares with a nurse that the friend is engaged to be married. The nurse knows that the friend's fiancé has tested positive for the human immunodeficiency virus (HIV). The nurse is legally obligated to:
1. advise the friend to postpone the marriage indefinitely.
2. inform the friend of the fiancé's HIV infectious status.
3. recommend that the friend be tested for HIV antibodies.
4. safeguard information in the fiancé's health history.

5. Several years ago, a client with an abdominal aortic aneurysm prepared an advance directive indicating that the client did not want heroic measures performed to sustain life. The physician wrote a "do not resuscitate" order on his medical record. If the client loses consciousness and remains unresponsive, which nursing action is most appropriate?
1. Call his immediate next of kin
2. Call the local ambulance service
3. Have him transferred to the hospital
4. Notify his attending physician

6

Leadership Roles and Management Functions

Learning Objectives

On completion of this chapter, you will be able to:

1. Differentiate leadership and management.
2. Define three styles of leadership.
3. Outline the purpose of power in the leadership role.
4. Describe the role of the LPN/LVN in managing client care.
5. Distinguish delegation and supervision.
6. Compare responsibility and accountability.
7. Discuss problems that may occur with delegation and supervision.
8. Describe the role of the LPN/LVN in collaboration and advocacy.
9. Explain the role of the LPN/LVN in resource management.
10. Discuss methods to manage time effectively.

Licensed practical/vocational nurses (LPN/LVNs), in their role of providing care to clients, must have skills in organizing client care, supervising care provided by unlicensed personnel, collaborating with other healthcare personnel, managing time and resources, and being accountable for assigned client care. Although primarily educated to provide direct client care, LPN/LVNs need a basic understanding of management and supervisory principles to function in leadership roles in various healthcare settings. This chapter provides an overview of theory related to leadership and management, with a focus on the role of the LPN/LVN in delegation and supervision.

LEADERSHIP AND MANAGEMENT

In many ways, leadership and management are interrelated concepts; discussing one is impossible without reference to the other. These terms, however, are not synonymous, as the following paragraphs explain.

Leadership

Leadership involves qualities related to a person's character and behaviors, as well as roles within a group or organization. It requires that a person have the ability to guide and influence another person, group, or both to think in a certain way, achieve common goals, or provide inspiration for change. Marquis and Huston (2008, p.5) state that leaders:

- Often do not have delegated authority, but obtain their power through other means, such as influence
- Have a wider variety of roles than do managers
- May not be part of the formal organization
- Focus on group process, information gathering, feedback, and empowering others
- Emphasize interpersonal relationships
- Direct willing followers
- Have goals that may or may not reflect those of the organization

Any healthcare provider has the potential to be a leader in terms of influencing a group or exercising power in a particular situation. Accordingly, LPN/LVNs also may be leaders, informally or formally. For example, an LPN working on a medical-surgical unit may assume responsibility for organizing social events for fellow employees. A more formal leadership role would be acting as co-chairperson of the unit's staffing policy committee.

Management

Management entails assigned functions such as planning, organizing, directing, and controlling to meet specific objectives within an organization (Ellis & Hartley, 2008). The manager's overall goal is to coordinate and direct resources, which include work space, supplies, equipment, budgetary concerns, and services. In addition, managers direct and coordinate the work of assigned employees. Managers (1) are assigned a position in an organization; (2) have a legitimate and more formal source of power owing to the delegated authority that accompanies their position; (3) are expected to carry out specific functions, duties, and responsibilities; (4) emphasize control, decision-making, decision analysis, and results; (5) manipulate resources to meet organizational goals; and (6) direct willing and unwilling subordinates (Marquis & Huston, 2008). A key feature is the individual manager's responsibility and accountability for the accomplishment of tasks (Ellis & Hartley, 2008).

The Relationship of Leadership and Management

To be effective, leaders and managers must possess certain qualities (Marquis & Huston, 2008):

- An ability to gain respect of others through competence and shared goals
- Expertise in communication skills, both oral and written
- A capacity to motivate others to achieve a particular purpose or accomplish goals

Ideally, a good manager is also a good leader, and a good leader is a good manager. In reality, some managers do not possess good leadership skills, and some leaders are ineffective managers. People can learn to be effective leaders and managers. Improving and developing skills through education and experience enhance a person's ability to lead and manage.

Integrated leaders/managers have traits that distinguish them from just leaders or managers:

- Thinking in the long term
- Seeing the big picture
- Influencing others outside their own group
- Emphasizing vision, values, and motivation
- Being politically astute
- Embracing change and modification

In addition, integrated leaders/managers set reasonable goals, think positively, and are willing to take risks.

Leadership Styles

Lewin (1951) identified three prevalent leadership styles that managers use, either consciously or unconsciously, to accomplish certain goals and tasks. These styles vary in the amount of control that the manager exerts and the degree of input that subordinates have in the decision-making process. The three styles include the following:

- **Autocratic leadership** entails strong control by the manager over the work group. The manager gives and asks for little input from staff for decisions. Communication flows from top to bottom. The focus is on accomplishing tasks.
- **Democratic leadership** involves more participation in decision-making by the work group. Leaders with this style often see themselves as coworkers or colleagues, as opposed to superiors. They emphasize communication, consensus, and teamwork (Ellis & Hartley, 2008).
- **Laissez-faire leadership,** or permissive management, involves the least structure and control. The manager leaves the work group to set goals, make decisions, and take responsibility for their own management (Ellis & Hartley, 2008).

Table 6-1 provides information about the advantages and disadvantages of the three leadership styles. Each style may be effective, depending on the particular situation. A good leader can determine which approach is best for a particular circumstance. Ellis and Hartley (2008) refer to this ability as **multicratic leadership**. The multicratic leadership style combines the best of all styles, mediated by requirements of the situation at hand. The multicratic leader provides maximum structure when appropriate to the situation, asks for maximum group participation when needed, and gives support and encouragement to subordinates in all instances.

▶ Stop, Think, and Respond Exercise 6-1

A new LPN/LVN works on a long-term care unit where the nurse manager typically uses an autocratic style of leadership. What are the advantages and disadvantages of this style for the new LPN/LVN?

Power and Leadership

The leader/manager has the potential to provide guidance, direction, and support to coworkers. The leader/manager also exerts a certain power. **Power** is the ability to control, influence, or hold authority over an individual or group. People in leadership/management positions are in a position to exert power in an organization. If leadership is to be effective, a degree of power must support it.

Each type of power has a particular source or base (Table 6-2). The first type of power is *reward power,* which a person attains through the ability to grant favors or rewards. For example, organizational leaders have the ability to grant financial rewards or special favors.

Coercive or *punishment power* is the ability to threaten or punish someone who fails to meet expectations. In using such power, a manager may threaten undesirable schedules, denial of vacation time, or layoff if an employee is not compliant.

A manager exercises *legitimate power* through a designated position, which also may be referred to as *authority.* A manager has legitimate power by virtue of the management position.

TABLE 6-1 Advantages and Disadvantages of Leadership Styles

LEADERSHIP STYLE	ADVANTAGES	DISADVANTAGES
Autocratic	Tasks are accomplished without questions. Communication is directive and flows downward. Lines of authority and policies are clear. Decisions are made quickly. Autocratic leadership works best in bureaucracies and with employees who have limited education or training.	Subordinates have little input into decision- or policy-making and receive little feedback or recognition. Staff members are not invested in management's goals. Leaders may create hostility and dependency. Work is highly controlled and dictated.
Democratic	Subordinates contribute to decision- and policy-making. Staff members are invested in planning and accomplishing goals. Communication is mutual—back and forth. Employees receive regular feedback. Democratic leadership works well with competent and motivated employees.	Decisions may not occur in a timely way. Staff members may fail to acknowledge the manager's role. Employees do not recognize the need for urgent decisions that are made without staff input.
Laissez-faire	Coworkers can develop their own goals, make their own decisions, and take full responsibility for their actions. Managers provide support and freedom for employees. Subordinates perform at high levels because of their independence. Staff members share the process of making decisions for the group. Laissez-faire leadership works well with professional employees.	Employees receive little direction or guidance. Generally, decisions are not made because managers are unable or unwilling to make them Staff members do not receive feedback regarding their performance. Communication is limited to memos. Change is rare.

TABLE 6-2 Sources of Power

TYPE OF POWER	SOURCE OF POWER	EXAMPLE
Reward power	Ability to grant favors	Team leader making assignments
Coercive power	Fear	Head nurse scheduling vacations
Legitimate power	Position	Director of nursing
Expert power	Knowledge and skill	An LPN/LVN with 20 years' experience working on a medical unit
Referent power	Association with others	Shift supervisor
Informational power	Need for information to accomplish a goal	Merit raise information related to annual evaluations

Adapted from Marquis, B. L. & Huston, C. J. (2008). *Leadership roles and management functions in nursing: Theory and application.* (6th ed.). Philadelphia: Lippincott Williams & Wilkins.

Expert power results from knowledge, expertise, or experience in a particular area. Managers typically possess expert power through education and work experience.

Referent power concerns the power a person has because of his or her association with others who are powerful. For example, society perceives that physicians are powerful. A new physician may use this referent power to his or her advantage. Referent power also may be called *charismatic* or *connection power,* referring to personal characteristics, such as charisma, the way a person talks or acts, the people he or she associates with, or the organizations to which he or she belongs.

Another type of power is *informational power,* which exists when a person has information that others need to accomplish certain goals. Examples may relate to budget preparation, planning for educational events, or making changes in an organization.

Leaders and managers may exercise power to accomplish assigned tasks. They also must have the authority or legitimate right to direct and guide work. A nurse in an authorized position (e.g., team leader, charge nurse) can exert power in a positive way.

THE LPN/LVN AS LEADER/MANAGER

Usually, managers are appointed to or hired for a specific management position. In healthcare, however, the term *manager* may be used more broadly, in that nurses manage the care of clients. This role involves overseeing the care that a client receives. Other healthcare providers may actually care for the clients. In acute care settings, registered nurses (RNs) are assigned to a group of clients. An LPN/LVN and certified nursing assistant (CNA) may work with the RN and be responsible for certain aspects of client care. The RN, as the manager of care, ensures that the LPN/LVN and CNA complete all assigned tasks, assess the clients, and evaluate the effects of nursing interventions.

In other healthcare settings, the role of the LPN/LVN may be extended. For example, in long-term care settings LPN/LVNs may be team leaders and thus assigned to oversee the work of unlicensed assistive personnel (UAPs). In medical offices, an LPN/LVN may be the office manager, coordinating certain aspects of the office work, such as scheduling and coordinating work assignments. These roles require the LPN/LVN to delegate responsibility for certain tasks and then supervise the accomplishment of the work.

Primary Leadership and Management Functions

Primary functions of LPN/LVNs as leaders/managers include *delegation, supervision, responsibility,* and *accountability.*

Delegation

The National Council of State Boards of Nursing (NCSBN) (1995, p. 3) states that **delegation** is "transferring to a competent individual the authority to perform a selected nursing task in a selected situation. The nurse retains the accountability for the delegation." Delegation also is a means of accomplishing work through others (Marquis & Huston, 2008). The ability to guide, teach, and direct others is integral to the ability to delegate.

Hathaway (2005) differentiates between direct and indirect client care activities that may be delegated to UAPs. Direct care activities are those that assist clients to meet basic needs, including vital signs, weights, specimen collection, and ambulation. Indirect activities are more focused on environmental tasks, such as cleaning equipment, emptying trash or soiled linen receptacles, and delivering meal trays.

Nurses need to learn delegation skills. The NCSBN (1995) identified the Five Rights of Delegation:

1. Right task
2. Right circumstances
3. Right person
4. Right direction/communication
5. Right supervision/evaluation

Ellis and Hartley (2008) suggest that carrying out the five rights of delegation requires following certain steps similar to those of the nursing process:

* *Assess the situation*—know the client's needs, the skills of the UAPs, and the priorities. Match the UAPs' skills with the tasks to be completed.
* *Plan actions*—identify the UAPs who will best handle the delegated tasks.
* *Implement the plan*—communicate expectations clearly to UAPs, including what they need to do, what to watch for, and potential problems.
* *Evaluate the results*—ensure that tasks are completed according to standards.

Box 6-1 provides tips for delegating successfully. Part of succeeding at delegating involves the process of supervision.

Supervision

Supervision is the process of guiding, directing, evaluating, and following up on tasks delegated to others (NCSBN, 1995). Delegation and supervision are tightly connected, because once a nurse has delegated a task, he or she is obligated to supervise the person assigned to that task. In reviewing the steps of delegation described in the previous section, supervision begins when the LPN/LVN implements the plan. The implementation step includes giving instructions about what needs to be done and when. The nurse must include any

---

BOX 6-1	**Tips for Delegating Successfully**

Know the abilities of unlicensed assistive personnel (UAPs)
Plan ahead to prevent problems
Match tasks to be accomplished to the skills of UAPs
Communicate expectations and directions clearly
Trust the UAP to complete the task
Supervise the UAP to determine progress in completing the task
Assess results
Provide positive feedback to the UAP as appropriate

Adapted from Ellis, J. R. & Hartley, C. L. (2004). *Managing and coordinating nursing care* (4th ed.). Philadelphia: Lippincott Williams & Wilkins.

---

specific issues, such as telling the UAP that a client must complete morning care before going for physical therapy at 10:00 AM. In addition, the nurse needs to tell the UAP about any potential problems, such as a client who may experience dizziness when getting up secondary to antihypertensive medications.

Supervision also is necessary throughout the implementation step. The LPN/LVN must check with UAPs during the shift to assess if tasks are complete, what the outcome is, if something has changed that may interfere with the work, or if the UAP is having problems accomplishing the task safely.

The evaluation step of delegation also includes supervision of the UAP, in that the LPN/LVN ensures that the client received the appropriate care, that the client's needs were met, and that problems were addressed. Providing feedback to UAPs also is important, in terms of letting them know that they did a good job or asking questions about the client's response to the care provided.

Delegation and supervision imply that the people carrying out these functions assume responsibility and accountability for their actions as well as the actions of those to whom they delegate. The next section defines these concepts.

Responsibility and Accountability

Responsibility is a duty or assignment related to a specific job. It means being obligated to perform certain activities and duties. When a person is responsible for something, he or she is obligated to ensure that the task or job is completed (Ellis & Hartley, 2008).

Accountability means being answerable for the consequences of one's actions or inactions. The term *liability* (see Chap. 5) is closely associated with accountability, because of the legal implications. Tasks an LPN/LVN delegates to a UAP remain the responsibility of the LPN/LVN, who must ensure that the task is appropriate for the UAP and that the UAP has the knowledge and skills to complete the task. The LPN/LVN is accountable for determining if the task is accomplished and if there are any issues associated with completing or not completing the task. In addition, the LPN/LVN also is accountable for evaluating the results of the tasks. The UAP is responsible for performing the actual task.

▶ **Stop, Think, and Respond Exercise 6-2**

An LPN is the team leader for 20 clients on a long-term care unit. She delegates to an experienced UAP the task of feeding supper to an older client. When the UAP feeds this client, the client begins to cough and choke, aspirating some food. The client eventually develops pneumonia and must be hospitalized for 1 week. Who is responsible for this incident?

Challenges to Leading and Managing

LPN/LVNs may experience some problems with delegation and supervision of tasks. In part this is because LPN/LVNs may not be well prepared for the role of team leader. Schools of practical/vocational nursing traditionally have focused primarily on the direct caregiver role. In turn, employers may not plan for LPN/LVNs to be team leaders or other managers of care, but out of necessity place LPN/LVNs in these roles. Other factors that may interfere with effective delegation and supervision are as follows:

- Reluctance to delegate from fear of overloading a co-worker or the desire to do everything
- Inability to move out of the role of direct caregiver—"It is easier to do it myself"
- Miscommunication regarding specific directions and desired outcomes
- Desire to be liked by coworkers, which interferes with ability to delegate, supervise, or both

In addition, LPN/LVNs are not strictly supervisors, in that they do not have the authority to hire or fire. They may have responsibility for overseeing and directing the care that UAPs provide, but they do not have the responsibility for disciplining them.

Solutions for improving one's ability to delegate and direct UAPs include obtaining education for this role. In addition, LPN/LVNs must focus on client care needs first. In this way, the LPN/LVN ensures that clients receive appropriate care and that tasks are carried out efficiently and in a caring manner. If an LPN/LVN remains responsible and accountable for his or her actions, it assists him or her to delegate and direct responsibly.

Other Functions

Although LPN/LVNs as team leaders have the primary responsibility of delegating tasks to UAPs, other functions are important for the LPN/LVN leader/manager. These functions include collaboration, advocacy, resource management, and time management.

Collaboration

Collaboration involves a team effort to achieve client care outcomes. Although RNs often direct collaborative efforts, LPN/LVNs are responsible for directing the care of UAPs. As a team member and leader, LPN/LVNs maintain open and effective communication with all team members. They also assist in solving problems related to client care. LPN/LVNs may contribute to decisions about client care and unit activities by participating in client care conferences and unit meetings. Lastly, collaborative behavior for the LPN/LVN involves participating in the management of the unit by following the appropriate channels of communication and supporting the group in collaborative efforts.

Advocacy

Advocacy means promoting the cause of another person or organization. In healthcare, advocates support the needs of a client or organization. Nurses in general act on behalf of their clients. Ethically, nurses support a client's right to be autonomous and to make informed decisions (American Nurses Association, 2004). LPN/LVNs function as client advocates by (Ellis & Hartley, 2004):

- Understanding the rights of all clients
- Remaining informed about diagnoses, treatments, prognoses, and choices
- Contributing to the provision of information and education
- Supporting the client's decisions
- Communicating with other professionals

Resource Management

Resource management, the responsibility of all who work in healthcare, means using resources, which include not only actual money but supplies, equipment, buildings, and personnel, optimally. Nurses who provide direct care may not have a direct role in formulating budgets, but they are responsible for controlling the use of resources and recognizing when resources are inadequate. In addition, they must know the costs of resources and the importance of using cost-effective measures when caring for clients.

Many factors are related to the rising costs of healthcare (Box 6-2). In general, new technologies increase costs, which leads to the need for better facilities and, it is hoped, better outcomes for client care. Related costs are salaries for healthcare personnel, newer and more expensive medications, and equipment. As a result of increased costs, healthcare providers are expected to be more cost-conscious. Cost-conscious measures include prudent use of expensive supplies, knowledgeable operation of medical equipment, careful monitoring of clients to reduce potential complications and lengths of stay, heightened awareness of practicing measures that reduce costs, essential knowledge of all costs of caring for clients, and deliberate reduction of waste of limited resources.

BOX 6-2 **Factors Involved in Rising Healthcare Costs**

Higher prices for new technology
New construction of facilities
Increased survival rate of clients (leads to more costly care)
Growing older population who require healthcare
Rising salaries of healthcare personnel
Higher prices for medications
Increased costs for medical equipment

Adapted from Ellis, J. R. & Hartley, C. L. (2008). *Nursing in today's world: Challenges, issues, and trends* (9th ed.). Philadelphia: Lippincott Williams & Wilkins.

LPN/LVNs also may be involved in controlling costs by participation in a client acuity system. Acute care and long-term care facilities may use an acuity system to determine staffing needs. Acuity measures the degree of a client's illness and what care is required to meet the client's needs. Often systems use categories to designate the level of care needed. For example, one category may reflect the need for complex dressing changes, another the need for special monitoring, such as neurologic checks. Each category has assigned points—at the end, the points are totaled to ascertain the acuity level of the client. This information may then be used to determine what nursing staff is needed to provide adequately for the needs of the unit (Ellis & Hartley, 2004).

Time Management

Time is an essential resource, particularly in today's fast-paced healthcare environment. **Time management** involves organizing time, as well as delegating tasks to other personnel and essentially optimizing available time. Marquis and Huston (2008) outline three basic steps for managing time. In the first step, the nurse makes time to plan and establish priorities. The second step involves completing the highest-priority task and moving from completing one task to beginning another. The final step requires that the nurse reassess and reprioritize tasks based on any changes.

The onset of managed care increased the focus on efficiency and productivity. Making the most of one's time is an important skill that takes effort to achieve. Although on chaotic days it may seem that nothing works, those who are most effective at managing time will have the most success in accomplishing the work that needs to be done. New nurses usually need to learn to organize their time. The following techniques are useful in learning to manage time:

- Assess expectations for the shift. Do so in a chart that identifies specific periods (e.g., 30-minute increments). This also can be done after a shift to determine how one spent time that particular day and how it might help to organize another shift.
- Use a worksheet to identify specific tasks and important assessments that need to be done for that particular shift. This works very well with multiple client assignments. Organize the worksheet according to each client. Many nurses refer to this as a "to do" list or "brain sheet." They use the worksheet not only to identify tasks, but also to write quick notes to jog their memories for further tasks or assessments.
- Prioritize tasks that need to be accomplished (Box 6-3). Reprioritize as needed.
- Write things down to remember later for charting and reporting. Many nurses use their worksheet as a report sheet for the oncoming shift.
- Develop efficiency and the ability to multitask, which means engaging in more than one task at a time. For example, if a client requests pain medication and you need to assess his roommate's vital signs, bring the needed equipment as well as pain medication.
- Delegate appropriate tasks to appropriate personnel.

Most people readily admit that they do not always make good use of their time and then have to scramble to complete

---

BOX 6-3 **Criteria for Setting Priorities**

1. Items critical to maintaining life: Think in terms of your cardiopulmonary resuscitation basics.
   - Essential assessment
   - Airway management
   - Breathing support
   - Circulation needs
   - Neurologic stability
2. Critical symptom management: What is important to the client?
   - Pain management
   - Relief of nausea
   - Relief of diarrhea
   - Relief of severe anxiety
3. Items needed to progress in health restoration: What orders has the physician written? What nursing plans have been developed?
   - Medication and fluid administration
   - Completing treatments
   - Preventing complications
   - Meeting nutritional needs
4. Items needed to move toward self-care
   - Teaching
   - Contacting referral needs
   - Meeting psychosocial needs
   - Creating comfort and feelings of well-being
   - Bathing
   - Changing linens

Adapted from Ellis, J. R. & Hartley, C. L. (2004). *Managing and coordinating nursing care* (4th ed.). Philadelphia: Lippincott Williams & Wilkins.

BOX 6-4 **Time Wasters**

Poor planning
Inability to delegate
Procrastination
Socializing
Unwillingness to say no
Poor communication
Inefficient use of time
Failure to write things down
Haste
Repetitive paperwork
Unclear direction
Management by crisis

---

tasks. Box 6-4 identifies some "time wasters." These essentially include an inability to plan, procrastination, chatting, allowing low-priority tasks to take precedence, inability to delegate appropriately, and difficulty saying no. Assessing what wastes one's time is an important step in using time more effectively.

CRITICAL THINKING EXERCISES

1. An LPN is a team leader on a skilled care unit. When she returns from her dinner break, the UAP reports the following:
- One client vomited after receiving her 6 PM medications.
- A family member is upset that his mother pulled out her feeding tube and that it has not been replaced.
- A client's catheter seems to be leaking.
- A physician wants to order medications for the new client who had hip replacement surgery 2 weeks ago. Prioritize these tasks—indicate what the LPN should attend to and what she can delegate.

2. An LVN is planning to change jobs from an acute care setting to a long-term care facility. He is concerned about his role in the new job as a team leader. He knows that he will be working with UAPs. What should he know about his role in delegating tasks to UAPs if he takes this new job?

3. An experienced LPN works nights at a rehabilitation hospital. As a charge nurse, the LPN is reluctant to delegate to the two UAPs working with her, because she is afraid the work will not be done right. As a result, this LPN is frequently stressed and feeling like she cannot keep up. What strategies could she use to better utilize the UAPs and feel better about delegation of tasks?

4. The LVN provides appropriate direction as she delegates a task to the UAP. However, the UAP makes an error that causes injury to the client. Who is responsible?

NCLEX-STYLE REVIEW QUESTIONS

1. The RN delegates a wound irrigation and dressing change to the LVN. The LVN has never done this particular type of wound irrigation but is hesitant to seek help. Which right of delegation did the RN neglect?
1. Right task
2. Right circumstances
3. Right person
4. Right communication

2. An LPN expresses interest in leadership opportunities at the long-term care facility where she works. In recognition of the LPN role, which of the following are appropriate? Select all that apply.
1. Apply for staff development position
2. Chair staff education committee for unlicensed personnel
3. Serve as night shift team leader
4. Volunteer to organize staff holiday gatherings
5. Write formal evaluations of co-assigned UAPs

3. The LPN on the day shift is assigned with a UAP to care for 12 clients on a skilled care unit. Which of the following tasks is most appropriate for the LPN to delegate to the UAP?
1. Assess the incision on a new client with a knee replacement
2. Assist a newly admitted client to the bathroom
3. Check the glucose level on a client who is difficult to arouse
4. Take vital signs on all of the assigned clients

4. A practical nursing student, in reviewing the different leadership styles, correctly states that a manager who is very task-focused and often writes memos and directives to the staff regarding what needs to be done or what has not been done is most likely a(n):
1. Autocratic leader
2. Democratic leader
3. Laissez-faire leader
4. Multicratic leader

5. A new LVN has been working on a medical unit for several months. The LVN has learned that many of the RNs on the unit have power because of their experience and knowledge. This type of power is called:
1. coercive
2. expert
3. legitimate
4. reward

UNIT 2
Client Care Concerns

7

Nurse–Client Relationships

Learning Objectives

On completion of this chapter, you will be able to:

1. List four roles that nurses perform within the nurse–client relationship.
2. Describe three phases in a nurse–client relationship.
3. Differentiate between verbal, nonverbal, and therapeutic communication.
4. Give examples of therapeutic and nontherapeutic communication techniques.
5. List and explain five components of nonverbal communication.
6. Name and explain the four proxemic zones.
7. Explain what is meant by a client's "comfort zone."
8. Differentiate between task-oriented and affective touch.
9. Explain the learning styles of cognitive, affective, and psychomotor learners.
10. Describe variables that affect learning.
11. Compare informal with formal learning.
12. Discuss guidelines for teaching adult clients.

The word *relationship* refers to an association between two or more people. Nurses form relationships with clients, families, and community groups. This chapter explores the scope of the nurse–client relationship, provides guidelines for effective interpersonal communication, and identifies principles for client teaching.

SCOPE OF THE NURSE–CLIENT RELATIONSHIP

The term *relationship*, in this chapter, is used in its strictest sense—that is, the association between nurses and their clients. The **nurse–client relationship** exists during the period when the nurse interacts with clients, sick or well, to promote or restore their health, help them to cope with their illness, or assist them to die with dignity. Communicating therapeutically, listening empathetically, sharing information, and providing client education are among the most basic processes that occur in the context of the nurse–client relationship. As in any effective relationship, each party has unique responsibilities to the other (Box 7-1).

Nursing Roles Within the Nurse–Client Relationship

The nurse–client relationship requires the nurse to respond to the client's needs. The National Council of State Boards of Nursing, which develops the national licensing examination for practical nurses (NCLEX-PN), identifies four categories of client needs as the structure for its test plan. These categories include (1) safe, effective care environment, (2) health promotion and maintenance, (3) psychosocial integrity, and (4) physiologic integrity. These content areas within nursing practice are consistently applied regardless of the stage in the client's life span or the setting for healthcare delivery.

To meet client needs, nurses perform four basic roles: caregiver, educator, collaborator, and delegator. Table 7-1 illustrates how these basic nursing roles correspond to the NCLEX-PN test plan's client needs categories.

The Nurse as Caregiver

A **caregiver** is one who performs health-related activities that a sick person cannot perform independently. The nurse's caregiving skills help to restore wellness, especially during an acute illness, or to maintain as much function and independence as possible for a client with chronic physical or mental health problems.

Traditionally, nurses have been providers of physical care; however, caring also involves a close emotional relationship. Contemporary nurses understand that illness and injuries cause feelings of insecurity that may threaten a person's ability to cope. Consequently, the nurse becomes the client's guide, companion, and interpreter. The supportive relationship that develops establishes trust and reduces fear and worry.

Nurses use **empathy**, an intuitive awareness of what the client is experiencing, to perceive the client's emotional state and need for support. Empathy helps the nurse become effective in providing for the client's needs while remaining compassionately detached.

▶ **Stop, Think, and Respond Exercise 7-1**

When you are assigned to one or more clients during clinical experience, what kinds of caregiving skills do you perform?

BOX 7-1 Nurse–Client Responsibilities

Nursing Responsibilities
Possess current knowledge
Be aware of unique age-related differences
Perform technical skills safely
Be committed to the client's care
Be available and courteous
Allow client to participate in decisions
Remain nonjudgmental
Advocate on the client's behalf
Provide explanations in language that is easily understood
Promote independence

Client Responsibilities
Identify current problem
Describe desired outcomes
Answer questions honestly
Provide accurate historic and subjective data
Participate to the fullest extent possible
Be open and flexible to alternatives
Comply with the therapeutic regimen
Keep follow-up appointments

The Nurse as Educator

An **educator** is one who provides information. Nurses offer health teaching that is pertinent to each client's needs and knowledge base. Some examples include explanations about diagnostic test procedures, self-administration of medications, techniques for managing wound care, and restorative exercises such as those performed after a mastectomy.

When it comes to treatment decisions, the nurse avoids giving advice, reserving the right of each person to make his or her own choices on matters affecting personal health and illness care. Instead, the nurse shares information on potential alternatives, allows the client the freedom to choose, and supports the client's ultimate decision.

Because nursing is considered a practice "without walls" (i.e., extending beyond the original treatment facility), nurses are resources for information about health services available in the community. This type of information empowers clients to become involved with self-help groups or those that offer rehabilitation, financial assistance, or emotional support.

The Nurse as Collaborator

A **collaborator** is one who works with others to achieve a common goal. Usually, many people are involved in a

TABLE 7-1 Integration of NCLEX-PN Test Categories with Nursing Roles

CATEGORY	SUBCATEGORIES	NURSING ROLE
Safe, Effective Care Environment	Coordinated Care *Example:* Using assistive personnel in client care	• Collaborator • Delegator
	Safety and Infection Control *Example:* Controlling exposure to sources of radiation and hazardous substances	• Caregiver • Collaborator • Educator
Health Promotion and Maintenance	*Example:* Facilitating the transition from independent living to living with assistance	• Caregiver • Collaborator • Educator
	Example: Minimizing risk factors related to the development of acute or chronic illnesses	• Educator • Caregiver • Collaborator
Psychosocial Integrity	*Example:* Using principles of therapeutic communication	• Caregiver • Collaborator
	Example: Promoting the expression of feelings within established boundaries	• Caregiver • Collaborator
Physiologic Integrity	Basic Care and Comfort *Example:* Encouraging fluid intake	• Caregiver • Educator • Collaborator • Delegator
	Pharmacologic Therapies *Example:* Identifying therapeutic and nontherapeutic reactions to medications	• Caregiver • Educator
	Reduction of Risk Potential *Example:* Performing blood glucose finger sticks	• Caregiver • Delegator • Collaborator
	Physiologic Adaptation *Example:* Maintaining a patent airway	• Caregiver • Delegator • Collaborator

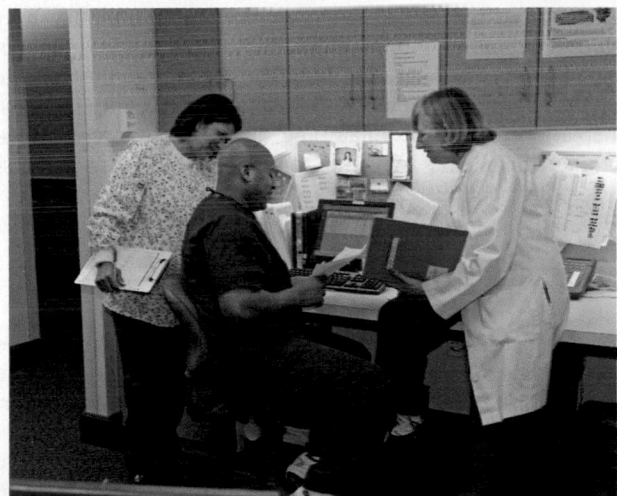

FIGURE 7-1. Collaboration may involve many members of the healthcare team.

client's care (Fig. 7-1). The most obvious example of collaboration occurs between the nurse who is responsible for managing care and those to whom the care is delegated. Collaboration also takes place when the nurse and physician share information and when they exchange information with other healthcare workers, such as the dietitian, physical therapist, respiratory therapist, and discharge planner.

Stop, Think, and Respond Exercise 7-2

Which healthcare workers might be involved in managing the care of a client with a stroke?

The Nurse as Delegator

A **delegator** is one who assigns a task to someone. Before the nurse assumes the role of delegator, he or she must know what tasks are appropriate for particular healthcare workers. It is unsafe to delegate a task to someone who does not have the knowledge or expertise to perform it correctly. Once a task has been assigned, it is still the delegator's responsibility to check that the task has been performed and to determine the resulting outcome. For example, if a nurse asks a nursing assistant to change a client's position, the nurse must verify that the assistant has completed the job and obtain other pertinent information such as the condition of the client's skin. If the delegated task is not performed or is performed incorrectly, the nurse is held accountable for the inadequate client care.

Stop, Think, and Respond Exercise 7-3

What tasks might a staff nurse delegate to a student nurse?

Phases of the Nurse–Client Relationship

The nurse–client relationship progresses through three phases: the introductory phase, the working phase, and the

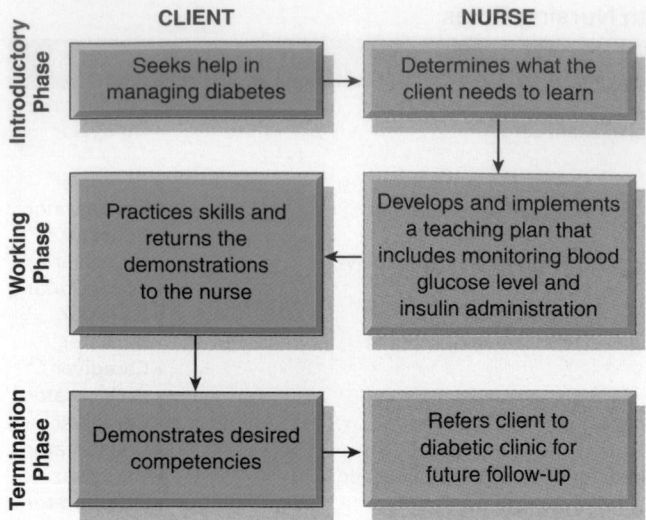

FIGURE 7-2. Examples of activities related to phases of the nurse–client relationship.

terminating phase. Figure 7-2 gives an example of the activities that occur in each of the three phases.

Introductory Phase

The **introductory phase** starts when the nurse and the client get acquainted and the client identifies one or more health problems for which he or she is seeking care. Both the nurse and client bring preconceived ideas about the other to the initial interaction, and these assumptions eventually are confirmed or dismissed. Initial contact may begin with an exchange of names and a handshake if appropriate. Before calling a person by his or her first name, the nurse should obtain permission or wait to be invited to use a more familiar form of address, which some cultures reserve for family and close friends. The nurse demonstrates courtesy, active listening, empathy, competence, and appropriate communication skills to convey that he or she values the client. Nurses demonstrate partnership and advocacy in the client's healthcare by:

- Treating each client as a unique person
- Respecting the client's feelings
- Striving to promote the client's physical, emotional, social, and spiritual well-being
- Encouraging the client to participate in problem-solving and decision-making
- Accepting that a client has the potential for change
- Communicating in terms and language that the client understands
- Using the nursing process to individualize the client's care
- Involving those persons to whom the client turns for support, such as family and friends, when providing care
- Implementing healthcare techniques that are compatible with the client's value system and cultural heritage

 Gerontologic Considerations

- An appreciation of the older adult as an individual with unique needs and concerns is the foundation of a positive nurse–client relationship. Avoid using terms of endearment (honey, sweetie) and plural identity ("Let's take our medicine"), which can be perceived as patronizing or disrespectful.

- Take time to listen actively to the older adult and allow ample time for responses to questions; remember that the health history of an older adult may span more than 80 years.

- Involving support persons such as family or friends may be particularly important when establishing a relationship with the older client, especially if his or her memory is impaired.

Working Phase

The **working phase** involves mutually planning the client's care and putting the plan into action. Both the nurse and the client participate. Each shares in performing those tasks that will lead to the desired outcomes identified by the client. During the working phase, attending to a client's personal dietary preferences demonstrates a respect for the unique characteristics of each person, which enhances the nurse–client relationship. The nurse supports the client's independence by allowing the client to pace his or her own care, even when this requires more time. Doing too much for the client is as harmful as doing too little. Allowing independence in self-care and decision-making promotes self-esteem and dignity.

Terminating Phase

The **terminating phase** occurs when the nurse and client mutually agree that the client's immediate health problems have improved and the nurse's services are no longer necessary.

Regression, evidenced by increased reliance on nursing assistance or the reemergence of physical symptoms, may indicate an underlying fear of having to assume independent responsibility for self-care. Initially, the nurse must ensure that the client is not developing health-related complications. Thereafter, a compassionate and a caring attitude helps to facilitate the client's transition to independent living or transfer to other healthcare services.

COMMUNICATION

Communication is an exchange of information. It involves both sending and receiving messages between two or more individuals. It is followed by feedback indicating that the information is understood or needs further clarification (Fig. 7-3).

The Joint Commission (2008) has developed National Patient Safety Goals, some of which relate specifically to communication:

- Encourage clients' active involvement in their own care as a client safety strategy.
- Define and communicate the means for clients and their families to report concerns about safety and encourage them to do so.
- Improve the effectiveness of communication among caregivers.

Understanding principles of communication is essential for developing an effective nurse–client relationship.

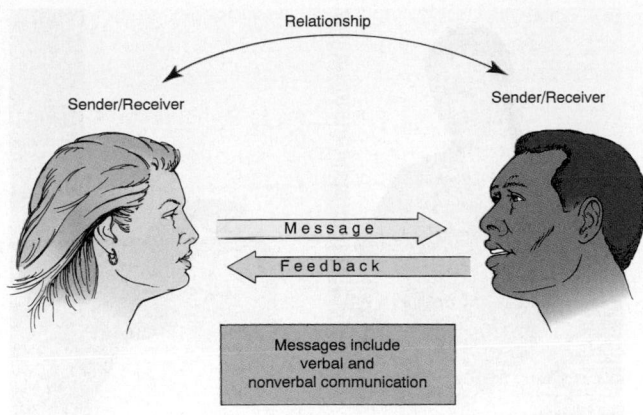

FIGURE 7-3. Communication is a two-way process.

Verbal Communication

Verbal communication is communication that uses words. It includes speaking, reading, and writing. The following variables affect verbal communication between clients and nurses and other healthcare workers:

- Attention and concentration
- Language compatibility
- Verbal skills
- Hearing and visual acuity
- Motor functions involving the throat, tongue, and teeth
- Noise and distracting activity
- Interpersonal attitudes
- Literacy
- Cultural similarities
- Listening

Listening is as important during communication as speaking. In contrast to **hearing**, which is perceiving sounds, **listening** is an activity that includes attending to and becoming fully involved in what the client says. Empathetic listening implies that the nurse attempts to perceive the client's emotions and meanings. When the nurse conveys empathy to clients, it helps him or her to feel both understood and valued. Empathetic listening often is demonstrated through nonverbal means.

When communicating with most American clients, it is best to position oneself at the client's level and make frequent eye contact (see cultural exceptions in Chap. 8). Nodding and encouraging the client to continue with comments, such as "Yes, I see," convey interest in what the client is saying. The nurse guards against sending messages that indicate boredom, such as looking out a window or interrupting a comment.

 Gerontologic Considerations

- Potential sensory changes in older clients can pose a barrier to verbal communication. Older adults tend to lose the ability to hear at high-pitched ranges, so it is best to lower the voice pitch when speaking, use a normal volume, and clearly enunciate consonants, especially at the

beginning and ending of words. Communicate with hearing-impaired adults by using the client's preferred method of enhancing communication, such as writing, pictures, or sign language.

- When an older adult repeatedly tells the same story or asks the same question, make an effort to determine if there is a hidden or unspoken fear or concern that the older adult is too apprehensive to discuss.

Nonverbal Communication

Nonverbal communication is the exchange of information without using words. It is what is not said. Nonverbal communication consists of components such as kinesics, paralanguage, proxemics, touch, and silence.

Kinesics

Kinesics refers to body language, or those collective nonverbal techniques that include facial expressions, postures, gestures, and body movements. Even clothing style and accessories (e.g., jewelry) can affect the context of communication. Table 7-2 lists examples of nonverbal behaviors and their meanings.

Knowledge of kinesics is important for the nurse who is being evaluated by his or her clients and visa versa. The following are suggestions to create a positive impression during a nurse–client interaction:

> ▶ **Stop, Think, and Respond Exercise 7-4**
>
> *What nonverbal message is communicated when a person wears a white lab coat, a ring on the third finger of the left hand, or a badge and gun?*

- Stand tall
- Relax arms, legs, and feet; do not cross any body part

TABLE 7-2 Examples of Body Language and Interpretations

BODY LANGUAGE	INTERPRETATION(S)
Positive	
Tilt of head	Interested
Open hands	Sincere
Brisk, erect walk	Confident
Hand to cheek	Contemplative
Rubbing hands	Anticipatory
Steepled fingers	Authoritative
Nod	Agreement
Negative	
Arms crossed	Blocking; oppositional
Clenched jaw	Angry; antagonistic
Downcast eyes	Remorseful; bored
Rubbing nose	Doubtful; deceitful
Drumming fingers	Impatient
Fondling hair	Insecure
Frown	Disagreement
Stroking chin	Stalling for time
Shifting from foot to foot	Desire to get away
Looking at watch	Bored

- Maintain eye contact approximately 60% to 70% of the time or as much as is appropriate for the culture (see Chap. 8); in a group, focus on the last person who spoke
- Keep your head level both horizontally and vertically
- Lean forward slightly to demonstrate interest and attention
- Keep the arms where they can be seen
- Strike a balance in arm movements, being neither too demonstrative nor too restrained
- Keep the legs as still as possible

Paralanguage

Paralanguage refers to vocal sounds (not actually words) that communicate a message. Some examples include drawing in a deep breath to indicate surprise, clucking the tongue to show disappointment, and whistling to get someone's attention. Crying, laughing, and moaning are additional forms of paralanguage. Vocal inflections, volume, pitch, and rate of speech add yet another dimension to communication.

Proxemics

Proxemics refers to the use of space when communicating. In general, four proxemic zones are common when Americans communicate. The zones include **intimate space, personal space, social space,** and **public space** (Table 7-3).

Most Americans tolerate strangers being 2 to 3 feet from them. Determining the circumference of a person's **comfort zone,** the area that when intruded does not create anxiety, is important because physical closeness is common during nursing care. Approaches that relieve a client's anxiety about being close include explaining beforehand how a nursing procedure will be performed and ensuring that the client is properly draped.

Touch

Touch is a tactile stimulus produced by personal contact with another person or object. In the context of nursing, touch is either task-oriented, affective, or both (Fig. 7-4). **Task-oriented touch** involves the personal contact that is required when performing nursing procedures. **Affective touch** is used to demonstrate concern or affection. Its intention is to

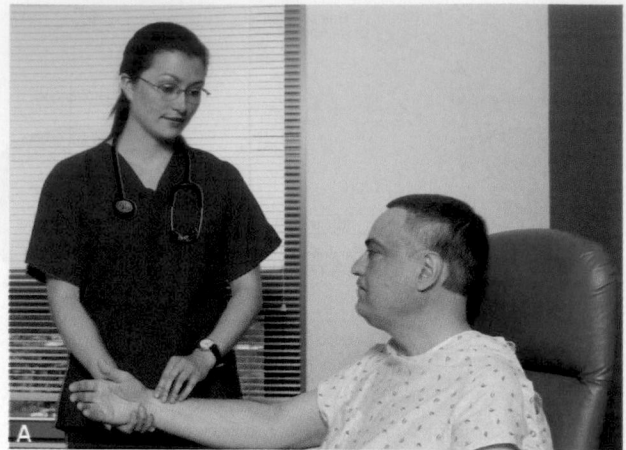
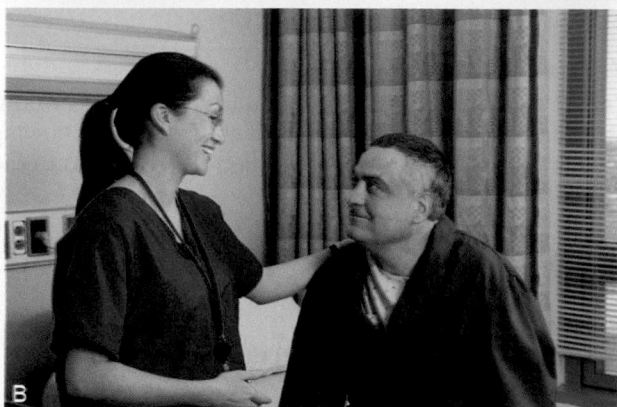

FIGURE 7-4. Types of touch: **(A)** Task-oriented touch. **(B)** Affective touch.

communicate caring and support. Most people respond positively to being touched; however, a nurse should use affective touching cautiously because there is a great deal of response variations among individuals. In general, nurses use affective touch therapeutically when a client is lonesome; uncomfortable; near death; anxious, insecure, or frightened; disoriented; disfigured; semiconscious or comatose; visually impaired; or sensory deprived.

 Gerontologic Considerations

- There is scant evidence to support the use of touch in the older adult. Therefore, touch should be used purposefully to reinforce verbal messages or in a manner that is culturally appropriate to convey concern or support. However, older adults may perceive touch as culturally inappropriate or offensive. Frailty or vulnerability may also impact the client's perception of touch; therefore, nursing judgment must be used.

Silence

Silence is the art of remaining quiet. One of its therapeutic uses is to encourage a client's verbal communication. Other therapeutic uses include providing a personal presence and a brief period during which clients can process information or respond to a question.

TABLE 7-3 Proxemic Zones

ZONE	DISTANCE	PURPOSE
Intimate space	Within 6 inches	Lovemaking Confiding secrets Sharing confidential information
Personal space	6 inches to 4 feet	Interviewing Physical assessment Therapeutic interventions involving touch Private conversations
Social space	4 to 12 feet	Teaching one-on-one Group interactions Lecturing Conversations that are not intended to be private
Public space	12 or more feet	Giving speeches Gatherings of strangers

TABLE 7-4 Therapeutic Communication Techniques

TECHNIQUE	USE	EXAMPLE
Broad opening	Relieves tension before getting to the real purpose of the interaction	"Wonderful weather we're having."
Giving information	Provides facts	"Your surgery is scheduled at noon."
Direct questioning	Acquires specific information	"Do you have any allergies?"
Open-ended questioning	Encourages the client to elaborate	"How are you feeling?"
Reflecting	Confirms that the nurse is following the conversation	*Client:* "I haven't been sleeping well." *Nurse:* "You haven't been sleeping well."
Paraphrasing	Restates what the client has said to demonstrate listening	*Client:* "After every meal, I feel like I will throw up." *Nurse:* "Eating makes you nauseous, but you don't actually vomit."
Verbalizing what has been implied	Shares how the nurse has interpreted a statement	*Client:* "All the nurses are so busy." *Nurse:* "You're feeling that you shouldn't ask for help."
Structuring	Defines a purpose and sets limits	"I have 15 minutes. If your pain is relieved, I could go over how your test will be done."
Giving general leads	Encourages the client to continue	"Uh, huh," or "Go on."
Sharing perceptions	Shows empathy for how the client is feeling	"You seem depressed."
Clarifying	Avoids misinterpretation	"I'm afraid I don't quite understand what you're asking."
Confronting	Calls attention to manipulation, inconsistencies, or lack of responsibility	"You're concerned about your weight loss, but you didn't eat any breakfast."
Summarizing	Reviews information that has been discussed	"You've asked me to check on increasing your pain medication and getting your diet changed."
Silence	Allows time for considering how to proceed or arouses the client's anxiety to the point that it stimulates more verbalization	

Therapeutic Communication

Communication occurs on a social or a therapeutic level. **Therapeutic communication** refers to using verbal and nonverbal communication to promote a person's physical and emotional well-being. Techniques that are helpful are identified in Table 7-4.

▶ *Stop, Think, and Respond Exercise 7-5*

Give an example of a therapeutic response to the following statement made by a client: "My family didn't visit me last evening."

When the client is quiet and uncommunicative, the nurse must avoid assuming that the client has no problems or understands everything. On the other hand, it is never appropriate to probe or press an unwilling client to communicate. It is best to wait for a response; reserved clients may share their feelings and concerns after they feel that the nurse is sincere and trustworthy.

The nurse also must respond delicately to a vocal and emotional client. For instance, when clients are angry or cry, the best nursing approach is to allow them to express their emotions without fear of retaliation or censure.

Although nurses have the best intentions of interacting therapeutically with clients, some fall into traps that block or hinder therapeutic communication. Table 7-5 lists common examples of nontherapeutic communication.

 Gerontologic Considerations

- Encourage the older client to reminisce. Ask about past events and relationships associated with positive experiences and feelings. Giving older adults an opportunity to talk about earlier times in their lives reinforces their value and unique identity. Be alert to the possibility that reminiscing may evoke painful memories or unresolved developmental tasks.

Communicating with Special Populations

Some clients, such as those who are verbally impaired, deaf, or cannot communicate in English, have special communication needs that must be met to ensure client safety. Nurses and other healthcare providers must find ways to help these clients effectively communicate their health problems and needs, give informed consent, or understand teaching about health practices that will impact their recovery or health maintenance. Regardless of the barrier, The Joint Commission is adamant that healthcare workers facilitate communication with all clients.

Communicating with Verbally Impaired Clients

There are instances when nurses and clients cannot communicate verbally despite the fact that each is proficient in English.

TABLE 7-5 Nontherapeutic Communication Techniques

TECHNIQUE AND CONSEQUENCE	EXAMPLE	IMPROVEMENT
Giving False Reassurance		
Trivializes the client's unique feelings and discourages further discussion	"You've got nothing to worry about. Everything will work out just fine."	"Tell me about your specific concerns."
Using Clichés		
Provides worthless advice and curtails exploring alternatives	"Keep a stiff upper lip."	"It must be difficult for you right now."
Giving Approval or Disapproval		
Holds the client to a rigid standard; implies that future deviation may lead to subsequent rejection or disfavor	"I'm glad you're exercising so regularly." "You should be testing your blood sugar each morning."	"Are you having any difficulty fitting regular exercise into your schedule?" "Let's explore some ways that will help you test your blood sugar each morning."
Agreeing		
Does not allow the client flexibility to change his or her mind	"You're right about needing surgery immediately."	"Having surgery immediately is one possibility. What others have you considered?"
Disagreeing		
Intimidates the client; makes the person feel foolish or inadequate	"That's not true! Where did you get an idea like that?"	"Maybe I can help clarify that for you."
Demanding an Explanation		
Puts the client on the defensive; the client may be tempted to make up an excuse rather than risk disapproval for an honest answer	"Why didn't you keep your appointment last week?"	"I see you couldn't keep your appointment last week."
Giving Advice		
Discourages independent problem-solving and decision-making; provides a biased view that may prejudice the client's choice	"If I were you, I'd try drug therapy before having surgery."	"Share with me the advantages and disadvantages of your options as you see them."
Defending		
Indicates such a strong allegiance that any disagreement to the contrary is not acceptable	"Ms. Johnson is my best nursing assistant. She wouldn't have let your light go unanswered that long."	"I'm sorry you had to wait so long."
Belittling		
Disregards how the client is responding as an individual	"Lots of people learn to give themselves insulin."	"You're finding it especially difficult to stick yourself with a needle."
Patronizing		
Treats the client condescendingly, as less than capable of making an independent decision	"Are we ready for our bath yet?"	"Would you like your bath now, or should I check with you later?"
Changing the Subject		
Alters the direction of the discussion to a topic that is safer or more comfortable	*Client:* "I'm so scared that a mammogram will show I have cancer." *Nurse:* "Tell me more about your family."	"It is a serious disease. What concerns you the most?"

For example, clients who have had a stroke sometimes experience **expressive aphasia**, an inability to utilize verbal language skills. Clients who have artificial airways, such as an endotracheal or tracheostomy tube, or who have their jaws wired following facial trauma cannot speak. Nevertheless, communication is still a nursing priority as mandated by The Joint Commission's National Patient Safety Goals.

The nurse may provide the verbally impaired client with a tablet and pencil or "magic slate," although this approach is time consuming. In some cases, the client may not have the use of the hands or fine motor skills to use a writing device. Other various communication tools are available to facilitate meeting the communication needs of verbally impaired clients. For example, the client may prefer to point to common phrases, spell with the alphabet, and identify numbers on a communication board (Fig. 7-5).

Communicating with Deaf Clients

A person who is **deaf** is unable to hear well enough to use hearing as a means of processing information; whereas a person who is **hard of hearing** has some hearing and is able to use it for communication purposes. If the deaf client can read and write, writing can facilitate communication. However, written communication may not be useful for all clients.

Many deaf clients, especially those who were born deaf or lost their hearing at a very early age, have learned to use American Sign Language (ASL). ASL uses signs made by hand movements and **fingerspelling**, an alphabetical substitute for words that have no sign (Fig. 7-6). However, the healthcare agency may not have anyone available who is proficient in ASL. To overcome this barrier, some hospitals use a **webcam**, a video camera that allows viewing via the Internet. The webcam allows **video interpreting**, in which

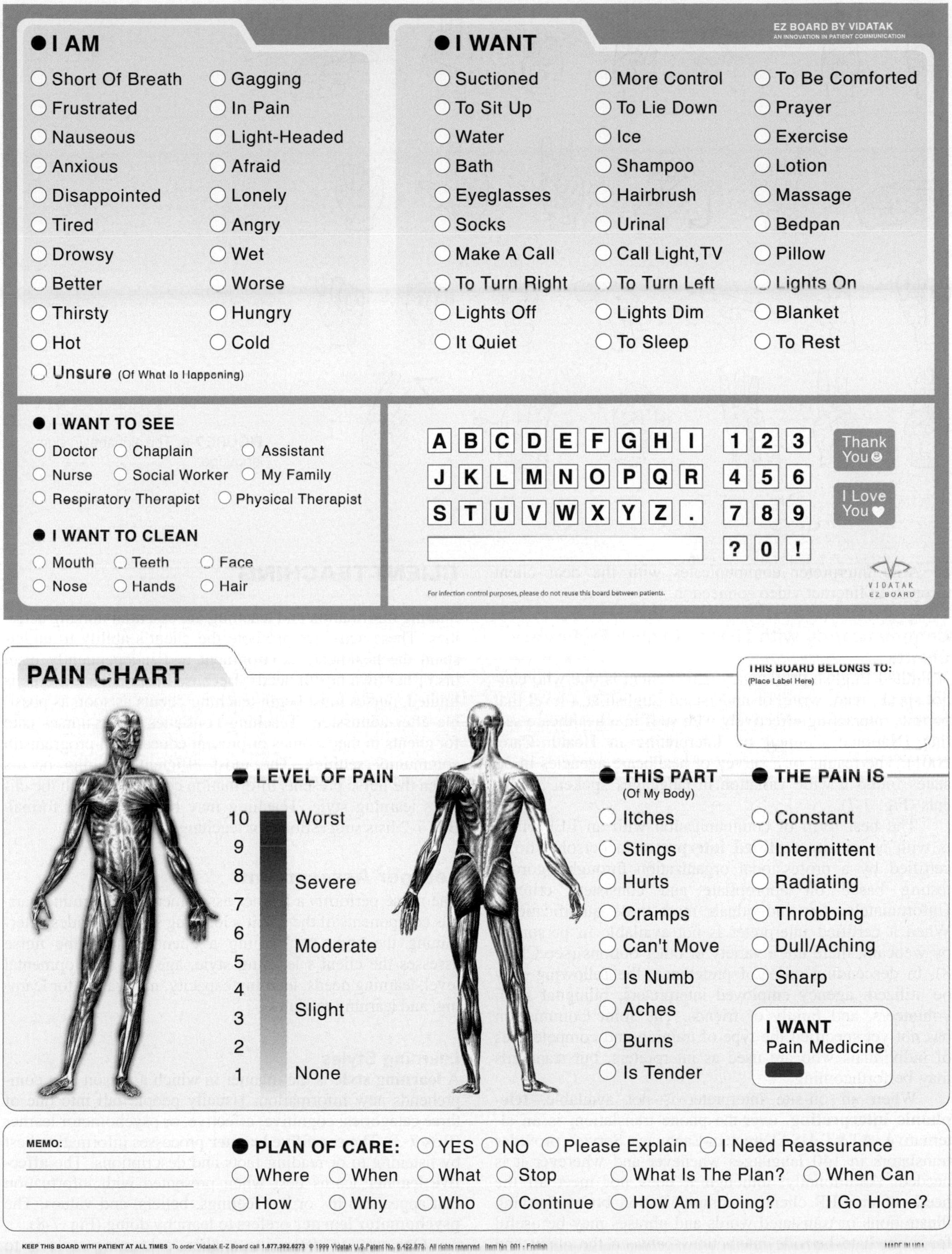

● I AM

- ○ Short Of Breath ○ Gagging
- ○ Frustrated ○ In Pain
- ○ Nauseous ○ Light-Headed
- ○ Anxious ○ Afraid
- ○ Disappointed ○ Lonely
- ○ Tired ○ Angry
- ○ Drowsy ○ Wet
- ○ Better ○ Worse
- ○ Thirsty ○ Hungry
- ○ Hot ○ Cold
- ○ **Unsure** (Of What Is Happening)

● I WANT

EZ BOARD BY VIDATAK
AN INNOVATION IN PATIENT COMMUNICATION

- ○ Suctioned ○ More Control ○ To Be Comforted
- ○ To Sit Up ○ To Lie Down ○ Prayer
- ○ Water ○ Ice ○ Exercise
- ○ Bath ○ Shampoo ○ Lotion
- ○ Eyeglasses ○ Hairbrush ○ Massage
- ○ Socks ○ Urinal ○ Bedpan
- ○ Make A Call ○ Call Light,TV ○ Pillow
- ○ To Turn Right ○ To Turn Left ○ Lights On
- ○ Lights Off ○ Lights Dim ○ Blanket
- ○ It Quiet ○ To Sleep ○ To Rest

● I WANT TO SEE

- ○ Doctor ○ Chaplain ○ Assistant
- ○ Nurse ○ Social Worker ○ My Family
- ○ Respiratory Therapist ○ Physical Therapist

● I WANT TO CLEAN

- ○ Mouth ○ Teeth ○ Face
- ○ Nose ○ Hands ○ Hair

A	B	C	D	E	F	G	H	I	1	2	3
J	K	L	M	N	O	P	Q	R	4	5	6
S	T	U	V	W	X	Y	Z	.	7	8	9

| | ? | 0 | ! |

Thank You ☺
I Love You ♥

VIDATAK EZ BOARD

For infection control purposes, please do not reuse this board between patients.

PAIN CHART

THIS BOARD BELONGS TO:
(Place Label Here)

● LEVEL OF PAIN

- 10 Worst
- 9
- 8 Severe
- 7
- 6
- 5 Moderate
- 4
- 3 Slight
- 2
- 1 None

● THIS PART (Of My Body)

- ○ Itches
- ○ Stings
- ○ Hurts
- ○ Cramps
- ○ Can't Move
- ○ Is Numb
- ○ Aches
- ○ Burns
- ○ Is Tender

● THE PAIN IS

- ○ Constant
- ○ Intermittent
- ○ Radiating
- ○ Throbbing
- ○ Dull/Aching
- ○ Sharp

I WANT
Pain Medicine

MEMO: _____

● PLAN OF CARE: ○ YES ○ NO ○ Please Explain ○ I Need Reassurance
○ Where ○ When ○ What ○ Stop ○ What Is The Plan? ○ When Can
○ How ○ Why ○ Who ○ Continue ○ How Am I Doing? I Go Home?

KEEP THIS BOARD WITH PATIENT AT ALL TIMES To order Vidatak E-Z Board call 1.877.392.6273 © 1999 Vidatak U.S. Patent No. 9,422,875. All rights reserved. Item No. 001 - English   MADE IN USA

FIGURE 7-5. A client who is verbally impaired due to a stroke or intubation can communicate his or her needs to the nurse using a communication board. (Courtesy of Vidatak, LLC. Los Angeles, CA 90069.)

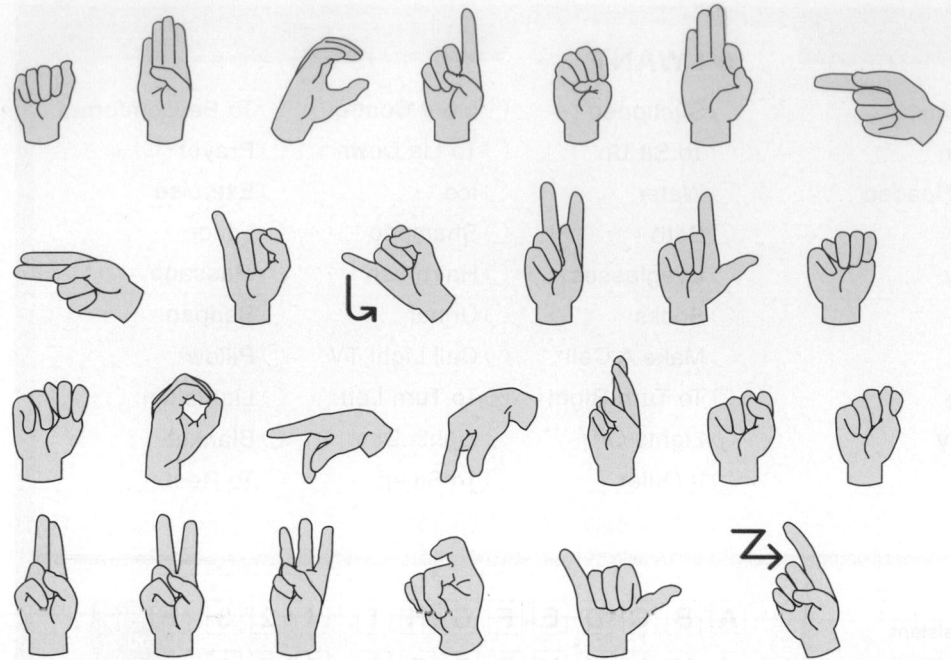

FIGURE 7-8. The alphabet in sign language.

an ASL interpreter communicates with the deaf client through an Internet video connection.

Communicating with Limited English Proficiency Clients

A limited English proficiency (LEP) client is one who cannot speak, read, write, or understand English at a level that permits interacting effectively with staff in a healthcare setting (National Council on Interpreting in Health Care, 2001). The results of a survey of healthcare agencies in 32 states found a wide variation in languages spoken by clients (Fig. 7-7).

The best form of communication with an LEP client is with an on-site **certified interpreter**, a person who is certified by a professional organization through rigorous testing based on appropriate and consistent criteria. Unfortunately, few individuals meet these qualifications. When a certified interpreter is not available in person or by webcam, there are a variety of other options (see Chap. 8). In descending order of preference, the following may be utilized: agency employed interpreters, bilingual staff, volunteers, and family or friends. The Joint Commission has not yet specified the type of training and competencies of individuals who are used as interpreters, but standards may be forthcoming.

When an on-site interpreter is not available, **telephonic interpreting**, over-the phone translation, is an alternative. AT&T USADirect In-Language Service provides translators in 140 languages whenever and wherever it is needed. Additionally, although it does not meet all the needs of an LEP client, a communication board showing illustrations or translated words and phrases may be useful for immediate bedside interactions between the client and nursing staff.

CLIENT TEACHING

Sharing information and teaching are essential nursing activities. These activities promote the client's ability to understand the healthcare environment and independently meet his or her own health needs. Because hospitalization time is limited, nurses must begin teaching clients as soon as possible after admission. Teaching continues while nurses care for clients in their homes or present educational programs in community settings. The most efficient teaching occurs when the nurse presents information compatible with the client's learning style. Teaching may be informal or formal. Box 7-2 lists suggestions for teaching adult clients.

Learner Assessment

The nurse performs a learner assessment to determine various components of the client's learning status. Besides determining the style of learning a client prefers, the nurse assesses the client's learning style, age and developmental level, learning needs, learning capacity, motivation for learning, and learning readiness.

Learning Styles

A **learning style** is the manner in which a person best comprehends new information. Usually people fall into one of three categories: cognitive, affective, or psychomotor learner (Box 7-3). The **cognitive learner** processes information best by listening to or reading facts and descriptions. The **affective learner** learns best when presented with information that appeals to his or her feelings, beliefs, and values. The **psychomotor learner** prefers to learn by doing (Fig. 7-8).

One way to determine a client's learning style is to ask, "When you learned to add fractions, what helped you

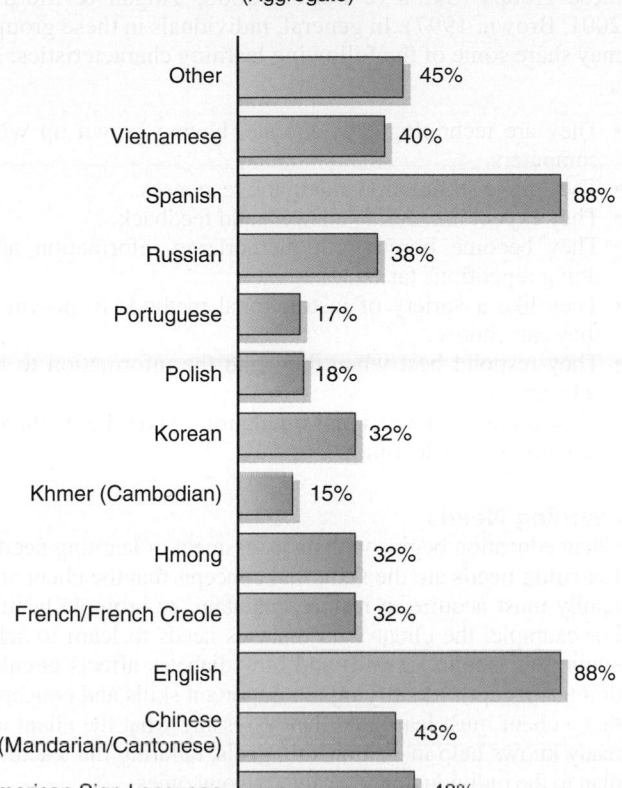

Hospital Reported Languages Spoken by Client (Aggregate)

Language	%
Other	45%
Vietnamese	40%
Spanish	88%
Russian	38%
Portuguese	17%
Polish	18%
Korean	32%
Khmer (Cambodian)	15%
Hmong	32%
French/French Creole	32%
English	88%
Chinese (Mandarian/Cantonese)	43%
American Sign Language	48%

% of Hospitals (n=60)

FIGURE 7-7. A survey of hospitals in 32 states identified Spanish and American Sign Language as the two most commonly spoken languages other than English. (From Wilson-Stronks, A., & Galvez, E. [2007]. *Hospitals, language, and culture: A snapshot of the nation.* The Joint Commission and The California Endowment. Available at: http://www.jointcommission.org/NR/rdonlyres/E64E5E89-5734-4D1D-BB4D-C4ACD4BF8BD3/0/hlc_paper.pdf Accessed March 2009.)

most: listening to the teacher's explanation, recognizing the value of fractions in cooking or carpentry, or working on sample problems?" Although most people favor one style of learning, presenting information through a combination of the three styles tends to optimize learning.

Age and Developmental Level

Nurses and all those who provide instruction must be aware of the basic learning characteristics of children, adults, older adult learners, and those learners that are developmentally compromised. Currently, there are three major categories:

- **Pedagogy** is the science of teaching children or those with cognitive ability comparable to children (although it often refers to the teaching of all individuals).
- **Andragogy** is the science of teaching adult learners.
- **Gerogogy** is the science of teaching older adults.

Many clients with health problems are in their later years. Box 7-4 offers tips for tailoring client teaching to

---

BOX 7-2 Teaching Adult Clients

- Identify the value or purpose for learning new information
- Determine if the client is comfortable at the moment
- Make sure the client is wearing glasses or using a hearing aid if needed
- Reduce noise and distractions in the environment
- Sit at eye level (unless doing group teaching) and face the client(s)
- Use short sentences of 10 words or fewer
- Avoid speaking rapidly
- Minimize technical terms and medical jargon; define words whenever necessary
- Use words that a seventh- to ninth-grader would understand
- Present at least one but no more than three new ideas at each teaching session
- Review frequently
- Use the active form of the verb rather than passive (e.g., "Wipe straight down the center of the incision," rather than "The incision is wiped down the center")
- Use examples with which the learner can identify
- Relate new information to prior learning
- Build in a learner performance evaluation, such as asking the client to repeat or paraphrase prior information, demonstrate a skill, or apply the information to a hypothetical situation, such as "What would you do if … ?"
- End teaching if the client cannot remain attentive

BOX 7-3 Activities That Promote Learning According to Styles

Cognitive Learners
Listing
Identifying
Naming
Describing
Summarizing
Selecting

Affective Learners
Advocating
Supporting
Accepting
Promoting
Internalizing
Valuing

Psychomotor Learners
Assembling
Changing
Emptying
Filling
Adding
Removing

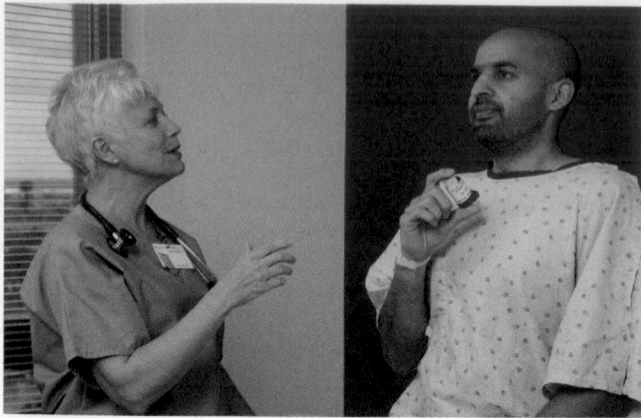

FIGURE 7-8. A psychomotor learner learns best by doing. If the client can demonstrate what the nurse has taught, learning has occurred.

older adults. Nurse educators are also advised to prepare themselves to teach young adults who belong to "Generation X", and "Generation Y" also known as the Net Generation. Generation X refers to those born between 1961 and 1981, and the Net Generation, sometimes referred to as "cyberkids" were born after 1981. Technology and imposed independence as a consequence of growing up in single-parent households or homes in which both parents

---

BOX 7-4 | Considerations for Teaching Older Adults

- Older adults have a lifetime of past experiences that can be used as a foundation for new learning.
- Before beginning a teaching session, ask the older adult about the need for glasses or a hearing aid or both. Make sure that glasses are clean and/or the hearing aid is in good working order and turned on.
- Choose printed materials that positively portray persons of similar age.
- Avoid using printed materials that are cluttered with extensive information.
- Be sure that printed materials are of sufficient size for easy reading. Such materials usually should be in at least 14-point type for older adults.
- Booklets, pamphlets, and brochures that are printed in black on white or cream matte paper improve visual clarity.
- Healthy older adults maintain cognitive abilities and can learn new information. They do, however, learn more effectively when they are allowed to progress at their own pace, when information is hooked into prior knowledge, and when content is presented in chunks of information to promote recall.
- Learning motor skills may be more difficult for older adults because of physiologic changes. They may need more time to learn new activities or modifications in the equipment required for the skill.
- Asking the older adult to explain practices used to maintain health can provide insight into various cultural practices to be integrated in a health teaching plan (see Chap. 9).

---

work have greatly affected the learning characteristics of these groups (Skiba & Barton, 2006; Tulgan & Martin, 2001; Brown, 1997). In general, individuals in these groups may share some of the following learning characteristics:

- They are technologically literate, having grown up with computers.
- They crave stimulation and quick responses.
- They expect immediate answers and feedback.
- They become bored with memorizing information and doing repetitious tasks.
- They like a variety of instructional methods from which they can choose.
- They respond best when they find the information to be relevant.
- They prefer visualizations, simulations, and other methods of participatory learning.

Learning Needs
Client education begins with an assessment of learning needs. **Learning needs** are the skills and concepts that the client and family must acquire to restore, maintain, or promote health. For example, the client with diabetes needs to learn to self-administer insulin (a skill) and how diabetes affects circulation (a concept). Identifying the important skills and concepts that a client must learn and then assessing what the client already knows help in establishing goals, tailoring the teaching plan to the individual, and evaluating outcomes.

Learning Capacity
Learning capacity refers to a person's intellectual ability to understand, remember, and apply new information. Illiteracy, sensory deficits, and a shortened attention span require special adaptations when implementing client teaching.

 Pharmacologic Considerations

- Some medications dull mental ability and make concentration and communication more difficult. Keep in mind that this can affect the client's ability to learn new material and to remember specific details taught during a teaching session.

Motivation
Motivation is the desire to acquire new information. Learning occurs at an accelerated rate when a person has a purpose or reason for mastering it. Some motivating forces include restoring independence, preventing complications, facilitating discharge, and returning to or remaining in the comfort of home.

Learning Readiness
Learning readiness pertains to the optimal time for learning. Ideally, it occurs when a client is in a state of physical and psychological well-being. For example, a client who is in pain, uncomfortably warm or cold, anxious, or depressed is not in the best condition for learning. In these situations, it is best to restore comfort first and then attend to teaching.

Informal and Formal Teaching

Informal teaching is unplanned. It occurs spontaneously, usually at the client's bedside or while caring for the client at home. **Formal teaching** requires a plan to avoid being haphazard. A **teaching plan** is the organized arrangement of content in a specific time frame. It facilitates reaching goals, providing essential information, and ensuring the client's comprehension before he or she assumes responsibility for self-care. Developing a plan and implementing it gradually and sequentially avoids overwhelming the client with new information or learning skills that are difficult to perform.

CRITICAL THINKING EXERCISES

1. Change the nontherapeutic interaction in the following example to one that is therapeutic:

    Client: "I'm having second thoughts about having this breast reduction surgery."

    Nurse: "You'll be happy with the results when it's over."

2. Studies have shown that older adults are not touched with the same frequency as clients in other age groups. Discuss reasons for this.

3. A client with a health problem does not speak English very well. How might you meet this client's communication needs?

4. What approaches should the nurse take when teaching an older adult with diabetes about his disease and its management?

NCLEX STYLE REVIEW QUESTIONS

1. Which one of the following is characteristic of the introductory phase of a nurse–client relationship?
    1. Developing goals with the client
    2. Gathering health-related data
    3. Performing nursing procedures
    4. Teaching the client about self-care

2. Which of the following therapeutic communication techniques is being demonstrated when the nurse says, "You seem depressed"?
    1. Paraphrasing
    2. Giving a general lead
    3. Sharing perceptions
    4. Clarifying

3. Which of the following would be the least desirable approach for communicating with a limited English proficiency (LEP) client?
    1. Utilize a certified interpreter
    2. Ask a family member to translate
    3. Request the services of a bilingual employee
    4. Contact a telephonic interpreter

4. After teaching a client how to perform breathing exercises, the best method for the nurse to evaluate the effectiveness of the teaching is to do which of the following?
    1. Request that the client explain the importance of breathing exercises.
    2. Ask the client to perform the breathing exercises as they were taught.
    3. Ask the client if he is performing the breathing exercises as required.
    4. Monitor the client's respiratory rate several times a day

5. Which of the following outcomes best supports that a nurse's care giving skills have been effective?
    1. Clients make their own choices about healthcare.
    2. Clients receive information about potential alternatives.
    3. Clients become empowered and involved with self-help groups.
    4. Clients with chronic physical problems maintain independence.

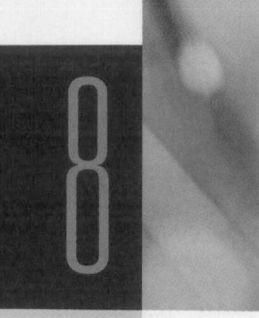

8

Cultural Care Considerations

Words To Know

biocultural ecology
cultural competence
culture
ethnicity
ethnocentrism
generalization
health beliefs
health practices
minority
race
stereotyping
subculture
transcultural nursing

Learning Objectives

On completion of this chapter, you will be able to:

1. Define terms related to culture.
2. List the five population groups delineated in the United States.
3. Differentiate race from ethnicity and culture.
4. Contrast stereotyping and generalization.
5. Describe how cultural background and practices influence actions and behaviors.
6. Name three views that societies use to explain illness or disease.
7. Discuss biocultural assessment.
8. Describe cultural assessment.
9. Explain the meaning and characteristics of transcultural nursing.
10. List at least five ways to demonstrate culturally competent nursing care.

Healthcare providers are becoming increasingly aware that high-quality care involves greater knowledge and appreciation of different linguistic and cultural backgrounds. Healthcare facilities in most large cities and many rural and suburban areas serve diverse populations. Providers and clients bring their respective cultural backgrounds and expectations to any healthcare situation (Diversity Rx, 2003). Thus, nurses must develop **cultural competence**, the ability to understand the client's worldview as well as their own and how these worldviews affect nursing care. This chapter provides information about cultural concepts, clinical variations among different ethnic and racial groups, and communication issues for various cultures. Knowledge of cultural differences and the ability to adapt to each client's cultural needs are crucial to providing quality care.

CULTURAL CONCEPTS

To deliver culturally competent care, nurses must understand terms related to culture. They also must view each person as a unique human being who may have a similar or different frame of reference as the nurse.

Culture

Sir Edward Tyler, a British anthropologist, first used the term *culture* in 1871. He stated that culture includes knowledge, beliefs, art, morals, laws, customs, and other capabilities and habits. The term **culture** provides a means for understanding people's values and beliefs, including those that relate to health practices. Four basic concepts characterize culture (Smeltzer et al., 2008): culture is (1) learned from birth through language and socialization; (2) shared by members of the same cultural group; (3) influenced by specific conditions related to environment, technology, and availability of resources; and (4) dynamic and ever-changing.

Subculture

The United States is often referred to as a *melting pot,* implying that culturally diverse groups are assimilated in one society. Subcultures, however, are readily apparent. **Subculture** refers to a particular group that shares characteristics identifying the group as a distinct entity (Smeltzer et al., 2008). For example, African Americans, Hispanic Americans, and Native Americans each share physical characteristics, language, and ancestry within their own group. These groups may have more subcultures related to specific place of origin, such as Latinos or Chicanos within the Hispanic American group. Other ways to categorize subcultures include region, religion, age, sex, social class, political party, ethnic, racial or cultural identity, and occupation.

Minority

The term **minority** describes a group of people who differ from the majority in a society in terms of cultural characteristics, physical characteristics, or both. Because people from the minority group are perceived as "different," the majority group may treat them unfairly. The United States defines five population groups: white, black, Hispanic, Asian/Pacific Islander, and American Indian/Alaskan Native. Whites still are considered the majority; the other groups are referred to as *ethnic minorities.* Other minorities are based on sex or religion. The defining characteristics for a minority group are not based on numbers but rather on powerlessness and lack of control. For example, women in the United States outnumber men, but women remain in lower-paying jobs and less powerful positions, and thus still are considered a minority.

Ethnicity

Ethnicity is the bond or kinship that people feel with their country of birth or place of ancestral origin. It provides a sense of identity. People demonstrate pride in their ethnic heritage by valuing certain physical characteristics, giving children ethnic names, wearing unique items of clothing, appreciating folk music and dance, or eating native food.

Race

The term *race* often is confused with ethnicity and culture. **Race** refers to biologic differences in physical features, such as skin color, bone structure, and eye shape. Many people associate physical differences, particularly skin color, with culture. Although ethnic and racial groups overlap, nurses must not equate skin color and other physical features with culture. Doing so may lead to erroneous assumptions that all people with certain physical attributes share essentially the same culture and ethnicity. This attitude leads to stereotyping.

Stereotyping

Stereotyping means assuming that all people in a particular cultural, racial, or ethnic group share the same values and beliefs, behave similarly, and are basically alike. For example, a nurse who thinks stereotypically may assign a client to a staff member who is of the same culture as the client, simply because the nurse assumes that all people of that culture are alike. This same nurse also may believe that clients with the same skin color have similar social situations. Because stereotypes are preconceived ideas unsupported by facts, they may not be real or accurate. In fact, they can be dangerous because they are dehumanizing and interfere with accepting others as unique individuals.

 Gerontologic Considerations

- Age may also be considered a cultural subgroup because older adults have shared experiences and resultant values and beliefs. *Ageism* is the stereotyping of older adults' behavior or vulnerability based on an individual's prior experiences or anticipation of behaviors. Ageism may lead to discrimination against older persons or impact nurses' beliefs regarding the delivery of care resources (Morris, 2007).

Generalization

Distinguishing between stereotyping and generalization is important. Stereotyping has an end point; the assumption prevents one from seeing another person as unique. **Generalization**, however, acknowledges common trends in a group while recognizing that more information is needed. As explained by Galanti (2000, p. 1), "If I meet a Mexican woman named Maria and assume that she has a large family, I am stereotyping her. But if I say to myself, 'Mexicans tend to have large families; I wonder if Maria does?' then I am generalizing." Cultural generalizations do not describe each client but provide a broad pattern of beliefs and behaviors for clients from a particular cultural group. This knowledge may assist healthcare providers to provide appropriate care. Nevertheless, generalization can lead to stereotyping, of which nurses must remain cognizant. Increased awareness will assist them to see each client as a unique person.

> ### ▶ Stop, Think, and Respond Exercise 8-1
>
> *You overhear a nurse talking about a client admitted with diabetes and a leg ulcer. The nurse says, "It figures he doesn't do what the doctors say—he's been in this country for 10 years and still can't speak English well. Those people are just stupid!" How would you respond?*

Ethnocentrism

Ethnocentrism is the belief that one's own ethnic heritage is the "correct" one and superior to others. Nurses are human and certainly enter the nursing profession with their own ethnocentrism. They must be aware that their way is not the only or best way. Clients will sense that a nurse feels superior if he or she approaches with a patronizing or condescending attitude. Clients bring their own values and practices and are not ignorant simply because they have different beliefs. Nurses must appreciate that their values and beliefs are not better than those of their clients—they simply are different.

Other Culture-Related Terms

Acculturation involves the process of adapting to or taking on the behaviors of another group. *Cultural blindness* is an inability to recognize the values, beliefs, and practices of others because of strong ethnocentric preferences. *Cultural imposition* is an inclination to impose one's cultural beliefs, values, and patterns of behavior on persons from a different culture. *Cultural taboos* are activities governed by rules of behavior that a particular cultural group avoids, forbids, or prohibits (Smeltzer et al., 2008).

CULTURALLY INFLUENCED CHARACTERISTICS

Cultural upbringing influences a person's actions and behaviors. Socially acceptable conduct for one person may be unacceptable for another. Cultural background affects a person's actions and reactions to his or her environment. When considering cultural background, there is the danger of stereotyping. Issues such as personal space, touch, time, diet, verbal behaviors, and beliefs about the cause of illness are unique for each individual but may be culturally influenced.

Eye Contact

Nurses are taught to maintain eye contact with clients when they are speaking with them, but respecting and understanding behavior and providing a comfortable climate for clients are important considerations. The physical act of making eye contact may be culturally influenced. Anglo-Americans typically value direct eye contact or "looking a person straight in the eye" while speaking. Such eye contact, however, may offend Asian Americans, Native Americans, and other cultural groups who view lingering eye contact as an invasion of privacy. Others, such as Hispanic clients, may avoid eye contact with authority figures as a sign of respect.

Space and Distance

People are not always aware of personal space needs until such needs are threatened. Healthcare situations, such as providing personal care or performing intricate procedures, reduce the accepted personal space, along with causing personal discomfort. Furthermore, nurses often provide comfort and support through close physical proximity, but such closeness may threaten some clients. Nurses must observe how clients position themselves and respect their desire for space as much as possible. Simple explanations of the need for physical proximity during clinical procedures and personal care alleviate the discomfort that some clients may experience.

Space and distance are also factors affecting interactions between nurses and clients. For example, Latinos are characteristically more comfortable sitting close to interviewers and letting interactions slowly unfold. Asian Americans may feel comfortable positioned more than an arm's length from the interviewer.

Touch

There are great cultural differences in the use of touch. For example, some Native Americans may interpret the Anglo-American custom of a strong handshake as offensive. They may be more comfortable with just a light passing of the hands. Arab culture prohibits male healthcare providers from physically examining women. In Asian American culture, touching the head is impolite because the spirit rests there. Orthodox Jewish women highly value their modesty and must keep their heads and limbs covered (Smeltzer et al., 2008). Nurses need to respect and adapt care to honor these and other differences related to touch.

Time

Throughout the world, people view clock time and social time differently (Giger & Davidhizar, 2008). *Clock time* implies the orderly division of time into years, months, weeks, days, hours, minutes, and seconds. Calendars, clocks, sunrises, tides, and moons define clock time. *Social time* is based more on cultural habits, meals, celebrations, and other events and is related to punctuality and waiting. Aspects of social time vary among cultures. For example, some cultures highly value punctuality. A client from such a culture may be on time for an appointment and then have to wait, increasing his or her frustration with the healthcare system. Clients from other cultures may place priority more on activities, such as family needs, and less on punctuality for appointments. Recognizing that clients have different perceptions of time assists the nurse to provide more sensitive care.

Diet

The relationship between food-related behaviors and culture is complex (Box 8-1). Basically, food is a means of survival—it relieves hunger, promotes health, and prevents disease. Its social meanings encompass love, togetherness, and celebration. Food also has other connotations in terms of its use to reward or punish, relieve stress, and delineate social classes. Culture often dictates the types of food and how frequently a person eats, the types of utensils he or she uses, and the status assigned to particular individuals (e.g., who eats first, who gets the most to eat). Religious practices also impose certain rules and restrictions, such as fasting,

BOX 8-1	**Selected Examples of Cultural Meanings of Food**

- Critical life force for survival
- Relief of hunger
- Peaceful coexistence
- Promotion of health and healing
- Prevention of disease or illness
- Expression of caring for another
- Interpersonal closeness or distance
- Promotion of kinship and familial alliances
- Solidification of social ties
- Celebration of life events (e.g., birthday, marriage)
- Expression of gratitude or appreciation
- Recognition of achievement or accomplishment
- Business negotiations
- Information exchange
- Validation of social, cultural, or religious ceremonial functions
- Way to generate income
- Expression of affluence, wealth, or social status

BOX 8-2 Prohibited Foods and Beverages for Selected Religious Groups

Hinduism
All meats
Animal shortenings

Islam
Alcoholic products and beverages (including extracts, such as vanilla and lemon)
Animal shortenings
Gelatin made with pork, marshmallow, and other confections made with gelatin
Pork

Judaism (*Note:* Not Necessarily Practiced by all Jewish Groups)
Blood by ingestion (e.g., blood sausage, raw meat)
(*Note:* Blood by transfusion is acceptable.)
Mixing dairy products and meat dishes at same meal
Pork
Predatory fowl
Shellfish and scavenger fish (e.g., shrimp, crab, lobster, escargot, catfish) (*Note:* Fish with fins and scales are permissible.)
Note: Packaged foods contain labels identifying *kosher* ("properly preserved" or "fitting") and *pareve* (made without meat or milk) items.

Mormonism (Church of Jesus Christ of Latter-Day Saints)
Alcohol
Beverages containing caffeine stimulants (coffee, tea, colas, and selected carbonated soft drinks)
Tobacco

Seventh-Day Adventism
Certain seafood, including shellfish
Fermented beverages
Pork
Note: Optional vegetarianism is encouraged.

Adapted from Smeltzer, S. C., Bare, B. G., Hinkle, J. L. & Cheever, K. H. (2008). *Brunner & Suddarth's Textbook of Medical–Surgical Nursing* (11th ed.). Philadelphia: Lippincott Williams &Wilkins.

Nutrition Notes 8-1
The Culturally Diverse Client

● Culture defines what food is; how it is obtained, stored, prepared, and served; when it is eaten; differences in food habits based on age, sex, and status; and food's meaning. In any cultural or ethnic group, food habits can vary greatly. Generalizations are intended only as a guide.

● African Americans are at increased risk for hypertension, stroke, diabetes, and obesity. Limiting fat, sodium, and excess calories may help prevent or treat these disorders. Because lactose intolerance is common, calcium intake may be inadequate. In the South, "soul food" refers to both cooking style (barbecued or fried) and particular foods consumed (e.g., pork, greens).

● Throughout Latin America, Indian and Spanish cultures and local food availability influence food practices. Obesity, diabetes, and hypertriglyceridemia are common among Latino Americans. Calcium intake may be inadequate because milk intake often is low.

● The traditional Asian diet is plant-based; common foods include rice, noodles, flat bread, potatoes, vegetables, nuts, seeds, beans, and soy foods. It is low in fat, saturated fat, and cholesterol, and rich in fiber and nutrients. Meat serves more as a condiment than as a main entrée. Preparing food usually takes longer than cooking it. Moderation is valued and obesity is rare. Lactose intolerance is common. Because of the extensive use of soy sauce, limiting sodium intake is difficult.

● Native Americans/Alaskan Natives represent a heterogeneous group of more than 500 tribes and villages. Eating patterns and habits are widely diverse and influenced by cultural and religious beliefs, geography, and food availability. Although staples vary among tribes, corn, squash, and beans are used extensively. Many plant foods also are used in traditional medicinal practices. Obesity, diabetes, and lactose intolerance are common among Native Americans.

eliminating some foods, and observing rituals (e.g., Passover seder; Box 8-2). There are implications for healthcare when a client is diagnosed with diabetes, hypertension, or other disorders that require dietary adjustments. Nurses must consider cultural and religious food preferences/requirements when instructing clients about the dietary restrictions related to a specific condition (Nutrition Notes 8-1).

Verbal Communication Patterns

General communication patterns are found among the major U.S. subcultures. The nurse must carefully observe or tactfully question clients about communication preferences and tailor the interview accordingly.

Anglo-Americans usually are open to providing personal health information and expressing positive and negative feelings. Asian Americans tend to control their emotion

and not reveal that they are physically uncomfortable (Giger & Davidhizar, 2008), especially when among people with whom they are unfamiliar. Similarly, Latino men may not show feelings or readily discuss symptoms because they may interpret doing so as less than manly (Andrews & Boyle, 2008). Male Latino behavior can be attributed to *machismo*, the belief that virile men are physically strong and must deal with emotions privately. Thus, many Latino men in general are protective and authoritarian when it comes to women and children. They expect to be consulted in decision-making when a family member is the primary client.

Many Native Americans are rather private and may hesitate to share much personal information with strangers. They also may fear encounters with non-Native American healthcare providers because of the long history of the careless treatment of Native Americans. They may interpret questioning as prying or meddling. Nurses should be patient and listen carefully. In Native American cultures, listening is a valued skill, whereas impatience is seen as disrespectful

(Lipson, Minarik, & Dibble, 2005). Some Native Americans may be skeptical of Anglo-American nurses who write down what clients say because Native Americans preserve their history through the oral tradition. If possible, writing notes after instead of during the interview may be helpful. Navajos, currently the largest tribe of Native Americans, feel that no person has the right to speak for another; they may refuse to comment on a family member's health problems.

Some clients may distrust healthcare personnel because of negative past experiences. For example, the U.S. healthcare system has a history of victimizing some African Americans as unknowing research subjects or denying them appropriate access to healthcare. Because of such experiences, African Americans may hesitate to give any more information than they are asked. They may not trust healthcare professionals to do the right thing. Nurses can show professionalism by introducing themselves and respectfully addressing clients by their last names, preceded by Mr., Mrs., or Ms. Following up thoroughly with requests is essential, as are respecting privacy and asking open-ended rather than direct questions until trust is established.

Other cultures may view healthcare professionals as authority figures. Clients from these backgrounds may feel uncomfortable asking questions. For example, Asian cultures consider it disrespectful to disagree with a person of authority or one who is more educated. They may consider it rude to imply that the person in authority did not teach properly or explain in enough detail. Asian Americans may not openly disagree with physicians and nurses because of their respect for harmony. Their reticence can conceal a potential for noncompliance when a particular therapeutic regimen is unacceptable from their perspective.

Language

Communication with someone who speaks a different language presents unique challenges. With many different cultural groups living in the United States, many do not speak English or have learned it as their second language and do not speak it well. Others may communicate fairly well in English but are unfamiliar with English medical terminology. In addition, most people prefer to speak in their native tongue, especially when under stress. Because more than 150 languages are spoken in the United States, it is unlikely that nurses can converse easily with most non–English-speaking clients.

When the client speaks a different language, nurses should use a translator, preferably one of the same sex as the client. Caution is needed when asking family members to interpret; embarrassment and lack of medical knowledge can result in miscommunication. Even when a nurse from one culture and a client from another speak the same language, the way they do so may cause miscommunication. An accepted pattern during verbal interactions for one may be unusual, rude, or offensive to the other. Understanding that unique cultural characteristics are related to verbal and nonverbal communication can facilitate the transition to culturally sensitive care. An interpreter is invaluable, but the nurse's actions, cultural respect, and nonverbal communication techniques will promote acceptance and cooperation. Box 8-3 outlines additional communication techniques.

BOX 8-3 **Communicating With Non–English-Speaking Clients**

When Clients Speak No English
- Learn a second language, especially one spoken by a large ethnic population serviced by the health agency.
- Speak words or phrases in the client's language, even if it is not possible to carry on a conversation.
- Refer to an English/foreign language dictionary for bilingual vocabulary words.
- Construct a loose-leaf folder or file cards with words in one or more languages spoken by clients in the community.
- Develop a list of employees or individuals to contact in the community who speak a second language and are willing to act as translators; in an extreme emergency, international telephone operators may be able to provide assistance.
- Select a translator who is the same sex as the client and approximately the same age, if possible.
- Look at the client, not the translator, when asking questions and listening to the client's response.

When English is a Second Language
- Determine if the client speaks or reads English, or both.
- Speak slowly, not loudly, using simple words and short sentences.
- Avoid using technical terms, slang, or phrases with a double or colloquial meaning, such as "Do you have to use the john?"
- Ask questions that can be answered by a "yes" or "no."
- Repeat the question without changing the words, if the client appears confused.
- Give the client sufficient time to process the question from English to the native language, and respond back in English.
- Rely heavily on nonverbal communication, and pantomime if necessary.
- Avoid displaying impatience.
- Ask the client to "read this line," to determine the client's ability to follow written instructions, which are provided in English.

Health Beliefs and Health Practices

A person's beliefs about health and illness and how illness is treated are strongly influenced by culture. **Health beliefs** are a person's ideas about what causes illness, the role of the sick person, how to restore health, and how one stays healthy. **Health practices** are the actions a person takes to maintain or restore health based on their health beliefs.

In general, societies use three views to explain illness or disease (Smeltzer et al., 2008):

- *Biomedical or scientific perspective:* This view, shared by many healthcare personnel, embraces a cause-and-effect philosophy of human body functions. An example is the belief that bacterial or viral organisms cause meningitis.
- *Naturalistic or holistic perspective:* This view espouses that human beings are only one part of nature. Natural balance or harmony is essential for health. Native Americans are one group who share this view. Many Asian groups

embrace *Yin/Yang theory,* which promotes the idea that energy forces exist between organisms and objects in the universe. The balance between these forces is health. Another example is the *hot/cold theory,* which says that diseases should be treated by adding or subtracting heat or cold or dryness or moisture to restore balance. Many Hispanic, African American, and Arab groups embrace beliefs based on the hot/cold theory.

- *Magico-religious perspective:* Supernatural forces dominate. Examples include faith healing in some Christian faiths and voodoo or witchcraft in some Caribbean cultures.

Nurses may disagree with a client's health/illness beliefs; however, they must appreciate these beliefs to assist the client to achieve healthcare goals.

 Gerontologic Considerations

- Access to healthcare may be more difficult for older adults due to transportation issues or limited resources, thereby increasing the likelihood of reverting to past health behavior practices, seeking nonprofessionals for health advice, or using alternative therapies.

▶ ***Stop, Think, and Respond Exercise 8-2***

Hot/cold theory proposes that illnesses caused by heat or cold must be treated with substances having the opposite property. A Puerto Rican client believes she has arthritis because she rinsed her hands in cold water after washing dishes in hot water. She believes that if she eats "hot" foods (e.g., chili peppers), the symptoms will subside. How would you respond?

ASSESSMENT CONSIDERATIONS

Biocultural Assessment

When assessing any client, the nurse must consider general appearance and obvious physical characteristics, components that make up biocultural assessment. Andrews and Boyle (2008) delineate four areas for consideration:

- *Physical appearance:* age, sex, level of consciousness, facial features, and skin color, including evenness of tone, pigmentation, intactness, and lesions or other abnormalities
- *Body structure:* stature, nutrition, symmetry, posture, position, and overall body build or contour
- *Mobility:* gait and range of motion
- *Behavior:* facial expression, mood and affect, fluency of speech, ability to communicate, appropriateness of word choice, grooming, and attire or dress

Biocultural ecology is an area of study that examines biologic cultural differences, with a particular emphasis on adaptation and homeostasis (Giger & Davidhizar, 2008). This research has a focus on "A direct relationship between race and body structure, skin color, other visible physical characteristics, enzymatic and genetic variations, electrocardiographic patterns, susceptibility to disease, nutritional preferences and deficiencies, and psychological characteristics" (Giger & Davidhizar, 2008, p. 147). Safe and competent nursing care relies on research that determines such things as different reactions to drugs because of racial variations in drug metabolism, and susceptibility to disease due to genetic distinctions.

Table 8-1 provides a brief overview of some biocultural variations to consider in nursing assessment. Table 8-2 lists biocultural aspects of selected diseases. Nurses should access more complete sources when caring for clients from culturally diverse backgrounds.

 Pharmacologic Considerations

- Biologic and physiologic variations among clients may influence the absorption and metabolism of drugs. Be alert to any variations in drug action or the appearance of unusual adverse drug reactions, which may or may not be related to the person's inherited characteristics.

Cultural Assessment

A cultural nursing assessment is a "systematic appraisal or examination of individuals, families, groups, and communities in terms of their cultural beliefs, values, and practices" (Smeltzer et al., 2008, p. 135). The nurse should include cultural characteristics along with health practices and beliefs in any initial assessment (Box 8-4).

Assessing Cultural Heritage

Cultural ignorance can profoundly affect access to quality healthcare. It can provide the motivation for expanding one's knowledge base about different cultures. Recognizing all the areas in which cultural differences subtly manifest themselves is important. Examples include communication patterns; hygiene practices, including feelings about modesty and accepting help from others; use of special clothing or amulets; food preferences; management of symptoms such as pain, constipation, and depression; rituals surrounding birth and death; spiritual or religious orientation, especially as related to healthcare; family relationships, including expectations of older adults and children; and patterns of interacting with healthcare providers (Lipson, Minarik & Dibble, 2005).

 Gerontologic Considerations

- In many African American families, a grandmother or an older aunt is considered the matriarch (female head or leader). It may be appropriate to include this person in teaching sessions or ask if the client would like this person to be present.

- Aging Asians tend to be cared for by and live with one of their children. Suggesting the placement of an aging parent in a nursing home may be considered rude.

- Illnesses, especially those that cause obvious physical changes or dependence on a woman for care, may threaten an aging male Latino's self-image and security.

TABLE 8-1 Biocultural Variations

	ASSESSMENT	VARIATIONS
Skin	Normal colors vary widely; melanin accounts for the shades and tones. Establish baseline tone to note future differences.	*Mongolian spots* are irregular areas of deep-blue pigmentation usually found in the sacral and gluteal areas of children of African, Asian, or Latin descent. They are not to be confused with bruising. *Vitiligo* are unpigmented skin patches. *Cyanosis* is difficult to assess in dark-skinned persons. Assess other factors such as respiratory rate, use of accessory muscles, and nasal flaring. People of Mediterranean descent normally have a dark blue tone around the mouth.
Jaundice	Jaundice is best observed in the sclera; establish normal scleral pigmentation.	African Americans, Filipino Americans, and other groups have heavy deposits of conjunctival fat, which contains carotene and may resemble jaundice.
Pallor	Generalized pallor is best observed in mucous membranes, lips, and nailbeds; nailbeds and conjunctiva are better to assess the pallor of anemia.	Dark-skinned clients may not have underlying red tones and exhibit pallor more as yellowish-brown or ashen-gray skin tones.
Erythema	Localized inflammation is characterized by reddened skin, which may not show in dark-skinned clients. Also assess for increased warmth, tautness, or edema.	Conditions such as carbon monoxide poisoning, in which flushing is present, may be observed in the lips of dark-skinned clients.
Skin changes/ normal aging	Light skin tends to show the effects of aging/sun exposure earlier; African Americans, Asian Americans, and Alaskan Natives wrinkle later than whites.	Healthcare providers frequently assess age inaccurately, based on their own cultural assumptions (e.g., African-American nurses often overestimate the age of white clients).
Secretions	Apocrine and eccrine sweat glands are important in fluid balance and thermoregulation. When skin flora contaminates sweat, odor results.	Alaskan Natives sweat less than whites on their trunks and extremities but more on their faces.
Eyes	Biocultural differences are common in eye color and structure. Asians have characteristic epicanthal eye folds.	Dark irises are associated with darker retinas and poorer night vision.
Skeletal system	The long bones of African Americans are longer and more dense; hence, this population has a low incidence of osteoporosis. Bone density of Asians and Alaskan Natives is less than in whites.	Many variations occur among all groups.
Laboratory tests	Biocultural variations occur in some laboratory results, such as hemoglobin/hematocrit, cholesterol, and blood glucose levels.	Be familiar with variations and their clinical significance.
Drug responses	Genetic or environmental factors may influence differences in pharmacokinetics.	Clients may respond differently to the same drug. For example, mydriatic drugs (drugs that cause eye dilation) produce less dilation in dark-colored eyes than in light-colored eyes.

Assessing Health Beliefs and Practices

As described earlier, both health beliefs and practices are perpetuated and influenced by strong cultural affiliations. To discover a client's health beliefs and practices, the nurse will find it useful to ask specific questions (see Box 8-4). Assessment of these factors helps identify the client's beliefs about his or her health or illness; recognize health-seeking behaviors on which to capitalize to promote health; view the situation from the client's perspective; distinguish behaviors that do not contribute to health restoration, maintenance, or promotion; perceive issues that can compromise the treatment plan; and establish a mutually agreed-on plan of care (McSweeney et al., 1997).

Pharmacologic Considerations

- Folk-healing beliefs and practices are important aspects of healing; almost all cultures and ethnic groups have traditional folk remedies. These preparations have pharmacologic actions that can affect physiology and cause drug interactions. Noncompliance with a prescribed pharmaceutical regimen may be a problem for clients who use folk remedies unless healthcare providers find ways to incorporate at least some of these remedies into the treatment regimen.

TABLE 8-2 Biocultural Aspects of Disease

DISEASE	CONSIDERATIONS
Alcoholism	Native Americans have twice the rate of whites. Chinese and Japanese Americans have decreased alcohol tolerance.
Anemia	Incidence is high among Vietnamese Americans because of infestations among immigrants and low-iron diets.
Arthritis	Incidence is increased among Native Americans.
Asthma and bronchitis	Incidence is six times greater for Native American infants than the rest of the population.
Cancer	The incidence of nasopharyngeal cancer is high among Chinese and Native Americans. Breast cancer is 1½ times more likely in African American women than white women. Esophageal cancer is the second leading cause of death for African American men aged 35 to 54 years. Filipino Hawaiians have the highest rate of liver cancer. The incidence of stomach cancer is twice as high in African American men than in white men. The incidence of cervical cancer is 120% higher in African American women than white women, and that of uterine cancer is 53% lower in African American than in white women. African American men have the highest incidence of prostate cancer in all groups.
Colitis	Incidence is increased in Japanese Americans.
Diabetes mellitus	Incidence is much higher in Filipino, Hispanic, and Native Americans than whites and African Americans.
Influenza	Death rate is increased among Native Americans 45 years of age and older.
Ischemic heart disease	This condition is responsible for 32% of heart-related deaths in Native Americans. African Americans have the highest related mortality rates.
Lactose intolerance	Incidence is increased in African, Chinese, and Hispanic Americans.
Myocardial infarction	This is the leading cause of heart disease in Native Americans, accounting for 43% of deaths. Incidence is decreased in Japanese Americans.
Otitis media	Incidence in school-aged Navajo children is 7.9%, versus 0.5% in whites. Up to one third of Alaskan Natives younger than 2 years of age have chronic otitis media. Incidence is increased among bottle-fed Native American and Alaskan Native infants.
Pneumonia	Death rate is increased among Native Americans 45 years of age and older.
Renal disease	Incidence is decreased in Japanese Americans.
Sickle cell anemia	Incidence is increased in African Americans.
Trachoma	Incidence is increased in Native American and Alaskan Native children.
Tuberculosis	Incidence is increased in Native Americans.
Ulcers	Incidence is decreased in Japanese Americans.

TRANSCULTURAL NURSING

Transcultural nursing, founded by Madeline Leininger (1977), is considered a specialty in nursing. It refers to nursing care that is provided within the context of another's culture. Its characteristics are (1) accepting each client as an individual, (2) possessing knowledge of health problems that affect particular cultural groups, (3) assessing cultural background and health beliefs and practices, and (4) planning care compatible with the client's health belief system.

Leininger (1991) theorizes that *culturally congruent care* (care that fits a person's cultural values) assists a client to achieve better health outcomes. If a nurse respects a client's cultural values and beliefs, he or she can better teach diet modifications or lifestyle changes that promote healthier outcomes without insulting or patronizing the client. For example, clients of Middle Eastern cultures do not normally drink milk beyond childhood. They do, however, eat yogurt and also a goat or sheep cheese called *feta*. For such clients who need to increase calcium intake, nurses can inform them that these foods provide needed calcium.

Developing Transcultural Sensitivity

Increasing one's awareness that the United States is a multicultural nation is a first step toward transcultural nursing.

Examining personal beliefs, communication habits, and healthcare practices is another. The following recommendations will help to develop a growing expertise in culturally sensitive nursing care:

- Learn to speak a second language.
- Use techniques for facilitating interactions: sit within the client's comfort zone and make appropriate eye contact.
- Become familiar with physical differences among ethnic groups.
- Be aware of biocultural aspects of disease (see Table 8-2).
- Perform physical assessments, using appropriate techniques that will provide accurate data.
- Perform cultural and health-beliefs assessment and plan care accordingly.
- Consult the client about ways to solve health problems.
- Never ridicule a cultural belief or practice, verbally or nonverbally.
- Integrate cultural practices that are helpful or harmless into the plan of care.
- Modify or gradually change unsafe practices.
- Avoid removing religious medals or clothing that hold symbolic meaning for the client; if this must be done, keep them safe and replace them as soon as possible.
- Provide food that is customarily eaten.

BOX 8-4 **Performing a Cultural Assessment**

Cultural Characteristics

The nurse asks about or observes for the following cultural characteristics:

• Where was the client born? How long has the client lived in this country?
• What is the client's ethnic background? Does the client identify strongly with others from the same cultural background? Does the client live in a neighborhood with others of the same ethnic or cultural background?
• To whom does the client turn for support? Who is the head of the family? Is he or she involved in decision-making about the client?
• What is the client's primary language and literacy level?
• What is the client's religion, and is it important in his or her daily life? Are there religious rituals related to sickness, death, or health that the client observes?
• Has the client sought the advice of traditional healers?
• What are the client's communication styles? Does the client avoid eye contact and maintain physical distance? Is the client open and verbal about symptoms?
• What are the client's food preferences or restrictions?
• Does the client participate in cultural activities such as dressing in traditional clothing and observing traditional holidays and festivals?

Health Beliefs and Practices

The nurse should ask the following specific questions about beliefs and practices in the initial assessment:

• What have you done in the past and what do you do now to maintain health?
• How do these activities help you maintain your health?
• What practices could you add to help promote health?
• What is your definition of good health?
• Do you have any difficulties with performing activities that will restore, maintain, or promote health?
• What do you call your health problem?
• What do you think has caused this problem?
• Why do you think it started when it did?
• What does this problem do to you?
• What are the difficulties that this health problem has caused you, personally, in your family, or at work?
• What do you fear most about this health problem?
• What kind of treatment do you think will help? What are the most important results you hope to get from this treatment?

Adapted from Lipson, J. G., Minarik, P.A. & Dibble, S. L., [2005]. *Culture and clinical care.* San Francisco UCSF Nursing Press, and McSweeney, J. C., Allan, J. D., & Mayo, K. [1997]. Exploring the use of explanatory models in nursing research and practice. *Image: Journal of Nursing Scholarship, 29,* 243–248.

• Advocate routine screening for diseases to which clients may be genetically or culturally prone.
• Facilitate rituals by whomever the client identifies as a healer within his or her belief system.
• Apologize if cultural traditions or beliefs are violated.

Being Culturally Competent

Providing culturally competent care is a process by which the nurse consistently endeavors to work within the cultural context of the client and his or her family and community (Andrews & Boyle, 2008). In doing so, the nurse must avoid stereotyping clients based on race or culture. The nurse also must listen to clients, acknowledge and respect their beliefs about health and illness, recognize culturally influenced health behaviors, communicate in a culturally sensitive manner, and adapt care to reflect cultural needs.

All individuals grow up with an ethnocentric perspective. The ethnocentrism reflects lack of knowledge and experience. Nurses must personally evolve from an ethnocentric viewpoint and develop a multicultural perspective that includes knowledge of their own as well as other cultures. They also must acknowledge any personal biases to develop a nonjudgmental attitude toward all clients. Developing strategies to avoid *cultural imposition* is absolutely pivotal (Andrews & Boyle, 2008).

The culturally competent nurse accepts each client as a unique individual. The first ethical principle in the American Nurses Association (ANA) Code of Ethics for Nurses states that "The nurse, in all professional relationships, practices with compassion and respect for the inherent dignity, worth, and uniqueness of every individual, unrestricted by considerations of social or economic status, personal attributes, or the nature of health problems" (ANA, 2001). This principle extends to providing culturally competent care to all individuals.

CRITICAL THINKING EXERCISES

1. How could a culturally sensitive nurse prepare for the home care of a non–English-speaking client from Pakistan (or some other foreign country)?
2. How could a culturally sensitive nurse respond to a pregnant woman who wears a chicken bone around her neck to protect her unborn child from birth defects?
3. You are assigned with a nursing assistant to care for a client who is Jewish. His care plan states that he practices religious dietary restrictions. The nursing assistant will be helping the client with his meals. What factor is most important to tell the nursing assistant before she feeds this client?
4. You are working in a health clinic. A recent immigrant to the United States is often late for appointments. What could you suggest to this client that may assist her to be on time for future appointments?

NCLEX-STYLE REVIEW QUESTIONS

1. Which of the following recommendations is the best choice for the nurse to provide to an African American client to manage disorders for which this population is at risk?
   1. Increase sodium intake
   2. Decrease water intake
   3. Limit saturated fat intake
   4. Increase protein intake

2. The nurse includes principles of good body mechanics in the discharge teaching plan of the client who has undergone spinal surgery. The client, however, speaks very little English. Which teaching method provides the best information regarding body mechanics for the non-English speaking client?
1. Have the client watch a video
2. Speak slowly while looking at the client
3. Use colorful pictures or diagrams
4. Write the instructions on paper

3. The LPN, reporting at change of shift to the RN, states that the client, originally from a Middle Eastern country, is driving the staff crazy with dietary requests. She states: "You know how demanding those people can be." The RN recognizes that this type of comment is an example of:
1. Ethnicity
2. Ethnocentrism
3. Generalization
4. Stereotyping

4. A client from Japan who does not speak English arrives at a clinic. He is accompanied by his wife and daughter, who speak English and offer to interpret for their husband/father. The nurse states that she prefers for a male interpreter to assist with interpretation for which of the following reasons? Select all that apply.
1. The client may not want to discuss his problems with his wife present.
2. The nurse will be reluctant to ask questions of a sexual nature.
3. The family may be embarrassed to answer some questions.
4. The wife may not understand the questions asked.

5. The nurse needs to obtain a history and assessment of a new Asian American client. This client may be offended by which of the following actions by the nurse?
1. The nurse asks the client to speak more loudly.
2. The nurse maintains minimal direct eye contact.
3. The nurse sits to the side of the client while asking questions.
4. The nurse touches the client's head as a gesture of empathy.

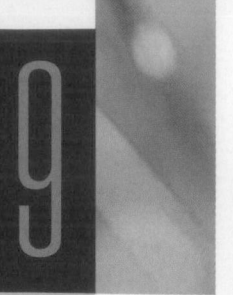

9

Complementary and Alternative Therapies

Words To Know

acupuncture
Adequate Intake
alternative therapy
apitherapy
aromatherapy
Ayurvedic medicine
biofeedback
biologically based practices
Chinese medicine
chiropractic
complementary therapy
conventional (allopathic) medicine
electromagnetic therapy
energy medicine
Estimated Average Requirement
ethnobotanicals
herbal therapy
homeopathy
humor
hypnosis
imagery
integrative medicine
manipulative and body-based therapies
massage therapy
medical systems
mind–body medicine
naturopathy
prebiotic
probiotic
recommended dietary allowance
reflexology
reiki
shiatsu
spiritual healing
tai chi
Tolerable Upper Intake Level
whole medical systems
yoga

Learning Objectives

On completion of this chapter, you will be able to:

1. Differentiate between the terms *complementary therapy, alternative therapy,* and *integrative medicine.*
2. Give five reasons that individuals choose to use complementary and alternative therapies.
3. List five categories of complementary and alternative therapies that the National Center for Complementary and Alternative Medicine investigates.
4. Describe the basic beliefs of three examples of alternative whole medical systems: Ayurvedic medicine, Chinese medicine, and Native American medicine.
5. Identify four examples of practices that use the mind to promote or restore physical health.
6. Describe four examples of biologically based practices.
7. Name anatomic structures that are the focus of manipulative and body-based therapies, and give examples of these therapies.
8. Describe techniques that are used in energy medicine.
9. Discuss the role nurses can play in relation to complementary and alternative therapies.

Many people in the United States, both native and foreign born, are assuming responsibility for their health. Many are using both **conventional (allopathic) medicine**, those practices that embody traditional Western treatment of diseases, and nontraditional interventions known as complementary and alternative therapies (CAT) or complementary and alternative medicine (CAM). The latter have often been characterized as non-orthodox practices that have no scientific basis for their effectiveness. However, there is a growing consensus that complementary and alternative therapies deserve further research.

Consequently, physicians and nurses, who are partners in healthcare, are now investigating and, in some cases, incorporating those broader approaches to managing and treating various disorders. Following a national conference in 1996 sponsored by the National Institutes of Health and the Uniformed Services University of the Health Sciences, it was felt that nursing and medical educators should provide information about complementary and alternative therapies in their standard curricula (Gaydos, 2001). This chapter provides an overview of various therapies that are undergoing scientific investigation and are being used without definitive biomedical explanations.

COMPLEMENTARY THERAPY, ALTERNATIVE THERAPY, AND INTEGRATIVE MEDICINE

The National Center for Complementary and Alternative Medicine (NCCAM) is a research unit in the National Institutes of Health. NCCAM defines a **complementary therapy** as one used *in addition to* conventional medical treatment. In contrast, an **alternative therapy** is one used *instead of* conventional medical treatment. Combining conventional medicine with complementary or alternative therapy is referred to as **integrative medicine**.

Use of Complementary and Alternative Therapies

According to the Committee on the Use of Complementary and Alternative Medicine in the United States (2005), about one-third of adults in the United States use some form of complementary and alternative medicine, but less than 40% share that information with their physician or other healthcare providers. Nearly three out of four adults over the age of 50 use some kind of alternative medicine, a rate that is higher than among any other population group in the United States (Ohio State University, 2004).

The increased interest in and use of CAM are attributed to one or more of the following reasons (Hospice and Palliative Nurses Association, 2000):

- Dissatisfaction with conventional medicine
- Desire to become more active in decision-making and self-care
- Increasing numbers of people with chronic, incurable conditions
- Difficulty meeting the rising costs of healthcare
- Growth of culturally diverse groups who do not share traditional American health beliefs and practices

 Gerontologic Considerations

- Older adults who are more likely to use alternative medicine reported that they were in poor health, chronic pain, and had problems with daily activities such as carrying groceries, eating, and bathing (Ohio State University, 2004).

Research

The goals of the NCCAM are to (1) study complementary and alternative therapies scientifically, (2) educate scientists and healthcare providers on the nature and principles of complementary and alternative therapies, and (3) distribute the results of research findings to whomever is interested in the information.

In spite of the absence of empirical evidence for the efficacy of some CAM modalities, the principle of "First, do no harm" should prevail. That is, if the CAM practice is not dangerous or unhealthy, it should be tolerated or even supported if it provides person with what they perceive as intrinsic benefits.

MODALITIES FOR COMPLEMENTARY AND ALTERNATIVE THERAPIES

The NCCAM subdivides complementary and alternative therapies into five general groups:

- Whole medical systems
- Mind–body medicine
- Biologically based practices
- Manipulative and body-based therapies
- Energy medicine

Whole Medical Systems

From a conventional American standpoint, **whole medical systems** are those alternative systems of healing theory and practice that evolved from other cultures. Some examples of non-Western medical systems include Ayurvedic medicine practiced in India, traditional Chinese medicine, and Native American medicine in the United States. Some examples of whole medical systems, such as naturopathy and homeopathy, had their origins in Europe and developed in parallel fashion, yet separately, in Western cultures. **Naturopathy** considers disease an aberration in natural healing; **homeopathy** proposes that the remedy for an illness should be one that produces symptoms similar to the disease itself.

What most Americans categorize as *alternative medical systems,* however, is considered *traditional* by the indigenous culture of origin, meaning that their system of healing existed before the beginning of modern medicine. Table 9-1 compares differences between alternative medical systems and conventional medical systems. The common thread among alternative medical systems is (1) the belief that one's body has the power to heal itself, and (2) that healing involves the mind, body, and spirit (National Center for Complementary and Alternative Medicine, 2007f).

Ayurvedic Medicine

Ayurvedic medicine has its roots in India and is the oldest system of medicine in the world. It is based on spiritual practices that developed among Tibetan monks. The object of Ayurvedic medicine is to help person become unified with nature to develop a strong body, clear mind, and tranquil spirit. One belief is that the *prana,* or the life force, moves through various centers in the body called *chakras* (Fig. 9-1). The Ayurvedic doctor prescribes modalities such as yoga, herbal medicine, fasting and eating cleansing foods, meditation, and massage to maintain or restore the dynamic flow of the *prana.*

Chinese Medicine

Although the term **Chinese medicine** is used, this medical system also includes contributions from Japan, Korea, and other Southeast Asian countries. Chinese medicine proposes that health is the outcome of balancing *yin* and *yang,* opposite forces that must remain equalized to maintain *qi* (or *chi*), life's energy force (similar to the *prana* in Ayurvedic medicine). Forces that alter *qi,* either by depleting or obstructing it, cause illness. Correcting an imbalance between two attributes such as motion and stillness or hot and cold restores harmony and health. Treatment measures such as acupuncture, herbal remedies, diet, exercise, and massage are used to restore *qi.*

TABLE 9-1 Differences Between Alternative and Conventional Medical Systems

ALTERNATIVE MEDICAL SYSTEMS	CONVENTIONAL MEDICAL SYSTEMS
Originated approximately 1500 BC or earlier	Originated with Hippocrates in approximately 5 BC
Believe that health results from harmony among the person, his or her environment (nature, universe), and energy force	Believe that health results from normal physiologic function
Focus on maintaining a healthy state	Focus on treating illness or injury
Do not correlate symptoms of disease with any specific organ or anatomic location	Correlate symptoms with the organ or location of the person's disorder
Identify with and are sensitive to cultural traditions	Recognize cultural differences but may not incorporate the client's beliefs into the treatment regimen
Incorporate religious principles	Do not reject spirituality, but do not apply any religious significance to a person's illness or recovery
Rely heavily on medicinal plants	Rely on manufactured pharmaceuticals
Accept the efficacy of treatment approaches based not on specific scientific explanation but rather traditional use	Demand scientific evidence for the mechanisms of treatment and replication of results through unbiased research
Do not have established educational standards for practitioners	Require practitioners to have formal education beyond college
Do not regulate practice	Require formal licensure for practice

Native American Medicine

Traditional Native American medicine views disease as resulting from disharmony with Mother Earth, possession by an evil spirit, or violation of a taboo. Followers rely on a *shaman,* a person in the tribal community who is both a medicine man (or woman) and a spiritual figure with the extraordinary ability to heal. The shaman has the power to achieve an altered state of consciousness to journey to the spirit world or assume the persona of another life form, such as an eagle or mountain lion.

Native American medicine believes that the shaman obtains knowledge from a higher power during a trance-like state, which is accompanied by chanting, drumming, dancing, and, in some cases, consuming psychoactive botanicals. The knowledge allows the shaman to determine the cause and remedies for sick person. Remedies may include herbs, meditation, fasting, and sweating. The shaman may fashion a talisman, a symbolic figure, that the sick person wears around the neck or another body location to ward off evil spirits or exorcise bad spirits.

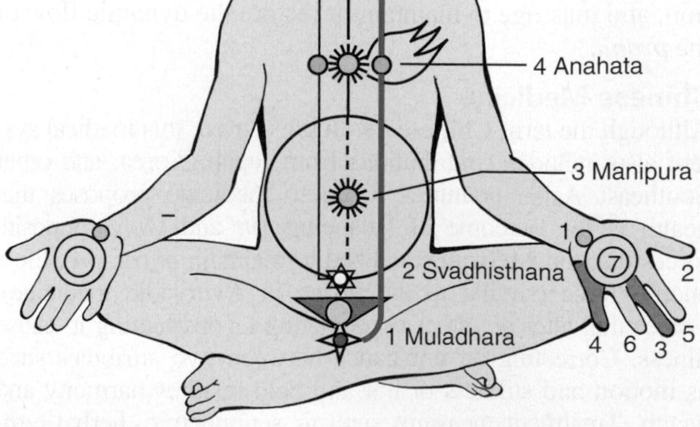

▶ **Stop, Think, and Respond Exercise 9-1**

Which alternative medical system is associated with the following examples: (a) yoga, (b) acupuncture, and (c) wearing a talisman?

Mind–Body Medicine

Mind–body medicine uses techniques that rely on the power of the brain, emotions, social interactions, and spiritual factors to alter body functions or symptoms. Many practices that were once categorized as alternative medicine (e.g., biofeedback, imagery, humor, hypnosis) are now becoming accepted as conventional medical treatments. Spiritual healing is a mind–body technique that the medical community has not yet entirely accepted as legitimately therapeutic. Most mind–body interventions have few physical risks, can be taught easily, and have provided evidence of positive effects (National Center for Complementary and Alternative Medicine, 2007e).

Biofeedback

Biofeedback is a technique in which an individual voluntarily controls one or more physiologic functions, such as body temperature, heart rate, blood pressure, and brain waves. Initially, clients are attached to a machine that translates a physiologic activity, such as heart rate, into a pulsating waveform, digital numbers, or audible sound. While receiving feedback from the machine, clients try to alter a particular function (e.g., decrease heart rate). If the machine's signal changes, it helps them determine if they are successful. Eventually, clients do not need to rely on the response from the device; they can alter their physiology at will. Biofeedback is currently being used in the United States to reduce hypertension and rapid heart rates, manage pain, abort seizures, relieve migraine headaches, and produce

FIGURE 9-1. The chakras and channels of energy.

7 Sahasrara
6 Ajna
5 Vishuddha
4 Anahata
3 Manipura
2 Svadhisthana
1 Muladhara

dilation of peripheral blood vessels in individuals with vascular disorders.

Imagery

Imagery is a psychobiologic technique that uses the mind to visualize a positive physiologic effect. When using imagery, clients conjure up mental images of their body waging and winning a battle with the disease process. For example, clients might visualize their body producing white blood cells in large numbers. They then imagine the white cells destroying cancer cells. Laboratory values of white cell counts taken before and after such imagery sessions often show that the numbers of white blood cells dramatically increase.

Humor

Humor can be used therapeutically. Laughter stimulates the immune system by increasing the number of white blood cells and lowering cortisol, which suppresses immune function. Laughter can cause the release of neuropeptides (endorphins and enkephalins). Norman Cousins (1979) shared his own pain-relieving and healing experiences using humor in his book *Anatomy of an Illness.*

Hypnosis

Hypnosis is a therapeutic intervention that facilitates a physiologic change through the power of suggestion. Hypnotism has been used to help person overcome habits such as smoking, relieve chronic pain, and extinguish irrational fears. Research is needed to find out how hypnotism works and why not everyone can be hypnotized.

> ### ▶ Stop, Think, and Respond Exercise 9-2
>
> *Which mind–body technique uses electronic equipment that converts physiologic data into sensory output that a person learns to consciously alter?*

Spiritual Healing

Spiritual healing restores health through a higher power (God or some other metaphysical force). An intermediary person may channel the healing force, acting strictly as a facilitator. Sometimes healing occurs through the sick person's prayers or those said by others on his or her behalf. In "hopeless" cases, some would call the healing a miracle; however, spiritual healing is not limited to miracles. Among his many books, such as *Prayer is Good Medicine* (1996) and *Healing Words: The Power of Prayer and the Practice of Medicine* (1993), the physician Larry Dossey notes that prayer-like thoughts offered from a distance have increased the healing rate of surgical wounds and sped the recovery of clients who have had surgery.

Biologically Based Practices

Biologically based practices use natural products such as dietary supplements, aromatherapy, and animal-derived extracts such as bee venom.

Dietary Supplements

The health food industry lobbied federal legislators in the early 1990s to "preserve the consumer's right to choose dietary supplements" (Barrett, 2000). As a result, the Dietary Supplement Health and Education Act of 1994 (DSHEA) was passed. DSHEA defines a "dietary supplement" as something that supplies one or more dietary ingredients, including vitamins, minerals, amino acids, herbs, and other substances (Nutrition Notes 9-1).

Vitamin and Mineral Supplements

Vitamin and mineral supplements are considered more legitimate for health than other biologically based practices. Scientists who advise the Food and Nutrition Board, a committee within the National Academy of Sciences, establish Dietary Reference Intakes, a set of four separate reference values used to plan and evaluate diets. The **Estimated Average Requirement** is the intake that meets the estimated need of 50% of individuals in a specific group (National Academy of Sciences, 2006). The **Recommended Dietary Allowances** (RDAs) represent the levels of essential nutrients necessary to meet the needs of most healthy persons. Special populations such as pregnant women, older adults, and people with medical disorders may have different RDA requirements. When there are insufficient data to determine the RDA, an **Adequate Intake** (AI) is set; it is the amount of a nutrient thought to meet or exceed requirements. The **Tolerable Upper Intake Level** (UL) is the highest level of daily nutrient intake that is likely to pose no risk of adverse health effects. The nutrient with the greatest risk for toxicity is vitamin A, especially for children and pregnant women.

Probiotics and Prebiotics

Additional types of supplements include probiotics and prebiotics. **Probiotics** are microorganisms that exert beneficial health effects, such as *Lactobacillus acidophilus*, which can lower the frequency or duration of diarrhea. **Prebiotics** include nondigestible food ingredients such as dietary fiber that beneficially stimulate or inhibit bacteria in the colon (Schrezenmeir & deVrese, 2001).

Herbal Supplements

The use of herbal supplements is based on **herbal therapy**, a technique for using plants to treat diseases and disorders. Herbal therapy techniques have mostly been handed down orally from generation to generation. For centuries, humans have used **ethnobotanicals**, plants that grow in a region where specific groups of people live, for food, clothing, shelter, and medicine. The particular plants that are used by the Chinese, Indians, Native Americans, and other groups are different in various world locales, but their general purposes are largely the same. The use of plants and herbs is commonly referred to as *folk medicine* because the benefits are

 Nutrition Notes 9-1
The Client Taking Dietary Supplements

- The Office of Dietary Supplements publishes online fact sheets for individual dietary supplements that includes what the supplement is used for, results of scientific research, potential side effects, cautions, and references. They are available at www.ods.od.nih.gov.
- After a dietary supplement is marketed, it is up to the FDA to prove danger rather than being up to the manufacturer to prove safety. Check the FDA Web site at www.cfsan.fda.fda.gov/~dms for consumer advisories on supplements not to use.

largely anecdotal rather than based on scientific investigation. However, the use of plants in medicine is not unique. In conventional medicine, approximately 25% of prescription drugs are derived from plants. Drugs manufactured from plant sources usually contain one or more extracts from the plant or a synthesized, molecularly similar structure.

Herbalists argue that using only parts of a plant changes the effects that are achieved from using the whole plant. Consequently, interest in self-treatment using herbs has been renewed (Table 9-2). Clients can use herbs in a variety of forms: liquified juice, mashed paste, steeped teas, compressed powders, fermented liquid, sweetened syrups, tinctures, liniments, and salves.

Herbal therapy is not regulated like pharmaceutical drugs are in the United States. Because herbs are classified as dietary supplements, they are not held to the same standards of unified dosages, safety, and efficacy as drugs. Manufacturers of herbal preparations, however, cannot claim that the herbal product prevents or treats a disease because that automatically places the substance in the category of a drug, which is highly regulated. To avoid federal regulation, labels on herbal products can make structure or function claims, such as "boosts stamina," as long as they also contain a

disclaimer that the U.S. Food and Drug Administration (FDA) has not evaluated the product.

As the NCCAM studies herbs more scientifically, more than anecdotal information will become available. Until then, Dr. Roberta Lee, Director of Education at the Beth Israel Center for Health and Healing in New York, advises consumers of herbs to (1) find out what they are using, (2) not use a product if information is unavailable, (3) use the lowest dose initially, (4) increase the dose gradually, and (5) never exceed the maximum dose. Even herbs have possibly lethal side effects. Consulting with a physician before using herbs and disclosing that information before any medication is prescribed are best. Use of herbs also is not recommended for pregnant or lactating women, infants, and children younger than 6 years of age.

 Pharmacologic Considerations

- Clients taking anticoagulants such as warfarin or aspirin must carefully consider the risks for spontaneous bleeding if taking herbs with anticoagulation properties such as ginkgo, ginger, or ginseng (Kuhn, 2002).

TABLE 9-2 Popular Herbs Used in the United States

HERB	BOTANICAL NAME	CLAIM FOR USE	PRECAUTIONS
Chamomile	*Chamomilla recutita*	Relieves digestive disorders	Avoid if allergic to ragweed, asters, chrysanthemums, or members of the daisy family.
Echinacea	*Echinacea augstifolia*	Boosts immune function and speeds healing	Avoid if allergic to plants in the daisy family; prolonged use may reduce effects.
Ephedra	*Ephedra vulgaris*	Relieves asthma, stimulates the central nervous system, promotes weight loss, increases energy	Action is similar to that of amphetamine; ephedra can cause tachycardia, headache, hypertension, seizures, insomnia, chest pain, decreased intestinal motility, and death from stroke or heart attack.
Garlic	*Allium sativum*	Lowers blood pressure, thins the blood	Possible side effects include intestinal gas; combining garlic with aspirin or other anticoagulants can prolong bleeding.
Ginkgo	*Ginkgo biloba*	Improves memory	Possible side effects include gastrointestinal distress, headaches, and allergic reactions; use with caution if taking aspirin or other blood-thinning drugs.
Ginseng	*Panax gensema*	Increases energy and helps in dealing with stress	Use may raise blood pressure and serum glucose level and can increase the growth of estrogen-dependent cancer.
Kava	*Piper methysticum*	Reduces stress and anxiety	Large doses can produce an intoxicating effect; long-term use can lead to dry, scaly skin.
St. John's Wort	*Hypericum perforatum*	Treats mild depression	Use may cause sensitivity to light; interactions with other drugs can be dangerous.
Saw palmetto	*Serenoa repens*	Relieves enlargement of the prostate gland	Avoid tea versions because the herb dissolves poorly; nausea and gastrointestinal distress are possible.
Valerian	*Valerian officinalis*	Relieves anxiety and insomnia	Possible side effects include blurred vision, excitability, and changes in heartbeat if taken in large doses or for more than 2 weeks.

- Certain herbs may decrease blood glucose levels, whereas some may enhance the effects of cardiac glycosides. The client should read labels on over-the-counter medications for any known contraindications with herbal use, or consult a pharmacist.

- The U.S. FDA (2004) has warned consumers to avoid purchasing Actra-Rx (also known as Yilishen), a product promoted as a dietary supplement for treating erectile dysfunction and enhancing sexual performance for men because it contains sildenafil (Viagra), a prescription drug that can pose a serious health risk for some users.

Aromatherapy

Most people agree that they positively or negatively associate odors of certain substances with various people, places, or feelings. **Aromatherapy** is the use of scents to alter emotions and biologic processes. For therapeutic uses, scents from botanical oils of lavender, peppermint, and the like are released by adding them to bath water, permeating the air where they are inhaled, or rubbing them on the skin. The olfactory nerves carry the scented molecules to the limbic system. The limbic system is the brain area used for learning, memory, and emotions. Once the limbic system is stimulated, it can trigger physiologic and psychological responses through neurotransmitters such as serotonin, endorphins, or norepinephrine, released by the hypothalamus. The neurotransmitters can, in turn, affect nervous, endocrine, and immune system functions. Some believe that aromatherapy can help control blood pressure and hormone secretions; relieve pain, depression, and anxiety; or promote higher states of alertness. More research is needed to validate the physiologic actions of various scents, evaluate how best to use them, and determine why one type of aroma affects people differently.

▶ **Stop, Think, and Respond Exercise 9-3**

Discuss particular scents and the images or feelings they create for you. For example, the smell of the ocean may make you happy because of the pleasant memories that you associate with a holiday or former residence. On the other hand, the antiseptic smell of the dentist's office may create feelings of anxiety or fear because you associate it with discomfort.

Apitherapy

Apitherapy is the medicinal use of bee venom. To date, apitherapy has been used as an alternative for treating various inflammatory conditions of the joints such as rheumatoid arthritis and osteoarthritis. It is also used to treat multiple sclerosis, a neurologic condition. Although reports of the use of bee venom have dated from the mid-1800s, interest in apitherapy gained momentum around 1920. Bee venom does contain various enzymes that may stimulate the adrenal glands and induce the release of cortisol, an anti-inflammatory and immunosuppressant hormone. Physicians currently consider apitherapy an unconventional treatment, however, and do not recommend its use or support a client's request for it. Nevertheless, experiments sponsored by the International Pain Institute have demonstrated relief of symptoms among research volunteers (Won, Hong, & Kim, 2007).

Under the supervision of the NCCAM, further study may validate (1) if bee venom therapy is effective; (2) if so, which types of disorders respond best when apitherapy is used; (3) which yields better results: the actual sting of the bee or chemically prepared apitoxin (bee venom); (4) how many stings or what apitoxin concentrations are necessary to achieve positive results; and (5) beside discomfort and potential allergic reactions, any other side effects to consider.

Manipulative and Body-Based Therapies

Manipulative and body-based therapies are those healing methods that focus on the structures and systems of the body, including the bones and joints, the soft tissues, and the circulatory and lymphatic system (NCCAM, 2007d). These methods use manipulation and movement to improve health and restore biologic functions. Some examples include massage therapies (including reflexology and shiatsu), chiropractic, yoga, and tai chi.

Massage Therapy, Reflexology, and Shiatsu

Massage therapy involves applying pressure and movement to stretch and knead soft body tissues. Massage therapists use the warmth of their hands, elbows, and forearms and lubricating oils to stimulate circulation and relieve physical and psychological tension. The benefits of massage include relief from discomfort and improved mobility or functional use of affected parts of the body.

▶ **Stop, Think, and Respond Exercise 9-4**

Discuss physiologic and emotional responses that you have experienced during and after receiving a backrub or a similar type of massage.

Reflexology is a complementary health practice in which manual pressure is applied to the feet and hands. The International Academy of Advanced Reflexology and those who practice reflexology claim that locations in the extremities contain reflex centers composed of more than 7000 nerve endings linked to body organs and tissues (Telepo, 2007). When pressure is applied to a reflex area, for instance in the foot (Fig. 9-2), the impulse travels from peripheral nerves to the spinal cord and brain. As a result, reflexologists believe that reconditioning or reprogramming the neural reflex improves the body's ability to facilitate natural healing.

Shiatsu is a Japanese word that means "finger pressure." Shiatsu has many similarities to acupressure and acupuncture because practitioners apply pressure to acupoints in various body meridians (energy channels; Fig. 9-3). Each meridian correlates with an organ or its function. Acupoints are locations along the meridians where Chinese medicine believes the body's life force, or *qi*, moves. Unblocking and strengthening *qi* rebalance the body's energy and restore health.

Chiropractic

Chiropractic theory proposes that subluxation (malalignment) of the spinal vertebrae alters nerve activities that regulate body functions in distant organs. To treat various disorders, chiropractors, who are the single largest group of alternative complementary therapy practitioners in the

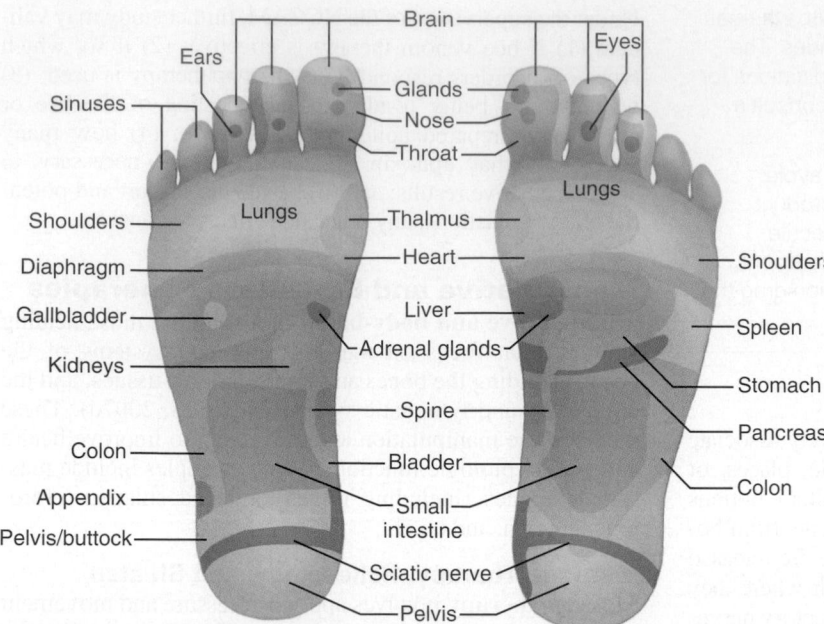

FIGURE 9-2. Reflex areas in the foot.

United States, perform spinal manipulation as a generic method for curing neuromuscular disorders and a host of other diseases. According to William T. Jarvis (2001, p. 2), "chiropractors have not shown that impinging a spinal nerve alters an impulse beyond the zone of impingement, nor have they shown that disrupting a nerve impulse produces disease." Despite the criticisms from Jarvis and many members of the American Medical Association (AMA), millions of people continue to seek chiropractic treatment with some improvement in their symptoms. Chiropractic treatment is further legitimized because (1) many health insurance policies cover it, (2) the federal government provides Medicare and Medicaid reimbursement for it, and (3) the costs are an approved medical income tax deduction (Jarvis, 2001).

Some feel that chiropractic is a form of pseudomedicine that has attracted clients who are disgruntled with the outcomes of conventional medical care. Critics continue to suggest that there is no reason to justify practitioners who use "one cure" for all ailments. In fact, some hold that this type of philosophy can delay appropriate medical treatment. Many agree that spinal manipulation should be limited to medically trained specialists such as osteopaths, orthopedists, and physiatrists, physicians who specialize in rehabilitation. But until the NCCAM conducts further scientific research, emotions and conjecture rather than facts will continue to fuel the controversy.

 Gerontologic Considerations

- Of the following six types of alternative medicine: chiropractic, acupuncture, massage, breathing exercises, herbal medicine, and meditation, 43% of surveyed older adults reported using chiropractic the most and acupuncture the least (Ohio State University, 2004). Older adults in various ethnic groups may prefer particular types of CAM therapies (Cherniack et al., 2008).

Yoga and Tai Chi

Yoga was developed in India, and **tai chi** has its origins in China. Both incorporate techniques that combine mental and physical exercises for the purpose of integrating body and mind. There are several branches of yoga; hatha yoga is the

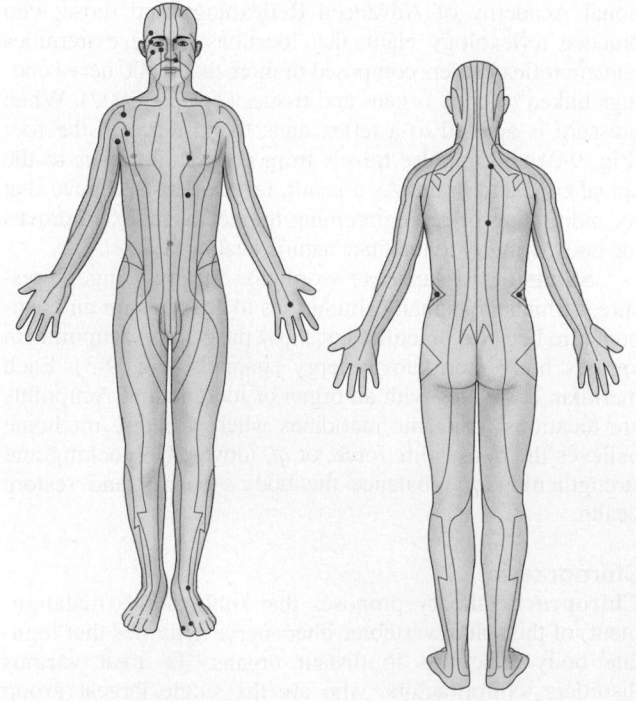

FIGURE 9-3. Locations of acupuncture meridians in the body.

most commonly practiced in the United States. Advocates of hatha yoga attribute the following benefits to its practice:

- Relaxation and centeredness
- Relief of headaches, insomnia, anxiety, and pain
- Increased musculoskeletal flexibility
- Improved breathing
- Overall contentment

The Chinese believe that tai chi exercises restore *qi* or *chi*. The exercises require standing and shifting body weight from one foot to another while performing a series of slow, choreographed arm movements. To obtain full advantage of the physical exercise, it should be accompanied by slow, controlled breathing and visualization of energy circulating throughout the body.

Proponents believe that tai chi exercises tone the whole body without the exertion and cardiac risks associated with other aerobic forms of physical exercise, restore health, and prevent disease. In China, where a slightly different form of tai chi called *qi gong* is practiced, there are reports that people develop psychokinetic powers, the ability to move objects and people without touching them.

Energy Medicine

Energy medicine is a field of alternative and complementary therapies in which techniques are used that claim to manipulate electromagnetic fields in the body. This may involve the use of mechanical vibration, laser beams, and electromagnetic forces of measurable wavelengths and frequencies (NCCAM, 2007c). Some examples include reiki, acupuncture, and techniques involving magnets and electricity.

Reiki

Reiki (pronounced "ray-key") shares many features with what Westerners may call "therapeutic touch" and spiritual healing. Reiki is a Japanese method of healing that was introduced to the Western world in the 1800s. *Rei* means "spirit" and *ki* is translated like *qi* or *chi*. Those who use reiki believe that *ki* promotes health and healing. They further believe that when *ki* is blocked and a person is ill, a reiki practitioner can channel energy—not from his or her own body, but from the universe—to the sick person's body. Once *ki* is restored, healing occurs.

The practitioner transfers the energy in the universe by laying-on of hands. Direct contact between the practitioner and client is the usual method of healing; however, healing can also occur from a distance, because the Japanese believe that the spirit is not confined by time or space. In other words, the practitioner and ill person can be geographically separate. The practitioner then moves his or her hands on an object that symbolically represents the sick person while visualizing the transmission of energy. The belief is that the recipient draws in the energy, which goes where it is needed.

Acupuncture

Acupuncture is a healing therapy in which a needle is placed in one or more acupoints to unblock *qi*. Acupuncture is considered a form of energy therapy because its ultimate goal is to restore the balance and free flow of energy in the body. Some acupuncturists take the technique one step further by manipulating the needles with an electrical current. When used in this manner, it is referred to as *electroacupuncture*.

Electromagnetic Therapy

Electromagnetic therapy promotes healing using electricity, magnets, or both. Microcurrent therapy, using low-intensity electrical currents to alter cellular physiology, is currently used to treat nonhealing fractures and to relieve pain. Magnetism is used diagnostically with MRI. Despite the use of electromagnetic therapies, several questions are yet unanswered: (1) how do these two forces produce healing; (2) what is the explanation for the anecdotal reports of symptom relief among people who wear magnets; and (3) if electromagnetic healing is validated, for what disorders is it best used?

The theory of electromagnetism is based on the physiologic principle that cellular membranes emit electrical currents. This electrical energy can be recorded using electrocardiograms, EEGs, and electromyelograms. Science also has confirmed that nerve stimulation causes the resting membrane potentials of cells to change to action potentials. Furthermore, a magnet can change the direction of an electrical current by separating charged ions. Consequently, speculation is that electromagnetic therapy (1) affects the cell membrane by changing the ion exchange of electrolytes such as calcium, sodium, and potassium; (2) stimulates the release of endorphins, naturally produced morphine-like chemicals, or other neurotransmitters through the cell's membrane; or (3) rebalances the electromagnetic field in the body.

Although questions about the what, why, and how of electromagnetic therapy remain largely unanswered, its use has been unscientifically expanded to include static magnet therapy and pulsed magnetic field therapy. Static magnet therapy refers to wearing stationary magnets, which are stronger than everyday refrigerator-type magnets, directly on the body. The static magnets are incorporated in bracelets, necklaces, belts, wraps, and even mattress pads. Pulsed magnetic field therapy uses devices that apply very low frequency electricity (50 Hz) to body areas at intervals of 25 pulses per second for 600 seconds (10 minutes) followed by an interval of rest. Supposedly, the pulsing effect produces rising and falling levels in the body's magnetic field.

Electromagnetic therapeutic devices continue to be used haphazardly for a host of unrelated conditions such as fibromyalgia, postpolio syndrome, peripheral neuropathy, multiple sclerosis, depression, epilepsy, and urinary incontinence. Research as to whether beneficial results can be attributed entirely to the placebo effect or if there is a legitimate scientific basis to its efficacy is long overdue.

NURSING MANAGEMENT OF COMPLEMENTARY AND ALTERNATIVE THERAPIES

Because nursing is a holistic practice, it is essential to integrate both conventional medical therapies and those complementary and alternative techniques that have demonstrated beneficial evidence-based outcomes. For those techniques that are still investigational, the nurse should teach the client regarding potential risk(s); however, it is important to respect and advocate for a client's choice of nontraditional medicine in combination with conventional medical treatment as long as there is no potential for harm.

Nursing can play a pivotal role in assisting clients to make knowledgeable choices about their healthcare by:

- Learning about complementary and alternative medicine.
- Assisting the client to obtain full disclosure about potential treatment options.
- Examining research findings to determine benefits and risks of complementary and alternative therapies.
- Empowering clients to assume autonomy for healthcare decisions.
- Supporting clients' choices as long as they are not potentially harmful.
- Preparing for possible untoward effects that may occur with nontraditional techniques.
- Avoiding the implementation of interventions that violate the legal scope of nursing practice.

CRITICAL THINKING EXERCISES

1. What information is appropriate to offer a person who is interested in using herbs and botanicals for health-related benefits?
2. A woman who is experiencing menopausal symptoms has been advised by her physician to avoid hormone replacement treatment. Why might this woman and others in a similar situation turn to alternative therapies?
3. Discuss how prayer could be considered a complementary or alternative therapy.
4. Individuals such as Dr. Thomas Dooley (1927–1961), a humanitarian American physician in Laos, and Mother Teresa (1910–1997), an Albanian nun who worked among the sick and dying in India, integrated conventional medicine with traditional cultural practices. Discuss possible reasons why they were able to gain the trust of their "clients," even though the Laotians and Indians were unfamiliar with conventional medicine.

NCLEX-STYLE REVIEW QUESTIONS

1. A client is interested in Ayurvedic medicine and asks the nurse to explain this modality and its beliefs about what facilitates health. Which of the following elements would the nurse discuss? Select all that apply.
   1. *Yin* and *yang* balance
   2. Strong body
   3. Meditation
   4. Clear mind
   5. Tranquil spirit
2. A client tells his nurse that he is considering acupuncture for treatment of his anxiety. Which statement should alert the nurse that the client does not understand the purpose of acupuncture?
   1. "Acupuncture will help restore my peace of mind."
   2. "I need to focus on restoring a healthy state of mind."
   3. "My doctor has recommended a reliable acupuncturist."
   4. "My life's energy force is not in balance."
3. Which of the following is a valid conclusion on the part of a nurse who researched alternative and conventional medical systems?
   1. Alternative medical systems are insensitive to cultural traditions.
   2. Alternative medical systems are not regulated by governmental standards.
   3. Conventional medical systems focus on maintenance of a healthy state.
   4. Conventional medical systems rely primarily on herbal supplements.
4. A client recently diagnosed with lung cancer asks the nurse to provide an explanation of using imagery to fight her disease. The nurse is correct in making which of the following statements?
   1. "The mind uses mental pictures to promote a positive physical outcome."
   2. "The power of suggestion will help you to make physical changes."
   3. "This process provides you with feedback when you try to alter oxygen levels."
   4. "This technique helps to stimulate the immune system."
5. When a client is admitted to the hospital, what questions should the nurse ask that are related to current medications the client is taking? Select all that apply.
   1. "Are you allergic to any medications or foods?"
   2. "Do you take any herbal supplements?"
   3. "Have your doctors prescribed any medications?"
   4. "When is the last time you took some medication?"

10

End-of-Life Care

Words To Know

acceptance
anger
anticipatory grieving
bargaining
denial
depression
hospice
near death experience
nearing death awareness
palliative treatment
respite care
waiting for permission phenomenon

Learning Objectives

On completion of this chapter, you will be able to:

1. Define attitudes of society and healthcare workers toward death.
2. Discuss outcomes of informing a client about a terminal illness.
3. Explain how clients and families can maintain hopefulness during a terminal illness.
4. Name emotional reactions the dying client experiences.
5. Identify how the dying client can ensure that others carry out his or her wishes for terminal care.
6. Describe physical phenomena that occur during the dying process.
7. Summarize psychological events that dying clients have reported.
8. Describe nursing management of the dying client and the family.

According to DeSpelder and Strickland (2001, p. 5), "Of all human experiences, none is more overwhelming in its implications than death. Yet, for most of us, death remains a shadowy figure whose presence is only vaguely acknowledged." Earlier in the 20th century, many people died in their homes, surrounded by family and loved ones. Later, it became more common to die in a hospital or nursing home. In the 1970s, the hospice movement began to promote care of dying clients at home or in hospice settings, providing a more dignified and supportive climate.

Increased technology and aggressive treatment have, in some ways, distorted the reality of dying and death for healthcare providers. For some, death signifies a failure to save lives and act as healers. Death, however, is a natural and universal experience, a part of life, and a component of healthcare. Healthcare providers must acknowledge death as the final stage of growth and development (Kübler-Ross, 1975). They also must explore their own mortality and feelings about dying and death. This is the only way that they can then provide care and comfort to dying clients and their families.

Education about death helps healthcare professionals to be better informed about dying and death and to incorporate this knowledge into the care they give clients. Nurses who care for dying clients share emotional pain with them and their families. Denying death creates a barrier to becoming involved with clients and families and interferes with personal growth.

Death can occur in any healthcare setting; therefore, facing the death of clients is necessary for nurses. It is not partial to a particular age group or population. Death can be slow and tortuous or very sudden and unexpected. Preparing clients and their families for an expected death is usually very different from caring for grieving family members after an unexpected death. Recognizing that nursing care always requires sensitivity and compassion for clients, families, and significant others is an essential component of quality care.

SUPPORTING THE DYING CLIENT

Although most people recognize that death is inevitable, they do not spend time getting ready until actually faced with the prospect. Factors the nurse needs to consider when caring for dying clients include informing clients, sustaining hope, assisting clients and families with emotional reactions, and recognizing clients' rights to make final decisions.

Informing the Dying Client

Nurses honor dying clients' right to know the seriousness of their condition. The physician usually is responsible for informing clients of the nature and gravity of their illness. Even though some informed clients react negatively at first, outcomes of being truthful include the following:

- The nurse–client relationship is based on honesty rather than on the false pretense that recovery will occur.
- The clients' autonomy and right to determine how to spend the rest of their life are upheld.
- Clients can complete unfinished business—prepare for and arrange legal and personal affairs and complete any remaining tasks or goals.
- Clients can use inner resources and determination to survive and prolong life, often referred to as the "will to live."
- Meaningful communication between clients and family members is promoted.

All members of the healthcare team must know what the client has been told regarding his or her prognosis. Lack of this knowledge greatly interferes with the nurse–client relationship. For example, the nurse may avoid all but the most superficial topics of conversation out of uncertainty about how to respond if asked "Am I going to die?" Some nurses feel that, regardless of how others might try to conceal the truth, most clients gradually recognize clues that their illness is terminal. Avoidance alone tends to confirm their suspicions that they are dying. When uninformed clients are given the opportunity, they may give hints of their awareness of approaching death. Some may even indicate they are ready to discuss dying. If nurses reply to comments by saying "Don't talk like that," they convey a message that the subject of dying is uncomfortable for the nurse. Often, clients will then avoid the subject in all future interactions.

Sustaining Hope

Nurses must recognize the value of communicating a spirit of hopefulness. Hopefulness means that dying clients have a right to believe that the healthcare team will make their remaining days meaningful, use whatever treatment and comfort measures are appropriate, and dignify the approaching death. Both nurses and clients, however, should not confuse hope with unrealistic optimism. When clients learn that their condition is terminal, they must also understand that the healthcare team remains dedicated to providing **palliative treatment**, which is treatment that reduces physical discomfort but does not alter a disease's progression (Box 10-1).

Assisting With Emotional Reactions

Although each dying client responds to terminal illness in unique ways, studies show a common emotional pattern.

Elisabeth Kübler-Ross, a physician who studied death and dying extensively, describes a series of five reactions—(1) denial, (2) anger, (3) bargaining, (4) depression, and (5) acceptance—that dying clients often demonstrate. Clients do not always follow these stages in order. Some regress and then move forward again. Others may be in several stages at once (e.g., a client who is angry as well as depressed).

The first stage, **denial**, is a psychological coping mechanism (see Chap. 67) in which a person refuses to believe certain information. Dying clients usually first deny that the diagnosis is accurate. A common response is "No, not me—there must be some mistake." They may imagine that test results are erroneous or reports have been confused. Denial of the diagnosis may be followed by a refusal to accept that the condition is terminal.

During the second stage, **anger**, clients ask "Why me?" Clients may say "I'm still young. My children still need me. Why did I get this disease?" They may displace this anger onto others, such as the physician, nurses, family, or even God. They may express such anger in less obvious ways, such as complaining about their care or blaming anyone and everyone for the slightest aggravation.

The third stage, **bargaining**, is an attempt to postpone death. Usually the client makes a secret bargain with God or some higher power. Clients attempt to negotiate a delay in dying until after a particularly significant event. They may say, "If I can just live until my daughter graduates from high school, I will accept death when it eventually comes."

The fourth stage is marked by **depression**. As clients realize the reality of their situation, they may mourn their potential losses, such as separation from their loved ones, the inability to fulfill their future goals, or loss of control.

In the fifth stage, **acceptance**, dying clients accept their fate and make peace spiritually and with those to whom they are close. Clients may begin to detach themselves from activities and acquaintances and seek to be with only a small circle of relatives or friends.

Gerontologic Considerations

- Although older adults require as much emotional support as do young or middle-aged dying clients, ageism may involve the myth that all older adults are ready to die because future life has no meaning or personal value has diminished. Markson identified that individual perspectives related to death vary according to social circumstances and prior life experiences; many older adults continue to have life goals and expectations and are not ready to die (Miller, 2009).

▶ ***Stop, Think, and Respond Exercise 10-1***

A client has learned that he has a terminal illness. He pleads with God to allow him to live long enough to see the birth of his first grandchild. What is this stage called? What may have preceded this stage?

BOX 10-1 **Five Principles of Palliative Care**

1. Palliative care respects the goals, likes, and choices of the dying person and his or her loved ones … helping them to understand the illness and what can be expected from it, and to figure out what is most important during this time.
2. Palliative care looks after the medical, emotional, social, and spiritual needs of the dying person … with a focus on making sure he or she is comfortable, not left alone, and able to look back on his or her life and find peace.
3. Palliative care supports the needs of family members … helping them with the responsibilities of caregiving and even supporting them as they grieve.
4. Palliative care helps to gain access to needed healthcare providers and appropriate care settings … involving various kinds of trained providers in different settings, tailored to the needs of the client and his or her family.
5. Palliative care builds ways to provide excellent care at the end of life … through education of care providers, appropriate health policies, and adequate funding from insurers and the government.

(Used with permission. The Robert Wood Johnson Foundation, Last Acts Palliative Care Task Force. [1999]. Five Principles of Palliative Care. Special supplement to *Advances*, 2, 3.)

Supporting Final Decisions

During this emotional turmoil, dying clients often must make some difficult decisions. The nurse presents options of where and how terminal care may be provided, respects client and family choices, and facilitates their preferences. As long as dying clients remain competent (retain the ability to understand the consequences of their choices), they have the right to request or refuse a variety of options. Problems arise when clients become incompetent before indicating their wishes about terminal care; at such times, they may become victims of decisions they would ordinarily oppose.

Dying clients or their families can control their destiny. Under a federal law called The Patient Self-Determination Act, passed in 1990, all healthcare facilities in the United States funded by Medicare must inform clients on admission of their right to refuse medical treatment and their right to prepare advance directives. *Advance directives* provide the client with the opportunity to write down his or her wishes in a living will or legally designate someone to have medical durable power of attorney (see Chap. 5). Most agencies supply the necessary forms.

A *living will* is a written or printed statement describing a person's wishes concerning her or his medical care when death is near (see Fig. 5-4 in Chap. 5). Usually, a living will describes a desire to avoid being kept alive by artificial means or the use of heroic measures. It is not a legal document and, as such, is not binding under the law. Rather, it serves as an informal directive, which others may or may not feel compelled to follow. Many physicians try to abide by their clients' wishes, however, if they are known or stated in writing.

A *medical durable power of attorney* or healthcare proxy is the person the client designates to make medical decisions on the client's behalf when the client no longer can do so. It allows competent clients to identify exactly what life-sustaining measures they want implemented, avoided, or withdrawn, and offers reassurance that others will carry out their wishes. The appointee cannot exercise this authority at any other time or in any other matters. For obvious ethical reasons, the client's physician or other healthcare workers may not be designated as durable power of attorney. When a medical durable power of attorney document exists, the client brings it to the institution at admission, and a photocopy is attached to the chart.

CARE OPTIONS FOR THE DYING CLIENT

Some terminally ill clients spend their last days in an acute care setting, using the best technology and resources available. Others prefer to be at home, with or without assistance from hospice home care. Others choose a hospice or extended care facility. Culture and family tradition may influence these choices (Table 10-1). Regardless of the setting, clients need to know that their symptoms, particularly pain, will be controlled and that they will be a part of the planning process for their care.

Home Care

In the early stages of a terminal illness, clients usually remain at home. Nurses often coordinate community services and secure needed home equipment. Many clients experience greater emotional and physical comfort in their own home. They have greater security and personal integrity in a familiar environment. Family members also may experience fewer feelings of guilt when they are involved in caring for the client. In addition, children can interact more frequently and may be helped to understand death with less fear.

A negative factor of home care is the burden it places on the primary caregiver. If prolonged, the role of primary caregiver can be very isolating and physically exhausting because the responsibility for providing care continues 24 hours a day, day after day. Home care nurses periodically need to assess the toll on the caregiver's physical and emotional health. They may arrange **respite care**, or care for the caregiver, to provide periodic relief.

Hospice Care

In 1967, Dr. Cicely Saunders founded St. Christopher's Hospice in Sydenham, England. This hospice has served as a model for hospice care in the United States. A **hospice** is a facility for the care of terminally ill clients, who can live out their final days with comfort, dignity, and meaningfulness. Hospice care emphasizes helping clients live however they wish until they die. Clients receive services that relieve their physical symptoms and emotional distress and promote spiritual support. Pain is liberally controlled.

In the United States, facilities have implemented the hospice philosophy in various ways. In general, most hospice clients, who usually have 6 months or less to live, receive care in their own homes. A multidisciplinary team of hospice professionals and volunteers provides support to the dying client and caregivers. Services include personal care, homemaking services, companionship, and support

TABLE 10-1 Cultural Diversity and Death

ETHNIC GROUP	ROLE OF FAMILY	ENVIRONMENT	PREPARATION OF THE BODY
African American	Family members may expect healthcare providers to communicate with oldest family member. Public displays of emotion are acceptable.	Family members frequently care for dying older adults at home. They may believe that a death in the home will bring the family bad luck.	Family members often expect the healthcare team to clean and prepare a loved one's body. They may consider organ donation a taboo but may agree to an autopsy.
Chinese American	Family members may prefer that the client not be told of terminal illness or imminent death and may prefer to tell the client themselves.	Some believe that dying in the home brings the family bad luck. Others believe that the client's spirit may get lost if the client dies in the hospital. Family members may make use of special amulets or cloths.	Some family members prefer to wash the client themselves. They may believe that the body should be kept intact; organ donation and autopsy are uncommon.
Filipino American	Family members may want healthcare providers to communicate with the head of the family, out of the family's presence. Public displays of emotion are acceptable.	Terminally ill clients may prefer to die at home. If the family is Catholic, they may ask that a priest perform the "sacrament of the sick" and may use religious objects, such as rosary beads and prayer.	Family members may want to wash the body and are likely to want time for all family members to say goodbye. They may not permit organ donation or autopsy.
Hispanic or Latino American	Family members may expect extended family members to care for ill loved ones, sharing information and decision-making. They may consider wailing as a sign of respect.	Dying in a hospital may not be desirable. Some believe that the client's spirit will get lost there. Special amulets, religious objects such as rosary beads and prayer are used.	Relatives may help with care of the body, and are likely to want time to say goodbye. Organ donation and autopsy are uncommon.

Adapted from Mazanec, P., & Tyler, M. K. (2003). Cultural considerations in end-of-life care. *American Journal of Nursing, 134*(3), 53.

programs for family members and significant others, including individual counseling during and after the death of the client (grief counseling). Box 10-2 outlines eligibility criteria for hospice care, and Box 10-3 lists home hospice care services covered by Medicare/Medicaid.

Institutionally Based Palliative Care

Some institutions provide palliative care to terminally ill clients who cannot maintain independent living. This care also may be referred to as hospice care. These units may be located in hospitals, long-term care facilities, or other, separate facilities. Nurses and other healthcare personnel give 24-hour care. Factors that influence the decision to use institutionally based palliative care include the following:

- The client's weakness or immobility causes him or her to require more assistance than can be provided at home.
- The client cannot manage elimination needs.
- The client has uncontrolled or inadequately controlled pain or nausea.
- The family cannot provide adequate care.
- The client requires too complex and demanding care.
- The caregiver is too exhausted to provide care.

Many of the rules that govern traditional hospital and long-term care are relaxed for palliative care units. Visiting hours and ages of visitors are not restricted. In addition, the

---

BOX 10-2 **Eligibility Criteria for Hospice Care**

General
- Serious, progressive illness
- Limited life expectancy
- Informed choice of palliative care over cure-focused treatment

Hospice-Specific
- Presence of a family member or other caregiver continuously in the home, when the client is no longer able to safely care for him/herself (some hospices have created special services within their programs for clients who live alone, but this varies widely)

Medicare and Medicaid Hospice Benefits
- Medicare Part A: Medical assistance eligibility
- Waiver of traditional Medicare/Medicaid benefits for the terminal illness
- Life expectancy of 6 months or less
- Physician certification of terminal illness
- Care must be provided by a Medicare-certified hospice program

(From Smeltzer, S. C., Bare, B. G. Hinkle, J. L., & Cheever, K. H. [2008]. *Brunner & Suddarth's textbook of medical–surgical nursing* [11th ed.]. Philadelphia: Lippincott Williams & Wilkins.)

BOX 10-3 **Home Hospice Services Covered Under the Medicare/Medicaid Hospice Benefit**

Routine Home Care Level

- Nursing care: Provided by or under the supervision of a registered nurse, available 24 hours a day
- Medical social services
- Physician's services
- Counseling services, including dietary counseling
- Home health aide/homemaker
- Physical/occupational/speech therapists
- Volunteers
- Bereavement follow-up (for up to 13 months after the death of the client)
- Medical supplies for the palliation of the terminal illness
- Medical equipment for the palliation of the terminal illness
- Medications for the palliation of the terminal illness

(From Smeltzer, S. C., Bare, B. G., Hinkle, J. L. & Cheever, K. H. [2008]. *Brunner & Suddarth's textbook of medical–surgical nursing* [11th ed.]. Philadelphia: Lippincott Williams & Wilkins.)

family is encouraged to bring in personal items for the client to enjoy and value.

 Gerontologic Considerations

- Many frail older adults with chronic conditions, especially cognitive decline, die in long-term care settings. By 2040, one in four persons is expected to die in a long-term care facility (Matzo & Sherman, 2004), necessitating education of long-term care staff regarding special end-of-life needs.

Acute Care

Hospitals offer acute care with a 24-hour staff of nurses and other medical personnel, readily available resuscitative equipment, and access to a greater variety of medications than those in long-term care. This form of terminal care, however, is probably the most expensive. In this setting, the time and attention afforded to the supportive care of dying clients may be limited.

SIGNS OF APPROACHING DEATH

Although death is unique for each individual, common physical and psychological events occur when death is approaching.

Physical Events

Death usually occurs gradually over hours or days. Cells deteriorate from an underlying lack of sufficient oxygen, which leads to multisystem failure. The following are signs of impending death that alert the nurse that the client will die shortly:

- *Cardiac dysfunction.* Failing cardiac function is one of the first signs that a client's condition is worsening. At first, heart rate increases in a futile attempt to deliver oxygen to cells. The apical pulse rate may reach 100 or more beats/minute. Cardiac output, the amount of blood the heart pumps per minute, may decrease, because a fast heart rate impairs the heart's ability to fill with blood. This may diminish the heart's own oxygen supply, which causes the heart rate to decrease and blood pressure to fall.
- *Peripheral circulation changes.* Reduced cardiac output compromises peripheral circulation, and impaired cellular metabolism produces less heat. The skin becomes pale or mottled, nail beds and lips may appear blue, and the client may feel cold.
- *Pulmonary function impairment.* Failure of the heart's pumping function causes fluid to collect in the pulmonary circulation. Breath sounds become moist. Oxygen does not diffuse very well, and the client cannot exhale carbon dioxide adequately, compounding the state of generalized hypoxia (low oxygenation).
- *Central nervous system alterations.* With hypoxia, the brain is less sensitive to accumulating levels of carbon dioxide; therefore, the client may experience periods of apnea (no breathing). Pain perception may be diminished, the client may stare blankly through partially open eyes, and the senses may become impaired, although hearing tends to remain intact. Eventually, the client becomes insensitive to all but extreme pressure.
- *Renal impairment.* Low cardiac output causes urine volume to diminish and toxic waste products to accumulate.
- *Gastrointestinal disturbances.* Peristalsis slows, causing gas and intestinal contents to accumulate. This buildup may stimulate the vomiting center, resulting in nausea and vomiting.
- *Musculoskeletal changes.* Reflexes become hypoactive. The client loses urinary and rectal sphincter muscle control, causing incontinence of urine and stool. The jaw and facial muscles also relax. As the tongue falls to the back of the throat, respirations become noisy. The accumulation of secretions in the respiratory tract, coupled with noisy respirations, is referred to as the death rattle. A brief period of restlessness may occur just before death.

Psychological Events

If they have reached the stage of acceptance, some terminally ill clients look forward to dying because it will end their suffering. Some clients, however, seem to forestall dying when they feel that their loved ones are not yet prepared to deal with their death. This has been described as the **waiting for permission phenomenon**, because death often occurs shortly after a significant family member communicates that he or she is strong enough and ready to "let go." Nurses must support family members at this time, because family members may feel as though they have given up and let their loved one down.

    Near death experiences, in which a person almost dies but is resuscitated, have been reported for some time. People who experience near death report similar events, such as:

- Floating above their bodies
- Moving rapidly toward a bright light

- Seeing familiar people who have already died
- Feeling warm and peaceful
- Being told that it is not time yet for them to die
- Regretting having to return to their resuscitated body

Nearing death awareness is a phenomenon characterized by a dying client's premonition of the approximate time or date of death. In addition, just before death, clients may reach out, point, or open their arms as if to embrace someone or call them by name.

NURSING MANAGEMENT FOR END-OF-LIFE CARE

Nursing care of dying clients focuses on providing palliative care to the client and supporting family members and significant others. Client comfort is the primary goal, with the major long-term goal being that the client will die with dignity. Other client goals include control of pain, maintenance of basic physiologic functions, relief of fears and anxieties, completion of unfinished business, and acceptance of death. Having the client's family remain cohesive and supportive is another goal, as is providing a safe and secure environment. See Nursing Care Plan 10-1.

Assessing Needs

Initially, nurses focus assessment on the client's basic physical needs, such as pain, breathing, nutrition, hydration, and elimination. They then include the psychosocial and spiritual needs of the client and family. Nurses must try not to repeat unnecessary assessments so as to allow the client to rest. They can make frequent checks without being physically intrusive. This frequency provides security, so that the client does not feel abandoned.

Controlling Pain

The primary objective of pain control for dying clients is to block pain without suppressing level of consciousness or breathing. The nurse usually gives pain medications on a routine schedule around the clock to avoid causing intense discomfort followed by a period of heavy sedation. Regular dosing sustains a plateau of continuous pain relief and prevents exhausting the client, who must use additional energy to cope with severe pain (see Chap. 11). The nurse also reassures the client that frequent use of narcotic analgesia will not cause addiction. The physician may prescribe other medications such as mild tranquilizers or antidepressants to reduce fear and anxiety. This is important because fear and anxiety can exacerbate pain. Other techniques such as imagery, humor, and progressive relaxation are useful in potentiating the effects of pain medication.

Facilitating Breathing

Placing the client in a Fowler's position may help ease difficulty with breathing. If the client cannot cough and raise secretions, the nurse gently suctions the client. Suctioning will not clear the lungs or ease breathing if the client has pulmonary edema (fluid in the lungs from heart failure). In this case, the physician may prescribe a sedative to relieve the anxiety created by the feeling of suffocation. Oxygen eventually may be used.

Nutrition Notes 10-1
The Client at the End of Life

- Good nutrition becomes a quality-of-life issue for dying clients.
- Eating favorite foods with a mealtime companion may stimulate appetite and promote a sense of comfort. Loss of appetite and weight, however, may be inevitable.
- Force feeding a dying client orally or through a tube may cause nausea and serves no useful purpose.
- Assure family members that decreased appetite and altered gastrointestinal function are normal parts of the dying process.

Administering Food and Fluids

If the client can take oral fluids and food, the nurse offers nourishment frequently in small amounts and serves it at the appropriate temperature. He or she encourages the family to bring in foods that the client likes or have been a tradition in the family's diet (Nutrition Notes 10-1).

Difficulty in swallowing, gastric and intestinal distention, and vomiting create a potential for aspiration of fluids, as well as a decrease in food intake. The nurse administers medications for controlling nausea and vomiting 1 hour or so before meals. The nurse and family should not insist that the client eat or drink if these symptoms cannot be controlled. The nurse reports weight loss and inadequate intake so the team can consider alternative nutritional and fluid administration routes. If drooling occurs, the nurse may elevate and turn the client's head to the side or suction the oral cavity.

Pharmacologic Consideration

- Morphine and meperidine (Demerol), which are used to control pain, can cause nausea and vomiting by direct stimulation of the emetic chemoreceptors located in the medulla.

Regulating Temperature

Skin temperature drops as death nears; the client may describe feeling cold. The nurse can give the client cotton socks, light blankets, and other light clothing if the client feels chilled. Gentle massaging of the arms and legs also may help because it transfers body heat from the hands to the skin surface and improves circulation. Touch also provides support and communicates personal concern.

Maintaining Skin and Tissue Integrity

A drop in blood pressure and rapid heart failure lead to poor tissue and organ perfusion. The nurse protects the client's skin from breakdown by changing the client's position at least every 2 hours. Poor tissue perfusion may cause inadequate drug absorption and decrease the effectiveness of drugs administered intramuscularly; in such cases, the nurse must

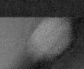

NURSING CARE PLAN 10-1 | Care of the Dying Client

Assessment

In addition to performing physical assessments of the dying client:

- Assess feelings of the client and family about losses, isolation, grief, hopelessness, and distress.

- Assess family and client communication and coping patterns, strengths, and supports.
- Assess spiritual and cultural beliefs and practices.
- Assess family's ability to provide care at home.

Nursing Diagnosis: **Anticipatory Grieving** related to functional losses and impending death

Expected Outcome: Client will verbalize grief and identify support systems.

Interventions	Rationales
Provide opportunities for client and family to share feelings.	These opportunities allow client and family to discuss anticipated losses.
Assist dying client to focus on the moment, review assets, and maintain relationships.	Doing so helps client to remain connected to his or her world.
If appropriate, encourage client to take care of any unfinished business.	Doing so assists client to heal spiritually and move on.
Identify support systems. Refer client and family to support groups and other resources.	Contact with such groups and resources promotes positive bereavement experiences.

Evaluation of Expected Outcome

Client and family can grieve and become reconciled to impending death.

Nursing Diagnosis: **Compromised Family Coping** related to client's inability to provide support to family and loved ones

Expected Outcome: Client and family verbalize resources to help deal with the situation.

Interventions	Rationales
Assist family to use coping skills that have been effective in other situations.	Coping skills decrease stress and strengthen use of resources.
Encourage family members to identify strengths and express feelings.	These measures help family members to draw on one another's strengths and share feelings, which increases coping.
Involve client and family in planning care.	Such involvement encourages feelings of control.
Refer family to appropriate resources.	They can help the client deal with stressors such as child care, financial needs, and other needs.

Evaluation of Expected Outcome

Client and family demonstrate use of other resources to increase coping with impending loss.

Nursing Diagnosis: **Fear** related to physical pain and concern that needs will not be met

Expected Outcome: Client will express trust that needs will be met.

Interventions	Rationales
Discuss client's fears with client and family.	Such discussion provides an opportunity to empathize with and provide accurate information for the client.
Encourage client to make decisions about care.	Doing so gives client some control and decreases fear that needs will not be met.
Plan care with client and family that addresses fears.	Addressing fears enhances feelings of control.
Discuss pain management program, including adjuncts to medication that promote comfort (see Chap. 11).	Information about pain management decreases fear of physical pain.

Evaluation of Expected Outcome

Client participates in decisions about care and expresses confidence that needs will be met.

Nursing Diagnosis: **Readiness for Enhanced Spiritual Well-being** related to desire to achieve harmony of mind, body, and spirit

Expected Outcome: Client will express feelings of hope.

(care plan continues on page 94)

NURSING CARE PLAN 10-1 **Care of the Dying Client** (Continued)

Interventions	Rationales
Provide client time to meditate, pray, and contemplate changes in health status.	Clients need time to be alone when health needs are changing.
Help client develop and accomplish short-term goals and tasks.	Such accomplishment increases self-esteem and self-worth.
Help client to find reasons to live and look forward.	Doing so promotes positive attitudes and ability to live for the moment.
Provide requested religious materials, books, or music.	They assist client to incorporate reading, music, imagery, or meditation into daily routine and spiritual life.
Provide privacy for client to pray with others or for members of his or her faith to visit.	Doing so demonstrates respect for and sensitivity to the client.

Evaluation of Expected Outcome

Client demonstrates spiritual well-being as evidenced by statements of hope, purpose, and trust in his or her faith.

---

consult with the physician. Drugs for raising blood pressure, improving tissue and organ perfusion, and correcting cardiac or circulatory problems may also be ordered.

Assisting with Self-Care and Activity

Dying clients may not tolerate physical activity well. The nurse may need to assist with personal hygiene. The client needs to be clean, well groomed, and free of unpleasant odors to promote dignity and self-esteem. The nurse gives oral care and ice chips, because mouth breathing makes the oral mucous membranes and lips dry. Petroleum jelly helps keep the lips lubricated. The nurse avoids glycerin applications because they tend to pull fluid from the tissue and eventually accentuate the drying problem.

Promoting Sleep

A disturbance in sleep pattern may occur because of anxiety, fear, pain, or other environmental stimuli, such as bright lights and disturbing noise. For this reason, nurses must cluster necessary activities to avoid awakening the client and to protect the client from a steady stream of healthcare workers or visitors. When possible, it is helpful to turn off or dim the lights at night and keep noise to a minimum. The radio, television, or recordings of the client's favorite music may mask the continuous hum of equipment and monitors.

Facilitating Elimination

The nurse can promote normal elimination by offering a bedpan or assisting the client to the bathroom or bedside commode. Incontinence of the bowel or bladder may occur because of the client's disease process or because the client is near death. The client needs absorbent pads when he or she has lost bowel or bladder control. The nurse assists with thorough cleaning. The client may need an indwelling or external catheter, particularly if skin breakdown is a problem.

Addressing Fear, Social Isolation, Hopelessness, and Powerlessness

Because the dying client tends to become isolated from others, the nurse must spend time with him or her apart from the time necessary to provide physical care. It is important for nurses to be flexible and to interrupt physical care if and when the client indicates a need for companionship, support, and communication. During unplanned, spontaneous moments, clients often discuss fears or concerns that nurses should not ignore or rush. The nurse can communicate interest and a willingness to listen by sitting down, leaning forward in the client's direction, and making direct eye contact. Nodding, responsive comments such as "Yes," or brief periods of silence encourage the client to continue verbalizing.

 Gerontologic Considerations

- The older adult may view dying as a natural part of life and therefore be more accepting of death than younger persons. Some older adults may fear prolonged illness, dependency, abandonment, loss of cognitive ability, or the unknown more than death itself.

Facilitating Grieving

Grieving is a painful yet normal reaction that helps clients cope with loss and leads to emotional healing. **Anticipatory grieving** occurs before death, often when the dying client and family begin to consider the impact of their potential loss. People express grief in a variety of ways: some become depressed and cry, some are angry and hostile, and some develop physical symptoms, such as anorexia and insomnia. Family members may withdraw emotionally from the dying client because they find the experience too painful, whereas others draw closer, realizing they have only a short time to be with their loved one. The nurse is responsible for facilitating the grieving process and helping the client and family deal with their emotions. To do this, nurses may empathetically share perceptions of what the client and family is experiencing by saying something like "It must be a very helpless feeling." Once the client and family sense they can speak freely, the nurse needs to listen in a nonjudgmental manner and avoid criticism or giving advice.

 Gerontologic Consideration

- Physical manifestations of grieving in older adults can include confusion, which may be falsely diagnosed as dementia.

Addressing Spiritual Distress

Religious beliefs and cultural customs influence attitudes about death. Clients may find great comfort and support from their religious faith and may want someone associated with their religion to visit. If clients indicate such a desire, the nurse notifies appropriate clergy. If asked, the nurse may pray with clients or assist as indicated. When clients are too ill to express their wishes, the nurse must ask the family about spiritual care.

Promoting Family Coping

People often find it difficult to communicate frankly with a dying person. Failure to verbalize feelings, express emotions, and show tenderness for the dying person is often a source of regret for grieving relatives. Therefore, families must feel that they can express their feelings with nurses who are compassionate listeners. If nurses encourage family members and listen to them in their frank communication, family members may feel more prepared to carry on a similarly honest dialogue with the dying client. Once they mutually express feelings and break communication barriers, both relatives and the client often experience comfort in their meaningful relationship.

If possible, the family should have a room where they can talk with other relatives, cry, and rest. For emotional support, the nurse may sit with the family for a short time, express concern for their welfare, and listen to their concerns. The nurse explains measures taken to provide comfort and pain relief for the dying client. Families may find it helpful for the nurse to explain that as death draws near, the dying client may appear to become detached and unaware of those nearby, and may slip into unconsciousness before death. The nurse is likely to be with the dying client and family at the moment of death. Some families may want to remain for a time with the body of the deceased. Therefore, the nurse allows a period of privacy before giving postmortem care. If family members or relatives seem unusually distraught, the nurse remains with them until a clergy member or other family member or friend arrives to be with them.

 Gerontologic Consideration

- Older adults who have outlived most of their family may die alone, without support from family members, relatives, or close friends. The nurse may be the only person to give close emotional support during the final hours of life. Including older adults in as many aspects of care as possible helps maintain self-esteem and personal dignity.

CRITICAL THINKING EXERCISES

1. Describe how nursing care of a young adult dying from acquired immunodeficiency syndrome (AIDS) might differ from the nursing care of an older adult dying from pneumonia.

2. A client with treatable cancer expresses a desire to go to Mexico, where they offer coffee enemas and injections with sheep urine as a cure. How would you respond? Would your response change if the client's cancer were untreatable? Why?

3. If a client wanted to die at home, how would you help the family prepare for terminal home care?

4. A client you are caring for is entering a palliative care unit in a long-term care facility. He is concerned that the nurses there will not adequately treat his pain. What could you say to reassure him?

NCLEX-STYLE REVIEW QUESTIONS

1. Which of the following interventions should a nurse perform when drooling occurs in a dying client?
  1. Elevate and turn the client's head to the side.
  2. Help the client sit on a chair upright.
  3. Place the client in the Fowler's position.
  4. Move the client from sitting to supine.

2. When the client with colon cancer does not respond to medical treatment, the physician asks the nurse to accompany him when he tells the client that nothing else can be done. Which nursing action is most helpful in assisting the client with terminal disease deal with his impending death?
  1. Allow the client privacy to think by himself.
  2. Encourage the client to talk about how he is feeling.
  3. Provide the client with literature on death and dying.
  4. Suggest that the client get a second opinion.

3. A client was told by his physician that he is terminally ill. The client tells the nurse that if he can live until his oldest daughter's wedding in three months that he will accept his situation and go peacefully. This behavior is best described in which stage of the grieving process?
  1. Denial
  2. Anger
  3. Bargaining
  4. Depression
  5. Acceptance

4. A hospice nurse is implementing the plan of care for a client with terminal cancer. Which interventions are most important to implement? Select all that apply.
  1. Ask the client if he has accepted his impending death.
  2. Assess the client's vital signs frequently.
  3. Discuss the client's financial concerns.
  4. Encourage the client to express any fears.
  5. Insist that the client try to eat his dinner.

5. A family whose loved one has chosen to die at home with hospice care asks how they will know when their loved one is close to death. The nurse is correct when she tells them which of the following? Select all that apply.
  1. Client appears to be in pain
  2. Client's muscles are tight and tense
  3. Extremities feel warm
  4. Respirations sound noisy
  5. Skin appears cool and mottled

UNIT 3
Foundations of Medical—Surgical Nursing

11

Pain Management

Learning Objectives

On completion of this chapter, you will be able to:

1. Define the term *pain*.
2. Compare nociceptive pain with neuropathic pain.
3. Give characteristics distinguishing acute from chronic pain.
4. Describe four phases of pain transmission.
5. Differentiate between pain perception, pain threshold, and pain tolerance.
6. Describe essential components of pain assessment.
7. Explain why assessing pain is difficult.
8. Give examples of tools for assessing the intensity of pain.
9. Discuss the Joint Commission's standards on pain assessment and pain management.
10. Explain pain management, and list five techniques commonly used.
11. Name categories of drugs used to manage pain.
12. Describe methods of administration for analgesic drugs.
13. Discuss the issues of addiction, tolerance, and physical dependence associated with pain medication.
14. List examples of noninvasive techniques used to manage pain.
15. Identify two surgical procedures performed on clients with intractable pain.
16. List at least three nursing diagnoses, besides Acute Pain and Chronic Pain, that are common among clients with pain.
17. Discuss the nursing management of clients with pain.
18. Describe information pertinent to teach clients and family about pain management.

P ain is a privately experienced, unpleasant sensation usually associated with disease or injury. Pain also has an emotional component referred to as *suffering*. Extensive research is being conducted to discover more about various types of pain, pain transmission, and treatment. This chapter discusses the problem of pain and the role of nursing in pain management.

TYPES OF PAIN

Pain can be classified into categories according to (1) its source or (2) its onset, intensity, and duration. When classified according to its source, pain can be categorized as either nociceptive or neuropathic. When classified according to its onset, intensity, and duration, pain can be categorized as either acute or chronic.

Nociceptive Pain

Nociceptive pain is the noxious stimuli that are transmitted from the point of cellular injury over peripheral sensory nerves to pathways between the spinal cord and thalamus, and eventually from the thalamus to the cerebral cortex of the brain (Fig. 11-1). Nociceptive pain is subdivided into somatic and visceral pain.

Somatic Pain

Somatic pain is caused by mechanical, chemical, thermal, or electrical injuries or disorders affecting bones, joints, muscles, skin, or other structures composed of connective tissue. *Superficial somatic pain*, also known as *cutaneous pain* (such as that from an insect bite or a paper cut), is perceived as sharp or burning discomfort. *Deeper somatic pain* such as that caused by trauma (e.g., a fracture) produces localized sensations that are sharp, throbbing, and intense. Dull, aching, diffuse discomfort is more common with long-term disorders such as arthritis.

Visceral Pain

Visceral pain arises from internal organs such as the heart, kidneys, and intestine that are diseased or injured. Causes for visceral pain are varied and include ischemia (reduced arterial blood flow to an organ), compression of an organ (as may be the case from a tumor), intestinal distention with gas, or contraction (spasm) as occurs with gallbladder or kidney stones. Visceral pain usually is diffuse, poorly localized, and accompanied by autonomic nervous system symptoms such as nausea, vomiting, pallor, hypotension, and sweating. **Referred pain** is a term used to describe discomfort that is perceived in a general area of the body, but not in the exact site where an organ is anatomically located (Fig. 11-2).

Neuropathic Pain

Neuropathic pain is pain that is processed abnormally by the nervous system (McCaffery & Pasero, 1999). It results from damage to either the pain pathways in peripheral nerves or pain processing centers in the brain. One theory is that activation of receptors for *N*-methyl-D-aspartate (NMDA) sensitizes pain circuits in the spinal cord and brain. An example of neuropathic pain is *phantom limb pain* or *phantom limb sensation*, in which individuals with an amputated arm or leg perceive that the limb still exists and that sensations such as burning, itching, and deep pain are located in tissues that have been surgically removed. Other examples include pain that is experienced by people with spinal cord injuries, strokes, diabetes, and herpes zoster (shingles).

Cancer pain may be either nociceptive or neuropathic. Nociceptive pain occurs when a tumor creates pressure in the organ or on adjacent tissue from its increased size. Neuropathic pain occurs when drugs or radiation used to treat the cancerous tumor cause nerve damage.

Acute Pain

Acute pain is discomfort that has a short duration (from a few seconds to less than 6 months). It is associated with tissue trauma, including surgery, or some other recent identifiable etiology. Although severe initially, acute pain eases with healing and eventually disappears. The gradual reduction in pain promotes coping with the discomfort because there is a reinforcing belief that the pain will resolve in time.

Acute and chronic pain both result in physical and emotional distress. Both also may be interrupted by pain-free periods, but that is where the similarities end.

Chronic Pain

The characteristics of **chronic pain**, discomfort that lasts longer than 6 months, are almost totally opposite from those of acute pain (Table 11-1). Chronic pain sufferers may have periods of acute pain, which is referred to as **breakthrough pain**. The longer pain exists, the more far-reaching its effects on the sufferer (Box 11-1). Others begin to show negative reactions to the chronic pain sufferer, such as (American Pain Society, 1999):

- Saying they are tired of hearing about the pain
- Ignoring the sufferer's concerns and complaints
- Getting angry with the sufferer
- Suggesting that the pain has a psychological basis

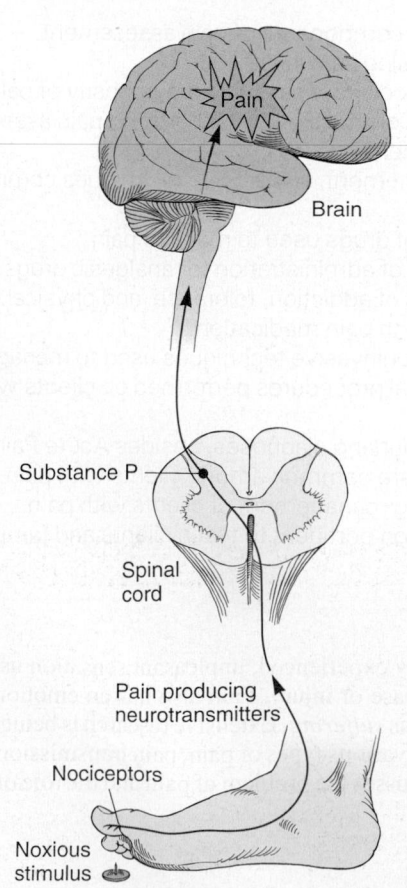

FIGURE 11-1. Nociceptive pain transmission pathway.

Brain

Substance P

Spinal cord

Pain producing neurotransmitters

Nociceptors

Noxious stimulus

Pain

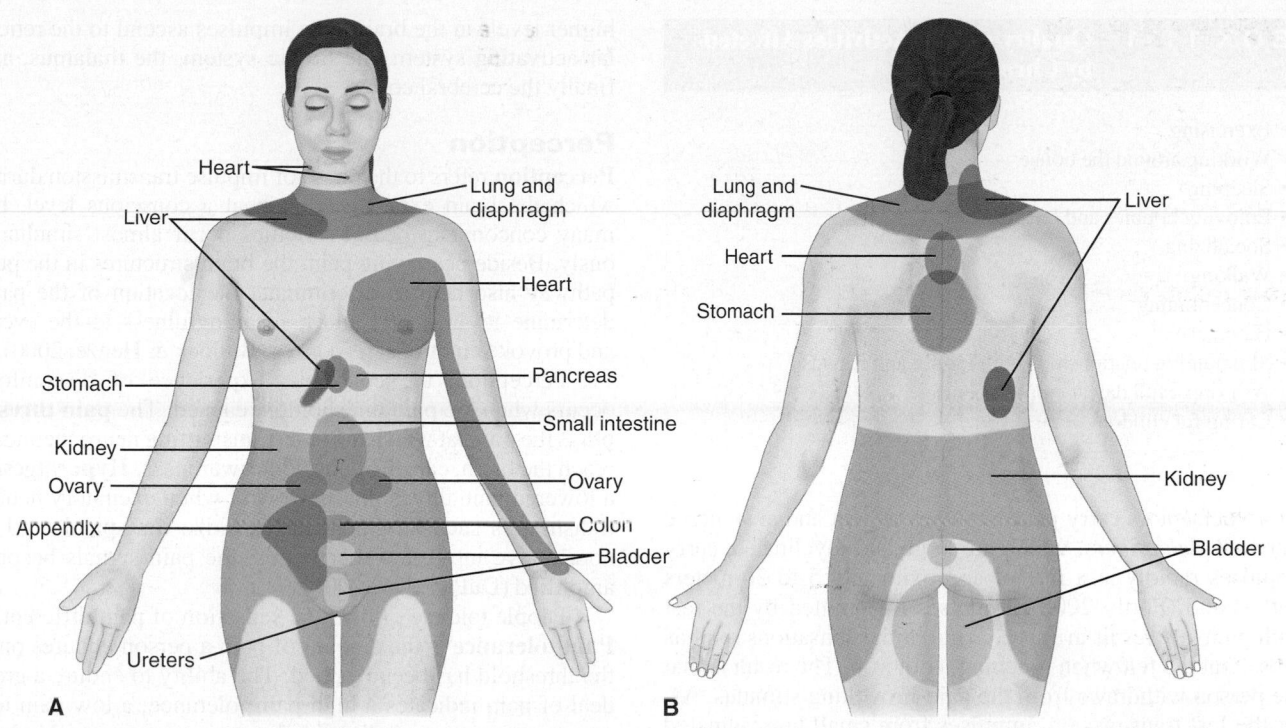

FIGURE 11-2. Common areas of referred pain.

- Telling the sufferer that he or she is using the pain to manipulate others for selfish purposes
- Criticizing the sufferer for using drugs as a "crutch"
- Suggesting that the person with chronic pain is addicted to analgesic medication

Gerontologic Considerations

- At least 70% of individuals over 65 years of age experience chronic pain, primarily due to osteoarthritis and neuralgia (Davis et al., 2002). Any chronic or recurrent pain can affect the cognitive, emotional, and physical functional abilities of an older adult client (Buckalew et al., 2008).

PAIN TRANSMISSION

The transmission of pain takes place in four phases: transduction, transmission, perception, and modulation (Fig. 11-3).

Transduction

Transduction is the conversion of chemical information in the cellular environment to electrical impulses that move toward the spinal cord. This phase is initiated by cellular disruption during which affected cells release various chemical mediators such as prostaglandins, bradykinin, serotonin, histamine, and substance P. The chemicals that are released by the damaged cells stimulate specialized pain receptors located in the free nerve endings of peripheral sensory nerves called **nociceptors**.

TABLE 11-1 Characteristics of Acute and Chronic Pain

ACUTE PAIN	CHRONIC PAIN
Recent onset	Remote onset
Symptomatic of primary injury or disease	Uncharacteristic of primary injury or disease
Specific and localized	Nonspecific and generalized
Severity associated with the acuity of the injury or disease process	Severity out of proportion to the stage of the injury or disease
Lasts less than 6 months	Lasts longer than 6 months
Responds favorably to drug therapy	Responds poorly to drug therapy
Requires gradually decreased drug therapy	Requires increasing drug therapy
Diminishes with healing	Persists beyond healing stage
Suffering decreases	Suffering intensifies
Associated with sympathetic nervous system responses such as hypertension, tachycardia, restlessness, anxiety	Absence of autonomic nervous system responses; manifests depression and irritability

- Exercising
- Working around the house
- Sleeping
- Enjoying hobbies and leisure time
- Socializing
- Walking
- Concentrating
- Having sex
- Maintaining relationships with family and friends
- Working a full day at employment
- Caring for children

Nociceptors carry pain impulses by fast and slow nerve fibers. *A-delta fibers*, which are large and myelinated, carry impulses rapidly at a rate of approximately 5 to 30 meters per second (Porth, 2006). Impulses transmitted by the fast pain pathway result in sharp, acute initial sensations such as those that are felt when touching a hot iron. The result is that the person withdraws from the pain-provoking stimulus. After the fast transmission, impulses from small unmyelinated fibers known as *C-fibers* carry impulses at a slower rate of 0.5 to 2 meters per second. They are responsible for the throbbing, aching, or burning sensation that persists after the immediate discomfort.

Transmission

Transmission is the phase during which peripheral nerve fibers form synapses with neurons in the spinal cord. The pain impulses move from the spinal cord to sequentially higher levels in the brain. The impulses ascend to the reticular activating system, the limbic system, the thalamus, and finally the cerebral cortex.

Perception

Perception refers to the phase of impulse transmission during which the brain experiences pain at a conscious level, but many concomitant neural activities occur almost simultaneously. Beside perceiving pain, the brain structures in the pain pathway also help to discriminate the location of the pain, determine its intensity, attach meaningfulness to the event, and provoke emotional responses (Bullock & Henze, 2000).

Perception, the conscious experience of discomfort, occurs when the pain threshold is reached. The **pain threshold** is the point at which the pain-transmitting neurochemicals reach the brain, causing conscious awareness. **Hyperalgesia**, a lowered pain threshold, may occur when excitatory neurotransmitters such as glutamate sensitize the spinal cord to nociceptive input. In other words, the pain signals become amplified (DuPen et al., 2007).

People tolerate or bear the sensation of pain differently. **Pain tolerance** is the amount of pain a person endures once the threshold has been reached. The ability to endure a great deal of pain indicates a high pain tolerance; a low pain tolerance refers to very little ability to endure pain. Various factors can affect pain tolerance. For example, fatigue diminishes the ability to cope with pain and heightens the perception of pain. Anticipatory fear, the expectation of pain such as that accompanying an injection or root canal procedure, can lower pain tolerance. Concurrently dealing with multiple or accumulating stressors and depression decreases a person's ability to tolerate pain. Pain intolerance also is associated with social isolation or feeling socially abandoned. Cultural beliefs and values affect how a person

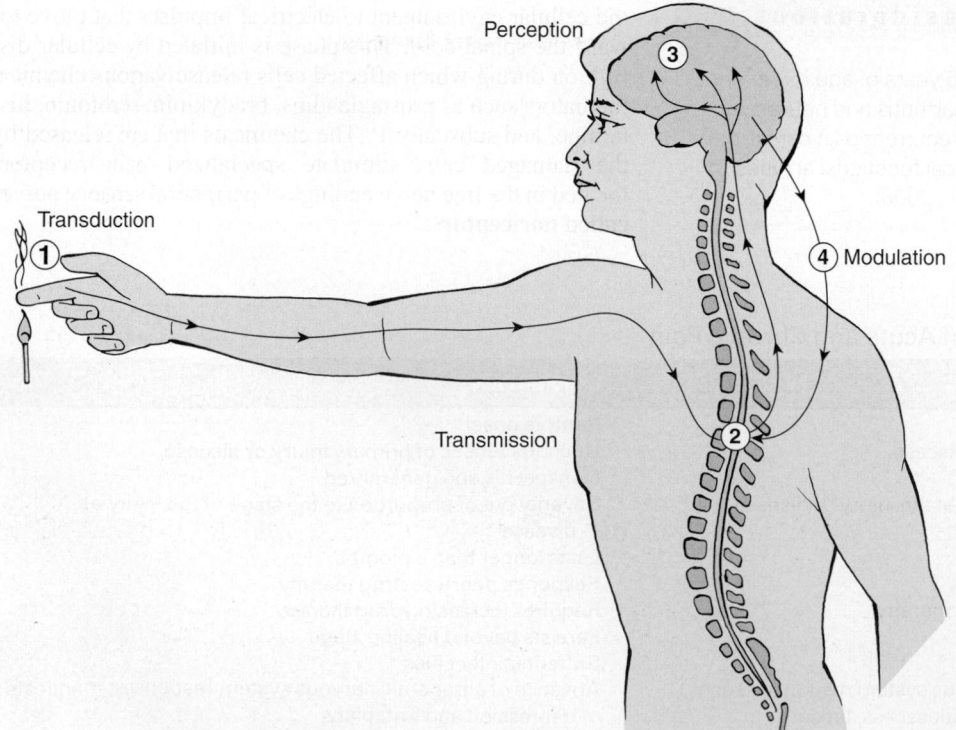

FIGURE 11-3. The phases of pain transmission.

deals with pain; some may be stoic, while others may be verbally and physically demonstrative in response to pain.

Research indicates that there are also gender differences in pain tolerance (Edwards et al., 2004; Jackson et al., 2002; Berkley, 1997). Men tend to report lower pain intensity and demonstrate higher pain tolerance; women tend to rate their pain at higher levels and report pain in more body regions than men. Some believe that estrogen increases pain perception (National Institute of Neurological Disorders and Stroke, 2007). These gender differences must be viewed with caution, because they may be examples of learned responses rather than physiologic differences.

 Gerontologic Considerations

- Some people assume that pain sensitivity and perception decrease with aging. Such an assumption can cause inaccurate assessment and undertreatment, leading to unnecessary suffering in older adults. All older clients should be asked about pain. Multiple factors may contribute to pain in older adults, causing difficulty determining individual causes (Ferrell, 2005).

Modulation

Modulation is the last phase of pain impulse transmission, during which the brain transmits a response down the spinal nerves to the point where the pain transmission originated to alter the pain experience. At this point, the painful sensation is reduced with the release of pain-inhibiting neurochemicals such as endogenous opioids, which are discussed later in this chapter, and gamma-aminobutyric acid (GABA).

PAIN ASSESSMENT

There is no perfect way to determine if pain exists and how severe it is. Margo McCaffery, a nursing expert on pain, states, "Pain is whatever the person says it is, and exists whenever the person says it does" (McCaffery & Beebe, 1989). Individuals in pain may demonstrate a variety of nonverbal behaviors such as:

- Positioning to avoid pain or being resistant to repositioning
- Rocking, fidgeting, or squirming
- Protective or guarding gestures
- Clenched jaw
- Frowning

- Sleep disturbances: increased sleep due to exhaustion or decreased sleep due to repeated awakening
- **Allodynia**, an exaggerated pain response due to increased sensitivity to stimuli such as air currents, pressure of clothing, vibration
- Loss of interest in eating
- Moaning, crying, or sighing
- Emotional irritability
- Impaired thinking, confusion, or combativeness
- Reduced social interactions

A pain assessment includes the client's description of its onset, quality, intensity, location, and duration (Table 11-2). In addition, nurses assess for accompanying symptoms, such as nausea or dizziness, and what makes the pain better or worse. The American Pain Society has proposed that pain assessment should be considered the fifth vital sign. In other words, the nurse should check and document the client's pain every time he or she assesses the client's temperature, pulse, respirations, and blood pressure.

 Gerontologic Considerations

- Some older adults may be reluctant to report pain; they may prefer to describe pain as discomfort, burning, or aching. Cognitively impaired older adults may be unable to report pain; comparison of current behavior with previous behavior patterns and reports from caregivers can help in assessing pain in these clients. Pain may manifest as agitation, aggression, withdrawal, or changes in behavior, positioning, or sleep patterns. The client's use of distraction techniques such as television viewing or reading does not indicate he or she is not experiencing pain.

Assessment Biases

Despite the fact that the client is the only reliable source for quantifying pain, nurses do not respond consistently to the client's description of pain intensity with pain-relieving interventions. According to McCaffery and Ferrell (1999), "Most nurses expect someone in severe pain to *look* as if he hurts." Neither behavior nor other physiologic data such as vital signs, however, are reliable indicators of pain. Responses to pain and coping techniques are learned, and clients may express them in a variety of ways. If a client's expressions of pain do not match the nurse's expectations, pain management may not be readily forthcoming. Consequently, the client's pain may be undertreated.

TABLE 11-2 Basic Components of Pain Assessment

CHARACTERISTIC	DESCRIPTION	EXAMPLES
Onset	Time or circumstances under which the pain appeared	After eating, while shoveling snow, during the night
Quality	Sensory experiences and degree of suffering	Throbbing, crushing, agonizing, annoying
Intensity	Magnitude of the pain, such as moderate, severe; or a quantifying scale, such as from 0 to 10	None, slight, mild; a level of "7"
Location	Anatomic site	Chest, abdomen, jaw
Duration	Time span of the pain	Continuous, intermittent, hours, weeks, months

Assessment Tools

Because there are no reliable objective indicators for pain, assessment tools are necessary. Common assessment tools for quantifying pain intensity include a numeric scale, a word scale, and a linear scale (Fig. 11-4). Clients identify how their pain compares with the choices on the assessment tool. One tool is not better than another. A numeric scale is commonly used when assessing adults. When using the numerical rating scale, the client is asked to identify how much pain they are having by choosing a number from zero (no pain) to 10 (the worst pain imaginable). The Wong-Baker FACES scale is best for pediatric, culturally diverse, and mentally challenged clients (Fig. 11-5). It uses pictures and short descriptive phrases. The FACES scale is available in English as well as 10 foreign languages: Spanish, French, German, Italian, Portuguese, Japanese, Chinese, Vietnamese, Romanian, and Bosnian. Children as young as 3 years of age can use the FACES scale.

> ### Stop, Think, and Respond Exercise 11-1
>
> *When assessing the pain of two postoperative clients, each tells the nurse that her incisional pain is a "10" using the numeric scale, in which "0" equals no pain and "10" is the most pain the person has ever felt. One of the clients is lying quietly in bed watching television. The other is restless and has placed both hands over the incisional area. Both have medical orders for 50 to 75 mg of meperidine intramuscularly (IM) every 3 to 4 hours as needed for pain. Both clients received 75 mg of meperidine IM 3 hours ago. What is the best nursing action at this time?*

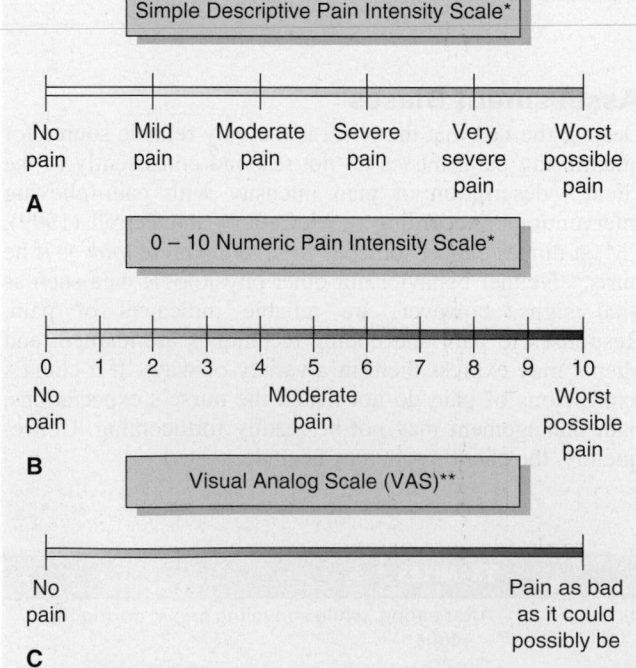

Pain intensity scales

Simple Descriptive Pain Intensity Scale*

| No pain | Mild pain | Moderate pain | Severe pain | Very severe pain | Worst possible pain |

A

0 – 10 Numeric Pain Intensity Scale*

0 1 2 3 4 5 6 7 8 9 10
No pain / Moderate pain / Worst possible pain

B

Visual Analog Scale (VAS)**

No pain / Pain as bad as it could possibly be

C

* If used as a graphic rating scale, a 10-cm baseline is recommended.

** A 10-cm baseline is recommended for VAS scales.

FIGURE 11-4. Pain assessment tools: (**A**) word scale, (**B**) numeric scale, and (**C**) linear scale.

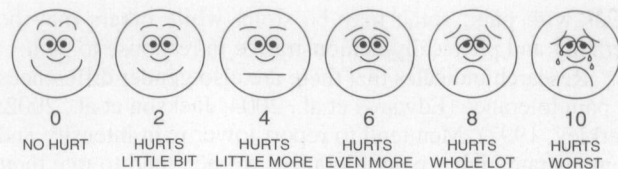

| 0 | 2 | 4 | 6 | 8 | 10 |
| NO HURT | HURTS LITTLE BIT | HURTS LITTLE MORE | HURTS EVEN MORE | HURTS WHOLE LOT | HURTS WORST |

FIGURE 11-5. Wong-Baker FACES Pain Rating Scale. Instructions: Explain to the person that each face is for a person who feels happy because he has no pain (hurt) or sad because he has some or a lot of pain. *Face 0* is very happy because he does not hurt at all. *Face 1* hurts just a little bit. *Face 2* hurts a little more. *Face 3* hurts even more. *Face 4* hurts a whole lot. *Face 5* hurts as much as you can imagine, although you do not have to be crying to hurt this bad. Ask the person to choose the face that best describes how he or she is feeling. Rating scale is recommended for persons age 3 years and older. (From Hockenberry, M. J., Wilson, D., Winkelstein, M.L. [2005]. *Wong's Essentials of Pediatric Nursing* [7th ed., p. 1259]. St. Louis: Mosby. Used with permission.)

Assessment Standards

In August 1999, the Joint Commission established pain assessment and management standards. All accredited healthcare organizations have been mandated to comply with these standards since 2001 (Joint Commission, 2000b). Table 11-3 lists components of an initial comprehensive pain assessment. Other aspects that are incorporated in the standards include the following:

- Everyone cared for in an accredited hospital, long-term care facility, home healthcare agency, outpatient clinic, or managed care organization has the right to assessment and management of pain.
- Pain is assessed using a tool that is appropriate for the person's age, developmental level, health condition, and cultural identity.
- Pain is regularly reassessed throughout healthcare delivery.
- Pain is treated in the healthcare agency or the client is referred elsewhere.
- Healthcare workers are educated regarding pain assessment and management.
- Clients and their families are educated about effective pain management as an important part of care.
- The client's choices regarding pain management are respected.

PAIN MANAGEMENT

Pain management refers to the techniques used to prevent, reduce, or relieve pain. The following are five general techniques for achieving pain management:

1. Blocking brain perception
2. Interrupting pain-transmitting chemicals at the site of injury
3. Combining analgesics with adjuvant drugs
4. Substituting sensory stimuli over shared pain neuropathways
5. Altering pain transmission at the level of the spinal cord

Any one or a combination of these techniques may be used.

Drug Therapy

Drug therapy is the cornerstone for managing pain. The World Health Organization (WHO) recommends following

TABLE 11-3 The Joint Commission's Components of a Comprehensive Pain Assessment*

COMPONENT	FOCUS OF ASSESSMENT
Intensity	Rating for present pain, worst pain, and least pain using a consistent scale
Location	Site of pain or identifying mark on a diagram
Quality	Description in client's own words
Onset	Time the pain began
Duration	Period that pain has existed
Variations	Pain characteristics that change
Patterns	Repetitiveness or lack thereof
Alleviating factors	Techniques or circumstances that reduce or relieve the pain
Aggravating factors	Techniques or circumstances that cause the pain to return or escalate in intensity
Present pain management regimen	Approaches used to control the pain and results and effectiveness
Pain management history	Past medications or interventions and responses; manner of expressing pain; personal, cultural, spiritual, or ethnic beliefs that affect pain management
Effects of pain	Alterations in self-care, sleep, dietary intake, thought processes, lifestyle, and relationships
Person's goal for pain control	Expectations for level of pain relief, tolerance, or restoration of functional abilities
Physical examination of pain	Assessment of structures that relate to the site of pain

*If clients have pain in more than one area, assessment data are collected for each.

a three-tiered approach, according to the client's pain intensity and response to selected drug therapy (Fig. 11-6). A fourth step being considered for clients with pain associated with cancer may include nerve blocks, analgesics administered *intrathecally* (in the subarachnoid or epidural spaces of the spine), electrical stimulation in the spinal cord, and neurosurgical analgesic techniques (Miguel, 2000). Examples of neurosurgical analgesic techniques are discussed later in this chapter.

Opioid and opiate **analgesics** such as morphine and meperidine (Demerol) are controlled substances referred to as *narcotics*. They interfere with pain perception centrally (at the brain). Nonopioid analgesics are not narcotics; they relieve pain by altering neurotransmission at the peripheral level (site of injury) (Drug Therapy Table 11-1).

 Gerontologic Considerations

- Pain is the number one complaint of older Americans, and one in five older adults takes an analgesic regularly (NINDS, 2007). However, many older adults may not be able to afford pain medications. It has been reported that 25% of older adults skip doses or split their doses of prescribed medications to "make them go further" (Barry, 2003).

- A reduced dose of analgesics, especially opioid analgesics, may be prescribed for the older adult initially; the initial dose may be one-half to two-thirds the usual adult dose. Older adults experience a higher peak effect and longer duration of pain relief from an opioid. The risk of increased accumulation of narcotics, benzodiazepines, and/or antidepressants also increases the potential for falls from sedation and changes in cognitive functioning.

- Because constipation is a common side effect of opioid use, a bowel regimen to prevent constipation should be started when any older adult is treated with opioids.

- Older adults taking medications for multiple chronic and/or acute conditions have an increased susceptibility to drug reactions and interactions. Older adults taking nonsteroidal anti-inflammatory drugs (NSAIDs) are at increased risk for renal toxicity and gastrointestinal problems.

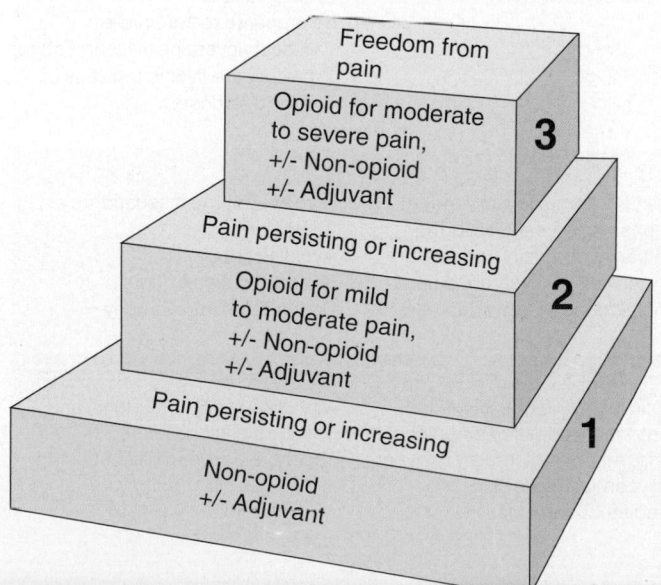

FIGURE 11-6. World Health Organization (WHO) analgesic ladder. (©World Health Organization. Redrawn with permission.)

 Pharmacologic Considerations

- Clients should not use an over-the-counter analgesic agent, such as aspirin, ibuprofen, or acetaminophen, consistently to treat chronic pain without first consulting a physician.

- Clients who take pain medications, especially aspirin or other NSAIDs, on a regular basis should inform the primary healthcare provider or dentist before any procedure because these drugs can cause undesirable side effects such as bleeding.

DRUG THERAPY TABLE 11-1 Analgesic Drug Therapy

Drug Category and Examples	Mechanism of Action	Side Effects	Nursing Considerations
Opioid analgesics *morphine sulfate, oxycodone (Roxicodone), hydromorphone (Dilaudid), meperidine (Demerol), fentanyl patch (Duragesic), tramadol (Ultram)*	Bind with opiate receptors in the central nervous system	Sedation, euphoria, nausea, vomiting, constipation, paralytic ileus, respiratory depression, urinary retention, physical dependence, hypotension	Do not administer if respirations are less than 12/minute. Encourage clients to cough and deep breathe to avoid atelectasis. Monitor for excessive sedation. Monitor bowel activity; begin bowel regimen to prevent constipation. Maintain safety precautions such as keeping side rails up and call bell within reach. Instruct client to call for assistance before ambulating. Administer before pain is severe to increase effectiveness. Change a fentanyl transdermal patch every 72 hours.
Nonopioid analgesics nonsteroidal anti-inflammatory drugs (NSAIDs): *ibuprofen (Motrin), naproxen (Naprosyn), indomethacin (Indocin)*	Inhibit the production of prostaglandins that increase sensitivity to pain	Nausea, gastritis and ulcers, increased bleeding, bone marrow depression, rash, anaphylactic reactions, renal impairment	Administer with food. Inform client of potential side effects, and instruct client to take orally as prescribed. Caution clients not to take more than one category of NSAID at a time.
Aspirin	Inhibits prostaglandin synthesis, producing analgesic effects	Nausea, gastritis, dizziness, tinnitus, occult bleeding, increased clotting time	Give with food. Report any side effects, including bleeding gums or bruising easily
miscellaneous nonopioid/non-NSAID analgesics: *acetaminophen (Tylenol)*	Analgesic for mild to moderate pain; mechanism of action unknown for nonopioid/non-NSAIDs used for pain management	Liver toxicity, bone marrow depression, hypoglycemia, kidney failure, rash due to hypersensitivity	Limit daily dosage to no more than 4 grams to avoid liver toxicity. Monitor serum drug levels with chronic use. Be prepared to administer N-acetylcysteine (Mucomyst) to protect the liver in the case of toxic overdose.
Antidepressants *Tricyclic antidepressants: amitriptyline (Elavil)*	Block the reuptake of serotonin and norepinephrine	Sedation, confusion, dry mouth, constipation, nausea, orthostatic hypotension, urinary retention, tachycardia, palpitations, bone marrow depression	Give at bedtime if sedation is a problem. Avoid alcohol. Report any side effects. Do not stop drug abruptly.
Corticosteroids *dexamethasone (Decadron), prednisone (Deltasone)*	Reduce pain with an inflammatory component; control nausea	Peptic ulcer, weight gain, fluid retention, impaired wound healing, masking of infection, hyperglycemia, fragile skin, redistribution of fat	Monitor weight, vital signs, and serum glucose level. Taper doses when discontinuing.

DRUG THERAPY TABLE 11-1 Analgesic Drug Therapy (continued)

Drug Category and Examples	Mechanism of Action	Side Effects	Nursing Considerations
Anticonvulsants *carbamazepine (Tegretol), clonazepam (Klonopin), gabapentin (Neurontin), lamotrigine (Lamictal)*	Suppress neuronal firing	Sedation, dizziness, impaired gait, weight gain, nausea, hepatotoxicity, bone marrow suppression, rash	Give with food or milk. Monitor blood counts and liver function tests. Protect from falls and injury. Taper dosage after long-term therapy.
Psychostimulants *methylphenidate (Ritalin)*	Counteract sedation; increase activity and appetite	Nervousness, insomnia, tachycardia, hypertension, weight loss, reduced red and white blood cell counts	Give before 6:00 PM to prevent insomnia. Monitor vital signs and weight. Avoid caffeine or other stimulants such as decongestants. Review results of blood tests.
Miscellaneous adjuvants *5% lidocaine local anesthetic skin patch*	Inhibit sodium ion channels, stabilizing neuronal cell membranes and inhibiting nerve impulse initiation and conduction	Localized redness and swelling at the patch site Allergic reactions in those who are sensitive to amide anesthetics. Use with caution in those taking antiarrhythmic drugs	Apply as many as 3 patches simultaneously to intact skin for 12 hours and remove for 12 hours; overdose can occur if the dose and time of application are increased. Patches can be cut without interfering with drug delivery. Provide cold applications over painful area when the patch is off. Dispose of used patches to avoid accidental contact with residual drug on patch by children and pets. Can combine with other analgesic drugs because lidocaine provides a local rather than systemic effect. Apply to area of pain no more than 3 to 4 times a day.
capsaicin cream (Zostrix)	Exact mechanism of action unknown	Temporary burning, redness, blistering at the application site. Severe allergic reactions	Instruct client to wash hands after use and avoid contact with the eyes. Do not cover with a tight bandage. Discontinue use if pain persists or worsens after 2 to 4 weeks of use.
synthetic marijuana (dronabinol, Marinol)	Multiple CNS effects; used to relieve chronic pain, nausea and vomiting associated with cancer, chemotherapy, anorexia, and weight loss	Drowsiness, difficulty concentrating, distorted vision, increased appetite, feelings of unreality, blurred vision, dry mouth Contraindicated in breast-feeding women	Never exceed 20 mg/day. Keep refrigerated. Assist client when rising from a lying or sitting position. Avoid combining with sedatives or other central nervous system depressants.

Methods of Administration

Analgesic drugs are administered by oral, rectal, transdermal, or parenteral (injected) routes, including a continuous infusion that may be instilled into the spinal canal or self-administered intravenously by clients. When changing from a parenteral to an oral route, it is best to administer an **equianalgesic dose**, an oral dose that provides the same level of pain relief as when the drug is given by a parenteral route (Table 11-4).

 Gerontologic Considerations

- Analgesics given intramuscularly to older adults are less effective because of older adults' diminished muscle mass.

Patient-Controlled Analgesia

Patient-controlled analgesia (PCA) allows clients to self-administer their own narcotic analgesic by means of an intravenous pump system (Fig. 11-7). The client infuses the drug by pressing a hand-held button. The dose and time intervals between doses are programmed into the device to prevent accidental overdose.

Intraspinal Analgesia

In intraspinal analgesia, a narcotic or local anesthetic is infused into the subarachnoid or epidural space of the spinal cord through a catheter inserted by a physician. Nurses do not administer intraspinal analgesia. The intraspinal analgesic is administered several times per day or as a continuous low-dose infusion. This method of analgesia relieves pain with minimal systemic drug effects. When used for clients who require long-term analgesia, there is less chance of affecting the subcutaneous tissues with repeated injections that may eventually lessen drug absorption.

Addiction, Tolerance, and Physical Dependence

Addiction refers to a repetitive pattern of drug seeking and drug use to satisfy a craving for a drug's mind-altering or mood-altering effects. Although opioid drugs can result in addiction, fewer than 1% of clients who are in need of drugs for pain relief, even for 6 months or longer, become addicted (McCaffery & Ferrell, 1999). Unfortunately, the fear of addiction causes many clients to refuse or self-limit pre-

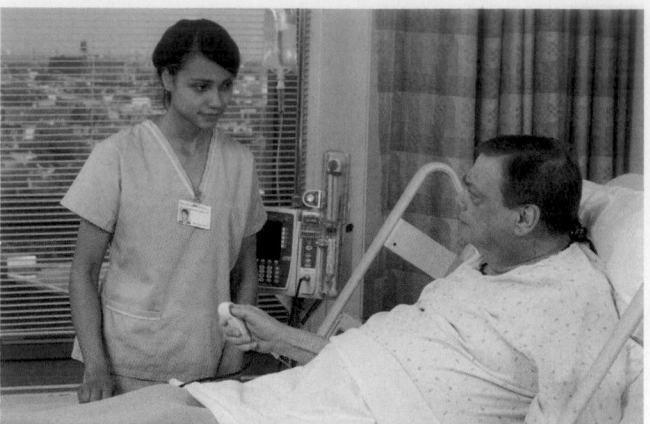

FIGURE 11-7. Patient-controlled analgesia (PCA) allows the client to self-administer medication to control pain.

scribed drug therapy. It also causes some nurses to administer subtherapeutic doses. Both actions are counterproductive to therapeutic outcomes. In addition, clients with severe, unrelieved pain may be falsely labeled as being addicted because they are focused on receiving analgesics, when in reality they are only seeking relief from unrelenting discomfort.

 Gerontologic Considerations

- Older adults may avoid taking medication, especially opioids, out of fear of addiction or drug side effects. Nurses can educate older clients about opioids, facts about addiction, and effective treatment options for any breakthrough pain or side effects such as constipation.

Although addiction rarely develops, tolerance is common. **Tolerance** is a condition in which a client needs increasingly larger doses of a drug to achieve the same effect as when the drug was first administered. Although responses to drug therapy differ among individuals, tolerance may not develop until a client has taken an opioid drug regularly for 4 weeks or more (McCaffery & Ferrell, 1999). The development of tolerance is not an indication of addiction. Rather, the client's request for pain-relieving drugs more often is a consequence of poor pain control, not drug-seeking for what some may think are the drug's pleasurable effects. The most appropriate nursing action is to consult with the physician regarding a need for an increased dose of the drug and not to reduce its dosage or frequency of administration. As a rule of thumb, an ineffective dose should be increased by 25% to 50% (McCaffery & Ferrell, 1999).

Because opioids depress the respiratory center in the brain, some nurses fear giving larger and larger doses of narcotic analgesics. In reality, respiratory depression is rare in those receiving opioids for prolonged periods of time. However, even if large doses of opioid analgesics coincidentally hasten death, the primary intention for their administration is controlling pain. The Hospice and Palliative Nurses Association (2004) and other professional

TABLE 11-4 Examples of Adult Equianalgesic Doses

DRUG	PARENTERAL DOSE	ORAL DOSE
morphine sulfate	10 mg q 3–4 h	30 mg q 3–4 h
meperidine (Demerol)	100 mg q 3 h	300 mg q 2–3 h
hydromorphone (Dilaudid)	1.5 mg q 3–4 h	7.5 mg q 3–4 h
pentazocine (Talwin)	60 mg q 3–4 h	150 mg q 3–4 h

Adapted from Carr, C. B.,Jacox, A. K., Chapman, C. R., etal. (1992; February). Acute pain management: *Operative or medical procedures and trauma. Clinical Practice Guideline No. 1.* (AHCPR Pub. 92-0032). Rockville, MD: Agency for Health Care Policy and Research.

organizations, therefore, acknowledge that it is an ethically acceptable intervention.

▶ *Stop, Think, and Respond Exercise 11-2*

A medical order states: meperidine hydrochloride 50–100 mg IM q3h prn for pain. If a client does not experience adequate pain relief after receiving 50 mg, what dose should the physician order to be more effective?

Just as tolerance is not a characteristic of addiction, neither is physical dependence. **Physical dependence** means that a person experiences physical discomfort, known as **withdrawal symptoms**, when a drug that he or she has taken routinely for some time is abruptly discontinued (see Chap. 71). To avoid withdrawal symptoms, drugs that are known to cause physical dependence are discontinued gradually. The dosage or the frequency of their administration is lowered over 1 week or longer.

Adjuvant Drug Therapy

Adjuvant drugs are medications that are ordinarily administered for reasons other than treating pain. When adjuvant drugs are combined with opioid and nonopioid analgesics, they may achieve any or all of the following: (1) improvement of analgesic effect without an increased analgesic dosage; (2) control of concurrent symptoms, such as inflammation, that worsen the pain; and (3) moderation of side effects of analgesics, such as nausea or sedation. Examples of adjuvant drugs used to manage pain include tricyclic antidepressants, corticosteroids, anticonvulsants, and psychostimulants (see Drug Therapy Table 11-1).

Nondrug Interventions

Several nondrug interventions can be used to help manage pain (see Chap. 9). Some, such as applications of heat and cold, are independent nursing measures or may require collaboration with the client's physician. Others, such as transcutaneous and percutaneous electrical nerve stimulation, acupuncture, and acupressure, are administered by individuals who have specialized training and expertise. The latter interventions are more likely to be used for clients with chronic pain or those for whom acute pain management techniques have been unsuccessful or are contraindicated.

Research is ongoing to determine how nondrug interventions relieve pain. Some question whether their effectiveness is the result of the placebo effect (see Chap. 67) or something more physiologic. McCaffery and Pasero (1999, p. 22) report that "the brain can accommodate a limited number of sensory signals. When individuals use techniques such as distraction, relaxation, and imagery to control pain, they direct their attention away from the pain sensation." Some believe that these techniques stimulate the visual portion of the brain's cortex in the right hemisphere, where abstract concepts and creative activities take place. In response, the body releases neurotransmitters such as GABA and serotonin that calm the body and promote emotional well-being. This may explain how some adjuvant drugs for pain relief such as anticonvulsants and antidepressants effect their actions.

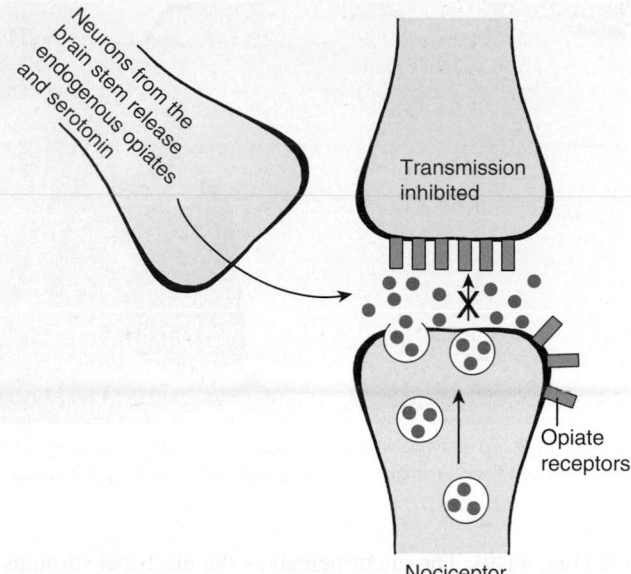

FIGURE 11-8. Endogenous opiates block receptors on nerves that transmit pain impulses toward the brain.

Techniques such as electrical nerve stimulation, acupuncture, and acupressure may work by stimulating sensory nerve fibers that conduct tactile or vibratory sensations over pathways shared for transmitting pain. The result is inhibition of pain transmission. Others speculate that these and other nondrug methods such as massage relieve pain by releasing **endogenous opiates** such as endorphins and enkephalins. Endogenous opiates are natural morphine-like substances in the body that modulate pain transmission by blocking receptors for substance P (Fig. 11-8).

Heat and Cold

Applications of heat and cold (thermal therapy) are well-established techniques for relieving pain. Pain associated with injury is best treated initially with cold applications such as an ice bag or chemical pack. The cold decreases vasodilation which reduces localized swelling, which may be useful for minor or moderate pain.

 Gerontologic Considerations

- Careful monitoring of heat application is necessary for older adults experiencing diminished sensation due to risk for burns. Monitoring is also required for application of cold packs to prevent hypothermia.

Transcutaneous Electrical Stimulation

Transcutaneous electrical nerve stimulation (TENS) is a pain management technique that delivers bursts of electricity to the skin and underlying nerves. It is safe for managing acute and chronic pain, and does not produce systemic side effects or addiction. The electricity is delivered from a battery-operated TENS unit through electrode patches that are placed at appropriate sites, such as directly over the affected area, at areas along a nerve pathway, or at points distal to the painful

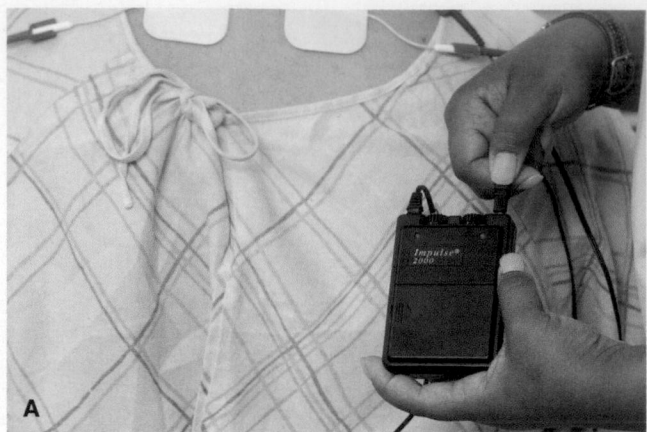 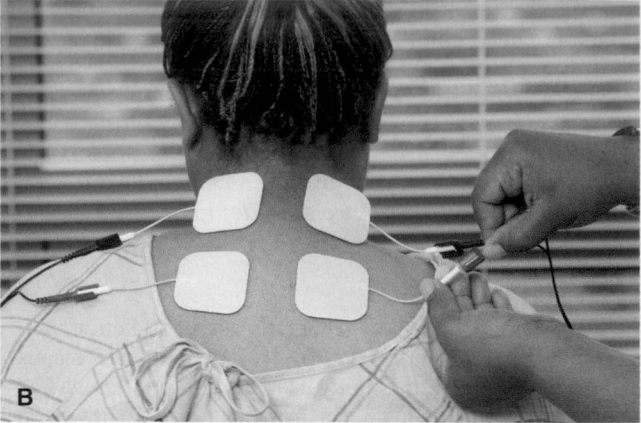

FIGURE 11-9. To activate various sensory nerves, a transcutaneous nerve stimulation (TENS) unit (**A**) may be placed close to the pain source. The TENS unit floods the gates in the spinal cord, blocking pain perception. Site of placement (**B**) depends on the pain's location.

area (Fig. 11-9). The client perceives the electrical stimulus as a pleasant tapping, tingling, vibrating, or buzzing sensation. Placement sites, intensity of electrical current, rate of electrical bursts, and duration can be changed according to the client's response.

Acupuncture and Acupressure

Acupuncture is a pain management technique in which long, thin needles are inserted into the skin. Acupressure uses tissue compression, rather than needles, to reduce pain. The location for needle placement and pressure is based on 2000-year-old traditions practiced in Chinese medicine (see Chap. 9). Relief of pain, especially chronic transmission pathway, is not permanent, and repeated treatments are almost always necessary.

Although both techniques have been demonstrated to prevent or relieve pain, their exact mechanism is not completely understood. Some speculate that the twisting, vibration, and pressure are forms of cutaneous stimuli that close the gates to pain-transmitting neurochemicals. Another theory is that acupuncture and acupressure stimulate the body to release endorphins and enkephalins.

Percutaneous Electrical Nerve Stimulation

One of the newest innovations in acute and chronic pain management is percutaneous electrical nerve stimulation (PENS), a form of electroacupuncture (see Chap. 9). It combines the use of acupuncture needles with TENS. The practitioner inserts the needles in soft tissue, and an electrical stimulus is conducted through the needles. PENS is considered superior to TENS in providing pain relief because the needles are located closer to nerve endings. PENS therapy is administered for 30 minutes three times a week for a total of 3 weeks (Hseih & Lee, 2002). The technique has been successful in research trials on clients with low back pain, pain caused by the spread of cancer to bones, shingles (acute herpes zoster viral infection), neuropathic pain among clients with diabetes or hemiplegia, and migraine headaches.

Other Noninvasive Techniques

Various other techniques are used alone or in addition to more traditional pain management techniques. Some include imagery, biofeedback, humor, breathing exercises and progressive relaxation, and distraction (see Chap. 9). In addition, in some situations (e.g., clients with severe burns), hypnosis is used. Hypnosis is a technique in which a person assumes a trance-like state during which perceptions are altered. During hypnosis, a suggestion is made that a person's pain will be eliminated or that the client will experience the sensation in a more pleasant way.

Co-therapies also may include physical or occupational therapy and counseling. Physical therapy can help to strengthen muscles weakened by disuse. Occupational therapy may help inactive clients relearn to perform physical tasks without aggravating their preexisting condition. Psychological counseling can help clients deal with depression and anxiety associated with pain.

Spinal Surgery Techniques

Intractable pain, pain that does not respond to analgesic medications, noninvasive measures, or nursing management, requires more drastic measures. Neurosurgical procedures that provide pain relief include rhizotomy and cordotomy.

Rhizotomy

A rhizotomy is a surgical procedure on the spine that involves a laminectomy (see Chap. 39) followed by sectioning of the posterior (sensory) nerve root just before it enters the spinal cord. Sectioning a spinal nerve prevents sensory impulses from entering the spinal cord and going to the brain, resulting in a permanent loss of sensation in the area supplied by the sectioned nerve. More than one nerve may need to be sectioned to produce the desired results. Chemical rhizotomy (using chemicals such as alcohol or phenol to destroy the nerve) or percutaneous rhizotomy (using radiofrequency waves to destroy pain fibers) are alternatives that may provide the same result. Rhizotomy usually is reserved for terminally ill clients.

Cordotomy

A cordotomy is an interruption of pain pathways in the spinal cord. The procedure includes a laminectomy and destruction of sensory nerve tracts in the vertebral column, thus preventing sensory nerve impulses from going to the brain. Loss of sensation is permanent. A percutaneous cervical cordotomy is basically the same procedure as a cordotomy but is performed under local anesthesia. It carries less risk and usually is better tolerated by terminally ill clients. Guided by fluoroscopy, the surgeon inserts a needle through the skin (percutaneous) in the neck (cervical) near the mastoid process. Movement of the needle interrupts pain pathways.

Nursing Management

The nurse performs a comprehensive assessment of each client's pain on admission as mandated by The Joint Commission (see Table 11-3). Regularly thereafter, the nurse determines the onset, quality, intensity, location, and duration of the client's pain. He or she explains the tool for assessing a client's pain so the client understands how to self-report his or her level of pain when the assessment tool is used again. Giving assurance that pain management is a nursing and agency priority is essential throughout the client's care. The nurse informs the client of available pain management techniques and incorporates any preferences or objections to interventions for pain management that the client may have when establishing a plan of care.

The nurse collaborates with each client about his or her goal for a level of pain relief and implements interventions for achieving the goal. The nurse never doubts or minimizes the client's description of pain or need for pain relief. If a client's goal for pain relief is not reached, the nurse collaborates with members of the health team for other approaches that may do so. Scheduling the administration of analgesics every 3 hours, rather than on an as-needed (prn) basis, often affords a uniform level of pain relief. Pro-

Nutrition Notes 11-1
The Client Receiving Drug Therapy for Pain

- Administering pain medications 30 to 45 minutes before meals may relieve pain and enable the client to consume an adequate nutritional intake.
- Small, frequent meals may help maximize intake in clients with drug-related or pain-related anorexia. Solicit food preferences.
- A high-fiber diet (i.e., a diet rich in whole grain breads and cereals, fresh fruits, and vegetables) along with increased fluids may help ease constipation, a possible side effect of opioids.

viding a client with equipment to self-administer analgesics, as with a PCA pump, also promotes a more consistent level of pain relief.

When medications are administered, the nurse monitors for and implements measures for managing side effects (see Drug Therapy Table 11-1). Problems that may develop with opioid and opiate therapy include Risk for Impaired Gas Exchange related to respiratory depression, Constipation related to slowed peristalsis, Risk for Injury related to drowsiness and unsteady gait, Risk for Imbalanced Nutrition: Less than Body Requirements related to anorexia and nausea, Risk for Deficient Fluid Volume related to reduced oral intake, and Disturbed Sleep Pattern (excessive or interrupted sleep) related to depression of the central nervous system. Some general nutrition considerations are listed in Nutrition Notes 11-1.

Client and Family Teaching 11-1
Pain

The nurse encourages the client and family to:

- Discuss with the physician what to expect from the disorder, injury, or its treatment.
- Talk with the physician about any concerns that relate to drug therapy.
- Share information about what drugs or pain-relieving techniques have and have not been helpful during previous episodes.
- Identify drug allergies to avoid adverse effects.
- Inform the physician about other medications being taken to avoid drug–drug interactions.
- Take prescribed drugs exactly as directed and report untoward effects.
- Avoid taking over-the-counter drugs unless the physician has been consulted; follow label directions for administration.
- Avoid alcohol and sedative drugs if the analgesic causes sedation.
- Keep analgesic drugs out of the reach of children; request childproof caps.
- Never share medications with others or take someone else's medications for pain.

BOX 11-2 **Nursing Responsibilities for Managing Pain**

- Assess for pain on a frequent and regular basis
- Respond quickly to a client's or family's report of pain
- Acknowledge the client's pain
- Explain available options for managing pain
- Encourage the client's participation in pain management decisions
- Respect the client's choice for managing the pain
- Implement measures to relieve pain in a timely manner
- Evaluate the effectiveness of an intervention
- Advocate on the client's behalf if pain is unrelieved or insufficiently relieved
- Provide pain-relieving alternatives
- Communicate with healthcare members concerning approaches and outcomes of a client's pain management

NURSING CARE PLAN 11-1 The Client With Acute Pain

Assessment

- Determine the following:
  - Source of client's pain; when it began; its intensity, location, characteristics, and related factors such as what makes the pain better or worse
  - How client's pain interferes with life, such as diminishing the ability to meet his or her own needs for hygiene, eating, sleep, activity, social interactions, emotional stability, concentration, and so forth
  - At what level client can tolerate pain

- Pain-related behaviors such as grimacing, crying, moaning, and assuming a guarded position
- Measure vital signs.
- Perform a physical assessment, taking care to gently support and assist client to turn as you examine various structures. Use light palpation in areas that are tender. Show concern when assessment techniques increase client's pain.
- Postpone nonpriority assessments until client's pain has been reduced.

Nursing Diagnosis: Acute Pain related to cellular injury or disease as manifested by stating, "I'm in severe pain"; rating pain at 10 using a numeric scale; pointing to the lower left abdominal quadrant; describing the pain as "continuous, throbbing, and starting this morning" without any known cause

Expected Outcomes: Client will rate the pain intensity at his or her tolerable level of "5" within 30 minutes of implementing a pain management technique.

Interventions	Rationales
Assess client's pain and its characteristics at least every 2 hours while awake and 30 minutes after implementing a pain management technique.	Quick interventions prevent or minimize pain.
Modify or eliminate factors that contribute to pain such as a full bladder, uncomfortable position, pain-aggravating activity, excessively warm or cool environment, noise, and social isolation.	Multiple stressors decrease pain tolerance.
Determine client's choice for pain relief techniques from among those available.	Encourage and respect client's participation in decision-making.
Administer prescribed analgesics or alternative pain management techniques promptly.	Suffering contributes to the pain experience and can be reduced by eliminating delays in nursing response.
Advocate on client's behalf for higher doses of prescribed analgesics or addition of adjuvant drug therapy if pain is not satisfactorily relieved.	Joint Commission standards mandate for nurses and other healthcare workers to facilitate pain relief for clients.
Administer a prescribed analgesic before a procedure or activity that is likely to result in or intensify pain.	Prophylactic interventions facilitate keeping pain at a manageable level.
Plan for periods of rest between activity.	Fatigue and exhaustion interfere with pain tolerance.
Reassure client that there are many ways to modify the pain experience.	Suggesting that there are additional untried options helps alleviate frustration or despair that there is no hope for pain relief.
Assist client to visualize a pleasant experience.	Imaging interrupts pain perception.
Help client focus on deep breathing, relaxing muscles, watching television, putting together a puzzle, or talking to someone on the phone.	Diverting attention to something other than pain reduces pain perception.
Apply warm or cool compresses to a painful sensory site.	Flooding the brain with alternative stimuli closes the spinal gates that transmit pain.
Gently massage a painful area or the same area on the opposite side of the body (contralateral massage).	Massage promotes the release of endorphins and enkephalins that moderate the sensation.
Promote laughter by suggesting that client relate a humorous story or watch a video or comedy of his or her choice.	Laughter releases endorphins and enkephalins that promote a feeling of well-being.

Evaluation of Expected Outcomes

- Client reports that pain is gone or at a tolerable level of "5" within 30 minutes.
- Client perceives the pain experience realistically and copes effectively.
- Client participates in self-care activities without undue pain.

The nurse may administer adjuvant drugs or implement nondrug alternatives for pain management to enhance the effect of opioid and nonopioid analgesics or as a substitute when drug side effects jeopardize the client's safety. When planning for the client's discharge from the healthcare agency, the nurse includes interventions for pain relief to facilitate a comfortable transition to the next level of care. Box 11-2 summarizes nursing responsibilities for managing pain.

An important component of pain management is client and family teaching (see Client and Family Teaching 11-1). Nursing Care Plan 11-1 details the nursing care of a client with acute pain.

CRITICAL THINKING EXERCISES

1. What questions should the nurse ask when a client states he or she has pain?
2. Discuss how acute pain after surgery is different from pain experienced by a client with chronic back pain.
3. Discuss nursing interventions that are appropriate if a client does not experience adequate pain relief from a prescribed analgesic.
4. What actions should a nurse take if a client he or she assumes to be in pain cannot verbalize discomfort?
5. If a client has an order for morphine sulfate 5 mg IM q 3 to 4 hours prn and ibuprofen (Motrin) 800 mg po tid prn and has not experienced pain relief 2 hours after receiving the morphine, what could the nurse do?

NCLEX-STYLE REVIEW QUESTIONS

1. A client has developed physical dependence on an opioid drug for pain relief. Which of the following interventions is appropriate first?
   1. Immediately discontinue all drug therapy.
   2. Replace the opioid with a nonopioid drug.
   3. Gradually decrease the dosage and frequency of the opioid.
   4. Increase the dosage but decrease the frequency of the opioid.
2. A postoperative client requests pain medication. Following the administration of morphine sulfate, which information is most important for the nurse to collect?
   1. Color and temperature of the skin
   2. Presence of bowel sounds
   3. Rate and depth of respirations
   4. Rhythm and force of the heart rate
3. A client comes to the emergency department because of severe upper abdominal pain. The client reports that it came on suddenly a few hours ago, and nothing thus far has relieved it. The nurse observes that the client is curled in a fetal position and is rocking back and forth. Which action would best assist the nurse in further assessing the client's pain?
   1. Ask the client to rate the pain on a scale from 0 to 10
   2. Determine if the client can stop moving about
   3. Give the client a prescribed pain-relieving drug
   4. Observe if the client is breathing heavily.
4. A client with metastatic cancer of the pancreas has an advance directive that requests no aggressive treatment. The client is referred for hospice care. If there is a physician's order for pain medication every 3 to 4 hours as necessary, which action by the hospice nurse is most appropriate in order to provide the client with maximum comfort at this time?
   1. Administer the medication every 3 hours
   2. Ask the physician to prescribe a high dose
   3. Give the medication immediately upon request
   4. Give the medication when the pain is severe
5. A client who has had chronic back pain for two months is going to be treated with transcutaneous electrical nerve stimulation (TENS). The nurse correctly describes the electrical stimulus as feeling like which of the following?
   1. Hard knocking feeling
   2. Intermittent burning reaction
   3. Pleasant tingling sensation
   4. Small shock to the affected area

12

Infection

Words To Know

bacteremia
carrier
community-acquired infections
culture
emerging infectious diseases
epidemic
fomites
host
chain of infection
leukocytosis
means of transmission
microorganisms
multidrug resistance
nonpathogens
nosocomial infections
opportunistic infections
pandemic
pathogens
phagocytosis
portal of entry
portal of exit
prion
reemerging infectious diseases
reservoir
sensitivity
sepsis
septicemia
severe sepsis
standard precautions
superinfections
susceptibility
transmission-based precautions
virulence
zoonotic pathogens

Learning Objectives

On completion of this chapter, you will be able to:

1. Describe types of infectious agents and list examples.
2. Differentiate between nonpathogens and pathogens.
3. Describe the six components of the chain of infection.
4. List factors that increase susceptibility to infection.
5. Explain the difference between mechanical and chemical defense mechanisms.
6. Describe events during the inflammatory process.
7. Differentiate localized from generalized infections.
8. List reasons why clients in healthcare agencies are at increased risk for infection.
9. Explain nursing actions to prevent or control transmission of infection in the hospital and in the community.
10. Describe measures to take if a needlestick injury occurs.
11. Name diagnostic tests ordered for clients suspected of having an infectious disorder.
12. Discuss the medical management of clients with infectious disorders.
13. Describe nursing care for the client with a potential or actual infection.

nfections have always plagued humankind. This chapter discusses the causes of infections, their transmission, methods for preventing and controlling infections, and techniques for managing the care of clients with infections.

INFECTIOUS AGENTS AND INFECTIOUS DISORDERS

Infection is the invasion of the body with agents that have the potential to cause disease. Infectious disorders are conditions that result from these infectious agents. Some infectious agents cause *communicable* or *contagious diseases*, infectious disorders that can be transmitted from one person to another. Examples include measles, streptococcal sore throat, sexually transmitted infections, and tuberculosis.

Types of Infectious Agents

Types of infectious agents include microorganisms and prions. **Microorganisms**, commonly called *germs*, are so small they can be seen only with a microscope. Infectious microorganisms include bacteria, viruses, fungi, rickettsiae, protozoans, mycoplasmas, helminths, and prions.

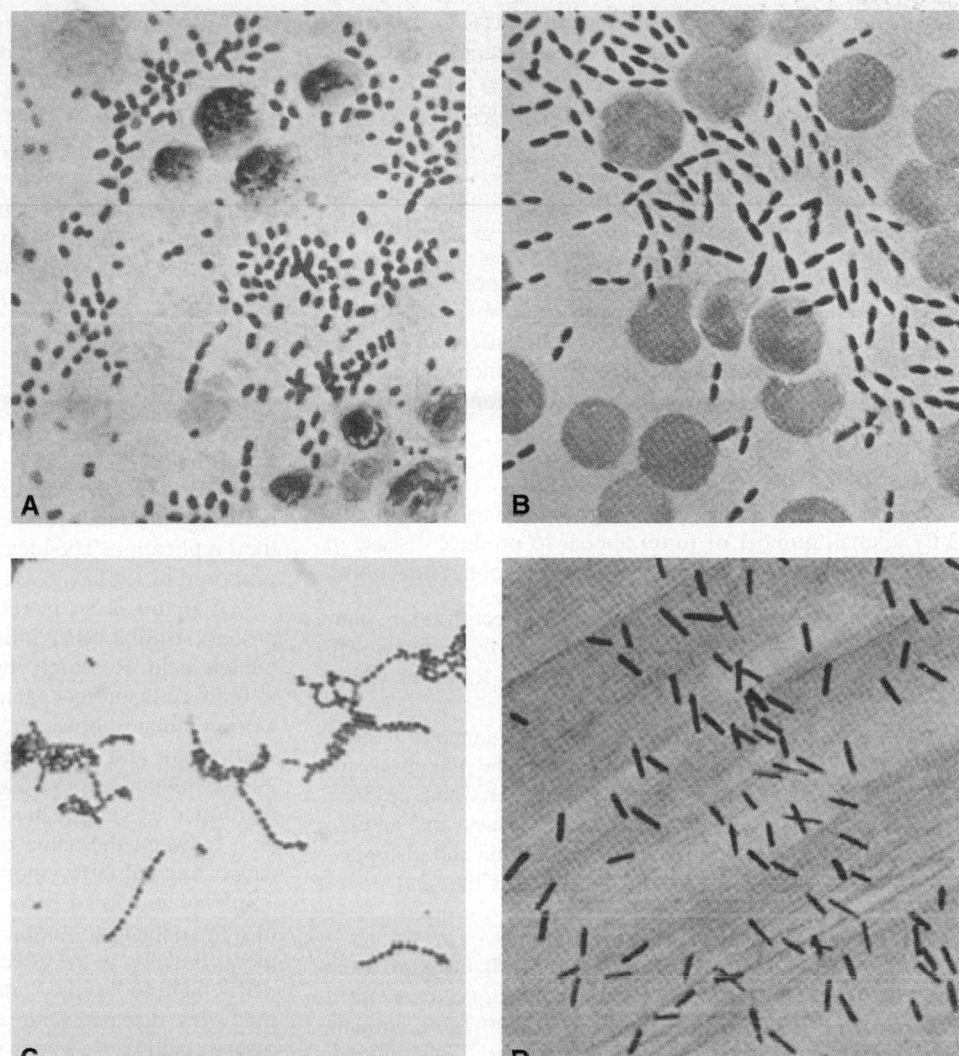

FIGURE 12-1. A sampling of microscopic bacteria demonstrating a variety of shapes and sizes: **(A)** bacilli known as *Yersinia pestis*; **(B)** diplococci known as *Streptococci pneumoniae*; **(C)** diplococci identified with Gram stain; **(D)** bacilli known as *Escherichia coli*. (From Public Images Library, Centers for Disease Control and Prevention. Available at: http://phil.cdc.gov.)

Bacteria

Bacteria are single-celled microorganisms. They appear in various shapes (Fig. 12-1). Round bacteria are called cocci and are further classified by how they grow. Staphylococci are round bacteria that grow in clusters; streptococci are round bacteria that grow in chains; and diplococci are round bacteria that grow in pairs. Rod-shaped bacteria are called bacilli. Spiral-shaped bacteria are called spirochetes.

Bacteria may be aerobic or anaerobic. *Aerobic bacteria* require oxygen to grow and multiply, whereas *anaerobic bacteria* grow and multiply in an atmosphere that lacks oxygen.

Some bacteria, such as *Staphylococcus aureus*, *Streptococcus pneumoniae*, and *Escherichia coli*, are developing **multidrug resistance**, the ability to remain unaffected by antimicrobial drugs such as antibiotics. Causes of antibiotic resistance, a consequence of bacterial mutations that interfere with the mechanism of antibiotic action, are related to the following:

• Inappropriate prescription of antibiotics for viral (rather than bacterial) infections

• Less than full client compliance with antibiotic drug regimens

• Prophylactic (preventive) administration of antibiotics without infection

• Environmental dispersal of antibiotic solutions that intermingle with microorganisms, such as when partially empty intravenous (IV) bags are deposited in waste containers or droplets are released when purging IV tubing or removing air from syringes used to inject antibiotics

• Administration of antibiotics to livestock, leaving traces of drug residue after slaughter

Infections with multidrug-resistant microorganisms are very difficult to destroy with pharmacologic agents. Thus, the potential for death from such infections is increased.

Viruses

Viruses are so small that they can be seen only with high-powered electron microscopes. They also are filterable, meaning they pass through very small barriers. Viruses are divided into two types: (1) those whose nucleic acid is composed of deoxyribonucleic acid (DNA), and (2) those whose nucleic acid is composed of ribonucleic acid (RNA). Viruses use the metabolic and reproductive materials of living cells or tissues to grow and reproduce. Viruses may survive, albeit not very long, outside a living organism or host, but they cannot reproduce outside the host because they lack their own genetic components for this.

Some viral infections, such as the common cold, are minor and *self-limiting*; that is, they terminate with or without medical treatment. Others, such as those that cause rabies, poliomyelitis, and viral hepatitis, are more serious and may be fatal. Occasionally, viruses are dormant in a living host, reactivate periodically, and cause the infection to recur. An example is the herpes simplex virus, which causes periodic outbreaks of cold sores (fever blisters) long after the initial infection (see Chap. 56).

Fungi

Fungi are divided into two basic groups: yeasts and molds. Only a small number of fungi appear to produce disease in humans. There are three types of fungal (mycotic) infections:

- *Superficial* (dermatophytoses), which affect the skin, hair, and nails; examples include *tinea corporis*, or ringworm, and *tinea pedis*, also known as athlete's foot (see Chap. 65)
- *Intermediate*, which chiefly affect subcutaneous tissues; an example is *candidiasis*, which affects the mucous membrane in the mouth, pharynx, or vagina (see Chap. 56)
- *Deep* (systemic), which affect deep tissues and organs; examples include pneumocystis pneumonia and histoplasmosis, both of which affect the lungs (see Chap. 35)

Rickettsiae

Rickettsiae resemble but are different from bacteria. Like viruses, they invade living cells and cannot survive outside a living organism or host. Arthropods (invertebrate animals with a segmented body, an external skeleton, and jointed, paired appendages) transmit rickettsial diseases. Examples of arthropods include fleas, ticks, lice, mosquitoes, and mites. Some rickettsial diseases that are spread by arthropods include Lyme disease, malaria, West Nile virus, eastern equine encephalitis, Rocky Mountain spotted fever, and bubonic plaque.

Protozoans

Protozoans are single-celled organisms classified according to their motility (ability to move). Some possess *amoeboid motion*, meaning that they extend their cell walls and their intracellular contents flow forward. Others move by means of *cilia*, hair-like projections, or *flagella*, whip-like appendages. Still others have little or no independent movement. *Giardia* is a protozoan-transmitted intestinal disorder that results in severe diarrhea.

Mycoplasmas

Mycoplasmas are single-celled microorganisms that lack a cell wall and, therefore, are pleomorphic (assume many shapes). They are similar to but not related to bacteria. They primarily infect the surface linings of the respiratory, genitourinary, and gastrointestinal (GI) tracts. Infections can range from pneumonia to urethritis (inflammation of the urethra). Some believe that mycoplasmas are a co-factor in various

other diseases such as Gulf War syndrome, chronic fatigue syndrome, and Crohn's disease (Chaps. 34 and 46) (Baseman & Tully, 1997).

Helminths

Helminths are infectious worms. Some are microscopic; others are easily visible. They are divided into three major groups: nematodes or roundworms, such as pinworms that infect the colon and rectum; cestodes or tapeworms; and trematodes, also known as flukes or flatworms. Some helminths enter the body in the egg stage, whereas others spend the larval stage in an intermediate host and then enter the human host. The organisms mate and reproduce in the infected host and are then excreted, after which the cycle begins again.

Prions

Until recently, the scientific community believed all infectious agents contained nucleic acid (DNA or RNA), enabling their replication. The idea of an atypical infectious agent was proposed in 1967.

A **prion** is an infectious particle made up entirely of protein. Unlike other infectious agents, it does not contain nucleic acid. Research suggests that normal prions, present in brain cells, protect against dementia (see Chap. 72). When a prion mutates, however, it is capable of becoming an infectious agent and changing other normal prion proteins into similar mutant copies. The mutant prions, which can either be formed by genetic predisposition or acquired by transmission between the same or similar infected animal species, cause transmissible spongiform encephalopathies (TSEs). TSEs are so named because the brain becomes spongy (full of holes), the brain tissue withers, and uncoordinated movements develop in the affected person or animal. Examples of TSEs include bovine spongiform encephalopathy (BSE) or mad cow disease, scrapie in sheep, and Creutzfeldt-Jakob disease (CJD). Research is ongoing to determine if mutant prions contribute to Alzheimer's disease (see Chap. 72), Parkinson's disease, and Huntington's disease (see Chap. 37), or if clients with these disorders lack sufficient or have ineffective prions.

Mutant prions have been transmitted from sheep to cattle when cattle are fed waste parts of slaughtered infected sheep. Although one form of CJD is known to be inherited, a new-variant form has developed in humans who have consumed beef infected with BSE in Europe. To prevent the transmission of new-variant CJD, infected animals are destroyed, and potentially infected animal tissues are banned from human consumption. The Centers for Disease Control and Prevention (2007, 2001) advises Americans traveling to Europe to avoid eating beef or beef products or to eat solid pieces of muscle meat from beef rather than ground meat products, which may contain tissues with infectious prions. Following the discovery of a BSE-infected Canadian cow in Washington State in 2003 and a Texas cow suspected of having BSE in 2004, the Food and Drug Administration (FDA) has also taken actions to strengthen the public health protection of people within the United States from acquiring this disease (U.S. Food and Drug Administration, 2004). Additionally, the American Red Cross adopted a new policy placing restrictions on blood donations to prevent the potential for collecting prion-contaminated blood (Meckler

& Ricks, 2001). The policy bans blood collection from anyone who has lived in the United Kingdom for a total of 6 months or longer between 1980 and 1996, lived in various countries in Europe including while serving in the military since 1980, or received a blood transfusion in the United Kingdom.

Characteristics of Infectious Agents

Not all microorganisms and prions are dangerous. Some are **nonpathogens** because they generally are harmless to healthy humans. For example, nonpathogens in the intestine help synthesize vitamin B_{12}, biotin, vitamin K, and folic acid. **Pathogens**, on the other hand, have a high potential to cause infectious diseases. Given the right circumstances, however, both pathogens and nonpathogens can cause infections.

Once infectious agents invade the body, one of three events occurs: (1) the body's immune defense mechanisms eliminate them (see Chap. 33), (2) they reside in the body without causing disease, or (3) they cause an infection or infectious disease. Factors that influence whether a microorganism becomes a pathogen and whether an infection develops are the type of microorganism and its characteristics and the components of the chain of infection.

INFECTION TRANSMISSION

The six components involved in the transmission of microorganisms are described as the **chain of infection**. All components in the chain of infection must be present to transmit an infectious disease from one human or animal to a susceptible host (Fig. 12-2): an infectious agent, an appropriate reservoir, exit route, means of transmission, portal of entry, and susceptible host.

Infectious Agent

Characteristics of the infectious agent that must be present include the ability to move or be moved from one place to another, **virulence** (power to produce disease), an adequate number of agents, and the ability to invade a host.

Reservoir

A **reservoir** is the environment in which the infectious agent can survive and reproduce. It may be human, animal, or nonliving, such as contaminated food and water. A human or animal that harbors (or is the reservoir of) an infectious microorganism but does not show active evidence of infectious disease is a **carrier**. Nonliving reservoirs are **fomites**.

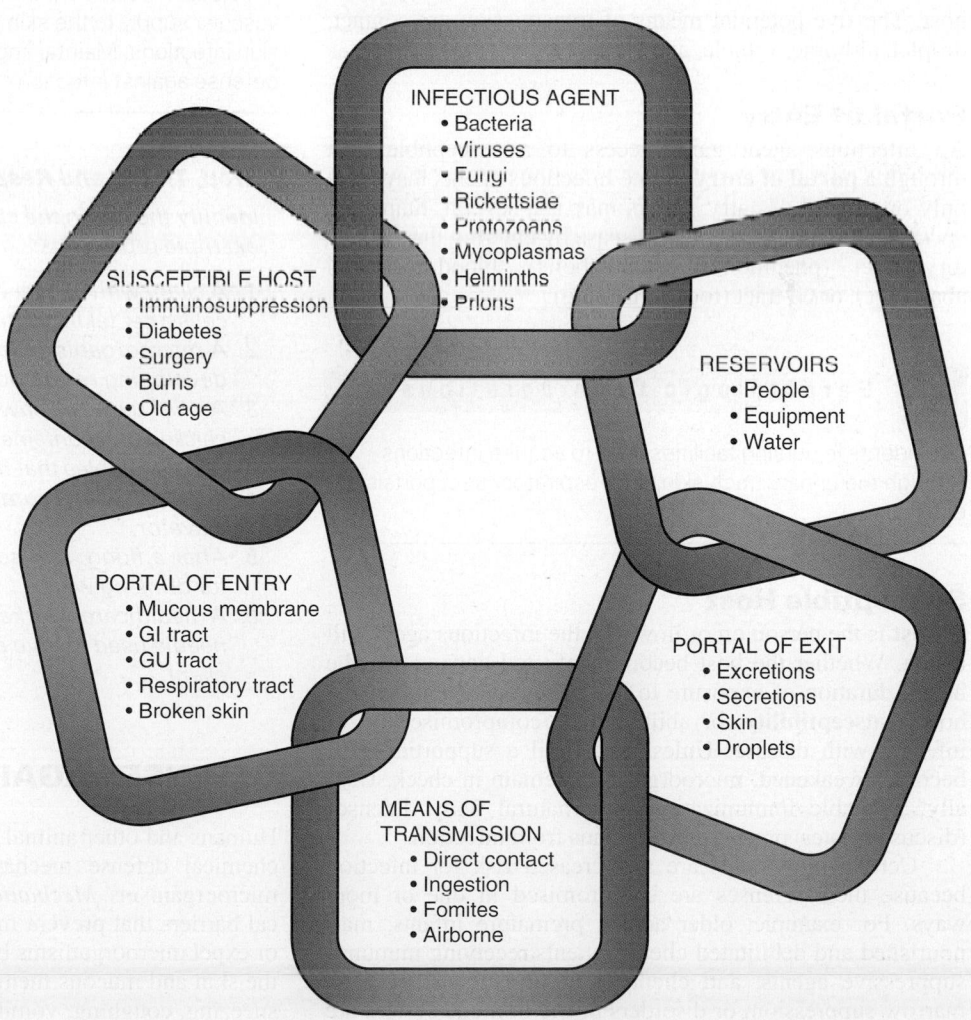

FIGURE 12-2. The chain of infection. (GI, gastrointestinal; GU, genitourinary.)

TABLE 12-1 Common Means of Transmission

ROUTE OF TRANSMISSION	DESCRIPTION	EXAMPLE
Contact		
Direct	Infected person to susceptible person	Sexual intercourse
Indirect	Contaminated substance to susceptible person	Handling a contaminated paper tissue
Droplet	Spray of moist particles within a 3-foot radius of infected person	Sneezing, coughing, talking
Airborne	Suspension and transport on air currents beyond 3 feet	Inhalation of microorganisms attached to dust particles
Vehicle	On or in contaminated food, water, objects, or equipment	Eating or drinking tainted products
Vector	Infected animal or insect to susceptible person	Transfer from bites of mosquitoes, bats, or ticks

Portal of Exit

The **portal of exit** is the route by which the infectious agent escapes from the reservoir. Examples include the respiratory, GI, or genitourinary tract; the skin and mucous membranes; and blood and other body fluids.

Means of Transmission

A microorganism's **means of transmission** refers to how it is transferred or moved from its reservoir to the susceptible host. The five potential means of transmission are contact, droplet, airborne, vehicle, and vector (Table 12-1).

Portal of Entry

An infectious agent gains access to a susceptible host through a **portal of entry**. Some infectious agents may have only one portal of entry; others may use several. Staphylococci, for example, can cause disease by entering the respiratory tract (pneumonia), skin (boils), blood (internal abscesses), or GI tract (food poisoning).

Gerontologic Considerations

- Residents in nursing facilities tend to acquire infections through the urinary tract, skin, and respiratory tract portals of entry.

Susceptible Host

A **host** is the person on or in whom the infectious agent will reside. Whether the host becomes infected depends on the host's duration of exposure to the infectious agent and the host's **susceptibility**, or ability to be compromised by or infected with disease. Unless and until a supporting host becomes weakened, microorganisms remain in check. Usually, available immunizations and natural body defenses (discussed later) protect most humans from infection.

Certain individuals are at increased risk for infection because their defenses are compromised in one or more ways. For example, older adults, premature infants, malnourished and debilitated clients, clients receiving immunosuppressive agents, and clients with impaired skin, bone marrow suppression, or disorders of the immune system are especially susceptible to virulent and nonvirulent strains of microorganisms.

Gerontologic Considerations

- Older adults with chronic conditions are at an increased risk for infections, especially infections that are resistant to antibiotics. In addition, thinning, drying, and decreases in vascular supply to the skin predispose the older person to skin infections. Maintaining intact skin is an excellent first-line defense against infection.

▶ ***Stop, Think, and Respond Exercise 12-1***

Identify the link in the chain of infection that each example represents:

1. *A client with cancer cannot produce sufficient blood cells after taking anticancer drugs.*
2. *A microorganism becomes especially virulent after developing resistance to multiple antibiotics.*
3. *A chef uses an unwashed counter to cut both raw chicken that contains infectious microorganisms and raw vegetables that he will incorporate into a salad.*
4. *A person with a common cold sneezes in a crowded elevator.*
5. *After a flood, raw sewage contaminates an aquifer for drinking water.*
6. *A healthcare worker receives a puncture from a needle used to give an injection to an HIV-positive client.*

DEFENSES AGAINST INFECTION

Humans and other animal species have both mechanical and chemical defense mechanisms to prevent infection with microorganisms. *Mechanical defense mechanisms* are physical barriers that prevent microorganisms from gaining entry or expel microorganisms before they multiply. Examples are the skin and mucous membranes, physiologic reflexes (e.g., sneezing, coughing, vomiting), and macrophages. *Chemical defense mechanisms* destroy or incapacitate microorganisms with naturally produced biologic substances. Examples include enzymes, antibodies, and secretions.

Mechanical Defenses

Skin and Mucous Membranes
The first line of defense against invading microorganisms is unbroken skin and mucous membranes, which separate underlying body tissues from environmental microorganisms. The normal flora (e.g., microorganisms) found on the skin compete with pathogens for nutrients, slowing pathogenic growth in these areas. In addition, the skin, which is acidic (because of the acetic acid in perspiration), creates an undesirable medium for pathogenic multiplication.

Mucus, a sticky substance secreted from mucous membranes, traps microorganisms and debris on its surface. For example, vaginal mucous membrane secretions favor the growth of nonpathogenic acid-producing bacteria, known as *Doederlein's bacilli*. The acid environment is unfavorable for the multiplication of pathogenic bacteria and fungi. A change in vaginal pH or destruction of the normal flora, however, can promote the development of a vaginal infection (see Chap. 53).

Physiologic Reflexes
If microorganisms gain entry, sneezing, coughing, and vomiting can forcefully expel them. Coughing is promoted by cilia in the upper respiratory tract that beat upward.

Macrophages
Macrophages are specialized cells that make up the *mononuclear phagocyte* system, formerly known as the reticuloendothelial system (see Chap. 33). They are located throughout body tissues and in the liver (*Kupffer's cells*), spleen, and lymphoid tissue (e.g., tonsils). Their primary function is **phagocytosis**, the ingestion of cells and foreign material, including microorganisms.

Chemical Defenses

Enzymes
Lysozyme (e.g., muramidase), an enzyme capable of splitting (lysing) the cell wall of some gram-positive bacteria, is present in tears, saliva, mucus, skin secretions, and some internal body fluids (e.g., gastric juices). Lysozyme is *bactericidal* (destroys bacteria) and thus defends against some pathogenic bacteria.

Antibodies
Antibodies, complex proteins also referred to as *immunoglobulins*, form when macrophages consume microorganisms and display the microorganisms' distinct cellular markers from their surfaces. Antibodies work with other white blood cells (WBCs) by rendering microorganisms more easily ingested (phagocytized) in one of several ways: by *lysing* (dissolving or reducing size) them, *neutralizing* their *toxins* (poisons that some microorganisms release), *opsonizing* (coating) them, *agglutinating* (clumping) them, or *precipitating* (solidifying) them.

Secretions
The WBCs and other cells produce *interferon*, another chemical protein, in response to viral infections and other factors. Interferon appears to trigger infected cells to manufacture an antiviral protein. Because it also appears to inhibit cell reproduction, interferon is being used in the adjunctive treatment of some cancers and viral disorders with positive results.

PATHOPHYSIOLOGY OF INFECTION

Despite the various defense mechanisms, humans continue to succumb to infections. Regardless of the specific process, all infections share some common pathophysiologic characteristics. Most infections remain localized. Some lead to sepsis and complications such as septic shock.

Localized Infection
The initial localized reaction to an invading microorganism activates the inflammatory process (Fig. 12-3). The cellular response results in leakage of fluid, colloids, and ions from the capillaries into the tissues between the cells, producing swelling (Fig. 12-4). An ensuing vascular response produces redness and heat, whereas a chemical response causes pain. WBCs—neutrophils, macrophages, monocytes, and lymphocytes—move to the injury site to destroy the toxins produced by the pathogens and to remove debris from the area.

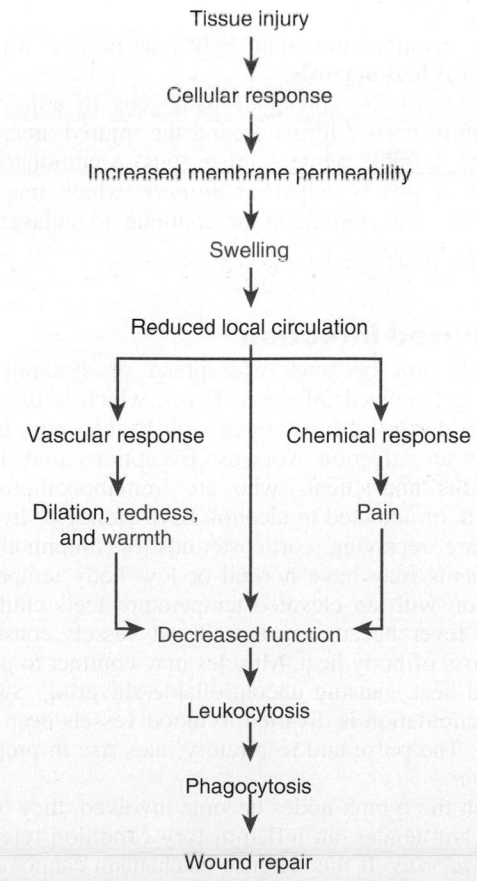

FIGURE 12-3. The inflammatory process.

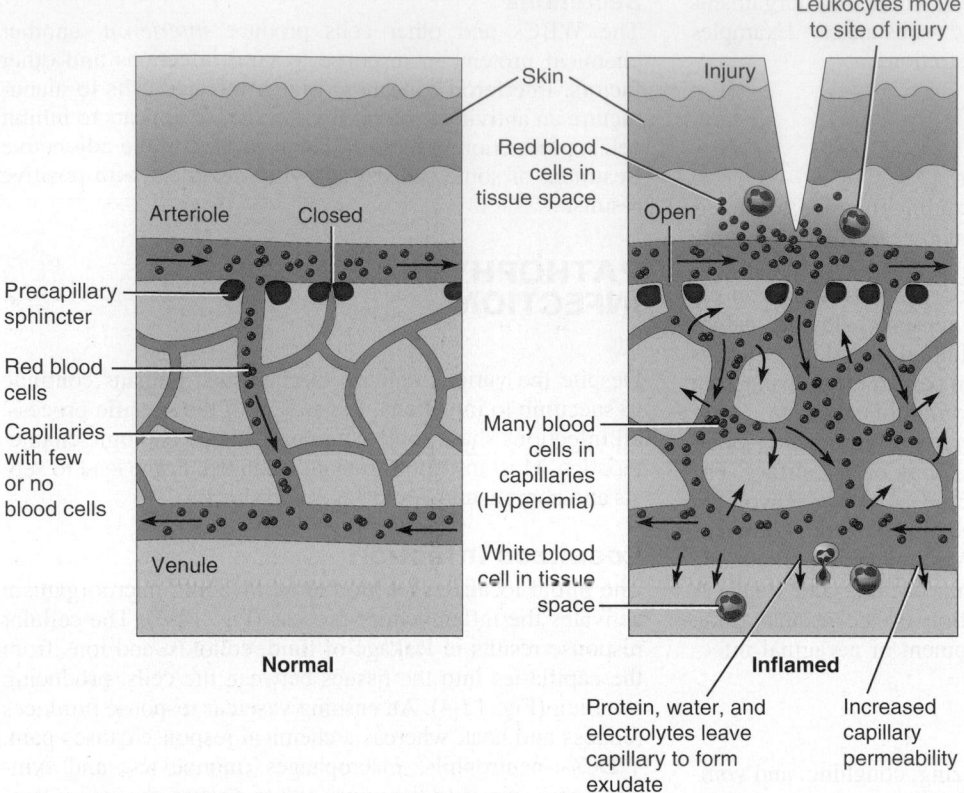

FIGURE 12-4. Vascular changes in acute inflammation. (From Premkumar, K. [2004]. *The massage connection: Anatomy and physiology.* Baltimore: Lippincott Williams & Wilkins.)

The body manufactures more WBCs as needed, a process referred to as **leukocytosis**.

To prevent the spread of pathogens to adjacent tissues, a fibrin barrier forms around the injured area. Inside the barrier, a thick, white exudate (pus) accumulates. This collection of pus is called an *abscess*, which may break through the skin and drain or continue to enlarge internally (Fig. 12-5).

Generalized Infection

If the infection becomes widespread or systemic, it is termed a generalized infection. Fever, which is the body's attempt to destroy the pathogen with heat, occurs in most people as an infection worsens. Exceptions may include older adults and clients who are immunocompromised, debilitated, or addicted to alcohol; have kidney or liver failure; or are receiving corticosteroids or immunotherapy. These clients may have normal or low body temperature. The person with an elevated temperature feels chilled despite the fever because surface blood vessels constrict to prevent loss of body heat. Muscles may contract to produce additional heat, causing uncontrollable shivering. Sweating stops as circulation is diverted to blood vessels deep within the body. The pulse and respiratory rates rise in proportion to the fever.

When the lymph nodes become involved, they become enlarged and tender, an inflammatory condition referred to as *lymphadenitis*. If this defense mechanism cannot contain the infection, the microorganisms begin to travel from node to node (see Chap. 32). Because the lymphatic system drains into the venous system, the microorganisms may eventually reach the bloodstream, causing a condition called **bacteremia** or **septicemia**.

Sepsis

Septicemia may lead to **sepsis**, a systemic inflammatory response syndrome resulting from infection. The pathophysiology of sepsis varies, depending on the virulence of the pathogen and condition of the host. Two or more of the following characterize sepsis:

- Temperature greater than 100.4°F (38°C) or less than 96.8°F (36°C)
- Heart rate greater than 90 beats per minute
- Respiratory rate greater than 20 breaths per minute or $Paco_2$ less than 32 mm Hg
- WBC count greater than 12,000 cells/mm³ or 10% immature (band) forms

The body uses an inflammatory response to suppress the infectious process. Once the proinflammatory mechanisms achieve a beneficial effect, the body releases anti-inflammatory mediators to restore homeostasis.

Severe Sepsis

An estimated 750,000 people per year in the United States develop **severe sepsis**, a disorder associated with organ dysfunction, hypotension, and hypoperfusion manifested by lactic acidosis, oliguria, and acute alteration in mental status (Porth, 2007). Basically, the system of proinflammatory mechanisms remains unchecked in severe sepsis. The

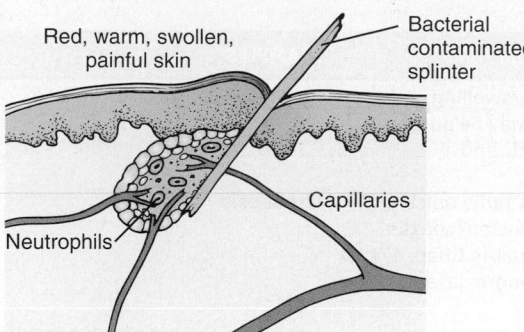

A Inflammation
Capillary dilation, fluid exudation, neutrophil migration

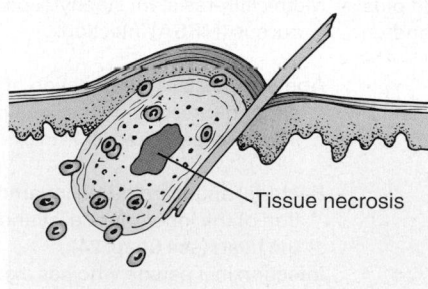

B Suppuration
Development of suppurative or purulent exudate containing degraded neutrophils and tissue debris

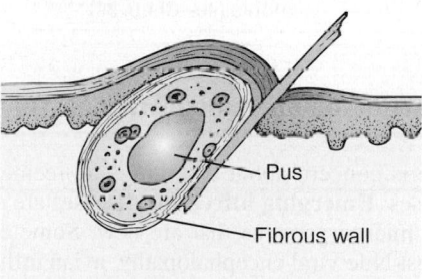

C Abscess formation
Walling off of the area of purulent (pus) exudate to form an abscess

FIGURE 12-5. Abscess formation. **(A)** Bacterial invasion and development of inflammation. **(B)** Continued bacterial growth, neutrophil migration, liquefaction tissue necrosis, and development of a purulent exudate. **(C)** Walling off of the inflamed area with its purulent exudate to form an abscess. (From Porth, C. M. [2007]. *Essentials of pathophysiology: Concepts in altered health states* [2nd ed.]. Philadelphia: Lippincott Williams & Wilkins.)

proinflammatory response promotes coagulation of blood (microvascular clots) and suppression of fibrinolysis, the process by which clots are dissolved. Systemic microvascular clotting leads to multiple organ failure because it interferes with delivery of oxygen to cells.

Some believe that severe sepsis results from deficiency of a substance called *protein C*, an inhibitor of coagulation. Protein C may also be responsible for interrupting the inflammatory cycle.

Although sepsis and severe sepsis are treated with one or more antimicrobial drugs, severe sepsis remains quite lethal. Many with severe sepsis develop septic shock (see Chap. 17) and die. A drug called *drotrecogin alfa* (Xigris) has been approved by the FDA for the sickest individuals with severe sepsis (Gillis, 2001). Xigris is a recombinant form of human protein C. According to the company that developed Xigris, the drug has reduced the death rate for severe sepsis from 44% to 29% (Eli Lilly and Company, 2007).

TYPES OF INFECTIONS

Infections can be described in terms of site (localized or generalized), source (community-acquired or nosocomial), and duration (acute or chronic/subacute). They may be further described by circumstances of infection (secondary or opportunistic). Table 12-2 explains these terms used to describe infections. The following sections discuss some of these types, as well as the concern regarding emerging and reemerging infectious diseases.

Community-Acquired Infections
Community-acquired infections, which are acquired in the community setting, are infectious communicable diseases, meaning that they are transmitted from one infected person or reservoir to another. Besides general systemic signs of infection (see Table 12-2), community-acquired diseases produce clusters of signs and symptoms that reflect dysfunction of the organs or tissues that the microorganisms have invaded. For example, a person with TB (see Chap. 21) develops a cough, lung congestion, and compromised gas exchange. A person with meningitis (see Chap. 37) develops a stiff neck, headache, arching of the back, and possibly seizures.

Nosocomial Infections
Nosocomial infections are infections acquired while receiving care in a healthcare agency that were not active, incubatory, or chronic at admission. They occur for many reasons. Hospitalized clients are more susceptible to infections than well people because they are exposed to pathogens in the healthcare environment, may have incisions or invasive equipment (e.g., IV lines) that compromise skin integrity, or may be immunosuppressed from poor nutrition, their disease process, or its treatment. Also, because healthcare personnel are in frequent and direct contact with many clients who harbor various microorganisms, the risk for transmitting pathogenic microorganisms between and among clients is high. Visitors also may introduce pathogens into the healthcare environment, as may equipment (e.g., wheelchairs) and facilities shared among several people (e.g., common bathrooms).

 Gerontologic Considerations

- Infections are often transmitted to vulnerable older adults through hospital equipment reservoirs such as indwelling urinary catheters, humidifiers, and oxygen equipment, or through incisional sites such as those for intravenous tubing, parenteral nutrition, or tube feedings. Handwashing, standard

TABLE 12-2 Types of Infections

TYPE	DESCRIPTION	COMMON SIGNS AND SYMPTOMS	EXAMPLES
Localized	Confined to a small area	Pain, redness, warmth, swelling, collection of fluid that may be purulent, swollen lymph nodes, and leukocytosis	Furuncle (boil)
Generalized	Systemic or widespread in one or more organs	Fever, chills, shivering, rapid pulse and respirations, hypotension (see discussion of septic shock in Chap. 17), headache, fatigue, anorexia, and marked leukocytosis	Urosepsis
Community-acquired	Transmitted from one infected species to another	Same as generalized plus organ-specific or disease-specific manifestations (e.g., rash with chickenpox, diarrhea with dysentery)	Influenza, chickenpox, tuberculosis
Nosocomial	Acquired in a healthcare agency and not present before admission	Same as localized and generalized plus additional manifestations depending on the infected tissue	Methicillin-resistant staphylococcus aureus (MRSA) infection
Acute	Sudden onset with serious and sometimes life-threatening manifestations	Symptoms appear suddenly	Appendicitis, an inflammation of the appendix secondary to a localized infection (see Chap. 46)
Chronic or subacute	An extended infection that resists treatment		Bacterial endocarditis, an inflammation of the inner muscle layer of the heart (see Chap. 24)
Secondary	A complication of some other disease process that occurred first		Infection in a person who has experienced severe burns
Opportunistic or superinfection	Occur among immuno-compromised hosts		Yeast infections in the mouth, bladder infections, gastroenteritis, and *Pneumocystis carinii* pneumonia (see Chap. 35)

precautions, and use of proper aseptic technique are essential preventive measures. Daily assessment for any signs of infection is imperative. Healthcare providers who are ill should take sick leave rather than expose susceptible older clients to infectious organisms.

Opportunistic Infections

In **opportunistic infections**, also called **superinfections**, nonpathogenic or remotely pathogenic microorganisms take advantage of favorable situations and overwhelm the host. For example, a prescribed antibiotic sometimes can upset biologic checks and balances. Although the antibiotic destroys one pathogen, other pathogens that the antibiotic does not affect grow and proliferate. Usually, however, common pathogens cause infections. Opportunistic infections commonly occur among immunocompromised clients.

Pharmacologic Considerations

- When a client is taking an antibiotic, a superinfection can result from overgrowth of microorganisms not affected by the drug. This can lead to a serious and potentially life-threatening diarrhea called *pseudomembranous colitis*. Report fever, abdominal cramps, and severe diarrhea immediately.

Emerging and Reemerging Infectious Diseases

Currently, there is concern about emerging and reemerging infectious diseases. **Emerging infectious diseases** are disorders caused by microorganisms that are new. Some examples include West Nile viral encephalopathy, avian influenza (bird flu), Lyme disease, Ebola hemorrhagic fever, and hantavirus pulmonary syndrome, all of which are transmitted by **zoonotic pathogens** that are spread from microorganisms to animals and then to humans. **Reemerging infectious diseases** are caused by microorganisms that have had a resurgence in the last 2 decades within and beyond a geographic range. Infectious diseases that are reemerging include tuberculosis, malaria, and influenza.

Gerontologic Considerations

- Older adults who had TB as children can experience reactivation of the disease if they become debilitated or experience a serious illness.

Collectively, emerging and reemerging infectious diseases are spreading because of (1) mutations among existing organisms, (2) increased world travel, (3) ecologic changes in human and animal habitats, (4) antimicrobial resistance, and (5) worldwide transport of animals and food products for human use. If unchecked, emerging and reemerging infectious diseases may cause **epidemics**, widespread infection in a confined geographic area, or **pandemics**, an infectious disorder that spreads to many different parts of the world in a relatively short amount of time.

INFECTION CONTROL AND PREVENTION

Precautions and Asepsis

Nurses and other healthcare personnel must take precautions to control infections when caring for all clients, regardless of diagnosis or infection status. These precautions are called **standard precautions**, measures for reducing the risk of transmitting pathogens from both recognized and unrecognized sources of infection (Box 12-1). Healthcare providers also must apply principles of medical asepsis, such as hand hygiene (Nursing Guidelines 12-1).

For clients known to be or suspected of being infected with highly transmissible pathogens, nurses and other healthcare personnel must also follow **transmission-based precautions** (Table 12-3). Because these precautions may isolate a client, it is important to consider the client's decreased social contact and lack of environmental stimulation. This isolation may increase confusion in older adults.

Prevention and Control of Nosocomial and Community-Acquired Infections

In addition to standard and transmission-based precautions and principles of medical asepsis, recommendations from the healthcare agency's infection-control committee provide further guidance to prevent and control nosocomial infections. Such committees usually consist of representatives from various areas and departments, such as medical staff, nursing service, clinical laboratories, pathology, operating room, housekeeping, and dietary service. Their responsibilities include conducting *surveillance*, the process of detecting, reporting, and recording nosocomial infections; educating personnel about methods to reduce nosocomial infections; providing guidelines for prevention of infectious diseases; and investigating outbreaks of nosocomial infections. Infection-control guidelines usually establish policies for pre-employment and postemployment health examinations, sterilization procedures and methods, disposal of garbage and biologic wastes, and housekeeping techniques; designate precautions to follow for specific infections; and define procedures for managing contaminated materials such as linens, equipment, and supplies used in the care of infectious clients.

Many community-acquired infections have been contained or eliminated because of advances in the prevention and treatment of infectious diseases. These advances include the discovery and use of antibiotics, the development of immunizing agents, guidelines for the proper disposal of human wastes, legislation controlling the preparation and sale of foods, immunization programs, and public education. Local, state, and federal public health agencies and the World Health Organization (WHO) cooperate in the detection and control of communicable diseases. Their combined efforts have reduced the incidence of many infectious

---

BOX 12-1 | Standard Precautions

- Wear clean gloves when touching:

  - Blood, body fluids, secretions, excretions, and items containing these body substances
  - Mucous membranes
  - Nonintact skin

- Perform handwashing immediately:

  - When there is direct contact with blood, body fluids, secretions, excretions, and contaminated items
  - After removing gloves
  - Between client contacts

- Wear a mask, eye protection, and face shield during procedures and client care activities that are likely to generate splashes or sprays of blood, body fluids, secretions, and excretions.
- Wear a cover gown during procedures and client care activities that are likely to generate splashes or sprays of blood, body fluids, secretions, or excretions or cause soiling of clothing.
- Remove soiled protective items promptly when the potential for contact with reservoirs of pathogens is no longer present.
- Clean and reprocess all equipment before reuse by another client.
- Discard all single-use items promptly in appropriate containers that prevent contact with blood, body fluids, secretions, and excretions; contamination of clothing; and transfer of microorganisms to other clients, healthcare workers, and the environment.
- Handle, transport, and process linens soiled with blood, body fluids, secretions, and excretions in such a way as to prevent skin and mucous membrane exposures, contamination of clothing, or transfer to other clients, healthcare workers, and the environment.
- Prevent injuries with used needles, scalpels, and other sharp devices by:

  - Never removing, recapping, bending, or breaking used needles
  - Never pointing the needle toward a body part
  - Using a one-handed "scoop" method, special syringes with a retractable protective guard or shield for enclosing a needle, or blunt-point needles
  - Depositing disposable and reusable syringes and needles in puncture-resistant containers

- Use a private room or consult with an infection control professional for the care of clients who contaminate the environment, or who cannot or do not assist with appropriate hygiene or environmental cleanliness measures.

---

diseases and virtually eliminated others (e.g., smallpox). To help prevent and control community-acquired infections, nurses encourage childhood and adult immunizations, vaccines that stimulate the body to produce antibodies against a specific disease organism. (Recommended immunization schedules are available on the website of the Centers for Disease Control and Prevention, www.cdc.gov.) Apathy,

NURSING GUIDELINES 12-1

Performing Hand Hygiene

- Use an alcohol-based handrub containing 60% to 95% ethanol or isopropanol for hand hygiene unless the hands are grossly contaminated (Fig. A). Alcohol-based handrubs are the most efficacious agents for reducing the number of bacteria on the hands (CDC, 2002).
- When using lathered soap for hand hygiene, rub vigorously for 15 seconds or longer if the hands are visibly soiled (Fig. B).
- Rinse soap from the wrists toward the fingers using running water. Directing the flow of rinse water toward the fingers avoids transferring microorganisms to cleaner skin areas.
- Use a paper towel to turn off a hand-operated faucet to avoid recontamination of the hands.
- Perform hand hygiene:

  - When arriving at and leaving work
  - Before and after contact with each client
  - Before and after handling equipment
  - Before and after gloving
  - Before and after collecting specimens
  - Before preparing medications
  - After administering medications
  - Before serving trays or feeding clients
  - Before eating
  - After toileting, hair combing, or performing other hygiene
  - After cleaning a work area

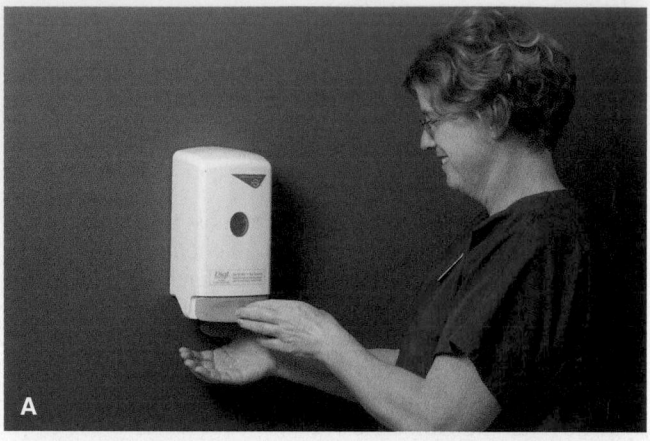

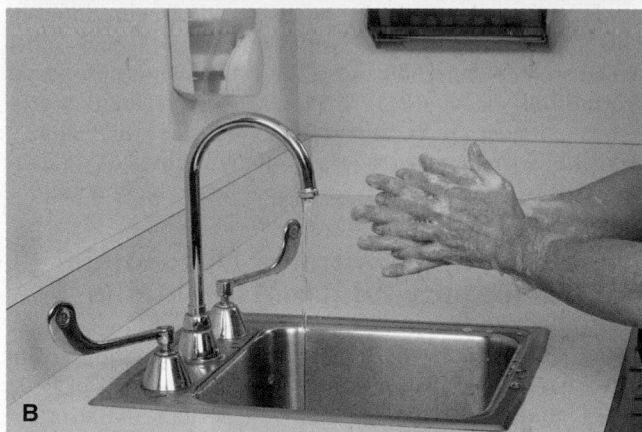

religious beliefs, fear that immunizations will cause illness, or inability to afford healthcare, however, can pose potential barriers to obtaining immunizations. Immunizations protect all people—children as well as adults who may not have developed sufficient immunity.

Gerontologic Considerations

- Pneumonia and influenza combined are the fifth leading cause of death in adults over the age of 65. While the older adult's immune response to active immunization may decrease (Eickhoff, 2005), immunizing the older adult for pneumococcal pneumonia and influenza can reduce morbidity and mortality.

Additional nursing measures to prevent infection transmission include the following:

- Wear a clean uniform; the Department of Health in the U.K. is requesting that nurses put on a clean uniform upon arriving at work and change before going home. Uniforms with sleeves no longer than elbow length are also advised

to facilitate adequate hand hygiene (Now cardigans look…, 2007).
- Do not wear hand or arm jewelry
- Avoid artificial nails and keep natural nails short and free of chipped nail polish
- Remain home when ill
- Advise sick visitors to refrain from contact with the client
- Protect immunosuppressed clients from pathogens
- Educate clients and families about ways to prevent infections at home (Client and Family Teaching 12-1)

Prevention of Infection from Needlestick Injuries

One of the greatest threats to healthcare workers is the potential for acquiring blood-borne infectious diseases such as hepatitis B virus (HBV) infection and acquired immunodeficiency syndrome (AIDS). Following standard precautions reduces this risk. Gloves, however, are not impervious to penetration by sharp objects (e.g., needles) that may contain blood. Despite following policies and precautions for avoiding blood-borne pathogens and using new needleless access devices on IV lines, needlestick injuries continue to occur.

TABLE 12-3 Transmission-Based Precautions

TYPE OF PRECAUTION	LOCATION	PROTECTION	EXAMPLES OF DISEASES
Airborne	Private room Negative air pressure* Room air is discharged to environment or filtered before being circulated	Follow Standard Precautions. Wear a mask for airborne pathogens or particulate air filter respirator in the case of TB. Place a mask on the client if transport is required.	TB Measles Chickenpox
Droplet	Private room, or in a room with similarly infected client(s) or one with at least 3 feet between the client and other client(s) or visitors	Follow Standard Precautions. Wear a mask when entering the room, but especially when within 3 feet of the infected client. Place a mask on the client if transport is required.	Influenza Rubella Streptococcal pneumonia Meningococcal meningitis
Contact	Private room, or in a room with similarly infected client(s), or consult with an infection control professional if the above options are not available	Follow Standard Precautions. Don gloves before entering the room. Remove gloves before leaving the room. Change gloves after contact with infective material. Perform handwashing with an antimicrobial agent immediately after removing gloves. Wear a gown when entering the room if your clothing could touch the client or items in the room, or if the client is incontinent, has diarrhea, an ileostomy, or a colostomy, or wound drainage not contained by a dressing. Avoid transporting the client, but, if required, use precautions that minimize transmission. Clean bedside equipment and client care items daily. Use items such as a stethoscope, sphygmomanometer, and other assessment tools exclusively for the infected client, and terminally disinfect them when precautions are no longer necessary.	Drug-resistant GI, respiratory, skin, or wound infections Acute diarrhea Draining abscess

TB, tuberculosis.

*Negative air pressure pulls air from the hall into the room when the door is opened, as opposed to positive air pressure, which pulls room air into the hall.

From Centers for Disease Control and Prevention. (2007). Guideline for isolation precautions: Preventing transmission of infectious agents in healthcare settings. Available at: http://www.cdc.gov/ncidod/dhqp/gl_isolation.html. Accessed January 2008.

Should an injury occur, healthcare workers are advised to follow postexposure recommendations:

- Report the injury to one's supervisor immediately.
- Document the injury in writing.
- Identify the person or source of blood, if possible.
- Obtain the HIV and HBV statuses of the source of blood, if it is legal to do so. Unless the client gives permission, testing and revealing HIV status are prohibited.
- Obtain counseling on the potential for infection.
- Receive the most appropriate postexposure prophylaxis.
- Be tested for disease antibodies at appropriate intervals.
- Receive instructions on monitoring potential symptoms and medical follow-up.

▶ Stop, Think, and Respond Exercise 12-2

The Centers for Disease Control and Prevention estimates that 2 million clients in U.S. hospitals develop nosocomial infections and that healthcare workers of all disciplines consistently fail to adhere to adequate hand hygiene practices (Houghton, 2006). What are some reasons that healthcare workers are lax in this basic method for preventing infection?

CARE OF THE CLIENT WITH INFECTION

Signs and Symptoms

Signs and symptoms vary depending on whether the infection remains localized, becomes generalized, or develops into sepsis (see Table 12-2). Manifestations for specific infections are discussed in relevant chapters in this text. Regardless of the type of infection, however, the infection process follows a similar course (Table 12-4).

 Gerontologic Considerations

- Symptoms of infections may be subtle or atypical among older adults. Older adults tend to have lower normal or baseline temperature, so a temperature that would typically be considered to be in the normal range may actually be elevated for the older adult. Common manifestations of infections in older adults include changes in behavior and mental status. Once established, infections are more likely to have a rapid course and life-threatening consequences.

Client and Family Teaching 12-1
Reducing Infections

To reduce potential infections, the nurse teaches the following measures:

- Perform frequent handwashing, especially before eating, after using the toilet, and after contact with nasal secretions.
- Bathe and perform other personal hygiene (e.g., oral care) daily.
- Keep the home environment clean; household bleach diluted 1:10 or 1:100 is an excellent disinfectant.
- Keep immunizations current. Tetanus vaccine is recommended every 10 years, influenza vaccine is repeated yearly, and one dose of pneumococcal pneumonia vaccine lasts a lifetime.
- Investigate the need for vaccinations, water purification techniques, and foods to avoid when traveling outside the United States.
- Eat the recommended servings from My Pyramid and use safe food handling practices.
- Use and immediately discard disposable paper tissues rather than reuse cloth handkerchiefs.
- Avoid sharing washcloths, drinking cups, and other personal care items.
- Follow safe sex practices.
- Stay home from work or school when ill rather than expose others to infectious pathogens.
- Avoid crowds and public places during local outbreaks of influenza.
- Follow posted infection control instructions when visiting hospitalized family members and friends.
- Understand that antibiotic therapy is not appropriate for every infectious disease, but when it is, take the full dose for the prescribed period.

TABLE 12-4 The Course of An Infectious Disease

STAGE	CHARACTERISTIC
Incubation period	The infectious agent reproduces. The host displays no recognizable symptoms; however, the infectious agent may exit the host at this time and infect others.
Prodromal stage	Initial symptoms appear; they may be vague and nonspecific. Possible symptoms include mild fever, headache, and loss of usual energy.
Acute stage	Symptoms become severe and specific to the affected tissue or organ. For example, tuberculosis is manifested by respiratory symptoms.
Convalescent stage	Symptoms subside as the host overcomes the infectious agent.
Resolution	The pathogen is destroyed. Health improves or is restored.

Diagnostic Tests

A thorough history and physical examination are essential for the diagnosis of an infectious disease. Diagnosis of some infectious diseases, however, requires additional tests and laboratory examinations to identify the microorganism.

White Blood Cell Count and Differential

Elevation in the number and type of WBCs, whose main function is phagocytosis, indicates an inflammatory and possibly infectious process. Although a total WBC count provides important information, a differential—one that indicates the percentage of WBC subtypes—is even more valuable. Elevated neutrophils, the largest subtype of WBCs, indicate that the body is in the early stages of responding to an invading pathogen. As the number of neutrophils becomes depleted, bone marrow produces additional cells called *band cells* (bands) that eventually mature and replace them. Elevated monocytes, the largest-sized subtype of WBCs, are the body's second line of defense.

Culture and Sensitivity Test

A **culture** identifies bacteria in a specimen taken from a person with symptoms of an infection. The source of the specimen may be body fluids or wastes, such as blood, sputum, urine, or feces, or the *purulent exudate*, collection of pus, from an open wound. The specimen is cultured, which involves placing a small amount of it in or on a special growth medium (Fig. 12-6). The specimen is incubated for a specific period (usually 48 to 72 hours), and then examined microscopically. To facilitate examination, it is stained or dyed (colored). One stain is the Gram stain. Those bacteria that absorb the color of the stain are classified as *gram positive*; those that do not are classified as *gram negative*. A coagulase test also may be used to test the microorganisms for pathogenicity or virulence. When a culture is reported as *coagulase positive*, it is more virulent than a culture of the same microorganism that produces a negative (*coagulase-negative*) response.

Sensitivity studies are done to determine which antibiotic inhibits the growth of a nonviral microorganism and will be most effective in treating the infection.

Examination for Ova and Parasites

Most ova (eggs) and parasites (those that live at the expense of the host) are intestinal worms. Therefore, the client's stool is examined for evidence of any forms in the infecting microorganism's life cycle. Usually, three random stools are collected from a bedpan, not the toilet. Urine and toilet paper may alter the specimen and therefore must be disposed of separately. Clients suspected of having intestinal ova and parasites should perform scrupulous handwashing to avoid reinfecting themselves and others.

Skin Tests

Skin testing determines the presence of a specific active or inactive infection. Diseases for which skin testing may be done include histoplasmosis, mumps, TB, diphtheria, and coccidioidomycosis. The material for skin testing is injected intradermally. The reaction is read after a specified period (usually 48 to 72 hours). The size of the *induration* (hard, elevated tissue), not including the surrounding area of

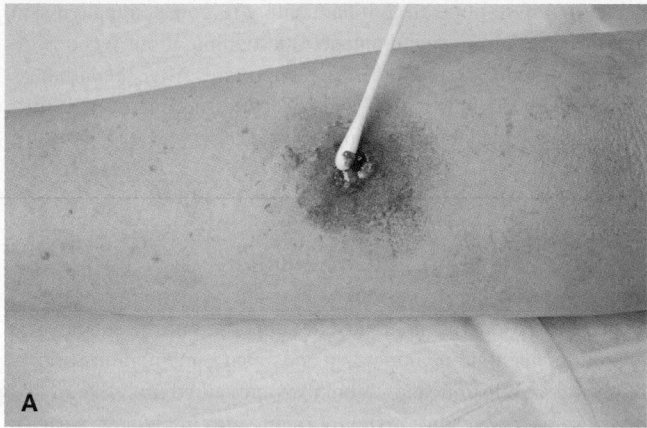

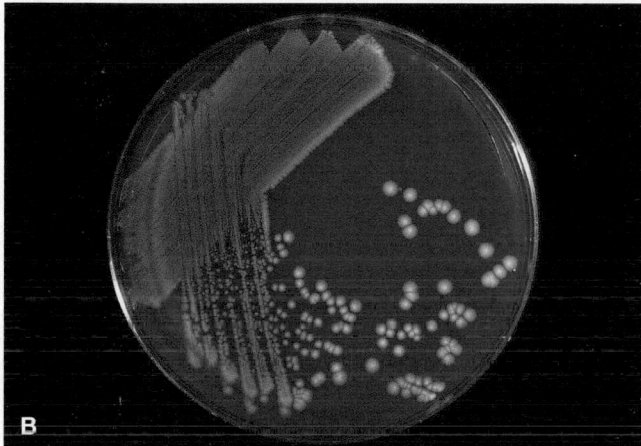

FIGURE 12-6. Bacterial culture. **(A)** A sterile culture swab is inserted in a wound to obtain a sample of exudates. **(B)** Variability of the macroscopic appearance of bacteria cultured on solid, agar-containing medium. (Part **B** from Porth, C. M. [2007]. *Essentials of pathophysiology: Concepts of altered health states* [2nd ed.]. Philadelphia: Lippincott Williams & Wilkins.)

erythema (redness), is measured in millimeters (mm). The measurement determines whether the reaction is significant. For example, a tuberculin skin test is considered positive if the induration is 15 mm or greater in persons with no known risk factors for TB; smaller measurements are significant in certain risk groups, such as immunocompromised clients.

Immunologic Tests
Immunologic tests determine the presence of *antigen* (substances that stimulate an immune response) and antibody reactions (see Chap. 33). For example, *agglutination* tests, such as the cold agglutinins test, may reveal the presence of high antibody titers confirming immunity to rubella (measles). *Precipitation tests*, such as the C-reactive protein test and erythrocyte sedimentation rate, produce elevated rates in some inflammatory diseases. *Complement fixation* tests, when results are elevated, indicate an inflammatory process. *Immunofluorescence* tests identify immunoglobulins, antibodies formed by the immune system.

Other Tests
Depending on the disease, other diagnostic tests may be used. Radiography (plain films or contrast studies), computed tomography (CT) scanning, and magnetic resonance

imaging (MRI) may be used to locate abscesses, identify displacement of organs or structures that may indicate abscess formation, and detect changes in tissues in areas such as the bones or lungs.

Medical Management
In some cases, supportive therapy such as rest, fluids, adequate nutrition, and antipyretics (e.g., aspirin or acetaminophen [Tylenol]) for a significantly elevated fever may be advised while the infectious disease runs its course. If the etiology is responsive to drug therapy, antimicrobials (e.g., antibiotics, sulfonamides, antiviral drugs) are prescribed.

Infected wounds may be *debrided*, a process of removing dead and damaged tissue. Wound irrigations, hydrotherapy (whirlpool), and application of wet-to-dry dressings may accomplish the same objective.

Treatment of a primary condition may relieve the infectious process. Bone marrow transplantation or administration of drugs that boost WBC production, such as filgrastim (Neupogen), may help immunosuppressed clients.

Pharmacologic Considerations

- When administering antibiotics, observe the client for adverse drug effects. Nausea, vomiting, anorexia, diarrhea, and rash are adverse effects of some antibiotics but also are symptoms associated with some infectious diseases. An accurate history and physical examination at the time of admission and ongoing documentation of the client's symptoms help distinguish between symptoms related to the infectious disease and those possibly caused by antibiotic therapy.

- Administer antibiotics on time and regularly around-the-clock to maintain therapeutic blood levels.

- With rectal administration of an antipyretic drug, the suppository is inserted high in the rectum. Check the client in 30 minutes to ensure that the suppository has not been expelled.

Nursing Management
Nursing management for the client with a potential or actual infection focuses on preventing or controlling the transmission of infection among clients, visitors, and healthcare workers and preventing complications. Some nursing actions include:

- Maintaining the client's skin integrity
- Monitoring vital signs, especially temperature and pulse rate
- Promoting adequate nutrition and hydration
- Regulating blood sugar within normal limits; sugar supports the growth of microorganisms
- Inspecting the client's body for signs of redness, swelling, and purulent drainage
- Reviewing white blood cell counts and reporting elevations above normal
- Obtaining cultures and transmiting them immediately to the laboratory

Nutrition Notes 12-1
The Client with Infection

- Malnutrition is the main cause of a suppressed immune system; ensuring that older adults are well nourished and that they maintain their body weight is one of the best ways to protect their aging immune systems.
- Fever is a major determinant of caloric needs during infection. Basal metabolic rate (BMR) increases 7% for each degree Fahrenheit that the temperature is above normal. For instance, the BMR for a person with a temperature of 103.6°F is increased 35% (5°F above normal × 7% = 35% increase). This translates into an extra 350 to 700 calories needed per day, based on an average BMR of 1000 to 2000 calories per day.
- Protein needs can increase to 1.5 to 2.0 g/kg of body weight for severe infections (normal protein requirement is 0.8 g/kg). Milk, milk drinks, and commercial supplements may be used to add significant proteins and calories.
- Fluid needs depend on the severity of fever and any complicating factors (e.g., diarrhea, vomiting, excessive sweating). Encourage the intake of ice water, broth, fruit juices, milk, popsicles, and gelatin. Clients should avoid tea, coffee, and carbonated beverages containing caffeine, which promote diuresis.
- Acutely ill clients may accept and tolerate a full liquid diet with in-between-meal supplements better than solid food. Advance the diet as tolerated to maximize intake.
- For clients who require transmission-based precautions, meals are served on disposable dinnerware. The tray is made as attractive as possible to encourage eating. Uneaten food is disposed of in the toilet, and plastic containers are deposited in sealed bags before removal.

- Keeping fresh wounds intact and covered for 24 to 48 hours
- Following aseptic principles when changing dressings
- Disposing of soiled substances in a waterproof container
- Administering antimicrobial drugs as prescribed
- Promoting urination to avoid catheterization
- Encouraging coughing and deep breathing to clear secretions from the airways

Nursing Process for the Client With a Potential or Actual Infection

Assessment

Obtain the client's history, paying particular attention to information that might suggest exposure to someone with an infectious illness or other reservoirs of infection, immunization status, recent travel to a foreign country, treatment with antimicrobial or immunosuppressive drugs, and current medical disorders. Weigh the client to gain information about nutritional status and measure vital signs to detect temperature, heart and respiratory rates, and blood pressure. A head-to-toe physical assessment helps detect manifestations of an inflammatory response, impaired skin, and evidence of unusual drainage. Questioning about feelings of lassitude (tiredness) and anorexia is important. After preparing the client for diagnostic tests and collecting specimens, monitor the results of the laboratory findings and observe the response to skin tests.

Diagnosis, Planning, and Interventions

Implement measures to prevent or interrupt components of the chain of infection. Examples include supporting nutrition and hydration, maintaining intact skin and mucous membranes, and following aseptic principles. Administer prescribed drug therapy and observe for evidence of improvement. Also implement measures that promote comfort (e.g., reducing fever).

Diagnoses, expected outcomes, and interventions for clients with infections include the following:

▶ **Risk for Infection** related to compromised defense mechanisms

▶ **Expected Outcomes:** Client will remain free of infection.

- Follow hand hygiene guidelines (see Nursing Guidelines 12-1). *Hand hygiene remains the single most important measure to prevent the spread of infection. It reduces the number of transient and resident microorganisms.*
- Advise the client to avoid touching any areas of impaired skin. *Hands contain microorganisms that clients can transfer to tissue and blood vessels beneath impaired skin.*
- Monitor food intake; offer nutritious supplements if appetite is suppressed (Nutrition Notes 12-1). *Sufficient intake helps restore biologic defense mechanisms (e.g., adequate WBCs, wound healing).*
- Keep dressings clean, dry, and intact. *They act as barriers to environmental microorganisms.*
- Use surgical asepsis when changing dressings or inserting or changing invasive equipment (e.g., urinary catheters, IV access devices). *Pathogens can enter from several different routes.*
- Use a prescribed topical antimicrobial or one approved by the agency during wound care. *Antimicrobials reduce microorganisms at the site of impaired skin.*
- Administer prescribed systemic antimicrobial medications. *Antibiotics may be ordered prophylactically (i.e., to reduce the potential for infection).*
- Monitor for signs of superinfection: diarrhea, vaginal discharge, and inflammation of oral mucous membranes. *Antibiotic therapy may cause microorganisms to overgrow elsewhere in the body.*

▶ **Potential Complication:** Sepsis

▶ **Expected Outcomes:** The nurse will manage and minimize sepsis.

- Follow transmission-based precautions (see Table 12-3). *They interfere with the ways a particular pathogen is spread.*
- Monitor vital signs every 4 hours or as ordered medically. *Changes may be the earliest indication of sepsis.*

- Observe the client's mental status. *Changes in mental activity accompany sepsis.*
- Check skin color and observe for signs of impaired circulation or bleeding. *Microvascular clots accompany sepsis; disseminated intravascular coagulation may develop from alterations in the clotting mechanisms.*
- Administer antimicrobials as prescribed. *Systemic antimicrobial therapy may be necessary to prevent, control, and eliminate an infection.*
- Report hypotension and signs of organ dysfunction to the physician. *Severe sepsis may lead to septic shock and death.*

Evaluation of Expected Outcomes

Expected outcomes include a WBC count below 10,000 cells/mm^3, body temperature less than 99°F, no purulent drainage from impaired skin, wound culture free of virulent pathogens, and no signs of superinfection. Changes in vital signs, mental status, and leukocyte count are detected early. The infection resolves and does not progress to septic shock.   ●

CRITICAL THINKING EXERCISES

1. Use the chain of infection illustrated in Figure 12-2 to trace the viral transmission of a common cold from one person to another.
2. Give a specific example of how pathogens are spread among clients and healthcare workers, and then identify techniques for preventing their transmission.
3. Select any community-acquired infection and identify the type of microorganism that causes it and its usual reservoir, portal of exit, means of transmission, and portal of entry.
4. Develop a list of suggestions for improving hand hygiene practices in healthcare agencies.

NCLEX-STYLE REVIEW QUESTIONS

1. When monitoring a client with an infection for the development of sepsis, which of the following signs should the nurse report immediately? Select all that apply.

   1. Temperature greater than 100.4°F (38°C)
   2. Heart rate greater than 90 beats per minute
   3. Respiratory rate less than 20 breaths per minute
   4. Paco$_2$ greater than 32 mm Hg
   5. WBC count less than 12,000 cells/mm^3

2. When changing a sterile dressing, which nursing action violates the principles of surgical asepsis?

   1. The nurse cleans the wound from the outer edge toward the center.
   2. The nurse dons clean gloves to remove the soiled dressing.
   3. The nurse performs handwashing before donning sterile gloves.
   4. The nurse places the soiled dressing in a moisture-resistant bag.

3. A client with tuberculosis (TB) is in a private room on a medical unit. A diagnosis of TB requires the use of airborne precautions. What must the nurse wear when entering the client's room?

   1. Face mask
   2. Isolation gown
   3. Particulate air filter respirator
   4. Sterile gloves

4. A client with drug-resistant wound infections will most likely require which type of precautions by healthcare personnel?

   1. Airborne
   2. Contact
   3. Droplet
   4. Standard

5. The client tells the nurse that the doctor identified a nosocomial infection affecting the bladder and kidneys. Which of the following statements provides the best explanation of a nosocomial infection for the client?

   1. "Your infection is affecting more than one organ and may become widespread."
   2. "Your infection is related to the wound infection you came in with."
   3. "This infection is confined just to the bladder."
   4. "This infection was acquired while you were hospitalized."

13

Intravenous Therapy

Learning Objectives

On completion of this chapter, you will be able to:

1. Explain common indications for intravenous (IV) therapy.
2. Differentiate between crystalloid and colloid solutions and give examples of each.
3. Describe the difference between isotonic, hypotonic, and hypertonic solutions.
4. Explain the difference between whole blood, packed cells, blood products, and plasma expanders.
5. Describe nursing responsibilities for preparing intravenous solutions, selecting tubing, and selecting an infusion technique.
6. Identify nursing responsibilities when preparing the client for IV therapy.
7. Describe nursing actions involved in performing a venipuncture, including sites and devices commonly used.
8. Explain the equipment that must be replaced during IV therapy.
9. List complications of IV therapy and signs and symptoms for which the nurse monitors.
10. Explain how the nurse discontinues IV therapy.
11. Discuss the purpose of a medication lock.
12. Describe the nursing process for the client requiring IV therapy.
13. Discuss the purpose of total parenteral nutrition, and name one solution often administered concurrently.
14. Explain special considerations for blood transfusion therapy, including the equipment used, blood compatibility, and complications.

I ntravenous (IV) therapy is the parenteral administration of fluids and additives into a vein. State nurse practice acts specify the qualifications for LPNs/LVNs who can administer or participate in IV therapy; only nurses who meet these qualifications and receive appropriate training can administer this particular therapy. All registered nurses can administer IV therapy. IV administration demands skillful administration techniques, close observation of the client, and several specific nursing considerations, all of which are discussed in this chapter.

INDICATIONS FOR INTRAVENOUS THERAPY

IV therapy is used to maintain or restore fluid balance when oral replacement is inadequate or impossible, to maintain or replace electrolytes, to administer water-soluble vitamins, to administer drugs, to provide a source of calories and nutrients, and to replace blood and blood products.

Intravenous therapy may be used to administer medications, because drugs given by the IV route have a more rapid effect than other routes of administration. Only drugs labeled for IV use are given by this route. Administering a drug intravenously may be indicated in the following circumstances:

- A rapid drug effect is required
- Oral intake is restricted
- A client cannot swallow
- Gastrointestinal absorption is impaired
- A continuous therapeutic blood level is desired.

 Pharmacologic Considerations

- Before adding a drug to an IV solution, read the label on the container carefully or check the literature. Some medications require special dilution or the use of specific diluents, or have warnings regarding the maximum dose allowed. After the drug is added, the solution container should be labeled with the name and dose of the drug, the date and time, and the name of the nurse who added the drug.

IV therapy designed to meet nearly all the caloric and nutritional needs of a client is called **total parenteral nutrition (TPN)**. Clients who are severely malnourished or cannot consume food or liquids for a long time may require TPN.

Special considerations for administering IV therapy for TPN and blood transfusions are discussed later in this chapter.

TYPES OF INTRAVENOUS SOLUTIONS

The two types of IV solutions are crystalloid and colloid solutions. **Crystalloid solutions** consist of water and uniformly

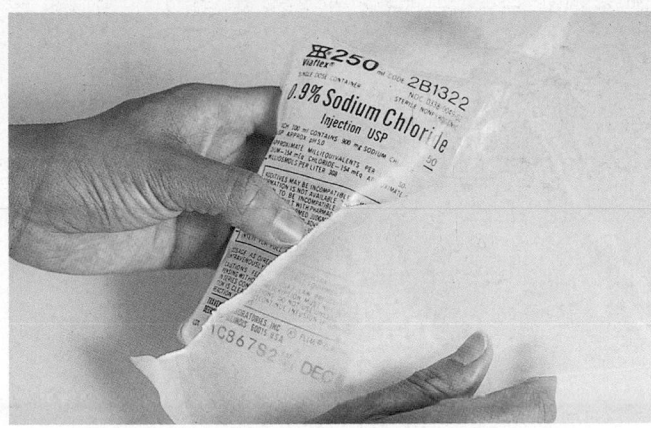

FIGURE 13-1. Crystalloid solution. (Photo © B. Proud.)

dissolved crystals such as salt (sodium chloride) or sugar (glucose, dextrose) (Fig. 13-1). **Colloid solutions** consist of water and molecules of suspended (undissolved) substances such as blood cells and blood products.

Crystalloid Solutions

Crystalloid solutions are divided into isotonic, hypotonic, and hypertonic solutions (Table 13-1). These terms refer to the concentration of dissolved substances in relation to the plasma into which they are instilled. When crystalloid solutions are administered to clients, the concentration influences the osmotic distribution of body fluid (Fig. 13-2).

Isotonic Solutions

An **isotonic solution** contains the same concentration of dissolved substances as is normally found in plasma. Isotonic solutions are administered to maintain fluid balance when clients temporarily cannot eat or drink. Because of its equal

TABLE 13-1 Types of Crystalloid Solutions

SOLUTION	COMPONENTS	SPECIAL COMMENTS
Isotonic Solutions		
0.9% Saline, also called normal saline (NS)	0.9 g Sodium chloride/100 mL water	Contains sodium and chloride in amounts physiologically equal to those in plasma
5% Dextrose in water, also called D_5W	5 g Dextrose (glucose/sugar)/100 mL water	Isotonic when infused, but the glucose is metabolized quickly, leaving a solution of dilute water
Ringer's solution or lactated Ringer's	Water and a mixture of sodium, chloride, calcium, potassium, bicarbonate, and, in some cases, lactate	Replaces electrolytes in amounts similarly found in plasma; lactate, when present, helps maintain acid-base balance
Hypotonic Solutions		
0.45% Sodium chloride, also called half-strength saline	0.45 g Sodium chloride/100 mL water	Contains a smaller proportion of sodium and chloride than found in plasma, causing it to be less concentrated in comparison
5% Dextrose in 0.45% saline	5 g Dextrose and 0.45 sodium chloride/ 100 mL water	The sugar provides a quick source of energy, leaving a hypotonic salt solution
Hypertonic Solutions		
10% Dextrose in water, also called $D_{10}W$	10 g Dextrose/100 mL water	Contains twice the concentration of glucose found in plasma
3% Saline	3 g Sodium chloride/100 mL water	The high concentration of salt in the plasma dehydrates cells and tissue
20% Dextrose in water	20 g Dextrose/100 mL water	Rapidly increases the concentration of sugar in the blood, causing a fluid shift to the intravascular compartment

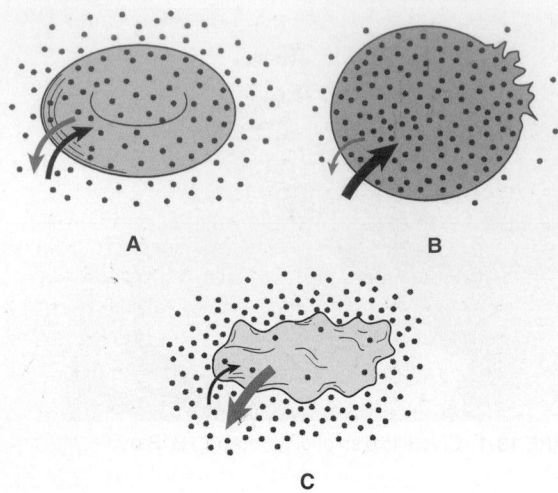

FIGURE 13-2. Osmotic distribution of fluid. (**A**) In *isotonic solutions*, cells maintain normal size because of fluid balance. (**B**) In *hypotonic solutions*, body fluids shift out of the blood vessels and into cells and the interstitial space. The cells fill with fluid and may burst. (**C**) In *hypertonic solutions*, the fluid is pulled from the cells and the interstitial tissues into the vascular space.

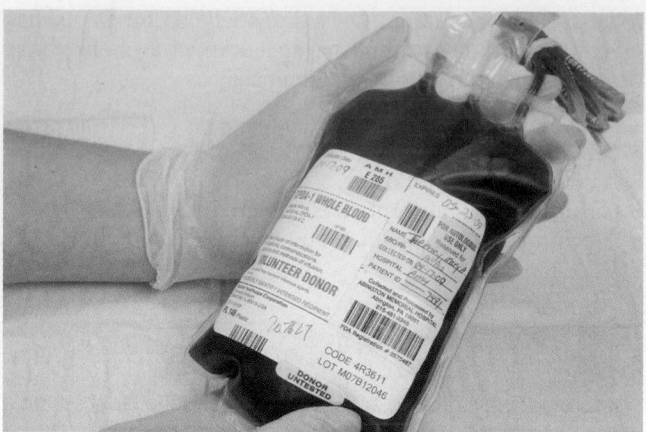

FIGURE 13-3. Unit of whole blood.

concentration to plasma, an isotonic solution causes no appreciable redistribution of body fluid on administration.

Hypotonic Solutions

A **hypotonic solution** contains fewer dissolved substances compared with plasma. Hypotonic solutions effectively rehydrate clients experiencing fluid deficits; therefore, they are administered to clients experiencing fluid losses in excess of fluid intake, such as those who have diarrhea or are vomiting. Because a hypotonic solution is dilute, the water in the solution passes through the semipermeable membrane of blood cells, causing them to swell. This swelling can temporarily increase blood pressure because it expands the circulating volume. The water also may pass through capillary walls and become distributed in other body cells and interstitial spaces.

Hypertonic Solutions

A **hypertonic solution** is more concentrated (contains more dissolved substances) than body fluid. Consequently, it draws fluid into the intravascular compartment from the more dilute areas in the cells and interstitial spaces. Hypertonic solutions are not used very frequently except when it is necessary to reduce cerebral (brain) edema, expand circulatory volume rapidly, or administer nutrition parenterally.

Colloid Solutions

Colloid solutions are used to replace circulating blood volume because the suspended molecules in the solutions pull fluid from other fluid compartments in the body. Examples include blood (whole blood and packed cells), blood products such as albumin, and solutions known as plasma expanders.

Blood

Whole blood and packed cells probably are the most commonly administered colloid solutions. One unit of **whole blood** (Fig. 13-3) contains approximately 475 mL of blood cells and plasma, with 60 to 70 mL of preservative and anticoagulant added. Whole blood is administered when clients need fluid restoration as well as blood cells. **Packed cells** have most of the plasma (fluid) removed and are preferred for clients who need cellular replacements but do not need and may be harmed by the administration of additional fluid. Such clients include those who have an inadequate oral intake of fluid and clients at risk for congestive heart failure (see Chap. 29).

Blood Products

Several types of solutions contain **blood products**, components extracted from blood (Table 13-2). Blood products are administered to clients who need specific blood substances but not all the fluid and cellular components in whole blood.

Plasma Expanders

Plasma expanders are nonblood solutions, such as dextran 40 (Rheomacrodex) and hetastarch (Hespan), that pull fluid

TABLE 13-2 Types of Blood Products

BLOOD PRODUCT	DESCRIPTION	PURPOSE FOR ADMINISTRATION
Platelets	Disk-shaped cellular fragments that promote coagulation of blood	Restores or improves the ability to control bleeding
Granulocytes	Types of white blood cells	Improves the ability to overcome infection
Plasma	Serum without blood cells	Replaces clotting factors or increases intravascular fluid volume by increasing colloidal osmotic pressure
Albumin	Plasma protein	Pulls third-spaced fluid by increasing colloidal osmotic pressure
Cryoprecipitate	Mixture of clotting factors	Treats blood-clotting disorders such as hemophilia

into the vascular space. They are used as an economical and virus-free substitute for blood and blood products when treating clients with hypovolemic shock.

ADMINISTERING INTRAVENOUS THERAPY

Selecting and Preparing Equipment

Equipment commonly used when administering IV therapy includes the solution, IV tubing, and an IV pole or infusion device. A fluid warmer may be used to raise the temperature of parenteral solutions when it is beneficial to ensure stable body temperature. The nurse selects and prepares the fluid that will be administered, chooses appropriate tubing, and decides on an infusion technique.

Preparing Intravenous Solutions

Crystalloid solutions are stored in plastic bags containing volumes of 1000, 500, 250, 100, and 50 mL. Only a few solutions are in glass containers. The physician specifies the type of solution, additional additives, and the volume to infuse over a specific period. To reduce the potential for infection, standard practice is to replace IV solutions every 24 hours even if the total volume in a container has not been instilled. Before preparing the solution, the nurse inspects the container and determines that the type of solution is the one prescribed, the solution is clear and transparent, the expiration date has not elapsed, no leaks are apparent, and a separate label is attached identifying the type and amount of drugs added to the original solution.

Selecting Intravenous Tubing

IV tubing consists of a spike for piercing the container of solution, a drip chamber for holding a small amount of fluid, a length of plastic tubing with one or more ports for instilling IV medications or additional solutions, and a roller or slide clamp for regulating the rate of the infusion (Fig. 13-4). Despite the common components, the nurse selects from various options in tubing design:

- Primary, secondary, or Y-administration tubing
- Vented or unvented tubing
- Drop size options (macrodrip or microdrip tubing)
- Filtered or unfiltered tubing

Primary, Secondary, or Y-Administration Tubing

Primary tubing is used to administer a large volume of IV solution over a long period or a small volume through a medication lock (discussed later). Primary tubing usually is quite long to span the distance from the solution, which hangs several feet above the infusion site, to the site itself. **Secondary tubing**, which is shorter, is used to administer smaller volumes of solution through a port in the primary tubing in a relatively short time. Y-administration tubing, used to administer whole blood or packed cells, is discussed later.

Vented Versus Unvented Tubing

IV tubing may be vented or unvented (Fig. 13-5). **Vented tubing** draws air into the container of solution and is used for administering solutions packaged in glass containers to facilitate their flow. **Unvented tubing** does not draw air into the container of solution and is used for solutions packaged in plastic bags.

Drop Size

The opening through which fluid passes from the solution container into the drip chamber determines the **drop size**. Tubing manufacturers design the drop size to deliver large-sized drops (**macrodrip tubing**) or small-sized drops (**microdrip tubing**). The nurse determines which to use. When a solution infuses by gravity at a fast rate such as over 100 mL/hr, it usually is easier to count fewer larger drops than to count many smaller ones. When the rate must be infused very precisely or at a slow rate, smaller drops are preferred.

Microdrip tubing, regardless of the manufacturer, delivers a standard volume of 60 drops (gtt)/mL. Macrodrip tubing, however, varies in the drop size. Common **drop factors**, the ratio of drops per milliliter, are 10, 15, and 20 gtt/mL. The nurse determines the drop factor, which is important in calculating the gravity infusion rate, by reading the package label.

Most intravenous solutions are infused using an electronic infusion device (discussed later). The drop size is of

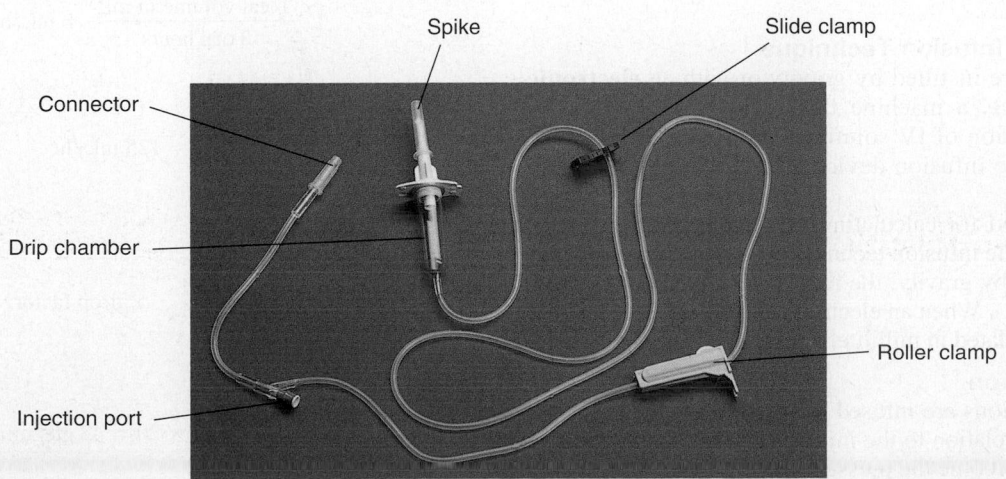

FIGURE 13-4. Basic components of intravenous tubing. (Courtesy of Abbott Laboratories, North Chicago, IL.)

Spike

Slide clamp

Connector

Drip chamber

Roller clamp

Injection port

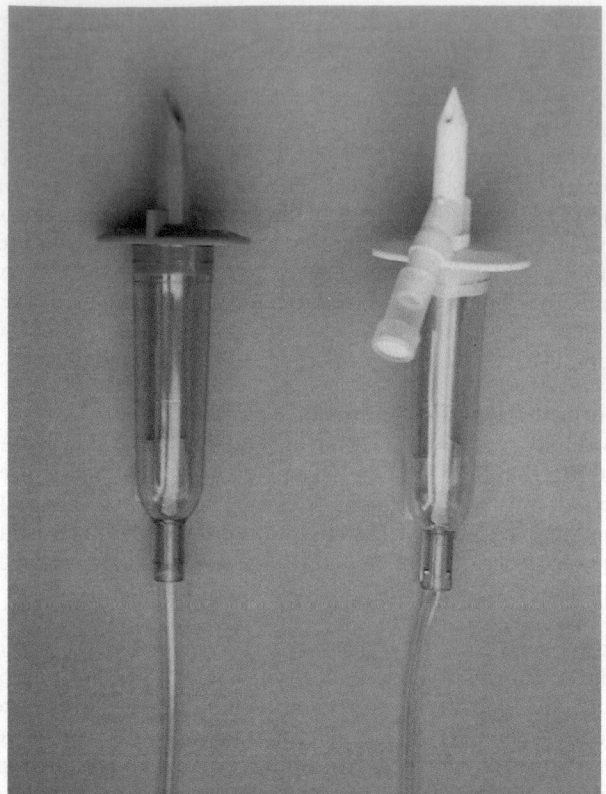

FIGURE 13-5. (*Left*) vented tubing and (*right*) unvented tubing. (Photo © Ken Timby.)

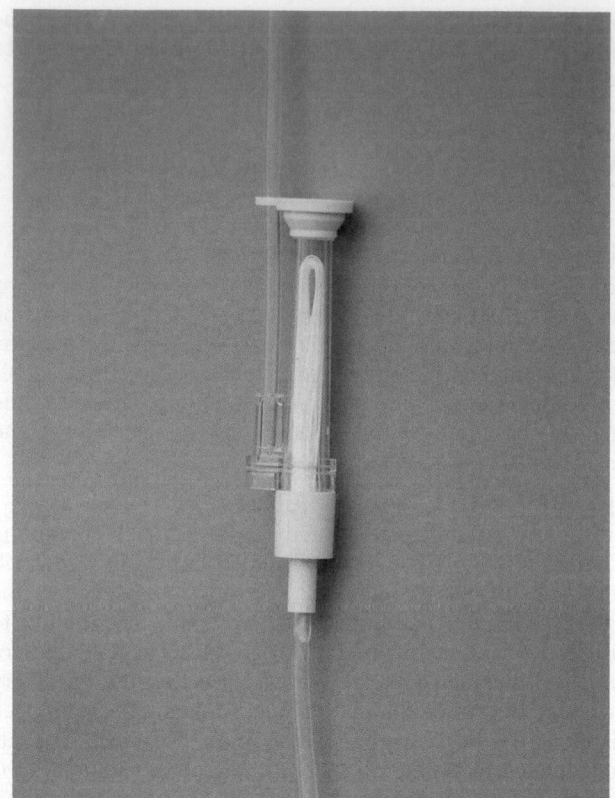

FIGURE 13-6. An in-line filter. (Photo © Ken Timby.)

no consequence with infusion devices because the rates are programmed electronically in milliliters per hour.

Filters

An **in-line filter** (Fig. 13-6) is a device that removes air bubbles as well as undissolved drugs, bacteria, and large molecules from the infusing solution. Filtered tubing is used when administering TPN, blood and packed cells, and solutions to immunosuppressed or pediatric clients.

Another factor that may affect the type of tubing selected is the technique that will be used to administer the IV solution.

Selecting an Infusion Technique

IV solutions are instilled by gravity or with an **electronic infusion device**, a machine that regulates and monitors the administration of IV solutions. In some cases, the use of an electronic infusion device affects the type of tubing used.

The method for calculating the rate of infusion varies depending on the infusion technique (Box 13-1). If the solution is infused by gravity, the rate is calculated in drops per minute (gtt/min). When an electronic infusion device is used, the rate is calculated in milliliters per hour (mL/h).

Gravity Infusion

When IV solutions are infused by gravity, the height of the IV solution in relation to the infusion site influences the rate of flow. To overcome the pressure in the client's vein, which is higher than atmospheric pressure, the nurse must elevate

the solution at least 18 to 24 inches (45–60 cm) above the infusion site. The higher the solution, the faster it infuses, and vice versa. The nurse uses the roller clamp to adjust the rate of flow. In some cases he or she may apply a **pressure infusion sleeve** around the bag of solution. The sleeve exerts

---

BOX 13-1 **Calculating Infusion Rates**

When using an electronic infusion device:

$$\frac{\text{Total volume in mL}}{\text{Total hours}} = \text{mL/hr}$$

Example:

$$\frac{1000 \text{ mL}}{8 \text{ hr}} = 125 \text{ mL/hr}$$

When infusing by gravity:

$$\frac{\text{Total volume in mL}}{\text{Total time in minutes}} \times \text{drop factor*} = \text{gtt/min}$$

Example:

$$\frac{1000 \text{ mL}}{480 \text{ min}} \times 20 = 42 \text{ gtt/min}$$

*The macrodrip drop factor varies among manufacturers.

a squeezing action around the solution bag to facilitate rapid infusion.

Electronic Infusion Devices

Electronic infusion devices are machines programmed to deliver a preset volume per hour and sound audible and visual alarms if the infusion is not progressing at the preprogrammed rate (Fig. 13-7). They also produce an audible sound when the infusion container is nearly empty, air is inside the tubing, or an obstruction or resistance to delivering the fluid occurs. The two general types of electronic infusion devices are infusion pumps and volumetric controllers.

Infusion Pumps. An **infusion pump** is a device that exerts positive pressure to infuse solutions. Infusion pumps usually require special tubing that contains a cassette for creating sufficient pressure to push fluid into the vein. The machine adjusts the pressure according to the resistance it meets. This feature accounts for one of its major disadvantages: if the catheter or needle within the vein becomes displaced, the pump may continue to infuse fluid into the tissue.

Volumetric Controllers. A **volumetric controller** is a device that infuses IV solutions by gravity by compressing the tubing at a certain frequency to infuse the solution at a precise preset rate. Volumetric controllers may or may not require special tubing. Some models allow the nurse to program the infusion of more than one solution. In some cases, when one container of fluid finishes infusing, the controller automatically shifts to infuse another.

Gerontologic Considerations

- Monitor responses to IV infusions closely, since the older adult may be unable to tolerate the same volumes or rates of infusion as younger adults, especially if respiratory, cardiac, or renal disorders are present.

▶ **Stop, Think, and Respond Exercise 13-1**

The physician orders an IV infusion of 1000 mL of 5% dextrose in water that will infuse over 8 hours. The nurse asks you to collect the fluid infusion supplies. What will you assemble?

Preparing the Client

The nurse explains the purpose of the IV therapy to clients at their level of understanding. It is best to do so before bringing the equipment to the client's room. The nurse tries to make the explanation as clear, concise, and informative as possible without causing the client undue anxiety. He or she also allows time to answer the client's questions. The nurse may address the following points: the reason that the client needs IV therapy, about how long the procedure will take, the site to be used, the amount of discomfort that normally accompanies insertion of the needle or catheter, and any instructions regarding limitation of activities.

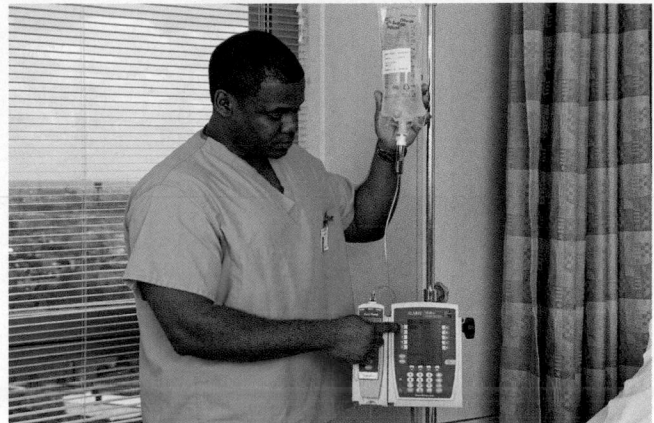

FIGURE 13-7. Electronic infusion devices are programmed to deliver a preset volume of IV solution per hour.

Performing a Venipuncture

A **venipuncture** is the method for gaining access to the venous system by piercing a vein with one of a variety of devices. Venipunctures are performed by nurses who are trained to do so. The nurse assesses the client to detect alterations in fluid volume and implements the physician's orders for IV fluid therapy. While the client undergoes fluid therapy, the nurse monitors to detect an increase, decrease, or rapid shift from one fluid compartment to another. The nurse follows the agency's infection-control policies as they relate to IV fluid therapy, uses aseptic techniques when caring for the venipuncture site or changing equipment, and gathers data as they relate to the presence of an infection.

For all venipunctures, the following items are necessary: venipuncture device; gloves; tourniquet; antiseptic swabs to clean the skin; antiseptic ointment, depending on the length of time that the site will be used and whether the site will be covered with a gauze dressing; a dressing; tape for securing the catheter or needle; tubing; and solution. An armboard or splint may be needed to prevent dislodging of the venipuncture device.

Gerontologic Considerations

- Rigidity of veins and poor skin turgor may make venipuncture in the older client more difficult. Use of a tourniquet may cause venous distention distal to the occlusion, increasing the risk of venous collapse. Place a soft cloth or material between the skin and tourniquet to avoid trauma or damage to the older adult's skin.

Venipuncture Sites

IV therapy is administered through peripheral venous sites or central veins. Short-term **peripheral venous sites** are superficial veins of the arm and hand (antecubital fossa, or inner elbow; dorsum, or back, of the hand; and forearm veins; Fig. 13-8). They are the most common sites for infusing IV fluids. Scalp veins may be used in infants. Veins in the foot are avoided because infusions in the lower extremities restrict mobility and increase the risk for forming blood

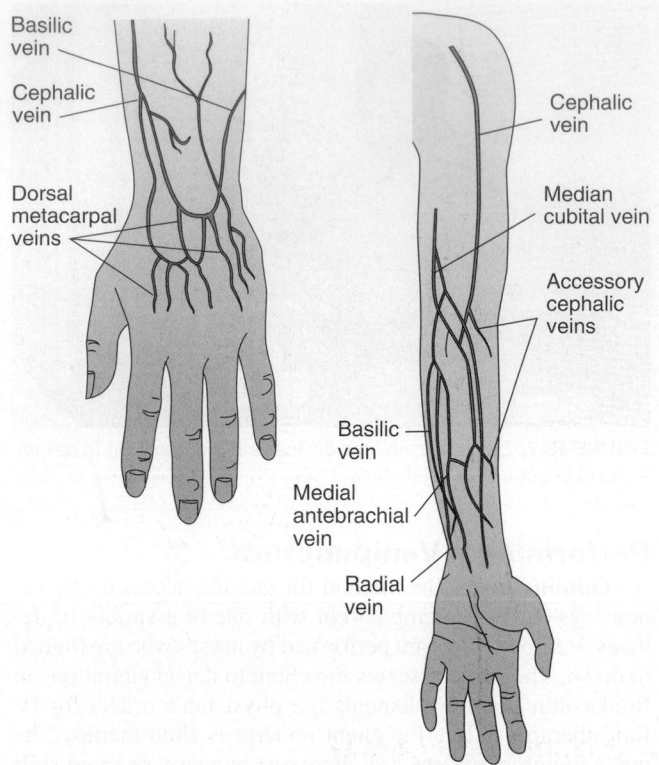

FIGURE 13-8. Venipuncture sites.

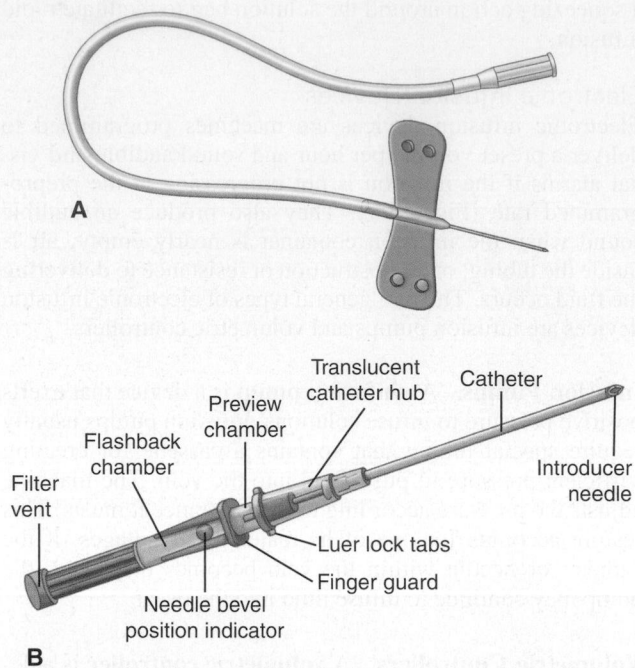

FIGURE 13-9. Examples of venipuncture devices. **(A)** Butterfly needle. **(B)** Over-the-needle catheter.

clots. **Central venous sites** are those that deliver solutions into a large central vein, such as the superior vena cava.

Selection of a vein depends on several factors, such as the client's age, condition of the veins, duration of IV therapy, IV solution ordered, size of venipuncture device, and client cooperation.

Venipuncture Devices
Peripheral Venous Access Devices
Several devices are used for accessing a vein: a butterfly needle, an over-the-needle catheter (most commonly used; Fig. 13-9), or a through-the-needle catheter. All of these types of venipuncture devices come in various diameters or gauges; the larger the gauge number, the smaller the diameter. The diameter of the venipuncture device always should be smaller than the vein into which it will be inserted to reduce the potential for occluding blood flow. The 18-, 20-, or 22-gauge venipuncture devices are the sizes most used for adults.

A **midline catheter** is another type of peripherally inserted venous access device (Fig. 13-10). It is 7 to 8 inches long, but only 3 to 6 inches of the catheter are inserted from just above or below the antecubital area in the basilic, cephalic, or median cubital vein until the tip rests in the upper arm just short of the axilla (Larouere, 2000b). Midline catheters are best suited for clients who have limited peripheral veins or who require an extended period of IV fluid therapy (Intravenous Nurses Society, 2006). This type of catheter can be used for up to 4 weeks before it requires replacement, which makes it ideal for use in the home healthcare setting.

When a peripherally inserted catheter extends from a superficial vein to the proximal end of the axillary or subclavian vein, it is referred to as a midclavicular catheter,

which can be used for 2 to 3 months. All three of these types (peripheral, midline, and midclavicular) are considered to be peripheral venous access devices because the tip remains distal to a central vein (i.e., the vena cava). Therefore, their use is confined to administering IV solutions and medications that would be given through a short-term peripheral venous access device.

There is current controversy about using a midclavicular catheter. Research has shown that when this catheter is placed near but not actually within the superior vena cava,

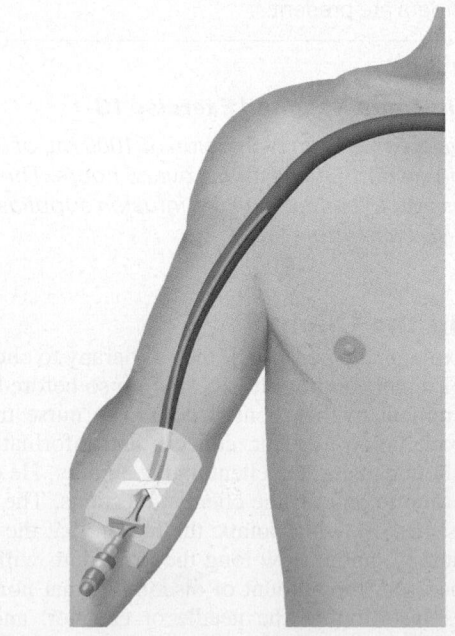

FIGURE 13-10. Placement of midline catheter insertion.

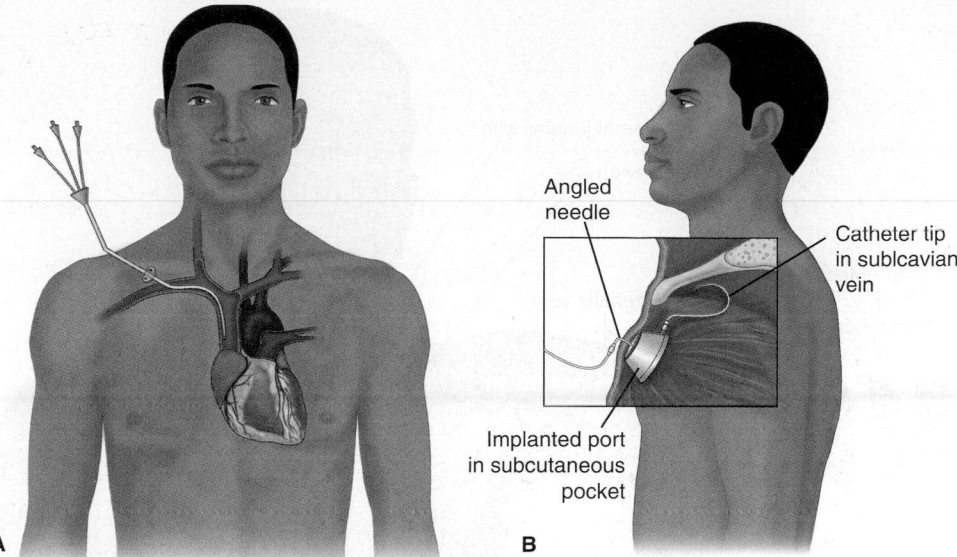

FIGURE 13-11. (**A**) Placement of triple-lumen nontunneled percutaneous central venous catheter. (**B**) Placement of an implanted port with the tip in the subclavian vein. Angled needle is inserted through skin and rubber septum into port.

Angled needle

Catheter tip in sublcavian vein

Implanted port in subcutaneous pocket

A

B

there is an increased incidence of thrombosis. Nurses should be alert for shortness of breath or pain in the chest, shoulder, or arm used for the insertion; these symptoms may indicate a developing thrombus. In addition, midclavicular catheters have the potential for venous spasm during removal that can lead to catheter tearing (Cook, 2007).

Midline and midclavicular sites should not be used to administer antineoplastic (cancer) chemotherapy, TPN (see later discussion), solutions with a pH less than 5 or greater than 9, solutions with an osmolality greater than 500 mOsm/L, rapid, high-volume infusions, or high-pressure bolus injections (Larouere, 2000a).

Central Venous Access Devices

A physician inserts a central venous catheter into the jugular or subclavian vein until the tip is located just above the heart (Fig. 13-11). Specially trained nurses insert a long catheter, called a *peripherally inserted central catheter* (PICC) or a *long line,* peripherally to a similar location (Fig. 13-12). Central venous catheters are inserted when providing TPN, monitoring central venous pressure, or administering concentrated or irritating IV solutions; when peripheral veins have collapsed; or when long-term IV therapy or thrombophlebitis (inflammation of a vein) and infiltration have reduced the availability of peripheral veins. After insertion of the catheter, a chest radiograph is taken to confirm catheter placement and to rule out an accidental puncture of the pleural membrane which can cause a pneumothorax (see Chap. 22).

▶ *Stop, Think, and Respond Exercise 13-2*

A client with cancer has a central venous catheter through which he receives antineoplastic drugs. Why is the medication infused through a central venous catheter and filtered tubing?

Replacing Equipment

Replacing equipment is important to reduce the potential for infection. Solutions are replaced when they finish infusing or every 24 hours, whichever comes first. Most IV tubing is changed every 72 hours, but the exact parameters depend on agency policy. Some exceptions include tubing used to administer TPN and intermittent secondary infusions. Y-administration tubing used to administer blood can be reused one time for a second unit that immediately follows the first. Medication locks (discussed later) and venipuncture devices are replaced every 7 hours or immediately if evidence of complications develops. Central catheters remain in the same site indefinitely.

Monitoring for Complications

Several complications are associated with the infusion of IV solutions. Any time the integrity of the skin is compromised with a venous access device such as a catheter or needle, the client is at risk for infection. Because the venous access device traumatizes the vein wall and disturbs the flow of blood cells in the vein, there is a potential for **phlebitis**, inflammation of the vein (Fig. 13-13), and thrombus formation (development of a clot). If the clot breaks free, it may travel to the lungs and cause a pulmonary embolism, which can be fatal. A bolus of air traveling through the venous system to the lungs is just as serious. If the venous access device fails to remain in the vein, fluid infiltrates the tissue, causing localized edema. Last, circulatory overload can develop if the volume of infusing solution exceeds the heart's ability to circulate it effectively.

 Pharmacologic Considerations

- If they infiltrate, some IV medications, such as dopamine (Intropin), can cause severe tissue damage in addition to

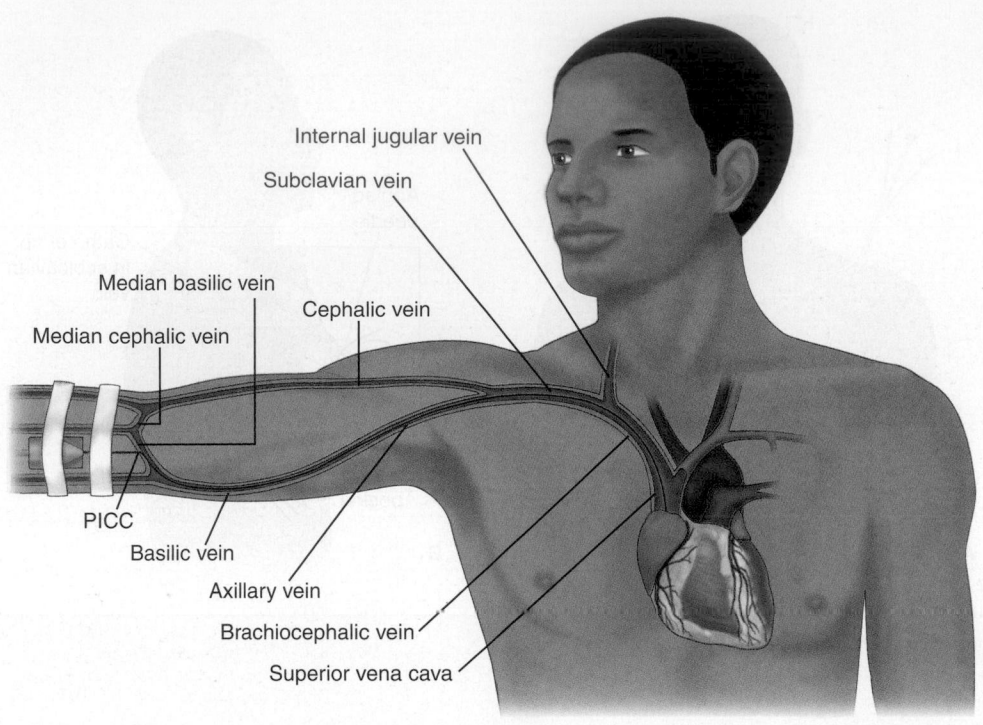

Internal jugular vein

Subclavian vein

Median basilic vein

Cephalic vein

Median cephalic vein

PICC

Basilic vein

Axillary vein

Brachiocephalic vein

Superior vena cava

FIGURE 13-12. Placement of peripherally inserted central catheter (PICC).

causing localized edema. Phentolamine (Regitine) is kept available should dopamine infiltrate. Report infiltration to the physician as soon as possible.

Inspecting the venipuncture site routinely and observing for signs of infection, infiltration, phlebitis, and thrombus formation are important nursing interventions. Table 13-3 identifies the causes and manifestations of these complications and appropriate nursing actions to take should they occur. The nurse documents site appearance daily in the client's medical record. A common practice is to change the dressing over the venipuncture site every 24 to 72 hours

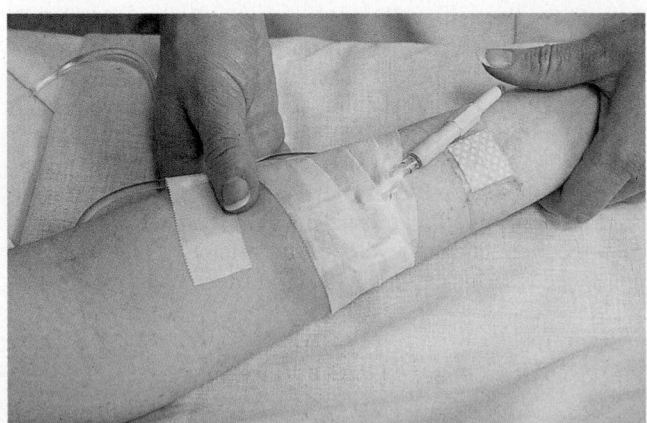

FIGURE 13-13. Checking inflammation surrounding infusion site. (Photo © B. Proud.)

according to the agency's infection-control policy or immediately if complications develop.

Gerontologic Considerations

- Older adults, especially those with chronic conditions, are at risk for fluid overload and electrolyte imbalances; observe for signs and symptoms. Also observe confused or disoriented clients frequently as excessive movement or pulling on the IV line may dislodge the venipuncture device.

Discontinuing Intravenous Therapy

IV infusions are discontinued when the solution has infused and no more is scheduled to follow (Nursing Guidelines 13-1). Alternatively, the venipuncture device may be temporarily capped and kept patent with the use of a **medication lock**, which is a sealed chamber that allows intermittent access to a vein. The nurse inserts the lock into the venipuncture device (Fig. 13-14). Flushing the lock with saline or heparinized saline keeps the vein patent. Medication locks are used when the client no longer needs continuous infusions, needs intermittent IV medication administration, or may need emergency IV fluids or medications.

Pharmacologic Considerations

- Read labels carefully on vials containing flush solutions for medication locks. One reason for compliance with The Joint

TABLE 13-3 Complications of Intravenous Therapy

COMPLICATION	SIGNS AND SYMPTOMS	CAUSE(S)	ACTION
Infection	Swelling, discomfort, redness at site, drainage from site	Growth of microorganisms	Change site Apply antiseptic and dressing to previous site Report findings
Circulatory overload	Elevated blood pressure, shortness of breath, bounding pulse, anxiety	Rapid infusion Reduced kidney function Impaired heart contraction	Slow the IV rate Contact the physician Elevate the client's head Give oxygen
Infiltration (extravasation)	Swelling at the site, discomfort, decrease in infusion rate, cool skin temperature at the site	Displacement of the venipuncture device	Restart the IV Elevate the arm
Phlebitis	Redness, warmth, and discomfort along the vein	Administration of irritating fluid Prolonged use of the same vein	Restart the IV Report the findings Apply warm compresses
Thrombus formation	Swelling, discomfort at site, slowed infusion	Stasis of blood at the catheter, needle tip, or vein	Restart the IV Report the findings Apply warm compresses
Pulmonary embolus	Sudden chest pain, shortness of breath, anxiety, rapid heart rate, drop in blood pressure	Movement of previously stationary blood clot	Stay with the client Call for help Administer oxygen
Air embolism	Same as pulmonary embolus	Failure to purge air from the tubing Disconnected tubing from central venous catheter	Same as for pulmonary embolus, but also place the client's head lower than the feet Position the client on left side

Commission's 2005 National Patient Safety Goals is that deaths occurred when potassium chloride was used incorrectly to flush a lock or central venous catheter. Now all concentrated electrolytes, such as vials of potassium chloride, are removed from client care units (Joint Commission Resources, 2004).

 NURSING GUIDELINES 13-1

Discontinuing an Intravenous Infusion

- Wash your hands.
- Clamp the tubing and remove the tape holding the dressing and venipuncture device in place.
- Don clean gloves.
- Gently press a dry, sterile gauze square over the site (use of an alcohol swab interferes with blood clotting).
- Remove the venipuncture device by pulling it out without hesitation, following the course of the vein.
- Continue to apply pressure to the site for 30 to 45 seconds while elevating the forearm to control bleeding.
- Cover the site with a dressing or bandage.
- Remove gloves and wash your hands.
- Record the time the IV infusion was discontinued, the amount of fluid infused, and the appearance of the venipuncture site.

Nursing Process for the Client Requiring IV Therapy

Assessment

Before initiating fluid therapy, gather clinical data related to fluid status (see Chap. 16). Examples include vital signs; body weight; color, volume, and specific gravity of urine; skin turgor; characteristics of oral mucous membranes; respiratory effort; and level of consciousness. Also review laboratory test results such as blood cell count and hematocrit and serum electrolyte levels. Identify the purpose(s) for administering IV fluid therapy.

Before performing the venipuncture, ask the client to identify the nondominant hand. The nondominant hand or forearm is preferred unless there are contraindications to its use, such as having had a breast and lymph nodes removed on that side or having had vascular surgery for kidney dialysis. If the client cannot respond, assume that the client is right-handed because that is more common. To determine which vein is most appropriate, first assess the size and condition of the veins in the hand or wrist area. If they are exceptionally small, tortuous, or traumatized by previous venipunctures, inspect veins in more proximal areas, trying to avoid the veins in the antecubital fossa, where the elbow bends, if at all possible. Read the label on the IV fluid at least three times to confirm that it is the volume and type of solution the physician has ordered.

After performing the venipuncture, monitor the IV site for swelling, warmth, pain, and induration (hardening). Assess at least

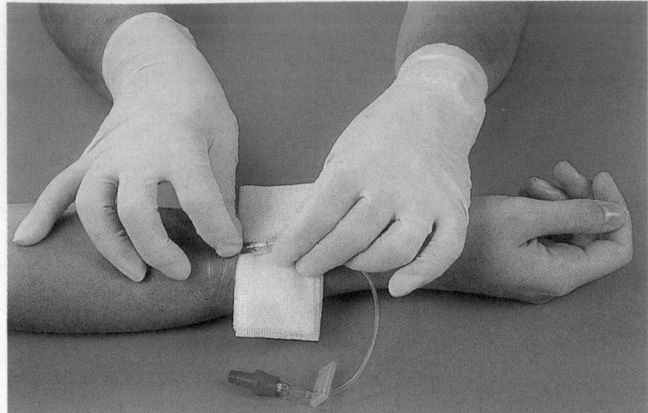

FIGURE 13-14. Attaching a lock device with extension tubing to the IV catheter hub. (Photo © B. Proud.)

hourly the rate at which fluid is infusing and the client's condition. Examine the electronic infusion device, if one is used, to ensure that it is correctly programmed and functioning properly. Throughout fluid therapy, measure intake and output volumes to determine trends in fluid balance. Auscultate lung sounds and heart sounds each shift or more often to evaluate the client's capacity to circulate the infusing fluid without complications. Inspect the venipuncture site at least once a day for signs of inflammation or infection, and observe the condition of the dressing, which should be dry and intact.

Diagnosis, Planning, and Interventions

▸ **Risk for Imbalanced Fluid Volume** related to rate of infusion that exceeds circulatory capacity or a shift in a fluid compartment

▸ **Expected Outcomes:** (1) Fluid volume will be maintained or restored. (2) Client will not experience cardiopulmonary complications secondary to the IV infusion of fluid.

- Calculate the rate of fluid infusion accurately, and correctly regulate the drip rate or program the electronic infusion device with the prescribed hourly infusion volume. *Errors in calculating or regulating the prescribed rate of fluid infusion can compromise the heart's ability to circulate the fluid or delay restoration of fluid balance.*
- Monitor the time strip on the container of IV solution hourly. *Reading the time strip is a quick method for determining if fluid is infusing at the predetermined hourly rate.*
- Respond when an electronic infusion device sounds an alarm. *Audible alarms call attention to a problem associated with the infusion of IV fluid.*
- Inspect the site where the fluid is infusing for signs of localized edema. *Parenteral fluid should be instilled in the vein; local edema suggests that the fluid is entering interstitial spaces, where it is more slowly absorbed.*
- Maintain an accurate intake and output record. *Fluid intake should approximate fluid output.*
- Note the amount of fluid the client takes orally and report when the combined volume of oral and parenteral fluid exceeds 3000 mL in 24 hours. *Normal adult fluid intake generally is 1500 to*

3000 mL/24 hours. *Volumes that exceed 3000 mL/day may be excessive unless the client is dehydrated or losing large volumes of fluid simultaneously.*
- Reassess fluid status at regular intervals according to the client's acuity level. *Changes in weight (e.g., 2 lbs in 24 hours), elevated blood pressure, dyspnea or adventitious lung sounds, abnormal heart sounds, peripheral edema, intake that significantly exceeds output, distended neck veins, anxiety, or diminished level of consciousness suggest excessive fluid volume.*

▸ **Risk for Infection** related to disrupted skin integrity secondary to venipuncture and presence of a venous access device

▸ **Expected Outcome:** Client will remain free of localized or generalized infection.

- Follow agency protocol for changing IV sites and venipuncture devices. *To avoid infection, the standard of care is to change IV sites every 48 to 72 hours. Clients with a suppressed immune system may require the use of tubing with a bacterial filter and more frequent site changes.*
- Check the initial date of use on the IV fluid container and tubing, and change equipment according to the agency's infection-control policies. *Infection-control policies usually advise changing IV solution containers every 24 hours; IV tubing can be used for up to 72 hours provided solution is continuously infusing through it. Nurses change tubing for intermittent infusions more frequently.*
- Use aseptic technique when changing IV site dressings, tubings, and solution containers. *Preventing or reducing the entrance of bacteria in the venipuncture site or vascular system decreases the potential for infection.*
- Assess for signs and symptoms of infection such as redness, warmth, tenderness, and purulent drainage at the venipuncture site; elevated temperature; and an increased white blood cell count. Discontinue the IV infusion and remove the venipuncture device if signs and symptoms of infection exist. *Removing the venipuncture device enables the impaired skin to heal and restores the barrier to microorganisms.*
- Document and report assessments that relate to an infection; follow agency protocols for obtaining a culture of the wound and its drainage. *Local antimicrobial therapy or systemic antibiotic therapy may be indicated in some cases of infection.*
- Elevate the extremity and apply warm compresses if an infection is suspected. *Elevation promotes venous circulation and reduces swelling. Warmth dilates blood vessels, relieves discomfort, and facilitates a reduction in local edema.*
- Restart the IV infusion in another site, preferably in the opposite upper extremity. *Fluid therapy should not be interrupted if it is still necessary.*

▸ **Risk for Imbalanced Nutrition: Less than Body Requirements** related to an inadequate nutritional intake from crystalloid solutions without oral nutrition

▸ **Expected Outcome:** The client will have adequate nutrition to meet the needs for growth and repair of tissue.

Nutrition Notes 13-1
The Client Receiving Intravenous Fluid Therapy

● When administered parenterally, dextrose provides 3.4 cal/g, not 4 cal/g as with carbohydrates consumed orally. Therefore, 1 L of 5% dextrose in water (D_5W), which contains 50 g dextrose, provides a total of 170 calories; 3 L of D_5W infused over 24 hours provides only 510 calories.

● Because simple IV solutions (i.e., dextrose in water) are nutritionally and calorically inadequate, it is best to avoid maintaining clients on them longer than 1 to 2 days.

• Weigh the client daily. *Although short-term weight changes usually relate to fluids, long-term weight loss may indicate inadequate caloric intake (Nutrition Notes 13-1).*

• Monitor laboratory test results such as blood cell count and hemoglobin, albumin, and transferrin levels. *A drop in specific laboratory findings indicates insufficient protein to ensure their normal production or replacement.*

• Implement the physician's orders to provide TPN if it becomes necessary. *TPN provides the client with protein, vitamins, and minerals as well as glucose and water. Intermittent fat emulsions complete the requirements for adequate nutrition.*

Evaluation of Expected Outcomes

Expected outcomes are that the client's fluid status is improved or maintained within normal, with approximately equal intake and output volumes and normal vital signs. Breathing remains quiet and effortless, with no signs of localized or generalized edema. The IV site is not red, tender, or warm, and shows no drainage. The client's body temperature remains within normal range. The client uses the extremity with minimal inconvenience from the IV infusion. He or she maintains pre-illness weight. Blood cell count and hemoglobin, albumin, and transferrin levels are within normal limits. ●

BOX 13-2 Candidates for Total Parenteral Nutrition

Candidates for TPN include clients:

• Who have not eaten for 5 days and are not likely to eat during the next week
• Who have had a 10% or more loss of body weight
• Exhibiting self-imposed starvation (anorexia nervosa)
• With cancer of the esophagus or stomach
• With postoperative GI complications
• With acute inflammatory bowel disease
• With major trauma or burns
• With liver and renal failure

▶ *Stop, Think, and Respond Exercise 13-3*

A client had surgery 2 days ago, at which time he lost approximately 500 mL of blood. After surgery, he is not allowed to have anything orally because he has a nasogastric tube connected to suction. In the meantime, he has also developed diarrhea, a side effect that the physician attributes to the parenteral antibiotic he is receiving. When you assess this client, his blood pressure is 104/62 mm Hg, much lower than his admission blood pressure of 132/86 mm Hg. His skin is dry and tents when you assess turgor; his urine output has been 350 mL over the past 8 hours, and the urine appears dark yellow.

1. *What additional information would you gather to assess the client's fluid status?*
2. *If IV fluids are administered, which type of solution is most appropriate to use and why?*

SPECIAL CONSIDERATIONS FOR INTRAVENOUS THERAPY

Total Parenteral Nutrition

The physician may order TPN for a client who is severely malnourished or cannot consume food or liquids for a long time (Box 13-2). TPN uses a solution of nutrients to meet the client's caloric and nutritional needs. The composition of a TPN solution is individualized according to the client's nutritional requirements and medical condition. Because concentrations of protein, carbohydrate, and fat are standard in standard volumes, however, individualization is somewhat limited.

TPN solutions, which are extremely concentrated (hypertonic), are instilled into the central circulation, where they are diluted in a fairly large volume of blood. Because of their immediate dilution, TPN solutions do not dehydrate cells.

A lipid emulsion is sometimes administered intermittently with TPN. An **emulsion** is a mixture of two liquids, one of which is insoluble in the other, and an emulsifier, which stabilizes the mixture by keeping one of the liquids dispersed in the other. Lipid emulsions contain fat from soybean and safflower oils, phospholipids from egg yolks that act as emulsifying agents, and glycerol to make the solution isotonic. Lipid emulsions provide essential fatty acids and are often used to meet 20% to 30% of the client's total calorie needs. However, lipid emulsions may be contraindicated in clients with elevated triglyceride levels

Before TPN is initiated, the physician gains access to the central circulation using a central venous catheter. Trained nurses administer TPN using filtered tubing and an electronic infusion device (Nursing Guidelines 13-2).

For clients receiving TPN at home or as a supplement to an inadequate oral diet, cyclical TPN is most often used. Cyclical TPN is infused in cycles over 10 to 16 hours, followed by 8 to 14 hours of rest. Cyclical TPN offers the client more mobility, especially if infused during the night, and has the advantage of allowing enzyme and hormone levels to drop

NURSING GUIDELINES 13-2

Administering Total Parenteral Nutrition

- Weigh client daily.
- Use tubing that contains a filter; however, bypass the filter when administering lipid emulsions to prevent large fat molecules from obstructing the filter.
- Label the tubing used for TPN to ensure that it is used exclusively for TPN and not IV medications or blood products.
- Change TPN tubings daily.
- Tape all connections in the tubing to prevent accidental separation and the potential for an air embolism.
- Clamp the central catheter whenever separating the tubing from its catheter connection.
- Use an electronic infusion device to administer TPN.
- Infuse initial TPN solutions gradually (e.g., 25–50 mL/hr); increase rate according to the agency's standard of care or the physician's medical orders.

- Monitor blood glucose levels regularly to assess the client's ability to metabolize the concentrated glucose.
- Administer insulin on a sliding scale according to blood glucose levels.
- Wean client from TPN gradually to avoid a sudden drop in blood glucose level.
- Infuse IV lipids three times a week.
- Monitor the following laboratory test results to evaluate the nutritional status of the client receiving TPN and lipids: serum transferrin, serum osmolality, cholesterol, triglycerides, electrolytes, blood urea nitrogen (BUN), and urine creatinine.

to normal during the rest periods. To give the body time to adjust to the decreasing glucose load (and prevent rebound hypoglycemia), the infusion should be tapered near the end of each cycle. The nurse should monitor the client's blood glucose level, because the glucose levels in TPN can cause hyperglycemia.

Blood Transfusion

Blood that is administered usually comes from nonautologous donors, meaning that it comes from a person other than the person who will receive the blood. Blood contains cells and additives and preservatives that enable it to be stored in a refrigerated state for approximately 1 month without clotting. For these reasons, administering blood intravenously requires special considerations.

Blood Transfusion Equipment

Because blood contains cells in addition to water, it is generally infused through a 16- to 20-gauge (preferably an 18-gauge) catheter. Blood is administered through **Y-administration tubing** (Fig. 13-15). This tubing contains two branches: one for blood and one for isotonic (normal) saline. The two branches extend above a filter that removes blood clots and cellular debris. The normal saline infuses before and after the blood infuses, or during the infusion if a transfusion reaction occurs.

Pharmacologic Considerations

- Never add medications to whole blood or to the saline solution used to start the transfusion. Allergic reactions are possible when blood is administered. If medications were added to the blood or saline, it would be impossible to tell if the allergic reaction occurred in response to the blood or to the medication.

Blood Compatibility

Before blood is administered, it must be examined to make sure the donor and recipient blood types are compatible. Blood is typed according to the **ABO system**. Everyone has one of four blood types: A, B, AB, or O. Red blood cells of types A, B, and AB blood have a protein on their surface called an antigen. Type A blood has antigen A; type B has antigen B, type AB has both antigen A and antigen B. Type O has neither A nor B antigens.

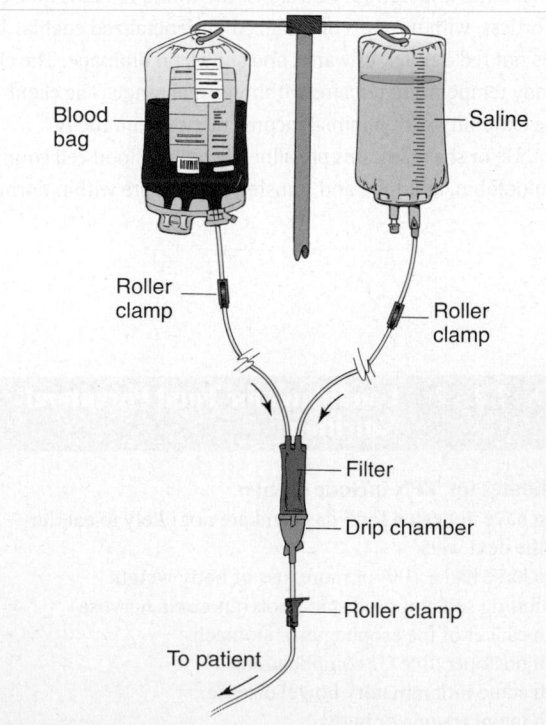

FIGURE 13-15. Blood administration set using Y-administration tubing.

The blood type is important when transfusing blood because antibodies in the blood plasma will react against transfused blood cells that have a different antigen on their surface. For example, if a person who has type A blood receives type B blood, anti-B antibodies will destroy the transfused blood cells carrying antigen B, with life-threatening consequences. Because type O blood has neither A nor B antigens on its surface, type O can be given to a person with any type of blood. For this reason, people with type O blood are referred to as **universal donors**. However, a person with type O blood cannot receive a type other than type O because anti-A and anti-B antibodies will attack the cells in the donated blood. Persons with type AB blood can receive AB, A, B, or O blood because they do not have anti-A or anti-B antibodies. Consequently, persons with type AB blood are called **universal recipients**.

Some blood cells have an additional protein surface marker known as the **Rh factor**. It acquired its name because the protein was first discovered in rhesus monkeys. Approximately 85% of humans have this additional protein on their blood cells, which makes them Rh positive (+). Those who lack the protein are Rh negative (−). The Rh factor acts as an antigen that will cause a fatal reaction if given to a person with Rh-negative blood. On the other hand, a person with Rh-positive blood will not be affected by type compatible blood that is Rh negative, because it does not have the antigenic protein on the cells' surface.

Whole blood and packed cells are typed and crossmatched in the laboratory before administration to ensure that the donor's and recipient's blood types and Rh factor are compatible (Table 13-4).

Each client that needs a blood transfusion has an additional identification bracelet that is attached when the laboratory draws a sample of blood for typing and cross matching. Before a blood transfusion is initiated, two nurses must check the identifying numbers on the bracelet to confirm that they match the numbers on the unit of blood from the blood bank.

▶ **Stop, Think, and Respond Exercise 13-4**

What blood type(s) are compatible for a client with an AB Rh-positive blood type, a client with an O Rh-negative blood type, and a client with a B Rh-positive blood type?

Complications of Blood Transfusion

Clients who receive blood are at risk for the same complications as those receiving crystalloid fluids. They also face additional risks, however.

A **transfusion reaction** is an untoward event at the time that blood is being administered. One of the most life-threatening transfusion reactions is an incompatibility reaction that occurs when the donor and recipient blood types are incorrectly matched. In this instance, the recipient's antibodies destroy the donor cells. Although an incompatibility reaction occurs once in approximately 25,000 blood transfusions, it accounts for more than 50% of reported transfusion-related deaths (Ting, 2002a). An acute incompatibility reaction occurs within minutes of infusing the donor blood. Milder

TABLE 13-4 Blood Groups and Compatible Types

BLOOD GROUPS	PERCENTAGE OF POPULATION	COMPATIBLE BLOOD TYPES
A	41%	A and O
B	9%	B and O
O	47%	O
AB	3%	AB, A, B, and O
Rh+	85% Whites	Rh+ and Rh−
	95% African Americans	Rh− only
Rh−	15% Whites	
	5% African Americans	

allergic reactions such as hives and itching or a febrile response may occur if the recipient is sensitive to noncellular substances in the donor blood. Delayed reactions, which are milder than incompatibility reactions, can occur weeks to months after a transfusion. Delayed reactions are more likely the result of an immune response against the antigens of the Rh component of blood cells.

Because serious transfusion reactions generally occur within the first 5 to 15 minutes of the infusion, many healthcare agencies require that a nurse remains with and monitors the client during this critical time. Because a transfusion reaction can occur at any time, however, nurses monitor clients frequently throughout a transfusion for signs of a reaction or other complications associated with receiving blood (see later discussion). Clients are instructed to call for assistance if they feel unusual while receiving the infusion of blood. In cases of a suspected transfusion reaction, it is appropriate to stop the infusion of blood and infuse a solution of normal saline while continuing to assess the client.

Nonimmune complications also are possible after blood transfusion. Clients may become septic if pathogens have grown and multiplied in the stored blood or during the interim when blood is being infused. A universal standard is to keep the blood refrigerated until just before use and to infuse the blood in 4 hours or less to prevent a septic reaction from bacterial contamination. Some clients have shaking chills and a fever during a septic or febrile reaction. Monitoring the client's temperature before, during, and after a blood transfusion is necessary to determine if chilling is the result of an emerging complication or of infusing cold blood.

Reduced levels of serum calcium can produce symptoms in clients who receive massive transfusions of blood over a very short time. Citrate, which is added to the donor blood, binds with calcium in the recipient's blood, causing hypocalcemia.

Blood-borne infections such as hepatitis A, B, and C and human immunodeficiency virus (HIV) infection also can be transmitted through blood from infected donors. Donors are asked questions about their infection history, foreign travel, and risk behaviors when being screened before donating blood. Donated blood also is tested for hepatitis virus and HIV antibody levels. Although it is impossible to guarantee that all donated blood is free of blood-borne pathogens, the incidence of transmission is much smaller than it was at one time.

TABLE 13-5 Complications of Blood Transfusion

COMPLICATION	SIGNS AND SYMPTOMS	CAUSE(S)	ACTIONS
Incompatibility reaction	Hypotension, rapid pulse rate, difficulty breathing, back pain, flushing	Mismatch between donor and recipient blood groups	Stop the infusion of blood Infuse the saline at a rapid rate Call for assistance Administer oxygen Raise the feet higher than the head Be prepared to administer emergency drugs Send first urine specimen to laboratory Save the blood and tubing
Febrile reaction	Fever, shaking chills, headache, rapid pulse, muscle aches	Allergy to foreign proteins in the donated blood	Stop the blood infusion Start the saline Check vital signs Report findings
Septic reaction	Fever, chills, hypotension	Infusion of blood that contains microorganisms	Stop the infusion of blood Start the saline Report findings Save the blood and tubing
Allergic reaction	Rash, itching, flushing, stable vital signs	Minor sensitivity to substances in the donor blood	Slow the rate of infusion Assess the client Report findings Be prepared to give an anti-histamine
Moderate chilling	No fever or other symptoms	Infusion of cold blood	Continue the infusion Cover and make the client comfortable
Circulatory overload	Hypertension, difficulty breathing, moist breath sounds, bounding pulse	Large volume or rapid rate of infusion; inadequate cardiac or kidney function	Reduce the rate of infusion Elevate the head Give oxygen Report findings Be prepared to give a diuretic
Hypocalcemia (low calcium)	Tingling of fingers, hypotension, muscle cramps, convulsions	Multiple blood transfusions containing anticalcium agents	Stop the blood infusion Start saline Report findings Be prepared to give antidote, calcium chloride
HIV and hepatitis B virus transmission	Opportunistic infections; elevated antibody titers, abnormal blood cell counts or liver enzyme levels	Blood collected from infected donors that passed screening examinations	Encourage autologous (self) blood collection if possible

Table 13-5 provides an overview of potential complications from blood transfusion and specific nursing actions.

To avoid the use of publicly donated blood, some surgeons administer salvaged blood. **Salvaged blood** is blood collected from a client during a surgical procedure and reinfused while surgery is being performed or shortly thereafter. Salvaging blood involves using a device known as a cell saver system. In this system, blood drains from the surgical site into a collection device; a reservoir sends debris into a separate waste container, and salvaged blood is reinfused intravenously to the client. Salvaged blood is commonly reclaimed during cardiothoracic and orthopedic joint replacement surgery. Using salvaged blood eliminates the potential for transmission of blood-borne diseases, provides type-specific blood, and frees stored blood in the blood bank so that it is available to other clients who may require a blood transfusion.

CRITICAL THINKING EXERCISES

1. Determine the rate of infusion for 1000 mL of solution ordered to infuse by gravity over 10 hours. You have tubing with a drop factor of 15 gtt/mL. Explain how you determine if the solution is infusing according to the calculated rate.
2. How is the administration of IV fluid different for an older adult compared with an individual who is middle age or younger?
3. If a unit of type A Rh-negative blood is obtained from the blood bank for administration to a client who is type A Rh positive, what action is appropriate?
4. What action is appropriate if the site where an intravenous fluid is infusing appears swollen and feels cool and tender when palpated?

5. Explain whether it would be better to infuse 1000 mL of IV solution in 8 hours using a gravity infusion method or an electronic infusion device for a client who is confused and restless.

NCLEX-STYLE REVIEW QUESTIONS

1. For which of the following clients would IV lipid emulsions be contraindicated?
   1. A client with a cardiac disorder
   2. A client with migraine headaches
   3. A client with acute pancreatitis
   4. A client with a urinary tract infection
2. If a client is to receive 1000 mL of Dextrose 5% and Normal Saline (D5NS) in 8 hours, the nurse accurately checks that the infusion pump administers an hourly volume of
   1. 50 mL
   2. 100 mL
   3. 125 mL
   4. 150 mL
3. During the night, a client is startled and continues to worry about an alarm that sounded from his electronic intravenous infusion pump. Which nursing intervention is most appropriate to relieve the client's anxiety at this time?
   1. Explain why the alarm sounded.
   2. Give a prescribed tranquilizer.
   3. Infuse the solution by gravity.
   4. Provide a midnight snack.
4. When discontinuing the administration of intravenous fluid, which nursing action is essential?
   1. Donning clean gloves
   2. Weighing the client daily
   3. Pulling the privacy curtain
   4. Taking vital signs
5. An older adult with metastatic cancer of the esophagus is undergoing palliative treatment that includes total parenteral nutrition (TPN) through a central subclavian catheter. Which nursing assessment is essential for evaluating the client's response to the TPN?
   1. Measure the arterial pulse pressure
   2. Monitor the capillary blood glucose
   3. Obtain an apical-radial pulse rate
   4. Test the urine's specific gravity

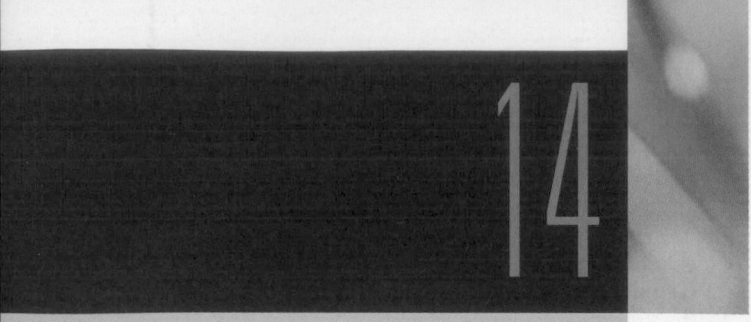

Perioperative Care

Words To Know
ambulatory surgery
anesthesia
anesthesiologist
anesthetist
dehiscence
embolus
evisceration
intraoperative
malignant hyperthermia
paralytic ileus
perioperative
phlebothrombosis
postoperative
preoperative
procedural sedation
surgical asepsis
thrombophlebitis

Learning Objectives

On completion of this chapter, you will be able to:

1. Describe why surgical procedures may be performed.
2. Differentiate the phases of perioperative care.
3. Outline preoperative assessments needed to identify surgical risk factors.
4. List components of a preoperative teaching plan.
5. Describe physical preparation of the client for surgery.
6. List preoperative medications that may be ordered.
7. Discuss psychosocial preparation of the client for surgery, including strategies for alleviating clients' preoperative anxiety.
8. Compare types of anesthesia.
9. Describe the roles and functions of the surgical team members.
10. Describe nursing management of the intraoperative client.
11. Discuss assessments needed to prevent postoperative complications.
12. Describe standards of care, nursing diagnoses, and common interventions for general surgical clients in the later postoperative period.

Clients undergo surgery for a variety of reasons (Table 14-1). No matter how minor, surgery causes stress and poses risks for complications for the client. Many variables, such as the procedure performed, age of the client, and coexisting medical conditions determine the care clients need before, during, and after surgery. However, administering anesthesia and disrupting physiologic processes (i.e., through creation of the surgical wound and the operation itself) subject all clients undergoing surgery to a common set of problems. These problems require standardized, in addition to individualized, assessments and interventions. As much as possible, clients require comprehensive education before and after surgery. Table 14-2 categorizes surgery in terms of urgency.

Traditionally, any surgical procedure required admitting the client to the hospital. However, many diagnostic or short therapeutic surgical procedures—such as bone marrow biopsy, endoscopy, or cardiac catheterization—are now performed in outpatient settings and ambulatory surgical centers. **Ambulatory surgery**, sometimes referred to as *same-day* or *outpatient surgery,* is defined as surgery that requires fewer than 24 hours of hospitalization. These short-term admissions may be as brief as 1 to 2 hours or extend to overnight. Ambulatory surgical units are located either in a hospital or in a separate building that the hospital owns. Others are freestanding, privately owned facilities not affiliated with a hospital.

The increase in the number of ambulatory surgical procedures is related to advances in surgical techniques and methods of anesthesia, prospective reimbursement, managed care, and changes in Medicare and Medicaid provisions (Smeltzer et al., 2008). A client admitted for ambulatory surgery must meet the following criteria:

TABLE 14-1 Reasons for Surgery

TYPE OF SURGERY	PURPOSE	EXAMPLES
Diagnostic	Removal and study of tissue to make a diagnosis	Breast biopsy Biopsy of skin lesion
Exploratory	More extensive means to diagnose a problem; usually involves exploration of a body cavity or use of scopes inserted through small incisions	Exploration of abdomen for unexplained pain Exploratory laparoscopy
Curative	Removal or replacement of defective tissue to restore function	Cholecystectomy Total hip replacement
Palliative	Relief of symptoms or enhancement of function without cure	Resection of a tumor to relieve pressure and pain
Cosmetic	Reshape normal body structures or improve appearance or change a physical feature	Rhinoplasty Cleft lip repair Mammoplasty
Preventive or prophylactic	Removal of tissue that does not yet contain cancer cells, but has a high probability of becoming cancerous in the future	Prophylactic bilateral oopherectomy (removal of both ovaries)
Reconstructive	Repair or reconstruct physical deformities and abnormalities caused by traumatic injuries, birth defects, developmental abnormalities, or disease	Breast reconstruction following mastectomy Cleft lip repair

- The client is not critically ill.
- The surgical procedure is not extensive and does not require many hours of general anesthesia.
- The client has few, if any, coexisting and disabling illnesses.
- Recovery is expected to be quick, with minimal specialized care after surgery.
- The client or family can provide adequate postoperative care.

Regardless of the setting, nursing goals when caring for surgical clients are to minimize clients' anxiety, prepare them for surgery, monitor for complications during surgery, and assist in a speedy, uncomplicated recovery. **Perioperative** is a term used to describe the entire span of surgery, including before and after the actual operation. The three phases of perioperative care are as follows:

1. **Preoperative:** begins with the decision to perform surgery and continues until the client reaches the operating area
2. **Intraoperative:** includes the entire surgical procedure until transfer of the client to the recovery area

3. **Postoperative:** begins with admission to the recovery area and continues until the client receives a follow-up evaluation at home or is discharged to a rehabilitation unit

Each phase requires specific assessments and nursing interventions.

PREOPERATIVE CARE

Time for preoperative assessment, nursing diagnoses, and evaluation of nursing management may be limited when a client is admitted for ambulatory surgery or shortly before surgery. Recognition of the client's immediate preoperative needs is important, however, and preparation for surgery still requires the nursing process.

Assessment

Preoperative care requires a complete assessment of the client (Box 14-1). The assessment varies, depending on the

TABLE 14-2 Categories of Surgery Based on Urgency

CLASSIFICATION	CONDITIONS	EXAMPLES
Emergency	Immediate; condition is life-threatening, requiring surgery at once	Gunshot wound Severe bleeding Small bowel obstruction
Urgent	Within 24 to 30 hours; client requires prompt attention	Kidney stones Acute gallbladder infection Fractured hip
Required	Planned for a few weeks or months after decision; client requires surgery at some point	Benign prostatic hypertrophy Cataracts Hernia without strangulation
Elective	Client will not be harmed if surgery is not performed but will benefit if it is performed	Revision of scars Vaginal repairs
Optional	Personal preference	Cosmetic surgery

(Adapted from Smeltzer, S. C., Bare, B. G., Hinkle, J. L., & Cheever, K. H., 2008. *Brunner and Suddarth's textbook of medical-surgical nursing*, 11th ed. Philadelphia: Lippincott Williams & Wilkins.)

BOX 14-1 Preoperative Assessment

Review Preoperative Laboratory and Diagnostic Studies
- Complete blood count
- Blood type and crossmatch
- Serum electrolytes
- Urinalysis
- Chest x-ray
- Electrocardiogram
- Other tests related to procedure or client's medical condition (e.g., prothrombin time, partial thromboplastin time, blood urea nitrogen, creatinine, other radiographic studies)

Review Client's Health History and Preparation for Surgery
- History of present illness and reason for surgery
- Past medical history
  Medical conditions—acute and chronic
  Previous hospitalizations and surgeries
  Any past problems with anesthesia
  Allergies
  Present medications
  Substance use: alcohol, tobacco, street drugs
- Review of systems

Assess Physical Needs
- Ability to communicate
- Vital signs

- Level of consciousness
  Confusion
  Drowsiness
  Unresponsiveness
- Weight and height
- Skin integrity
- Ability to move/ambulate
- Level of exercise
- Prostheses
- Circulatory status

Assess Psychological Needs
- Emotional state
- Level of understanding of surgical procedure and preoperative and postoperative instructions
- Coping strategies
- Support system
- Roles and responsibilities

Assess Cultural Needs
- Language—need for an interpreter
- Particular customs related to surgery, privacy, disposal of body parts, and blood transfusions

urgency of the surgery and whether the client is admitted the same day of surgery or earlier. For any preoperative client, however, the nurse must make every effort to gather as much data as possible.

On admission, the nurse reviews preoperative instructions, such as diet restrictions and skin preparations, to ensure the client has followed them. If the client has not carried out a specific portion of the instructions, such as withholding foods and fluids, the nurse immediately notifies the surgeon. He or she identifies the client's needs to determine if the client is at risk for complications during or after the surgery. General risk factors are related to age; nutritional status; use of alcohol, tobacco, and other substances; and physical condition (Table 14-3).

When surgery is not an emergency, the nurse performs a thorough history and physical examination. He or she assesses the client's understanding of the surgical procedure, postoperative expectations, and ability to participate in recovery. The nurse also considers the client's cultural needs, specifically as they relate to beliefs about surgery, personal privacy, disposal of body parts, blood transfusions, and presence of family members during the preoperative and postoperative phases (see Chap. 8).

If the surgical procedure is an emergency, the nurse may have to omit some tasks because of the client's condition or need for rapid preparation. There may not be time to perform a thorough assessment or write a complete care plan. Assessment of the surgical client is essential, but the situation dictates the extent of this process.

▶ **Stop, Think, and Respond Exercise 14-1**

A client who is admitted for knee replacement surgery is 100 lb overweight. What are the potential postoperative concerns?

Surgical Consent

Before surgery, the client must sign a surgical consent form or operative permit. When signed, this form indicates that the client consents to the procedure and understands its risks and benefits as explained by the surgeon. Box 14-2 describes the criteria needed for valid informed consent. If the client has not understood the explanations, the nurse notifies the surgeon before the client signs the consent form. Clients must sign a consent form for any invasive procedure that requires anesthesia and has risks of complications.

If an adult client is confused, unconscious, or not mentally competent, a family member or guardian must sign the consent form. If the client is younger than 18 years of age, a parent or legal guardian must sign the consent form. Persons younger than age 18 years of age, living away from home and supporting themselves, are regarded as emancipated minors and sign their own consent forms. In an emergency, the surgeon may have to operate without consent. Healthcare personnel, however, make every effort to obtain consent by telephone, telegram, or fax. Each nurse must be familiar with agency policies and state laws regarding surgical consent forms.

TABLE 14-3 Surgical Risk Factors and Potential Complications

VARIABLE	POTENTIAL COMPLICATION
Age	
Very young—Immaturity of organ systems and regulatory mechanisms	Respiratory obstruction, fluid overload, dehydration, hypothermia, and infection
Older adults—Multiple organ degeneration and slowed regulatory mechanisms	Decreased metabolism and excretion of anesthetics and pain medications, fluid overload, renal failure, formation of blood clots, delayed wound healing, infection, confusion, and respiratory complications
Nutritional Status	
Malnourished—Low weight and nutrient deficiencies	Fluid and electrolyte imbalances, cardiac dysrhythmias, delayed wound healing, wound infections
Obese—Stressed cardiovascular system, decreased circulation, decreased pulmonary function	Atelectasis, pneumonia, blood clots, delayed wound healing, wound infection, delayed metabolism and excretion of anesthetics and pain medication
Substance Abuse	
Altered respiratory function, nutritional status, or liver function	Atelectasis, pneumonia, altered effectiveness of anesthetics and pain medications, drug interactions, drug withdrawal
Medical Problems	
Immune—Allergies and immunosuppression secondary to corticosteroid therapy, transplants, chemotherapy, or diseases such as AIDS	Adverse reactions to medications, blood transfusions, or latex; infection
Respiratory—Acute and chronic respiratory problems and history of tobacco use	Atelectasis, bronchopneumonia, respiratory failure
Cardiovascular—Hypertension, coronary artery disease, peripheral vascular disease	Hypotension, hypertension, fluid overload, congestive heart failure, shock, dysrhythmias, myocardial infarction, stroke, blood clots
Hepatic—Liver dysfunction	Delayed drug metabolism leading to drug toxicity, disrupted clotting mechanisms leading to excessive bleeding or hemorrhage, confusion, increased risk of infection
Renal—Kidney disease, chronic renal insufficiency, renal failure	Fluid and electrolyte imbalances, congestive heart failure, dysrhythmias, delayed excretion of drugs leading to drug toxicity
Endocrine—Diabetes	Hypoglycemia, hyperglycemia, hypokalemia, infection, delayed wound healing

Clients must sign the consent form before receiving any preoperative sedatives. When the client or designated person has signed the permit, an adult witness also signs it to indicate that the client or designee signed voluntarily. This witness usually is a member of the healthcare team or an employee in the admissions department. The nurse is responsible for ensuring that all necessary parties have signed the consent form and that it is in the client's chart before the client goes to the operating room (OR).

Preoperative Teaching

Teaching clients about their surgical procedure and expectations before and after surgery is best done during the preoperative period. Clients are more alert and free of pain at this time. Clients and family members can better participate in recovery if they know what to expect. The nurse adapts instructions and explanations to the client's ability to understand. When clients understand what they can do to help themselves recover, they are more likely to follow the

---

BOX 14-2 **Criteria for Valid Informed Consent**

Voluntary Consent
Valid consent must be freely given, without coercion.

Incompetent Client
Legal definition: Individual who is *not* autonomous and cannot give or withhold consent (e.g., individuals who are cognitively impaired, mentally ill, or neurologically incapacitated)

Informed Subject
Informed consent should be in writing. It should contain the following:
• Explanation of procedure and its risks

• Descriptions of benefits and alternatives
• An offer to answer questions about procedure
• Instructions that the client may withdraw consent
• A statement informing the client if the protocol differs from customary procedure

Client Able To Comprehend
Information must be written and delivered in language understandable to the client. Questions must be answered to facilitate comprehension if material is confusing.

(From Smeltzer, S. C., Bare, B. G., Hinkle, J.L. & Cheever, K.H. [2008]. *Brunner & Suddarth's textbook of medical-surgical nursing* [11th ed.]. Philadelphia: Lippincott Williams & Wilkins, p. 485.)

preoperative instructions and work with healthcare team members.

Information to include in a preoperative teaching plan varies with the type of surgery and the length of the hospitalization. The following are examples of information to include in preoperative teaching:

- Preoperative medications—when they are given and their effects
- Postoperative pain control
- Explanation and description of the postanesthesia recovery room or postsurgical area
- Discussion of the frequency of assessing vital signs and use of monitoring equipment

The nurse also explains and demonstrates deep-breathing and coughing exercises, use of incentive spirometry, how to splint the incision for breathing exercises and moving, position changes, and feet and leg exercises.

In addition, the nurse must inform the client about intravenous (IV) fluids and other lines and tubes. Sometimes IV fluids are initiated before surgery, along with indwelling catheters or nasogastric tubes. When clients receive demonstrations, it is important that they practice these skills and provide an opportunity for the nurse to assess whether they understood the instructions. Preoperative teaching time also gives clients the chance to express any anxieties and fears and for the nurse to provide explanations that will help alleviate those fears.

When clients are admitted for emergency surgery, time for detailed explanations of preoperative preparations and the postoperative period is unavailable. If the client is alert, however, the nurse provides brief explanations. During the postoperative period, explanations will be more complete. Family members require as many preoperative explanations as possible.

The purpose of adequate preoperative teaching/learning is for the client to have an uncomplicated and shorter recovery period. He or she will be more likely to deep breathe and cough, move as directed, and require less pain medication. The client and family members will demonstrate sufficient knowledge of the surgical procedure, preoperative preparations, and postoperative procedures, and can participate fully in the client's care.

 Gerontologic Considerations

- Diminished abilities to hear, see, and understand may interfere with preoperative and postoperative teaching. Nurses may need to repeat explanations and demonstrations, and include family members or significant others. Removal of assistive devices such as eye glasses or hearing aids before surgical procedures may cause sensory deprivation or contribute to confusion.

Physical Preparation

Preparing a client for surgery is an essential element of preoperative care. Depending on the time of admission to the hospital or surgical facility, the nurse may perform some of the physical preparation, which includes the following:

- *Skin preparation:* Skin preparation depends on the surgical procedure and the policies of the surgeon or institution. The goal is to decrease bacteria without compromising skin integrity. For planned surgery, the client may be asked to cleanse the particular area with detergent germicide soap for several days before surgery. Hair usually is not removed before surgery unless it is likely to interfere with the incision. In that case, the hair is removed with electric clippers at the time of surgery.
- *Elimination:* The nurse may need to insert an indwelling urinary catheter preoperatively for some surgeries, particularly of the lower abdomen. A distended bladder increases the risk of bladder trauma and difficulty in performing the procedure. The catheter keeps the bladder empty during surgery. If a catheter is not inserted, the nurse instructs the client to void immediately before receiving preoperative medication. Enemas or laxatives may be ordered to clean out the lower bowel if the client is having abdominal or pelvic surgery. A clean bowel allows for accurate visualization of the surgical site and prevents trauma to the intestine or accidental contamination by feces to the peritoneum. A cleansing enema or laxative is prescribed the evening before surgery and may be repeated the morning of surgery.
- *Food and fluids:* The physician gives specific instructions about how long before surgery food and fluids are to be withheld, often at least 8 to 10 hours before surgery. After midnight the night before surgery, the client usually is not allowed to have anything by mouth (NPO). Many ambulatory surgical centers, however, allow clear fluids up to 3 or 4 hours before surgery. Before these times, the nurse encourages the client to maintain good nutrition to help meet the body's increased need for nutrients during the healing process. Adequate intake of protein and ascorbic acid (vitamin C) is especially important in wound healing.
- *Care of valuables:* The nurse encourages the client to give valuables to a family member to take home. If this is not possible, however, the nurse itemizes the valuables, places them in an envelope, and locks them in a designated area. The client signs a receipt, and the nurse notes their deposition on the client's chart. If the client is reluctant to remove a wedding band, the nurse may slip gauze under the ring, then loop the gauze around the finger and wrist or apply adhesive tape over a plain wedding band. The client also removes eyeglasses and contact lenses, which the nurse places in a safe location or gives to a family member.
- *Attire/grooming:* Usually clients wear a hospital gown and a surgical cap in the OR. Hair ornaments and all makeup and nail polish must be removed. If the client is having minor surgery performed under local anesthesia in a room separate from the general surgical suites, the nurse instructs the client on what clothing and cosmetics to remove and provides appropriate hospital attire. The physician may order thigh-high or knee-high antiembolism stockings or order the client's legs to be wrapped in elastic bandages before surgery to help prevent venous stasis during and after the surgery. Removal of cosmetics assists the surgical team to observe the client's lips, face, and nail beds for cyanosis, pallor, or other signs of decreased

oxygenation. If a client has acrylic nails, one usually is removed to attach a pulse oximeter, which measures oxygen saturation (see Chap. 19).

* *Prostheses:* Depending on agency policy and physician preference, the client removes full or partial dentures. Doing so prevents the dentures from becoming dislodged or causing airway obstruction during administration of a general anesthetic. Some anesthesiologists prefer that well-fitting dentures be left in place to preserve facial contours. If dentures are removed, the nurse usually places them in a denture container and leaves them at the client's bedside or places them with the client's belongings. Other prostheses, such as artificial limbs, also are removed, unless otherwise ordered.

Preoperative Medications

The anesthesiologist frequently orders preoperative medications. Common preoperative medications include the following:

* *Anticholinergics,* which decrease respiratory tract secretions, dry mucous membranes, and interrupt vagal stimulation
* *Histamine$_2$-receptor antagonists,* which decrease gastric acidity and volume
* Opioids which decrease the amount of anesthesia needed, help reduce anxiety and pain, and promote sleep
* *Sedatives,* which promote sleep, decrease anxiety, and reduce the amount of anesthesia needed
* *Tranquilizers,* which reduce nausea, prevent emesis, enhance preoperative sedation, preoperative anxiety, slow motor activity, and promote induction of anesthesia

Drug Therapy Table 14-1 provides more information about dosages and the desired and adverse effects of preoperative medications.

Before administering preoperative medications, the nurse checks the client's identification bracelet, asks about drug allergies, obtains blood pressure (BP) and pulse and respiratory rates, asks the client to void, and makes sure the surgical consent form has been signed. The nurse also reviews with the client what to expect after receiving the medications. Immediately after giving the medications, the nurse instructs the client to remain in bed; he or she places side rails in the up position and ensures that the call button is within easy reach.

 Pharmacologic Considerations

- Preoperative medication is given precisely at the time prescribed by the anesthesiologist. If the preoperative medication is given too early, the optimum potency will be reached before it is needed; if the drug is given too late, its action will not begin before the anesthesia is initiated.

- If the client experiences acute anxiety before surgery, the physician may prescribe a tranquilizer or sedative. Notify the physician if the medication does not appear to be effective.

- The evening before surgery, a sedative drug may be ordered to ensure rest. Document the effects of the medication on the client's chart.

Psychosocial Preparation

Preparing the client emotionally and spiritually is as important as doing so physically. Psychosocial preparation should begin as soon as the client is aware that surgery is necessary. Anxiety and fear, if extreme, can affect a client's condition during and after surgery. Anxious clients have a poor response to surgery and are prone to complications. Many clients are fearful because they know little or nothing about what will happen before, during, and after surgery. Careful preoperative teaching and listening by the nurse about what will happen and what to expect can help allay some of these fears and anxieties. The nurse also must assess methods the client uses for coping. Religious faith is a source of strength for many clients; therefore, nurses facilitate contact with a client's clergyperson or the hospital chaplain if requested.

Preoperative Checklist

Most clients are transported to the OR on a stretcher. To provide privacy, safety, and warmth, the nurse covers the client with a blanket and fastens restraint straps around the client. Before the client leaves the room, the nurse records all necessary information on the client's chart: vital signs, weight, preoperative medications administered, procedures performed, whether the client has voided, disposition of valuables and dentures, and pertinent observations.

Most hospitals or surgical facilities use a preoperative checklist to ensure that all assessments and procedures for the client are complete before surgery. A checklist usually includes the following:

* *Assessment:* includes the identification and allergy bracelet; identification of allergies; list of current medications; last time the client ate or drank; disposition of valuables, dentures, or prostheses; removal of makeup and nail polish; and wearing of hospital attire
* *Preoperative medications:* includes route and time administered
* *IV:* includes location, type of solution, and rate
* *Preoperative preparations:* includes, as appropriate, skin preparation; indwelling urinary catheter or nasogastric tube insertion; times and results of enemas or douches; application of antiembolism stockings or wraps; and time and amount of last voiding
* *Chart:* includes surgical consent signed and on chart; history and physical completed by physician and on chart; old records with chart; and ordered test results on chart (e.g., electrocardiogram, complete blood count, urinalysis, type and screen or type and crossmatch for blood transfusions)
* *Other information:* as required by agency policy
* *Signature(s):* of nurse and other personnel involved with preparing the client for surgery and transporting the client to the OR

When the preoperative checklist is complete, the client is ready to go to the operating suite. Personnel from the OR assist in the transfer of the client to the stretcher and then to the OR or surgical holding area.

There is an increased emphasis on making sure that the right client has the right procedure at the right site. To prevent "wrong site, wrong procedure, wrong person surgery,"

DRUG THERAPY TABLE 14-1 Preoperative Medications

Drug Category and Examples	Mechanisms of Action	Side Effects	Nursing Considerations
Anticholinergics atropine sulfate, scopolamine, glycopyrrolate (Robinul)	Decreases oral, respiratory, and gastric secretions Prevents laryngospasm and reflex bradycardia	Dry mouth; tachycardia; excessive CNS stimulation (tremor, restlessness, confusion), followed by excessive CNS depression (coma, respiratory depression); constipation; paralytic ileus; urinary retention; ocular effects: mydriasis, blurred vision, photophobia	Inform client that a dry mouth may occur, but to refrain from taking oral fluids. Immediately after administering the medications, instruct client to remain in bed. Place side rails in the up position, and ensure the call button is in easy reach.
Antiemetics droperidol (Inapsine), promethazine (Phenergan)	Reduces nausea, prevents emesis, and enhances preoperative sedation	Dry mouth; urinary retention; hypotension, including orthostatic hypotension; extrapyramidal reactions—dyskinesia, dystonia, akathisia, parkinsonism	Inform client that drowsiness may occur about 20 minutes after administration.
Tranquilizers (hypnotics) diazepam (Valium), flurazepam (Dalmane), lorazepam (Ativan)	Reduces preoperative anxiety and promotes induction of anesthesia	Depression of breathing	Inform client that drowsiness will occur about 20 minutes after administration. Immediately after administering the medication, instruct client to remain in bed. Place side rails in the up position, and ensure the call button is in easy reach.
Sedatives midazolam (Versed), barbiturates: phenobarbital (Nembutal), secobarbital (Seconal)	Promotes sleep, decreases anxiety, and promotes the use of anesthesia	Depression of breathing; may produce coughing, sneezing, and laryngospasm	Inform client that drowsiness will occur about 20 minutes after administration. Immediately after administering the medication, instruct client to remain in bed. Place side rails in the up position, and ensure the call button is in easy reach. Because these drugs require injection, they are not useful for children, who have small veins.
Opioids (narcotics) morphine, meperidine (Demerol)	Reduces anxiety and pain, promotes sleep, and decreases amount of anesthesia needed	May slow rate of respiration, hypotension, dizziness, nausea, vomiting, constipation	Inform client that drowsiness will occur about 20 minutes after administration. Immediately after administering the medication, instruct client to remain in bed. Place side rails in the up position, and ensure the call button is in easy reach.

CNS, central nervous system.

The Joint Commission (2003) established a universal protocol to achieve this goal (Box 14-3).

Nursing Process for Preoperative Care

Assessment

Assess the client's physical and psychological status, as described earlier in this section.

Diagnosis, Planning, and Interventions

▶ **Anxiety** related to upcoming surgery, results of surgery, and postoperative pain

▶ **Expected Outcome:** Client will express feelings of anxiety.

- Ask what concerns the client has about the upcoming surgery. *Such discussion provides specific information about the client's fears.*
- Provide appropriate explanations for preoperative procedures and postoperative expectations. *Clients experience less anxiety if they know what to expect.*

BOX 14-3 **Universal Protocol for Preventing Wrong Site, Wrong Procedure, Wrong Person Surgery**

Preoperative Verification Process
- *Purpose*: To ensure that all of the relevant documents and studies are available before the start of the procedure; that they have been reviewed; and that they are consistent with each other, with the client expectations, and with the team's understanding of the intended client, procedure, site, and, as applicable, any implants. Missing information or discrepancies must be addressed before starting the procedure.
- *Process*: An ongoing process of information gathering and verification, beginning with the determination to do the procedure, continuing through all settings and interventions involved in the preoperative preparation of the patient, up to and including the "time out" just before the start of the procedure.

Marking the Operative Site
- *Purpose*: To identify unambiguously the intended site of incision or insertion.

- *Process*: For procedures involving right/left distinction, multiple structures (such as fingers and toes), or multiple levels (as in spinal procedures), the intended site must be marked such that the mark will be visible after the client has been prepped and draped.

"Time Out" Immediately Before Starting the Procedure
- *Purpose*: To conduct a final verification of the correct client, procedure, site and, as applicable, implants.
- *Process*: Active communication among all members of the surgical/procedure team, consistently initiated by a designated member of the team, conducted in a "fail-safe" mode; i.e., the procedure is not started until any questions or concerns are resolved.

The Joint Commission (2003). Available at http://www.jointcommission.org/NR/rdonlyres/E3C60. Accessed May 6, 2008.

- Maintain as much contact as possible with the client. *Being present and approachable encourages communication.*

▶ Deficient Knowledge related to preoperative procedures and postoperative expectations

▶ Expected Outcome: Client will verbalize understanding of preoperative and postoperative procedures.

- Assess client's level of knowledge about the perioperative plans. *Building on a client's knowledge assists in reinforcing instructions and helps to correct false information.*
- Use audiovisual aids to present information. *Verbal reinforcement of other forms of instruction promotes learning.*
- Include family members or significant others in preoperative instructions. *These people help in reinforcing instructions and providing support to the client.*

Evaluation of Expected Outcomes

The client reports minimal anxiety. He or she demonstrates knowledge of the preoperative instructions and demonstrates postoperative exercises. ●

INTRAOPERATIVE CARE

The intraoperative period begins when the client is transferred to the operating table. The surgical team is responsible for the client's care during this time.

Anesthesia

Anesthesia is the partial or complete loss of the sensation of pain with or without loss of consciousness. Surgical procedures are performed with general, regional, or local anesthe-

sia. Procedural sedation may also be used for ambulatory surgery.

General Anesthesia

General anesthesia acts on the central nervous system to produce loss of sensation, reflexes, and consciousness. Vital functions such as breathing, circulation, and temperature control are not regulated physiologically when general anesthetics are used. General anesthetics are administered as IV, intramuscular (IM), inhaled (Fig. 14-1), or rectal medications. Four stages are used to describe the induction of general anesthesia (Smeltzer et al., 2008):

- *Stage 1, Beginning anesthesia:* This short period is crucial for producing unconsciousness. The client experiences dizziness, detachment, a temporary heightened sense of awareness to noises and movements, and a sensation of "heavy" extremities and being unable to move them. Inhaled or IV anesthetics are used to produce this phase. When the client becomes unconscious, his or her airway is secured with an endotracheal tube.
- *Stage 2, Excitement:* During this stage the client may struggle, shout, talk, sing, laugh, or cry. He or she may make uncontrolled movements, so team members must protect the client from falling or other injury. Quick and smooth administration of anesthesia can prevent this phase.
- *Stage 3, Surgical anesthesia:* In this stage the client remains unconscious through continuous administration of the anesthetic agent. This level of anesthesia may be maintained for hours with a range of light to deep anesthesia.
- *Stage 4, Medullary depression:* This stage occurs when the client receives too much anesthesia. The client will have shallow respirations, weak pulse, and widely dilated

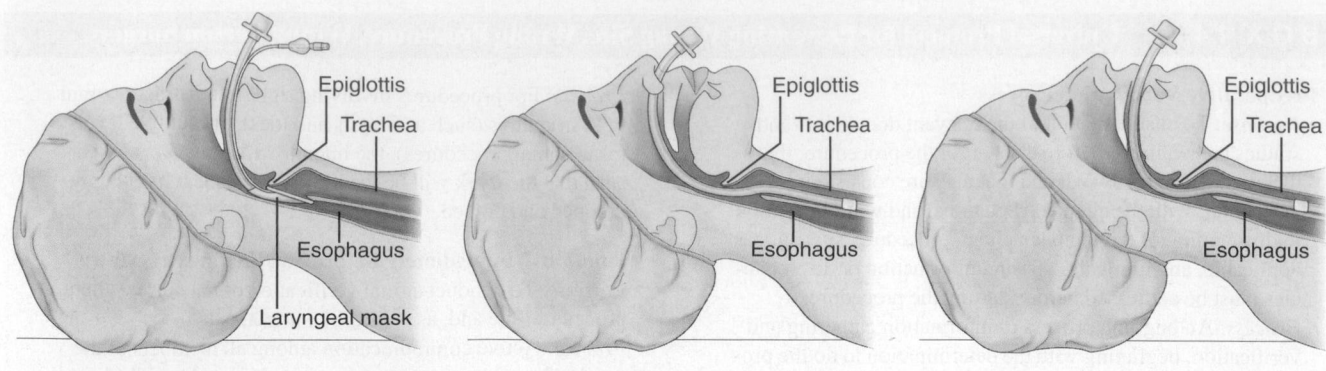

A Laryngeal mask airway (LMA)   **B** Intranasal intubation   **C** Oral intubation

FIGURE 14-1 Inhaled anesthetic delivery methods: (**A**) laryngeal mask, (**B**) nasal endotracheal catheter (in position), and (**C**) oral endotracheal intubation (tube in position with cuff inflated).

pupils unresponsive to light. Without prompt intervention, death can occur.

Usually, with smooth administration of general anesthesia, there is no major division between the first three stages, and the fourth stage does not occur. Throughout the duration of and recovery from anesthesia, team members closely monitor the client for effective breathing and oxygenation, effective circulatory status, including BP and pulse within normal ranges, effective regulation of temperature, and adequate fluid balance. When anesthetics are carefully withdrawn at the end of a surgical procedure, the client will wake enough to follow commands and breathe independently. The endotracheal tube used for inhaled anesthetics may be removed before the client leaves the OR. The recovery period can be brief or long. Many effects of general anesthesia take some time for the client to eliminate completely. Usually clients do not remember much about the initial recovery period.

Regional Anesthesia

Regional anesthesia uses local anesthetics to block the conduction of nerve impulses in a specific region (Table 14-4). The client experiences loss of sensation and decreased mobility to the specific anesthetized area. He or she does not lose consciousness. Depending on the surgery, the client may be given a sedative before the local anesthetic to promote relaxation and comfort during the procedure. Types of regional anesthesia include local anesthetics, spinal anesthesia, and conduction blocks.

Advantages of regional anesthesia include less risk for respiratory, cardiac, or gastrointestinal complications. There may be issues related to allergic responses and toxicity (overdose). Team members must monitor the client for signs of allergic reactions, changes in vital signs, and toxic reactions. In addition, they must protect the anesthetized area from injury while sensation is absent. The client is at risk for injuries and burns.

TABLE 14-4 Types of Regional Anesthesia

TYPE OF REGIONAL ANESTHESIA	ANESTHETIC USES AND EFFECTS	EXAMPLES
Local anesthesia	Administered topically or by local infiltration when medicine is injected into and under the epidural surface of the area to be treated Provides local loss of sensation Used primarily for dental, eye, and minor surgeries	procaine (Novocaine) lidocaine (Xylocaine) bupivacaine (Marcaine) dibucaine (Nupercaine) ropivacaine (Naropin)
Spinal anesthesia	Local anesthetic injected into the subarachnoid space of the lumbar area (usually L4 or L5), which contains cerebrospinal fluid Anesthetizes spinal nerves as they exit the spinal cord Used for surgery involving the abdomen, perineum, and lower extremities	procaine (Novocaine) lidocaine (Xylocaine) tetracaine (Pontocaine) ropivacaine (Naropin)
Epidural block	Local anesthetic injected into the extradural space near the spinal cord, anesthetizing several spinal nerves at once Although similar to spinal anesthesia, headache that frequently follows usually not present; greater technical competence, however, is required	Same as above; opioids such as morphine or fentanyl may be added to enhance the anesthetic effect and to provide analgesia when the block has worn off
Peripheral nerve block	Local anesthetic injected in a specific body region and directed at a particular nerve or group of nerves Peripheral nerve blocks named according to region in which anesthetic is injected; examples are brachial plexus block, ulnar nerve block, and sciatic nerve block Requires a high level of technical competence	lidocaine (Xylocaine) mepivacaine (Carbocaine) bupivacaine (Marcaine) ropivacaine (Naropin)

Procedural Sedation

For many ambulatory surgery procedures, clients are sedated but not unconscious. *Sedation* refers to a pharmacologically induced state of relaxation and emotional comfort. *Analgesia* is the absence or relief of pain. **Procedural sedation** (formerly known as *conscious sedation*) describes a state in which the client is free of pain, fear, and anxiety and can tolerate unpleasant procedures; the client maintains independent cardiorespiratory function and the ability to respond to verbal commands and tactile stimulation. IV anesthesia usually is used to induce procedural sedation. If other routes are used, the client must have venous access for treatment of possible adverse effects, such as anaphylaxis.

The presedation evaluation determines which clients are suitable for administration of sedative medications. It is similar to the preoperative evaluation. The nurse considers past adverse reactions to sedative medication. The client's age and weight help determine the amount of medication he or she will need.

Gerontologic Considerations

- Acute confusion in older adult clients may be associated with anticholinergics, antiemetics, antihistamines, benzodiazepines, and narcotics (AJN, 2004). Also, the mechanisms of medication clearance in older adults may be prolonged, leading to risk of overdose. Therefore, older adults usually receive smaller doses of preoperative, intraoperative, and postoperative medications, especially those that affect the central nervous, cardiovascular, and renal systems.

The three phases of the sedation process are as follows:

1. Titration of sedative medications, which is the administration of multiple small doses of medication until the desired drug effect is achieved
2. Performance of the diagnostic or therapeutic procedure
3. Recovery phase

In each phase, the client requires careful monitoring for complications. Levels of sedation range from slight drowsiness to anesthesia. Unpredictable absorption, metabolism, and excretion of medications make the client vulnerable to complications of undersedation or oversedation. Increased vigilance is necessary during titration of medications and recovery phases. At these times, the client has the greatest potential to become more deeply sedated because there is no painful stimulus. Even when the client does not seem to be sedated at the end of the procedure, late sedation may develop from continued drug uptake, delayed excretion, pharmacodynamics, or lack of stimulation.

Nurses who care for clients receiving sedation must be aware of the effects, side effects, and desired doses of sedative. Benzodiazepines, opioids, sedative-hypnotics, and barbiturates are the drug classes used in procedural sedation (Drug Therapy Table 14-2). These drugs can cause nausea, dizziness, euphoria or depression, flushed skin, coughing, jerking movements, and unusual eye and tongue movements. Although harmless, such side effects can frighten clients. Because virtu-ally all sedative medications carry a risk of respiratory depression, the nurse also must be prepared for respiratory or cardiopulmonary arrest.

Antagonists, also called *reversal drugs,* reverse the effects of opioids or benzodiazepines. Drugs from this class should be readily available whenever narcotics or benzodiazepines are used. If reversal drugs are required, the nurse *must* observe the client for an extended period, because the reversal effects nearly always are shorter than the effects of the drugs being reversed. This may result in resedation. Naloxone (Narcan) reverses opioids; flumazenil (Romazicon) reverses benzodiazepines.

Surgical Team

The surgical team consists of an anesthesiologist or anesthetist, surgeon and his or her assistants, and intraoperative nurses.

The **anesthesiologist** is a physician who has completed 2 years of residency in anesthesia. This person is responsible for administering anesthesia to the client and for monitoring the client during and after the surgical procedure. The anesthesiologist assesses the client before surgery, writes preoperative medication orders, informs the client of the options for anesthesia, and explains the risks involved.

The **anesthetist** may be a medical doctor who administers anesthesia but has not completed a residency in anesthesia, a dentist who administers limited types of anesthesia, or a registered nurse (RN) who has completed an accredited nurse anesthesia program and passed the certification examination (Certified Registered Nurse Anesthetist [CRNA]). The anesthesiologist supervises the anesthetist. The anesthetist may assess the client before surgery, discuss options for anesthesia, write preoperative medication orders, administer anesthesia, and monitor the client during and after surgery. The anesthesiologist and anesthetist are not sterile members of the surgical team, meaning that they wear OR attire but they do not wear sterile gowns or work within the sterile field.

Anesthesiologists or anesthetists classify clients according to their general physical status and assign a risk potential (Smeltzer et al., 2008). They use the American Society of Anesthesiologists' (ASA) Physical Status Classification System (Box 14-4).

The *surgeon* heads the surgical team. He or she is a physician, oral surgeon, or podiatrist with specific training and qualifications. The surgeon is responsible for determining the surgical procedure required, obtaining the client's consent, performing the procedure, and following the client after surgery.

Surgical assistants are classified as either first, second, or third assistants. The *first assistant* assists in the surgical procedure and may be involved with the client's preoperative and postoperative care. He or she may be another physician, a surgical resident, or an RN who has appropriate approval and endorsement from the American Operating Room Nurses (AORN) and the American College of Surgeons. Second or third assistants are RNs, licensed practical or vocational nurses (LPNs/LVNs), or surgical technologists who assist the surgeon and first assistant. All assistants are sterile members of the surgical team—they wear sterile gloves and gowns over OR attire and work within the sterile field.

Intraoperative nurses include the *scrub nurse* and *circulating nurse.* The scrub nurse wears a sterile gown and

DRUG THERAPY TABLE 14-2 Agents Used to Sedate Clients for Diagnostic and Therapeutic Procedures

Drug Category and Examples	Mechanisms of Action	Side Effects	Nursing Considerations
Opioids *meperidine hydrochloride (Demerol), morphine sulfate, fentanyl (Sublimaze)*	Bind to various opioid receptors, producing analgesia and sedation (opioid agonist)	Respiratory and CNS depression, hypotension, nausea, vomiting, constipation, histamine release, headache, restlessness, tachycardia, seizures, increased intracranial pressure, decreased urination, rash, hives, pain at injection site, bronchospasm, laryngospasm	Use with caution in clients with asthma, hepatic or renal disorders, or seizure disorders. These drugs are useful for sedation during painful procedures. They may cause hypotension in clients with acute myocardial infarction.
Benzodiazepines *midazolam hydrochloride (Versed), diazepam (Valium), lorazepam (Ativan)*	Bind to benzodiazepine receptors	Respiratory depression, cardiac arrest, hypotension, bradycardia, tachycardia, nausea, vomiting, bronchospasm, laryngospasm, blurred vision, diplopia, pain and local reaction at injection site, hiccups, amnesia, paradoxical excitement	Use with caution in clients with hypersensitivity reactions to other opioid agonists. Respiratory depression may persist beyond period of analgesia. Do not use in clients with increased intracranial pressure. Theophylline may antagonize the sedative effects of midazolam. Adverse effects increase when these drugs are administered with narcotics. These drugs cause profound retrograde amnesia and have no analgesic effect.
Sedative-hypnotics *chloral hydrate*	Exact mechanism of action unknown	Respiratory depression, nausea, vomiting, diarrhea, hallucinations, rash, urticaria, paradoxical excitement, fever, headache, confusion	Use with caution in clients with congestive heart failure, renal impairment, pulmonary disease, or hepatic failure. Do not use in clients with narrow-angle glaucoma, hepatic or renal impairment, gastritis, peptic ulcer disease, or severe cardiac disease.
Barbiturates *pentobarbital (Nembutal)*	Alter sensory cortex, cerebellar, and motor activities	Respiratory depression, laryngospasm, cardiac dysrhythmias, bradycardia, hypotension, CNS excitement or depression, pain or thrombophlebitis at injection site, hallucinations	Use can result in false-positive urine glucose with Clinitest method. Do not give to clients with marked liver impairment or porphyria. Use with caution in clients with hypovolemic shock, congestive heart failure, hepatic impairment, or respiratory or renal dysfunction.

CNS, central nervous system.

gloves and assists the surgical team by handing instruments to the surgeon and assistants, preparing sutures, receiving specimens for laboratory examination, and counting sponges and needles. The circulating nurse wears OR attire but not a sterile gown. Responsibilities include obtaining and opening wrapped sterile equipment and supplies before and during surgery, keeping records, adjusting lights, receiving specimens for laboratory examination, and coordinating activities of other personnel, such as the pathologist and radiology technician.

BOX 14-4 American Society of Anesthesiologists (ASA) Physical Status Classification System

Anesthetists and anesthesiologists use the American Society of Anesthesiologists Physical (P) Status Classification System to describe the client's general status and identify potential risks during surgery. There are six classes of physical status:

- **P1**—a normal healthy client
- **P2**—a client with mild systemic disease that does not limit activities, such as controlled hypertension or controlled diabetes without target organ damage
- **P3**—a client with severe systemic disease that does limit activities, such as stable angina or diabetes with target organ damage
- **P4**—a client with severe systemic disease that is a constant threat to life, such as severe heart failure or end-stage renal disease
- **P5**—a moribund client who is not expected to survive without the operation or other intervention
- **P6**—a client declared brain-dead whose organs are being removed for donation

If the procedure is an emergency, the physical status classification is followed by an E (e.g., ASA Class P2E).

(From O'Donnell, J. M., Bragg, K., & Sell, S. [2003]. Procedural sedation. *Nursing 2003, 33*[4], 38.)

The Operating Room Environment

The OR or surgical suite environment is physically isolated from other areas of the hospital or surgical clinic. This restricts access to the area to only authorized OR personnel and surgical clients. In the surgical suite, air is filtered and positive pressure is maintained to reduce the number of possible microbes that can cause infection. Three designated zones help to separate clean and contaminated areas and decrease the presence of microbes (AORN, 2002):

- Unrestricted zone—street clothes are allowed
- Semi-restricted zone—personnel are required to wear scrub clothes and caps
- Restricted zone—personnel are required to wear scrub clothes, caps, shoe covers, and masks

Surgical suites are designed to be efficient, in that the needed equipment and supplies are immediately available for use. Usually the furniture is made of stainless steel for easy cleaning and disinfecting. The temperature in the OR is kept below 70° F to provide a cooler environment that does not promote bacterial growth, to offer more comfort for OR personnel working in bright lights and wearing OR attire, and to maintain a temperature that enhances client comfort and safety.

OR personnel wear specific attire that decreases the opportunity for microbial growth. They strictly adhere to rules about where to change clothes and what to wear in the OR, including protective attire (Box 14-5). In addition, OR personnel must report any symptoms of infection they are experiencing, because colds, sore throats, and skin infections are potential sources of infection to the client.

BOX 14-5 Operating Room Attire

- *Scrubs* include tops, pants with cuffs, and jackets with cuffs. Changing rooms are located near the OR; personnel change into OR attire before entering the OR and take OR attire off when they leave.
- *Masks* are worn at all times in the OR; personnel change masks between surgical procedures or if masks become wet.
- *Headgear* is worn to cover the hair and hairline. Beards also must be covered.
- *Shoes* should be comfortable. Agencies vary in specific requirements. Shoe covers also are worn over the shoes. The conductive covers provide an electrical ground.

Nursing Management

Nursing management during the intraoperative period depends on routine tasks performed during surgery as well as on variables such as type of surgery performed, type of anesthesia used, client's age and condition, and any complications. Asepsis in the OR is the responsibility of all OR personnel. **Surgical asepsis** prevents contamination of surgical wounds. The risk of infection is high because of the break in skin integrity from the surgical incision. The client's own pathogens, plus those found in the OR, create an unsafe environment if personnel neglect to uphold strict aseptic technique. Thus, they strictly follow asepsis protocols to protect the client as much as possible. The client's safety and protection during surgery are essential.

Intraoperative Assessment

Assessment of the client in the OR is based largely on the type or extent of surgery, the client's age, and any preexisting conditions. Depending on circumstances, assessment before the administration of the anesthetic may include the following:

- BP and pulse and respiratory rates
- Level of consciousness
- General physical condition
- Presence of catheters and tubes
- Review of client's chart, including a signed operative permit, administration of preoperative medications (time, dose, client response), voiding, skin preparation, carrying out other preoperative orders, and laboratory and diagnostic tests.

▶ *Stop, Think, and Respond Exercise 14-2*

A client was told not to take his morning medications on the day of surgery. When he arrives at the OR, he informs the RN that he took his morning diuretic by mistake a few hours ago. What implications does this have for his care during surgery?

Prevention of Intraoperative Complications

Nurses who work in the OR assess the client continuously and protect the client from potential complications, including:

- *Infection:* Strict aseptic technique is absolutely necessary before and during surgery. If a nurse notes a break in technique, he or she immediately notifies the surgeon and OR personnel. Clients are also at risk for the retention of foreign objects in the wound. The scrub nurse and circulating nurse count surgical instruments, gauze sponges, and sharps to prevent this problem. The circulating nurse records the counts on the intraoperative record.

- *Fluid volume excess or deficit:* The anesthesiologist usually adds fluids to the IV lines, but the circulating nurse also may perform this function. The circulating nurse is responsible for recording and keeping a running total of IV fluids administered. If the client has an indwelling catheter, the nurse measures urine output during surgery.

- *Injury related to positioning:* The OR staff positions the client on the OR table according to the type of surgery. Careful positioning and monitoring help to prevent interruption of blood supply secondary to prolonged pressure, nerve injury related to prolonged pressure, postoperative hypotension, dependent edema, and joint injury related to poor body alignment.

- *Hypothermia:* During the procedure, the client may be at risk for hypothermia related to the low temperature in the OR, administration of cold IV fluids, inhalation of cool gases, exposure of body surfaces for the surgical procedure, opened incisions/wounds, and prolonged inactivity. For some surgeries, the body temperature is deliberately lowered to make the procedure safer (Smeltzer et al., 2008).

- *Malignant hyperthermia:* **Malignant hyperthermia** (MH) inherited disorder occurs when body temperature, muscle metabolism, and heat production increase rapidly, progressively, and uncontrollably in response to stress and some anesthetic agents. There are two tests that indicate if a client is susceptible to MH: skeletal muscle biopsy, which determines muscle contractile qualities, and a blood test for a genetic mutation linked to MH. Certain anesthetic agents trigger uncontrolled calcium release within skeletal muscle cells, which leads to muscle rigidity and a hypermetabolic state (Dixon & O'Donnell, 2006). Signs and symptoms include jaw muscle rigidity, rapidly rising temperature, elevated $Paco_2$ and serum potassium levels, metabolic acidosis, tachycardia, tachypnea, diaphoresis, mottled skin, hypotension, irregular heart rate, decreased urine output and eventual kidney failure, and, if untreated, cardiac arrest. Prevention of malignant hyperthermia is essential because the mortality rate is high. Clients at risk include "those with bulky, strong muscles, a history of muscle cramps or muscle weakness and unexpected temperature elevation and an unexplained death of a family member during surgery that was accompanied by a febrile response" (Smeltzer et al., 2008, p. 517). The circulating nurse closely monitors the client for signs of hyperthermia. If the client's temperature begins to rise rapidly, anesthesia is discontinued and the OR team implements measures to correct physiologic problems, such as fever or dysrhythmias.

 Gerontologic Considerations

- An age-related loss of elasticity of blood vessels may place the older client at higher risk for injury related to prolonged surgical positioning. Therefore, pressure relief is needed every 1.5 to 2 hours based on the skin assessment of blanching. Presence of chronic conditions such as arthritis may necessitate special positioning. Chronic health conditions and age-related physical changes (e.g., cardiac, renal, respiratory, immunologic conditions) may also increase the risks associated with surgical procedures.

Nursing Process for the Client Undergoing Procedural Sedation

The client undergoing procedural sedation requires special considerations for intraoperative nursing management.

Assessment

Before sedation, the nurse gathers important client data, records baseline vital signs and oximeter readings, and provides education to clients and their families. Education includes instructions specific to the procedure, preparations for the procedure, likely sensations (pain, discomfort, cramping, gagging, nausea), and common side effects of medications.

During sedation, the nurse continuously evaluates the client. Monitoring during all phases includes assessment of heart rate, respiratory rate, BP, oxygen saturation, and level of consciousness. The nurse monitors cardiac rhythm in clients who are at risk for dysrhythmias or cardiovascular compromise. If vital signs deviate significantly during sedation, the nurse collects additional information to help determine if those deviations are secondary to an adverse reaction to the sedation or to the procedure itself. When the client shows signs of distress (i.e., deviation in vital signs, respiratory compromise), the nurse immediately reports these signs to the physician and provides interventions such as suctioning, gentle tactile stimulation, or administration of oxygen. He or she continues to monitor the client's response until the level of consciousness and vital signs are at baseline. The nurse documents these observations at intervals specified by the institution.

Diagnosis, Planning, and Interventions

▶ **Risk for Ineffective Breathing Patterns** related to effect of sedative medications

▶ **Expected Outcome:** Client will demonstrate a normal breathing pattern.

- Position client in an upright or semi-Fowler's position. *These positions facilitate lung expansion.*
- Observe for signs and symptoms of distress related to inappropriate head position (stridor, increased respiratory effort); reposition head as indicated. *Early intervention prevents further complications.*
- Encourage client to take deep breaths and cough at least every hour. *Deep breathing and coughing improve oxygenation and assist in clearing the effects of anesthesia.*

▶ **Risk for Injury** related to sedation

▶ **Expected Outcome:** Client will remain safe and free of injury.

- Provide safety by preventing client from falling out of bed, stretcher, or recliner; assisting with ambulation; and carefully monitoring all activities. *Clients recovering from sedation may have impaired judgment and reflexes; the nurse must protect them from injury.*

- Monitor client for return to presedation level of consciousness. *Until client is fully responsive, he or she continues to be at risk for injury.*
- Discharge client to the care of a person who has received instructions regarding client safety. *Sedative effects may last for several more hours; the client requires continued care after discharge.*

Evaluation of Expected Outcomes

The client has a patent airway and effective breathing patterns. He or she experiences no threats to safety. ●

POSTOPERATIVE CARE

The postoperative period designates the time that the client spends recovering from the effects of anesthesia. Factors such as the client's age and nutritional status, preexisting diseases, type of surgery, and length of anesthesia may affect the duration, type, and extent of nursing management.

Transport of the Client

Immediately after the surgical procedure is complete, the client is transported to the postanesthesia care unit (PACU), also known as the *postanesthesia recovery room,* located near the OR. The nursing staff there is specifically knowledgeable in the care of clients recovering from anesthesia. Specialized equipment is available to monitor and treat the client. Surgical and anesthesia personnel are immediately available for any emergencies.

Nursing Management

Immediate Postoperative Period

When clients are transferred from the OR to the PACU, the anesthesiologist or anesthetist is responsible for the client's safety. Critical considerations include maintaining an intact surgical site (incision), observing for potential vascular changes, and keeping the client warm. Position of the client is also important so that the incision is not compromised, drains do not obstruct, and the client does not experience *orthostatic hypotension.* The nurse receiving the client from the OR needs the following information (Smeltzer et al., 2008):

- Medical diagnosis and surgical procedure done
- Past medical history and allergies
- Age, general condition, airway status, and current vital signs
- Anesthetic agents and medications given during surgery
- Complications during surgery
- Any pathology found and if so whether family members are informed
- Amounts of fluids and blood administered and amounts of fluids and blood lost
- Any tubes, catheters, etc.
- Any other pertinent information needed to care for the client

The most important aspect of nursing management is close observation and monitoring of the client during emergence from anesthesia.

Initial Postoperative Assessment

Initial postoperative assessments include airway patency; effectiveness of respirations; presence of artificial airways, mechanical ventilation, or supplemental oxygen; circulatory status; vital signs; wound condition, including dressings and drains; fluid balance, including IV fluids, output from catheters and drains, and ability to void; level of consciousness; and pain. The nurse's major responsibilities during the client's PACU stay are to ensure a patent airway; help maintain adequate circulation; prevent or assist with the treatment of shock; maintain proper position and function of drains, tubes, and IV infusions; and monitor for potential complications.

An important assessment is determining how the client is recovering from anesthesia. A useful assessment tool is the Aldrete scale, which rates the client's mobility, respiratory status, circulation, consciousness, and pulse oximetry (Table 14-5). A score of 9 or greater indicates that the client has recovered from anesthesia.

 Gerontologic Considerations

- A major adverse reaction to anesthesia in older adults is decreased mental functioning, which can manifest with symptoms similar to delirium or dementia.

TABLE 14-5 Modified Aldrete Scale for Assessing Recovery from Anesthesia

	SCORE*		
	0	1	2
Activity	Unable to move extremities voluntarily or on command	Able to move two extremities voluntarily or on command	Able to move all extremities voluntarily or on command.
Respiration	Apneic	Dyspnea or limited breathing	Able to breathe deeply and cough freely
Circulation	BP +/− 50 mm Hg of preanesthesia level	BP +/− 20-49 mm Hg of preanesthesia level	BP +/− 20 mm Hg of preanesthesia level
Consciousness	Unresponsive	Arousable with verbal stimuli	Fully awake
SpO₂	< 90% with supplemental oxygen	Needs supplemental oxygen to maintain > 90%	> 92% on room air

* Add the scores for all criteria for a total score; a score of 9 or greater on this modified Aldrete scale means that the client has recovered from anesthesia.
Source: Halliday, A. (2006). Shades of sedation. *Nursing 2006, 36*(4), p. 40.

Prevention of Postoperative Complications

Hemorrhage. Hemorrhage can be internal or external. If the client loses a lot of blood, he or she will exhibit signs and symptoms of shock (see Chap. 17). The nurse inspects dressings frequently for signs of bleeding and checks the bedding under the client, because blood may pool under the body and be evident on the bedding. If bleeding is internal, the client may need to return to surgery for ligation of the bleeding vessels. Blood transfusions may be necessary to replace lost blood. When bleeding occurs, the nurse notes the amount and color on the chart. Bright red blood signifies fresh bleeding; dark, brownish blood indicates older blood. The nurse may need to reinforce soiled or saturated dressings. A written order is needed to change dressings. The nurse also must be aware of any wound drains and the type and amount of drainage expected. If such drainage is expected, the nurse explains to the client that the drainage is normal and does not indicate a complication. He or she places incontinence pads under the client if drainage occurs.

Shock. Fluid and electrolyte loss, trauma (both physical and psychological), anesthetics, and preoperative medications all may contribute to shock. Signs and symptoms include pallor, fall in BP, weak and rapid pulse rate, restlessness, and cool, moist skin (see Chap. 17). Shock must be detected early and treated promptly because it can irreversibly damage vital organs such as the brain, kidneys, and heart.

Narcotics are not administered to a client in shock until a physician evaluates the client, who should remain supine. Some physicians advocate elevating the legs to enhance the flow of venous blood to the heart. Treatment of shock varies and depends on the cause, if known. Blood, plasma expanders, parenteral fluids, oxygen, and medications such as adrenergic agonists may be used (see Chap. 17).

Hypoxia. Factors such as residual drug effects or overdose, pain, poor positioning, pooling of secretions in the lungs, or obstructed airway predispose the client to hypoxia (decreased oxygen). Oxygen and suction equipment must be available for immediate use. The nurse observes the client closely for signs of cyanosis and dyspnea. Breathing may be obstructed if the tongue falls back and blocks the nasopharynx. If this occurs, the nurse pulls the lower jaw and inserts an oropharyngeal airway (Fig. 14-2). Positioning the client on his or her side also may relieve nasopharyngeal obstruction. Restlessness, crowing or grunting respirations, diaphoresis, bounding pulse, and rising BP may indicate respiratory obstruction. If a client cannot breathe effectively, mechanical ventilation is used.

Aspiration. Danger of aspiration from saliva, mucus, vomitus, or blood exists until the client is fully awake and can swallow without difficulty. Suction equipment must be kept at the client's bedside until the danger of aspiration no longer exists. The nurse closely observes the client for difficulty swallowing or handling of oral secretions. Unless contraindicated, the nurse places the client in a side-lying position until the client can swallow oral secretions.

Later Postoperative Period

The later postoperative period begins when the client arrives in the hospital room or postsurgical care unit. Because the nurse can anticipate, prevent, or minimize many postoperative problems, he or she must approach the care of the client systematically.

Ongoing Assessments

Assessment during this period includes respiratory function; general condition; vital signs; cardiovascular function and fluid status; pain level; bowel and urinary elimination; and dressings, tubes, drains, and IV lines.

Respiration. The nurse focuses on promoting gas exchange and preventing atelectasis. Hypoventilation related to anesthesia, postoperative positioning, and pain is a common problem. Preoperative and postoperative instructions include teaching the client to deep breathe and cough, and how to splint the incision to minimize pain. Clients who have abdominal or thoracic surgery have greater difficulty taking deep breaths and coughing. Some clients require supplemental oxygen. Nursing management to prevent postoperative respiratory problems includes early mobility, frequent position changes, deep breathing and coughing exercises, and use of incentive spirometer.

Hiccups (*singultus*) also may interfere with breathing. They result from intermittent spasms of the diaphragm and may occur after surgery, especially abdominal surgery. They may be mild and last for only a few minutes. Prolonged hiccups not only are unpleasant but also may cause pain or discomfort. They may result in wound dehiscence or evisceration, inability to eat, nausea and vomiting, exhaustion, and fluid, electrolyte, and acid-base imbalances. If hiccups persist, the nurse needs to notify the physician.

Circulation. The nurse must assess the client's BP and circulatory status frequently. Although problems with postoperative bleeding decrease as the recovery time advances, the client is still at risk for bleeding. Some clients experience syncope when moving to an upright position. To prevent this (and the danger of falling), the nurse helps the client to move slowly to an upright or standing position.

The client also is at risk for impaired venous circulation related to immobility. When clients lie still for long periods without moving their legs, blood may flow sluggishly through the veins (venous stasis). Venous stasis predisposes the client to venous inflammation and clot formation in the veins (**thrombophlebitis**), or clot formation with minimal or absent inflammation (**phlebothrombosis**). These two conditions are most common in the lower extremities. If the clot travels in the bloodstream (an **embolus**), it may obstruct

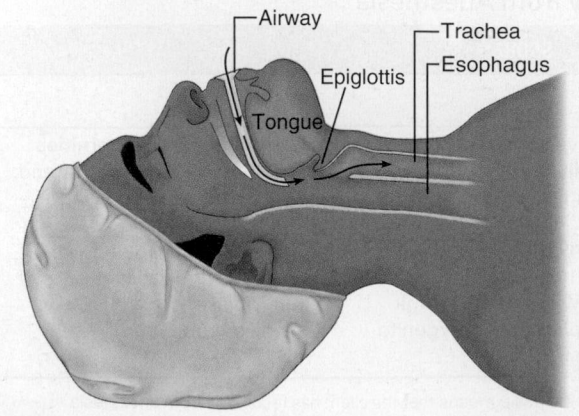

FIGURE 14-2 Oropharyngeal airway in place.

Pharmacologic Considerations

- The use of PCA does not eliminate the need for frequent observation of the client for effectiveness of the analgesic.

- Closely monitor the client receiving narcotic analgesics for adverse effects, such as respiratory depression, decreased BP, nausea, excessive drowsiness, agitation, or hallucinations. Bring these findings to the physician's attention immediately. Naloxone (Narcan) can be given to counteract narcotic-induced respiratory depression.

- Antiemetics such as promethazine (Phenergan) or prochlorperazine (Compazine) can potentiate the hypotensive effects of opioids.

circulation to a vital organ, such as the lungs, and cause severe symptoms and possibly death.

To prevent venous stasis and other circulatory complications, the nurse encourages the client to move his or her legs frequently and do leg exercises. The nurse also does not place pillows under the client's knees or calves unless ordered. He or she avoids placing pressure on the client's lower extremities, applies elastic bandages or antiembolism stockings as ordered, ambulates the client as ordered, and administers low-dose subcutaneous heparin every 12 hours as ordered.

Pain Management. Most clients experience pain after an operation, and a range of postoperative analgesics usually are ordered. Postoperative pain reaches its peak between 12 and 36 hours after surgery and diminishes significantly after

NURSING GUIDELINES 14-1

Resuming Oral Fluids After Surgery

- Most clients can begin to take fluids within 4 to 24 hours after surgery (except when surgery involves the GI tract). Check physician's orders to ensure that fluids can be given.
- If not allowed oral fluids, provide the client with mouth rinses and a cool, wet cloth or ice chips against the lips to relieve dryness.
- Before giving fluids, assess that the client has recovered sufficiently from anesthesia to swallow. Ask the client to try swallowing without drinking anything. If the client can do so, offer a small sip of water or a few ice chips.
- Give only a few sips of water or ice chips at a time. Introduce fluids slowly and give them in small amounts to prevent vomiting. The client can take fluids through a straw so he or she does not have to sit up. Once the client can sit up, however, straws are discouraged because clients tend to swallow air as well, which can lead to abdominal distention and gastric discomfort.
- If the client vomits, reassure him or her that it should cease shortly. Offer mouthwash to remove the taste of anesthetics and vomitus. Administer antiemetics as indicated.

48 hours. Pain creates varying degrees of anxiety and emotions. If accompanied by great fear, the degree of pain can increase. Clients must receive pain and discomfort relief. When patient-controlled analgesia (PCA) is used, clients administer their own analgesic (see Chap. 11).

The nurse assesses for adverse effects of analgesics, timing of the medication in relation to other activities, effects of other comfort measures, contraindications, and source of the pain. The need for pain medications depends on the type and extent of the surgery, and the client. Pain unrelieved by medication may signal a developing complication, which underscores the need for a thorough assessment of the cause and type of pain (see Chap. 11).

Gerontologic Considerations

- Medications such as narcotics and barbiturates may cause confusion and disorientation in older adults, even when given in standard doses. The respiratory depressive effects of narcotics may also be increased in older adults.

Fluids and Nutrition. IV fluids usually are administered after surgery. Length of administration depends on the type of surgery and the client's ability to take oral fluids. The nurse monitors the IV fluid flow rate and adjusts it as needed. He or she also assesses for signs of fluid excess or deficit (see Chap. 16) and notifies the physician of any such signs.

Many clients complain of thirst in the early postoperative recovery period. Because anesthesia slows peristalsis, ingesting liquids before bowel activity resumes can lead to nausea and vomiting. Pain medications also may cause nausea and vomiting. Nursing Guidelines 14-1 includes factors to consider before resuming oral fluids.

Once peristalsis has returned and the client is tolerating clear liquids, the nurse helps the client to increase dietary intake. Dietary progression (from clear liquids to a full, solid diet) often depends on the type of surgery, the client's progress, and physician preference. IV fluids usually are discontinued when the client can take oral fluids and food, and nutritional needs are met (Nutrition Notes 14-1).

▶ **Stop, Think, and Respond Exercise 14-3**

Postoperatively the client complains of nausea. What is an important nursing action?

Skin Integrity/Wound Healing. A surgical incision is a wound or injury to skin integrity. Initially the client may have a wound or incisional drain, which is a tube that exits from the peri-incisional area into either a dressing or portable wound suction device. Figure 14-3 depicts three types of wound devices: Penrose, Jackson-Pratt, and Hemovac drains.

When assessing the wound, the nurse inspects for approximation of the wound edges, intactness of staples or sutures, redness, warmth, swelling, tenderness, discoloration, or drainage. He or she also notes any reactions to the tape or dressings. The first phase of wound healing is the

Nutrition Notes 14-1
The Postoperative Client

- Progress the diet as soon as possible after surgery to promote an adequate oral intake.
- Encourage clients who are anorexic or nauseated to consume small, frequent feedings. They may tolerate high-protein, low-fat liquids better than traditional meals.
- If possible, schedule pain medications enough in advance to allow the client a pain-free mealtime.
- Normal weight loss during the early postoperative period is about half a pound daily. Weight gain during this period signifies fluid accumulation.
- Protein, calories, vitamins A and C, and zinc are important for wound healing and immune system functioning; actual requirements depend on the client's nutritional status, extent of surgery, and development of complications.
- Unlike the stomach, which does not regain motility for 24 to 48 hours after surgery, the small intestine resumes peristalsis and the ability to absorb nutrients within several hours after surgery.
- If the client is malnourished, hypermetabolic, or not expected to resume an oral intake within a few days, a needle-catheter jejunostomy tube may be inserted during surgery so enteral feedings can be given.

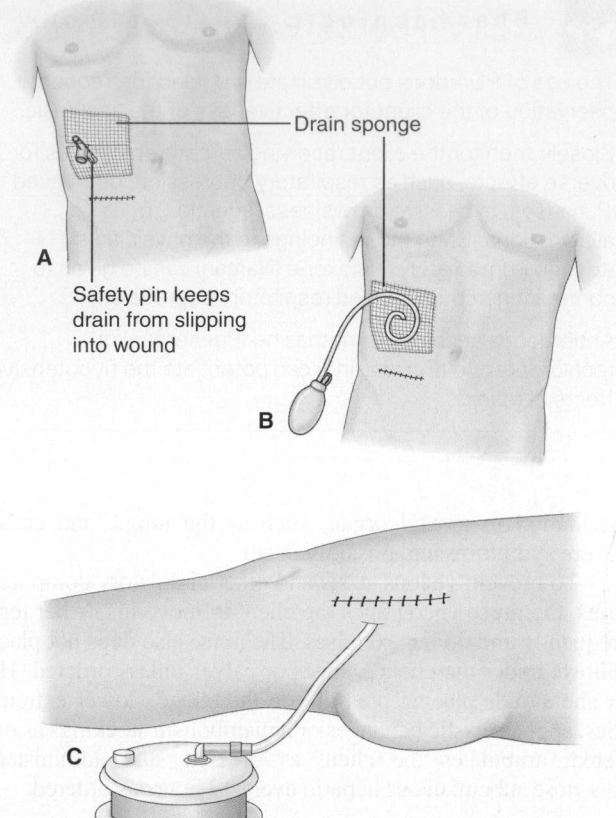

FIGURE 14-3 Types of surgical drains. (**A**) Penrose, (**B**) Jackson-Pratt, and (**C**) Hemovac.

inflammatory stage, which is when a blood clot forms, swelling occurs, and phagocytes ingest the debris from damaged tissue and the blood clot. This phase lasts 1 to 4 days. The second phase is the *proliferative phase,* in which collagen is produced and granulation tissue forms. It occurs over 5 to 20 days. The last phase is referred to as the *maturation* or *remodeling phase* and lasts from 21 days to several months and even 1 to 2 years. During this phase, the tensile strength of the wound increases through synthesis of collagen by fibroblasts and lysis by collagenase enzymes.

In addition, surgical wounds are formed aseptically, depending on the nature of the incision and the underlying condition. There are three modes of wound healing (Fig. 14-4):

- *Primary intention:* The wound layers are sutured together so that wound edges are well approximated. This type of incision usually heals in 8 to 10 days, with minimal scarring.
- *Secondary intention:* Granulating tissue fills in the wound for the healing process. The skin edges are not approximated. This method is used for ulcers and infected wounds. This type of wound healing is slow, although new products, such as antimicrobial underdressings or calcium alginate dressings, promote healing.
- *Tertiary intention:* The approximation of wound edges is delayed secondary to infection. When the wound is drained and cleaned of infection, the wound edges are sutured together. The resulting scar is wider than that with primary intention.

The key to healing is adequate blood flow. Poor blood supply to the wound delays healing, as can excessive tension or pulling on wound edges. The nurse must be alert for signs and symptoms of impaired circulation, such as swelling, coldness, absence of pulse, pallor, or mottling, and report them immediately. Other factors that interfere with healing include malnutrition, impaired inflammatory and immune responses, infection, foreign bodies, and age. Obesity may also contribute to poor wound healing, secondary to impaired oxygenation, hyperglycemia, immobility, and nutritional deficits. Studies show that obese clients are more likely to have wound infections, as well as dehiscence, pressure ulcers, and deep tissue injury (Baugh, 2007). Excess fat prolongs the length of surgery and necessitates the use of more forceful retraction (holding surgical openings open with instruments), which contributes to tissue damage. It also adds to pressure on wound edges, decreasing blood flow and increasing the danger of dehiscence.

GerontologicConsiderations

- A thinning of the skin and loss of subcutaneous tissue accompany the aging process. This may lead to poor wound healing, tissue breakdown caused by excessive pressure on a part, or inadequate development of granulation tissue in healing wounds. Additionally, older adults may have a diminished immunologic response, leading to a higher risk for infection.

PRIMARY INTENTION

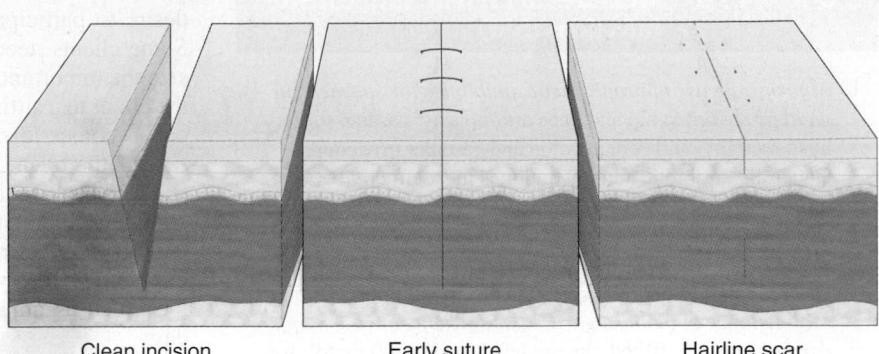

Clean incision   Early suture   Hairline scar

SECONDARY INTENTION

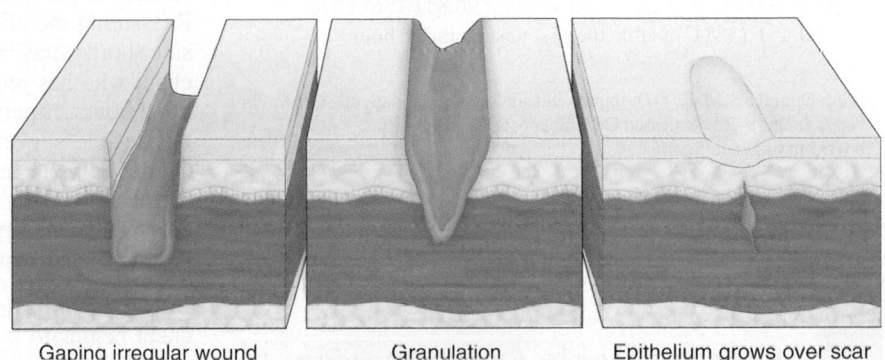

Gaping irregular wound   Granulation   Epithelium grows over scar

TERTIARY INTENTION

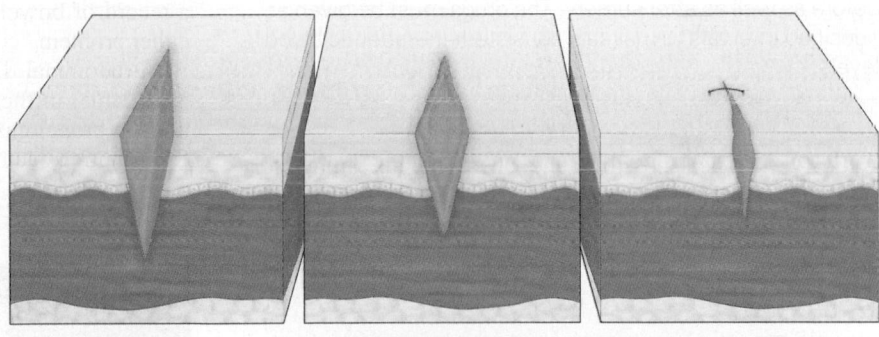

Wound   Increased granulation   Late suturing with wide scar

FIGURE 14-4 Types of wound healing.

The nurse must be careful when changing dressings to avoid damaging new tissue as well as causing the client unnecessary discomfort. Using normal saline to soak packings and dressings that adhere to the wound bed may ease removal.

The nurse closely monitors the client for signs and symptoms of wound infection, such as increased incisional pain; redness, swelling, and heat around the incision; purulent drainage; fever and chills; headache; and anorexia. Treatment of wound infections includes antibiotics, wound care, and measures to promote healing such as adequate nutrition and rest. Surgical site infections (SSIs) account for almost 20% of hospital-acquired infections (Daniels, 2007). A national partnership of healthcare organizations called Surgical Care Improvement Project (SCIP) seeks to prevent SSIs through the appropriate preoperative use of prophylactic antibiotics, hair removal methods, controlling glucose

levels in cardiac surgical clients, and maintaining normal temperatures in clients having colon surgery. Box 14-6 provides a brief overview of these recommendations.

Other complications of wound healing are dehiscence and evisceration. Wound **dehiscence** (Fig. 14-5*A*) is the separation of wound edges without the protrusion of organs. **Evisceration** (Fig. 14-5*B*) occurs when the wound completely separates and organs protrude. These complications are most likely to occur within 7 to 10 days after surgery. Risk factors for wound disruption are identified in Box 14-7.

The client may complain of something "giving way." Pinkish drainage may appear suddenly on the dressing. If wound disruption is suspected, the nurse places the client in a position that puts the least strain on the operative area. If evisceration occurs, the nurse places sterile dressings moistened with normal saline over the protruding organs and tissues. For any wound disruption, the nurse notifies the physician immediately.

Postoperative wound care also must include teaching the client and family members about wound care, while in the hospital and when discharged (Client and Family Teaching 14-1).

Pharmacologic Considerations

- Antibiotics to prevent or fight infection may be ordered before as well as after surgery. The drugs must be given at specified intervals to maintain consistent therapeutic blood levels.

Activity. When possible, the client begins ambulatory activities shortly after surgery. Factors such as pain toler-ance, response to analgesics, general physical condition, and desire to participate affect the client's ability to be active. Some clients need encouragement. The nurse must emphasize the importance of increasing activities. He or she assists the client to a sitting position at the side of the bed. If the client becomes dizzy longer than momentarily, the nurse returns the client to a supine position. When the client can stand, the nurse assists and supports the client. The nurse continues to assist with ambulation until the client can walk without help. Some clients experience moderate to severe fatigue after surgery. For these clients, the nurse spaces activities such as ambulation and personal care throughout the day.

If the client has received regional anesthesia, activity may initially be restricted. At first, the client experiences numbness and a feeling of heaviness in the anesthetized area. Reassuring the client that numbness is typical and will subside shortly may be necessary. Unless ordered otherwise, the client who has received spinal anesthesia remains flat for 6 to 12 hours. If permitted, the nurse turns the client from side to side at least every 2 hours. As the anesthesia wears off, the client begins to have a "pins-and-needles" sensation in the anesthetized parts and to feel pain in the operative area. Clients who develop a headache after spinal anesthesia may have to remain lying flat for a longer period.

Bowel Elimination. Constipation may develop after the client begins to take solid food. Causes of this constipation include inactivity, diet, and narcotic analgesics. Some clients may experience diarrhea as a result of diet, medications such as antibiotics, or the surgical procedure. The nurse maintains a record of bowel movements and notifies the physician of either problem.

Abdominal distention results from the accumulation of gas (flatus) in the intestines because of failure of the intestines to propel gas through the intestinal tract by peristalsis. Contributing factors include manipulation of the intestines

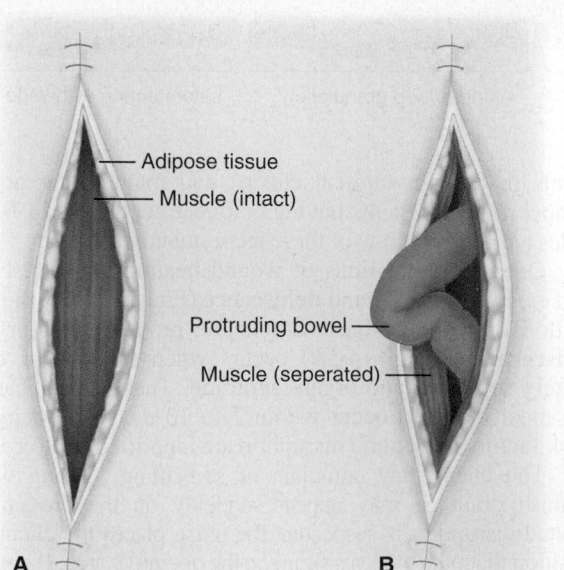

FIGURE 14-5 (A) Wound dehiscence. **(B)** Wound evisceration.

Client and Family Teaching 14-1
Care of Postoperative Wounds/Incisions

The nurse teaches the client and family member the following information.

While Sutures Are Still Present

- Keep wound/incision clean and dry.
- Follow physician instructions about bathing and showering.
- Do not remove dressing and/or splint unless instructed to do so.
- Follow instructions for changing the dressing and cleaning the wound/incision.
- Report any signs of infection:
  - Redness exceeding 1/2 inch surrounding the wound/incision
  - Red streaks in skin near wound/incision
  - Pus, discharge, foul odor
  - Chills or temperature above 100°F (37.5°C)
- If there is soreness or pain at the site of the wound/incision, apply an ice pack or cold-water pack. Do not use a wet pack. Take pain medications according to directions.
- If swelling is present, elevate the affected part to or above the level of the heart.

After Sutures Are Removed

- Follow directions regarding the level of activity allowed.
- Keep suture line clean and dry.
- Wash, dry, and apply dressing as directed.
- Wound edges may look slightly raised and red — this is normal.
- If the wound/incision site looks red and thick and is painful to touch 8 weeks after sutures are removed, contact the physician (excessive collagen may have formed).

(Adapted from Smeltzer, S. C., Bare, B. G., Hinkle, J.L. et al. [2008]. *Brunner & Suddarth's textbook of medical-surgical nursing* [11th ed.] Philadelphia: Lippincott Williams & Wilkins.)

during abdominal surgery, inactivity after surgery, interruption of normal food and fluid intake, swallowing of large quantities of air, and anesthetics and medications given during or after surgery. If the symptoms are mild, they can be treated with nursing measures. The nurse encourages and assists clients who are permitted out of bed to ambulate. Sometimes walking, plus privacy in the bathroom, enable the client to expel the gas. The nurse encourages clients to change position frequently and to eat as normally as possible within the allowed dietary limits. If discomfort is severe or not relieved promptly by nursing measures, the nurse must contact the physician.

Sometimes a serious condition called **paralytic ileus** occurs in which the intestines are paralyzed and, thus, peristalsis is absent. Fluids, solids, and gas do not move through the intestinal tract. Bowel sounds are absent, the abdomen is distended, and abdominal pain often is severe. Vomiting also may occur. If the client complains of severe abdominal pain,

assessment includes inspecting the abdomen for distention, palpating for rigidity, and auscultating for bowel sounds. If bowel sounds are absent or abnormal or the abdomen is distended or rigid, the nurse notifies the physician immediately. A nasogastric tube usually is inserted and food and fluids withheld until bowel sounds return.

Acute gastric dilatation, a condition in which the stomach becomes distended with fluids, is a complication similar to paralytic ileus. The client may regurgitate small amounts of liquid, the abdomen appears distended, and as the condition progresses, symptoms of shock may develop. Treatment includes inserting a nasogastric tube, applying suction, and removing the gas and fluid. Some surgeons routinely use suction of the gastrointestinal tract to prevent paralytic ileus and acute gastric dilatation.

Urinary Elimination. Some clients experience difficulty voiding after surgery, particularly lower abdominal and pelvic surgery. Operative trauma in the region near the bladder may temporarily decrease the voiding sensation. Fear of pain also causes tenseness and difficulty voiding. If the client has an indwelling catheter, the nurse monitors urine output frequently. If the client does not have a catheter, the nurse assesses the client's ability to void and measures urine output. If the client cannot void within 8 hours after surgery, the nurse notifies the physician unless catheterization orders are in place. Signs and symptoms of bladder distention include restlessness, lower abdominal pain, discomfort or distention, and fluid intake without urinary output.

Psychosocial Status. Many clients experience anxiety and fear after surgery, as well as an inability to cope with changes in body image, lifestyle, and other factors. The nurse assesses what the client is experiencing and how the client is dealing with those issues. Many clients need referrals for counseling, support groups, and social services. The nurse acts as an effective listener, identifies areas of concern, and works with other healthcare professionals to assist the client and family to work through the problems.

Box 14-8 summarizes the potential complications that clients may experience postoperatively.

Gerontologic Considerations

- Older adults are more prone to postoperative complications such as shock, atelectasis, pneumonia, paralytic ileus, gastric dilatation, and venous stasis. The increased risk is due to age-related changes in metabolism of anesthetics and vulnerability of organ systems, as well as chronic illness. Cognitive changes may be an indication of urinary track infection.

Client and Family Teaching and Discharge
Before discharge, the client needs to receive instructions on how to carry out treatments at home. The nurse conveys the discharge instructions verbally and in writing. The nurse evaluates clients to determine their ability to carry out their care and to determine their specific needs, such as the need for:

- Supervised home care (e.g., visiting nurse, other healthcare agencies and personnel)

BOX 14-8 Potential Postoperative Complications

Respiratory
Atelectasis
Pneumonia
Pulmonary embolism
Aspiration
Cardiovascular
Shock
Thrombophlebitis
Urinary
Acute urine retention
Urinary tract infection
Neurologic
Delirium
Stroke
Gastrointestinal
Constipation
Paralytic ileus
Bowel obstruction
Functional
Weakness
Fatigue
Functional decline
Wound
Infection
Dehiscence
Evisceration
Delayed healing
Hemorrhage
Hematoma

- Supplies (e.g., dressings, tape, ostomy supplies, crutches)
- Special dietary needs
- Adjustments to the living environment (e.g., special bed, portable commode, wheelchair access)

Because sedative medications affect memory for events surrounding their administration, the nurse must review discharge instructions with an adult who will be responsible for the client after discharge. He or she instructs the client not to drink alcoholic beverages for a specified period after the procedure and to resume prescription and nonprescription medications when appropriate. The nurse must instruct the client about when it is appropriate to begin taking pain medications, because they may have an additive effect with the sedative medications that were administered. Client and Family Teaching Box 14-2 outlines key information to teach postoperatively.

For clients who have undergone ambulatory surgery, surgical units use outcome criteria to determine if the client's condition is stable and if he or she can safely leave the hospital or outpatient setting. These criteria include that the client

- Has stable cardiovascular function and a patent airway.
- Is easily aroused.
- Has intact protective reflexes.
- Can talk.
- Can sit up unaided.
- Is adequately hydrated.

Client and Family Teaching 14-2 Postoperative Instructions

The nurse develops a teaching plan to meet the client's needs. Points may include the following:

- Follow physician's instructions about cleaning the incision, applying the dressing, bathing, diet, and physical activity.
- Notify physician of any of the following: chills or fever; drainage from the incision (some drainage may be expected in certain cases); foul odor or pus from the incision; redness, streaking, pain, or tenderness around the incision; other symptoms not present at discharge (e.g., vomiting, diarrhea, cough, or chest or leg pain)
- Take medications as prescribed, including pain medications. Do not omit or change the dose unless the physician advises to do so.
- Do not take nonprescription medications unless approved by the physician.
- Follow dietary advice and drink fluids liberally, unless directed otherwise.
- Do not drive or operate machinery until cleared by the physician.
- Keep all postoperative appointments.
- Tell the physician about any problems during recovery.

Gerontologic Considerations

- If an older adult lives alone or with a spouse who is experiencing functional decline, additional considerations must be given to discharge planning. This client may require the services of relatives or friends, a public health nurse, a visiting nurse, or home healthcare personnel during the recovery period. In some instances, admitting the client to a skilled nursing facility for rehabilitation is necessary.

Nursing Process for Standards of Postoperative Care

Nurses must follow standards of care for postoperative clients. The following material provides commonly used nursing diagnoses and interventions in postoperative care. It does not provide a complete list but contains minimum standards for the general surgical client. Other standards may also apply.

Standard I: Respiratory function is maintained.

▶ **Risk for Altered Respiratory Function and PC: Atelectasis/Pneumonia** related to immobility, effects of anesthesia and analgesics, and pain

▶ **Expected Outcome:** Client will have clear lungs and full and unlabored respirations.

- Monitor respiratory rate and characteristics.
- Auscultate lung sounds once a shift or more often if indicated.
- Help client turn and deep breathe every 1 to 2 hours.
- Reinforce use of incentive spirometer.
- Show client how to splint incision before coughing.

- Assess client's ability to mobilize secretions; suction if necessary.
- Administer oxygen as ordered.
- Refrain from administering narcotic analgesics if respiratory rate is less than 12 breaths/minute.
- Encourage early ambulation.

Standard II: Circulatory function is maintained.

▶ PC: Fluid/Electrolyte Imbalance

▶ **Expected Outcome:** The nurse will manage imbalances in fluid and electrolytes.

- Assess vital signs and monitor laboratory values.
- Ensure that IV fluids are infusing at the prescribed rate and that the IV site is patent.
- Monitor postoperative intake and output for at least 48 hours or until all drains and tubes have been removed, client is tolerating oral intake, and urine output is normal.
- Report discrepancies in intake and output, hypotension, dizziness, palpitations, or abnormal laboratory values. (See Chap. 16 for additional information on management of fluid and electrolyte imbalance.)

▶ PC: Hemorrhage and Hypovolemic Shock

▶ **Expected Outcome:** The nurse will manage and minimize hemorrhage and shock.

- Monitor for signs or symptoms of shock: tachycardia, hypotension, decreased urine output, cold, clammy skin, and restlessness.
- Keep head of bed flat unless contraindicated.
- Maintain patent IV line.
- Assess surgical site for excessive external bleeding.
- Reinforce dressing or apply pressure if bleeding is frank.
- Monitor for internal bleeding: peri-incisional hematoma and swelling, abdominal distention if abdominal surgery was performed, excessive bloody output in wound-drainage collection devices, falling hemoglobin and hematocrit levels, orthostatic hypotension, and signs of impending shock. (See Chap. 17 for additional information on management of shock.)
- Report findings immediately.

Standard III: Pain and discomfort are recognized and effectively treated.

▶ Pain related to surgical incision and manipulation of body structures

▶ **Expected Outcome:** Client will experience relief of pain.

- Assess pain level using an established scale (visual or numerical).
- Determine source of pain (e.g., incision, body position, flatus, IV lines or drainage tubes, distended bladder).
- Provide pain medication and evaluate effectiveness 30 minutes after administration.
- Reposition client to improve comfort.
- Teach client nonpharmacologic methods of pain relief: breathing exercises, relaxation techniques, and distraction (see Chap. 11).

▶ Altered Comfort (nausea and vomiting) related to effects of anesthesia or side effects of narcotics

▶ **Expected Outcome:** Client will report increased comfort and relief of nausea and vomiting.

- Encourage client to breathe deeply to help eliminate inhaled anesthetics.
- Help client sit up and turn head to one side while vomiting to avoid aspiration.
- Record intake and output.
- Offer small sips of flat ginger ale or cola, or ice chips if permitted.
- Administer antiemetics as ordered.
- Provide mouth care and fresh linens after vomiting.
- Monitor intake and output and assess for signs or symptoms of dehydration or electrolyte imbalance (see Chap. 16).

▶ Risk for Sleep Pattern Disturbance related to difficulty in assuming comfortable position secondary to surgery, unusual environment, noise, and interruptions

▶ **Expected Outcome:** Client will report enhanced sleep pattern.

- Identify factors contributing to poor sleep (noise, room temperature, position, daytime sleeping, hospital routines).
- Reduce environmental distractions—use night lights, close door.
- Schedule nursing activities to coincide with client's schedule.
- Teach client progressive relaxation techniques and deep-breathing exercises to facilitate sleep.
- Provide back rub.
- Assist with hygiene; provide clean gown and linens.
- Limit daytime sleeping; encourage increased daytime activity.
- Collaborate with physician about sleeping medication if other methods fail.

Standard IV: Client safety is maintained.

▶ Risk for Injury related to decreased alertness secondary to effects of anesthesia and pain medication

▶ **Expected Outcome:** Client will remain free of injury.

- Place bed in low position and elevate side rails.
- Place call bell within reach.
- Ensure that tubings are long enough or properly secured to allow for movement. Inspect drainage tubes for kinks.
- Ensure that all equipment is functioning properly.
- Provide emesis basin, tissues, ice chips (if allowed), bedpan, and urinal within easy reach.
- Instruct clients to call for assistance with any activity.

Standard V: Wound healing is promoted and wound management is provided.

▶ Risk for Infection related to break in skin integrity (surgical incision, wound drainage devices)

▶ **Expected Outcome:** Wound healing is uncomplicated, as shown by intact edges, granulation tissue, and lack of induration or swelling at site.

- Inspect surgical site and peri-incisional drain sites for signs or symptoms of infection (redness, warmth, tenderness, separation of wound edges, purulent drainage).

- Wash hands before and after dressing changes; follow aseptic or sterile technique.
- Change wet dressings frequently (surgeon usually does first dressing change).
- Use skin barrier to protect skin and wound from irritating drainage.
- Avoid using excessive tape.
- Keep drainage tube exit sites clean.
- Prevent excess tension on drainage tubes by securing tubes to dressing.
- Empty collection devices frequently to promote drainage; note characteristics of drainage.
- Teach client to splint wound when coughing or changing position.

Standard VI: Complication potential is continuously assessed, and any complications are immediately and effectively treated.

▶ PC: Deep Vein Thrombosis

▶ **Expected Outcome:** The nurse will manage and minimize risk of phlebitis/thrombosis.

- Reinforce need to perform leg exercises every hour while awake.
- Instruct client not to cross legs or prop pillow under knees.
- Apply compression and antiembolic stockings as ordered.
- Monitor for signs and symptoms of thrombophlebitis: calf pain, tenderness, warmth, or redness; swelling of the extremity; low-grade fever. Notify physician of any such signs or symptoms, and maintain bed rest until client can be further evaluated.
- Ambulate or encourage client to ambulate for a few minutes each hour while awake.
- Help client avoid prolonged sitting and poorly fitting, constrictive antiembolic hose.
- Do not massage calves or thighs.
- Administer anticoagulant medication as ordered; monitor laboratory values for therapeutic levels.

▶ PC: Acute Urinary Retention

▶ **Expected Outcome:** The nurse will manage and minimize risk of urinary retention.

- Assess for bladder distention, discomfort, and urge to void.
- Encourage client to try to void within the first 4 hours after surgery.
- Assess volume of first voided urine to determine adequacy of output (voiding frequent, small amounts indicates retention of urine with elimination of overflow only).
- If client has difficulty voiding in the bedpan or using the urinal in bed, stand male clients (if allowed) and ambulate female clients to bathroom (if allowed).
- If client cannot void within 8 hours of surgery, consult with physician regarding instituting intermittent catheterization until voluntary voiding returns.

▶ PC: Paralytic Ileus

▶ **Expected Outcome:** The nurse will manage and minimize risk for developing postoperative paralytic ileus.

- Assess bowel sounds every shift or more often if indicated.
- Assess returning bowel function as evidenced by passage of flatus or stool.
- Maintain NPO status until bowel sounds return.
- Report large amounts of emesis (more than 300 mL).
- Provide client with moistened gauze to wet lips and tongue until oral intake is allowed.
- Assist with passage of nasogastric tube, if ordered.

Standard VII: Gastrointestinal function is maintained.

▶ Risk for Colonic Constipation related to effects of anesthesia, surgery (manipulation of abdominal organs), side effects of narcotics, and decreased intake of fluids and fiber

▶ **Expected Outcome:** Client will have regular bowel movements.

- Once bowel sounds have returned and client resumes oral intake, encourage intake of sufficient fluids and fiber.
- Encourage ambulation to promote peristalsis.
- Encourage use of bathroom if possible. Provide privacy if client must use bedside commode or bedpan.
- Administer bulk-forming laxatives or stool softeners prophylactically if ordered.
- Notify physician if client has had no bowel movement within 2 to 3 days after surgery.

Standard VIII: Self-care and mobility are encouraged as appropriate.

▶ Activity Intolerance related to decreased mobility and weakness secondary to anesthesia and surgery

▶ **Expected Outcome:** Client will regain strength and activity tolerance.

- Encourage progressive activity.
- Help client dangle legs over bedside the evening of surgery or the next morning, if allowed, followed by sitting out of bed for 15 minutes (or more if tolerated).
- Progress to ambulation in room and hallway.
- Collaborate with client in establishing goals to increase ambulation.
- Help client with hygiene the evening of surgery; encourage increased self-care as appropriate.
- Schedule regular rest periods.

Standard IX: Psychosocial needs are recognized and effectively managed.

▶ Anxiety related to unfamiliar environment, loss of privacy, threat to biologic integrity, and fear secondary to illness and surgery

▶ **Expected Outcome:** Client will share anxieties and report increased psychological comfort.

- Ask client to rate anxiety level on a scale of 0 (none) to 10 (unbearable).

- Explore reasons for anxiety (concerns about health, financial status, family coping, effects on independence). Provide information and reassurance.
- Provide referrals if appropriate.
- Encourage client to use anxiety-reduction techniques (see Chap. 68).
- Determine how to modify the environment to improve relaxation (e.g., close or open curtains, reduce noise, move client closer to nurses' station).
- Assess anxiety level after interventions.

Standard X: Discharge instructions, including follow-up care and home health services, are provided.

▶ **Risk for Ineffective Management of Therapeutic Regimen** related to incomplete knowledge of wound care, activity and diet restrictions, medications, reportable signs and symptoms, and follow-up care

▶ **Expected Outcome:** Client or family will demonstrate ability to provide wound care, restate specific instructions regarding diet and activity, and identify signs and symptoms of complications and needed follow-up care. (Carpenito, 2008; Nettina, 2005)

- Explain, demonstrate, and provide written instructions about care of surgical wound.
- Observe the client or family performing care.
- Discuss signs and symptoms of wound infection, and instruct client and family to contact healthcare provider if they develop.
- Describe and provide written instructions about activity restrictions and when to resume normal activity.
- Include information on walking, bending, lifting, climbing stairs, bathing, showering, driving, and engaging in sexual activity.
- Explain need for adequate nutrition and fluids and how to manage constipation, which can result from decreased intake, decreased activity, and narcotic pain relievers.
- Review all medications, including dose, route of administration, intended effect, side effects, and duration of prescription.
- Review signs and symptoms of complications such as shortness of breath, fever, productive cough, weakness, new or unusual pain, pain unrelieved by medication, calf tenderness and swelling, and wound drainage.
- Evaluate client's and family's understanding of discharge instructions. ●

CRITICAL THINKING EXERCISES

1. The nurse is checking to ensure that a client's surgical consent form is signed and on the chart the evening before surgery. When the nurse assesses this client, the client reports that he is uncertain about having the surgery and does not understand what is expected or its long-term consequences. What steps should the nurse take? What must the nurse document?

2. A client reports to the nurse that her family has lost several family members unexpectedly during surgery. The client is very scared about her upcoming surgery. What actions should the nurse take? What should the nurse document?

3. It is the fifth day of a client's postoperative period (5 days postop). He complains of incisional pain, feeling warm, and nausea. What assessments should the nurse make? What should he or she document?

4. What concerns should nurses have when caring for postoperative clients with a history of smoking at least one pack of cigarettes per day for many years?

NCLEX-STYLE REVIEW QUESTIONS

1. A teenage client will require surgery to realign the bones in a fractured tibia sustained while backpacking with a youth group. In this case, from whom is it most appropriate to obtain consent to perform the surgical procedure?
   1. The client
   2. The client's parent
   3. The client's physician
   4. The client's youth leader

2. A surgical client experiences abdominal incisional discomfort when coughing postoperatively. Which nursing intervention is most appropriate for reducing the client's discomfort?
   1. Administer an analgesic soon after coughing.
   2. Apply light pressure to the incision with a pillow.
   3. Have the client lie supine before trying to cough.
   4. Tell the client to flex both knees while coughing.

3. A postoperative client asks the nurse to explain the purpose of the Penrose drain positioned in his abdomen. The best explanation is that an open wound drain is used to do which of the following?
   1. Decrease the formation of scar tissue
   2. Provide a means for irrigating the wound
   3. Release accumulating intestinal gas
   4. Remove fluid from the surgical area

4. If a postoperative client is on a clear liquid diet, which food item is most appropriate to provide?
   1. A bowl of ice cream
   2. A cup of creamed soup
   3. A dish of gelatin
   4. A glass of milk

5. A postoperative client asks the nurse why performing leg exercises is important. The nurse is correct in stating that leg movement that involves contracting and relaxing leg muscles helps to prevent which of the following?
   1. Developing varicose veins
   2. Formation of blood clots
   3. Loss of muscle strength
   4. Swelling of the extremities

15

Disaster Situations

Learning Objectives

On completion of this chapter, you will be able to:

1. Define *disaster* and give two general examples.
2. Identify three categories of human disasters that may result from acts of terrorism.
3. Name three methods by which a radiologic disaster could be created.
4. Explain the difference between external and internal radiation contamination.
5. Name three substances used to prevent or reduce radiologic organ damage.
6. List possible indications of a bioterrorism attempt.
7. Name three biologic agents likely to be used as weapons of mass destruction.
8. List possible indications of a chemical terrorism attempt.
9. Name four types of chemical agents that may be used to create a human disaster.
10. List four triage categories that emergency workers use to prioritize victims' need for treatment.
11. Provide examples of collaborative problems and nursing diagnoses that the nurse may be required to manage following a disaster.

An emergency department (ED) is the location for managing extraordinary events that require a rapid response (Gebbie & Qureshi, 2002). An ED is typically busy caring for clients who have experienced myocardial infarctions, motor vehicle collisions, sports-related injuries, and other acute conditions. However, a disaster exponentially increases an ED's stress and chaos.

The American Red Cross defines a **disaster** as "a threatening … event of such destructive magnitude and force as to dislocate people, separate family members, damage or destroy homes, and injure or kill people" (Willshire, Hassmiller, & Wodicka, 2004). The magnitude of the disaster is related to the causal event. Disasters overwhelm emergency and healthcare services.

There are essentially two types of disasters: (1) *natural disasters* such as earthquakes, floods, and hurricanes, and (2) *human disasters*, which may be intentionally or unintentionally caused, such as explosions, fires, and acts of terrorism. Both types of disaster may result in mass trauma and disruptions of services. Although nurses have always played an integral role in natural disaster relief efforts, nursing skills are an essential component in the Department of Homeland Security's plan for preparing and defending the United States against the global threat of terrorism. In the event that a disaster may occur, the nurse provides suggestions that may be beneficial for temporary survival (Client and Family Teaching 15-1).

Client and Family Teaching 15-1
Preparing for a Disaster

The nurse teaches the following points for disaster preparedness:

● Keep a 7-day supply of medications and extra hearing aids or eyeglasses on hand at all times in case of a disaster.
● Store a supply kit with a flashlight, battery-operated radio, and extra batteries in case of loss of electricity.
● Keep a supply of canned or dried packaged food and bottled water on hand.
● In the event of biologic, chemical, or radiologic disaster, avoid consuming fresh food or water from the faucet because these items also might be contaminated with pathogens, chemicals, or fallout.
● Affix a tag to a pet's collar with a name, address, and phone number in case the pet is rescued and taken to an animal shelter.
● Create a network of person who could provide support during and after a disaster, especially if older or disabled.

The focus of this chapter is the role nurses play when three types of human disasters occur: (1) bombings, which may result in radiation exposure, (2) biologic disasters, and (3) chemical disasters. The actual or potential threat from these three forms of human disasters recently has been attributed to terrorists, people whose objective is to manipulate the politics and policies of a country by frightening and maiming its civilian population.

BOMBS AND RADIOLOGIC DISASTERS

Bombings accounted for nearly 70% of all terrorist attacks in the United States and its territories between 1980 and 2001 according to the U.S. Federal Bureau of Investigation (CDCa, 2005). Post-explosion injuries generally cause penetrating and blunt trauma. However, if the blast includes a radioactive substance, it will also have life-threatening consequences for people, animals, and the environment. Harmful levels of **gamma (ionizing) radiation**, energy released from unstable atoms, can penetrate, damage, and destroy body cells.

Types of Radiologic Disasters

Radiologic disasters, those in which people, animals, and the environment are exposed to radiation, can occur in the following ways:

• Explosion of a dirty bomb
• Damage to or human error in a nuclear power plant
• Nuclear blast

The significance of resulting danger depends on the type of radiologic event and the distance of person from its center.

Dirty Bomb

A **dirty bomb** is a conventional explosive device (e.g., dynamite) that spreads small amounts of radiation in the

form of powder or pellets. The greater danger is from the explosion; the radiation dispersed is a secondary danger to those in the immediate area of the blast and others downwind who may inhale the radioactive dust and smoke. Another consequence is the fear and perhaps mass hysteria resulting from such an attack. Healthcare workers focus attention on legitimate victims and those referred to as the **worried well**, unaffected people who believe they are at risk for physical consequences.

Nuclear Power Plant Disaster

Nuclear power plants use radioactive materials as a source of fuel to create electrical energy for consumers. The devices that initiate, control, and sustain the nuclear reactions as well as spent fuel are potential concerns for the escape of radiation. Accidents involving a nuclear power plant occurred at Three Mile Island, Pennsylvania, in 1979 and Chernobyl in the Ukraine in 1986.

The U.S. Nuclear Regulatory Commission (NRC) oversees civilian use of nuclear materials to ensure adequate protection of public health and safety. The chairman of the NRC has indicated that nuclear power plants can resist damage from hurricanes, tornadoes, earthquakes, and the impact of a small plane. However, nuclear power plants have not been built to withstand a crash from a large airliner like those used in the September 11, 2001, terrorist attack. Although the risk of radiologic sabotage is lower in the U.S. than in other countries with less rigorous regulations, the Government Accounting Office (2006) has recommended that the NRC evaluate and implement measures to strengthen the defense of nuclear power plants against terrorists seeking to cause the release of radioactive materials. The NRC currently requires states with a population within 10 miles of a commercial nuclear plant to have immediate access to a supply of **potassium iodide** (prophylaxis for protecting the thyroid gland from absorption of radiation) and to provide a place for shelter during a power plant accident (Boston Public Health Commission, 2005).

Nuclear Blast

A **nuclear blast** is an explosion that produces an intense wave of heat, light, air pressure, and radiation. The explosion creates a fireball and mushroom cloud that contains radioactive material and vaporized particles. When the vapor cools, it condenses and drops back to earth, whereupon it is known as **fallout**. Wind currents can carry the fallout long distances (CDC, 2003a).

The consequences for survivors of a nuclear blast include severe burns, trauma from debris, blindness, radiation sickness, and cancer, all of which result from external and internal radiologic contamination. **External radiologic contamination** occurs from exposure to fallout on the skin, hair, and clothing. **Internal radiologic contamination** occurs when fallout enters an open wound, is inhaled via contaminated air, or is consumed through contaminated food and water.

Assessment Findings

The appearance of burns (see Chap. 66) and trauma are obvious. What is unseen is perhaps even more devastating. Invisible gamma radiation penetrates the body and can be

BOX 15-1 Manifestations of Acute Radiation Syndrome

- Nausea, vomiting, and diarrhea within minutes to days of exposure
- Dehydration
- Weakness
- Swelling, itching, and redness of skin
- Blisters in the mouth and throat
- Open sores on the skin
- Hair loss
- Bone marrow dysfunction
- Infections
- Bleeding from the nose, mouth, and gums

eliminated in blood, sweat, urine, and feces. Consequently, a contaminated person can contaminate others through contact with body fluids or surfaces he or she touches.

Based on the experiences of those involved in the bombings of Hiroshima and Nagasaki, Japan, during World War II and those exposed to radiation at Chernobyl, many people develop **acute radiation syndrome** (ARS) (Box 15-1). ARS may result in death in as little as 10 hours and the potential for death may last up to 5 weeks (Boston Public Health Commission, 2005). The chance of surviving ARS depends on the dose of gamma radiation a person receives.

Long-term effects experienced by those exposed to radiologic disasters include thyroid cancer, leukemia, and non-Hodgkin's lymphoma (see Chaps. 50, 30, and 31). In addition, genetic effects have been seen among infants conceived shortly before or subsequent to radiologic disasters. Some of these include major congenital malformations, stillbirths, impaired growth and development, and shorter life expectancies from the development of various types of cancer (Neel, 2002).

Medical and Nursing Management

The most immediate concern is to limit external and internal exposure to radiation. The amount of radiation increases and decreases with the time people spend near the source, how near or far from the source they are, and any shielding that they use as a barrier. Lead is necessary to protect against gamma radiation.

Once exposure is limited, the next concern is to reduce radiologic organ damage by administering substances that interfere with organ concentration or speed up the removal of the radioactive substance.

Limiting External Contamination

External contamination can be limited in the following ways:

- Stay indoors and go to a centrally located room or basement with as few windows as possible; turn off all fans, air-conditioners, and forced-air heating units.
- If outside, remove all or at least outer clothing and shoes before entering the house or a public shelter. (Removing all garments can eliminate 90% of external radioactive contamination.)
- Place clothing and shoes inside a plastic bag.

- Shower/wash with soap and water.
- Temporarily seal windows and doors with duct tape or plastic sheeting for a few hours.
- Tune the radio to an emergency response network for further information.
- If directed to evacuate:
  - Go to the specified emergency shelter.
  - Keep car windows closed and the ventilation system turned off.
  - Bring medications and a change of clothes; most emergency shelters will not accept pets.

Limiting Internal Contamination

Internal contamination can be limited by:

- Covering the mouth and nose with a scarf, handkerchief, or other cloth
- Drinking only bottled water
- Consuming canned, dried, and packaged food products
- Avoiding the inhalation of tobacco products

Reducing Radiologic Organ Damage

Taking substances called potassium iodide, Prussian blue, and diethylenetriamine pentaacetate can prevent or reduce radiologic organ damage.

Potassium iodide (KI) prevents radioactive iodine from reaching the thyroid gland by saturating the gland with non-radioactive iodine. Radioactive iodine may be released in a nuclear power plant disaster or nuclear blast. A high dose of radioactive iodine can lead to thyroid cancer within a few years of exposure. The person must take KI as soon as possible up to 24 hours after exposure. It limits or protects only the thyroid gland; it does not interfere with radiologic effects on other organs.

Prussian blue is a dye used to treat internal contamination with ingested radioactive cesium, a chemical element produced by a nuclear reactor or nuclear blast. Prussian blue promotes the excretion of cesium by trapping it in the intestine and preventing its absorption. It reduces the half-life of cesium by almost 23% from 8 days to 3 days, thus limiting the time of radiation exposure. The CDC has stockpiled Prussian blue in case of an emergency. It is administered 3 to 4 times a day for up to 150 days, depending on the extent of contamination.

Diethylenetriamine pentaacetate (DTPA) is an injectable salt or inhalant spray containing calcium (Ca-DTPA) or zinc (Zn-DTPA) and is used to treat internal contamination with radioactive substances such as plutonium. It is most effective if given within the first 24 hours of exposure, but DTPA may still provide beneficial effects for days to weeks after contamination (CDC, 2005).

 Pharmacologic Considerations

- Potassium iodide should not be given to someone allergic to iodine without consulting a physician. Prussian blue capsules can be opened and mixed with food or liquids if swallowing intact capsules is difficult for the client. Co-ingesting food with Prussian blue increases its effectiveness. Prussian blue will turn the mouth, teeth, and stools blue temporarily (Hussar, 2005).

- Ca-DTPA should not be administered to those with kidney disease or bone marrow depression, children younger than 18 years, or those who are pregnant or suffering from hemochromatosis.

> **Stop, Think, and Respond Exercise 15-1**
>
> *Which type of radiation is the most dangerous? What three methods can be used to limit exposure to it?*

BIOLOGIC DISASTERS

A **biologic disaster** is one in which pathogens or their **toxins** (pathologic substances produced by microorganisms) cause harm to many humans and other living species. Examples of biologic disasters include the outbreak of bubonic plague in Eurasia in the 12th century and the influenza epidemic in the United States during the early 20th century. Although these disasters occurred naturally, the current concern is the deliberate use of biologic agents as weapons of mass destruction. Box 15-2 lists incidents that suggest the use of a bioterrorist agent.

Three agents likely to be used in bioterrorist warfare include anthrax, botulism, and smallpox. These agents pose a high threat because they are (1) stable and simple to mass produce, (2) easy to deliver to a large population, (3) associated with high mortality, and (4) likely to cause public fear (Chettle, 2002).

ANTHRAX

Anthrax is a spore-forming bacterium known as *Bacillus anthracis*. Anthrax is fairly easy to promulgate because in its spore form, it is inactive and causes disease only when inhaled, ingested, or introduced into nonintact skin. Once inside the body, the spores multiply and produce toxins. Anthrax sent in powdered form within letters delivered by the U.S. Postal Service caused 22 infections and 11 deaths among Americans in 2001 (Centers for Disease Control and Prevention [CDC], 2003b). Most forms of anthrax are not transmitted from human to human. Standard Precautions, measures for reducing the risk of transmitting pathogens (see Chap.

BOX 15-2 Indications of Bioterrorism

- High outbreak of similar symptoms among previously healthy people
- Increased numbers of sick people seeking healthcare
- Atypical incidence of illness for the time of year and geographic location
- Clusters of sick people from a shared locale
- Unusual mortality rates among people following a brief illness
- Unexplained deaths or illness among domestic and wild animals

Adapted from Chettle, C. C. (2002). "Preparing for bioterrorism: Nurses on the front line." Available at: http://www2.nursingspectrum.com/CE/Self-Study_modules/tools/print.html?ID=375. Accessed November 2007.

---

12), are sufficient when caring for clients infected with anthrax.

Assessment Findings

The most serious form of anthrax develops upon inhalation. At the onset, it may be mistaken for a cold or flu, but if misdiagnosed and untreated, the infection progresses into severe respiratory distress and almost certain death. Ingesting the bacteria is slightly less lethal, with symptoms of nausea, vomiting, diarrhea, and abdominal pain as anthrax infects the gastrointestinal tract, circulatory system, and mesenteric lymph nodes. Skin infection is the least deadly form and the only one that may be transmitted by direct contact. It is characterized by painless lesions usually on the head, hands, and arms that develop into black-centered blisters that eventually ulcerate (Fig. 15-1).

Medical and Nursing Management

When anthrax is diagnosed by culturing blood, stool, and wound exudate, it is treated fairly successfully with antibiotic therapy. The preferred antibiotic is ciprofloxacin (Cipro) or levofloxacin (Levaquin), both of which are fluoroquinolones; the treatment lasts 4 weeks or longer for an inhalant infection. Although the infection responds to doxycycline (Vibramycin), a tetracycline, it is not used initially because the bacteria have demonstrated the ability to develop tetracycline-resistant forms.

A vaccine has been developed to prevent infection with anthrax, but currently only military personnel and at-risk civilians are being targeted as recipients. The vaccine requires a series of 6 doses over 18 months (Stilp, 2005).

BOTULISM

Botulism is a disease that develops from the neurotoxin produced by *Clostridium botulinum*, an anaerobic bacterium (see Chap. 12). The pathogen is generally food-borne, but it also can be acquired through inhalation. People infected with

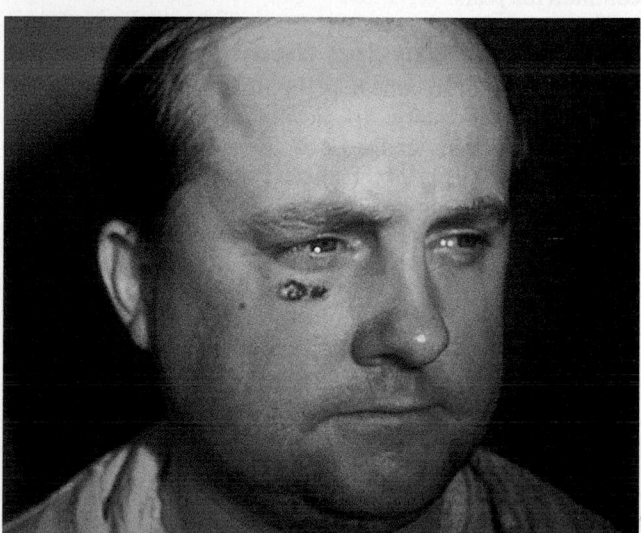

FIGURE 15-1 Appearance of anthrax skin lesion. (Courtesy of the Public Health Image Library, Centers for Disease Control and Prevention.)

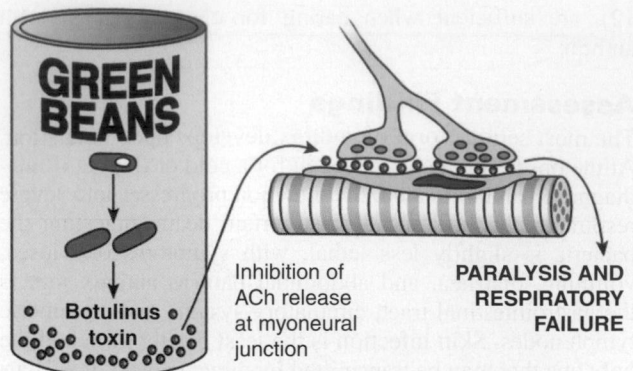

FIGURE 15-2 Botulinum toxin inhibits acetylcholine at the myoneural junction, causing paralysis and respiratory failure. (From Rubin, R. & Strayer, D. S., Eds. [2008]. *Rubin's pathology: Clinicopathologic foundations of medicine* [5th ed.]. Baltimore: Lippincott Williams & Wilkins.)

botulinum toxin are not a risk to others; there have been no reports of person-to-person transmission. If used as a weapon of mass destruction, the pathogen most likely would be spread via toxin-contaminated food or aerosolization.

Assessment Findings

The botulinum toxin blocks acetylcholine, a parasympathetic neurotransmitter. Acetylcholine is responsible for the transmission of neural impulses to muscles. Blockage of acetylcholine results in paralysis of motor and autonomic nerves (Fig. 15-2). Early signs of botulism can be characterized by "4Ds": diplopia (double vision), dysarthria (difficulty speaking), dysphonia (vocal changes, such as hoarseness), and dysphagia (difficulty swallowing) (Stilp, 2005). There also may be drooping of the eyes and generalized muscular weakness. The greatest potential for lethality occurs with paralysis of the respiratory muscles. Even when a person survives, respiratory difficulty and muscular weakness may continue for years.

Medical and Nursing Management

Generally, initial treatment of botulism follows a clinical, rather than a laboratory, diagnosis. Tests on serum, gastric, and fecal specimens tend to be too time consuming to justify a delay in treatment. Mechanical ventilation is required to support breathing for 2 to 3 months. If large numbers of people were to become acutely ill simultaneously as a consequence of bioterrorism, the numbers of ventilators available in any particular agency would likely become exhausted quickly.

An antitoxin is available from the state's public health department or the CDC. Nevertheless, a near-9% hypersensitivity develops among recipients of the antitoxin, necessitating a preadministration skin test to reduce a potential adverse effect (CDC, 1999).

Although a preexposure vaccine given in a series of three injections over 3 months has been developed, it too is associated with a risk for a severe allergic response known as anaphylaxis (see Chap. 34). Protection with the vaccine is short-lived, requiring yearly booster injections.

SMALLPOX

Smallpox is a highly contagious disease caused by the variola virus. The disease acquired its name because of the raised bumps that appear on the face and body.

The World Health Organization proclaimed eradication of smallpox in 1980 following the success of aggressive vaccination programs. Believing that smallpox had been conquered, the United States stopped administering routine childhood vaccinations in 1972 (CDC, 2004a). The status of immunity among adults vaccinated prior to that date is unknown. Consequently, estimates are that nearly 2 billion susceptible people could die if the smallpox virus that has been stored in a small number of laboratories around the world was released as a bioterrorist act (Chettle, 2002). The projected death rate is estimated at 30% of those eventually infected (CDC, 2004a).

Smallpox can be spread in three ways: (1) direct contact with an infected person, (2) contact with body fluids or contaminated objects (e.g., bedding) that contain the live virus, or (3) exposure to an aerosol containing the virus. Terrorists would most likely use the aerosol method. Although aerosolized smallpox virus may not survive longer than 24 hours, if the virus infects even one person, it poses a public health threat.

Assessment Findings

A person infected with smallpox may be asymptomatic for the first 7 to 14 days. A few days before the rash develops, the person becomes noticeably ill with a fever as high as 101° to 104°F. The fever subsides temporarily with the onset of the rash, but rises again until the rash resolves.

Smallpox may be mistaken for chickenpox (*varicella*), although the outbreak and progression of the rash are opposite in these illnesses (Fig. 15-3). The rash associated with smallpox begins on the face and progresses to the extremities, including the palms and soles, with few lesions on the trunk. The rash of chickenpox begins heavily on the trunk and spreads lightly to the face and extremities, but tends to be missing or sparse on the palms and soles. Smallpox lesions are generally all in the same stage of development, but successive crops of chickenpox macules and papules appear every few days. Table 15-1 provides a timeline for the course of a smallpox infection, the progression of signs and symptoms, and the stages at which the disease is contagious.

Although smallpox may be a differential diagnosis based on the clinical signs and symptoms, laboratory culture from lesions on the skin confirms the infection. Because smallpox is a virus, the collected specimen must be grown within live cells and examined with an electron microscope. Healthcare providers must alert local and state health departments as well as the CDC when they suspect cases of smallpox.

Medical Management

Because of the high potential for widespread mortality, any person suspected of having smallpox will be under strict contact transmission-based (isolation) precautions in a room under negative air pressure (CDC, 2001). Caregivers use both airborne and droplet precautions to control the respiratory spread of the virus (see Table 12-1). They wear gloves

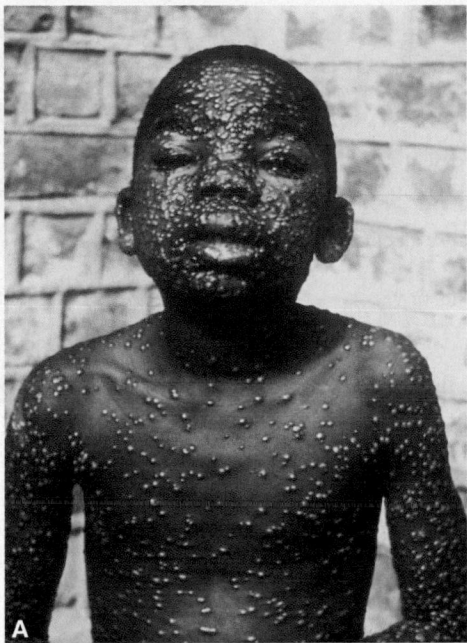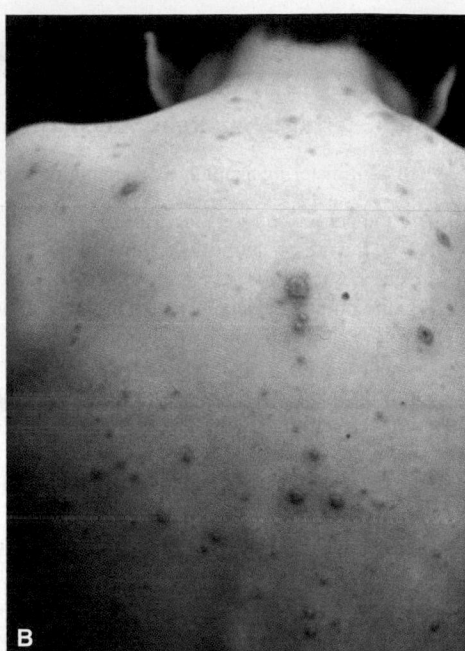

FIGURE 15-3 Smallpox may be mistaken for chickenpox. **(A)** Characteristic lesions of smallpox; the rash begins on the face and progresses to the extremities. **(B)** Characteristic lesions of chickenpox; the rash begins on the trunk and spreads lightly to the face and extremities. (Images courtesy of the Public Health Image Library, Centers for Disease Control and Prevention.)

as a barrier against contact with the lesions. Care providers also autoclave or incinerate linens and clothing that are presumably contaminated (Stilp, 2005). Those in close contact with the smallpox victim require vaccination and monitoring for a rise in temperature. If they develop a fever within 17 days of exposure to the victim, they will be isolated as well.

Smallpox has no specific treatment. Supportive measures such as fluid therapy, antipyretics, and antibiotics for secondary bacterial infections reduce symptoms and help prevent death. New antiviral agents, such as cidofovir (Vistide), are being developed. Laboratory studies of cidofovir, presently used to treat viral infections such as cytomegalovirus (CMV), suggest that it also may be effective against smallpox (CDC, 2004).

The U.S. government is proactively stockpiling sufficient smallpox vaccine to administer potentially to everyone in the country. It may take up to 12 hours for the vaccine to arrive at any needed destination, however, which could be problematic in the event of a wide-scale attack. The smallpox vaccine is effective in preventing infection if administered within 3 days of exposure to the virus; however, in most cases, the exposed person may be unaware that he or she has been exposed. The vaccine is useless for a person who is already symptomatic. Both a vaccine and *vaccinia immune-globulin* (VIG), a method of providing passive immunity (see Chap. 33) can be used for those who may be at risk of side effects from the smallpox vaccine, can be administered to those still asymptomatic but whose exposure exceeds 3 days. Vaccination is contraindicated

TABLE 15-1 Course of Smallpox Infection

APPROXIMATE TIMELINE	DEVELOPMENT OF DISEASE	STATE OF CONTAGION
Day 1–17	No evidence of symptoms	Not contagious

Day 19–21	Onset of symptoms:
	  High fever
	  Headache
	  Body aches
	  Malaise
		Potentially contagious

Day 22–24	Rash appears on the tongue and in the mouth. Rash proceeds to develop on the face and spreads to the arms, legs, and feet. The rash becomes raised papules. The papules fill with fluid, with a depressed central area resembling a navel.	Most contagious
Day 25–29	The papules become pustules that are round and firm, as though embedded with pellets.	Remains contagious
Day 30–34	Pustules begin to crust and scab.	Remains contagious
Day 35–40	Scabs are shed over a 3-week period, leaving pitted scars.	Remains contagious
After day 40	Scabs have resolved.	No longer contagious

Adapted from CDC (2004). "Smallpox disease overview." Available at: http://www.bt.cdc.gov/agent/smallpox/overview/disease-facts.asp. Accessed February 4, 2008.

NURSING GUIDELINES 15-1

Administering a Smallpox Vaccination

When administering a smallpox vaccination, the nurse will:

- Use the deltoid site for vaccination.
- Avoid the use of alcohol as a skin disinfectant because alcohol inactivates the virus.
- Dip the bifurcated needle once into the multidose vial of vaccine to create a tiny drop at the tip.
- Hold the needle perpendicular to the site.
- Pierce the skin rapidly in a 5-mm area at least three times, or the number identified on the vial, to cause a trace of blood to appear (see figure to the right).
- Dab the site with dry sterile gauze and discard in an infection-control receptacle.
- Cover the site of the vaccination with loose gauze followed by adhesive tape.

Adapted from CDC (2004). Smallpox vaccination method. Available at: http://emergency.cdc.gov/agent/smallpox/vaccination/vaccination-method.asp. Accessed December 2008.

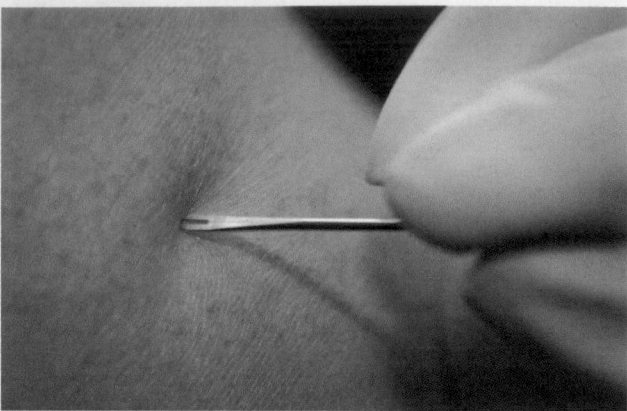

A bifurcated needle is used to administer a smallpox vaccination. (Courtesy of Public Health Image Library, Centers for Disease Control and Prevention.)

for pregnant women, those who are immunosuppressed, and those with eczema. No one who has been exposed to smallpox will be vaccinated forcibly, but they may be placed in isolation for at least 18 days to monitor for symptoms (CDC, 2004).

Nursing Management

Nurses would play a major role in vaccinating the public during a potential or actual outbreak of smallpox (Nursing Guidelines 15-1). They would also teach anyone vaccinated for smallpox how to care for the vaccination site (Client and Family Teaching 15-2).

Client and Family Teaching 15-2
Caring for a Smallpox Vaccination Site

The nurse teaches the client and family to do the following:

- Avoid scratching or rubbing the site of vaccination.
- Keep the site covered with a gauze dressing
- Place a waterproof cover over the site when bathing.
- Change the gauze dressing every 1 to 2 days or if it becomes wet.
- Discard the soiled dressing, waterproof covering, and scab, when it is shed, in a sealable plastic bag.
- Wash hands thoroughly or use an alcohol-based handrub after touching the site or dressings, clothing, towels, or sheets in contact with the site.
- Separate and wash clothes, towels, and bed linens that come in contact with the vaccination site in hot water, detergent, or bleach.
- Call a healthcare provider if there are concerns about the vaccination site.
- Have the site checked 7 days following the vaccination.

Adapted from CDC (2004). Smallpox vaccination method. Available at: http://emergency.cdc.gov/agent/smallpox/vaccination/vaccination-method.asp. Accessed December 2008.

▶ *Stop, Think, and Respond Exercise 15-2*

Which of the three biologic agents discussed in this chapter can be transmitted from human to human, thus necessitating the use of transmission-based (isolation) precautions when caring for victims?

CHEMICAL DISASTERS

Chemical disasters result from the release of toxic man-made substances with a potential for causing mass casualties. Release of chemical agents among a population may occur either through an industrial accident or during transport. Terrorists also can use chemical agents as weapons. Examples of extremely toxic chemicals include nerve agents, cyanide, respiratory toxins, and blistering agents.

Detecting a chemical accident or attack is difficult because most chemical agents are liquids that vaporize quickly with either no odors or odors that may be attributed to other substances (e.g., garlic, onions). Box 15-3 lists some indications of a chemical release.

NERVE AGENT POISONING

Nerve agents, the most toxic of all chemical agents, are potent organophosphate compounds that cause fatal consequences by inhibiting acetylcholinesterase. Acetylcholinesterase is an enzyme that inactivates acetylcholine, a neurotransmitter of the parasympathetic (cholinergic) nervous system. Consequently, in cases of attacks with nerve agents, the functions of the parasympathetic nervous system will be active without any potential for disinhibition.

One example of a nerve agent is the commonly used insecticide malathion. Malathion is highly toxic to insects, but not to humans or the environment when applied following the

- Numerous dead animals such as birds, domestic pets, fish, or insects in a confined area
- Dead or dying vegetation
- Sick, dying, and dead humans, especially indoors or downwind
- Unexplained odor atypical for the location
- Fog-like or low-lying cloud in the atmosphere
- Abandoned devices that could be used for spraying chemicals

Adapted from: "Criminal/terrorist use of chemical/biological agents," Available at: http://www.rcmp-learning.org/docs/ecdd1022.htm. Accessed February 2008.

labeled directions (U.S. Environmental Protection Agency, 2007). If released in large quantity or indiscriminately, however, it could be toxic to large numbers of people. Dangerous nerve agents such as **sarin**, which was released in a Tokyo subway in 1995, are 100 to 150 times more potent.

Assessment Findings

People exposed to a nerve agent vapor may develop symptoms within a few seconds; if exposed to a liquid form, they may show symptoms in minutes to hours. Clusters of symptoms develop when the nicotinic and muscarinic receptors of cholinergic nerves are stimulated. Box 15-4 lists these clusters of symptoms and the mnemonics (aids to remembering lists) to help remember them. The mnemonic for muscarinic-receptor stimulation is DUMBELS, and the mnemonic for nicotinic-receptor stimulation is MTWHF, almost the same sequence as the days of the week. The effects of nerve agent poisoning depend on the route and amount of exposure. Clients may experience mild or moderate effects as late as 18 hours following dermal exposure. Death may occur within 10 minutes of inhalation if antidotes are not administered.

BOX 15-4 | **Signs and Symptoms of Nerve Agent Toxicity**

Muscarinic Stimulation
D: Diarrhea
U: Urination
M: Miosis (pupil constriction)
B: Bradycardia, bronchorrhea, bronchospasm
E: Emesis
L: Lacrimation
S: Salivation, secretions, sweating

Nicotinic Stimulation
M: Mydriasis (pupil dilation)
T: Tachycardia
W: Weakness
H: Hypertension
F: Fasciculations (muscle twitching)

Source: U.S. Army Medical Research Institute of Chemical Defense. (2001). *Medical management of chemical casualties handbook,* 4th ed. McLean, VA: International Medical Publishing, Inc.

Medical Management

Two drugs given to manage the effects of nerve agent toxicity are atropine sulfate, which counteracts excess acetylcholine at muscarinic sites, and pralidoxime chloride (2-PAM), which reactivates acetylcholinesterase (Sidell, 2002). Diazepam (Valium) may be needed to control possible seizures. Atropine is administered every 5 to 10 minutes until hypersecretion ceases and breathing is adequate.

Nursing Management

Supportive measures include moving the victim(s) to fresh air and administering oxygen-assisted ventilation via a bag-valve mask to avoid cross-contamination. Clothing that may contain nerve agent residue is removed with gloves and deposited in a sealed container. Areas of skin exposure are washed with a solution containing bleach and flushed with plain water.

CYANIDE POISONING

Cyanide is a solid salt or volatile liquid chemical that causes death in minutes. It is used currently in gas chambers to execute prisoners. The Nazis used cyanide known as Zyklon B to exterminate Jews in gas chambers of concentration camps during World War II. The mechanism of cyanide's action is the inhibition of an enzyme, cytochrome oxidase, needed for oxygen metabolism and cellular energy.

The gas that forms with release of cyanide is colorless and may have a faint odor of "bitter almonds." Inhalation, especially in an enclosed space, is the most deadly type of poisoning. Cyanide also can be ingested by eating foods laced with it, or in accidental poisoning when consuming various industrial chemicals that break down into a cyanide-containing by-product. An example is the compound used to remove artificial fingernails (CDC, Facts about cyanide, 2004b). Cyanide also can be absorbed through the skin.

Assessment Findings

Cyanide poisoning is manifested primarily by toxic effects to the heart and brain. Following inhalation of cyanide, people generally develop tachycardia and cardiac dysrhythmias, rapid breathing, low blood pressure, restlessness, dizziness, headache, loss of consciousness, and respiratory failure. Despite impaired ventilation, the victim does not appear cyanotic. Ingestion of cyanide causes nausea, weakness, and dizziness shortly before more lethal symptoms.

Medical and Nursing Management

Nurses and other healthcare personnel must wear protective garments and respirator masks if the victim's clothing contains cyanide. They remove such contaminated clothing and place it in a sealed container while resuscitation proceeds.

They administer one or all of the following antidotes: amyl nitrite, sodium nitrite, and sodium thiosulfate. Amyl nitrite promotes the formation of methemoglobin, which combines with cyanide to form nontoxic cyanmethemoglobin. Nursing Guidelines 15-2 provides information on administering amyl nitrite.

If a victim does not respond to amyl nitrite, additional treatment with sodium nitrite is necessary. Sodium nitrite,

NURSING GUIDELINES 15-2

Administering Amyl Nitrite

To give amyl nitrite to a victim of cyanide poisoning, the nurse proceeds as follows:

- Break an ampule of amyl nitrite into a piece of cloth or gauze square.
- Insert the cloth or gauze containing amyl nitrite into an oxygen mask.
- Place the oxygen mask with 100% concentration of oxygen and the cloth containing amyl nitrite over the victim's nose and mouth for 15 seconds.
- Remove the mask every 15 seconds.
- Continue the sequence of applying and removing the mask 5 or 6 times.
- Use a fresh ampule of amyl nitrite every 3 minutes until the client regains consciousness; a total of 1 to 4 ampules may be needed.

Source: "Cyanide: Health effects and treatment plan for medical professionals." Available at: http://www.airproducts.com/NR/rdonlyres/F5FDBEE4-BB14-49F4-BA85-47A23036A3B5/0/CyanideMP.doc. Accessed February 4, 2008.

administered intravenously for at least 5 minutes, attracts cyanide from the heme group of cytochrome oxidase. Intravenous sodium thiosulfate is given following sodium nitrite. It produces thiocyanate, a nontoxic substance that detoxifies cyanide (Air Products and Chemicals, Inc., no date). Most clients can be revived in 1 to 2 hours.

Pharmacologic Considerations

- Amyl nitrite increases intraocular and intracranial pressure. It should be used with caution in people with glaucoma, recent head injury, or hemorrhagic stroke.

- Methemoglobin can cause cyanosis and hypotension if it exceeds 15% to 30% in an adult. If amyl nitrite is administered in the recommended doses, toxic levels of methemoglobin should not develop.

RESPIRATORY TOXIN POISONING

Respiratory toxins are chemical agents that primarily cause pulmonary edema when inhaled. Two common examples are **chlorine** and **phosgene**, liquids that become gases when released in the atmosphere. When vaporized, the gas settles and remains close to ground level for some time.

Chlorine is used in households and commercially as a cleaning agent; it is effective in reducing the growth of microorganisms in water and pools. Phosgene has multiple industrial uses and helps produce polyurethane, insecticides, and solvents. Phosgene is a by-product when Freon, a gas used in refrigerators and air conditioners, burns (Slepski,

2005). Both chemicals are used widely and therefore available for legitimate or possible terrorist purposes.

Assessment Findings

As a liquid, chlorine can damage the skin and mucous membranes of the eyes and nose. When chlorine combines with water, it forms hydrochloric acid. On wet skin, chlorine produces a dermal injury similar to frostbite or thermal burns. Liquid phosgene is injurious internally if the liquid contaminates food or water. Both chlorine and phosgene, however, are more hazardous to large numbers of people in their gaseous form.

Exposure to these respiratory toxins leads to tearing, coughing, bronchospasms, and laryngospasms with airway obstruction from localized swelling. Phosgene actually breaks down alveolar tissue. Death occurs as fluid infiltrates the pulmonary air spaces and terminal bronchioles interfering with gas exchange.

Medical and Nursing Management

The consequences of exposure to chlorine or phosgene are related to the amount, route, and length of chemical exposure. The most immediate measure taken to avoid fatality requires assisting victims to fresh air on higher ground. Emergency workers remove the victim's clothing, double bagging it if possible. Skin exposed to the chemical is washed with copious amounts of water and soap and as little delay as possible. Contact lenses, if worn, are removed, and the eyes are rinsed with plain water for at least 15 minutes. Drinking water or inducing vomiting is contraindicated to avoid secondary injuries and potential aspiration. After immediate first aid, ventilation is supported mechanically until the client can breathe effectively without assistance. Victims who seem improved must be assessed for up to 48 hours to detect a delayed onset of symptoms. Following recovery from the acute event, victims may develop chronic bronchitis and emphysema.

BLISTERING AGENTS

Blistering agents, also known as **vesicants**, are chemicals that damage exposed skin and mucous membranes on contact. If inhaled, blistering agents also can damage respiratory tissues. Two examples of vesicants that have been used in chemical warfare include sulfur mustard (referred to as "mustard gas" during World War I) and lewisite, which was developed during World War I but never used. Some speculated that the Iraqi government under Saddam Hussein had stockpiled vesicants, which is why the U.S. military wore protective hoods, masks, and suits during the early phase of Iraq War.

In addition to being a contactant, vesicants can penetrate fabric. When in contact with skin, these chemicals combine with perspiration to form a solution that penetrates the skin and becomes anchored to dermal cells, forming blisters via enzymatic protein digestion. Some chemical enters the circulation and potentially can affect major internal organs. For example, vesicants damage the DNA of rapidly growing cells, which may explain why nitrogen mustard continues to be a chemotherapeutic agent for cancer (Armada & Mendelson, 2002).

Assessment Findings

Skin reaction with sulfur mustard is almost immediate but occurs hours later with lewisite. The skin itches and becomes red and blistered like sunburn. The blisters come together to form large, dome-shaped lesions filled with clear or yellow fluid that eventually rupture. The impaired skin creates the potential for infection. Inhalation of the vesicant is almost sure to cause death within 24 hours from airway obstruction with blisters within the respiratory passages. Other potential long-term effects include cancer, blood dyscrasias, infertility, and fetal abnormalities, most likely from biologic damage to the victim's DNA (Armada & Mendelson, 2002).

Medical and Nursing Management

A person exposed to a vesicant must be decontaminated immediately, preferably within 1 to 2 minutes, by personnel who also must protect themselves from becoming cross-contaminated. Personnel perform decontamination similarly to that for a person exposed to a respiratory toxin; that is, removing and bagging all clothing followed by washing or showering the victim extensively. Personnel irrigate the victim's eyes with water and apply topical analgesic, antibiotic, and lubricant.

Only one vesicant antidote is available, and it is effective only for lewisite. The antidote, known as dimercaprol, or British anti-lewisite (BAL), is most effective if given as soon as possible after exposure. It also can be used to treat heavy metal poisoning from arsenic, mercury, or gold.

Care for the skin lesions is similar to burn wound management (see Chap. 66). Damaged skin may take several months to heal and longer if the wound becomes infected. Breathing is supported with mechanical ventilation. Blood transfusions or administration of colony stimulating factors such as erythropoietin (Epogen, Procrit) and filgrastim (Neupogen) may be necessary if bone marrow function becomes suppressed.

▶ **Stop, Think, and Respond Exercise 15-3**

For which agent are the following antidotes used: amyl nitrite, atropine sulfate, and dimercaprol?

Nursing Process for the Client in a Disaster Situation

Nurses are just one group of healthcare providers involved in a disaster. Others include police; fire fighters; emergency medical technicians and paramedics; and local, state, and federal disaster workers under the direction of the American Red Cross, the Federal Emergency Management Agency (FEMA), and the Department of Health and Human Services. Many nurses are involved in triage activities as well as caring for victims in shelters or EDs.

Assessment

Assess as many victims as possible at the scene of the disaster to manage time efficiently and to avoid overwhelming valuable resources. Wear protective garments and start with the closest victim, working outward from there. Begin by assessing a victim's airway, breathing, and circulation. Cut off clothing in a sequence from head to foot. Logroll the client to examine the body's posterior surface. Following a head-to-toe examination, use one of four categories in the standard triage system to prioritize victims' needs for treatment: *immediate, delayed, minimal,* and *expectant* (Table 15-2). Ideally, tag the victims after assessing them to prevent duplication of assessments by another nurse or emergency worker (Fig. 15-4).

Diagnosis, Planning, and Interventions

▶ **PC:** Severe hypoxia, cardiogenic shock, hemorrhage, major trauma

▶ **Expected Outcome:** The nurse will manage and minimize life-threatening but survivable injuries.

• Provide comfort and emotional support to victims in an expectant triage category; reassess them again after managing those in the immediate triage category. Do not totally abandon victims in the expectant category; transport them for treatment when resources become available. *Victims who have injuries that are treatable are the priority for attention, but those who may soon die should not be neglected.*

• Administer first aid to victims in the immediate triage category by keeping the airway open, loosely covering an open chest wound, controlling bleeding, and splinting fractures; facilitate

TABLE 15-2 Triage Categories

CATEGORY	COLOR COORDINATE	DESCRIPTION	EXAMPLES
Immediate	Red	Life-threatening, but survivable if rapid medical attention is provided	Significant hemorrhage, pneumothorax, partial- or full-thickness burns of the face and neck
Delayed	Yellow	Serious, but stable enough to survive if treatment is delayed 6-8 hours	Penetrating abdominal wound, fractures, partial- or full-thickness burns not involving the head
Minimal	Green	Minor injuries that can wait longer for treatment	Minor lacerations, superficial burns, contusions
Expectant	Black	Soon to die; lack of spontaneous respirations after opening the airway	Head injury with a Glasgow Coma Score less than 8, multisystem trauma, partial- or full-thickness burns over 85% of body surface

Personal Property/
Evidence Tag

*Attach stub or seal inside
personal property
or evidence bag*

☐ Personal property
☐ Evidence tag

Dest _____

Patient Destination
and Transport Unit

*Remove this stub after arrival at
hospital and keep until attached
to patient care report*

Unit _____

PEEL AND STICK TO ◯ PATIENT CHART

RESPIRATIONS	**PERFUSION**	**MENTAL STATES**
R ☐ Yes ☐ No	P ☐ Pulse ☐ No	M ☐ Can Do ☐ Can't Do

Move ANYONE ambulatory	⇨ MINOR
No respiration after head tilt	⇨ DECEASED
Respirations <u>OVER</u> 30	⇨ IMMEDIATE
No radial pulse or capillary refill over 2 seconds	⇨ IMMEDIATE
Unable to follow simple commands	⇨ IMMEDIATE
Everyone else	⇨ DELAYED

☐S	☐L	☐U	☐D	☐G	☐E	☐M
Salivation	Lacrimation	Urination	Defecation	GI Distress	Emesis	Miosis

NAAK AUTO INJECTOR ☐1 ☐2 ☐3 ☐4 ☐5

☐ Dry decon
☐ Gross decon
☐ Technical decon
Decon solution _____

Circle
nature of
contaminant

☢ Chemical Agent

Vitals

Time	B/P	Pulse	Resp	O₂ Sat.

Medications

Time	Medication	Dose	Route

IV Location _____ Ga. _____ Solution: _____ Rate: _____

Airway adjunct: _____ Size: _____ Depth. _____

DECEASED

IMMEDIATE
LIFE THREATENING INJURIES

DELAYED
NON-LIFE THREATENING INJURIES

MINOR
MINOR INJURIES

UNINJURED
DOCUMENTED BY OFFICIAL

DISASTER TRIAGE TAG ◯

☐ Allergies _____

1. Abrasion
2. Amputation
3. Avulsion
4. Bleeding
5. Contusion
6. Puncture
7. Laceration
8. Pain
9. Deformity
10. Swelling
11. Other

Burn Reference
Head-9%   Child/Abd.
Arms-9% each   Front-10%
Legs-10% each   Rear-10%

Place related minor of guardian labels here.

VICTIM DEMOGRAPHICS

Sex   ☐ Information unavailable
☐ M
☐ F   Age _____ DOB _____ Wt. _____ ☐ Lb.
                                                    ☐ Kg.

Name _____

Address _____

City _____ St _____ Zip _____

Phone _____

SSN _____

Religion _____

Triage		Other
Treat		Other
Trans		Other

DECEASED

IMMEDIATE
LIFE THREATENING INJURIES

DELAYED
NON-LIFE THREATENING INJURIES

MINOR
MINOR INJURIES

UNINJURED
DOCUMENTED BY OFFICIAL

FIGURE 15-4 An example of a triage tag that identifies a person's category by color code and includes additional identifying information.

transport to a treatment facility. *Stabilizing a client in the immediate triage category helps facilitate a better outcome where more advanced medical services are available.*

- Direct victims with injuries that can withstand a delay in treatment for up to 10 hours to a separate waiting area. *Delaying treatment for stable victims helps to avoid overwhelming advanced treatment facilities needed for victims in critical condition.*
- Delegate the care of those with minimal health needs to volunteers with first aid skills. *Assistive personnel can manage victims with minor injuries with negligible consequences.*

▸ **Impaired Skin Integrity** related to prior or concurrent trauma or thermal or chemical burns as manifested by a disruption in epidermal and dermal tissue

▸ **Expected Outcome:** The client's skin will become intact.

- Cleanse the wound using Standard Precautions. *Cleansing reduces pathogens; Standard Precautions protect the nurse from contact with pathogens.*
- Apply a semiocclusive dressing over the wound. *A moist wound increases the rate of epithelialization.*

▶ Risk for Infection, Risk for Radiologic Contamination* related to possible exposure to a biologic agent or exposure to gamma radiation.

▶ Expected Outcome: Clients in the triage and treatment area will have their risk for infection reduced and their risk for internal radiologic contamination minimized.

- Restrict public access to clients who are nauseated, vomiting, or experiencing diarrhea. *Separating infected from uninfected people helps reduce spread of contamination.*
- When providing client care, wear personal protective equipment such as gloves, mask, gown, eye protection, or a self-contained respirator and vapor-protective suit, depending on the potential pathogen. *Personal protective equipment can prevent the transmission of an infectious agent to the nurse and others.*
- Double bag and dispose of all clothing and body waste in biohazard containers. *Confining sources of possible pathogens and radiologic contaminants reduces the potential for direct and indirect contact.*
- Have victims shower and change clothes; irrigate or wash open wounds with soap and water. *Cleansing the skin helps to reduce the transition from external to internal radiologic contamination.*
- Bandage any decontaminated wound with a sterile waterproof dressing. *A waterproof dressing acts as a barrier to the entrance of pathogens or external radiologic contaminants.*
- Administer a prescribed colony-stimulating agent such as filgastrim (Neupogen). *Exposure to high-dose gamma radiation suppresses bone-marrow production of white blood cells. Filgastrim promotes white blood cell production, making victims of radiologic contamination less susceptible to infections.*
- Immunize against smallpox or administer vaccinia immune-globulin if smallpox has been released. *A smallpox vaccination given early enough will prevent susceptible people from acquiring this infection. Vaccinia immune globulin provides passive immunity.*

▶ Ineffective Coping related to lack of information and fear of personal danger

▶ Expected Outcome: The client will cope effectively as evidenced by expressing emotions appropriately and cooperating with directives from disaster workers.

- Minimize panic by providing information on the type and extent of the disaster. *Coping effectively depends on acquiring accurate information to facilitate a realistic perception of the disaster.*
- Reassure the client that he or she will receive care and shelter. *Relieving insecurity facilitates a sense that the situation is under control.*
- Encourage the client to express feelings and concerns. *Verbalizing allows an opportunity for clarifying misperceptions, obtaining answers to questions, and putting fears in perspective.*
- Listen nonjudgmentally to the victim recount the horror that he or she has just experienced. *Convey that a victim is not atypical and feels similar to normal people who have lived through an abnormal event.*
- Reunite family members or provide information concerning their whereabouts and condition. *Family members are the strongest links to emotional support.*

Evaluation of Expected Outcomes

The nurse assesses triaged victims accurately and gives them appropriate treatment. The client's impaired skin is clean and covered with a dressing. Risks for infection and contamination are prevented or reduced. The client copes effectively with the physical and emotional trauma of having survived a disaster.

*Risk for Radiologic Contamination is not on the NANDA taxonomy list of nursing diagnoses at this time. ●

CRITICAL THINKING EXERCISES

1. Discuss why smallpox would be a particularly dangerous choice as a potentially lethal weapon of mass destruction.
2. Which triage category should the nurse assign to victims with the following assessment data?
   - Victim A is conscious; clothing is bloody; pulse is 110 and weak; respirations are 40 breaths per minute.
   - Victim B is alert and crying; an obvious deformity of the arm suggests a fracture; pulse and respirations are rapid but within normal range.
   - Victim C is unresponsive; respirations are 4 breaths per minute after opening the airway; gurgling is heard with each respiration.
   - Victim D is conscious and hysterical; there is evidence of abrasions on exposed skin; the person pleads to be transported in an emergency vehicle for further treatment.
3. Discuss why triage does not mean "first come, first served."
4. What are indications of a terrorist attempt, and what are the actions a victim should take when suspicious of such an attempt?

NCLEX-STYLE REVIEW QUESTIONS

1. Why does the nurse need to administer pralidoxime chloride to a victim of a nerve agent attack?
   1. To protect against effects of blistering agents
   2. To reactivate acetylcholinesterase
   3. To protect thyroid glands from radiation
   4. To provide antibiotic protection
2. An emergency department (ED) receives a report of an overturned truck that was transporting liquid chlorine. What preparation should the nursing staff make first for potential admissions to the ED?
   1. Contact the nursing supervisor for additional staff to care for multiple clients.
   2. Notify respiratory therapy staff of possible need for ventilatory support for affected clients.
   3. Call the physical therapist to initiate chest physical therapy for clients with breathing issues.
   4. Call the cardiac care physician on call to assess clients for heart damage.

3. When teaching a class about potential exposure to radiation, the nurse tells the students that it is important to minimize external contamination. Which actions best accomplish this? Select all that apply.
   1. Do not go to a shelter.
   2. Keep contaminated clothes nearby.
   3. Seal windows with plastic sheeting and duct tape.
   4. Stay indoors until danger has passed.
   5. Wash liberally with soap and water.

4. Because of the danger of widespread contagion and mortality if there is an outbreak of smallpox, which of the following nursing actions should be done first for a client suspected of having smallpox?
   1. Incinerating contaminated linens and clothing
   2. Placing client on strict and thorough isolation precautions.
   3. Reporting the suspicion to the local Public Health Department.
   4. Vaccinating family members and others in close contact with client.

5. In a disaster situation, nurses triage clients needing immediate attention as those who:
   1. Have a compound fracture of the left femur
   2. Have a significant head injury with low response level
   3. Have full-thickness burns on the face and neck
   4. Have multiple lacerations and superficial burns

UNIT 4
Caring for Clients with Multisystem Disorders

16

Caring for Clients with Fluid, Electrolyte, and Acid-Base Imbalances

Words To Know

acidosis
acids
active transport
alkalosis
anion gap
anions
baroreceptors
bases
bicarbonate–carbonic acid buffer system
cation
Chvostek's sign
circulatory overload
compensation
dehydration
dependent edema
electrolytes
extracellular fluid
facilitated diffusion
filtration
generalized edema
hemoconcentration
hemodilution
hypervolemia
hypovolemia
interstitial fluid
intracellular fluid
intravascular fluid
ions
natriuretic peptides
osmoreceptors
osmosis
passive diffusion
pitting edema
renin-angiotensin-aldosterone system
serum osmolality
skin tenting
third-spacing
Trousseau's sign

Learning Objectives

On completion of this chapter, you will be able to:

1. List three chemical substances that are components of body fluid.
2. Name the two main fluid locations in the human body and two subdivisions.
3. Give the average fluid intake per day for adults.
4. List four ways in which the body normally loses fluid.
5. Identify five processes by which water and dissolved chemicals are relocated in the body.
6. Name three mechanisms that help regulate fluid and electrolyte balance.
7. List two types of fluid imbalance.
8. Explain the difference between hypovolemia and dehydration.
9. Explain hemoconcentration and hemodilution.
10. Identify assessment findings of and nursing interventions for hypovolemia.
11. List and identify the differences in three types of edema.
12. Identify assessment findings of and nursing interventions for hypervolemia.
13. Explain third-spacing and medical techniques for relocating this fluid.
14. List factors that contribute to electrolyte loss and excess.
15. Name four electrolyte imbalances that pose a major threat to well-being.
16. Discuss the nursing management of clients with electrolyte imbalances.
17. Discuss the role of acids and bases in body fluid.
18. Explain pH and identify the normal range of plasma pH.
19. Identify two chemicals and two organs that play major roles in regulating acid-base balance.
20. Give the names of two major acid-base imbalances and subdivisions of each.
21. List three components of arterial blood gas findings used to determine acid-base imbalances.
22. Discuss the nursing management of clients with acid-base imbalances.

Body fluids consist of water and chemicals, including electrolytes, acids, and bases. **Electrolytes** are substances that carry an electrical charge when dissolved in fluid. **Acids** are substances that release hydrogen into fluid, and **bases** are substances that bind with hydrogen. The delicate balance of fluids, electrolytes, acids, and bases is ensured by an adequate intake of water and nutrients, physiologic mechanisms that regulate fluid volume, and chemical processes that buffer the blood to keep its pH nearly neutral. This chapter discusses fluid, electrolyte, and acid-base balance and the disorders that occur when there are imbalances.

FLUID AND ELECTROLYTE BALANCE

Body Fluid Compartments

About 60% of the adult human body is water. Put another way, for every 100 lb of body weight, approximately 60 lb is water. Most body water is located within cells (**intracellular fluid**). The rest is outside cells (**extracellular fluid**). Extracellular fluid includes the water between cells (**interstitial fluid**) and in the plasma (serum) portion of blood (**intravascular fluid;** Fig. 16-1). The volume of fluid in each location varies with age and sex (Table 16-1).

Intake and Output

In healthy adults, oral fluid intake averages about 2500 mL/day; however, it can range between 1800 and 3000 mL/day, with a similar volume of fluid loss. A standard formula for calculating daily fluid intake is as follows (Mentes, 2004):

- 100 mL/kg for the first 10 kg of weight, plus
- 50 mL/kg for the next 10 kg of weight, plus
- 15 mL/kg per remaining kilograms of weight

The primary sources of body fluid are food and liquids. As fluid volume increases, the body loses fluid, primarily through urination, in a proportionate volume to maintain or restore equilibrium. Other mechanisms of fluid loss include bowel elimination, perspiration, and breathing. Losses from sweat and the vapor in exhaled air are referred to as *insensible*

losses because they are, for practical purposes, unnoticeable and unmeasurable (Fig. 16-2).

▶ **Stop, Think, and Respond Exercise 16-1**
Using the formula for calculating fluid intake requirements according to weight, how much oral fluid per day is considered adequate for a client who weighs 176 lb?

Distribution of Fluids and Electrolytes

Translocation (movement back and forth) of fluid and exchange of chemicals—including electrolytes, acids, and bases—is continuous in and among all areas where water is located. Physiologic processes govern the movement and relocation of fluids and chemicals at the cellular level. These processes include osmosis, filtration, passive and facilitated diffusion, and active transport.

Osmosis

Osmosis is the movement of water through a *semipermeable membrane,* one that allows some but not all substances in a solution to pass through, from a dilute area to a more concentrated area. *Tonicity* refers, in this case, to the quantity (concentration) of substances dissolved in the water. The power to draw water toward an area of greater concentration is referred to as *osmotic pressure. Colloids,* large-sized substances such as serum proteins (e.g., albumin, globulin, fibrinogen) and blood cells, do not readily pass through cell and tissue membranes. They contribute to fluid concentration and act as a force for attracting water—a property referred to as *colloidal osmotic pressure.*

Fluid distribution through osmosis occurs in the following ways. If the solute concentration is higher in the cell, water is drawn through the membrane into the cell from the interstitial space. The process continues until the concentration is the same (*isotonic*) on both sides of the membrane. The reverse also is true: if the solute concentration is higher in the interstitial space, water is pulled into the interstitial space from the cell (Fig. 16-3).

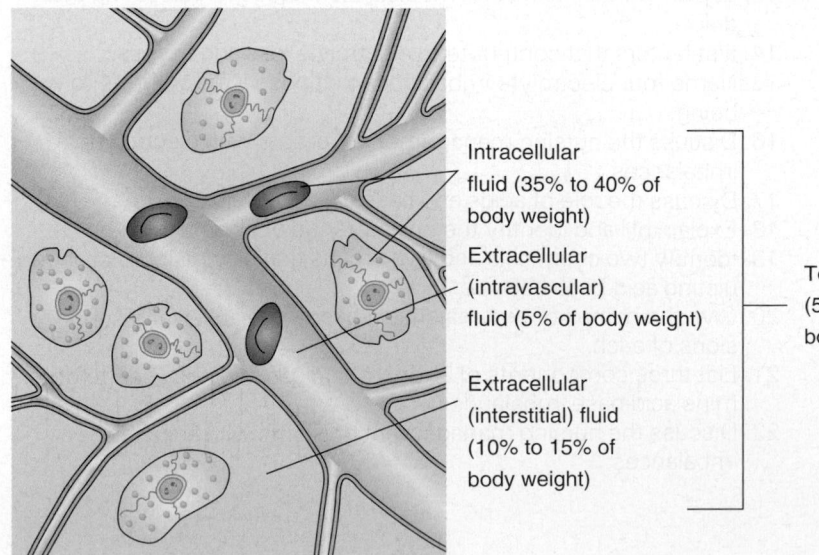

Intracellular fluid (35% to 40% of body weight)

Extracellular (intravascular) fluid (5% of body weight)

Extracellular (interstitial) fluid (10% to 15% of body weight)

Total body fluid (50% to 60% of body weight)

FIGURE 16-1. Distribution of body fluid at the cellular level. Total body fluid represents 50% to 60% of body weight in an average adult. Location of body fluid at the cellular level.

TABLE 16-1 Percentages of Body Fluid According to Age and Sex

FLUID COMPARTMENT	INFANTS	MALE ADULTS	FEMALE ADULTS	OLDER ADULTS
Intravascular	4%	4%	5%	5%
Interstitial	25%	11%	10%	15%
Intracellular	48%	45%	35%	25%
Total	77%	60%	50%	45%

Filtration

Filtration promotes the movement of fluid and some dissolved substances through a semipermeable membrane according to pressure differences. It relocates water and chemicals from an area of high pressure to an area of lower pressure. For example, fluid is under higher pressure at the arterial end than at the venous end of capillaries. Filtration causes the fluid and some dissolved substances (e.g., oxygen) to move into the interstitial space. Most of the water is then reabsorbed at the venous end of the capillaries by colloidal osmotic pressure (Fig. 16-4). Filtration also affects how the kidneys excrete fluid and wastes and then selectively reabsorb water and other chemicals that need to be conserved. The kidneys filter about 180 L of fluid from the blood each day; all but 1 to 1.5 L is reabsorbed.

Diffusion

Passive diffusion is a physiologic process by which dissolved substances (e.g., electrolytes) move from an area of high concentration to an area of lower concentration through a semipermeable membrane. Passive diffusion, like osmosis, remains fairly static (unchanged) once equilibrium occurs. In **facilitated diffusion**, certain dissolved substances require assistance from a carrier molecule to pass through a semipermeable membrane. For example, the carrier substance insulin facilitates the distribution of glucose molecules inside cells.

Active Transport

Active transport requires an energy source, a substance called *adenosine triphosphate* (ATP), to drive dissolved chemicals from an area of low concentration to an area of higher concentration—the opposite of passive diffusion. An example of active transport is the sodium-potassium pump system. Its function is to move potassium from lower concentrations in the extracellular fluid into cells where potassium is highly concentrated. The pump also moves sodium, which is in lower amounts in the cells, to extracellular fluid, where it is more abundant (Fig. 16-5). Metabolic disorders that diminish ATP, such as hypoxia, seriously affect normal cellular functions by impairing the distribution of chemicals in intracellular and extracellular fluid. Any significant change in fluid volume or its distribution can disrupt normal body functioning.

> ▶ **Stop, Think, and Respond Exercise 16-2**
>
> *If a client takes an oral potassium supplement or receives potassium in an intravenous solution, for example 20 mEq in 1000 mL of solution, which physiologic process relocates the potassium within cells?*

Mechanisms of Fluid and Electrolyte Regulation

Under normal conditions, several mechanisms maintain normal fluid volume and electrolyte concentrations. They include those promoted by osmoreceptors (i.e., the release or inhibition of antidiuretic hormone [ADH]), the renin-angiotensin-aldosterone system, and the secretion of atrial natriuretic peptide (ANP).

Osmoreceptors

Fluid volume is regulated primarily by the excretion of water in the form of urine and the promotion of thirst. These processes are in turn regulated in the hypothalamus by **osmoreceptors**, specialized neurons that sense the **serum osmolality**, or concentration of substances, in blood. When the blood becomes overly concentrated, osmoreceptors stimulate the hypothalamus to synthesize ADH, released by the

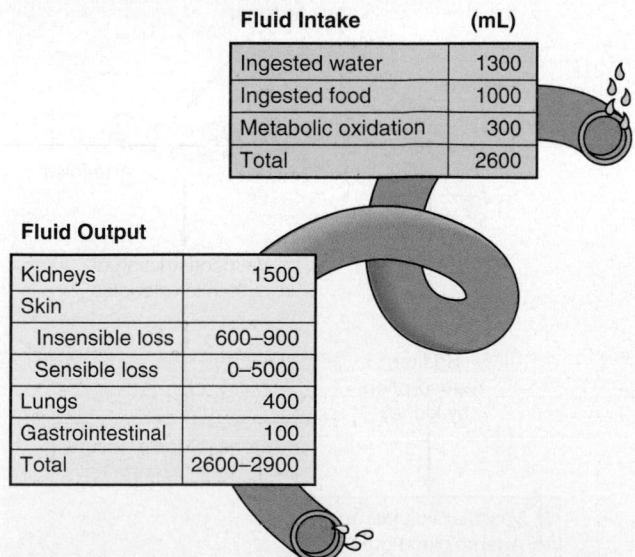

Fluid Intake	(mL)
Ingested water	1300
Ingested food	1000
Metabolic oxidation	300
Total	2600

Fluid Output

Kidneys	1500
Skin	
Insensible loss	600–900
Sensible loss	0–5000
Lungs	400
Gastrointestinal	100
Total	2600–2900

FIGURE 16-2. In the healthy person, fluid intake and output are about equal. The amounts indicated are average daily fluid sources and losses.

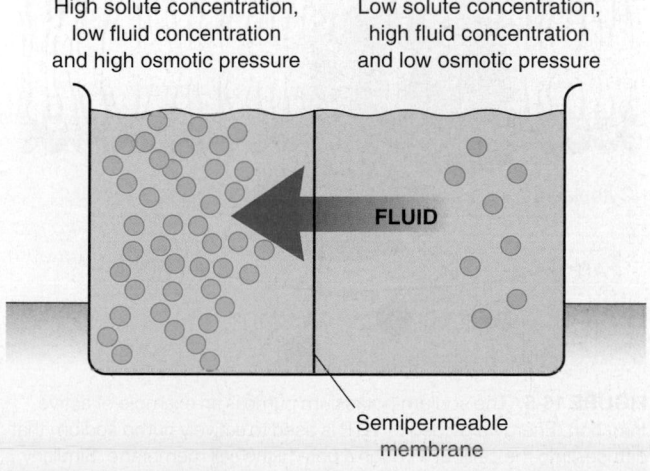

High solute concentration, low fluid concentration and high osmotic pressure

Low solute concentration, high fluid concentration and low osmotic pressure

FLUID

Semipermeable membrane

FIGURE 16-3. Osmosis.

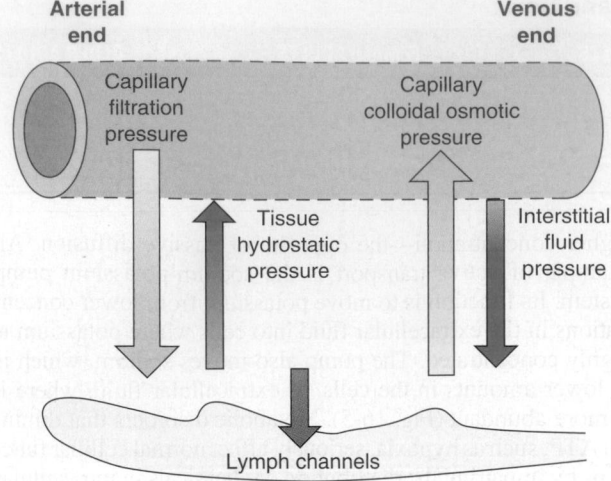

FIGURE 16-4. Fluid exchange at the capillary level.

posterior lobe of the pituitary gland. Release of ADH inhibits urine formation by increasing reabsorption of water from the distal and collecting tubules in the nephrons of the kidneys. The reabsorbed water restores normal serum osmolality, increases circulating blood volume, improves cardiac output, and maintains blood pressure (BP).

Osmoreceptors also are sensitive to changes in blood volume and BP through information relayed by baroreceptors. **Baroreceptors** are stretch receptors in the aortic arch and carotid sinus that signal the brain to release ADH when blood volume decreases by 10%, systolic BP falls below 90 mm Hg, or the right atrium is underfilled (National Heart, Lung, and Blood Institute, 2006; Veijo & Nicolaus, 1999). They signal the brain to suppress ADH when blood volume increases, systolic BP rises, or the right atrium is overfilled.

Osmoreceptors also trigger thirst, a mechanism that promotes increased intake of oral fluid. A person senses thirst when

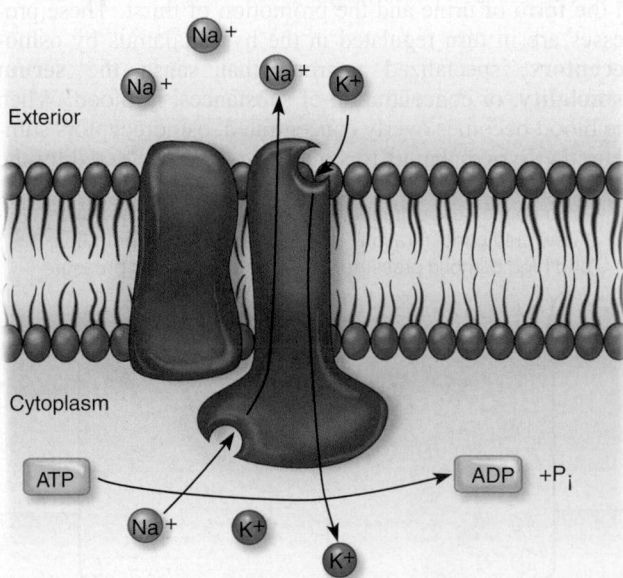

FIGURE 16-5. The sodium-potassium pump is an example of active transport. Energy provided by ATP is used to actively pump sodium that diffuses into the cell out through a pore in the cell membrane. Similarly, the pump actively replaces potassium that diffuses from the cell.

extracellular volume decreases by approximately 700 mL, an amount that equals about 2% of body weight (Edwards, 2001).

Renin-Angiotensin-Aldosterone System

The **renin-angiotensin-aldosterone system** is a chain of chemicals released to increase both BP and blood volume. It is triggered by the *juxtaglomerular apparatus,* a ring of pressure-sensing cells that surround the arterioles leading to each glomerulus in the kidneys. When the volume of arterial blood supplying the glomeruli is reduced, the juxtaglomerular cells release renin. Renin begins the transformation of angiotensinogen to angiotensin I to angiotensin II. Angiotensin II causes vasoconstriction and raises BP; it also stimulates release of aldosterone from the adrenal cortex. Aldosterone causes the kidneys to reabsorb sodium, which in turn increases blood volume and BP (Fig. 16-6).

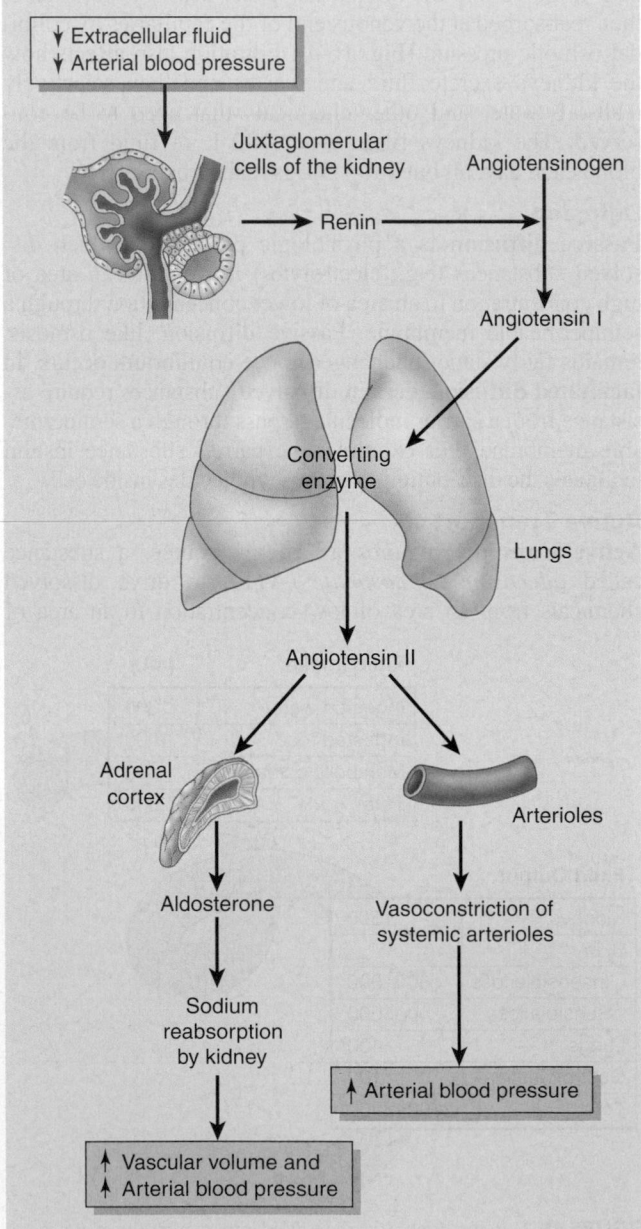

FIGURE 16-6. Control of blood pressure by the renin-angiotensin-aldosterone system.

Natriuretic Peptides

Natriuretic peptides are hormone-like substances that act in opposition to the renin-angiotensin-aldosterone system (Hill, 2002). Currently, three natriuretic peptides have been identified: (1) atrial natriuretic peptide (ANP), produced by the heart's atrial muscle; (2) brain natriuretic peptide (BNP), synthesized in the ventricles of the heart, despite originally being attributed to the brain; and (3) C-type natriuretic peptide (CNP), which actually is made in the brain. ANP and BNP are released in response to overstretching of the atrial and ventricular walls. They reduce blood volume by inhibiting the release of renin, aldosterone, and ADH. Consequently, urine production increases due to excretion of sodium in urine (see Chap. 28).

FLUID IMBALANCES

Fluid imbalance is a general term describing any of several conditions in which the body's water is not in the proper volume or location. Common fluid imbalances include hypovolemia, hypervolemia, and third-spacing.

HYPOVOLEMIA

Hypovolemia (fluid volume deficit) refers to a low volume of extracellular fluid. Dissolved chemical substances, such as electrolytes, are usually similarly depleted. Clients at risk for hypovolemia include those who are lethargic, depressed, or vomiting; have dementia, a fever, difficulty swallowing, or diarrhea; cannot speak to communicate their needs; eat poorly (i.e., less than 50% of their food); require assistance to drink because of weakness, paralysis, or limited range of motion; take diuretics, laxatives, or drugs that inhibit cell hydration (e.g., drugs with anticholinergic properties); or receive tube feedings without additional instillations of water.

Dehydration results when the volume of body fluid is significantly reduced in both extracellular and intracellular compartments. In dehydration, all fluid compartments have decreased volumes; in hypovolemia, only blood volume is low.

Gerontologic Considerations

- The most common fluid imbalance in older adults is dehydration. Because of reduced thirst sensation that often accompanies aging, older adults tend to drink less water. Use of diuretic medications, laxatives, or enemas may also deplete fluid volume in older adults. Chronic fluid volume deficit can lead to other problems, such as electrolyte imbalances.

Pathophysiology and Etiology

Factors that contribute to hypovolemia include inadequate fluid intake; fluid loss in excess of fluid intake such as with hemorrhage, prolonged vomiting or diarrhea, wound loss (as with burn injury), or profuse urination or perspiration; and translocation of fluid to compartments where it is trapped, such as the abdominal cavity or interstitial spaces (e.g., third-spacing). When circulatory volume is decreased, blood pressure falls and the heart compensates by increasing the heart rate to maintain adequate cardiac output (see Chap. 22). BP falls with postural changes, or it may become severely lowered when blood is rapidly lost. **Hemoconcentration**, a high ratio of blood components in relation to watery plasma, increases the potential for blood clots and urinary stones and compromises the kidney's ability to excrete nitrogen wastes. Hypovolemia eventually depletes intracellular fluid, which can affect cellular functions. One example is the change in mentation that usually occurs.

Assessment Findings

One of the earliest symptoms of hypovolemia is thirst. Other signs and symptoms are listed in Table 16-2. Evidence of

TABLE 16-2 Signs and Symptoms of Fluid Volume Deficit and Excess

ASSESSMENT	FLUID DEFICIT	FLUID EXCESS
Weight	Weight loss ≥2 lb/24 hr	Weight gain ≥2 lb/24 hr
Blood pressure	Low	High
Temperature	Elevated	Normal
Pulse	Rapid, weak, thready	Full, bounding
Respirations	Rapid, shallow	Moist, labored
Urine	Scant, dark yellow	Light yellow
Stool	Dry, small volume	Bulky
Skin	Warm, flushed, dry	Cool, pale, moist
Skin turgor	Poor, tents	Pitting & dependent edema
Mucous membranes	Dry, sticky	Moist
Eyes	Sunken	Swollen
Lungs	Clear	Crackles, gurgles
Breathing	Effortless	Dyspnea, orthopnea
Energy	Weak	Fatigues easily
Jugular neck veins	Flat	Distended
Cognition	Reduced	Reduced
Mental state	Sleepy	Anxious

hemoconcentration is reflected in elevated hematocrit level and blood cell counts, a consequence of water deficiency. Urine specific gravity is high. Serum electrolyte levels tend to remain normal because they are depleted in proportion to the water loss (Porth, 2007). Central venous pressure (CVP; see Chap. 29) is below 2 to 3 mm Hg.

Medical Management

Fluid deficit is restored by treating its etiology, increasing the volume of oral intake, administering intravenous (IV) replacing fluids (see Chap. 13), and controlling fluid losses.

Nursing Management

The nurse gathers assessment data that provide evidence of fluid status (Nursing Care Plan 16-1). If they reflect a fluid deficit, he or she plans measures to restore fluid balance (Nursing Guidelines 16-1) and evaluates the outcomes of interventions. In addition, the nurse teaches clients who have a potential for hypovolemia and their families to:

- Respond to thirst because it is an early indication of reduced fluid volume.
- Consume at least 8 to 10 (8 ounce) glasses of fluid each day, and more during hot, humid weather.
- Drink water as an inexpensive means to meet fluid requirements.
- Avoid beverages with alcohol and caffeine, because they increase urination and contribute to fluid deficits.
- Do not restrict salt or sodium intake.
- Rise slowly from a sitting or lying position to avoid dizziness and potential injury.

Gerontologic Considerations

- Because aging causes skin to lose elasticity, assessing skin turgor may be ineffective to detect fluid volume deficit in older adults. If assessing skin turgor in older clients, use the skin of the forehead or sternum.

HYPERVOLEMIA

Hypervolemia (fluid volume excess) means there is a high volume of water in the intravascular fluid compartment.

Pathophysiology and Etiology

Hypervolemia is caused by fluid intake that exceeds fluid loss, such as from excessive oral intake or rapid IV infusion of fluid. It also is a consequence of heart failure (see Chap. 28) when the heart cannot adequately distribute fluid to the kidneys for filtration. It also can result from inadequate fluid elimination, as may accompany kidney disease (see Chap. 58). Fluid retention (reduced fluid loss) also can occur secondary to excessive salt intake (sodium chloride), adrenal gland dysfunction (see Chap. 50), or administration of corticosteroid drugs such as prednisolone (Delta-Cortef).

Clients at risk for hypervolemia include those who:

- Have altered cardiac or kidney function.
- Have increased ADH production, which sometimes accompanies brain trauma.
- Are receiving corticosteroid therapy, large rapid volumes of IV fluid, or IV colloid solutions (e.g., albumin).
- Consume oral fluids to excess, such as clients with schizophrenia who can develop water intoxication.
- Ingest highly salted food or foods that contain large amounts of sodium.

Hypervolemia can lead to **circulatory overload**, a fluid volume that exceeds what is normal for the intravascular space and can potentially compromise cardiopulmonary function. The excess volume raises BP and causes the heart to increase its force of contraction.

Assessment Findings

Signs and Symptoms

Early signs of hypervolemia (see Table 16-2) are weight gain, elevated BP, and increased breathing effort. As the excess fluid volume is distributed to the interstitial space, **pitting edema**, indentations in the skin after compression, may be noted (see Fig. 16-7). Pitting edema usually does not occur, however, until there is a 3-L excess in the intravascular volume. There may be evidence of **dependent edema** (edema in body areas most affected by gravity, such as the feet, ankles, sacrum, or buttocks) in clients confined to bed. Rings, shoes, and stockings may leave marks in the skin. The jugular neck veins may appear prominent when the client sits. Eventually, fluid congestion in the lungs leads to moist breath sounds.

Diagnostic Findings

The blood cell count and hematocrit level are low as the result of **hemodilution**, a reduced ratio of blood components to watery plasma. Urine specific gravity is also low, reflecting the larger proportion of water. CVP is elevated above its normal range of 2 to 6 mm Hg.

Medical Management

The condition causing the fluid excess is treated. Oral and parenteral fluid intake is restricted. Diuretics, drugs that promote urinary excretion, are prescribed. Salt and sodium intake is limited.

Nursing Process for the Client With Hypervolemia

Assessment

Obtain baseline weight and weigh the client daily thereafter on the same scale and at the same time before breakfast, in similar clothing. A 2-lb weight gain in 24 hours indicates that the client is retaining 1L of fluid. Maintain accurate intake and output records, and report significant differences in the two measurements. Auscultate the lungs to detect abnormal breath sounds. Determine if an S_3 heart sound is present and inspect the neck veins to assess for distention (see Chap 22). Measure BP, heart rate, and respiratory rate regularly. Note the client's activity tolerance. To detect pitting edema, gently press the skin over a bony area, such as the tibia or

NURSING CARE PLAN 16-1 | **The Client With Hypovolemia**

Assessment

- Look for gross sources of fluid loss: vomiting, diarrhea, bleeding, wound drainage, GI suctioning, and diaphoresis.
- Weigh client daily at the same time, on the same scale, and dressed similarly. Report a loss of 2 lb (1 kg) or more in 24 hours (a 2-lb loss equals 1 L of body fluid).
- Note medications. Daily diuretic therapy or chronic laxative use may promote excess fluid losses.
- Record vital signs regularly; the frequency depends on client's acuity level. Check for postural hypotension (a drop in systolic pressure of 15 mm Hg immediately after client rises from a sitting or recumbent position). Increased insensible losses may cause or result from elevated body temperature.
- Ask if client is thirsty.
- Examine skin for dryness. Assess turgor (elasticity) by lifting the skin over the sternum, inner thigh, or forehead each shift.

- Skin tenting, skin that remains elevated and is slow to return to underlying tissue, indicates dehydration.
- Observe the tongue for furrowing (linear lines), and look for dry oral mucous membranes.
- Determine cognition by performing a Mini-Mental Status Examination (see Chap. 67).
- Examine urine. Urine that is dark yellow, has a strong odor, or has a specific gravity of 1.020 or more indicates low fluid volume.
- Monitor blood test results for hemoconcentration (high hematocrit level and blood cell counts).
- Keep a daily record of fluid intake and output. Report output that is less than 500 mL per 24 hours or less than 50 mL if measuring hourly volumes.
- Observe if client has the strength, ability to swallow, and mental capacity to drink fluid without assistance.

Nursing Diagnosis: Deficient Fluid Volume related to fluid loss greater than intake as manifested by vomiting and diarrhea secondary to gastroenteritis, oral intake of 500 mL, fluid loss of 1700 mL in previous 24 hours, concentrated urine, postural hypotension, tachycardia, and dry mucous membranes

Expected Outcome: Client will have a fluid intake of at least 1500 mL per 24 hours and urine output within 500 mL of oral intake (i.e., at least 1000 mL per 24 hours).

Interventions	Rationales
Withhold solid food for 8 hours.	Solid food can irritate gastric mucosa.
Provide dilute mouthwash or weak salt water as an oral rinse after vomiting.	An oral rinse reduces the unpleasant aftertaste of emesis that may trigger additional vomiting.
Empty the emesis basin and change linens soiled with vomitus.	The sight and smell of emesis perpetuate the cycle of vomiting.
Encourage slow, deep breaths when the client experiences waves of nausea.	Breathing distracts the client from the nausea until the reversed peristaltic action passes.
Avoid jarring the bed or activities that require movement on the client's part.	The vestibular center in the ear is sensitive to movement of the head and can stimulate the vomiting center (as in motion sickness).
Administer prescribed antiemetics according to the physician's written orders.	Antiemetics may inhibit the vomiting center directly or help control vomiting by other mechanisms (e.g., slowing GI peristalsis).
Provide sips of liquids like weak tea, flat carbonated soft drinks, and water as often as the client can tolerate them.	Small volumes of fluids that are not strongly flavored or highly carbonated are less likely to cause nausea or distend the stomach.
Progress fluid selection to include gelatin, bouillion, Gatorade, or Pedialyte when the client can tolerate fluids identified earlier.	These products provide glucose, sodium, chloride, and other electrolytes.
Eliminate dairy products if the client is lactose intolerant.	Clients who do not produce lactase, the enzyme that aids in milk digestion, develop cramps and diarrhea when they consume dairy products.
Offer dry crackers or toast if the client retains fluids.	Solid foods in readily digestible carbohydrates are tolerated better than other types of food.
Administer prescribed antidiarrheals as medically ordered.	They reduce the frequency and consistency of watery stools by adsorbing excess liquid from and soothing the bowel and slowing bowel motility.
Increase to a low-residue diet, starting with the BRAT (bananas, rice, applesauce, toast) diet when diarrhea is controlled.	Low-residue foods reduce stool bulk and slow GI transit time; the BRAT diet contains foods that are high in pectin, which helps make stools firm.

Evaluation of Expected Outcomes:

Intake is 1500 mL and output is 1750 mL, 500 mL of which is emesis. Episodes of vomiting and diarrhea are reduced. BP is stable at 110/68 mm Hg in both lying and sitting positions. Urine is medium yellow. Client is tolerating clear fluids, saltines, and dry white toast.

NURSING GUIDELINES 16-1

Managing Fluid Volume Deficit

- Inform client that he or she must increase consumption of oral fluids. Set a target goal for intake per hour, shift, and 24-hour period; a goal of 3000 to 4000 mL is not excessive for dehydrated clients. Schedule the bulk of fluid intake at meals and when the client is awake (i.e., more intake during daytime than throughout the night).
- Offer at least 180 mL of fluid when administering oral medications.
- Implement a "sip 'n go" plan by which anyone entering the room offers the client at least 60 mL of fluid (Mentes, 2004).
- Obtain a list of fluids the client prefers; include gelatin, popsicles, ice cream, and sherbet if they are allowed.
- Provide various liquids, replace with a fresh supply periodically, and ensure they are an appropriate temperature.

- Modify fluid containers to accommodate for client's strength and physical skills (e.g., cups with handles, covered cups with an opening for the mouth or insertion of a straw).
- Offer small volumes frequently, rather than expecting the client to consume a large volume at once.
- Thicken watery fluid with a commercial thickener if the client has difficulty swallowing.
- Relieve nausea, vomiting, mouth discomfort, and other problems that interfere with drinking.
- Ensure that clients prone to low fluid volume have fasting tests done expeditiously to reduce the time they are without food or fluids.
- Evaluate goals by recollecting assessment data and analyzing trends, especially in intake and output totals. Report results to the physician, especially if collaborative efforts fall short.

1+ Pitting Edema

- Slight indentation (2 mm)
- Normal contours
- Associated with interstitial fluid volume 30% above normal

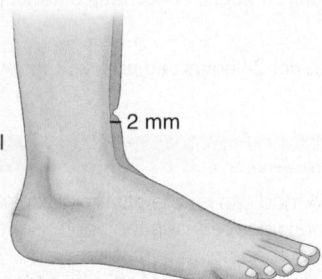

2+ Pitting Edema

- Deeper pit after pressing (4 mm)
- Lasts longer than 1+
- Fairly normal contour

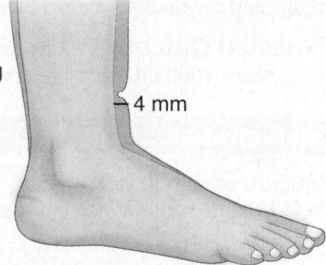

3+ Pitting Edema

- Deep pit (6 mm)
- Remains several seconds after pressing
- Skin swelling obvious by general inspection

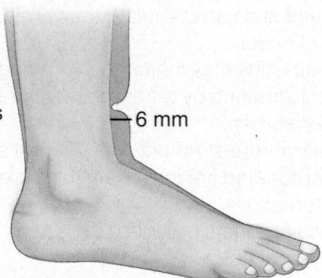

4+ Pitting Edema

- Deep pit (8 mm)
- Remains for a prolonged time after pressing, possibly minutes
- Frank swelling

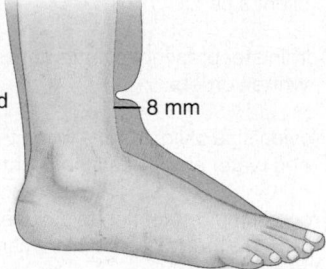

Brawny Edema

- Fluid can no longer be displaced secondary to excessive interstitial fluid accumulation
- No pitting
- Tissue palpates as firm or hard
- Skin surface shiny, warm, moist

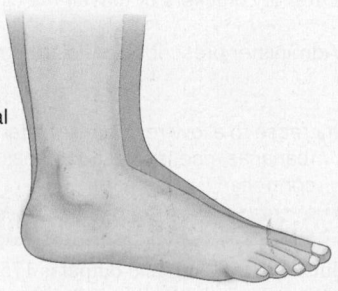

FIGURE 16-7. Grading edema is somewhat subjective; assessment findings may vary depending on the clinician. These criteria are offered to assist in documentation.

dorsum of the foot, for up to 5 seconds and observe the results (see Fig. 16-7). Inspect edematous skin for cracks and breakdown.

Diagnosis, Planning, and Interventions

Implement prescribed interventions such as limiting sodium and water intake and administering ordered medications that promote fluid elimination. Elevating the client's head can relieve labored breathing. Take measures to prevent skin breakdown in cases of peripheral edema. Reassessment is necessary to determine if planned interventions have restored fluid volume balance.

Also perform necessary teaching with the client and family. Show common containers and indicate the volume that each holds. Instruct clients to avoid foods that are high in salt or sodium (Box 16-1). Teach how to read food labels and look for the words *salt, sodium,* and other sources of sodium such as baking soda or baking powder. Provide information concerning diuretic drug therapy. List ways to determine if fluid excess is recurring or has resolved.

▶ **Excess Fluid Volume** related to intake that exceeds fluid loss (or reduced fluid loss in relation to intake)

▶ **Expected Outcome:** Fluid status will return to normal, as evidenced by weight loss, reduced edema, BP within normal limits, and urine output of at least 2000 mL/day.

- Assess vital signs, daily weight, intake and output, breath sounds, and location and extent of edema as often as necessary. *Focused assessments help determine if interventions are reducing or eliminating the problem.*
- Use guidelines established by the physician for restricting oral fluid. *Limiting fluid intake helps reduce the volume absorbed into the vascular system.*
- Develop a plan with the client for distributing the allotted oral volume over 24 hours. *Involving the client in care promotes compliance and demonstrates that healthcare professionals value and respect the client's preferences.*
- Ration fluid so the client can consume approximately 20% to 25% at times other than meals (Mentes, 2004). *The client should be able to consume some fluid whenever thirsty; restricting fluids to meals only is inappropriate.*

BOX 16-1   Foods High in Salt or Sodium

- Processed meats (hot dogs and cold cuts)
- Most fast food choices
- Most frozen convenience meals
- Salted and smoked fish
- Cheeses, especially processed varieties
- Powdered cocoa and hot chocolate mixes
- Canned vegetables
- Foods preserved in brine (pickles, olives, sauerkraut)
- Tomato and tomato vegetable juices
- Canned soup and instant soups or bouillon
- Boxed casserole mixes
- Salted snack foods
- Seasonings: catsup, gravy mixes, soy sauce, monosodium glutamate (MSG), pickle relish, tartar sauce, mustard, horseradish, barbecue sauce, steak sauce

---

- Collaborate with the dietitian to modify the diet to meet salt/sodium restrictions and to avoid sweet or dry foods. *The higher the concentration of sodium (salt) in the blood, the greater the serum osmolality, with a proportionate increase in fluid volume. Sweet or dry food increases a client's desire to consume fluid.*
- Administer prescribed diuretics. *They promote sodium excretion and water elimination.*
- Prepare client and assist with medical interventions such as dialysis (see Chap. 58). *Dialysis uses principles of osmosis and filtration to promote fluid elimination from the blood.*

▶ **Altered Comfort: Dry Mouth and Thirst** related to restricted oral fluid

▶ **Expected Outcomes:** (1) Client's mouth will be moist despite fluid restrictions. (2) Client will state that thirst is tolerable.

- Provide supplies for frequent oral hygiene. *Keeping the mouth clean and moist reduces discomfort.*
- Substitute ice chips for oral liquids. *The volume of melted ice is half that of solid ice. Holding ice chips in the mouth gives the psychological impression of consuming more fluid. Because melting ice chips stay in the mouth longer than water, they promote the sensation that larger volumes are being ingested.*
- Instruct client to wet the mouth with a measured volume of fluid in a squeezable squirt bottle or spray atomizer. *Squirting or spraying water in the oral cavity moisturizes the surface of the oral mucous membranes with a small volume of fluid and reduces dryness and thirst.*

▶ **Risk for Impaired Skin Integrity** related to compromised circulation secondary to edema

▶ **Expected Outcome:** The client's skin will remain intact.

- Change client's position every 2 hours. *Doing so relieves pressure on capillaries. If capillary pressure falls below 32 mm Hg for more than 2 hours, the skin and underlying tissue are deprived of oxygenated blood, predisposing the client to cell death and skin breakdown.*
- Evaluate client's skin blanching at area of contact with bed or chair by applying light finger pressure. *Light finger pressure should cause brief blanching followed by prompt skin capillary refill. Prolonged blanching may indicate lack of sufficient blood pressure or circulatory volume; this finding may necessitate more frequent position changes than every 2 hours.*
- Keep client's legs elevated higher than the heart. *Doing so facilitates return of venous blood to the heart. Improved circulation reduces metabolic waste products and their toxic effects.*
- Encourage ambulation or isometric bed exercises within client's level of tolerance. *Activity increases respiratory and heart rates; muscle contraction promotes venous return to the heart. All these factors improve delivery of oxygenated blood to the skin and other body cells and removal of metabolic wastes.*
- Apply elastic stockings. *They support valves in the veins and prevent fluid from pooling in dependent areas like the feet and ankles.*

Evaluation of Expected Outcomes

Expected outcomes are a daily weight loss of approximately 1 lb, decreased edema from previous assessments, clear lungs, and unlabored respirations. Laboratory values for red blood cells, hematocrit, urine specific gravity, and electrolytes return to normal. Elevations in BP or heart rate resolve. Oral mucous membranes are moist, and the client reports that the distribution of oral fluids controls thirst within a tolerable level. The client shows no evidence of skin breakdown, with reduced or eliminated edema. The toes and feet are warm. Blood returns to the nailbed within 2 to 3 seconds after release of the compressed area. ●

THIRD-SPACING

Third-spacing describes the translocation of fluid from the intravascular or intercellular space to tissue compartments, where it becomes trapped and useless. It is associated with the loss of colloids, as may accompany *hypoalbuminemia* (low level of albumin in the blood) or burns, and severe allergic reactions that alter capillary and cellular membrane permeability. Fluid translocation follows the shift in osmotic pressure to other locations. If the translocation depletes fluid volume in the intravascular area, it can lead to hypotension, shock, and circulatory failure (see Chap. 17).

Assessment Findings

The client manifests signs and symptoms of hypovolemia with the exception of weight loss. Fluid volume remains relatively unchanged, but the percentages in various locations are altered. There may be signs of localized enlargement of organ cavities (such as the abdomen) if they fill with fluid, a condition referred to as *ascites* (see Chap. 47). There may be **generalized edema** in all the interstitial spaces, which sometimes is called *brawny edema* or *anasarca* (see Fig. 16-7). Results of laboratory blood tests and urine specific gravity are borderline normal or reveal evidence of hemoconcentration. CVP is below normal, as are other hemodynamic measurements (pressure as it relates to intravascular volume; see Chap. 29).

Medical Management

The medical priority is to restore circulatory volume in clients with hypotension and eliminate the trapped fluid. This is done by administering IV solutions—sometimes at rapid rates—and blood products, such as albumin, to restore colloidal osmotic pressure. Administration of albumin pulls the trapped fluid back into the intravascular space. When this occurs, clients who were previously hypovolemic can suddenly become hypervolemic. An IV diuretic may be ordered to reduce the potential for circulatory overload.

Nursing Management

Nursing care combines the assessment techniques for detecting both hypovolemia and hypervolemia. Policies and practices vary concerning how much responsibility LPN/LVNs may assume with regard to IV fluid therapy and administration of IV medications (see Chap. 13).

ELECTROLYTE IMBALANCES

Electrolytes are in both intracellular and extracellular water. They include **ions**, positively and negatively charged particles, such as potassium, magnesium, sodium, phosphate, sulfate, calcium, chloride, bicarbonate, protein, and organic acids. Sodium, calcium, and chloride ion concentrations are higher in extracellular fluid, whereas potassium, magnesium, and phosphate concentrations are higher in the cells. These differences are responsible for electrical potentials that develop across cell membranes and perhaps for the degree of cell membrane permeability.

Electrolyte imbalances occur when there is a deficit or an excess of electrolytes or when electrolytes are translocated to any one or more fluid compartments. A loss or gain in fluid usually is accompanied by a similar change in electrolytes. Electrolyte imbalances are identified primarily by measuring their levels in the serum (watery portion of blood).

Electrolyte deficits sometimes result from inadequate intake of food that provides their natural source. Other causes include administering IV solutions that contain none, or only some, needed electrolytes and conditions that deplete water and substances dissolved therein (e.g., vomiting, diarrhea). Administration of certain medications (e.g., diuretics) also depletes electrolytes.

Factors that contribute to excess electrolytes include an overabundance of orally consumed or parenterally administered electrolytes, kidney failure, and endocrine (glandular) dysfunction, especially of the pituitary gland or adrenal cortex. Electrolytes move from within cells into serum when cell membranes are damaged, such as in crushing injuries or burns. Sodium, potassium, calcium, and magnesium deficits or excesses are of particular concern.

 Gerontologic Considerations

- Several factors can lead to fluid and electrolyte imbalances in older adults. Decreased renal function in older adults can cause an inability to concentrate urine. Enema use can also potentially cause fluid and electrolyte imbalance. Laxatives draw fluid into the intestine and may cause fluid depletion if not administered with water. A poor appetite, erratic meal patterns, inability to prepare nutritious meals, or financial circumstances may influence nutritional status, resulting in fluid and electrolyte imbalances.

SODIUM IMBALANCES

Sodium (Na^+), the chief **cation** (positively charged electrolyte) in extracellular fluid, is essential for maintaining normal nerve and muscle activity, regulating osmotic pressure, and preserving acid-base balance. The principal role of sodium is to regulate and distribute fluid volume in the body. Normal concentration ranges from 135 to 145 mEq/L. Lower than normal serum sodium level is *hyponatremia;* higher than normal serum sodium level is *hypernatremia.*

Hyponatremia

Causes of hyponatremia include profuse diaphoresis, excessive ingestion of plain water or administration of nonelectrolyte IV fluids, profuse diuresis, loss of GI secretions (e.g., in prolonged vomiting, GI suctioning, draining fistulas), and Addison's disease (see Chap. 50).

Manifestations include mental confusion, muscular weakness, anorexia, restlessness, elevated body temperature, tachycardia, nausea, vomiting, and personality changes. If the deficit is severe, symptoms are more intense, and convulsions or coma can occur. In such cases, the serum sodium level is below 135 mEq/L.

When possible, the underlying cause is corrected. Treatment of mild deficits includes oral administration of sodium (foods high in sodium, water to which salt has been added, and salt tablets). For severe deficits, administration of IV solutions containing sodium chloride (see Chap. 13) are prescribed.

Hypernatremia

Hypernatremia is excess sodium in the blood. Causes include profuse watery diarrhea, excessive salt intake without sufficient water intake, high fever, decreased water intake (e.g., in older adults, debilitated, unconscious, or developmentally delayed clients), excessive administration of solutions that contain sodium, excessive water loss without an accompanying loss of sodium, and severe burns.

Hypernatremia results in thirst; dry, sticky mucous membranes; decreased urine output; fever; a rough, dry tongue; and lethargy, which can progress to coma if the excess is severe. In such cases, the serum sodium level is above 145 mEq/L.

Treatment depends on the cause and includes oral administration of plain water or IV administration of a hypotonic solution, such as 0.45% sodium chloride or 5% dextrose (see Chap. 13). In mild cases, sodium intake may be restricted until laboratory test results are normal.

Gerontologic Considerations

- Older adults are at increased risk for hyponatremia related to the kidneys' inability to excrete water and the sluggish renin-angiotensin-aldosterone response. Hypernatremia is also common in older adults; it may be manifested as confusion. In addition, older adults should be taught that prolonged laxative use can lead to hypernatremia and hypermagnesemia (discussed later).

Nursing Management for Sodium Imbalances

Nursing management includes early detection, especially in clients at risk for hyponatremia or hypernatremia. The nurse apportions oral fluids according to target volumes, maintains accurate intake and output measurements, assesses vital signs every 1 to 4 hours, and closely monitors the infusion of IV fluids. He or she implements prescribed dietary restrictions or supplements (Nutrition Notes 16-1). The nurse gathers data that indicate increased or decreased symptoms and notifies the physician if symptoms worsen or laboratory values show a significant change.

Nutrition Notes 16-1
The Client with a Sodium Imbalance

● Under normal circumstances, the body maintains sodium balance over a wide range of intakes by regulating urinary sodium excretion.
● A rule of thumb guideline for determining if a food is high or low in sodium is to look at the % Daily Value (DV) on the Nutrition Facts label. If an item provides ≤ 5% of the DV for sodium, it is considered low in sodium. If it provides ≥ 20%, that food is high in sodium.
● Because salt and sodium compounds are used extensively in food processing and manufacturing, processed and convenience foods are estimated to account for 75% of the sodium in the average American diet. Naturally occurring sources of sodium (e.g., in milk, meats, certain vegetables) provide 10%. The remaining 15% comes from salt added during cooking and at the table.

Pharmacologic Considerations

- Drugs containing sodium, such as some antacids, laxatives, and NSAIDs containing sodium salicylate, are given cautiously to clients with edema, congestive heart failure, or renal dysfunction.

▶ **Stop, Think, and Respond Exercise 16-3**
Which sodium imbalance is likely in a client who manifests mental confusion, muscular weakness, anorexia, restlessness, elevated body temperature, tachycardia, nausea, vomiting, and personality changes?

POTASSIUM IMBALANCES

The potassium cation (K^+) is the chief electrolyte found in intracellular fluid. Potassium has the same functions intracellularly as sodium has extracellularly. A deficit of potassium in the blood is called *hypokalemia;* an excess is called *hyperkalemia.*

Hypokalemia

Potassium-wasting diuretics such as furosemide (Lasix), ethacrynic acid (Edecrin), hydrochlorothiazide (HydroDIURIL) contribute to hypokalemia. Loss of fluid from the GI tract (as with severe vomiting or diarrhea, draining intestinal fistulae, or prolonged suctioning) also causes potassium deficit. Large doses of corticosteroids, IV administration of insulin and glucose, and prolonged administration of nonelectrolyte parenteral fluids can deplete potassium.

Hypokalemia causes fatigue, weakness, anorexia, nausea, vomiting, cardiac dysrhythmias (abnormal heart rate or rhythm, especially in people receiving cardiac glycosides such as digitalis preparations), leg cramps, muscle weakness, and paresthesias (abnormal sensations). Severe cases result in hypotension, flaccid paralysis, and even death from cardiac or respiratory arrest. Hypokalemia produces characteristic changes in the electrocardiogram (ECG) waveform (Fig. 16-8). The serum potassium level is below 3.5 mEq/L. Symptoms may not develop, however, until the serum potassium level is below 3.0 mEq/L.

Treatment includes elimination of the cause (when possible). The physician may substitute a potassium-sparing diuretic such as spironolactone (Aldactone) for one that causes excretion of potassium. Mild hypokalemia is treated by increasing oral intake of potassium-rich foods or using a prescribed potassium oral replacement such as K-Lor, K-Lyte, or Klorvess. Severe hypokalemia is treated with IV administration of solutions containing a potassium salt, such as potassium chloride.

Hyperkalemia

Hyperkalemia can occur with severe renal failure, in which the kidneys cannot excrete potassium; severe burns; administration of potassium-sparing diuretics; overuse of potassium supplements, salt substitutes or some diet sodas (which contain potassium instead of sodium), or potassium-rich foods; crushing injuries; Addison's disease; and rapid administration of parenteral potassium salts.

Symptoms include diarrhea, nausea, muscle weakness, paresthesias, and cardiac dysrhythmias. The serum potassium level is above 5.5 mEq/L. Hyperkalemia also causes

unique changes in ECG waveforms (see Fig. 16-8C) that can forewarn of sudden cardiac death.

Treatment depends on the cause and severity. Mild hyperkalemia is treated by decreasing the intake of potassium-rich foods or discontinuing oral potassium replacement until laboratory values are normal. Severe hyperkalemia is treated by intravenously administering a combination of regular insulin and glucose that temporarily shifts serum potassium into cells within 30 minutes of administration (Garth, 2007). A slower-acting method of reducing an elevated serum potassium level is the oral or rectal administration of a cation-exchange resin such as sodium polystyrene sulfonate (Kayexalate). Peritoneal dialysis or hemodialysis, techniques for removing toxic substances from the blood, also may be used (see Chap. 58).

Nursing Management for Potassium Imbalances

The nurse assesses clients for conditions with the potential to cause potassium imbalances, identifies signs and symptoms associated with potassium imbalances, monitors laboratory findings measuring serum potassium, administers medications that restore potassium balance, and evaluates the client's response to medical therapy. He or she consults with the physician when a client is receiving prolonged IV fluid therapy without added potassium. If IV potassium is ordered, it must be diluted in an IV solution and administered at a

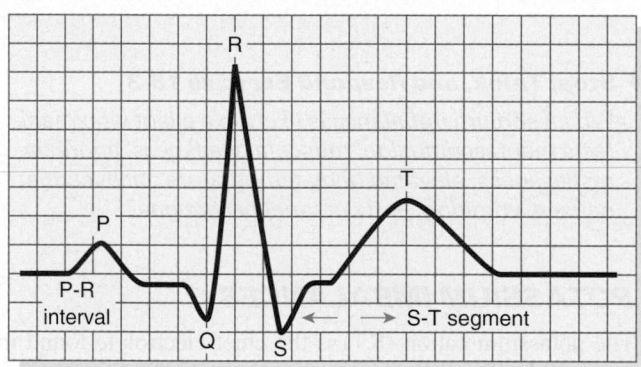

A

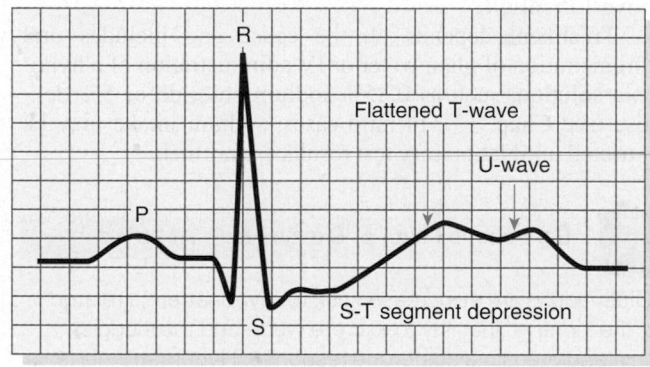

B

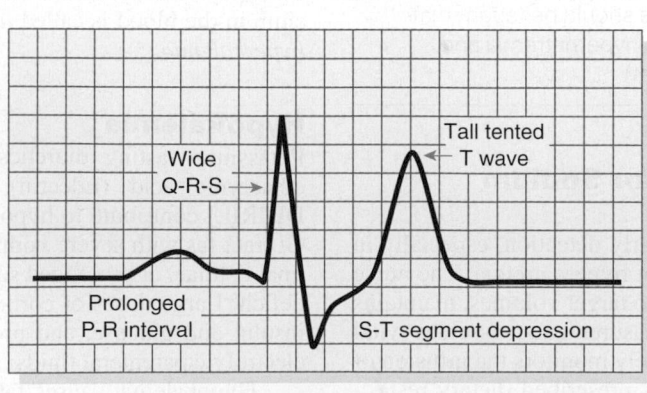

C

FIGURE 16-8. Effects of potassium on ECG. (**A**) Normal tracing. (**B**) Serum potassium level below normal (hypokalemia) results in ST segment depression, flattened T wave, and a U wave. (**C**) High potassium level (hyperkalemia) produces prolonged PR interval; widened QRS; ST segment depression; and a tall, peaked T wave. (From Porth, C. [2007]. *Essentials of pathophysiology: Concepts of altered health states.* Philadelphia: Lippincott Williams & Wilkins).

rate below 10 mEq/hour. The nurse observes the infusion frequently to verify it is being administered at the appropriate rate. He or she also informs clients at risk for potassium imbalances and their families about:

- Medications that cause urinary excretion of potassium, such as non-potassium-sparing diuretics
- Food sources of potassium: vegetables, dried peas and beans, wheat bran, bananas, oranges, orange juice, melon, prune juice, potatoes, and milk
- Taking oral potassium supplements shortly after meals or with food to avoid GI distress; effervescent tablets or liquids are taken with a full glass of water

 Pharmacologic Considerations

- Potassium should never be administered to a client with insufficient kidney function.

- Therapeutic doses of potassium are administered orally or are diluted in large volumes of intravenous fluid; they are *never* administered in a concentrated strength by IV. When given as an intravenous bolus, potassium depresses heart contraction, causing bradycardia (slow heart rate) and cardiac arrest.

- Clients may experience burning along the vein with IV infusion of potassium in proportion to the infusion's concentration. If the client can tolerate the fluid, consult with the physician about diluting the potassium in a larger volume of IV solution.

- In clients receiving a digitalis preparation, monitor closely for digitalis toxicity, which can accompany potassium and magnesium deficits.

CALCIUM IMBALANCES

Most of the body's calcium (Ca^{++}) is found in the bones and teeth. A small percentage (about 1%) is in the blood. The parathyroid glands regulate the serum calcium level. Calcium is necessary for blood clotting; smooth, skeletal, and cardiac muscle function; and transmission of nerve impulses. Vitamin D is needed for calcium absorption in the intestine. *Hypocalcemia* occurs when the serum calcium level is lower than normal; *hypercalcemia* occurs when the level is higher than normal.

Hypocalcemia

Causes of hypocalcemia include vitamin D deficiency, hypoparathyroidism, severe burns, acute pancreatitis, certain drugs such as corticosteroids, rapid administration of multiple units of blood that contain an anticalcium additive, intestinal malabsorption disorders, and accidental surgical removal of the parathyroid glands.

Hypocalcemia is evidenced by tingling in the extremities and the area around the mouth (*circumoral paresthesia*), muscle and abdominal cramps, positive **Chvostek's sign** (spasms of the facial muscles when the facial nerve is tapped; Fig. 16-9A), carpopedal spasms referred to as **Trousseau's sign** (Fig. 16-9B), mental changes, laryngeal spasms with airway

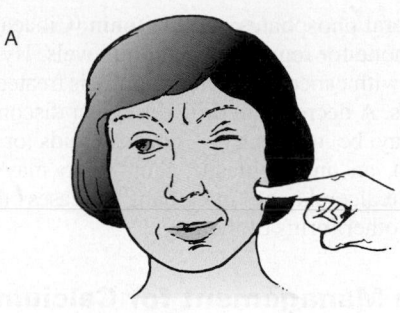
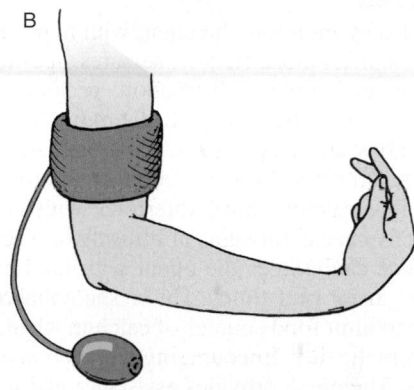

FIGURE 16-9. Signs of hypocalcemia. **(A)** Chvostek's sign, unilateral spasm of facial muscles, is elicited by tapping over the facial nerve, which lies approximately 2 cm anterior to the earlobe. **(B)** Trousseau's sign is evidenced by a spasm of the fingers, hand, and wrist when a blood pressure cuff is inflated to a level between the client's systolic and diastolic blood pressure for 3 minutes. (From *Lippincott manual of nursing practice*, 8th ed. [2006]. Philadelphia: Lippincott Williams & Wilkins.)

obstruction, *tetany* (muscle twitching), seizures, bleeding, and cardiac dysrhythmias. The client has hypocalcemia if the total serum calcium level is below 8.8 mg/dL (normal range, 9 to 11 mg/dL) or the ionized calcium level is below 4.4 mg/dL (normal range, 4.4 to 5.4 mg/dL).

Treatment includes administration of oral calcium and vitamin D for mild deficits and IV administration of a calcium salt, such as calcium gluconate, for severe hypocalcemia.

Hypercalcemia

Hypercalcemia is associated with parathyroid gland tumors, multiple fractures, Paget's disease, hyperparathyroidism, excessive doses of vitamin D, prolonged immobilization, some chemotherapeutic agents, and certain malignant diseases (multiple myeloma, acute leukemia, lymphomas).

Hypercalcemia causes deep bone pain, constipation, anorexia, nausea, vomiting, polyuria, thirst, pathologic fractures, and mental changes such as decreased memory and attention span. Chronic hypercalcemia can promote the formation of kidney stones. The total serum calcium level is above 10 mg/dL, and the ionized calcium level is above 5.4 mg/dL.

Treatment includes determining and correcting the cause when possible. Mild hypercalcemia is treated by increasing oral fluid intake and limiting calcium consumption until laboratory findings are normal. Acute hypercalcemia is treated by administering one or more of the following: IV sodium chloride solution (0.45% or 0.9%) and a diuretic such as furosemide (Lasix) to increase calcium excretion in the urine; oral phosphates; or calcitonin (Cibacalcin), a synthetic hormone for regulating calcium levels. Hypercalcemia associated with cancer or chemotherapy is treated on an individual basis. A decrease in drug dosage or discontinuation of therapy may be necessary. Corticosteroids or plicamycin (Mithracin), an antineoplastic agent, also may be used to treat hypercalcemia of malignant diseases that do not respond to other forms of therapy.

Nursing Management for Calcium Imbalances

The nurse closely monitors the client with hypocalcemia for neurologic manifestations (tetany, seizures, spasms), cardiac dysrhythmias, and airway obstruction, because emergency interventions may be necessary. If the deficit is severe, seizure precautions are necessary. Clients with severe muscle cramping remain on bed rest for comfort and to avoid falls. Because a low calcium level interferes with clotting, the nurse routinely checks for signs of bruising or bleeding.

The nurse encourages the client with mild hypercalcemia to drink many oral fluids. He or she collaborates with the dietitian to limit food sources of calcium when calcium is restricted from the diet. Encouraging ambulation as tolerated is important. The nurse provides assistance and instructs the client to wear shoes to avoid falls that may result in pathologic fractures.

A teaching plan for the client with hypocalcemia or hypercalcemia includes the following points:

- Follow the physician's recommendations regarding the addition or restriction of calcium to the diet. Milk, yogurt, and hard cheese are rich sources of dietary calcium. Non-dairy sources are turnip and mustard greens, collards, kale, broccoli, canned fish with bones, and calcium-fortified orange juice.
- Lactose-free milk and nonprescription lactase enzymes are available for lactose-intolerant clients.
- Take prescribed or physician-recommended drugs as directed; do not exceed or omit a dose.

 Pharmacologic Considerations

- Calcium replacement is given cautiously to clients with kidney stones because high calcium levels in the kidney tubules may contribute to additional stone formation.

MAGNESIUM IMBALANCES

Magnesium (Mg^{++}) is found in bone cells and specialized cells of the heart, liver, and skeletal muscles. Only a small percentage of the total magnesium in the body is found in extracellular fluid. Magnesium is involved in the transmission of nerve impulses and muscle excitability and activates several enzyme systems, including the functioning of B vitamins and use of potassium and calcium. A lower-than-normal serum level of magnesium is *hypomagnesemia;* higher than normal is *hypermagnesemia.*

Hypomagnesemia

Conditions that can result in hypomagnesemia include chronic alcoholism, diabetic ketoacidosis, severe renal disease, severe burns, severe malnutrition, pregnancy-induced hypertension, intestinal malabsorption syndromes, excessive diuresis (drug induced), hyperaldosteronism (see Chap. 50), and prolonged gastric suction. Physical stress or high intake of calcium, protein, or alcohol may increase the need for magnesium.

Signs and symptoms include tachycardia and other cardiac dysrhythmias, neuromuscular irritability, paresthesias of the extremities, leg and foot cramps, hypertension, mental changes, positive Chvostek's and Trousseau's signs (see Fig. 16-9), dysphagia (difficulty swallowing), and seizures. The serum magnesium level is below 1.3 mEq/L (normal range, 1.3 to 2.1 mEq/L).

Treatment includes administration of oral or parenteral magnesium salts or the addition of magnesium-rich foods to the diet. Magnesium is found in green leafy vegetables, whole grains (especially wheat germ and bran), nuts, cocoa, chocolate, nuts, soybeans, seafood, and dried peas and beans. A severe magnesium deficit is treated with IV administration of magnesium sulfate.

Hypermagnesemia

Hypermagnesemia can be a consequence of renal failure, Addison's disease, excessive use of antacids or laxatives that contain magnesium, and hyperparathyroidism.

Clients with hypermagnesemia experience flushing, warmth, hypotension, lethargy, drowsiness, *bradycardia,* muscle weakness, depressed respirations, and coma. The serum magnesium level is above 2.1 mEq/L.

Treatment includes decreasing oral magnesium intake or discontinuing administration of parenteral replacement. In severe hypermagnesemia, hemodialysis may be necessary. If respiratory failure occurs, mechanical ventilation is essential.

Nursing Management for Magnesium Imbalances

The nurse closely observes clients with hypomagnesemia for dysrhythmias and early signs of neuromuscular irritability, which he or she reports to the physician immediately. If administering IV magnesium sulfate, the nurse checks BP frequently because such administration can produce vasodilation and subsequent hypotension. Calcium gluconate is kept available as an antidote for an adverse reaction during administration of magnesium sulfate. If dysphagia occurs, the nurse consults with the physician and dietitian about alternatives or modifications to dietary management.

Vital signs of clients with actual or potential hypermagnesemia require close monitoring. The nurse notifies the physician immediately of significant changes, especially in respiratory rate, rhythm, or depth.

Teaching points include the following:

- Check with the physician, pharmacist, or nurse concerning antacids or laxatives that contain magnesium.
- If use of an antacid or laxative is allowed, follow the physician's recommendations regarding the frequency of use.

Pharmacologic Consideration

- When administering electrolytes to correct or prevent a deficiency, measure the dose carefully and give only as directed by the prescriber because these agents are potentially dangerous.

▶ *Stop, Think, and Respond Exercise 16-4*

Identify the electrolyte imbalance each client is most likely manifesting:

Client A is nauseous and weak. The ECG shows a U wave.
Client B has muscle twitching and tingling around the mouth.
Client C is thirsty, lethargic, and excreting only scant urine.

ACID-BASE BALANCE

In addition to water and electrolytes, body fluid also contains acids and bases. One of the chief acids is carbonic acid (H_2CO_3). An example of a base, sometimes referred to as an alkaline substance, that neutralizes acids is bicarbonate (HCO_3). Acid and base content influence the pH of body fluid. The symbol *pH* refers to the amount of hydrogen ions in a solution; pH can range from 1, which is highly acidic, to 14, which is highly basic. A pH of 7 is neutral. The more hydrogen ions in a solution, the more acidic it is. Acidity is indicated by a pH below 7. The degree of alkalinity is identified by a pH above 7. Normal plasma pH is 7.35 to 7.45, or slightly alkaline. The body maintains the normal plasma pH by two mechanisms: chemical regulation and organ regulation.

Chemical Regulation

Chemical regulation occurs through one or more buffering systems by which hydrogen ions are either added or eliminated. Adding hydrogen ions increases acidity; removing them promotes alkalinity. The major chemical regulator of plasma pH is the **bicarbonate–carbonic acid buffer system**. A ratio of 20 parts bicarbonate to 1 part carbonic acid maintains normal plasma pH.

Organ Regulation

The lungs and kidneys facilitate the ratio of bicarbonate to carbonic acid. Carbon dioxide (CO_2) is one of the components of carbonic acid:

$$CO_2 + H_2O \text{ (water)} = H_2CO_3 \text{ (carbonic acid)}$$

The lungs regulate carbonic acid levels by releasing or conserving CO_2 by increasing or decreasing the respiratory rate, volume, or both. The kidneys assist in acid-base balance by retaining or excreting bicarbonate ions. If an imbalance in acids or bases occurs, these regulatory processes are accelerated, which is referred to as **compensation**.

ACID–BASE IMBALANCES

An imbalance in acids or bases is life-threatening. Death occurs quickly if plasma pH is outside the range of 6.8 to 7.8

(Sherwood, 2007). Arterial blood gas (ABG) results are the main tool for measuring blood pH, CO_2 content ($PaCO_2$), and bicarbonate. An acid-base imbalance may accompany a fluid and electrolyte imbalance.

There are essentially two types of acid-base imbalances: acidosis and alkalosis (Fig. 16-10). **Acidosis** means excessive accumulation of acids or excessive loss of bicarbonate in body fluids. **Alkalosis** means excessive accumulation of bases or loss of acid in body fluids. Either can stem from metabolic or respiratory alterations. There are four subtypes: metabolic acidosis, metabolic alkalosis, respiratory acidosis, and respiratory alkalosis.

METABOLIC ACIDOSIS

Metabolic acidosis is a condition that results in decreased plasma pH because of increased organic acids (acids other than carbonic acid) or decreased bicarbonate. Organic acids increase during periods of anaerobic metabolism, when cells attempt to produce ATP without oxygen. Anaerobic metabolism is much less efficient than aerobic (with oxygen) metabolism and produces by-products such as lactic acid. It occurs during shock and cardiac arrest. Acids also increase in starvation and diabetic ketoacidosis (see Chap. 51), as fatty acids accumulate because the body cannot use glucose for energy. Accumulation of acids also may follow renal failure because the kidneys cannot reabsorb bicarbonate to buffer the blood. They also accumulate with aspirin (acetylsalicylic acid) overdosage or profuse diarrhea. Another cause of acid accumulation is loss of intestinal fluid through wound drainage, in which bicarbonate can be lost in disproportionate amounts.

Assessment Findings

Signs and Symptoms

Metabolic acidosis is accompanied by deep and rapid breathing (*Kussmaul's breathing*), a compensatory mechanism to rid the body of CO_2 and thus prevent carbonic acid from forming. The client may experience anorexia, nausea, vomiting, headache, confusion, flushing, lethargy, malaise, drowsiness, abdominal pain or discomfort, and weakness.

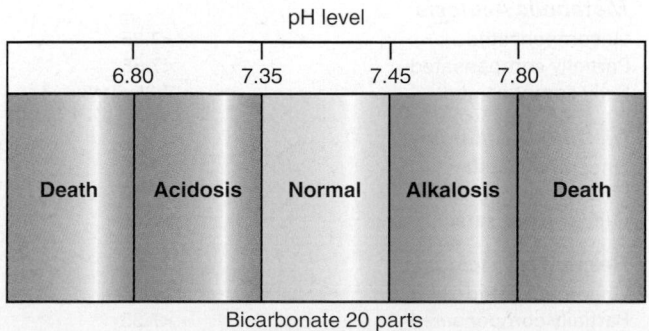

pH level

| 6.80 | 7.35 | 7.45 | 7.80 |

| Death | Acidosis | Normal | Alkalosis | Death |

Bicarbonate 20 parts
Carbonic acid 1 part

FIGURE 16-10. Acid-base balance and imbalances. Note that *acidosis* is used to describe the condition when pH is between 6.8 and 7.35. *Alkalosis* describes the condition when pH is between 7.45 and 7.80. When the pH exceeds these limits in either direction, death can occur.

Dangerous cardiac dysrhythmias can develop, and the force of cardiac contractions can be weakened. In severe stages, stupor and coma occur, and death may follow shortly.

Diagnostic Findings

The ABG values usually show decreased pH and plasma bicarbonate (HCO_3). Initially, $PaCO_2$ is normal, a condition referred to as an *uncompensated state*. As the rapid and deep breathing becomes effective, $PaCO_2$ decreases. Until pH returns to normal, it is referred to as a *partially compensated state*. When pH returns to normal, it is referred to as a *fully compensated state*, even though HCO_3 and $PaCO_2$ values are abnormal (Table 16-3). In a fully compensated state, regardless of the initial imbalance and current abnormal values, the client is out of danger.

The anion gap also is used to identify metabolic acidosis. The **anion gap** is the difference between sodium and potassium cation (positive ion) concentrations and the sum of chloride and bicarbonate **anions** (negative ions) in the extracellular fluid. The measured cations usually exceed the measured anions; the gap reflects the remaining unmeasured anions, such as phosphates, sulfates, organic acids, and proteins (Porth, 2004). The normal anion gap is 12 ± 4 mEq/L. An anion gap that exceeds 16 mEq/L indicates, but is not absolutely diagnostic for, metabolic acidosis. Low or negative anion gaps are relatively rare (Martin, 1999).

The measurement of all base buffers—sometimes referred to as the base excess or deficit—is used to identify acid-base imbalances. The base buffers include bicarbonate, phosphate, protein, and hemoglobin. To determine if the base is in excess or deficit, the laboratory determines the amount of a fixed acid or base that is necessary to reach a pH of 7.4 in a sample of the client's blood (Porth, 2004). The normal range is ± 3.0 mEq/L. A base deficit indicates metabolic acidosis; a base excess indicates metabolic alkalosis.

Medical Management

Treatment includes eliminating the cause and replacing fluids and electrolytes that may have been lost. IV bicarbonate is administered for severe metabolic acidosis.

▶ **Stop, Think, and Respond Exercise 16-5**

Calculate the anion gap using the following measurements, and indicate those that are signs of metabolic acidosis.

> Sodium (Na^+): 165 mEq/L
> Potassium (K^+): 4.0 mEq/L
> Chloride (Cl^-): 112 mEq/L
> Bicarbonate (HCO_3): 32 mEq/L

METABOLIC ALKALOSIS

Metabolic alkalosis results in increased plasma pH because of accumulated base bicarbonate or decreased hydrogen ion concentrations. Factors that increase base bicarbonate include excessive oral or parenteral use of bicarbonate-containing drugs or other alkaline salts, a rapid decrease in extracellular fluid volume (e.g., in diuretic therapy), and loss of hydrogen and chloride ions (e.g., in vomiting, prolonged gastric suctioning, hypokalemia, hyperaldosteronism). The result is retention of sodium bicarbonate and increased base bicarbonate.

 Gerontologic Considerations

- Older adults may avoid consulting a physician for the management of gastric hyperacidity and self-treat with household baking soda (sodium bicarbonate) as an inexpensive substitute for a commercial antacid. Overuse of sodium bicarbonate may lead to metabolic alkalosis.

TABLE 16-3 Arterial Blood Gas Trends in Acid-Base Imbalances

CONDITION	pH	HCO₃	PaCO₂
Acid-base balance	7.35–7.45	22–26 mEq/L	35–45 mm Hg
Metabolic Acidosis			
Uncompensated	<7.35	<22 mEq/L	Normal
Partially compensated	<7.35	<22 mEq/L	<35 mm Hg
Fully compensated	7.35–7.45	<22 mEq/L	<35 mm Hg
Metabolic Alkalosis			
Uncompensated	>7.45	>26 mEq/L	Normal
Partially compensated	>7.45	>26 mEq/L	>45 mm Hg
Fully compensated	>7.45	>22 mEq/L	>45 mm Hg
Respiratory Acidosis			
Uncompensated	<7.35	Normal	>45 mm Hg
Partially compensated	<7.35	>26 mEq/L	>45 mm Hg
Fully compensated	7.35–7.45	>26 mEq/L	>45 mm Hg
Respiratory Alkalosis			
Uncompensated	7.45	Normal	<35 mm Hg
Partially compensated	7.45	<22 mEq/L	<35 mm Hg
Fully compensated	7.35–7.45	<22 mEq/L	<35 mm Hg

Assessment Findings

Clients in metabolic alkalosis can manifest anorexia, nausea, vomiting, circumoral paresthesias, confusion, carpopedal spasm, hypertonic reflexes, and tetany. The respiratory rate and volume decrease in a compensatory effort to produce more carbonic acid to increase and restore the acidic level in the blood. Initially, ABGs show increased pH and HCO_3 and normal $PaCO_2$ levels (see Table 16-3). As compensatory respiratory mechanisms result in slower and shallower breathing, the $PaCO_2$ level is elevated; eventually, pH may return to normal.

Medical Management

Treatment involves eliminating the cause. The physician may prescribe potassium (as a potassium salt) if hypokalemia is present. In hypokalemia, hydrogen ions shift to the intracellular space to ensure the appropriate level of cations, the intracellular shift of hydrogen raises blood pH. Administering potassium allows hydrogen to return to the intravascular space and reestablishes a normal blood pH (Yaseen, 2007).

Treatment may also involve prescribing sodium chloride. When sodium is reabsorbed in the kidney tubules, hydrogen ions are excreted, contributing to a state of alkalosis. Maintaining an adequate sodium level reduces the excretion of hydrogen ions and offsets the rising pH.

RESPIRATORY ACIDOSIS

Respiratory acidosis, which may be either acute or chronic, is caused by excess carbonic acid, which causes the blood pH to drop below 7.35. Conditions that predispose to respiratory acidosis include pneumothorax, hemothorax, pulmonary edema, acute bronchial asthma, atelectasis, hyaline membrane disease or other forms of respiratory distress in the newborn, pneumonia (see Chap. 21), some drug overdoses, and head injuries. Chronic respiratory acidosis is associated with disorders such as emphysema, bronchiectasis, bronchial asthma, and cystic fibrosis.

Assessment Findings

Acute respiratory acidosis is associated with extreme respiratory insufficiency. The client may make frantic efforts to breathe, breathe slowly or irregularly, or stop breathing. Expiratory volumes are decreased. Lung sounds may be moist or absent in some lobes. Tachycardia usually is present, and cardiac dysrhythmias can develop. In later stages, *cyanosis,* a dusky appearance to the skin, may be evident. The accumulation of CO_2 leads to behavioral changes (mental cloudiness, confusion, disorientation, hallucinations), tremors, muscle twitching, flushed skin, headache, weakness, stupor, and coma. Responses to chronic respiratory acidosis are less prominent and can include an increased breathing effort, lack of energy, reduced activity, dull headache, and weakness.

ABG values show a decreased pH and an increased $PaCO_2$ above 45 mm Hg. As the kidney attempts to compensate, which may take 2 to 3 days, the HCO_3 rises, followed by a return to normal pH if full compensation occurs (see Table 16-3).

Gerontologic Considerations

- Poor respiratory exchange as the result of decreased lung expansion from inactivity, remaining in the same position for prolonged periods, thoracic skeletal changes, or chronic lung disease may lead to chronic respiratory acidosis.

Medical Management

Treatment is individualized, depending on the cause of the imbalance and whether the condition is acute or chronic. Mechanical ventilation may be necessary to support respiratory function. IV sodium bicarbonate is administered when ventilation efforts do not adequately restore a balanced pH. Heart rate and rhythm are monitored to detect sudden cardiac changes. In less acute situations, treatment may include the administration of pharmacologic agents, such as bronchodilators and antibiotics, to improve breathing. Airway suctioning may be necessary if the client is too weak to cough secretions.

RESPIRATORY ALKALOSIS

Respiratory alkalosis results from a carbonic acid deficit that occurs when rapid breathing releases more CO_2 than necessary with expired air. *Tachypnea* (rapid breathing) may result from acute anxiety, high fever, thyrotoxicosis (overactive thyroid), early salicylate (aspirin) poisoning, *hypoxemia* (low oxygen in the blood), or mechanical ventilation.

Assessment Findings

The most obvious manifestation is an increased respiratory rate. Accompanying symptoms include lightheadedness, numbness and tingling of the fingers and toes, circumoral paresthesias, sweating, panic, dry mouth, and, in severe cases, convulsions. The ABG values indicate a pH above 7.45 and a $PaCO_2$ below 35 mm Hg. If the kidney compensates by excreting bicarbonate ions, the HCO_3 falls below 22 mEq to restore pH (see Table 16-3).

Medical Management

Treatment aims to correct the cause of the rapid breathing. Having the client breathe into a paper bag held over the nose and mouth and rebreathe expired air may be useful temporarily. Sedation may be necessary when extreme anxiety is the cause of tachypnea.

NURSING MANAGEMENT FOR ACID-BASE IMBALANCES

The nurse carefully documents all presenting signs and symptoms to provide accurate baseline data. He or she monitors laboratory values; compares ABG findings with previous results (if any); and reports current results to the physician as soon as they are obtained. The same applies to abnormal electrolyte levels. The nurse maintains accurate intake and output records to monitor fluid status. He or she implements prescribed medical therapy, such as administering fluid and electrolyte replacements, suctioning the airway, maintaining mechanical ventilation, and monitoring cardiac rate and rhythm (see Chaps. 20 and 21). The nurse administers cardiopulmonary resuscitation whenever necessary.

CRITICAL THINKING EXERCISES

1. Describe the relationship of water to imbalances in electrolytes, acids, and bases.
2. Explain the action that occurs when an intravenous bolus of potassium is used to execute criminals by lethal injection.
3. Which respiratory acid/base imbalance do you think is more common? Support your answer.
4. What imbalances are likely to occur among athletes, and what steps are taken to help avoid serious consequences?

NCLEX-STYLE REVIEW QUESTIONS

1. A client is concerned about consuming sufficient water. If the client weighs 80 kg, how much fluid intake is adequate in a day?
   1. About 8 L
   2. About 2.5 L
   3. About 800 mL
   4. About 3.5 L
2. Results of a client's ECG show a tall T wave. For which of the following electrolytes would the nurse suspect an imbalance?
   1. Potassium
   2. Magnesium
   3. Calcium
   4. Sodium
3. The hypertensive client will begin taking furosemide (Lasix), a potassium-wasting diuretic every day. The nurse knows that teaching regarding the need for potassium-rich foods is successful when the client makes which of the following statements?
   1. "I can have a daily serving of gelatin."
   2. "I need to have more fruits like bananas and nectarines."
   3. "I will add more servings of broiled white fish."
   4. "I will eat more pasta and cheese."
4. A client has been taking aluminum and magnesium hydroxide (Maalox), an antacid, for many days because of gastric discomfort. The nurse suspects that the client's magnesium level is elevated because of which symptoms? Select all that apply.
   1. Bradycardia
   2. Hyperventilation
   3. Hypotension
   4. Insomnia
   5. Shivering
5. Which client statement following a subtotal thyroidectomy is most indicative that the client is experiencing hypocalcemia?
   1. "I don't have much of an appetite."
   2. "I feel so weak when I ambulate."
   3. "Light seems to bother my eyes."
   4. "My lips feel numb and tingly."

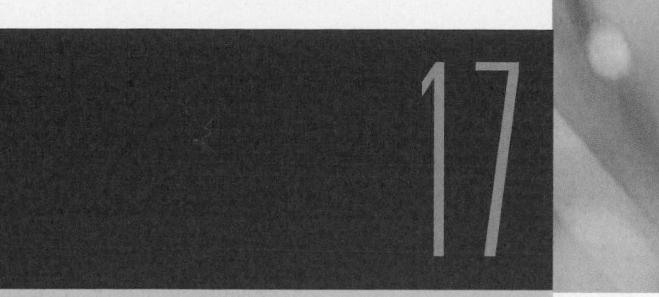

17

Caring for Clients in Shock

Learning Objectives

On completion of this chapter, you will be able to:

1. Define shock.
2. Name four general categories of shock.
3. Identify the subcategories of distributive shock.
4. List pathophysiologic consequences of shock.
5. Name the three stages of shock.
6. Identify three physiologic mechanisms that attempt to compensate for shock.
7. Discuss signs and symptoms manifested by clients in shock.
8. Name three diagnostic measurements used when monitoring clients in shock.
9. Give three medical approaches for treating shock.
10. List complications of shock.
11. Discuss the nursing management of clients with shock.

This chapter discusses shock and its various types, pathophysiologic consequences, and assessment findings, which may vary according to type. It also presents the medical and nursing management of clients in shock.

SHOCK

Shock is a life-threatening condition that occurs when arterial blood flow and oxygen delivery to tissues and cells are inadequate. Shock develops as a consequence of one of three events: (1) blood volume decreases, (2) the heart fails as an effective pump, or (3) peripheral blood vessels massively dilate (Collins, 2000). The body implements compensatory mechanisms to counteract the effects of shock. When compensatory mechanisms become ineffective, shock progresses until therapeutic measures are implemented. If physiologic and therapeutic measures are inadequate, organs are damaged and death may follow.

Types of Shock

The four main categories of shock are hypovolemic, distributive, obstructive, and cardiogenic, depending on the cause (Chavez & Brewer, 2002; Smeltzer et al., 2008) (Table 17-1). More than one type of shock can develop simultaneously.

Hypovolemic Shock

In **hypovolemic shock**, the most common type of shock, the volume of extracellular fluid is significantly diminished, primarily because of lost or reduced blood or plasma (serum; see Chap. 16). Because the intravascular, interstitial, and intracellular fluid volumes are interdependent, a

TABLE 17-1 Types of Shock

TYPE	CAUSE	ILLUSTRATION	EXAMPLES
Hypovolemic shock	Decreased blood volume with decreased filling of the circulatory system		Hemorrhage (frank and internal) Extreme diuresis Severe diarrhea or vomiting Dehydration Third-spacing
Distributive shock *Neurogenic* *Septic* *Anaphylactic*	Enlargement of the vascular compartment and redistribution of intravascular fluid from arterial circulation to venous or capillary areas		Neurogenic: Spinal cord injury Septic: Toxic reaction to gram-negative bacterial infection Anaphylactic: Severe allergic reaction
Obstructive shock	Impaired filling of heart with blood due to mechanical impediment		Cardiac tamponade (see Chap. 23) Dissecting aneurysm Tension pneumothorax (see Chap. 21)
Cardiogenic shock	Decreased force of ventricular contraction		Myocardial infarction (see Chap. 25) Cardiac dysrhythmia (see Chap. 26)

Illustrations from Porth, C. M. (2007). *Essentials of pathophysiology: Concepts of altered health states.* (2nd ed.) Philadelphia: Lippincott Williams & Wilkins.

loss from one location results in a similar depletion in the others. Thus, a deficit of intravascular volume (plasma) reduces the net circulating volume. Hypovolemic shock can develop when overall fluid volume is depleted from significant bleeding, such as during surgery, after trauma, or after delivery of an infant. It also may result from significant fluid loss, as with burns, large draining wounds, reduced fluid intake, suctioning, or disorders in which fluid losses exceed fluid intake, such as diabetes insipidus (see Chap. 50).

Symptoms are not evident until there is a 15% to 30% (750 mL to 1500 mL) loss of fluid volume. Marked deterioration occurs when there is a 30% to 40% (1500 mL to 2000 mL) volume depletion. When the volume deficit is more than

40% (more than 2000 mL), the situation becomes life-threatening (Kleinpell, 2007).

Distributive Shock

Distributive shock is sometimes called *normovolemic shock* because the amount of fluid in the circulatory system is not reduced, yet the fluid circulation does not permit effective tissue perfusion. Vasodilatation, a prominent characteristic of distributive shock, increases the space in the vascular bed. Central blood flow is reduced because peripheral vascular or interstitial areas exceed their usual capacity. Three types of distributive shock are neurogenic, septic, and anaphylactic shock.

Neurogenic Shock

Neurogenic shock, the rarest type of shock, results from an insult to the vasomotor center in the medulla of the brain or to the peripheral nerves that extend from the spinal cord to the blood vessels. Injury to the spinal cord or head or overdoses of opioids, opiates, tranquilizers, or general anesthetics can cause neurogenic shock. The tone of the sympathetic nervous system is impaired, resulting in decreased arterial vascular resistance, vasodilatation, and hypotension. Because blood remains distributed in the periphery, the heart does not fill adequately, cardiac output is reduced, tissue perfusion is compromised, cells are deprived of oxygen and switch to anaerobic metabolism, and metabolic acidosis develops from an increase in lactic acid.

Septic Shock

Septic shock, also called *toxic shock*, has the highest mortality rate of the various types of shock. Approximately 40% to 60% of those who develop septic shock die despite aggressive treatment (Chamberlain, 2004). It is associated with overwhelming bacterial infections (see Chap. 12). Septic shock is preceded by a **systemic inflammatory response syndrome** (SIRS), an inflammatory state without a proven source of infection (Box 17-1). SIRS progresses to sepsis when symptoms of SIRS are present and an infection is proven. Severe sepsis is a pre-septic shock condition that develops when sepsis is combined with organ hypoperfusion (see Chap. 12). Once septic shock, which is accompanied by hypotension, develops, the client may deteriorate to the point of **multiple organ dysfunction syndrome**, a complication of overwhelming inflammation that results in massive cellular, tissue, and organ injury.

Septic shock occurs most commonly in clients with gram-negative bacteremia (bacteria in the blood) caused by such pathogens as *Escherichia coli*, species of *Pseudomonas*, and gram-positive drug-resistant *Staphylococcus aureus* and streptococcal species. **Endotoxins**, harmful chemicals released by bacterial cells, are probably the major cause of septic shock. They trigger an immune response in which vasoactive chemicals, such as cytokines (see Chap. 33), dilate the blood vessels and increase capillary permeability, causing vascular fluid to shift to the interstitium. Unlike other forms of shock, clients with septic shock have an elevated leukocyte count and initially manifest a fever accompanied by warm, flushed skin and a rapid, bounding pulse. As septic shock progresses, however, affected clients eventually develop cold, pale or mottled skin and hypotensive symptoms, findings common with other forms of shock.

Anaphylactic Shock

Anaphylactic shock is a severe allergic reaction that follows exposure to a substance to which a person is extremely sensitive(see Chap. 34). Common allergic substances include bee venom, latex, fish, nuts, and penicillin. The body's immune response to the allergic substance causes mast cells in the connective tissues, bronchi, and gastrointestinal tract to release histamine and other chemicals. The results are vasodilatation, increased capillary permeability accompanied by swelling of the airway and subcutaneous tissues, hypotension, and hives or an itchy rash.

Obstructive Shock

Obstructive shock occurs when there is interference with the circulation of blood into and out of the heart, compromising the volume of blood that enters and leaves the heart en route to the lungs and tissues. Any condition that fills the thoracic cavity with fluid, air, or tissue can lead to obstructive shock. Examples include increased fluid or blood in the pericardial sac (cardiac tamponade; see Chap. 23); air that accumulates between the layers of pleura (tension pneumothorax; see Chap. 21); or abdominal tissue, fluid, or air that crowds the diaphragm, as in an enlarged liver and ascites (see Chap. 47), thus reducing the size of the thorax.

Cardiogenic Shock

In **cardiogenic shock**, heart contraction is ineffective, which reduces **cardiac output**, the volume of blood ejected from the left ventricle per minute. A myocardial infarction (MI) with subsequent heart failure (see Chaps. 25 and 28) is a leading cause of cardiogenic shock.

 Gerontologic Considerations

Older adults, particularly those with cardiac disease, are prone to cardiogenic shock. They also have a decreased percentage of body water and are more likely to develop hypovolemic shock. Due to a decreased immune response, which hinders the body's ability to fight infection, older adults may be at higher risk for developing septic shock.

▶ **Stop, Think, and Respond Exercise 17-1**

Indicate the type of shock each client is most likely experiencing:

- *Client A has had an MI and cardiac arrest; paramedics resuscitated him. He is now having difficulty breathing, a rapid heart rate, and chest pain. Urine output is 50 mL in the last 4 hours.*
- *Client B was involved in a motor vehicle collision. Paramedics note a substantial bruise on his right upper thigh, which is much larger than his left upper thigh. Based on assessment findings and a distorted alignment of the right leg, they suspect a fractured pelvis or femur. They also suspect a ruptured spleen because the client has abdominal tenderness. He is hypotensive with pale and cool skin.*
- *Client C was pruning roses when a bee stung her. Within minutes she had difficulty breathing and lost consciousness. Her neighbor called 911. Paramedics note that the client is hypotensive, tachycardic, and barely able to breathe.*

Stages and Pathophysiology

Regardless of the type, many complex events accompany shock, which usually progresses through three stages: (1) compensation, (2) decompensation, and (3) irreversible (Fig. 17-1).

BOX 17-1 | **Criteria for Systemic Inflammatory Response Syndrome**

SIRS is diagnosed when two or more of the following are present when there is a strong suspicion of inflammation such as microbial infection, pancreatitis, multiple trauma, and others:

- Heart rate greater than 90 beats per minute
- Body temperature less than 36°C (96.8°F) or greater than 38°C (100.8°F)
- Respiratory rate over 20 breaths per minute or partial pressure of carbon dioxide ($PaCO_2$) on blood gas measurement of less than 32 mm Hg (normal is 35–45 mm Hg)
- White blood cell count less than 4000 cells/mm^3 or greater than 12000 cells/mm^3 or the presence of more than 10% immature neutrophils.

Source: Paterson, R.L., Webster, N.R. (2000). *Sepsis and the systemic inflammatory response syndrome.* Available at: http://www.rcsed.ac.uk/Journal/vol45_3/4530010.htm. Accessed November 2007.

Compensation Stage

The **compensation stage** is the first stage of shock, during which several physiologic mechanisms attempt to stabilize the spiraling consequences. If these mechanisms are successful, homeostatic stability potentially can be achieved. If natural or medical means can reverse shock, the chances of uncomplicated recovery are greatly improved. As shock progresses, positive outcomes are less predictable. Compensatory mechanisms include the release of catecholamines; activation of the renin-angiotensin-aldosterone system; and production of antidiuretic and corticosteroid hormones.

Catecholamines

Catecholamines are neurotransmitters that stimulate responses via the sympathetic nervous system (Table 17-2). To compensate in shock, the sympathetic nervous system releases endogenous catecholamines, epinephrine and norepinephrine, into the circulation. The adrenal medulla secretes epinephrine, whereas the endings of sympathetic nerve fibers secrete norepinephrine. Epinephrine and norepinephrine increase heart rate and myocardial contractility, which may be counterproductive in cardiogenic shock because it increases a demand for oxygen by an already compromised heart. Venous return to the right atrium subsequently increases, as does blood sent to the lungs. Bronchial dilatation increases the amount of oxygenated air entering the lungs, followed by a more efficient exchange of oxygen and carbon dioxide (CO_2).

Renin-Angiotensin-Aldosterone System

The **renin-angiotensin-aldosterone system** is a mechanism that restores blood pressure (BP) when circulating volume is diminished (see Fig. 16-6 in Chap. 16). In response to low renal (kidney) blood perfusion, the juxtaglomerular cells release renin, an enzymatic hormone in the nephrons of the kidneys. Release of renin causes a series of chemical reactions that eventually produce angiotensin II, a potent

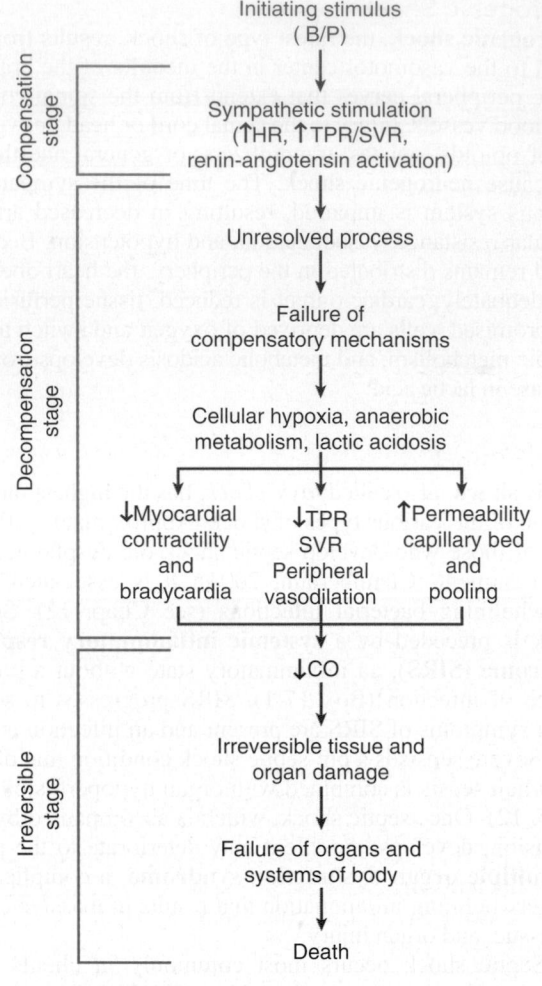

FIGURE 17-1. Stages of shock. B/P = blood pressure; CO = cardiac output; HR = heart rate; SVR = systemic vascular resistance; TPR = total peripheral resistance.

vasoconstrictor that raises BP. Angiotensin II also stimulates the hypothalamus to signal the adrenal cortex via the pituitary gland to release aldosterone, a mineralocorticoid that promotes reabsorption of sodium and water by the kidneys, which serves to increase blood volume.

Antidiuretic Hormone and Corticosteroid Hormones

Low blood volume also stimulates the pituitary to secrete **antidiuretic hormone** (ADH), also known as *vasopressin,* and **adrenocorticotropic hormone** (ACTH). ADH promotes reabsorption of water that the kidneys would ordinarily excrete. ACTH stimulates the adrenal glands to secrete **corticosteroid hormones**, which include glucocorticoids and mineralocorticoids. *Glucocorticoids* help the body respond to stress. *Mineralocorticoids,* such as aldosterone, conserve sodium and promote potassium excretion. Thus, they play an active role in controlling sodium and water balance. Both ADH and corticosteroid hormones promote fluid reabsorption and retention.

TABLE 17-2 Effects of Endogenous Catecholamines

EFFECT	CONSEQUENCES
Constriction of arterioles of skin, mucous membranes, subcutaneous tissues	Sends blood to larger blood vessels supplying vital organs
Dilatation of arterioles of skeletal muscles	Increases blood supply to skeletal muscles
Dilatation of coronary arteries	Increases oxygen to myocardium
Increased contractile ability of myocardium	Increases amount of blood leaving the left ventricle each time ventricle contracts (cardiac output)
Increased heart rate	Increases blood supply to body, especially vital organs
Bronchial dilatation	Increases amount of air entering the lungs on inspiration
Release of glycogen stored in the liver	Provides energy

Decompensation Stage

The **decompensation stage** occurs as compensatory mechanisms fail. The client's condition spirals into cellular hypoxia, coagulation defects, and cardiovascular changes.

Cellular Hypoxia

Hypoxia refers to decreased oxygen reaching the cells. Hypoxic cells are forced to switch from aerobic metabolism to **anaerobic metabolism**, a less efficient mechanism for meeting energy requirements. As the energy supply falls below the demand, pyruvic and lactic acids increase, causing metabolic acidosis. The structural integrity of cells is impaired because without sufficient adenosine triphosphate (ATP), the energy source for operating the sodium and potassium pumps, sodium and water enter the cell and potassium exits into the extracellular fluid (Fig. 17-2). Eventually, the cells swell and rupture, disrupting their ability to carry out electrochemical processes. Lysosomes, the cellular structure for breaking down cellular waste, leak enzymatic fluid and contribute to further cellular destruction. Gradually, significant numbers of cells are damaged.

Coagulation Defects

As cells become damaged, an inflammatory response ensues. Platelets become sticky and accumulate in the blood vessels of the volume-depleted client, predisposing him or her to the formation of microemboli. Clots further compromise the ability of the red blood cells (RBCs) to deliver oxygen throughout the body. Cell and organ death is potentiated.

Cardiovascular Changes

Impaired myocardial cells cannot maintain sufficient heart rate and force of contraction to circulate blood efficiently. Subsequently, brain cells in the medulla can no longer sustain the stimulus for vasoconstriction. The blood vessels

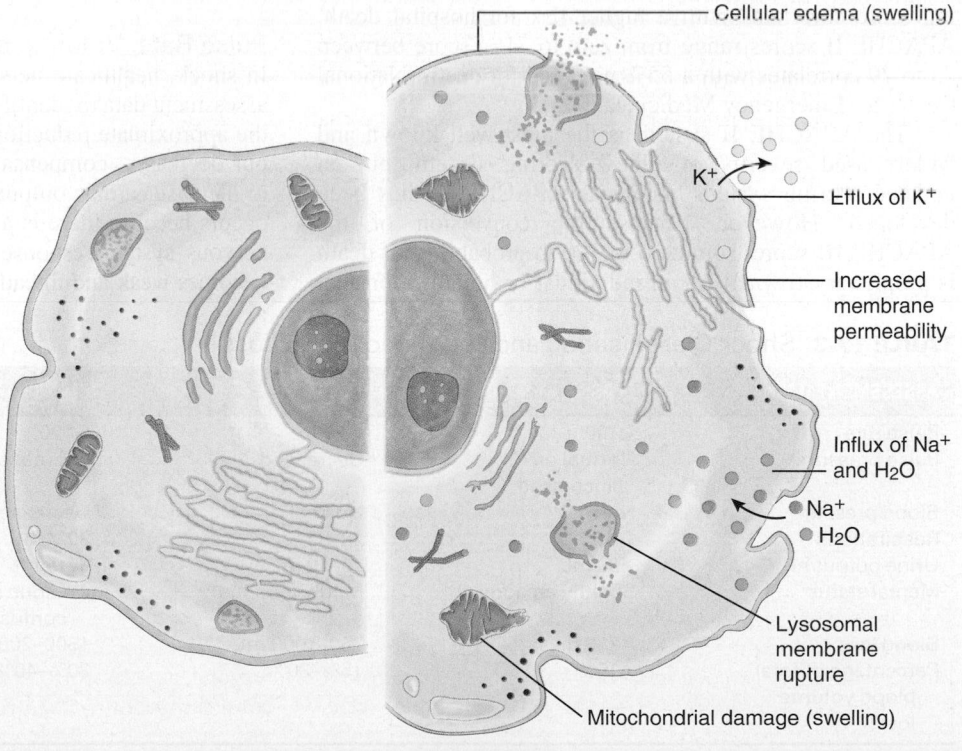

FIGURE 17-2. Cellular effects of shock. The cell swells, the cell membrane becomes more permeable, and fluids and electrolytes seep out of and into the cell. Mitochondria and lysosomes are damaged, and the cell dies.

Cellular edema (swelling)

K$^+$ Efflux of K$^+$

Increased membrane permeability

Influx of Na$^+$ and H$_2$O

Na$^+$
H$_2$O

Lysosomal membrane rupture

Mitochondrial damage (swelling)

Normal Cell   **Effects of Shock - cell damage -**

dilate, blood pools in the periphery or leaks into the interstitium, cardiac output decreases, and BP falls. Clinical signs are more obvious and include bradycardia, hypotension, confusion, lethargy, decreased urine production, cold, pale skin, and reduced peristalsis. Aggressive interventions are necessary to prevent the irreversible stage of shock and ensure the client's survival.

Irreversible Stage

The **irreversible stage** occurs when significant cells and organs become damaged. The client's condition reaches a "point of no return" despite treatment efforts. The client no longer responds to medical interventions. Multiple systems begin to fail. When the kidneys, heart, lungs, liver, and brain cease to function, death is imminent.

Assessment Findings

Signs and Symptoms

The nurse monitors the client for evidence that blood volume or circulation is becoming compromised. Although shock can develop quickly, early signs and symptoms are evident during the decompensation stage. Critical assessments include vital signs, characteristics of peripheral pulses, and changes in mentation, skin, and urine output (Table 17-3).

Some healthcare personnel use a scoring system known as APACHE II, which stands for **A**cute **P**hysiology, **A**ge, and **C**hronic **H**ealth **E**valuation, to arrive at a number that reflects the severity of the client's status and predicts the potential outcome of care. The physiologic data include vital signs, results from laboratory tests such as arterial pH, serum sodium, potassium, creatinine, white blood cell count, hematocrit, and Glasgow Coma Score. The point value increases according to age and health problems. An increasing score correlates with a higher risk for hospital death. APACHE II scores range from zero to 71; a score between 25 to 29 correlates with a 55% potential for death (National Center for Emergency Medicine, 2004).

The APACHE II system is the most well known and widely used severity of illness scoring system, but an updated scoring system known as APACHE III has been developed. However, because the conversion of the APACHE III score from zero to 300 to probability of death is proprietary (owned by an individual or organization that restricts its use), the system is not widely used (Hall, Schmidt, & Wood, 2005).

Arterial Blood Pressure

In shock, both systolic and diastolic arterial BPs fall because cardiac output decreases or the vascular bed increases. Hypotension may be rapid and sudden or slow and insidious. For the normotensive (normal BP) adult, the systolic BP is slightly less than 120 mm Hg. A systolic BP of 90 to 100 mm Hg indicates impending shock, whereas 80 mm Hg or below indicates shock. If it is difficult to auscultate BP but a peripheral pulse can be palpated, the BP is at least 80 mm Hg (Collins, 2000).

To determine the presence of shock, the client's previous BP must be known. Regardless of the numeric figure, a significant and progressive fall in BP from baseline is serious. For example, a BP of 120/82 mm Hg usually is considered normal; however, if an individual with an original BP of 190/112 mm Hg has a BP of 120/ 82 mm Hg, shock is developing. The nurse must make the physician aware of any trends such as a significant fall below the client's usual systolic BP, or any trend in progressively decreasing BP. Direct BP monitoring (intra-arterial) is more accurate than indirect monitoring—the usual, auscultatory method using a BP cuff (see Chap. 22)—but it is implemented primarily in critical care areas.

Pulse Pressure

Pulse pressure is the numeric difference between systolic and diastolic BP. If a client has a BP of 120/80 mm Hg, the pulse pressure is 40 mm Hg. A pulse pressure between 30 and 50 mm Hg is considered normal, with 40 mm Hg being a healthy average. In shock, the pulse pressure tends to narrow (decrease) as the falling systolic pressure nears the diastolic pressure.

Pulse Rate, Volume, and Rhythm

In shock, healthcare personnel use the pulse rate and other assessment data to identify the severity of shock and estimate the approximate reduction in blood volume. As cardiac output decreases, compensatory tachycardia initially develops to increase cardiac output. In neurogenic shock, bradycardia occurs because there is a loss of compensatory sympathetic nervous system response (Kleinpell, 2007b). Pulse volume becomes weak and thready as circulating volume diminishes.

TABLE 17-3 Shock Classification and Estimated Blood Loss

ASSESSMENT DATA	CLASS I	CLASS I	CLASS II	CLASS IV
Pulse rate	<100	>100	>120	>140
Pulse pressure	Normal or increased	Decreased	Decreased	Decreased
Blood pressure	Normal	Normal	Decreased	Decreased
Respirations	14–20	20–30	30–40	>35
Urine output/hr	≥30 mL	20–30 mL	5–15 mL	Negligible
Mental status	Slightly anxious	Mildly anxious	Anxious and confused	Confused and lethargic
Blood loss	≤750 mL	750–1000 mL	1500–2000 mL	≥2000 mL
Percentage of total blood volume lost*	≤15%	15%–30%	30%–40%	≥40%

*Estimates are based on an adult male weighing 70 kg.

(Adapted from American College of Surgeons. [1993] *Advanced trauma life support for physicians*. Chicago: Author.)

In the later stages, the pulse may be slow and imperceptible. Pulse rhythm may change from regular to irregular. Hypoxia, especially when it affects heart tissue, is a leading cause of dangerous cardiac dysrhythmias such as ventricular fibrillation (see Chap. 26).

Respirations

In shock, tissues receive less oxygen. In response, the body tries to obtain more oxygen by breathing faster. Rapid respirations help move blood in the large veins toward the heart. Respirations are shallow, and the client may be heard grunting. In early stages, the client is hungry for air, but in profound shock as death nears, the respiratory rate decreases.

Temperature

Heat-regulating mechanisms are depressed in shock, and added diaphoresis increases heat loss. With the possible exception of septic shock, subnormal body temperature is characteristic.

Mentation

Altered cerebral function often is the first sign of inadequate oxygen delivery to the tissues. Mild anxiety, increasing restlessness, agitation, and confusion can accompany shock. As the condition deteriorates, the client becomes listless and stuporous, ultimately losing consciousness.

Skin

In all but the early stages of septic and neurogenic shock, the skin is cold and clammy. As peripheral blood vessels constrict to direct blood from the skin to more vital organs (heart, kidneys, brain), the skin becomes pale. Eventually the skin may appear mottled (i.e., a mix of pale and cyanotic areas lacking any uniform color). Capillary filling longer than 3 seconds and cyanosis, especially of the nailbeds, lips, and earlobes, indicate oxygen deficiency. In clients with highly pigmented skin (such as African Americans), cyanosis is more accurately detected by inspecting the conjunctiva and oral mucous membranes. Lack of cyanosis, however, does not prove the absence of hypoxia because cyanosis is one of the last signs to appear.

Urine Output

Reduced cardiac output decreases renal blood flow, which leads to decreased urine output. Vasoconstriction, the physiologic response to shock, also contributes to markedly reduced renal blood flow. In many instances, the rate of urine formation is an important indicator of the status of a client in shock (see Table 17-3). When shock is quickly reversed, urine output usually returns to normal. Continued **oliguria** (decreased urine formation) indicates renal damage, caused by reduced blood flow to the kidneys.

▶ *Stop, Think, and Respond Exercise 17-2*

Which stage of shock is characterized by the following physiologic changes?

1. Client is unconscious, with a slow pulse, systolic BP of 85 mm Hg, and mottled skin color.
2. Client is alert and oriented, with tachycardia but normal BP and skin color.
3. Client is somewhat disoriented, with BP lower than earlier assessment and pale skin.

Diagnostic Findings

Arterial blood gas (ABG), central venous pressure, and pulmonary artery pressure measurements can support a diagnosis of shock. They also are used to monitor response to treatment.

Arterial Blood Gas (ABG) Measurements

ABG specimens are drawn from a direct arterial puncture or an indwelling arterial catheter (see Chap. 29). In shock, the partial pressure of oxygen in arterial blood (PaO_2, normally 80 to 100 mm Hg) falls below 60 mm Hg. The partial pressure of CO_2 in arterial blood ($PaCO_2$) may be normal, decreased with hyperventilation, or increased with hypoventilation. or decreased. A pulse oximeter, sometimes used to monitor oxygenation continuously, measures the amount of oxygen bound to hemoglobin, or the saturated oxygen (SpO_2) level, which normally is 95% to 100%. If the SpO_2 level is above 90%, it can be assumed that the PaO_2 is 60 mm Hg or above.

Central Venous Pressure

Central venous pressure (CVP) is the pressure of the blood in the right atrium or venae cavae. It distinguishes relationships among hemodynamic variables in shock: venous return, quality of right ventricular function, and vascular tone. CVP measurements, especially trends in readings, are useful in the management of a client in shock (see Chap. 29). Normal CVP is 2 to 7 mm Hg or 4 to 10 cm H_2O, depending on how it is measured. In hypovolemic shock, the CVP is lower than normal due to a low blood volume; in cardiogenic shock, it usually is above normal because there is venous congestion due to low cardiac output. The trend in CVP measurements is more helpful than isolated readings.

Pulmonary Artery Pressure

Although CVP measurements can indicate the status of right ventricular function, they do not provide information about left ventricular function. Because left ventricular function is more pertinent to circulation than right, knowing fluid pressures on the left side of the heart is more meaningful. To assess left ventricular function, a two-, three-, or four-lumen catheter is inserted into the vena cava and advanced through the right atrium and right ventricle into the pulmonary artery (Fig. 17-3). The catheter is connected to a monitor from which the *pulmonary artery pressure* (PAP) or *pulmonary capillary wedge pressure* (PCWP) is measured (see Chap. 29). Normal PAP ranges from 20 to 30 mm Hg systolic and from 8 to 12 mm Hg diastolic. Normal PCWP ranges from 4 to 12 mm Hg. In shock, PAP measurements usually are low because they reflect the low volume of blood in the arterial system.

Medical Management

Aggressive treatment of conditions that predispose to shock may prevent it. Once shock develops, treatment depends on its type and level and usually includes one or more of the following: intravenous (IV) fluid therapy, vasopressor drug therapy, and mechanical devices that restore blood circulation to cells.

Intravenous Fluid Therapy

IV fluids are prescribed to restore intravascular volume. The total volume, type of solution(s), and rate of administration vary according to the etiology of shock. Usually, a ratio of 3:1 is followed; that is, 3 L of fluid is administered for every 1 L of fluid lost. This amount stabilizes the client, replaces the deficit, and provides a reserve to prevent shock from

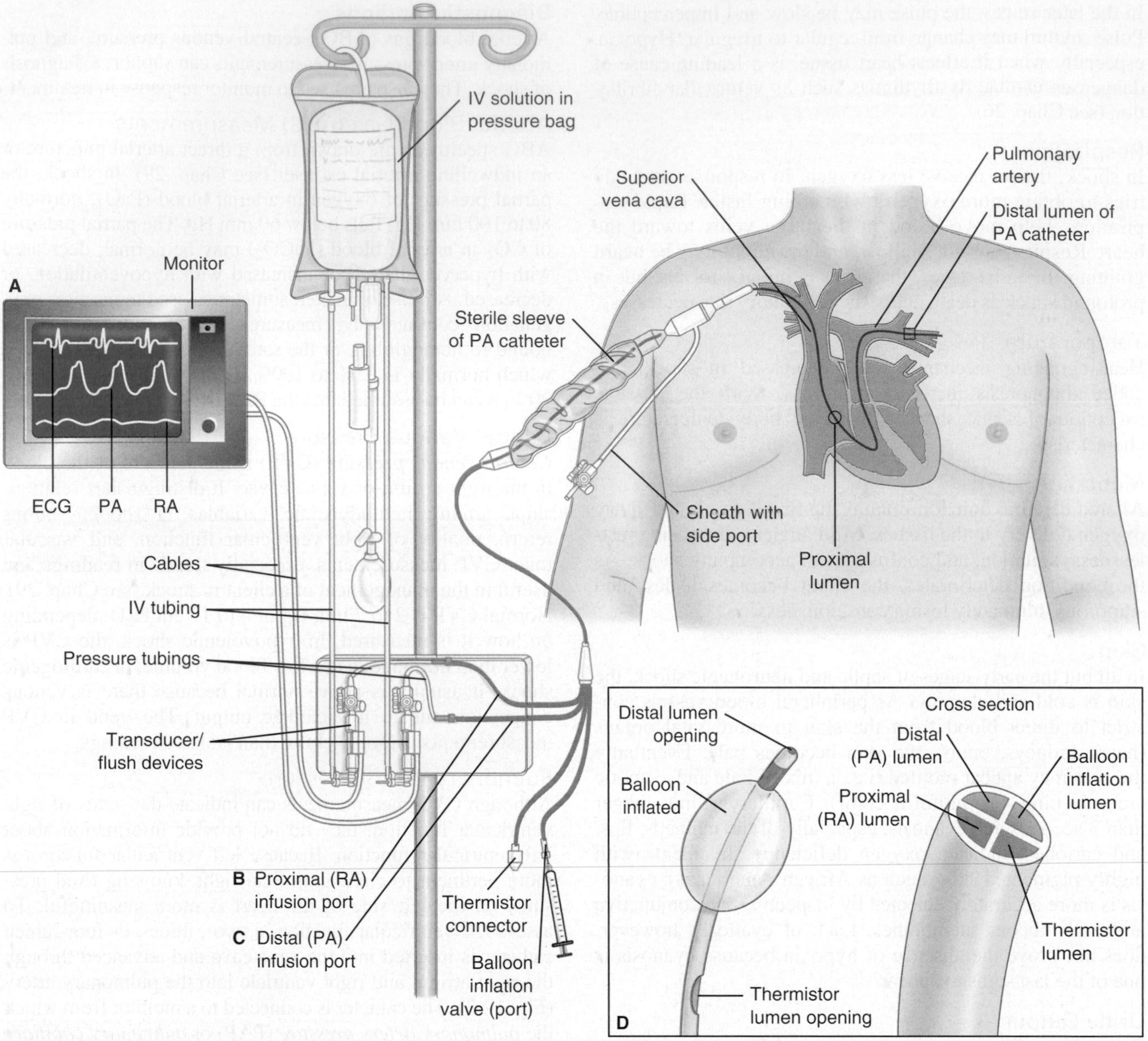

A

Monitor

ECG   PA   RA

Cables

IV tubing

Pressure tubings

Transducer/
flush devices

B Proximal (RA)
infusion port

C Distal (PA)
infusion port

Thermistor
connector

Balloon
inflation
valve (port)

IV solution in
pressure bag

Superior
vena cava

Sterile sleeve
of PA catheter

Pulmonary
artery

Distal lumen of
PA catheter

Sheath with
side port

Proximal
lumen

D

Distal lumen
opening

Balloon
inflated

Thermistor
lumen opening

Cross section

Distal
(PA) lumen

Proximal
(RA) lumen

Balloon
inflation
lumen

Thermistor
lumen

FIGURE 17-3. Example of a pulmonary artery (PA) catheter and pressure monitoring system. (**A**) Bedside cardiac monitoring. (**B**) Right atria (RA) or central venous pressure monitoring system connected to proximal infusion lumen hub. (**C**) PA monitoring system connected to distal infusion lumen hub. Each system is attached to pressurized IV fluid, a transducer with stopcock and flush device, and pressure tubing. A cable attaches each transducer to the bedside monitor. (**D**) Magnified view of distal end of PA catheter with cross-section of catheter lumen.

recurring. Initially, as much as 250 to 500 mL may be infused in 1 hour. Solutions may include crystalloid solutions, those containing dissolved substances such as sodium, other electrolytes, or glucose in water; colloid solutions, those containing proteins (such as albumin) to increase osmotic pressure; and blood and blood products if blood loss has been major (see Chap. 13).

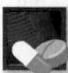 **Pharmacologic Considerations**

- Ringer's lactate and 0.9% sodium chloride (isotonic solutions) commonly are used to treat hypovolemic shock.

To ensure oxygenation of tissues, especially in cases of hemorrhage or if the hemoglobin level is 7 g/dL or less, administering whole blood or packed RBCs is best. One unit of RBCs can increase an adult's hemoglobin by 1 g/dL (American National Red Cross, 2007). Clients who are alert and capable of making informed decisions but refuse blood transfusions on the basis of religious beliefs (e.g., Jehovah's Witnesses) require bloodless alternatives and measures that conserve blood and its oxygen-carrying capacity. Such measures include the following:

- Drawing the minimum volume of blood for laboratory analysis
- Restricting movement and activity to only that which is essential

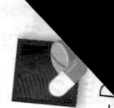

- Reinfusing the client's own blood that has been collected in a closed-circuit cell saver
- Using lasers and electrocautery devices to minimize bleeding during surgery
- Administering pharmacologic agents such as erythropoietin to stimulate the bone marrow to manufacture RBCs
- Administering cryoprecipitate, factor VIII, and thrombin to promote *hemostasis,* control of bleeding using substances in the body's natural coagulation process

Drug Therapy

Medical management of shock is extremely complex; drugs are carefully titrated and used alone or in combination to improve cardiovascular status (Drug Therapy Table 17-1).

Adrenergic drugs are the main [...] shock. **Vasopressors**, drugs with [...] increase peripheral vascular resis[...] ples include dopamine (Introp[...] ophed), and metaraminol (A[...] administered after fluid therapy [...] fluid volume; otherwise, the va[...] ther impair cellular circulation, which already is comp[...] mised by the effects of angiotensin. If infusions of first-line vasopressors such as dopamine and norepinephrine become ineffective, vasopressin may be used. Vasopressin, also known as antidiuretic hormone, causes contraction of arterial smooth muscles, raises blood pressure, and diverts blood to vital organs.

DRUG THERAPY TABLE 17-1   Agents to Treat Shock

Drug Category and Examples	Mechanism of Action	Side Effects	Nursing Considerations
Vasopressor Agents (Alpha-Adrenergic Activity)			
norepinephrine (Levophed), metaraminol (Aramine), phenylephrine (Neo-Synephrine)	Increase peripheral vascular resistance and raise BP	Headaches, restlessness, palpitations, tremors, nausea, vomiting, anxiety, dizziness	Protect from light. Monitor BP closely during administration. Monitor intake and output. Avoid abrupt withdrawal of these medications.
Positive Inotropic Agents (Beta-Adrenergic Activity)			
dobutamine (Dobutrex), isoproterenol (Isuprel), milrinone (Primacor), amrinone (Inocor)	Strengthen cardiac contraction and increase cardiac output	Headache, tremors, nervousness, fatigue, palpitations, nausea, vomiting, anxiety, flushing	Inform client to report anginal pain. Observe for dysrhythmias. Monitor BP, pulse, respirations, intake, output, and weight.
digoxin (Lanoxin)	Increase contraction of cardiac muscle	Visual disturbances, diaphoresis, confusion	Take apical pulse for 1 full minute before giving. Note rate and rhythm. Withhold if pulse is below 60 or above 110 beats/min. Do not administer with an antacid. Monitor serum levels for possible toxicity.
Combined Alpha- and Beta-Adrenergic Activity			
epinephrine (Adrenalin), dopamine (Intropin)	Strengthen myocardial contraction, increase cardiac rate and output	Nervousness, anxiety, tremors, headache, weakness, nausea, vomiting, palpitations	Protect from light. Do not use discolored solutions. Monitor BP, pulse, respirations, intake, and output. Check blood glucose levels, which may increase.
Non-adrenergic Vasoconstrictor			
vasopressin (antidiuretic hormone)	Increases arterial blood pressure and improves organ perfusion when norepinephrine and dopamine are ineffective	Decreased cardiac output, intestinal ischemia, hypertension and rebound hypotension when discontinued, angina in clients with coronary artery disease, water intoxication, pulmonary edema	Assess baseline vital signs and monitor throughout infusion. Doses greater than 0.04Units/minute may lead to cardiac arrest. Keep emergency medications, such as nitroglycerin and antiarrhythmics, available in case angina, myocardial infarction, or dysrhythmias develop. Monitor urine output and specific gravity. Assess levels of consciousness and mentation for signs of water intoxication.

Drugs with beta-adrenergic activity that increase heart rate and improve the force of heart contraction are **positive inotropic agents** (*inotropic* means affecting the force of muscular contraction). Digoxin (Lanoxin), isoproterenol (Isuprel), dobutamine (Dobutrex), milrinone (Primacor), and amrinone (Inocor) are examples.

Many drugs have combined alpha- and beta-adrenergic effects. Epinephrine is an example and is the drug of choice in anaphylactic shock. Dopamine also has combined actions. Anaphylactic shock also may be treated with an antihistamine, ACTH, or adrenal corticosteroids to counter the allergen. Other drug categories, such as antidysrhythmics and drugs that reduce peripheral vascular resistance, such as calcium channel blockers, angiotensin-converting enzyme inhibitors, and vasodilators such as the nitrates, are appropriate for cardiogenic shock.

In 2001, the U. S. Food and Drug Administration approved drotrecogin alfa (Xigris) for the treatment of severe sepsis. When given to the sickest septic clients, drotrecogin alfa reduced the death rate from 44% to 29% (Eli Lilly and Company, 2007). The prognosis is even better the earlier the drug is given. Drotrecogin alfa is a recombinant form of a human protein that has antithrombotic, profibrinolytic, and anti-inflammatory effects. The combination of actions prevents microcirculatory problems that decrease blood flow and oxygen to cells and combats the profound hypotension associated with the inflammatory response. Serious bleeding is a side effect that can be managed with blood transfusions.

Mechanical Devices

Mechanical devices help improve cardiac output or redistribute blood. Those used in the treatment of cardiogenic shock include the intra-aortic balloon pump (IABP) and ventricular assist device (VAD; see Chap. 28). First responders (paramedics) use a pneumatic antishock garment (PASG), also called *military antishock trousers* (MAST), which redistributes blood from the lower extremities to the central circulation. The use of PASGs, however, is somewhat controversial because (1) incorrect application or removal is life-threatening, (2) poor outcomes have occurred when such garments have been used indiscriminately to manage types of shock other than hypovolemic, and (3) their application lengthens the time between the field treatment of the client and transport to a trauma center (Peitzman et al., 2007).

Currently, there are two justifications for their use: (1) to control hemorrhage and hypotension resulting from pelvic fractures, and (2) to compensate for severe hypovolemia after intra-abdominal trauma en route to the operating room (National Association of EMS Physicians, 2000). Consensus is that PASGs are contraindicated in uncontrolled hemorrhage outside the area covered by the garment, pulmonary edema, rupture of the diaphragm, dysfunction of the left ventricle, intrathoracic hemorrhage, and severe injuries of the central nervous system.

Although there are reservations concerning PASGs, a new type of antishock garment known as Dyna Med Anti-Shock Trousers (DMAST) has been developed in cooperation with the National Aeronautics and Space Administration (NASA) Research Center. In contrast to PASGs, the DMAST is noninflatable, uses lower pressures to promote central circulation, and can be applied in less than 60 seconds (Fig. 17-4).

Prognosis and Complications

When shock is treated adequately and promptly, the client usually recovers. Recovery may be tenuous, however, because of secondary complications, which almost always result directly from tissue hypoxia and organ **ischemia**, reduced oxygenation. Life-threatening complications include kidney failure, neurologic deficits, bleeding disorders such as disseminated intravascular coagulation, acute respiratory distress syndrome (see Chap. 21), stress ulcers, and sepsis that can lead to multiple organ dysfunction (see Chap. 12).

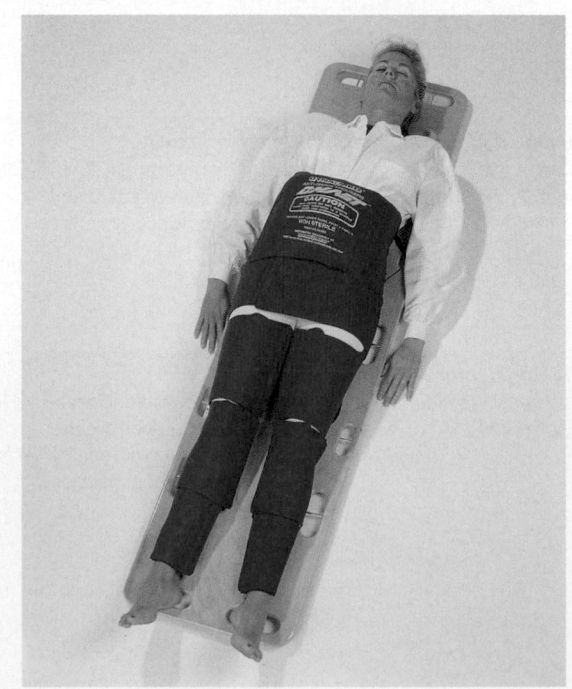

FIGURE 17-4. Dyna Med Anti-Shock Trousers (DMAST).

Nursing Process for the Client in Shock

Regardless of the cause, prolonged shock is incompatible with life. In few instances is the careful attention to nursing practices and principles more important than in the management of a client in impending or actual shock.

Assessment

Assess for early signs of shock and report such findings to the physician immediately. Check vital signs on initial contact and frequently thereafter to closely monitor the client's condition. An automatic BP device may be substituted for manual assessments. Observe skin color and temperature and assess the rate and quality of radial and peripheral pulses. Monitor urine output and determine respiratory rate and effort to detect evidence of dyspnea or airway obstruction resulting from edema, which accompanies anaphylactic shock. Inspect for bleeding or other causes that may explain the developing symptoms of shock. Determine level of consciousness and orientation status regularly to detect changes. In cases of suspected cardiogenic shock, auscultate the chest for abnormal lung and heart sounds. Check laboratory test results for evidence of low RBCs and hemoglobin, findings that correlate with hypovolemic shock. An elevated white blood cell count supports septic shock. Analysis of ABG findings is essential for evidence of hypoxemia and metabolic acidosis. Elevated serum lactate levels suggest lactic acidosis precipitated by sepsis and septic shock. Apply a pulse oximeter to monitor SpO_2. Monitor the results of coagulation tests such as platelet counts, the international normalized ratio, prothrombin time, and partial thromboplastin time.

Diagnosis, Planning, and Interventions

Implement measures to control bleeding, other fluid losses, or fluid maldistribution, and to promote blood circulation to the brain and vital organs. Support of breathing is necessary to ensure adequate blood oxygenation. Use measures to maintain normal body temperature and implement medical therapy as directed. Other care includes, but is not limited to, the following:

▶ **Decreased Cardiac Output** related to (specify) blood loss, impaired fluid distribution, impaired circulation, inadequate heart contraction, massive vasodilatation

▶ **Expected Outcome:** Cardiac output will be of adequate volume, as evidenced by heart rate between 60 and 100 beats/minute, systolic BP near 119 mm Hg, urine output greater than 35 to 50 mL/hour, alert mental status, and warm, dry skin.

- Restrict activity to total rest. *Rest decreases cellular oxygen requirements, which already are compromised in shock. Inactivity reduces heart rate, allowing the heart to fill with more blood between contractions. The force of heart contraction, which promotes cardiac output, is related to myocardial stretch as the heart fills with blood.*
- Establish at least one and preferably two IV sites with large-gauge catheters. *Access to the intravascular fluid compartment ensures quick replacement of circulating fluid. Cardiac output depends on circulating volume and adequate contraction of heart muscle. Emergency medications usually are administered*

by the IV route. *If the client is volume depleted, IV fluid therapy with or without whole blood or packed cells may be necessary.*

- Administer IV fluids or blood products at the prescribed rate, ensuring patency of the IV catheter(s). *IV fluids replace fluid lost or trapped in the interstitial space. Administration of whole blood or packed cells increases tissue and cellular oxygenation. IV fluids are delivered through a high-volume infusion device at 1 L in 10 to 15 minutes in severe hemorrhage; type O negative blood is transfused until type-specific blood is available (Weil, 2007).*
- Administer prescribed vasopressor or inotropic drugs. *They can raise BP, increase the force of heart contraction, and promote blood circulation to the kidneys to ensure waste excretion.*
- Measure fluid intake and compare with voided urine output; obtain a medical order for insertion of an indwelling catheter if hourly urine output measurements are necessary. *Urine output above 35 to 50 mL/hour or 500 mL/day indicates that kidney perfusion is sufficient to ensure the excretion of toxic wastes. Urinary volume aids in the evaluation of the effectiveness of therapeutic interventions.*

▶ **Impaired Tissue Perfusion** related to reduced cardiac output secondary to blood loss, heart failure, altered body fluid distribution, vasodilatation, and bradycardia secondary to neurologic trauma or adverse effects from central nervous system depressants

▶ **Expected Outcomes:** (1) Systolic BP will be at least 90 mm Hg, with hourly urine output 50 mL or greater. (2) Peripheral pulses will be strong. (3) Capillary refill time will be between 2 and 3 seconds. (4) Skin will be warm. (5) Client will be alert and oriented.

- Control frank bleeding by applying direct pressure to the site. *Pressure compresses the area and slows blood loss from the vascular system.*
- Maintain client in a supine position with legs elevated 12 inches (higher than the heart) unless there is head injury, heart failure, increased intracranial pressure, possible spinal cord injury, or dyspnea. *Elevating the legs promotes blood perfusion to heart, lungs, and brain.*
- In cases of shock accompanied by lung congestion, raise client's upper body to approximately 45° and lower extremities approximately 15°. *Elevating the upper body lowers the diaphragm and provides more room for lung expansion and gas exchange. Elevating the head reduces intracranial pressure. Elevating the legs promotes blood perfusion to heart, lungs, and brain.*
- Administer oxygen by the medically prescribed method and percentage. *Administration at higher percentages than in room air increases the oxygen bound to hemoglobin and dissolved in blood so that cells can maintain aerobic metabolism.*
- Collaborate with the physician about alternative techniques to control internal bleeding such as esophageal gastric balloon tamponade with a Sengstaken-Blakemore tube (see Chap. 48) used to manage bleeding esophageal varices. *An internally inflated balloon is used to apply internal pressure to esophageal and gastric areas of venous bleeding that are impossible to reach manually.*
- Increase the rate of IV fluid infusion if BP falls during deflation of the PASG. *Increasing the circulating fluid volume maintains BP.*

- Implement measures to reduce the work of the heart in cardiogenic heart failure, such as administering diuretics, vasodilators, and antidysrhythmics. *A heart in failure is best supported by reducing the volume it must circulate, decreasing the arterial resistance that it must overcome to eject blood, and slowing the heart to reduce its oxygen requirements.*
- Prepare the client in cardiogenic shock for insertion of an intra-aortic balloon pump (IABP) or ventricular assist device (VAD). *Mechanically supporting or enhancing natural heart contractions improves cardiac output and tissue perfusion (see Chap. 29).*
- Immobilize possible spinal injuries and splint fractures. *Reducing complications from trauma can minimize the potential for neurogenic and hypovolemic shock.*

▶ **Impaired Gas Exchange** related to edema of the airway secondary to a severe allergic reaction leading to anaphylactic shock

▶ **Expected Outcomes:** (1) SpO$_2$ level will be at least 90%, PaO$_2$ will be 80 to 100 mm Hg, and PaCO$_2$ will be 35 to 45 mm Hg. (2) Airway will be patent, respiratory rate will be no more than 24 breaths/minute at rest, and breathing will be quiet and effortless.

- Assist with the insertion of an artificial airway and ventilatory support (see Chap. 21). *Intubation facilitates maintenance of a patent airway; artificial ventilation ensures that respiratory gases enter and leave the lungs.*
- Suction the airway when secretions compromise gas exchange. *Suctioning removes fluid that occupies space in the airways needed for the movement and exchange of gases.*
- Administer prescribed adrenergic, bronchodilating, anti-inflammatory, and antihistamine medications. *Drug therapy helps to improve the potential for gas exchange.*

▶ **Hypothermia** related to hemorrhage

▶ **Expected Outcome:** Body temperature will be restored to normal range.

- Keep client dry and covered. *Measures that prevent evaporation and heat loss from radiation interfere with the loss of body heat.*
- Raise the room temperature to approximately 80°F. *Using the physics of convection, warming the environment can raise body temperature.*
- Place client on a warming blanket or direct warming lights to the client's body. *Conduction and radiation transfer heat.*
- Keep client's head covered with a turban made of stockinette or other material. *Body heat is lost in significant amounts from the head; covering the head reduces heat loss.*
- Warm IV solutions and blood products. *Warmed infusions raise the temperature of tissues where they are circulated.*
- Warm the humidified air that is mixed with oxygen during mechanical ventilation. *Inhalation of warmed air increases core body temperature.*

▶ **Hyperthermia** related to altered temperature regulation secondary to sepsis

▶ **Expected Outcome:** Body temperature will be reduced to normal range.

- Administer prescribed antipyretics. *They block the production of prostaglandins, which elevate the temperature set point within the hypothalamus.*
- Place client on a cooling mattress. *Contact with a cool surface lowers body temperature.*
- Control shivering. *Shivering increases body heat through the contraction of skeletal and pilomotor muscles in the skin.*
- Administer a tepid sponge bath. *Body temperature is lowered when the heat of the skin vaporizes water.*
- Administer prescribed antibiotics. *They reduce or destroy pathogens responsible for sepsis.*

Evaluation of Expected Outcomes

Vital signs are stable. Tissue perfusion is satisfactory, as evidenced by adequate urine output; strong, palpable peripheral pulses; warm, dry skin; and intact sensorium. Capillary refill is immediate. ABGs are within normal range. Blood pH is between 7.35 and 7.45. The client is normothermic. ●

CRITICAL THINKING EXERCISES

1. Which types of shock usually are accompanied by warm skin rather than cool skin?
2. In which type of shock does the client manifest a slow rather than a rapid heart rate?
3. Although all forms of shock are serious, which type of shock do you feel would have the best outcome? Support your answer with rationales.
4. Explain reasons that make septic shock the type of shock with the highest mortality.

NCLEX-STYLE REVIEW QUESTIONS

1. A nurse stops to assist at a severe car accident and notes a large pool of blood under the body of a victim. Which type of shock is the client most likely to develop?
   1. Hypovolemic shock
   2. Anaphylactic shock
   3. Septic shock
   4. Distributive shock
2. Which of the following are signs manifested by a client in most types of shock? Select all that apply.
   1. Flushed, warm skin
   2. Low urine output
   3. Bradycardia
   4. Tachypnea
   5. Hypotension
   6. Weak pulse
3. A nursing home resident is admitted to the hospital with a diagnosis of septic shock. If the physician ordered all of the following, the nurse is most correct in reviewing which laboratory test because it is most indicative of septic shock?
   1. Red blood cell count
   2. White blood cell count
   3. Arterial blood gas results
   4. Prothrombin time

4. Which of the following factors is most essential for the nurse to assess to determine the presence of shock?
1. Client's age
2. Client's weight
3. Client's previous blood pressure
4. Client's previous pulse pressure

5. A client in septic shock has been diagnosed with hyperthermia. Which of the following nursing interventions is most appropriate?
1. Keep the client dry and covered.
2. Keep the client's head covered.
3. Give prescribed vasopressor or inotropic drugs.
4. Administer a tepid sponge bath.

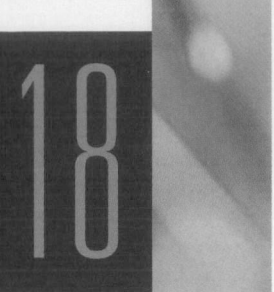

18

Caring for Clients with Cancer

Words To Know

alopecia
antineoplastic
apheresis
benign
brachytherapy
cancer
carcinogenesis
carcinogens
chemotherapy
engraftment
extravasation
gene therapy
immunotherapy
leukopenia
malignant
metastasis
myelosuppression
neoplasms
neutropenia
oncology nursing
radiation therapy
stomatitis
thrombocytopenia
tumor-specific antigen
vesicants
xerostomia

Learning Objectives

On completion of this chapter, you will be able to:

1. Discuss the pathophysiology and etiology of cancer.
2. Compare benign and malignant tumors.
3. Name factors that contribute to the development of cancer.
4. Identify the warning signs of cancer.
5. Describe ways to reduce risks of cancer.
6. Explain methods for diagnosing cancer.
7. Describe systems for staging and grading malignant tumors.
8. Differentiate various treatments and methods for managing cancer.
9. Discuss various adverse effects that occur with cancer treatments and methods used to treat those effects.
10. Describe emotions associated with the diagnosis of cancer.
11. Use the nursing process as a framework for caring for clients with cancer.

Cancer is characterized by abnormal, unrelated cell proliferation. Cancerous tumors invade healthy tissues and compete with normal cells for oxygen, nutrients, and space. The nursing specialty related to care of clients with cancer is **oncology nursing**. However, nurses in all settings care for clients of all ages with cancer, a complex and challenging endeavor. A diagnosis of cancer is frightening to most people, although reactions depend on the particular diagnosis, location, stage, treatment, effects on bodily functions, and prognosis.

UNDERSTANDING CANCER

Pathophysiology

The cell is the basic structural unit in plants and animals. Differentiated cells work together to perform specific functions. Cell regeneration occurs through cell division and reproduction. Abnormal changes in cells develop for many reasons. These abnormal cells reproduce in the same way as normal cells, but they do not have the regulatory mechanisms to control growth. Thus, abnormal cell growth proliferates in an uncontrolled and unrestricted way.

New growths of abnormal tissue are called **neoplasms** or *tumors*. Table 18-1 classifies tumor cells. The first part of the tumor's name indicates the particular cell or tissue. The suffix *-oma* indicates it is a tumor. Four main tumor classifications according to tissue type are *carcinomas* (cancers originating from epithelial cells), *lymphomas* (cancers originating from organs that fight infection), *leukemias* (cancers originating from organs that form blood), and *sarcomas* (cancers originating from connective tissue, such as bone or muscle). Tumors also are classified according to their cell of origin and whether their growth is **benign**, not invasive or spreading, or **malignant**, invasive and capable of spreading (Table 18-2).

TABLE 18-1 Classification of Tumor Cells

ORIGIN	MALIGNANT	BENIGN
Skin	Basal cell carcinoma	
	Squamous cell carcinoma	Papilloma
	Malignant melanoma	Nevus (mole)
Epithelium	Adenocarcinoma	Adenoma
Muscle	Myosarcoma	Myoma
Connective tissue		
Fibrous tissue	Fibrosarcoma	Fibroma
Adipose (fatty) tissue	Liposarcoma	Lipoma
Cartilage	Chondrosarcoma	Chondroma
Bone	Osteosarcoma	Osteoma
Nerve tissue	Neurogenic sarcoma	Neuroma
	Neuroblastoma glioblastoma	Ganglioneuroma glioma
Bone marrow	Multiple myeloma leukemia	

Benign tumors remain at their site of development. They may grow large, but their growth rate is slower than that of malignant tumors. They usually do not cause death unless their location impairs the function of a vital organ, such as the brain. On the other hand, malignant tumors have uncontrolled growth and, unless completely removed, are likely to undergo **metastasis** (spreading). Cancer can metastasize by direct extension to adjacent tissues, from lymph vessels into the tissues adjacent to lymphatic vessels, by transport from blood or lymph systems, and by diffusion within a body cavity. Specific malignant cells also have a special affinity for binding with molecules in certain tissues (Smeltzer et al., 2008). The *primary site* is the area where malignant cells first form. The *secondary* or metastatic sites are regions to which cancer cells have spread. These malignant cells seed on the surfaces of other body tissues/organs. Metastasis is one of cancer's most discouraging characteristics because even one malignant cell can give rise to a metastatic lesion in a distant part of the body. Metastatic tumors are treated aggressively when possible to improve quality of life and lengthen survival time. Cancer is known to spread to the lymph nodes that drain the tumor area. When a malignant tumor is removed, lymph node dissection usually also is done, along with a wide excision of the tumor.

Carcinogenesis is the process of malignant transformation (Smeltzer et al., 2008). The initial (*initiation*) process involves **carcinogens** (factors that contribute to the development of cancer; see discussion below) that alter the genetic structure of DNA within the cells. Repeated exposure to carcinogens (*promotion*) transforms the genetic information so that cells begin to produce mutant cell populations. The final step involves malignant behavior (*progression*), in which malignant cells demonstrate an ability to invade adjacent tissues and metastasize.

Etiology

Cancer is the second leading cause of death in the United States, where one half of all men and one third of all women will develop cancer at some point during their lives (American Cancer Society, 2007). Lung cancers account for the most

TABLE 18-2 Characteristics of Benign and Malignant Neoplasms

CHARACTERISTICS	BENIGN	MALIGNANT
Cell characteristics	Well-differentiated cells that resemble normal cells of the tissue from which the tumor originated	Undifferentiated cells that often bear little resemblance to the normal cells of the tissue from which they arose
Mode of growth	Grows by expansion and does not infiltrate the surrounding tissues; usually encapsulated	Grows at the periphery and sends out processes that infiltrate and destroy the surrounding tissues
Rate of growth	Rate of growth is usually slow	Rate of growth is variable and depends on level of differentiation; the more anaplastic the tumor, the faster the growth
Metastasis	Does not spread by metastasis	Gains access to the blood and lymphatic channels and metastasizes to other areas of the body
General effects	Is usually a localized phenomenon that does not cause generalized effects unless its location interferes with vital functions	Often causes generalized effects, such as anemia, weakness, and weight loss
Tissue destruction	Does not usually cause tissue damage unless it interferes with blood flow	Often causes extensive tissue damage as the tumor outgrows its blood supply or encroaches on blood flow to the area; may also produce substances that cause cell damage
Ability to cause death	Does not usually cause death unless its location interferes with vital functions	Usually causes death unless growth can be controlled

From Porth, C.M. (2008). *Pathophysiology: Concepts of altered health states* (8th ed.). Philadelphia, PA: Lippincott Williams & Wilkins.

cancer-related deaths in both men and women. Common cancers in men include prostate, lung, and colon. Breast, lung, and colon cancer most commonly affect women.

Damage to cellular deoxyribonucleic acid (DNA) causes cancer cells to develop. In many cases, the body repairs such damage; in cancer cells, the DNA remains damaged. Inherited cancers occur when the damaged DNA is passed to the next generation. Carcinogens include chemical agents, environmental factors, dietary substances, viruses, defective genes, and medically prescribed interventions.

Chemical agents in the environment are believed to account for 75% of all cancers. The effects of tobacco smoke and nicotine, as well as chewing tobacco, are related to cancers of the lung, mouth, throat, neck, esophagus, pancreas, cervix, and bladder. Prolonged exposure to chemicals such as asbestos and coal dust is associated with some cancers. Chemical substances in workplaces can cause cancer. Potential chemical substances include aromatic amines and aniline dyes; pesticides and formaldehydes; arsenic, soot, and tars; asbestos; benzene; betel nut and lime; cadmium; chromium compounds; nickel and zinc ores; wood dust; beryllium compounds; and polyvinyl chloride (Smeltzer et al., 2008). Organs most affected are the lungs, liver, and kidneys, because they are involved with biotransformation and excretion of chemicals.

Environmental factors include prolonged exposures to sunlight, radiation, and pollutants. Electromagnetic fields from microwaves, power lines, and cellular phones are other possible carcinogens, although study results related to such factors are conflicting. People who live in the vicinity of nuclear power plants appear to have a higher incidence of leukemia, multiple myeloma, and lung, bone, breast, or thyroid cancers.

Gerontologic Considerations

- Prolonged, cumulative exposure of older adults to sunlight over many years may contribute to an increased risk for skin cancers such as basal cell and squamous cell carcinomas.

Diet is an important variable. What a person fails to consume is as important as what he or she does consume (Box 18-1). Foods high in fat and those smoked or preserved with salt, alcohol, or nitrates are associated with an increased cancer risk. Foods believed to reduce cancer risk are high in fiber, cruciferous (e.g., cabbage, broccoli), and high in carotene (e.g., winter squash, carrots, and cantaloupe). Vitamins A, C, and E also seem to have anticancer value. There is some evidence that obesity is associated with endometrial and postmenopausal breast cancers, as well as colon, gallbladder, and kidney cancers (Smeltzer et al., 2008).

Viruses and bacteria are implicated in many cancers. The cell changes that a virus incorporates into the genetic information may cause cancerous cells to form. An example of a viral connection to cancer is Kaposi's sarcoma, which is associated with human immunodeficiency virus (HIV; see Chap. 35). *Helicobacter pylori* (see Chap. 45) is associated with gastric cancers.

Defective genes are responsible for diverse cancers. Some types of leukemia, retinoblastoma (an eye tumor in

---

BOX 18-1 **Diet Modifications for Reducing the Risk of Cancer**

- Decrease intake of red meat.
- Increase the number of servings of cruciferous vegetables such as broccoli, cabbage, and cauliflower.
- Reduce intake of processed meats that contain nitrites and nitrates as preservatives.
- Increase fiber intake.
- Decrease fat intake to 20%–30% of total daily calories.
- Increase intake of foods rich in vitamins A and C, such as fruits and yellow and leafy green vegetables.
- Reduce alcohol intake to no more than two drinks per day for men and one drink per day for women. (A drink is defined as 12 ounces of beer, 5 ounces of wine, or 1½ ounces of 80-proof distilled spirits).

From the American Cancer Society, 2008. *Common questions about diet and cancer.* Available at: http://www.cancer.org/docroot/PED/content/PED_3_2X_Common_Questions_About_Diet_and_Cancer.asp. Accessed June 2008.

---

children), and skin cancer are associated with genetic factors. Breast, prostate, and colorectal cancers are also associated with defective genes.

Medically prescribed interventions such as immunosuppressive drugs, hormone replacements, and anticancer drugs have been associated with increased incidence of cancer in people or their offspring exposed in utero.

The immune system is a major factor in the prevention or development of cancer. An intact immune system fights cancer in the following ways:

- Recognizing tumor-associated antigens (responsible for cellular changes)
- Producing macrophages and T lymphocytes that work to eliminate malignant cells
- Generating interferon in response to a viral invasion—has some ability to fight malignant cells
- Making antibodies that help to resist malignant cells
- Producing natural killer cells that destroy malignant cells

If the immune system fails to recognize malignant cells or is not stimulated in any way to fight cancer cells, tumor growth is not inhibited. Malignant cells survive and proliferate.

Assessment Findings

Signs and Symptoms

Cancer is insidious (slow growing). It initially may cause no symptoms or signs or it may be vague. This factor underscores the importance of educating clients about prevention and self-examination so that cancer can be diagnosed as early as possible. Seven warning signals of cancer should be familiar to all:

1. A change in bowel habits or bladder function
2. Sores that do not heal
3. Unusual bleeding or discharge
4. Thickening or lump in the breast or other body parts
5. Persistent indigestion or difficulty swallowing
6. A change in a wart or mole
7. A persistent nagging cough or hoarseness

Box 18-2 describes possible warning signs of specific cancers.

Better education has improved awareness of both warning signals and factors that may influence cancer development. Public education focuses on periodic physical examinations and cancer-screening programs. Healthcare providers must emphasize and teach self-examination of the breasts, testicles, and skin. Avoidance of factors that predispose people to cancer and early detection of cancer increase the chances of cure. Box 18-3 describes healthy habits that reduce cancer risk.

▶ *Stop, Think, and Respond Exercise 18-1*

Review the general warning signs for cancer and the possible warning signs for specific cancers. If you were caring for a client who complained of chronic fatigue, abdominal bloating, and intermittent constipation, what further information is needed?

BOX 18-2 | **Possible Warning Signs of Specific Types of Cancers**

- *Bladder and Kidney*: Blood in urine; pain and burning with urination; increased frequency of urination.
- *Breast*: Lump(s), thickening, and/or other physical changes in the breast; itching, redness, and/or soreness of the nipples not associated with breast-feeding or menstruation.
- *Cervical and Uterine*: Bleeding between menstrual periods; unusual discharge; painful menstrual periods; heavy periods.
- *Colon*: Rectal bleeding; blood in stool; changes in bowel habits (persistent diarrhea and/or constipation).
- *Endometrial*: Same signs as for cervical and uterine cancers above.
- *Laryngeal*: Persistent cough; hoarse throat.
- *Leukemia*: Paleness; fatigue; weight loss; repeated infections; easy bruising; bone and joint pain; nosebleeds.
- *Lung*: A persistent cough; sputum with blood; heavy chest and or chest pain.
- *Lymphoma*: Enlarged, rubbery lymph nodes; itchy; night sweats; unexplained fever and/or weight loss.
- *Mouth and Throat*: A chronic ulcer of the mouth, tongue, or throat that does not heal.
- *Ovarian*: Often no obvious symptoms until it is in later stages of development.
- *Prostate*: Weak and interrupted urine flow; continuous pain in lower back, pelvis, and/or upper thighs.
- *Skin*: Tumor or lump under the skin, resembling a wart or an ulceration that never heals; moles that change color or size; flat sores; lesions that look like moles
- *Stomach*: Indigestion and pain after eating; weight loss; blood in vomit.
- *Testicular*: Lump(s); enlargement of a testicle; thickening of the scrotum; sudden collection of fluid in the scrotum; pain and discomfort in a testicle or in the scrotum; mild ache in the lower abdomen or groin; enlargement or tenderness of the breasts.

BOX 18-3 | **Healthy Lifestyle Habits That Reduce the Risk of Cancer**

- Learn and regularly practice self-examination techniques.
- See physician or nurse practitioner regularly.
- Include periodic colon examinations, mammograms, Pap smears, testicular examinations, and prostate-specific antigen testing as indicated.
- Eat a healthy diet (see Box 18-1).
- Abstain from smoking or using tobacco products.
- Avoid overexposure to the sun; use sunscreen with SPF of 15 or greater.
- Maintain weight within suggested limits.
- Exercise regularly.
- Practice safety in the workplace to avoid exposure to chemicals and radiation.
- Limit alcohol intake.

Diagnostic Findings

A client's history, physical examination, and diagnostic studies contribute to the diagnosis of cancer. In some cases, physical examination findings are unremarkable, but the client's history is suspect. In addition, the client is evaluated for risk factors. Many diagnostic studies are used to establish a diagnosis of cancer. The physician, using information obtained during the history and physical examination, selects tests that help to establish a diagnosis.

Laboratory Tests

Specific cancers alter the chemical composition of blood and other body fluids. Specialized tests have been developed for *tumor markers*, specific proteins, antigens, hormones, genes, or enzymes that cancer cells release (Table 18-3). Normally, tumor markers are not present in or not found in large quantities in the blood.

Other laboratory tests may be useful in establishing a diagnosis. Although abnormal values do not directly indicate a malignant process, they may help to formulate a total clinical picture. For example, a complete blood count may indicate anemia in a client with possible colon cancer. Occult blood in the stool may indicate colorectal cancer.

Radiologic and Imaging Tests

Radiographic Studies. Radiographs, commonly known as x-rays, are plain films that use contrast media or specialized equipment to detect tumors in specific organs. A *contrast medium* is a substance that highlights, outlines, or provides more detail than shown in a plain film. A barium enema is an example of a study done with contrast medium.

Computed Tomography. The computed tomography (CT) scan provides three-dimensional cross-sectional views of tissues to determine tumor density, shape, size, volume, and location, as well as highlighting blood vessels that feed the tumor. The views are made through a computer and can be enlarged for better viewing. CT is useful in diagnosing many types of cancer.

Magnetic Resonance Imaging. Producing detailed sectional images, magnetic resonance imaging (MRI) uses magnetic fields to differentiate diseased tissue from healthy

TABLE 18-3 Some Specific Tumor Markers

MARKER	NORMAL VALUE	SIGNIFICANCE
Alpha-fetoprotein (α-FP)	20 ng/mL	Serum globulin normally secreted by liver cells in embryonic life. High levels seen in carcinomas of testicles, pancreas, and liver but may be elevated in acute viral hepatitis.
Carcinoembryonic antigen (CEA)	0.0–3.4 ng/mL	Glycoprotein found in fetal pancreas, liver, and colon. Increased antibody titers found in serum of persons with breast cancer, pancreatic, liver, kidney, and colon cancers. Also may be elevated in pancreatitis, acute renal failure, pneumonia, ulcerative colitis, cigarette smokers, and for no apparent reason.
Prostate-specific antigen (PSA)	Female: <0.5 ng/mL Male: 0.0–4 ng/mL	Protein tumor-specific antigen expressed from prostatic tissues, markedly increased in prostatic cancer, slightly increased in benign prostatic hyperplasia, prostatitis, prostate surgery.
CA 15-3	0–30 U/mL	Glycoprotein elevated in metastatic breast cancer; a smaller percentage is elevated in primary breast cancer, but the marker may be elevated in benign breast disease and gastrointestinal disease.
CA 19-9	0–37 U/mL	Antibody developed against tumor-associated antigens from gastrointestinal and pancreatic cancers. Shows greater specificity for pancreatic cancer than CEA.
CA 125	0–35 U/mL	Antibody developed against tumor-associated antigen, a glycoprotein found on the surface of ovarian cancer cells; also may be elevated during pregnancy, pelvic inflammatory disease; and in endometriosis.
CA 27. 29	0–38 U/mL	Membrane antigen for breast cancer screening; when associated with other marker tests, positive predictive values improve.
Human chorionic gonadotropin (hCG)	<5 mIU/mL	Glycoprotein used in diagnosis and monitoring of gestational trophoblastic diseases such as hydatidiform mole, invasive mole, and choriocarcinoma.

tissue and to study blood flow. It helps to visualize tumors hidden by bone or other structures.

Nuclear Scans. Clients ingest or receive intravenous (IV) radioisotopes (also known as tracers). After specific time intervals, images are taken of tissues that are affected by cancer or other diseases; the images distinguish tissues or portions of tissues that absorb more or less of the tracer. "Hot spots" show on an image of a tumor that has increased concentrations of the tracer, whereas "cold spots" can be the image of a tumor that has decreased concentration of the tracer. Examples of specific types of nuclear scans include the following:

- *Positron Emission Tomography.* The positron emission tomography (PET) scan uses computed cross-sectional images of increased concentrations of radioisotopes in malignant cells. It provides information about the biologic activity of the cells and assists in differentiating benign and malignant processes and responses to treatment. PET is principally used for brain, lung, colon, liver, and pancreatic cancers. A newer imaging machine incorporates PET scanning with CT scanning, allowing for better details related to increased cellular activity and thus improving the ability to locate tumors.

- *Radioimmunoconjugates.* Monoclonal antibodies, labeled with radioisotopes and injected intravenously, accumulate at the tumor site. Scanners may then visualize the tumor. These studies are particularly useful for colorectal, breast,

ovarian, head, and neck tumors. They also may be used for lymphomas and melanomas.

Ultrasound. Ultrasound uses high-frequency sound waves to detect abnormalities of a body organ or structure. The sound wave reflections (echoes) are projected on a screen and may be recorded on film. These studies help differentiate solid and cystic tumors of the abdomen, breasts, pelvis, and heart.

Fluoroscopy. Fluoroscopy studies moving body structures with the use of a continuous x-ray beam that passes through the body part being examined. The views are transmitted to a monitor so that both the body part and its motion are examined. An example of fluoroscopy is a barium study.

Other Studies

Biopsy. Tissue samples excised from the body are directly examined microscopically for malignant or premalignant processes. Tissue samples may be obtained during surgery, via insertion of a biopsy needle under local anesthesia, or by endoscopic procedures. A biopsy provides the most definitive method for diagnosing cancer. More information related to biopsies is provided in the surgery section.

Frozen Section. During some surgeries, when a tumor or node is removed, it is taken to the pathologist for immediate examination. The specimen is quickly frozen and then sliced into very thin pieces so that it may be examined under a

TABLE 18-4 TNM Staging System and Classification

SYMBOL	MEANING
T	Tumor
TX	Primary tumor cannot be measured
T0	No evidence of primary tumor
Tis	Carcinoma in situ
T1, T2, T3, T4	Progressive increase in tumor size and extension; the higher the number, the larger the tumor and the greater the extension
N	Regional lymph nodes
NX	Regional lymph nodes cannot be assessed clinically
N0	No regional lymph node involvement
N1, N2, N3	Increase in regional lymph node involvement; the higher the number, the greater the lymph node involvement
M	Distant metastasis
MX	Cannot be assessed
M0	No distant metastasis found
M1	Distant metastasis present
Example: T2, N1, M0	Indicates the primary tumor has grown and spread to regional lymph nodes but has not metastasized
GX	Grade cannot be evaluated
G1	Well-differentiated grade (the cancer cells look very similar to normal cells)
G2	Moderately well-differentiated grade
G3, G4	Poorly to very poorly differentiated grade or undifferentiated grade; G4 is linked to the worst outcome

microscope. Once the preliminary findings are known, the surgeon decides the type of surgery needed. Healthcare providers make the client aware of the possibilities before surgery.

Endoscopy. Fiberoptic instruments are flexible tubes that contain optical fibers, which enable light to travel in a straight line or at various angles and illuminate the area being examined. Specific body areas can be examined with gastroscopy, bronchoscopy, and colonoscopy. Tissue biopsies may be done if a malignancy is suspected.

Cytology. Microscopic examination of cells from various body areas may be used to diagnose malignant or premalignant disorders. Cells are obtained by needle aspiration, scraping, brushing, or sputum. An example of a cytologic test is the Papanicolaou (Pap) smear used to diagnose changes in the endometrium, cervix, and vagina (see Chap. 53).

 Gerontologic Considerations

- Normal changes of aging and/or chronic conditions may complicate cancer screening and treatment decisions in older adults. In addition, the client's values and preferences should be included for an honest discussion of anticipated risks/benefits of cancer screening and treatments. Evidence indicates that older adults receive less aggressive therapies than younger adults, leading to questions about possible ageist beliefs of healthcare providers (Oncology Nursing Society and Gerontology Ontologic Consortium, May 2007).

Staging of Tumors

Tumors are staged and graded based upon how they tend to grow and the cell type before a client is treated for cancer. The American Joint Committee on Cancer developed a staging system referred to as the TNM classification. *T* indicates the size of the tumor, *N* stands for the involvement of regional lymph nodes, and *M* refers to the presence of metastasis (Table 18-4). Once the TNM descriptions are established, they are grouped together in a simpler set of stages that include tumor size, evidence of metastasis, and lymph node involvement:

- *Stage 0:* The cancer is *in situ*, which means the malignant cells are confined to the layer of cells in which they began, with no signs of metastasis.
- *Stages I, II, and III:* Higher numbers indicate that the tumor is of greater size and/or the spread of cancer is to nearby lymph nodes and/or organs near the primary tumor.
- *Stage IV:* Cancer has invaded or metastasized to other organs of the body.

Grading of tumors involves the differentiation of the malignant cells. Basically there are two classifications: differentiated and undifferentiated. Cancer cells are evaluated in comparison with normal cells. *Well-differentiated* cells are those that most closely resemble the tissue of origin. *Undifferentiated cells* bear little resemblance to the tissue of origin. Cell differentiation is graded from I to IV. The higher the number, the less differentiated is the cell type. Tumors with poorly differentiated cells are graded IV; these tumors are very aggressive and unpredictable, and the prognosis usually is not good. Grade IV tumors do not respond well to cancer treatments.

TREATMENT OF CANCER

Three basic methods are used to treat cancer: (1) surgery, (2) radiation therapy, and (3) chemotherapy. Other methods, such as bone marrow transplantation and stem cell transplants, are used for selected cancers. Immunotherapy, gene therapy, and other alternative therapies also may be used. Cancer frequently is treated with a combination of therapies using standardized protocols.

Surgery

Surgery continues to be a primary method for diagnosing, staging, and treating cancer. Newer and less invasive surgical techniques allow for removal of tumors while preserving as much normal tissue and function as possible (American Cancer Society, 2008). Surgery may range from tumor excision alone to extensive excision, including removal of the tumor and adjacent structures such as bone, muscle, and lymph nodes. The type and extent of surgery depend on the extent of the disease, actual pathology, client's age and physical condition, and anticipated results. When tumors are confined and have not invaded vital organs, the surgery is more likely to be curative and is referred to as the *primary treatment*. In some cases, the entire tumor cannot be removed but as much of it as possible is removed, which is referred to as *debulking* or *cytoreductive surgery*.

Two types of excisions are generally done. The first is *local excision,* in which the tumor is removed along with a small margin of healthy tissue. The other type is *wide* or *radical excision,* which removes the primary tumor, lymph nodes, any involved adjacent structures, and surrounding tissues that pose a risk for metastasis. *Diagnostic and staging procedures* are also done to obtain tissue samples used to determine cell type and the extent of the cancer. Box 18-4 describes common biopsy methods.

Salvage surgery is done when there is a local recurrence of cancer. It usually is more extensive. For example, a cancerous tumor may be removed from the breast (lumpectomy). If a tumor reappears, a mastectomy most likely will be done.

Prophylactic or preventive surgery may be done if the client is at considerable risk for cancer. According to Smeltzer et al. (2008), prophylactic surgery may be done when there is a family history or genetic predisposition, ability to detect surgery at an early stage, and client acceptance of the postoperative outcome. Examples of prophylactic surgery include mastectomy and hysterectomy. Clients who choose prophylactic surgery require careful preoperative counseling and teaching so that they are fully aware of the consequences of surgery.

Surgery that helps to relieve uncomfortable symptoms or prolong life is considered *palliative*. Some palliative surgeries are used to remove excess fluid and increase comfort, such as *paracentesis* (removal of fluid from the abdominal cavity) and *thoracentesis* (removal of fluid from the chest). Surgical procedures used to relieve pain include nerve blocks, placement of epidural catheters for administration of epidural analgesics, and placement of venous access devices for administration of parenteral analgesics.

Reconstructive or *plastic surgery* may be done after extensive surgery to correct defects caused by the original surgery. Some surgeries are disfiguring or so profound that the client may have difficulty adjusting to body changes. In these cases, radiation therapy may be a better option. Other surgical interventions include the following:

- *Cryosurgery*—uses liquid nitrogen to freeze tissue, which destroys cells
- *Electrosurgery*—uses electric current to destroy tumor cells
- *Laser* (light amplification by stimulated emission of radiation) *surgery*—uses photoablation and photocoagulation lasers to aim light and energy aimed directly at an exact tissue location and depth to vaporize cancer cells, destroying tissue or sealing tissues or vessels.
- *Mohs surgery (formerly called chemosurgery)*—involves shaving off one thin layer of skin, layer-by-layer. Each layer is examined microscopically. Surgery ends when all cells look normal. *Chemosurgery* involves the use of topical chemicals as layers are removed, but is not part of Mohs surgery.
- *Stereotactic radiosurgery (SRS)*—uses a single high dose of radiation therapy and very precise administration for some types of brain, head, and neck tumors (see discussion in next section)

Perioperative care is discussed in Chapter 14. Specific surgeries are addressed in separate chapters.

Radiation Therapy

Radiation therapy uses high-energy ionizing radiation, such as high-energy x-rays, gamma rays, and radioactive particles (alpha and beta particles, neutrons, and protons) to destroy cancer cells, shrink tumors, and relieve symptoms. Radiation destroys cells by breaking a strand of the DNA molecule in the cell, thereby preventing the cell from growing and dividing. Cell death can occur immediately or when the cell can no longer reproduce.

The goal of radiation therapy is to destroy malignant, rapidly dividing cells without permanently damaging surrounding healthy tissues. Although radiation therapy may also destroy some normal cells, rapidly reproducing malignant cells are more sensitive to radiation; it affects cells undergoing mitosis (cancer cells) more than cells in slower growth cycles (normal cells). Radiation therapy may be applied externally or internally, both with curative and palliative intent. Nearly 60% of all clients with cancer receive some form of radiation; about 60% of those clients are cured (Washington & Leaver, 2004).

External Radiation Therapy

External radiation therapy or external beam radiation uses high-energy x-rays aimed at a specific body location. Higher energy levels are used to achieve deeper penetration into the body. A treatment plan is developed and customized for each

---

BOX 18-4   Common Biopsy Procedures

Fine needle aspiration biopsy: A very thin needle attached to a syringe is used to extract a small amount of tissue from a tumor. Ultrasound or other imaging method may be used to guide the needle into the tumor.

Core needle biopsy: The procedure is similar to fine needle aspiration, but a slightly larger needle is used to remove some tissue. More tissue can be obtained, assuring a more accurate diagnosis.

Excisional or incisional biopsy: An incision is made to remove the entire tumor (excisional biopsy) or a small part of the tumor (incisional biopsy). The procedures can often be done with local or regional anesthesia.

client. Various types of external radiation may be used (Box 18-5), including (Smeltzer et al., 2008):

- Kilovoltage therapy devices—used for superficial lesions
- Linear accelerators and betatron machines—use higher energy x-rays to treat tumors that are deeper and spare damage to the skin
- Gamma rays—also of higher energy to deliver radiation to deeper structures
- Intraoperative radiation therapy (IORT)—used in the operating room to deliver a high-fraction single dose of radiation directly to the exposed tumor; avoids radiation exposure to skin and other tissues

External radiation therapy enables treatment of large body areas, targeting the tumor and nearby lymph nodes. Clients usually have daily radiation treatments over several weeks on an outpatient basis. Their skin is marked with a marker or tattoo to identify the reference points for the treatment plan. Clients are instructed not to wash off these

---

BOX 18-5 Types of External Radiation Therapy Procedures

Stereotactic Radiosurgery/Stereotactic Radiation Therapy (SRS)
A device called a *gamma knife* delivers large, precise radiation doses to a small tumor area. Although there is no actual surgery, the gamma knife is referred to as "surgery" because of its accuracy. Currently, this type of radiation therapy is used on brain tumors. The head must be immobilized. Angiography, CT, or MRI locates the tumor. It is hoped that this method will eventually be used on other types of cancer.

Three-Dimensional Conformal Radiation Therapy (3D-CRT)
Special computers precisely map the cancer's location. A plastic mold or cast keeps the body part stabilized so that radiation beams can be more accurately aimed from several directions. It is hoped that radiation damage to normal tissues will decrease as the radiation dose to the cancer increases.

Intensity Modulated Radiation Therapy (IMRT)
Technology similar to 3D-CRT aims photon beams from several directions. The intensity can be adjusted, allowing for a higher dose to the tumor but less to the normal tissue. The person being treated must remain absolutely still; thin casts or molds are used.

Intraoperative Radiation Therapy (IORT)
Radiation therapy is delivered directly to the tumor during surgery. It usually is used on abdominal and pelvic cancers or those cancers that are most likely to recur. IORT reduces damage to normal tissues because they can be moved out of the way during surgery and protected from radiation. The advantage is that higher doses of radiation can be delivered. The disadvantage is that clients must move from the operating room (OR) to the radiation therapy department and then back to the OR to complete the surgery.

Adapted from American Cancer Society (2008): *What's new in radiation therapy?* Available at: http://www.cancer.org/docroot/ETO/content/ETO_1_4X_Whats_new_in_radiation_therapy.asp. Accessed June 2008.

---

markings until the therapy is complete. Clients are not radioactive when receiving external beam radiation therapy.

Gerontologic Considerations

- The skin of older adults often is dry. They may experience intense itching and dryness during and after radiation therapy; therefore, additional treatment of skin problems may be necessary. Inspect the skin frequently for signs of breakdown, excessive scratching, and infection.

Internal Radiation Therapy

Internal radiation therapy (**brachytherapy**) refers to short-distance therapy. It involves the direct application of a radioactive source on or within a tumor and can deliver a high dose of radiation to a small area. The advantage of brachytherapy is that it delivers a high dose of radiation to a specific tumor, applying less radiation to adjacent normal tissues. It may be used alone or combined with surgery, chemotherapy, and external radiation therapy. The most common methods of brachytherapy include interstitial implants, intracavitary implants, and systemic therapy.

Interstitial implants and intracavitary implants use *sealed radiation sources* in the forms of needles, seeds, wires, catheters, ribbons, or capsules. In interstitial radiation therapy, the radioactive source is inserted directly into a tumor or into tissue near the tumor, such as a tumor in the head or neck. For intracavitary implants, the radioactive source is placed directly in the body cavity and an applicator holds it in place. When the implants are removed, no radioactivity is left in the body. In some cases, seeds are left in permanently, such as with prostate or brain cancer (Nevidjon & Sowers, 2000). The radioactivity of the seeds decays over several weeks or months, depending on the radioactive element's *half-life* (the time for 50% of the isotope to lose its radioactivity). Clients usually go home if they have permanent implants. Clients must stay away from other people for a few days while the radiation is most active. After the implant, they must restrict close contact with children or pregnant women to 5 minutes and no closer than 6 feet for 2 months.

A client must be hospitalized when receiving sealed radiation sources because he or she will emit radiation during therapy. Specific orders for treatment and precautions to be taken, as well as the type and dosage of the radioactive substance, time and area of insertion, type of applicator used, and when to remove the material are noted in the client's chart. If any orders are unclear, the nurse should contact the radiation oncologist or radiation safety officer. Box 18-6 lists safety measures when a client is receiving sealed radiation therapy. Everyone involved in the client's care must recognize the necessity to limit radiation exposure. The degree of possible hazard depends on the type and amount of radioactive material used. Usually, no special precautions are required when a small amount of a radioactive substance is used for diagnostic studies. If necessary, the radiation oncologist specifies precautions, informs personnel, and posts a radiation sign (Fig. 18-1).

Systemic internal radiation therapy uses *unsealed radiation sources* (radiation in a suspension or solution or

---

BOX 18-6 **Safety Measures for Protecting Healthcare Personnel and Visitors From Excessive Exposure to Radiation**

- Client is placed in private room; some rooms have walls that are lined with lead.
- Standardized sign (see Fig. 18-1) is placed on door to designate the room as a radiation room.
- Anyone entering the room must have knowledge of the precautions required. Children younger than age 18 and pregnant women are never permitted in the room.
- Healthcare personnel limit time spent in the room and limit distance from source of radiation by working as far from the source of radiation as possible.
- The physician and radiation safety personnel are notified if the sealed sources become dislodged.
- When the client has unsealed sources, gloves must be worn at all times. Policies regarding disposal of body fluids and contaminated articles such as dressings must be adhered to.

---

radiopharmaceutical therapy), such as iodine-131. These sources may be administered orally, intravenously, or into a body cavity. Various body parts take up these sources in doses sufficient to treat cancer or, if received in small amounts, to diagnose cancer. This type of radiation has systemic effects and is excreted primarily in urine, but also through saliva, sweat, and feces. As an example, the half-life for iodine-131 is 8.05 days (Nevidjon & Sowers, 2000). To reduce exposure, clients are asked to:

- Wash hands carefully after going to the bathroom.
- Flush toilet several times after each use.
- Use separate eating utensils and towels.
- Wash laundry separately.
- Drink plenty of fluids to help flush radioactive substances away.
- Avoid kissing and sexual contact.

A more recently developed method of brachytherapy, known as Selective Internal Radiation Therapy (SIRT),

FIGURE 18-1. International radiation symbol. (From International Atomic Energy Agency [IAEA], www.iaea.org.)

delivers millions of microscopic radioactive beads via a hepatic pump targeted directly to the malignant tissue to treat tumors from the inside out. The surrounding tissue is relatively unaffected. This type of therapy is effective for shrinking tumors of the liver and improving quality of life.

Expected side effects may result from the destruction of normal cells in the area being irradiated and are specific to the anatomic site treated. They include the following:

- **Alopecia** (hair loss)
- Erythema (local redness and inflammation of the skin)
- Desquamation (shedding of epidermis, which can be dry or moist)
- Alterations in oral mucosa, including **stomatitis** (inflammation of the mouth), **xerostomia** (dryness of the mouth), change or loss in taste, and decreased salivation
- Anorexia (loss of appetite)
- Nausea and vomiting
- Diarrhea
- Cystitis (inflammation of the bladder)
- Pneumonitis (inflammation of the lungs)
- Fatigue
- **Myelosuppression** (depression of bone marrow function) if marrow-producing sites are irradiated, resulting in anemia (decreased red blood cells, hemoglobin, or volume of packed red blood cells), **leukopenia** (decreased white blood cell count), and **thrombocytopenia** (decreased platelet count)

Effects of radiation are cumulative. Often the client experiences chronic or long-term side effects after completing therapy. Many times these effects result from decreased blood supply and normal tissue destruction. The changes are irreversible. Possible effects include fibrosis (abnormal formation of scar tissue) in the small intestine, lungs, and bladder; cataracts; disturbances in blood cell formation; sterility; and new cancers.

 Pharmacologic Considerations

- Drugs may be ordered for other adverse effects during radiation therapy: aspirin or acetaminophen for fever, antibiotics for infection, and various ointments and creams (applied exactly as prescribed) for skin irritation.

Radiation Safety

The National Committee on Radiation Protection and Measurements publishes guides for radiation safety. The effects of long-term and short-term exposures must be considered. The latent period between the exposure and the accumulated biologic effect often is long, and great care is taken to protect occupationally exposed workers from radiation injury that can accumulate over years. Pregnant women should avoid exposure to radioactive substances. Nursing Guidelines 18-1 provide standard interventions for clients receiving radiation therapy. When nurses provide information, clients need to know the type and duration of treatment, what is required of the client, possible side effects, skin and mouth care, nutritional and dietary

NURSING GUIDELINES 18-1

Managing Clients Receiving Radiation Therapy

- Provide information regarding the safety of radiation: effects on others, effects on tumor, and side effects related to radiation.
- Teach client about the actual procedure of external or internal radiation therapy.
- Explain the need for optimal nutritional intake.
- Perform additional client and family teaching related to protecting the skin and mucous membranes (see Client and Family Teaching 18-1).
- Protect the skin from irritation.
- Assess skin and mucous membranes for changes, particularly the areas being treated. Effects of radiation on skin include redness, tanning, peeling, itching, hair loss, and decreased perspiration.
- Cleanse the client's skin with mild soap (be careful not to wash radiation marks) and tepid water.

- Moisturize with mild, water-based lubricant lotions.
- Maintain intact oral mucous membranes.
- Assess lesions—culture as necessary.
- Monitor client for signs of bone marrow suppression: decreased leukocyte, erythrocyte, and platelet counts.
- Assess for signs of bleeding; assess lesions and culture as necessary.
- Monitor for signs and symptoms related to area of irradiation: cerebral edema, malabsorption, pleural effusion, pneumonitis, esophagitis, cystitis, and urethritis.
- Encourage client to share fears and anxieties related to radiation therapy.
- Inform client that fatigue is a common effect of radiation therapy.

concerns, and precautions needed. Client and Family Teaching 18-1 provides additional teaching points.

When radioisotopes are used to treat cancer, three safety principles must always be kept in mind: time, distance, and shielding (where applicable).

Time
Time refers to the length of exposure. The less time spent in the vicinity of a radioactive substance, the less radiation is received. Healthcare personnel must plan carefully and work quickly and efficiently to spend minimal time at the bedside. Clients are placed in private rooms. Healthcare personnel who are involved in the care of the client wear dosimeter badges. Careful psychological preparation helps the client accept the limited amount of nursing time. Visitors are limited to 30 minutes per day.

Distance
Distance refers to the length in feet between the person entering the room and the radioactive source (client). The inverse square law applies to radiation exposure. The rate of exposure varies inversely to the square of the distance from the source (client). For example, nurses standing 4 feet from the source of radiation receive 25% of the radiation they would receive if they stood 2 feet from the source. Visitors must maintain a distance of at least 6 feet from the client.

Shielding
Shielding is the use of any type of material to decrease the radiation that reaches an area. The material usually used is lead, such as lead-lined gloves and lead aprons. Other materials, such as concrete walls, are capable of shielding.

Chemotherapy

Chemotherapy uses **antineoplastic** agents to treat cancer cells locally and systemically. These agents may be used alone or combined with other therapies to cure cancer, prevent it from metastasizing, slow its growth, destroy tumor cells that have metastasized, or relieve symptoms.

Client and Family Teaching 18-1
Radiation Therapy

The nurse instructs clients who receive radiation therapy on an outpatient basis as follows:

- Be aware that effects of radiation on skin include redness, tanning, peeling, itching, hair loss, and decreased perspiration.
- Avoid using ointments or creams on the area receiving radiation therapy unless prescribed or instructed to by a physician or radiation therapist.
- Wear loose, cotton clothing to avoid irritating the irradiated areas of skin.
- Avoid extremes of heat or cold, including heating pads, heat lamps, ultraviolet light, diathermy, whirlpool, sauna, steam baths, or direct sunlight.
- Protect skin from sun exposure, chlorine, and wind.
- Report any blistering.
- If receiving radiation to the head or scalp, avoid shampooing with harsh shampoos (baby or mild shampoo is acceptable), tinting, permanent waving, hair dryers, curling irons, and any hair products or treatments unless approved by the physician or radiation therapist.
- Bathe carefully. Avoid using soap and friction over the irradiated area. Do not wash off skin markings because they serve as guides for setting and adjusting the treatment machine over the area to be radiated.
- Shave with an electric razor.
- Report oral burning, pain, open lesions, or problems with swallowing; use nonalcoholic mouthwash.
- Brush with soft toothbrush and avoid electric toothbrushes.
- Floss gently; use WaterPik cautiously.
- Keep lips moist with lip balm.
- Avoid alcoholic beverages, very hot drinks and foods, highly seasoned foods, acidic foods, and tobacco products.

Antineoplastic agents work by interfering with cellular function and reproduction. They are classified according to their relationship to cell division and reproduction. Healthy and malignant cells follow a cell-cycle pattern, which involves division of the cell and reproduction of two identical daughter cells. There are distinct phases:

- G1 phase—A growth phase during which ribonucleic acid (RNA) and protein synthesis occur.
- S phase—RNA synthesis is complete, and DNA synthesis occurs.
- G2 phase—Another growth phase in which DNA synthesis is complete, and cell mitosis begins.
- M phase—Mitosis or cell division takes place.
- G0 phase—This is a dormant or resting phase, which can occur after mitosis and during the G1 phase.

Cell Cycle–Specific Drugs

Antineoplastic drugs are most effective during cell division. Cell cycle–specific drugs are used to treat rapidly growing tumors because they attack cancer cells when they enter a specific phase of cell reproduction. Most chemotherapeutic agents affect cells in the S phase by interfering with RNA and DNA synthesis. Others are more specific to the M phase. Chemotherapy is administered in multiple, repeated doses to produce a greater cell kill and to halt the growth of tumor cells. Examples of cell cycle–specific agents are topoisomerase I inhibitors, antimetabolites, mitotic spindle poisons, and some of the miscellaneous agents (Drug Therapy Table 18-1).

Cell Cycle–Nonspecific Drugs

Cell cycle–nonspecific drugs are effective during any phase of the cell cycle, whether reproducing or resting. They are used for large, slow-growing tumors. The amount of drug given is more important than the frequency. Cell cycle–nonspecific drugs have more prolonged effects on cells, which results in cell damage and destruction. They often are given in combination with cell cycle–specific drugs, and also may be combined with or follow radiation therapy. Examples of cell cycle–nonspecific agents are alkylating agents, antitumor antibiotics, nitrosoureas, hormones, and some of the miscellaneous agents (see Drug Therapy Table 18-1).

Routes and Devices for Administration of Chemotherapy

Chemotherapeutic drugs are administered by several routes. The most common are the oral and IV routes, but they also may be given intramuscularly, intraperitoneally, intraarterially, intrapleurally, topically, intrathecally, or directly into a cavity. Dosage is based on the client's total body surface area, prior responses to chemotherapy and other therapies, function of the major organs, and the client's health status. IV administration is monitored closely to prevent the drug from leaking into surrounding tissues, referred to as **extravasation**. Inspecting the site daily for signs of thrombophlebitis, such as tenderness, pain, swelling, and induration, is also important. Most antineoplastic agents can be very irritating. Blistering and tissue necrosis are possible effects of extravasation. If a client complains of burning or pain during the chemotherapy infusion, the drug must be discontinued.

Vesicants are particularly damaging antineoplastics, in that they cause tissue necrosis of underlying tendons, nerves, and blood vessels. Sloughing and ulceration of the skin may be so severe that the client needs skin grafts. If vesicants are being administered, there are protocols for treating the extravasation (Box 18-7). In addition, there are safety issues for the nurse who administers chemotherapy (Box 18-8).

Various vascular devices are used to administer chemotherapy and are particularly beneficial for long-term chemotherapy. The client does not have to endure repeated venipunctures. In addition, they are beneficial when a client has poor veins. One method used is the insertion of venous access devices, which are special catheters inserted into a peripheral or central vein so that the catheter tip is located in the superior vena cava or right atrium. Examples include peripheral indwelling catheters (PIC lines), peripherally inserted central catheters (PICC lines), and external catheters (Hickman catheters, Broviac catheters). Another type is the implanted vascular access device (IVAC), also referred to as a *port*. A metal or plastic port encloses a self-sealing silicone rubber septum. The port is surgically implanted subcutaneously. A silicone catheter attached to the port is threaded subcutaneously to the right atrium. To access the port, a needle is inserted in the self-sealing septum of the port.

Chemotherapy infusion pumps are used for some cancers. They provide constant infusion of an antineoplastic drug directly into the cancerous organ. A small pump (similar in size to a hockey puck) is surgically implanted subcutaneously in the abdomen or attached externally.

Adverse Effects of Chemotherapy

Some clients experience little discomfort or few adverse effects. Others have a wide range of symptoms. The tissues most susceptible to chemotherapy are those with rapidly growing cells, such as epithelial tissue, hair follicles, and bone marrow. Chemotherapy can potentially harm all body systems. Common adverse effects associated with chemotherapy are as follows:

- Nausea and vomiting are common during the first 24 hours after chemotherapy administration; use of concurrent antiemetics helps to reduce the incidence and severity.
- Stomatitis and mouth soreness or ulceration may result from destruction to the epithelial layer.
- Alopecia develops because chemotherapy affects rapidly growing cells of the hair follicles.
- Myelosuppression results from inhibition of the manufacture of red and white blood cells and platelets. Severe anemia, bleeding tendencies, leukopenia, **neutropenia** (decreased neutrophils), and thrombocytopenia are possible if bone marrow depression is profound. Blood transfusions may be necessary, as well as protection of the client from infections.
- Fatigue results from the aforementioned effects, the chemotherapy itself, and the increased metabolic rate that accompanies cell destruction.

Antineoplastic drugs are potentially toxic. Nurses must be thoroughly familiar with their adverse effects and toxicity. The dose or length of treatment depends, in some cases, on the client's response to therapy.

DRUG THERAPY TABLE 18-1 Antineoplastic Agents

Drug Category and Examples	Mechanism of Action	Cell Cycle Specificity	Side Effects*
Alkylating Agents busulfan, carboplatin, chlorambucil, cisplatin, cyclophosphamide, dacarbazine, hexamethyl melamine, ifosfamide, melphalan, nitrogen mustard, thiotepa	Alter DNA structure by misreading DNA code, initiating breaks in the DNA molecule, cross-linking DNA strands	Cell cycle–nonspecific	Bone marrow suppression, nausea, vomiting, cystitis (cyclophosphamide, ifosfamide), stomatitis, alopecia, gonadal suppression, renal toxicity (cisplatin)
Nitrosoureas carmustine (BCNU), lomustine (CCNU), semustine (methyl CCNU), streptozocin	Similar to the alkylating agents; cross the blood–brain barrier	Cell cycle–nonspecific	Delayed and cumulative myelosuppression, especially thrombocytopenia; nausea, vomiting
Topoisomerase I Inhibitors irinotecan, topotecan	Induce breaks in the DNA strand by binding to enzyme topoisomerase I, preventing cells from dividing	Cell cycle–specific	Bone marrow suppression, diarrhea, nausea, vomiting, hepatotoxicity
Antimetabolites 5-azacytidine, cytarabine, edatrexate fludarabine, 5-fluorouracil (5-FU), FUDR, gemcitabine, hydroxyurea, leustatin, 6-mercaptopurine, methotrexate, pentostatin, 6-thioguanine	Interfere with the biosynthesis of metabolites or nucleic acids necessary for RNA and DNA synthesis	Cell cycle–specific (S phase)	Nausea, vomiting, diarrhea, bone marrow suppression, proctitis, stomatitis, renal toxicity (methotrexate), hepatotoxicity
Antitumor Antibiotics bleomycin, dactinomycin, daunorubicin, doxorubicin (Adriamycin), idarubicin, mitomycin, mitoxantrone, plicamycin	Interfere with DNA synthesis by binding DNA; prevent RNA synthesis	Cell cycle–nonspecific	Bone marrow suppression, nausea, vomiting, alopecia, anorexia, cardiac toxicity (daunorubicin, doxorubicin)
Mitotic Spindle Poisons Plant alkaloids. etoposide, teniposide, vinblastine, vincristine (VCR), vindesine, vinorelbine	Arrest metaphase by inhibiting mitotic tubular formation (spindle); inhibit DNA and protein synthesis	Cell cycle–specific (M phase)	Bone marrow suppression (mild with VCR), neuropathies (VCR), stomatitis
Taxanes: paclitaxel, docetaxel	Arrest metaphase by inhibiting tubulin depolymerization	Cell cycle–specific (M phase)	Bradycardia, hypersensitivity reactions, bone marrow suppression, alopecia, neuropathies
Hormonal Agents androgens and antiandrogens, estrogens and antiestrogens, progestins and antiprogestins, aromatase inhibitors, luteinizing hormone–releasing hormone analogs, steroids	Bind to hormone receptor sites that alter cellular growth; block binding of estrogens to receptor sites (antiestrogens); inhibit RNA synthesis; suppress aromatase of P450 system, which decreases estrogen level	Cell cycle–nonspecific	Hypercalcemia, jaundice, increased appetite, masculinization, feminization, sodium and fluid retention, nausea, vomiting, hot flashes, vaginal dryness
Miscellaneous Agents asparaginase, procarbazine	Unknown or too complex to categorize	Varies	Anorexia, nausea, vomiting, bone marrow suppression, hepatotoxicity, anaphylaxis, hypotension, altered glucose metabolism

*Note special nursing consideration: Any chemotherapy drug administered via IV route is accompanied by a high risk for thrombophlebitis. Assess the IV site daily for tenderness, pain, swelling, and induration.

BOX 18-7 Treatment of Extravasation

General Measures
- Stop administration of drug.
- Leave needle in place.
- Gently aspirate residual drug and blood into tubing or needle.
- Inject neutralizing solution such as sodium thiosulfate, hyaluronidase, or sodium bicarbonate to reduce tissue damage. Selection of neutralizing agent depends on vesicant.

Vesicant-Specific Measures
- Doxorubicin
  - Elevate and rest extremity.
  - Apply topical cooling for 24 hours.
  - Give hydrocortisone as ordered.
- Nitrogen mustard
  - Apply cold compresses.
  - Administer thiosulfate as ordered.
- Vinca alkaloids (vinblastine, vincristine, vindesine)
  - Apply warm compresses.
  - Do not apply ice—increases skin toxicity.
  - Administer hyaluronidase as ordered.
- Mitomycin
  - Apply ice.
  - Administer dimethylsulfoxide (DMSO) as ordered.

Pharmacologic Considerations

- If stomatitis pain is severe, an analgesic may be prescribed, or topical agents may be prescribed to promote eating.

- Monitor the client taking an antineoplastic agent for symptoms of gout, which include increased uric acid levels, joint pain, and edema. Allopurinol may be prescribed to decrease the uric acid level. Encourage the client to increase fluid intake (up to 2000 mL/day) if his or her condition permits.

- Most antineoplastic agents are teratogenic. Female clients taking these drugs must use birth control measures throughout therapy. If a client suspects pregnancy, she must notify the primary healthcare provider immediately.

BOX 18-8 Safety Measures When Administering Chemotherapy

- Prepare chemotherapy in designated biologic safety area.
- Use gloves when handling chemotherapy drugs and excretions from clients receiving chemotherapy.
- Wear disposable long-sleeved gowns when preparing and administering chemotherapy.
- Use Luer-lok fittings on IV tubing used in delivering chemotherapy.
- Dispose of all equipment used in chemotherapy preparation and administration in designated containers.
- Dispose of all chemotherapy wastes as hazardous materials.

NURSING GUIDELINES 18-2

Managing Clients Receiving Chemotherapy

- Monitor client for symptoms of anaphylactic reaction: urticaria (hives), pruritus (itching), sensation of lump in throat, shortness of breath, wheezing.
- Assess for electrolyte imbalances (see Chap. 16).
- Prevent extravasation of vesicant drugs. Implement measures to treat extravasation of vesicant medications if it occurs (see Box 18-7).
- Assess for signs of bone marrow depression: decreased white and red blood cell, granulocyte, and platelet counts.
- Assess for signs of bleeding and infection.
- Monitor for signs of renal insufficiency:

  - Elevated urine specific gravity
  - Abnormal electrolyte values
  - Insufficient urine output (<30 mL/hour)
  - Elevated blood pressure, BUN (blood urea nitrogen), and serum creatinine
- Inform client about the reasons for nausea and vomiting.
- Administer antiemetics before and during administration of chemotherapy, or as indicated.
- Assess oral mucosa for dryness, redness, swelling, lesions, ulcerations, viscous (sticky) saliva, or white patches.

Nursing Management
Nursing management of the client receiving chemotherapy varies depending on the drug, dose administered, and route used (Nursing Guidelines 18-2). Client teaching is an important nursing responsibility (Client and Family Teaching 18-2). In addition, there are recommended safety procedures that nurses must follow when caring for clients receiving chemotherapy (Box 18-9).

▶ Stop, Think, and Respond Exercise 18-2
You are assigned to a client who was recently diagnosed with lung cancer. Surgery is planned, followed by chemotherapy. Your client says that he has heard that large doses of vitamin C would contribute to postoperative healing and also would enhance chemotherapy. He asks if he should begin megadoses of vitamin C. How should you respond?

Bone Marrow and Peripheral Blood Stem Cell Transplantation
Cancers that are very sensitive to high doses of chemotherapy and radiation therapy may be treated with stem cell transplantation. *Stem cell transplantation* replaced the older method of obtaining bone marrow from donors. Stem cells refer to young (immature) cells called *hematopoietic (blood-forming) stem cells*. They are used to replace bone marrow destroyed by cancer or cancer treatments. For some types of cancer, such as leukemia, the white blood cells from the donor identify any remaining cancer cells and destroy them. In addition, the new stem cells develop into healthy

Client and Family Teaching 18-2
Chemotherapy

The nurse instructs clients receiving chemotherapy on an outpatient basis to:

- Keep all appointments for chemotherapy treatments.
- If hair loss is anticipated, purchase a wig, cap, or scarf before therapy begins. Hair usually begins to grow again within 4 to 6 months after therapy; new growth may have a slightly different color and texture.
- Make the following dietary modifications:
  - Eat small, frequent meals.
  - Eat slowly.
  - Eat cool, bland foods and liquids.
  - Suck on hard candy during chemotherapy if taste alterations occur.
  - Avoid hot or very cold liquids, food with fat and fiber, spicy foods, and caffeine.
- Increase fluid intake to 2500 to 3000 mL/day (unless contraindicated or advised by physician).
- Report excessive fluid loss or gain, change in level of consciousness, increased weakness or ataxia (lack of muscle coordination), paresthesia (numbness, prickling, or tingling), seizures, persistent headache, muscle cramps or twitching, nausea and vomiting, or diarrhea.
- Have periodic evaluations and examinations as recommended.

---

blood cells, settling into bone marrow and producing new blood cells, a process referred to as **engraftment**. For adults, stem cells are generally obtained from bone marrow or peripheral blood. Umbilical cord blood is also a source for children, but inadequate for adults. There are three types of stem cell transplants: autologous, allogeneic, and syngeneic.

BOX 18-9 **Safety Precautions When Caring for Clients Receiving Chemotherapy**

- Use protective equipment (gloves and gowns) when handling body fluids; wear a face shield if splashing is possible.
- Encourage clients to use toilets if possible. In addition, ask male clients to sit to void instead of standing to reduce splashing.
- Protect the skin of incontinent clients with moisture-barrier products to the perineal and perirectal area.
- Flush toilets with lids down to avoid aerolization of chemotherapeutic agents.
- Dispose of contaminated equipment and linens in appropriate, leak-proof, and puncture-proof containers.
- Dispose of all chemotherapy wastes as hazardous materials.
- Maintain chemotherapy precautions for 48 hours postadministration of chemotherapy

(Adapted from Polovich, M. White, J. M. & Keller, L.O. Eds. [2005]. *Chemotherapy and biotherapy: Guidelines and recommendations for practice.* [2nd ed.]. Pittsburgh, PA: Oncology Nursing Society.)

Autologous Stem Cell Transplantation

Autologous stem cell transplants come from the client himself or herself, either from bone marrow or circulating blood. The stem cells are removed before other cancer treatments and frozen to be reinfused after cancer treatment is complete. Clients having autologous stem cell transplants do not require immunosuppressant drugs. There is a risk, however, that tumor cells are present in the stem cells and therefore the blood may be treated with chemotherapy prior to reinfusion.

Allogeneic Stem Cell Transplantation

Allogeneic stem cell transplantation uses stem cells from a donor whose tissue type matches the client's. The donor can donate to additional stem cells if required, because they are usually obtained from peripheral blood. Donor stem cells produce immune cells that can destroy any remaining cancer cells. Engraftment may not occur with allogeneic transplantation. Recipients are also prone to infections carried by the donor, although donors are carefully screened. Another risk is graft-versus-host disease (GVHD), in which the donor cells produce new immune cells that attack the recipient's body. Allogeneic transplants are primarily used for cancers affecting blood, such as leukemia, and other bone marrow disorders.

A newer type of allogeneic transplant is called a *reduced-intensity transplant*, also called a *non-myeloablative transplant* or *mini-transplant*. Clients having this type of transplant have reduced doses of chemotherapy and/or radiation therapy. The donor cells are then able to assist in the destruction of tumor cells and with time replace the recipient's own bone marrow cells. This method is most effective in clients whose disease is slower-growing and less extensive.

Syngeneic Stem Cell Transplantation

Syngeneic stem cell transplantation is rarely done because it is possible only if the client has an identical twin with identical tissue type. Syngeneic stem cell transplant does not cause GVHD, a distinct advantage. However, all cancer cells must be destroyed prior to transplantation, because the donor stem cells cannot destroy any remaining cancer cells.

Nursing Management

Nursing management for the client receiving any form of stem cell transplantation is crucial. Before the procedure, the nurse thoroughly evaluates the client's physical condition, organ function, nutritional status, complete blood studies (including assessment for past antigen exposure such as HIV, hepatitis, or cytomegalovirus), and psychosocial status.

Prior to receiving stem cells, clients usually undergo intensive chemotherapy and possibly whole-body radiation. Because a large amount of tissue is treated, nausea, vomiting, diarrhea, and stomatitis are common. In addition, until transplanted stem cells begin to multiply and make new blood cells, usually within two to six weeks, these clients have no physiologic means to fight infection, which makes them very prone to infection. They are at high risk for dying from sepsis and bleeding before engraftment. Nurses must monitor clients closely and take measures to prevent infection. Clients also are at risk for bleeding, renal complications, and liver damage.

After stem cell transplantation, the nurse closely monitors the client for at least 3 months because complications related to the transplant are still possible. Getting blood counts back to normal may take 6 to 12 months. Infections are possible, as is GVHD. The client's immune system is deficient because of the chemotherapy, radiation therapy, and decreased blood counts. Throughout the entire process, the nurse assesses the client's psychological status. Clients experience many mood swings and need support and assistance throughout this process. Their families and significant others also require support. See Nursing Guidelines 18-3.

Immunotherapy

Immunotherapy either uses the client's own immune system to stimulate the body's natural immunity to restrict and destroy cancer cells or involves receiving immune system components to do the same. Many of these treatments are new and in trial phases and are not widely used. Research demonstrates that the body's natural immunity, a process of surveillance, recognition, and attack on foreign cells, is a defense against cancer (see Chap. 33). The purpose of immunotherapy is to manipulate the natural immune response by restoring, modifying, stimulating, or augmenting the natural defenses.

Results of immunotherapy vary. Some clients respond well; others have little or no response. Usually, immunotherapy is not instituted until surgery, radiation therapy, and chemotherapy have failed. The three types of immunotherapy include nonspecific immunotherapy, monoclonal antibody immunotherapy, and cancer vaccines.

Nonspecific Immunotherapy

Nonspecific immunotherapy uses nonspecific agents such as bacille Calmette-Guérin (BCG) or *Corynebacterium parvum* to act as antigens to stimulate an immune response. When these agents are injected into a client, the goal is for the stimulated immune system to destroy malignant growths. These agents are useful in treating localized melanoma and localized bladder cancer (Smeltzer et al., 2008). Adjuvants are substances used in addition to the primary treatment to boost the immune system and enhance the main treatment.

Cytokines, another type of nonspecific immunotherapy, are substances that immune system cells produce to enhance the immune system. Common types of cytokines are interferons, interleukin-2, colony-stimulating factors, and tumor necrosis factor (Table 18-5). In general, they stimulate the immune system or assist in inhibiting tumor growth. Side effects include flulike symptoms, gastrointestinal (GI) disturbances, alopecia, and low blood counts (Nevidjon & Sowers, 2000).

Monoclonal Antibody Immunotherapy

Monoclonal antibody immunotherapy uses monoclonal antibodies (MAbs or MoAbs). Previously, MAbs were produced entirely by injecting specific tumor cells into mice. The tumor cells acted as antigens to which the mice produced antibodies. The antibody-producing cells were fused with a cancer cell that then produced more antibodies in a culture medium. These cells are referred to as *hybridomas*. The desired antibodies were harvested from the hybridomas, and purified and prepared for use in humans. However, in some

NURSING GUIDELINES 18-3

Managing Clients Receiving Stem Cell Transplantation

- Assess client's nutritional status.
- Monitor for signs and symptoms of infection and renal insufficiency (see Nursing Guidelines 18-2).
- Assess for signs and symptoms of graft-versus-host disease (GVHD): irritability, pulmonary infiltration, hepatitis, enlarged spleen, enlarged lymph nodes, anemia, sepsis, diarrhea, maculopapular rash, and skin desquamation.
- Implement Standard Precautions and use protective isolation as needed.
- Assist with thorough hygiene.
- Review information related to prevention of infection, signs of rejection, importance of adherence to medical regimens and follow-up, medication instructions, and dietary needs.
- Encourage client to discuss anxieties and fears.
- Provide ongoing information about recovery phase and status of recuperation.

people the immune system sensed the mice antibodies as foreign and mounted an allergic response against them. The technology has evolved so that human antibody proteins can be used instead of mice antibody proteins, which has lessened the likelihood of an allergic response.
MAbs have several uses:

- Diagnostic—radioactive substances are attached to the MAbs to detect tumors (radioimmunodetection)
- To purge remaining tumor cells from blood or bone marrow for clients who are having a peripheral stem cell transplant
- Cancer therapy—used directly to destroy tumor cells

The goal is for the MAbs to overwhelm and destroy the tumor cells. Some MAbs are currently treating non-Hodgkin's lymphoma, some types of metastatic breast cancer, and some forms of leukemia. More recently some MAbs have been approved for the treatment of colorectal cancer and lung cancers. More research is being done to treat other types of cancer.

Cancer Vaccines

The development of cancer vaccines is relatively new and mostly still in clinical trials. The vaccines that are approved for use in the United States include the human papillomavirus (HPV), which may help prevent women from getting cervical cancer. Vaccines not yet approved are being developed to boost the immune system's ability to attack a cancer that already exists.

Hyperthermia

Hyperthermia or thermal therapy uses temperatures greater than 106.7°F (41.5°C) to destroy tumor cells. Heat is in the form of radio waves, ultrasound, microwaves, magnetic waves, hot water baths, or immersion in hot wax. Methods of delivery include extracorporeal circulators, probes, or infusion of heated chemotherapeutic agents into the blood or

TABLE 18-5 Cytokines

CYTOKINES	HOW PRODUCED	FUNCTION	USE
Interferons	Naturally occurring protein molecules produced in response to viral infections	Stimulate immune system, inhibit tumor cell growth, or both	Used to treat hairy cell leukemia, chronic myelogenous leukemia, melanoma, Kaposi's sarcoma, non-Hodgkin's lymphoma, and sometimes renal carcinoma and hematologic malignancies
Interleukins	Produced by lymphocytes and monocytes About 15 types have been identified	Signal and coordinate other cells of the immune system	Interleukin-2 (IL-2) approved for renal cell cancer and metastatic melanoma May be used in combination with chemotherapy
Hematopoietic growth factors (colony-stimulating factors)	Hormone-like substances produced by the immune system	Stimulate production of blood cells: neutrophils, RBCs, lymphocytes, platelets, erythrocytes, monocytes, and macrophages	Do not treat cancers but instead treat the toxic effects of cancer treatments on bone marrow; allow higher doses of chemotherapy with less suppression of bone marrow function Higher doses of chemotherapy may be given with less suppression of bone marrow function.
Tumor necrosis factor (TNF)	Naturally produced by macrophages, lymphocytes, astrocytes, and microglial cells of the brain	Exact mechanism of action not understood—appears to stimulate other cells in the immune response and directly kills tumor cells	Research is being done in the treatment of melanoma, lung and renal cancers, and sarcomas

directly into a cancerous organ. A client also may be immersed in heated water or paraffin. Tumor cells are more sensitive to the harmful effects of high temperatures for several reasons (Smeltzer et al., 2008):

- Malignant cells cannot repair themselves.
- Many tumor cells lack sufficient blood supply to provide the increased need for oxygen required during hyperthermia.
- The tumor blood vessels are inadequate for dispersing heat.
- Hyperthermia appears to stimulate the immune system.

Hyperthermia is combined with other therapies. When used with radiation therapy, the tumor cells are more sensitive to the radiation and cannot repair themselves at all. Hyperthermia alters cell membrane permeability so that uptake of chemotherapy is increased. It enhances the function of immunotherapeutic agents. Clients receiving hyperthermia may experience local burns and tissue damage, electrolyte imbalances, fatigue, GI disturbances, and neuropathies.

Photodynamic Therapy

Photodynamic therapy (PDT) or phototherapy uses a photoactive drug, porfimer (Photofrin) that, when administered intravenously, is stored in higher concentrations in malignant tissues. Several days later, laser light applied to the tumor activates the drug and destroys the malignant cells. Damage to healthy tissues is minimal (Smeltzer et al., 2008; Smith, 2004). This type of therapy requires a commitment from clients to protect their eyes and skin from sunlight and bright indoor light for at least 30 days after receiving the porfimer. Failure to comply can result in a severe sunburn-like reaction that may require hospitalization to treat pain, dehy-

dration, and local skin care. This therapy is currently used to treat lung cancer.

Gene Therapy

Scientists have theorized that many cancers result from gene alterations. Strategies to confront this problem include **gene therapy**, which involves replacing altered genes with correct genes, inhibiting defective genes, and introducing substances that destroy genes or cancer cells (Smeltzer et al., 2008). Scientists predict that gene therapy will play a significant role in the future prediction, diagnosis, and treatment of cancer. It is currently being investigated in the treatment of brain tumors, melanoma, and renal, breast, ovarian, lung, and colon cancers.

Apoptosis or "Programmed Cell Death"

Apoptosis is a new approach to cancer treatment currently under investigation. Research demonstrates that many types of cancer cells need an anti–cell-death molecule (called BCL-2) to survive. Theorists conclude that specifically designed drugs could inhibit the BCL-2 molecules; cancer cells then would die. Apoptosis is a normal process that rids the body of cells that are no longer needed or are damaged or abnormal in some way. Although cancer cells are abnormal and have damaged DNA, the BCL-2 molecules block the self-destruct checks. Future research will focus on developing drugs that silence the BCL-2 molecules.

Clinical Trials

Clinical trials provide methods to test new treatments for specific cancers. The trials may involve a new drug, a new combination of existing drugs, or new therapies. The process for new treatments to become accepted practice is lengthy. Before testing on humans, there is testing on laboratory animals to ascertain safety and effectiveness. After animal testing, there are four phases:

1. Phase I—Treatment is given to a small group of people to determine dosing, schedule for treatment, and toxicity. Participants usually are clients for whom standard treatment has been ineffective. Clients are fully aware of the trial's experimental nature.
2. Phase II—Treatment is given to a larger group of clients to further determine effectiveness with specific cancers and to get better information about dosing, side effects, and toxicity. Clients are similar to the clients selected for phase I.
3. Phase III—If the treatment appears effective in phase II, then a larger number of clients are selected and compared with clients receiving accepted treatments for a particular type of cancer. At this point, the new treatment has had significant testing and review.
4. Phase IV—In this phase, there is further testing of newly accepted treatments for other uses, dosing, and toxicity.

Complementary and Alternative Therapies

Complementary and alternative therapies includes imagery, medicinal therapy, special diets, and mystical and spiritual approaches (Table 18-6). Alternative therapy also refers to treatments that are not proven to be effective in treating a particular disease but are used instead of conventional treatments. Examples include hydrogen peroxide therapy, hydrazine sulfate, and Essiac tea (American Cancer Society, 2007).

It is difficult for healthcare professionals to condone unconventional therapies because many of the methods do not have a scientific foundation. There also are legal and ethical implications if healthcare personnel participate in unaccepted treatments. Information that they provide to clients must be factual and understandable. Although some alternative methods have successfully augmented conventional treatments, many methods have no positive effects and indeed some actually are harmful.

NURSING MANAGEMENT OF THE CLIENT WITH CANCER

Managing the care of clients with cancer is challenging. The diagnosis itself implies multiple problems, and the treatments result in many secondary problems. This care requires a comprehensive plan designed to meet or assist the client and family's needs (Nursing Care Plan 18-1).

Pain is a major problem for clients with cancer (see Chap. 11). Sources of pain include bone metastasis; nerve compression; obstructed blood vessels, lymph systems, or organs; inflammation; ulceration; infection; or necrosis. Pain ranges from dull and aching to sharp, unrelenting, and throbbing.

Clients with cancer also experience fatigue, which is a frequent side effect of cancer treatments that rest fails to relieve. Fatigued clients are constantly weary, lack energy, and often feel too weak to carry out normal activities. The nurse must assess the client for other stressors that contribute to fatigue, such as pain, nausea, fear, and lack of adequate support. The nurse works with other healthcare team members to treat the client's fatigue.

Another major problem for clients with cancer is infection. Many factors predispose clients with cancer to infection: impaired skin and mucous membranes, chemotherapy, radiation therapy, and other therapies, the malignancy itself, malnutrition, medications, invasive catheters and IV lines, contaminated equipment, age, chronic illness, and prolonged hospitalization (Smeltzer et al., 2008). Clients should avoid crowds and people with colds, flu, or other infectious diseases. Nurses must provide scrupulous care to clients with cancer and monitor for signs and symptoms of infection, including fever, elevated white blood cell counts, pain, redness, swelling, and drainage.

See Nutrition Notes 18-1 for nutrition considerations. Other potential issues that clients with cancer face are as follows:

- Bleeding—may result from bone marrow suppression, medications that interfere with coagulation and platelet function, or both

TABLE 18-6 Complementray and Alternative Methods of Cancer Treatment

METHOD	DESCRIPTION
Imagery, relaxation techniques, stress reduction exercises, yoga, biofeedback, massage, and music therapy	These methods are used to reduce pain, promote relaxation, and enhance conventional treatment methods based on beliefs that there is a link between the immune system and cancer and that these methods boost the immune system's ability to fight the cancer cells.
Medicinal agents	Many "cures" for cancer have been concocted from plants, herbs, flowers, and fluids of humans and animals. Although a few merit scientific investigation, many are considered quackery. The use of vitamins, minerals, proteins, and other ingredients is advocated for treatment of many cancers and prevention or treatment of side effects.
Special diets	Many diet regimens are advocated as treatment for certain cancers or as adjuncts to treatment. Examples include organic foods, macrobiotic diets, and particular foods that reportedly kill cancer cells.
Spiritual methods	These methods are derived from powers of faith that people believe will help them to overcome cancer. Examples include faith healing, laying on of hands, and prayer.

Nutrition Notes 18-1
The Client with Cancer

- Improving the client's nutritional status not only improves quality of life, but may make cancer cells more susceptible to treatment. Good nutrition also promotes rehabilitation, may lessen the effects of treatment, and may increase the chances of survival. Conversely, poor nutritional status may potentiate the toxicity of cancer treatments.
- Malnutrition is not an inevitable consequence of cancer; once established, however, it can be difficult to reverse. To prevent malnutrition, it usually is more effective to increase the nutrient density of foods consumed rather than to expect a client to eat more food. Fortifying casseroles, beverages, cereals, and other foods with skim-milk powder, whole milk, cheese, cream cheese, peanut butter, eggs, butter, and honey increases density without increasing volume. Small, frequent feedings also are beneficial.
- Side effects of cancer and cancer therapies can devastate the client's ability to eat, which may change daily or as often as with each meal. Clients with nausea fare better with low-fat foods and "dry" meals (taking liquids between meals). Clients receiving chemotherapy should avoid eating or drinking for 1 to 2 hours after treatment to avoid nausea.
- Clients with anorexia should consume small, frequent meals. Encourage clients to view eating as part of therapy, not a voluntary activity.
- Clients with vomiting need to replenish fluids by taking water or flat beverages every 10 to 15 minutes.
- Clients who develop taste alterations from chemotherapy often complain that meat tastes "bad" or "rotten." Offer cold protein alternatives such as cheese, cottage cheese, protein beverages, and sandwiches. Assure the client that eating meat is not the only way to consume adequate protein. Sucking on hard candy during chemotherapy infusion may prevent a bitter or metallic taste.
- Clients with fatigue should rest before meals and avoid items that require a lot of chewing.
- Clients with difficulty swallowing should use gravies and sauces liberally. They may tolerate semisolid foods better than liquids. They should avoid extremely hot foods.
- A high fluid intake is necessary to promote excretion of chemotherapeutic drugs. Water, milk, fruit juices, and high-protein beverages are all good choices; clients should avoid beverages containing caffeine and limit soft drinks, which are high in empty calories.
- Clients with a sore mouth should avoid highly seasoned foods, acidic juices, salty items, and coarse breads and cereals. They may tolerate cold food and beverages better than warm items. For clients receiving palliative care, do not force feedings, weigh clients, or use nutritional support.

- Impaired skin integrity—may result from chemotherapy, radiation therapy, surgery and other invasive procedures, nutritional deficits, and incontinence
- Hair loss
- Alterations in body image

- Changes in psychological and mental status
- Grieving—coping with a cancer diagnosis and treatments is frequently overwhelming

Gerontologic Considerations

- The risk for infection with cancer may be increased in older clients because of age-related changes in the immune response. Older adults may have problems with nutrition and adequate fluid intake, possibly complicated by normal aging changes in taste sensation and appetite, especially if stomatitis occurs. Additional skin care problems and complications related to inactivity may be present. Assessment of functional abilities is crucial to determine increased fall risk. Also, because older adults are more prone to electrolyte imbalance, excessive vomiting during or after cancer treatments may result in a serious electrolyte disturbance.

Although cancer is not necessarily fatal, it does change a person's life in many ways. For those clients facing long and intense treatments and for those with few options for treatment, nurses must be supportive and guide them to resources (Smeltzer et al., 2008).

Psychological Support

The diagnosis of cancer is frightening and frequently overwhelming. Psychological support is as important as medical treatments and physical care. Clients have many reactions, ranging from anxiety, fear, and depression to feelings of guilt related to viewing cancer as a punishment for past actions or failure to practice a healthy lifestyle. They also may express anger related to the diagnosis and their inability to be in control. Clients have the right to know their diagnosis, treatment plan, and prognosis so they can make informed decisions. A client may never accept a cancer diagnosis. When provided with adequate information and supported psychologically, however, clients are more likely to face their diagnosis and be involved with their care and treatment. Families and significant others also require support.

Client and Family Teaching

Clients and their families or significant others require education to understand the diagnostic procedures, make treatment choices, participate in preventing complications, and recognize side effects and other adverse signs. Teaching focuses on:

- Medications, treatments, and procedures
- Adverse effects associated with treatment
- Possible changes in body image or function
- Resources for support
- Follow-up needed after discharge from the hospital

When developing a plan for client and family teaching, the nurse must consider facts such as the type of malignancy, treatment given, proposed treatments, client's condition, and effectiveness of the family support system. These facts will determine the areas to discuss in more detail. The nurse should be aware of any explanations or information that

NURSING CARE PLAN 18-1   The Client With Cancer

Assessment

- Assess client's level of understanding about the diagnosis, treatment, and follow-up care.
- Determine the client's strengths, coping mechanisms, response to diagnosis, and emotional and physical support systems.

- Evaluate the family's response to illness.
- Check client's overall physical condition, energy and pain levels, and nutritional and fluid status.

Nursing Diagnosis: Anxiety related to diagnosis, prognosis, treatments, changes in health status

Expected Outcome: Client demonstrates decreased anxiety.
    Refer to Chapter 68 for nursing interventions.

Evaluation of Expected Outcomes

Client and family share anxieties about diagnosis and care.

Nursing Diagnosis: Fatigue related to side effects of treatments, weakness from cancer, and physical and psychological stress

Expected Outcomes: (1) Client will participate in daily care as much as possible. (2) Client will identify measures to conserve and improve energy.

Interventions	Rationales
Identify energy level by asking client to evaluate it on a scale of 0 (not tired) to 10 (totally exhausted).	Such identification establishes current level of fatigue.
Plan care around energy level and include rest periods.	Rest reduces physical stress and conserves energy.
Encourage adequate protein and calorie intake.	It increases activity tolerance.
Encourage use of relaxation techniques and mental imagery.	They promote relaxation and reduce psychological stress.

Evaluation of Expected Outcomes

(1) Client can participate in care without becoming exhausted. (2) Client can identify need for rest.

Nursing Diagnosis: Anticipatory Grieving related to potential loss and altered role status

Expected Outcomes: Client will identify and verbalize feelings. Client will continue to make future-oriented plans, even if one day at a time. Client will verbalize understanding of the dying process.
    Refer to Chapter 10 for nursing interventions.

Evaluation of Expected Outcomes

(1) Client expresses feelings of guilt, anger, or sorrow. (2) Client plans for future one day at a time.

Nursing Diagnosis: Chronic Pain related to disease, metastasis, effects of surgery and treatments

Expected Outcomes: Client will report pain relief. Client will use relaxation methods and other alternatives to reduce pain and discomfort.
    Refer to Chapter 11 for nursing interventions.

Evaluation of Expected Outcomes

Client states that pain medications are effective.

Nursing Diagnosis: Disturbed Body Image related to side effects of treatments, weight loss, and changes in appearance

Expected Outcomes: Client will verbalize understanding of changes in appearance. Client will demonstrate coping methods and adaptation to changes he or she is experiencing.

Interventions	Rationales
Explore strengths and resources with client.	Emphasizing strengths promotes a positive self-image.
Discuss possible changes in weight and hair loss. Suggest that the client select a wig before hair loss occurs.	Planning for an event such as weight or hair loss decreases anxiety associated with a change in appearance.

NURSING CARE PLAN 18-1   **The Client With Cancer** (Continued)

Interventions	Rationales
Acknowledge client's anger, sadness, or depression.	Body image changes cause anxiety and other feelings; acknowledging such feelings assists the client to cope.
Refer client to a support group or counseling.	Support groups and counseling allow the client to share feelings and to recognize that he or she is not alone.

Evaluation of Expected Outcomes

Client states acceptance of change or loss and demonstrates ability to adjust.

Nursing Diagnosis: Imbalanced Nutrition: Less than Body Requirements related to loss of appetite, difficulty swallowing, side effects of chemotherapy, or obstruction by tumor

Expected Outcomes: Client will increase dietary intake. Client will demonstrate understanding of the need for adequate intake of nutrients and fluids.

Interventions	Rationales
Monitor daily food intake.	Such monitoring provides baseline data.
Encourage intake of sufficient calories, nutrients, and fluids (see Nursing Guidelines 18-2), offering small, frequent meals and fluids.	These measures reduce the sensation of fullness and decrease the stimulus to vomit.
Administer antiemetics as ordered before meals.	They are more effective when given before nausea.
Monitor laboratory studies for signs of dehydration, biochemical imbalances, and malnutrition.	Such monitoring reveals evidence of imbalances and assists in making needed interventions.

Evaluation of Expected Outcomes

Client demonstrates minimal weight loss and verbalizes necessity to have adequate intake.

Nursing Diagnosis: Impaired Skin Integrity and **Impaired Oral Mucous Membranes** related to immunologic deficits, effects of chemotherapy and radiation therapy, poor nutrition, immobility, and altered oral flora

Expected Outcome: Client will demonstrate measures to prevent complications from skin or tissue impairment or to promote tissue or skin healing.
  Refer to Chapter 12 for interventions.

Evaluation of Expected Outcomes

Client manages treatment for skin impairment and has minimal impairment of oral mucous membranes.

---

other healthcare providers give to the client and family. He or she also must allow time for clients to express their feelings or discuss home care. Doing so also helps identify issues the client or family does not understand.

Care of the Terminally Ill Client

Nursing management of the terminally ill client can be both physically and emotionally difficult. It must include both client and family. The nurse must carry out tasks gently to reduce the possibility of pain and discomfort and to keep the client as comfortable as possible. He or she pays attention to controlling pain, providing adequate fluid and nutrition, keeping the client warm and dry, and controlling odors (when present). An important part of nursing care is to help the client maintain dignity, despite an illness that often requires dependence on others for activities of daily living. See Chapter 10 for more information on nursing and hospice care.

CRITICAL THINKING EXERCISES

1. A client with endometrial cancer has been told that she will be treated with internal radiation therapy. Discuss what information to include in her teaching plan.

2. A client has been receiving chemotherapy while in the hospital. The RN identified a nursing diagnosis of Risk for infection related to altered immunologic response. As the LPN caring for this client, what steps should you take to minimize the client's risk of infection?

3. A client tells you that she is afraid of losing her hair related to treatment for cancer. What strategies may assist her with coping with her alopecia?

4. Often clients are most fearful of pain and pain control options when dealing with cancer. What would reassure this client?

NCLEX-STYLE REVIEW QUESTIONS

1. A client diagnosed with cancer comes to the clinic after receiving a combination of radiation and chemotherapies. She complains of nausea, vomiting, and diarrhea. The nurse should initially assess for signs and symptoms related to which of the following?
   1. Fatigue
   2. Dehydration
   3. Infection
   4. Anemia

2. At a routine clinic visit, the nurse weighs a client who has cancer and finds that he has lost 25 pounds since beginning cancer treatment. The best suggestion the nurse can make to increase the client's caloric intake is to eat which of the following?
   1. Red meat
   2. Larger portions
   3. Foods high in fat
   4. Small, frequent meals

3. A nurse instructs a group of young adults at a community center about behaviors that can decrease the risk of cancer. Which information is most applicable for this age group?

   1. Avoid smoking and prolonged sun exposure.
   2. Schedule yearly mammograms or prostate examinations.
   3. Perform self-examination techniques four times per year.
   4. Eat a diet low in salt and fat.

4. A client newly diagnosed with cancer receives external radiation therapy. Which nursing instruction regarding bathing is most appropriate?
   1. Use a soft washcloth to wash the irradiated skin.
   2. Avoid getting the irradiated skin wet.
   3. Use alcohol instead of soap on the irradiated skin.
   4. Cover the reddened irradiated area with clear plastic.

5. A client is receiving chemotherapy for cancer. After several treatments, blood studies demonstrate that the client is experiencing bone marrow suppression. The LPN can expect that the client will exhibit which of the following signs and symptoms? Select all that apply.
   1. Easy bruising
   2. Bleeding from gums
   3. Bone pain
   4. Headaches
   5. Fatigue

UNIT 5
Caring for Clients with Respiratory Disorders

19

Introduction to the Respiratory System

Words To Know

adenoids
alveoli (sing. alveolus)
bronchi (sing. bronchus)
bronchioles
carina
cilia
diaphragm
diffusion
epiglottis
ethmoidal sinuses
frontal sinuses
glottis
hilum
interstitium
larynx
lungs
maxillary sinuses
mediastinum
nasal septum
nasopharynx
oropharynx
paranasal sinuses
parietal pleura
perfusion
pharynx
pleura
pleural space
respiration
sphenoidal sinuses
thoracentesis
tonsils
trachea
turbinates (conchae)
ventilation
visceral pleura
vocal cords

Learning Objectives

On completion of this chapter, you will be able to:

1. Describe the structures of the upper and lower airways.
2. Explain the normal physiology of the respiratory system.
3. Differentiate respiration, ventilation, diffusion, and perfusion.
4. Describe oxygen transport.
5. Define forces that interfere with breathing, including airway resistance and lung compliance.
6. Identify elements of a respiratory assessment.
7. List diagnostic tests that may be performed on the respiratory tract.
8. Discuss preparation and care of clients having respiratory diagnostic procedures.

The respiratory system provides oxygen for cellular metabolic needs and removes carbon dioxide (CO_2), a waste product of cellular metabolism. Respiratory disorders and diseases are common, ranging from mild to life-threatening. Disorders that interfere with breathing or the ability to obtain sufficient oxygen greatly affect respiratory and overall health status.

RESPIRATORY ANATOMY

The respiratory system (Fig. 19-1) is divided into the upper airway and lower airway.

Upper Airway

The upper airway consists of the nose, sinuses, turbinates, pharynx, and larynx.

Nose

Nasal bones and cartilage support the external nose. The nares are the external openings of the nose. The internal nose is divided into two cavities separated by the **nasal septum.** Each nasal cavity has three passages created by the projection of turbinates or conchae from the lateral walls. The vascular and ciliated mucous lining of the nasal cavities warms and humidifies inspired air. Mucus secreted from the nasal mucosa traps

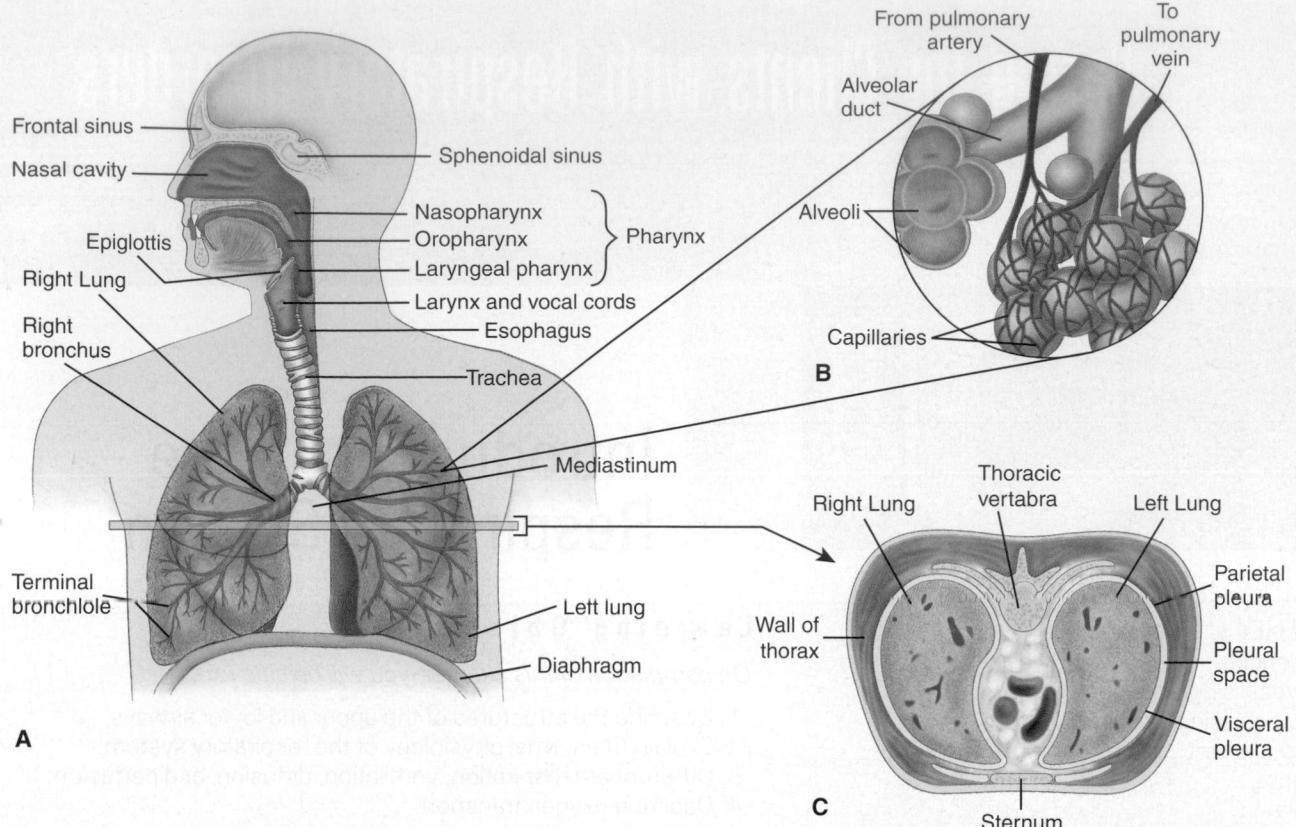

FIGURE 19-1. Major structures of the respiratory system. (**A**) Overview. (**B**) Alveoli (air sacs) of the lungs and the blood capillaries. (**C**) Transverse section through the lungs.

small particles (e.g., dust, pollen). **Cilia** (fine hairs) move the mucus to the back of the throat. This movement helps prevent irritation to and contamination of the lower airway. The nasal mucosa also contains olfactory sensory cells that are responsible for the sense of smell.

The olfactory area lies at the roof of the nose. The cribriform plate forms part of the roof of the nose and the floor of the anterior cranial fossa. Trauma or surgery in this area carries the risk of injuring or causing infection in the brain.

Paranasal Sinuses

The **paranasal sinuses** are extensions of the nasal cavity located in the surrounding facial bones (Fig. 19-2). They lighten the weight of the skull and give resonance to the voice. There are four pairs of these bony cavities. The two **frontal sinuses** lie in the frontal bone that extends above the orbital cavities. The ethmoid bone, located between the eyes, contains a honeycomb of small spaces called the **ethmoidal sinuses**. The **sphenoidal sinuses** lie behind the nasal cavity. The **maxillary sinuses** are found on either side of the nose in the maxillary bones. The maxillary sinuses are the largest sinuses and the most accessible to treatment.

The lining of the sinuses is continuous with the mucous-membrane lining of the nasal cavity. Mucus traps particles that cilia sweep toward the pharynx. Immunoglobulin A (IgA) antibodies in the mucus protect the lower respiratory tract from infection.

Turbinate Bones (Conchae)

The **turbinates** (or **conchae**) are bones that change the flow of inspired air to moisturize and warm it better. As air is inhaled, the turbinates deflect it toward the roof of the nose. They have a large, moist, and warm mucous-membrane surface that can trap almost all dust and microorganisms. They also contain sensitive nerves that detect odors or induce sneezing to remove irritating particles, such as dust or soot.

Pharynx

The **pharynx**, or throat, carries air from the nose to the larynx, and food from the mouth to the esophagus. The pharynx is divided into three continuous areas: the **nasopharynx** (near the nose and above the soft palate), the **oropharynx** (near the mouth), and the *laryngeal pharynx* (near the

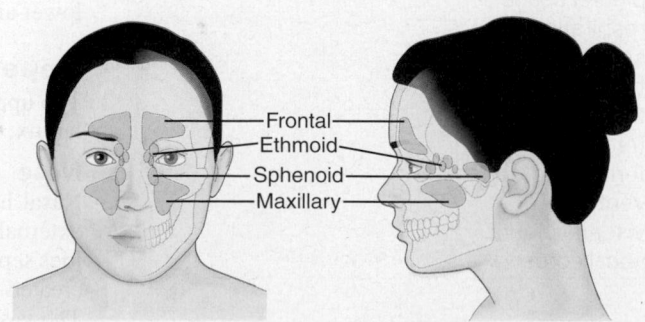

FIGURE 19-2. The paranasal sinuses.

larynx). The nasopharynx contains the adenoids and openings of the eustachian tubes. The eustachian tubes connect the pharynx to the middle ear and are the means by which upper respiratory infections spread to the middle ear. The oropharynx contains the tongue. The muscular nature of the pharynx allows for closure of the epiglottis during swallowing and relaxation of the epiglottis during respiration.

Tonsils and **adenoids**, which do not contribute to respiration but instead protect against infection, are found in the pharynx. Palatine tonsils consist of two pairs of elliptically shaped bodies of lymphoid tissue. They are located on both sides of the upper oropharynx. Adenoids, or pharyngeal tonsils, also composed of lymphoid tissue, are found in the nasopharynx. Chronic throat infections often lead to removal of the tonsils and adenoids. In adults, adenoids may shrink and become nonfunctional.

Larynx

The **larynx**, or voice box, is a cartilaginous framework between the pharynx and trachea. Its primary function is to produce sound. The larynx also protects the lower airway from foreign objects because it facilitates coughing.

Important structures in the larynx include the **epiglottis**, a cartilaginous valve flap that covers the opening to the larynx during swallowing; the **glottis**, an opening between the vocal cords; and the **vocal cords**, folds of tissue in the larynx that vibrate and produce sound as air passes through. The pharynx, palate, tongue, teeth, and lips mold the sounds made by the vocal cords into speech. Table 19-1 reviews laryngeal structures.

Lower Airway

The lower respiratory airway consists of the trachea, bronchi, bronchioles, lungs, and alveoli (see Fig. 19-1). Accessory structures include the diaphragm, rib cage, sternum, spine, muscles, and blood vessels.

Trachea

The **trachea** is a hollow tube composed of smooth muscle and supported by C-shaped cartilage. The cartilaginous rings

TABLE 19-1. Structures of the Larynx

STRUCTURE	DESCRIPTION
Epiglottis	Valve flap of cartilage that covers the opening of the larynx during swallowing
Glottis	Opening between the vocal cords in the larynx
Thyroid cartilage	Largest cartilage in the trachea; part of it forms the Adam's apple
Cricoid cartilage	Only complete cartilaginous ring in the larynx, located below the thyroid cartilage
Arytenoid cartilages	Used in vocal cord movement with the thyroid cartilage
Vocal cords	Ligaments controlled by muscular movement that produce vocal sounds

(Adapted from Smeltzer, S. C. Bare, B. G. Hinkle, J. L., & Cheever, K. H. [2008]. *Brunner & Suddarth's textbook of medical–surgical nursing* [11th ed.]. Philadelphia: Lippincott Williams & Wilkins.)

are incomplete on the posterior surface. The trachea transports air from the laryngeal pharynx to the bronchi and lungs.

Bronchi and Bronchioles

The trachea bifurcates (divides) at the **carina** (lower end of the trachea) to form the left and right **bronchi**. Stimulating the carina causes coughing and *bronchospasm* (spasm of the bronchial smooth muscle, leading to narrowing of the lumen). The right mainstem bronchus is shorter, more vertical, and larger than the left mainstem bronchus. Aspiration of foreign objects is more likely in the right mainstem bronchus and right upper lung. Mucous membrane continues to line this portion of the respiratory tract. Cilia sweep mucus and particles toward the pharynx.

The right and left mainstem bronchi divide into three secondary right bronchi and two secondary left bronchi. Each secondary bronchus supplies air to the three right lobes and two left lobes of the lung. The entrance of the bronchi to the lungs is called the **hilus**. The bronchi branch, enter each lobe, and continue to branch to form smaller bronchi and finally terminal **bronchioles** (smaller subdivisions of bronchi).

Lungs and Alveoli

The **lungs** are paired elastic structures enclosed by the thoracic cage. They contain the **alveoli**, small, clustered sacs that begin where the bronchioles end. Adult lungs contain approximately 300 million alveoli, which form most of the pulmonary mass. Each alveolus consists of a single layer of squamous epithelial cells. Capillaries surround these thin-walled alveoli and are the site of exchange of oxygen and CO_2.

The epithelium of the alveoli consists of the following types of cells:

- Type I cells—line most alveolar surfaces
- Type II cells—produce *surfactant*, a phospholipid that alters the surface tension of alveoli, preventing their collapse during expiration and limiting their expansion during inspiration
- Type III cells—destroy foreign material, such as bacteria

The **interstitium** lies between the alveoli and contains the pulmonary capillaries and elastic connective tissue. Elastic and collagen fibers allow the lungs to have *compliance*, the ability to expand. Lung expansion creates a negative or subatmospheric pressure, which keeps the lungs inflated. If air gets into the space between the lungs and the thoracic wall, the lungs will collapse.

 Gerontologic Considerations

- As adults age, the cartilage of the nasal septum increases in length and may harden, resulting in air flow changes such as septal deviations, leading to risk for obstructive apnea. Although the number of alveoli remains stable with age, the alveolar walls become thinner and contain fewer capillaries, resulting in decreased gas exchange. The lungs also lose elasticity, diminishing lung expansion and increasing dead space. Muscle tone, the cough reflex, and the number of cilia decrease. These changes place older adults at increased risk for respiratory disease.

Accessory Structures

The **diaphragm** separates the thoracic and abdominal cavities. On inspiration, the respiratory muscles contract. The diaphragm also contracts and moves downward, enlarging the thoracic space and creating a partial vacuum. On expiration, the respiratory muscles relax, and the diaphragm returns to its original position.

The **mediastinum** is a wall that divides the thoracic cavity into two halves. This wall has two layers of **pleura**, a saclike serous membrane. The **visceral pleura** covers the lung surface, whereas the **parietal pleura** covers the chest wall. Serous fluid within the **pleural space** separates and lubricates the visceral and parietal pleurae. The remaining thoracic structures are located between the two pleural layers.

RESPIRATORY PHYSIOLOGY

The main function of the respiratory system is to exchange oxygen and CO_2 between the atmospheric air and the blood and between the blood and the cells. This process is called **respiration**. Other terms related to respiration are defined in Table 19-2.

Ventilation

Ventilation is the actual movement of air in and out of the respiratory tract. Air must reach the alveoli for gas to be exchanged. This process requires a patent airway and intact and functioning respiratory muscles. Pressure gradients between atmospheric air and the alveoli enable ventilation. Air flows from an area of higher pressure to an area of lower pressure.

Mechanics of Ventilation

During inspiration, the diaphragm contracts and flattens, which expands the thoracic cage and increases the thoracic cavity. The pressure in the thorax decreases to a level below atmospheric pressure. As a result, air moves into the lungs.

TABLE 19-2. Terms Related to Respiration

TERM	DEFINITION
Ventilation	Movement of air into and out of the lungs sufficient to maintain normal arterial oxygen and carbon dioxide tensions
Inspiration	Movement of oxygen into the lungs
Expiration	Removal of carbon dioxide from the lungs
Diffusion	Transfer of a substance from an area of higher concentration or pressure to an area of lower concentration or pressure; exchange of oxygen and carbon dioxide across the alveolar-capillary membrane and at the cellular level
Perfusion	Flow of blood in the pulmonary circulation
Distribution	Delivery of atmospheric air to the separate gas exchange units in the lungs

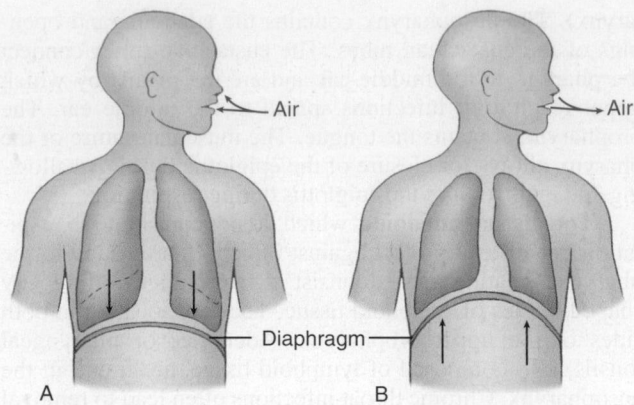

FIGURE 19-3. The mechanics of ventilation: (**A**) inspiration, (**B**) expiration.

When inspiration is complete, the diaphragm relaxes, and the lungs recoil to their original position. The size of the thoracic cavity decreases, increasing the pressure to levels greater than the atmospheric pressure. Air then flows out of the lungs into the atmosphere (Fig. 19-3).

Neurologic Control of Ventilation

Several mechanisms control ventilation. The respiratory centers in the medulla oblongata and pons control rate and depth. Central chemoreceptors in the medulla respond to changes in CO_2 levels and hydrogen ion concentrations (pH) in the cerebrospinal fluid. They convey a message to the lungs to change the depth and rate of ventilation. Peripheral chemoreceptors in the aortic arch and carotid arteries respond to changes in the pH and levels of oxygen and CO_2 in the blood. Table 19-3 describes other neurologic controls of ventilation.

Diffusion

Diffusion is the exchange of oxygen and CO_2 through the alveolar-capillary membrane. Concentration gradients determine the direction of diffusion. During inspiration, the concentration of oxygen is higher in the alveoli than in the capillaries. Therefore, oxygen diffuses from the alveoli to the capillaries and is carried to the arteries. The concentration of oxygen in the arteries is higher than that in the cells; thus, oxygen diffuses into the cells.

As cellular CO_2 gradients increase, CO_2 diffuses from the cells into the capillaries and then into the venous circulatory system. As CO_2 travels to the pulmonary circulation, its concentration is higher there than in the alveoli. Therefore, CO_2 diffuses into the alveoli.

Alveolar Respiration

Alveolar respiration determines the amount of CO_2 in the body. Increased CO_2, which is present in body fluids primarily as carbonic acid, causes the pH to decrease below the normal 7.4. Decreased CO_2 causes the pH to increase above 7.4. The pH affects the rate of alveolar respiration by a direct action of hydrogen ions on the respiratory center in the medulla oblongata.

The kidneys contribute to maintaining normal pH by excreting excess hydrogen ions, which in turn keep serum

TABLE 19-3. Neurologic Control of Respiration

CONTROL	DESCRIPTION
Hering-Breuer reflex	Stretch receptors located in the alveoli are activated during inspiration, so that inspiration is inhibited and lungs are not overdistended.
Proprioceptors	Exercise stimulates breathing. Movement activates proprioceptors located in the muscles and joints and increases ventilation.
Baroreceptors	These receptors in the aortic and carotid bodies respond to changes in arterial blood pressure (BP). Elevated arterial BP causes a reflex hypoventilation; lowered BP causes a reflex hyperventilation.

bicarbonate levels near normal. The lungs and kidneys combine to maintain the ratio of carbonic acid to bicarbonate at 1:20, fixing the pH at approximately 7.4.

In a critically ill client, various homeostatic mechanisms compensate for alterations. In an attempt to maintain normal pH, two mechanisms may occur:

- The lungs eliminate carbonic acid by blowing off more CO_2. They also conserve CO_2 by slowing respiratory volume and reabsorbing bicarbonate (HCO_3).
- The kidneys excrete more bicarbonate.

A client's condition remains compensated if the carbonic acid-to-bicarbonate ratio remains 1:20.

Disturbances in pH that involve the lungs are considered respiratory. Disturbances in pH involving other mechanisms are termed *metabolic*. At times, respiratory and metabolic disturbances coexist (see Chap. 16).

▶ **Stop, Think, and Respond Exercise 19-1**

Explain the differences between ventilation and respiration.

Transport of Gases

Oxygen transport occurs in two ways: (1) a small amount is dissolved in water in the plasma, and (2) a greater portion combines with hemoglobin in red blood cells (RBCs; oxyhemoglobin). Dissolved oxygen is the only form that can diffuse across cellular membranes. As this oxygen crosses cellular membranes, oxygen from the hemoglobin rapidly replaces it. Large amounts of oxygen are transported in the blood as oxyhemoglobin. The formula for this process is $O_2 + Hgb \rightarrow HgbO_2$.

CO_2 diffuses from the tissue cells to the blood. Bicarbonate ions are then transported to the lungs for excretion. Most of the CO_2 enters the RBCs, although some combines with hemoglobin to form carbaminohemoglobin. Most of the CO_2 combines with water in the cells and exits as bicarbonate ions (HCO_3^-), which the plasma transports to the kidneys. A small portion remains in the plasma and is called

carbonic acid. The formation of carbonic acid yields hydrogen ions (H^+). The amount of hydrogen ions determines the pH, which also determines the amount of CO_2 for the lungs to excrete. Refer to Chapter 16 for a review of acid-base balance. Briefly, acid-base imbalances are compensated in the following ways:

- Respiratory acidosis—kidneys retain more HCO_3 to raise the pH
- Respiratory alkalosis—kidneys excrete more HCO_3 to lower pH
- Metabolic acidosis—lungs "blow off" CO_2 to raise pH
- Metabolic alkalosis—lungs retain CO_2 to lower pH

Pulmonary Perfusion

Perfusion refers to blood supply to the lungs, through which the lungs receive nutrients and oxygen. The two methods of perfusion are the bronchial and pulmonary circulation.

Bronchial Circulation

The bronchial arteries, which supply blood to the trachea and bronchi, arise in the thoracic aorta and intercostal arteries. The bronchial arteries also supply the lungs' supporting tissues, nerves, and outer layers of the pulmonary arteries and veins. This circulation returns either to the left atrium through the pulmonary veins or to the superior vena cava through the bronchial and azygos veins.

The bronchial circulation does not supply the bronchioles or alveoli unless pulmonary circulation is interrupted. In that event, it will supply those areas, but the bronchioles and alveoli cannot perform their function of gas exchange (Bullock & Henze, 2000).

Pulmonary Circulation

The pulmonary artery transports venous blood from the right ventricle to the lungs. It divides into the right and left branches to supply the right and left lungs. The blood circulates through the pulmonary capillary bed, where diffusion of oxygen and CO_2 occurs. The blood then returns to the left atrium through the pulmonary veins.

Pulmonary circulation is referred to as a *low-pressure system* (Smeltzer et al., 2008). This means that gravity, alveolar pressure, and pulmonary artery pressure affect pulmonary perfusion. A person in an upright position has less perfusion to the upper lobes. If a person is in a side-lying position, perfusion is greater to the dependent side. In addition, increased alveolar pressure can cause pulmonary capillaries to narrow or collapse, affecting gas exchange. Decreased pulmonary artery pressure results in decreased perfusion to the lungs. Clients with lung and cardiovascular diseases may have decreased pulmonary perfusion.

Ventilation/Perfusion Ratio

A client's cardiopulmonary status involves several factors; in particular, the client's ventilation/perfusion ratio (V/Q ratio) indicates the effectiveness of airflow within the alveoli (ventilation) and the adequacy of gas exchange within the pulmonary capillaries (perfusion) (Ayers & Lappin, 2004). Figure 19-4 depicts normal and abnormal V/Q ratios and their implications.

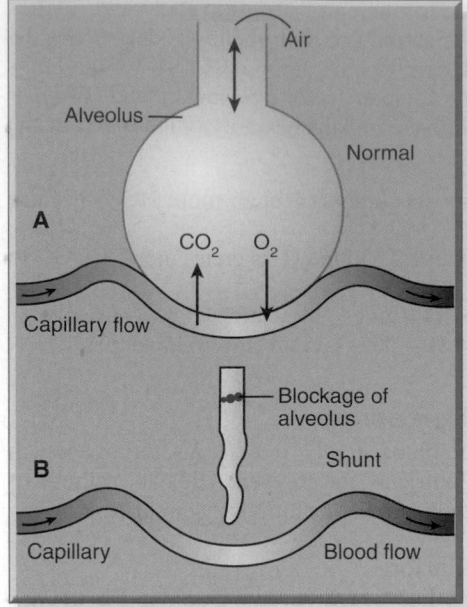
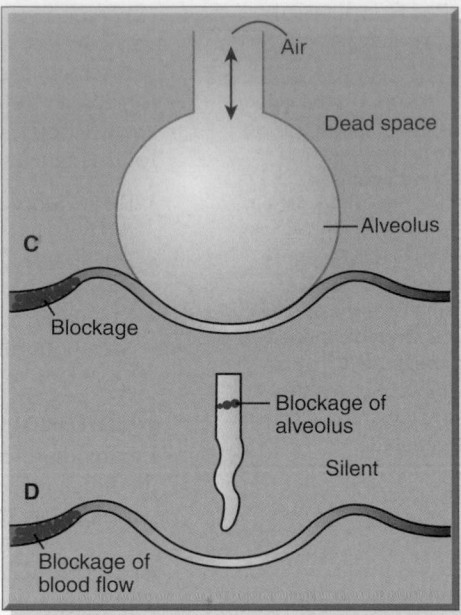

FIGURE 19-4. (**A**) Normal ventilation/perfusion (V/Q) ratio is 1:1 (ventilation matches perfusion). (**B**) When perfusion exceeds ventilation, a shunt exists. (**C**) When ventilation exceeds perfusion, dead space results. (**D**) In the absence of ventilation and perfusion, or with limited ventilation and perfusion, a condition known as a silent unit occurs.

Problems in Respiratory Physiology

The respiratory system usually has sufficient reserves to maintain the normal partial pressures or tension of oxygen and CO_2 in the blood during times of stress. Respiratory insufficiency develops if there is too much interference with ventilation, diffusion, or perfusion. Abnormalities in these processes can lead to hypoxia, hypoxemia, hypercapnia, and hypocapnia (Table 19-4).

Several factors influence the work of breathing. Pressures needed to overcome the forces interfering with breathing determine the respiratory effort needed. Forces that interfere with breathing include airway resistance and lung compliance.

Airway resistance is related to airway diameter, rate of air flow, and speed of gas flow. As the rate of breathing increases, so does the resistance. A narrowed airway results from increased or thick mucus, bronchospasm, or edema. Conditions that may alter bronchial diameter and affect airway resistance include contraction of bronchial smooth muscle (e.g., asthma); thickening of bronchial mucosa (e.g., chronic bronchitis); airway obstruction by mucus, a tumor, or a foreign body; and loss of lung elasticity (e.g., emphysema).

Decreased surfactant, fibrosis, edema, and atelectasis (alveolar collapse) affect lung compliance. Greater pressure gradients are needed when lungs are stiff.

TABLE 19-4. Conditions Related to Abnormalities in Ventilation, Perfusion, Diffusion, and Distribution

CONDITION	DESCRIPTION
Hypoxia	Decreased oxygen in inspired air
Hypoxemia	Decreased oxygen in the blood
Hypercapnia	Increased carbon dioxide in the blood
Hypocapnia	Decreased carbon dioxide in the blood

ASSESSMENT

Assessment of the respiratory system includes obtaining information about physical and functional issues related to breathing. It also means clarifying how these issues may affect the client's quality of life.

History

Often a client seeks medical attention because of respiratory problems related to one or more of the following: dyspnea (labored or difficult breathing), pain on inspiration, increased or more frequent cough, increased sputum production or change in the color/consistency of the mucus, wheezing, or hemoptysis (blood in the sputum). The nurse obtains information about the client's general health history and his or her family history. He or she asks the client about the frequency of respiratory illnesses, allergies, smoking history, nature of any cough, sputum production, dyspnea (Box 19-1), and wheezing. Questioning the client about respiratory treatments or medications (prescription and over-the-counter) is essential. In addition, the nurse inquires about last pulmonary tests (chest radiograph, tuberculosis test). He or she includes questions about occupation, exercise tolerance, pain, and level of fatigue.

Physical Examination

The physical examination begins with a general examination of overall health and condition. Clients with respiratory problems may show signs of shortness of breath when speaking, or they may have a certain posture or position to facilitate breathing. Other observations include skin color; level of consciousness; mental status; respiratory rate, depth, effort, and rhythm; use of accessory muscles; and shape of the chest and symmetry of chest movements. Extremities are

- What makes you short of breath?
- Do you cough when you are short of breath?
- Do you have other symptoms when you are short of breath?
- Do you get short of breath suddenly or gradually?
- When do you usually have difficulty breathing?
- Can you lie flat in bed?
- Do you get short of breath when you rest? With exercise? Running? Climbing stairs?
- How far can you walk before you get short of breath?

TABLE 19-5. Common Abnormalities of the Chest

CONTROL	DESCRIPTION
Kyphosis	Exaggerated curvature of the thoracic spine; congenital anomaly or associated with injuries and osteoporosis
Scoliosis	Lateral S-shaped curvature of the thoracic and lumbar spine
Barrel chest	Anteroposterior diameter increases to equal the transverse diameter; chest is rounded; ribs are horizontal; sternum is pulled forward; associated with emphysema and aging
Funnel chest	Also known as *pectus excavatum;* the sternum is depressed from the second intercostal space—more pronounced with inspiration; a congenital anomaly
Pigeon chest	Also known as *pectus carinatum;* the sternum abnormally protrudes; the ribs are sloped backward; a congenital anomaly

assessed for finger clubbing, a condition in which the tips of the fingers or toes are enlarged because the soft tissue beneath the nail beds is increased. Although it is not always clear why this occurs, it may be related to levels of proteins that stimulate blood vessel growth or to genetic factors. Finger clubbing seems to occur with some lung diseases such as lung cancer, but not with others such as asthma; it can also occur with congenital heart, liver, and thyroid diseases.

The nurse inspects the nose for signs of injury, inflammation, symmetry, and lesions. He or she examines the posterior pharynx and tonsils with a tongue blade and light and notes any evidence of swelling, inflammation, or exudate, as well as changes in color of the mucous membranes. The nurse also notes any difficulty with swallowing or hoarseness.

A physician or nurse practitioner inspects the larynx either directly with a laryngoscope or indirectly with a light and laryngeal mirror. Both procedures require a local anesthetic to suppress the gag reflex and reduce discomfort.

The nurse inspects and gently palpates the trachea to assess for placement and deviation from the midline. He or she notes any lymph node enlargement. The nurse also examines the anterior, posterior, and lateral chest walls for lesions, symmetry, deformities, skin color, and evidence of muscle weakness or weight loss. Checking the contour of the chest walls is important. Normally the anteroposterior diameter of the chest wall is half the transverse diameter; however, some pulmonary conditions (e.g., emphysema) change the chest dimensions.

An experienced examiner palpates the chest wall to detect tenderness, masses, swelling, or other abnormalities (Table 19-5). Tactile or vocal *fremitus* (vibrations from the client's voice transmitted to the examiner's fingers) depends on the capacity to feel sound through the fingers and palm placed on the chest wall. The palpable vibrations occur when the client speaks. The examiner uses the palmar surfaces of the fingers and hands to palpate and asks the client to repeat "99" as the examiner moves his or her hands. If the client is healthy and thin, the fremitus will be highly palpable. Conditions that affect fremitus include a thick or muscular chest wall (decreased fremitus), lung diseases such as emphysema and pneumonia (increased fremitus), and fluid, air, or masses in the pleural space (decreased fremitus).

The experienced examiner performs percussion of the chest wall to assess normal and abnormal sounds. With the client sitting, the examiner places his or her middle finger on the chest wall and taps that finger with the middle finger of the opposite hand. Table 19-6 describes the types of sounds heard with percussion.

The nurse auscultates breath sounds from side to side, moving from the upper to the lower chest (Fig. 19-5). He or she listens anteriorly, laterally, and posteriorly. Normal breath sounds include the following:

- Vesicular sounds—Produced by air movement in bronchioles and alveoli, these sounds are heard over the lung fields; they are quiet and low pitched, with long inspiration and short expiration.

TABLE 19-6. Sounds Heard with Chest Wall Percussion

SOUND	DESCRIPTION	IMPLICATIONS
Flat	High pitch, little intensity, decreased duration	Heard during percussion of a solid area, such as a mass or pleural effusion
Dull	Medium pitch, medium intensity, medium duration	Heard when no air or fluid is in the lung (e.g., atelectasis, lobar pneumonia)
Tympanic	High pitch, loud intensity, long duration	Normal sounds heard over stomach and bowel; abnormal sounds heard over lungs, such as in a pneumothorax
Resonant	Low pitch, loud intensity, long duration	Normal lung sounds
Hyperresonant	Lower pitch, very loud, longer duration	Abnormal sounds that occur when free air exists in the thoracic cavity (e.g., emphysema, pneumothorax)

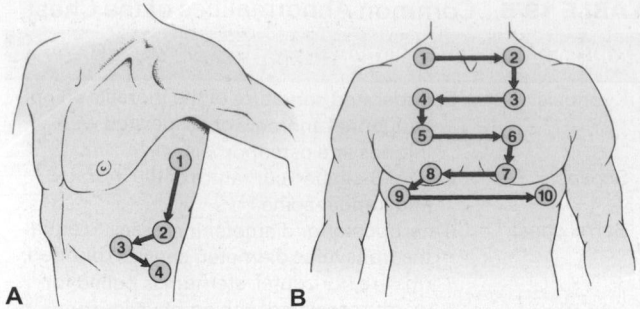

FIGURE 19-5. (**A**) Each side of the chest is auscultated and compared. (**B**) The anterior chest is systematically examined over each lung field.

TABLE 19-7. Normal Values for Arterial Blood Gases

BLOOD GAS	NORMAL VALUE
pH, hydrogen ion concentration, acidity or alkalinity of the blood	7.35–7.45
PaO_2, partial pressure of oxygen in arterial blood	80–100 mm Hg
$PaCO_2$, partial pressure of carbon dioxide in arterial blood	35–45 mm Hg
HCO_3, bicarbonate ion concentration in the blood	22–26 mm Hg
SaO_2, arterial oxygen saturation or percentage of the oxygen-carrying capacity of the blood	95%–100%

- Bronchial sounds—Produced by air movement through the trachea, these sounds are heard over the trachea and are loud with long expiration.
- Bronchovesicular sounds—These normal breath sounds are heard between the trachea and upper lungs; pitch is medium with equal inspiration and expiration.

Adventitious or abnormal breath sounds are categorized as crackles or wheezes. *Crackles* (formerly called *rales*) are discrete sounds that result from the delayed opening of deflated airways. They resemble static or the sound made by rubbing hair strands together near one's ear. Sometimes they clear with coughing. They may be present because of inflammation or congestion. Crackles that do not clear with coughing may indicate pulmonary edema or fluid in the alveoli.

Wheezes may be sibilant (hissing or whistling) or sonorous (full and deep). Sibilant wheezes (formerly called *wheezes*) are continuous musical sounds that can be heard during inspiration and expiration. They result from air passing through narrowed or partially obstructed air passages and are heard in clients with increased secretions. Sonorous wheezes (formerly called *rhonchi*) are lower pitched and are heard in the trachea and bronchi. Friction rubs are heard as crackling or grating sounds on inspiration or expiration. They occur when the pleural surfaces are inflamed and do not change if the client coughs.

Diagnostic Tests

Arterial Blood Gases

Oxygenation of body tissues depends on the amount of oxygen in arterial blood. Arterial blood gases (ABGs) determine the blood's pH, oxygen-carrying capacity, and levels of oxygen, CO_2, and bicarbonate ion. Blood gas samples are obtained through an arterial puncture at the radial, brachial, or femoral artery. A client also may have an indwelling arterial catheter from which arterial samples are obtained.

ABGs frequently are ordered when a client is acutely ill or has a history of respiratory disorders. If the partial pressure of oxygen in arterial blood (PaO_2) is decreased, body tissues do not receive sufficient oxygen. Table 19-7 presents the descriptions and measures of normal ABGs. Clients with respiratory disorders can neither get oxygen into the blood nor get CO_2 out of the blood. Some conditions that affect ABGs are as follows:

- Hyperventilation during collection of ABGs, causing elevated PaO_2
- Hypoventilation with neuromuscular disease, chronic obstructive pulmonary disease (COPD), or insufficient oxygen in the atmosphere, causing decreased PaO_2
- Elevated $PaCO_2$ in clients with COPD, inadequate ventilation with a mechanical ventilator, or decreased respiratory rates
- Decreased $PaCO_2$ in clients who are nervous or anxious or have a condition that causes hyperventilation or a rapid respiratory rate

Pulse oximetry is a noninvasive method that uses a light beam to measure the oxygen content of hemoglobin (SaO_2). The monitoring device attaches to the client's earlobe or fingertip and connects to the oximeter monitor. The monitor registers wavelengths of light passing through the earlobe or fingertip and uses them to calculate the arterial oxygen saturation. Normal values are 95% or higher (Nursing Guidelines 19-1).

Pulmonary Function Studies

Pulmonary function studies measure the functional ability of the lungs. These studies are done to diagnose pulmonary conditions and to assess preoperative respiratory status. They also may be used to determine the effectiveness of bronchodilators or to screen employees who work in environments that are hazardous to pulmonary health. Measurements of pulmonary function are obtained with a spirometer and include:

- Tidal volume—volume of air inhaled and exhaled with a normal breath
- Inspiratory reserve volume—maximum volume of air that normally can be inspired
- Expiratory reserve volume—maximum volume of air that normally can be exhaled by forced expiration
- Residual volume—volume of air left in the lungs after maximal expiration
- Vital capacity—maximum amount of air that can be expired after maximal inspiration
- Forced vital capacity—amount of air exhaled forcefully and rapidly after maximal inspiration
- Inspiratory capacity—maximum amount of air that can be inhaled after normal expiration

NURSING GUIDELINES 19-1

Performing Pulse Oximetry

- Explain the procedure to the client.
- Assess potential sensor sites for quality of circulation, edema, tremor, restlessness, nail polish, or artificial nails.
- Review the medical history for data indicating vascular or other pathology (e.g., anemia, carbon monoxide poisoning).
- Check prescribed medications for vasoconstrictive effects.
- Assess client's understanding of pulse oximetry.
- Position the sensor so that the light emission is directly opposite the detector.
- Observe the numeric display, audible sound, or waveform on the oximeter.
- Set the high and low alarms according to the manufacturer's directions.

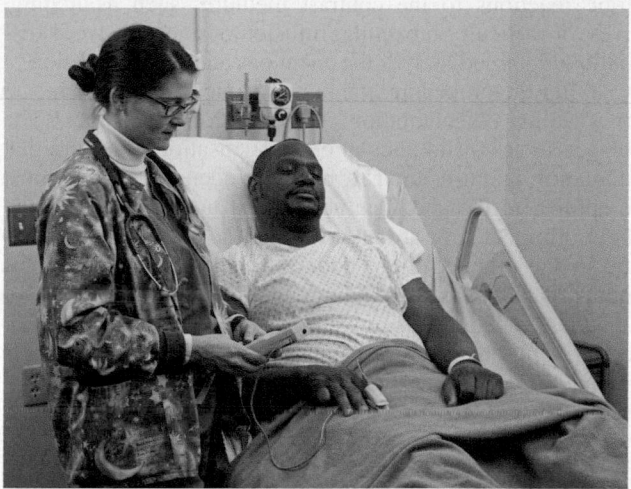

Portable pulse oximetry unit, used to measure oxygen saturation (SpO_2) of arterial blood.

- Functional residual capacity—amount of air left in the lungs after a normal expiration
- Total lung capacity—total volume of air in the lungs when maximally inflated

Pulmonary function results vary according to age, sex, weight, and height. The maximum lung capacities and volumes are best achieved when the client is sitting or standing. The test should not be performed within 2 hours after a meal. The nurse explains the procedure to the client and instructs him or her to wear loose-fitting clothing. A nose clip prevents air from escaping through the client's nose when blowing into the spirometer. Bronchodilators may be used after the initial spirometry to see if there is any improvement or response with the inhaled medication. Although the test is simple, the client may be tired afterward.

Sputum Studies

Sputum specimens are examined for pathogenic microorganisms and cancer cells. Culture and sensitivity tests are done to diagnose infections and prescribe antibiotics. Negative results on the examination of sputum smears do not always indicate the absence of disease, so collection of sputum for successive days may be necessary. Sputum is collected by having the client expectorate a specimen (Nursing Guidelines 19-2), by suctioning the client, or during a bronchoscopy (see later discussion).

Radiography

Chest radiographs show the size, shape, and position of the lungs and other structures of the thorax. Physicians use chest radiography to screen for asymptomatic disease and to diagnose tumors, foreign bodies, and other abnormal conditions. Fluoroscopy enables the physician to view the thoracic cavity with all its contents in motion. It more precisely diagnoses the location of a tumor or lesion. Computed tomography scanning or magnetic resonance imaging may be used to produce axial views of the lungs to detect tumors and other lung disorders during early stages.

Pulmonary Angiography

Pulmonary angiography is a radioisotope study that allows the physician to assess the arterial circulation of the lungs, particularly to detect pulmonary emboli. A catheter is introduced into an arm vein and threaded through the right atrium and ventricle into the pulmonary artery. Contrast medium is rapidly injected into the femoral artery, and radiographs are taken to see the distribution of the radiopaque material.

During pulmonary angiography, the nurse obtains data about the client's level of anxiety and knowledge of the procedure. The nurse provides explanations and reinforces the client's understanding. The client will experience a feeling of pressure on catheter insertion. When the contrast medium is infused, the client will sense a warm, flushed feeling and an urge to cough.

 NURSING GUIDELINES 19-2

Collecting a Sputum Specimen

- Explain the procedure to the client.
- Collect a sputum specimen early in the morning or after an aerosol treatment.
- Collect the specimen in a sterile specimen container.
- Instruct the client to rinse the mouth with tap water.
- Instruct the client to take several deep breaths, cough forcefully, and expectorate into the container.
- Collect at least 1 to 3 mL ($^1/_2$ teaspoon).
- Deliver the specimen to the laboratory as soon as possible. The container should be transported in a sealed plastic bag with requisition.

The nurse must determine if the client has any allergies, particularly to iodine, shellfish, or contrast dye. During the procedure, the nurse monitors for signs and symptoms of allergic reactions to the contrast medium, such as itching, hives, or difficulty breathing. Infusion of contrast dye is discontinued immediately if the client has an allergic reaction.

After the procedure, the nurse inspects the puncture site for swelling, discoloration, bleeding, or hematoma. The nurse assesses distal circulation and sensation to ensure that circulation is unimpaired. If bleeding occurs, pressure must be applied to the site. The nurse must notify the physician about diminished or absent distal pulses, cool skin temperature in the affected limb, poor capillary refill, client complaints of numbness or tingling, and bleeding or hematoma. The client remains on bed rest for 2 to 6 hours after the procedure. The pressure dressing, applied after the catheter is removed, remains in place for this period.

Lung Scans

Several types of lung scans may be done for diagnostic purposes: the perfusion and ventilation scan, referred to as a V-Q scan; the gallium scan; or the positron emission tomography (PET) scan. The V-Q scan requires the use of radioisotopes and a scanning machine to detect patterns of blood flow through the lungs and patterns of air movement and distribution in the lungs. V-Q scans are particularly useful in diagnosing pulmonary emboli. They are also used to diagnose lung cancer, COPD, and pulmonary edema.

A radioactive contrast medium is administered intravenously for the perfusion scan and by inhalation as a radioactive gas for the ventilation scan. Before the perfusion scan, nurses must assess the client for allergies to iodine. During the procedure, the radiologist asks the client to change positions. During inhalation, the client may need to hold his or her breath for short periods as scanning images are obtained. The client must receive adequate explanations before the procedure to reduce anxiety. The nurse must reassure the client that the amount of radiation from this procedure is less than that used during a chest radiograph.

A gallium scan is used to determine if any inflammatory conditions exist within the lungs or if abscesses, adhesions, or tumors are present. Clients receive an intravenous injection of gallium, a radioisotope, and then have scans taken at various intervals up to 48 hours after the gallium injection. The scan shows gallium uptake by the lung tissues.

A PET scan also uses radioisotopes with advanced technology that allows the examiner to differentiate normal and abnormal tissue and view metabolic changes within the lung tissue. This scan can evaluate malignancies by showing blood flow and other functioning of organs and tissues.

Bronchoscopy

Bronchoscopy allows for direct visualization of the larynx, trachea, and bronchi using a flexible fiberoptic bronchoscope. The physician introduces the bronchoscope through the nose or mouth or through a tracheostomy or artificial airway. Bronchoscopy is used to diagnose, treat, or evaluate lung disease; obtain a biopsy of a lesion or tumor; obtain a sputum specimen; perform aggressive pulmonary cleansing; or remove a foreign body.

Bronchoscopy is very frightening to clients, who require thorough explanations throughout the procedure. For at least 6 hours before the bronchoscopy, the client must abstain from food or drink to decrease the risk of aspiration. Risk is increased because the client receives local anesthesia, which suppresses the swallow, cough, and gag reflexes.

The client receives medications before the procedure—usually atropine to dry secretions and a sedative or narcotic to depress the vagus nerve. This consideration is important because if the vagus nerve is stimulated during the bronchoscopy, hypotension, bradycardia, or dysrhythmias may occur. Other potential complications include bronchospasm or laryngospasm secondary to edema, hypoxemia, bleeding, perforation, aspiration, cardiac dysrhythmias, and infection. Nursing Care Plan 19-1 provides more information about nursing care.

Laryngoscopy

Laryngoscopy provides direct visualization of the larynx using a laryngoscope. It is done to diagnose lesions, evaluate laryngeal function, and determine any inflammation. Physicians also may dilate laryngeal strictures and biopsy lesions. Refer to the preceding section on bronchoscopy and to Nursing Care Plan 19-1 for more information.

Mediastinoscopy

Mediastinoscopy provides visualization of the mediastinum and is done under local or general anesthesia. The physician makes an incision above the sternum and inserts a mediastinoscope. With this procedure, the physician can visualize lymph nodes and obtain biopsy samples. Possible complications include dysrhythmias, myocardial infarction, pneumothorax, and bleeding.

Thoracoscopy

Thoracoscopy allows for examination of the pleural cavity. Small incisions are made into the pleural cavity through an intercostal space. An endoscope is inserted to visualize a specific area (Fig. 19-6). The location selected is based on other clinical and diagnostic findings. If fluid is present, the examiner aspirates it and sends it for culture and cellular studies. Biopsies also may be done. A chest tube may be inserted following the procedure (see Chap. 21). Thoracoscopy is done to evaluate pleural effusions and pleural disease, and for staging of tumors. Future potential exists for laser treatment of pulmonary nodules and other growths. This technique is less invasive than thoracotomy procedures (Smeltzer et al., 2008) (see Chap. 21).

Thoracentesis

A small amount of fluid lies between the visceral and parietal pleurae. When excess fluid or air accumulates, the physician aspirates it from the pleural space by inserting a needle into the chest wall. This procedure, called **thoracentesis**, is performed with local anesthesia. Thoracentesis also may be used to obtain a sample of pleural fluid or a biopsy specimen from the pleural wall for diagnostic purposes, such as a culture and sensitivity or microscopic examination. Bloody fluid usually suggests trauma. Purulent fluid is diagnostic for infection. Serous fluid may be associated with cancer, inflammatory conditions, or heart failure. When thoracentesis is done for therapeutic reasons,

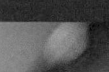

NURSING CARE PLAN 19-1 | The Client Undergoing a Bronchoscopy

Assessment

- Assess level of anxiety and understanding of the procedure.
- Obtain baseline vital signs.
- Assess lung sounds.
- Ask client if he or she wears dentures and when he or she last ate or drank.
- Check record to ensure that the consent form is signed and witnessed.

Nursing Diagnosis: Fear related to lack of knowledge about what to expect during and after procedure

Expected Outcome: Client will exhibit coping behaviors and follow instructions.

Interventions	Rationales
Acknowledge client's fear.	Validating fear communicates acceptance.
Provide simple explanations about the procedure after determining what the client knows and his or her misconceptions.	Acknowledging misconceptions provides a starting point. Adults learn more readily when teaching is based on their previous knowledge and experience. Understanding helps to alleviate fear.
Inform client that he or she will receive medications to alleviate anxiety, reduce secretions, and block the vagus nerve.	Information reduces fear and anxiety.
Explain that a tube will be inserted through the nose and throat and into the lungs and that the medication will assist the client.	Thorough explanations reinforce understanding and reduce fear.
Tell client that after the procedure, food and fluids are withheld until the cough reflex returns.	Preoperative sedation and local anesthesia impair the cough reflex and swallowing for several hours.
Inform client that the throat will be irritated and sore for a few days, and that he or she may cough up blood-tinged mucus.	Knowledge about expected signs and symptoms reduces fear after the procedure.

Evaluation of Expected Outcome

Client tolerates procedure without untoward effects, follows instructions, and states that fear is minimal.

Nursing Diagnosis: Risk for Aspiration related to diminished gag reflex

Expected Outcomes: (1) Client will maintain a patent airway. (2) Risk of aspiration will decrease.

Interventions	Rationales
Assess cough and gag reflexes.	Depressed cough or gag reflex increases risk of aspiration.
Keep client NPO until the gag reflex returns (usually 2 to 8 hours).	NPO status reduces the risk of aspiration.
Keep suction equipment available.	If the client aspirates, suctioning helps to maintain a patent airway.
Place client in semi-Fowler's position with the head to one side.	Proper positioning decreases the risk of aspiration.
Encourage client to expectorate secretions frequently into an emesis basin.	Expectoration reduces the risk of aspiration.
After the gag reflex returns, offer sips of water or ice chips initially, then progress the diet to soft foods.	Beginning with sips of water or ice chips ensures that the gag reflex has returned. The client can most easily swallow soft foods.

Evaluation of Expected Outcomes

Airway remains patent. Client does not experience aspiration.

PC. Pneumothorax: dysrhythmia, bronchospasm

Expected Outcome. The nurse will manage and minimize potential complications.

Interventions	Rationales
Monitor vital signs and respiratory status, comparing against baseline assessment data.	Comparison helps the nurse determine if the client is experiencing any respiratory distress.
Observe for symmetric chest movements.	Decreased or asymmetric chest expansion is a sign of pneumothorax.
Report hemoptysis, stridor, or dyspnea immediately.	These findings indicate respiratory distress and probable pneumothorax.

Evaluation of Expected Outcome

Client experiences no postprocedure complications.

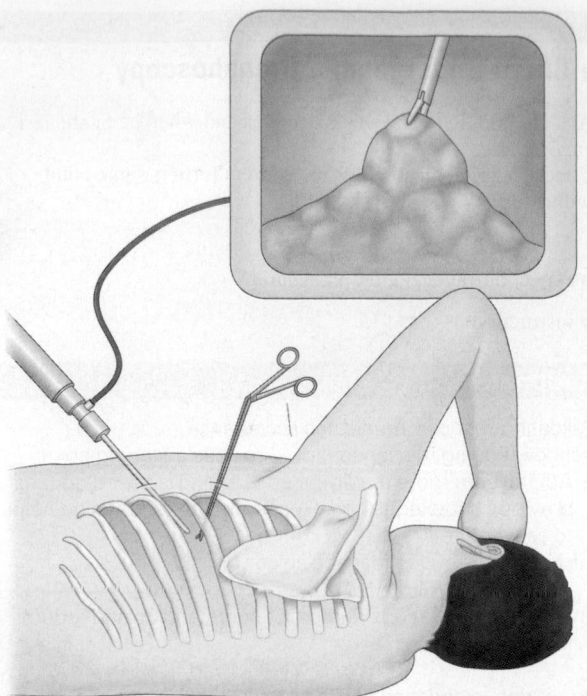

FIGURE 19-6. Endoscopic thorascopy. Like bronchoscopy, thorascopy uses fiberoptic instruments and video cameras to visualize thoracic structures. Unlike bronchoscopy, thorascopy usually requires the surgeon to make a small incision before inserting the endoscope. Thorascopy is used to exercise tissue for biopsy, evaluate pleural disease, and stage tumor.

1 to 2 L of fluid may be withdrawn to relieve respiratory distress. Medication may be instilled directly into the pleural space to treat infection.

Thoracentesis is done at the bedside or in a treatment or examining room. The client either sits at the side of the bed or examining table or is in a side-lying position on the unaffected side. If the client is sitting, a pillow is placed on a bedside table, and the client rests her or his arms and head on the pillow. The physician determines the site for aspiration by radiography and percussion. The site is cleaned and anesthetized with local anesthesia. When the procedure is complete, a small pressure dressing is applied. The client remains on bed rest and usually lies on the unaffected side for at least 1 hour to promote expansion of the lung on the affected side. A chest radiograph is done after the procedure to rule out a pneumothorax (also called collapsed lung; see Chap. 21). Complications that can follow a thoracentesis are pneumothorax, subcutaneous emphysema (air in subcutaneous tissue), infection, pulmonary edema, and cardiac distress. Nursing Guidelines 19-3 outlines the nurse's role in assisting with thoracentesis.

▶ **Stop, Think, and Respond Exercise 19-2**

Your client had a thoracentesis 2 hours ago. He begins to complain of feeling short of breath and is very anxious. What should you assess?

NURSING GUIDELINES 19-3

Assisting with Thoracentesis

- Explain the procedure to the client.
- Reassure the client that he or she will receive local anesthesia. Explain that the client will still experience a pressure-like pain when the needle pierces the pleura and when fluid is withdrawn.
- Assist client to an appropriate position (sitting with arms and head on padded table or in side-lying position on unaffected side).
- Instruct client not to move during the procedure, including no coughing or deep breathing.
- Provide comfort.
- Inform client about what is happening.
- Maintain asepsis.
- Monitor vital signs during the procedure—also monitor pulse oximetry if client is connected to it.
- During removal of fluid, monitor for respiratory distress, dyspnea, tachypnea, or hypotension.
- Apply small sterile pressure dressing to the site after the procedure.
- Position client on the unaffected side. Instruct client to stay in this position for at least 1 hour and to remain on bed rest for several hours.
- Check that chest radiography is done after the procedure.
- Record the amount, color, and other characteristics of fluid removed.

- Monitor for signs of increased respiratory rate, asymmetry in respiratory movement, syncope or vertigo, chest tightness, uncontrolled cough or cough that produces blood-tinged or frothy mucus (or both), tachycardia, and hypoxemia.

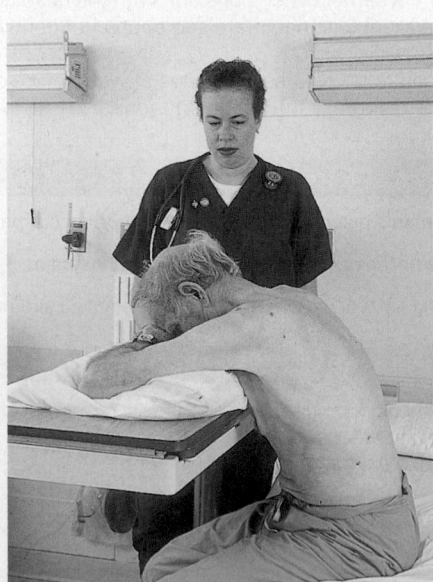

Client positioning for thoracentesis

NURSING MANAGEMENT

In addition to the nursing management of individual tests, clients require informative and appropriate explanations of any diagnostic procedures they will experience. Nurses must remember that, for many of these clients, breathing may in some way be compromised. Energy levels may be decreased. For that reason, explanations should be brief yet complete and may need to be repeated. The nurse also must help ensure adequate rest periods before and after the procedures. After invasive procedures, the nurse must carefully assess for signs of respiratory distress, chest pain, blood-streaked sputum, and expectoration of blood. He or she needs to repeat post-procedure expectations to help reduce the client's anxiety and to ensure the best possible recovery.

CRITICAL THINKING EXERCISES

1. Lung disease can impact a client's quality of life. For what psychosocial issues may the client with lung disease be at risk?
2. Your client had a bronchoscopy and just returned back to your unit. What are the most important assessments that need to be made?
3. There are many respiratory diseases and conditions. What are common signs of respiratory disease?
4. What factors do you think contribute to lung disease?

NCLEX-STYLE REVIEW QUESTIONS

1. A client comes to the doctor's office describing shortness of breath and strange breath sounds when inhaling deeply. Upon auscultation of the lung fields, sibilant wheezes are noted. The nurse is most correct in stating that wheezes result from which of the following?
   1. Air passing through narrowed passages
   2. Air escaping through a pneumothorax
   3. Air collecting in the pleural cavity
   4. Air between visceral and parietal pleurae

2. The nurse is giving instructions to a client having pulmonary angiography. Which of the following statements is the best evidence that the client understands the nurse's instructions about what will take place during the diagnostic procedure? Select all that apply.
   1. "I may feel some pressure at the site."
   2. "I may have bleeding at the site following the procedure."
   3. "I will be able to go to the bathroom when I return from the test."
   4. "I will sense a warm, flushed feeling and an urge to cough when the dye is injected."

3. A client has undergone thoracentesis and has been ordered to undergo a chest radiograph. Which of the following would the nurse identify for the client as the rationale for the radiograph?
   1. To evaluate for pulmonary edema
   2. To rule out emphysema
   3. To assess for any cardiac distress
   4. To check for pneumothorax

4. Which of the following nursing interventions is most important during a lung scan?
   1. Reassure the client about the amount of radiation from the procedure.
   2. Coach the client to hold his or her breath at times during the procedure.
   3. Administer sedative or narcotic as per orders before the procedure.
   4. Aid the client to rest arms and head on a pillow during the procedure.

5. A nurse is auscultating the lung sounds of a the client who came to the clinic for a physical exam. There is not any history of lung disease. The nurse expects to hear:
   1. adventitious breath sounds
   2. bronchial breath sounds
   3. bronchovesicular breath sounds
   4. vesicular breath sounds

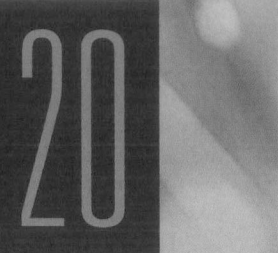

20 Caring for Clients with Upper Respiratory Disorders

Words To Know

adenoidectomy
adenoiditis
aphonia
coryza
deviated septum
epistaxis
hemoptysis
hypertrophied turbinates
laryngitis
laryngoscopy
laryngospasm
nasal polyps
peritonsillar abscess
pharyngitis
polysomnography
rhinitis
rhinorrhea
sinusitis
sleep apnea syndrome
stridor
tonsillectomy
tonsillitis
tracheostomy
tracheotomy

Learning Objectives

On completion of this chapter, you will be able to:

1. Describe nursing care for clients experiencing infectious or inflammatory upper respiratory disorders.
2. Discuss assessment data required to provide nursing care to clients with structural disorders of the upper airway.
3. Describe airway problems a client may experience following trauma or obstruction to the upper airway.
4. Identify risk factors that contribute to the development of laryngeal cancer.
5. Identify the earliest symptom of laryngeal cancer.
6. Discuss treatments for laryngeal cancer.
7. Describe measures used to promote alternative methods of communication for clients with a laryngectomy.
8. Discuss psychosocial issues that clients may experience following a laryngectomy.
9. Relate treatment modalities for clients experiencing short-term or long-term problems with airway management.
10. Identify possible reasons for and nursing management of a tracheostomy.
11. Explain why a client may require endotracheal intubation.

Disorders of the upper airway range from common colds to cancer. The severity depends on the nature of the disorder and the client's physiologic response. Most people experience common colds and sore throats and find them more inconvenient than serious. For others, even the most common disorders of the upper respiratory airway are of great concern because other physical problems compound their effects.

INFECTIOUS AND INFLAMMATORY DISORDERS

The most common upper airway illnesses are infectious and inflammatory disorders. The average person experiences three to five upper respiratory infections (URIs) each year. For some individuals, URIs develop into bronchitis or pneumonia, which involves more serious symptoms and may require antibiotics or other treatments (see Chap. 21).

RHINITIS

Rhinitis is inflammation of the nasal mucous membranes. It also is referred to as the *common cold,* or **coryza**. Rhinitis may be acute, chronic, or allergic, depending on the cause. The most common cause is the rhinovirus, of which more than 100 strains exist. Colds are rapidly spread by inhalation of droplets and direct contact with contaminated

DRUG THERAPY TABLE 20-1 Agents to Treat Upper Respiratory Disorders

Drug Category and Examples	Mechanism of Action	Side Effects	Nursing Considerations
Antitussives dextromethorphan (Benylin), guaifenesin (Robitussin)	Act on the central nervous system to raise the cough threshold and dampen cough reflex.	Drowsiness, constipation, GI upset, headache	For use with nonproductive coughs. Encourage client to speak with healthcare provider if known chronic condition exists. Read label and follow manufacturers' recommendations for dosage. Seek healthcare provider if cough continues or becomes productive.
Decongestants pseudoephedrine	Affect the autonomic nervous system to relieve nasal congestion.	Nervousness, insomnia, headache, dry mouth	Many are over-the-counter products, so encourage client to speak with healthcare provider if there are known chronic conditions. Encourage increased fluid intake and follow the proper manufacturer's directions for administration.
Antihistamines diphenhydramine (Benadryl), cetirizine (Zyrtec) *Claritin Allegra* (handwritten)	Block the actions of histamine at the H$_1$-receptor. *dries out secretions* (handwritten)	Dry mouth, headache, drowsiness, dizziness, urinary retention, nausea, hypersensitivity reaction, hypotension	Contraindicated in clients with certain heart conditions. Encourage clients to increase fluid intake. May cause drowsiness; advise caution when driving if unaware of individual reactions.
Anti-inflammatories intranasal glucocorticoids, fluticasone propionate (Flonase)	When sprayed on local tissues in the nasal mucosa, decrease the secretions of inflammatory mediators and reduce tissue edema.	Transient nasal irritation, burning, sneezing, or dryness	Educate client on proper administration of nasal spray to avoid swallowing medication, and instruct to rinse mouth after use. May take 2 to 4 weeks to reach maximum effectiveness. Report nosebleeds or irritation lasting more than a few doses.

articles (e.g., telephone receivers, doorknobs). Allergic rhinitis is a hypersensitive reaction to allergens, such as pollen, dust, animal dander, or food. Rhinitis is usually not a serious condition; however, it may lead to pneumonia and other more serious illnesses for debilitated, immunosuppressed, or older clients.

Symptoms associated with rhinitis include sneezing, nasal congestion, **rhinorrhea** (clear nasal discharge), sore throat, watery eyes, cough, low-grade fever, headache, aching muscles, and malaise. With the common cold, these symptoms continue for 5 to 14 days. A sustained elevated temperature suggests a bacterial infection or infection in the sinuses or ears. Symptoms of allergic rhinitis will persist as long as the client is exposed to the specific allergen.

For most clients, treatment for rhinitis is minimal. Unless specific bacteria are identified as the cause of the infection, antibiotics are not used. Clients may be advised to use antipyretics, such as acetaminophen or nonsteroidal analgesics, for fever. Decongestants such as pseudoephedrine may be recommended for severe nasal congestion. For clients experiencing a prolonged cough, antitussives may be ordered. Saline gargles are useful for a sore throat, as is

saline spray for nasal congestion and prevention of crusting. For allergic rhinitis, antihistamines are often used. An example of a first-generation antihistamine is diphenhydramine (Benadryl). Newer antihistamines include loratadine (Claritin), fexofenadine (Allegra), and cetirizine (Zyrtec). Combination decongestants and antihistamines may also be helpful. An example of this is brompheniramine/pseudoephedrine (Dimetapp). Medications that desensitize or suppress immune responses, such as cromolyn (Nasalcrom) or intranasal glucocorticosteroids, such as fluticasone (Flonase) may also be prescribed for allergic rhinitis (Drug Therapy Table 20-1).

Pharmacologic Considerations

- In multiple-ingredient cold preparations, one or more drug ingredients may be contraindicated in certain disorders (e.g., glaucoma, heart disease, hypertension, prostatic enlargement). Encourage clients with these diseases who are taking prescription drugs to consult a physician before using nonprescription drugs to treat a cold.

- Some cold tablets contain antihistamines that thicken nasal secretions. Although this action may temporarily decrease the discomfort of profuse nasal secretions, thickened secretions can block the drainage openings of the sinus cavity, lead to failure of the sinuses to drain adequately, and become a focus for continuing infection.

The nurse teaches the client simple measures to treat rhinitis (Client and Family Teaching 20-1). Teaching clients about URIs helps prevent them and minimizes potential complications. Maintaining a healthy lifestyle of adequate rest and sleep, proper diet, and moderate exercise is the best prevention (Nutrition Notes 20-1). Another important preventive factor is frequent handwashing, which greatly reduces the spread of infection.

Gerontologic Considerations

- The common cold may be potentially serious for older adults, especially when they have other diseases such as a chronic respiratory disorder or heart disease. Advise older clients to see a healthcare provider if cold symptoms are severe or breathing is difficult.

SINUSITIS

Sinusitis is inflammation of the sinuses. The maxillary sinus is affected most often. Sinusitis can lead to serious complications, such as infection of the middle ear or brain.

Pathophysiology and Etiology

The principal causes are the spread of an infection from the nasal passages to the sinuses and the blockage of normal sinus drainage (Fig. 20-1). Interference with sinus drainage predisposes a client to sinusitis because trapped secretions readily become infected. Impaired sinus drainage may result from allergies (which cause edema of the nasal mucous membranes), nasal polyps, or a deviated septum.

Client and Family Teaching 20-1
Treating Rhinitis

For all types of rhinitis:

● Rest as much as possible.
● Increase fluid intake to assist in liquefying secretions.
● Use a vaporizer to help liquefy secretions.
● Blow nose with mouth open slightly to equalize pressure.
● Wash hands frequently to avoid spreading infection.
● Use over-the-counter medications as directed; be aware of possible side effects, especially interactions with food and alcohol.

For allergic rhinitis:

● Be tested for allergen sensitivity.
● Avoid specific allergens.
● Use antihistamines and decongestants as ordered.

Nutrition Notes 20-1
The Client with Rhinitis

● A review of the research shows that vitamin C modestly shortens the duration of a cold by less than 1 day per cold when daily intake is at least 1000 mg/day (the RDA is 75 mg/day for women and 90 mg/day for men). The placebo effect is credited for reducing the number of colds in people who thought they were taking vitamin C supplements but were actually receiving a placebo.
● Evidence on the effectiveness of zinc lozenges in shortening the duration of colds is inconclusive.

Measures that help reduce the incidence or severity of sinusitis include eating a well-balanced diet, getting plenty of rest, engaging in moderate exercise, avoiding allergens, and seeking medical attention promptly if a cold persists longer than 10 days or nasal discharge is green or dark yellow and foul smelling.

Assessment Findings

Signs and symptoms depend on which sinus is infected. They include headache, fever, pain over the affected sinus,

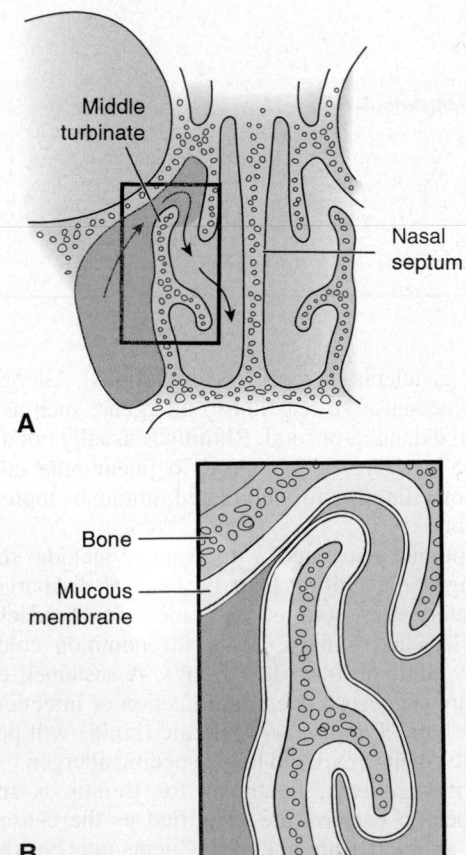

FIGURE 20-1. Edema can obstruct sinus drainage. (**A**) The maxillary sinuses normally drain through the openings that lie under the middle turbinates. The openings for the drainage are near the upper portion of the sinus. (**B**) Edema, which commonly accompanies upper respiratory infections, can obstruct the openings and prevent normal sinus drainage.

nasal congestion and discharge, pain and pressure around the eyes, and malaise. A nasal smear or material obtained from irrigation of the sinus for culture and sensitivity testing identifies the infectious microorganism and appropriate antibiotic therapy. Transillumination and radiographs of the sinuses may show a change in the shape of or fluid in the sinus cavity. A thorough history, including an allergy history, usually confirms the diagnosis.

Medical and Surgical Management

Acute sinusitis frequently responds to conservative treatment designed to help overcome the infection. Saline irrigation of the maxillary sinus may be done to remove accumulated exudate and promote drainage. Such irrigation is accomplished by insertion of a catheter through the normal opening under the middle concha. Antibiotic therapy is necessary for severe infections. Vasoconstrictors, such as phenylephrine nose drops, may be recommended for short-term use to relieve nasal congestion and aid in sinus drainage.

Surgery is often indicated for chronic sinusitis. Endoscopic sinus surgery helps provide an opening in the inferior meatus to promote drainage. More radical procedures, such as the Caldwell-Luc procedure and external sphenoethmoidectomy, are done to remove diseased tissue and provide an opening into the inferior meatus of the nose for adequate drainage.

Nursing Management

If the client is receiving medical treatment, the nurse informs him or her that use of mouthwashes and humidification, as well as increased fluid intake, may loosen secretions and increase comfort. He or she instructs the client to take nasal decongestants and antihistamines as ordered.

If the client has had sinus surgery, the nurse institutes standards for postoperative care (see Chap. 14). He or she observes the client for repeated swallowing, a finding that suggests possible hemorrhage. One risk of sinus surgery is damage to the optic nerve. Thus, the nurse assesses postoperative visual acuity by asking the client to identify the number of fingers displayed. The nurse monitors the client's temperature at least every 4 hours. He or she assesses for pain over the involved sinuses, a finding that may indicate postoperative infection or impaired drainage. The nurse administers analgesics as indicated and applies ice compresses to involved sinuses to reduce pain and edema.

The postsurgical client will have nasal packing and a dressing under the nares ("moustache" dressing or "drip pad"). Because nasal packing forces the client to breathe through the mouth, the nurse encourages oral hygiene and gives ice chips or small sips of fluids frequently. Such measures alleviate the dryness caused by mouth breathing. The nurse changes the drip pad as needed and reports excessive drainage. Postoperative client and family teaching includes telling the client not to blow the nose, lift objects more than 5 to 10 lbs, or do the Valsalva maneuver for 10 to 14 days postoperatively. The nurse urges the client to remain in a warm environment and to avoid smoky or poorly ventilated areas.

▶ **Stop, Think, and Respond Exercise 20-1**

A neighbor tells you that she is taking antibiotics for an acute sinus infection. She states that she has severe pain in her sinuses and wonders what she can do other than take analgesics. What advice might you give?

PHARYNGITIS

Pharyngitis, inflammation of the throat, is often associated with rhinitis and other URIs (Fig. 20-2). Viruses and bacteria cause pharyngitis. The most serious bacteria are the group A streptococci, which cause a condition commonly referred to as *strep throat*. Strep throat can lead to dangerous cardiac complications (endocarditis and rheumatic fever) and harmful renal complications (glomerulonephritis). Pharyngitis is highly contagious and spreads via inhalation of or direct contamination with droplets.

The incubation period for pharyngitis is 2 to 4 days. The first symptom is a sore throat, sometimes severe, with accompanying *dysphagia* (difficulty swallowing), fever, chills, headache, and malaise. Some clients exhibit a white or exudate patch over the tonsillar area and swollen glands. A throat culture reveals the specific causative bacteria. Rapid identification methods, such as the Biostar or the Strep A optical immunoassay (OIA), are available to diagnose group A streptococcal infections. These tests are done in clinics and physician offices. Standard 24-hour throat culture and sensitivity tests identify other organisms.

Early antibiotic treatment is the best choice for pharyngitis to treat the infection and help prevent potential complications. Penicillin or its derivatives are generally the antibiotics of choice. Clients sensitive to penicillin receive erythromycin. The antibiotic regimen is 7 to 14 days.

TONSILLITIS AND ADENOIDITIS

Tonsillitis is inflammation of the tonsils, and **adenoiditis** is inflammation of the adenoids. These conditions generally occur together—the common diagnosis is tonsillitis. Although both disorders are more common in children, they also may be seen in adults.

Pathophysiology and Etiology

The tonsils and adenoids are lymphatic tissues and common sites of infection. Primary infection may occur in the tonsils and adenoids, or the infection can be secondary to other URIs. Chronic tonsillar infection leads to enlargement and partial upper airway obstruction. Chronic adenoidal infection can result in acute or chronic infection in the middle ear (otitis media). If the causative organism is group A

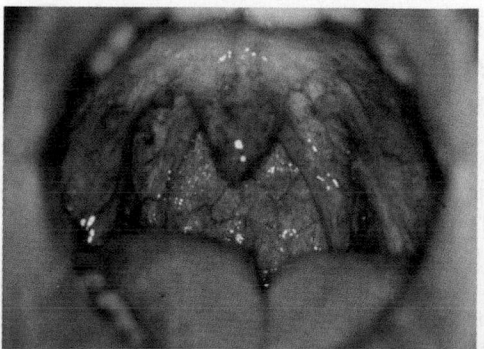

FIGURE 20-2. Pharyngitis—inflammation without exudate. (From Bickley, L. S. & Szilagyi, P.G. [2007]. *Bates' guide to physical examination and history taking*, 9th ed. Philadelphia: Lippincott Williams & Wilkins.)

streptococcus, prompt treatment is needed to prevent potential cardiac and renal complications.

Assessment Findings

Sore throat, difficulty or pain on swallowing, fever, and malaise are the most common symptoms. Enlarged adenoids may produce nasal obstruction, noisy breathing, snoring, and a nasal quality to the voice. Visual examination reveals enlarged and reddened tonsils. White patches may appear on the tonsils if group A streptococci are the cause. A throat culture and sensitivity test determines the causative microorganism and appropriate antibiotic therapy.

Medical and Surgical Management

Antibiotic therapy, analgesics such as acetaminophen, and saline gargles may be used to treat the infection and associated discomfort. Chronic tonsillitis and adenoiditis may require **tonsillectomy**, operative removal of the tonsils, and **adenoidectomy**, operative removal of the adenoids. The criteria for performing these procedures are repeated episodes of tonsillitis, hypertrophy of the tonsils, enlarged obstructive adenoids, repeated purulent otitis media, hearing loss related to serous otitis media associated with enlarged tonsils and adenoids, and other conditions (e.g., asthma, rheumatic fever) exacerbated by tonsillitis. Tonsillectomy and adenoidectomy are generally done as outpatient procedures.

Nursing Process for the Client Undergoing Tonsillectomy and Adenoidectomy

Assessment

Assess the client's understanding of the procedure and obtain baseline vital signs. Ask if the client wears dentures and when the client last had food or drink. Pay special attention to laboratory results for hematocrit, platelet count, and clotting time because of the high risk for postoperative hemorrhage. Ask the client about bleeding tendencies and recent use of aspirin, nonsteroidal anti-inflammatory drugs (NSAIDs), or other medications that prolong bleeding time. Some herbal supplements, such as feverfew or gingko, may

also prolong bleeding, so it is also important to ask about the use of these supplements.

Diagnosis, Planning, and Intervention

Following surgery, implement the postoperative standards described in Chapter 14. Additional nursing care is discussed as follows and in Client and Family Teaching 20-2.

▶ **Risk for Aspiration** related to impaired swallowing secondary to throat surgery and reduced gag reflex secondary to anesthesia

▶ **Expected Outcomes:** (1) Client will maintain a patent airway with clear breath sounds. (2) Client will expectorate secretions and vomitus as needed.

● After surgery, position client, until alert, on either side with emesis basin to catch drainage or vomitus. *Retained secretions/vomitus can obstruct airway and cause aspiration.*
● Assess gag reflex and ability to swallow. *A depressed gag reflex and inability to swallow increase the risk for aspiration.*
● Elevate head of bed 45° when client is fully awake. *This position decreases surgical edema and increases lung expansion.*
● Monitor respiratory rate, rhythm, and effort at least every hour. *Increased respiratory rate, decreased breath sounds, or both indicate an increased respiratory effort, possibly related to a partially obstructed airway, aspiration, or both.*
● Auscultate breath sounds for crackles at least every hour. *Aspiration of small amounts may occur without evidence of coughing or respiratory distress.*
● Encourage client to spit secretions/vomitus into the emesis basin. *Removal of secretions/vomitus promotes a clear airway and prevents aspiration.*
● Assess for lethargy, behavior changes, or disorientation. *Decreased level of consciousness indicates poor air exchange.*
● Have oral suction equipment available. *Prompt oral suctioning removes secretions/vomitus from the mouth, preventing aspiration.*

▶ **Risk for Impaired Tissue Integrity** related to injury to the suture line

▶ **Expected Outcome:** Client will maintain an intact suture line.

● Monitor client for bloody drainage from mouth or frequent swallowing. *These findings indicate increased bleeding from suture site and require immediate attention.*
● Instruct client not to cough, clear throat, blow nose, or use a straw in the first few postoperative days. *These actions increase pressure on the suture line and may cause disruption and bleeding.*
● Instruct client to avoid carbonated fluids and fluids high in citrus content. *Such fluids are caustic to the surgical site and may traumatize tissue, disrupting the suture line.*
● Encourage client to first try ice chips, then small sips of cold fluids, and then popsicles and full liquids as tolerated. *Gradual introduction of increasingly thick fluids provides client with an opportunity to slowly try swallowing, without disrupting the suture line.*

- Add soft food, such as gelatin and sherbet, as tolerated, after the first 24 hours postoperatively. *As the diet advances, small amounts of soft foods are less likely to traumatize the suture line.*

▶ Acute Pain related to the surgical incision in the throat

▶ Expected Outcomes: Client will acknowledge relief from pain medications and demonstrate improved ability to swallow.

- Anticipate the need for pain relief, medicating client as ordered. *Early treatment of pain assists to decrease its intensity.*
- Apply ice collar as ordered. *Cold reduces swelling and inflammation in the soft tissues surrounding the surgical incision. The ice pack will help to control bleeding, reduce edema and inflammation, and block pain receptors.*
- Encourage client to gently gargle with warm saline three to four times daily. *Gentle gargling cleanses the surgical site and helps reduce inflammation and pain, remove thick mucus, and improve swallowing.*

Evaluation of Expected Outcomes

Client maintains a clear airway and can expectorate secretions and vomitus. He or she experiences minimal postoperative bleeding. The suture line remains intact. Client states relief of pain and that he or she can swallow.

▶ *Stop, Think, and Respond Exercise 20-2*

What is the most serious complication of a tonsillectomy? Why?

PERITONSILLAR ABSCESS

A **peritonsillar abscess** is an abscess that develops in the connective tissue between the capsule of the tonsil and the constrictor muscle of the pharynx. It may follow a severe streptococcal or staphylococcal tonsillar infection. Clients with a peritonsillar abscess experience difficulty and pain with swallowing, fever, malaise, ear pain, and difficulty talking. On visual examination, the affected side is red and swollen, as is the posterior pharynx. Drainage from the abscess is cultured to identify the microorganism. Sensitivity studies determine the appropriate antibiotic therapy.

Immediate treatment of a peritonsillar abscess is recommended to prevent the spread of the causative microorganism to the bloodstream or adjacent structures. Penicillin or another antibiotic is given immediately after a culture is obtained and before results of the culture and sensitivity tests are known. Surgical incision and drainage of the abscess are done if the abscess partially blocks the oropharynx. A local anesthetic is sprayed or painted on the surface of the abscess, and the contents are evacuated. Repeated episodes may necessitate a tonsillectomy.

Nursing management of the client undergoing drainage of an abscess includes placing the client in a semi-Fowler's position to prevent aspiration. An ice collar may be ordered to reduce swelling and pain. The nurse encourages the client to drink fluids. He or she observes the client for signs of respiratory obstruction (e.g., dyspnea, restlessness, cyanosis) or excessive bleeding.

LARYNGITIS

Laryngitis is inflammation and swelling of the mucous membrane that lines the larynx. Edema of the vocal cords frequently accompanies laryngeal inflammation. Laryngitis may follow a URI and results from spread of the infection to the larynx. Other causes include excessive or improper use of the voice, allergies, and smoking.

Hoarseness, inability to speak above a whisper, or **aphonia** (complete loss of voice) are the usual symptoms. Clients also complain of throat irritation and a dry, nonproductive cough. The diagnosis is based on the symptoms. If hoarseness persists more than 2 weeks, the larynx is examined (**laryngoscopy**). Persistent hoarseness is a sign of laryngeal cancer and thus merits prompt investigation. Treatment involves voice rest and treatment or removal of the cause. Antibiotic therapy may be used if a bacterial infection is the cause. If smoking is the cause, the nurse encourages smoking cessation and refers the client to a smoking-cessation program.

STRUCTURAL DISORDERS

EPISTAXIS

Pathophysiology and Etiology

Epistaxis, or nosebleed, is a common occurrence. It is not usually serious but can be frightening. Nosebleeds are the rupture of tiny capillaries in the nasal mucous membrane. They occur most commonly in the anterior septum, referred to as *Kiesselbach's plexus.* Causes of nosebleed include trauma, rheumatic fever, infection, hypertension, nasal tumors, and blood dyscrasias. Epistaxis that results from hypertension or blood dyscrasias is likely to be severe and difficult to control. Those who abuse cocaine may have frequent nosebleeds. Foreign bodies in the nose and deviated septum contribute to epistaxis, along with forceful nose blowing and frequent or aggressive nose picking.

Assessment Findings

Inspection of the nares, using a nasal speculum and light, reveals the area of bleeding. The examiner uses a tongue blade to check the back of the throat and a laryngeal mirror to view the area above and behind the uvula.

Medical and Surgical Management

The severity and location of the bleeding determine the treatment. One or a combination of the following therapies may be used:

- Direct continuous pressure to the nares for 5 to 10 minutes with the client's head tilted slightly forward
- Application of ice packs to the nose
- Cauterization with silver nitrate, electrocautery, or application of a topical vasoconstrictor such as 1:1000 epinephrine
- Nasal packing with a cotton tampon
- Pressure with a balloon inflated catheter—inserted posteriorly for a minimum of 48 hours

Nursing Management

The nurse monitors vital signs and assesses for signs of continued bleeding. He or she may initiate measures to control

Client and Family Teaching 20-3
Epistaxis

The nurse instructs clients experiencing epistaxis to do the following:

- Apply pressure to the nares with two fingers. Breathe through the mouth and sit with the head tipped forward slightly to prevent blood from running down the throat.
- Do not swallow blood; spit out any blood oozing from the area. Do not blow the nose. If blood has been swallowed, the client may see diarrhea and black, tarry stools for a few days.
- Do not attempt to remove nasal packing or to cut the string anchoring the packing.
- Take pain medications as ordered. Do not use aspirin or ibuprofen products until bleeding is controlled.
- Notify the physician if bleeding persists or if any respiratory problems develop.

---

bleeding, such as applying pressure and ice packs. Other treatments require a physician's order. The client experiencing epistaxis is usually anxious and requires reassurance. If underlying conditions are the cause, the nurse refers the client for medical follow-up. He or she may also recommend humidification, use of a nasal lubricant to keep the mucous membranes moist, and avoidance of vigorous nose blowing and nose picking, or other nose trauma. Client and Family Teaching 20-3 outlines teaching about the treatment of severe nosebleed.

NASAL OBSTRUCTION

Obstruction of the nasal passage interferes with air passage. Three primary conditions lead to nasal obstruction: a deviated septum, nasal polyps, and hypertrophied turbinates.

Pathophysiology and Etiology

A **deviated septum** is an irregularity in the septum that results in nasal obstruction. The deviation may be a deflection from the midline in the form of lumps or sharp projections or a curvature in the shape of an "S." Marked deviation can result in complete obstruction of one nostril and interference with sinus drainage. A deviated septum may be congenital, but often it results from trauma.

Nasal polyps are grapelike swellings that arise from the nasal mucous membranes. They probably result from chronic irritation related to infection or allergic rhinitis. They obstruct nasal breathing and sinus drainage, ultimately leading to sinusitis. Most are benign and tend to recur when removed.

Hypertrophied turbinates are enlargements of the nasal conchae, three bones that project from the lateral wall of the nasal cavity. The hypertrophy, which results from chronic rhinitis, interferes with air passage and sinus drainage, and eventually leads to sinusitis.

Assessment Findings

Symptoms include a history of sinusitis, difficulty breathing out of one nostril, frequent nosebleeds, and nasal discharge. Clients usually report difficulty breathing through one or both sides of the nose. Inspection with a nasal speculum reveals a left or right deviation of the nasal septum, the number and location of the polyps, or enlarged turbinates.

Medical and Surgical Management

A submucous surgical resection or septoplasty may be necessary to restore normal breathing and to permit adequate sinus drainage for the client with a deviated septum. This procedure involves an incision through the mucous membrane and removal of the portions of the septum that cause obstruction. After this procedure, both sides of the nasal cavity are packed with gauze, which remains in place for 24 to 48 hours. A moustache dressing or drip pad is applied to absorb any drainage.

Rhinoplasty, reconstruction of the nose, may also be done at the same time. This procedure enhances the client's appearance cosmetically and corrects any structural nasal deformities that interfere with air passage. The surgeon makes an incision inside the nostril and restructures the nasal bone and cartilage. As with septoplasty, the nasal cavity is packed with gauze, and the nose is taped. Application of a nasal splint maintains the shape and structure of the nose and reduces edema. The splint remains in place for at least 1 week.

Treatment for polyps includes a steroidal nasal spray to reduce inflammation or direct injection of steroids into the polyps. If nasal obstruction is severe, the surgeon performs a *polypectomy,* the removal of polyps with a nasal snare or laser under local anesthesia. The polyps are examined microscopically to rule out malignant disease.

Hypertrophied turbinates are often treated with the application of astringents or aerosolized corticosteroids to shrink them close to the nose. Occasionally, one of the turbinates may be surgically removed (*turbinectomy*).

Nursing Management

Surgery for correction of nasal obstruction is usually done on an outpatient basis. The nurse provides thorough explanations throughout the procedures to alleviate anxiety. It is particularly important to emphasize that nasal packing will be in place postoperatively, necessitating mouth breathing. The application of an ice pack will reduce pain and swelling.

Placing the client in a semi-Fowler's position promotes drainage, reduces edema, and enhances breathing. The nurse inspects the nasal packing and dressings frequently for bleeding and asks the client to report excessive swallowing, which can indicate bleeding. Ongoing monitoring of vital signs is necessary, as is providing oral hygiene and saline mouth rinses (when permitted) to keep mucous membranes moist. The nurse tells the client that feeling or hearing a sucking noise when swallowing is normal and will resolve when the nasal packing is removed. Client and Family Teaching 20-4 lists additional teaching measures.

Client and Family Teaching 20-4
Surgery for Nasal Obstruction

Teaching measures for clients having surgery to relieve nasal obstruction include preparing the postoperative client for edema and discoloration around the eyes and nose that will disappear after a few weeks. The nurse also instructs the client to do the following to prevent bleeding:

● Do not bend over.
● Do not blow nose.
● If sneezing, keep mouth open.
● Avoid contact with nose or surrounding tissue.
● Keep head elevated with an extra pillow when lying down.
● Avoid heavy lifting.
● Do not use aspirin, ibuprofen, alcohol, or tobacco products.

TRAUMA AND OBSTRUCTION OF THE UPPER AIRWAY

FRACTURES OF THE NOSE

A nasal fracture usually results from direct trauma. It causes swelling and edema of the soft tissues, external and internal bleeding, nasal deformity, and nasal obstruction. In severe nasal fractures, cerebrospinal fluid, which is colorless and clear, may drain from the nares. Drainage of cerebrospinal fluid suggests a fracture in the cribriform plate.

The diagnosis of a nasal fracture may be delayed because of significant swelling and bleeding. As soon as the swelling decreases, the examiner inspects the nose internally to rule out a fracture of the nasal septum or septal hematoma. Both conditions require treatment to prevent destruction of the septal cartilage. If drainage of clear fluid is observed, a Dextrostix is used to determine the presence of glucose, which is diagnostic for cerebrospinal fluid. Radiography studies are done to ascertain any other facial fractures.

Medical and Surgical Management

If the fracture is a lateral displacement, pressure applied to the convex portion of the nose reduces the fracture. Cold compresses control the bleeding. If the fracture is more complex, surgery is done after the swelling subsides, usually after several days. The surgeon applies a splint postoperatively to maintain the alignment.

Nursing Management

Nursing management is similar to that for nasal obstruction. The nurse instructs the client to keep the head elevated and to apply ice four times a day for 20 minutes to reduce the swelling and pain. He or she gives analgesics as ordered to alleviate pain. Postoperatively, the nurse assesses the client for airway obstruction, respiratory difficulty (i.e., tachypnea, dyspnea), dysphagia, signs of infection, pupillary responses, level of consciousness, and periorbital edema. In addition,

the nurse helps reduce the client's anxiety by answering questions and offering reassurance that the bruising and swelling will subside and sense of smell will return.

▶ **Stop, Think, and Respond Exercise 20-3**

On your way to class you see a woman suddenly slip on ice and fall on her face. As you approach, she gets to a sitting position. She is wearing a scarf. Blood is pouring from her nose, and your initial impression is that the nose appears deformed. What actions should you take?

LARYNGEAL TRAUMA AND LARYNGEAL OBSTRUCTION

Pathophysiology and Etiology

Laryngeal trauma occurs during motor vehicle accidents when the neck strikes the steering wheel or other blunt trauma occurs in the neck region. Endoscopic and endotracheal intubations are other possible causes. Although uncommon, a fracture of the thyroid cartilage is also traumatic to the larynx.

Laryngeal obstruction is an extremely serious and often life-threatening condition. Some causes of upper airway obstruction include edema from an allergic reaction, severe head and neck injury, severe inflammation and edema of the throat, and aspiration of foreign bodies.

Assessment Findings

Signs and Symptoms

Laryngeal trauma causes neck swelling, bruising, and tenderness. If the tissues surrounding the larynx are greatly swollen, the client will exhibit **stridor**, a high-pitched, harsh sound during respiration, indicative of airway obstruction. The client also has dysphagia, hoarseness, cyanosis, and possible **hemoptysis** (expectoration of bloody sputum).

Total obstruction prevents the passage of air from the upper to the lower respiratory airway; choking clients will clutch their throats—the universal distress sign for choking. Unless total obstruction is relieved immediately, death occurs from respiratory arrest. Partial obstruction results in difficulty breathing.

Diagnostic Findings

Laryngoscopy reveals the extent of trauma and internal swelling. Radiographs and oxygenation studies will be performed after a patent airway has been established.

Medical and Surgical Management

Maintenance of a patent airway is crucial. If the client has aspirated a foreign body, the Heimlich maneuver is performed to force the object out of the upper respiratory passages (Nursing Guidelines 20-1). Allergic reactions resulting in severe inflammation and edema may be treated with epinephrine or a corticosteroid and possibly intubation. Severe obstruction requires an emergency *tracheostomy* (surgical opening into the trachea).

NURSING GUIDELINES 20-1

The Heimlich Maneuver for Dislodging an Airway Obstruction

- Ask the person if he or she is choking. (Note: Hands crossed at the neck is the universal sign of choking.)
- Assess ability to speak and cough. If the person cannot talk or cough, say that you can help and place your arms around his or her waist.
- Make a fist with one hand and place the thumb toward the victim above the umbilicus.
- Hold your fist with the other hand and thrust upward into the abdomen. Repeat thrusts.
- If the object is dislodged and the victim can cough effectively, encourage him or her to do so to eject the object.
- If the object is not ejected or coughed out and the victim loses consciousness, lower the victim to the ground.
- Straddle the victim's body and place the heel of one hand on top of the other. Position the hands midway between the umbilicus and the xiphoid process.
- Deliver thrusts and repeat.
- Open the mouth to assess if the object can be swept out with a hooked finger (do not sweep the mouth in children).
- If the airway remains obstructed, repeat the procedure.

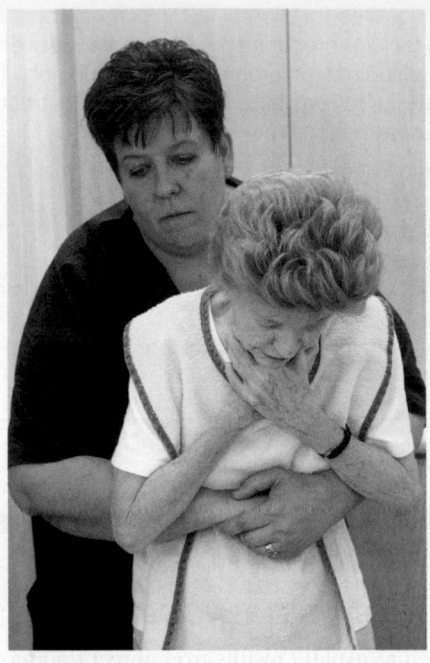

Heimlich maneuver on a conscious victim.

Nursing Process for the Client with Trauma to the Upper Airway

Assessment

Assess for air movement within the upper respiratory tract. Listen to lung sounds, monitor respiratory patterns, and look for signs of increased nasal swelling and bleeding and symptoms of laryngeal edema. Determine if the airway is obstructed.

Diagnosis, Planning, and Intervention

Partial or total obstruction of the upper airway requires immediate recognition and intervention. If present when a victim aspirates a foreign body, use the Heimlich maneuver (see Nursing Guidelines 20-1). If this maneuver fails to dislodge the object, a physician may perform an emergency tracheostomy. If edema is the cause of partial upper airway obstruction, oxygen can be given until a physician examines the client. Emergency drugs and a tracheostomy tray are made available for immediate use. Other measures are as follows:

▶ Ineffective Breathing Pattern related to partial obstruction of the upper airway secondary to trauma, nasal packing, bleeding, or edema

▶ Expected Outcomes: (1) Client will maintain a patent airway. (2) Client will demonstrate improved breath sounds.

- Assess airway patency at least every 2 hours. *Maintaining the airway is the highest priority.*
- Auscultate lungs for wheezing or decreased or absent breath sounds every 4 hours. *Wheezing may indicate increased airway resistance. Decreased or absent breath sounds indicate obstruction.*

- Assess respiratory effort, including respiratory rate, depth, nasal flaring, and use of accessory muscles. *Increased respiratory effort indicates respiratory difficulties.*
- Assess vital signs and monitor for changes at least every 4 hours. *Increased work of breathing will increase respiratory rate and heart rate.*
- Monitor arterial blood gases (ABGs). *Increasing $PaCO_2$ and decreasing PaO_2 indicate impending respiratory failure.*
- Position client in the semi-Fowler's position. *This position promotes maximum lung expansion and improved air exchange.*
- Apply ice to nasal area four times a day for 20 to 30 minutes. *Ice helps to reduce inflammation and bleeding.*
- Initiate CPR and prepare for possible airway intubation/tracheostomy if airway is completely obstructed. *Preparation for potential emergency assists to maintain the airway.*

▶ Anxiety related to airway obstruction, pain, injury, bleeding, or anticipation of medical or surgical treatments

▶ Expected Outcome: Client will communicate a decreased level of anxiety.

- Assess level of apprehension. *Anxiety increases with respiratory difficulties. Fear can interfere with ability to follow instructions.*
- Monitor for increased respiratory rate and irritability. *These signs indicate increased anxiety.*
- Provide brief explanations. *Increased anxiety impairs ability to focus.*
- Reassure client that he or she is safe—stay with client if necessary. *An anxious client will benefit from the nurse's calm and reassuring presence.*

- Assist client to practice anxiety-reducing methods such as relaxation or positive visualization. *Anxiety-reducing strategies assist client to feel that he or she has control.*

▶ Acute Pain related to injury, surgical incision, or both

▶ Expected Outcome: Client will verbalize relief of or reduced pain.

- Assess nature of pain: quality, severity, location, duration, and onset, what precipitated it, and if anything relieves it. *Pain assessment provides a qualitative description of the pain and a baseline of the client's experience.*
- Monitor vital signs, restlessness, or other signs related to pain. *These assessments give additional data for determining level of pain, particularly in clients who deny discomfort.*
- Evaluate response to analgesics and comfort measures such as ice packs and repositioning. *Such evaluation helps determine the need for changes to the treatment regimen.*

Evaluation of Expected Outcomes

The airway is free of obstruction, and breathing patterns improve. Client reports decreased anxiety and that pain has decreased in intensity and duration. ●

SLEEP APNEA SYNDROME

Sleep apnea syndrome, characterized by frequent, brief episodes of respiratory standstill during sleep, is classified according to respiratory muscle effort:

- Central—air movement is absent secondary to absence of ventilatory efforts; the brain malfunctions in its normal signal to breathe.
- Obstructive—air movement is absent secondary to pharyngeal obstruction; chest and abdominal movements are present; this is the most common form of sleep apnea.
- Mixed—combination of central and obstructive sleep apnea in one apneic episode

Pathophysiology and Etiology

According to the National Heart, Lung, and Blood Institute (NHLBI, 2008), more than 12 million Americans have obstructive sleep apnea, with half of those affected classified as overweight. Sleep apnea affects one out of 25 middle-aged men and one out of 50 middle-aged women. Women are more likely to have sleep apnea after menopause. In general, as people age, they are at higher risk for sleep apnea, with one out of 10 people over 65 years of age diagnosed with sleep apnea. Other factors that may predispose people to sleep apnea are ethnicity (African Americans, Hispanics, and Pacific Islanders are more likely to develop sleep apnea), heredity, and having smaller airways, allergies, or other conditions that contribute to increased congestion (NHLBI, 2008). Cigarette smokers are at increased risk, as are clients with any condition that reduces pharyngeal muscle tone: neuromuscular disease, use of sedative or hypnotic medications, and frequent and heavy intake of alcohol.

Obstructive sleep apnea results from a reduced diameter of the upper airway, which may develop when the upper airway collapses secondary to the normally reduced muscle tone during sleep. The repeated apneic spells have serious effects on the cardiopulmonary system. Clients with sleep apnea often have hypertension and are therefore at greater risk of cerebrovascular accident and myocardial infarction (MI), as well as heart arrhythmias and heart failure.

Gerontologic Considerations

- Large neck circumference and obesity and other comorbidities experienced by older adults increase the risk for sleep apnea.

Assessment Findings

During sleep, clients with obstructive sleep apnea snore loudly, with cessation of breathing for at least 10 seconds. These episodes may occur many times within one hour, from as few as five to thirty times, and up to a total of several hundred per night. Clients awaken suddenly as the partial pressure of oxygen (PaO$_2$) level drops, usually with a loud snort. Other symptoms include daytime fatigue, morning headache, inability to concentrate when awake, sore throat, enuresis, and erectile dysfunction. Partners may report that the client behaves differently and is not the same in personality and that the snoring progressively worsens. Box 20-1 reviews symptoms of sleep apnea.

Initial diagnosis is made according to the client's reported symptoms. To determine the nature of the sleep apnea, clients undergo **polysomnography**, which consists of tests that monitor the client's respiratory and cardiac status while he or she is asleep. Specifically, a polysomnogram records a client's brain activity, eye movement, muscle

BOX 20-1	Symptoms of Sleep Apnea

- Restless sleep
- Loud, heavy snoring—often interrupted by silence and then gasps
- Excessive daytime sleepiness—can occur while driving or working
- Morning headaches
- Loss of energy
- Trouble concentrating
- Irritability
- Forgetfulness
- Mood or behavior changes, including anxiety or depression
- Decreased interest in sex
- Systemic hypertension
- Dysrhythmias
- Enuresis

(National Heart, Lung & Blood Institute. [2008]. " Sleep apnea." Available at: http://www.nhlbi.nih.gov/health/dci/desease/sleepapnea/sleepapnea_whatis.html. Accessed July 4, 2008.)

movement, respiratory and heart rates; the amount of air that moves in and out of the lungs; and the oxygen concentration in the blood.

Medical and Surgical Management

Treatment for sleep apnea focuses on improving the quality of nighttime sleep and daytime wakefulness, as well as reducing risks for cardiovascular problems. Depending on the severity of sleep apnea, clients may change their lifestyle, including:

- Losing weight
- Quitting smoking
- Eliminating alcohol or other medications that depress respirations and contribute to an inability to maintain an open airway
- Using special pillows to keep clients in a side-lying position when sleeping
- Using allergy medications or saline nasal spray to reduce congestion and dryness

Another treatment is fitting the client for an oral appliance that assists in adjusting the lower jaw and tongue so that the airway remains open while the client is sleeping. A dentist or orthodontist fits the client for a custom-made oral appliance.

Additional treatment includes the use of noninvasive positive pressure ventilation (NPPV), which is the application of positive pressure via full-face mask, nasal mask, or cannula with supplemental oxygen to enhance ventilation. There are two commonly used types:

- Continuous positive airway pressure (CPAP)—provides constant airway pressure during inspiration and expiration
- Bilevel positive airway pressure (BIPAP)—provides two levels of pressure: inspiratory and expiratory airway pressures

With this treatment, the client receives airway pressure either through his or her own inspirations or by machine-initiated inspirations. A set number of breaths are delivered. Clients often are not compliant because they do not like the continuous pressure of CPAP or the varying pressures of BIPAP or do not like using equipment and oxygen every night. In addition, these methods do not completely eliminate the problem. A newer technology referred to as auto-titrating continuous positive airway pressure (APAP) automatically adjusts airway pressure as needed (Strohl & Wylie, 2004). Side effects of positive pressure ventilation include dry mouth, rhinitis, and sinus congestion.

If the cause of sleep apnea is obstructive, surgical procedures are done to relieve the obstruction. The most common surgery is *uvulopalatopharyngoplasty,* a surgical procedure to remove tissues in the throat, including the uvula, palate, and pharynx, to relieve obstruction.

Tracheostomy is a successful treatment. Clients may reject this option, however, because of the trauma, the seemingly barbaric nature of the procedure, and the alteration that it creates in appearance. Tracheostomy also may be technically difficult if the client is markedly obese. If a client chooses to have a tracheostomy, he or she may plug it during the day.

Medication sometimes is prescribed for central sleep apnea, and clients take such drugs at bedtime. The goal is to increase the respiratory drive and improve upper airway muscle tone. An example of a medication for this purpose is protriptyline (Vivactil, Triptil). Clients also may use low-flow oxygen at night to relieve hypoxemia.

Nursing Management

Clients with sleep apnea usually are anxious and require reassurance and adequate instruction about their condition. The nurse provides thorough explanations of the disease process, polysomnography, and treatments. He or she refers clients to self-help groups or to appropriate counseling for weight loss or alcohol and substance abuse issues. The nurse collaborates with respiratory therapists to instruct the client in the use of CPAP or other NPPV and furnishes the client with information about sleep apnea and its potential complications if not treated.

LARYNGEAL CANCER

With early detection, cancer of the larynx has great potential for cure. Preventive health measures focus on early consultation for persistent hoarseness and other changes in voice quality.

Pathophysiology and Etiology

Laryngeal cancer is most common in people 50 to 70 years of age. Men are affected more frequently than are women. The cause of laryngeal cancer is unknown. Carcinogens, such as tobacco, alcohol, and industrial pollutants, are associated with laryngeal cancer. In addition, chronic laryngitis, habitual overuse of the voice, and heredity may contribute. Most laryngeal malignancies are squamous cell carcinomas, that is, a malignancy arising from the epithelial cells lining the larynx. The tumor may be located on the glottis (true vocal cords), above the glottis (supraglottis or false vocal cords), or below the glottis (subglottis).

Assessment Findings

Signs and Symptoms

Persistent hoarseness (longer than two weeks) is usually the earliest symptom. At first the hoarseness is slight, and clients tend to ignore it. Later, the client notes a sensation of swelling or a lump in the throat, followed by dysphagia and pain when talking. The client may also complain of burning in the throat when swallowing hot or citrus liquids. If the malignant tissue is not removed promptly, symptoms of advancing carcinoma, such as dyspnea, weakness, weight loss, enlarged cervical lymph nodes, pain, and anemia develop. Halitosis or bad breath is also characteristic of laryngeal cancer. Clients also may complain of earaches.

Diagnostic Findings

Visual examination of the larynx (laryngoscopy) and biopsy confirm the diagnosis and identify the type of malignancy. In addition, computed tomography (CT) scanning and chest radiography are used to detect metastasis and to determine tumor size. The physician also assesses the mobility of the

TABLE 20-1. Descriptions of Laryngeal Surgery

SURGERY	DESCRIPTION	INDICATION	POSTOPERATIVE EXPECTATIONS
Partial laryngectomy	The affected vocal cord is removed; other structures remain intact	For early-stage laryngeal cancer when only one cord is involved	Voice will be hoarse; intact trachea; no problems with swallowing; high cure rate
Supraglottic laryngectomy	Hyoid bone, glottis, and false cords removed; radical neck dissection done on involved side; remaining structures left intact	For supraglottic tumors	Voice will be hoarse; postoperative tracheostomy until glottic airway functions; nutrition administered through nasogastric tube until surgical sites heal; recurrence is possible
Hemivertical laryngectomy	Thyroid cartilage of trachea is split at midline; one true cord and one false cord are removed along with arytenoid cartilage and half the thyroid cartilage.	When tumor extends beyond the vocal cord but is smaller than 1 cm	Client will have a tracheostomy and nasogastric tube after surgery until healed; voice will be hoarse and diminished; client will have an intact airway and the ability to swallow.
Total laryngectomy	Both vocal cords removed along with the hyoid bone, epiglottis, cricoid cartilage, and two or three rings of the trachea; the tongue, pharyngeal walls, and trachea remain intact; usually a radical neck dissection is done on the affected side.	When the cancer extends beyond the vocal cords	Permanent tracheal stoma; prevents aspiration. No voice but ability to swallow remains. Metastasis to cervical lymph nodes is common.
Radical neck dissection	The neck is opened from the jaw to the clavicle from the midline to the interior border of the trapezius muscle. The following are removed: subcutaneous and soft tissue, sternocleidomastoid muscle, jugular vein, and spinal accessory nerve innervates trapezius muscle—client's shoulder will droop after surgery as the trapezius muscle atrophies). A split-thickness skin graft is applied over the carotid artery.	When cancer has metastasized to cervical lymph nodes	Permanent tracheal stoma. No voice; ability to swallow remains. Client requires physical therapy for neck muscles, along with a prescribed exercise program.

vocal cords. Limited mobility indicates that the tumor growth is affecting the surrounding tissue, muscle, and airway.

Medical and Surgical Management

Treatment depends on factors such as the size of the lesion, the client's age, and metastasis. Medical treatment may include chemotherapy, which appears to have only minimal effects, and radiation therapy, either alone or with surgery.

Surgical treatment (Table 20-1) includes laser surgery for early lesions or a partial or total laryngectomy. In more advanced cases, total laryngectomy may be the treatment of choice. If the disease has extended beyond the larynx, a radical neck dissection (removal of the lymph nodes, muscles, and adjacent tissues) is performed. Laser surgery may also be used to relieve obstruction in more advanced cases.

A client with a total laryngectomy has a permanent tracheal *stoma* (opening) because the trachea is no longer connected to the nasopharynx. The larynx is severed from the trachea and removed completely. The only respiratory organs in use are the trachea, bronchi, and lungs. Air enters and leaves through the tracheostomy (Fig. 20-3). The client no longer feels air entering the nose. Because the anterior wall of the esophagus connects with the posterior wall of the larynx, it must be reconstructed. Tube feeding facilitates

healing by preventing muscle activity and irritation of the esophagus (see Chap. 45).

Loss of the ability to speak normally is a devastating consequence of laryngeal surgery. Clients with a malignancy of the larynx require emotional support before and after surgery and help in understanding and choosing an alternative method of speech. Some methods of alaryngeal speech used after a laryngectomy include the following:

- *Esophageal speech*—requires regurgitation of swallowed air and formation of words with lips; voice quality will be lower-pitched and gruff-sounding, but more natural
- *Artificial (electric) larynx*—a throat vibrator held against the neck that projects sound into the mouth; words are formed with the mouth
- *Tracheoesophageal puncture (TEP)*—a surgical opening in the posterior wall of the trachea, followed by the insertion of a prosthesis such as a Blom-Singer device (Fig. 20-4). Air from the lungs is diverted through the opening in the posterior tracheal wall to the esophagus and out the mouth. The client covers the stoma with his or her finger and forces air through the esophagus; this causes the walls of the throat to vibrate as the client speaks. It sounds more natural than an artificial larynx.

A speech pathologist works with the client to use an artificial speech device, learn esophageal speech, or speak

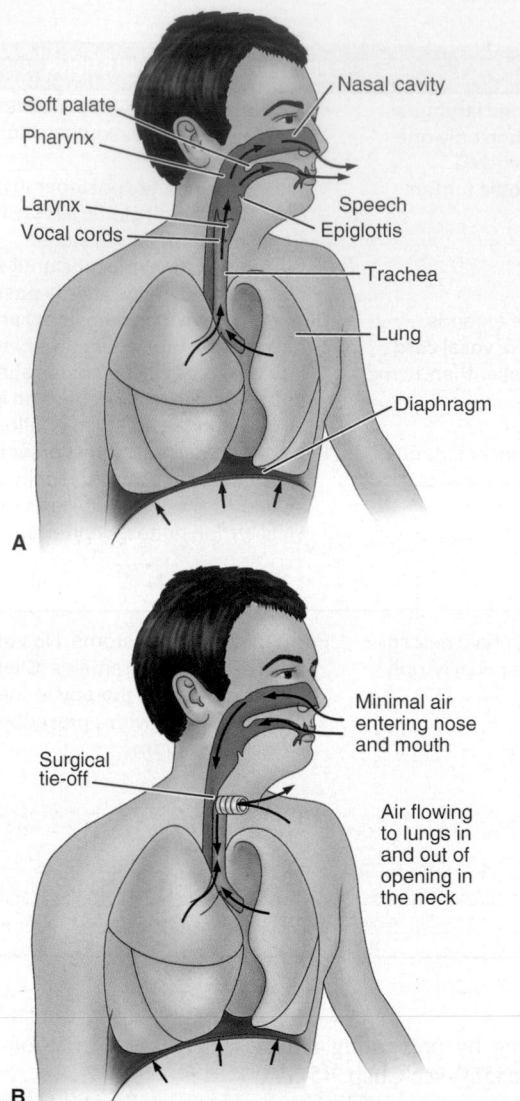

FIGURE 20-3. Total laryngectomy changes the airflow for breathing and speaking. (**A**) Normal airflow. (**B**) Airflow through a permanent tracheal stoma after total laryngectomy.

clearly with a prosthesis. Clients having a partial laryngectomy also may require speech therapy.

Nursing Process for the Client Undergoing Laryngeal Surgery

Assessment

Determine the client's level of understanding of the diagnosis, reason for surgery, and probable outcome. Assess for hoarseness, sore throat, dyspnea, dysphagia, pain, or burning in the throat. Ascertaining the client's level of anxiety is important, as is identifying coping strategies. Also assess the client's ability to communicate in ways other than speaking, such as abilities to read and write. Begin preoperative teaching, allowing the client to express fears about the surgery, diagnosis, and potential loss of voice postoperatively. Discuss alternative methods of communication and identify which

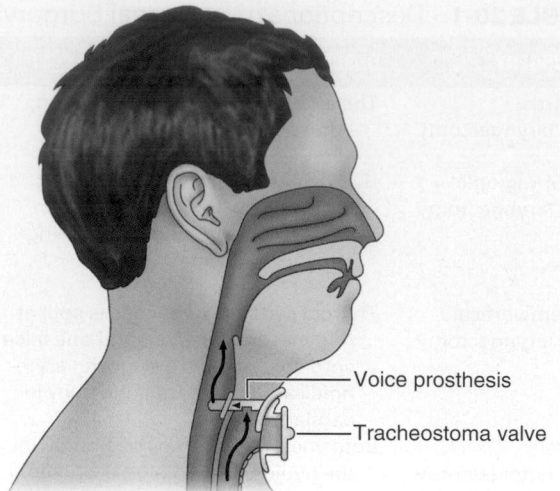

FIGURE 20-4. Schematic representation of tracheoesophageal puncture (TEP) speech. Air travels from the lung through a puncture in the posterior wall of the trachea into the esophagus and out the mouth. A voice prosthesis is fitted over the puncture site.

method the client prefers. After surgery, carefully assess for a patent airway and effective airway clearance.

Diagnosis, Planning, and Interventions

Care centers around preventing postoperative complications, managing pain, preventing wound infection, helping the client communicate, and fostering the client's ability to cope with changes in body image. Provide the client and family with the following postoperative instructions:

• Water should not enter the stoma because it will flow from the trachea to the lungs. Thus, avoid swimming, and take care when bathing. Avoid showers until experienced with care of the stoma, and then use a hand-held shower device if possible.
• Wear a scarf or gauze dressing over the stoma to make the opening less obvious.
• Avoid fabrics or dressings that fray to prevent small fibers from being drawn into the stoma.

In addition to the following diagnoses, outcomes, and interventions, refer to Chapter 14 for general postoperative care.

▶ **Ineffective Airway Clearance** related to surgical alterations of the airway

▶ **Expected Outcome:** Client will maintain effective airway clearance as evidenced by clear breath sounds, normal respirations, and effective cough.

• Position client in semi-Fowler's position. *This position provides optimal lung expansion and decreases edema in the surgical site.*
• Auscultate breath sounds and respiratory effort at least every 4 hours. *Initial and ongoing assessments provide a baseline for comparison.*
• Assess effectiveness of client's cough. *An effective cough promotes airway clearance.*
• Encourage deep breathing and coughing every 2 hours while client is awake. *These measures prevent atelectasis and promote effective gas exchange.*

- Monitor for restlessness, dyspnea, anxiety, and increased heart rate. *These signs indicate ineffective airway clearance.*
- Observe level of consciousness for signs of lethargy or disorientation. *These signs indicate poor gas exchange.*

▶ **Impaired Verbal Communication** related to removal of larynx and postoperative edema

▶ **Expected Outcome:** Client will communicate effectively with alternative methods.

- Frequently assess client's need to communicate. *Assessments alleviate client's anxiety.*
- Allow client time to communicate needs. *Adequate time promotes acceptance of client and decreases anxiety about ability to communicate.*
- Provide alternative methods of communication: paper and pen, wipe board, or word or picture board. *Having supplies available provides comfort to client.*
- Reinforce instructions regarding use of a voice prosthesis, electrolarynx, or esophageal speech. *Support and instruction help client to become more proficient with alternative speech methods.*

▶ **Imbalanced Nutrition: Less than Body Requirements** related to swallowing deficits

▶ **Expected Outcome:** Client will have adequate caloric and fluid intake as evidenced by increase in or maintenance of preoperative weight.

- Instruct client on need for enteral feedings if prescribed. *Enteral feedings are used until the suture line heals, usually 10 to 14 days postoperatively.*
- Provide meticulous mouth care every 4 hours. *Oral care keeps mouth fresh and promotes interest in caloric intake.*
- Introduce thick oral liquids initially and solid foods as tolerated. *Gradual advancement of the diet promotes ease in swallowing.*
- Reassure the client that the senses of taste and smell are diminished but will return as client accommodates to airway alterations. *Inhaled air passes directly into the trachea, bypassing the nose. Loss of ability to smell alters taste sensations and may lead to anorexia.*
- Monitor for signs of dysphagia. *Difficulty swallowing will decrease caloric content and lead to weight loss.*

▶ **Social Isolation** related to change in body image, tracheal stoma, and change in or loss of speech

▶ **Expected Outcome:** Client will demonstrate evidence of adjustment to changes and resume social interactions.

- Demonstrate acceptance of client's changed appearance. *Acceptance provides a sense of belonging and promotes positive self-esteem.*
- Encourage client to maintain or reestablish social relationships. *Social relationships reduce the sense of isolation and increase feelings of acceptance.*
- Provide time for client to express feelings about changes. *Allowing time for expression of feelings assists the client to cope with changes.*

- Refer client to support services such as the International Association of Laryngectomees, and arrange for visits from clients who have had a laryngectomy. *Rehabilitation is lengthy; support from others has a positive effect.*

Evaluation of Expected Outcomes

The client maintains a clear airway, effectively clearing secretions. He or she demonstrates effective alternative communication methods and maintains adequate caloric and fluid intake. The client maintains or establishes social interactions and copes with changes.

▶ *Stop, Think, and Respond Exercise 20-4*

Name three of the most common postoperative complications of laryngectomy.

TREATMENT MODALITIES FOR AIRWAY OBSTRUCTION OR AIRWAY MAINTENANCE

Clients with serious airway conditions require aggressive treatment to maintain an airway or relieve airway obstruction. This section discusses tracheostomy, tracheotomy, endotracheal intubation, and mechanical ventilation.

TRACHEOTOMY AND TRACHEOSTOMY

A **tracheotomy** is the surgical procedure that makes an opening into the trachea. A **tracheostomy** is a surgical opening into the trachea into which a tracheostomy or laryngectomy tube is inserted. A tracheostomy may be temporary or permanent. A permanent opening in the trachea is required for certain disorders, such as a laryngectomy for laryngeal cancer.

General Considerations

Tracheostomy tubes come in several sizes and differ from laryngectomy tubes in their length and diameter. A cuffed tracheostomy tube has a cuff on the lower end that is inflated with air to provide a snug fit (Fig. 20-5). The cuff prevents aspiration of liquids or escape of air when a mechanical ventilator is used. The physician specifies the amount of air to be injected into the cuff, usually to achieve a pressure between 20 and 25 mm H_2O. The amount of air determines the seating of the cuff in the trachea. The pressure in the cuff requires monitoring with a pressure gauge every 8 hours.

During the immediate postoperative period, the physician may change the tracheostomy tube every 3 to 5 days. To pass a tracheostomy tube into the tracheal opening, an obturator is placed in the tube to facilitate placement. Once the tracheostomy tube is in place, the obturator is removed. The outer tube is held snugly in place by tapes inserted in openings on either side of it and tied at the side of the client's neck.

The respiratory passages react to the creation of the new opening with inflammation and excessive mucus secretion. Copious respiratory secretions are life-threatening. The client cannot be left unattended during the immediate postoperative period because the secretions make frequent suctioning necessary. Additionally, inspired air passes directly into the trachea, bronchi, and lungs without becoming warmed and

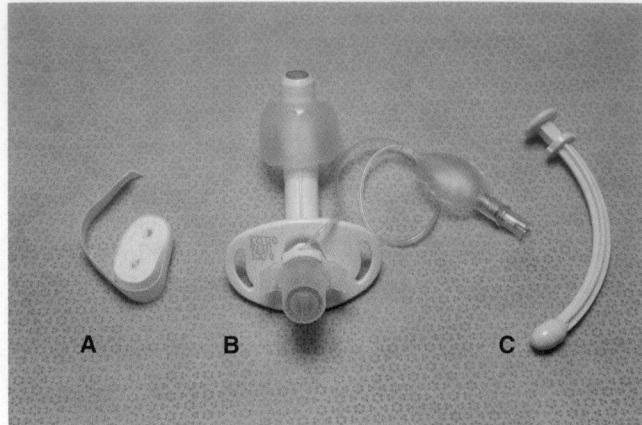

FIGURE 20-5. Cuffed tracheostomy components. (**A**) Tracheostomy ties. (**B**) Cuffed tracheostomy tube. The cuff at the lower end of the outer tracheostomy tube is inflated with air to provide a snug fit in the trachea. (**C**) Obdurator is used to guide placement of tracheostomy tube.

NURSING GUIDELINES 20-2

Suctioning the Client With a Tracheostomy

- Use sterile equipment (e.g., gloves, suction catheter, normal saline) and aseptic technique for tracheal suctioning.
- Place client in Fowler's position. Preoxygenate client for at least 1 to 2 minutes. Check that suction pressure is at a low setting.
- Open the suction kit, don gloves, lubricate a sterile, 10- to 14-French disposable catheter with sterile saline, and insert it into the lumen of the tube.
- Do not apply suction while the catheter is inserted down the trachea because this irritates the lining of the trachea.
- Begin intermittent suctioning while slowly withdrawing and rotating the catheter. Do not suction for more than 10 seconds at a time.
- Allow client to rest and deep breathe before repeating if more suctioning is necessary.
- Discard the suction catheter after use.

moistened by passing through the nose. Dry secretions can subsequently develop, which easily form crusts and can break off, obstruct the lower airway, and cause serious respiratory problems. Humidification by a mist collar is usually necessary to prevent drying and incrustation of the mucous membrane in the trachea and the main bronchus. The long-term and short-term complications of tracheostomy include infection, bleeding, airway obstruction resulting from hardened secretions, aspiration, injury to the laryngeal nerve, erosion of the trachea, fistula formation between the esophagus and trachea, and penetration of the posterior tracheal wall.

Nursing Management

After surgery, the nurse monitors vital signs and auscultates breath sounds. He or she assesses skin color, level of consciousness, and mental status. The nurse monitors for potential complications and checks airway patency frequently. Secretions can rapidly clog the inner lumen of the tracheostomy tube, resulting in severe respiratory difficulty or death by asphyxiation. If the airway is obstructed, the client becomes cyanotic, restless, and frightened.

To facilitate breathing during the immediate postoperative period, the nurse positions the client as ordered. When the client is fully awake and blood pressure is stable, the nurse elevates the head of the bed to about 45°. This position decreases edema and makes breathing easier.

The nurse inspects the tracheostomy carefully, ensuring that tapes are secure. If the tube is not tied securely, the client can cough it out, a serious occurrence if the edges of the trachea have not been sutured to the skin. This may be the case in a temporary tracheostomy. The nurse keeps a tracheal dilator at the bedside at all times. If the outer tube accidentally comes out, the nurse inserts the dilator to hold the edges of the stoma apart until the physician arrives to insert another tube. A tracheal tube must never be forced back in place. Use of force may compress the client's trachea (by pushing the tube alongside and compressing the trachea, rather than inserting the tube into the stoma). Such action could cause respiratory arrest.

The nurse suctions the client to remove secretions that can obstruct the airway (Nursing Guidelines 20-2). He or she avoids unnecessary suctioning to decrease trauma to the airway. When explaining the procedure, the nurse tells the client that the suction catheter will be inserted for only a few seconds. Keeping an extra tracheostomy tube of the same size at the bedside is essential, because an immediate change may be necessary if the tube becomes blocked with mucus that cannot be removed. The nurse provides routine tracheostomy care (Nursing Guidelines 20-3). He or she places a gauze dressing under the tube to absorb secretions. The hospital gown and bed linens must never cover the opening of the tracheostomy tube. Nursing Care Plan 20-1 describes additional care.

ENDOTRACHEAL INTUBATION AND MECHANICAL VENTILATION

An endotracheal tube (Fig. 20-6) is inserted through the mouth or nose into the trachea to provide a patent airway for clients who cannot maintain an adequate airway on their own. Examples include those with respiratory difficulty, comatose clients, those undergoing general anesthesia, and clients with extensive edema of upper airway passages.

General Considerations

An endotracheal tube can remain in place for up to 2 weeks. The cuff is inflated to provide a tight seal. The endotracheal tube is attached to a ventilator for control of respirations and ventilation of the lungs. Humidification is necessary, because air going to the lungs through an endotracheal tube does not pass through the moist mucous membranes of the upper airway.

There are several modes of mechanical ventilation, classified according to the manner in which they support

NURSING GUIDELINES 20-3

Providing Tracheostomy Care

- Maintain aseptic technique, washing hands before, during, and after the procedure.
- Position client in a supine or low Fowler's position.
- Using a clean glove, remove the soiled stomal dressing and discard it, glove and all, in an appropriate receptacle.
- Open the tracheostomy kit without contaminating the contents. Don sterile gloves—keep the dominant hand sterile. Pour hydrogen peroxide and normal saline into respective containers.
- Unlock the inner cannula by turning it counterclockwise. Remove it and place in hydrogen peroxide. Clean the inside and outside of the cannula with pipe cleaners.
- Rinse the cleaned cannula with normal saline. Tap the cannula and wipe the excess solution with sterile gauze.
- Replace the inner cannula and turn it clockwise within the outer cannula.
- Clean around the stoma with an applicator moistened with normal saline.
- Place a sterile dressing around the tracheostomy tube. Change the tracheostomy ties by placing the new ones on first, and

removing the soiled ones last. Tie the new ends securely, but not tightly, at the side of the neck.

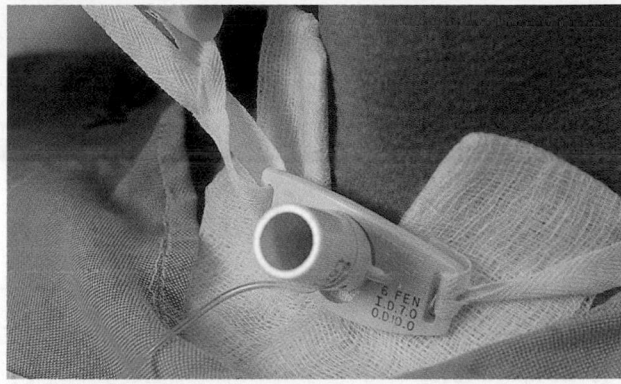

Securing a tracheostormy dressing.

ventilation. Two major classifications are negative-pressure and positive-pressure ventilators (Table 20-2). Positive-pressure ventilators are used more commonly. The major difference between the two types is that negative-pressure ventilators exert negative pressure, a pulling or sucking force, on the external chest, whereas positive-pressure ventilators inflate the lungs by exerting positive pressure, pushing air into the airway. Negative-pressure ventilators are used for clients with chronic respiratory failure related to neuromuscular disease such as poliomyelitis or myasthenia gravis. Positive-pressure ventilators require intubation and are used for clients with acute respiratory failure and primary lung disease, such as cystic fibrosis, or for clients who are comatose, are under general anesthesia, or have extensive upper airway edema. Complications related to mechanical ventilation include damage to the lungs, decreased lung expansion, and ventilator-associated pneumonia (VAP).

A new modality, referred to as airway pressure release ventilation (APRV), promotes spontaneous breathing in a ventilated client (Andrews & Habashi, 2006). In APRV, the ventilator cycles between higher and lower pressure levels of CPAP. This helps to open alveoli and promotes better gas exchange. Clients are more comfortable, requiring less sedation to maintain traditional mechanical ventilation. Because they are not sedated heavily while on APRV, clients also can maintain a cough reflex. Generally, clients on APRV have the potential for earlier removal (weaning) from the ventilator.

Accidental removal of an endotracheal tube must be prevented, because this can result in laryngeal edema or **laryngospasm** (spasm of the laryngeal muscles, resulting in narrowing of the larynx) and subsequent respiratory arrest. The inflated cuff and placement of tape around the tube

attached to the client's cheek secures the endotracheal tube. The proximal end of the tube is marked for determining if downward displacement has occurred.

The intubated client has the endotracheal tube removed when the vital capacity is adequate and the client can breathe without assistance. Blood gas studies also are used as a guideline for removal. Depending on hospital policy, the removal of an endotracheal tube may be done by the nurse, the respiratory therapist, or the doctor. Before removing the tube, emergency equipment for respiratory support must be available. The pharynx must be suctioned before the cuff is deflated to prevent the aspiration of secretions during removal of the tube. The tube usually is removed with the client in semi-Fowler's position. If laryngospasm occurs, air is administered by positive pressure. Reinsertion of the endotracheal tube by the physician or other trained personnel may be necessary if laryngospasm continues. Possible complications with the use of endotracheal intubation include ulceration and stricture of the trachea or larynx, atelectasis, and pneumonia.

Nursing Management

Major goals for the client with an intubation are to improve respirations, maintain a patent airway, and communicate needs to others. The nurse monitors vital signs periodically, depending on the client's condition and the reason for endotracheal tube insertion. Blood gas studies and pulse oximetry provide methods of ongoing evaluation of the client's respiratory status. The nurse reviews the results of these studies and reports changes to the physician.

The nurse observes the client at frequent intervals for response to respiratory support and complications

NURSING CARE PLAN 20-1 | The Client With a Tracheostomy

Assessment

- Monitor vital signs and auscultate breath sounds.
- Assess skin color, level of consciousness, and mental status.
- Monitor for potential complications.
- Assess frequently for a patent airway.
- Inspect tracheostomy frequently for placement and security of ties.

PC. **Hypoxia, Hemorrhage, Displaced Tracheostomy Tube, Accidental Extubation**

Expected Outcome. The nurse will prevent or manage complications of the tracheostomy.

Interventions	Rationales
Monitor for signs and symptoms of respiratory distress: difficulty breathing, diminished or absent breath sounds, use of accessory muscles, and asymmetric chest wall movements.	Early recognition of signs and symptoms of respiratory distress prevents further complications.
Assess for subcutaneous emphysema (air trapped in tissues) around the stoma, neck, and chest.	Injury or trauma to the airway can cause air to leak into surrounding tissues. Severe subcutaneous emphysema indicates significant leaking and potential airway obstruction.
Provide humidification.	A tracheostomy bypasses the nose; thus, inspired air is not warmed or humidified. Increased warmth and humidity thin and help remove secretions.
Keep tracheostomy ties secure but not too tight (one finger should slip easily under ties).	Ties maintain tube placement without damaging underlying skin or causing discomfort.
Monitor pulse oximetry or arterial blood gas results. Administer oxygen as needed.	Such monitoring ensures adequate oxygenation.

Evaluation of Expected Outcome

The nurse manages the client's care and prevents complications.

Nursing Diagnosis. **Risk for Ineffective Airway Clearance** related to increased secretions and possible occlusion of the inner cannula

Expected Outcome. Airway and tracheostomy tube will remain clear.

Interventions	Rationales
Provide warm, humidified air.	Such air prevents drying and crusting of secretions.
Suction as needed.	Suctioning clears secretions.
Maintain a patent airway. In cases of suspected obstruction: (1) suction the tracheostomy, (2) induce coughing, (3) change the inner cannula, and (4) position client to maximize respiratory effort.	These measures remove thick secretions and possible mucous plugs and promote lung expansion.

Evaluation of Expected Outcome

Client's airway and tracheostomy are patent.

Nursing Diagnosis. **Risk for Infection** related to loss of upper airway protection

Expected Outcome. Risk for infection will be reduced.

Interventions	Rationales
Monitor stoma for erythema, exudate, or odor.	Such findings may indicate infection.
Assess skin around stoma and under tracheostomy ties for signs of breakdown.	Intact skin prevents infection.
Monitor white blood cell (WBC) count.	Elevated WBCs may indicate infection.
Provide routine tracheostomy care every 8 hours and as necessary. Maintain sterile technique.	These measures prevent infection.
Position client so that secretions do not pool around the stoma.	Maintaining a clean and dry stoma prevents infection.

NURSING CARE PLAN 20-1   The Client With a Tracheostomy (Continued)

Evaluation of Expected Outcome

Client does not have any signs or symptoms of infection.

Nursing Diagnosis. Risk for Ineffective Management of Therapeutic Regimen related to lack of knowledge about tracheostomy care and home support

Expected Outcome. Client or caregiver will demonstrate skills appropriate for tracheostomy care.

Interventions	Rationales
Assess client's and caregiver's ability to provide adequate home care.	This assessment provides a baseline for teaching needs and referrals.
Begin teaching skills one at a time.	Step-by-step teaching provides time to absorb information.
Teach client how to suction airway, clean tube, change dressing and ties, provide stoma care, and reinsert tracheostomy tube. Have client demonstrate skills.	Demonstration of skills ensures that client or caregiver has adequate knowledge for home care.
Teach client or caregiver to check for signs and symptoms of infection.	Such measures prevent or enable early treatment of infection.
Refer client and caregiver to support groups and home care services.	Home care needs are planned for before discharge.

Evaluation of Expected Outcome

Client or caregiver demonstrates adequate skill in tracheostomy care and is sufficiently independent for discharge home.

---

associated with endotracheal intubation. He or she evaluates any change in mental status. Confusion may result from abnormal blood gas levels or electrolyte imbalances. Sudden restlessness or agitation may indicate obstruction of the endotracheal tube, which can be life-threatening. The nurse auscultates the lungs and observes the symmetric rise and fall of the chest every 30 to 60 minutes. If he or she cannot detect bilateral breath sounds, the nurse notifies the physician immediately.

Humidification is necessary to keep the inspired air moist. Clients with endotracheal intubation cannot cough, secretions are often thick and tenacious, and swallowing reflexes are depressed. An increase in $PaCO_2$ caused by

blockage of the endotracheal tube or malfunctioning of the ventilator may occur secondary to secretions or because the client is biting on the tube. Keeping the airway patent at all times is absolutely necessary, using the same suctioning technique as for a tracheostomy. If the client is biting on the tube, a bite block or oral airway may be used to keep the tube patent.

The nurse changes the client's position every 2 hours to prevent atelectasis. He or she gives oral care as needed to keep the mouth and lips free of crusts and mucus. The nurse suctions the oropharynx and mouth as needed and cleans the teeth with applicators. The nurse inspects the oral cavity frequently and reports any signs of oral bleeding to the physician.

The client may display anxiety or fear because of the tube, inability to speak, suctioning, and dependence on a machine for breathing. Each time suctioning is needed, the nurse reassures the client that the procedure takes only a short time. The client may attempt to remove or pull on the tube if he or she is awake or partially awake. Restraining the client may be necessary. The nurse should contact the physician if the client is extremely restless. Providing a "Magic Slate," wipe board, or pencil and paper to the client enables communication, as does asking questions that the client can answer by shaking the head yes or no.

Once the endotracheal tube is removed, the nurse places the client in a high-Fowler's or semi-Fowler's position to promote optimal chest and lung expansion. The posterior pharynx may be dry, and the voice may be hoarse. The nurse observes the client frequently for signs of laryngeal edema and increased respiratory distress. He or she immediately reports any sign of respiratory distress because reinsertion of the endotracheal tube may be necessary.

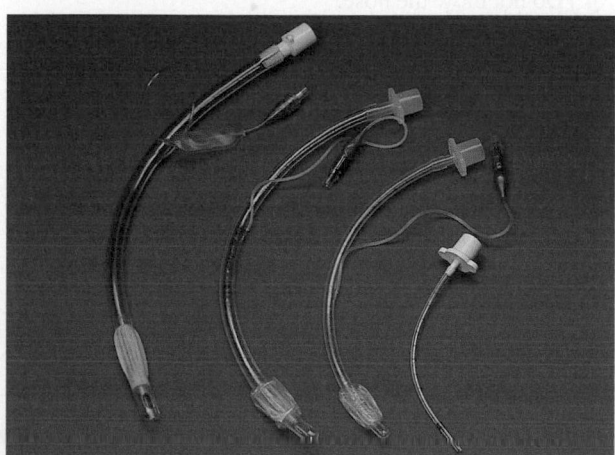

FIGURE 20-6. Endotracheal tubes.

TABLE 20-2. Types of Mechanical Ventilators

CLASSIFICATION	HOW USED
Negative pressure	Exerts negative pressure on chest; decreases intrathoracic pressure during inspiration, allowing air to flow into lungs; does not require intubation
	Used for clients experiencing chronic respiratory failure, such as in poliomyelitis, myasthenia gravis, muscular dystrophy, amyotrophic lateral sclerosis
Drinker respirator tank	Also known as the *iron lung;* a negative-pressure chamber; used extensively in the past for clients with poliomyelitis
Body wrap (pneumo-wrap) and chest cuirass (tortoise shell)	Requires a rigid cage or shell around the thorax to create a negative-pressure chamber
Positive pressure	Exerts positive pressure on airway to inflate lungs; expiration is passive
	Usually requires endotracheal or tracheal intubation
Pressure-cycled	Inspiration ends when a preset pressure is reached; cycle means that ventilator cycles on, delivers flow of air until a certain pressure is reached, and then cycles off
	Designed for short-term use because volume of air varies as client's airway resistance or compliance changes
Time-cycled	Controls respiration after a preset time; length of inspiration and flow rate of air regulate volume the client receives; usually used on newborns and infants
Volume-cycled	Delivers a preset volume of air with each inspiration; once volume is delivered, ventilator cycles off and client expires air passively
	Provides consistent adequate breaths despite airway resistance or changes in compliance; most commonly used ventilator for adults
Noninvasive	Ventilation delivered by face masks or other nasal devices; does not require intubation of any kind; used for clients with sleep-related breathing disorders or other chronic respiratory disorders

CRITICAL THINKING EXERCISES

1. A client with severe pharyngitis is diagnosed with a group A streptococcal infection. The physician prescribes penicillin. What discharge instructions should you give the client?

2. The LPN is assigned to assist the RN in the care of a client on a positive pressure ventilator. A primary nursing goal is for the client to maintain optimal gas exchange. What nursing actions would promote this?

3. Your client is scheduled for a partial laryngectomy. What information must you share to help prepare her for the postoperative period?

4. A client arrives at the emergency room with uncontrolled epistaxis. What actions should the RN instruct the LPN to take?

NCLEX-STYLE REVIEW QUESTIONS

1. Of the following instructions, which is most important for the nurse to teach the client to help loosen secretions and increase comfort during medical treatment for sinusitis?
1. Engage in normal activity.
2. Elevate the head of the bed by 45 degrees.
3. Increase fluid intake.
4. Blow the nose frequently.

2. A client is seen in a clinic for possible laryngeal cancer. In reviewing the client's record, the nurse will most likely see which of the following early complaints expressed by the client?
1. Enlarged lymph nodes in the neck
2. Persistent hoarseness for the last month
3. Difficulty swallowing hot liquids
4. Generalized discomfort in the neck

3. The nurse is providing postoperative care for a client who has undergone tonsillectomy. In which position will the nurse place the head of the bed when the client is fully awake?
1. Flat with the head elevated on a pillow
2. Slightly raised at a 15° angle
3. Raised at a 45° angle
4. Raised at a 90° sitting position

4. A client was seen in the emergency room with severe epistaxis. After the physician places a nasal packing, the bleeding is controlled. What should the nurse include as part of the discharge instructions? Select all that apply.
1. Keep nasal packing in place until seen for follow-up appointment
2. Continue taking baby aspirin as ordered
3. Swallow any oozing blood to avoid coughing.
4. Do not blow the nose.
5. Call physician if bleeding persists or becomes worse.

5. A client comes to the doctor's office stating that he has a lump in his throat and is afraid that it is cancer. Which initial question by the nurse addresses the earliest symptom of laryngeal cancer?
1. "Do you smoke or have you ever smoked?"
2. "Do you have a burning in your throat?"
3. "Do you have swollen lymph nodes?"
4. "Did you notice a persistent cough?"

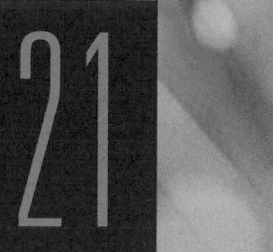

21 Caring for Clients with Lower Respiratory Disorders

Words To Know

acute bronchitis
asbestosis
asthma
atelectasis
bronchiectasis
chronic bronchitis
chronic obstructive pulmonary disease
cystic fibrosis
emphysema
empyema
flail chest
hemoptysis
influenza
lobectomy
lung abscess
orthopnea
pleural effusion
pleurisy
pneumoconiosis
pneumonectomy
pneumonia
pneumothorax
pulmonary contusion
pulmonary edema
pulmonary embolism
pulmonary hypertension
restrictive lung disease
segmental resection
septicemia
silicosis
subcutaneous emphysema
thoracotomy
tracheitis
tracheobronchitis
tuberculosis
wedge resection

Learning Objectives

On completion of this chapter, you will be able to:

1. Describe infectious and inflammatory disorders of the lower respiratory airway.
2. Identify critical assessments needed for a client with an infectious disorder of the lower respiratory airway.
3. Define disorders classified as obstructive pulmonary disease.
4. Discuss strategies for preventing and managing occupational lung diseases.
5. Describe the pathophysiology of pulmonary hypertension.
6. List risk factors associated with the development of pulmonary embolism.
7. Discuss conditions that may lead to acute respiratory distress syndrome.
8. Differentiate acute and chronic respiratory failure.
9. Explain the difficulties associated with early diagnosis of lung cancer.
10. Describe nursing assessments required for a client who experiences trauma to the chest.
11. Explain the purpose of chest tubes after thoracic surgery.
12. Describe preoperative and postoperative nursing management for clients undergoing thoracic care.

Various problems and disorders can compromise the ability of the lower respiratory tract to perform its primary functions of gas exchange and ventilation. If untreated, many of these disorders can lead to respiratory failure. Other disorders become chronic and affect the client's quality of life.

INFECTIOUS AND INFLAMMATORY DISORDERS

Infectious and inflammatory disorders of the lower airway are medically more serious than those of the upper airway. Inflammation and infection in the alveoli and bronchioles impair gas exchange. In addition, clients may experience greater difficulty in maintaining a clear airway secondary to retained secretions.

ACUTE BRONCHITIS
Pathophysiology and Etiology

Inflammation of the mucous membranes that line the major bronchi and their branches characterizes **acute bronchitis**. If the inflammatory process involves the trachea, it is referred to as **tracheobronchitis**. Typically, acute bronchitis begins as an upper respiratory infection (URI);

the inflammatory process then extends to the tracheobronchial tree. The secretory cells of the mucosa produce increased mucopurulent sputum.

Viral infections most commonly give rise to acute bronchitis. Clients with viral URIs are more vulnerable to secondary bacterial infections, which then may lead to acute bronchitis. Sputum cultures identify the causative bacterial organisms, the most common of which are *Haemophilus influenzae, Streptococcus pneumoniae,* and *Mycoplasma pneumoniae.* Fungal infections such as *Aspergillus* may be identified as the cause of acute bronchitis. Chemical irritation from noxious fumes, gases, and air contaminants also may induce acute bronchitis. A potential complication is bronchial asthma.

Assessment Findings

Signs and symptoms initially include fever, chills, malaise, headache, and a dry, irritating, and nonproductive cough. Later, the cough produces mucopurulent sputum, which may be blood-streaked if the airway mucosa becomes irritated with severe tracheobronchitis and coughing. Clients experience paroxysmal attacks of coughing and may report wheezing. Laryngitis and sinusitis complicate the symptoms. Moist, inspiratory crackles may be heard on chest auscultation. A sputum sample is collected for culture and sensitivity testing to rule out bacterial infection. A chest film also may be done to detect additional pathology, such as pneumonia.

Medical Management

Acute bronchitis usually is self-limiting, lasting for several days. Suggested treatment is bed rest, antipyretics, expectorants, antitussives (drugs used to prevent coughing), and increased fluids. Humidifiers assist in keeping mucous membranes moist because dry air aggravates the cough. If secondary bacterial invasion occurs, the previously mild infection becomes more serious, and usually is accompanied by a persistent cough and thick, purulent sputum. Secondary infections usually subside as the bronchitis subsides, but they may persist for several weeks. When a secondary infection is evident, the physician orders a broad-spectrum antibiotic when sputum culture results are available.

Pharmacologic Considerations

- The indiscriminate use of nonprescription cough medicines may cause more harm than good. Coughing is the mechanism the body uses to clear the respiratory passages of mucus; depressing the cough reflex may cause a pooling of secretions and lead to further problems. Clients with respiratory disease are advised to check with their physicians before using nonprescription antitussive preparations.

Nursing Management

The nurse auscultates breath sounds and monitors vital signs every 4 hours, especially if the client has a fever. He or she encourages the client to cough and deep breathe every 2 hours while awake and to expectorate rather than swallow sputum. Humidification of surrounding air loosens bronchial secretions. The nurse changes the bedding and the client's clothes if they become damp with perspiration and offers fluids frequently. The nurse, in an effort to prevent the spread of infection, teaches the client to wash the hands frequently, particularly when handling secretions and soiled tissues; cover the mouth when sneezing and coughing; discard soiled tissues in a plastic bag; and avoid sharing eating utensils and personal articles with others.

PNEUMONIA

Pneumonia is an inflammatory process affecting the bronchioles and alveoli. Although it usually is associated with an acute infection, pneumonia also can result from radiation therapy, chemical ingestion or inhalation, or aspiration of foreign bodies or gastric contents. Pneumonia, when combined with influenza, ranks as the eighth leading cause of death in the United States (American Lung Association, 2007).

Pathophysiology and Etiology

Pneumonia is classified according to its etiology. Bacterial pneumonias are referred to as *typical pneumonias.* Atypical pneumonias (Box 21-1) are those caused by mycoplasmas, *Legionella pneumophila* (the causative agent of Legionnaire's disease), chlamydiae, viruses, parasites, and fungi. *Mycobacterium tuberculosis* also may cause pneumonia. Viruses are the most common etiology, with influenza type A virus the usual causative organism. Bacterial pneumonias are less common but more serious. Causative bacterial organisms include *Streptococcus pneumoniae, Pneumocystis*

BOX 21-1 | **Atypical Pneumonias**

Mycoplasma pneumoniae
  Is the most common cause of atypical pneumonia
  Develops gradually, with a prolonged clinical course
  Is rarely fatal
Chlamydia pneumoniae
  Is a common cause of pneumonia and URIs
  Requires long-term treatment with broad-spectrum
    antibiotics
Chlamydia psittaci
  Causes psittacosis, a flulike disease progressing to
    irregular consolidation and interstitial pneumonia
  Is transmitted from birds and sheep
Legionella pneumophila
  Was first described at an American Legion convention in
    Philadelphia, Pennsylvania
  Is a fastidious bacterium that resides in aquatic
    environments
  Outbreaks traced to air conditioners and humidifiers
  Is rapid growing, causing inflammation and fibrin formation
    within the alveoli, and often complicated by empyema
  Symptoms include fever, cough, and chest pain, with a
    mortality rate of 10% to 20%

jiroveci, Staphylococcus aureus, Klebsiella pneumoniae, Pseudomonas aeruginosa, and *Haemophilus influenzae.*

Radiation pneumonia results from damage to the normal lung mucosa during radiation therapy for breast or lung cancer. Chemical pneumonia results from ingestion of kerosene or inhalation of volatile hydrocarbons (kerosene, gasoline, or other chemicals), which may occur in industrial settings. Aspiration pneumonia occurs when a person inhales a foreign body or gastric contents during vomiting or regurgitation. Hypoventilation of lung tissue over a prolonged period can occur when a client is bedridden and breathing with only part of the lungs. Bronchial secretions subsequently accumulate, which may lead to hypostatic pneumonia.

Pneumonia is also categorized according to its presenting symptoms. Bronchopneumonia means that the infection is patchy, diffuse, and scattered throughout both lungs. Lobar pneumonia means that the inflammation is confined to one or more lobes of the lung (Fig. 21-1).

Another classification of pneumonia refers to where the client acquired the inflammatory process (Table 21-1). There are four general categories. The first is community-acquired pneumonia (CAP), which means that the client contracted the illness in a community setting or within 48 hours of admission to a healthcare facility. Hospital-acquired pneumonia (HAP), or nosocomial pneumonia, occurs in a healthcare setting more than 48 hours after admission. Pneumonia in the immunocompromised host is a third category; this type includes *Pneumocystis jiroveci* pneumonia, fungal pneumonia, and pneumonia related to tuberculosis. The fourth category is aspiration pneumonia.

Organisms that cause pneumonia reach the alveoli by inhalation of droplets, aspiration of organisms from the upper airway, or, less commonly, seeding from the bloodstream. When organisms reach the alveoli, the inflammatory reaction is intense, producing an exudate that impairs gas exchange. Capillaries surrounding the alveoli become engorged and cause the alveoli to collapse (atelectasis), further impairing gas exchange and interfering with ventilation.

White blood cells (WBCs) move into the area to destroy the pathogens, filling the interstitial spaces. If untreated, consolidation occurs as the inflammation and exudate increase. Hypoxemia results from the inability of the lungs to oxygenate blood from the heart. Bronchitis, **tracheitis** (inflammation of the trachea), and spots of *necrosis* (death of tissue) in the lung may follow.

In atypical pneumonias, the exudate infiltrates the interstitial spaces rather than the alveoli directly. The pneumonia is more scattered, as described for bronchopneumonia. As the inflammatory process continues, it increasingly interferes with gas exchange between the bloodstream and lungs. Increased carbon dioxide (CO_2) in the blood stimulates the respiratory center, causing more rapid and shallow breathing.

Without an interruption of any type of pneumonia, the client becomes increasingly ill. If the circulatory system cannot compensate for the burden of decreased gas exchange, the client is at risk for heart failure. Death from pneumonia is most common in older adults and those weakened by acute or chronic diseases or disorders (e.g., acquired immunodeficiency syndrome [AIDS], cancer, lung disease) or prolonged periods of inactivity. Complications of pneumonia include congestive heart failure (CHF), **empyema** (collection of pus in the pleural cavity), **pleurisy** (inflammation of the pleura), **septicemia** (infective microorganisms in the blood), atelectasis, hypotension, and shock. In addition, septicemia may lead to a secondary focus of infection, such as endocarditis (inflammation of the endocardium), pericarditis (inflammation of the pericardium), and purulent arthritis. Otitis media (infection of the middle ear), bronchitis, or sinusitis also may complicate recovery, especially from atypical pneumonia.

 Gerontologic Considerations

- Older adults are at greater risk for pneumonia and may experience a higher acuity due to concomitant health problems, such as heart disease and diabetes. Vaccination against pneumococcal pneumonia is recommended for clients older than 50 years with a chronic or debilitating illness, those over age 65, and residents in long-term care facilities. Current guidelines recommend a booster dose if the initial immunization was 5 or more years ago. Older adults should also be advised to receive an annual influenza immunization.

Assessment Findings

Signs and Symptoms

Symptoms vary for the different types of pneumonia. The onset of bacterial pneumonia is sudden. The client experiences fever, chills, a productive cough, and discomfort in the chest wall muscles from coughing. There also is general malaise. The sputum may be rust colored. Breathing causes pain; thus, the client tries to breathe as shallowly as possible.

Viral pneumonia differs from bacterial pneumonia in that results of blood cultures are sterile, sputum may be more copious, chills are less common, and pulse and respiratory rates are characteristically slow. The course of viral pneumonia

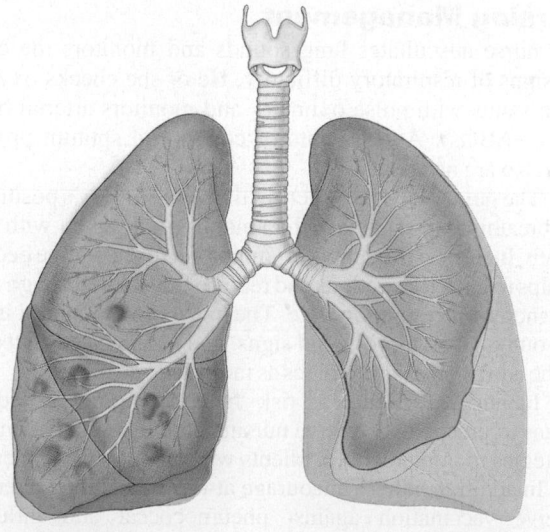

Bronchopneumonia   Lobar pneumonia

FIGURE 21-1. Distribution of lung involvement in bronchopneumonia and lobar pneumonia.

TABLE 21-1 Categories of Pneumonia

TYPE	ORGANISM RESPONSIBLE	COMMON CLINICAL MANIFESTATIONS	USUAL TREATMENT
Community-Acquired Pneumonia (CAP)			
Streptococcal pneumonia (pneumococcal)	*Streptococcus pneumoniae*	Abrupt or insidious onset; one or more lobes involved; flu-like symptoms; lobar infiltrates seen on x-ray; pleuritic and/or chest pain; often begins with a URI	Penicillins or alternative antibiotics such as cefotaxime, cephalosporin, erythromycin, or others
Haemophilus influenza	*Haemophilus influenzae*		
Legionnaire's disease	*Legionella pneumophila*		Treated based on symptoms
Mycoplasma pneumonia	*Mycoplasma pneumoniae*		
Viral pneumonia	Influenza virus types A, B, adenovirus, parainfluenza, cytomegalovirus, coronavirus		
Chlamydial pneumonia	*Chlamydia pneumoniae*		
Hospital-Acquired Pneumonia (HAP)			
Pseudomonas pneumonia	*Pseudomonas aeruginosa*	Diffuse consolidation on chest x-ray; fever; chills; productive cough; bacteremia; cyanosis; hypoxemia; clients have toxic appearance; can get lung abscesses	Antibiotics; antipseudomonal agents such as piperacillin; rifampin or gentamycin; third-generation cephalosporins
Staphylococcal pneumonia	*Staphylococcus aureus*		
Klebsiella pneumonia	*Klebsiella pneumoniae*		
Pneumonia in Immunocompromised Host			
Pneumocystis carinii pneumonia (PCP)	*Pneumocystis carinii*	Pulmonary infiltrates on chest x-ray; cough; dyspnea; hemoptysis; fever; night sweats; weight loss	Trimethoprim/sulfamethoxazole (TMP-SMZ); amphotericin B; rifampin; streptomycin
Fungal pneumonia	*Aspergillus fumigatus*		
Tuberculosis	*Mycobacterium tuberculosis*		

(Adapted from Smeltzer, S. C., Bare, B. G., Hinkle, J. L., & Cheever, K. H. 2008. *Brunner & Suddarth's textbook of medical-surgical nursing* [11th ed.]. Philadelphia: Lippincott Williams & Wilkins.)

usually is less severe than that of bacterial pneumonia. The mortality rate from viral pneumonia is low but rises when bacterial pneumonia occurs as a secondary infection. Many clients with viral pneumonia are weak and ill for a longer period than those with successfully treated bacterial pneumonia.

Diagnostic Findings

Auscultation of the chest reveals wheezing, crackles, and decreased breath sounds. The nail beds, lips, and oral mucosa may be cyanotic. Sputum culture and sensitivity studies can help to identify the infectious microorganism and effective antibiotics for treatment in cases of bacterial pneumonia. A chest film shows areas of infiltrates and consolidation. A complete blood count discloses an elevated WBC count. Blood cultures also may be done to detect any microorganisms in the blood.

A newer and more efficient method to diagnose pneumonia is called an electronic nose or "e-nose." The maker, Cyrano Sciences, Inc., calls this device the Cyranose 320. Although not yet fully approved by the U. S. Food and Drug Administration, this hand-held device senses and evaluates exhaled breath for various types of pneumonia and sinusitis. Tests indicate a 70% to 90% accuracy rate, which is similar to standard testing. The e-nose also provides diagnosis in approximately 40 minutes, whereas standard testing results are usually not available for several hours ("Sniffing out," 2004).

Medical Management

Medical management involves prompt initiation of antibiotic therapy for bacterial pneumonia, hydration to thin secretions, supplemental oxygen to alleviate hypoxemia, bed rest, chest physical therapy and postural drainage (techniques that involve manual pounding or clapping to loosen secretions and positioning of the client to drain and remove secretions from specific areas of the lungs), bronchodilators, analgesics, antipyretics, and cough expectorants or suppressants, depending on the nature of the client's cough. If a client is hospitalized, treatment is more vigorous, depending on the potential or actual complications. Fluid and electrolyte replacement sometimes is necessary secondary to fever, dehydration, and inadequate nutrition. If the client experiences severe respiratory difficulty and thick, copious secretions, he or she may require intubation along with mechanical ventilation.

Nursing Management

The nurse auscultates lung sounds and monitors the client for signs of respiratory difficulty. He or she checks oxygenation status with pulse oximetry and monitors arterial blood gases (ABGs). Assessments of cough and sputum production also are necessary.

The nurse places the client in the semi-Fowler's position to aid breathing and increase the amount of air taken with each breath. Increased fluid intake is important to encourage because it helps to loosen secretions and replace fluids lost through fever and increased respiratory rate. The nurse monitors fluid intake and output, skin turgor, vital signs, and serum electrolytes. He or she administers antipyretics as indicated and ordered.

Identifying clients at risk for pneumonia provides a means to practice preventive nursing care. Box 21-2 identifies strategies to implement for clients who are at risk for pneumonia. In addition, nurses encourage at-risk and elderly clients to receive vaccination against pneumococcal and influenza infections. Because the nursing care of clients with infectious lung disorders is similar regardless of the etiology, refer to "Nursing Process: Tuberculosis" for additional interventions.

BOX 21-2 Preventing Pneumonia

- Promote coughing and expectoration of secretions if client experiences increased mucus production.
- Change position frequently if client is immobilized for any reason.
- Encourage deep-breathing and coughing exercises at least every 2 hours.
- Administer chest physical therapy as indicated.
- Suction client if he or she cannot expectorate.
- Prevent aspiration in clients at risk.
- Prevent infections.
- Cleanse respiratory equipment on a routine basis.
- Promote frequent oral hygiene.
- Administer sedatives and opioids carefully to avoid respiratory depression.
- Encourage client to stop smoking and reduce alcohol intake.

PLEURISY

Pleurisy or *pleuritis* refers to acute inflammation of the parietal and visceral pleurae. During the acute phase, the pleurae are inflamed, thick, and swollen, and an exudate forms from fibrin and lymph. Eventually the pleurae become rigid. During inspiration, the inflamed pleurae rub together, causing severe, sharp pain.

Pathophysiology and Etiology

Pleurisy usually is a consequence of a primary condition, such as pneumonia or other pulmonary infections. The inflammatory process spreads from the lungs to the parietal pleura. Pleurisy also may develop with tuberculosis (TB), lung cancer, cardiac and renal diseases, systemic infections, or pulmonary embolism.

Assessment Findings

Respirations become shallow secondary to excruciating pain. Pleural fluid accumulates as the inflammatory process worsens. The pain decreases as the fluid increases because the fluid separates the pleurae. The client develops a dry cough, fatigues easily, and experiences dyspnea. A *friction rub* (coarse sounds heard during inspiration and early expiration) is heard during auscultation early in the disease process. As fluid accumulates, the pleural friction rub disappears. Decreased ventilation may result in atelectasis, hypoxemia, and hypercapnia.

Chest radiography shows changes in the affected area. Microscopic examination of sputum and a sputum culture may reveal pathogenic microorganisms. If a thoracentesis (removal of fluid from the chest; see Chap. 19) is performed, a pleural fluid specimen is sent to the laboratory for analysis. Occasionally the physician may perform a pleural biopsy.

Medical Management

The underlying condition dictates the treatment. Analgesic and antipyretic drugs provide relief for pain and fever. A nonsteroidal anti-inflammatory drug (NSAID) such as indomethacin (Indocin) provides analgesia and promotes more effective coughing. Severe cases may require a procaine intercostal nerve block.

Nursing Management

The client has considerable pain with inspiration; sneezing and coughing make the pain worse. The nurse instructs the client to take analgesic medications as prescribed. Heat or cold applications may provide some topical comfort. The nurse teaches the client to splint the chest wall by turning onto the affected side. The client also can splint the chest wall with his or her hands or a pillow when coughing. Providing emotional support is essential—the client is very anxious and needs reassurance.

PLEURAL EFFUSION

Pleural effusion is an abnormal collection of fluid between the visceral and parietal pleurae (Fig. 21-2). Under normal conditions, approximately 5 to 15 mL of fluid between the pleurae prevent friction during pleural surface movement. Pleural effusion may be a complication of pneumonia, lung cancer, TB, pulmonary embolism, and CHF. The amount of accumulated fluid may be so large that the lung partially collapses on the affected side. As a consequence, pressure is placed on the heart and other organs of the mediastinum.

Assessment Findings

Fever, pain, and dyspnea are the most common symptoms. Chest percussion reveals dullness over the involved area. The examiner may note diminished or absent breath sounds over the involved area when auscultating the lungs; he or she also may hear a friction rub. Chest radiography and computed tomography (CT) scan show fluid in the involved area. Thoracentesis sometimes is done to remove pleural fluid for analysis and examination for malignant cells.

Medical Management

The main goal of treatment is to eliminate the cause and relieve discomfort. Treatment includes antibiotics, analgesics,

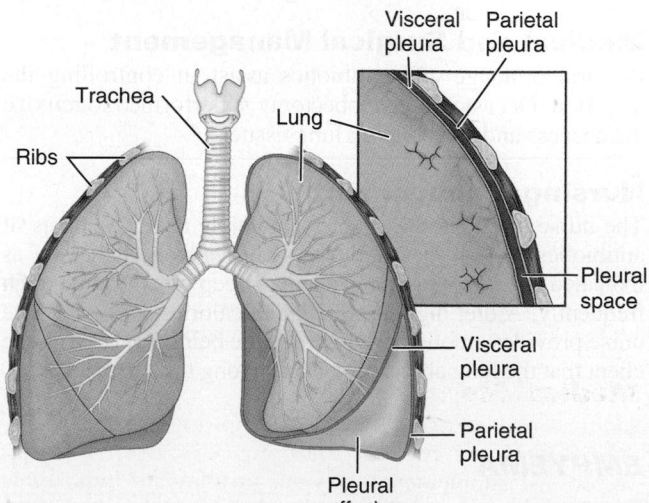

FIGURE 21-2. In pleural effusion, an abnormal volume of fluid collects in the pleural space.

cardiotonic drugs to control CHF (when present), thoracentesis to remove excess pleural fluid, insertion of a chest tube to promote drainage over a longer period, and surgery for cancer when present.

Nursing Management

If thoracentesis is needed, the nurse prepares the client for this procedure (see Nursing Guidelines 19-3 in Chap. 19). The client usually is frightened; thus, the nurse must provide support. If a client has a chest tube, the nurse monitors the function of the drainage system and the amount and nature of the drainage (see discussion later in the chapter).

LUNG ABSCESS

A **lung abscess** is a localized area of pus formation in the lung parenchyma. As the abscess increases, the tissue becomes necrotic. Later, the affected area collapses and creates a cavity. The infection can then extend into one or both bronchi and the pleural cavity.

Pathophysiology and Etiology

A lung abscess may develop from aspiration, bacterial pneumonia, or mechanical obstruction of the bronchi, such as with a tumor. Other causes include necrosis of lung tissue after an infection and necrotic lesions resulting from inhalation of dust particles. Clients with an impaired cough reflex or altered immune function are at risk for lung abscesses.

Assessment Findings

Signs and symptoms include chills, fever, weight loss, chest pain, and a productive cough. Sputum may be purulent or blood streaked. Finger clubbing may occur in chronic cases. Chest auscultation reveals dull or absent breath sounds in the area of the abscess. Chest radiography and CT scan usually locate the abscess. Results of blood and sputum cultures may be positive for pathogens. Chest percussion detects an area of dullness. In some instances, thoracentesis may be done, with the aspirated fluid sent to the laboratory for culture and sensitivity tests.

Medical and Surgical Management

Postural drainage and antibiotics assist in controlling the infection. Occasionally, a lobectomy is performed to remove the abscess and surrounding lung tissue.

Nursing Management

The nurse monitors the client for possible adverse effects of antibiotics. He or she administers chest physical therapy as indicated and encourages the client to deep breathe and cough frequently. A diet high in protein and calories is pivotal. The nurse provides emotional support, while being honest with the client that the lung abscess may take a long time to resolve.

EMPYEMA

Empyema is a general term used to denote pus in a body cavity. It usually refers, however, to pus or infected fluid in the pleural cavity (*thoracic empyema*). Empyema may follow chest trauma, such as a stab or gunshot wound, or a preexisting disease, such as pneumonia or TB. The pus-filled area may become walled off and enclosed by a thick membrane.

Assessment Findings

Fever, chest pain, dyspnea, anorexia, and malaise may accompany empyema. Chest auscultation reveals diminished or absent breath sounds over the affected area. The affected lung area is distinguished on a chest radiograph.

Medical and Surgical Management

Aspiration of purulent fluid by thoracentesis may be necessary to identify the microorganisms, remove pus or fluid, and select appropriate antibiotic therapy. Closed drainage may be used to empty the empyemic cavity. **Thoracotomy** (surgical opening of the thorax) is performed, and one or more large chest tubes are inserted, which are then connected to an underwater-seal drainage bottle. Open drainage, which necessitates the removal of a section of one or more ribs, may be used when pus is thick and the walls of the empyemic cavity are strong enough to keep the lung from collapsing while the chest is opened. One or more tubes may be placed in the opening to promote drainage. The wound is then covered by a large absorbent dressing, which is changed as necessary. The drainage of pus results in a drop in temperature and general symptomatic improvement.

Inadequately treated empyema may become chronic. A thick coating forms over the lung, preventing its expansion. *Decortication* (removal of the coating) and evacuation of the pleural space allow the lung to reexpand.

Nursing Management

Empyema takes a long time to resolve. The client requires emotional support during treatment. The nurse teaches the client to do breathing exercises as prescribed.

INFLUENZA

Influenza (flu) is an acute respiratory disease of relatively short duration. The major strains of the flu virus are A, B, and C; the strains are related yet distinct from one another. Each virus can mutate and produce variants within the given strain. The variants are called *subtypes*. Viruses that cause influenza are transmitted through the respiratory tract.

Flu chiefly occurs in epidemics, although sporadic cases appear between them. Because the viruses change, antibodies produced by those who have had one case of flu are not effective against new subtypes, and a different antibody must be produced annually or during major epidemics. Most clients recover. Fatalities usually are related to secondary bacterial complications, especially among pregnant women, elderly or debilitated clients, and those with chronic conditions, such as cardiac disease and emphysema.

During a flu epidemic, the death rate from pneumonia and cardiovascular disease rises. According to the Centers for Disease Control and Prevention, each year 5% to 20% of the population in the United States is diagnosed with influenza; more than 200,000 people are hospitalized, and approximately 36,000 people die (CDC, 2008). Complications include tracheobronchitis, bacterial pneumonia, and

TABLE 21-2 Signs and Symptoms of Influenza

Incubation period	1–4 days
Onset	Sudden
	Abrupt onset of fever and chills
	Severe headache
	Muscle aches
Progression	Anorexia
	Weakness, apathy, malaise
	Respiratory symptoms:
	Sneezing
	Sore throat, laryngitis
	Dry cough
	Nasal discharge—rhinitis
	Conjunctival irritation
Duration	Fever may persist for 3 days; other symptoms usually continue for 7–10 days. Cough may persist longer.
Period of contagion	One day before symptoms begin through 5 days after the onset of illness

cardiovascular disease. Staphylococcal pneumonia is the most serious complication.

Table 21-2 lists signs and symptoms of flu that form the basis for diagnosis. Additional diagnostic studies, such as chest radiography and sputum analysis, may be performed to rule out other diseases.

Nursing management focuses on prevention. Annual flu vaccinations are recommended for healthcare workers and people at high risk for complications or for those exposed to many different people daily. Each year a new vaccine is developed from three different virus strains that are predicted to be present in the coming flu season. The standard flu vaccine is made from inactivated influenza vaccine and is administered intramuscularly. During the 2004–2005 flu season, another form called FluMist was developed, which is a live, attenuated influenza vaccine administered intranasally. It is currently approved for healthy children aged 2 to 5 years, who do not have a history of asthma and wheezing, and for healthy persons between the ages of 5 and 49 years who are not pregnant (CDC, 2008). FluMist is not recommended for the following groups:

- People with underlying medical conditions such as diabetes or renal dysfunction
- People with known or suspected immunodeficiency diseases or those receiving immunosuppressive therapy
- People with a history of Guillain-Barré syndrome

- Children or adolescents who regularly take aspirin
- Pregnant women
- People with a hypersensitivity to eggs
- Children less than 2 years of age
- Adults 50 years of age and older

Clients admitted to the hospital with flu need to be isolated from clients who do not have it. Nurses must maintain airborne transmission precautions when caring for those clients. If a community is experiencing an epidemic, hospitals and other healthcare facilities usually develop policies regarding visitation and admissions. Box 21-3 provides information on preventing an influenza outbreak in a healthcare facility.

PULMONARY TUBERCULOSIS

Pulmonary **tuberculosis** (TB) is a bacterial infectious disease primarily caused by *M. tuberculosis*. TB essentially affects the lungs, but it may also affect the kidneys and other organs. TB continues to be a worldwide health problem. It affects one third of the world's population and is the leading cause of death from infectious diseases and among people with human immunodeficiency virus (HIV) infection (World Health Organization [WHO], 2007). In the United States, as in much of the world, new cases of TB are slowly declining. Only in African countries is the incidence of new cases of

---

BOX 21-3 **Preventing Outbreaks of Influenza in Healthcare Settings**

To prevent outbreaks of influenza, healthcare settings take the following precautions in addition to Standard Precautions:

- Institute droplet precautions for air clients with suspected or confirmed influenza.
- Isolate clients with cases of suspected and confirmed influenza in private rooms, or place clients with possible pneumonia together and clients with confirmed pneumonia together.
- Administer antiviral prophylaxis according to current recommendations to all clients on an affected unit who do not appear

to have influenza and for whom it is not contraindicated to receive the antiviral.
- Administer the current inactivated influenza vaccine to unvaccinated clients and healthcare personnel.
- Offer antiviral prophylaxis to unvaccinated personnel who work on the affected unit.
- Do not allow visitors with symptoms of respiratory infection to visit the hospital.
- Encourage personnel with symptoms of respiratory infection to stay at home until they are well.

(Source: Goldrick, B. A. [2004]. Influenza 2004-2005: What's new with the flu? *American Journal of Nursing, 104*[10], 38.)

TB increasing, and this correlates with the higher incidence of HIV (2005). The WHO is committed to stopping tuberculosis throughout the world. Organizations such as the Bill and Melinda Gates Foundation (2008) have donated major funding for the development, testing, licensing, and distribution of at least one new TB vaccine within 10 years.

Gerontologic Considerations

- The incidence of tuberculosis in older adults is twice that of the general population; tuberculosis is most prevalent in those aged 65 or older residing in long-term care facilities. The current cohort of older adults may have initially acquired tuberculosis during childhood or World War II; the disease may be reactivated by aging or treatment changes influencing immunity (Ebersole et al., 2008).

Pathophysiology and Etiology

Tubercle bacilli are gram positive, rod shaped, acid-fast, and aerobic. Although they can live in the dark for months as spores in particles of dried sputum, exposure to direct sunlight, heat, or ultraviolet light destroys them in a few hours. They are difficult to kill with ordinary disinfectants and are destroyed by pasteurization, a process widely used in milk and milk products to prevent the spread of TB.

TB is transmitted most commonly through the inhalation of droplets produced by coughing, sneezing, and spitting from a person with active disease. Brief contact usually does not result in infection. In contrast to the number of people who have been infected with tubercle bacilli, only a small proportion ever becomes ill. Many factors predispose a client to the development of TB, including inadequate healthcare, malnutrition, overcrowding, and poor housing.

The classification of TB is based on the client's history, physical examination, skin test, chest x-ray, and microbiologic tests. The American Thoracic Society classifies tuberculosis in a systematic way to monitor the epidemiology and treatment. The classification is as follows (Smeltzer et al., 2008, p. 646):

- Class 0: no exposure; no infection
- Class 1: exposure; no evidence of infection
- Class 2: latent infection; no disease (e.g., positive PPD reaction but no clinical evidence of active TB)
- Class 3: disease; clinically active
- Class 4: disease; not clinically active
- Class 5: suspected disease; diagnosis pending

TB is characterized by stages of early infection (or primary TB), latency, and potential for recurrence after the primary disease (called *secondary TB*). The bacilli may remain dormant for many years and then reactivate, producing clinical symptoms of TB.

Early Infection

Tubercle bacilli, when inhaled, pass through the bronchial system and implant on the bronchioles or alveoli. Initially, the host has no resistance to this infection. *Phagocytes* (neutrophils and macrophages) engulf the bacilli, which continue to multiply. The bacilli also spread through the lymphatic channels to the regional lymph nodes and subsequently to the circulating blood and distant organs. Eventually, the cellular immune response limits further multiplication and dissemination of the bacilli.

Immune Activation

When immune activation occurs (usually a full response occurs within 2 weeks), a characteristic tissue reaction results in formation of a granuloma, referred to as the *Ghon tubercle,* from epithelial cells merging with the macrophages. Lymphocytes surround the Ghon tubercle, of which the central portion undergoes necrosis. This caseous necrosis has a cheesy appearance and may liquefy and slough into the connecting bronchus, producing a cavity. It also may enter the tracheobronchial system, promoting airborne transmission of infectious particles.

Healing of the Primary Lesion

Healing of the primary lesion occurs through resolution, fibrosis, and calcification. The granulation tissue of the primary lesion becomes more fibrous and creates a scar around the tubercle. This is referred to as the *Ghon complex* and is visible on radiography.

Latent Period

As the lesion heals, the infection enters a latent period that can persist for many years or even an entire lifetime without producing clinical symptoms. If the immune response has been inadequate, however, the affected person eventually will develop clinical disease. Clients at particular risk are those with HIV infection or diabetes and those on chemotherapy or long-term steroids. Only a small percentage of those infected with TB actually develop clinical symptoms.

Secondary Tuberculosis

Secondary TB usually involves reactivation of the initial infection. The person already has had an immune response, and thus the lesions that form tend to remain in the lungs. The course of this phase usually is as follows:

1. Acute local inflammation and necrosis occur.
2. Infected lung tissue becomes ulcerated.
3. Tubercles cluster together and become surrounded by inflammation.
4. Exudate fills the surrounding alveoli.
5. The client develops bronchopneumonia.
6. TB tissue becomes caseous and ulcerates into the bronchus.
7. Cavities form.
8. Ulcerations heal, with scar tissue left around cavities.
9. Pleurae thicken and retract.

The course of TB becomes a cyclical one of inflammation, bronchopneumonia, ulceration, cavitation, and scarring. The TB gradually spreads throughout the lung fields and into the rest of the respiratory structures, as well as to other organs through the lymph system. A client may experience periods of exacerbation, followed by remissions.

Assessment Findings

Signs and Symptoms

The onset of TB is insidious, and early symptoms vary. An infected person may be asymptomatic until the disease is advanced. As symptoms develop, they often are vague and can be overlooked, particularly because they are systemic. Fatigue, anorexia, weight loss, and a slight, nonproductive cough are all symptoms attributable to overwork, excessive smoking, or poor eating habits. They also, however, are early symptoms of TB. Low-grade fever, particularly in the late afternoon, and night sweats are common as the disease progresses. The cough typically becomes productive of mucopurulent and blood-streaked sputum. Marked weakness, wasting, **hemoptysis** (expectoration of blood or bloody sputum), and dyspnea are characteristics of later stages. Chest pain may result from spread of the infection to the pleurae.

Diagnostic Findings

Diagnostic tests chiefly consist of the tuberculin skin test, chest radiography, CT scan, magnetic resonance imaging (MRI), and analyse of sputum and other body fluids. The tuberculin skin test, or Mantoux test, determines if a client has been infected with *M. tuberculosis* (Nursing Guidelines 21-1). A positive tuberculin skin test result is evidence that a TB infection has existed at some time somewhere in the body, but does not necessarily indicate active disease. The chief value of tuberculin skin tests lies in case finding. All long-term care facilities are required to test each resident on admission for TB.

Microscopic examination of sputum and other body fluids identifies the bacilli and is ordered when TB is suspected, during and after a course of drug therapy for TB, and after surgical removal of a diseased lobe of the lung. The client is instructed to cough deeply so that the specimen does not consist mainly of saliva. Most clients find that it is easier to raise sputum when they first awaken. It may be necessary to collect specimens on several consecutive days (see Nursing Guidelines 19-2 in Chap. 19).

Gastric lavage, gastric aspiration, or bronchoscopy may be used to determine the presence of the tubercle bacilli, particularly when a client has had difficulty raising a sputum specimen for examination. Tubercle bacilli may reach the stomach from the lungs when the client raises sputum but swallows rather than expectorates it. When invasion of other body areas by tubercle bacilli is suspected, specimens are obtained to confirm the diagnosis.

Medical and Surgical Management

In many cases, drugs have speeded recovery and provided a chance to arrest TB in clients with advanced lesions; however, they do not guarantee a cure. Their usefulness lies in their ability to retard the growth and multiplication of tubercle bacilli, thus giving the body a chance to overcome the disease. Two factors make drug therapy less than ideal: drug toxicity and the tendency of the tubercle bacilli to develop drug resistance. Combined therapy with two or more drugs decreases the likelihood of drug resistance, increases the tuberculostatic action of the drugs, and lessens the risk for toxic drug reactions (Drug Therapy Table 21-1).

Pharmacologic Considerations

- Isoniazid (INH) is used in combination with other antitubercular drugs and alone as a prophylactic to prevent the spread of TB. For example, INH may be given to household members and close associates of those recently diagnosed with TB.

Resistance of the bacilli to drugs is an important factor in the lack of response to medical treatment. Drug therapy usually is carried out while the client is at home. Regular

NURSING GUIDELINES 21-1

Performing a Mantoux Test

- Draw up 0.1 mL of intermediate-strength purified protein derivative (PPD) in a tuberculin syringe ($^1/_2$-inch 26- to 27-gauge needle).
- Prepare the injection site on the inner aspect of the forearm, approximately halfway between the elbow and wrist.
- Hold the syringe bevel up, almost parallel to the forearm.
- Inject the PPD to form a pronounced wheal, which indicates proper intradermal injection (Fig. A).
- Record the site, name of PPD, strength, lot number, and date and time of test.
- Read the test site 48 to 72 hours after injection by palpating the site for induration. If induration is present, measure it at its greatest width (Fig. B). Erythema (redness) without induration is not significant. If erythema is present with induration, read the induration only. Interpret the test results as follows:

Negative reaction—0- to 4-mm induration; no follow-up needed

Questionable reaction—5- to 9-mm induration; if the client is aware of contact with someone with active tuberculosis, this reaction is seen as significant

Positive reaction—10 mm or greater induration

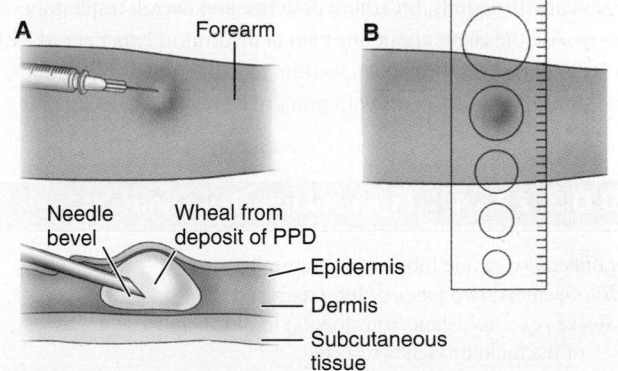

DRUG THERAPY TABLE 21-1 Drug Regimen For Tuberculosis

Treatment Period	Drugs Prescribed	Length of Drug Therapy
Initial treatment	isoniazid (INH) rifampin (RIF) pyrazinamide (PZA) (These three medications now in a combination tablet.)	INH, RIF, PZA for 4 months INH and RIF for additional 2 months
Suspected drug resistance	isoniazid (INH) rifampin (RIF) pyrazinamide (PZA) ethambutol (EMB) or streptomycin (SM)	If sensitive, continue INH and RIF for 6 more months. If resistant to INH, use other drugs for 6 months. If resistant to RIF, use other drugs for 12–18 months
Prophylactic treatment	isoniazid (INH) May use pyridoxine (vitamin B$_6$) to minimize side effects	6–12 months

visits to the physician's office or clinic for follow-up care are necessary for assessment of response to therapy. Culture and sensitivity tests may be performed, and the adverse effects of the drugs are evaluated.

When the disease is located primarily in one section of the lung, that portion may be removed by **segmental resection** (removal of a lobe segment) or **wedge resection** (removal of a wedge of diseased tissue). If the diseased area is larger, **lobectomy** (removal of a lobe) may be performed. In some cases, the lung is so diseased that **pneumonectomy** (removal of an entire lung) is necessary (Box 21-4).

Nursing Process for the Client with Pulmonary Tuberculosis

Assessment

Assess breath sounds, breathing patterns, and overall respiratory status. Ask the client about any pain or discomfort experienced with breathing. Inspect the client's sputum for color, viscosity, amount, and signs of blood. Clients with primary TB may have complaints

BOX 21-4 Types of Lung Resections

Lobectomy: single lobe of lung removed
Bilobectomy: two lobes of lung removed
Sleeve resection: cancerous lobe(s) removed and a segment of the main bronchus resected
Pneumonectomy: removal of entire lung
Segmentectomy: segment of lung removed
Wedge resection: removal of small, pie-shaped area of the segment
Chest wall resection with removal of cancerous lung tissue: for cancers that have invaded the chest wall

(Adapted from Smeltzer, S. C., Hinkle, J. C., & Cheever, K. H., Bare, B. G, 2008. *Brunner and Suddarth's textbook of medical-surgical nursing* [11th ed.]. Philadelphia: Lippincott Williams & Wilkins.)

related to fatigue, weakness, anorexia, weight loss, or night sweats. Clients with secondary TB may report chest pain and a cough that produces mucopurulent or blood-tinged mucus or blood. They also may report a low-grade fever.

Diagnosis, Planning, and Interventions

Antitubercular drug regimens extend for long periods and without interruption because healing is slow and interrupted treatment increases drug resistance. The primary focus of nursing management is encouraging the client to adhere to the prescribed medication regimen and teaching.

Instruct the client to take medications exactly as prescribed, closely observing the time interval between each dose. Clients must not skip doses or take more than the amount prescribed. Clients need to complete the entire course of drug therapy to control infection. Continuous therapy is essential because lapses in taking the prescribed drugs can result in reactivation of the infection. Advise clients to notify the physician if symptoms worsen or sudden chest pain or dyspnea develops. Clients also should drink plenty of fluids, discontinue smoking immediately, and avoid exposure to second-hand smoke. They need to eat a balanced diet with ample protein and calories to promote healing and maintain weight.

Other nursing care includes the following diagnoses, outcomes, and interventions.

▶ **Ineffective Airway Clearance** related to pain with coughing, inability to cough, and abnormal respirations

▶ **Expected Outcome:** Client will effectively clear secretions.

- Assess cough, noting the attributes of the secretions: color, consistency, amount, and presence of blood. *Coughing usually becomes more frequent with increased expectorant; hemoptysis occurs in advanced TB.*
- Encourage client to drink 3 to 4 L/day. *This amount liquefies and thins secretions and facilitates expectoration.*
- Humidify inspired air. *Humidified air maintains moisture to assist in liquefying secretions.*

- Encourage deep breathing and coughing every 2 hours while awake. *These measures promote lung expansion and mobilization of secretions.*
- Place client in semi-Fowler's position. *This position improves breathing and assists client to expectorate mucus.*
- Provide instructions about postural drainage. *Postural drainage facilitates airway drainage and clearance.*

▶ **Acute Pain** related to chest expansion secondary to lung infection/inflammation

▶ **Expected Outcome:** Client will manage pain with analgesics and use of splinting techniques when coughing.

- Assess pain level. *This information provides a baseline for treatment and evaluation.*
- Evaluate effectiveness of pain relief measures. *Such evaluation helps the nurse to determine if measures are effective or other therapies are necessary.*
- Administer analgesics as indicated. *Proper pain assessment and appropriate analgesic administration provide more effective pain control.*
- Instruct client in splinting techniques for use during coughing. *Proper splinting decreases pain and facilitates expectoration of secretions.*

▶ **Activity Intolerance** related to general weakness, respiratory difficulties, fever, and severity of illness

▶ **Expected Outcome:** Client will demonstrate increased activity tolerance.

- Encourage rest periods, particularly before meals, performing activities of daily living (ADLs), and exercise. *Rest reduces fatigue and spaces activities.*
- Prioritize necessary tasks, eliminating nonessential tasks. *Prioritization of tasks promotes rest.*
- Assist client with activities as required. *Giving assistance reduces client's energy expenditure, but allows him or her choices.*
- Keep equipment (e.g., telephone, tissues, wastebasket, bedside commode) close to client. *Keeping needed items close by reduces energy expenditure.*
- Encourage active range-of-motion (ROM) exercises three times a day. *Active ROM exercises maintain muscle strength and joint ROM.*

▶ **PC: Side Effects of Medication Therapy** hepatitis, neurologic changes, gastrointestinal (GI) upset

▶ **Expected Outcome:** Nurse will assist client to minimize side effects of medications.

- Instruct client to take medication 1 hour before or 2 hours after meals. *Food interferes with medication absorption.*
- Instruct clients taking isoniazid (INH) to avoid foods with tyramine and histamine (e.g., tuna, aged cheese, red wine, soy sauce, yeast extracts). *INH, when combined with these foods, may cause lightheadedness, flushing, hypotension, headache, and other symptoms.*
- Ask if client is taking any beta blockers or oral anticoagulants. *Rifampin increases the metabolism of beta blockers and oral*

anticoagulants. *Dosages may need to be adjusted or medications changed.*
- Inform the client who wears contact lenses that rifampin may color them. *The client may prefer to wear glasses while taking rifampin.*
- Monitor for side effects related to medication regimen. For hepatitis, check liver enzymes. For kidney function, check blood urea nitrogen and serum creatinine levels. For neurologic changes, look for hearing loss and neuritis. Also check for skin rash. *Early identification of side effects promotes prompt treatment of side effects and adjustments in medications.*

Evaluation of Expected Outcomes

The client manages secretions with effective coughing, increased fluid intake, and appropriate postural drainage. He or she reports adequate pain relief and can tolerate increased amounts of time out of bed and perform most ADLs. The client adheres to treatment regimen and schedules tests for liver and kidney function. ●

▶ ***Stop, Think, and Respond Exercise 21-1***

A client diagnosed with TB lives in a four-room apartment with his wife. What precautions must the couple follow?

OBSTRUCTIVE PULMONARY DISEASES

Obstructive pulmonary disease describes conditions in which airflow in the lungs is obstructed. Resistance to inspiration is decreased, whereas resistance to expiration is increased, so that the expiratory phase of respiration is prolonged (Bullock & Henze, 2000). **Chronic obstructive pulmonary disease (COPD)** is an umbrella term for chronic lung diseases that have limited airflow in and out of the lungs. Symptoms of COPD include chronic cough and expectoration, dyspnea, shortness of breath, wheezing, and impaired expiratory airflow. Bronchiectasis, atelectasis, chronic bronchitis, and emphysema, although not categorized as COPD, involve chronic impairment of airflow. Asthma also is an obstructive disorder that is more episodic and usually more acute than COPD. Sleep apnea syndrome also can have obstructive causes (see Chap. 20). Cystic fibrosis also has obstructive characteristics and is included in this section.

BRONCHIECTASIS

Bronchiectasis is found in clients with COPD and is characterized by chronic infection and irreversible dilatation of the bronchi and bronchioles. Causes include bronchial obstruction by tumor or foreign body, congenital abnormalities, exposure to toxic gases, and chronic pulmonary infections. When clearance of the airway is impeded, an infection can develop in the walls of the bronchus or bronchioles. The structure of the wall tissue subsequently changes, resulting in formation of saccular dilatations, which collect purulent material. Airway clearance is further impaired, and the purulent material remains, causing more dilatation, structural damage, and more infection.

Assessment Findings

Clients with bronchiectasis experience a chronic cough with expectoration of copious amounts of purulent sputum and possible hemoptysis. The coughing worsens when the client changes position. The amount of sputum produced during one paroxysm varies with the stage of the disease, but it can be several ounces. When the sputum is collected, it settles into three distinct layers: the top layer is frothy and cloudy, the middle layer is clear saliva, and the bottom layer is heavy, thick, and purulent. Clients also experience fatigue, weight loss, anorexia, and dyspnea.

Chest radiography and bronchoscopy demonstrate the increased size of the bronchioles, possible areas of atelectasis, and changes in the pulmonary tissue. Sputum culture and sensitivity tests identify the causative microorganism and effective antibiotics to control the infection. Pulmonary function studies also may be done.

Medical Management

Treatment of bronchiectasis includes drainage of purulent material from the bronchi; antibiotics, bronchodilators, and mucolytics to improve breathing and help raise secretions; humidification to loosen secretions; and surgical removal if bronchiectasis is confined to a small area.

Nursing Management

Nursing management focuses on instructing the client in postural drainage techniques, which help the client mobilize and expectorate secretions. The positions for the client to assume depend on the site or lobe to be drained. Figure 21-3 shows positions that drain specific segments of all lobes of the lungs. The client remains in each position for 10 to 15 minutes. Chest percussion and vibration may be performed during this time. When complete, the client coughs and expectorates the secretions. This procedure may be repeated. The nurse provides oral hygiene after treatment.

ATELECTASIS

Clients with COPD are at greater risk for developing **atelectasis**, the collapse of alveoli (Fig. 21-4). Atelectasis may involve a small portion of the lung or an entire lobe. When alveoli collapse, they cannot perform their function of gas exchange. Atelectasis occurs secondary to aspiration of food or vomitus, a mucous plug, fluid or air in the thoracic cavity, compression on tissue by tumors, an enlarged heart, an aneurysm, or enlarged lymph nodes in the chest. Ill clients may experience atelectasis when on prolonged bed rest, when unable to breathe deeply or cough and raise secretions, or both.

Assessment Findings

The amount of involved lung tissue determines the extent of the symptoms. Small areas of atelectasis may cause few symptoms. With larger areas, cyanosis, fever, pain, dyspnea, increased pulse and respiratory rates, and increased pulmonary secretions may be seen. Although crackling may be auscultated over the affected areas, usually breath sounds are absent. A chest radiograph reveals dense shadows, indicating collapsed lung tissue. Sometimes the radiograph results are inconclusive. ABG and pulse oximetry results may be abnormal.

Client and Family Teaching 21-1
Using an Incentive Spirometer

The nurse instructs the client as follows:

1. Sit upright unless contraindicated.
2. Mark the goal for inhalation.
3. Exhale normally.
4. Place mouthpiece in mouth, sealing lips around it.
5. Inhale slowly until predetermined volume has been reached.
6. Hold breath for 2 to 6 seconds.
7. Exhale normally.
8. Repeat the exercise 10 to 20 times per hour while awake, or as ordered.
9. Do not rush during the procedure. Slow down if dizziness is experienced.

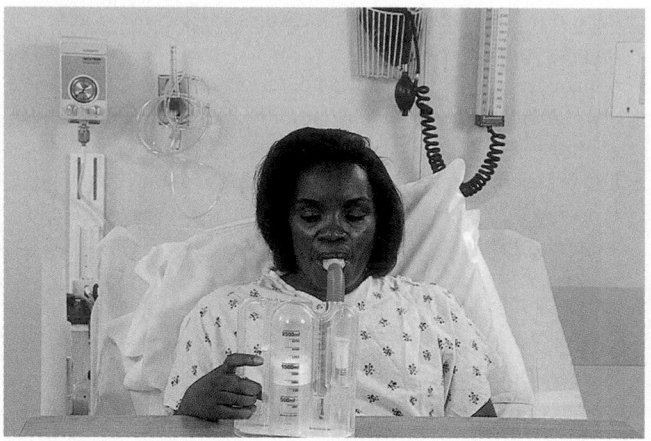

Medical Management

Treatment includes improving ventilation, suctioning, and deep breathing and coughing to raise secretions. Bronchodilators and humidification assist in loosening and removing secretions. Oxygen is administered for dyspnea. Removal of the cause of atelectasis helps to correct the condition.

Nursing Management

Nursing care focuses on preventing atelectasis (Box 21-5), especially when the client is at risk because of failure to aerate the lungs properly. Postoperative deep breathing and coughing can prevent atelectasis. If atelectasis occurs, the nurse encourages the client to take deep breaths and cough at frequent intervals and instructs the client in the use of an incentive spirometer (Client and Family Teaching 21-1).

CHRONIC BRONCHITIS

Chronic bronchitis is a prolonged (or extended) inflammation of the bronchi, accompanied by a chronic cough and excessive production of mucus for at least 3 months each year for 2 consecutive years. This serious health problem develops gradually and may go untreated for many years until the disease is well established.

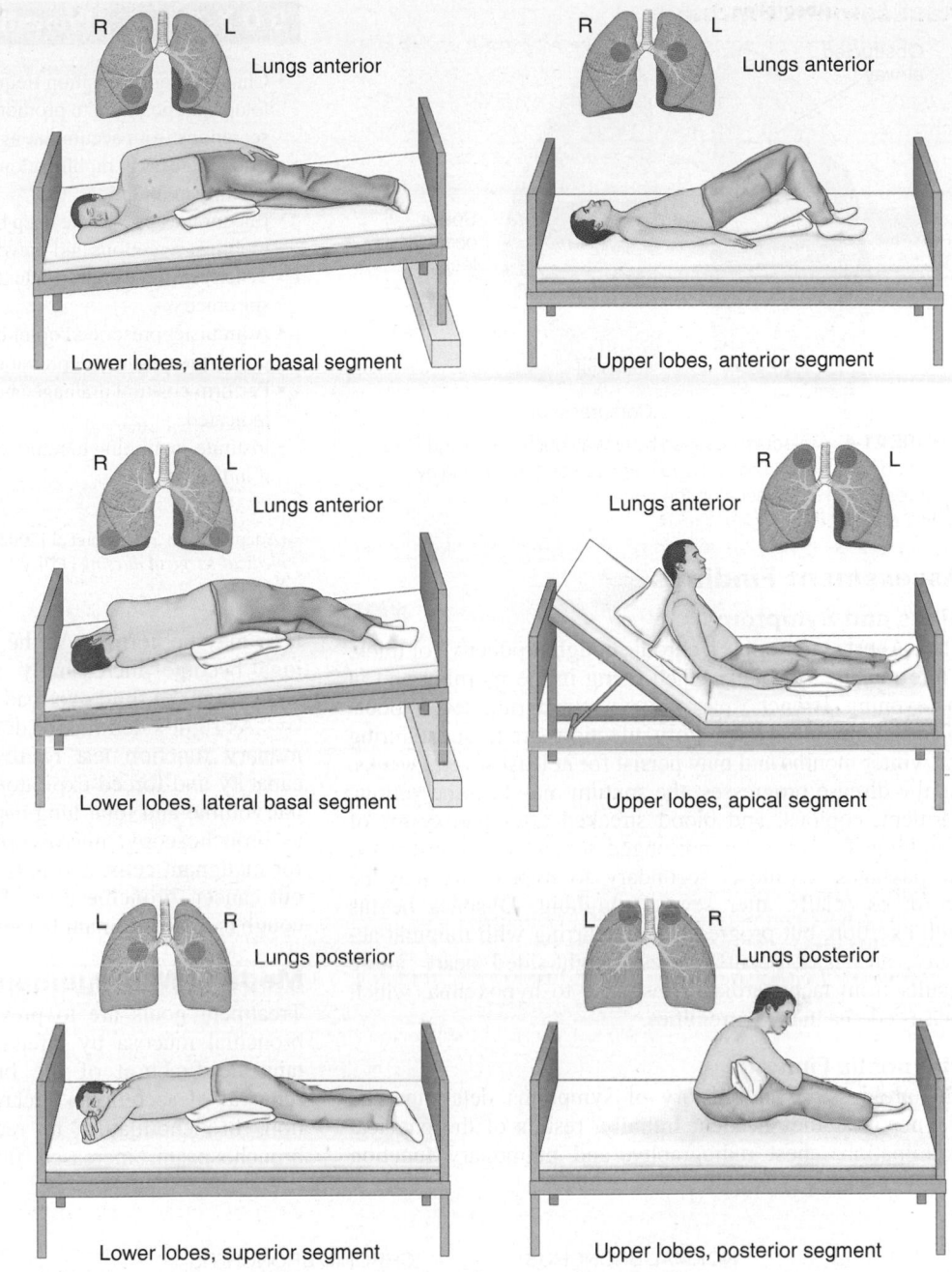

R L
Lungs anterior

Lower lobes, anterior basal segment

R L
Lungs anterior

Upper lobes, anterior segment

R L
Lungs anterior

Lower lobes, lateral basal segment

R L
Lungs anterior

Upper lobes, apical segment

L R
Lungs posterior

Lower lobes, superior segment

L R
Lungs posterior

Upper lobes, posterior segment

FIGURE 21-3. Lung areas to be drained and the best postural drainage positions for them.

Pathophysiology and Etiology

Chronic bronchitis is characterized by hypersecretion of mucus and recurrent or chronic respiratory tract infections. As the infection progresses, the ability of the cilia that line the airway to propel secretions upward becomes significantly altered. Secretions remain in the lungs and form plugs in the smaller bronchi. These plugs become areas for bacterial growth and chronic infection, which increases mucous secretion and eventually causes areas of focal tissue death. Airway obstruction results from the bronchial inflammation (Fig. 21-5).

Multiple factors are associated with chronic bronchitis. Its development may be insidious or follow a long history of bronchial asthma or an acute respiratory tract infection, such as influenza or pneumonia. Air pollution and smoking are significant factors.

Chronic bronchitis may develop at any age, but it appears most commonly in middle age after years of untreated, low-grade bronchitis. Diagnosis is based on evaluation of the duration of symptoms, determination of how the disease process began, and history of occupational health hazards, pulmonary disease, and smoking.

▶ *Stop, Think, and Respond Exercise 21-2*

Your client with acute bronchitis smokes two packs of cigarettes per day. What would you advise this client?

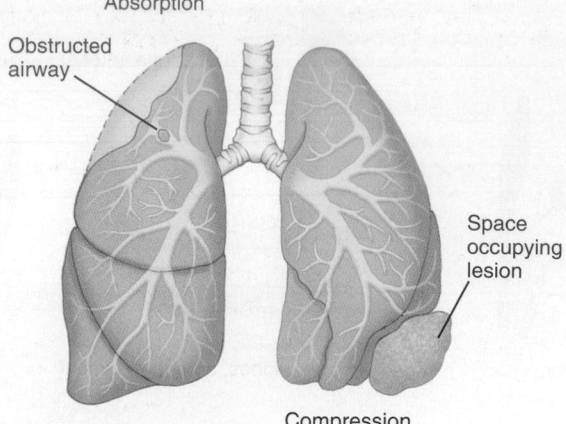

FIGURE 21-4. Atelectasis caused by airway obstruction and absorption of air from the involved lung area on the *left* and by compression of lung tissue on the *right*.

<div class="box">

BOX 21-5 **Preventing Atelectasis**

- Change client's position frequently, especially from supine to upright position, to promote ventilation and prevent secretions from accumulating.
- Encourage early mobilization from bed to chair, followed by early ambulation.
- Encourage appropriate deep breathing and coughing to mobilize secretions and prevent them from accumulating.
- Teach/reinforce appropriate technique for incentive spirometry.
- Administer prescribed opioids and sedatives judiciously to prevent respiratory depression.
- Perform postural drainage and chest percussion, if indicated.
- Institute suctioning to remove tracheobronchial secretions, if indicated.

(Adapted from Smeltzer et al.[2008]. *Brunner & Suddarth's textbook of medical-surgical nursing* [11th ed.]. Philadelphia: Lippincott Williams & Wilkins.)

</div>

Assessment Findings

Signs and Symptoms

The earliest symptom is a chronic cough productive of thick, white mucus, especially when rising in the morning and in the evening. Bronchospasm may occur during severe bouts of coughing. Acute respiratory infections are frequent during the winter months and may persist for at least several weeks. As the disease progresses, the sputum may become yellow, purulent, copious, and blood streaked after paroxysms of coughing. Expiration is prolonged secondary to obstructed air passages. Cyanosis secondary to hypoxemia may be noted, especially after severe coughing. Dyspnea begins with exertion, but progresses to occurring with minimal activity, and later occurs at rest. Right-sided heart failure results from tachycardia in response to hypoxemia, which causes edema in the extremities.

Diagnostic Findings

The progression and history of symptoms determine the diagnostic studies needed. Initially, results of the physical examination, chest radiography, and pulmonary function tests may be normal. As the disease progresses, these findings become increasingly abnormal. Chest radiography shows signs of fluid overload and consolidation in the lungs.

As right-sided failure develops, the heart enlarges. Pulmonary function test results demonstrate decreased vital capacity and forced expiratory volume and increased residual volume and total lung capacity. Diagnostic studies such as bronchoscopy, microscopic examination of the sputum for malignant cells, and lung scan may be necessary to rule out cancer, bronchiectasis, TB, or other diseases in which cough is a predominant feature.

Medical Management

Treatment goals are to prevent recurrent irritation of the bronchial mucosa by infection or chemical agents, maintain the function of the bronchioles, and assist in the removal of secretions. Treatment includes smoking cessation, bronchodilators to reduce airway obstruction and bronchospasm, increased fluid intake, maintenance of a

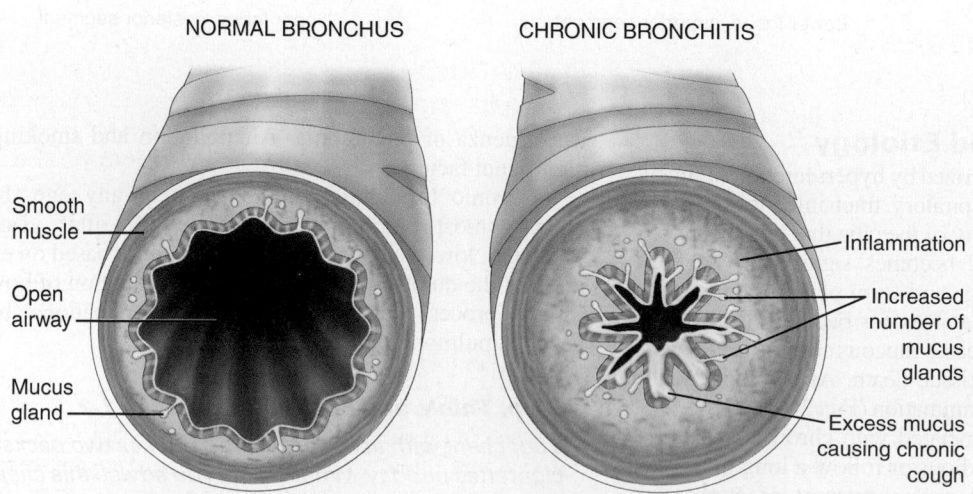

NORMAL BRONCHUS   CHRONIC BRONCHITIS

Smooth muscle
Open airway
Mucus gland

Inflammation
Increased number of mucus glands
Excess mucus causing chronic cough

FIGURE 21-5. Pathophysiology of chronic bronchitis as compared with normal bronchus. The bronchus in chronic bronchitis is narrowed and has impaired air flow due to multiple mechanisms: inflammation, excess mucus production, and potential smooth muscle constriction (bronchospasm).

well-balanced diet, postural drainage to remove bronchial secretions, steroid therapy if other treatment is ineffective, change in occupation if work involves exposure to dust and chemical irritants, filtration of incoming air to reduce sputum production and cough, and antibiotic therapy.

Nursing Management

Nursing management focuses on educating clients in managing their disease. The nurse helps clients identify ways to eliminate environmental irritants. Such measures include smoking cessation, occupational counseling, monitoring air quality and pollution levels, and avoiding cold air and wind exposure that can cause bronchospasm.

Preventing infection is another important aspect of care. The nurse instructs clients to avoid others with respiratory tract infections and to receive pneumonia and flu immunizations. He or she teaches the client to monitor sputum for signs of infection. The nurse also teaches the proper use of aerosolized bronchodilators and corticosteroids.

Metered-dose inhalers (MDI) are pressurized devices that contain an aerosolized powder of specific medications. When the client pushes on the pressurized canister, an exact amount of medication is delivered via inhalation. Clients need instruction regarding the use of a MDI (Client and Family Teaching 21-2). It may be difficult for clients to coordinate the equipment and the need to inhale forcibly as the medication is released. For that reason, spacers (holding chambers) are added to hold the medication, allowing the client to inhale slowly and deeply and with more control to receive the full dose of the inhaled medication. There are also other types of inhalers specific to particular medications; each requires thorough client instruction.

The nurse instructs the client in postural drainage techniques and measures to improve overall health, such as eating a well-balanced diet, getting plenty of rest, and engaging in moderate aerobic activity. For clients with lung disease, dyspnea, not heart rate, should determine the amount of aerobic activity. In other words, clients should exercise at the pace and for the length of time they can tolerate without dyspnea. Refer to nursing management of emphysema for nursing diagnoses and additional interventions.

PULMONARY EMPHYSEMA

Emphysema is a chronic disease characterized by abnormal distention of the alveoli. The alveolar walls and capillary beds also show marked destruction. This process of destruction occurs over a long period. By the time of diagnosis, damage to the lungs usually is permanent. Emphysema is a common cause of disability and the most common obstructive lung disorder.

Pathophysiology and Etiology

In emphysema, the alveoli lose elasticity, trapping air that the client normally would expire. On microscopic examination, the alveolar walls are broken down, forming one large sac instead of multiple, small air spaces. The capillary beds, previously located within the alveolar walls, are destroyed, and fibrous scarring replaces much of the tissue. Formation

Client and Family Teaching 21-2
Using a Metered-Dose Inhaler (MDI)

The nurse provides the following instructions:

1. Attach the stem of the canister into the hole of the mouthpiece so that the inhaler looks like an "L." If a spacer is used, attach the spacer to the mouthpiece on one end and to the MDI on the other end.
2. Shake the canister to distribute the drug in its pressurized chamber.
3. Exhale slowly through pursed lips.
4. Seal lips around the mouthpiece or hold inhaler a few inches from mouth.
5. Compress the canister between thumb and fingers and slowly inhale; if not using a spacer, you must compress the canister and inhale at the same time.
6. Release the pressure on the canister, but continue inhaling as much as possible. Inhalation should be for 3 to 5 seconds.
7. Withdraw the mouthpiece.
8. Hold breath for a few seconds.
9. Exhale slowly through pursed lips.
10. If second dose is required, wait for a few seconds before repeating procedure.

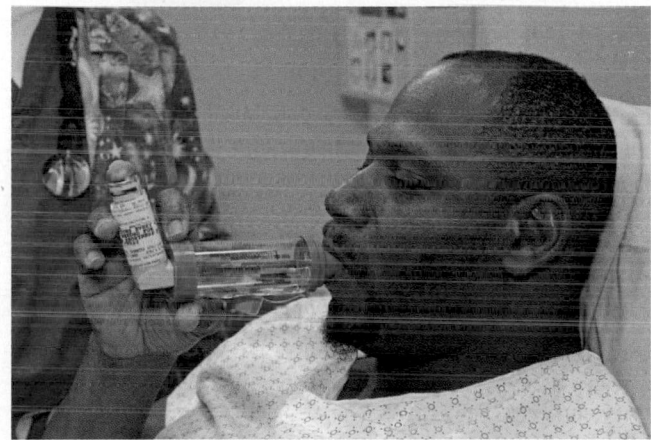

Metered-dose inhaler with spacer.

of fibrous tissue and destruction of the alveoli prevent the proper exchange of oxygen and CO_2 during respiration.

As the disease progresses, large air sacs (bullae, blebs) may be seen over the lung surface. These sacs can rupture, allowing air to enter the thorax (**pneumothorax**) with each respiration. In this case, emergency thoracentesis is performed to remove the air from the thoracic cavity. A chest tube may be inserted to keep additional air from entering. Recurrent episodes of pneumothorax may require surgery to correct the problem (see section on Thoracic Surgery).

Assessment Findings

Signs and Symptoms

Shortness of breath with minimal activity is called *exertional dyspnea* and often is the first symptom of emphysema. As the disease progresses, breathlessness occurs even at rest. A

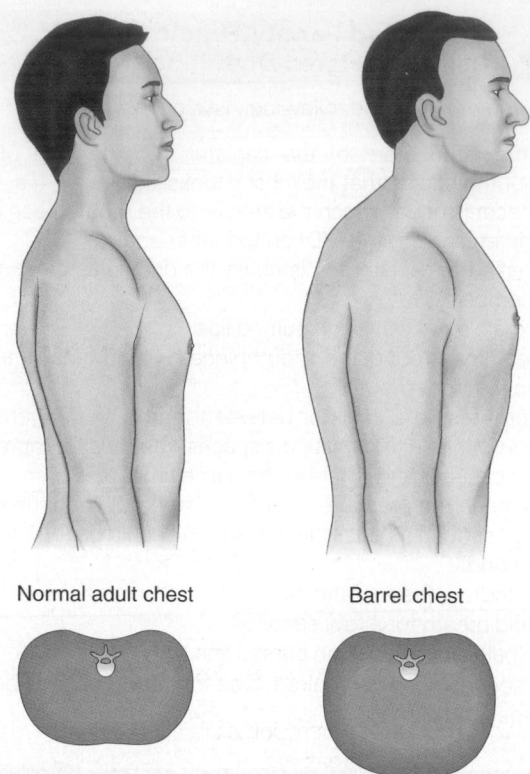

Normal adult chest   Barrel chest

FIGURE 21-6. Profile and anteroposterior diameter of normal adult chest (*left*) and barrel chest (*right*), as seen in emphysema.

chronic cough invariably is present and productive of muco-purulent sputum. Inspiration is difficult because of the rigid chest cage, and the chest is characteristically barrel shaped (Fig. 21-6).

The client uses the accessory muscles of respiration (muscles in the jaw and neck and intercostal muscles) to maintain normal ventilation. Expiration is prolonged, difficult, and often accompanied by wheezing. In advanced emphysema, respiratory function is markedly impaired. Clients with advanced emphysema characteristically appear drawn, anxious, and pale. They speak in short, jerky sentences. When sitting up, they often lean slightly forward and are markedly short of breath. The neck veins may distend during expiration.

In advanced emphysema, memory loss, drowsiness, confusion, and loss of judgment may result from the markedly reduced oxygen that reaches the brain and the increased CO_2 in the blood. If the disorder goes untreated, the CO_2 content in the blood may reach toxic levels, resulting in lethargy, stupor, and, eventually, coma. This condition is called *carbon dioxide narcosis*. Lung auscultation reveals decreased breath sounds, wheezing, and crackles. Heart sounds are diminished or muffled. Visual inspection shows a barrel-chested person breathing through pursed lips and using the accessory muscles of respiration.

Diagnostic Findings

Chest radiography, fluoroscopy, and CT scanning demonstrate hyperinflated lung fields. Results of pulmonary function studies show a marked decrease in overall function, including increased total lung capacity and residual volume and decreased vital capacity and forced expiratory volume. ABG analysis usually reveals hypoxemia and respiratory acidosis.

Medical Management

The goals of medical management include improving the client's quality of life, slowing the disease progression, and treating the obstructed airways. Treatment includes the following measures:

- Bronchodilators to dilate airways by decreasing edema and spasms and improving gas exchange
- Aerosol therapy with nebulized aerosols for deep inhalation of bronchodilators and mucolytics in the tracheobronchial tree
- Supplemental oxygen may be prescribed
- Antibiotics
- Corticosteroids on a limited basis to assist with bronchodilation and removal of secretions
- Physical therapy to increase ventilation—deep breathing, coughing, chest percussion, vibration, and postural drainage

If the prescribed treatment regimen does not help the client, progressive loss of sleep, appetite, weight, and physical strength is likely. As the disease progresses, the client may need to curtail physical activities.

Nursing Management

Clients with emphysema may require supplemental oxygen. It is important to monitor oxygen levels as well as carbon dioxide ($PaCO_2$) levels, because some clients with emphysema tend to have chronic hypercapnia (elevated $PaCO_2$). For this group, when supplemental oxygen is administered, the hemoglobin is saturated with oxygen and unable to carry carbon dioxide. This results in increased hypercapnia (Smeltzer et al., 2008).

The safest method of oxygen administration is by nasal catheter or cannula, with the oxygen flow rate set at no more than 2 to 3 L/min. If the client's color improves but his or her level of consciousness decreases, the nurse discontinues oxygen administration and notifies the physician; the client may be approaching a state of respiratory arrest.

Therapeutic breathing exercises effectively use the diaphragm (diaphragmatic breathing), thus relieving the compensatory burden on the muscles of the upper thorax. The nurse teaches the client to let the abdomen rise when taking a deep breath and to contract the abdominal muscles when exhaling. Clients can feel the correct way to do this by placing one hand on the chest and the other on the abdomen: during abdominal breathing, the chest should remain quiet and the abdomen should rise and fall with each breath.

Other exercises include blowing out candles at various distances and blowing a small object, such as a pencil or piece of chalk, along a tabletop. The nurse encourages the client to exhale more completely by taking a deep breath and then bending the body forward at the waist while exhaling as fully as possible. Pursed-lip breathing (i.e., breathing with the lips pursed or puckered on expiration) helps to control the respiratory rate and depth and slows expiration. This maneuver may decrease dyspnea and in turn reduce the anxiety that often is associated with breathing difficulties.

In addition, client education is aimed at helping clients adjust to their current level of disability and to the potential for increased disability in the future. The primary goal is to prevent or delay the progression of emphysema. Clients who are motivated will profit more from available treatments and

Client and Family Teaching 21-3
Following a Treatment Regimen for Emphysema

The nurse teaches the client strategies to slow the disease progression:

- Success of treatment depends on strict adherence to the treatment regimen.
- Take medication exactly as prescribed. Observe the time intervals between medications. Do not skip doses or take more than what is prescribed.
- Maintain close medical supervision.
- Contact the physician if adverse drug effects occur, drugs fail to relieve symptoms, new symptoms appear, symptoms become more severe, or signs or symptoms of respiratory infection develop.
- Drink extra fluids as indicated, unless fluids are restricted.
- Avoid respiratory irritants and people with respiratory infections.
- Eat a well-balanced diet.
- Perform breathing exercises as prescribed.
- Take frequent rests during the day. Space activities to prevent fatigue and shortness of breath.
- Avoid dry-heated areas that can aggravate symptoms.
- Humidify inspired air during the winter months.

Nutrition Notes 21-1
The Client With Emphysema

- Malnutrition among clients with emphysema is multifactorial
  - Shortness of breath and difficulty breathing impair the ability to chew and swallow.
  - Inadequate oxygenation of GI cells causes anorexia and gastric ulceration.
  - Slowed peristalsis and digestion contribute to loss of appetite.
  - Labored breathing increases calorie requirements.
  - Eating is not a priority among clients who are anxious about breathing.
- To correct malnutrition, a high-protein, high-calorie diet is indicated, but an excessive calorie intake is avoided because it increases respiratory stress by increasing carbon dioxide output.
- Small, frequent feedings of nutrient-dense foods help maximize intake and lessen fatigue; concentrated liquid supplements are beneficial.
- Encourage ample fluid intake. Fluids consumed between meals instead of with meals are less likely to interfere with food intake.
- Obese clients with emphysema are encouraged to lose weight to improve breathing.

make the best use of their remaining pulmonary function. Client and Family Teaching 21-3 outlines strategies to slow disease progression. Refer also to Nutrition Notes 21-1.

Nursing Process for the Client With Obstructive Pulmonary Disease

Assessment

Assess the client's respiratory status, including respiratory effort, rate, and pattern. Determine whether the client has diminished breath sounds and prolonged expiration. Observe for evidence of dyspnea at rest, as well as accentuated accessory neck muscles and barrel-shaped chest. Ask the client about tolerance for activity and check the characteristics of secretions: consistency, quantity, color, or odor. Other important assessment data are the client's ability to expectorate secretions, signs and symptoms of infection, and what the client does to relieve pulmonary symptoms.

Diagnosis, Planning, and Interventions

▶ **Ineffective Airway Clearance** related to bronchoconstriction, increased mucus production, and ineffective cough

▶ **Expected Outcome:** Client will maintain a patent airway and adequate airway clearance.

- Auscultate breath sounds at least every 8 hours. *Findings may indicate airway obstruction secondary to mucous plug, increasing airway resistance, or fluid in larger airways.*
- Encourage client to cough and clear secretions; suction as needed. *These measures promote airway clearance and improve ventilation.*

- Perform postural drainage with percussion and vibration twice a day as indicated. *Postural drainage assists in mobilizing secretions for expectoration.*
- Observe for dyspnea, restlessness, increased anxiety, or use of accessory muscles. *Such findings indicate possible airway obstruction or ineffective clearance of secretions.*
- Increase fluid intake to 3 L/day if not contraindicated. (Right-sided or left-sided cardiac failure is a contraindication.) Humidify inspired air. *These measures keep secretions moist and easier to expectorate.*
- Instruct client in early signs of infection: increased sputum production, changes in sputum color and consistency, fever, increased coughing, and increased dyspnea. *Early recognition prevents an infection from progressing to a potentially lethal process.*
- Administer bronchodilators by nebulizer or MDI as indicated. *Bronchodilators open airways, facilitating breathing and expectoration of secretions.*
- Teach and encourage the use of diaphragmatic and pursed-lip breathing. *These techniques improve ventilation and mobilize secretions.*

▶ **Impaired Gas Exchange** related to prolonged expiration, loss of lung tissue elasticity, and atelectasis

▶ **Expected Outcome:** Client will maintain optimal gas exchange.

- Promote more effective breathing patterns through optimal positioning, pursed-lip breathing, and use of abdominal muscles. *High Fowler's position promotes better lung expansion; turning side to side promotes aeration of lung lobes; pursed-lip* breathing and other methods open airways and provide for better exhalation.

- Administer oxygen as prescribed. *Clients with COPD chronically retain CO_2 and depend on hypoxic drive as the stimulus for breathing; accurate oxygen administration is essential for preventing cessation of breathing.*
- Monitor level of consciousness and mental status. *Problems with mentation indicate inadequate oxygenation.*
- Monitor results of ABGs and pulse oximetry. *Changes in these findings indicate respiratory deterioration and provide an opportunity for early interventions.*

▶ PC: Atelectasis

▶ **Expected Outcome:** Nurse will manage and minimize atelectasis.

- Instruct client to do deep-breathing and coughing exercises, incentive spirometry, or both. *These techniques promote lung expansion.*
- Encourage client to use abdominal muscles when breathing. *Diaphragmatic breathing promotes lung expansion.*

Evaluation of Expected Outcomes

The client's airway is free of secretions; breath sounds are clear. ABG and pulse oximetry results are within baseline values, and client remains alert and responsive. The client has no signs or symptoms of atelectasis and demonstrates the ability to do pulmonary exercises and abdominal breathing as instructed. ●

ASTHMA

Asthma is usually a reversible obstructive disease of the lower airway. Inflammation of the airway and hyper-responsiveness of the airway to internal or external stimuli characterize asthma. The incidence of asthma is increasing, particularly in children and adolescents. Asthma affects almost one fifth of the population at some time in their lives. Asthma may be fatal, but for most people it causes disruptions in school and work attendance and affects choices in careers and activities.

Pathophysiology and Etiology

There are two types of asthma: *allergic asthma* (extrinsic), which occurs in response to allergens, such as pollen, dust, spores, and animal dander; and *non-allergic asthma* (intrinsic), associated with factors such as upper respiratory infections, emotional upsets, and exercise. Many clients experience *mixed asthma,* which has characteristics of allergic and non-allergic asthma.

Acute asthma results from increasing airway obstruction caused by bronchospasm and bronchoconstriction, inflammation and edema of the lining of the bronchi and bronchioles, and production of thick mucus that can plug the airway (Fig. 21-7). The airways in people with asthma are hyper-reactive in response to stimuli. Allergic asthma causes the immunoglobulin E (IgE) inflammatory response (see Chap. 33). These antibodies attach to mast cells within the lungs. Reexposure to the antigen causes the antigen to attach to the antibody, releasing mast cell products such as

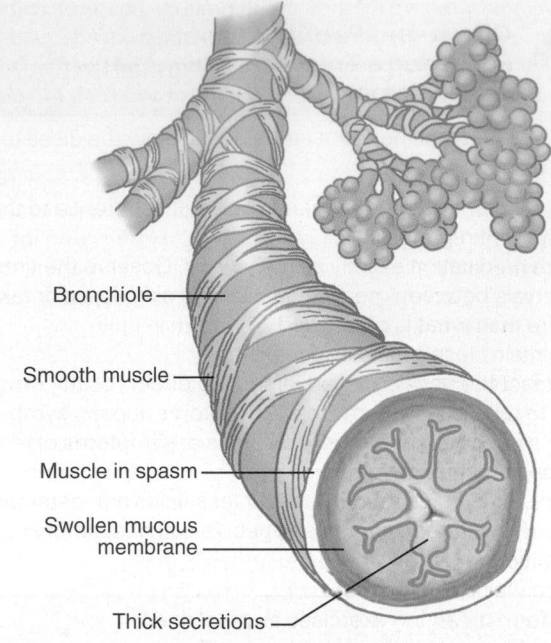

Bronchiole

Smooth muscle

Muscle in spasm

Swollen mucous membrane

Thick secretions

FIGURE 21-7. Bronchial asthma. Muscle spasms, mucosal edema, and thick secretions obstruct the bronchiole on expiration.

histamine. The manifestations of asthma become evident as this occurs. Other types of asthma are hyper-responsive to the inflammatory changes.

Because alveoli cannot expel air, they hyperinflate and trap air in the lungs. The client breathes faster, blowing off excess CO_2. Although the client tries to force the air out, the narrowed airway makes it difficult. Wheezing usually is audible with expiration, resulting from air being forced out of the narrowed airway. Other pathophysiologic changes include interference with gas exchange, poor perfusion, possible atelectasis, and respiratory failure if inadequately treated.

Asthma may develop at any age. There appears to be a significant relationship between bronchiolitis (inflammation of the bronchioles) in the first year of life and development of asthma in early childhood. Asthma may be limited to occasional attacks, with the client symptom free between attacks.

Assessment Findings

Signs and Symptoms

Asthma is typified by paroxysms of shortness of breath, wheezing, and coughing and the production of thick, tenacious sputum. Duration of acute episodes varies; it may be brief (less than 1 day) or extended (lasting for several weeks).

Most clients are aware of the wheezing and report it as one of their symptoms. Every breath becomes an effort. During an acute episode, the work of breathing greatly increases, and the client may suffer from a sensation of suffocation. The client frequently assumes a classic sitting position, with the body leaning slightly forward and the arms at shoulder height. This position facilitates chest expansion and more effective excursions of the diaphragm. Because life depends on the power to breathe, fear and anxiety often accompany and also intensify the symptoms.

Marked prolongation of the expiratory phase of respiration accompanies the effort to move trapped air. Coughing commences with the onset of the attack but is ineffective in the early stage. Only as the attack begins to subside can the client expectorate large quantities of thick, stringy mucus. The skin usually is pale. During a severe attack, the nurse may observe cyanosis of the client's lips and nail beds. Perspiration typically is profuse during an acute attack. After spontaneous or drug-induced remission of the episode, examination of the lungs commonly shows normal findings. Sometimes an acute attack intensifies and progresses to status asthmaticus (persistent state of asthma), which can be life-threatening.

Diagnostic Findings

Chest auscultation reveals expiratory and sometimes inspiratory wheezes and diminished breath sounds. Results of pulmonary function studies, especially of forced expiratory volume, may be abnormal, with total lung capacity and functional residual volume increased secondary to trapped air. The forced expiratory volume and forced vital capacity are decreased. During acute attacks, blood gases show hypoxemia. The partial pressure of carbon dioxide ($PaCO_2$) level may be elevated if the asthma becomes worse, but usually the $PaCO_2$ level is decreased because of the rapid respiratory rate. A normal $PaCO_2$ level in the latter part of an asthma attack may indicate impending respiratory failure.

Medical Management

Symptomatic treatment is given at the time of the attack. Long-term care involves measures to treat as well as to prevent further attacks. An effort must be made to determine the cause. If the history and diagnostic tests indicate allergy as a causative factor, treatment includes avoidance of the allergen, desensitization, or antihistamine therapy. Oxygen usually is not necessary during an acute attack because most clients are actively hyperventilating. Oxygen may be necessary if cyanosis occurs.

Pharmacologic management is often classified as rescue therapy and maintenance therapy. Rescue-therapy medications treat acute episodes of asthma, whereas maintenance therapy is a daily regimen designed to prevent and control symptoms. Many medications are taken through MDIs. Drug Therapy Table 21-2 lists medications used for both types of therapy.

Humidification of inspired air is valuable because dehydration of the respiratory mucous membrane may lead to

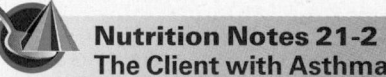

Nutrition Notes 21-2
The Client with Asthma

- Encourage clients with asthma to consume adequate calories and protein to optimize health and resist infection.
- Large meals may aggravate asthma by distending the stomach; small frequent meals may be better tolerated.
- Certain vitamins and minerals are important for immune function, especially vitamins A, C, B$_6$, and the mineral zinc, and should be liberally consumed.
- Food allergens that may trigger asthma include milk, eggs, seafood, and fish.

asthmatic attacks. Use of steam or cool vapor humidifiers also has proved effective. Liquefaction of the secretions promotes more effective clearing of the airways and a rapid return to normal. Air conditioners may filter offending allergens as well as control temperature and humidity.

Pharmacologic Considerations

- Bronchodilators are used to manage acute breathing disorders, such as acute asthma attacks or reversible bronchospasm. Examples of bronchodilators include adrenergic drugs, such as epinephrine, isoproterenol (Isuprel), and terbutaline (Bricanyl), and the xanthine derivatives, such as theophylline and aminophylline. When theophylline or aminophylline is used, serum theophylline levels should be maintained in the therapeutic range of 10 to 20 micrograms (mcg)/mL. Levels over 20 mcg/mL are associated with toxicity.

Nursing Management

During asthma attacks, clients are extremely anxious. The nurse reassures the client that someone will remain with him or her during the acute phase. The nurse administers oxygen if indicated and puts the client in a sitting position. Rest and adequate fluid intake are important. Increased fluid intake makes secretions less tenacious and replaces the fluids lost through perspiration. Thus, the nurse keeps fluids within easy reach and encourages the client to drink them. The nurse checks the intravenous (IV) site frequently for signs of extravasation. This monitoring is especially important during an acute attack because restlessness can result in catheter dislodgment. The nurse observes for adverse drug effects, especially when the client is receiving epinephrine or other adrenergic agents, which may cause palpitations, nervousness, trembling, pallor, and insomnia.

Clients with asthma must demonstrate understanding of the following (Smeltzer et al., 2008):

- Asthma as a chronic inflammatory disease
- Role of inflammation and bronchoconstriction
- Action and purpose of medications
- How to avoid triggers for asthma attacks
- Use of metered-dose inhalers
- Use of peak-flow monitoring
- When and how to obtain medical assistance

The nurse assesses the client's level of understanding of these topics and provides education as needed.

The nurse determines whether the client has a peak flow meter and obtains one for the client if needed. The peak flow meter measures the peak expiratory flow rate (PEFR), which is the point of highest flow during forced expiration. The nurse instructs the client in using the peak flow meter to monitor the degree of asthma control (Client and Family Teaching 21-4). The client can use the peak flow meter to assess the effectiveness of medication or breathing status. The nurse tells the client to seek care if readings fall below baseline and teaches the correct use of inhalers. He or she also helps the client to identify

DRUG THERAPY TABLE 21-2 Drug Therapy for Asthma

Drug Category and Examples	Mechanism of Action	Side Effects	Nursing Considerations
Rescue Therapy			
Short-Acting Beta Agonists albuterol (Ventolin)	Dilate the smooth muscles of the bronchioles, reduce muscle spasm, and therefore increase the size of the airway	Restlessness, apprehension, anxiety, fear, central nervous system stimulation, nausea, dysrhythmias, sweating, flushing, paradoxical airway resistance with repeated excessive use	Ensure that client understands technique for administering inhalers. Teach client not to exceed recommended dose and to report chest pain, dizziness, irregular heart rate, difficulty breathing, productive cough, or failure to achieve relief.
Anticholinergics ipratropium bromide (Atrovent)	Decrease vagal tone to airways, resulting in bronchodilation	Nervousness, dizziness, headache, nausea, cough, palpitations, exacerbation of glaucoma, and urinary retention	Demonstrate proper use of inhaler. Teach client to report eye pain or visual changes, rash, difficulty voiding.
Maintenance Therapy			
Long-Acting Beta Agonists formoterol (Foradil Aerolizer) salmeterol (Serevent)	Dilate the smooth muscles of the bronchioles, reduce muscle spasm, and therefore increase the size of the airway	Restlessness, apprehension, anxiety, fear, central nervous system stimulation, nausea, dysrhythmias, sweating, flushing, paradoxical airway resistance with repeated excessive use	Educate client that the difference between short- and long-acting beta agonists is the duration of medication effectiveness; otherwise, the drugs are very similar.
Inhaled Corticosteroids triamcinolone (Azmacort)	Decrease inflammatory response	Inhalants*: oral, laryngeal, and pharyngeal irritations and fungal infections. Common side effects are hoarseness, dry mouth, cough, and sore throat.	Teach client not to use during an acute asthma attack and not to use more often than prescribed. If using an aerosolized bronchodilator, administer the bronchodilator first. Instruct client to rinse mouth after inhalation. Teach client not to discontinue medication abruptly.
Mast Cell Inhibitors inhaled cromolyn (Intal)	Prevent the release of mast cell products, promoting bronchodilation and decreasing inflammation; ineffective in acute attacks, but very therapeutic if taken regularly	Dizziness, nausea, throat irritation	Educate client not to use during an acute attack, to follow manufacturer's instructions for administration, and not to discontinue abruptly.
Leukotriene Modifiers montelukast (Singulair)	Mediate the inflammatory response, reduce inflammation and ease bronchoconstriction	Headache, nausea, diarrhea	Teach client that the medication is not for acute use; it has delayed onset. Medication is to be taken as prescribed, even during symptom-free periods.

*Corticosteroids administered by other routes and in higher dosages are associated with multiple adverse effects.

Client and Family Teaching 21-4
Using a Peak Flow Meter

To determine peak flow, the nurse instructs the client as follows:

- Sit upright in bed or chair or stand and inhale as deeply as possible.
- Form a tight seal around the mouthpiece with lips.
- Exhale forcefully and quickly.
- Note the reading.
- Repeat these steps two more times; write the highest of the three numbers in the asthma record.
- After 2 to 3 weeks of asthma therapy, determine your best or usual individual peak flow.
- Monitor the peak flow readings according to three zones
  - Green zone—80% to 100% of your best or usual peak flow; indicates asthma is under good control
  - Yellow zone—50% to 80% of your best or usual peak flow; indicates the asthma symptoms are getting worse
  - Red zone—less than 50% of your best or usual peak flow; indicates increasingly dangerous condition.
- Depending on the zone, take actions as instructed by healthcare providers.

triggering events such as dust, smoking, emotional upset, or exposure to irritants such as cleaning fluids or insecticides. The nurse teaches the client relaxation techniques and therapeutic breathing techniques, as discussed previously in the section on the nursing management of emphysema.

Stop, Think, and Respond Exercise 21-3

Your client has asthma caused by extrinsic factors, particularly dust. How can this client reduce asthma attacks?

CYSTIC FIBROSIS

Cystic fibrosis (CF) is an inherited multisystem disorder that affects infants, children, and young adults. It obstructs the lungs, leading to major lung infections, as well as obstructing the pancreas. In the past, children with CF did not survive much beyond adolescence. Although CF remains a serious childhood disease, new treatments and therapies are enabling clients with CF to live longer and are improving their lives in terms of quality and productivity.

Pathophysiology and Etiology

CF results from a defective autosomal recessive gene. A person with CF inherits a defective copy of the CF gene from both parents. A person who is a carrier has one normal copy of the gene and one defective copy. When two carriers give birth to a child, the child has a 25% chance of having CF, a 50% chance of being a carrier, and a 25% chance of not being a carrier. The genetic mutation causes dysfunction of the exocrine glands, involving the mucus-secreting and eccrine sweat glands. Resulting major abnormalities include the following:

- Faulty transport of sodium and chloride in cells lining organs, such as the lungs and pancreas, to their outer surfaces
- Production of abnormally thick, sticky mucus in many organs, especially the lungs and pancreas
- Altered electrolyte balance in the sweat glands

The genetic defect causes inadequate synthesis of a protein (CF gene product) referred to as the *CF transmembrane conductance regulator* (CFTR). CFTR molecules are located in the cells lining the ducts of the exocrine glands, particularly the lungs, pancreas, intestine, and sweat ducts. Clients with CF cannot synthesize adequate CFTR to regulate the combination of water and electrolytes with exocrine secretions and mucus. Subsequently, thick, viscous secretions and protein plugs eventually block the ducts of the exocrine glands. Eventually, ducts may become fibrotic and convert into cysts (Bullock & Henze, 2000).

Assessment Findings

Signs and Symptoms

Clients usually exhibit signs and symptoms in infancy or early childhood. Some individuals, however, do not have signs of the disease until late childhood or adolescence. Clinical manifestations differ related to the degree of organ involvement and the progression of the disease. The three major reasons to suspect CF in children are respiratory symptoms, failure to thrive, and foul-smelling, bulky, greasy stools. In newborns, the first clinical sign may be a meconium ileus (impacted meconium in the intestines). Another sign may be salty-tasting skin.

Respiratory symptoms become very common and include frequent respiratory infections, ranging from URIs with increased cough and purulent sputum to the production of thick, tenacious mucus. Finger clubbing is common. Hemoptysis also may occur as blood vessels are damaged in the lungs, secondary to frequent coughing and constant efforts to clear mucus.

Children also experience malabsorption of fats and fat-soluble vitamins, secondary to impaired pancreatic function. They have difficulty gaining weight. Risk for bowel obstruction, cholecystitis, and cirrhosis is increased.

Diagnostic Findings

The standard and most reliable diagnostic test for CF is the pilocarpine iontophoresis sweat test. Up to 20 years of age, levels higher than 60 mEq/L are diagnostic, and those between 50 and 60 mEq/L are highly suggestive for CF.

Chest radiography demonstrates widespread consolidation, fibrotic changes, and overaerated lungs. Some clients also have areas of collapse. Pulmonary function tests assist in determining current function as well as progression of the disease.

Radiographic studies of the GI system show fibrous abnormalities. In 80% of those with CF, tests for pancreatic enzymes in duodenal contents fail to show evidence of trypsin (Bullock & Henze, 2000). Feces show steatorrhea (fat in stools).

Medical and Surgical Management

Treatment depends on the stage of the disease and the extent of organ involvement; it aims at relieving the symptoms.

Respiratory treatment includes promoting the removal of the thick sputum through postural drainage, chest physical therapy with vigorous percussion and vibration, breathing exercises, hydration to help thin secretions, bronchodilator medications, nebulized mist treatments with saline or mucolytic medications, and prompt treatment of lung infections with antibiotics. Inhaled antibiotics, such as tobramycin, are being used successfully and have the benefit of decreasing systemic absorption. For some clients, ibuprofen, an anti-inflammatory, has been instrumental in slowing the rate at which lung function decreases; other clients are benefiting from azithromycin, an antibiotic that preserves and improves lung function (Cystic Fibrosis Foundation, 2007).

When the digestive system is involved, clients take pancreatic enzyme replacements (such as Pancrease) with all meals and snacks to aid with the absorption of protein, fat, and fat-soluble vitamins. Clients also take multivitamins and fat-soluble vitamin supplements and follow a high-protein, high-calorie diet. A liberal sodium intake is recommended to replace sodium lost through sweat.

Clients with end-stage lung disease sometimes receive a lung transplant. In some cases, clients may receive a liver transplant as well. If successful, the transplants greatly extend the client's life.

Other new treatments are in various stages of implementation and investigation. These include mucous-thinning drugs that reduce lung infections, NSAIDs, inhaled antibiotics, drugs to stimulate cells to secrete chloride and thin mucus, and gene therapy. The potential for clients with CF to live longer increases every year. Current research is focused on treating not only the symptoms but also the causes of CF (Cystic Fibrosis Foundation, 2007).

Nursing Management

Nursing care of clients with CF focuses on preventing complications and promoting as normal a lifestyle as possible. It is important that the client prevent respiratory infections by avoiding people with colds or flu like symptoms, particularly in the fall and winter months. Strict adherence to a vigorous pulmonary toilet (cleansing) is essential for the client with CF who has significant respiratory involvement. Components include chest physical therapy (including postural drainage, percussion, and vibration) two to four times daily, deep-breathing and coughing exercises, nebulized treatments, and medications. New methods, such as high-frequency chest wall oscillation through the use of an inflatable vest, may better clear secretions from the lungs. Attached to an air-pulse generator, the vest rapidly inflates and deflates to gently compress and release the chest wall, creating coughlike forces and increasing airflow in the lungs. In a 10- to 30-minute session, the airflow moves mucus toward larger airways, where the client can clear them by coughing, huffing, or suctioning (Rueling & Adams, 2003).

Clients also need to recognize early signs and symptoms of infection, which include low-grade temperature, increased mucus production, increased cough, and change in color of secretions (white to yellow to greenish). Clients must begin antibiotics as soon as infection occurs to prevent the infection from getting worse. Preventing or minimizing infection prevents or slows lung damage. Some clients are on prophylactic antibiotic therapy to decrease the occurrence of infections. This form of treatment is not common because of the threat of developing antibiotic-resistant infections, which can be deadly for clients with CF. Clients may be taught to administer IV antibiotics at home.

For the client with CF who has significant GI involvement, the nurse must review the client's diet. Collaboration with dietitians can ensure that the client has a diet high in calories, with appropriate amounts of carbohydrates, fats, and proteins. It is essential for the client to take his or her pancreatic enzymes (Cotazym, Creon, or Pancrease), which aid in the digestion of carbohydrates, fats, and proteins. The nurse reminds the client to take the pancreatic enzymes before or during all meals and snacks.

Young adults with CF usually are very knowledgeable about their condition. Nurses must respect their knowledge and allow them to determine their schedule for treatments and procedures. The nurse provides support for clients' efforts in self-care. He or she refers the client as requested to other healthcare professionals, such as dietitians and respiratory and physical therapists, as needed.

OCCUPATIONAL LUNG DISEASES

Exposure to organic and inorganic dusts and noxious gases over a long period can cause chronic lung disorders. **Pneumoconiosis** refers to a fibrous inflammation or chronic induration of the lungs after prolonged exposure to dust or gases. It specifically refers to diseases caused by the inhalation of silica (**silicosis**), coal dust (black-lung disease, miners' disease), or asbestos (**asbestosis**). The resulting effect is referred to as **restrictive lung disease**, which means that the lungs have decreased volume and inability to expand completely. Although these conditions are not malignant, they may increase the client's risk for development of malignancies. Table 21-3 describes these specific conditions in more detail.

The primary focus is prevention, with frequent examination of those who work in areas of highly concentrated dust or gases. Laws require work areas to be safe in terms of dust control, ventilation, protective masks, hoods, industrial respirators, and other protection. Workers are encouraged to practice healthy behaviors, such as quitting smoking.

Dyspnea and cough are the most common symptoms of occupational lung diseases. Those exposed to coal dust may expectorate black-streaked sputum. The diagnosis is based on the history of exposure to dust or gases in the workplace. A chest radiograph may reveal fibrotic changes in the lungs. The results of pulmonary function studies usually are abnormal.

Treatment typically is conservative because the disease is widespread rather than localized. Surgery seldom is of value. Infections, when they occur, are treated with antibiotics. Other treatment modalities include oxygen therapy if severe dyspnea is present, improved nutrition, and adequate rest. Many people with advanced disease are permanently disabled.

Nursing management of clients with occupational lung diseases is basically the same as for clients with emphysema. Many clients require a great deal of emotional support because these diseases may result in permanent disability at a relatively young age.

TABLE 21-3 Occupational Lung Diseases

OCCUPATIONAL LUNG DISEASE	PATHOPHYSIOLOGY AND ETIOLOGY	SIGNS AND SYMPTOMS
Coal miner's pneumoconiosis	Referred to as black lung disease, this condition is caused by inhalation of coal dust and other dusts. Initially, lungs clear particles by phagocytosis and transport out of the lungs. When dust inhalation becomes too great, macrophages collect in the bronchioles, leading to clogging of the airways with dusts, macrophages, and fibroblasts. This results in local emphysema and eventually massive blackened lung lesions. Coal macules eventually form, seen as black dots on radiography.	Chronic cough—sputum production Dyspnea Large amounts of sputum containing black fluid (melanoptysis) Respiratory failure
Silicosis	This illness results from inhalation of silica dust and is seen in workers involved with mining, quarrying, stone-cutting, and tunnel building. Silica particles inhaled into the lungs cause nodular lesions that enlarge and form dense masses over time. The results are loss of lung volume and restrictive and obstructive lung disease.	Shortness of breath Hypoxemia Obstruction of airflow Right-sided heart failure Edema
Asbestosis	This illness results from inhalation of asbestos dust. Laws restrict asbestos use, but old materials still contain asbestos. Asbestos fibers enter the alveoli and cause fibrous tissue to form around them. Pleura also have fibrous changes and plaque formation. Results are restrictive lung disease, decreased lung volume, and decreased gas exchange.	Dyspnea Chest pain Hypoxemia Anorexia and weight loss Respiratory failure

PULMONARY CIRCULATORY DISORDERS

PULMONARY ARTERIAL HYPERTENSION

Pulmonary arterial hypertension refers to continuous high pressure in the pulmonary arteries and results from heart disease, lung disease, or both. It does not become clinically apparent until the client is quite ill. Diagnosis is difficult without invasive testing. Clients with pulmonary arterial hypertension experience difficulty breathing and usually present as quite ill.

Pathophysiology and Etiology

Resistance to blood flow in the pulmonary circulation causes pulmonary arterial hypertension. The pressure in the pulmonary arteries increases, which in turn increases the workload of the right ventricle. Normal pulmonary arterial pressure is approximately 25/10 mm Hg. In pulmonary arterial hypertension, the pressure rises above 40/15 mm Hg and can be higher as the disease progresses.

Primary pulmonary arterial hypertension, which exists without evidence of other disease, is a rare condition. Although the cause is not apparent, there appears to be a familial tendency. "It occurs most often in women 20 to 40 years of age and is usually fatal within 5 years of diagnosis" (Smeltzer et al., 2008, p. 659). Secondary pulmonary arterial hypertension accompanies other heart and lung conditions, most commonly COPD.

Complex mechanisms cause pulmonary arterial hypertension. In primary pulmonary arterial hypertension, the inner lining of the pulmonary arteries thickens and hypertrophies, followed by increased pressure in the pulmonary arteries and vascular bed (Fig. 21-8). In secondary pulmonary arterial hypertension, alveolar destruction causes increased resistance and pressure in the pulmonary vascular bed. In both types of pulmonary arterial hypertension, the increased resistance and pressure in the pulmonary vascular bed results in pulmonary artery hypertension. Consequently, strain is placed on the right ventricle, resulting in enlargement and possible failure.

Assessment Findings

The most common symptoms of primary and secondary hypertension are dyspnea on exertion and weakness. In clients with secondary pulmonary arterial hypertension, additional symptoms are those of the underlying cardiac or respiratory disease: chest pain, fatigue, distended neck veins, **orthopnea** (difficulty breathing while lying flat), and peripheral edema.

An electrocardiogram (ECG) may show right ventricular hypertrophy or failure. Results of ABG analysis are abnormal. Cardiac catheterization demonstrates elevated pulmonary arterial pressures. The results of pulmonary function studies show an increased residual volume but a decreased forced expiratory volume. Echocardiography may show various abnormalities, such as left ventricular dysfunction and tricuspid valve insufficiency. A ventilation-perfusion scan or pulmonary angiography may be done to determine any defects in the pulmonary vessels, such as a pulmonary embolism.

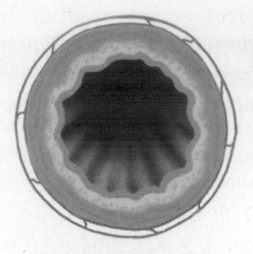

A. Normal. Pulmonary arteriole is normally thin and distensible.

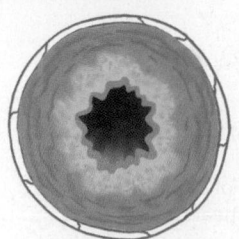

B. Pulmonary hypertension (early). Mild pulmonary hypertension is characterized by thickening of the medial (muscular) layer.

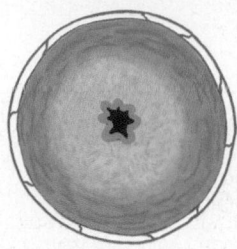

C. Pulmonary hypertension (late). Severe pulmonary hypertension exhibits extensive intimal fibrosis and medial thickening.

FIGURE 21-8. Progression of pulmonary hypertension.

Medical Management

Treatment of primary pulmonary arterial hypertension includes the administration of vasodilators and anticoagulants. Primary pulmonary arterial hypertension has a poor prognosis; therefore, some affected clients are considered candidates for heart-lung transplantation. Treatment of secondary pulmonary arterial hypertension includes management of the underlying cardiac or respiratory disease. Oxygen therapy commonly is used to increase pulmonary arterial oxygenation. If right-sided heart failure is present, other treatments include medications such as digitalis to improve cardiac function, rest, and diuretics.

Nursing Management

Nursing management focuses on recognizing signs and symptoms of respiratory distress. The nurse can reduce the body's need for oxygen by preventing fatigue, assisting with ADLs, and administering oxygen, when needed.

PULMONARY EMBOLISM

Pulmonary embolism involves the obstruction of one of the pulmonary arteries or its branches. The blockage is the result of a thrombus that forms in the venous system or right side of the heart.

Pathophysiology and Etiology

An embolus is any foreign substance, such as a blood clot, air, or particle of fat that travels in the venous blood flow to the lungs. The clot moves to and occludes one of the pulmonary arteries, causing infarction (necrosis or death) of lung tissue distal to the clot. Scar tissue later replaces the infarcted area.

Clots usually form in the deep veins of the lower extremities or pelvis and become the source for pulmonary emboli. Emboli also may arise from the endocardium of the right ventricle when that side of the heart is the site of a myocardial infarction (MI) or endocarditis. A fat embolus usually occurs after a fracture of a long bone, especially the femur. Other conditions that cause pulmonary emboli include recent surgery, prolonged bed rest, trauma, the postpartum state, and debilitating diseases. Three conditions, referred to as *Virchow's triad,* predispose a person to clot formation: venostasis, disruption of the vessel lining, and hypercoagulability (Bullock & Henze, 2000).

Assessment Findings

When a small area of the lung is involved, signs and symptoms usually are less severe and include pain, tachycardia, and dyspnea. The client also may have fever, cough, and blood-streaked sputum. Larger areas of involvement produce more pronounced signs and symptoms, such as severe dyspnea, severe pain, cyanosis, tachycardia, restlessness, and shock. Sudden death may follow a massive pulmonary infarction when a large embolism occludes a main section of the pulmonary artery.

Serum enzymes typically are markedly elevated. A chest radiograph may show an area of atelectasis. An ECG rules out a cardiac disorder such as MI, which produces some of the same symptoms. In addition, a lung scan, CT scan, or pulmonary angiography may be performed to detect the involved lung tissue. Ultrasonography and impedance plethysmography are other imaging studies that help to confirm the presence of lower extremity deep vein thrombosis (see Chap. 23).

Medical and Surgical Management

Treatment of a pulmonary embolism depends on the size of the area involved and the client's symptoms. IV heparin may be administered to prevent extension of the thrombus and the development of additional thrombi in veins from which the embolus arose. IV injection of a thrombolytic drug (one that dissolves a thrombus) such as urokinase, streptokinase, or tissue plasminogen activator also may be used (see Chap. 25). Anticoagulants commonly are given after thrombolytic therapy. Other measures used to treat symptoms of pulmonary emboli include complete bed rest, oxygen, and analgesics.

Pulmonary embolectomy, using cardiopulmonary bypass to support circulation while the embolus is removed, may be necessary if the embolus is lodged in a main pulmonary artery. The insertion of an umbrella filter device (Greenfield filter) in the vena cava prevents recurrent episodes of pulmonary embolus. The umbrella filter is inserted by an applicator catheter inserted into the right internal jugular vein and threaded downward to an area below the renal arteries. Another surgical treatment is the placement of Teflon clips on the inferior vena cava. These clips create narrow channels in the vena cava, allowing blood to pass through on its return to the right side of the heart but keeping back large clots.

BOX 21-6 Preventing the Formation of Pulmonary Emboli

Help client practice active and passive leg exercises.

Instruct client to pump muscles (tense and relax) to improve circulation in lower extremities.

Assist client to ambulate as early as possible after a procedure.

Teach client to:

- Wear support hose/elastic hose as directed
- Avoid constrictive clothing
- Avoid sitting for long periods or with legs crossed
- Drink fluids liberally unless contraindicated
- When traveling, move lower legs and feet while sitting, change positions as able, do not cross legs, and ambulate if able

Nursing Management

The best management of pulmonary emboli is through prevention of deep vein thrombosis (DVT) (Box 21-6). When determining the client's potential for DVT, it is important to note the client's ability to engage in activity such as leg exercises and ambulation. Clients on bed rest are encouraged to do active and/or passive leg exercises. Physicians may order clients to wear elastic compression stockings or use intermittent compression systems such as Venodyne. In addition, the nurse assesses the client for signs of localized calf tenderness, swelling, increased warmth, or prominence of superficial veins in one or both lower extremities, and history of DVT, all of which may indicate the presence of DVT (see Chap. 23).

 Gerontologic Considerations

- Vascular changes of aging and chronic vascular diseases cause alterations in arterial and venous lumen, increasing the risk of deep vein thrombosis. The nurse should assess the older client's history of cardiovascular disease, level of activity, hydration status, and constricting clothing such as tight-fitting hose or socks.

Pulmonary embolism almost always occurs suddenly, and death can follow within 1 hour. Obviously, early recognition of this problem is essential. The nurse starts an IV infusion as soon as possible to establish a patent vein before shock becomes profound. He or she administers vasopressors such as dopamine or dobutamine as ordered to treat hypotension. The nurse provides oxygen for dyspnea and analgesics for pain and apprehension. Close monitoring of vital signs is necessary, as is observing the client at frequent intervals for changes. The nurse institutes continuous ECG monitoring because right ventricular failure is a common problem.

Areas for the nurse to monitor include fluid intake and output, electrolyte determinations, and ABGs. The nurse assesses the client for cyanosis, cough with or without hemoptysis, diaphoresis, and respiratory difficulty. He or she monitors blood coagulation studies (e.g., partial thromboplastin time, prothrombin time) when anticoagulant or thrombolytic therapy is instituted.

The nurse assesses the client for evidence of bleeding and relief of associated symptoms. Because clients with pulmonary emboli are discharged on oral anticoagulants, they require instruction related to checking for signs of occult bleeding, taking medication exactly as prescribed, reporting missed or extra doses, and keeping all appointments for follow-up blood tests and office visits.

▶ Stop, Think, and Respond Exercise 21-4

A 54-year-old woman recently experienced thrombophlebitis in her left calf, probably related to prolonged bed rest after a motor vehicle collision. The thrombophlebitis resolved without complications. She is no longer taking anticoagulants. She expresses concerns about having clots in the future. What should she do?

PULMONARY EDEMA

Pulmonary edema is accumulation of fluid in the interstitium and alveoli of the lungs. Pulmonary congestion results when the right side of the heart delivers more blood to the pulmonary circulation than the left side of the heart can handle. The fluid escapes the capillary walls and fills the airways. A client with pulmonary edema experiences dyspnea, breathlessness, and a feeling of suffocation. In addition, he or she exhibits cool, moist, and cyanotic extremities. The overall skin color is cyanotic and gray. The client has a continual cough productive of blood-tinged, frothy fluid. This condition requires emergency treatment. (See Chap. 28 for a discussion of cardiogenic pulmonary edema.)

RESPIRATORY FAILURE

Respiratory failure describes the inability to exchange sufficient amounts of oxygen and CO_2 for the body's needs. Even when the body is at rest, basic respiratory needs cannot be met. The ABG values that define respiratory failure include a PaO_2 less than 50 mm Hg, a $PaCO_2$ greater than 50 mm Hg, and a pH less than 7.25.

Respiratory failure is classified as acute or chronic. Acute respiratory failure occurs suddenly in a client who previously had normal lung function. In chronic respiratory failure, the loss of lung function is progressive, usually irreversible, and associated with chronic lung disease or other disease.

Pathophysiology and Etiology

Table 21-4 describes precipitating factors that can result in respiratory failure. Acute respiratory failure is a life-threatening condition in which alveolar ventilation cannot maintain the body's need for oxygen supply and CO_2 removal. The result is a fall in arterial oxygen (hypoxemia) and a rise in arterial CO_2 (hypercapnia), detected by ABG analysis. Ventilatory failure develops when the alveoli cannot adequately expand, when neurologic control of respirations is impaired, or when traumatic injury to the chest wall occurs.

TABLE 21-4 Factors that Precipitate Respiratory Failure

PRECIPITATING FACTOR	EXAMPLE
Pulmonary infection—especially with COPD	Bacterial, viral, or fungal pneumonia
Trauma	Motor vehicle collision
	Gunshot/knife wound
	Burns
Infection	Sepsis
	Wound infection
Cardiovascular event	Myocardial infarction
	Aortic aneurysm
	Pulmonary embolism
Allergic reaction	Transfusion reaction
	Drug allergy
	Bee sting or other venom
Pulmonary aspiration	Vomitus
	Near drowning
Surgical procedure	Abdominal or thoracic surgery
Drug reaction	Overdose of barbiturates or narcotics
	Reaction to anesthesia
Mechanical factor	Pneumothorax
	Pleural effusion
	Abdominal distention
Iatrogenic factor	Endotracheal intubation
	Failure to clear tracheobronchial secretions
Neuromuscular disorders	Guillain-Barrè syndrome
	Multiple sclerosis
	Muscular dystrophy

The most common diseases leading to chronic respiratory failure are COPD and neuromuscular disorders. The underlying disease accounts for the pathology that is seen when the respiratory system fails. Gas exchange dysfunction occurs over a long period. Symptoms of acute respiratory failure are not apparent in chronic respiratory failure because the client experiences chronic respiratory acidosis over a long period. Refer to the section on COPD for discussion of diagnostic findings, medical management, and nursing management of chronic respiratory failure.

Assessment Findings

Apprehension, restlessness, fatigue, headache, dyspnea, wheezing, cyanosis, and use of the accessory muscles of respiration are seen in clients with impending respiratory failure. If the disorder remains untreated, or if treatment fails to relieve respiratory distress, confusion, tachypnea, cyanosis, cardiac dysrhythmias and tachycardia, hypotension, CHF, respiratory acidosis, and respiratory arrest occur.

The client's symptoms, history (e.g., surgery, known neurologic disorder), and ABG results form the basis for a diagnosis of respiratory failure. Additional tests include chest radiography and serum electrolyte determinations.

Medical Management

Treatment of respiratory failure focuses on maintaining a patent airway (in cases of upper respiratory airway obstruction) by inserting an artificial airway, such as an endotracheal or a tracheostomy tube. Additional treatments include administration of humidified oxygen by nasal cannula, Venturi mask, or rebreather masks (Fig. 21-9). Respiratory failure is managed with mechanical ventilation using intermittent positive-pressure ventilation. When possible, the underlying cause of respiratory failure is treated.

Nursing Management

Because symptoms often occur suddenly, recognition is important. The nurse must notify the physician immediately and obtain emergency resuscitative equipment.

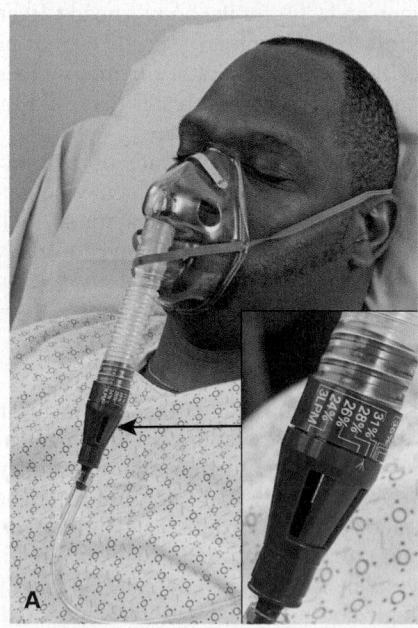
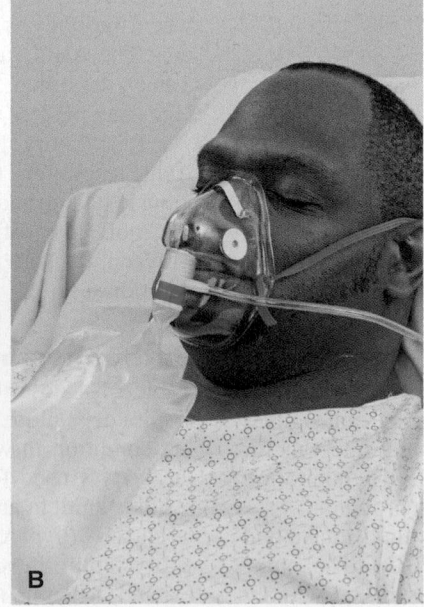
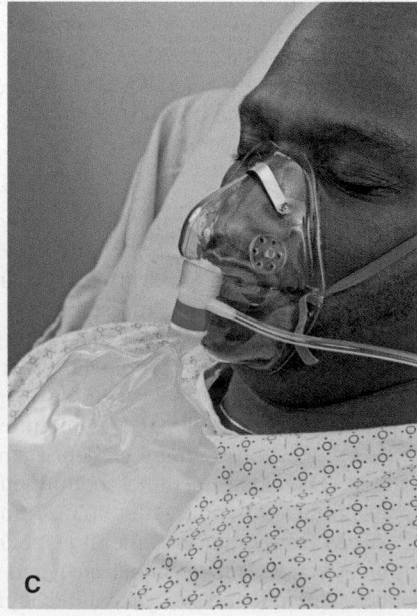

FIGURE 21-9. Types of oxygen masks. (**A**) Venturi mask. (**B**) Nonrebreather mask. (**C**) Partial rebreather mask.

Assessment and monitoring of respirations and vital signs are necessary at frequent intervals. The nurse must pay particular attention to respiratory rate and depth, signs of cyanosis, other signs and symptoms of respiratory distress, and the client's response to treatment. He or she monitors ABG results and pulse oximetry findings and implements strategies to prevent respiratory complications, such as turning and ROM exercises. The nurse provides explanations to the client and initiates measures to relieve anxiety.

ACUTE RESPIRATORY DISTRESS SYNDROME

Acute respiratory distress syndrome (ARDS), previously referred to as *adult respiratory distress syndrome,* is a clinical condition that occurs following other clinical conditions. The less severe form of this condition is referred to as acute lung injury (ALI). ARDS and ALI are not primary diseases. When it occurs, ARDS can lead to respiratory failure and death. It is referred to as *noncardiogenic pulmonary edema* (pulmonary edema not caused by a cardiac disorder—occurs without left-sided heart failure). Sudden and progressive pulmonary edema, increasing bilateral infiltrates seen on chest radiography, severe hypoxemia, and progressive loss of lung compliance characterize ARDS.

Pathophysiology and Etiology

Factors associated with the development of ARDS include aspiration related to near drowning or vomiting; drug ingestion/overdose; hematologic disorders such as disseminated intravascular coagulation or massive transfusions; direct damage to the lungs through prolonged smoke inhalation or other corrosive substances; localized lung infection; metabolic disorders such as pancreatitis or uremia, shock, trauma such as chest contusions, multiple fractures, or head injury; any major surgery; embolism; and septicemia (Smeltzer et al., 2008). The mortality rate with ARDS is high, particularly if the underlying cause cannot be treated or is inadequately treated.

The body responds to injury by reducing blood flow to the lungs, resulting in platelet clumping. The platelets release substances such as histamine, bradykinin, and serotonin, causing localized inflammation of the alveolar membranes. Increased permeability of the alveolar capillary membrane subsequently ensues. Fluid then enters the alveoli and causes pulmonary edema. The excess fluid in the alveoli and decreased blood flow through the capillaries surrounding them cause many of the alveoli to collapse (microatelectasis). Gas exchange decreases, resulting in respiratory and metabolic acidosis. ARDS also causes decreased surfactant production, which contributes to alveolar collapse. The lungs become stiff or noncompliant. Decreased functional residual capacity, severe hypoxia, and hypocapnia result.

Assessment Findings

Severe respiratory distress develops within 8 to 48 hours after the onset of illness or injury. In the early stages, few definite symptoms may be seen. As the condition progresses, the following signs appear: increased respiratory rate; shallow, labored respirations; cyanosis; use of accessory muscles; respiratory distress unrelieved with oxygen administration; anxiety; restlessness; and mental confusion, agitation, and drowsiness with cerebral anoxia.

Diagnosis is made according to the following criteria: evidence of acute respiratory failure, bilateral infiltrates on chest radiography, and hypoxemia as evidenced by PaO_2 less than 50 mm Hg with supplemental oxygen of 50% to 60%. Chest radiographs reveal increased infiltrates bilaterally. There is no evidence of left-sided heart failure (see Chap. 28), such as increased size of the left ventricle.

Medical Management

The initial cause of ARDS must be diagnosed and treated. The client receives humidified oxygen. Insertion of an endotracheal or a tracheostomy tube ensures maintenance of a patent airway. Mechanical ventilation usually is necessary, using positive end-expiratory pressure (PEEP), which provides pressures to the airway that are higher than atmospheric pressures. Mechanical ventilators usually raise airway pressure during inspiration and let it fall to atmospheric or zero pressure during expiration (intermittent positive-pressure ventilation). When PEEP is used, positive airway pressure is maintained on inspiration, expiration, and at the end of expiration (continuous positive-pressure ventilation). The client's pulmonary status, determined by ABG findings and pulse oximetry results, dictates the oxygen concentration and ventilator settings. Complications associated with the use of PEEP include pneumothorax and pneumomediastinum (air in the mediastinal space).

Hypotension results in systemic hypovolemia. Although the client experiences pulmonary edema, the rest of the circulatory volume is decreased. Pulmonary artery pressure monitors the client's fluid status and assists in determining the careful administration of IV fluids. Colloids such as albumin are used to help pull fluids in from the interstitium to the capillaries. Adequate nutritional support is essential (Nutrition Notes 21-3). Usually, the first choice is enteral feedings, but total parenteral nutrition may be necessary.

Nursing Management

Nursing management focuses on promotion of oxygenation and ventilation and prevention of complications. Assessing

Nutrition Notes 21-3
The Client With Respiratory Failure or Distress

- Although adequate protein and calories are important to support lung function, overfeeding is avoided because it causes overproduction of CO_2 and increases respiratory workload.
- Specially designed enteral formulas are available for clients with respiratory failure or distress; they are high in fat and low in carbohydrates to reduce CO_2 production. Studies have not confirmed their effectiveness in reducing respiratory distress.

and monitoring a client's respiratory status are essential. Potential complications include deteriorating respiratory status, infection, renal failure, and cardiac complications. The client also is anxious and requires explanations and support. In addition, if the client is on a ventilator, verbal communication is impaired. The nurse provides alternative methods for the client to communicate.

MALIGNANT DISORDERS

Tumors and growths affecting the respiratory system usually are malignant. Malignancies may be primary in that they arise from the lungs or mediastinum, or they can be secondary metastatic growths from other sites. Treatment of primary or secondary cancers usually does not stop progression of the disease (see Chap. 18). Disability, debilitation, and death are common outcomes from respiratory malignancies.

LUNG CANCER

Lung cancer is a very common cancer, particularly among cigarette smokers and those regularly exposed to second-hand smoke. It remains the number one cause of cancer-related deaths among men and women in the United States (American Cancer Society, 2007), with more Americans dying each year from lung cancer than from breast, prostate, and colorectal cancers combined. The incidence of lung cancer has markedly increased since the early 1980s, related to:

- More accurate methods of diagnosis
- The growing population of aging people
- The continued popularity of cigarette smoking
- Increased air pollution
- Increased exposure to industrial pollutants

Lung cancer is more common in men than in women. The rate of women dying from lung cancer continues to increase, however, and indeed is greater than the rate of women dying from breast cancer. Most clients are older than 40 years of age when diagnosed with lung cancer.

Pathophysiology and Etiology

The exact mechanism for the development of lung cancer is unknown; however, the link between irritants and lung cancer is well established. Prolonged exposure to carcinogens more than likely will produce cancerous cells. Smokers who quit reduce their risk of lung cancer to that of nonsmokers within 10 to 15 years.

Lung cancers are grouped in two overall categories: *non-small cell carcinomas*, which includes epidermoid or squamous cell carcinomas, large cell or undifferentiated type, and adenocarcinoma; and *small cell carcinoma*, also referred to as oat cell carcinoma. Many tumors begin in the bronchus and spread to the lung tissue, regional lymph nodes, and other sites, such as the brain and bone. Many tumors have more than one type of cancer cell. Table 21-5 differentiates between the major cell types of lung cancer.

The transformation of an epithelial cell in the airway initiates the growth of a lung cancer lesion. As the tumor grows, it partially obstructs the lumen of an airway or completely obstructs it, resulting in airway collapse distal to the tumor. The tumor may hemorrhage, causing hemoptysis (Bullock & Henze, 2000).

Assessment Findings

Signs and Symptoms
The cell type of the lung cancer, size and location of the tumor, and degree and location of metastasis determine the presenting signs and symptoms. A cough productive of

TABLE 21-5 Differentiation of Lung Cancers

CELL TYPE	PATHOLOGY	METASTASIS
Non-small Cell Carcinomas		
Epidermoid or squamous cell carcinomas (located in the bronchial tubes; 25% to 35% of all lung tumors)	These slow-growing tumors arise from bronchi and bronchioles and spread into the bronchial lumen, causing obstruction.	Well-differentiated epidermoid cells typically metastasize in the thorax, whereas poorly differentiated epidermoid cells metastasize to the small bowel.
Large cell (undifferentiated) carcinomas (found near the bronchial surface; 5% to 20% of all lung tumors)	These arise in peripheral bronchi and do not have well-defined growth patterns. They usually are diagnosed first as a bulky tumor mass.	These metastasize early, usually to the CNS.
Adenocarcinoma (arise from mucus glands; 25% to 35% of all lung tumors)	These occur in the peripheral lung tissue and lead to patchy growth throughout the lung fields. They typically invade the pleura, leading to malignant pleural effusion.	Early metastasis occurs to the brain, other lung tissue, bone, liver, and adrenal glands.
Small Cell Carcinoma		
Oat cell (10% to 25% of lung tumors)	This most malignant form of lung cancer arises from the bronchi. The tumor cells hypersecrete antidiuretic hormone, leading to hyponatremia.	Metastasis is early through the bloodstream and lymphatics to the mediastinum, liver, bone, bone marrow, CNS, adrenal glands, pancreas, and other endocrine organs.

CNS, central nervous system.

mucopurulent or blood-streaked sputum is a cardinal sign of lung cancer. The cough may be slight at first and attributed to smoking or other causes. As the disease advances, the client may report fatigue, anorexia, and weight loss. Dyspnea and chest pain occur late in the disease. Hemoptysis is common.

If pleural effusion occurs from tumor spread to the outside portion of the lungs, the client experiences dyspnea and chest pain. Other indications of tumor spread are symptoms related to pressure on nerves and blood vessels. Symptoms include head and neck edema, pericardial effusion, hoarseness, and vocal cord paralysis.

Diagnostic Findings
Early diagnosis of cancer of the lung is difficult because symptoms often do not appear until the disease is well established. The sputum is examined for malignant cells. Chest films may or may not show a tumor. A CT or PET scan or MRI is done if results from the chest radiograph are inconclusive, or to further delineate the tumor area.

Bronchoscopy may be done to obtain bronchial washings and a tissue sample for biopsy. Fine-needle aspiration under fluoroscopy or CT guidance may be done to aspirate cells from a specific area that is not accessible by bronchoscopy. A lung scan also may locate the tumor. A bone scan detects metastasis to the bone. The results of a lymph node biopsy may be positive for malignant changes if the lung tumor has metastasized. Mediastinoscopy provides a direct view of the mediastinal area and possible visualization of tumors that extend into the mediastinal space.

Medical and Surgical Management
The client's prognosis is poor unless the tumor is discovered in its early stages and treatment begins immediately. Because lung cancer produces few early symptoms, its mortality rate is high. Metastasis to the mediastinal and cervical lymph nodes, liver, brain, spinal cord, bone, and opposite lung is common.

Treatment depends on several factors. One major consideration is the classification and staging of the tumor. After classification of the tumor, the stage of the disease is determined. Staging refers to the extent and location of the tumor and the absence or presence and extent of metastasis (see Chap. 18). Other factors that determine treatment are the client's age and physical condition and other diseases or disorders, such as renal disease and CHF.

Surgical removal of the tumor offers the only possibility of cure and usually is successful only in the early stages of the disease. The type of lung resection (see Box 21-4) depends on the tumor's size and location.

Radiation therapy may help to slow the spread of the disease and provide symptomatic relief by reducing tumor size, thus easing the pressure exerted by the tumor on adjacent structures. In turn, pain, cough, dyspnea, and hemoptysis may be relieved. In a small percentage of cases, radiation may be curative, but for most, it is palliative. Complications associated with the use of radiation therapy include esophagitis, fibrosis of lung tissue, and pneumonitis.

Chemotherapy may be used alone or with radiation therapy and surgery. The principal effects of chemotherapy are to slow tumor growth and reduce tumor size and accompanying pressure on adjacent structures. Chemotherapy also is used to treat metastatic lesions. Most chemotherapeutic regimens use a combination of drugs rather than a single agent and, although not curative, often make the client more comfortable.

New treatments in various stages of development include the following (LungCancer.org, 2009):

- New chemotherapy regimens
- Monoclonal antibodies that target specific cancer proteins
- Photodynamic therapy that is a combination treatment with chemicals and light
- Lung cancer vaccines to stimulate an effective immune response

Nursing Management
Management of clients with lung cancer is essentially the same as that for any client with a malignant disease. See Chapter 18 for the nursing management of a client with cancer and Chapter 14 for perioperative care.

MEDIASTINAL TUMORS
Tumors of the mediastinum in adults often are malignant and metastatic. They are designated as anterior, middle, or posterior, according to their location on the mediastinum. The cause of these tumors is not known. Mediastinal tumors may be asymptomatic initially. When symptoms occur, they include chest pain, chest wall bulging, difficulty swallowing, dyspnea, and orthopnea. Symptoms are related to pressure of the tumor on other chest structures. Chest radiography, CT scan, MRI, mediastinoscopy, and biopsy of the lesion identify the tumor. Malignant tumors of the mediastinum almost always are inoperable but may respond to radiation therapy and chemotherapy. Benign tumors are operable.

> **Stop, Think, and Respond Exercise 21-5**
> Your 85-year-old neighbor tells you that he smoked for 25 years but quit 5 years ago. He has been experiencing a productive cough for 3 weeks. Occasionally he sees blood in the sputum. What can you advise him?

TRAUMA

All chest injuries are serious or potentially serious. A client with a chest injury must be observed for dyspnea, cyanosis, chest pain, weak and rapid pulse, and hypotension—all signs and symptoms of respiratory distress. Clients with a chest injury need to be examined by a physician as soon as possible.

FRACTURED RIBS

Fractured ribs are a common injury and may result from a hard fall or a blow to the chest. Fractured ribs usually are not considered serious, unless accompanied by other injuries.

Pathophysiology and Etiology
Automobile and household accidents are frequent causes of fractured ribs. Rib fractures are painful but not life-threatening. When a client experiences a fractured rib, other structures may be injured as well. For example, the sharp end of the broken rib may tear the lung or thoracic blood vessels. If

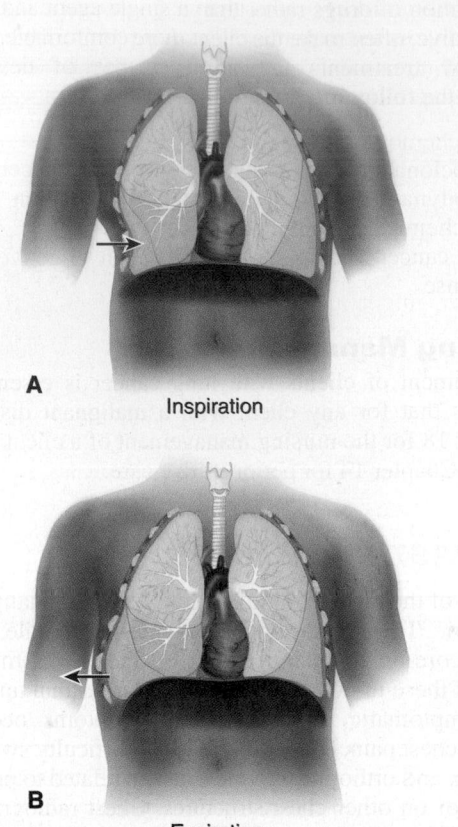

A
Inspiration

B
Expiration

FIGURE 21-10. Flail chest during inspiration and expiration.

the injury involves fractured ribs without complications, the client usually may return home after emergency treatment.

Flail chest occurs when two or more adjacent ribs fracture in multiple places (two or more) and the fragments are free-floating (Fig. 21-10). This affects the stability of the chest wall and results in impairment of chest-wall movement. A paradoxical movement develops: with inspiration the chest expands, but the free-floating segments move inward instead of outward. On expiration the free-floating segments move outward, interfering with exhalation. These movements affect intrathoracic pressures, significantly decreasing the movement of air. Many pathophysiologic phenomena occur as a result: increased dead space, reduced gas exchange, decreased lung compliance, retained airway secretions, atelectasis, and hypoxemia.

 Gerontologic Considerations

- Changes associated with aging or chronic conditions may increase older adults' risk for falls. Falls may cause fracture of one or more ribs, increasing susceptibility to pneumonia from decreased lung expansion.

Assessment Findings

Symptoms consist primarily of obvious trauma and severe pain on inspiration and expiration. The client experiences shortness of breath. With flail chest, the client has hypotension and inadequate tissue perfusion secondary to decreased cardiac output. Respiratory acidosis occurs because of increased CO_2. Chest radiographs (usually from several angles) are necessary to confirm the diagnosis.

Medical Management

Supporting the chest with an elastic bandage or a rib belt assists in immobilizing the rib fractures. These measures, however, can lead to decreased lung expansion followed by pulmonary complications such as pneumonia and atelectasis. Therefore, the use of these devices usually is limited to multiple rib fractures. Analgesics such as codeine may be prescribed for pain. Sometimes a regional nerve block is used to relieve pain.

Management of flail chest includes supporting ventilation, clearing lung secretions, and managing pain. Other treatment depends on the severity of the flail chest. If a **pulmonary contusion** (crushing bruise of the lung) also exists, fluids are restricted because of the damage to the pulmonary capillary bed. Antibiotics are given to prevent infection, which is common after this type of injury. Endotracheal intubation and mechanical ventilation may be necessary if a client's respiratory status is greatly compromised.

Nursing Management

With fractured ribs, the nurse may apply the immobilization device after the physician examines the client. In such a case, the nurse instructs the client about the application and removal of the rib belt or elastic bandage. He or she stresses the importance of taking deep breaths every 1 to 2 hours, even though breathing is painful. Nurses plan and implement care of clients with more severe injuries based on respiratory needs. The nurse assesses and monitors the client for signs of respiratory distress, infection, and increased pain.

BLAST INJURIES

Compression of the chest by an explosion can seriously damage the lungs by rupturing the alveoli. Death often results from hemorrhage and asphyxiation. Severe respiratory distress with outward evidence of chest trauma is apparent. **Subcutaneous emphysema** (air in subcutaneous tissues) is a common finding because the lungs or air passages have sustained an injury. This condition resembles a superficial swelling. Crepitation (a crackling sound) is heard or felt upon palpation and may be caused by air leaking around the chest wound. Diagnosis is based on symptoms and physical examination. Additional diagnostic tests, such as chest radiography and lung scan, may be necessary to identify foreign objects or air in the chest.

Treatment includes complete bed rest and oxygen administration. Thoracentesis to remove air or fluid may be necessary. Some clients may require surgery and the insertion of chest tubes if severe injury to lung tissue has occurred or if pneumothorax is present. When a client has suffered a blast injury, the most important nursing task is immediate recognition of respiratory distress. Victims of a blast injury are closely observed for early signs of respiratory distress.

PENETRATING WOUNDS

Gunshot and stab wounds are common types of penetrating wounds to the lungs. Penetrating wounds potentially affect cardiopulmonary function and may be life-threatening.

Pathophysiology and Etiology

Penetrating wounds are classified according to the velocity of the cause. Stab wounds from weapons such as knives or switchblades usually are low velocity because they involve a small area. Gunshot wounds may be low, medium, or high velocity, depending on the caliber of the gun, the distance from which the gun was fired, and the nature of the ammunition (Smeltzer et al., 2008).

Any type of penetrating wound to the chest is serious because of the opening into the thorax. On inspiration, the thorax normally is at negative pressure. The penetrating wound creates continuous and direct communication with the outside, which is at positive pressure. Thus, air enters the thoracic cavity, causing an open pneumothorax (Fig. 21-11). If not recognized and treated promptly, death may occur. If the wound is large, a sucking noise may be heard as air enters and leaves the chest cavity. Depending on the size of the wound, it takes seconds to hours before the lung collapses as the pressure in the thorax reaches atmospheric pressure. Many chest injuries involve both pneumothorax and *hemothorax*, the collection of blood in the pleural cavity.

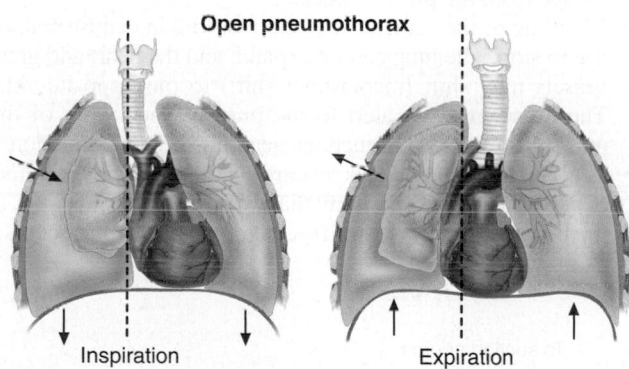

Open pneumothorax

Inspiration   Expiration

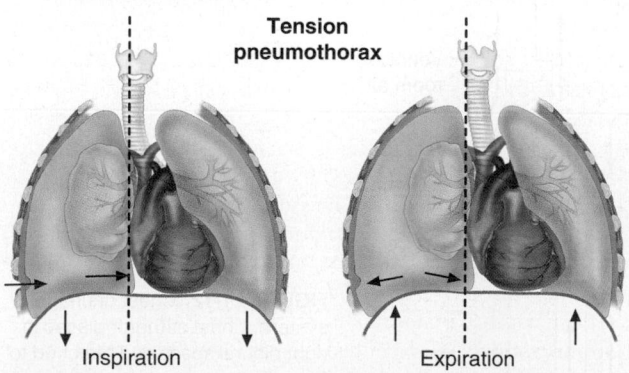

Tension pneumothorax

Inspiration   Expiration

FIGURE 21-11. In open or communicating pneumothorax (*top*), air enters the chest during inspiration and exits during expiration. In tension pneumothorax (*bottom*), air enters but does not leave the chest. As pressure increases, the heart, great vessels, and unaffected lung are compressed, while the mediastinal structures and trachea shift toward the opposite side of the chest.

Subcutaneous emphysema also may be present. Other possible trauma includes hemorrhage, lung contusion, damage to surrounding tissues, fractured ribs or other bones, and injury to the heart, blood vessels, or both.

Assessment Findings

Clients exhibit various signs and symptoms, depending on the location and extent of the penetrating wound; dyspnea, pain, and bleeding are common. Clients are at risk for respiratory distress and shock. It also is important that the client be thoroughly examined to ascertain if other injuries are present, such as more penetrating wounds, particularly in the abdominal area.

Diagnosis is based on the history of injury, physical examination, and auscultation of the lungs. Radiographs show the degree of lung collapse and the amount of air or blood in the thoracic cavity. The client's cardiopulmonary status is assessed through ABG analysis, pulse oximetry, and ECGs. CT scans or MRI may be necessary depending on the extent of the injuries.

Medical and Surgical Management

Airway management is the first concern. Once an airway is established, then other treatment begins. Thoracentesis is done to remove air and blood from the pleural space. A chest tube is inserted and attached to an underwater-seal drainage system. A thoracotomy may be required to repair the injury. Foreign bodies that entered the chest, such as a bullet or a knife, are surgically removed. Their presence in the wound may prevent or slow the entrance of air. Removal before the victim is transported to the hospital may result in continuous sucking of air into the chest, collapse of the lung, compression of the heart and opposite lung, and death. Surgical intervention may be necessary if there is bleeding from the chest tube or indications of injury to other organs or blood vessels.

Emergency treatment of pneumothorax caused by a penetrating wound includes the application of a tight pressure dressing over the injury site to prevent more air from entering the thorax. Immediate evaluation of the client's respiratory status is imperative. Oxygen is given until the physician examines and treats the injury. IV fluids, colloid solutions, or blood is administered to treat or prevent shock. An indwelling catheter is inserted to monitor urine output. A nasogastric tube is placed to prevent aspiration of stomach contents and to decompress the GI tract.

Nursing Management

Care of a client with a penetrating chest wound is similar to that of a client who has thoracic surgery. Refer to the nursing management of a client undergoing thoracic surgery in the next section.

THORACIC SURGERY

A thoracotomy is a surgical opening in the chest wall. It may be done to:

- Remove fluid, blood, or air from the thorax.
- Remove tumors of the lung, bronchus, or chest wall.
- Remove all or a portion of a lung (see Box 21-4).

- Repair or revise structures contained in the thorax, such as open heart surgery or repair of a thoracic aneurysm.
- Repair trauma to the chest or chest wall, such as penetrating chest wounds or crushing chest injuries.
- Sample a lesion for biopsy.
- Remove foreign objects such as a bullet or metal fragments.

A thoracentesis may be done as an emergency procedure to remove blood, fluid, or air from the chest. In some instances, it is necessary to perform a thoracotomy to insert chest tubes (tube thoracotomy) to remove air or fluid from the chest during the preoperative period.

Preoperative Nursing Management

Preparing clients for thoracic surgery includes assessment of vital signs and breath sounds, particularly noting the presence or absence of breath sounds in any area of the chest. The client's condition dictates the extent of the assessment and obtaining a history. If the surgery is an emergency, physical assessment may be limited to a general statement of the client's condition, a list of emergency measures and treatments done, and vital signs (see Chap. 14).

Postoperative Nursing Management

The opening of the thoracic cavity requires special postoperative nursing measures. A significant issue is the interference with normal pressures in the thoracic cavity. When the chest is opened, air from the atmosphere rushes in because of the negative pressure that exists in the thoracic cavity on inspiration. The entrance of air under atmospheric pressure causes the lungs to collapse and no longer expand or contract. The anesthesiologist ventilates the client during surgery.

After thoracic surgery, draining secretions, air, and blood from the thoracic cavity is necessary to allow the lungs to expand. A catheter placed in the pleural space provides a drainage route through a closed or underwater-seal drainage system (Fig. 21-12). Sometimes two chest catheters are

placed—one anteriorly and one posteriorly. The anterior catheter (usually the upper one) removes air; the posterior catheter removes fluid.

Chest tubes are securely connected to an underwater-seal system. The tube coming from the client always must be under water. A break in the system, such as from loose or disconnected fittings, allows air to enter the tubing and then the pleural space, further collapsing the lung. When chest tubes are inserted at the end of the surgical procedure, they are connected to an underwater-seal drainage system. All connections are taped carefully to minimize the possibility of air entering the closed system.

When caring for a client with chest tubes, the nurse should be aware of the following:

- Fluctuation of the fluid in the water-seal chamber is initially present with each respiration. Fluctuations cease when the lung reexpands. The time for lung reexpansion varies. Fluctuations also may cease if:
  - the chest tube is clogged.
  - the wall suction unit malfunctions.
  - a kink or dependent loop develops in the tubing.
- Bubbling in the water-seal chamber occurs in the early postoperative period. If bubbling is excessive, the nurse checks the system for leaks. If leaks are not apparent, the nurse notifies the physician.
- Bloody drainage is normal, but drainage should not be bright red or copious.
- The drainage tube(s) must remain patent to allow fluids to escape from the pleural space.
- Clogging of the catheter with clots or kinking causes drainage to stop. The lung cannot expand, and the heart and great vessels may shift (mediastinal shift) to the opposite side. The nurse must be alert to the proper functioning of the drainage system. Malfunctions need immediate correction.
- If a break or major leak occurs in the system, the nurse clamps the chest tube immediately with hemostats kept at the bedside. He or she notifies the physician if this occurs.

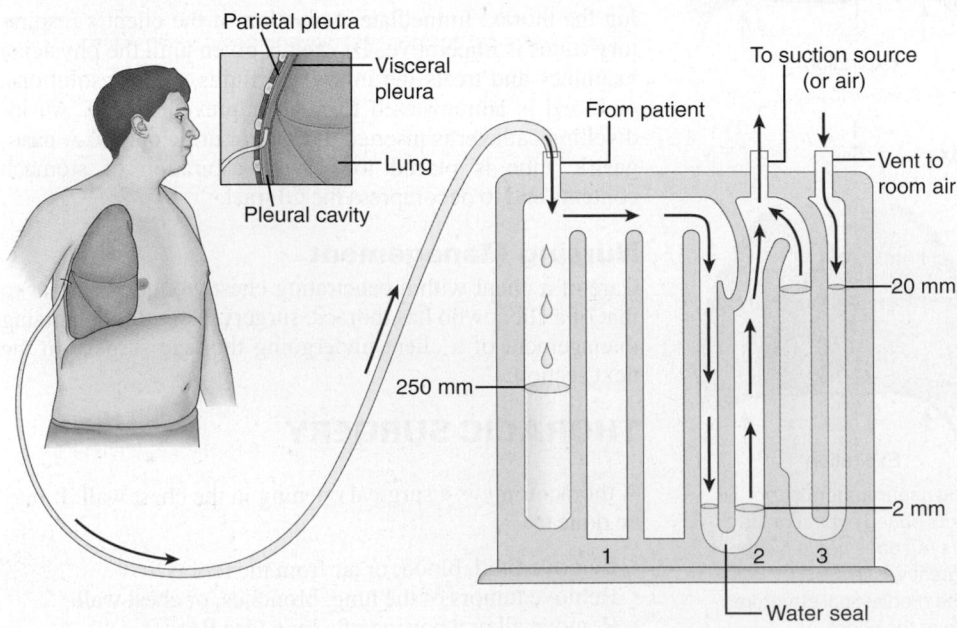

FIGURE 21-12. Chest drainage system. Chest catheter placed in right pleural space and attached to Pleur-Evac system with three chambers: (1) drainage collection chamber from client; (2) the water-seal chamber; and (3) the suction control chamber, attached to source of suction and vented to room air.

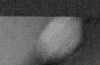

NURSING CARE PLAN 21-1 | The Client Recovering From Thoracic Surgery

Assessment

- Assess respirations: rate, depth, rhythm, and use of accessory muscles.
- Observe skin color, particularly for signs of cyanosis.
- Auscultate breath sounds at least every 4 hours.
- Evaluate mental status.
- Monitor heart rate and rhythm.
- Monitor results of ABGs, pulse oximetry, and other blood tests.
- Assess dressings and incisions for drainage or adherence.
- Check the chest tube drainage system.
- Assess level of pain.

Nursing Diagnosis: Impaired Gas Exchange related to decreased lung expansion, impaired lung function, and surgical procedure

Expected Outcome: Client will maintain optimal gas exchange.

Interventions	Rationales
Monitor vital signs every 15 minutes for at least 2 hours after return from postanesthesia care unit and then less frequently as condition stabilizes.	Such information provides baseline data and early indications of problems.
Reinforce preoperative instructions about deep breathing, coughing, and incentive spirometry. Remind client to do these exercises every 1 to 2 hours.	These exercises expand the alveoli, which prevents atelectasis.
Position client with the head of the bed elevated 30° to 40° initially. When the client can tolerate it, position him or her on the nonoperative side.	Such positioning promotes lung expansion and drainage from operative side.

Evaluation of Expected Outcome

Client demonstrates improved gas exchange, as evidenced by results of ABGs and pulse oximetry and improved efforts with incentive spirometry.

Nursing Diagnosis: Impaired Physical Mobility: Arm on Affected Side related to incisional pain, edema, and decreased strength

Expected Outcome: Client will demonstrate effective range-of-motion (ROM) on affected side.

Interventions	Rationales
Assess ROM in affected upper extremity within 24 hours by having the client raise arm laterally.	This assessment provides baseline data about ROM. During thoracotomy, chest muscles are incised, making ROM difficult after surgery.
Perform passive ROM exercises on affected arm four times a day.	These exercises increase mobility and promote renewed strength of affected arm.
Encourage client to use affected arm in activities of daily living (ADLs).	Gradual use of arm promotes movement of it.
Instruct client to move arms, slowly increasing movement and exercise as tolerated.	These measures promote mobility and begin to increase strength on affected side.
Increase exercise level after removal of chest tubes.	Removal of chest tubes decreases discomfort and assists client to move more freely.
Collaborate with physical therapists to plan therapy; reinforce instructions regarding exercise and discharge.	A full exercise plan will help client gain full ROM of affected upper extremity.

Evaluation of Expected Outcome

Client demonstrates increased ROM and better ability to perform ADLs independently.

Nursing Diagnosis: Deficient Fluid Volume related to surgical procedure, drains, and pain

Expected Outcome: Client will maintain adequate fluid volume.

Interventions	Rationales
Monitor and record intake and output hourly.	Such monitoring provides ongoing information about client's fluid status.
Assess skin turgor and mucous membranes for signs of dehydration.	These assessments provide baseline data about fluid status.
Monitor and document vital signs.	Tachycardia can occur with hypovolemia to maintain adequate cardiac output. Pulse may be weak with hypovolemia. Hypotension occurs with hypovolemia.

(care plan continues on page 298)

NURSING CARE PLAN 21-1   The Client Recovering From Thoracic Surgery (Continued)

Interventions	Rationales
Report urine output less than 30 mL/hour for 2 consecutive hours.	Urine output of less than 30 mL/hour for 2 or more hours indicates dehydration.
Monitor serum electrolyte and urine osmolality levels, reporting abnormal values.	Elevated hemoglobin, blood urea nitrogen, and urine specific gravity suggest fluid deficit.
Administer parenteral fluids as ordered, and maintain an accurate record of intravenous intake.	Parenteral fluids prevent dehydration.
Encourage client to drink at least 30 mL every hour.	This amount promotes adequate fluid intake.

Evaluation of Expected Outcome

Client is adequately hydrated as evidenced by urine output greater than 30 mL/hour, stable blood pressure and pulse, and normal skin turgor.

PC: Blood Loss; Hemorrhage

Expected Outcome: Nurse will manage and minimize blood loss.

Interventions	Rationales
Monitor and record vital signs.	Monitoring vital signs provides baseline data and information about changes in a client's status.
Assess chest tube drainage and dressings for signs of bleeding.	Bloody drainage from chest tubes may occur initially but should decrease. Increased blood in chest tubes, on dressings, or both indicates a bleeding problem that requires immediate intervention.
Anticipate or prepare client for return to surgery if bleeding is secondary to surgical procedure.	These measures are necessary to resolve the problem.
Increase parenteral fluids as ordered.	Increased parenteral fluid maintains an adequate circulating volume until bleeding stops.
Administer blood products as ordered.	Blood products replace lost blood and volume.

Evaluation of Expected Outcome

Nurse ensures the management of bleeding and its complications.

Immediate postoperative care includes following the standards outlined in Chapter 14. It also is essential that the nurse check the underwater-seal drainage system, noting the amount and color of drainage and any bubbling or fluctuation. The nurse assesses dressings for drainage and firm adherence to the skin. He or she inspects the skin around the dressings for signs of subcutaneous emphysema. The nurse assesses the client's color, neurologic status, and heart rate and rhythm; monitors respiratory rate, depth, and rhythm; and auscultates the chest for normal and abnormal breath sounds. He or she also assesses levels of pain and anxiety. Nursing Care Plan 21-1 and Client and Family Teaching 21-5 describe additional nursing management.

Pharmacologic Considerations

- When administering a narcotic to a client who has had thoracic surgery, count the respiratory rate before and 20 to 30 minutes after the client receives the medication. If the respiratory rate is below 10 breaths per minute at either time, notify the physician immediately.

Client and Family Teaching 21-5
Care After Thoracic Surgery

The nurse develops a teaching plan that includes instructions given by the physician as well as the following guidelines:

- Continue to perform arm exercises to prevent stiffness and pain.
- Eat a well-balanced diet, or follow the recommended diet.
- Take rest periods throughout the day until fatigue decreases.
- Practice breathing exercises, and take frequent deep breaths.
- Contact the physician if breathing is difficult; drainage, excessive redness, or pain develops around the incision; fever develops; or pain occurs elsewhere in the body.
- Avoid infection or irritants.
- Increase activities slowly and avoid fatigue.
- Take drugs as prescribed, and do not omit, increase, or decrease doses.

CRITICAL THINKING EXERCISES

1. A male client who underwent cholecystectomy (removal of the gallbladder) 2 days ago presses his call button. As you enter his room, he tells you that he is having trouble breathing and has chest pain. What brief questions would you ask the client before you call the physician?

2. A female client has a history of asthma. She arrives at the outpatient clinic and states that her chest feels tight and that she cannot "catch her breath." The nurse notes that this client is having trouble speaking. Immediate care of this client includes fluids, administration of bronchodilators, and relief of anxiety. When the client is stabilized and able to be discharged, the nurse wants to assure that the client can take steps to help prevent future asthmatic attacks. What information from the client does the nurse need to better provide appropriate discharge teaching?

3. A client who has AIDS develops pleurisy. His physician instructs him to perform deep-breathing and coughing exercises every 2 hours. What can you do to ease the client's pain and discomfort when he is performing these exercises?

4. A client who has bronchiectasis in his left lower lobe attends a pulmonary disease clinic. His physician instructs him to perform postural drainage by lying laterally on the bed, leaning from the waist, and lowering his head close to the floor. Two weeks later, the client tells you that he cannot tolerate this postural drainage position. Can you think of another way to perform postural drainage for the left lower lobe that may cause less discomfort?

NCLEX-STYLE REVIEW QUESTIONS

1. An elderly client is brought to the emergency department. Vital signs are T, 102°F; P, 88; R, 32; and BP, 160/86. Upon physical examination, the client is having difficulty breathing. Which of the following would be most appropriate for the nurse to do next?
1. Instruct the client to take slow, deep breaths.
2. Suction the client's pharynx of secretions.
3. Apply a pulse oximeter to the client's finger.
4. Help the client perform postural drainage.

2. A client comes to an urgent care clinic with pleurisy. The nurse is most correct in anticipating that which of the following will be the most common complaint from the client?
1. Thick, green sputum
2. Pain with each breath
3. Hot flashes with chills
4. Petechiae on the chest

3. The nurse is caring for a client with tuberculosis. A sputum sample is ordered for the next 3 consecutive days. The nurse is correct to schedule the sputum sample to be obtained at which of the following times?
1. Upon arising in the morning
2. Midmorning following breakfast
3. In the evening
4. At bedtime

4. A client with moderately controlled asthma needs to use a peak flow meter. The nurse instructing this client correctly tells the client that the peak flow meter is used to measure the:
1. amount of forced inspiration
2. depth of forced inhalation
3. highest flow with forced expiration
4. residual volume after exhalation

5. The LPN notes that the RN, in the care plan for a client who transferred from ICU 2 days post-op thoracic surgery, selected "Impaired gas exchange related to decreased lung expansion, impaired lung function, and surgical procedure." Which interventions are of primary importance for the care of this client? Select all that apply.
1. Thirty minutes after administering pain medication, ask the client to rate his pain on a scale of 1 to 10.
2. Assess the client's dressings and incisions for increased drainage.
3. Monitor client's temperature at least every 4 hours.
4. Remind the client to deep breathe and cough at least every 2 hours.
5. Reposition the client so that the head is elevated 30° to 40°.

22

Introduction to the Cardiovascular System

Learning Objectives

On completion of this chapter, you will be able to:

1. Describe the normal anatomy and physiology of the cardiovascular system.
2. Identify and describe focus assessment criteria when caring for a client with cardiovascular problems.
3. List common diagnostic tests used to evaluate the client with suspected heart disease.
4. Discuss the nursing management of a client undergoing cardiovascular diagnostic tests.

The function of the cardiovascular system is to supply body cells and tissues with oxygen-rich blood and eliminate carbon dioxide (CO_2) and cellular wastes. Damage and disease in the cardiovascular system greatly jeopardize a person's health. In fact, heart disease is the leading cause of death for adults in the United States. Many advanced treatments have been and are being created to treat heart disease. Human heart transplantation and the temporary use of an artificial heart are realities. Nevertheless, the primary focus remains preserving the natural heart by preventing heart disease.

ANATOMY AND PHYSIOLOGY

The cardiovascular system consists of the heart, the major blood vessels that empty into or exit directly from the heart, and a vast network of smaller peripheral blood vessels. The heart itself is about the size of a person's fist. It lies below and slightly to the left of the midline of the sternum in the mediastinum, a portion of the thoracic cavity that also contains the trachea and major blood vessels. The upper portion of the heart is the base, and the tip is the apex.

Heart Chambers
The heart is a four-chambered muscular pump (Fig. 22-1). The upper chambers, the right and left **atria** (singular, *atrium*), are receiving chambers for blood. The lower chambers, the right and left **ventricles**, are the heart's major pumping chambers. A thick **septum**, or wall, separates the

right side of the heart from the left side. The right atrium receives deoxygenated blood from the venous system, and the right ventricle pumps that blood to the lungs to be oxygenated. The left atrium receives oxygenated blood from the lungs, and the left ventricle pumps that blood to all the cells and tissues of the body. Therefore, the heart is a double pump—the right side facilitates pulmonary circulation, and the left side is responsible for systemic circulation.

Cardiac Tissue Layers

Three distinct layers of tissue make up the heart wall. The outer layer is the **epicardium**, which is composed of fibrous and loose connective tissue. The middle layer, the **myocardium**, consists of muscle tissue and is the force behind the heart's pumping action. The inner layer, the **endocardium**, is composed of a thin, smooth layer of endothelial cells. Folds of endocardium form the heart valves. The endocardium is in direct contact with the blood that passes through the heart.

The **pericardium** is a saclike structure that surrounds and supports the heart. Two membranous layers form the pericardium. The outer tougher layer is called the *parietal pericardium*. The inner serous layer is called the *visceral pericardium* (also called the *epicardium*), which adheres to the heart itself. The density of the parietal pericardium safeguards the heart from invasion by infectious microorganisms. Serous fluid fills the pericardial space between the two layers, lubricating the heart and reducing friction with each heartbeat (Fig. 22-2).

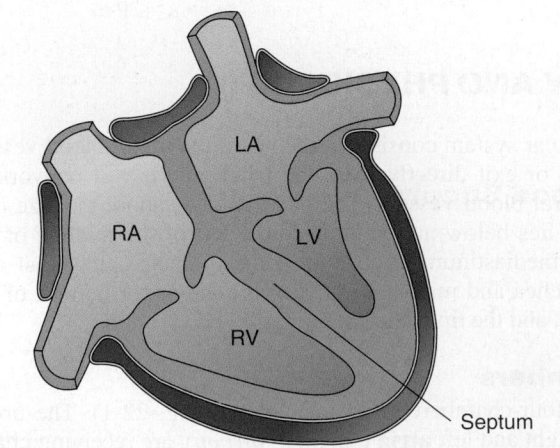

FIGURE 22-1. Cross section of the heart, showing the four chambers. *LA*, left atrium; *LV*, left ventricle; *RA*, right atrium; *RV*, right ventricle.

Heart Valves

The valves of the heart are membranous structures that ensure that blood passes through the heart in a one-way, forward direction. In a normal heart, the valves do not allow blood to backflow, or regurgitate, into the chamber from which it has come.

The two **atrioventricular (AV) valves** separate the atria from the ventricles. They prevent blood from returning to the atria when the ventricles contract. These valves are cusped, or leaflike. The valve between the right atrium and right ventricle is the **tricuspid valve**. The word *tricuspid* signifies that the valve has three cusps. The valve between the left atrium and left ventricle is the **bicuspid** (two-cusped) **valve**, also known as the **mitral valve**.

Attached to the tricuspid and mitral valves are cordlike structures known as *chordae tendineae*, which in turn attach to *papillary muscles*, two major muscular projections from the ventricles. When the ventricles contract, the papillary muscles also contract, applying tension to the atrioventricular valves. The contraction of the papillary muscles and the firm support of the chordae tendineae prevent eversion of the valves and regurgitation of blood back into the atria.

The other two valves, called the *semilunar valves* because they resemble portions of the moon, prevent blood from flowing back into the ventricles after the heart contracts. The valves are named for the blood vessel into which the blood is deposited. The valve between the right ventricle and pulmonary artery is the **pulmonic** (or pulmonary) **valve**. The valve between the left ventricle and aorta is the **aortic valve**. Contraction of the ventricles forces blood into the pulmonary artery and aorta. Relaxation follows, and the fall in pressure in the ventricles causes the pulmonic and aortic valves to close, preventing backflow into the ventricles.

▶ **Stop, Think, and Respond Exercise 22-1**

Where are the following cardiac valves located?—
(A) mitral valve; (B) tricuspid valve; and (C) pulmonic valve.

Arteries and Veins

Arteries carry oxygenated blood from the heart, and **veins** return deoxygenated blood to the heart. The smallest arteries are called **arterioles**, and the smallest veins are called **venules**. Arteries and arterioles are elastic and dilate or constrict to accommodate changes in blood flow. Veins have thinner walls than arteries because venous pressure is lower than

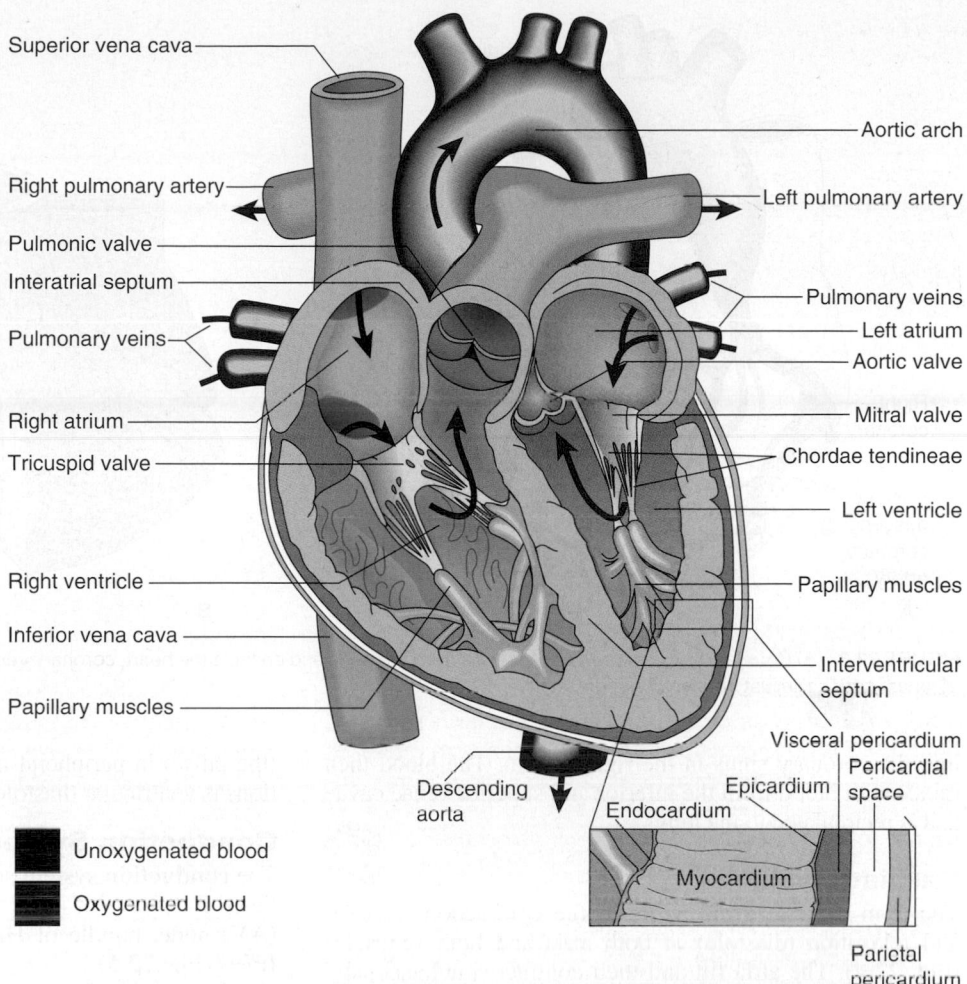

Superior vena cava

Right pulmonary artery

Pulmonic valve

Interatrial septum

Pulmonary veins

Right atrium

Tricuspid valve

Right ventricle

Inferior vena cava

Papillary muscles

Aortic arch

Left pulmonary artery

Pulmonary veins

Left atrium

Aortic valve

Mitral valve

Chordae tendineae

Left ventricle

Papillary muscles

Interventricular septum

Visceral pericardium

Pericardial space

Epicardium

Endocardium

Myocardium

Parietal pericardium

Descending aorta

Unoxygenated blood

Oxygenated blood

FIGURE 22-2. Structure of the heart. Arrows show the course of blood flow through the heart chambers.

arterial pressure. Despite being thinner, veins have larger diameters than corresponding arteries (Martini, 2006).

Arterioles branch into **capillaries**, which are microscopic vessels that form a connecting network between arterioles and venules. Capillaries are one cell layer thick and in direct contact with the cells of all tissues. This complex circulatory network delivers oxygen and metabolic substances to the cells. After this exchange, the venules and veins transport blood back to the heart.

Heart contraction moves blood from the heart into arteries and arterioles; skeletal muscle contraction compresses veins and propels blood back to the heart. Closure of successive sets of valves in veins keeps the blood from pooling under the influence of gravity.

Cardiopulmonary Circulation

The largest veins, the **inferior vena cava** and **superior vena cava**, bring venous (deoxygenated) blood from all areas of the body into the right atrium. The right atrium fills with blood, and the tricuspid valve opens. Blood then travels into the right ventricle and is pumped into the **pulmonary artery** (the only artery in an adult that carries deoxygenated blood). The pulmonary artery branches to deliver venous blood to the right and left lungs. The lungs exchange the oxygen in

inspired air for the CO_2 in the venous blood. The CO_2 is transferred into the alveoli and exhaled. The pulmonary veins then bring the oxygenated blood into the left atrium. The oxygenated blood flows out of the left atrium through the bicuspid, or mitral, valve and into the left ventricle. The left ventricle then pumps the blood through the aorta to all the body's cells and tissues.

▶ **Stop, Think, and Respond Exercise 22-2**

Give the next location of blood when it is in the following structures: (A) right ventricle; (B) inferior vena cava; (C) left ventricle; and (D) pulmonary veins.

Blood Supply to the Heart

The left and right **coronary arteries** supply oxygenated blood to cardiac muscle (Fig. 22-3). The openings to the coronary arteries, called the **coronary ostia** (singular, *ostium*), lie at the base of the aorta. When the left ventricle is filling with blood, the coronary ostia dilate and fill with blood. Thus, the myocardium is the first tissue of the body to receive oxygen-rich blood with each heartbeat.

After having distributed oxygenated blood to the myocardial cells, the coronary veins carry away the CO_2 produced by cellular metabolism. The coronary veins empty

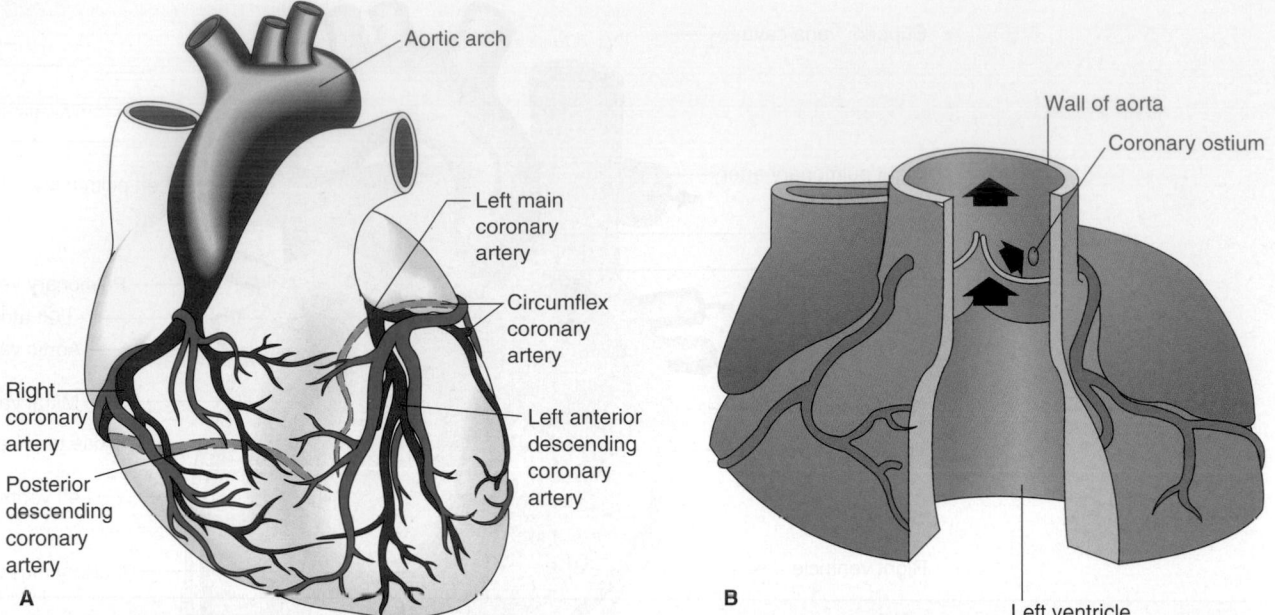

FIGURE 22-3. (**A**) Coronary arteries (*red vessels*) arise from the aorta and encircle the heart; coronary veins (*blue vessels*). (**B**) The orifices of the coronary arteries lie just beyond the aortic valve

into the coronary sinus in the right atrium. The blood then mixes with blood from the inferior and superior venae cavae and is recirculated to the lungs.

Cardiac Cycle

The term **cardiac cycle** refers to the contraction (systole) and relaxation (diastole) of both atria and both ventricles (Fig. 22-4). The atria fill and then contract simultaneously; as they relax, the ventricles contract and relax. The contraction of the left ventricle can be felt as a wavelike impulse

(the pulse) in peripheral arteries. The pause between pulsations is ventricular diastole.

Conduction System

The **conduction system** sustains the electrical activity of the heart. It consists of the sinoatrial (SA) node, atrioventricular (AV) node, bundle of His, bundle branches, and Purkinje fibers (Fig. 22-5).

The *SA node* is an area of nerve tissue located in the posterior wall of the right atrium. The SA node is called the

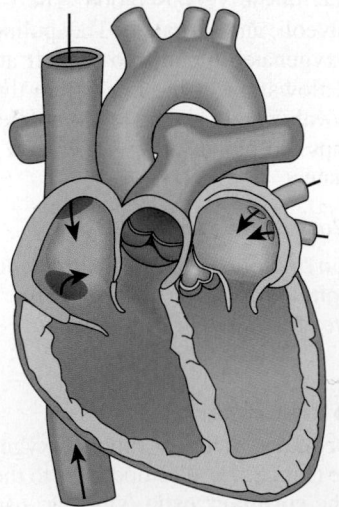

Atrial diastole
Atria fill with blood, which begins to flow into ventricles as soon as their walls relax.

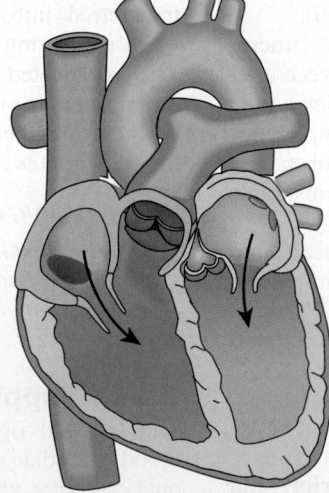

Ventricular diastole
Contraction of atria pumps blood into the ventricles.

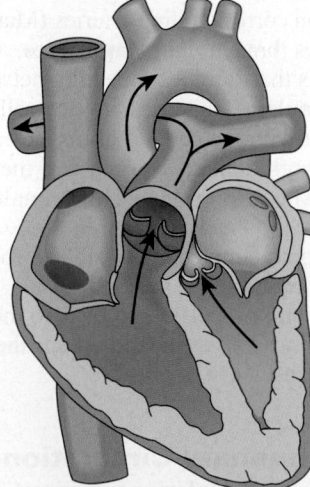

Ventricular systole
Contraction of ventricles pumps blood into the aorta and pulmonary arteries.

FIGURE 22-4. Pumping cycle of the heart. During atrial diastole, blood from the venae cavae and pulmonary veins fills the atria. During atrial systole, blood is delivered to the ventricles. When the ventricles contract, blood is pumped into the aorta and pulmonary arteries. (From Cohen, B.J. & Taylor, J.J. [2009]. *Memmler's structure and function of the human body.* [9th ed.]. Philadelphia: Lippincott Williams & Wilkins.)

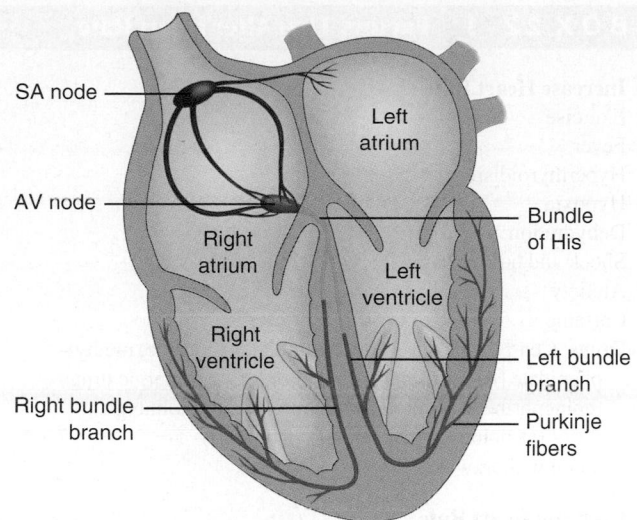

SA node

Left atrium

AV node

Right atrium

Bundle of His

Left ventricle

Right ventricle

Left bundle branch

Right bundle branch

Purkinje fibers

FIGURE 22-5. Electrical conduction system of the heart.

pacemaker of the heart because it initiates the electrical impulses that cause the atria and ventricles to contract. Normally, it produces between 60 and 100 impulses per minute; the average is approximately 72 impulses per minute. Other areas in the conduction pathway may initiate an electrical impulse if the SA node malfunctions, but they do so at rates slower than the SA node.

In the normal sequence of events, the cardiac impulse starts in the SA node. It spreads throughout the atria over intranodal and interatrial pathways. The waves of stimulation through the heart resemble the rings that a pebble makes when dropped into a pond. Once the cells in the atria are excited, they contract in unison. When the impulse reaches the *AV node*, it is delayed a few hundredths of a second. The impulse then stimulates the ventricles. While the ventricles fill with blood, the impulse travels from the AV node to the *bundle of His*, to the *right and left bundle branches*, and eventually to the *Purkinje fibers*. Then, both ventricles contract.

During diastole, while the myocardial cells are at rest, and before an impulse is generated, the cells are in a polarized state (**polarization**). Positive ions predominate outside myocardial cell membranes; negative ions predominate inside. When an electrical impulse is initiated, it spreads from cell membrane to cell membrane, causing a transfer of ions. The positive ions move inside the myocardial cell membranes, and the negative ions move outside. This process, which corresponds with cardiac muscle contraction, is called **depolarization**. It occurs first in the atria and then in the ventricles. Once depolarization has occurred, the ions realign themselves in their original position and wait for another electrical impulse. This process is called **repolarization**. Another normal cardiac impulse cannot be carried out until the ions are again in polarized alignment. The time during which the cells are resistant to electrical stimulation is called the **refractory period**.

Depolarization and repolarization produce electrical changes. Because body tissues conduct current easily, this electrical activity can be detected by electrodes placed on the external surface of the body. The detection of the energy is recorded by a machine known as the *electrocardiograph (ECG)* (discussed later in this chapter).

▶ *Stop, Think, and Respond Exercise 22-3*

Which part of the conduction system is known as the natural pacemaker because it initiates electrical impulses in normal heart conduction?

Regulation of Heart Rate

Heart rate fluctuates according to stimulation from the autonomic nervous system, baroreceptors, and chemoreceptors. The autonomic nervous system affects heart rate through sympathetic and parasympathetic nervous system innervation. When released by sympathetic nerve fibers, adrenergic neurotransmitters, such as norepinephrine and epinephrine, excite the SA and AV nodes in the conduction system, increasing heart rate. These same neurotransmitters also stimulate beta-adrenergic receptors in the atria and ventricles, increasing the force of myocardial contraction. Conversely, the heart rate slows when parasympathetic nerve fibers from the cardiac branches of the vagus nerve release the cholinergic neurotransmitter acetylcholine. Parasympathetic neurostimulation, however, usually does not affect the force of contraction.

Responses to **baroreceptors**, pressure-sensitive nerve endings in the walls of the atria and major blood vessels (e.g., vena cava, arch of the aorta, and carotid arteries), also affect the heart rate. The main function of baroreceptors is to sense the pressure from blood as it stretches vascular tissues containing the baroreceptors. If blood pressure (BP) decreases in the areas of the baroreceptors, such as when a person rises quickly from a lying or standing position, the baroreceptors send impulses to the brain stem to increase heart rate. An almost immediate reflexive response of accelerated heart contractions follows. The heart rate increases to compensate for the drop in BP. When the BP is stabilized, the heart rate returns to within a normal range.

Chemoreceptors, structures that are sensitive to the pH and CO_2 and oxygen levels of blood, are located in the carotid bodies, aortic bodies, and medulla of the brain (Fig. 22-6). They regulate sympathetic stimulation or inhibition. A fall in pH, rise in CO_2, and decrease in oxygen levels in the blood results in increased heart contraction. The heart rate returns to a more usual parameter when pH and CO_2 levels become normalized. Box 22-1 highlights additional factors that alter heart rate.

▶ *Stop, Think, and Respond Exercise 22-4*

What effect will each of the following have on heart rate?—(A) anxiety; (B) fever; (C) hypothyroidism; (D) caffeine; and (E) athletic conditioning.

Cardiac Output

Cardiac output is the amount of blood pumped out of the left ventricle each minute. In a healthy adult, cardiac output ranges from 4 to 8 L/min (the average is approximately 5 L/min). Volume varies according to body size. The heart

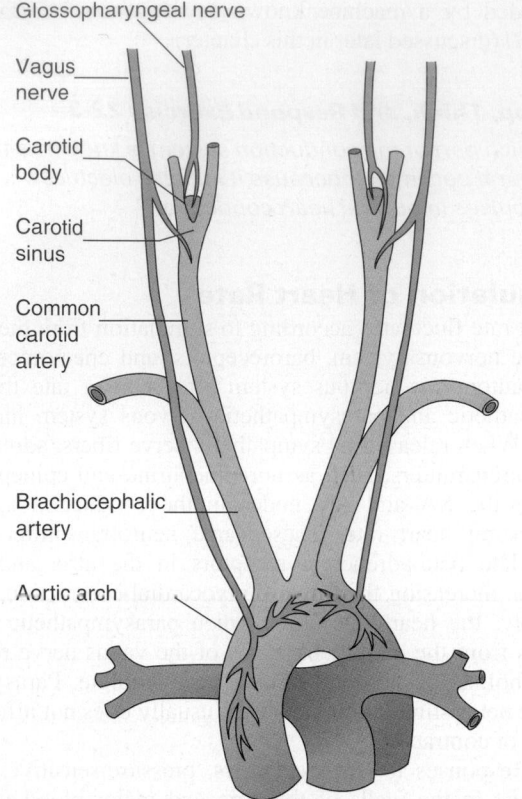

FIGURE 22-6. Location and innervation of the aortic arch and carotid sinus baroreceptors and the carotid body chemoreceptors. Chemoreceptors regulate sympathetic stimulation or inhibition. (From Chaffee, E. E. & Lytle, I. M. [1980]. *Basic physiology and anatomy* [4th ed.]. Philadelphia: J. B. Lippincott.)

Labels on figure:
- Glossopharyngeal nerve
- Vagus nerve
- Carotid body
- Carotid sinus
- Common carotid artery
- Brachiocephalic artery
- Aortic arch

BOX 22-1 **Factors That Alter Heart Rate**

Increase Heart Rate
Exercise
Fever
Hyperthyroidism
Hypoxia
Dehydration
Shock and hemorrhage
Anxiety
Caffeine
Drugs: Central nervous system stimulants (cocaine, methylphenidate [Ritalin], methamphetamine), adrenergic drugs (epinephrine, isoproterenol [Isuprel]), anticholinergic drugs (atropine, glycopyrrolate [Robinul])
Alcohol withdrawal

Decrease Heart Rate
Rest
Hypothermia
Hypothyroidism
Athletic conditioning
Drugs: Cardiac glycosides (digoxin [Lanoxin]), central nervous system depressants (morphine), calcium channel blockers (verapamil [Calan], nifedipine [Procardia]), beta-adrenergic blockers (atenolol [Tenormin], metoprolol [Lopressor], propranolol [Inderal])

▶ **Stop, Think, and Respond Exercise 22-5**

If a person's heart rate is 72 beats per minute (bpm), what is the cardiac output?

---

adjusts cardiac output to the body's changing needs. During active exercise, athletes may have a cardiac output that is five to seven times the normal amount. Cardiac output can be increased in two ways: by increasing the heart rate and by increasing the stroke volume. **Stroke volume** is the amount of blood pumped per contraction of the heart. The stroke volume averages about 65 to 70 mL. The following formula is used to calculate cardiac output:

$$\text{Cardiac output} = \text{heart rate} \times \text{stroke volume}$$

 Gerontologic Considerations

- Changes in cardiovascular structure and function that are seen in older adults are due to risk factors and lifestyle/ environmental influences (e.g., smoking, inadequate nutrition, lack of exercise) more often than the aging process itself. Include age, lifestyle, and environmental risk factors and influences in the assessment.

- The aging heart requires more time to return to baseline levels after stress. This inability to handle stress results from decreased cardiac output and contractile strength and delayed conduction in the heart.

ASSESSMENT OF THE CARDIOVASCULAR SYSTEM

History

The initial assessment includes the client's (or family member's) description of the symptoms the client experienced before and during admission. The history also includes the client's past medical history and family medical history. The family medical history is important because many cardiac disorders have a familial or genetic predisposition. If close blood relatives are no longer living, it is important to ask about the cause of death, age at death, and relationship to the client.

The nurse asks the client to identify prescription and nonprescription drugs that he or she is taking. Adverse effects or drug interactions can contribute to cardiac symptoms. Use of illicit drugs, like cocaine and methamphetamine, are also significant to the cardiac history. Drug and food allergies are noted because future diagnostic procedures may involve the administration of drugs or substances, such as radiopaque dyes.

 Pharmacologic Considerations

- Medications can affect BP and pulse rate and rhythm. When conducting a medication history, it is very important to obtain

NURSING GUIDELINES 22-1

Assessing Blood Pressure and Pulse for Postural Changes

- Have the client lie down for at least 3 minutes.
- Take the client's blood pressure and pulse.
- Assist the client to a sitting position.
- Be prepared to steady or assist the client should he or she become dizzy or faint.
- Reassess the blood pressure and pulse within 30 seconds after the client sits.
- Repeat the assessments with the client standing.
- Determine the difference in systolic and diastolic blood pressures in the upright position from that recorded in the previous position.
- Determine the difference in the heart rate from that recorded in the previous position.
- Conclude that the client manifests postural changes if the blood pressure is lower than 10 mm Hg from the previous measurement and the heart rate increases 10% or more from the previous measurement (Bickley, 2007).

a list of all prescription and nonprescription medications and medicinal herbs from the client or a family member.

Physical Examination

General Appearance

An appraisal of the client's general appearance may suggest problems that require further exploration. The client's nonverbal behavior and body position may indicate that he or she is anxious, depressed, in pain, or uncomfortable.

Pain

Poor circulation, a common problem in clients with cardiovascular disorders, causes ischemia (reduced blood supply) to body organs. A classic sign of ischemia is pain, which results from a lack of oxygen in the tissue. Chest pain is a manifestation of ischemia to the heart muscle. Leg pain, especially with activity, can indicate inadequate oxygenation to leg muscles.

When pain is present, the nurse evaluates it carefully. Obtaining as much information as possible is essential. Rapid treatment of pain is extremely important (see Chap. 11).

Vital Signs
Temperature

Fever is characteristic in some types of heart disease. It can accompany the inflammatory response when myocardial cells are damaged after an acute myocardial infarction (MI; heart attack) or infections such as rheumatic fever and bacterial endocarditis.

Pulse

When taking a client's pulse, the nurse notes its rate, rhythm, and quality. Pulse rhythm is the pattern of the pulsations and the pauses between them. A normal pulse is felt regularly with a similar length of pause. The pulse quality refers to its palpated volume. Pulse volume is described as feeling full, weak, or thready, meaning barely palpable. The nurse also determines any pulse deficit by counting the heart rate through auscultation at the apex while a second nurse simultaneously palpates and counts the radial pulse for a full minute. The difference, if any, is the pulse deficit.

Respiratory Rate

The nurse counts the respiratory rate for 60 seconds. He or she observes the character of the respirations, noting whether the client's breathing is effortless or labored (dyspneic), deep or shallow, noisy or quiet. The use of accessory muscles (neck or abdominal muscles) during respiration is an indication that the client is having difficulty breathing.

Blood Pressure

Cardiac disorders often are associated with changes in BP. If the client is not acutely ill, the nurse takes the BP with the client in the lying, sitting, and standing positions (orthostatic vital signs; Nursing Guidelines 22-1). These baseline determinations are necessary to monitor the effects of cardiovascular diseases and drugs that can alter the BP during position changes. To ensure an accurate assessment, the nurse selects the cuff width most appropriate for the diameter of the client's arm.

The nurse takes the BP in both arms on admission and at least once daily thereafter. He or she reports a marked difference in pressure between the left and right arms. When charting, the nurse identifies the arm used to measure the BP and the client's position at the time it was measured. The nurse questions the client about dizziness or lightheadedness when changing positions, such as rising from a sitting or lying position. These symptoms may indicate postural (or orthostatic) hypotension.

Cardiac Rhythm

The electrical activity that produces the heart rhythm can be observed continuously with bedside cardiac monitoring. Electrodes are attached to the chest and connected to a machine that displays the cardiac rhythm on an oscilloscope. The components of an ECG are discussed later in the chapter. A paper strip of the cardiac rhythm can be printed and attached to the client's record.

A cardiac monitor reveals the heart's electrical but not its mechanical activity. The healthcare provider must palpate a peripheral pulse or auscultate the apical heart rate to obtain this information. Comparing the heart rate and rhythm with the information displayed on the monitor is important because the ECG pattern may appear normal in some clients even when mechanical function is abnormal.

Cardiac **telemetry** sends ECG information over radio waves to a monitor that is distant from the client. Paramedics use telemetry to communicate information to personnel in the hospital emergency department. Telemetry also may be used when a client's condition is stable enough to allow transfer from a critical care unit but still requires continuous monitoring. When telemetry is used, the electrodes are attached to a battery pack, which is secured inside a pocket on the client's hospital gown or clothing.

Gerontologic Considerations

- Age-related changes in the conductive system include a decrease in the number of pacemaker cells and changes in their shape. An increase in fat deposits, collagen, and elastic fibers in the SA node leads to a higher risk for cardiac dysrhythmias.

- Abnormal rhythms are difficult to treat in the older adult because organs can be further compromised by the lack of adequate blood supply if other chronic conditions exist.

Heart Sounds
Normal Heart Sounds
Auscultation of the heart requires familiarization with normal and abnormal heart sounds. The first heart sound ("lub"), referred to as S_1, is the closing of the mitral and tricuspid valves. S_1 is heard loudest over the apex of the heart and occurs nearly simultaneously with the palpated pulse. The second heart sound ("dub"), referred to as S_2, is the closing of the aortic and pulmonic valves. S_2 is heard loudest with the stethoscope in the aortic area, which is at the second intercostal space to the right of the sternum (Fig. 22-7).

Abnormal Heart Sounds
All other heart sounds are abnormal and take considerable practice to recognize. A sound that follows S_1 and S_2 is called an S_3 heart sound or a ventricular gallop. When the three sounds are heard together, some say the cadence sounds like "Ken-tuck-y" or "lub-dub-dee." An S_3, although normal in children, often is an indication of heart failure in an adult. An extra sound just before S_1 is an S_4 heart sound, or atrial gallop. Some say this sound resembles the word "Ten-nes-see" or "lub-lub-dub." An S_4 sound often is associated with hypertensive heart disease.

In addition to heart sounds, auscultation may reveal other abnormal sounds, such as murmurs and clicks caused by turbulent blood flow through diseased heart valves. A friction rub may cause a rough, grating, or scratchy sound that is indicative of pericarditis (inflammation of the pericardium).

Peripheral Pulses
The nurse palpates the radial arteries and the major arteries of the leg bilaterally during the physical assessment (Fig. 22-8). He or she records the presence or absence of these pulses and their strength.

Skin
Many clients with cardiac disorders exhibit changes in skin color (e.g., cyanosis, pallor). A good light is necessary when assessing skin color. Cyanosis can be detected by carefully noting color changes in the oral mucous membranes as well as on the lips, earlobes, skin, and nail beds. In light-skinned clients, extreme pallor is easy to detect because the skin appears almost bloodless. In dark-skinned clients, a grayish cast to the skin usually indicates pallor.

The nurse inspects the arms and legs for variations in skin color and temperature and compares his or her bilateral findings with other areas of the body. Sparse hair growth on the legs and thick toenails can indicate poor

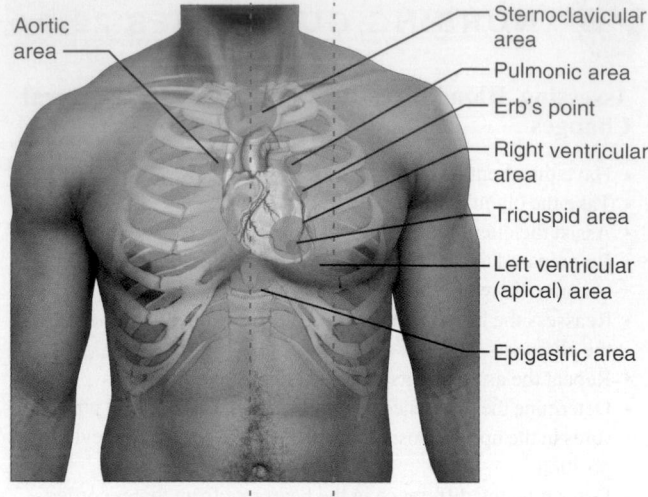

FIGURE 22-7. Areas assessed when evaluating heart function. Heart sounds can be auscultated in the aortic area, pulmonic area, Erb's point, tricuspid area, and apical area.

circulation. The nurse also notes any varicosities (enlargement of veins).

Peripheral Edema
Edema occurs when blood is not pumped efficiently or plasma protein levels are inadequate to maintain osmotic pressure. When blood has nowhere else to go, the extra fluid enters the tissues. Particular areas for examination are the dependent parts of the body, such as the feet and ankles. Other areas prone to edema are the fingers, hands, and over the sacrum. To assess for edema, the examiner gently presses his or her fingers into the skin and then quickly releases. If the marks of the fingers remain, the effect is termed *pitting edema*. Edema is evaluated on a scale of +1 to +4, depending on the depth of the pit and the amount of time it takes the pit to disappear (see Chap. 16). The higher the number, the more pronounced is the edema.

Weight
Weight gain can indicate edema. A rapid gain in weight often means that edema is increasing. Weight loss often

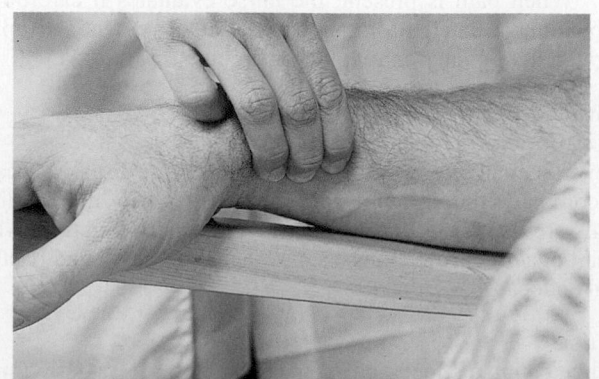

FIGURE 22-8. Proper placement of the fingers along the radial artery.

reflects the loss of excess fluid from the tissues and is used to evaluate the effectiveness of drug therapy, especially diuretics. If weight is recorded daily, the nurse weighs the client at the same time, with the same amount of clothing, using the same scale, each day. The weight is recorded as accurately as possible.

Jugular Veins

If the right side of the heart fails to pump efficiently, blood becomes congested in the neck veins. With the client sitting at a 45° angle, the client turns his or her head to the left or right so the nurse can inspect the external jugular vein. Distention of this vein usually indicates increased fluid volume and pressure in the right side of the heart (see Chap. 28).

Lung Sounds

If the left side of the heart fails to pump efficiently, blood backs up into the pulmonary veins and lung tissue. The nurse auscultates the lungs for abnormal and normal breath sounds. With left-sided congestive heart failure, auscultation reveals a crackling sound and possibly wheezes and gurgles. Wet lung sounds are accompanied by dyspnea and an effort to sit up to breathe. If uncorrected, left-sided heart failure is followed by right-sided heart failure because the circulatory system is a continuous loop.

Sputum

Clients with cardiac disease may have a productive or nonproductive cough. The nurse notes the type and frequency of the cough and the amount and appearance of the sputum. These findings can be important in diagnosing heart failure or other pulmonary complications.

Mental Status

Some clients with cardiac disorders may be alert and oriented; others may be confused and disoriented. Confusion or disorientation can result from a decrease in the oxygen supply to the brain (cerebral ischemia) as a result of poor circulation. Chest pain and impaired breathing can create anxiety. The nurse reports extremes of emotion or disturbances in thought processes to the physician because such effects could interfere with the client's safety, diagnostic testing, and prescribed therapy.

 Gerontologic Considerations

- Advanced vascular changes may lead to decreased perfusion to brain tissues, resulting in intermittent confusion and disorientation. As a confused and disoriented client does not always retain information, revised explanations or repeated communication may be needed during all phases of the nursing process.

Diagnostic Tests

Laboratory Tests

Various general laboratory tests are used in the diagnosis of heart disease and in monitoring the client's progress. Laboratory tests may be performed daily or every few days. They may be used to monitor the results of therapy. Blood chemistries, such as fasting blood glucose and serum electrolyte, cholesterol, and triglyceride levels, may be used as parts of the diagnostic process. Analysis of serum enzymes and isoenzymes may also be used. Serum cholesterol and lipid tests and isoenzyme analyses are discussed in more detail in Chapter 25. When tissues and cells break down, are damaged, or die, large quantities of certain enzymes are released into the bloodstream. Enzymes can therefore be elevated in response to cardiac or other organ damage.

Radiography and Radionuclide Studies

Chest radiography and fluoroscopy determine the size and position of the heart and condition of the lungs. These studies also are used to guide the insertion and confirm the placement of cardiac catheters and pacemaker wires. CT scanning and magnetic resonance imaging are used to determine heart size and detect lung involvement.

Radionuclides are radioactive chemical elements that are injected into and travel through the bloodstream. Their use sometimes is referred to as *nuclear cardiology*. The radionuclide technetium-99m is used to detect areas of myocardial damage. The radionuclide thallium-201 is used to diagnose ischemic heart disease during a stress test.

Magnetic Resonance Imaging (MRI)

Magnetic resonance imaging (MRI) is a diagnostic tool used to identify disorders that affect many different structures in the body without performing surgery. The principle underlying MRI is that many elements within the human body, such as hydrogen, are magnetic. The MRI machine's magnetic field excites the hydrogen atoms, creating a radio signal. The radio signal is converted to an image on a computer monitor. Because magnetism is used, clients undergoing an MRI are not exposed to radiation as would occur with tests involving x-rays.

Healthcare professionals are now using MRI to diagnose cardiac disorders. Cardiovascular MRI scanning can provide data about cardiac anatomy, function, blood flow, metabolism, and circulatory perfusion with a single examination (Darty et al., 2002). The image of blood within the heart appears white; dense tissues such as cardiac muscle and the valves are dark gray.

The client can undergo examination in a resting state, while actively exercising, or using medications to induce cardiac stress. MRI excludes those clients who have metallic implants, pacemakers, or implanted defibrillators. Preparation for a cardiac MRI includes starting intravenous infusions in one or two sites for the purpose of instilling fluids, contrast medium, and medications to accelerate the heart rate. The technician conducting the MRI informs the client that the machine produces loud knocking sounds during the test. To muffle the sounds, the technician can provide headphones and earplugs to the client. Some clients become claustrophobic within the MRI scanning chamber and can receive medication to relieve their anxiety; however, they must remain conscious to follow instructions regarding brief periods of breath holding during the test.

The nurse may need to administer medications to counteract allergic reactions or side effects of the drugs that increase the heart rate (stress) to a range that facilitates diagnostic measurements. Side effects that the client may experience include chest pressure, rapid heart rate, and

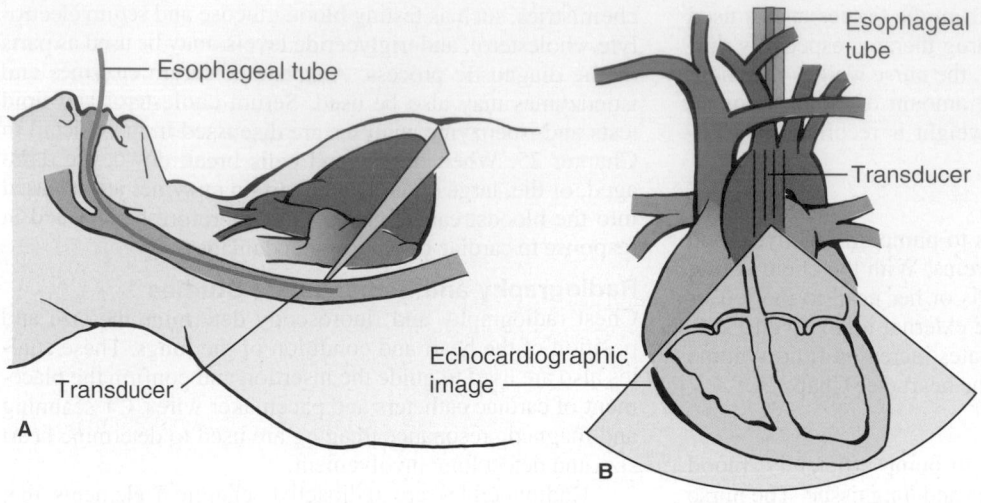

FIGURE 22-9. Transesophageal echocardiography. (**A**) An ultrasound transducer mounted on a flexible tube is passed into the esophagus. (**B**) When the transducer is at the level of the posterior heart, it transmits an image of the heart and its internal structures.

hypotension. The test is terminated if myocardial ischemia develops.

Echocardiography

Echocardiography uses ultrasound waves to determine the functioning of the left ventricle and to detect cardiac tumors, congenital defects, and changes in the tissue layers of the heart. High-frequency sound waves, which the human ear cannot hear, pass through the chest wall (transthoracic) and are displayed on an oscilloscope. The image is recorded and kept as a permanent record. This technique is also known as transthoracic echocardiography.

A second ultrasound technique is **transesophageal echocardiography** (TEE), which, as the name implies, involves passing a tube with a small transducer internally from the mouth to the esophagus (Fig. 22-9). From the esophagus, which lies behind the heart, the transducer can obtain images of the posterior heart and its internal structures. TEE provides superior views that are not possible using standard transthoracic echocardiography. It also is an adjunct for assessing intraoperative complications in the heart during cardiothoracic surgery. Clients whose chests are rotund or who are obese are candidates for TEE. Because the throat is anesthetized locally, the nurse cautions the client to avoid eating or drinking until sensation and the gag reflex return, which may take 1 hour or longer after removal of the tube containing the transducer.

Electrocardiography

Electrocardiography (ECG) is the graphic recording of the electrical currents generated by the heart muscle. During electrocardiography, color-coded electrodes matched to corresponding lead wires connect the client to the recording machine. The electrodes are coated with conductive gel and applied to the skin surface of the wrists, ankles, and chest (Fig. 22-10). A computerized ECG machine immediately interprets the tracings, or rhythm strips, which serve as a screening device. A physician later interprets the rhythm strips to aid in diagnosing heart disease (Fig. 22-11).

Resting electrocardiography is performed as a baseline before doing an exercise electrocardiography. Exercise electrocardiography is more diagnostic than resting electrocardiography because it demonstrates how the heart functions when subjected to activity.

Ambulatory Electrocardiography

Ambulatory ECG, or Holter monitoring, is the recording of an ambulatory client's cardiac rate and rhythm over 24 to 48 hours as the client performs daily activities. The Holter monitor, which is worn on a belt or carried on a shoulder strap, consists of a tape recorder connected to ECG leads attached to the client's chest (Fig. 22-12). During the test period, the client keeps a diary of activities and associated symptoms. At the end of the recording period, the monitor is returned to the hospital or physician and the tape is analyzed. The

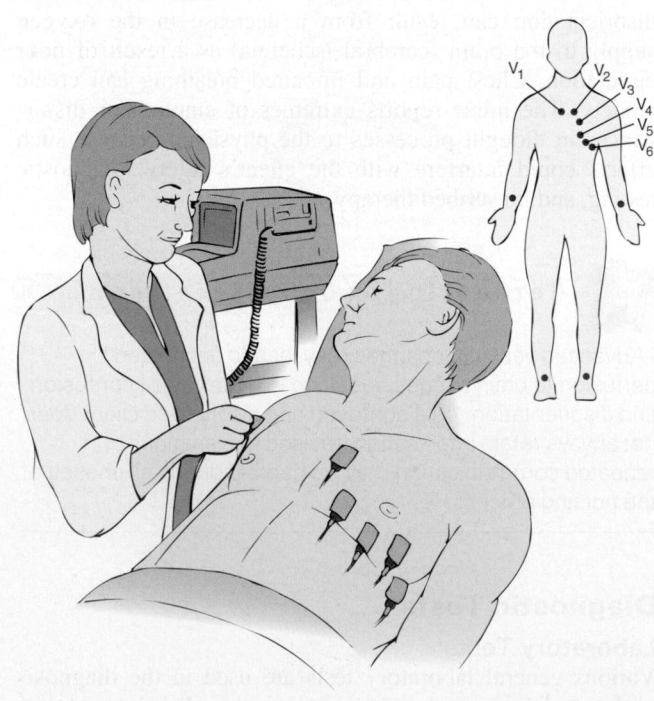

FIGURE 22-10. The nurse attaches electrodes to the client's chest and limbs before an ECG.

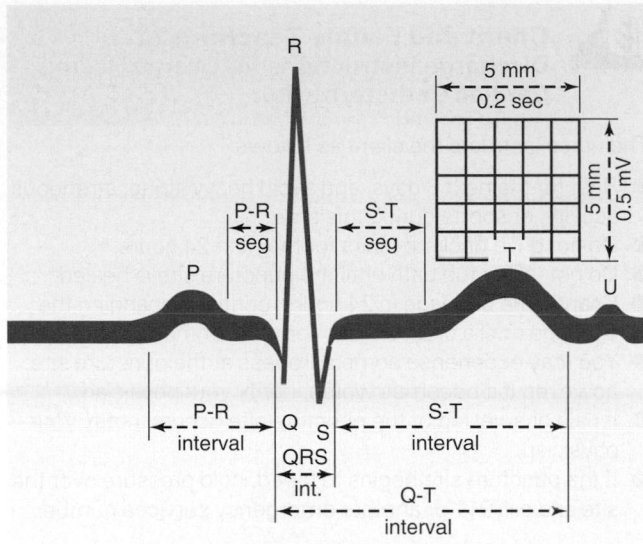

FIGURE 22-11. ECG and commonly measured complex components. Each small box represents 0.04 second on the horizontal axis and 1 mm or 0.1 millivolt on the vertical axis. The PR interval is measured from the beginning of the P wave to the beginning of the QRS complex; the QRS complex is measured from the beginning of the Q wave to the end of the S wave; the QT interval is measured from the beginning of the Q wave to the end of the T wave.

client's written notes are compared with the recorded information. Ambulatory ECG helps to detect dysrhythmias (rhythm abnormalities) and myocardial ischemia that occur sporadically during activity or rest.

Exercise Electrocardiography

During an **exercise electrocardiography**, also known as a stress test, the electrical activity of the heart is assessed with an ECG monitor while the client walks on a treadmill, pedals a stationary bicycle, or climbs up and down stairs (Fig. 22-13). The speed of the treadmill, the force required to pedal the bicycle, or the pace of stair climbing is gradually increased. The goal is to increase the heart's workload to reach a predetermined target heart rate. The client's heart rate and rhythm are monitored continuously, and ECG waveforms are recorded periodically. The client's BP and respiratory rate also are assessed. The client is instructed to report the onset of chest pain, dizziness, leg cramps, or weakness. The stress test is aborted if the client develops chest pain, severe dyspnea, elevated BP, confusion, or dysrhythmias. The physician interprets ECG tracings obtained during the test. Radionuclides also may be used during a stress test to provide additional information.

Drug-Induced Stress Testing

Drugs may be used to stress the heart for clients with sedentary lifestyles or those with a physical disability, such as severe arthritis, that interferes with exercise testing. Drugs such as adenosine (Adenocard), dipyridamole (Persantine), or dobutamine (Dobutrex) may be administered singularly or in combination by the IV route. The drugs dilate the coronary arteries, similar to the vasodilation that occurs when a

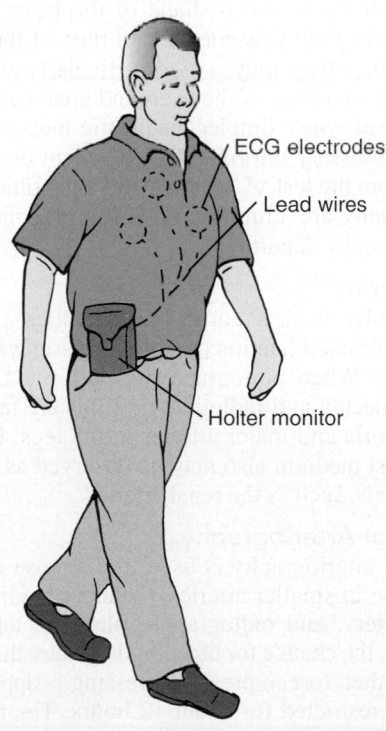

FIGURE 22-12. Ambulatory electrocardiography records the client's cardiac rate and rhythm during regular daily activities.

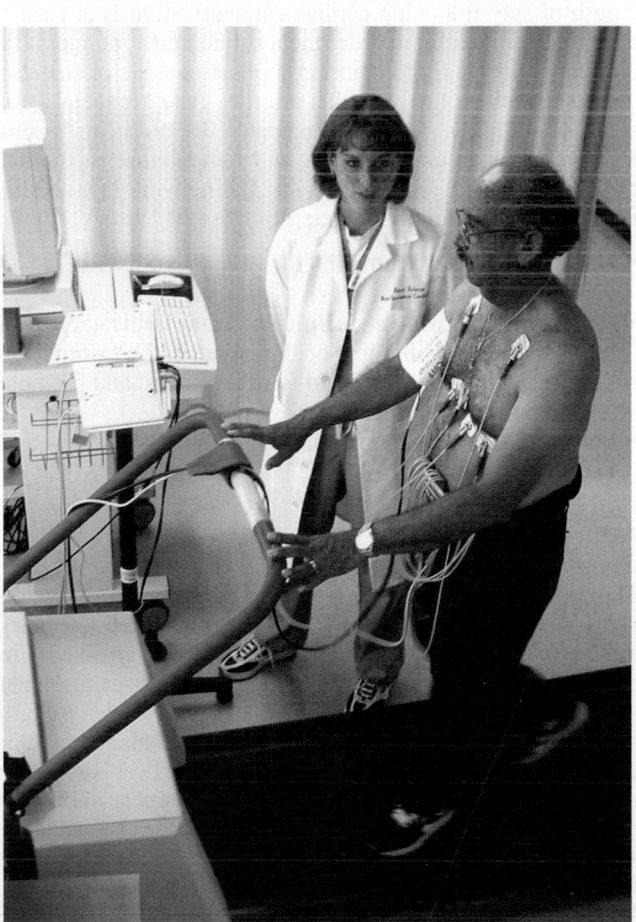

FIGURE 22-13. Treadmill exercise stress test. (Image © Texas Heart Institute, www.texasheart.org.)

person exercises to increase the heart muscle's blood supply. When thallium, a radionuclide, is injected a few minutes later, a scan of the heart can detect compromised blood flow, which indicates coronary artery disease, or evidence of well-perfused heart muscle.

Cardiac Catheterization

Cardiac catheterization is a diagnostic test performed in an operative setting. It can be done for a variety of purposes. In this procedure, a long, flexible catheter is inserted from a peripheral blood vessel in the groin, arm, or neck into one of the great vessels (inferior or superior vena cava which is attached to the heart) and then into the heart. Cardiac catheterization may be carried out on the left side of the heart by way of an artery or on the right side by way of a vein.

Before the procedure, the client needs to consult the physician about which prescribed medications to take or omit the day of the cardiac catheterization. Food and fluids usually are withheld; however, if the test is late in the day, light food may be permitted. Allergies must be identified; those of primary concern before a cardiac catheterization are iodine, shellfish, radiographic dye, and latex. IV fluids are administered before the test to maintain hydration and to administer any necessary medications. A sedative is administered before the test, but anesthesia is not necessary.

After the test, the catheter is removed and the site is covered with a pressure dressing to control bleeding. The usual length of stay following cardiac catheterization is at least 5 to 9 hours or overnight. After the test, the nurse monitors BP and pulse frequently to detect complications. He or she also checks the dressing over the insertion site frequently for signs of bleeding. The nurse palpates the pulse in various locations and checks the color and temperature in the extremity to confirm that blood is circulating well. Instructions for the client and family include:

- Keep the extremity straight for several hours and avoid movement.
- Report any warm, wet feeling that may indicate oozing blood, numbness, tingling, or sharp pain in the extremity.
- Drink a large volume of fluid to relieve thirst and promote the excretion of the dye.
- Follow discharge instructions for home care (Client and Family Teaching 22-1).

Arteriography
Coronary Arteriography

The most common use of a left-sided cardiac catheterization is to determine the degree of blockage of the coronary arteries by performing arteriography while the catheter is in place. An **arteriography** is a diagnostic procedure that involves instilling dye, referred to as *contrast medium*, into an artery. In this case, it is instilled into the catheter and deposited into each coronary artery. Occlusive heart disease is indicated if one or more coronary arteries appear narrow or do not fill. Clients with coronary artery disease who are considered candidates for invasive treatment procedures must undergo cardiac catheterization and coronary arteriography.

After removal of the catheter, the nurse inspects the insertion site for bleeding, tenderness, hematoma formation, and inflammation. The client remains on bed rest for the rest

Client and Family Teaching 22-1
Discharge Instructions for Clients Having Cardiac Catheterization

The nurse instructs the client as follows:

- Rest for the next 3 days, and avoid heavy lifting, strenuous activity, or sports during this time.
- Do not drive or climb stairs for the next 24 hours.
- Do not take a tub bath until the puncture site is healed.
- Change the bandage in 24 hours; continue changing the bandage until a crust or scab forms over the puncture site.
- You may experience some soreness at the puncture site; however, if it becomes worse, notify your physician.
- If pain or swelling of the puncture site occurs, notify your physician.
- If the puncture site begins to bleed, hold pressure over the site and call 911 or another emergency services number.

of the day. He or she must avoid flexion, or bending, of the arm or leg used for catheter insertion. Vascular assessments distal to the insertion site continue at frequent intervals. Absent distal peripheral pulses, cool toes, and pale or cyanotic arms and legs indicate arterial occlusion, usually from a blood clot. These signs as well as a rapid or irregular pulse rate indicate a medical emergency that the nurse must report immediately to the physician.

Angiocardiography

In **angiocardiography**, a radiopaque dye is injected into a vein, and its course through the heart is recorded by a series of radiographic pictures taken in rapid succession. The pictures reveal the size and shape of the heart chambers and great vessels and the sequence and time of their filling with dye. Angiocardiography is used particularly to diagnose congenital abnormalities of the heart and great vessels. It usually is performed when simpler diagnostic measures fail to provide the necessary information. The client fasts for at least 3 hours before the test. A sedative and an antihistaminic medication usually are administered before the client is taken to the radiography department.

Aortography

Aortography detects aortic abnormalities such as aneurysms (abnormal dilatation of a blood vessel wall) and arterial occlusions. When aortography is performed, contrast medium is injected and radiographic films are taken of the abdominal aorta and major arteries in the legs. Distribution of the contrast medium also may be observed as it circulates to other vessels, such as the renal arteries.

Peripheral Arteriography

Peripheral arteriography is used to diagnose occlusive arterial disease in smaller arteries. Contrast medium is injected into an artery, and radiographic films are taken. After the procedure, the chance for bleeding is greater than after a venipuncture; therefore, a pressure dressing is applied and client activity is restricted for about 12 hours. The nurse observes the client for bleeding and cardiac dysrhythmias and assesses the adequacy of peripheral circulation by frequently checking the peripheral pulses.

Nursing Process for the Client Undergoing Diagnostic Procedures of the Cardiovascular System

Assessment

For both outpatients and inpatients, perform a thorough initial assessment of clients undergoing diagnostic testing to establish accurate baseline data for use before, during, and after the procedure. Weigh the client and measure vital signs. If applicable, measure BP in both arms and compare findings. Assess apical and radial pulses, noting rate, quality, and rhythm. Check peripheral pulses in the lower extremities.

Ask the client to describe any symptoms. If the client is experiencing chest pain, a history of its location, frequency, and duration is necessary, as is a description of the pain, if it radiates to a particular area, what precipitates its onset, and what brings relief. Another important area of questioning is whether the client is experiencing pressure, fluttering, or palpitations in the chest. Ask if the client has episodes of dyspnea, dizziness, or fainting. Assess the lower extremities for edema and toes for color and temperature.

Auscultate heart and lung sounds and obtain family history of heart disease or other chronic diseases that are related to cardiovascular disorders such as diabetes mellitus. Identify current prescribed medications, herbal preparations, and over-the-counter drugs used for self-treatment. Assess the client for iodine or seafood allergy before beginning any diagnostic test requiring an iodinated contrast. A hypoallergenic nonionic contrast may be used if an allergy is suspected. Also determine the client's anxiety level and knowledge about the procedure.

Diagnosis, Planning, and Interventions

▶ **Anxiety** related to insecurity

▶ **Expected Outcome:** Anxiety will be reduced to whatever the client identifies as tolerable using a scale from 0 to 10.

• Greet client by name and introduce personnel involved in care. *Introductions are a common courtesy, promote personal involvement, and eliminate the feeling of being cared for by strangers.*

• Promote a relaxed environment by sitting during the interview, reducing unnecessary noise and activity, and giving client time to think and respond to questions. *A relaxed nurse promotes relaxation in the client. Rushing or exposing the client to sensory stimulation is likely to communicate and heighten anxiety.*

• Orient client to surroundings. *Familiarity with the testing area and equipment that will be used reduces fears that may be highly exaggerated.*

• Tell client when the test will begin and how long it will take. *Giving the client a time frame reduces anticipatory anxiety.*

• Keep client informed of unexpected delays. *Providing information decreases anxiety.*

• Remain in view of the client or establish some other means of contact for assistance such as a signal light. *Knowing that he or she can summon the nurse for questions or assistance is reassuring to the client.*

▶ **Deficient Knowledge** (test's purpose, performance, and after care) related to lack of prior experience or lack of recall

▶ **Expected Outcome:** Client and family will demonstrate sufficient knowledge with which to provide informed consent and perform self-care afterward.

• Assess client's and family's knowledge of the diagnostic procedure. *Clarifying any misconceptions or misinformation and building on what is already known are important interventions.*

• Provide both verbal and written information concerning the test's purpose, procedure, and after-care. *Written information enables the client to further process the verbal information and serves as a basis for recalling verbal instructions.*

• Use language that the client can easily understand. *Medical terminology that is not part of the client's vocabulary may heighten anxiety and intimidate the client to the extent that he or she may not ask further questions.*

• Ask client, family, or both to paraphrase information. *The ability to paraphrase provides evidence as to whether they understood information the nurse provided.*

▶ **Pain and Activity Intolerance** related to ischemia

▶ **Expected Outcomes:** (1) Pain will be relieved or controlled within a tolerable level during the diagnostic procedure. (2) Activity will be limited to that which avoids dyspnea or tachycardia.

• Assess pain level (see Chap. 11) frequently before, during, and after the diagnostic procedure. *Pain is a subjective symptom that the nurse can reliably assess only by asking the client to rate and describe it.*

• Allow for rest periods. *Rest reduces heart rate and demand for increased oxygenated blood.*

• Stop the procedure, assess vital signs, give a short-acting prescribed vasodilator such as nitroglycerin, and administer oxygen if chest pain occurs. *Monitoring and treating chest pain with prescribed interventions that improve blood flow to the heart are within the interdependent nursing domain.*

• Notify the physician if rest, oxygen, or prescribed medications do not provide relief. *Sustained chest pain may require medical assessment and additional interventions.*

▶ **Risk for Injury** related to untoward reactions during or after diagnostic tests

▶ **Expected Outcome:** The client's condition will remain stable during and after diagnostic tests.

• If diagnostic procedure is invasive, withhold food and fluids before procedure and until the client is stable and free from nausea and vomiting after the procedure. *Nausea, which precedes vomiting, can be triggered by gastric distension. Vomiting will require temporary interruption of the test and prolongs recovery if it occurs following the test.*

• Assess for dyspnea, hypotension or hypertension, cardiac dysrhythmias, mental changes, pain or discomfort, and cyanosis. *Post-test findings that differ significantly from pretest results are highly suggestive of a cause-and-effect relationship between the test's physiologic requirements and the client's response.*

- Implement nursing measures to stabilize the client, such as ensuring a patent IV access and administering oxygen and pre-scribed medications. *The nurse's role includes independent, interdependent, and dependent nursing actions.*

- Collaborate with the physician to restore client to a stable condition. *The physician's role is to manage complications medically; the nurse assists the physician.*

 Gerontologic Considerations

- The older adult who has renal impairment or is chronically dehydrated is at increased risk for complications during and after diagnostic studies requiring the use of a dye because the iodinated contrast is nephrotoxic. Interventions to hydrate should be considered prior to the test.

Evaluation of Expected Outcomes

The client is relaxed and feels secure. The test is performed uneventfully or the client is stabilized when complications are managed successfully. The client and family have an accurate understanding of the diagnostic testing process and discharge instructions.

CRITICAL THINKING EXERCISES

1. During admission, the nurse notes that the client has an irregular pulse rate. What aspect of cardiac anatomy and physiology is most likely contributing to the assessment data?

2. The function of which heart chamber is most important to maintain? Explain your answer.

3. What are consequences that may occur if cardiac output is decreased below normal?

4. What information is important for the nurse to communicate to a client who is scheduled for a cardiac diagnostic test?

NCLEX-STYLE REVIEW QUESTIONS

1. A client comes to the emergency department complaining of chest pain. Which question is most important for the nurse to ask initially?
   1. "When did your pain begin?"
   2. "Have you had this type of pain before?"
   3. "Do you have any food or drug allergies?"
   4. "Do you have pain in any other place?"

2. A hospitalized client takes an antihypertensive medication and complains of being light-headed when getting out of bed. Which nursing intervention is most appropriate at this time?
   1. Notify the client's primary care physician.
   2. Take the client's blood pressure while lying, sitting, and standing.
   3. Ask the client if this has happened before.
   4. Hold the client's medication until the client feels better.

3. When assessing heart sounds, place an "X" in the anatomic area that is best for ausculating an S_1 heart sound.

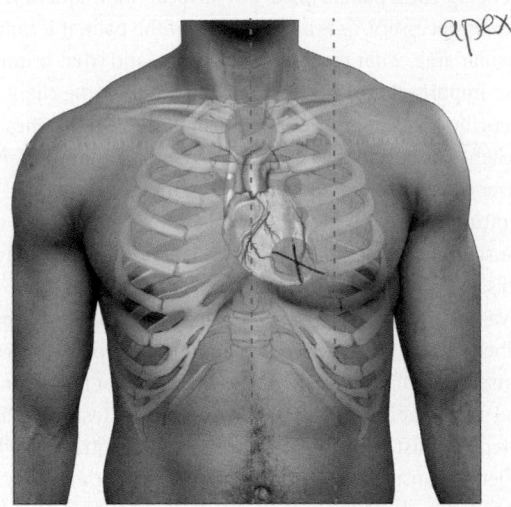

apex

4. Which client is most important for the nurse to assess for complications following a cardiac catheterization?
   1. A 75-year-old man with chronic kidney disease
   2. A 50-year-old woman who experiences occasional numbness and tingling in her hands
   3. A 25-year-old who complains of chest pain
   4. A 38-year-old with a family history of a bleeding disorder

5. Which of the following are indications that a client may have cardiac disease? Select all that apply.
   1. Unquenchable thirst
   2. Chest pain on exertion
   3. Hypertension
   4. Father died at age 48
   5. Presence of S_2 heart sound

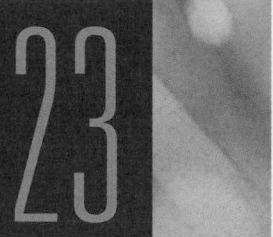

23

Caring for Clients with Infectious and Inflammatory Disorders of the Heart and Blood Vessels

Words To Know

cardiac tamponade
cardiomyopathy
decortication
deep vein thrombosis
effusion
emboli
Homans' sign
impedance plethysmography
infective endocarditis
intermittent claudication
Janeway lesions
murmur
myocardial disarray
myocarditis
myofibrils
Osler nodes
pericardiectomy
pericardiocentesis
pericardiostomy
pericarditis
petechiae
polyarthritis
postphlebitic syndrome
precordial pain
pulmonary embolus
pulsus paradoxus
rheumatic carditis
Roth's spots
sequelae (sing., sequela)
splinter hemorrhages
sympathectomy
syncope
thrombectomy
thromboangiitis obliterans
thrombophlebitis
vegetations
vena caval filter
vena caval plication
venography
ventriculomyomectomy
Virchow's triad

Learning Objectives

On completion of this chapter, you will be able to:

1. Identify three organisms that cause infectious conditions of the heart.
2. List four inflammatory conditions of the heart.
3. Describe treatment for inflammatory and infectious heart disorders.
4. Discuss the nursing management of clients with infectious or inflammatory heart disorders.
5. Name three types of cardiomyopathy.
6. Differentiate between thrombophlebitis and thromboangiitis obliterans.
7. List three interventions that reduce the risk of thrombophlebitis.
8. Discuss the nursing management of clients with inflammatory disorders of peripheral blood vessels.

The body uses many defense mechanisms to combat the effects of trauma, disease, and microorganisms. The inflammatory response, skin and mucous membranes, and immune system work together to protect the body's cardiovascular system. Despite these protective mechanisms, infectious and inflammatory disorders may compromise the heart and blood vessels.

 Gerontologic Considerations

- A decline in immune system function that occurs with age may lead to increased risk for infectious or inflammatory disorders of the cardiovascular system. Decreased inflammatory and immune responses may also prolong recovery from cardiovascular trauma, disease, or microorganisms.

INFECTIOUS AND INFLAMMATORY DISORDERS OF THE HEART

RHEUMATIC FEVER AND RHEUMATIC CARDITIS

Rheumatic fever is a systemic inflammatory disease that sometimes follows a group A streptococcal infection of the throat. **Rheumatic carditis** refers to the inflammatory cardiac manifestations of rheumatic fever in either the acute or later stage. Cardiac structures that usually are affected include the heart valves (particularly the mitral valve), endocardium, myocardium, and pericardium.

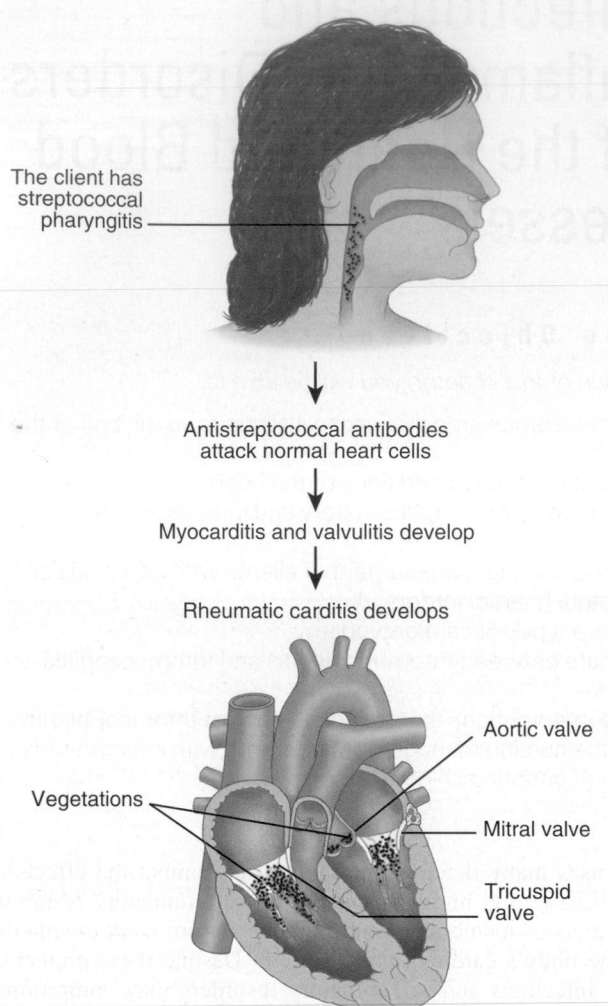

The client has streptococcal pharyngitis

↓

Antistreptococcal antibodies attack normal heart cells

↓

Myocarditis and valvulitis develop

↓

Rheumatic carditis develops

Aortic valve

Vegetations

Mitral valve

Tricuspid valve

FIGURE 23-1. Rheumatic carditis after group A streptococcal pharyngitis.

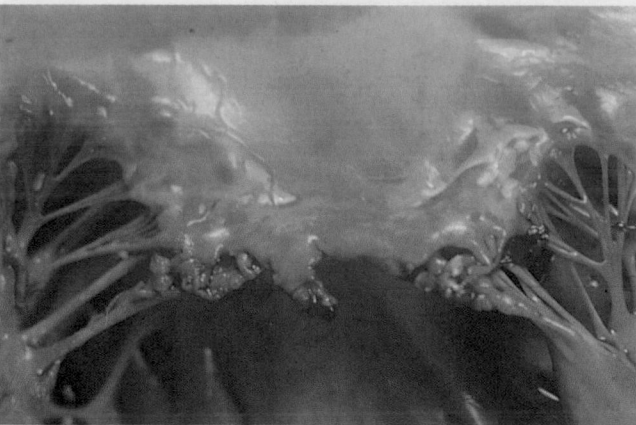

FIGURE 23-2. The mitral valve shows destructive vegetations. (From Rubin, E., et al. [2005]. *Rubin's pathology: Clinicopathologic foundations of medicine* [4th Ed.]. Philadelphia: Lippincott Williams & Wilkins.)

Pathophysiology and Etiology

The inflammatory symptoms of rheumatic carditis are believed to be induced by antibodies originally formed to destroy the group A beta-hemolytic streptococcal microorganisms. The antibodies, however, "mistakenly" cross-react against the proteins in the connective tissue of the heart, joints, skin, and nervous system (Fig. 23-1). This cross-reaction causes valvular damage and *pancarditis*, inflammation of all layers of the heart (endocardium, myocardium, and pericardium).

As the antibody response ensues, white blood cells (WBCs) migrate to the endocardium, causing inflammatory debris to accumulate as **vegetations** around the valve leaflets (Fig. 23-2). When the inflammatory process is relieved, fibrinous tissue replaces the damaged areas. This fibrinous tissue fuses or thickens valve leaflets and shortens the chordae tendineae; thus, the valves may lose their ability to open fully or close tightly (see Chap. 24). The fibrinous replacements also cause surface irregularities around the valves, making them prone to future colonization by blood-borne bacteria.

The antibodies also attack cardiac myosin, the muscle protein in myocardial tissue. Because myosin is instrumental in cardiac muscle contraction, rheumatic carditis may cause weakened heart contractions and heart failure (see Chap. 28). If the pericardium is involved, it becomes tough and leathery from accumulated fibrinous fluid that interferes with the heart's ability to stretch and fill with blood. *Tachydysrhythmias*, fast abnormal heart rhythms, develop to compensate for the decreased cardiac output (the volume of blood ejected from the left ventricle per minute). After the acute episode, most clients recover, but valvular changes remain.

Gerontologic Considerations

- Rheumatic heart disease may occur in the older adult who had rheumatic fever at an earlier age, or an acute episode may develop later in life.

Assessment Findings

Signs and Symptoms

Acute rheumatic fever is most common in children 2 to 3 weeks after a streptococcal infection. The **sequelae**, abnormal conditions that follow a disease, include carditis (inflammation of the layers of the heart), **polyarthritis** (inflammation of more than one joint), rash, subcutaneous nodules, and chorea characterized by involuntary grimacing and an inability to use skeletal muscles in a coordinated manner. Adults do not exhibit the same degree and range of symptoms as young children.

A mild fever, if untreated, continues for several weeks. The heart rate is rapid and the rhythm may be abnormal. A red, spotty rash referred to as erythema marginatum appears on the trunk but disappears rapidly, leaving irregular circles on the skin. Several joints, most commonly the knees, ankles, hips, and shoulders, become swollen, warm, red, and painful. The involvement migrates across joints. Sometimes marble-sized nodules appear around the joints. Central nervous system manifestations result in chorea. Cardiac complications may develop: a heart murmur suggests valve damage; a pericardial friction rub indicates pericarditis; and

BOX 23-1 **High-Risk Procedures for Clients With a History of Rheumatic Carditis or Infective Endocarditis**

Prophylactic antibiotic therapy is recommended before:
- Dental procedures associated with significant bleeding from hard or soft tissues, including tooth extraction, dental implant and reimplantation, teeth cleaning, scaling, periodontal surgery, root canal instrumentation, orthodontic band placement (initial), and intraligamentary local anesthetic injections
- Gastrointestinal procedures associated with a high rate of transient bacteremia, such as dilation of esophageal stricture, sclerotherapy of esophageal varices, biliary tract surgery or

instrumentation (e.g., endoscopic retrograde cholangiography), and operative procedures involving the intestinal mucosa
- Genitourinary surgery, instrumentation, or diagnostic procedures, especially in the presence of a urinary tract infection, such as transurethral resection of the prostate, cystoscopy, urethral dilation, and urethral catheterization
- Respiratory tract procedures that involve bronchoscopy with a rigid endoscope or surgery involving respiratory mucosa such as a tonsillectomy and adenoidectomy

(Adapted from Prevention of bacterial endocarditis: Recommendations by the American Heart Association. [On-line.] Available: http://www.americanheart. org/presenter.jhtml?identifier-11086.)

congestive heart failure (CHF) develops if the myocardium fails to compensate for functional demands.

Diagnostic Findings

No laboratory test is specific for the diagnosis of rheumatic fever. The results of laboratory tests such as an antistreptolysin O titer, erythrocyte sedimentation rate (ESR), and C-reactive protein are elevated, indicating an inflammatory process involving the streptococcal organism. Specific cardiac tests, such as electrocardiography (ECG) and echocardiography, may show structural changes in the valves, size of the heart, and the heart's ability to contract.

Medical and Surgical Management

Intravenous (IV) antibiotics are given. Penicillin is the drug of choice for group A streptococci, unless contraindicated because of an allergy. For clients who are allergic to the penicillin family of antibiotics, another antibiotic such as azithromycin (Zithromax), clindamycin (Cleocin), or vancomycin (Vancocin) may be prescribed. Cephalosporins such as cephalexin (Keflex) or cefadroxil (Duricef) may be prescribed if the client has not had a previous severe allergic reaction to penicillin. Bed rest may be indicated, depending on the client's condition. Aspirin is used to control the formation of blood clots around heart valves. Steroids are used to suppress the inflammatory response.

Concurrent treatment of rheumatic carditis depends on the extent of heart involvement. If minor, no treatment may be given; if heart failure or life-threatening dysrhythmias occur, extensive treatment is necessary. Surgery may be required to treat constrictive pericarditis and damage to heart valves. Prophylactic antibiotic therapy is recommended before future procedures that are associated with the dissemination of microorganisms that can lead to bacteremia and recurrence of endocarditis (Box 23-1).

Nursing Management

The nurse administers prescribed drug therapy and monitors for therapeutic and adverse effects. He or she plans diversional activities that require minimal activity, such as reading and putting puzzles together, to reduce the work of the myocardium and counteract the boredom of bed rest. Focused cardiac assessments help to track the progression or

Nutrition Notes 23-1
The Client with Rheumatic Carditis

- A full liquid diet is used in the initial treatment of rheumatic heart disease and is progressed as tolerated.
- Sodium is restricted if the client has edema or is treated with steroids.
- Anorexia and weight loss are common side effects of infections; calories and protein should be increased as needed to replenish losses.
- Fever increases fluid requirements.
- Encourage small, frequent feedings to maximize intake.

improvement of heart involvement. Clients with a history of rheumatic fever are susceptible to infective endocarditis (discussed next) and are told to take prophylactic antibiotics before any invasive procedure, including dental work. Additional nursing management depends on assessment data. Nutrition Notes 23-1 describes nutrition considerations.

▶ **Stop, Think, and Respond Exercise 23-1**

What information is important to give to parents whose children develop a severe sore throat?

INFECTIVE ENDOCARDITIS

Infective endocarditis (formerly called *bacterial endocarditis*) is inflammation of the inner layer of heart tissue as a result of an infectious microorganism (Fig. 23-3). Although clients with rheumatic carditis do develop endocarditis, it is initially considered an autoimmune response—not an infection—because no microorganism can be isolated from blood or other cultured specimens. Subsequent to the initial rheumatic carditis, however, the valvular changes increase the client's susceptibility to endocardial colonization by pathogens. In addition to clients who have recovered from rheumatic carditis, other susceptible clients include those who have nonrheumatic valve disease or artificial heart valves, repaired congenital heart defects, a prolapsed mitral

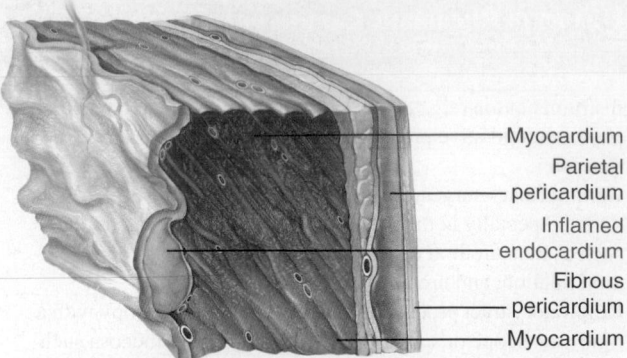

- Myocardium
- Parietal pericardium
- Inflamed endocardium
- Fibrous pericardium
- Myocardium

FIGURE 23-3. Tissue changes in endocarditis.

valve, or hypertrophic cardiomyopathy (discussed later); IV drug users; and immunosuppressed clients with central venous catheters.

Gerontologic Considerations

- The prevalence of infective endocarditis among older adults has increased, due in part to the increased number of prosthetic valve replacements, including replacements for older adults, and an increase in hospital-acquired bacteremia. Older males are eight times more likely to develop infective endocarditis than older females (Lakatta, 2006).

Pathophysiology and Etiology

The microorganisms that cause infective endocarditis include bacteria and fungi (Table 23-1). *Streptococcus viridans* and *Staphylococcus aureus* are the bacteria most frequently responsible for this disorder. They are found abundantly on the skin and mucous membranes of the mouth, nose, throat, and other cavities.

Most pathogens find their way into the bloodstream through trauma caused by invasive procedures involving mucous membranes or other tissues that harbor microorganisms. Although anyone can contract endocarditis, clients with a history of rheumatic carditis are especially susceptible. Prolonged IV therapy, insertion of cardiac pacemakers, cardiac catheterization, tracheal intubation, cardiac surgery, genitourinary instrumentation (Foley catheters and cystoscopy), and IV drug abuse create portals of entry for the causative microorganisms.

Once the microorganisms migrate to the endocardial surface, they attach to the vegetations composed of fibrin and platelets surrounding the heart valves, chordae tendineae, and papillary muscles. The microorganisms bury themselves in the vegetative mass, making them difficult to destroy with natural defenses or antibiotic therapy. The cycle continues with layer upon layer of imbedded microorganisms and fibrin/platelet deposits.

The endocardium on the left side of the heart is affected more often than on the right. The mitral valve is the most common location of vegetations and microbial deposits. If the valve leaflets erode and slough, blood leaks between the

TABLE 23-1 Microorganisms That Cause Endocarditis

MICROORGANISMS	DESCRIPTION
Streptococci	Account for 55% of cases of endocarditis
Group A beta-hemolytic	Attack normal or damaged heart valves and may cause rapid destruction
S. bovis	Related to GI malignancy
S. viridans	Tend to affect previously damaged heart valves
Staphylococci	Cause 30% of cases of endocarditis
S. aureus	Virulent strain with high mortality rate
S. epidermidis	Associated with dental procedures and valve replacements
S. faecalis	Cause both acute and subacute infections
	Associated with urologic instrumentation in men, bacteremia, respiratory tract infections, pneumonia, sinusitis, otitis media, and epiglottitis
Enterococci	Normal inhabitants of the GI tract, anterior urethra, and occasionally the mouth
E. faecalis and E. faecium	Relatively resistant to single antibiotics; require combination of antibiotic therapy for a minimum of 4 weeks
HACEK Group	Slow-growing gram-negative bacilli
Haemophilus parainfluenzae and	Require culture for 2 weeks or longer when initial culture is negative
Haemophilus aphrophilus	Cause subacute presentations
Aggregabactor	Associated with very large vegetations
actinomycetemcomitans	
Cardiobacterium hominis	
Eikenella corrodens	
Kingella kingae	
Fungi	Increased incidence in IV drug users
Candida	Risk increased with improper use of antibiotics and steroids
Gram-negative bacteria	May travel from GI or genitourinary tract
Escherichia coli	Increased risk in older adults
Klebsiella species	
Pseudomonas species	

GI, gastrointestinal.

heart chambers, diminishing the heart's efficiency as a pump. Heart failure often is a consequence. The vegetations can break off to form **emboli**, mobile masses of fibrin and clusters of platelets that circulate in the bloodstream. Emboli may occlude small blood vessels and interfere with an organ's blood supply.

Assessment Findings

Signs and Symptoms

Infective endocarditis can have an acute onset (less than 1 week) from a previously healthy state. The client presents with fever, chills, muscle aches in the lower back and thighs, and joint pain. Subacute infections progress more insidiously over weeks to months with more vague manifestations, such as headache, malaise, fatigue, and sleep disturbances. As the condition advances, purplish, painful nodules called **Osler nodes** may appear on the pads of the fingers and toes. Black longitudinal lines, called **splinter hemorrhages**, can be seen in the nails. There may be small, painless, red-blue macular lesions known as **Janeway lesions** on the palms of the hands and soles of the feet (Wisniewski, 2003). **Roth's spots**, white areas in the retina surrounded by areas of hemorrhage, may be detected. The spleen may be enlarged, and tenderness may be noted on abdominal palpation. A heart murmur may be present from malfunctioning valves. **Petechiae**, tiny, reddish hemorrhagic spots on the skin and mucous membranes, are signs of embolization. Pronounced weakness, anorexia, and weight loss are common. Symptoms can change suddenly if embolization or heart failure occurs. Emboli to the brain cause cerebrovascular accidents (see Chap. 38); emboli to the kidneys cause flank pain and renal failure (see Chap. 58); pulmonary emboli result in sudden chest pain and dyspnea (see Chap. 21). Clients with heart failure present with dyspnea, hypotension, and peripheral or pulmonary edema.

Diagnostic Findings

Anemia and slight leukocytosis are common findings. A series of three blood cultures collected over 1 to 24 hours usually identifies the microorganism circulating in the blood. Some cultured specimens require incubation for 3 weeks or more to identify accurately the infecting species. Occasionally the vegetations also can be cultured. Transesophageal echocardiography is more likely than transthoracic echocardiography to reveal the vegetations, altered valvular function, and impaired pumping quality of the ventricles. ECG may reveal abnormalities in heart rhythm if the vegetations involve a valve close to conduction tissue.

Medical and Surgical Management

High doses of an IV antibiotic to which the organism is susceptible are prescribed initially (Drug Therapy Table 23-1). Antibiotic therapy extends at least 2 to 6 weeks. It is resumed if the infection recurs after discontinuation of the drug. Bed rest is ordered initially. When the client begins to improve, bathroom privileges and increased activity are allowed. If a heart valve has been severely damaged and drug therapy does not adequately support the heart in failure, valve replacement may be necessary (see Chaps. 24 and 29).

Client and Family Teaching 23-1
Infectious and Inflammatory Heart Disorders

The nurse provides the following instructions:

● Continue regular follow-up care, because there will always be a risk for a reoccurrence
● If there is a history of rheumatic fever, congenital valve disorders, or prosthetic valve replacements, see a physician if fever, malaise, or other symptoms of infection occur
● There may be a need for antibiotics just before, and for a short time after, an event that might cause bacteremia, such as dental surgery
● If an antibiotic is prescribed, take the full dose for the full time because noncompliance with the drug regimen can hinder the complete destruction of the pathogen.

Nursing Management

Many clients cannot appreciate the danger of the disease without seeing external signs of the damage. The nurse gently but firmly reminds the client to limit activity. He or she continually assesses for changes in weight and pulse rate and rhythm and notes and reports new symptoms. The nurse administers prescribed antibiotics around the clock to sustain therapeutic blood levels of the medication at all times. He or she informs clients that periodic antibiotic therapy is a lifelong necessity because they will be vulnerable to the disease for the rest of their lives.

Client and Family Teaching 23-1 provides appropriate health information for clients who have infectious or inflammatory heart disorders.

▶ **Stop, Think, and Respond Exercise 23-2**

If a client asks why he or she has been advised to take an antibiotic such as penicillin before having dental work done, what information is appropriate to provide?

MYOCARDITIS

Pathophysiology and Etiology

Myocarditis is an inflammation of the myocardium (the muscle layer of the heart) (Fig. 23-4). A viral, bacterial, fungal, or parasitic infection causes most cases; a viral origin is most common in the United States. The usual viral agents are coxsackie viruses A and B, influenza A and B viruses, measles, adenovirus, mumps, rubella, rubeola, Epstein-Barr virus, and cytomegalovirus. The myocardium also can become inflamed from the toxins of microorganisms, chronic alcohol and cocaine abuse, radiation therapy, or autoimmune disorders. Clients with bulimia who use syrup of ipecac to facilitate purging can develop myocardial damage similar to viral myocarditis.

Whatever the damaging agent, an inflammatory response causes the cardiac muscle tissue to swell, which

DRUG THERAPY TABLE 23-1 Agents Used To Treat Endocarditis

Drug	Mechanism of Action	Side Effects	Nursing Considerations
penicillin G (Pfi-zerpen, Pen-tids, Wycillin, Bicillin)	Inhibits cell wall synthesis of organisms sensitive to penicillin G, killing the organisms	Allergic reaction: rash, fever, wheezing; possibly anaphylaxis and deaths Nausea, vomiting, diarrhea, abdominal pain, glossitis, stomatitis, gastritis, furry tongue	Be sure to check client's allergy history before administering. In acute care settings, retrieve the IV antibiotic solution from the refrigerator 15 minutes before administration. Evaluate the IV site for phlebitis before and after administration. Administer IM penicillin deep into the muscle mass.
nafcillin (Unipen)	Inhibits cell wall synthesis of organisms sensitive to nafcillin, killing the organisms	Lethargy, hallucinations, seizures, glossitis, stomatitis, gastritis, furry tongue, anemia, nephritis	Use cautiously in clients with renal disorders. If giving IM, alternate sites. Repeated use of the same site can result in atrophy Be sure to administer oral forms 1 hour before or 2 hours after meals. Do not administer with soft drinks or fruit juices.
gentamicin (Garamycin, Gentacidin)	Inhibits protein synthesis in gram-negative, susceptible strains Appears to disrupt function of bacterial cell membranes, killing the bacteria	Tinnitus, dizziness, vertigo, nausea, vomiting, palpitations, purpura, rash, fever, apnea, irreversible ototoxicity, nephrotoxicity	Give by IM route if possible. Ensure that the client receives adequate hydration throughout therapy. Monitor results of renal function tests, complete blood counts, and serum drug levels.
ceftriaxone (Rocephin)	Inhibits cell wall synthesis of bacteria sensitive to ceftriaxone, killing the organisms	Nausea, vomiting, diarrhea, anorexia, abdominal pain, flatulence, rash, fever, pain, superinfections	Advise clients to avoid alcohol and substances that contain alcohol to prevent a disulfiram-like reaction. Protect the drug from exposure to light. For clients with renal or hepatic impairment, monitor blood levels of the drug to prevent toxicity.
vancomycin (Vancocin)	Inhibits cell wall synthesis of bacteria sensitive to vancomycin, killing the organisms	Ototoxicity, nausea, nephrotoxicity, urticaria (hives)	When clients are receiving long-term therapy, continually monitor results of renal function tests. Advise the client not to discontinue the drug without notifying the physician.
rifampin (Rifradin)	Inhibits RNA polymerase activity in sensitive bacterial cells	Headache, drowsiness, fatigue, dizziness, heartburn, epigastric distress, eosinophilia, thrombocytopenia, rash, "flulike syndrome"	Administer this drug to a client with an empty stomach 1 hour before or 2 hours after meals. Advise client that this drug will color body fluids orange-red. Tell the client to report fever, chills, muscle and bone pain, fatigue, anorexia, yellow skin or eye, or unusual bruising, bleeding, rash, or itching.

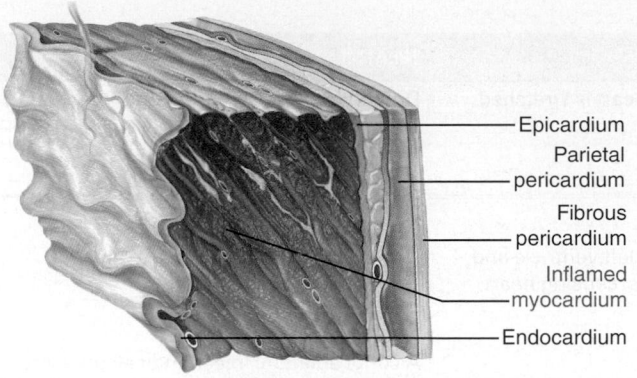

Epicardium
Parietal pericardium
Fibrous pericardium
Inflamed myocardium
Endocardium

FIGURE 23-4. Tissue changes in myocarditis.

interferes with the myocardium's ability to stretch and recoil. Cardiac output is reduced and blood circulation is impaired, predisposing the client to CHF (see Chap. 28). The myocardium becomes ischemic from a reduced supply of oxygenated blood, predisposing the client to tachycardia and dysrhythmias. Cardiomyopathy, evidenced as atypical changes in the myocardial wall, may develop as a complication of myocarditis and other disorders.

Pharmacologic Considerations

- Cardiac toxicity manifested by damage to the myocardium may develop in clients with cancer who are undergoing radiation and taking chemotherapy drugs such as doxorubicin (Adriamycin) and vinca alkaloids such as vincristine (Oncovin). Encapsulating the cardiotoxic drug in a small globule of fat called a liposome tends to shield the drug and reduce damage to the heart. Dexrazoxane (Zinecard),which blocks the formation of free radicals formed by doxorubicin, has also been used to manage cardiotoxicity.

Assessment Findings

Signs and Symptoms
Clients may complain of sharp stabbing or squeezing chest discomfort that resembles a myocardial infarction; however, sitting up relieves the pain. Accompanying manifestations include a low-grade fever, tachycardia, dysrhythmias, dyspnea, malaise, fatigue, and anorexia. The skin may be pale or cyanotic. If the heart's pumping activity becomes impaired, neck vein distention, ascites, and peripheral edema may be noted, indicating right-sided heart failure. Crackles may be heard in the lungs if the left side fails. An S_3 galloping rhythm or a pericardial friction rub may be heard.

Diagnostic Findings
Serum electrolyte levels and thyroid function studies help rule out other causes for the client's symptoms. The WBC count is slightly elevated. C-reactive protein, a nonspecific antigen–antibody test, is elevated in inflammatory conditions. Cardiac isoenzyme levels are elevated, and ECG results may be abnormal. Chest radiography shows overall

heart enlargement and fluid infiltration in the lungs. Echocardiography demonstrates structural and functional abnormalities in the ventricles, such as impaired motion of the ventricular wall and reduced ejection of blood from the heart. Radionuclide studies reveal areas where the myocardial wall is enlarged, thickened, or scarred. A myocardial biopsy may be done to obtain a definitive diagnosis.

Medical and Surgical Management
Management aims at treating the underlying cause and preventing complications. Antibiotics are prescribed if the infecting microorganism is bacterial. Bed rest, a sodium-restricted diet, and cardiotonic drugs (digitalis and related drugs) are prescribed to prevent or treat heart failure. In severe cases of cardiomyopathy, a heart transplant is necessary.

Nursing Management
The nurse monitors the client's cardiopulmonary status to assess for possible complications such as CHF or dysrhythmias. Assessments include vital signs, daily weights, intake and output, heart and lung sounds, pulse oximetry measurements, and dependent edema. The nurse also maintains the client on bed rest to reduce cardiac workload and promote healing. If the client has a fever, the nurse administers a prescribed antipyretic along with independent nursing measures such as minimizing layers of bed linens, promoting air circulation and evaporation of perspiration, and offering oral fluids. Administering supplemental oxygen relieves tachycardia that may develop from hypoxemia. The nurse elevates the client's head to promote maximal breathing potential. He or she uses a bedside cardiac monitor or telemetry unit to assess heart rhythm. The nurse uses cardiac rhythm analyses to determine if and when antidysrhythmic medications are necessary, or the client's response to their use.

CARDIOMYOPATHY

Cardiomyopathy is a chronic condition characterized by structural changes in the heart muscle. The three major types of cardiomyopathies are (1) dilated cardiomyopathy, (2) hypertrophic cardiomyopathy, and (3) restrictive cardiomyopathy (Table 23-2; Fig. 23-5). The International Society and Federation of Cardiology and the World Health Organization added two other types of cardiomyopathy to the list: arrhythmogenic right ventricular cardiomyopathy, which is inherited, and peripartum cardiomyopathy, which develops in women shortly before or after giving birth (Porth, 2006). The following discussion focuses on dilated, hypertrophic, and restrictive cardiomyopathies.

Pathophysiology and Etiology
In some cases, cardiomyopathy develops without explanation. In others, cardiomyopathy accompanies or follows another medical problem, such as myocarditis, connective tissue disorders such as systemic lupus erythematosus, muscular dystrophy, chronic alcoholism, or cancer chemotherapy.

Regardless of the cause, the heart muscle loses its ability to pump blood efficiently. When a client's medical history includes disorders that are bacterial or viral in origin, a

TABLE 23-2 Types of Cardiomyopathy

TYPE	CAUSES	DESCRIPTION	TREATMENT
Dilated	Viral myocarditis Autoimmune response Chemicals (e.g., chronic alcohol ingestion)	The cavity of the heart is stretched (dilated).	Drug therapy to minimize symptoms and prevent complications Abstinence from alcohol Salt restriction Weight loss Possible heart transplantation
Hypertrophic	Hereditary Unknown	The muscle of the left ventricle and septum thickens, causing heart enlargement.	Drug therapy to reduce heart rate and force of contraction Antidysrhythmic drugs Artificial pacemaker Alcohol ablation: injection of alcohol into an artery supplying the extra tissue to destroy excess heart muscle (currently experimental) Ventriculomyotomy, a surgical procedure to reduce muscle tissue
Restrictive	Deposits of amyloid Scleroderma, a connective tissue disorder Granulomatous tumors Hemochromatosis, iron stores in tissue Scar tissue that forms after a myocardial infarction	Heart muscle stiffens, which interferes with its ability to stretch and fill with blood.	No specific treatment; drugs such as diuretics and antihypertensives used to control symptoms

family history of early cardiac deaths, or any of several other conditions that correlate with heart involvement, the possibility of cardiomyopathy is considered. Some affected clients remain in stable condition for a long period before they develop disabling symptoms; others may be unaware of their condition until they experience a potentially fatal cardiac event such as a sudden dysrhythmia or heart failure.

Assessment Findings

Signs and Symptoms

The manifestations of cardiomyopathy vary slightly according to the type that develops. *Dilated cardiomyopathy*, the most common type, is accompanied by dyspnea on exertion and when lying down. The client feels fatigued and his or her legs swell. He or she may experience palpitations and chest pain.

Hypertrophic cardiomyopathy is associated with **syncope** (sudden loss of consciousness) or near-syncopal episodes, which the client may describe as "graying out." Clients also may feel fatigued, become short of breath, and develop chest pain. Many are asymptomatic, however, and the disorder is not discovered until the affected person dies or becomes acutely ill after strenuous exercise.

Restrictive cardiomyopathy, which is the least common type in the United States but more common in tropical locales of Africa, India, South and Central America, and Asia, has symptoms of exertional dyspnea, dependent edema in the legs, ascites (fluid in the abdomen), and hepatomegaly (enlarged liver).

A heart **murmur**, which is an atypical heart sound, may be the first abnormal sign detected in any type. Forceful heart contractions may be palpated over the left chest wall.

Diagnostic Findings

Cardiomyopathy sometimes is detected among asymptomatic clients during other diagnostic tests. For example, chest radiography may show heart enlargement. An exercise, chemical, or ambulatory ECG provides evidence of abnormal cardiac rhythm. Definitive diagnosis is determined by performing an echocardiogram and cardiac catheterization. Cardiac catheterization detects elevated pressures in the ventricles of the heart. In some cases, an endomyocardial biopsy is performed to obtain a specimen of heart tissue for microscopic examination. The biopsy may reveal **myocardial disarray** (Fig. 23-6), an alteration in the usual alignment of **myofibrils**, the contractile component of muscle tissue. The result is a lack of coordination during systole (ventricular contraction) and impaired diastole (ventricular relaxation) (Porth, 2006). Radionuclide studies show the heart muscle's inability to contract efficiently when stressed during exercise.

Medical and Surgical Management

Treatment depends on the type of cardiomyopathy (see Table 23-2). In general, diuretics, cardiac glycosides such as digitalis, and antihypertensives are prescribed to promote effective heart contraction and adequate cardiac output. Antidysrhythmics are used to manage abnormally conducted heart impulses. Anticoagulants are administered to prevent the formation of blood clots that may develop when blood pools in the heart chambers. Anti-inflammatory agents such

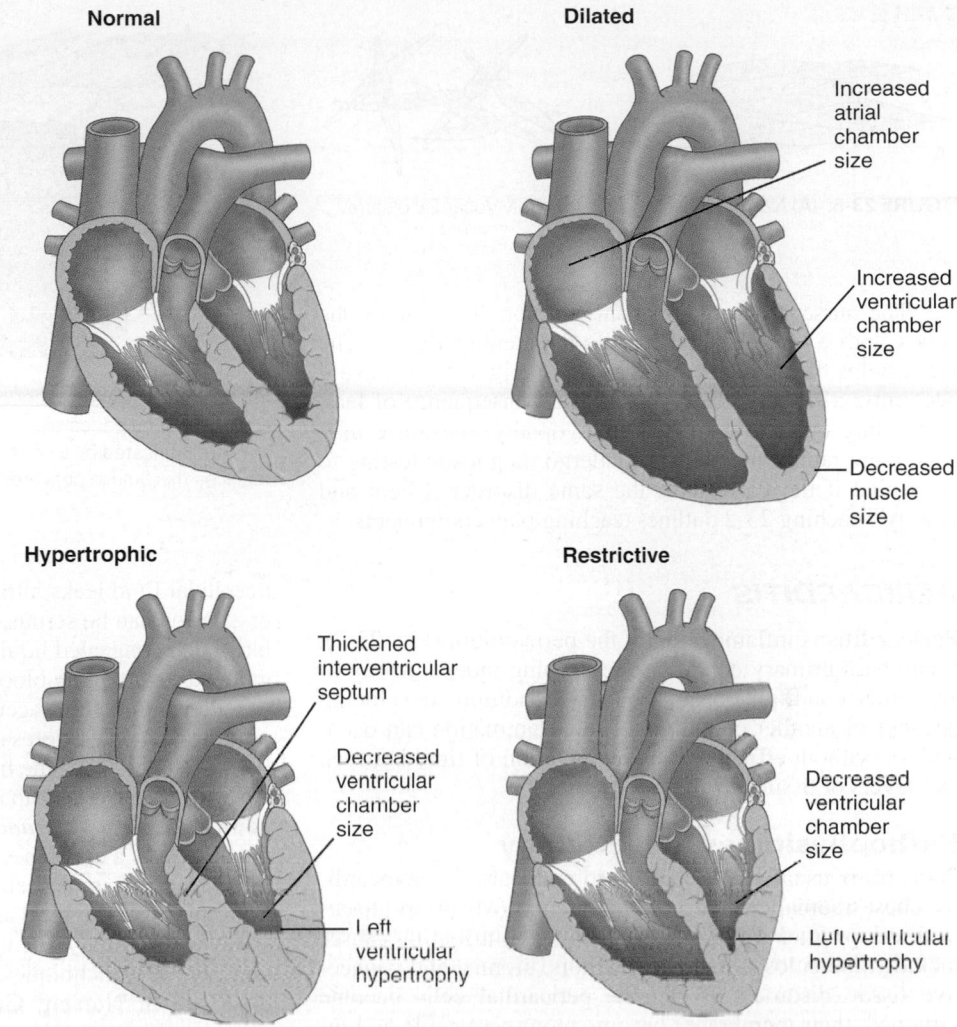

Normal

Dilated

Increased atrial chamber size

Increased ventricular chamber size

Decreased muscle size

Hypertrophic

Thickened interventricular septum

Decreased ventricular chamber size

Left ventricular hypertrophy

Restrictive

Decreased ventricular chamber size

Left ventricular hypertrophy

FIGURE 23-5. Types of cardiomyopathies: dilated, hypertrophic, and restrictive.

as corticosteroids are used in select clients to control cardiomyopathy caused by autoimmune connective tissue disorders. Dietary sodium is restricted to reduce fluid retention.

Drug therapy sometimes is accompanied by placement of an artificial pacemaker or implanted automatic defibrillator (see Chap. 26). Clients with hypertrophic cardiomyopathy may experience relief of symptoms when a **ventriculomyomectomy**, removal of thickened myocardial muscle from the septum, is performed. This surgical procedure enlarges the left ventricular chamber and allows a greater ejection of blood with each heart contraction. The mitral valve also may be replaced at the same time as the ventriculomyomectomy to correct the leakage of blood from the left atrium into the left ventricle (see Chap. 24). When there are no other alternatives for supporting the heart's pumping function, the client may become a candidate for heart transplantation (see Chap. 29). If clinical trials and FDA approval of a permanent artificial heart pump is successful, candidates for heart transplantation may be treated with this alternative.

Nursing Management

The nurse obtains a comprehensive medical and family history and asks the client to describe any symptoms. Outpatients may be attached to an ambulatory cardiac monitor; nurses teach such clients to keep a journal of their symptoms. The nurse performs a physical examination that includes taking vital signs, auscultating heart and lung sounds, and checking for peripheral edema and abdominal enlargement. He or she is especially alert for an irregular pulse, tachycardia, or reduced levels of oxygen saturation (SpO$_2$) on pulse oximetry, which may occur during postural changes or exercise. The nurse advocates for cardiac monitoring either at the bedside or by telemetry.

Oxygen is administered either continuously or when dyspnea or dysrhythmias develop. The nurse administers prescribed medications and collects data to evaluate their effectiveness. For example, if the client receives a diuretic, the nurse monitors intake and output, assesses weight, and checks for dependent edema regularly. He or she ensures that the client's activity level is reduced and sequences any activity that is slightly exertional between periods of rest.

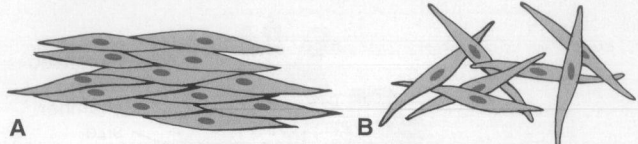

FIGURE 23-6. (**A**) Normal muscle structure. (**B**) Myocardial disarray

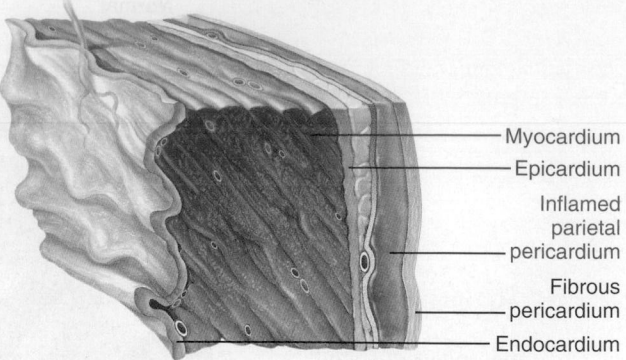

FIGURE 23-7. Tissue changes in pericarditis. Normally, the epicardium and pericardium slide over each other easily because they are lubricated by a small amount of fluid. Thicker material replaces this fluid in pericarditis.

The nurse supports the client emotionally as he or she copes with a chronic, perhaps life-threatening illness. The nurse helps the client identify realistic limitations, yet avoid becoming a self-restricted invalid as a consequence of fear. Depending on the type of cardiomyopathy, the nurse may encourage family members to undergo diagnostic testing to determine if they also have the same disorder. Client and Family Teaching 23-2 outlines teaching plan components.

PERICARDITIS

Pericarditis is inflammation of the pericardium (Fig. 23-7). It can be a primary condition (developing independently of any other condition) or a secondary condition (developing because of another condition). The inflammation can occur with or without **effusion**, the accumulation of fluid between two layers of tissue.

Pathophysiology and Etiology

Pericarditis usually is secondary to endocarditis, myocarditis, chest trauma, or myocardial infarction (MI; heart attack) or develops after cardiac surgery. Other contributing causes include tuberculosis, malignant tumors, uremia, and connective tissue disorders. When the pericardial cells become inflamed, their membranes become more permeable and in-

tracellular fluid leaks into the interstitial spaces. The exudate or effusion can be serous, resembling clear serum; fibrinous, like thick, congealed liquid; purulent, containing pus; or sanguineous, containing blood.

Pericardial fluid accumulation results in **cardiac tamponade**, acute compression of the heart. The pericardial fluid occupies space the heart needs to accommodate for filling with blood. The impaired filling is reflected by a condition called *pulsus paradoxus* or *paradoxical pulse*. **Pulsus paradoxus** is a difference of 10 mm Hg or more between the first Korotkoff sound heralding systolic blood pressure (BP) heard during expiration and the first that is heard during inspiration. Normally, the difference between the two is 4 to 5 mm Hg. The technique for detecting pulsus paradoxus is described in Nursing Guidelines 23-1. Pulsus paradoxus develops because of a greater reduction in the volume capacity of the left ventricle during inspiration, combined with an impaired ability of the left ventricle to expand because of the rigid pericardium. The smaller capacity reduces the stroke volume from the left ventricle. As cardiac tamponade progresses, stroke volume is diminished, cardiac output is compromised, and death may result if the condition continues uncorrected.

Client and Family Teaching 23-2
Cardiomyopathy

The nurse teaches the client with cardiomyopathy as follows:

- Achieve a healthy weight by following dietary instructions, limiting sodium to reduce fluid retention, and avoiding beverages containing caffeine, which contributes to tachycardia.
- Stop using tobacco products because nicotine is a vasoconstrictor and cardiac stimulant.
- Stay within your level of exercise tolerance or stop activity immediately if dyspnea or chest pain develops.
- Restrict driving or operating equipment if syncope is a common symptom.
- Keep appointments for medical follow-up to evaluate the status of the disease and symptom control.
- Receive the pneumonia vaccine and yearly influenza vaccinations to avoid pulmonary complications that may compromise cardiopulmonary function.
- For female clients, seek co-consultation with a cardiologist and an obstetrician if pregnancy is desired.

NURSING GUIDELINES 23-1

Assessment of Pulsus Paradoxus

- Advise client to breathe normally throughout the assessment.
- Inflate BP cuff 20 mm Hg above systolic pressure.
- Deflate the cuff slowly, noting that sounds are audible during expiration but not inspiration.
- Note when the first BP sound (Korotkoff's) is heard.
- Continue to deflate the cuff until BP sounds are heard during both inspiration and expiration.
- Measure the difference in mm Hg between the first BP sound heard during expiration and the first BP sound heard during both inspiration and expiration.

Assessment Findings

Signs and Symptoms

The typical signs and symptoms that accompany an inflammatory response, such as fever and malaise, are present. The client is dyspneic or complains of heaviness in the chest. One chief characteristic is **precordial pain** (pain in the anterior chest overlying the heart). It may be slight or severe and can be mistaken for esophagitis, indigestion, pleurisy, or MI. Moving and breathing deeply worsen the pain; sitting upright and leaning forward relieve it. In contrast, the pain of acute MI remains unchanged regardless of position, movement, or breathing. A pericardial friction rub, a scratchy, high-pitched sound, is a diagnostic sign. Heart sounds are difficult to hear because the accumulating fluid muffles them. Respiratory symptoms occur as the enlarged heart crowds the airway passages and lung tissue and respirations become rapid and labored. Hypotension is severe, and pulse quality is weak.

Diagnostic Findings

The ST segment of the ECG is elevated, but cardiac isoenzyme levels are normal (see Chap. 25). The heart may appear enlarged on chest radiography. Echocardiography demonstrates a wide gap between the pericardium and epicardium, indicating that the space is filled with fluid. Hemodynamic monitoring values are abnormal (see Chap. 29). Pericardial fluid may be cultured, but if the cause of the pericarditis is nonbacterial, the test results often are nondiagnostic. Because of the inflammatory nature of pericarditis, the WBC count and ESR often are elevated.

Medical and Surgical Management

MI (see Chap. 25) must be ruled out. Treatment of pericarditis depends on the underlying cause. Rest, analgesics, antipyretics, nonsteroidal anti-inflammatory drugs (NSAIDs), and sometimes corticosteroids are prescribed. **Pericardiocentesis**, needle aspiration of fluid from between the visceral and parietal pericardium, may be necessary when cardiac output is severely reduced. A small drainage catheter can be left in place. Needle aspiration is hazardous because the needle can puncture the myocardium, a branch of a coronary artery, or the pleura.

When pericardiocentesis and catheter drainage are inadequate, a **pericardiostomy**, a surgical opening or window, is made in the pericardium to allow the fluid to drain. Surgical treatment for constrictive pericarditis involves removing the pericardium (**pericardiectomy**) or removing the surface layer of the pericardium (**decortication**) to allow more adequate filling and contraction of the heart chambers.

Nursing Process for the Client With Pericarditis

Assessment

Ask the client about the incidence and nature of the pain and what worsens or relieves it. Assess for a pericardial friction rub by auscultating heart sounds while the client briefly holds his or her breath; a pericardial friction rub does not disappear when the client holds the breath. Note additional signs and symptoms that may further

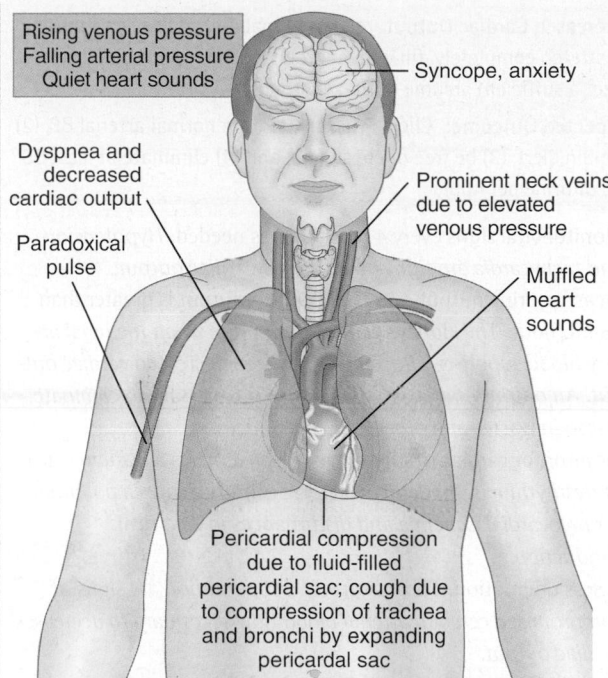

FIGURE 23-8. Signs and symptoms of cardiac tamponade.

suggest cardiac tamponade and decreased cardiac output, such as muffled heart sounds, pulsus paradoxus, jugular neck vein distention, persistent cough, dyspnea, fainting or near-fainting, anxiety, and changes in pulmonary function (Fig. 23-8).

Diagnosis, Planning, and Interventions

❧ Pain related to pericardial inflammation and decreased myocardial perfusion

❧ **Expected Outcomes:** Client will be free of pain or pain will be tolerable 30 minutes after nursing intervention.

- Assess pain status as often as vital signs. *Pain is considered the fifth vital sign. Whenever pain exists, the nurse must implement interventions targeted for its relief.*
- Assist client to a position of comfort such as sitting upright and leaning forward. *Only the outer layer of the lower parietal pericardium is sensitive to pain (Porth, 2006); some of the pain of pericarditis results from inflammation of surrounding structures. Sitting up and leaning forward positions the stretched pericardium away from the pleura, which relieves discomfort.*
- Administer anti-inflammatory drugs and analgesics as prescribed. *Reduced inflammation and pain transmission promote comfort.*
- Reassure the client that pericardial pain does not indicate an MI. *Anxiety increases heart rate and force of heart contraction, which contribute to pain. Clarifying the reality and significance of the pain may reduce the workload of the heart and acuity of discomfort.*

▶ Decreased Cardiac Output related to inability of the heart muscle to stretch completely, fill with appropriate amount of blood, and eject a sufficient volume during ventricular systole

▶ Expected Outcome: Client will (1) maintain normal arterial BP, (2) remain alert, (3) be free of chest pain, and (4) eliminate at least 35 mL of urine per hour.

- Monitor vital signs every 4 hours and as needed. *Hypotension and tachycardia are signs of decreased cardiac output.*
- Measure urine output every hour unless output is greater than 35 mL/hour. *The kidneys cannot form urine when the renal artery blood supply is reduced secondary to decreased cardiac output. An output of at least 35 mL/hour is necessary to eliminate nitrogen wastes and other toxic substances.*
- Monitor for cardiac dysrhythmias. *Hypoxemia is a leading cause of dysrhythmias. Inadequate cardiac output creates a potential for myocardial ischemia and disturbances in electrical conduction.*
- Assess orientation. *Confusion and disorientation are signs of compromised cerebral arterial blood flow secondary to decreased cardiac output.*
- Instruct the client to report chest pain. *It is a consequence of inadequate blood supply to the myocardium.*
- Maintain bed rest. *Activity increases the demand for myocardial oxygenation, which depends on cardiac output.*
- Administer supplemental oxygen as prescribed. *Giving more than the 20% oxygen that is present in room air helps to reduce hypoxemia that results from inadequate cardiac output.*
- Provide six small meals a day; avoid gas-forming foods. *Abdominal distention crowds the thoracic cavity and compresses the space the heart needs to fill with blood and the lungs need to fill with air.*
- Restrict caffeine and sodium. *Caffeine increases heart rate and sodium increases circulating blood volume, both of which increase myocardial work and the need for cardiac output.*
- Collaborate with the physician regarding a stool softener. *Bearing down during bowel movements interferes with cardiac filling and output. Stool softeners promote ease of eliminating stool.*
- Administer prescribed medications such as sedatives, anxiolytics, vasodilators, diuretics, and antidysrhythmics. *Reducing anxiety, keeping the client calm and quiet, reducing BP and volume, and facilitating normal heart conduction help avoid exceeding the heart's ability to eject an adequate cardiac output.*

▶ PC: Cardiac Tamponade

▶ Expected Outcome: The nurse will manage and minimize cardiac tamponade.

- Monitor for tachycardia, pulsus paradoxus, neck vein distention, cough, syncope, and muffled heart sounds every 4 hours and as needed. *This cluster of signs and symptoms accompanies cardiac tamponade, which interferes with filling volumes. Blood that cannot enter the heart accumulates in both venous and pulmonary circulation.*

- Have an emergency pericardiocentesis tray available. *Removing fluid from between the parietal and visceral pericardium relieves cardiac tamponade.*
- Reinforce the physician's explanation of a pericardiocentesis and witness the client's signature on a consent form. *Pericardiocentesis is an invasive procedure that requires informed consent from the client if he or she is alert or from whoever has durable power of attorney for healthcare.*
- Obtain baseline vital signs before pericardiocentesis. *They are used for comparison during and after the pericardiocentesis.*
- Measure, describe, and record the amount of pericardial fluid removed. *Documentation is a record of the client's care and outcomes of treatment.*
- Label all specimens for laboratory analysis and send them promptly to the laboratory. *Accurate information and prompt delivery facilitate diagnosis and appropriate treatment.*
- Cover the site of the pericardiocentesis with a sterile dressing and inspect the dressing for bleeding or leaking fluid. *Compromising the skin and underlying tissue creates a potential for blood and fluid loss as well as an entry site for microorganisms.*
- Reinforce the dressing if it becomes moist. *Moist gauze acts as a wick and pulls microorganisms from the skin surface toward the puncture wound and deeper tissue.*
- Continue to monitor vital signs until they are stable. *Continued assessments help identify complications so they can be treated early or validate a favorable response to therapy.*

Evaluation of Expected Outcomes

The client states pain is relieved. Vital signs are stable, and cardiac rhythm is normal. The client is alert and oriented. Urine output exceeds 35 mL/hour. Cardiac tamponade is managed. ●

▶ **Stop, Think, and Respond Exercise 23-3**

While caring for a client with pericarditis, you measure the client's BP and hear the first Korotkoff sound during expiration at 110 mm Hg. The sounds continue throughout auscultation, and you note that when the manometer is at 98 mm Hg, you hear sounds during both inspiration and expiration. Is this client manifesting pulsus paradoxus?

INFLAMMATORY DISORDERS OF THE PERIPHERAL BLOOD VESSELS

THROMBOPHLEBITIS

Thrombophlebitis is an inflammation of a vein accompanied by clot or thrombus formation. Although clots can form in any blood vessel, the veins deep in the lower extremities are most commonly affected. In such cases, the condition is referred to as **deep vein thrombosis** (DVT). Thrombi that form in or above the popliteal vein of the leg are at high risk for migration toward the pulmonary circulation; these cases are referred to as a **pulmonary embolus** (PE).

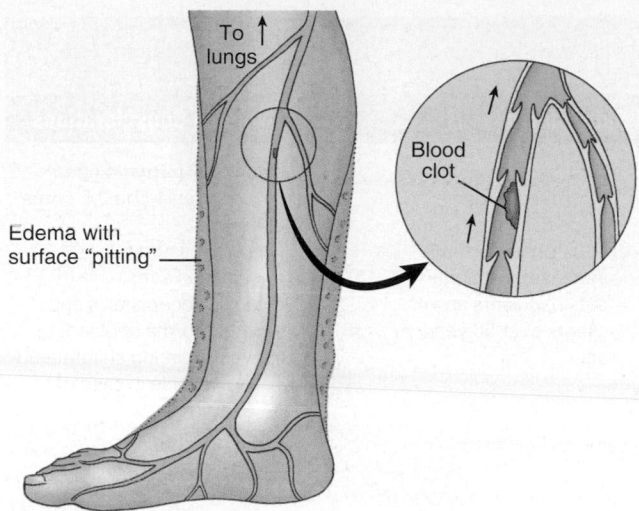

To lungs

Blood clot

Edema with surface "pitting"

FIGURE 23-9. Deep vein thrombosis accompanied by pitting edema.

Pathophysiology and Etiology

When the inner lining of a vein is irritated or injured, platelets clump together, forming a clot (Fig. 23-9). The clot interferes with blood flow, causing congestion of venous blood distal to the blood clot. Sometimes collateral vessels recirculate the blood blocked by the clot. Accumulated waste products in the blocked vessel irritate the vein wall, initiating an inflammatory response. The increased permeability of cells and the convergence of leukocytes and lymphocytes cause the area to swell, redden, and feel warm and tender.

The development of a PE may complicate thrombophlebitis if the clot in the extremity becomes mobile and moves in the venous circulation to the lungs (see Chap. 21). Despite appropriate and successful treatment of thrombophlebitis, some clients experience a vascular complication referred to as **postphlebitic syndrome** for up to 5 years after the initial episode (Church, 2000). For example, valvular impairment in the affected vein may follow the original thrombotic event. The incompetent valves are less efficient at returning venous blood to the heart. When venous pressure increases because of pooled blood, some fluid leaks from capillaries into subcutaneous tissue, causing leg ulcers.

Venous stasis (slowed circulation), altered blood coagulation, and trauma to the vein, referred to as **Virchow's triad**, predispose clients to thrombosis and thrombophlebitis. Factors that contribute to clot formation include inactivity, reduced cardiac output, compression of the veins in the pelvis or legs, and injury. Some IV drugs and chemicals also irritate the vein. Thrombi are prone to form in arm, subclavian, or jugular veins cannulated for extended IV use. Older adults with heart and blood vessel disease are susceptible to thrombophlebitis because of impaired mobility, reduced activity, and compromised circulation. Risk for clot formation is increased among women who take oral contraceptives, although the exact trigger is not known. Women who take oral contraceptives and smoke are at even higher risk.

Assessment Findings

Signs and Symptoms

Clients with thrombophlebitis often complain of discomfort in the affected extremity. Calf pain that increases on dorsiflexion of the foot is referred to as a positive **Homans' sign**. Heat, redness, and swelling develop along the length of the affected vein. Capillary refill takes less than 2 seconds because of venous congestion. The client often has a fever, malaise, fatigue, and anorexia.

Diagnostic Tests

Most cases of thrombophlebitis are diagnosed according to clinical findings alone. Doppler ultrasound is a noninvasive diagnostic technique for imaging blood flow through cardiovascular structures that may detect an area of venous obstruction. The results of Doppler ultrasound sometimes are difficult to interpret because there are so many collateral vessels, and deep veins are especially difficult to assess.

Venography, using radiopaque dye instilled into the venous system, indicates a filling defect in the area of the clot. It is important to assess the client's allergy history prior to a venography because some are hypersensitive to the dye. Following a venography, the vein is flushed and the client is instructed to drink extra fluids to promote dye excretion.

Impedance plethysmography (IPG) is the preferred test for diagnosing clots in deep veins. During IPG, a sensor records blood volume in the arm or leg before and after inflating a BP cuff to stop venous blood flow. If a clot is present, the blood volumes are nearly the same because the clot impairs venous return.

Medical and Surgical Management

Complete rest of the arm or leg is essential to prevent the thrombus from breaking free and floating in the circulation (embolus). Anticoagulant therapy with heparin, oral anticoagulants, or drugs that prevent platelet aggregation (clustering) are prescribed to decrease the incidence of future clot formation (Drug Therapy Table 23-2). With the advent of low-molecular-weight heparins such as enoxaparin (Lovenox), some clients with thrombophlebitis in which the thrombi are small are not hospitalized but treated at home. People with repeated episodes may be placed on oral anticoagulant therapy for 3 to 6 months. Continuous warm, wet packs are ordered to improve circulation, ease pain, and decrease inflammation.

Surgical intervention may be necessary when a clot occludes a large vein or the danger of a PE arises. **Thrombectomy**, the surgical removal of a clot, is performed if the clot interferes with venous drainage from a large vein such as the femoral vein. With danger of PE, surgery on the inferior vena cava may be necessary to reduce the possibility of a clot traveling from the legs to the lungs. Several surgical procedures may be performed on the vena cava: ligation, insertion of a vena caval filter, or plication. A **vena caval filter** (Fig. 23-10) is an umbrella-like filter inserted to trap emboli before they reach the heart and lungs. A **vena caval plication** is a procedure that changes the lumen of the vena

DRUG THERAPY TABLE 23-2 Anticoagulants

Drug	Mechanism of Action	Side Effects	Nursing Considerations
heparin sodium (Hepalean)	Inhibits thrombus and clot formation by blocking the conversion of pro-thrombin to thrombin and fibrinogen to fibrin	Hemorrhage, bruising, thrombocytopenia, alopecia, chills, fever Chance of hemorrhage increases with oral anticoagulants and in clients over 60 years of age	Monitor PTT test range between 1.5 to 2.5 times normal. Apply pressure to all IM injection sites. Monitor for epistaxis and other forms of bleeding. Have protamine sulfate readily available in case of overdose.
fondaparinux sodium (Arixtra, a synthetic derivative of heparin)	Same as heparin sodium	Same as heparin sodium	Administered only subcutaneously
low-molecular-weight heparin, enoxaparin (Lovenox), dalteparin (Fragmin), ardeparin (Normiflo)	Inhibits thrombus and clot formation by blocking clotting factors Xa and IIa	Bruising, hemorrhage, fever, pain, local irritation	Note that laboratory monitoring is not done. Provide devices like a soft toothbrush and electric razor to protect against bleeding. Ensure the availability of protamine sulfate in case of overdose. Ensure that the client avoids foods with vitamin K.
warfarin (Coumadin)	Interferes with the hepatic synthesis of vitamin K–dependent clotting factors	Nausea, alopecia, urticaria, dermatitis, prolonged bleeding	Monitor PT ratio or INR regularly to adjust dosage. Evaluate client regularly for signs of blood loss—petechiae, dark stools and urine, bruises, bleeding gums. Keep vitamin K on hand in case of overdose. Monitor WBC count before and during therapy to assess for neutropenia.
clopidogrel (Plavix)	Inhibits binding of fibrinogen and interactions of platelets	Diarrhea, nausea, vomiting, abdominal pain, neutropenia, phlebitis	Administer with food. Give with food.
aspirin	Inhibits platelet aggregation	Nausea, epigastric pain, occult blood loss, anaphylaxis, tinnitus, dizziness, increased risk of bleeding, especially with other anticoagulants	Advise client not to crush or chew enteric-coated or sustained-release tablets.
glycoprotein IIb/IIIa inhibitors: tirofiban (Aggrastat)	Binds to the platelet receptor glycoprotein, preventing fibrinogen from binding	Dizziness, weakness, bleeding, hypotension	Use in conjunction with heparin. Assess complete blood count, PT, aPTT, and active clotting time before and periodically during therapy.
direct thrombin inhibitors: argatroban (Acova, Novastan), bivalirudin (Angiomax)	Inhibit thrombin directly, binds with and inhibits thrombin that is free in the blood and thrombin bound in clots	Fever, nausea, allergic reactions, hepatic impairment, minor bleeding, back pain	Monitor for bleeding. Assess complete blood count, PT, aPTT. To this point is used with aspirin, administered by continuous IV infusion, and not suited for outpatient use.

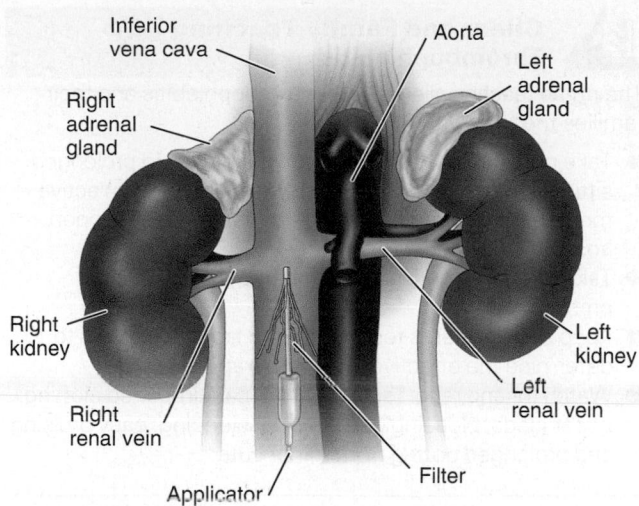

FIGURE 23-10. A permanently implanted vena caval filter is an umbrella-like filter that allows blood to circulate to the lungs but traps blood clots before they enter the pulmonary circulation. The filter is inserted with an applicator; the applicator is withdrawn when the filter fixes itself to the wall of the inferior vena cava.

cava from a single channel to several small channels through the use of a suture or Teflon clip.

Nursing Process for the Client With Thrombophlebitis

Assessment

Determine whether the client has a history of blood clots or other risk factors that predispose to thrombus formation, such as cardio-vascular disorders or recent surgery, especially repair of a hip frac-ture or hip joint replacement; self-imposed inactivity as a result of obesity or sedentary lifestyle; immobility from a medical condition, pain, or treatment regimen; current use of an oral contraceptive; use of tobacco products; dehydration that may decrease the fluid volume of blood; or recent trauma to an extremity.

Assess for Homans' sign by asking whether the client experien-ces pain or tenderness in the calf of the affected extremity when dorsiflexing the foot, or if movement causes or aggravates pain. Inspect the color, temperature, and capillary refill of extremities and measure the circumference of the leg (or arm) at various areas; compare the findings with the unaffected extremity. Regularly check for a low-grade fever. Consult with the client about chest pain and dyspnea, which are hallmarks of PE, a complication of thrombophlebitis. If drug therapy is prescribed, monitor the labora-tory test results associated with anticoagulant therapy.

 Pharmacologic Considerations

- Frequent monitoring of prothrombin time (PT) is important for clients taking the oral anticoagulant, warfarin (Coumadin), for venous thrombosis; PT should be 1.5 to 2.5 times the control value (12–15 seconds) to achieve the therapeutic effect of anticoagulant therapy. When PT is reported as an international normalized ratio (INR) factor, the normal range is 2.0 to 3.0.

- The anticoagulant heparin is measured in units and the dosage is regulated by venous clotting time determinations, such as a partial thromboplastin time (PTT) or activated partial thromboplastin time (aPTT). Optimum drug effect is reached when PTT and aPTT are 1.5 to 2.5 times normal.

- The risk of hemorrhage during heparin therapy is greater in clients 60 years of age or older.

Diagnosis, Planning, and Interventions

An important role is to prevent venous stasis and thrombophlebitis by promoting activity and exercise for at-risk clients (Fig. 23-11). Ankle-pumping exercises are imperative for clients on bed rest. For inactive clients, apply knee- or thigh-high elastic stockings or use a pneumatic venous compression device that alternately inflates and deflates to support vein walls and promote venous circulation (Fig. 23-12). Assist the client to change positions frequently and avoid restricting venous blood flow from prolonged sitting or bending the bed at the knees (Client and Family Teaching 23-3).

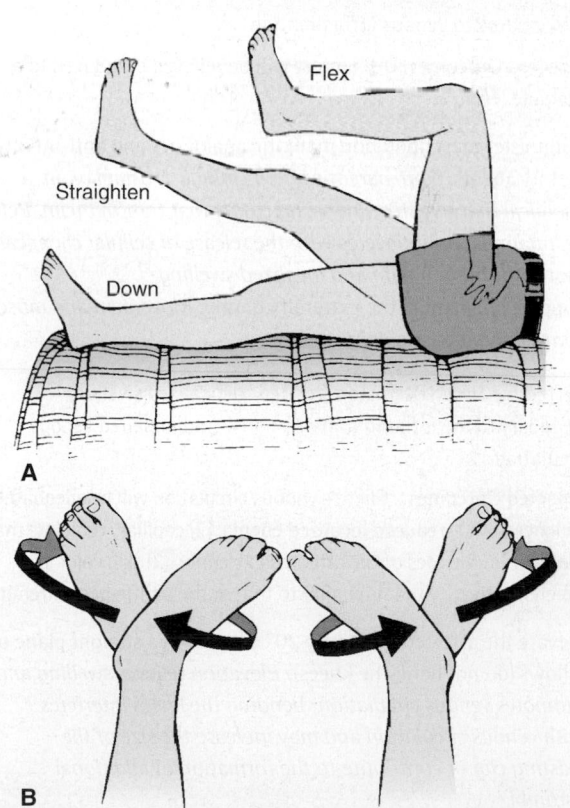

FIGURE 23-11. Leg exercises help prevent thrombophlebitis. **(A)** Have client raise the leg, bend the knee, and hold for 3 seconds. Repeat with each leg five times each hour. **(B)** Have client trace circles five times with each foot every hour.

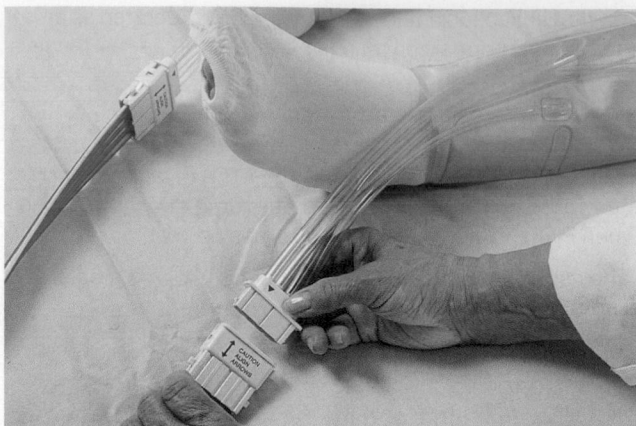

FIGURE 23-12. Pneumatic compression device.

 Gerontologic Considerations

-Encourage older clients who are inactive to move every hour during the day to promote circulation. Such movement is especially important during long car or airplane trips, and can be as simple as flexion and extension of the foot.

Additional nursing management includes the following measures.

▸ **Pain** related to venous inflammation

▸ **Expected Outcome:** Discomfort will be relieved or reduced to a tolerable level.

• Administer prescribed non-narcotic analgesics and anti-inflammatory agents. *Non-narcotic agents inhibit prostaglandin, a chemical that sensitizes nerve receptors that transmit pain. Relief of inflammation interferes with the release of cellular chemicals that contribute to pain and localized swelling.*

• Support and handle the extremity gently. *Movement and muscle contraction increase pain.*

▸ **Ineffective Tissue Perfusion** related to localized swelling secondary to the inflammatory response and impaired venous circulation

▸ **Expected Outcomes:** Client's venous circulation will be adequate as evidenced by (1) reduced localized edema, (2) capillary refill less than 3 seconds in the toes of the affected extremity, (3) skin color in affected extremity that is similar to that of the unaffected extremity.

• Elevate the affected extremity 20° or more in a straight plane on pillows (do not bend the knees). *Elevation relieves swelling and promotes venous circulation; bending the knees interferes with venous circulation and may increase the size of the existing clot or contribute to the formation of additional thrombi.*

• Apply warm, moist compresses to the area of discomfort or apply an aquathermia pad over protected skin at a setting of approximately 105°F (40.5°C). Remove compresses and reapply after 20 minutes or sooner if cooling occurs. Remove the

 Client and Family Teaching 23-3
Thrombophlebitis

The nurse teaches clients with thrombophlebitis and their families the following:

● Take measures to prevent recurrences: avoid prolonged sitting and crossing the legs at the knee, perform active movement, elevate the legs periodically, wear support hose, and drink fluids liberally

● Take long-term anticoagulant therapy exactly as prescribed

● Keep appointments for the ordered laboratory tests to determine the effectiveness of therapy

● Watch for and report signs that indicate impaired clotting: nosebleeds, bleeding gums, rectal bleeding, easy bruising, and prolonged oozing from minor cuts

aquathermia pad every 2 hours for 20 minutes to assess the skin. *Warmth dilates blood vessels, improves circulation, and relieves swelling, all of which relieve discomfort. Moist heat is more comforting than dry heat. Skin assessments are standard care to avoid injury.*

• Promote a liberal intake (2000–2500 mL/24 hours) of oral fluid unless contraindicated. *Adequate fluid volume dilutes blood cells in plasma and reduces the risk for platelet aggregation.*

▸ **PC: Pulmonary Embolus**

▸ **Expected Outcome:** The nurse manages and minimizes complications such as a PE.

• Maintain bed rest after the diagnosis of thrombophlebitis for approximately 1 week or until the physician discontinues activity restriction. *Restricting activity helps stabilize the blood clot to the vein wall and decreases the risk of its conversion to an embolus.*

• Administer prescribed anticoagulant therapy. *Depending on the prescribed drugs, medications that alter clotting factors or interfere with platelet aggregation prevent additional thrombi and subsequent emboli.*

• Instruct client to perform active leg exercises with the unaffected extremity at least five times each waking hour. *Exercise prevents venous stasis by promoting venous circulation toward the heart. Promoting venous blood flow prevents the formation of thrombi and subsequent potential for emboli in the unaffected extremity.*

• Apply elastic stockings to extremities if prescribed by the physician. *Elastic stockings support the valves in veins and reduce the potential for venous stasis and clot formation.*

• Monitor for dyspnea, tachypnea, cough, hypotension, abnormal lung sounds, or chest pain. *Abnormal results of focus assessments indicate cardiopulmonary complications such as a PE.*

• Elevate the head if dyspnea develops. *Head elevation lowers abdominal organs away from the diaphragm and facilitates increased inspiration of higher lung volumes to compensate for impaired oxygenation in the pulmonary circulation.*

- Prepare to administer oxygen by cannula or mask if dyspnea and chest pain occur. *Raising oxygen levels above 20% compensates for impaired oxygenation at the alveolar-capillary level.*
- Prepare to start an IV and administer parenteral narcotic analgesia and emergency medications by the IV route. *Drug therapy helps relieve severe chest pain and improve BP.*

▶ PC: Bleeding

▶ Expected Outcome: The nurse will manage and minimize blood loss.

- Monitor laboratory test findings that reflect coagulation status such as partial thromboplastin time (PTT), prothrombin time (PT), and international normalized ratio (INR); report values that exceed therapeutic levels. *With the exception of low-molecular-weight heparin, doses of anticoagulant drug therapy are adjusted according to laboratory test results.*
- Calculate dosages of anticoagulants carefully and administer drug therapy as prescribed. *Unfractionated heparin may be administered by IV infusion; the dose often is titrated according to PTT and may require periodic rate adjustments during the infusion. Oral and subcutaneous dosages of anticoagulants (except low-molecular-weight heparin) may be changed daily.*
- Keep antidotes for overdose of anticoagulants (protamine sulfate for unfractionated heparin and vitamin K [phytonadione, Aqua-Mephyton] for warfarin) available. *In extreme cases, it may be prudent to quickly reverse the effects of anticoagulant therapy.*
- Observe the client for blood in the urine or stool, easy bruising, bleeding gums, and excessive bleeding from minor cuts or scratches. *These findings are signs of impaired clotting and suggest that the client could easily bleed internally.*
- Provide the client with a soft-bristled toothbrush for oral hygiene; advise using an electric razor for shaving. *Reducing the potential for skin and soft tissue trauma decreases the possibility of bleeding.*
- Test stools, emesis, urine, and nasogastric drainage for blood. *Hemoccult testing may detect blood that is not obvious to the naked eye.*
- Protect the client from falls or other trauma. *An injury, even though ordinarily minor, may precipitate excessive or prolonged bleeding if the client is receiving anticoagulant therapy.*
- Perform neurologic assessments every 1 to 2 hours if the client experiences a head injury (see Chaps. 36 and 39). *Changes in level of consciousness, size and response of pupils to light, and verbal responses suggest intracranial bleeding.*
- Apply direct pressure to the site of external bleeding. *Pressure compresses vascular walls and decreases blood flow, providing time for an initial clot to form.*
- Place an ice pack at the site of prolonged oozing of blood. *Ice causes vasoconstriction and decreases the volume of blood loss.*
- Be prepared to administer IV fluid, blood, or blood products. *Parenteral fluids replace lost fluid volume; blood and blood products replace cells and fluid.*

Evaluation of Expected Outcomes

Expected outcomes include reduced or eliminated pain. Venous circulation improves and adequate blood flow to the heart is maintained; both extremities are comparable in size, temperature, and color. Passive Homans' sign is negative; a PE does not develop, or if it does, it is managed successfully. Bleeding is prevented or controlled. ●

THROMBOANGIITIS OBLITERANS (BUERGER'S DISEASE)

Thromboangiitis obliterans, also known as Buerger's disease, is inflammation of blood vessels associated with clot formation and fibrosis of the blood vessel wall. It affects primarily the small arteries and veins of the legs. It occasionally involves the arms.

Pathophysiology and Etiology

The cause of thromboangiitis obliterans has not been established. It is far more common in men than in women, and the onset usually is during young adulthood. Cigarette smoking aggravates the condition. The affected arteries are prone to spasms that constrict the arterial lumen. Inflammatory lesions are found in isolated segments intermixed among healthy areas of the same vessel. The lesions occlude blood flow through the vessel during exercise and at rest. Skin and soft tissue cells experience degrees of hypoxia and anoxia. Some cells die. The necrotic (dead) tissues slough, forming ulcerations. The extent may be so severe that gangrene results. Thrombophlebitis also may be present.

Assessment Findings

The client notes that one or both feet are always cold and may report numbness, burning, and tingling in some areas of the feet. **Intermittent claudication**, leg cramps after exercise, is a common symptom. Pain occurs at rest when circulation has been seriously impaired. The symptoms usually fluctuate in severity; remissions often follow attacks of acute distress.

Cyanosis and redness of the feet and legs sometimes occur. The skin frequently is a mottled purplish-red and appears thin and shiny, with sparse hair growth. Shallow, dry leg ulcers in various stages of healing may be seen. Black gangrenous areas may develop on the toes and heels (Fig. 23-13). The nails are thick. Peripheral pulses are present during rest but diminish or disappear with activity. Capillary refill is prolonged. Doppler ultrasound, IPG, and angiography help to evaluate the location and extent of vessel destruction.

Medical and Surgical Management

Tobacco in any form is restricted. Buerger-Allen exercises are ordered to stimulate and promote collateral circulation. Walking and active foot exercises are allowed as long as they do not cause pain. Analgesics are prescribed to ease discomfort. If leg ulcers develop, treatment may include moist dressings that are changed when the gauze becomes damp (i.e., wet-to-dry dressings) and topical antiseptics or antibiotic ointments.

Sympathectomy, the surgical interruption or suppression of some portion of the sympathetic nerve pathway, is

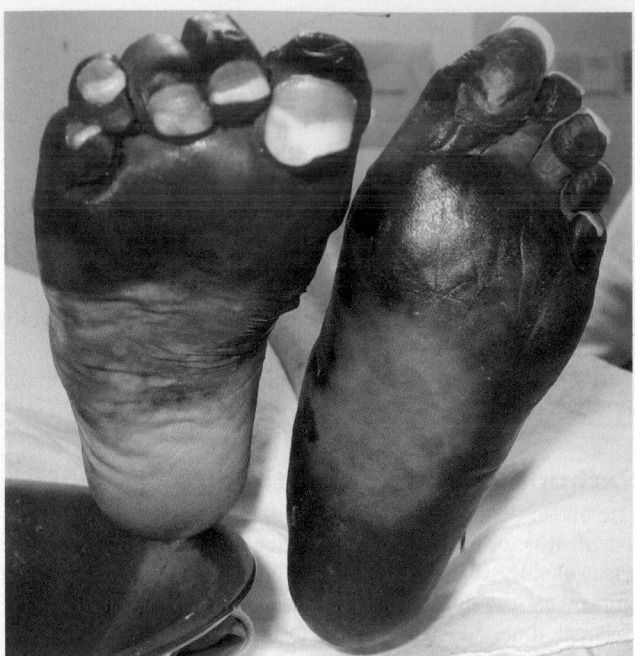

FIGURE 23-13. Thromboangiitis obliterans accompanied by gangrene. (Image provided by Stedman's).

performed to relieve vasospasm. If ulcerations occur, wound debridement (removal of necrotic tissue) and skin grafting may be required. If circulation becomes so impaired that gangrene results, amputation is necessary.

Pharmacologic Consideration

- Pentoxifylline (Trental) may be used to improve (but not cure) intermittent claudication. This drug decreases blood viscosity and improves blood flow. Common adverse reactions include nausea, dizziness, headache, and dyspepsia.

Nursing Management

The nurse takes a thorough history, including a smoking history and a review of symptoms and how long they have been present. He or she records the client's description of the type and degree of pain and factors that increase or decrease it. The nurse examines the affected areas for redness, swelling, and other color changes, such as cyanosis and mottling. He or she inspects the nails and skin for changes and notes the skin temperature above and below the affected area. The nurse also monitors the presence and quality of peripheral pulses and assesses capillary refill time.

The nurse instructs and supervises the client about Buerger-Allen leg exercises (Client and Family Teaching 23-4). When the client is not performing exercises, he or she must keep the legs horizontal or dependent. Elevating the legs increases ischemia and, therefore, contributes to pain. The nurse carries out meticulous wound care if leg or foot ulcers exist.

Client and Family Teaching 23-4
Performing Buerger-Allen Exercises

The nurse teaches the client to:

1. Lie flat in bed with both legs elevated above the level of the heart for 2 or 3 minutes.
2. Sit on the edge of the bed with the legs dependent, or lower than the head, for 3 minutes.
3. Exercise the feet and toes by moving them up, down, inward, and outward.
4. Return to the first position and hold it for about 5 minutes.
5. Repeat the exercises several times during one exercise period and perform them periodically throughout the day.

Hospitalization for acute problems or complications may occur, but the client must carry out most care at home. The nurse teaches the client self-care techniques and stresses the importance of smoking cessation and performing prescribed exercises consistently. He or she instructs clients to avoid caffeine, tobacco products, and over-the-counter drugs that cause vasoconstriction, such as nasal decongestants. The nurse advises the client to inspect the fingernails, toenails, and skin on the arms and legs daily. He or she teaches the client to clean the arms and legs daily; prevent trauma to the extremities; wear properly fitting shoes and stockings (or socks); and avoid prolonged exposure to the cold. When cold weather is unavoidable, the nurse advises the client to wear thick socks or insulated boots and gloves to protect against exposure to low temperatures.

CRITICAL THINKING EXERCISES

1. Of the three major inflammatory disorders of the heart, endocarditis, myocarditis, and pericarditis, which has the fewest long-term effects? Support your answer.
2. A client complains of intermittent claudication, pain when the legs are elevated, and cold, numb feet. The nurse notes several dry ulcerations of the feet. Does the client suffer from venous or arterial insufficiency? What additional assessment data must the nurse collect? What lifestyle habits might predispose the client to this disorder?
3. What health teaching is important for a client with a history of thrombophlebitis?
4. Which category of anticoagulant drug therapy would a client be most able to manage independently?

NCLEX-STYLE REVIEW QUESTIONS

1. A client comes to the emergency department complaining of dyspnea and heaviness in the chest. Pericarditis is suspected, and further investigation reveals severe precordial pain. When auscultating the client's chest, which of the following should the nurse anticipate hearing?
   1. A friction rub
   2. Well-defined S_1 and S_2 heart sounds
   3. Expiratory wheezing
   4. A bounding apical pulse

2. A client with thrombophlebitis receives instructions regarding this condition. Which statement made by the client indicates a need for further teaching?
   1. "When I go back to work, I need to change my position often."
   2. "I will need to take anticoagulants for a while."
   3. "I will notify the nurse if I have any trouble breathing."
   4. "When I feel cramping in my calf, I should rub it until the pain goes away."

3. A client is diagnosed with endocarditis. When obtaining the client's medical history, which question asked by the nurse is most important initially?
   1. "Have you recently been treated for strep throat?"
   2. "Have you recently had flu-like symptoms?"
   3. "Do you have any skin rashes?"
   4. "Have you had any recent cuts or bruises?"

4. Which of the following nursing interventions should a nurse perform when a client with cardiomyopathy receives a diuretic? Select all that apply.
   1. Monitor intake and output
   2. Administer oxygen
   3. Assess daily weight
   4. Check for dependent edema
   5. Maintain strict bed rest

5. The nurse checks the results of the partial thromboplastin time (PTT) of a client who has been receiving a daily subcutaneous dose of heparin. The client's PTT is 100 seconds; the normal PTT value is 60 to 70 seconds. Which of the following can the nurse expect when the PTT lab result is reported to the physician?
   1. The physician will order the same daily dose of heparin because the client's PTT level is within a therapeutic range.
   2. The physician will order a higher dose of heparin because the client is not adequately anticoagulated.
   3. The physician will order to withhold today's dose of heparin because the client's ability to clot is dangerously impaired.
   4. The physician will order protamine sulfate to counteract the effect of the heparin.

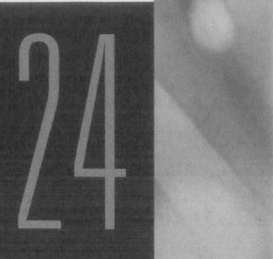

24

Caring for Clients with Valvular Disorders of the Heart

Words To Know

aortic regurgitation
aortic stenosis
balloon valvuloplasty
commissures
mitral regurgitation
mitral stenosis
mitral valve prolapse
mitral valve prolapse syndrome
point of maximum impulse
valvular incompetence
valvular regurgitation
water-hammer pulse

Learning Objectives

On completion of this chapter, you will be able to:

1. List five disorders that commonly affect heart valves.
2. Discuss assessment findings common among clients with valvular disorders.
3. Name three diagnostic tests used to confirm valvular disorders.
4. Identify consequences of valvular disorders.
5. Name five categories of drugs used to treat valvular disorders.
6. Give two examples of treatments other than drug therapy to correct valvular disorders.
7. Discuss nursing management of clients with valvular disorders.

Each heart structure helps to maintain normal cardiac function. The four cardiac valves—aortic, mitral, tricuspid, and pulmonic—promote the forward circulation of blood to sustain adequate cardiac output (Fig. 24-1). The structure and function of cardiac valves can be affected by malformations at birth, inflammatory and infectious disorders (see Chap. 23), age-related degeneration, structural damage after myocardial infarction (MI), or injury during an intracardiac procedure. The aortic and mitral valves, located on the left side of the heart, where fluid pressures are higher than on the right side, are most commonly affected. Less common are disorders involving the pulmonic and tricuspid valves. This chapter provides information on common valvular disorders and the medical and nursing management of clients who are affected.

DISORDERS OF THE AORTIC VALVE

The aortic valve has three cusps, or leaflets, and is described as a *semilunar* valve because each cusp appears like a half-moon. The left ventricle pumps blood from the heart through the aortic valve. When the left ventricle contracts, a nondiseased aortic valve opens to allow the unrestricted passage of oxygenated blood into the arterial vascular system. The coronary arteries supplying the myocardium are the first blood vessels perfused. After ejection of left ventricular blood, the aortic valve closes tightly to prevent backflow of blood. Two valvular conditions interfere with unidirectional blood flow from the left side of the heart: aortic stenosis and aortic regurgitation.

AORTIC STENOSIS

Stenosis means *narrowing*. **Aortic stenosis** is a narrowing of the opening in the aortic valve when the valve cusps become stiff and rigid. It is a common valvular disorder in the United States, especially among older adults.

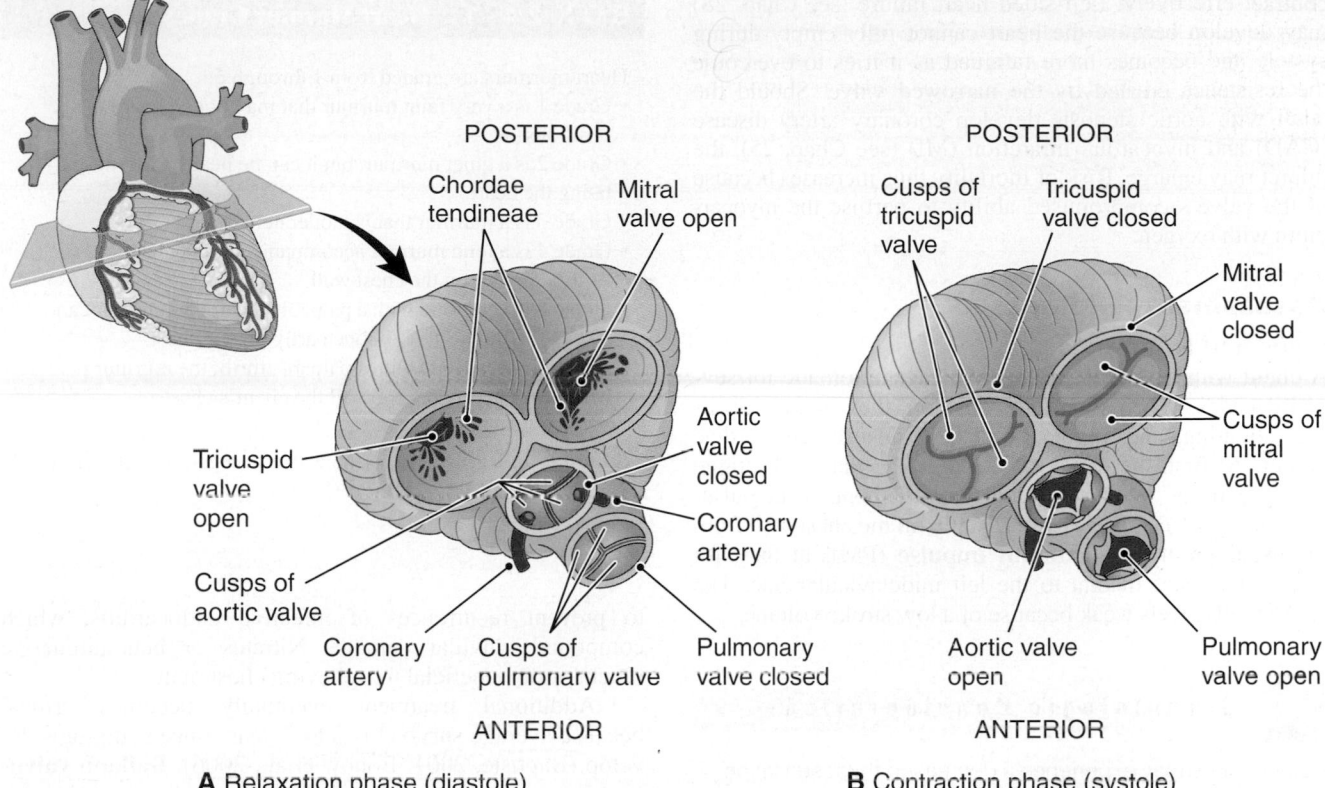

POSTERIOR

Chordae tendineae — Mitral valve open

Tricuspid valve open

Cusps of aortic valve

Coronary artery — Cusps of pulmonary valve — Pulmonary valve closed

Aortic valve closed

Coronary artery

ANTERIOR

A Relaxation phase (diastole)

POSTERIOR

Cusps of tricuspid valve — Tricuspid valve closed

Mitral valve closed

Cusps of mitral valve

Aortic valve open — Pulmonary valve open

ANTERIOR

B Contraction phase (systole)

FIGURE 24-1. Valves of the heart. **(A)** During diastole, the tricuspid and mitral valves are open and allow blood to flow freely from the atria to the ventricles. The aortic and pulmonary valves are closed. **(B)** When the ventricles contract (systole), the tricuspid and mitral valves close, preventing blood from returning to the atria. The pulmonary and aortic valves open as blood is ejected from the ventricles. (Adapted from Cohen, B. J. & Taylor, J. J. [2009]. Memmler's structure and function of the human body. [9th ed.]. Philadelphia: Lippincott Williams & Wilkins.)

Pathophysiology and Etiology

In older adults without predisposing cardiac conditions, narrowing of the aortic valve is an age related degenerative change from progressive calcium deposits in valve cells. In young adults, aortic stenosis usually is a later consequence of a congenital defect in which the valve has two instead of three cusps. At birth and throughout childhood, this defect does not produce symptoms. Symptoms appear after several decades, when the same calcification process that affects older adults causes the valves to harden. In others, aortic stenosis results directly from valvular damage related to rheumatic carditis and infective endocarditis (see Chap. 23).

Gerontologic Considerations

- Age-related effects, such as stiffening of the aorta and calcification and fibrotic thickening of the mitral and aortic valves, contribute to development of symptoms (e.g., increased systolic blood pressure, dangerous dysrhythmias) and complications (e.g., increased myocardial oxygen demand, heart failure, and alterations in cardiac output) in the older adult with valvular heart disease (Cheitlin, 2006).

The stiff, calcified valve cannot open properly and needs more force to push blood through its narrowed opening

(Fig. 24-2). The muscular wall of the left ventricle enlarges and thickens (*hypertrophies*) in response. The blood volume passing through the narrowed valve eventually becomes insufficient to nourish the myocardium and other organs. Exercise or any circumstance that increases heart rate can cause myocardial ischemia, affecting the heart's ability to

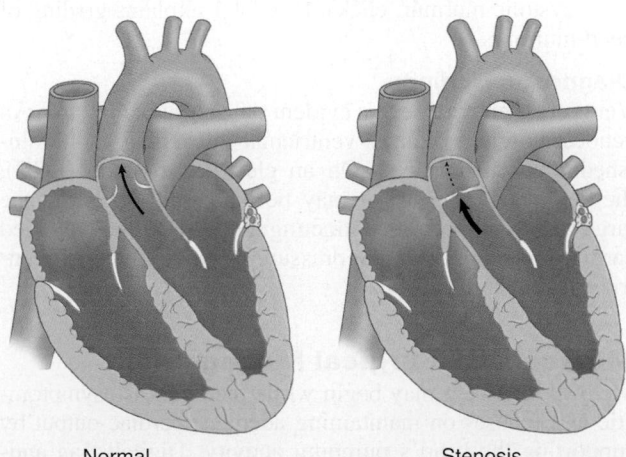

Normal   Stenosis

FIGURE 24-2. Aortic stenosis. Because blood cannot completely pass through the narrowed valve opening, blood pools in the left ventricle and cardiac output is reduced.

contract effectively. Left-sided heart failure (see Chap. 28) may develop because the heart cannot fully empty during systole and becomes more fatigued as it tries to overcome the resistance created by the narrowed valve. Should the adult with aortic stenosis develop coronary artery disease (CAD) and myocardial infarction (MI) (see Chap. 25), the infarct may enlarge. Risk of mortality thus increases because of the valve's compromised ability to perfuse the myocardium with oxygen.

Assessment Findings

Signs and Symptoms

A client with aortic stenosis may be asymptomatic for several decades. When symptoms develop, they include dizziness, fainting, and angina because of insufficient cardiac output. At first, the client experiences dyspnea and fatigue during activity. With ventricular enlargement, heart pulsations are displaced laterally or distally on the chest wall from the usual **point of maximum impulse** (PMI) at the fifth intercostal space medial to the left midclavicular line. The carotid pulse feels weak because of a low stroke volume.

Gerontologic Considerations

- Older adults may experience a decreased thirst sensation, increasing the risk for dehydration, which may result in fatigue and weakness that can be confused with symptoms of valvular disease.

The S_2 heart sound is split, that is, there is a definite separation between the sounds of the aortic valve and pulmonic valve closing. Usually, these sounds occur in unison or are so closely timed that they seem as one. While listening at the second intercostal space to the right and left of the sternum, the S_1 and split S_2 sounds like "lub-t-dub." The split persists throughout inspiration and expiration and does not disappear when the client sits up during auscultation. This finding distinguishes the split S_2 from a normal, physiologic splitting. Sometimes auscultation identifies other abnormal sounds (e.g., systolic murmur, click). Box 24-1 explains grading of heart murmurs.

Diagnostic Findings

Ventricular enlargement is evident on a chest radiograph. An echocardiogram validates ventricular thickening and diminished transvalvular size. On an electrocardiogram (ECG), the height of the R wave may be increased, reflecting the large mass and force of contracting muscle. During left-sided cardiac catheterization, the pressure of blood in the left ventricle is higher than usual.

Medical and Surgical Management

Medical treatment may begin while the client is asymptomatic and focuses on maintaining adequate cardiac output by supporting the heart's pumping activity. Digitalis, an antidysrhythmic drug particularly for atrial fibrillation with rapid ventricular response (see Chap. 26), and a diuretic may be prescribed. Sodium is restricted. Antibiotics are prescribed

BOX 24-1   **Heart Murmur Grades**

Heart murmurs are graded from 1 through 6:
- Grade 1 is a very faint murmur that may not be heard in all positions.
- Grade 2 is a quiet murmur, but it can be heard when auscultating the heart.
- Grade 3 is a murmur that is moderately loud.
- Grade 4 is a loud murmur accompanied by a palpable *thrill*, a vibration felt on the chest wall.
- Grade 5 is very loud with a palpable thrill; the murmur can be heard with the stethoscope partly off the chest.
- Grade 6 is very loud with a palpable thrill; the murmur is heard with the stethoscope off the client's chest.

Source: Todd, B.A., & Higgins, K. (2005). Recognizing aortic and mitral valve disease. *Nursing* 35(6): 58–63.

to prevent recurrences of infective endocarditis, which compound valvular damage. Nitrates or beta-adrenergic blockers are beneficial for relieving chest pain.

Additional treatment eventually becomes critical because average survival is 2 to 3 years once symptoms develop (Baptiste, 2001; Bonow et al., 2006). **Balloon valvuloplasty** is an invasive, nonsurgical procedure to enlarge a narrowed valve opening. A catheter with a deflated balloon is threaded through a peripheral blood vessel into the heart until the tip is located in the stenotic valve. When in position, the balloon is inflated to stretch the opening (see Fig. 24-4 for illustration of balloon valvuloplasty for mitral valve stenosis). Balloon valvuloplasty is considered temporary for clients whose conditions are too unstable for immediate surgery, yet whose symptoms cannot be adequately controlled more conservatively (Baptiste, 2001). The stretched valve opening tends to narrow again within 6 to 12 months (Bonow et al., 2006).

Surgical aortic valve replacement eventually becomes necessary. Ideally, aortic valve replacement is performed before the client reaches the late stages of heart failure (see Chap. 28). A coronary arteriogram is performed to identify CAD; if present, valve replacement and surgical measures to improve vascular supply to the myocardium may be performed at the same time.

Gerontologic Considerations

- Balloon valvuloplasty is used cautiously, if at all, in older adults because the stretching may fracture the aortic valve if it is calcified, as is often the case in older clients. Therefore, older adults are generally candidates for valve replacement surgery.

Nursing Management

The nurse monitors subjective and objective symptoms and explains the purposes and techniques of diagnostic tests. He

Nutrition Notes 24-1
The Client with a Valvular Heart Disorder

● Clients with valvular disorders often need to limit sodium intake because decreasing the volume of blood decreases cardiac workload.

● Because approximately 75% of sodium in the typical American diet comes from processed foods, encourage clients to substitute homemade foods for convenience products and prepared items. Foods to avoid include canned fish, meat, poultry, soup, vegetables, and vegetable juices; smoked and processed meats; sauerkraut; commercial mixes; instant rice and pasta mixes; casserole mixes; frozen dinners, entrées, pizzas, and vegetables with sauces; most fast foods; condiments such as catsup, relish, pickles, barbecue sauce, soy sauce, and Worcestershire sauce; and seasoning salts.

● Salt substitutes replace sodium with potassium or other minerals and may taste bitter. Low-sodium salt substitutes may contain up to half as much sodium as regular table salt. Clients should not use either type without a physician's approval.

● Clients with valvular disorders may need to restrict fluid because volume affects cardiac emptying. Foods that liquefy at room temperature (e.g., ice cream, ice milk, gelatin, ice pops, sherbet) are counted as liquids when fluid intake is restricted.

or she administers prescribed medications and monitors for therapeutic or adverse responses. The nurse institutes measures to ensure adequate cardiac output and tissue oxygenation. He or she assists the client to comply with dietary modifications to reduce fluid volumes and the work placed on the heart (Nutrition Notes 24-1). Nursing Care Plan 24-1 describes additional nursing management of a client with a valvular disorder.

AORTIC REGURGITATION

Aortic regurgitation occurs when the aortic valve does not close tightly and blood can leak backward. The valve's inability to close tightly is a condition called **valvular incompetence**.

Pathophysiology and Etiology

Valvular incompetence can result from damage to the valve cusps or papillary muscles. It may be a consequence of various disorders such as rheumatic carditis, endocarditis, syphilis, age-related stretching of the proximal aorta, and systemic inflammatory conditions. In 1997, the incidence of aortic and mitral regurgitation increased as a result of the use of fenfluramine (Pondimin) with phentermine (known as Fen-Phen), fenfluramine alone, and dexfenfluramine (Redux) alone for weight loss. Various researchers identified that 29% to 36% of clients who took these drugs developed valvular disorders (Bonow et al., 2006).

When blood is pumped through the incompetent aortic valve, some leaks backward (**valvular regurgitation**) into the left ventricle. This backflow reduces cardiac output and causes fluid overload in the left ventricle, which becomes chronically stretched, hindering its ability to pump effectively (see Chap. 28). High fluid pressure in the left ventricle causes the mitral valve to shut early, which interferes with left atrial emptying. The blood in the left atrium backs up into the pulmonary circulation. Left ventricular enlargement increases the heart's need for oxygen. When the coronary arteries cannot supply the heart muscle with enough oxygen because of decreased cardiac output, the myocardium becomes ischemic and the client experiences angina. Dizziness, dyspnea on exertion, confusion, and left ventricular failure may develop.

Assessment Findings

Signs and Symptoms

The client remains asymptomatic as long as the left ventricle can sustain adequate circulation. Tachycardia is one of the first signs. When valve damage affects the left ventricle, the client becomes aware of forceful heart contractions (palpitations). At first, palpitations occur only when lying flat or on the left side. In later stages, the client experiences dyspnea and chest pain.

During physical examination, skin may be flushed and moist, especially in the upper body. The radial pulse may be very strong, with quick, sharp beats followed by a sudden collapse of force, a characteristic called a **water-hammer pulse** or *Corrigan's pulse*. Often, pulse pressure is wide because systolic blood pressure (BP) tends to be extremely high, whereas diastolic BP usually remains low or normal. The enlarged heart displaces the PMI. The chest may heave or rock from the forceful contractions of the enlarged left ventricle. A heart murmur, caused by the turbulence of blood falling back through the dilated aortic valve, also may be heard.

Diagnostic Findings

Cardiac catheterization reveals high left ventricular pressure and backward movement of blood. A chest radiograph reveals heart enlargement, and the aortic valve appears dilated. The ECG presents with tall R waves; depressed ST segments indicate myocardial ischemia. A radionuclide scan comparing blood flow through the heart at rest and during exercise reveals the severity of the disease. Standard or transesophageal echocardiography provides images of atypical valvular and myocardial function. A CT or MRI scan may be performed if the echocardiographic images are inconclusive.

Medical and Surgical Management

Because aortic regurgitation is mild and only slowly progressive in most people, clients are sustained with cardiac glycosides (Drug Therapy Table 24-1) or beta blockers and diuretics. When taken appropriately, prophylactic antibiotics prevent recurrences of infective endocarditis. Clients are advised to modify their lifestyle to avoid excessive demands on the heart, such as those that may result from strenuous exercise and emotional stress.

NURSING CARE PLAN 24-1 | The Client With a Valvular Disorder

Assessment

Determine the following:

- Vital signs, noting tachycardia, rapid respirations, dyspnea, hypotension, or hypertension
- Any episodes of dizziness or fainting with or without confusion
- Chest pain and its characteristics
- Normal or abnormal lung and heart sounds

- Fluid intake and output
- Current weight and fluctuations during treatment
- Level of activity tolerance
- Social aspects (e.g., occupational activities) as they relate to physical energy requirements
- Knowledge of medical condition and current and future treatment protocols

Nursing Diagnosis: Risk for Decreased Cardiac Output related to diminished cardiac muscle contractility, tachycardia, and hypertension

Expected Outcome: Cardiac output will be adequate as evidenced by no chest pain, hypotension, or dizziness.

Interventions	Rationales
Monitor cardiac rhythm and rate.	Heart rate affects and tachydysrhythmias compromise cardiac output.
Measure urine output every 8 hours or more often if less than 500 mL/day.	Renal output reflects the heart's ability to perfuse the renal arteries.
Maintain client on bed rest.	Rest lowers heart rate, which increases diastolic filling volume.
Reduce anxiety by responding to requests for attention or assistance.	Relief of anxiety reduces tachycardia and hypertension.
Provide substitutes for dietary sources of caffeine and sodium.	Caffeine increases heart rate and promotes vasoconstriction; sodium contributes to fluid retention.
Promote ease in eliminating stool through such measures as increasing fiber and administering a prescribed stool softener.	Bearing down to eliminate stool interferes with cardiac filling; reduced cardiac filling decreases cardiac output.
Reduce any fever by changing to lighter or fewer bed linens, assisting with tepid sponge baths, or administering prescribed antipyretics.	Increased heart rate accompanies fever and adds to the heart's workload, which may compromise cardiac output.

Evaluation of Expected Outcome

Client is pain free; heart rate, BP, and urine output are within normal ranges. The client's sensorium is clear.

Nursing Diagnosis: Activity Intolerance related to decreased cardiac output

Expected Outcome: Client will tolerate activity without dyspnea or heart rate above 100 beats/min.

Interventions	Rationales
Provide complete or partial assistance with activities of daily living.	Activity taxes endurance and results in increased heart rate and blood pressure.
Allow adequate time for client to perform self-care.	Activity that is done without urgency is less physically demanding.
Intersperse periods of activity with rest.	Rest helps the heart recover from demands that increase its rate or force of contraction.

Evaluation of Expected Outcome

Client manages self-care and moderate activity without becoming breathless, hypotensive, or tachycardic.

Nursing Diagnosis: Pain related to myocardial ischemia

Expected Outcome: Pain will be reduced to client's self-described tolerance level within 30 minutes of a nursing intervention.

Interventions	Rationales
Provide rest immediately.	Rest slows the heart rate and decreases the myocardium's need for oxygen.
Administer oxygen temporarily.	Increasing inhaled oxygen concentration promotes myocardial cellular oxygenation.
Give prescribed short-acting nitrate or analgesic.	Nitrates cause vasodilatation and increase blood flow from the coronary arteries to the myocardium; analgesics block the transmission or perception of pain.

NURSING CARE PLAN 24-1 The Client With a Valvular Disorder (Continued)

Interventions	Rationales
Assist clients with mitral valve prolapse to lie flat and elevate the legs 90° for 3 to 5 minutes.	Elevating the legs facilitates volume changes in the heart.

Evaluation of Expected Outcome

Client is free of pain.

Nursing Diagnosis: **Risk for Infection** related to increased susceptibility secondary to previous endocardial inflammatory or infectious disorders

Expected Outcome: Client will remain free of infection as evidenced by normal temperature and white blood cell count.

Interventions	Rationales
Reassign care of client if designated caregiver has infectious symptoms, or have caregiver don protective garments (e.g., face mask) and change them frequently.	Reducing exposure to microorganisms associated with infective endocarditis minimizes the potential for infection and repeated valvular damage.
Perform conscientious hand hygiene.	Hand hygiene is the single most effective method to reduce infectious microorganisms.
Follow aseptic principles when changing dressings covering impaired skin and vascular insertion sites.	Impaired skin is an entrance site for microorganisms that may lead to bacteremia and repeated valvular damage.

Evaluation of Expected Outcome

Client does not acquire a nosocomial infection.

PC: **Heart Failure**

Expected Outcome: The nurse will monitor for, manage, and minimize heart failure.

Interventions	Rationales
Auscultate lung and heart sounds at least once per shift or more often if abnormal sounds are evident.	Crackles, rhonchi (gurgles), and an S_3 heart sound are signs of cardiopulmonary complications such as left-sided congestive heart failure.
Weigh client daily at the same time, with similar clothing, on the same scale.	A weight gain of 2 lb or more in 24 hours suggests fluid retention equal to 1 L.
Support compliance with prescribed sodium and fluid restrictions.	Such restrictions decrease the work and sustain the ability of the heart to contract efficiently.

Evaluation of Expected Outcome

The nurse documents appropriate assessment findings, reports critical information to the physician, and implements prescribed interventions.

Nursing Diagnosis: **Risk for Ineffective Management of Therapeutic Regimen** related to insufficient knowledge of self-care

Expected Outcome: Client will accurately describe discharge instructions.

Interventions	Rationales
Completely explain all treatments.	Client cannot implement interventions that are not explained.
Advise client to consult the physician about prophylactic antibiotic therapy before dental or invasive treatments.	Prophylactic antibiotics reduce the potential for recurrent endocarditis and additional valvular damage.
Caution against lifting heavy objects or straining at stool.	Bearing down with forced expiration through a closed glottis (Valsalva maneuver) increases BP, which predisposes the client to heart failure.
Teach client to recognize signs and symptoms of heart failure (see Chap. 28) and to report them immediately.	Early intervention facilitates an improved prognosis if a complication develops.
Advise client to avoid caffeine and over-the-counter medications that contain cardiac stimulants (e.g., decongestants).	They cause tachycardia and vasoconstriction, increasing the risk for myocardial ischemia, tachydysrhythmias, and heart failure.
Instruct client to avoid strenuous exercise and competitive sports.	Activity beyond tolerance and competition increase heart rate, BP, and cardiac risks.

Evaluation of Expected Outcome

Client accurately describes his or her disorder, methods for controlling symptoms, and precautions that reduce the risk for complications.

DRUG THERAPY TABLE 24-1 Agents to Treat Valvular Heart Disorders

Drug Category and Examples	Mechanism of Action	Side Effects	Nursing Considerations
Antibiotics penicillin G potassium (Pfizerpen)	Inhibit cell wall synthesis in susceptible organisms, causing cell death	Anaphylaxis, glossitis, gastritis, sore mouth, nausea, vomiting, diarrhea, rash, fever, superinfection, phlebitis	Ascertain if client is allergic to penicillin before administering. After administering first parenteral dose, monitor client's response for 30 minutes. Assess IV site for pain and signs and symptoms of phlebitis. Administer oral doses with a full glass of water to a client on an empty stomach.
Anticoagulants aspirin (ASA, acetylsalicylic acid) dipyridamole (Persantine) warfarin (Coumadin)	Prevent thrombi by interfering with various aspects of platelet function, primarily aggregation Prolongs clotting times by interfering with vitamin K-dependent clotting factors	Increased bleeding time, nausea, diarrhea, abdominal pain, GI bleeding (ASA), CNS effects (dipyridamole) Increased bleeding, nausea, leukopenia, alopecia, dermatitis, fever, rash	Instruct client to report any unusual or excessive bleeding. Monitor complete blood counts, PT and INR frequently. Advise that client wear a MedicAlert bracelet. Instruct client to report any unusual or excessive bleeding
Cardiac Glycosides digoxin (Lanoxin)	Increase cardiac output by slowing heart rate (negative chronotropic action) and increasing force of contraction (positive inotropic action)	Fatigue, generalized muscle weakness, agitation, hallucinations (toxic effects on heart may be life-threatening and require immediate attention), yellow-green halos around images, blurred vision, anorexia	Assess pulse rate before each dose. Withhold administration if pulse is <60 or >120 beats/min. Monitor serum potassium levels; ensure intake of potassium. Administer before meals to promote absorption.
Antiplatelets clopidogrel (Plavix)	Decrease clot production by interfering with platelet aggregation	Dizziness, diarrhea, nausea, abdominal pain, flu-like symptoms, bruising, bleeding, rash	Administer with food or meals. Monitor blood cell count, and assess for excessive bleeding. Relate need for regular, follow-up laboratory tests.
Antidysrhythmics quinidine (Quinaglute)	Alter the action potential of cardiac cells and interfere with heart's electrical excitability	Nausea, vomiting, diplopia, new dysrhythmias, hemolytic anemia, rash, tinnitus, headache	Monitor for new or worse dysrhythmias. Ensure reduced dosage in clients with hepatic or renal failure. Monitor blood counts during prolonged therapy. Monitor for signs of cinchonism (quinidine toxicity): ringing in the ears, headache, nausea, dizziness, fever.

When a client becomes symptomatic, replacement of the diseased aortic valve is considered (see Chap. 29). The less heart damage occurs before surgery, the better the outcome. If the aorta is diseased, the procedure is more involved because repair involves a vascular graft.

Pharmacologic Considerations

- Nonselective beta blockers can aggravate chronic obstructive pulmonary disease and contribute to hyperglycemia in insulin-dependent adults. Some diuretics deplete potassium, causing hypokalemia.

- Before administering beta blockers, take the client's apical pulse. If the heart rate is less than 60 beats/minute, withhold the drug and notify the primary healthcare provider.

- Closely monitor clients taking beta blockers for signs and symptoms of overdosage: bradycardia, severe dizziness, drowsiness, and bluish discoloration of the palms, fingernails, or both. Notify the primary healthcare provider immediately if these symptoms appear.

 Gerontologic Considerations

-Older adults may require lower doses of cardiac glycosides than younger clients because of age-related metabolic changes. The more medications older adults take, the more likely they are to have dangerous interactions. For older adults taking beta blockers, monitor the heart rate and BP closely; the adverse effects of bradycardia and hypotension can cause confusion and falls.

Nursing Management

The nurse prepares the client for diagnostic procedures and monitors responses. He or she reports changes in heart rate and rhythm, dyspnea, chest pain, and loss of consciousness to the physician immediately. The nurse administers prescribed medications and evaluates the client's response. Ensuring that physical activity is balanced according to the client's tolerance is important. Before discharge, the nurse explains the need for antibiotic therapy before medical and dental procedures and teaches how to assess BP regularly as well as methods to control hypertension. See Nursing Care Plan 24-1 for more information.

▶ *Stop, Think, and Respond Exercise 24-1*

A client with an aortic valvular disorder experiences chest pain while performing bathing and hygiene. What nursing actions are appropriate?

DISORDERS OF THE MITRAL VALVE

The mitral valve, which lies between the left atrium and left ventricle, is a bicuspid valve. The two cusps are attached on the ventricular surface to strands of fibrous tissue called *chordae tendineae*, which are projections from papillary muscles (see Fig. 22-2 in Chap. 22). The papillary muscles contract in unison with the ventricle, pull on the chordae tendineae, and prevent the cusps from ballooning into the left atrium. The functions of the mitral valve are to open widely to allow oxygenated blood to fill the left ventricle and close tightly to prevent blood from re-entering the left atrium after the left ventricle is filled. As long as the mitral valve remains structurally sound, blood exits the left ventricle through the aortic valve, where the aorta receives a 50- to 70-mL bolus

of oxygenated blood, referred to as the *stroke volume*. The valve may become rigid (stenotic), incompetent (inadequate closure), or prolapsed (floppy). Mitral valve prolapse is the most commonly diagnosed valvular disorder.

MITRAL STENOSIS
Pathophysiology and Etiology

Mitral stenosis means that the valve does not open properly to facilitate filling of the left ventricle (Fig. 24-3). It is primarily a sequela (a condition that follows a disease) of rheumatic carditis (see Chap. 23). Mitral stenosis worsens with each recurrence of endocarditis. The inflammation causes the cusps to stick together and form a thick, rigid, calcified scar at the **commissures**, the area where the cusps contact each other, and the chordae tendineae fuse and shorten. The mitral valve cannot open completely, leading to incomplete emptying of the left atrium. Pooled blood from incomplete emptying contributes to clot formation, which puts the client at risk for arterial emboli. The left atrium enlarges because it has to contract more forcibly to empty. Pressure from overfilling is conveyed backward through the blood vessels to the lungs, creating pulmonary hypertension and the potential for pulmonary edema (see Chap. 21). Pulmonary hypertension increases the work of the right ventricle as it pumps against the high pressure in the pulmonary vascular system.

Because blood flows in a circuit, the disease on the left side of the heart eventually affects the right side. The right ventricle may enlarge in response to its increased workload. When the contraction of the right ventricle can no longer overcome the pulmonary resistance, right-sided heart failure develops. Excess blood accumulates in the venous circulation, the liver becomes congested, and edema occurs in the legs.

Assessment Findings
Signs and Symptoms

It may take 20 to 40 years for a client who has had rheumatic fever to develop mitral stenosis. The normal valve opening is 4 to 5 cm^2; symptoms develop when the valve area is less than 2.5 cm^2 (Bonow et al., 2006). At that time, clients report fatigue and dyspnea after slight exertion. Symptoms become disabling approximately 10 years after onset; they are accentuated when unusual demands are placed on the heart (e.g., fever, emotional stress, pregnancy). Later, clients experience heart palpitations caused by *tachydysrhythmias* (rapid dysrhythmias). With the onset of pulmonary hypertension, clients may become more dyspneic at night and must sleep in a sitting position. They may develop a cough productive of pink, frothy sputum. Crackles heard in the bases of the lungs are a sign of pulmonary congestion.

Changes in heart sounds may be the earliest indication of mitral valve stenosis. S$_1$ may be extremely loud if the cusps are fused, or muffled or absent if the cusps have calcified and are immobile. A murmur, described as sounding like a rumbling underground train, can be heard at the heart's apex, especially when the client assumes a left lateral position. The systolic BP is low from reduced cardiac output. If backward pressure through the pulmonary circulation is

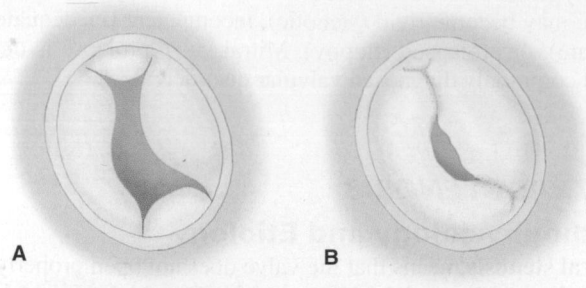

A   B

Normal mitral valve (open)   Mitral valve stenosis

FIGURE 24-3. (**A**) The normal mitral valve opens widely to allow blood to pass from the left atrium to the left ventricle. (**B**) Following what is generally an infectious process, the mitral valve leaflets become fused with scar tissue, causing a partially obstructed pathway for the passage of blood.

sufficient to affect the right ventricle, the client's face is flushed; neck vein distention is evident; the liver is enlarged; and there is peripheral edema.

Diagnostic Findings

A chest radiograph reveals an enlarged left atrium and mitral valve calcification. In advanced stages, evidence of fluid congestion in the lungs (pulmonary edema) is found. A standard or esophageal echocardiogram demonstrates decreased movement of the mitral valve cusps and changes in the size of the atrial chamber. On ECG, the P wave is notched, showing that the left atrium takes longer to depolarize than the right atrium because of its increased size.

Medical and Surgical Management

Antibiotic therapy is prescribed to prevent future episodes of infective endocarditis. Preventing or relieving the symptoms of heart failure is essential. A daily aspirin, dipyridamole (Persantine), or other oral anticoagulant may be ordered to avoid clot formation.

Pharmacologic Considerations

-Oral anticoagulant therapy requires close monitoring of prothrombin time (PT). Therapeutic PT levels are 1.5 to 2.5 times the control value. When the PT is reported as an international normalized ratio, the normal range is 2.0 to 3.0. The American College of Chest Physicians recommends an INR of 2.5 to 3.5 for clients with mechanical prosthetic valves (Baptiste, 2001).

Dysrhythmias (abnormal electrical impulse transmission through the conduction system), such as *atrial fibrillation* (quivering of the atrial muscle with insufficient force to pump blood), are treated with drugs or cardioversion. Cardioversion stops the heart momentarily to allow the sinoatrial node to reestablish itself as the pacemaker.

Commissurotomy is a surgical technique to separate the fused valve leaflets (see Chap. 29). However, not all clients

with mitral stenosis are suitable candidates for surgery. Those whose condition is so slight that it does not cause symptoms or so severe or of such long duration that profound changes in the heart and lungs have occurred usually are excluded. The earlier surgery is performed, the greater is the likelihood that it will relieve the symptoms.

Percutaneous balloon valvuloplasty, also called *valvotomy,* is a nonsurgical alternative. When percutaneous balloon valvuloplasty is performed, a catheter with an uninflated balloon is passed through the femoral vein and threaded into the right atrium. The septum is then punctured between the right and left atria. When the catheter is in the mitral valve, it is inflated (Fig. 24-4). Clients often are discharged on the same day as the procedure. The atrial puncture allows some blood to shunt from the left atrium to the right, but the opening usually closes within 6 months. Complications, although rare, include mitral regurgitation (discussed next), residual atrial-septal defect, perforation of the left ventricle, embolization, and MI. Management of the client after percutaneous balloon valvuloplasty includes the following:

- Echocardiogram within 72 hours to detect mitral regurgitation, left ventricular dysfunction, or pronounced atrial-septal defect
- Oral anticoagulation therapy within 1 to 2 days for clients who have a history of atrial fibrillation or instituted for others if atrial fibrillation develops in the future
- Prophylactic antibiotic protocols to prevent infective endocarditis
- Yearly medical follow-up that includes echocardiography, chest radiography, and ECG

Nursing Management

The nurse monitors the client's physical condition, prepares him or her for diagnostic testing, and provides post-treatment care. Discharge teaching includes information regarding drug therapy, activity modification, signs and symptoms of

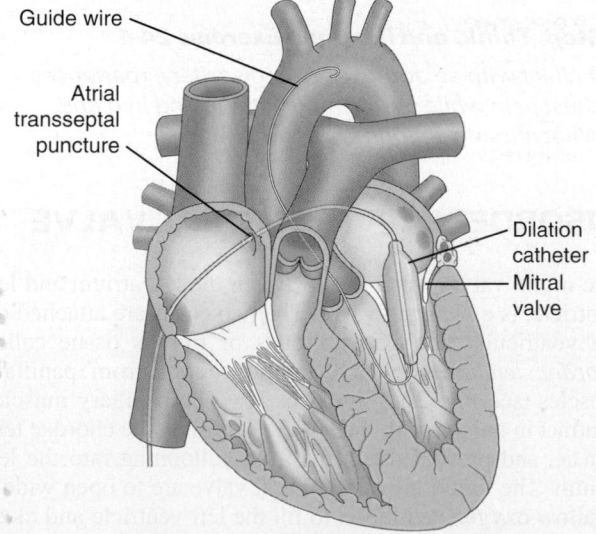

Guide wire

Atrial transseptal puncture

Dilation catheter

Mitral valve

FIGURE 24-4. Balloon valvuloplasty. Cross-section of heart illustrating dilation catheter placed through an atrial transseptal puncture and across the mitral valve. The guide wire extends from the aortic valve into the aorta for catheter support.

complications, and when to contact the physician. See Nursing Care Plan 24-1 for additional discussion.

MITRAL REGURGITATION (INSUFFICIENCY)

Mitral regurgitation, sometimes referred to as *mitral insufficiency*, occurs when the mitral valve does not close completely (Fig. 24-5). Some clients present with severe acute symptoms; others, whose heart muscle increases in size to compensate, remain asymptomatic or develop symptoms gradually over many years.

Pathophysiology and Etiology

Mitral regurgitation is associated with rheumatic carditis and mitral valve prolapse (discussed next). It also is linked with damage to the papillary muscles, impaired myocardial function after MI, connective tissue disorders, stretching of the valve opening from an enlarged left ventricle, and malfunction of a replaced valve. It also can develop after balloon valvuloplasty. Use of the weight loss drugs identified in the discussion of aortic regurgitation also has been associated with mitral valve regurgitation.

When the mitral valve becomes incompetent (i.e., does not close completely), blood flows backward into the left atrium during ventricular systole and leaks into the left ventricle during atrial diastole. The heart usually can compensate for a small amount of blood that is regurgitated backward and forward by increasing the size of the left ventricle and left atria. The larger size facilitates ejection of blood from the heart, in which case pulmonary congestion does not occur. If the regurgitation occurs rapidly, however, the heart is less able to compensate. Forward output from the left ventricle is diminished, and the client develops signs of cardiogenic shock (see Chap. 17). Accumulation of blood in the left atrium results in pulmonary congestion.

Assessment Findings

Signs and Symptoms

The client typically experiences chronic fatigue and dyspnea on exertion. He or she may notice heart palpitations caused by the forceful contraction of the left ventricle as it attempts to empty the excess blood from its chamber. The S_1 heart sound is diminished because of incomplete closure of the mitral valve. An S_3 heart sound, if heard, is an early sign of impending heart failure. Hypertension may develop when reduced cardiac output triggers the renin-angiotensin-aldosterone cycle. Tachycardia is a compensatory mechanism when stroke volume decreases. A loud, blowing murmur often is heard throughout ventricular systole at the heart's apex. If pulmonary congestion occurs, the client develops shortness of breath and moist lung sounds typical of left ventricular failure (see Chap. 28).

Diagnostic Findings

Standard transthoracic or transesophageal echocardiography is the best technique to identify structural changes in the mitral valve. Chest radiography shows enlarged chambers on the left side of the heart. Radionuclide angiography, an

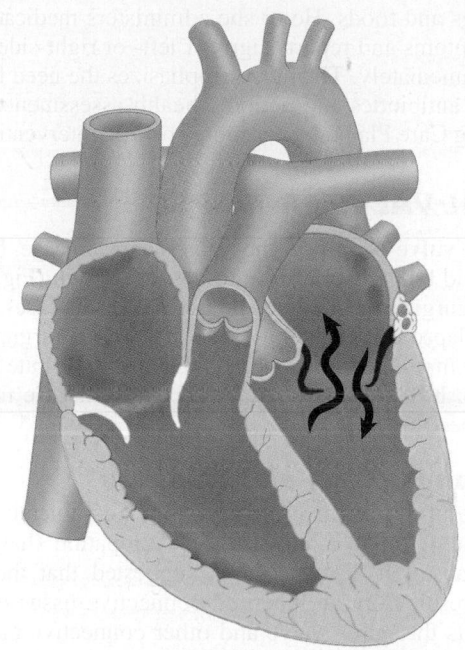

FIGURE 24-5. Mitral regurgitation (insufficiency). The incompetent atrioventricular valve allows blood to return to the left atrium.

imaging procedure using an intravenously injected radioactive substance, shows the heart's chambers in motion and provides information on the volume of regurgitated blood. ECG reflects cardiac enlargement, papillary muscle or chordae tendineae dysfunction, and various associated dysrhythmias (e.g., atrial fibrillation).

Medical and Surgical Management

Asymptomatic clients are monitored through physical examination and annual echocardiograms. Exercise is not limited until mild symptoms develop. An angiotensin-converting enzyme inhibitor such as quinapril (Accupril) reduces afterload, preserving the left ventricle's ability to eject blood effectively. Digitalis, calcium channel blockers, beta blockers, or other antidysrhythmic drugs control tachycardia. Some clients are given drugs to prevent intracardiac thrombi, a common complication of blood stasis that accompanies atrial fibrillation. Prophylactic antibiotics are prescribed to prevent recurrences of infective endocarditis. An intra-aortic balloon pump, which provides counterpulsation to the contraction of the left ventricle, can be used in an emergency to stabilize a client in left ventricular failure (see Chap. 28).

Surgery to correct mitral regurgitation includes *annuloplasty*, repair of the valve leaflets and their fibrous ring. The implantation of a biologic or prosthetic valve to restore unidirectional blood flow may accompany annuloplasty. Annuloplasty and valve replacement are discussed in Chap. 29.

Nursing Management

The nurse closely monitors BP, heart rate and rhythm, heart sounds, and lung sounds. He or she weighs the client to determine changes in fluid balance. If sodium is restricted, the nurse works with the client and dietitian to find palatable seasonings and foods. He or she administers medications to treat symptoms and reports signs of left- or right-sided heart failure immediately. The nurse emphasizes the need for prophylactic antibiotics and periodic health assessments. Refer to Nursing Care Plan 24-1 for more specific interventions.

MITRAL VALVE PROLAPSE

In **mitral valve prolapse**, the valve cusps enlarge, become floppy, and bulge backward into the left atrium (Fig. 24-6). Mitral regurgitation may occur, but not in all cases. Mitral valve prolapse is the leading cause of mitral regurgitation. It is more common in young women than men. Despite its high incidence, it is considered to be a benign disease for most affected people.

Pathophysiology and Etiology

The cause of mitral valve prolapse is not completely understood, and it often is classified as idiopathic (having no known cause). It also has been suggested that the tissue changes result from an inherited connective tissue disorder that affects the mitral valve and other connective tissues in the body. It has been observed that some clients develop mitral valve prolapse in association with CAD, although there is speculation that no etiologic relationship actually exists. There is, however, strong evidence that mitral valve prolapse accompanies the valvular changes of rheumatic carditis, and structural changes predispose the valve to further damage if infective endocarditis develops.

Some people develop **mitral valve prolapse syndrome**, symptoms that cannot be attributed to valvular disease alone. It is associated with autonomic nervous system dysfunction. This association may explain why some clients have increased levels of catecholamines (i.e., epinephrine, norepinephrine), abnormal catecholamine regulation, and decreased intravascular volume, which causes symptoms that mimic severe anxiety (tachycardia, palpitations, breathlessness, dizziness). Decreased circulatory volume may contribute to the client's symptomatology by triggering an abnormal renin-angiotensin-aldosterone response (see Chap. 17). Changes in the mitral valve tissue layers cause the cusps to distend. The billowing cusps stretch the papillary muscles as they balloon backward into the left atrium. The stretching of the papillary muscles causes local ischemia and atypical chest pain. As the papillary muscles provide less support to the mitral valve, valvular incompetence occurs. The left atrium and ventricle eventually may enlarge and subsequently progress to congestive heart failure.

Assessment Findings

Many clients with mitral valve prolapse are asymptomatic. When symptoms are present, they include chest pain, palpitations, and fatigue. The chest pain differs from that of angina: its onset does not correlate with physical exertion, its duration is prolonged, and it is not easily relieved. Some clients also experience symptoms that resemble anxiety or panic, such as a rapid and irregular heart rate, shortness of breath, light-headedness, difficulty concentrating, and fear that the symptoms indicate impending death. Auscultation of heart sounds reveals a characteristic "click" during ventricular systole caused by tightening of the chordae tendineae.

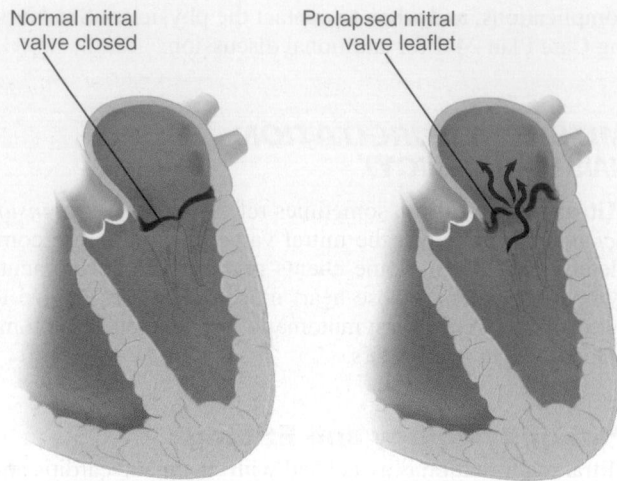

FIGURE 24-6. In mitral valve prolapse, the floppy valve leaflets bulge backward into the left atrium. This may allow blood to regurgitate, or move in retrograde fashion, from the left ventricle to the left atrium.

A systolic murmur is associated with mitral regurgitation. The presumptive diagnosis of mitral valve prolapse is strong if the murmur disappears or diminishes when the client squats during auscultation. Additional symptoms of mitral regurgitation also may be manifested.

Echocardiography shows abnormal movement of one or more mitral valve leaflets during systole. The ECG (resting, exercise, chemical, or ambulatory) is essentially normal, eliminating MI as a cause for the chest pain. ECG, however, may detect other causes.

Medical and Surgical Management

Many clients with mitral valve prolapse require no treatment except periodic antibiotic therapy before invasive procedures. Such drugs as digitalis, beta blockers, and calcium channel blockers control tachydysrhythmias; all but digitalis also control hypertension. Medications to reduce platelet aggregation (e.g., a single, daily, low-dose aspirin or ticlopidine [Ticlid]) are prescribed to prevent thrombus formation. If symptoms become severe, valve replacement is indicated.

Antianxiety medication may be prescribed to prevent symptoms related to the sympathetic nervous system among those with mitral valve prolapse syndrome. Such clients also are advised to avoid caffeine to prevent tachycardia and heart palpitations. To compensate for symptoms associated with hypovolemia, liberal fluid and adequate sodium intake is recommended. Because alcohol can suppress antidiuretic hormone (ADH), leading to loss of extracellular fluid, clients with mitral valve prolapse syndrome are advised to restrict or eliminate its use.

 Pharmacologic Consideration

- Beside contributing to increased fluid loss from inhibition of ADH, elimination of alcohol is also recommended because it interferes with metabolism of the anticoagulant warfarin and may contribute to the risk for bleeding (Baptiste, 2001).

Nursing Management

One measure to relieve chest pain is to have the client lie flat with the legs elevated and supported against a wall or couch at a 90° angle for 3 to 5 minutes to facilitate volume changes in the heart. Other recommendations include increasing activity when tachycardia occurs to eliminate the initiation of extra, ineffective beats; make up for reduced cardiac output; and lower levels of catecholamines. To relax or decrease shortness of breath, the nurse instructs the client to breathe deeply and slowly and then exhale through pursed lips. He or she advises the client to avoid caffeinated beverages and over-the-counter medications that contain stimulating chemicals to avoid contributing to an already rapid heart rate. If hypertension is not a problem, the nurse encourages the client to drink adequate fluid and continue moderate use of salt to maintain intravascular fluid volume. He or she discourages the use of alcohol because of its dehydrating effects and because withdrawal after chronic use can cause cardiac stimulation. The nurse warns clients who are prescribed minor tranquilizers not to stop the medication abruptly or they may experience stimulating withdrawal symptoms. Additional nursing management depends on other assessment data. See Nursing Care Plan 24-1.

▶ *Stop, Think, and Respond Exercise 24-2*

Explain why clients with valvular disorders may need exercise modifications.

CRITICAL THINKING EXERCISES

1. Compare and contrast stenosis and regurgitation of the aortic and mitral valves.
2. You are assisting a newly admitted client with a diagnosis of mitral stenosis into his hospital room. The person in the next bed is diagnosed with trachcobronchitis, has a humidifier at the bedside, and receives frequent aerosol breathing treatments. What is the potential problem? What measures are appropriate to correct it?
3. What effect would the administration of a vasodilator, such as nitroglycerin, have on a client with aortic stenosis?

4. Explain why angina, syncope, and exertional dyspnea are common symptoms of aortic stenosis.

NCLEX-STYLE REVIEW QUESTIONS

1. Which of the following topics would the nurse include in teaching the client with aortic regurgitation? Select all that apply.
   1. An exercise plan for weight loss
   2. Reasons for antibiotic therapy
   3. Ways to elevate the legs
   4. How to assess blood pressure regularly
   5. Methods to control hypertension
2. The nurse assesses the client diagnosed with aortic regurgitation. The nurse should notify the primary care physician of which of the following findings?
   1. The heart rate is above 120 beats per minute.
   2. The skin is pale and dry.
   3. The S_2 sounds are split.
   4. The point of maximum impulse is at the fifth intercostal space.
3. When auscultating the chest of a client diagnosed with mitral valve prolapse, what is the nurse most likely to hear?
   1. A clicking sound during systole
   2. Heart rate less than 60 beats per minute
   3. Moist breath sounds on inspiration
   4. Respiratory rate less than 12 per minute
4. Mitral valve regurgitation secondary to mitral valve prolapse is the admitting diagnosis for a client. The nurse should frequently assess for which complication?
   1. Thrombus formation
   2. Infection
   3. Decreased urine output
   4. Ascites
5. For which one of the following assessments should the nurse withhold a beta blocker such as atenolol (Tenormin) when caring for a client with a valvular disorder of the heart?
   1. The client's systolic blood pressure is 150 mm Hg.
   2. The client's heart rate is 56 beats per minute.
   3. The client has an S_2 heart sound.
   4. The client's heart rhythm is irregular.

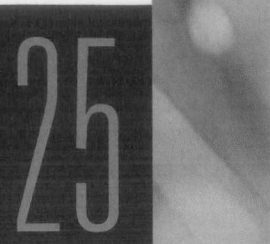

25

Caring for Clients with Disorders of Coronary and Peripheral Blood Vessels

Words To Know

acute coronary syndrome
aneurysm
angina pectoris
arteriosclerosis
atherectomy
atheroma
atherosclerosis
bruit
cardiac rehabilitation
cholesterol
collateral circulation
coronary artery disease
coronary occlusion
coronary stent
coronary thrombosis
electron beam computed tomography
embolus
enhanced external counter pulsation
high-density lipoprotein
homocysteine
hyperlipidemia
infarct
ischemia
laser angioplasty
lipid profile
low-density lipoprotein
neoangiogenesis
percutaneous transluminal coronary angioplasty
peripheral vascular disease
phlebothrombosis
phytoestrogens
plaque
subendocardial infarction
thrombolytic agents
thrombosis
thrombus
topical hyperbaric oxygen
transmural infarction
transmyocardial revascularization
varicose veins
vein ligation
vein stripping
venous insufficiency
venous reflux
venous stasis ulcer

Learning Objectives

On completion of this chapter, you will be able to:

1. Distinguish between arteriosclerosis and atherosclerosis.
2. List risk factors associated with coronary artery disease and discuss which can be modified.
3. Describe the symptoms, diagnosis, treatment, and nursing management of coronary artery disease.
4. Discuss the symptoms, diagnosis, treatment, and nursing management of myocardial infarction.
5. Discuss the symptoms, diagnosis, treatment, and nursing management of Raynaud's disease, thrombosis, phlebothrombosis, embolism, and venous insufficiency.
6. Discuss the symptoms, diagnosis, and treatment of varicose veins.
7. Describe nursing management of clients undergoing surgery for varicose veins.
8. Discuss the symptoms, diagnosis, treatment, and nursing management of clients with an aortic aneurysm.

Cardiovascular disease is the leading cause of death in the United States. Occlusive disorders of the coronary arteries and resulting complications are largely responsible for cardiac deaths. Occlusive disorders of peripheral blood vessels also contribute to morbidity and mortality. The most common causes of occlusive vascular diseases are arteriosclerosis, atherosclerosis, clot formation, and vascular spasm. Venous insufficiency and valvular incompetence also foster peripheral vascular disorders. This chapter discusses a variety of conditions that affect the coronary arteries and peripheral blood vessels.

ARTERIOSCLEROSIS

Arteriosclerosis refers to the loss of elasticity or hardening of the arteries that accompanies the aging process.

As cells in arterial tissue layers degenerate with age, calcium is deposited in the cytoplasm. The calcium causes the arteries to lose elasticity. As the left ventricle contracts, sending oxygenated blood from the heart, the rigid arterial vessels fail to stretch. The potential result is a reduced volume of oxygenated blood delivered to organs such as the myocardium, brain, kidneys, and extremities.

 Gerontologic Considerations

- The incidence of arteriosclerosis and other vascular disorders increases with age. General physiologic changes of aging predispose clients to vascular occlusive disease, especially as a result of atherosclerotic plaque formation. In addition, atherosclerosis is the most common cause of peripheral arterial problems in the older adult.

ATHEROSCLEROSIS

Atherosclerosis is a condition in which the lumen of arteries fill with fatty deposits called **plaque**. The plaque is chiefly composed of **cholesterol**, a fatty (lipid) substance. Atherosclerosis is a more modifiable contributor than arteriosclerosis to vascular disease. Therefore, it is the focus of attention and research into the mechanisms that contribute to plaque formation and its reduction to decrease vascular disease.

Pathophysiology and Etiology

Areas of atherosclerotic research include determining the mechanisms by which lipids are formed and metabolized, and the roles that body fat, obesity, infectious and inflammatory processes may play in contributing to higher risk factors for vascular diseases.

Hyperlipidemia

Hyperlipidemia, or high levels of blood fat, triggers atherosclerotic changes. Factors such as gender, heredity, diet, diseases such as metabolic syndrome (see Chap. 51), and inactivity individually or collectively contribute to hyperlipidemia. For example, some clients are genetically predisposed to produce cells with reduced numbers of receptors for binding with cholesterol; therefore, they are more likely to develop high lipid levels. Clients who consume a high-fat diet may saturate all available cholesterol receptors, which also results in hyperlipidemia. Obese people with metabolic syndrome who are prone to diabetes tend to have lower levels of *leptin*, which regulates energy metabolism, and *adiponectin*, a protein with anti-inflammatory effects (You et al., 2005). Above-normal cholesterol levels also have been linked to a by-product of methionine, an amino acid present in meat, called **homocysteine**. High levels of homocysteine also are implicated in thickening, narrowing, and scarring of arterial walls.

Infection

A current hypothesis is that atherosclerosis is linked to prior infections with *Chlamydia pneumoniae,* a bacterium that commonly causes respiratory infections (Prasad et al., 2002; Centers for Disease Control and Prevention [CDC], 2001). Research has shown that *C. pneumoniae* can infect smooth muscle and endothelial cells of arterial walls. Some evidence suggests that *C. pneumoniae* either accelerates the atherosclerotic process or destabilizes one that already exists, leading to an area of local inflammation. Scientists support their hypothesis with the finding that *C. pneumoniae* has been cultured from the **atheroma** (fatty mass) in the arterial wall. Furthermore, results of blood tests such as highly sensitive C-reactive protein (HS-CRP) levels and white blood cell (WBC) counts, which reflect inflammation and infection, are elevated among clients hospitalized for coronary events (Adam et al., 2002; Cushman, 2005). An elevated C-reactive

protein level recently has been added as a predictive cardiac risk factor unique to women (Ridker, 2007).

Recently conducted large clinical trials support the *C. pneumoniae* hypothesis and also suggest a connection between atheromatous plaque formation and other infectious microorganisms such as *Helicobacter pylori*, herpes simplex virus, and cytomegalovirus (Singh et al., 2005). However, research has not shown that antibiotic therapy plays a significant role in secondary prevention or improving long-term outcomes (Tarbutton & Mitra, 2007).

Inflammation

Published information in the *American Journal of Physiology, Endocrinology, and Metabolism* (You et al., 2005) indicates a relationship between body fat and the production of inflammatory and thrombotic (clot-facilitating) proteins. Researchers are finding that fatty tissue releases proinflammatory proteins: interleukin 6, tumor necrosis factor-alpha, and a third protein known as plasminogen activator inhibitor-1. The first pair of proteins is believed to promote the buildup of atherosclerotic plaque in blood vessels. The third interferes with the body's ability to dissolve blood clots that form within the vessels. This information suggests that decreasing obesity and body fat stores via exercise, dietary modification, or developing drugs that target proinflammatory proteins may reduce risk factors for heart disease.

Effect of Multiple Factors

Currently, it is safe to assume that multiple factors contribute to arteriovascular disease. A client with elevated lipid levels who also has other risk factors (cigarette smoking, stressful lifestyle, obesity, diabetes mellitus, hypertension, or a previous infection with *C. pneumoniae* or other microorganisms) is predisposed to the accelerated accumulation of fatty plaque beneath the intimal layer of the arteries.

When lipids accumulate, they are deposited under the endothelial cells of the tunica intima. The enlarging lesion elevates the endothelium of the artery wall and narrows the lumen (Fig. 25-1). Atherosclerotic vessels cannot produce endothelial-derived relaxing factors, which impairs the ability of the artery to dilate. As the subendothelial atheroma enlarges, the intimal layer may split and expose the lesion. As blood flows through the vessel, platelets become trapped in the roughened wall and initiate the clotting cascade. When the clot develops in a coronary artery, the resulting condition is called *coronary thrombosis.*

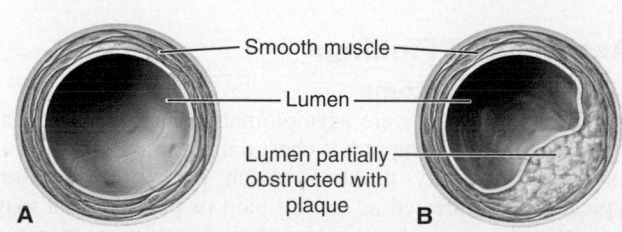

FIGURE 25-1. (A) Cross-section of a normal artery in which the lumen is fully patent, or open. **(B)** Cross-section of an atherosclerotic artery. (Images from Anatomical Chart Company.)

OCCLUSIVE DISORDERS OF CORONARY BLOOD VESSELS

Coronary occlusion is the closing of a coronary artery, which reduces or totally interrupts blood supply to the distal muscle area. Coronary artery disease precedes coronary occlusion, which, untreated, leads to myocardial infarction (MI). Symptoms usually do not occur until at least 60% of the arterial lumen is occluded.

CORONARY ARTERY DISEASE

Coronary artery disease (CAD) refers to arteriosclerotic and atherosclerotic changes in the coronary arteries supplying the myocardium. It may not be diagnosed until clients are in late middle age or older, but the vascular changes most likely begin much earlier. Although CAD occurs 10 to 15 years earlier in men than in women, the incidence rises in postmenopausal women and becomes similar to that in men thereafter. Women with a family history of cardiac disease present 7 years earlier than women with no family history. Women who smoke present 9 years earlier than female non-smokers and 4 years earlier than male smokers, suggesting that women who smoke have a greater gender susceptibility to CAD (Braun, 2007).

Gerontologic Considerations

- CAD is the most common cause of death in adults older than 65 years (Aronow, 2006).

Pathophysiology and Etiology

CAD results from many factors rather than a single cause. Several inherited and behavioral risk factors contribute to the development of CAD (Box 25-1).

At rest, ample blood flow may be maintained despite considerable CAD. The condition may go unrecognized, particularly among those with a sedentary lifestyle. During situations that increase myocardial oxygen demand (i.e., exercise, emotional stress), however, the compromised coronary arteries cannot adequately oxygenate the myocardium. When the myocardial tissue becomes *ischemic* (deprived of oxygen), clinical manifestations of CAD, such as **angina pectoris** (chest pain of cardiac origin) occur. Death of heart muscle does not accompany angina.

Assessment Findings

Signs and Symptoms

In mild CAD, clients are asymptomatic or complain of fatigue. The classic symptom is chest pain (angina) or discomfort during activity or stress. Such pain or discomfort typically is manifested as sudden pain or pressure that may be centered over the heart (precordial) or under the sternum (substernal). The pain may radiate to the shoulders and arms, especially on the left side, or to the jaw, neck, or teeth (Fig. 25-2). Some clients, especially women, experience more

BOX 25-1	Risk Factors for Coronary Artery Disease

Inherited
Male sex
Diabetes mellitus
Increased lipid levels
Genetic predisposition
Hypertension

Behavioral
Smoking
Sedentary lifestyle
Obesity
Competitive, aggressive personality
High-fat diet

atypical symptoms such as nausea, fatigue, and dizziness, which is often overlooked as significant for heart disease and consequently goes misdiagnosed. Some describe discomfort other than pain, such as indigestion or a burning, squeezing, or crushing tightness in the upper chest or throat. Table 25-1 highlights various types of angina. The American Heart Association now suggests the term **acute coronary syndrome** to describe any group of clinical symptoms compatible with acute myocardial **ischemia** (impaired oxygenation).

Some clients present with signs suggesting hyperlipidemia. They may be obese and hypertensive. An obese person with an apple-shaped body (carries most weight in the abdomen) is at higher risk for CAD than one with a pear-shaped body (carries most weight below the hips). The pulse may be high at rest and become irregular with exercise. An opaque white ring about the periphery of the cornea, called *arcus senilis* (Fig. 25-3), results from a deposit of fat granules but may be apparent only in older adults. *Xanthelasma,* a raised yellow plaque on the skin of the upper and lower eyelids (Fig. 25-4), suggests lipid accumulation. Although research is ongoing, some cardiologists indicate a relationship between a diagonal crease in the earlobe and the risk for CAD (Edston, 2006).

Diagnostic Findings

Diagnosis of coronary artery disease is a composite of lipid profile studies and electron beam computed tomography, discussed below, as well as exercise electrocardiography (ECG), cardiac catheterization, and arteriography, all of which are discussed in Chap. 22. ECG or stress testing may reveal ST segment depression, dysrhythmias, or exercise-induced hypertension. A nuclear stress test using a radionuclide such as thallium may be injected intravenously (IV) during and a few hours after exercise electrocardiography, followed by a heart scan. Narrowing of one or more coronary arteries is documented during coronary arteriography.

Lipid Profile Studies

A **lipid profile** is a group of tests that measure various blood fats. It is one indicator of a person's risk for cardiac and vascular disease. A lipid profile generally consists of measuring

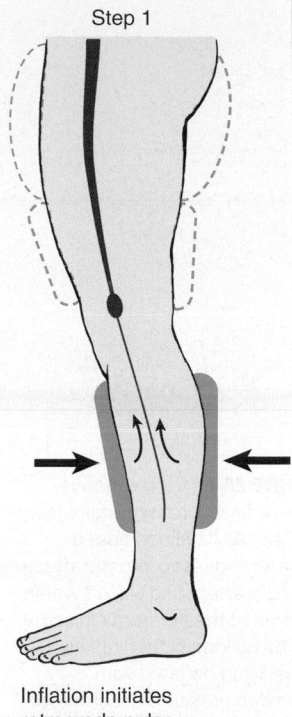

Step 1

Inflation initiates
retrograde pulse
wave

FIGURE 25-5. Inflation and defla...

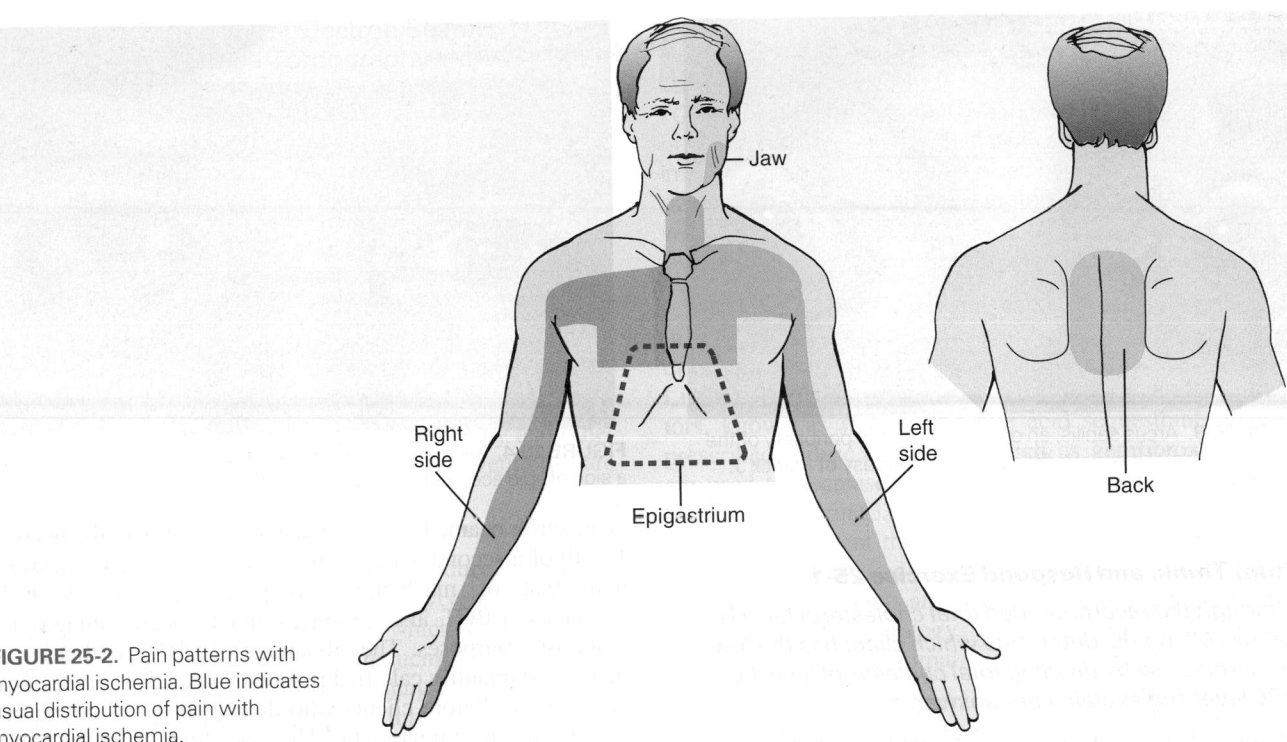

FIGURE 25-2. Pain patterns with myocardial ischemia. Blue indicates usual distribution of pain with myocardial ischemia.

form of passive exercise tha
collateral circulation, acc
blood.

Although the mechani
symptoms is not well under
the therapeutic results are m
son & Hui, 2000). Advan
frequency of angina and imp
vantages are that EECP is t
cians offer or refer clients f
interest from medical perso
third-party payers can better
less time-consuming treatme

Invasive Perfusion Techr
Invasive nonsurgical proced
coronary arteries include pe
nary angioplasty, coronary s
procedures include coronary
myocardial revascularization.

Percutaneous Translumi
For clients who fit specific
minal coronary angioplasty
to as *balloon angioplasty,* i
uses sedation and local anest
is inserted through the skin
artery into the diseased coro
passage of the catheter is mo
catheter is positioned in the
is inflated with carbon dioxi
to several minutes. Inflation

total serum cholesterol, low-density lipoprotein cholesterol, high-density lipoprotein cholesterol, and triglycerides. Cardiac risk increases when the level of total serum cholesterol is elevated. Another risk factor is an elevation of triglycerides, which are chains of fatty acids.

Proteins transport lipids (cholesterol) in the blood. **Low-density lipoprotein** (LDL) has a lower ratio of protein to cholesterol; **high-density lipoprotein** (HDL) is just the opposite—it has a higher ratio of protein to cholesterol. In clients with CAD, the level of LDL, which sometimes is referred to as "bad cholesterol" because it sticks to arteries, exceeds recommended amounts. The level of HDL, called "good cholesterol" because it carries cholesterol to the liver for removal, is lower than desirable (Table 25-2).

Cardiac risk can be estimated by dividing the total serum cholesterol level by the HDL level; a result greater than 5 suggests a potential for CAD. Depending on an assessment of risk factors, treatment for hyperlipidemia may begin when the LDL level ranges between 100 mg/dL and 130 mg/dL, with the goal being a level below 100 mg/dL.

TABLE 25-1 Types of Angina

	STABLE ANGINA	UNSTABLE ANGINA	VARIANT (PRINZMETAL'S) ANGINA	MICROVASCULAR ANGINA (CARDIAC SYNDROME X)
Causes	75% Coronary occlusion that accompanies exertion Elevated heart rate or BP Eating a large meal	Progressive worsening of stable angina, with more than 90% coronary occlusion	Arterial spasm in normal or diseased coronary arteries	Constriction of myocardial capillaries too small for standard cardiac tests to detect
Symptoms	Chest pain that lasts 15 minutes or less and may radiate Similar pain severity, frequency, and duration with each episode	Chest pain of increased frequency, severity, and duration poorly relieved by rest or oral nitrates Client at risk of MI within 18 months of angina's onset	Chest pain that occurs at rest (usually between 12 and 8 AM), is sporadic over 3 to 6 months, and diminishes overtime, ST elevation rather than depression on ECG	Prolonged chest pain that accompanies exercise and is not always relieved by medication
Treatment	Rest, sublingual nitrates, antihypertensives, lifestyle changes	Sedation, IV nitroglycerin, oxygen, antihypertensives, anticoagulant or antiplatelet therapy, revascularization procedures	Nitrates or calcium channel blockers	Heart-healthy habits and trials with medications like a nitrate, beta blocker, or calcium channel blocker

DRUG THERA

Drug Category and Examples
Vasodilators nitroglycerin
Beta-Adrenergic Blockers propranolol (Inderal)
Thrombolytics alteplase (Activase); recombinant tissue plasminogen activator (r-TPA)
Anticoagulants heparin sodium (Hepalean)
Calcium Channel Blockers diltiazem (Cardizem)
Diuretics furosemide (Lasix)

CHF, congestive heart failure;

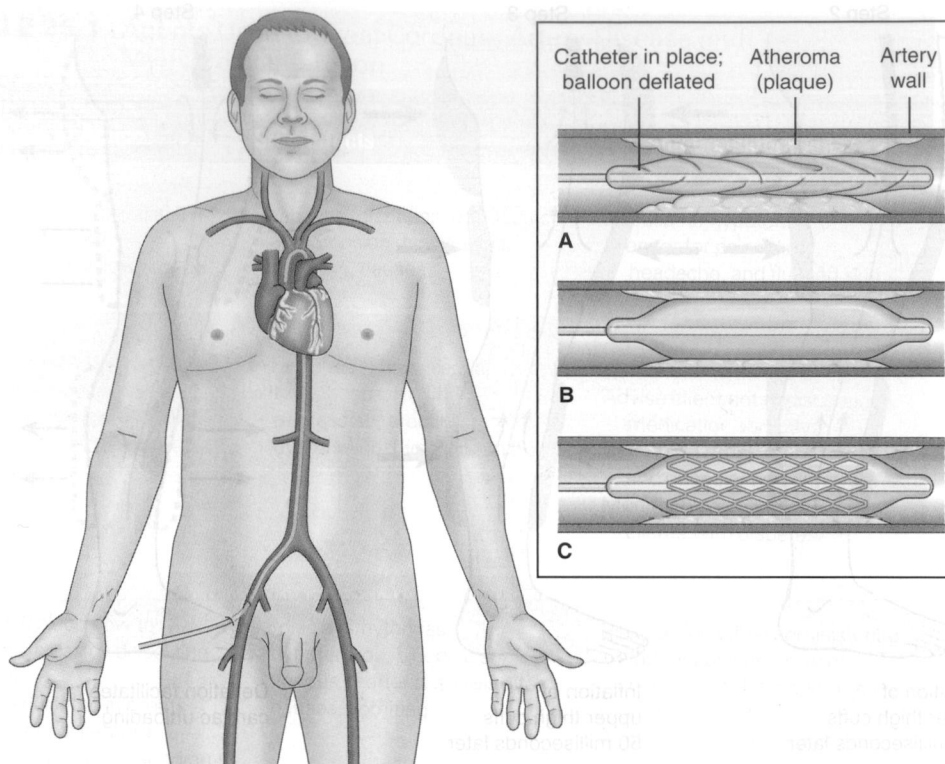

FIGURE 25-6. Percutaneous transluminal coronary angioplasty (PTCA). (**A**) A balloon-tipped catheter is passed into the affected coronary artery and placed within the area of the atheroma (plaque). (**B**) The balloon is then rapidly inflated and deflated with controlled pressure to compress the atheroma. (**C**) A stent is placed to maintain patency of the artery, and the balloon is removed.

Client and Family Teaching 25-1
Self-Care Following Percutaneous Transluminal Coronary Angioplasty

The nurse provides the following instructions before the client is discharged:

● Avoid lifting more than 10 lbs for at least 3 days if the groin was used for catheter insertion. Avoid lifting more than 1 lb for at least 3 days if a site in the upper extremity was used.
● Refrain from riding a bicycle, driving a vehicle, or mowing the lawn for at least 3 days.
● Refrain from sexual activity for 1 week.
● Shower rather than bathe until the cutaneous catheterization site heals.
● Clean the site with soap and water; eliminate any dressing.
● Relieve discomfort at the site with a mild analgesic such as acetaminophen (Tylenol); numbness at the site is temporary and not unusual.
● Expect to see a bruise, which may last 1 to 3 weeks, at the catheter insertion site.
● Report any signs of bleeding, infection or impaired circulation: fever, swelling, redness, bloody or purulent drainage, acute pain in the extremity, cold or pale skin.
● Notify the cardiologist immediately if there is pain or tightness in the chest, which could indicate obstructed blood flow through the coronary artery.

an improved technique for maintaining patency of previously obstructed arteries.

Atherectomy

Clients whose atherosclerotic plaque is no longer soft and pliable may benefit from an **atherectomy,** removal of fatty plaque. The plaque is removed by either inserting a cardiac catheter with a cutting tool at the tip (Fig. 25-7) or by

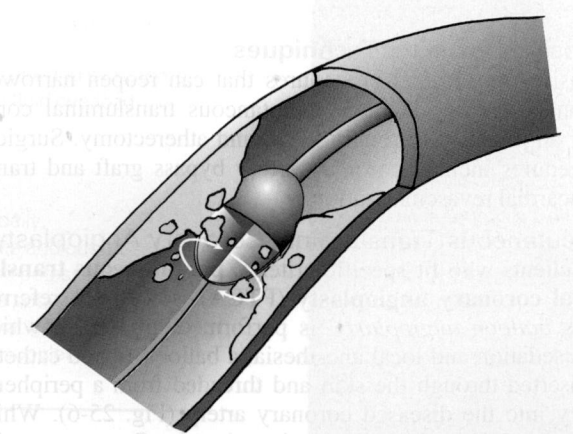

FIGURE 25-7. An atherectomy catheter removes plaque with either a circular blade or an abrasive material. This type of catheter is effective when plaque is hardened. Soft plaque can be compressed by a balloon catheter.

performing laser angioplasty. The following describes four atherectomy options:

- *Directional coronary atherectomy* shaves the plaque from the arterial wall and stores the particles in the catheter.
- *Transluminal extraction* uses a cardiac catheter with a spinning blade to separate plaque from the arterial wall and removes the debris with a vacuum attachment.
- *Percutaneous transluminal catheter rotational ablation* uses a rotating bur that spins at 200,000 revolutions per minute. Because the particles of freed plaque are smaller than red blood cells, phagocytes and the lymphatic system remove them.
- **Laser angioplasty** uses short pulses of light that vaporize plaque without creating heat that is intense enough to damage the arterial wall.

Atherectomy usually is followed by PTCA and placement of a stent.

Coronary Artery Bypass Graft Surgery

Coronary artery bypass graft (CABG) surgery (see Chap. 29) is a technique for revascularizing the myocardium. A section from a healthy leg vein or chest artery is used to reroute the flow of oxygenated blood from the aorta or a chest artery to below the obstruction in the diseased coronary artery. More than one graft may be necessary if several coronary arteries are occluded. The procedure is performed through a 10- to 12-inch midsternal incision, which is closed with wire, staples, or sutures. The heart is stopped during tra-

ditional CABG surgery, but blood is circulated through a heart-lung machine so that oxygen continues to be delivered to cells, tissues, and organs while CO_2 is removed. When the vascular reconnections are completed, heart function is restored. The client remains on a ventilator for approximately 24 hours. It may be several weeks before the client can return to work. Results after CABG surgery tend to last longer than PTCA, stenting, or atherectomy. Chapter 29 provides information about minimally invasive direct coronary artery bypass, an alternative to traditional CABG surgery.

Transmyocardial Revascularization

A **transmyocardial revascularization** (TMR) laser procedure, which improves oxygenation of myocardial tissue, may improve quality of life for clients with chest pain that does not respond to medication and who are not candidates for CABG surgery. TMR may be performed for the following reasons:

- The occluded coronary arteries are too narrow or distal to permit catheter insertion.
- There are so many occlusions that risks from a lengthy surgical procedure are unreasonable.
- The client has end-stage (seriously advanced) CAD, which increases the potential for life-threatening complications or death.

To access the heart, a thoracotomy incision is made between ribs on the left side of the chest. While the heart is visualized with transesophageal echocardiography, the laser

---

Nutrition Notes 25-1
The Client at Risk for Cardiovascular Disease

A healthy diet and lifestyle forms the cornerstone of cardiovascular disease prevention and treatment. The following recommendations for risk reduction are appropriate for all people over the age of 2; they may be intensified for clients with established cardiovascular disease:

- Attain or maintain healthy weight by balancing calorie intake with physical activity. Excess body weight increases LDL cholesterol levels, blood glucose levels, and blood pressure and lowers HDL levels.
- Consume an overall healthy diet rich in a variety of fruits and vegetables. Fruits and vegetables are rich in nutrients and fiber and low in calories.
- Select whole grains for at least half of all grain choices. Whole grains are rich sources of fiber; soluble fiber helps lower LDL cholesterol, and insoluble fibers are associated with lower CVD risk.
- Eat fatty fish at least twice a week. Fatty fish, such as salmon, swordfish, and king mackerel, provide omega 3 fatty acids that are associated with a reduced risk of both sudden death and death from coronary artery disease. A higher intake of fish may also displace the intake of red meats that are high in saturated fat.
- Limit the intake of saturated fat, trans fat, and cholesterol by choosing lean meats, using plant proteins, choosing

fat-free dairy products, and limiting the intake of partially hydrogenated fats found in stick margarines, shortenings, and commercially baked products. Diets low in saturated fat, trans fat, and cholesterol lower CVD risk mostly by lowering LDL cholesterol.
- Limit food and beverages high in added sugars, such as desserts, candy, and carbonated beverages. Added sugars are generally empty calories.
- Limit salt intake by eating and preparing foods with little or no salt. Generally, as salt intake increases, so does blood pressure.
- Drink alcohol in moderation, if at all. Moderate alcohol intake (less than 1 drink/day for women, 2 drinks/day for men) increases HDL cholesterol levels, but it is not recommended that people begin drinking for the purpose of reducing their risk of CVD.

Antioxidant supplements, such as those containing vitamin E, beta carotene, and selenium, are not recommended because clinical trials have failed to confirm beneficial effects from their use. People are urged to consume dietary sources of antioxidants, such as fruits, vegetables, whole grains, and vegetable oils.

probe is aimed at the beating heart. The probe makes 15 to 40 channels that are 1 mm deep and 1 cm apart from the epicardium, through the ischemic myocardium, to the endocardium. The channels that the laser creates allow the ischemic myocardium to absorb the oxygenated blood that seeps into the area. Therefore, the myocardium receives oxygen not from a coronary artery, but from the blood that seeps into the space between the cells. There are other hypotheses for the mechanism by which TMR relieves the client's symptoms. Some believe that it disrupts the myocardial nerve supply, which suppresses the ability to perceive anginal pain. Others suggest that the trauma stimulates **neoangiogenesis,** new growth of blood vessels, which results in additional collateral blood supply to the heart muscle.

Clients remain in the hospital for up to 1 week. Activity is restricted for several weeks to allow a safe period of healing. Because TMR relieves symptoms only, cardiac rehabilitation requires clients to continue to modify risk factors that caused CAD. Such modification means the client must eliminate smoking, follow a heart-healthy diet, and incorporate regular, moderate exercise. Variations in TMR also are being implemented. Sometimes TMR is performed with a percutaneously inserted catheter.

Nursing Management

The nurse assesses the characteristics of chest pain and administers prescribed drugs that dilate the coronary arteries or reduce the work of the heart. He or she encourages rest and administers oxygen to improve the available oxygen supply to the heart muscle. If drugs, rest, and oxygen do not relieve the pain, the nurse notifies the physician.

The nurse helps clients learn how to reduce modifiable CAD risk factors, which can improve not only cardiac health but also overall well-being. He or she explains that balancing caloric intake with physical activity to achieve or maintain healthy body weight can significantly reduce risks. The nurse arranges a consultation with a dietitian and provides written material about a heart-healthy diet (Nutrition Notes 25-1). He or she refers clients to smoking-cessation programs and discusses medications that can help (see Chap. 71).

The nurse teaches about the administration and side effects of antianginal drugs (Client and Family Teaching 25-2). He or she emphasizes that severe, unrelieved chest pain indicates a need to be examined by a physician without delay. The nurse advises the client to report changes in the usual pattern of angina, such as increased frequency or severity or occurrence with rest or during sleep.

The nurse informs clients about diagnostic tests or treatment procedures. The nurse who prepares the client for invasive, nonsurgical procedures performed with a percutaneous catheter cleanses and removes hair from skin insertion sites (one for the coronary catheter and the other for an arterial line through which blood pressure [BP] will be directly monitored). He or she withholds anticoagulant therapy before the procedure to decrease the chance of hemorrhage. The nurse monitors all vascular sites for bleeding after a procedure and assesses distal pulses. He or she observes mental status because cerebral emboli can occur. The nurse monitors urine output and administers analgesics for discomfort. He or she reports any of the following data immediately: severe chest pain, abnormal heart rate or rhythm, mental confusion or loss of consciousness,

---

Client and Family Teaching 25-2
Use of Short-Acting Nitroglycerin

The nurse discusses the following points with clients who are prescribed short-acting nitroglycerin and their families.

For sublingual nitroglycerin:

- Sit down and rest before self-administering nitroglycerin. Decreased activity may relieve chest pain; sitting will prevent injury should the nitroglycerin lower BP and cause fainting.
- Place one nitroglycerin tablet under the tongue if 2 to 3 minutes of rest fails to relieve pain.
- Expect to feel dizzy or flushed or to develop a headache.
- Let the tablet dissolve slowly; there should be slight tingling or burning under the tongue.
- Take a second nitroglycerin tablet in 5 minutes if chest pain is still present.
- Take a third nitroglycerin tablet in 5 more minutes if chest pain is still present.
- Call 911 if chest pain continues; do not drive to an emergency department. Discuss the chest pain with the physician if self-management relieved it or its usual characteristics changed.
- Keep a few nitroglycerin tablets in a dark, dry container with you at all times; consult with the pharmacist about a sealed metal container that you can wear around the neck.

- Do not place other medications in the container with the nitroglycerin.
- Replace nitroglycerin tablets every 6 months or after any container has been opened six times.

For nitroglycerin spray:

- Assume a sitting position.
- Hold the canister upright.
- Spray the nitroglycerin onto the tongue without inhaling.
- Close the mouth immediately afterward.
- Expect to feel dizzy or flushed or to develop a headache.
- Repeat spraying every 5 minutes for a second and third time if chest pain is unrelieved.
- Call 911 if chest pain continues.
- Discuss the chest pain with the physician if self-management relieved it or its usual characteristics changed.
- Expect a new canister of nitroglycerin to deliver approximately 200 doses.
- Check the amount of nitroglycerin in the canister by floating it in a bowl of water; the higher the canister floats, the less medication it contains. Obtain a reserve canister when the present canister shows signs of becoming empty.

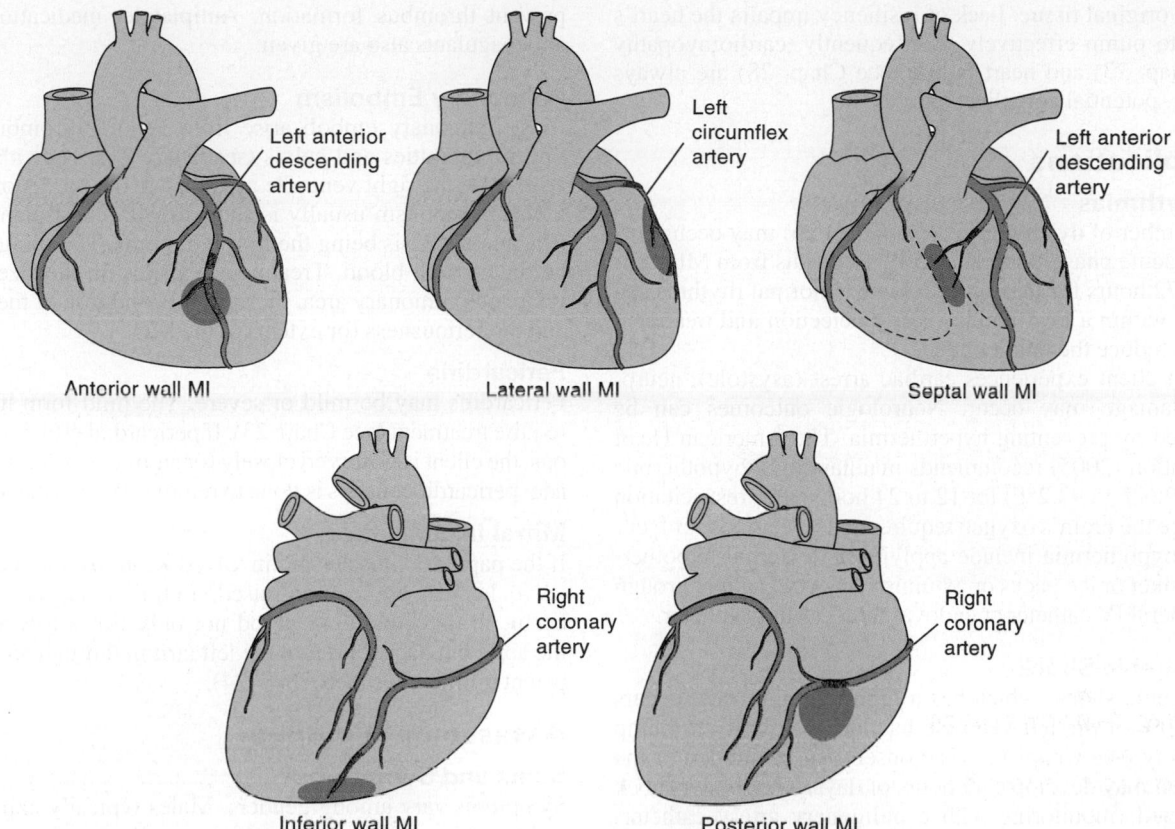

FIGURE 25-8. Zones of myocardial infarction (MI) based on the artery that becomes occluded.

hypotension, urine output of less than 30 to 50 mL/hour, or a cold, pulseless extremity. See Chapter 29 for the Nursing Process for the Client Undergoing Cardiac or Vascular Surgery.

MYOCARDIAL INFARCTION

An **infarct** is an area of tissue that dies (*necrosis*) from inadequate oxygenation. An MI, or heart attack, occurs when there is prolonged total occlusion of coronary arterial blood flow. The larger the necrotic area is, the more serious the damage. An infarct that extends through the full thickness of the myocardial wall is called a **transmural infarction** or Q-wave MI. A partial-thickness infarct is called a **subendocardial infarction** or a non-Q-wave MI. Each coronary artery supplies oxygenated blood to a different area of the myocardium. The location of the infarction depends on the area where the blood supply to the myocardium is interrupted by the respective occluded coronary artery (Fig. 25-8).

Pathophysiology and Etiology

The most common cause of MI is <u>coronary thrombosis,</u> the consequence of a blood clot located within a coronary artery. Thrombosis usually is secondary to arteriosclerotic and atherosclerotic changes. <u>Arterial spasms</u> also may cause an MI. Once an area of the myocardium has been damaged and destroyed, the cells in that area lose their special functions of automaticity, excitability, conductivity, contractility, and rhythmicity. Thus, dysrhythmias and heart failure are common consequences (see Chaps. 26 and 28).

Injury to the myocardium triggers the inflammatory response. Proinflammatory chemicals disrupt the permeability of cell membranes (see Chap. 12). The damaged cells release serum cardiac markers (intracellular enzymes) and electrolytes into the extracellular fluid. Loss of intracellular potassium and accumulation of lactic acid from anaerobic cellular metabolism affect depolarization and repolarization of myocardial cells. Dangerous dysrhythmias can develop during this time because the affected areas are electrically unstable.

The infarction process can take up to 6 hours. There are three zones of tissue damage:

1. The first zone consists of a central area of necrotic (dead) myocardial cells.
2. A second zone of injured cells, which may live if blood supply to the area is restored, surrounds the first zone.
3. The third zone is the ischemic area that will probably survive.

Thrombolytic drugs, called clot busters, are given during this 6-hour window of opportunity to reestablish blood flow and save as much myocardial tissue as possible.

Leukocytosis and slightly elevated body temperature follow in 3 to 7 days. New capillaries begin to grow to establish collateral circulation to the infarcted area; however, it takes 2 or 3 weeks before such flow is significant. A "cardiac patch" of collagen fibers begins to form within the first 2 weeks of the infarct, but it takes as long as 3 months for the scar to grow firm. The scar tissue is less effective than the myocardium it is replacing; it does not stretch and contract like the original tissue. Lack of resiliency impairs the heart's ability to pump effectively. Consequently, cardiomyopathy (see Chap. 23) and heart failure (see Chap. 28) are always lifelong, potential complications.

Complications

Dysrhythmias

Any number of dysrhythmias (see Chap. 26) may occur during the acute phase. More than 50% of deaths from MI occur within 72 hours for this reason. Some abnormal rhythms can be fatal within a few minutes. Early detection and treatment of them reduce the fatality rate.

If a client experiences cardiac arrest (asystole), neurologic damage may occur. Neurologic outcomes can be improved by preventing hyperthermia. The American Heart Association (2005) recommends maintaining a hypothermic state (89.6°F to 93.2°F) for 12 to 24 hours after resuscitation to reduce the brain's oxygen requirements. Methods for facilitating hypothermia include applying an external hypothermia blanket or ice packs or administering cold saline through a peripheral IV catheter or endovascular cooling catheter.

Cardiogenic Shock

Cardiogenic shock, which has a high mortality rate, occurs when 40% of the left ventricle has lost the ability to pump effectively (see Chap. 17). The onset may be sudden or the condition may develop over hours or days. The sooner shock is detected (monitoring with a pulmonary artery catheter) and treatment is instituted, the better the client's chances of survival. This complication has been successfully treated with medications, ventricular assist devices, and an intra-aortic balloon pump (see Chap. 28).

Ventricular Rupture

Ventricular rupture occurs when a soft necrotic area from a transmural or interventricular septal MI ruptures. Dyspnea, rapid right-sided heart failure, and shock result. *Hemopericardium* (blood in the pericardium) and cardiac tamponade follow. The prognosis is poor, although survival is possible.

Ventricular Aneurysm

A ventricular aneurysm is a bulging of the portion of the heart affected by the MI. This area of poorly contractile tissue predisposes the heart to failure. Blood trapped in the projection tends to form thrombi, which may be released into the arterial circulation. The aneurysm may burst, resulting in hemorrhage and death.

Arterial Embolism

Clots can form in the cavity of the ventricular aneurysm (mural thrombi), or tissue debris can break free. If clots enter the systemic arterial circulation, they may occlude a peripheral artery. Symptoms depend on the location of the affected artery. Arteriotomy (opening of an artery) and embolectomy (removal of an embolus) may be necessary; a client who has recently had an MI, however, is a poor surgical risk.

Venous Thrombosis

Venous thrombosis arises mostly in the veins of the lower extremities and pelvis. The use of antiembolism stockings and regular performance of foot and leg exercises help to prevent thrombus formation. Antiplatelet medications and anticoagulants also are given.

Pulmonary Embolism

Most pulmonary emboli arise from venous thrombi in the lower extremities and pelvis (see Chap. 21). They also may arise from the right ventricle after an MI. The onset of a pulmonary embolism usually is sudden, with chest pain, dyspnea, and cyanosis being the first symptoms. The sputum may be tinged with blood. Treatment depends on the size of the infarcted pulmonary area, the age and condition of the client, and the seriousness (or extent) of the MI.

Pericarditis

Pericarditis may be mild or severe. The mild form may not require treatment (see Chap. 23). If pericardial effusion develops, the client is observed closely for signs of cardiac tamponade; pericardiocentesis is done to remove excess fluid.

Mitral Insufficiency

If the papillary muscles are involved in an MI and the mitral valve leaflets are compromised, mitral regurgitation may occur. In this condition, blood not only flows forward into the aorta but backward into the left atrium through an incompetent mitral valve (see Chap. 24).

Assessment Findings

Signs and Symptoms

Symptoms vary among genders. Males typically experience sudden, severe chest pain, which usually is substernal and may radiate to the shoulder, arm, teeth, jaw, or throat. Women more often than men have more vague symptoms, such as unexplained fatigue, abdominal pain, and shortness of breath, which often leads to misdiagnosis of females in emergency departments (Ashton, 2007). Most clients are aware of the seriousness of their symptoms and are apprehensive. When chest pain is experienced, it is more severe and lasts longer than anginal pain. Some clients describe it as squeezing or crushing. Unlike anginal pain, rest and sublingual nitrates do not relieve MI pain. If untreated, it may last for several hours or 1 or 2 days. Finally, it becomes sore or achy before disappearing entirely. A few clients, such as older adults and diabetics, experience little or no pain and may never know that they had an MI until an ECG detects it weeks, months, or years later. Clients appear pale and diaphoretic. They may experience nausea and vomiting or be hypotensive and faint. Pulse is rapid and weak and may be irregular. Signs of left-sided heart failure (dyspnea, cyanosis, cough) may appear if left ventricular pumping is sufficiently impaired.

 Gerontologic Considerations

- Less than 50% of older adults report chest pain with acute MI, whereas approximately 80% of younger adults report chest pain. Older adults are more likely to have nonspecific symptoms such as dyspnea, confusion, syncope, epigastric distress, nausea, heartburn, or indigestion.

- Older adults delay seeking health care after the onset of presenting symptoms of acute MI more often than younger adults (Aronow, 2006).

TABLE 25-4 Serum Cardiac Markers After an Acute Myocardial Infarction

CARDIAC MARKER	CHARACTERISTICS
Myoglobin	Present as early as 2 hours after MI; peaks in 3 to 15 hours; returns to normal in 20 to 24 hours
Troponin T	Rises 3 to 4 hours after MI; peaks in 4 to 6 hours; returns to normal in several weeks
Troponin I	Rises 4 to 6 hours after MI; peaks in 14 to 18 hours; returns to normal in 6 to 7 days
CK-MB (creatine kinase)	Rises 4 to 12 hours after MI; peaks in 24 hours; returns to normal in 3 to 4 days
AST (aspartate aminotransferase)	Increases 6 to 12 hours after MI; peaks in 36 hours; returns to normal in 3 to 4 days
LDH_1 and LDH_2 (lactate dehydrogenase)	Rises 24 to 48 hours after MI; peaks in 3 to 6 days; returns to normal in 7 to 14 days. An LDH_1:LDH_2 ratio greater than 1.0 indicates myocardial damage.

Diagnostic Findings

Serum Enzymes and Isoenzymes

Laboratory tests to diagnose MI include a series of serum cardiac markers, substances that are released by damaged myocardial cells during an infarct (Table 25-4). When tissues and cells break down, are damaged, or die, great quantities of certain enzymes are released into the bloodstream. Enzymes are complex proteins produced by living cells that function as catalysts, substances capable of producing chemical changes without being changed themselves. An **isoenzyme** is one of several forms of the same enzyme that may exist in cells and is capable of being identified separately from others. The following serum cardiac markers are measured initially and every 8 hours for 24 hours to determine elevated levels:

- Myoglobin, a biomarker that rises in 2 to 3 hours after heart damage
- Troponin, and subunits known as troponin T and troponin I, enzymes in myocardial contractile tissue
- Creatine kinase (CK), formerly creatine phosphokinase, and its cardiospecific isoenzyme, CK-MB
- Lactate dehydrogenase (LDH) and isoenzymes LDH_1 and LDH_2
- Aspartate aminotransferase (AST), formerly called serum glutamic oxaloacetic transaminase (SGOT)

Troponin is present only in myocardial tissue; therefore, it is the gold standard for determining heart damage in the early stages of an MI. The other enzymes can be elevated in response to cardiac or other organ damage. Therefore, the isoenzymes CK-MB, LDH_1, and LDH_2 are evaluated for their cardiac specificity.

Miscellaneous Laboratory and Diagnostic Tests

The WBC count, C-reactive protein, and erythrocyte sedimentation rate increase on about the third day following MI because of the inflammatory response that the injured myocardial cells triggered. Blood glucose level may be elevated because of the body's response to a major stressor. After an MI, characteristic changes appear on the ECG within 2 to 12 hours. They may, however, take as long as 3 days to develop. These changes include T-wave inversion, ST segment elevation, and a Q wave (Fig. 25-9).

Medical Management

Treatment is directed toward reducing tissue hypoxia, relieving pain, treating shock (if present), and alleviating dys-

rhythmias if they occur. Because women are three times more likely to be misdiagnosed and erroneously discharged, they suffer a higher mortality rate than men following a myocardial infarction (Ashton, 2007).

Thrombolytic Therapy

The goal for administering **thrombolytic agents**, intravenous drugs that dissolve blood clots, is a "door to needle" time of 30 minutes. Drugs such as streptokinase and recombinant tissue plasminogen activator (t-PA) dissolve the thrombus occluding the coronary artery, restoring the circulation of oxygenated blood to the myocardium. If administered within the first 2 hours after the onset of symptoms, a MI can be greatly minimized. Even if the client is seen within 12 to 24 hours of the onset of the occlusion, reestablishing coronary artery blood flow can reduce the zone of necrosis (ACC/AHA [American College of Cardiology/American Heart Association], 2004). A thrombolytic can be administered within the specified timelines unless the client is disqualified on the basis of criteria that identify possible concomitant risks for neurological complications and bleeding (Box 25-2).

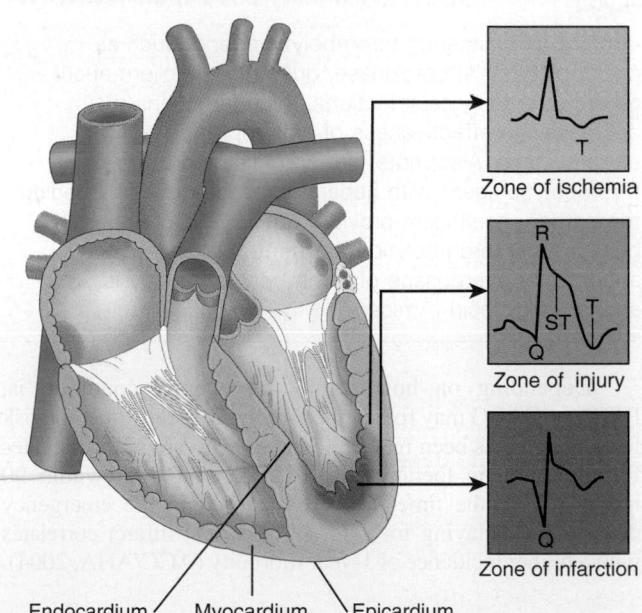

FIGURE 25-9. Characteristic ECG changes after an MI. T-wave inversion, ST segment elevation, and sometimes a Q wave are evidence of myocardial ischemia, injury, and infarction, respectively.

BOX 25-2 Contraindications for Thrombolytic Therapy

Absolute Contraindications

- Any prior intracranial hemorrhage
- Structural cerebral vascular lesion
- Malignant intracranial neoplasm
- Ischemic stroke within past 3 months
- Suspected aortic dissection
- Active bleeding (excluding menses)
- Significant closed head or facial trauma within past 3 months

Relative Contraindications

- Chronic, severe, poorly controlled hypertension
- Uncontrolled hypertension as evidenced by systolic BP < 180 mm Hg or diastolic BP < 110 mm Hg
- Ischemic stroke < 3 months ago, dementia or other intracranial pathology not covered in absolute contraindications
- Traumatic or prolonged CPR or major surgery within past 3 weeks
- Internal bleeding within past 2–4 weeks
- Noncompressible vascular punctures
- Prior exposure (< 5days) or prior allergic reaction if streptokinase is considered for use
- Pregnancy
- Active peptic ulcer
- Current use of anticoagulants

Source: ACC/AHA Guidelines for the Management of Patients with ST-Elevation Myocardial Infarction—Executive Summary (2004). Available at http://www.acc.org/qualityandscience/clinical/guidelines/stemi/exec_summ/index.htm. Accessed December 2007.

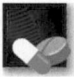

Pharmacologic Considerations

- Before administering thrombolytic agents such as anistreplase or streptokinase, question the client about recent streptococcal infections; such infections may decrease the effectiveness of anistreplase or streptokinase. Also, note that administration of a thrombolytic agent with heparin increases risk of bleeding; the primary healthcare provider usually discontinues the heparin until thrombolytic treatment is completed. An antidote for overdosage of thrombolytic therapy is aminocaproic acid (Amicar).

Depending on how stable the client's condition is, PTCA or CABG may follow thrombolytic therapy after the risk for bleeding has been reduced. Clients who are not candidates for thrombolytic therapy should undergo PTCA within 90 minutes from the time they are assessed in the emergency department; delaying for 2 to 3 hours post infarct correlates with a higher incidence of 1-year mortality (ACC/AHA, 2004).

Symptomatic Treatment

An intravenous (IV) infusion is initiated to provide fluid while eating is restricted. The IV route also is used to administer parenteral medications. Drug therapy includes analgesics for pain, nitrates or other vasodilating drugs to improve blood flow, diuretics to reduce circulating blood volume, sedatives to promote rest and reduce anxiety, anticoagulants to prevent additional thrombus formation, and drugs to treat dysrhythmias (see Drug Therapy Table 25-1). Oxygen is ordered to treat or prevent hypoxemia. Complete bed rest is prescribed initially but not recommended for uncomplicated MIs after the first 12 hours. Activity is adjusted according to the extent of the MI, complications, and response to therapy. When chest pain is controlled, a clear liquid diet is allowed and progressed to a heart-healthy diet thereafter (see Nutrition Notes 25-1). Clients who regularly consumed caffeine before an MI are allowed up to 400 mg/day, which equals two to four cups of coffee, without danger of increasing BP (ACC/AHA, 2004). A stool softener is prescribed to prevent increased BP from straining with the passage of stool. Permanent smoking cessation is imperative. The intra-aortic balloon pump may be used for clients who develop severe left ventricular failure (see Chap. 28).

Surgical Management

CABG surgery (see Chap. 29) is done to revascularize the myocardium surgically. In clients who are experiencing cardiogenic shock, a ventricular assist device may be implanted or cardiomyoplasty (a procedure for grafting skeletal muscle to the heart) or an alternative called a heart wrap may be used (see Chap. 28).

Cardiac Rehabilitation

After a significant cardiac event such as an MI or heart surgery, clients are encouraged to participate in a medically supervised **cardiac rehabilitation** program, which combines exercise and educational activities to speed recovery and reduce or prevent recurring episodes. Cardiac rehabilitation usually begins before discharge but continues on an outpatient basis. The plan is designed according to the client's unique needs. Some clients may achieve the goals of therapy by meeting two to three times a week for 1 hour or more over a few weeks. Other clients may require therapy for 3 to 4 months. Activities and educational topics include the following:

- Gradual exercise that increases according to the client's tolerance
- Establishment of physical limitations such as the maximum amount the client can lift
- Recognition and management of depression
- Medication regimen: importance of drug therapy, dose, time taken, adverse drug effects
- Smoking cessation
- When and how to resume sexual activity (Client and Family Teaching 25-3)
- Diet modifications, how to read food labels, what food labels indicate
- How to monitor pulse rate and BP
- Symptoms to report to a physician as soon as possible
- How to avoid or minimize stressors
- Importance of continued medical supervision

Client and Family Teaching 25-3
Sexual Guidelines After Myocardial Infarction

The nurse provides the following information to the client:

● Check with physician before resuming sexual activity.
● Avoid sex with anyone other than your usual partner.
● Avoid positions that require supporting your own weight.
● Get adequate rest before sexual intercourse.
● Have sex in the same environment as before the MI.
● Postpone sex for 2 to 3 hours after eating a heavy meal or consuming alcohol.
● Use a short-acting nitrate, if the physician approves, before intercourse.
● Begin with moderate sexual foreplay.
● Use medium water temperatures when bathing or showering before or after sexual activity.

Nursing Management

The detailed nursing management of a client experiencing an acute MI is discussed in Nursing Care Plan 25-1. Instructions for performing cardiopulmonary resuscitation (CPR) (discussed in the Nursing Care Plan) are presented in Nursing Guidelines 25-1.

OCCLUSIVE DISORDERS OF PERIPHERAL BLOOD VESSELS

Peripheral vascular disease is a term for disorders that affect blood vessels distant from the large central blood vessels supplying the myocardium or that circulate blood directly in and out of the heart. Common peripheral vascular disorders, which occlude blood flow by various mechanisms, include Raynaud's disease, thrombosis, phlebothrombosis, and embolism.

Gerontologic Considerations

- Many older adults have peripheral vascular insufficiency that is manifested in weak or absent pedal pulses; cold, clammy feet; thickened toenails; and shiny skin on the lower extremities.

- Discourage older adults from using electric heating devices; burns are more likely to occur because of decreased temperature perception resulting from impaired circulation. Thermal underwear and blankets are alternatives to electric blankets and heating pads.

RAYNAUD'S DISEASE

Raynaud's disease is characterized by periodic constriction of the arteries that supply the extremities. The disorder is most common in young women.

Pathophysiology and Etiology

Raynaud's disease is characterized by brief spasms of the arteries and arterioles in the fingers (most common site), toes, nose, ears, or chin. The spasms last approximately 15 minutes and cause temporary ischemia (impaired oxygenation) to the tissues. The vessels then dilate widely, apparently to compensate for the restriction. Patchy areas of necrosis occur with prolonged ischemia.

The underlying cause of Raynaud's disease is not entirely clear. In some clients, it seems *idiopathic* (no explainable reason); in others, it is secondary to connective tissue diseases, such as scleroderma, systemic lupus erythematosus, or rheumatoid arthritis (see Chap. 63).

The anatomy of the arteries and arterioles is normal. One theory explaining the vasospasms is impaired release of *prostaglandins* (chemicals stored in cellular membranes). Some prostaglandins cause vasoconstriction; others cause vasodilation. The type that accompanies an inflammatory response causes vasodilation.

Assessment Findings

Signs and Symptoms

Attacks are intermittent and of varying frequency but are especially common after exposure to cold. When the condition occurs in the hands, they become cold, blanched, and wet with perspiration. Numbness and tingling also may occur. The client may note awkwardness and fumbling, especially when attempting fine movements. After the initial pallor, the hands, especially the fingers, become deeply cyanotic and begin to ache. The hallmark symptoms of arterial insufficiency include ischemia, pain, and paresthesia. Placing the affected part in warm water or going to a warm area can relieve an attack. Eventually the vasospasm is relieved, and blood rushes to the affected part. The skin in the deprived areas becomes flushed, swollen, and warm, and the person has a sensation of throbbing pain.

In the early stages of the disease, the hands usually appear normal between attacks. The disease does not necessarily progress to cause severe disability. Symptoms often are mild and may even improve spontaneously. When the disease is severe and of long standing, cyanosis of the fingers persists between attacks and skin changes gradually develop. Painful ulcers and superficial gangrene may appear at the fingertips. The fingers are especially vulnerable to infection. Healing of even minor lesions often is slow and uncertain.

Diagnostic Findings

No specific laboratory studies can confirm Raynaud's disease. Diagnosis is made by a history of the symptoms and examination of the involved part. Laboratory blood tests are ordered to confirm or rule out an accompanying connective tissue disorder (see Chap 63).

Medical and Surgical Management

Treatment involves avoiding factors that precipitate attacks. Smoking is contraindicated because it causes vasoconstriction. Drug therapy with peripheral vasodilators, such as isoxsuprine (Vasodilan), may be attempted, but results usually are less favorable than desired. Other drugs, such as nifedipine (Procardia), are being used investigationally. An IV

NURSING CARE PLAN 25-1 The Client with Acute Myocardial Infarction

Assessment

Determine the following.

- Client's description of pain: location, type, duration, intensity using a scale of 0 to 10, and whether it radiates to other areas
- Vital signs every 30 minutes until stable and then every 4 hours and as needed (prn)
- Presence of nausea, vomiting, diaphoresis, anxiety
- Oxygen saturation level with pulse oximeter
- Cardiac rhythm via cardiac monitor or ECG

- Heart and lung sounds
- Presence and quality of peripheral pulses
- Results of serum cardiac markers
- A thorough history to establish baseline data about disorders such as diabetes mellitus, hypertension, recent streptococcal infection or allergic reaction to streptokinase, and findings that may disqualify the client from thrombolytic therapy
- Drug history for prescribed, over-the-counter, and herbal products

Nursing Diagnosis: Acute Pain related to diminished myocardial oxygenation

Expected Outcome: Pain will be within client's identified comfort level within 30 minutes.

Interventions	Rationales
Administer oxygen at 2 L/minute by nasal cannula or as prescribed.	Supplemental oxygen raises hemoglobin saturation and oxygen in plasma. Adequate myocardial oxygen diminishes angina.
Administer prescribed sublingual or spray nitroglycerin every 5 minutes, up to three doses, if pain is unrelieved.	Nitroglycerin dilates blood vessels, improving blood flow through coronary arteries, and lowers BP, which decreases cardiac afterload.
Administer prescribed IV morphine sulfate.	Morphine reduces pain perception and anxiety. Reduced anxiety decreases heart rate and BP, alleviating the heart's demand for oxygenation.

Evaluation of Expected Outcome

Pain is eliminated or reduced to a tolerable level.

Nursing Diagnosis: Anxiety or **Fear** related to perception of impending doom, concern over actual/potential lifestyle changes, worry concerning family situation

Expected Outcome: Client will report decreased anxiety and fear.

Interventions	Rationales
Allow client to express fears and anxiety.	Sharing feelings with a supportive person tends to relieve or reduce emotional distress.
Explain all procedures before performing them.	Information eliminates the element of surprise or misinterpretation of nursing activities.
Carry out procedures in a calm, relaxed manner.	A client who senses confidence in the nurse may experience less apprehension.
Promote uninterrupted blocks of time for rest, sleep, or visits with family members.	Physical rest and support from others promote the ability to cope.
Check client frequently, and answer call lights promptly.	Knowing that help is quickly available can relieve fear.
Acknowledge grief over perceived or actual changes in lifestyle.	Dealing with reality facilitates grieving.
Administer prescribed sedatives and anxiolytic drugs as indicated.	They block sympathetic nervous system responses, which reduce anxiety and fear.

Evaluation of Expected Outcome

Anxiety is reduced as evidenced by normal heart rate and BP, no nervous activity, and self-reported tolerance of stressors.

PC: Hemorrhage related to thrombolytic therapy

Expected Outcome: The nurse will monitor to detect, manage, and minimize bleeding.

Interventions	Rationales
Observe closely for bleeding during thrombolytic therapy and until sufficient half-lives reduce pharmacodynamic effects.	The client is at risk for bleeding when thrombolytic drugs change plasminogen to plasmin.
Check for blood in stool or urine, bruising, epistaxis, abdominal pain, or altered neurologic status.	Thrombolytic drugs dissolve blood clots and interfere with their formation.

NURSING CARE PLAN 25-1   The Client with Acute Myocardial Infarction (Continued)

Interventions	Rationales
Avoid intramuscular, IV, and arterial punctures during therapy and until the risk for excessive bleeding has subsided.	Controlling bleeding may be difficult while an active level of thrombolytic drug remains in the bloodstream.
Keep client on bed rest; pad the side rails if agency policy mandates.	Trauma can cause excessive blood loss.
Have aminocaproic acid (Amicar) available as an antidote for bleeding.	Aminocaproic acid is an antiplasmin agent that inhibits plasminogen activator.

Evaluation of Expected Outcome

Client shows no evidence of bleeding.

PC: Dysrhythmias related to reperfusion of myocardium with thrombolytic therapy and instability of the conduction system

Expected Outcome: The nurse will monitor to detect, manage, and minimize dysrhythmias.

Interventions	Rationales
Place client on a cardiac monitor and closely observe for dangerous dysrhythmias.	A cardiac monitor continuously displays heart rate and rhythm; it sounds an alarm to call attention to a dysrhythmic event.
Be prepared to perform CPR if a life-threatening dysrhythmia or asystole occurs.	CPR provides basic life support (Nursing Guidelines 25-1).
Assist with endotracheal intubation, defibrillation, and administration of antidysrhythmic drugs.	Advanced cardiac life support may resuscitate a client.

Evaluation of Expected Outcome

Dysrhythmias are controlled.

---

infusion of prostaglandin E may provide temporary relief. *Sympathectomy* (cutting peripheral sympathetic nerves) may be performed; however, because of disappointing results, the procedure is performed less frequently than in the past. Gangrenous areas are amputated.

Nursing Management

Once an episode of pain occurs, there are several ways that the attack can be aborted. If warming the hands in water is impossible, the nurse encourages the client to imagine warming them in some way such as holding them near a roaring fire. The mind can alter the physiology of blood flow. Another technique is to teach clients to imitate the exercise snow skiers use called the McIntyre maneuver: while standing, clients swing their arms behind and then in front of their bodies at a rate of about 180 times per minute. The swinging motion distributes blood to the distal areas of the fingers.

Teaching for clients with Raynaud's disease and their family members is important. The nurse instructs clients to avoid situations that contribute to ischemic episodes. He or she explains that injuries may heal slowly. If clients smoke, they must stop because nicotine causes vasoconstriction and

NURSING GUIDELINES 25-1

Performing Cardiopulmonary Resuscitation (CPR)

- Attempt to arouse client by shaking and calling his or her name.
- Notify emergency personnel if client does not respond.
- Open airway with head-tilt, chin-lift.
- Remove objects or emesis from the mouth.
- Ascertain whether client is breathing by looking and listening for air.
- If client is not breathing, pinch his or her nose shut and give 2 rescue breaths through the mouth, using a one-way valve pocket mask, if available.
- Feel for a carotid pulse. If absent, administer cardiac compressions at a rate of 30 compressions to 2 breaths for both one- and two-rescuer resuscitation of adults and single rescuer resuscitation of infants to the age of puberty. Use a ratio of 15

compressions to 2 breaths for two rescuers of infants to the age of puberty. Give 100 compressions per minute.
- Check effectiveness of CPR after 4 cycles of 15 compressions to 2 breaths (pupils responding to light, pulse at carotid artery, improved skin color).
- Use an automatic electronic defibrillator (AED) if available.
- Continue with CPR between or in lieu of defibrillation if an AED is not available.
- Do not interrupt CPR for more than 6 to 7 seconds.

(Adapted from Guidelines for cardiopulmonary resuscitation and emergency cardiovascular care (2005). Available at: http://circ.ahajournals.org/cgi/content/full/112/24_suppl/IV-1.)

increases the frequency of episodes. The nurse advises clients to wear wool socks and mittens during cold weather. Clients should avoid over-the-counter decongestants, cold remedies, and drugs for symptomatic relief of hay fever because of their vasoconstrictive qualities. The nurse advises clients to wear work gloves during household chores such as gardening and washing dishes to prevent accidental injury. He or she informs clients how to perform nail care to avoid injury, such as soaking the hands or feet before trimming nails, trimming nails straight across, and seeing a podiatrist for the treatment of corns or calluses. If a sympathectomy is done, the nurse emphasizes that the areas of altered sympathetic stimuli no longer perspire. He or she instructs the client that applying cream to prevent excessive skin dryness may be helpful.

THROMBOSIS, PHLEBOTHROMBOSIS, AND EMBOLISM

A **thrombus** is a stationary clot. **Thrombosis** is a state in which a thrombus has formed in a blood vessel. Thrombophlebitis is an inflammation of a vein accompanied by clot or thrombus formation (see Chap. 23). **Phlebothrombosis** is the development of a clot within a vein without inflammation. Phlebothrombosis and thrombophlebitis have similar symptoms and treatment. An **embolus** is a moving mass (clot) of particles, either solid or gas, in the bloodstream.

Pathophysiology and Etiology

Thrombosis in the venous system most often occurs in the lower extremities and usually is associated with disorders or circumstances that cause venous stasis (inactivity, immobility, or trauma to a blood vessel). Orthopedic surgical procedures increase the incidence of deep vein thrombosis (DVT) of the lower extremities. Atherosclerosis, endocarditis, pooling of blood in a ventricular aneurysm, and dysrhythmias such as atrial fibrillation can precipitate arterial thrombosis and subsequent embolization. When a thrombus forms or an embolus reaches a blood vessel too small to permit its passage, blood flow is partly or totally occluded.

Assessment Findings

Signs and Symptoms

When an arterial clot is present, symptoms arise from ischemia to the tissues that depend on the obstructed vessel for their oxygenated blood supply. With total occlusion, the extremity suddenly becomes white, cold, and extremely painful. Arterial pulsations are absent below the obstructed area. Numbness, tingling, or cramping also may be present, and surrounding blood vessels spasm. Loss of sensation and ability to move the part follows. Symptoms of shock frequently result if a large vessel is obstructed. When a small vessel is occluded, symptoms of ischemia, such as pallor and coldness, occur but are less severe. Unless blood flow is restored, gangrene develops (see Fig. 23-13 in Chap. 23).

Clients with phlebothrombosis may have few, if any, symptoms because inflammation is absent. Signs and symptoms of DVT usually include mild fever and pain, swelling, and tenderness of the affected extremity. A positive *Homans' sign,* pain on dorsiflexion of the foot, may be pres-

ent. A thrombus may become a mobile embolus and lodge in a distal blood vessel, such as the pulmonary capillaries, causing symptoms related to the organ to which circulation has become impaired. (See discussions of pulmonary embolism in Chap. 21 and cerebral embolism in Chap. 38).

Diagnostic Findings

Arteriography or venography (also called *phlebography*) using a contrast dye identifies the point of obstruction. Doppler ultrasonography is used to detect abnormalities in peripheral blood flow. Plethysmography measures volume changes in the venous or arterial system.

Medical and Surgical Treatment

Treatment depends on whether an artery or a vein is occluded and the degree of occlusion (partial or complete).

Arterial Occlusive Disease

If an artery is completely occluded, treatment cannot be delayed. The physician may order an immediate IV injection of heparin to prevent the development of further clots or the extension of those already present. An attempt may be made to improve circulation by administering vasodilating drugs. A sympathetic nerve block (injection of a local anesthetic into the sympathetic ganglia) may relieve vasospasm. Narcotics may relieve pain and ease the client's apprehension. A thrombolytic agent may be prescribed if the client has experienced a pulmonary embolism or the embolus is occluding a large arterial vessel. If circulation to the extremity cannot be restored, a thrombectomy, embolectomy, *endarterectomy* (removal of the lining of an artery), or CABG is necessary. Nursing management of thrombectomy, embolectomy, endarterectomy, and CABG is discussed in Chapter 29.

Venous Occlusive Disease

Venous thrombosis is treated with bed rest, elevation of the extremity, local heat, analgesics for pain, and intermittent subcutaneous injections or continuous IV heparin therapy, followed by oral anticoagulants once the heparin has achieved a therapeutic effect. DVT may necessitate surgical removal of the clot (*thrombectomy*).

Nursing Management

The nurse obtains a history of symptoms and identifies characteristics of the pain. He or she assesses for Homans' sign by having the client dorsiflex each foot. The nurse examines the extremities and compares skin color, temperature, capillary refill time, and tissue integrity; he or she also measures each calf. The nurse palpates peripheral pulses or uses a Doppler ultrasound device if pulses cannot be palpated. He or she marks the location of each peripheral artery with a soft-tipped pen to facilitate its relocation. The nurse immediately reports any change in the quality of a peripheral pulse or its sudden absence. Outlining any color change (line of demarcation) above or below the occluded area with a soft-tipped pen is useful to establish a baseline for future comparison.

The nurse monitors the client's response to anticoagulation therapy. If heparin is administered, the nurse assesses IV infusions hourly. He or she monitors partial thromboplastin time (PTT), prothrombin time (PT), and international normalized ratio (INR) when concurrent oral anticoagulation is prescribed. These values help determine therapeutic response and daily dosage. The nurse is alert for signs of bleeding and keeps protamine sulfate on hand for reversing heparin and vitamin K on hand for reversing oral anticoagulants. Additional nursing management is directed at increasing arterial or venous blood flow, relieving pain, and preventing complications.

Thorough teaching before discharge is essential. To prevent a recurrence of thrombosis, phlebothrombosis, or embolism, the nurse informs clients to avoid prolonged periods of inactivity (especially sitting), elevate the legs periodically, and walk or do isometric leg exercises frequently if sitting is unavoidable. He or she recommends wearing antiembolism stockings to prevent venous stasis (especially if the client has venous leg ulcers). The nurse instructs the client to apply these stockings before assuming a dependent position or after elevating the extremities for several minutes. The client needs to remove and reapply antiembolism stockings twice a day or as recommended by the physician. The nurse informs those who must take continued anticoagulants to observe for signs of unusual bleeding and keep appointments for laboratory tests.

VENOUS INSUFFICIENCY

Venous insufficiency is a peripheral vascular disorder in which the flow of venous blood is impaired through deep or superficial veins (or both). The condition usually affects the lower extremities, most often the medial aspect of the leg or around the ankle.

Pathophysiology and Etiology

Venous insufficiency may be a consequence of varicose veins (discussed later) or valvular damage from a previous venous thrombosis. When the forward movement of venous blood is affected, venous congestion develops from the accumulating blood volume. Increased hydrostatic fluid pressure causes fluid to leave the veins and enter interstitial spaces. Localized edema is evident; the skin becomes shiny and hard. The fluid-filled space acts as a barrier between the cells in the surrounding tissue and their capillary blood supply. Consequently, cells are subjected to accumulating amounts of CO_2. As unoxygenated cells die, they release inflammatory chemicals that cause *dermatitis,* inflammation of the dermis layer of skin. The skin becomes red and "hot." Hemoglobin from blood cells also escapes into the extravascular space, causing the tissue to appear dark brown, deep purple, or black. Serous fluid oozes from the skin when there is no outlet for vascular or lymphatic circulation. Eventually the skin becomes impaired. A lesion referred to as a **venous stasis ulcer** forms (Fig. 25-10). Without adequate circulation, healing is retarded. Some ulcers may be present for years. The skin is fragile and easily retraumatized in the process of healing. Secondary infections often occur in the ulceration.

Assessment Findings

Signs and Symptoms

The foot or feet appear swollen. Testing for pitting is difficult because the congested fluid cannot be displaced. Superficial veins are dilated and obvious during inspection. Skin color is not uniform; there usually is a red or darkly pig-

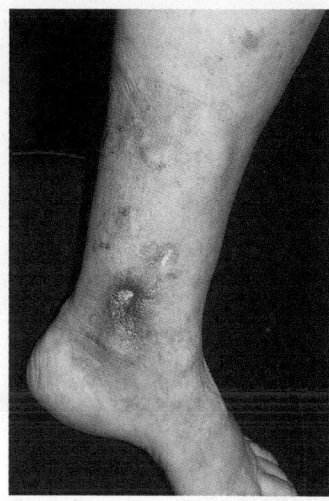

FIGURE 25-10. Ulcer from venous stasis. (From Goodheart, H. P. [2003]. *Goodheart's photoguide of common skin disorders* [2nd ed.]. Philadelphia: Lippincott Williams & Wilkins.)

mented area. If a lesion is present, its margin usually is irregular. Serous fluid may have collected in a pocket beneath the skin, or the area has beads of fluid on its surface that return after being wiped away. If an infection is present, the drainage may change from clear to opaque. Most clients report moderate pain. Pedal and tibial pulses may be difficult to palpate because of the congestion of venous fluid.

Diagnostic Findings

Doppler ultrasound demonstrates a reversed direction of blood flow, indicating valvular incompetence in superficial or deep veins. *Photoplethysmography,* a diagnostic test for venous pathology, measures light that is not absorbed by hemoglobin and consequently is reflected back to the machine. When clients with venous insufficiency undergo photoplethysmography during exercise and rest, light reflection is greater during rest, showing that the client has decreased oxygen-bound hemoglobin and an increased volume of **venous reflux** (downward flow of venous blood). Air plethysmography measures venous pressure by filling a cuff with air after it is applied to the calf while the client is supine with the legs elevated. When the client stands, the pressure is measured again and venous pressure increases, indicating an increased volume of venous reflux.

Medical and Surgical Management

A major goal of therapy is to promote venous circulation. This is accomplished by applying elastic compression stockings, such as *Jobst* stockings, that maintain venous pressure at 40 mm Hg. The client wears the stockings at all times except when lying down. Because older adults may have difficulty applying elastic compression stockings, the physician may apply a nonelastic gauze dressing soaked in zinc paste and glycerine known as an *Unna boot.* Pneumatic compression pump therapy, similar to EECP, also may be implemented. The compression pump promotes venous blood flow more efficiently than compression stockings but is more expensive and time-consuming. Furthermore, it interferes with performance of daily activities during its use. Mild analgesics are recommended for pain. Vascular surgery can

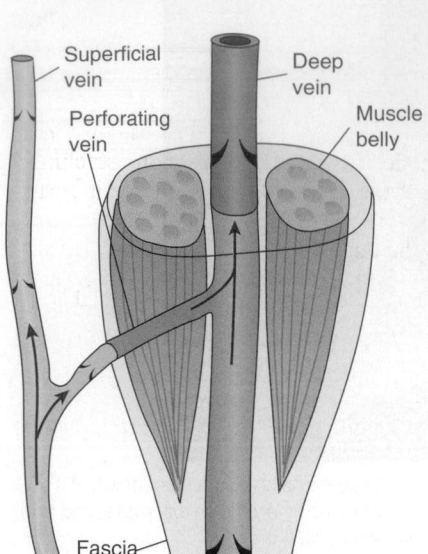

A Muscles relaxed

Superficial vein

Deep vein

Perforating vein

Muscle belly

Fascia

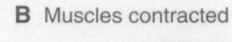

B Muscles contracted

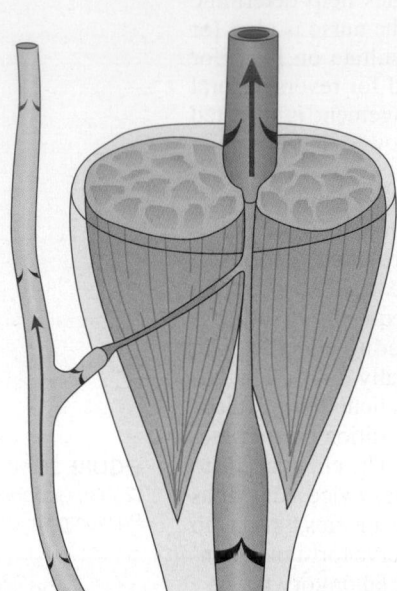

FIGURE 25-11. The skeletal muscle pumps and promotes blood flow in the deep and superficial calf vessels. Most perforating veins lie below the knee. When the calf muscle is relaxed (**A**), blood moves from the superficial to the deep veins. Muscle contraction (**B**) propels blood in the deep veins toward the heart; closure of the venous valves prevents backflow. (From Margolis, D. J. [1992]. Management of venous ulcerations. *Hospital Practice, 27*(5), 37. ©1992, The McGraw-Hill Companies.)

be performed in which the valves in larger veins are repaired or incompetent valves are bypassed using a length of vein with healthy valves from elsewhere in the body.

A stasis ulcer is managed by keeping the skin and ulcer clean with soap and water or a diluted solution of a disinfectant such as Hibiclens. Necrotic tissue is debrided. Any infection is treated by applying Silvadene, an antibacterial cream, or an antibiotic ointment. The wound is covered with an occlusive transparent dressing such as Tegaderm that traps moisture, which speeds healing. Chronic, nonhealing skin lesions also are treated with **topical hyperbaric oxygen** (THBO) therapy. This approach delivers oxygen above atmospheric pressure directly to the wound rather than to the full body as with other disorders such as carbon monoxide poisoning. Oxygen accelerates the healing process. THBO is applied by covering the area with an inflatable boot that confines the oxygen at low hyperbaric pressure at the wound site. The boot remains in place for approximately 90 minutes a day for 4 consecutive days. The treatment is repeated after 3 days of nontreatment in a cycle over 8 to 10 weeks.

Nursing Management

The nurse assesses the appearance of the extremities and quality of circulation. If an ulcer is present, he or she measures it and describes its appearance. The nurse asks the client to rate his or her pain and administers an analgesic if warranted. He or she measures the diameter of the calf and ankle and the length of the leg from heel to knee to obtain accurately fitting compression stockings. The nurse helps apply the stockings each morning before the client lowers the legs to the floor. He or she implements wound care according to physician directives.

The nurse teaches the client to do the following:

- Purchase more than one pair of compression stockings so one pair is worn while the other pair is laundered.
- Dry elastic stockings by laying them flat rather than hanging them, which stretches elastic.

- Lose weight if necessary.
- Elevate the legs periodically for at least 15 to 20 minutes.
- Walk or do isometric calf muscle pumps hourly to promote venous circulation.
- Raise the foot of the bed to promote venous drainage during sleep.
- Avoid morning showers or sitting in front of a fire because heat dilates blood vessels and contributes to venous congestion.
- Wear shoes with laces rather than slippers or sandals to reduce pooling of blood in the feet.

DISORDERS OF BLOOD VESSEL WALLS

VARICOSE VEINS

Varicose veins or varicosities are dilated, tortuous veins. Both sexes suffer equally from this disorder. The saphenous leg veins commonly are affected because they lack support from surrounding muscles. Varicose veins also may occur in other body parts, such as the rectum (hemorrhoids) and esophagus (esophageal varices).

Pathophysiology and Etiology

Varicose veins have a familial tendency. The valves of the veins become incompetent in early adulthood, resulting in varicosities. In others, anything that constricts or interferes with venous return contributes to the formation of varicose veins. Prolonged standing compromises venous return as blood pools distally with gravity. Obesity and pressure on blood vessels from an enlarging fetus, liver, or abdominal tumor contribute to venous congestion. Thrombophlebitis may lead to varicose veins because the inflammatory process may damage vein valves.

Normally, the action of leg muscles during movement and exercise aids venous return (Fig. 25-11). When valves in veins become incompetent, blood accumulates rather than being propelled efficiently to the heart. The congestion stretches the veins. Over time, they cannot recoil and remain chronically distended. Venous hypertension then forces some fluid to move into the interstitial spaces of surrounding tissue. Venous congestion and local edema may diminish arterial blood flow, impairing cellular nutrition. Even minor skin or soft tissue injuries easily become infected and ulcerated. The healing of such lesions is slow and uncertain.

Assessment Findings

Signs and Symptoms

Often the condition first manifests itself when other factors impair venous return. The legs feel heavy and tired, particularly after prolonged standing. The client may say that activity or elevation of the legs relieves the discomfort. The leg veins look distended and tortuous and can be seen under the skin as dark blue or purple, snakelike elevations. The feet, ankles, and legs may appear swollen. The skin may be slightly darker in the areas of impaired circulation. There may be signs of skin ulcerations in various stages of healing. Capillary refill may be abnormal.

Diagnostic Findings

The Brodie-Trendelenburg test is performed for diagnostic purposes. The client lies flat and elevates the affected leg to empty the veins. A tourniquet is then applied to the upper thigh, and the client is asked to stand. If blood flows from the upper part of the leg into the superficial veins when the tourniquet is released, the valves of the superficial veins are considered incompetent. Ultrasonography and venography also are used to detect impaired blood flow.

Medical and Surgical Management

Treatment of mild varicose veins includes exercising (walking, swimming), losing weight (if needed), wearing elastic support stockings, and avoiding prolonged periods of sitting or standing. The defective vein may be sclerosed or occluded by injecting a chemical that sets up an inflammation in the vein wall. Eventually adhesions form, and blood flow must find an alternate route through collateral veins.

Surgical treatment for severe or multiple varicose veins consists of vein ligation with or without vein stripping. A **vein ligation** is a procedure in which the affected veins are ligated (tied off) above and below the area of incompetent valves, but the dysfunctional vein remains. For better results, a **vein stripping** is performed; in this procedure the ligated veins are severed and removed. The entire great saphenous vein, which extends from the groin to the ankle, or the small saphenous vein may be removed.

Nursing Management

The nurse assesses the skin, distal circulation, and peripheral edema. He or she asks the client to rate the level of discomfort and ability to do active and isometric leg exercises. See Chapter 20 for routine perioperative care.

When the client returns from surgery with a gauze dressing covered by elastic roller bandages on the operative leg(s), the nurse monitors for swelling in the operative leg(s) and its effect on circulation. He or she removes and rewraps the roller bandage to facilitate blood flow. The nurse inspects the dressing for signs of active bleeding. In the immediate postoperative period, the nurse elevates the foot of the bed to aid venous circulation to the heart and reminds the client to alternately contract and relax the lower leg muscles. If active exercise is inadequate, the nurse consults with the physician about using pneumatic venous compression stockings, which cover the leg from foot to thigh and periodically inflate and release air, simulating isometric muscle contraction. The nurse helps the client ambulate as soon as possible to promote venous circulation, reduce edema, and prevent venous thrombosis. When bleeding is no longer a problem, the nurse applies elastic antiembolism stockings in place of the elastic roller bandage. He or she provides adequate fluid to decrease potential thrombosis.

When teaching the client and family, the nurse identifies factors that impair venous circulation: wearing elastic girdles or tight belts, using round garters or rolling and twisting nylon stockings, standing or sitting for prolonged periods, and sitting with the knees crossed. He or she describes appropriate foot and nail care to facilitate tissue integrity. The nurse explains that any open areas on the feet or lower legs require examination and treatment by the physician. He or she recommends active or isometric exercises and elevation of the extremities frequently during the day. The nurse demonstrates how to apply and remove elastic support stockings. He or she refers the client to the dietitian if weight loss is indicated.

ANEURYSMS

An **aneurysm** is stretching and bulging of an arterial wall. Aneurysms of the aorta (aortic arch, thoracic, abdominal) are the most common, but aneurysms can be found in other arteries, such as those in the legs and brain.

Pathophysiology and Etiology

Arteriosclerosis, hypertension, trauma, or a congenital weakness can affect the elasticity of the *tunica media* (middle layer of the artery wall), causing part of the vessel to bulge. Once formed, some aneurysms lay down layers of clots, blocking the vessel until blood flow stops. Most aneurysms enlarge until they rupture. Loss of a large volume of arterial blood leads to shock and death if not controlled. Some aneurysms tear and leak blood into surrounding cavities, such as the thorax or abdomen. Blood in a dissecting aneurysm is unavailable to arteries that branch off the aorta. When blood flow decreases or stops, tissue necrosis occurs.

Assessment Findings

Signs and Symptoms

Many aneurysms go unnoticed until found during physical examination or the client has a massive hemorrhage. Some cause pain, discomfort, and symptoms related to pressure on nearby structures. For example, a thoracic aortic aneurysm can cause bronchial obstruction, *dysphagia* (difficulty swallowing), and dyspnea. An abdominal aortic aneurysm can produce nausea and vomiting from pressure exerted on the intestines, or it may cause back pain from pressure on the vertebrae or spinal nerves. Most clients are hypertensive. A pulsating mass may be felt or even seen around the umbilicus or to the left of midline over the abdomen. A **bruit** (purring or blowing sound) can be auscultated over the mass. Circulation to tissue may be impaired.

Symptoms of a dissecting aneurysm vary and depend on whether a branching artery has been occluded or a tear has occurred in the aortic wall. Many clients become suddenly and acutely ill. Difference in the BPs of the left and right arms may be marked, or the BPs of the left and right legs may be unequal. Severe pain and signs of shock usually are present, but symptoms can be less severe in some instances. Because symptoms vary, diagnosis may be difficult.

Diagnostic Findings

Radiographs can demonstrate aneurysms when the arterial wall contains calcium deposits. Aortography identifies the size and exact location of the aneurysm.

Medical and Surgical Management

Medical treatment includes administering antihypertensive drugs to keep BP within normal range. Aneurysms are treated surgically whenever possible; no other cure exists. They are repaired by bypass or replacement grafting (see Chap. 29). A dissecting or ruptured aneurysm is a surgical emergency.

Nursing Management

The nurse helps control hypertension by keeping activity and stress to a minimum. The client should avoid straining during bowel movements, coughing, and holding the breath while changing positions. The nurse monitors BP, pulse, hourly urine output, skin color, level of consciousness, and characteristics of pain for signs of hemorrhage or dissection. He or she prepares the client for diagnostic testing and surgical interventions. Afterward, the nurse monitors for shock and adequate tissue perfusion. See Chapter 29 for nursing management of a client undergoing cardiovascular surgery.

CRITICAL THINKING EXERCISES

1. A client presents in the emergency department complaining of substernal chest pain. He has a history of angina. What assessment criteria will help you differentiate between an anginal attack and an MI? What diagnostic tests will confirm an MI?

2. What are some possible reasons women are often misdiagnosed and erroneously treated at the time of an MI?

3. A client with Raynaud's disease relates that she has difficulty reducing attacks during the winter. What client teaching is indicated? How can the client reduce the ischemic episodes?

4. A client who has had a ligation of varicose veins returns to her room after surgery. What assessments are a priority? How can you teach the client to reduce the incidence of further varicose vein formation?

NCLEX-STYLE REVIEW QUESTIONS

1. A client's lipid panel indicates an LDL of 182 mg/dL. Which of the following is an accurate analysis of the laboratory result?
   1. The client's LDL is desirable because it is < 200 mg/dL.
   2. The client's LDL is optimal; lifestyle habits should be continued.
   3. The client's LDL is high; lifestyle changes should be encouraged.
   4. The client's LDL is borderline optimal; regular reassessment is recommended.

2. The nurse advises a client recovering from an MI to decrease dietary fat and salt. Which choices would the nurse encourage in the client's diet?
   1. Oatmeal and apple juice
   2. Bacon and scrambled eggs
   3. Pepperoni pizza and beer
   4. Cheeseburger and french fries

3. A client is given a prescription for sublingual nitroglycerin to be taken when chest pain develops. Which of the following instructions from the nurse are appropriate? Select all that apply.
   1. Place the tablet in the pouch between your cheek and gum.
   2. You may feel dizzy within minutes of taking the medication.
   3. Experiencing a headache is a sign of nitroglycerin toxicity.
   4. Take another tablet in 5 minutes if chest pain is unrelieved.
   5. Replace your supply of nitroglycerin tablets at least every month.

4. Which of the following discharge instructions for self-care should the nurse provide to a client who has undergone a percutaneous transluminal coronary angioplasty (PTCA)? Select all that apply.
   1. Take tub baths to promote healing at the catheter insertion site.
   2. Clean the catheter insertion site with soap and water each day.
   3. Replace the dressing over the catheter insertion site daily.
   4. Refrain from driving for at least three days after the procedure.
   5. Resume sexual activity after the procedure at any time.

5. A client with venous stasis in the lower extremities complains to the nurse that the elastic compression stockings are "too tight." Which response by the nurse is most appropriate?
   1. "I'll remove them and remeasure your extremities."
   2. "I will call the doctor and see about discontinuing them."
   3. "Do you feel numbness and tingling in your toes?"
   4. "I'll request a larger pair of stockings."

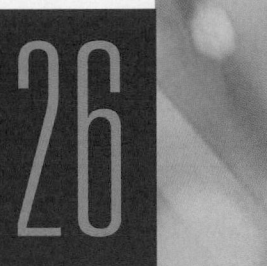

26

Caring for Clients with Cardiac Dysrhythmias

Words To Know

asystole
atrial fibrillation
atrial flutter
automatic implanted cardioverter defibrillator
bigeminy
bradydysrhythmia
chemical cardioversion
couplets
defibrillation
demand (or synchronous) mode pacemaker
dysrhythmia
ectopic pacemaker site
elective electrical cardioversion
electrophysiology study
fixed-rate (or asynchronous) mode pacemaker
heart block
Maze procedure
multifocal PVCs
pacemaker
premature atrial contraction
premature ventricular contraction
radiofrequency catheter ablation
R-on-T phenomenon
sinus bradycardia
sinus tachycardia
supraventricular tachycardia
tachydysrhythmias
transcutaneous pacemaker
transvenous pacemaker
ventricular fibrillation
ventricular tachycardia

Learning Objectives

On completion of this chapter, you will be able to:

1. Name and describe common cardiac dysrhythmias.
2. Identify medications to control or eliminate dysrhythmias.
3. Explain the purpose and advantages of elective cardioversion.
4. Explain when defibrillation is used to treat dysrhythmias.
5. Discuss the purpose for implanting an automatic internal cardiac defibrillator.
6. Name various types of artificial pacemakers and the purpose for their use.
7. Describe nursing management of the client with a dysrhythmia treated by drug therapy, elective cardioversion, defibrillation, or pacemaker insertion.

ardiac rhythm refers to the pattern (or pace) of the heartbeat. The conduction system of the heart and the inherent rhythmicity of cardiac muscle produce a rhythm pattern, which greatly influences the heart's ability to pump blood effectively. Basic cardiac conduction and electrocardiogram (ECG) waveforms are discussed in Chapter 22. The usual cardiac rhythm is called *normal sinus rhythm* (Box 26-1; Fig. 26 1). An ECG is used to identify normal and abnormal cardiac rhythms.

This chapter gives a comprehensive overview of various dysrhythmias. A **dysrhythmia** (also called an *arrhythmia*) is a conduction disorder that results in an abnormally slow or rapid heart rate or one that does not proceed through the conduction system in the usual manner. Cardiac output, the volume of blood ejected from the heart per minute, may be greatly compromised when a rhythm disturbance develops.

Some dysrhythmias do not require treatment; others require immediate intervention because they are potentially fatal. The most common cause of dysrhythmias is ischemic heart disease (see Chap. 25). Drug therapy, electrolyte disturbances, metabolic acidosis, hypothermia, and degenerative age-related changes are other conditions that cause dysrhythmias.

▶ **Stop, Think, and Respond Exercise 26-1**

   Describe the characteristics of normal sinus rhythm.

CARDIAC DYSRHYTHMIAS

Cardiac dysrhythmias may originate in the atria, atrioventricular node, or ventricles.

Dysrhythmias Originating in the Atria

Examples of dysrhythmias originating in the sinus node of the right atrium include sinus bradycardia and sinus tachycardia. Atrial dysrhythmias that develop in sites outside the sinus node yet within the atria include premature atrial contractions, supraventricular tachycardia, atrial flutter, and atrial fibrillation.

Sinus Bradycardia

Sinus bradycardia is a dysrhythmia that proceeds normally through the conduction pathway but at a slower than usual rate (≤60 beats/min; Fig. 26-2). Healthy athletes and others who are physically fit often have heart rates below 60 beats/minute; however, this example of sinus bradycardia reflects a well-toned heart conditioned through regular exercise. A heart rate slower than 60 beats/minute is pathologic in clients with heart disorders, increased intracranial pressure, hypothyroidism, or digitalis toxicity. The danger in sinus bradycardia is that the slow rate may be insufficient to maintain cardiac output. Atropine sulfate, a cholinergic blocking agent, is given intravenously (IV) to increase a dangerously slow heart rate.

Pharmacologic Considerations

- A dose of 0.5 to 1.0 mg of atropine sulfate may be given every 1 to 2 hours. A maximum of 2.0 mg is given IV.

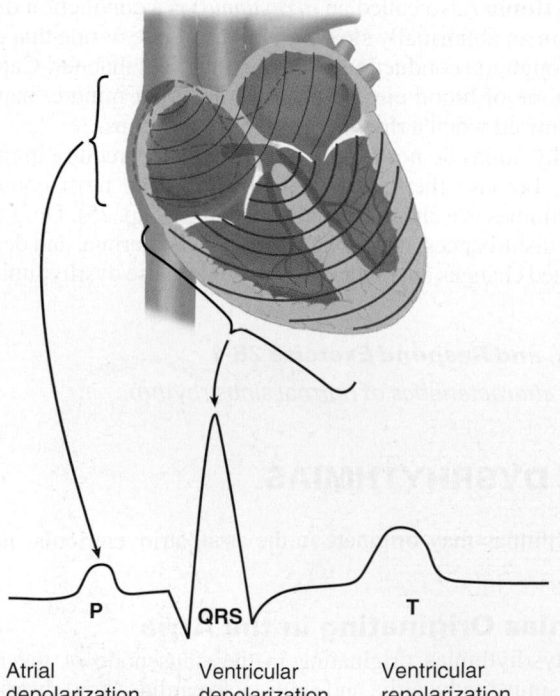

P	QRS	T
Atrial depolarization	Ventricular depolarization	Ventricular repolarization

FIGURE 26-1. Normal conduction and ECG waveforms.

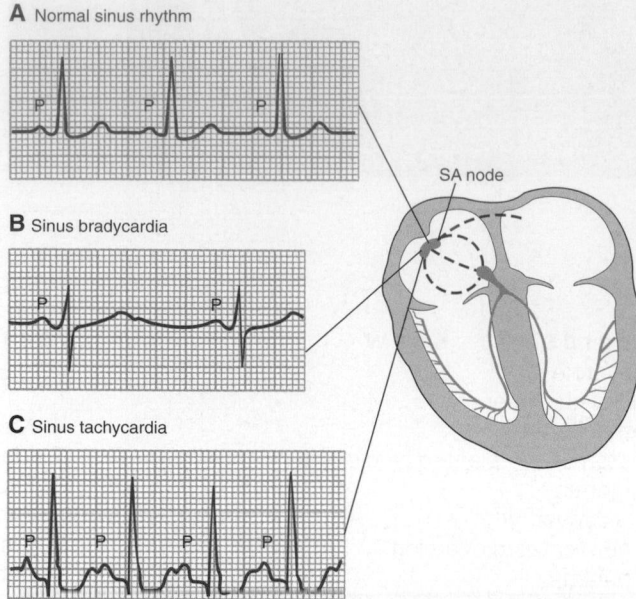

A Normal sinus rhythm

B Sinus bradycardia

C Sinus tachycardia

SA node

FIGURE 26-2. (**A**) In sinus rhythm, the SA node initiates impulses (P waves) 60 to 100 times/min. (**B**) In sinus bradycardia, the SA node initiates impulses at 40 to 60 times/min. (**C**) In sinus tachycardia, the SA node initiates impulses at 100 to 150 times/min.

Isoproterenol (Isuprel), a beta-adrenergic blocker, is also used to treat severe bradycardia. When either drug is administered, closely monitor the pulse rate for drug response.

Sinus Tachycardia

Sinus tachycardia is a dysrhythmia that proceeds normally through the conduction pathway but at a faster than usual rate (100–150 beats/min; see Fig. 26-2). It occurs in clients with healthy hearts as a physiologic response to strenuous exercise, anxiety and fear, pain, fever, hyperthyroidism, hemorrhage, shock, or hypoxemia.

Premature Atrial Contractions

Occasionally, neural tissue in the atrial conduction system initiates an early electrical impulse called a **premature atrial contraction** (PAC), which is identified by an irregularity in the underlying rhythm (Fig. 26-3). The P wave of the waveform may look similar to other conducted impulses or may differ slightly because it is initiated somewhere in the

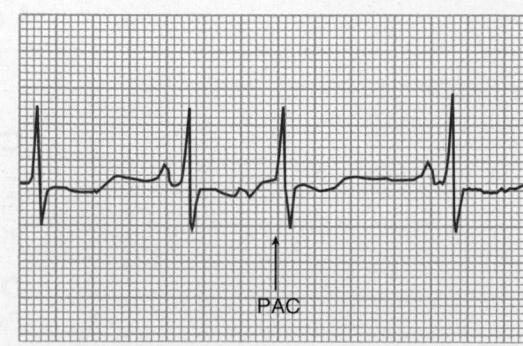

PAC

FIGURE 26-3. Normal sinus rhythm with one premature atrial contraction (PAC).

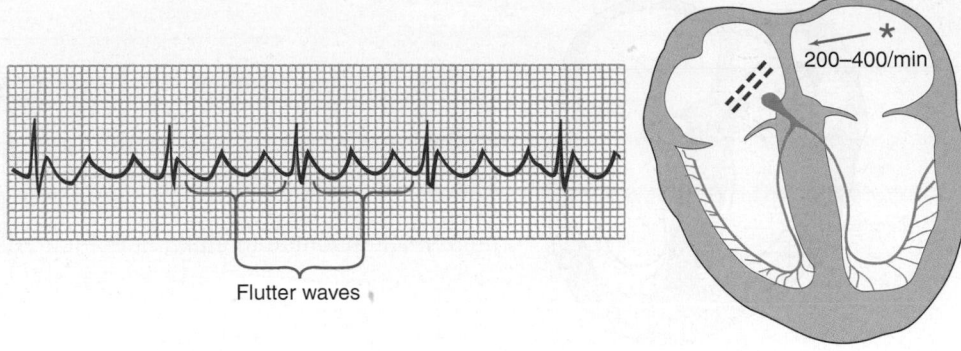

FIGURE 26-4. Atrial flutter produces sawtooth flutter waves. Most of the atrial impulses are not conducted to the ventricles.

atria other than the sinoatrial (SA) node. PACs can occur for various reasons: consumption of caffeine, use of nicotine or other sympathetic nervous system stimulants, or in response to heart disease or metabolic disorders such as hyperthyroidism. When PACs are isolated or infrequent, there is no cause for alarm. Eliminating the cause usually controls PACs. Occasionally, the **ectopic pacemaker site,** one that initiates an electrical impulse independently of the SA node, can lead to more serious dysrhythmias such as supraventricular tachycardia.

Supraventricular Tachycardia

Supraventricular tachycardia (SVT) is a dysrhythmia in which the heart rate has a consistent rhythm, but beats at a dangerously high rate (≥150 beats/min). Diastole is shortened and the heart does not have sufficient time to fill. Cardiac output drops dangerously low and heart failure can occur, especially in clients with preexisting heart disease or damage. Clients with coronary artery disease (CAD) and SVT can develop chest pain because coronary blood flow cannot meet the increased need of the myocardium for oxygen imposed by the fast rate. Besides tachycardia and angina, hypotension, syncope, and reduced renal output are signs and symptoms of low cardiac output and impending heart failure. Digitalis, adrenergic blockers, and calcium channel blockers are used to slow the heart rate.

Atrial Flutter

Atrial flutter (Fig. 26-4) is a disorder in which a single atrial impulse outside the SA node causes the atria to contract at an exceedingly rapid rate (200–400 contractions/min). The atrioventricular (AV) node conducts only some impulses to the ventricle, resulting in a ventricular rate that is slower than

the atrial rate. The atrial waves in atrial flutter have a characteristic sawtooth pattern.

Atrial Fibrillation

In **atrial fibrillation,** several areas in the right atrium initiate impulses resulting in disorganized, rapid activity. The atria quiver rather than contract (Fig. 26-5). The ventricles respond to the atrial stimulus randomly, causing an irregular ventricular heart rate, which may be too infrequent to maintain adequate cardiac output. One of the chief complications of atrial fibrillation is the formation of blood clots within the atria that may become emboli if they enter the circulation. Heparin is generally prescribed initially if the dysrhythmia persists longer than 48 hours. Clients with persistent atrial fibrillation may be prescribed an oral anticoagulant such as dicumarol (Coumadin) or a daily aspirin to prevent the potential for a stroke or if there is a potential for its reoccurrence.

 Gerontologic Considerations

- Atrial fibrillation increases the risk for stroke by 1.5% in people 50 to 59 years of age and by 30% in those 80 to 89 years of age (Lazar & Clark, 2007). Therefore, the need to restore normal sinus rhythm is critical.

Ibutilide (Corvert) is an antidysrhythmic drug used to convert new-onset atrial fibrillation into sinus rhythm; flecainide (Tambocor) and propafenone (Rythmol) also are used to treat and prevent atrial fibrillation. Use of drugs to

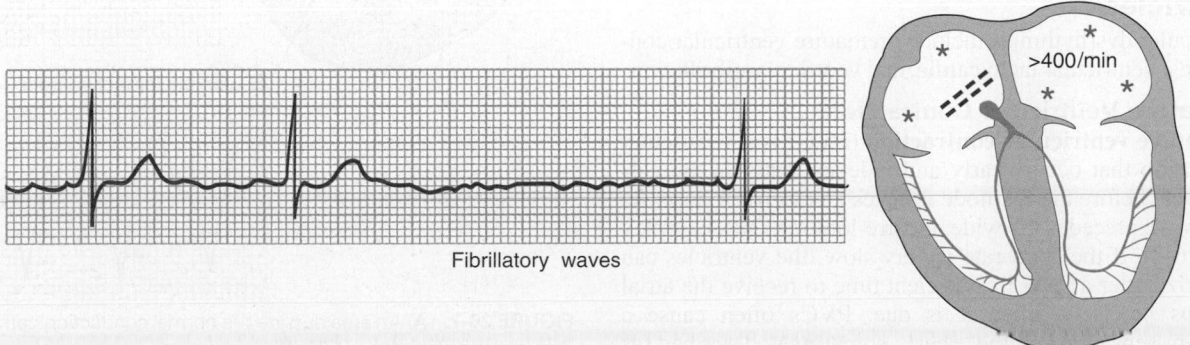

FIGURE 26-5. In atrial fibrillation, there are no identifiable P waves. The atrial impulses look like a fine undulating line.

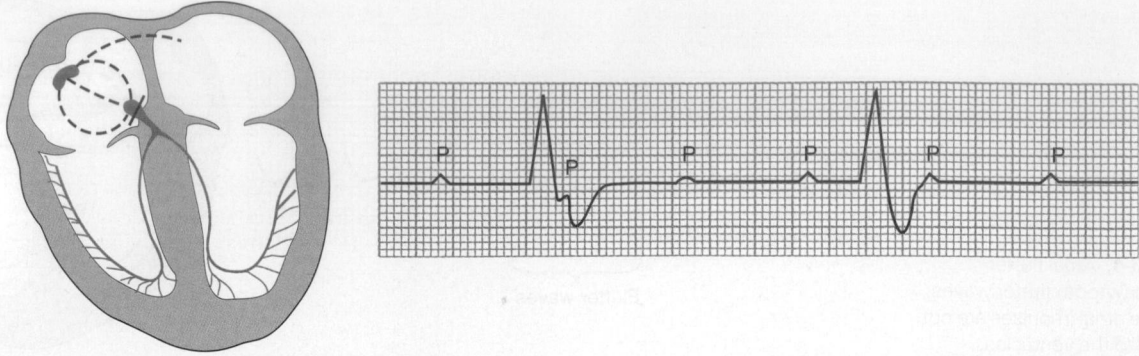

FIGURE 26-6. In heart block, SA-initiated impulses are delayed at the AV node or fail to progress altogether. In this example of complete heart block, the ventricles are beating independently of the atria.

eliminate a dysrhythmia is referred to as **chemical cardioversion**. Atrial fibrillation also is treated with elective cardioversion (discussed later) or digitalis if the ventricular rate is not too slow. Clients with atrial fibrillation who are not candidates for cardioversion and fail to respond to conventional measures may be candidates for a surgical intervention referred to as the **Maze procedure**. During the Maze procedure, the surgeon creates a new conduction pathway that eliminates the rapid firing of ectopic pacemaker sites in the atria. Some individuals with atrial fibrillation continue to experience chronic atrial fibrillation or episodic events.

Dysrhythmia Originating in the Atrioventricular Node: Heart Block

Heart block refers to disorders in the conduction pathway that interfere with the transmission of impulses from the SA node through the AV node to the ventricles. Heart block may be first degree, second degree, or third degree (also called *complete heart block*). In first- and second-degree heart block, the impulse is delayed. In complete heart block (Fig. 26-6), the atrial impulse never gets through, and the ventricles develop their own rhythm independent of the atrial rhythm. In complete heart block, the ventricular rate is slow (30–40 beats/min). Pacemaker insertion (discussed later) is the treatment for complete heart block.

▶ *Stop, Think, and Respond Exercise 26-2*

Discuss the consequences of a slow heart rate and low cardiac output.

Dysrhythmias Originating in the Ventricles

Ventricular dysrhythmias include premature ventricular contractions, ventricular tachycardia, and ventricular fibrillation.

Premature Ventricular Contractions

Premature ventricular contraction (PVC) is a ventricular contraction that occurs early and independently in the cardiac cycle before the SA node initiates an electrical impulse. No P wave precedes the wide, bizarre-looking QRS complex (Fig. 26-7). If the heart rate is very slow, the ventricles can repolarize after a PVC in sufficient time to receive the atrial stimulus precisely when it is due. PVCs often cause a flip-flop sensation in the chest, sometimes described as "fluttering." Associated signs and symptoms include pallor,

nervousness, sweating, and faintness. Many people experience occasional PVCs, which usually are harmless. They may be related to anxiety, stress, fatigue, alcohol withdrawal, or tobacco use. Although PVCs normally are not associated with a specific heart disorder, those whom they frequently trouble should consult a physician. A thorough examination is important to ensure no heart disease exists.

In the presence of acute heart injury, such as after cardiac surgery or with acute myocardial infarction (MI), PVCs in certain patterns suggest myocardial irritability and are precursors of lethal dysrhythmias (Fig. 26-8):

- Six or more PVCs per minute
- Runs of **bigeminy** (every other beat is a PVC)
- Two PVCs in a row (**couplets**)
- Runs of PVCs (three or more in a row)
- **Multifocal PVCs** (originating from more than one location)
- A PVC whose R wave falls on the T wave of the preceding complex (**R-on-T phenomenon**)

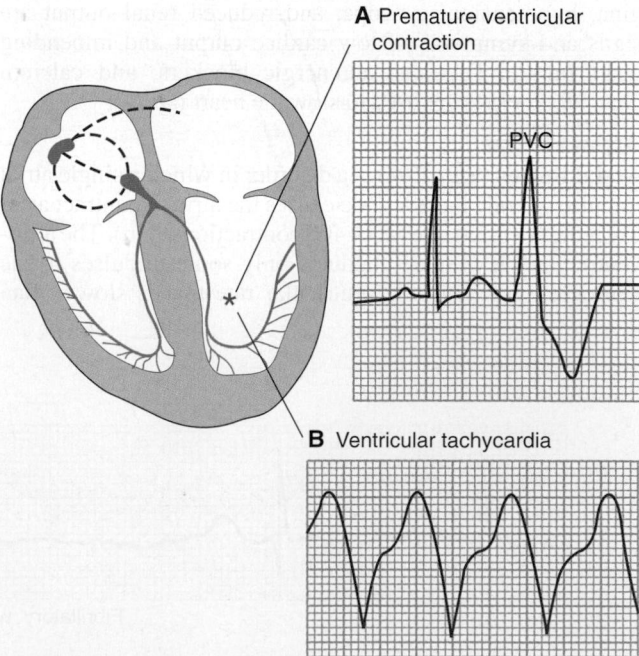

A Premature ventricular contraction

PVC

B Ventricular tachycardia

FIGURE 26-7. (A) An area outside the normal conduction pathway in the ventricles initiates a PVC. **(B)** Continuous generation of impulses results in ventricular tachycardia.

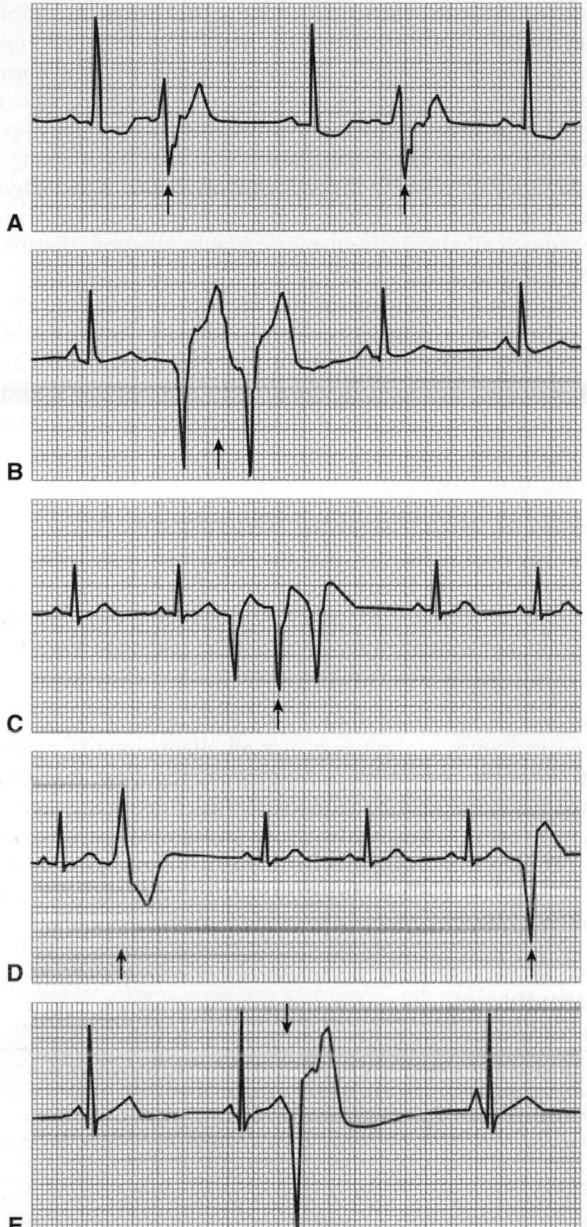

FIGURE 26-8. Dangerous forms of PVCs: (**A**) bigeminal, (**B**) couplets, (**C**) run, (**D**) multifocal, and (**E**) R-on-T phenomenon.

When dangerous PVCs occur, the client is given an IV bolus of lidocaine (Xylocaine) followed by an IV infusion of the drug.

Pharmacologic Considerations

- Administration of lidocaine can have serious adverse effects, including convulsions and cardiac arrest. An airway should be readily available. If hypotension or additional dysrhythmias occur during administration, adjust the IV infusion to the slowest possible rate until the physician can examine the client.

Ventricular Tachycardia

Ventricular tachycardia is caused by a single, irritable focus in the ventricle that initiates and then continues the same repetitive pattern (see Fig. 26-7). The ventricles beat very fast (150–250 beats/min), and cardiac output is decreased. Depending on how long the dysrhythmia is present, the client may lose consciousness and become pulseless. Ventricular tachycardia sometimes ends abruptly without intervention but often requires defibrillation. It may progress to ventricular fibrillation.

Ventricular Fibrillation

Ventricular fibrillation (Fig. 26-9) is the rhythm of a dying heart. PVCs or ventricular tachycardia can precipitate it. The ventricles do not contract effectively and there is no cardiac output. Ventricular fibrillation is an indication for cardiopulmonary resuscitation (CPR) and immediate defibrillation.

Pathophysiology and Etiology of Cardiac Dysrhythmias

Many clinical states predispose clients to dysrhythmias. One of the most common causes of serious dysrhythmias is myocardial ischemia, lack of oxygenated blood to the heart muscle, which can occur secondary to CAD, congestive heart failure, inadequate ventilation, and shock. The conduction system also is susceptible to disturbances from anxiety, pain, endocrine disorders, electrolyte imbalances, valvular heart disease, placement of invasive catheters in the heart, and drug effects. Because of the altered rate and rhythm, all dysrhythmias affect the heart's pumping action and cardiac output to some degree.

Gerontologic Considerations

- Age increases the risk for dysrhythmias, because with aging the cells in the SA node decrease in number and accumulate fat and calcium which compromise their function. In older adults, stress, exercise, or illness may cause dysrhythmias and other cardiac disorders such as heart failure and myocardial ischemia. (Age-related changes in the cardiac conduction system are identified in Chapter 22.)

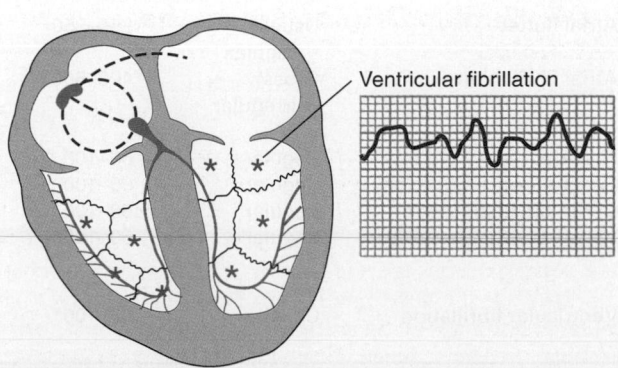

FIGURE 26-9. During ventricular fibrillation the ventricles quiver, as shown by a wavy line.

Assessment Findings

Signs and Symptoms

A client whose dysrhythmia causes decreased cardiac output is likely to feel weak and tired, experience anginal pain, or faint. Some clients with **tachydysrhythmias** (abnormally fast rhythms) describe palpitations or flutterings in their chest. Blood pressure (BP) usually is low. Pulse is irregular or difficult to palpate; the rate is unusually fast or slow. The apical and radial pulse rates may differ. The skin may be pale and cool. The client may be disoriented and confused if the brain is not adequately oxygenated, or there may be loss of consciousness and even clinical death.

Diagnostic Findings

A monitor rhythm strip or 12-lead ECG can identify dysrhythmias. Electrophysiology studies can locate their origin. An **electrophysiology study** is a procedure that enables the physician to examine the electrical activity of the heart, produce actual dysrhythmias by stimulating structures in the conduction pathway, determine the best method for preventing further dysrhythmic episodes, and, in some cases, eradicate tissue in the area of the heart that is producing the dysrhythmia.

The test is performed by passing three flexible wire electrode catheters into veins in the neck and groin. The catheters are then advanced into the heart in each of the following locations: right atrium, bundle of His, and right ventricle. The electrode catheters monitor and record the heart's rhythm. The physician can use these same catheters to reproduce the abnormal heart rhythm that the client usually experiences by stimulating areas in the conduction system. When the dysrhythmia is produced, the physician uses several drugs to evaluate each one's efficacy at restoring normal heart rhythm. The outcome of the trial drugs helps determine how to relieve the client's symptoms medically. The normal heart rhythm also may be restored with electrical shocks. With the catheters in place, the physician may use the opportunity to prevent the dysrhythmia from ever reoccurring by delivering electricity to the area that originates the dysrhythmia. The electricity destroys the pathogenic tissue with a procedure called radiofrequency catheter ablation, discussed later in this chapter.

Preparation, management, and recovery for the client undergoing an electrophysiology study are similar to those for a client undergoing a heart catheterization (see Chap. 22). Usually, the client is monitored for a full day and discharged the following day if no bleeding or vascular complications occur.

Medical and Surgical Management

Some dysrhythmias are not life-threatening and may not require treatment. Many are treated with drug therapy and electrical modalities such as elective electrical cardioversion, defibrillation, or temporary or permanent pacing (Table 26-1).

Drug Therapy

Oral and IV antidysrhythmic drugs are used to treat clients with dysrhythmias; however, not all clients require medication. Usually, long-term antidysrhythmic drug therapy is based on the degree of hemodynamic compromise and the potential for the client to develop a life-threatening dysrhythmia. During resuscitation efforts, one or more of the various drugs used in cardiac emergencies is administered (Drug Therapy Table 26-1).

TABLE 26-1 Characteristics and Treatment of Selected Dysrhythmias

DYSRHYTHMIA	RHYTHM	ATRIAL RATE (BEATS/MIN)	VENTRICULAR RATE (BEATS/MIN)	TREATMENT
Sinus bradycardia	Regular	<60	<60	None unless symptomatic; atropine
Sinus tachycardia	Regular	100–150	100–150	None unless symptomatic; treat underlying disease
Premature atrial contraction	Irregular	60–100	60–100	None or treat underlying cause, if known
Supraventricular tachycardia	Regular	150–250	150–250	Valsalva maneuver, unilateral carotid massage, immersion of face in ice water, administration of IV adenosine, cardioversion, radiofrequency ablation
Atrial flutter	Usually regular	250–350	75–175	Cardioversion, digitalis, quinidine, propranolol, verapamil
Atrial fibrillation	Grossly irregular	400–600	100–160	Digitalis, quinidine, cardioversion, verapamil, ibutilide, flecainide, amiodarone, anticoagulant
First-degree AV block	Regular	60–100	60–100	None unless symptomatic
Second-degree AV block	Regular	60–100	30–100	Pacemaker
Complete heart block	Regular	60–100	<40	Pacemaker
Ventricular tachycardia	Regular	60–100*	150–300	Lidocaine, procainamide, bretylium, cardioversion, defibrillation if pulseless
Ventricular fibrillation	Chaotic	60–100*	400–600	Defibrillation preceded by or followed with epinephrine

*Rate may not be distinguishable.

(Adapted from Kelley, W. N. [2004]. *Textbook of internal medicine* [4th ed.]. Philadelphia: Lippincott Williams & Wilkins.)

DRUG THERAPY TABLE 26-1 Antidysrhythmics

Drug Category and Examples	Mechanism of Action	Side Effects	Nursing Considerations
Class I Antidysrhythmics: Sodium Channel Blockers			
Class IA (moderate block)			
procainamide hydrochloride (Pronestyl)	Slow electrical conduction, suppressing ventricular dysrhythmias	Hypotension, GI upset, rash; potential immune system problems with long-term use	Monitor cardiac rhythm and BP frequently.
Class IB (weak block)			
lidocaine hydrochloride (Xylocaine)	Suppress ventricular dysrhythmias by decreasing ventricular excitability	Dizziness, fatigue, drowsiness, nausea, vomiting, vision changes, seizures, hypotension	Monitor cardiac rhythm and vital signs. Keep life support equipment available.
Class IC (pronounced block)			
flecainide (Tambocor)	Strong blocker of fast NA$^+$ channels; slows conduction velocity in Purkinje fibers and AV node	Blurred vision, dizziness, headache, nausea, conduction disturbances, and ventricular dysrhythmias	Teach client to take exactly as prescribed and to report adverse reactions immediately. Monitor cardiac rhythm and BP.
Class II Antidysrhythmics			
Beta-adrenergic blockers			
isoproterenol (Isoprel)	Reduce calcium entry and depress depolarization to suppress dysrhythmias	Fatigue, insomnia, drowsiness, erectile dysfunction or decreased libido, bradycardia, confusion	Monitor cardiac rhythm and condition. Monitor for hyperglycemia. Monitor older clients for cognitive dysfunction, depression, and hallucinations.
Class III Antidysrhythmics			
Potassium channel blockers			
amiodarone (Cordarone)	A class III drug that also possesses classes I, II, and IV effects. Used to treat life-threatening recurrent ventricular dysrhythmias that do not respond to adequate doses of other antidysrhythmics.	Pulmonary toxicity, dyspnea, dry cough, hypotension, bradycardia, dysrhythmias, fever, nausea, vomiting, abnormal liver function test, discoloration of skin, possibly CHF.	Teach client to report adverse reactions immediately. Monitor closely for respiratory compromise; clients need chest x-ray and pulmonary function test after use of drug.
bretylium tosylate (Bretylol)	Inhibit the release of norepinephrine Used for ventricular dysrhythmias resistant to other antidysrhythmic agents	Nausea, vomiting, anorexia, profound hypotension, pain at IV site	Monitor cardiac rhythm and BP continuously. Keep client recumbent.
Class IV Antidysrhythmics			
Calcium channel blockers			
verapamil hydrochloride (Calan)	Suppress tachydysrhythmias by inhibiting the movement of calcium across cell membranes; reduce myocardial contractility	Dizziness, headache, bradycardia, hypotension, heart block	Monitor BP, heart rate, rhythm, and output. Keep client flat for 1 hr after administration. Have equipment for cardioversion and pacing available.
Miscellaneous Antidysrhythmics and Drugs Used in Cardiac Resuscitation			
Vasopressors			
epinephrine hydrochloride (Adrenalin)	Increase heart rate, force of contraction, and BP Used in asystole	Hypertension, dysrhythmias, pallor, oliguria	Administer every 5 min during cardiac resuscitation. Monitor vital signs and cardiac rhythm.
Cholinergic Antagonists			
atropine sulfate	Block the effects of vagus nerve stimulation Increase heart rate Used for bradydysrhythmias	Palpitations, tachycardia, urinary retention	Monitor for therapeutic and adverse effects. Document heart rate before and after administration.

(drug table continues on

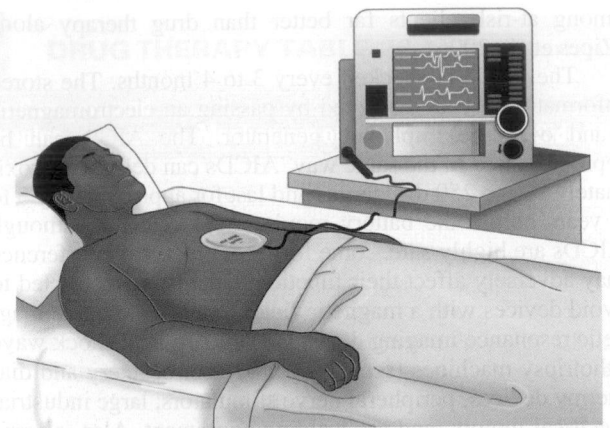

FIGURE 26-12. Transcutaneous pacemaker with electrode pads connected to the anterior and posterior chest walls.

Temporary Pacemakers

The three types of temporary pacemakers are transcutaneous, transvenous, and transthoracic. An external **transcutaneous pacemaker** is an emergency measure for maintaining adequate heart rate. It uses disposable, self-adhering leads applied to the chest (Fig. 26-12). The heart rate is paced from an external generator. Use of a transcutaneous pacemaker is temporary until either a transvenous or permanent pacemaker can be placed or the client is stabilized with medication.

A **transvenous pacemaker** is a temporary pulse-generating device that sometimes is necessary to manage transient bradydysrhythmias such as those that occur during acute MIs or after coronary artery bypass graft surgery, or to override tachydysrhythmias. The electrical lead is introduced through the subclavian, external or internal jugular, or cephalic vein and threaded first into the right atrium, then into the right ventricle (Fig. 26-13). It may be inserted at the bedside. Fluoroscopy and a cardiac monitor are used to determine the correct placement of the tip of the pacemaker lead.

The leads of a *transthoracic pacemaker* are inserted during open-heart surgery. They extend from the chest incision. If the client requires cardiac pacing during postoperative recovery, the leads are connected to a temporary pacing unit.

Permanent (Implanted) Pacemaker

An **implanted pacemaker** is a totally implanted electrical device used to manage a chronic bradydysrhythmia. The most frequent indication for inserting a permanent pacemaker is complete or second-degree heart block accompanied by a slow ventricular rate. Occasionally, permanent pacing is used to treat certain tachydysrhythmias that do not respond to treatment or whose treatment results in bradycardia.

The lead of an implanted pacemaker is inserted transvenously, and the pacing threshold, voltage, and rate are set. One type of pacemaker has leads in both the right atrium and right ventricle (dual chamber); the lead of a single-chamber pacemaker is in either the right atrium or right ventricle. The implantable pacemaker generator, which is about the size of a half-dollar coin and three times as thick, is then positioned under the skin below the right or left clavicle (Fig. 26-14). The small incision is closed with sutures. PVCs are more frequent during the early postimplantation period, and drug therapy may be ordered to suppress this dysrhythmia.

Power for the pacemaker is provided by mercury, lithium, or nuclear-powered (plutonium) batteries. The mercury battery has the shortest life (5–7 years); the nuclear-powered has the longest (8–10 years). Externally charged batteries also are used. Pacemaker batteries do not fail suddenly. The physician regularly monitors the status of their power. When the battery is nearing its end, the entire generator is replaced and the leads are connected to the new generator. After the pacemaker is inserted, the client is reassessed in 3 months and every 6 months thereafter. If the client redevelops original symptoms or suddenly shows dyspnea, vertigo, syncope, unexplained fatigue, edema in upper or lower extremities, muscle twitching, or extended hiccupping develop in the interim, the pacemaker is checked over the telephone. Routine telephone checks are scheduled every 2 to 4 months for the first 3 years and every month thereafter. If a problem develops, the pacemaker is reprogrammed with an external wand just like the AICD.

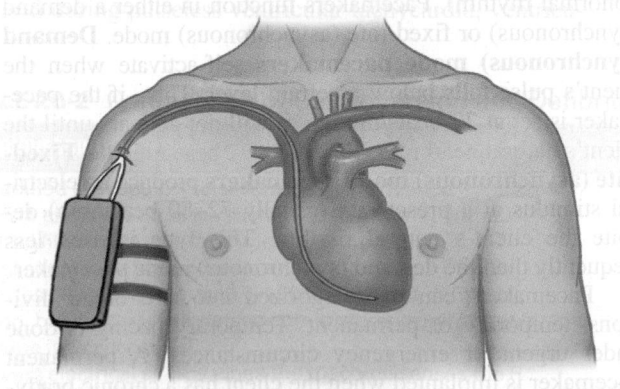

FIGURE 26-13. A transvenous pacemaker.

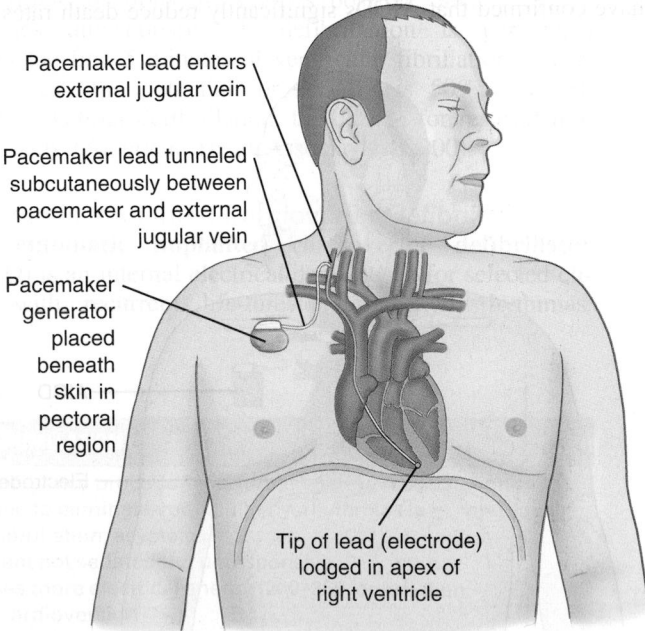

Pacemaker lead enters external jugular vein

Pacemaker lead tunneled subcutaneously between pacemaker and external jugular vein

Pacemaker generator placed beneath skin in pectoral region

Tip of lead (electrode) lodged in apex of right ventricle

FIGURE 26-14. A permanent pacemaker uses an implanted transvenous pacing electrode and pacemaker generator.

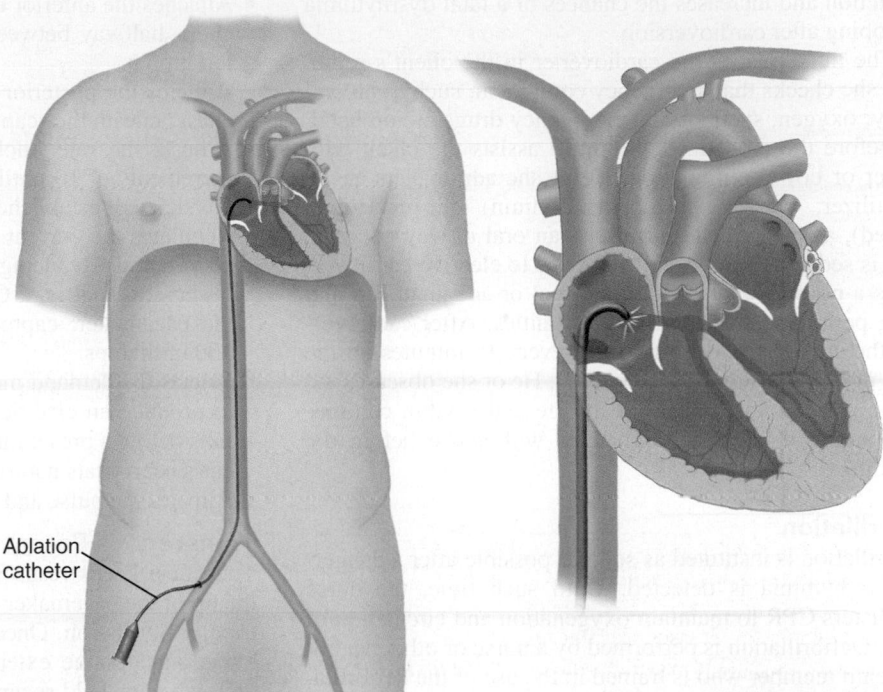

Ablation
catheter

FIGURE 26-15. A catheter is guided to the heart, and radiofrequency catheter ablation destroys the defective conducting tissue.

Radiofrequency Catheter Ablation

Radiofrequency catheter ablation is a procedure in which a heated catheter tip destroys dysrhythmia-producing tissue. A catheter is threaded transvenously into the heart, initially for electrophysiology studies. Once the location of the dysrhythmia-generating tissue is identified, electrical energy is sent to the catheter tip (Fig. 26-15). The heat destroys the errant tissue, allowing impulse conduction to travel over appropriate pathways. Accompanying risks include bleeding from the insertion site, perforation of the catheterized vein, and vascular complications such as thrombus formation. When the catheter is in the heart itself, it may pierce the myocardium, leading to pericardial tamponade. It is also possible for the heated tip to obliterate normal conductive tissue, requiring a permanent pacemaker to ensure heart contraction.

Nursing Management

Clients with symptomatic dysrhythmias require careful monitoring and documentation of symptoms. Clients with serious dysrhythmias are potentially unstable, making frequent rhythm analyses important. Administering and monitoring the effects of antidysrhythmic drugs are key nursing responsibilities. Drugs given to restore or control cardiac rhythm are powerful, and their therapeutic levels often are close to toxic levels. Many of these drugs cause unwanted side effects and are contraindicated in certain conditions. The nurse assists with medical procedures that help to restore normal sinus rhythm and manages postprocedural care. He or she provides health teaching that promotes the client's ability to maintain safe self-management after discharge. Clients with cardiac risk factors should avoid drinking more than 6 ounces of beer or wine per day; during alcohol withdrawal, catecholamines are released and may cause dangerous dysrhythmias.

 Pharmacologic Considerations

- Drug toxicity can occur even when normal doses of digitalis and cardiac glycosides are administered. Signs of toxicity include anorexia, nausea, vomiting, visual disturbances (e.g., halos around dark objects, objects appear green or yellow), diarrhea, abdominal discomfort, and dysrhythmias such as bradycardia, and tachycardia. Withhold the drug and notify the physician if the heart rate is less than 60 beats/minute.

- Digitalis toxicity usually is treated by discontinuing the preparation, which allows digitalis levels to return to normal within a short time. If digoxin levels are severely elevated to a life-threatening level, 800 mg of the digitalis antidote, digoxin immune fab (Digibind), is given IV over 30 minutes.

Elective Electrical Cardioversion

Prior to electrical cardioversion, the client may be anticoagulated to reduce the risk of thrombus formation and embolization. When the partial thromboplastin time (PTT) or international normalized ratio (INR) is within a therapeutic range, the nurse prepares the client for electrical cardioversion similarly to preparing a client for a surgical procedure. He or she verifies that a consent form has been signed. Food and oral fluids are restricted. The nurse ensures a patent IV line. He or she consults the physician to determine if scheduled drugs are to be temporarily withheld or additional drugs to decrease anxiety are to be administered. The physician may order a sedative 30 to 60 minutes before the procedure. Digitalis and diuretics are withheld for 24 to 72 hours before cardioversion; it is believed that the presence of these drugs in myocardial cells decreases the ability to restore normal conduction and increases the chances of a fatal dysrhythmia developing after cardioversion.

The nurse places the cardioverter in the client's room. He or she checks that emergency equipment, such as an oral airway; oxygen; suction; and emergency drugs are on hand. Just before the procedure, the nurse assists the client with bladder or bowel elimination. He or she administers an IV tranquilizer, usually diazepam (Valium) or midazolam (Versed), as prescribed and inserts an oral airway once the client is sedated. The desired response to elective cardioversion is a normal sinus rhythm, normal or adequate BP, and strong peripheral pulses in all extremities. After cardioversion, the nurse monitors vital signs every 15 minutes for the first 1 or 2 hours and then as ordered. He or she observes the cardiac monitor to evaluate heart rate and rhythm continuously and compares ECG changes with those before the procedure.

Defibrillation

Defibrillation is instituted as soon as possible after a dangerous dysrhythmia is detected. Until such time, the nurse administers CPR to maintain oxygenation and circulation of blood. Defibrillation is performed by a nurse or other healthcare team member who is trained in the use of the defibrillator (Nursing Guidelines 26-1).

After successful defibrillation, the nurse frequently monitors level of consciousness, ECG pattern, BP, and pulse and respiratory rates. He or she reviews laboratory results, such as arterial blood gas analyses and serum electrolyte levels. The nurse checks the paddle application sites for redness and impaired skin integrity. The defibrillator is kept on standby because repeat defibrillation may be necessary. Even when cardiac activity is restored, the possibility remains that oxygen deprivation has affected one or more organs. The nurse monitors urine output to detect kidney failure and assesses for motor weakness or paralysis, memory impairment, and level of consciousness to detect for possible effects from cerebral anoxia.

Pacemakers

Transcutaneous Pacemaker

When initiating the use of a transcutaneous pacemaker, the nurse:

- Attaches the anterior electrode patch to the left side of the chest, halfway between the xiphoid process to below the left nipple.
- Adheres the posterior electrode patch to the left posterior chest beneath the scapula and lateral to the spine.
- Adjusts the rate knob beginning at 40 beats/minute in increments of 10 until reaching the rate prescribed by the physician or established by agency policy.
- Regulates the current knob, which has a capacity starting at zero and advancing to 120 milliamps until capturing is observed—that is, a QRS complex follows each spike of the pacemaker; capturing usually occurs between 50 to 100 milliamps.
- Selects the demand mode, which programs the pacemaker to produce an electrical stimulus whenever the heart rate falls below a preset rate but remains inactive when the client's heart beats naturally at an adequate rate.
- Palpates the pulse and observes the client's response.

Transvenous Pacemaker

The nurse keeps resuscitation equipment close by because the tip of the pacemaker lead can mechanically provoke ventricular fibrillation. Once the pacemaker lead is inserted, the nurse attaches the external end to the external pacemaker unit, which is held securely to the client's forearm by means of tape or other anchoring device. The nurse positions the unit so that no tension is on the pacemaker lead. He or she checks the connection several times each day because an improper connection or displacement of the wire from the terminal results in pacemaker malfunction. If the client is confused or restless and movement disturbs the external pacemaker or its lead, the nurse notifies the physician. Only grounded electrical equipment is used in the room. This means that all electrical plugs must have three prongs.

If the client is on a cardiac monitor, an alarm sounds if the client's heart rate drops below the lowest level set on the alarm system. The drop in heart rate may result from battery failure, internal dislodgment of the pacemaker lead, or a break in the pacemaker lead. The battery of an external pacemaker is easily replaced; the nurse keeps one or more spare batteries readily available. The nurse reports dislodgment of the pacemaker lead or a broken wire to the physician immediately so that the pacemaker can be repositioned or replaced by a new one.

NURSING GUIDELINES 26-1

Performing Defibrillation

When performing defibrillation, the nurse:

- Determines that there is no breathing or pulse
- Checks the ECG rhythm
- Facilitates CPR until the client is prepared for defibrillation
- Applies gel or saline pads to the skin of the upper right chest near the sternum and apical area
- Charges the paddles to 200 joules of energy while stating "Charging"
- Selects the nonsynchronized mode on the defibrillator (the synchronized mode is used for cardioversion)

- Places the paddles on the chest over the gel or pads with firm pressure
- Shouts "All clear" to ensure that no one is in contact with the client or the bed
- Presses the discharge buttons on each paddle with the thumbs while stating "Shocking now"
- Evaluates the postdefibrillation cardiac rhythm
- Repeats defibrillation using 200 joules one more time and 360 joules for subsequent defibrillation attempts if there is no improvement in the cardiac rhythm
- Continues CPR as IV medications are administered and between defibrillation attempts

Permanent Pacemaker

The nurse places the client with an internal pacemaker on a cardiac monitor and examines the rhythm strip for the pacemaker's characteristic electrical artifact or "spike," identified by a thin, straight stroke. Absence of the spike with a demand pacemaker setting means that the natural pacemaker, the SA node, initiates the impulse. With a fixed-rate pacemaker, there is a spike each time the heart is stimulated. The location of the spike in the series of waveforms is important to note. The nurse reports any deviation from the expected pattern. Absence of the spike in a fixed-rate pacemaker may mean faulty monitoring equipment or, more seriously, failure to pace. Other complications include infection, perforation of the ventricular myocardium by the tip of the pacemaker lead, and development of dysrhythmias. Postimplantation instructions for the client include the following:

- Avoid strenuous movement especially of the arm on the side where the pacemaker is inserted.
- Keep the arm on the side of the pacemaker lower than the head except for brief moments when dressing or performing hygiene.
- Delay for at least 8 weeks such activities as swimming, bowling, playing tennis, vacuum cleaning, carrying heavy objects, chopping wood, mowing or raking, and shoveling snow.
- Avoid sources of electrical interference similar to those problematic for people with AICDs.

Client and Family Teaching 26-1 highlights maintenance and care instructions for clients with permanent pacemakers.

Client and Family Teaching 26-1
Permanent Pacemakers

The nurse instructs clients with permanent pacemakers and their families as follows:

- Maintain follow-up care.
- Report if the suture line becomes inflamed or sore.
- Avoid injury to the area where the pacemaker is inserted.
- Follow the physician's advice regarding lifting, sports, and exercise.
- Palpate the pulse and count the rate for a full minute daily or when feeling ill.
- Obtain and wear a MedicAlert bracelet or tag identifying that a pacemaker is implanted.
- Be cautious of situations that can cause pacemaker malfunction: gravitational force during airplane departures or landings, bumpy car rides, high-tension wires, shortwave radio transmissions, telephone transformers, and nuclear magnetic resonance imaging. Move to another location and check the pulse rate if dizziness or palpitations occur.
- Request hand scanning during airport security checks; some pacemakers trigger alarms.
- Maintain at least 6 inches between a cellular phone and the pacemaker generator or 12 inches if the cellular phone transmits over 3 watts.
- Check with the physician concerning transtelephonic pacemaker checks or when a pacemaker battery change will be necessary in the future.

Nursing Process for the Client With a Dysrhythmia

Assessment

Review the client's medical history, including allergy and drug history. In addition to performing a general cardiovascular assessment (see Chap. 22), note trends in heart rate, cardiac rhythm, BP, level of consciousness, urinary output, and physiologic changes in response to activity. If hemodynamic monitoring devices such as an arterial line, central venous pressure monitoring system, or pulmonary artery catheter are used (see Chap. 29), analyze the results of pressure readings and measurements of cardiac output. Record any symptoms the client reports, such as dizziness, fainting, or chest pain. Determine the level of the client's knowledge about drug therapy or other supportive treatment measures such as elective cardioversion or use of an AICD or a pacemaker.

Diagnosis, Planning, and Interventions

▶ **Decreased Cardiac Output** related to ineffective heart contraction secondary to dysrhythmia or ineffective response to treatment measures

▶ **Expected Outcome:** Client will maintain adequate cardiac output as evidenced by stable vital signs; no chest pain, dizziness, or syncope; and urinary output of at least 1500 mL per 24 hours.

- Maintain physical and emotional rest. *Rest reduces tachycardia and may relieve the consequences of a tachydysrhythmia.*
- Provide supplemental oxygen for dyspnea, chest pain, or syncope. *Supplemental oxygen by inhalation diffuses at the alveolar-capillary level and increases oxygen concentration in the blood, making more oxygen available for cellular metabolism.*

▶ **PC:** Life-Threatening Dysrhythmia

▶ **Expected Outcome:** The nurse will monitor to detect dysrhythmias and manage and minimize any that occur.

- Monitor cardiac rhythm continuously. *Cardiac monitors display real-time heart rate and rhythm and alert the nurse to potentially life-threatening dysrhythmias.*
- Ensure a patent IV access. *Emergency medications are usually given by the IV route.*
- Administer antidysrhythmic drugs as prescribed. *They restore normal sinus rhythm by interfering with ectopic pacemaker sites.*
- Prepare client for elective cardioversion or use of a temporary pacemaker (see earlier discussion). *An alert client will be less anxious when given an explanation of the purpose and techniques for measures to restore normal cardiac rhythm.*
- Summon the team who will provide advanced cardiac life support measures such as defibrillation, and administer CPR. *CPR provides supportive breathing and circulates blood by heart compression to facilitate resuscitation. Advanced cardiac life support provides endotracheal intubation, positive pressure ventilation, and electrical defibrillation to enhance the potential for resuscitation (see earlier discussion for specifics on defibrillation).*

▶ Risk for Ineffective Management of Therapeutic Regimen related to unfamiliarity with treatment measures

▶ **Expected Outcome:** Client will describe ways to manage self-care before discharge.

- Explain the action, side effects, dosage, route, administration, and importance of medications used to control the dysrhythmia. *Thorough understanding promotes safety and adherence.*
- Teach client the technique for palpating and counting the radial pulse. *An accurate pulse assessment helps the client evaluate his or her response to treatment measures.*
- Identify the guidelines for withholding specific drugs and reporting symptoms to the physician. *Communication enhances early intervention when complications develop.*
- Provide information about the precautions required with an AICD or a pacemaker. *Electrical interference and magnetization can impair the function of these devices.*
- Stress the importance of continued medical follow-up. *Regular medical consultations ensure that the client's condition remains stable or facilitate early modifications to treatment.*

Evaluation of Expected Outcomes

Expected outcomes are the restoration and maintenance of adequate cardiac output. Any life-threatening dysrhythmias are effectively treated. The client and family accurately relate the treatment plan and postdischarge care. ●

CRITICAL THINKING EXERCISES

1. A client for whom an antidysrhythmic drug has been prescribed returns for a follow-up examination. How would you determine if the client has followed the drug therapy regimen?
2. What information is essential to document when helping to resuscitate a client who has experienced a cardiac arrest?
3. Describe similarities and differences between an implanted pacemaker and an automatic implanted cardioverter defibrillator (AICD).

4. Many individuals purchase and self-medicate with ubiquinone (Coenzyme Q10, CQ10, CoQ, vitamin Q10) as a form of complementary or alternative therapy. It accounted for more than $200 million in sales in the United States (Bonadker & Guarneri, 2005). Discuss the use of this substance in relation to cardiovascular disease.

NCLEX-STYLE REVIEW QUESTIONS

1. A client in the intensive care unit (ICU) is noted to have ventricular fibrillation. Which nursing action is most appropriate initially?
   1. Performing immediate defibrillation
   2. Preparing the client for pacemaker insertion
   3. Assessing the client for electrolyte imbalance
   4. Taking temperature, pulse, and blood pressure
2. What evidence indicates to the nurse that a client with a dysrhythmia has insufficient cardiac output? Select all that apply.
   1. Hypotension
   2. Confusion
   3. Decreased urine output
   4. Labored respirations
   5. Thready pulse
   6. Flushed skin
3. Atropine sulfate 0.5 mg is prescribed. The supplied dosage is 0.4 mg per mL. Calculate the volume to prepare.
4. Which of the following interventions are necessary when caring for a client with a transvenous pacemaker?
   1. Keep the resuscitation equipment at a distance.
   2. Use only grounded electrical equipment in the room.
   3. Check the connection of the unit once a day.
   4. Monitor the client's vital signs every 15 minutes.
5. Which of the following nursing interventions is required when caring for a client undergoing elective electrical cardioversion?
   1. Restrict food and fluids before the procedure.
   2. Continue to administer digitalis daily.
   3. Perform CPR until cardioversion is successful.
   4. Monitor the pulse pressure every 15 minutes.

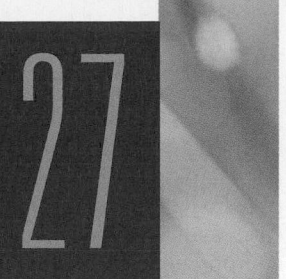

27

Caring for Clients with Hypertension

Words To Know
accelerated hypertension
diastolic blood pressure
essential hypertension
hypernatremia
hypertension
hypertensive cardiovascular disease
hypertensive heart disease
hypertensive vascular disease
malignant hypertension
natriuretic factor
papilledema
prehypertension
secondary hypertension
stage 1 hypertension
stage 2 hypertension
systolic blood pressure
white-coat hypertension

Learning Objectives

On completion of this chapter, you will be able to:

1. Identify the two physiologic components that create blood pressure.
2. List factors that influence blood pressure.
3. List three structures that physiologically control arterial pressure.
4. Explain systolic and diastolic arterial pressure.
5. Define hypertension and identify groups at risk for it.
6. Differentiate essential and secondary hypertension.
7. Identify causes of secondary hypertension.
8. List consequences of chronic hypertension.
9. Discuss the assessment findings in hypertension.
10. Discuss the medical and nursing management of the client with hypertension.
11. Differentiate between accelerated and malignant hypertension.
12. Identify potential complications of uncontrolled malignant hypertension.
13. Discuss the medical and nursing management of the client with malignant hypertension.

This chapter provides information about the physiology that underlies normal blood pressure, the ranges in normal and abnormal blood pressure measurements, the consequences of sustained, elevated blood pressure or **hypertension**, and medical and nursing interventions that help to lower blood pressure measurements to healthier levels.

PHYSIOLOGY OF BLOOD PRESSURE

Blood pressure (BP) is the force produced by the volume of blood in arterial walls. It is represented by the formula:

$$BP = CO \text{ (cardiac output)} \times PR \text{ (peripheral resistance)}$$

The measured BP reflects the ability of the arteries to stretch and fill with blood, the efficiency of the heart as a pump, and the volume of circulating blood. Blood pressure is affected by age, body size, diet, activity, emotions, pain, position, gender, time of day, and disease states. Studies of healthy persons show that BP can fluctuate within a wide range and remain normal. Thus, obtaining several measurements for comparison is important.

When measured, arterial blood pressure, the pressure during systole and diastole, is expressed as a fraction. The top number is the systolic BP; the bottom number is the diastolic BP. Normal BP for adults ranges from 100/60 to 119/79 mm Hg. The autonomic nervous system, the kidneys, and various endocrine glands regulate arterial pressure. BP tends to increase with age, most likely from arteriosclerotic and atherosclerotic changes in blood vessels or other effects of chronic diseases such as diabetes and renal dysfunction. Screening of BP is an important method for identifying people at risk for heart failure, renal failure, and stroke. Those at highest risk are older adults, African Americans, and clients with diabetes mellitus.

Systolic Blood Pressure

Systolic blood pressure is determined by the force and volume of blood that the left ventricle ejects during systole and the ability of the arterial system to distend at the time of ventricular contraction. The arterial walls are normally elastic and yield to the force and volume of ventricular contraction. In older clients, systolic BP may be elevated because of loss of arterial elasticity (arteriosclerosis). Narrowing of the arterioles, either from arteriosclerosis or some other mechanism causing vasoconstriction, increases peripheral resistance, which in turn increases systolic BP. This resistance can be compared to the narrowing of a tube, such as a drinking straw. The narrower the lumen is, the greater the pressure needed to move liquid through it.

Diastolic Blood Pressure

Diastolic blood pressure reflects arterial pressure during ventricular relaxation. It depends on the resistance of the arterioles and the diastolic filling times. If arterioles are resistant (constricted), blood is under greater pressure.

HYPERTENSIVE DISEASE

Approximately 50 million people, or 1 in 4 adults, in the United States have high blood pressure. Because hypertension places people at risk for heart disease, heart failure (see Chap. 28), stroke, and kidney disease, healthcare professionals have revised guidelines for identifying hypertension. What once was considered normal blood pressure measurements, a systolic pressure of 120 and diastolic pressure of 80, are now the lower ranges of prehypertension (Table 27-1). **Prehypertension** is defined as a systolic blood pressure of 120 to 139 mm Hg or a diastolic blood pressure between 80 and 89 mm Hg (National Heart, Lung, and Blood Institute, 2003).

The term *hypertension*, sustained elevations in systolic or diastolic blood pressure that exceed prehypertension levels, now subdivides into two categories. **Stage 1 hypertension,** as defined by The Joint National Committee on Prevention, Detection, Evaluation, and Treatment of High Blood Pressure (2003), is systolic blood pressure of 140 to 159 mm Hg or a diastolic blood pressure between 90 and 99 mm Hg. **Stage 2 hypertension** is systolic blood pressure that equals or exceeds 160 mm Hg or a diastolic pressure that equals or exceeds 100 mm Hg.

When elevated BP causes a cardiac abnormality, the term **hypertensive heart disease** is used. When vascular damage is present without heart involvement, the term **hypertensive vascular disease** is used. When both heart disease and vascular damage accompany hypertension, the appropriate term is **hypertensive cardiovascular disease**.

ESSENTIAL AND SECONDARY HYPERTENSION

Hypertension is further divided into two main categories: essential (primary; idiopathic) and secondary. **Essential hypertension,** about 95% of cases, is sustained elevated BP with no known cause. **Secondary hypertension** is elevated BP that results from or is secondary to some other disorder.

Some people experience **white-coat hypertension,** a term describing elevated BP that develops during evaluation by medical personnel, who traditionally have worn a white coat. This hypertension most likely results from anxiety that is accompanied by a surge of epinephrine and norepinephrine, powerful neurohormones that cause vasoconstriction. To confirm or exclude this phenomenon, the BP is measured a second time before the client leaves the agency. In cases of white-coat hypertension, this subsequent measurement is likely to be normal. If the client remains hypertensive, he or she is advised to check BP regularly, either at home with the help of a family member, at a public-service location in the community (e.g., pharmacy), or at the office of the primary physician. The client is advised to bring the record of BP measurements to his or her medical appointments.

Pathophysiology and Etiology

The exact cause of essential hypertension is unknown. BP often increases with age; hypertension may run in families. Essential hypertension affects African Americans at a higher rate than it does other ethnic groups. Obesity, inactivity, smoking, excessive alcohol intake, and ineffective stress management are risk factors.

Research into specific factors that contribute to the development of essential hypertension continues. For instance, it is well documented that **hypernatremia** (elevated serum sodium level) increases blood volume, which raises BP. A low serum potassium level, however, actually may cause sodium retention as the kidneys try to maintain a balanced number of cations (positively charged electrolytes) in body fluid. Scientists are also investigating the role of calcium in hypertension because serum calcium levels are low in some hypertensive clients.

Essential hypertension also may develop from alterations in other body chemicals. Defects in BP regulation may result from an impairment in the renin-angiotensin-aldosterone

TABLE 27-1 Classification of Blood Pressure in Adults 18 Years or Older

BP CLASSIFICATION	SYSTOLIC BP, mm Hg		DIASTOLIC BP, mm Hg
Normal	<120	*and*	<80
Prehypertension	120–139	*or*	80–89
Stage 1 hypertension	140–159	*or*	90–99
Stage 2 hypertension	≥160	*or*	≥100

mechanism (see Chap. 16). Renin is a chemical that the kidneys release to raise BP and increase vascular fluid volume in response to renal hypoperfusion. For people with a heightened stress response, hypertension may be correlated with a higher than usual release of catecholamines, such as epinephrine and norepinephrine, which elevate BP. Last, some researchers theorize that a deficiency of **natriuretic factor,** a hormone produced by the heart, results in an elevation of blood pressure because its role is to promote the excretion of sodium by the kidneys (see Chap. 16).

Secondary hypertension may accompany any primary condition that affects fluid volume or renal function or causes arterial vasoconstriction. Predisposing conditions include kidney disease, pheochromocytoma (a tumor of the adrenal medulla), hyperaldosteronism (increased secretion of mineralcorticoid by the adrenal cortex), atherosclerosis, use of cocaine or other cardiac stimulants (e.g., weight-control drugs, caffeine), and use of oral contraceptives.

Regardless of whether a person has essential or secondary hypertension, the accompanying organ damage and complications are the same. Hypertension causes the heart to work harder to pump against the increased resistance. Consequently, the size of the heart muscle increases. When the heart no longer can pump adequately to meet the body's metabolic needs, heart failure occurs (see Chap. 28). The extra work and the greater mass increase the heart's need for oxygen. If the myocardium does not receive sufficient oxygenated blood, myocardial ischemia occurs and the client experiences angina.

In addition to its direct effects on the heart, high BP damages the arterial vascular system. It accelerates atherosclerosis. Furthermore, the increased resistance of the arterioles to the flow of blood causes serious complications in other body organs, including the eyes, brain, heart, and kidneys. Hemorrhage of tiny arteries in the retina may cause marked visual disturbances or blindness. A cerebrovascular accident (stroke) may result from hemorrhage or occlusion of a blood vessel in the brain. Myocardial infarction (MI) may result from occlusion of a branch of a coronary artery. Impaired circulation to the kidneys may result in renal failure.

 Gerontologic Considerations

- High blood pressure in older adults may go undiagnosed; therefore, the older adult should be encouraged to have blood pressure checks at least every 6 months.

Assessment Findings

Signs and Symptoms

Clients with hypertension may be asymptomatic. The onset of hypertension, considered "the silent killer," often is gradual. It can exist for years but be discovered only during a routine physical examination or when the client experiences a major complication. As the BP becomes elevated, clients may identify symptoms such as a throbbing or pounding headache, dizziness, fatigue, insomnia, nervousness, nosebleeds, and blurred vision. Angina or dyspnea may be the first clue to hypertensive heart disease.

The most obvious finding during a physical assessment is a sustained elevation of one or both BP measurements. The pulse may feel bounding from the force of ventricular contraction. Clients may be overweight. They may have a flushed face from engorgement of superficial blood vessels. Peripheral edema may be present. An ophthalmic examination may reveal vascular changes in the eyes, retinal hemorrhages, or edema of the optic nerves, known as **papilledema**.

Diagnostic Findings

Diagnostic tests are performed to determine the extent of organ damage. Electrocardiography, echocardiography, and chest radiography may reveal an enlarged left ventricle. A multiple gated acquisition (MUGA) scan, a test that detects how well or inefficiently the heart pumps, can detect heart failure that may be associated with hypertension (see Chap. 28). Blood tests may show elevated blood urea nitrogen and serum creatinine levels, indicating impaired renal function, findings that excretory urography (intravenous pyelography [IVP]) may further validate. Fluorescein angiography, an ophthalmologic test using IV dye, often reveals leaking retinal blood vessels.

If the cause of hypertension is a renal vascular problem, renal arteriography demonstrates narrowing of the renal artery. If the cause is related to dysfunction of the adrenal gland, a 24 hour collected urine specimen detects elevated catecholamines. Blood studies reveal elevated cholesterol and triglyceride levels, indicating that atherosclerosis is an underlying factor.

Medical Management

The primary objective of therapy for hypertension is to lower the BP and prevent major complications. Treatment recommendations depend on the stage of the client's hypertension (see Table 27-1). Nonpharmacologic interventions are used for clients with prehypertension. Weight reduction, decreased sodium intake (Box 27-1), moderate exercise, and reduced contributing factors (e.g., smoking, alcohol use) may return the BP to normal levels. Table 27-2 identifies the potential benefits that are possible with lifestyle changes alone.

Currently, it is believed that in persons older than 50 years of age, reducing the systolic pressure below 140 mm Hg is more important than decreasing the diastolic blood pressure. Once the systolic blood pressure is controlled below 140 mm Hg, a reduction in the diastolic blood pressure generally follows. In clients with higher risk for hypertensive complications, as in clients with diabetes or chronic kidney disease, the goal is to reduce blood pressure to <130/80 mm Hg.

When drug therapy is needed, treatment decisions depend on the stage of hypertension and compelling indications (Fig. 27-1; Table 27-3). Clients who require drug therapy may be treated initially with one drug, usually a thiazide diuretic. However, most people with hypertension will need two or more antihypertensive medications to reduce their blood pressure to target level (Drug Therapy Table 27-1). If the BP remains elevated with two drug combinations, a third or fourth antihypertensive agent may be added. Secondary hypertension often resolves by treating its cause.

BOX 27-1 Recommendations for Limiting Sodium

- Consume less than 2300 mg of sodium per day or no more than 1500 mg for those who are salt sensitive (American Heart Association, 2009). One teaspoon of table salt equals 2300 mg of sodium.
- Because the sodium content of prepared foods can vary greatly among different brands, read Nutrition Facts Labels to compare the sodium content. Any food that provides more than 20% of the Daily Value of sodium in one serving is considered very high in sodium.
- Prepare food from "scratch" without adding salt, as opposed to purchasing premade, convenience, or packaged foods, which usually are highly salted.
- Substitute unsalted, no salt, sodium-free, low sodium, or reduced sodium products for regular salted products.

- Choose fresh or plain, frozen vegetables. If canned vegetables are chosen, drain and rinse before eating.
- Avoid or limit consumption of hot dogs, ham, bacon, and processed meat products, which often contain sodium nitrate as a preservative.
- Substitute healthy snacks such as fresh or dried fruit for those that are salted.
- Experiment with seasonings such as lemon, garlic, and onion powder as alternatives to salt.
- Eliminate or restrict items that contain significant sodium such as pickles, green olives, sauerkraut, mustard, catsup, barbecue sauce, pizza sauce, canned soup, and packaged mixes.

(Adapted from U.S. Department of Agriculture and U.S. Department of Health and Human Services. [2005]. Dietary guidelines for Americans. [On line.] Available at: http://www.health.gov/DIETARYGUIDELINES/dga2005.document/pdf/DGA2005.pdf.)

 Pharmacologic Considerations

- A possible adverse effect of all antihypertensive drugs is postural hypotension, which can lead to falls. Teaching should include tips for managing syncope and dizziness.

- Monitor angiotensin converting enzyme (ACE) inhibitors cautiously in clients with renal or hepatic impairment and older adults. A sudden drop in BP may occur during the first 1 to 3 hours after the initial dose of an ACE inhibitor; administration of IV normal saline may manage the hypotensive episode.

- ACE inhibitors may cause a persistent cough until the medication is discontinued.

 Gerontologic Considerations

- Older adults are at increased risk for development of hypokalemia from diuretic drugs. Lower doses of potassium wasting diuretics or the use of potassium sparing diuretics can control hypertension and minimize the risk of hypokalemia.

Nursing Process for the Client With Hypertension

Assessment

Take the BP initially in both arms with the client in a supine, sitting, and then standing position, using an appropriately sized cuff

TABLE 27-2 Lifestyle Changes and Benefits to Blood Pressure

MODIFICATION	RECOMMENDATION	AVERAGE SYSTOLIC BLOOD PRESSURE REDUCTION RANGE*
Weight reduction	Maintain normal body weight (body mass index: 18.5–24.9 kg/m^2).	5–20 mm Hg/10 kg
DASH eating plan	Adopt a diet rich in fruits, vegetables, and low-fat dairy products, with reduced content of fats, red meat, sweets, and sugar-containing beverages.	8–14 mm Hg
Dietary sodium restriction	Reduce dietary sodium intake to 100 mmol per day (2.3 g sodium or 6 g sodium chloride). (A further reduction to 1.5 g sodium/day would be ideal.)	2–8 mm Hg
Aerobic physical activity	Engage in regular aerobic physical activity (e.g., brisk walking) at least 30 minutes per day, most days of the week.	4–9 mm Hg
Moderation of alcohol consumption	Men: Limit to ≤ 2 drinks per day. Women and lighter weight persons: Limit to ≤ 1 drink per day. (1 drink = 12 oz beer, 5 oz wine, 1.5 oz 80-proof whiskey)	2–4 mm Hg

*Effects are dose and time dependent.

(From U.S. Department of Health and Human Services, National Institutes of Health, National Heart, Lung, and Blood Institute, *Reference Card From the Seventh Report of the Joint National Committee on Prevention, Detection, Evaluation, and Treatment of High Blood Pressure (JNC 7)*, NIH Publication No. 03-5231, May 2003.)

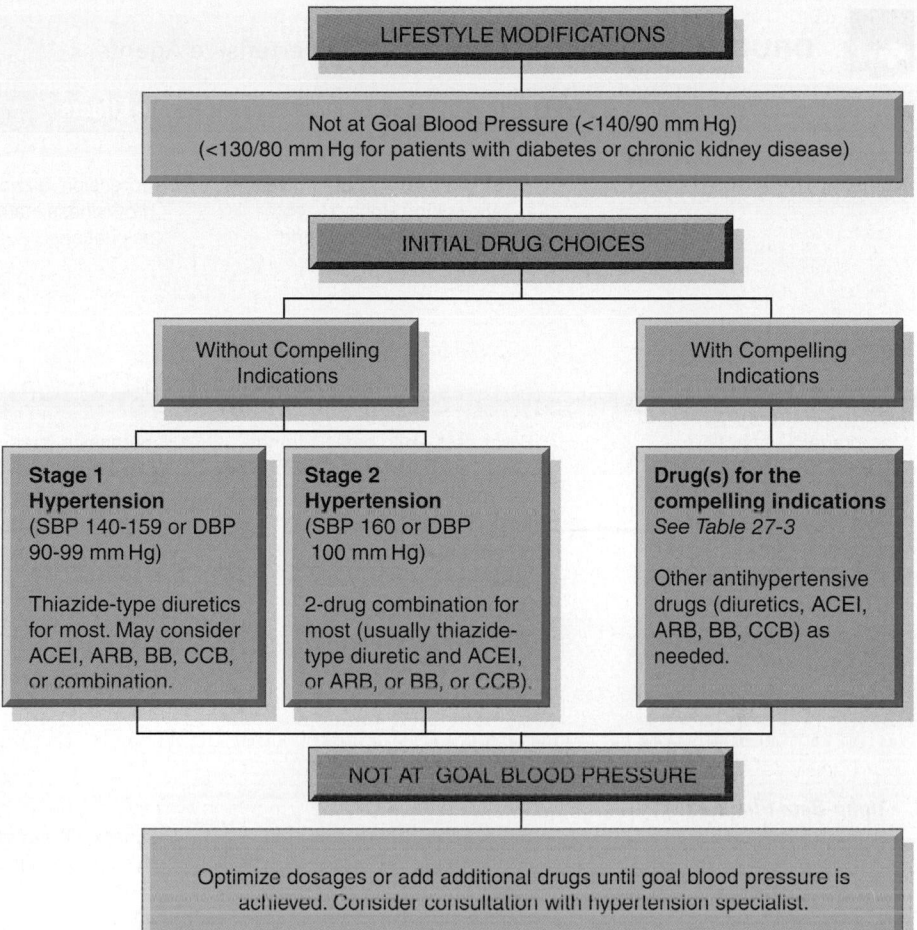

LIFESTYLE MODIFICATIONS

Not at Goal Blood Pressure (<140/90 mm Hg)
(<130/80 mm Hg for patients with diabetes or chronic kidney disease)

INITIAL DRUG CHOICES

Without Compelling Indications

With Compelling Indications

Stage 1 Hypertension (SBP 140-159 or DBP 90-99 mm Hg)

Thiazide-type diuretics for most. May consider ACEI, ARB, BB, CCB, or combination.

Stage 2 Hypertension (SBP 160 or DBP 100 mm Hg)

2-drug combination for most (usually thiazide-type diuretic and ACEI, or ARB, or BB, or CCB).

Drug(s) for the compelling indications See Table 27-3

Other antihypertensive drugs (diuretics, ACEI, ARB, BB, CCB) as needed.

NOT AT GOAL BLOOD PRESSURE

Optimize dosages or add additional drugs until goal blood pressure is achieved. Consider consultation with hypertension specialist.

FIGURE 27-1. Algorithm for treatment of hypertension. (From National Heart, Lung, and Blood Institute. *Seventh Report of the Joint National Committee on Prevention, Detection, Evaluation, and Treatment of High Blood Pressure.* [2003]. Bethesda, MD: National Institutes of Health. Available at: http://www.nhlbi.nih.gov/guidelines/hypertension/phycard.pdf. Retrieved October 2008.)

(Table 27-4). Thereafter, use the same arm and place the client in the same position each time a reading is taken. Ask questions to determine if the client is following the treatment regimen. Perform additional cardiac assessments (see Chap. 22), depending on the client's medical history and current symptoms.

Diagnosis, Planning, and Interventions

Teach the client about nonpharmacologic and pharmacologic methods for restoring and maintaining BP at or below goal levels, as well as techniques for self-management (Client and Family

TABLE 27-3 Compelling Indications for Individual Drug Classes

COMPELLING INDICATION	INITIAL THERAPY OPTIONS
Heart failure	THIAZ, BB, ACEI, ARB, ALDO ANT
Post-myocardial infarction	BB, ACEI, ALDO ANT
High CVD risk	THIAZ, BB, ACEI, CCB
Diabetes	THIAZ, BB, ACEI, ARB, CCB
Chronic kidney disease	ACEI, ARB
Recurrent stroke prevention	THIAZ, ACEI

Key: *ACEI* = angiotensin converting enzyme inhibitor, *ALDO ANT* = aldosterone antagonist, *ARB* = angiotensin receptor blocker, *BB* = beta blocker, *CCB* = calcium channel blocker, *THIAZ* = thiazide diuretic

Client and Family Teaching 27-1 Hypertension

The nurse instructs as follows:

● Adhere to the treatment regimen even if you have few, if any, symptoms and feel well. Hypertension is a chronic condition requiring lifelong management and treatment.
● Learn to regularly monitor BP using a home sphygmomanometer or arrange for monitoring by a community agency that provides this service at no or low cost.
● Keep a log of BP measurements for follow-up visits.
● Comply with the treatment regimen involving diet, exercise, and drug therapy.
● Consult cookbooks published or endorsed by the American Heart Association, American Diabetes Association, or other reliable sources for "heart smart" recipes.
● Follow directions for medications; never increase, decrease, or omit a prescribed drug unless first conferring with the primary care provider.
● Report adverse effects from medications to the prescribing provider. Get medical approval before taking nonprescription drugs. Inform all physicians and dentists of medications that you are taking.
● Avoid tobacco and beverages containing caffeine or alcohol, unless permitted by the provider.

DRUG THERAPY TABLE 27-1 Antihypertensive Agents

Drug Category and Examples	Mechanism of Action	Side Effects	Nursing Considerations
Alpha-Adrenergic Blockers prazosin (Minipress)	Relax vascular smooth muscle by blocking alpha$_1$ receptor sites for epinephrine and norepinephrine	Hypotension, dizziness, drowsiness, nausea, palpitations	Administer first dose just before bedtime to reduce potential for syncope. Monitor client for postural hypotension. Caution client to change positions slowly.
Beta-Adrenergic Blockers propranolol (Inderal)	Block beta$_1$- and beta$_2$-adrenergic receptors Decrease renin levels	Hypotension, bradycardia, bronchospasm, CHF, depression, erectile dysfunction, hypoglycemia	Administer with meals. Advise client not to discontinue medication abruptly. Monitor for fluid retention, rash, and difficulty breathing. Monitor blood glucose level in clients with diabetes. Some drugs are contraindicated in clients with chronic respiratory disorders.
Alpha-Beta Blockers labetalol (Normodyne)	Block alpha-, beta$_1$-, and beta$_2$-adrenergic receptors	Dizziness, GI symptoms, dyspnea, cough, erectile dysfunction, decreased libido	Administer with meals. Caution client to avoid discontinuing drug therapy abruptly and to inform anesthesiologist of use before surgery to avoid drug interactions.
Diuretics *thiazide diuretic:* chlorothiazide (Diuril)	Inhibit reabsorption of sodium in distal convoluted tubules	Hypokalemia, dizziness, hypotension, allergic reactions, hyperglycemia, hyperuricemia, photosensitivity	Monitor blood pressure, blood sugar, serum electrolytes, uric acid; assess weight, intake and output
loop diuretic: furosemide (Lasix)	Promote sodium and water excretion, thus reducing circulating blood volume	Dizziness, dehydration, blurred vision, anorexia, diarrhea, nocturia, polyuria, thrombocytopenia, orthostatic hypotension, hypokalemia	Weigh client daily. Measure intake and output. Monitor serum potassium level. Advise client to replace lost potassium with bananas, orange juice, or prescribed supplement.
ACE Inhibitors captopril (Capoten), quinapril (Accupril)	Block ACE from converting angiotensin I to angiotensin II (a potent vasoconstrictor) Promote fluid and sodium loss and decrease peripheral vascular resistance	Tachycardia, hypotension, GI irritation, pancytopenia, proteinuria, rash, cough, dry mouth, hyperkalemia	Excretion is reduced in clients with renal failure. First-dose hypotension is common in older adults. Administer 1 hour before or 2 hours after meals. Monitor serum potassium blood urea nitrogen and creatinine.

DRUG THERAPY TABLE 27-1 Antihypertensive Agents (continued)

Drug Category and Examples	Mechanism of Action	Side Effects	Nursing Considerations
Angiotensin Receptor Blockers losartan (Cozaar)	Block effects of angiotensin II Relax vascular smooth muscle Increase salt and water excretion Reduce plasma volume	Orthostatic hypotension; GI disturbances; hyperkalemia; respiratory congestion; swelling of face, lips, eyelids, tongue in hypersensitive persons	Assess BP for postural changes. Monitor serum potassium levels. Observe for allergic reactions when drug therapy begins.
Calcium Channel Blockers nifedipine (Procardia XL), verapamil (Isoptin)	Decrease BP by dilating coronary and peripheral arteries	Hypotension, dizziness, CHF, edema, atrioventricular block, nausea	Check BP and heart rate before each dose. Withhold drug in cases of hypotension. Observe for signs and symptoms of CHF and fluid overload.

ACE, angiotensin-converting enzyme; *BP,* blood pressure; *CHF,* congestive heart failure; *GI,* gastrointestinal.

Teaching 27-1). Collaborate with a dietitian to provide information on dietary modifications such as Dietary Approaches to Stop Hypertension, also referred to as the DASH diet (Nutrition Notes 27-1). Additional nursing management follows on p. XX.

▶ **Risk for Decreased Cardiac Output** related to excessive or prolonged systemic vascular resistance

▶ **Expected Outcome:** Client will maintain an adequate cardiac output as evidenced by reduced BP to normal or goal levels, heart rate between 60 and 100 beats/minute, effortless breathing, clear lung sounds, alert mental status, and urine output that approximates or slightly exceeds intake.

- Promote physical rest. *Rest decreases BP and reduces the resistance that the heart must overcome to eject blood.*
- Relieve emotional stress. *Reduced stress decreases production of neurotransmitters that constrict peripheral arterioles.*
- Instruct client to avoid bearing down against a closed glottis (Valsalva maneuver). *Straining or bearing down against a closed glottis momentarily increases BP.*
- Encourage compliance with salt/sodium restrictions. *Doing so decreases blood volume and improves the potential for greater cardiac output.*

- Recommend smoking cessation. *Nicotine raises heart rate, constricts arterioles, and reduces the heart's ability to eject blood.*
- Enforce prescribed fluid restrictions. *Reduced oral fluid ultimately decreases circulating blood volume and systemic vascular resistance.*
- Help client reduce or eliminate caffeine and tobacco. *Caffeine and nicotine increases heart rate and causes vasoconstriction.*
- Administer prescribed antihypertensives. *They use various mechanisms to control BP, including increasing urine elimination, blocking production of angiotensin, and dilating blood vessels.*

▶ **Risk for Injury** related to syncope and dizziness secondary to side effect of antihypertensive drugs

▶ **Expected Outcome:** The client will be injury free.

- Monitor postural changes in BP by assessing client while he or she is lying, sitting, and standing. *A 20 mm Hg fall in systolic blood pressure or a 10 mm Hg fall in diastolic blood pressure within 3 minutes of assuming an upright position indicates postural hypotension (Pickering et al., 2005). Assessment validates whether the drop in BP is significant.*

TABLE 27-4 Recommended Bladder Dimensions For Blood Pressure Cuffs

ARM CIRCUMFERENCE AT MIDPOINT* (CM)	CUFF NAME	BLADDER WIDTH (CM)	BLADDER LENGTH (CM)
22–26	Small adult	12	22
27–34	Adult	16	30
35–44	Large adult	16	36
45–52	Adult thigh	16	42

*Midpoint of arm is defined as half the distance from the acromion to the olecranon processes.
(Source: American Heart Association. [2005]. Recommendations for blood pressure measurement in humans and experimental animals. *Circulation* 111:697–716.)

Nutrition Notes 27-1
The Client with Hypertension

- Losing weight without reducing sodium intake lowers BP, even if the client does not attain ideal weight and regardless of the degree of excess weight. Ideally, BMI should be < 25 kg/m². Preventing weight gain in those with a normal weight is vitally important.

- The DASH diet, a total diet approach to preventing or treating hypertension, has been shown to significantly lower blood pressure in both normotensive and hypertensive people and in all major risk groups. The diet is rich in fruit, vegetables, and low-fat dairy products and emphasizes whole grains, poultry, fish, and nuts. Fat, red meat, sweets, and sugar-containing beverages are restricted. Nutritionally, the diet is high in potassium, magnesium, calcium, and fiber and slightly high in protein. The diet's effectiveness likely comes from several factors, not just one food or nutrient.

- Subsequent studies have shown that lowering the sodium content of a DASH diet further improves its effectiveness in lowering blood pressure. Although the relationship between sodium and blood pressure is direct and progressive, the benefits of lowering sodium intake are generally greater in African Americans; middle-aged and older adults; and those with hypertension, diabetes, or chronic kidney disease. While 1.5 g/day of sodium may be ideal, 2.3 g/day is a more realistic goal.

- The DASH eating plan contains:

  - 6 to 8 servings of grains, with whole grains recommended for most grain choices
  - 4 to 5 servings of vegetables
  - 4 to 5 servings of fruit
  - 2 to 3 servings of low-fat or nonfat dairy products
  - 6 ounces or less of lean meat, poultry, and fish
  - 4 to 5 servings of nuts per week
  - 2 to 3 servings of added fat per day,
  - 5 or fewer servings of sweets and added sugars per week

- As appropriate, ensure the signal cord is in the client's reach and advise him or her to use it whenever getting out of bed. *Nursing personnel can prevent injury if they assist clients.*

- Encourage client to rise slowly from a sitting or lying position. *Gradual changes in position provide time for the heart to increase its rate of contraction to resupply oxygen to the brain.*

- Help client to sit or lie down if he or she is dizzy. *The support of a chair or bed reduces the potential for falling.*

Evaluation of Expected Outcomes

Expected outcomes are that adequate cardiac output is maintained or improved when systolic BP is below 140 mm Hg or 130 mm Hg for those with diabetes or chronic kidney disease or diastolic BP is below 90 mm Hg or 80 mm Hg for those with diabetes or chronic kidney disease. The client does not experience syncope or fall from postural changes in BP. ●

▶ Stop, Think, and Respond Exercise 27-1

A neighbor asks you to take her BP. The measurement is 160/90 mm Hg. What questions will you ask? What recommendations will you make for follow-up?

ACCELERATED AND MALIGNANT HYPERTENSION

Accelerated hypertension and malignant hypertension are more serious forms of elevated BP that develop in clients with either essential or secondary hypertension. **Accelerated hypertension** describes markedly elevated BP, accompanied by hemorrhages and exudates in the eyes. If untreated, accelerated hypertension may progress to **malignant hypertension,** which describes dangerously elevated BP accompanied by papilledema.

Pathophysiology and Etiology

Accelerated hypertension and malignant hypertension occur in clients with undiagnosed hypertension or in those who fail to maintain follow-up or comply with medical therapy. Accelerated hypertension and malignant hypertension usually have abrupt onset; if untreated, severe symptoms and complications follow rapidly. Malignant hypertension is fatal unless BP is quickly reduced. Even with intensive treatment, the kidneys, brain, and heart may be permanently damaged.

Consequences are life-threatening when the BP in the vascular system becomes extremely elevated. Some arterial blood vessels already may have ruptured or will soon. Retinal hemorrhages can lead to blindness. A stroke occurs if vessels in the brain rupture and bleed. If an aneurysm has developed in the aorta from chronic hypertension, it may burst and cause hemorrhage and shock. Cardiac effects include left ventricular failure with pulmonary edema or MI. Renal failure also may be forthcoming if the pressure is not reduced.

Assessment Findings

Signs and Symptoms

Some clients may present with confusion, headache, visual disturbances, seizures, and, possibly, coma. The sudden, marked rise in BP may cause chest pain, dyspnea, and moist lung sounds. Renal failure is evidenced by less than 30 mL/hour of urine. The onset of sudden, severe back pain accompanied by hypotension (abnormally low BP) indicates that an aortic aneurysm is dissecting or has ruptured (see Chap. 25).

Systolic BP is 160 mm Hg or higher, diastolic BP is 100 mm Hg or higher, or both. The optic disk (nerve) appears to bulge forward into the posterior chamber from swelling of the brain. The retinal blood vessels are obscured where they radiate from the bulging disk, making identification of their continuous pathway difficult. The retinas may show flame-shaped hemorrhages or fluffy white exudates.

Diagnostic Findings

Diagnostic studies that may reveal abnormalities include computed tomographic scan, positron emission tomography scan, and magnetic resonance imaging. Reduced BP is a priority, and these neurologic tests may be postponed while emergency treatment measures are instituted.

Medical Management

In true hypertensive emergencies, the goal is to lower the BP within 1 to 2 hours by using potent IV drugs, such as diazoxide (Hyperstat IV), nitroprusside (Nitropress), nitroglycerin, or labetalol (Normodyne). If the client's condition is not extremely critical, other alternative antihypertensive drugs, such as nifedipine (Procardia), verapamil (Isoptin), captopril (Capoten), and prazosin (Minipress), are prescribed for oral administration. Oxygen is ordered to reduce hypoxia-induced tachycardia.

Nursing Management

The nurse implements medical orders promptly to ensure that BP is lowered as quickly and safely as possible. He or she mixes drugs with IV solution after carefully calculating the dosage. The nurse administers the medicated solution with an infusion pump or controller and titrates the rate of infusion according to the client's response and the parameters set by the physician. He or she checks the site and progress of the infusion at least hourly. The nurse applies an automatic BP recording machine to the arm to measure the BP every few minutes, or assesses the BP directly if using an arterial catheter. The nurse reports a systolic BP of 160 mm Hg or higher or a diastolic BP of 115 mm Hg or higher immediately. While awaiting medical orders, the nurse restricts client activity and monitors the client closely for neurologic, cardiac, and renal complications. He or she keeps emergency equipment and drugs ready in case complications develop. See "Nursing Process for the Client With Hypertension" for additional nursing management.

CRITICAL THINKING EXERCISES

1. On admission, a client's BP is 210/112 mm Hg in a supine position. What additional data would be pertinent to collect before reporting the finding to the nurse in charge and physician?
2. To which community resources in your locale would you refer a client with hypertension for support or care after discharge?
3. A nurse takes a blood pressure on an obese client using an adult-size cuff. What error in blood pressure measurement is likely to result?
4. What response is appropriate when a client with hypertension divulges that she does not take prescribed antihypertensive medications because she does not experience any symptoms?

NCLEX-STYLE REVIEW QUESTIONS

1. At a community center, the nurse instructs men and women about the signs and symptoms of hypertension. Of the following people who are present at the discussion, whose blood pressure is most important for the nurse to assess?
   1. A 75-year-old African-American man
   2. A 50-year-old executive who lifts weights
   3. A 35-year-old woman who weighs 120 pounds
   4. A 60-year-old man who is being treated for a dysrhythmia
2. While getting blood pressure checked, a client asks the nurse why it is important to control hypertension. Which nursing response is most accurate?
   1. Sustained hypertension predisposes to narrowing of the cardiac valves.
   2. Sustained hypertension decreases the life span of many blood cells.
   3. Sustained hypertension leads to the formation of venous blood clots.
   4. Sustained hypertension compromises blood flow to many vital organs
3. When obtaining a health history from a client, which finding is most suggestive that the client is hypertensive?
   1. The client experiences occasional heart palpitations.
   2. The client has observed blood in his urine.
   3. The client has had unexplained nosebleeds.
   4. The client has difficulty sleeping all night.
4. A client diagnosed with hypertension begins drug therapy using an antihypertensive agent. The nurse instructs the client's spouse to remove any objects in the home that can lead to falls. The nurse knows that the teaching has been successful when the client restates which of the following?
   1. "Antihypertensive drugs can lead to hypotension, resulting in falls."
   2. "Blurred vision is a common side effect of antihypertensive therapy."
   3. "Fatigue and weakness are manifestations of antihypertensive medications."
   4. "Antihypertensives can contribute to muscle weakness and joint instability."
5. The hypertensive client's physician recommends following a low-sodium diet. What is the best evidence that the client understands the dietary restriction?
   1. The client avoids seasoning with onion powder.
   2. The client uses maple syrup instead of sugar.
   3. The client eliminates the use of soy sauce.
   4. The client drinks skim rather than whole milk.

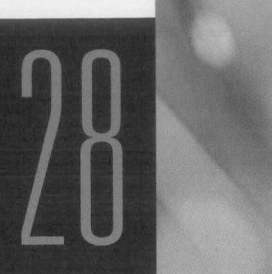

28

Caring for Clients with Heart Failure

Words To Know

acute heart failure
afterload
aldosterone
angiogenesis
ß-type natriuretic peptide
cardiac resynchronization therapy
cardiomyoplasty
chronic heart failure
congestive heart failure
cor pulmonale
digitalization
ejection fraction
exertional dyspnea
heart failure
hemoptysis
intra-aortic balloon pump
left-sided heart failure
multiple gated acquisition (MUGA) scan
myocardial oxygen demand
orthopnea
paroxysmal nocturnal dyspnea
preload
pulmonary vascular bed
right-sided heart failure
ventricular assist device

Learning Objectives

On completion of this chapter, you will be able to:

1. Discuss the pathophysiology and etiology of heart failure.
2. Distinguish between acute and chronic heart failure.
3. Identify differences between left-sided and right-sided heart failure.
4. Describe the symptoms, diagnosis, and treatment of left-sided and right-sided heart failure.
5. Discuss the nursing management of clients with heart failure.
6. Discuss the pathophysiology, etiology, symptoms, diagnosis, and treatment of pulmonary edema.
7. Discuss the nursing management of clients with pulmonary edema.

The heart is a double pump: the right side pumps deoxygenated blood to the lungs for oxygenation, and the left side pumps oxygen-rich blood into the systemic circulation (see Chap. 22). This process provides a continuous supply of oxygen and nutrients for cellular metabolism and a mechanism to eliminate carbon dioxide (CO_2) and metabolic wastes. Disturbances in one part of the heart, if they are severe or last long enough, eventually affect the entire circulation. This chapter discusses the pathophysiology of heart failure, and the medical and nursing management for clients who develop it.

HEART FAILURE

Heart failure is the inability of the heart to pump sufficient blood to meet the body's metabolic needs. An estimate of the heart's efficiency as a pump is its **ejection fraction,** the percentage of blood the left ventricle ejects when it contracts. Normally, a healthy heart ejects 55% or more of the blood that fills the left ventricle during diastole. As the heart fails, the amount of ejected blood decreases (Table 28-1). The heart's ejection fraction is measured using an echocardiogram (see Chap. 22) or multiple gated acquisition scan (discussed later).

The term **congestive heart failure** (CHF) describes the accumulation of blood and fluid in organs and tissues from impaired circulation.

Types

One way to classify heart failure is by how it develops: acute or chronic. Another way to classify it is by location: right-sided or left-sided.

Acute and Chronic Heart Failure

Acute heart failure is a sudden change in the heart's ability to contract. It can cause life-threatening symptoms and pulmonary edema (discussed later). **Chronic heart failure** occurs when the heart's ability to pump effectively is gradually compromised and its impaired contractility remains prolonged. The New York Heart Association (NYHA) further

TABLE 28-1 Assessment of Left Ventricular
Ejection Fraction

EJECTION FRACTION	EVALUATION OF FUNCTION
≥55%	Normal
45%–55%	Mildly reduced
35%–45%	Moderately reduced
<35%	Severely reduced

classifies chronic heart failure based on the amount of activity restriction it imposes; their four functional stages of chronic heart failure are as follows (Heart Failure Society of America, 2006):

- *Class I* (Mild): Ordinary physical activity does not cause undue fatigue, palpitations, or dyspnea. The client does not experience any limitation of activity.
- *Class II* (Mild): The client is comfortable at rest, but ordinary physical activity results in fatigue, heart palpitations, or dyspnea.
- *Class III* (Moderate): There is marked limitation of physical activity. The client is comfortable at rest, but less than ordinary activity causes fatigue, heart palpitations, or dyspnea.
- *Class IV* (Severe): The client is unable to carry out any physical activity without discomfort. Symptoms of cardiac insufficiency occur at rest. Discomfort is increased if any physical activity is undertaken.

The American Heart Association and the American College of Cardiology also use criteria to describe four stages of heart failure. The scale ranges from Stage A, in which there are no current symptoms, but the client has one or more risk factors (such as hypertension or diabetes) that predispose to heart failure, to Stage D, in which there is advanced structural heart disease and marked symptoms at rest despite maximal medical therapy. The two classification systems differ in that there is no comparable class in the NYHA classification for Stage A (Brookes, 2004).

Left-Sided and Right-Sided Heart Failure

Because the heart is a double pump, it is possible for either the left or right ventricle (or both) to become impaired. The terms left-sided (left ventricular) heart failure and right-sided (right ventricular) heart failure describe the location of the pumping dysfunction. **Left-sided heart failure** results from various conditions that impair the left ventricle's ability to eject blood into the aorta. **Right-sided heart failure** occurs when the right ventricle fails to eject its total diastolic filling volume into the pulmonary artery, causing congestion of blood in the venous vascular system. The major cause of right-sided heart failure is left-sided heart failure. Chronic obstructive pulmonary disease (COPD) also contributes to the development of right-sided heart failure.

Pathophysiology and Etiology

Two mechanisms can cause heart failure. The primary reason for failure of either the left or right ventricle is inability of the heart muscle to contract because of direct damage to the muscular wall. Myocardial infarction (MI) usually

affects the pumping ability of the left or right ventricle and frequently contributes to acute heart failure. Acute heart failure may immediately follow an MI or develop some time after the initial episode. The second mechanism occurs when the pumping chambers enlarge and weaken, as in cardiomyopathy and hypertension, making it impossible for the ventricles to eject all the blood they receive.

Left-Sided Heart Failure

When the left ventricle fails, the heart muscle cannot contract forcefully enough to expel blood into the systemic circulation (cardiac output). Blood subsequently becomes congested in the left ventricle, left atrium, and finally the pulmonary vasculature. The fluid accumulates and creates congestion in the **pulmonary vascular bed** (the capillary network surrounding the alveoli). Increased pulmonary vascular bed pressure causes fluid to move from the pulmonary capillaries into the alveoli. Gas exchange is impaired, cells become hypoxic (a state of insufficient oxygen), and CO_2 accumulates in the blood.

Hypertension, tachydysrhythmias, valvular disease, cardiomyopathy, and renal failure can contribute to chronic heart failure. These conditions reduce cardiac output by:

1. Increasing afterload or systemic vascular resistance. **Afterload,** the force that the ventricle must overcome to empty its diastolic volume, increases with arterial hypertension, aortic stenosis, pulmonary hypertension, or excessive blood volume from renal failure.
2. Reducing ventricular ejection volume because diastole, during which the ventricle fills with blood (**preload**), is shortened as a result of a tachydysrhythmia.
3. Causing a loss of elasticity in the muscle as a result of cardiomyopathy

Gerontologic Considerations

- Age-related vascular changes can lead to heart failure by interfering with the blood supply to the heart muscle and causing the heart to become fatigued while pumping blood through vessels that have become narrow and inflexible.

Right-Sided Heart Failure

When right ventricular failure develops, the right ventricle cannot forcefully contract and push the blood into the pulmonary artery. As a result, congestion of blood and backflow accumulate first in the right ventricle, then in the right atrium, the superior and inferior vena cavae, and subsequently the venous vasculature. MIs that affect the right ventricle also can cause right ventricular failure. Clients with chronic respiratory disorders tend to develop right-sided failure as a consequence of cor pulmonale. **Cor pulmonale** is a condition in which the heart (*cor*) is affected secondarily by lung damage (*pulmonale*). Pulmonary disease impairs exchange of oxygen and CO_2 in the alveoli, leading to increased CO_2 in the blood. By an unknown mechanism, pulmonary arterial vasoconstriction occurs. Prolonged pulmonary arterial vasoconstriction results in *pulmonary hypertension* (elevated pressure in the pulmonary arterial system; see

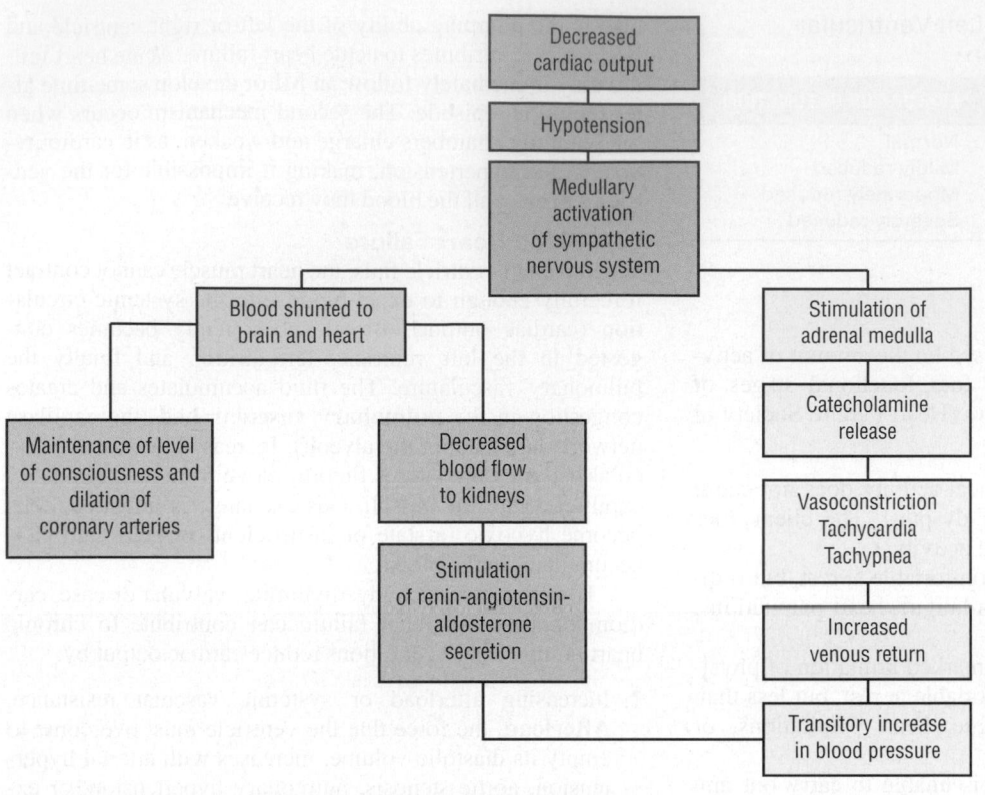

FIGURE 28-1. Compensatory mechanisms of the sympathetic nervous system. Decreased cardiac output triggers a series of compensatory mechanisms in the body in an effort to maintain level of consciousness and blood pressure.

Chap. 21). With pulmonary hypertension, the right ventricle is forced to pump against a high pressure gradient. Subsequently, the right ventricle enlarges and weakens under the increased workload, leading to failure. When the right ventricle fails to empty completely, blood is trapped in the venous vascular system. Eventually, the fluid is forced to move in retrograde fashion into the interstitial spaces and cells of other organs and tissues of the body.

Compensatory Mechanisms

The body can compensate for changes in heart function that occur over time (Fig. 28-1). When cardiac output falls, the body uses certain compensatory mechanisms designed to increase stroke volume and maintain blood pressure (BP). These compensatory mechanisms can temporarily improve the client's cardiac output but ultimately fail when contractility is further compromised.

As cardiac output falls, the client becomes hypotensive. The low BP stimulates the sympathetic nervous system to release catecholamines (e.g., epinephrine, norepinephrine) to raise heart rate and BP. The increased force and contraction of the heart maintain the client's BP but increase **myocardial oxygen demand** (the amount of oxygen the heart needs to perform its work). Epinephrine also causes blood vessels to constrict in an effort to raise BP. As the sympathetic nervous system is stimulated, the body shunts more blood to the vital organs of the brain and heart, decreasing blood supply to the kidneys. The kidneys secrete renin in response to decreased blood flow, which initiates the renin-angiotensin-aldosterone mechanism. Renin activates angiotensin. Angiotensin causes vasoconstriction and increases

BP. Angiotensin also stimulates the adrenal gland to secrete **aldosterone,** a hormone that causes retention of sodium and water to increase BP by increasing the amount of blood returning to the heart. Sensing an increase in fluid pressure within the heart, the ventricles secrete a neurohormone known as β**-type natriuretic peptide** (BNP). BNP is cardioprotective. Its function is to decrease blood pressure by increasing the excretion of sodium and water and promoting arterial dilation. It achieves its effects by counteracting renin, angiotensin, and aldosterone.

Ultimately, if compensatory mechanisms fail to restore homeostasis, the client's status is compromised by increased blood volume that the heart must pump and overwhelming the resistance the heart must overcome from arterial constriction. As cardiac output falls, the body's cells become deprived of oxygen and switch from aerobic metabolism to the less efficient anaerobic metabolism. Anaerobic metabolism results in an accumulation of lactic acid, which lowers blood pH and can eventually cause metabolic acidosis.

Assessment Findings

Signs and Symptoms

The severity of symptoms depends on the body's ability to adjust to the decreased cardiac output. Initial signs and symptoms reflect the ventricle of the heart that is experiencing dysfunction. Usually when a client has chronic heart failure, he or she develops signs and symptoms of both right-sided and left-sided heart failure. Box 28-1 highlights the clinical differences between left-sided and right-sided heart failure.

Signs and Symptoms of Left and Right Ventricular Failure

Left-Sided Failure
Fatigue
Paroxysmal nocturnal dyspnea
Orthopnea
Hypoxia
Crackles
Cyanosis
S_3 heart sound
Cough with pink, frothy sputum
Elevated pulmonary capillary wedge pressure

Right-Sided Failure
Weakness
Ascites
Weight gain
Nausea, vomiting
Dysrhythmias
Elevated central venous pressure
Jugular vein distention

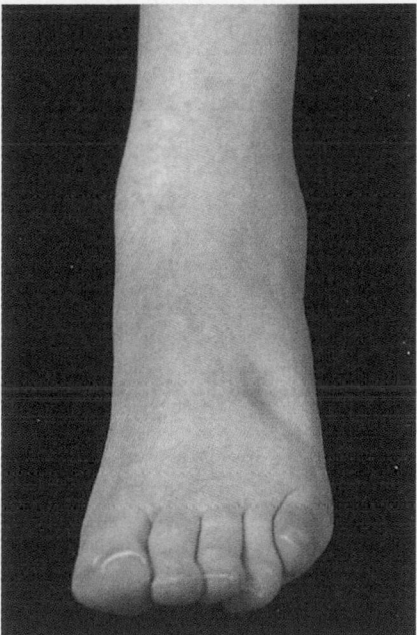

FIGURE 28-2. Example of pitting edema.

Left-Sided Heart Failure

Left-sided heart failure produces hypoxemia as a result of reduced cardiac output of arterial blood and respiratory symptoms. Many clients notice unusual fatigue with activity. Some find **exertional dyspnea** (effort at breathing when active) to be the first symptom. Inability to breathe unless sitting upright (**orthopnea**) or being awakened by breathlessness (**paroxysmal nocturnal dyspnea**) may prompt the client to use several pillows in bed or to sleep in a chair or recliner. Pulse may be rapid or irregular. BP may be elevated from sympathetic nervous system stimulation. A cough, **hemoptysis** (blood streaked sputum), and moist crackles on auscultation are typical respiratory findings. Urine output is diminished. If acute left-sided heart failure with pulmonary edema develops, the client suddenly becomes hypoxic, restless, and confused.

 Gerontologic Considerations

- Dyspnea on exertion is the earliest symptom of heart failure in many older clients. Confusion or anxiety are other early symptoms of decreased oxygenation from heart failure.

Right-Sided Heart Failure

The client with right-sided heart failure may have a history of gradual unexplained weight gain from fluid retention. *Dependent pitting edema* (excess fluid volume in the interstitial space in body areas affected by gravity) in the feet and ankles can be observed (Fig. 28-2). This type of edema may seem to disappear overnight but really is temporarily redistributed by gravity to other tissues, such as the sacral area. Fluid may distend the abdomen (ascites), and the liver may be enlarged (hepatomegaly). Jugular veins often are distended from increased central venous pressure (Nursing Guidelines 28-1).

Enlarged abdominal organs often restrict ventilation, creating dyspnea. Clients may observe that rings, shoes, or clothing have become tight. Accumulation of blood in abdominal organs may cause anorexia, nausea, and flatulence.

▶ *Stop, Think, and Respond Exercise 28-1*

Which type of heart failure is evidenced by the following assessment findings?

- *Client A has swollen ankles. His clothes fit poorly, and he has purchased larger pants and shirts. When he is weighed, he remarks that he has gained 10 lb in the last month, but his diet has not changed. He says he feels "full," can't eat as much as usual, and "works hard" to breathe.*
- *Client B becomes breathless while changing into a gown before the assessment. She reports sleeping better when sitting up in a recliner. Her cough is "wet." She is tachycardic and says she has noticed less frequent urination.*

Diagnostic Findings
Left-Sided Heart Failure

Chest radiography shows cardiac enlargement and fluid accumulation in the lungs. An echocardiogram can reveal the increased size of the left ventricle and ineffective pumping of the heart. A **multiple gated acquisition (MUGA) scan**, also called a *gated blood pool scan*, measures a decrease in the ejection fraction. A MUGA scan is the most accurate noninvasive test that measures the left ventricle's ejection fraction during rest and activity. When a MUGA scan is performed, the client receives an injection with an intravenous radioisotope that concentrates within the red blood cells in approximately 20 to 30 minutes. A gamma camera can identify the cells once they are radioactive. The client is then attached to a cardiac monitor, and the gamma camera

NURSING GUIDELINES 28-1

Estimating Central Venous Pressure

Central venous pressure (CVP) is the pressure produced by venous blood in the right atrium. CVP measurement and monitoring are discussed in Chap. 29. To estimate CVP, the nurse measures the height of jugular vein distention:

1. Obtain a centimeter ruler.
2. Help client to lie flat.
3. Slowly elevate head of bed to 45°.
4. Locate the sternal angle by placing two fingers at the sternal notch and sliding them down the sternum until they reach a bony prominence.
5. Estimate venous pressure by measuring the vertical distance from the sternal angle (0 cm) to the level of jugular vein distention (cm above 0).
6. Add 5 cm to the ruler measurement to estimate CVP. CVP is elevated more than 12 to 15 cm H_2O in clients who have right ventricular heart failure. A more accurate measurement of CVP is obtained by using a central venous catheter.

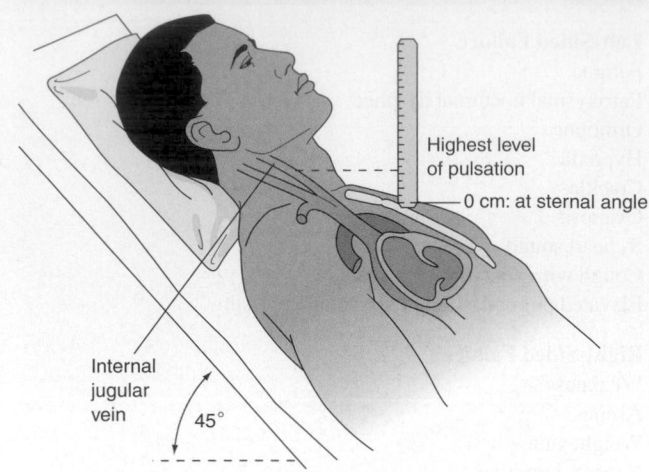

takes images as the blood passes through the heart and major blood vessels (Fig. 28-3). The client must lie very still at intermittent times during the 45-minute test. Diuretics are contraindicated the morning of a test to avoid any interruptions for urination. Clients also are medicated to relieve a cough that may cause movement during the test. Although allergic reactions to the intravenous chemical can occur, they are rare.

At first, arterial blood gas (ABG) analysis may reveal respiratory alkalosis as a result of rapid, shallow breathing. Later, there is a shift to metabolic acidosis as gas exchange becomes more impaired. Serum sodium levels may be elevated. Elevated blood urea nitrogen indicates impaired renal perfusion. If the client is seriously ill, a pulmonary artery catheter may be inserted for hemodynamic monitoring. Cardiac output can be measured by the pulmonary artery catheter. Cardiac output is diminished in left-sided heart failure, and pulmonary artery pressure and pulmonary capillary wedge pressure measurements are elevated. The BNP levels are above 100 picograms (pg)/mL (a picogram is a billionth of a gram) (Box 28-2).

Right-Sided Heart Failure
A chest radiograph, electrocardiogram (ECG), and echocardiography reveal right ventricular enlargement. A lung scan and pulmonary arteriography can confirm cor pulmonale. Liver enzymes are elevated if the liver is impaired.

Medical Management
Medical management of both left-sided and right-sided heart failure is directed at reducing the heart's workload and improving cardiac output, primarily through dietary modifications, drug therapy, and lifestyle changes. A low-sodium diet is prescribed, and fluids may be restricted. Activity is limited according to the condition's severity. Sedatives or tranquilizers reduce dyspnea and relieve anxiety. In acute or worsening heart failure, a device for resynchronizing the

heart's contraction or an intra-aortic balloon pump that provides mechanical circulatory support may be used to support left ventricular function.

Drug Therapy
Drug therapy with one or more medications aims at improving cardiac output (Drug Therapy Table 28-1). Digoxin is the primary drug used to slow and strengthen the heart. The method of giving large doses of digoxin at the beginning of therapy to build up therapeutic blood levels of the drug is termed **digitalization**. The apical heart rate is assessed for a full minute before every administration and is documented in the medication administration record. Digitalis drugs are withheld if the heart rate is less than 60 or more than 120 beats/minute until a physician is consulted. In acute heart failure or pulmonary edema (discussed later), the physician may prescribe a potent inotropic agent, one that increases the

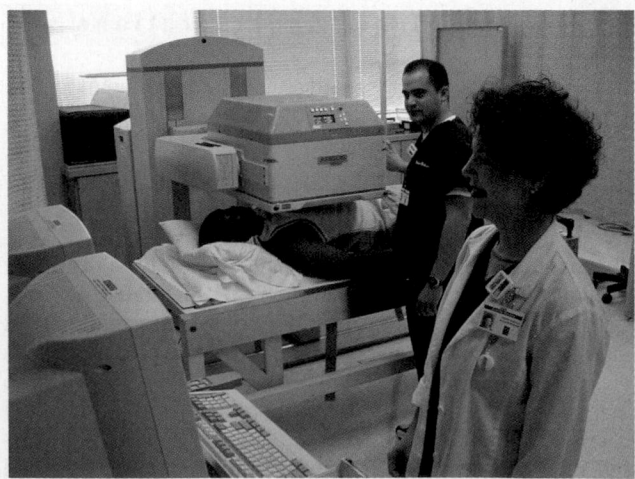

FIGURE 28-3. Technicians conduct a multiple gated acquisition (MUGA) scan. (Image © Texas Heart Institute, www.texasheart.org.)

force of contraction, thereby improving stroke volume. Examples include dopamine (Intropin) and dobutamine (Dobutrex). Nesiritide (Natrecor), which is human BNP, is given as a short-term infusion to clients in severe heart failure to decrease the fluid load on the heart and improve cardiac function.

Diuretic therapy helps reduce the heart's work load by decreasing the exertion required to overcome afterload. Thiazide diuretics such as hydrochlorothiazide (Hydro-DIURIL) can manage many cases of mild heart failure. Severe heart failure usually requires a loop diuretic such as furosemide (Lasix). These drugs increase sodium and therefore water excretion, but they also increase potassium excretion. If a client becomes hypokalemic, digitalis toxicity is more likely; it is evidenced by loss of appetite; nausea or vomiting; rapid, slow, or irregular heart rate; or sudden disturbance in color vision. Low serum potassium levels and signs of digitalis toxicity must be reported to the physician. The blood level of digitalis is measured if there is a question concerning its concentration.

Pharmacologic Considerations

- Digitalis preparations are potent and may cause various toxic effects. The margin between a therapeutic and toxic effect is narrow. Observe clients for signs of digitalis toxicity throughout client care. Teach the client about the signs and symptoms of electrolyte and water loss and the importance of adhering to the prescribed medication schedule. Also instruct the client to eat foods high in potassium or take a prescribed potassium supplement.

Gerontologic Considerations

- Age-related changes in the gastrointestinal, renal, and hepatic systems may alter drug metabolism and necessitate careful monitoring for therapeutic or adverse effects related to digitalis preparations. Older adults are at increased risk for toxicity because of the decreased ability of the kidneys to excrete the drug.

Vasodilators also reduce afterload. Clients with a history of heart failure may receive a drug such as an angiotensin-converting enzyme (ACE) inhibitor (e.g., captopril

[Capoten]) or some other category of drug that causes vasodilatation. ACE inhibitors such as captopril, fosinopril (Monopril), enalapril (Vasotec), and ramipril (Altace) may also be used to treat heart failure in clients who have not responded to digitalis and diuretics.

Clinical trials continue on a synthetic peptide compound termed chrysalin (TP508). Its purpose is to promote **angiogenesis,** regeneration of myocardial blood vessels, stimulate healing of diabetic foot ulcers, and accelerate bone growth in fractures and surgical procedures such as spinal fusion. Its developers envision that it can be used to improve the prognosis for clients in early stages of heart failure or in combination with a ventricular assist device (see later discussion) in later-stage heart failure.

▶ **Stop, Think, and Respond Exercise 28-2**

A client with a possible bowel obstruction has a history of chronic heart failure. He has been taking digoxin (Lanoxin) at home. What nursing actions are appropriate?

Cardiac Resynchronization Therapy

Cardiac resynchronization therapy (CRT) is a new technique that restores synchrony in the contractions of the right and left ventricles. CRT is used primarily for clients whose heart failure is caused by dilated cardiomyopathy (see Chap. 23). It is achieved with a biventricular pacemaker. The biventricular pacemaker is inserted transvenously similarly to a traditional pacemaker, with electrical leads in the right atrium and right ventricle and the battery placed beneath the skin of the chest. It has an additional internal third lead, however, that is placed outside the left ventricle. The dual ventricular leads stimulate the right and left ventricles to contract at the same time. When the ventricles contract simultaneously, the force of contraction improves, and more blood is ejected with each heartbeat.

Intra-Aortic Balloon Pump

If cardiogenic shock (see Chap. 17) accompanies acute left ventricular heart failure, an **intra-aortic balloon pump** (IABP) may be used. An IABP acts as a temporary, secondary mechanical circulatory pump to supplement the ineffectual contraction of the left ventricle. It is inserted as a catheter into the left femoral artery and threaded up to the descending aortic arch (Fig. 28-4). The IABP is connected to a machine that inflates the balloon portion during ventricular diastole and deflates during systole, a process known as *counterpulsation.* Inflation of the IABP increases coronary artery, renal artery, and myocardial perfusion. Deflation actually keeps the aorta distended so that cardiac output is improved; the work of the left ventricle is decreased, and peripheral organs are more adequately perfused with oxygenated blood. The IABP is intended for only a few days' use.

Surgical Management

When medical treatment alone is unsuccessful, clients may require surgical treatment options such as the insertion of a ventricular assist device, cardiomyoplasty, or an implantable artificial heart. Human heart transplantation is discussed in Chapter 29.

DRUG THERAPY TABLE 28-1 Agents To Treat Heart Failure

Drug Category and Examples	Mechanism of Action	Side Effects	Nursing Considerations
Cardiac Glycosides digoxin (Lanoxin)	Increase cardiac output by slowing heart rate (negative chronotropic action) and increasing force of contraction (positive chronotropic action)	Fatigue, generalized muscle weakness, anorexia, nausea, vomiting, yellow-green halos around visual images, dysrhythmias	Monitor pulse rate before each dose. Withhold if pulse is <60 or >120 beats/min. Provide dietary sources of potassium.
Diuretics *loop diuretic:* furosemide (Lasix)	Promote sodium and water excretion, thus reducing circulating blood volume and decreasing heart's workload	Dizziness, dehydration, blurred vision, anorexia, diarrhea, nocturia, polyuria, thrombocytopenia, orthostatic hypotension, hypokalemia	Weigh client daily. Measure intake and output. Monitor serum potassium levels. Replace lost potassium with bananas, orange juice, or prescribed supplement.
thiazide diuretic: chlorothiazide (Diuril)	Increase urine production and output, decreasing total blood volume and the overall heart's workload	Electrolyte imbalances, potassium loss in urine, orthostatic hypotension	Monitor for dizziness and lightheadedness. Monitor laboratory values for electrolytes. Weigh the client daily and report weight changes of greater than 2 lbs. in a 24-hour period. Replace lost potassium with appropriate diet options or a supplement.
Vasodilators nitroglycerin	Improve stroke volume by reducing afterload; reduce preload by dilating veins and arteries	Headache, dizziness, orthostatic hypotension, tachycardia, flushing, nausea, hypersensitivity	Assess for hypotension. Monitor for headache and flushed skin.
ACE Inhibitors captopril (Capoten)	Block ACE from converting angiotensin I to angiotensin II (a potent vasoconstrictor); promote fluid and sodium loss and decrease peripheral vascular resistance	Tachycardia, hypotension, GI irritation, pancytopenia, proteinuria, rash, cough, dry mouth, hyperkalemia, increased BUN and creatinine	Excretion is reduced in clients with renal failure. First-dose hypotension is common in older adults. Administer 1 hr before or 2 hr after meals.
Nonglycoside Inotropic Agents dobutamine (Dobutrex) dopamine (Intropin) amrinone (Inocor)	Relieve cardiogenic shock by strengthening force of myocardial contraction and increasing cardiac output	Headache, hypertension, tachycardia, angina, nausea	Monitor for increased heart rate, elevated BP, and dysrhythmias.
hBNP nesiritide (Natrecor)	Peptide hormone that acts on the kidneys to increase the excretions of sodium and water and reduce blood pressure.	Severe hypotension, vasodilation.	Administered IV only and requires continuous monitoring. Only for use in clients with acutely decompensated heart failure.

ACE, angiotensin-converting enzyme; *BP*, blood pressure; *BUN*, blood urea nitrogen; *GI*, gastrointestinal.

Ventricular Assist Device

Some clients awaiting heart transplants are treated with a **ventricular assist device** (VAD), which is an auxiliary heart pump that supplements the heart's ability to eject blood. If the VAD supports left ventricular function, it is referred to as a *left ventricular assist device* or LVAD, which is designed to be used for weeks to months. Some clients have relied on LVADs for more than 1 year. The natural heart remains in place and continues to function at whatever capacity is possible. Most LVADs use an outflow and inflow cannula to carry blood from the left ventricle into the aorta (Fig. 28-5). They are battery operated through an external power source worn about the waist. By assisting the weak, ineffective left ventricle, LVADs maintain cardiac output at normal volumes. The Thoratec VAD is a double-assist device that can be used for left-sided, right-sided, or biventricular heart

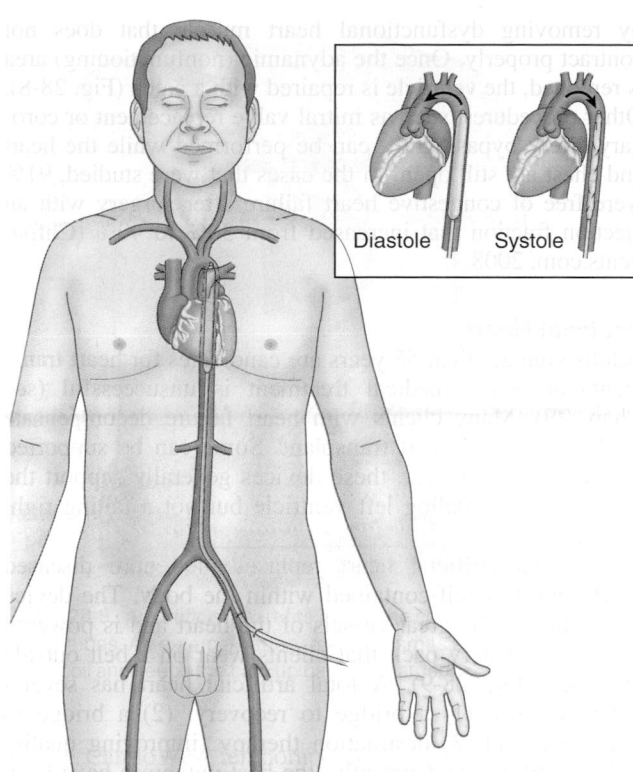

Diastole   Systole

FIGURE 28-4. The intra-aortic balloon pump (IABP).

failure. It requires a large external driver to power the device, necessitating continuous hospitalization for its use. The trend is to develop miniaturized devices, which internally measure 1 × 3 inches and weigh less than 4 ounces. Clients can easily manage smaller models, making it possible for some to return home until heart transplantation.

Cardiomyoplasty

Cardiomyoplasty is a surgical procedure in which the client's own chest muscle (latissimus dorsi) is grafted to the aorta and wrapped around the heart. An electrical stimulator placed in a subcutaneous pouch triggers skeletal muscle contraction (Fig. 28-6). The contraction acts as a counterpulsation mechanism similar to the IABP. It augments the ineffective myocardial muscle contraction.

A ventricular containment procedure, sometimes referred to as a "heart wrap," may be performed. In this procedure, a polyethylene/polyester support mesh device (Fig. 28-7), which some have likened to pantyhose, serves as an alternative to the cardiomyoplasty procedure. The heart wrap is pulled over the heart and sutured in place. The wrap supports the heart and reverses heart remodeling (i.e., restores

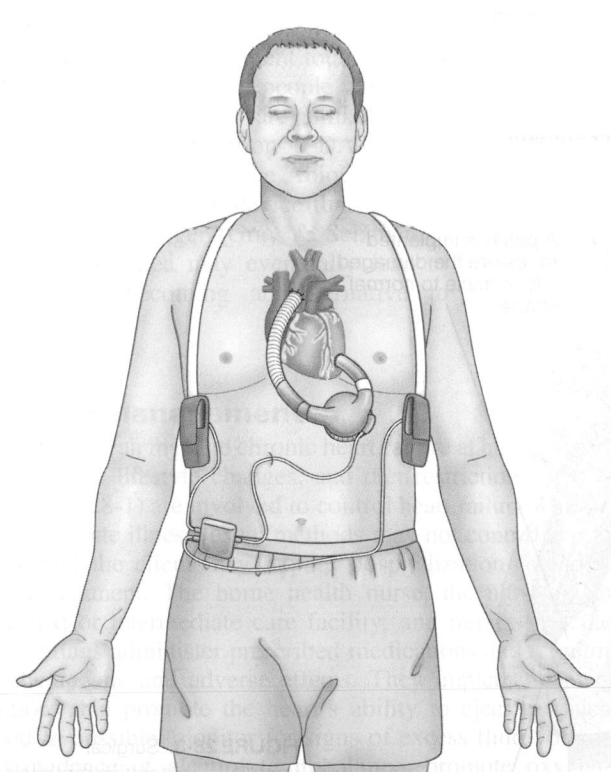

FIGURE 28-5. The LVAD pump weighs 1.5 lb. It is implanted below the diaphragm; its battery pack is carried outside the body. Tubes connect the pump to the left ventricle and aorta.

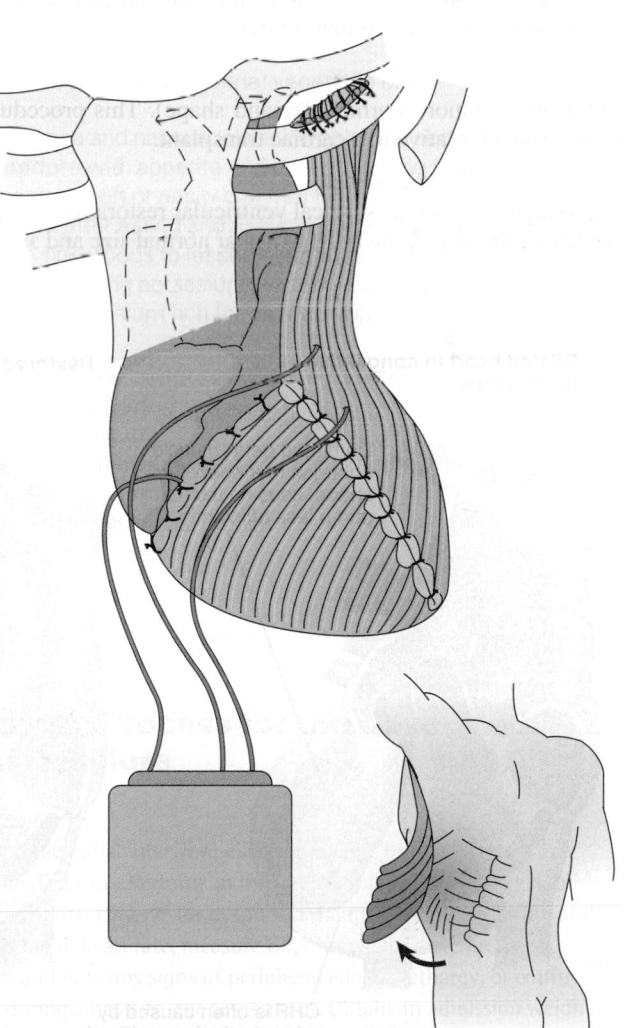

FIGURE 28-6. In cardiomyoplasty, the latissimus dorsi muscle is dissected and wrapped around the heart itself.

Client and Family Teaching 28-1
Heart Failure

The nurse instructs about the disease process, meaning of the term *failure*, signs and symptoms of impending CHF (weight gain, ankle swelling, fatigue, dyspnea), and importance of taking all medications regularly. He or she also covers the following points:

- Measure pulse and blood pressure daily.
- Check weight at the same time each day using the same scale; consult a physician if you gain more than 2 lb in 24 hours.
- Schedule rest periods to reduce or eliminate fatigue and dyspnea.
- Increase activities such as walking when able to do so without dyspnea or fatigue.
- Identify and avoid occasions that produce stress.
- Elevate the legs while sitting.
- Follow the diet prescribed by the physician.
- Avoid extreme heat, cold, or humidity.
- Report a heart rate less than 60 or more than 120 beats/minute before taking digitalis.
- Contact the physician if symptoms return or swelling in the legs, ankles, or feet suddenly increases.
- Maintain follow-up care.

---

laboratory test results of serum electrolytes, because drug therapy with certain diuretics depletes potassium blood levels. Initiate intake and output measurements and evaluate fluid volumes at least every 8 hours. Measure abdominal girth to determine if the client is developing ascites or responding to therapeutic measures. Note respiratory difficulties during activity and rest. Question the client about nocturnal dyspnea (asking how many pillows the client normally uses for sleep) and listen for crackles on auscultation of lungs. While auscultating the chest, listen for additional heart sounds. Monitor oxygenation status with pulse oximetry or review the results of ABG studies.

Diagnosis, Planning, and Interventions

▶ **Decreased Cardiac Output** related to ineffective ventricular contraction, tachycardia, reduced stroke volume, hypertension, and increased vascular volume

▶ **Expected Outcome:** Client will have increased cardiac output as evidenced by heart rate between 60 to 100 beats/minute, urinary output between 1500 to 3000 mL/day, systolic BP below 120 mm Hg, diastolic BP below 80 mm Hg, and no mental confusion.

- Assess apical heart rate before administering a cardiac glycoside (digitalis) or other drug that slows heart rate. *Cardiac output is related to heart rate and stroke volume. Withhold a cardiac glycoside until the physician is consulted when the heart rate is less than 60 or more than 120 beats/minute.*
- Administer prescribed medications such as cardiac glycosides (digitalis), diuretics, and antihypertensives. *Cardiac glycosides slow heart rate and increase force of contraction. Diuretics*

decrease afterload by reducing circulating fluid volume. Antihypertensives promote vasodilation, thus reducing afterload. One or a combination of these drugs reduces the workload of the left ventricle.

- Promote rest. *Rest reduces heart contraction (ventricular work). Increasing diastole helps increase the volume in the ventricles (preload) and the ejected volume (stroke volume).*
- Avoid activities that engage the Valsalva maneuver, such as straining with bowel elimination or using the arms to pull and reposition oneself. *The Valsalva maneuver increases intrathoracic pressure, reduces right atrial filling, triggers tachycardia, and increases BP.*
- Prepare client or assist with procedures that improve cardiac output, such as the insertion of a biventricular pacemaker, cardiomyoplasty, LVAD, IABP, or artificial mechanical heart. *Improving the heart's force of contraction or stroke volume improves cardiac output.*

▶ **Excess Fluid Volume** related to reduced renal function secondary to increased antidiuretic hormone and aldosterone production and reduced cardiac output

▶ **Expected Outcome:** Fluid volume will be reduced as evidenced by reduced weight and peripheral edema, normal BP measurements, increased urine output, and no adventitious lung sounds.

- Administer prescribed diuretic. *Diuretics promote the excretion of sodium and water.*
- Provide sodium-restricted diet as prescribed. *Sodium attracts water; reduced sodium decreases water retention.*
- Apportion oral fluid according to prescribed limitations. *Limiting oral fluid intake reduces circulating volume.*

▶ **Risk for Impaired Gas Exchange** related to pulmonary congestion secondary to left ventricular dysfunction

▶ **Expected Outcome:** Client will maintain adequate gas exchange as evidenced by clear lung sounds, decreased work of breathing, pulse oximeter reading above 90%, partial pressure of arterial oxygen (PaO_2) between 80 and 100 mm Hg, partial pressure of arterial CO_2 ($PaCO_2$) between 35 and 45 mm Hg, and blood pH between 7.35 and 7.45.

- Maintain client in a high Fowler's, semi-Fowler's, or orthopneic position. *Elevating the upper body maximizes lung expansion by decreasing pressure on the diaphragm.*
- Administer supplemental oxygen therapy as prescribed to maintain the pulse oximetry level (SpO_2) at or above 90%. *If SpO_2 is at or above 90%, PaO_2 usually is high enough to maintain plasma levels of oxygen in less-than-critical ranges.*
- Avoid gas-forming foods. *Gas that accumulates in the intestine increases the volume in the abdominal cavity. Expansion of the intestine can crowd the diaphragm and interfere with inspired volumes of air.*
- Offer small, frequent feedings. *Preventing stomach distention increases the space in the thoracic cavity for lung expansion.*
- Limit physical activity. *Activity requires increased oxygen for cellular metabolism.*

▶ Activity Intolerance related to hypoxemia secondary to decreased cardiac output

▶ **Expected Outcome:** Client will tolerate activity associated with daily living without becoming breathless, hypertensive, or tachycardic.

- Space activities of daily living (ADLs) between periods of rest. *Rest reduces oxygen deficits.*
- Keep personal items within easy reach. *Reduced exertion decreases oxygen expenditure.*
- Gradually increase activity and self-care as condition improves. *Tolerance for activity increases after a therapeutic response to the treatment regimen.*

▶ PC: Hypokalemia related to excretion of potassium secondary to diuretic therapy

▶ **Expected Outcome:** The nurse will monitor for evidence of hypokalemia and prevent or manage low serum potassium levels.

- Monitor for clinical signs of hypokalemia: fatigue, muscle weakness, and abnormal sensations such as tingling or numbness. *Potassium is necessary for normal nerve and muscle activity; neuromuscular changes, anorexia, nausea, and vomiting are signs of a low potassium level.*
- Observe the ECG, cardiac monitor, or cardiac rhythm strip for a U wave or cardiac dysrhythmia. *A U wave is associated with hypokalemia. The heart is a muscle that may develop a dysrhythmia if the potassium level is not within normal range.*
- Provide foods and beverages that are good sources of potassium, such as bananas and orange juice, within the client's dietary and fluid restrictions. *Dietary intake of foods and beverages that are rich in potassium affects serum potassium levels (see Nutrition Notes 28-1).*
- Administer a prescribed potassium supplement. *It ensures potassium replacement.*

Evaluation of Expected Outcomes

Expected outcomes are that BP and heart rate return to baseline, with no evidence of excess fluid. Respirations are unlabored, and lungs are clear. Fluid intake approximates output. The client can participate in ADLs within his or her level of tolerance. Serum potassium level remains within or is restored to normal range. ●

CARDIOGENIC PULMONARY EDEMA

Pulmonary edema is fluid accumulation in the lungs, which interferes with gas exchange in the alveoli. It represents an acute emergency and is a frequent complication of left-sided heart failure. Cardiac dysrhythmias and cardiac or respiratory arrest are associated complications. The following discussion focuses on cardiogenic pulmonary edema, which develops as a result of heart disease in general and heart failure more specifically. Noncardiogenic pulmonary edema, also referred to as *acute respiratory distress syndrome*, develops when a pulmonary embolism, infection, or blast injury alters the pulmonary capillary membrane; it is discussed in Chapter 21.

Pathophysiology and Etiology

In cardiogenic pulmonary edema, the left ventricle becomes incapable of maintaining sufficient output of blood with each contraction. The right ventricle continues to pump blood toward the lungs, however, and the left ventricle has difficulty emptying. There is retrograde fluid accumulation in the left atrium and pulmonary veins. The pulmonary capillaries and alveoli become engorged with blood. The lungs rapidly fill with fluid, and acute respiratory distress develops. As CO_2 accumulates, respiratory rate and depth increase. Without treatment, hyperventilation becomes insufficient to prevent respiratory acidosis. Metabolic acidosis follows.

Assessment Findings

Clients with acute pulmonary edema exhibit sudden dyspnea, wheezing, orthopnea, restlessness, cough (often productive of pink, frothy sputum), cyanosis, tachycardia, and severe apprehension. Respirations sound moist or gurgling. If a pulmonary artery catheter is in place, the pulmonary artery and pulmonary capillary wedge pressures are elevated, and cardiac output is reduced. While the body responds with arterial vasoconstriction, it may temporarily sustain adequate BP; however, the client eventually becomes hypotensive and peripheral pulses disappear. Chest radiographs show pulmonary infiltration with fluid. ABGs indicate severe hypoxemia (low PaO_2), hypercapnia (high $PaCO_2$), and a pH below 7.35.

Medical Management

Because pulmonary edema can be fatal, lung congestion needs to be relieved as quickly as possible. Supplemental oxygen or mechanical ventilation is used to support breathing. Inotropic medications, which improve myocardial contractility, are administered to relieve symptoms. If the cause of heart failure and pulmonary edema can be corrected surgically (e.g., a mitral valve disorder), the client is supported medically while being prepared for surgery.

Oxygenation

To facilitate gas exchange, oxygen is administered. A mask rather than nasal cannula is needed to deliver the maximum percentages of oxygen. If respiratory failure occurs, the client is intubated and oxygen is administered under continuous positive airway pressure or with mechanical ventilation with positive end-expiratory pressure.

Drug Therapy

Inotropic agents, such as dopamine (Intropin), dobutamine (Dobutrex), and amrinone (Inocor), or digitalis are administered IV to improve the force of ventricular contraction. To reduce myocardial oxygen consumption, drugs that reduce venous return to the heart (diuretics) and promote vasodilatation (nitrates, ACE inhibitors, calcium channel blockers) are prescribed. IV morphine sulfate often is given to lessen anxiety. Morphine seems to help relieve respiratory symptoms by depressing higher cerebral centers, thus relieving anxiety and slowing respiratory rate. Morphine also promotes muscle relaxation and reduces the work of breathing.

Invasive Measures

If the client does not respond to drug therapy and oxygenation, additional interventions such as the insertion of an IABP, biventricular pacemaker, or LVAD are used to sustain life. Cardiomyoplasty, use of an artificial heart, and subsequent heart transplantation are further treatments.

Nursing Management

Effective resolution of pulmonary edema requires both medical and nursing management. The nursing diagnoses, interventions, and expected outcomes for clients with pulmonary edema are similar to those for clients experiencing heart failure. Clients with pulmonary edema need close assessment in an intensive care unit.

The nurse establishes an IV line immediately (if one is not already in place) for medication administration. Because of the severity of symptoms and respiratory compromise, he or she administers IV diuretics and inotropic agents. The nurse monitors the therapeutic and adverse effects of medication therapy. Bedside ECG monitoring is standard, as are continuous pulse oximetry and automatic BP and pulse measurements approximately every 15 to 30 minutes. Critically ill clients may have a pulmonary artery catheter inserted to measure the pressure readings in the heart chambers and to estimate cardiac output. A urinary catheter is inserted to evaluate response to diuretics. The nurse assesses for proper placement/adherence of electrodes and ascertains that electronic monitoring equipment is functioning properly.

The client receives oxygenation to maintain normal blood gases. If the client requires mechanical ventilation, the nurse suctions the airway as needed, provides frequent mouth care, and establishes an alternative method for verbal communication.

Pharmacologic Considerations

- Observe the effectiveness of drug therapy and any adverse effects in clients who are receiving emergency drug therapy for acute pulmonary edema. Many medications given for this disorder are IV drugs and occasionally are administered in large doses (hence the importance of client observation).

CRITICAL THINKING EXERCISES

1. Discuss how the care of a client with right-sided heart failure differs from the care of a client with left-sided heart failure.
2. A client diagnosed with heart failure presents with the following assessment data: temperature 99.1°F, pulse 100 beats/minute, respirations 42 breaths/minute, BP 110/50 mm Hg; crackles in both lung bases; nausea; pulse oximeter reading of 89%; enlarged, soft abdomen. Which assessment findings need immediate attention? Why?
3. While making a home visit to evaluate the status of a client who is being treated for heart failure, what assessment data suggests that the client's treatment regimen is effective?
4. A client with heart failure is on a low-sodium diet. While reviewing the modifications in the client's diet before discharge, what information indicates that the client understands which foods should be avoided or limited for sodium restriction?

NCLEX-STYLE REVIEW QUESTIONS

1. A client comes to the clinic complaining of shortness of breath, pink-tinged sputum, and a cough. The nurse suspects left-sided heart failure. Which assessment finding further confirms the diagnosis?
   1. Moist crackles in the lung fields
   2. Bradycardia less than 60 beats/minute
   3. Blood pressure 90/60 mm Hg
   4. Increased urine output
2. A client with left-sided heart failure is admitted to the hospital for treatment. Which nursing intervention is the first action the nurse should take?
   1. Administer 3 L O_2 per nasal cannula.
   2. Give a loading dose of digoxin (Lanoxin).
   3. Draw blood for baseline electrolytes.
   4. Assess for distended neck veins.
3. Prior to giving a client the morning dose of digoxin (Lanoxin), the nurse determines that the apical pulse is less than 55 beats/minute. Which nursing action is the priority?
   1. Call the physician and report the finding.
   2. Hold the drug and assess for toxic effects.
   3. Take the client's blood pressure.
   4. Recheck the pulse in 30 minutes.
4. Which of the following instructions is most important to include in the teaching plan for a client with right-sided heart failure?
   1. Count pulse rate every hour.
   2. Eat three meals per day.
   3. Maintain bed rest.
   4. Elevate the legs while sitting.
5. A client with chronic heart failure takes a daily thiazide diuretic. The client asks the nurse why it is important to consume potassium-rich foods on a daily basis. What is the best response?
   1. Consuming potassium-rich foods replaces what is lost in your urine.
   2. Potassium promotes the excretion of excess fluid by your kidneys.
   3. Potassium improves the therapeutic action of your diuretic.
   4. Your thiazide diuretic may cause significant hypocalcemia.

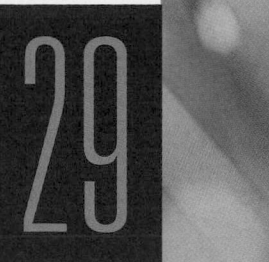

29

Caring for Clients Undergoing Cardiovascular Surgery

Words To Know
annuloplasty
cardiac index
cardioplegia
cardiopulmonary bypass
central venous pressure
commissurotomy
coronary artery bypass
embolectomy
endarterectomy
extracorporeal circulation
left ventricular end-diastolic pressure
myocardial revascularization
nomogram
pulmonary capillary wedge pressure
thrombectomy
valvuloplasty

Learning Objectives

On completion of this chapter, you will be able to:

1. Describe the purpose of cardiopulmonary bypass and its disadvantages.
2. Name indications for cardiac surgery.
3. Describe how coronary artery blood flow is surgically restored.
4. Name four surgical procedures for revascularizing the myocardium.
5. Identify techniques to correct valvular disorders.
6. Describe two methods for controlling bleeding from heart trauma.
7. List five problems associated with heart transplantation.
8. List three types of surgery performed on central or peripheral blood vessels.
9. Discuss the nursing management of clients undergoing cardio-vascular surgery.

Cardiovascular surgery is performed to correct and treat various cardiac and vascular disorders discussed in earlier chapters in this unit. This chapter describes the operative procedures and management of clients undergoing surgery to revascularize the myocardium, repair or replace cardiac valves, repair a ventricular aneurysm, remove heart tumors, manage heart trauma, and replace the heart with one from a human donor.

CARDIAC SURGICAL PROCEDURES

Before the 1950s, few attempts at cardiac surgery were made. Initially, hypothermia and crude mechanisms for oxygenating blood outside the body were used. In the 1960s, the technique for mechanically circulating and oxygenating blood outside the body, called **extracorporeal circulation** or **cardiopulmonary bypass**, was developed (Fig. 29-1). Removing blood from the venae cavae, circulating it through an oxygenator, and returning it to the aorta or femoral artery provides a nearly bloodless area while the beating heart is stopped.

Although most forms of cardiac surgery use cardiopulmonary bypass, some new surgical techniques have eliminated its use. Surgery on the beating heart without cardiopulmonary bypass reduces the potential for negative "pump" consequences (Box 29-1).

Myocardial Revascularization

Myocardial revascularization refers to surgical techniques that improve the delivery of oxygenated blood to the myocardium for clients who have coronary artery disease (CAD). These techniques are used when less invasive methods such as an atherectomy or percutaneous transluminal coronary angioplasty (PTCA) are not treatment options

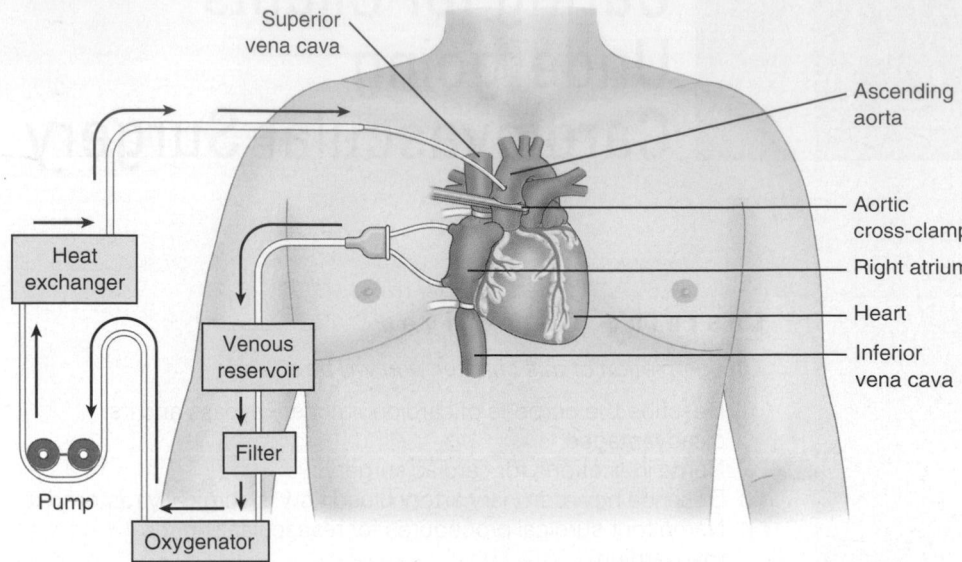

FIGURE 29-1. The cardiopulmonary bypass system. Cannulae are placed into the superior and inferior venae cavae to divert blood from the body and into the bypass system. The pump creates a vacuum and pulls blood into the venous reservoir. The filter clears the blood of air bubbles, clots, and particulates. The blood then passes through the oxygenator, to the pump, and to the heat exchanger, which regulates the blood's temperature. The blood is then returned to the body.

(see Chap. 25). (Chapter 25 also discusses transmyocardial revascularization [TMR].) **Coronary artery bypass** surgery improves myocardial oxygenation by bypassing or detouring around the occluded portion of one or more coronary arteries with a relocated blood vessel. A coronary artery bypass is performed when (1) the client has multiple coronary artery occlusions, (2) the atheromas are calcified and noncompressible, or (3) the anatomic location of the occlusion(s) interferes with the safe insertion of a coronary artery catheter.

The saphenous vein in the leg is the vessel most often used for grafting in coronary artery bypass. It is harvested by making a long incision on the medial aspect of the leg or by removing the vein endoscopically through one to three small (1-inch) leg incisions (Fig. 29-2). An endoscopically removed vein results in less muscle and tissue damage, decreased pain, and reduced scarring. Alternative graft vessels include the following:

- The internal mammary and internal thoracic arteries in the chest
- The basilic and cephalic veins in the arm
- The radial artery in the arm
- The gastroepiploic artery from the stomach, in some cases.

BOX 29-1 **Disadvantages of Cardiopulmonary Bypass**

- Long operative period (6 hours)
- Necessity for anticoagulation
- Hypotension
- Need for postoperative blood replacement
- Overall decline in mental function, perhaps because of an inflammatory response triggered by blood circulating through plastic tubing or gaseous bubbles in the circulated blood
- Risk for stroke, dysrhythmias, and renal failure

Although used less often than the saphenous vein, internal mammary artery (IMA) grafts have 90% or greater patency, which results in better survival rates, fewer reoperations, and fewer cardiac events for up to 10 years after surgery. Grafts using the saphenous vein tend to develop progressive atherosclerosis that compromises long-term patency (American College of Cardiology/American Heart Association Task Force, 2004).

Techniques for performing coronary bypass surgery include conventional coronary artery bypass graft (CABG), off-pump coronary artery bypass (OPCAB), minimally invasive direct coronary artery bypass (MIDCAB), and port access coronary artery bypass (PACAB). Table 29-1 compares these methods for performing myocardial revascularization.

Conventional Coronary Artery Bypass Graft (CABG)

CABG is the most conventional technique for performing coronary artery bypass and the eighth most common type of

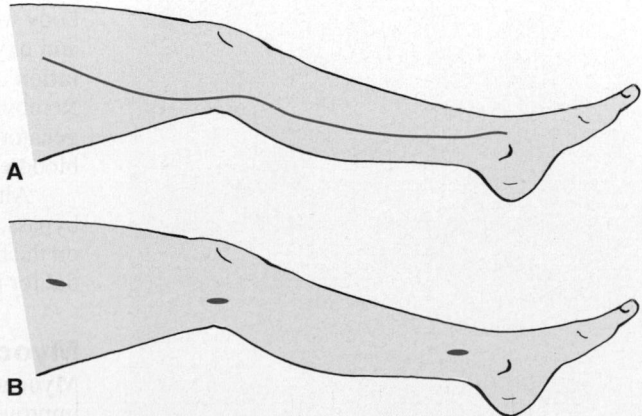

FIGURE 29-2. Two methods for harvesting the saphenous vein. **(A)** Traditional surgery requires a long incision in the leg. **(B)** Endoscopic removal involves one to three 1-inch incisions.

TABLE 29-1 Comparison of Surgical Myocardial Revascularization Techniques

	CONVENTIONAL CABG	MIDCAB	PACAB	OPCAB
Length of incision	12″	4″	(3) ⅓″ (1) 1″	8–12″
Duration of hospitalization	7–10 days	4–6 days	3–4 days	6–10 days
Time for full recovery	6–10 weeks	2–4 weeks	2–3 weeks	4–6 weeks
Maximum number of grafted arteries	5	1–2	4	4
Years in clinical practice*	45 years	11 years	12 years	9 years
Cost	$35,000–45,000	~40% less than conventional CABG	~15% less than conventional CABG	~25% less than conventional CABG
Operation on beating heart	No	Yes	No	Yes
Use of cardiopulmonary bypass	Yes	No	Yes	No
Time in surgery	3–6 hours	2–3 hours	2 hours	2–5 hours
Operative mortality rate	2.9%	1.5%	1.0%	0.8%

*Since 2008.

(Source: Biomedical Department, Brown University, Providence, Rhode Island, 2008.)

surgery in the U.S. (Clinical Procedures, 2004). The technique involves a long (approximately 12-inch) mid-chest incision, use of a cardiopulmonary bypass machine, and **cardioplegia** (stopping the heart) during surgery. During CABG, the surgeon attaches one end of a vessel such as a harvested portion of the saphenous vein or other distant vessel to the aorta and the other end below the occlusion in the coronary artery (Fig. 29-3). One or several occluded areas can be bypassed during the surgical procedure, which is referred to as a *double, triple,* or *quadruple* bypass depending on the number of vessels that are grafted.

As an alternative, the distal end of the internal mammary or internal thoracic artery can be reattached below the occlusion on the anterior surface of the heart while leaving the proximal end in its natural location. The advantage of using chest arteries is that doing so avoids making a second operative incision elsewhere on the body. The disadvantage is that the portion of the chest arteries available for graft use is shorter than other graft vessels.

Off-Pump Coronary Artery Bypass (OPCAB)

OPCAB, which has been performed since early 2000, is very similar to conventional CABG except that it does not involve the use of a cardiopulmonary bypass machine. Instead, the surgeon keeps the heart beating at a slow rate with drugs such as adenosine (Adenocard) and esmolol (Brevibloc). The OPCAB chest incision is approximately 8 to 10 inches, somewhat less than in a conventional CABG procedure. Instruments that lift and stabilize the heart facilitate the surgeon's ability to graft vessels on the anterior, lateral, and posterior walls of the beating heart (Fig. 29-4).

Advocates note that OPCAB reduces the risks associated with using the coronary bypass machine and decreases

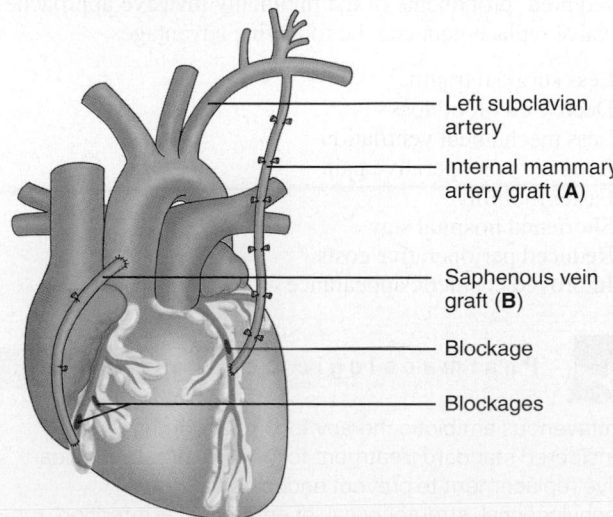

FIGURE 29-3. Coronary artery bypass grafts using (**A**) internal mammary artery and (**B**) saphenous vein.

Left subclavian artery
Internal mammary artery graft (**A**)
Saphenous vein graft (**B**)
Blockage
Blockages

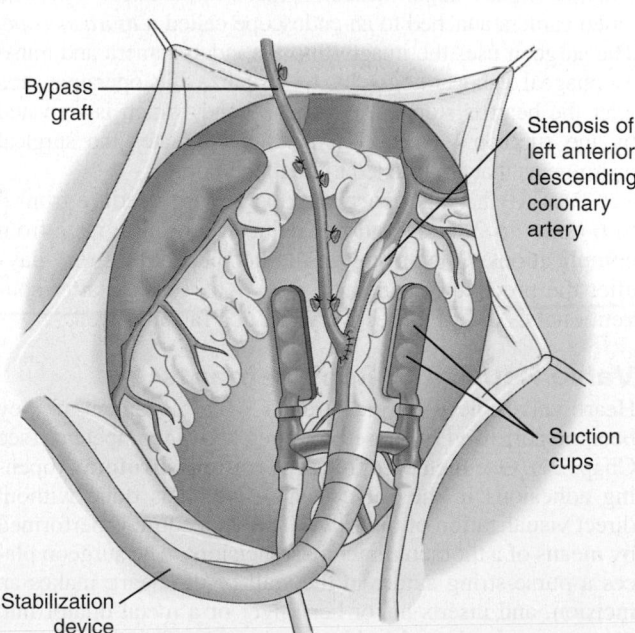

FIGURE 29-4. Example of stabilizer device used for off-pump coronary artery bypass (OPCAB).

Bypass graft
Stenosis of left anterior descending coronary artery
Suction cups
Stabilization device

postoperative recovery time spent in the hospital. Until more OPCAB procedures are performed, however, it is too early to determine if the long-term success is as good as or better than with conventional CABG.

Minimally Invasive Direct Coronary Artery Bypass (MIDCAB)

A MIDCAB is another example of a "beating heart" procedure. It is called *minimally invasive* because the incision, which is made between the ribs, is only about 3 to 5 inches long. Because the incision is small, the surgeon uses an endoscope to view the heart while grafting the vessels. Some surgeons are learning to use a robotic instrument inside the chest cavity rather than their hands.

This type of procedure is limited to grafting only one or two vessels on the anterior surface of the heart in clients who are not obese or whose coronary arteries are not heavily calcified. Despite these limitations, the MIDCAB procedure shortens the surgical time and postoperative recovery period, eliminates the risks of cardiopulmonary bypass, and is cosmetically more acceptable because of the smaller scar.

Port Access Coronary Artery Bypass (PACAB)

PACAB is a coronary artery bypass technique that uses the cardiopulmonary bypass machine attached to the femoral artery and vein rather than the great vessels of the heart. A triple lumen vascular catheter is inserted: one lumen allows occlusion of blood flow through the aorta, the second removes blood from the left ventricle, and the third delivers the solution that stops the heart from beating.

PACAB eliminates the long sternal incision common in conventional CABG. The surgeon gains access to the heart through several small incisions on the left lateral chest near the axilla. Metal tubes approximately the diameter of a pencil are then inserted through the incisions (Fig. 29-5). It is through these tubes, or ports, that surgical instruments are inserted. Another slightly larger incision is made in the chest to insert a video camera attached to an endoscope called a *thoracoscope*. The surgeon uses the image from the video camera and transesophageal echocardiography to visualize the operative area after the heart is stopped. A robotic hand, which is activated by the surgeon's voice command, manipulates the surgical instruments that are inserted through the ports.

PACAB has shortened the operative procedure from 3 to 6 hours to 2 hours and has reduced mortality rates from complications. Clients stay in the hospital only 2 to 3 days after the procedure, compared with 7 to 10 days after conventional CABG. Full recovery is much faster as well.

Valve Repairs or Replacements

Heart valves need surgical repair or replacement if they become narrowed (stenosed) or stretched (incompetent) (see Chap. 24). One method of repair is **commissurotomy** (opening adhesions in the valve cusps), which is done without direct visualization of the valve. This procedure is performed by means of a thoracotomy (chest incision). The surgeon places a purse-string suture in the wall of the heart, makes an incision, and inserts his or her finger or a metal dilator into the narrowed valve, stretching its opening. The surgeon then pulls the purse-string suture tight to prevent blood from escaping. Another less invasive technique is *balloon*

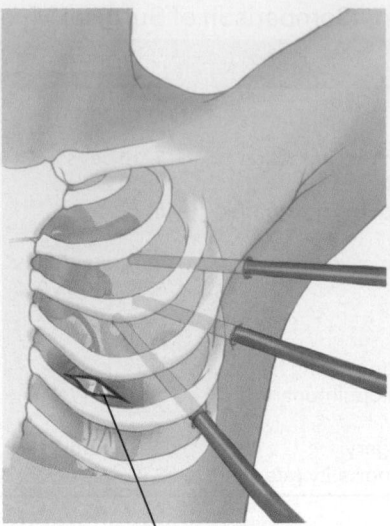

thoracic incision

FIGURE 29-5. In a PACAB technique, the surgeon makes three small incisions in the chest near the axilla. He or she inserts surgical instruments through the ports and an endoscope through a larger incision. The surgeon then views the surgical field.

valvuloplasty, which uses a balloon catheter to stretch the stenosed valve (see Chap. 24). Cardiopulmonary bypass is not required for minimally invasive techniques, but it usually is kept available for immediate use if complications develop or direct visualization is required to repair the valve.

Other methods of repair include **valvuloplasty** (valve repair) and **annuloplasty** (repair of the fibrous ring that encircles the valve). These procedures surgically tighten an incompetent valve (Fig. 29-6).

If a valve cannot be repaired and needs to be replaced, the diseased valve can be excised and replaced with a mechanical valve or a bioprosthetic valve (Fig. 29-7; Table 29-2). Surgeons also use minimally invasive approaches when replacing heart valves. Some of these approaches are performed through a mini-sternotomy, or parasternal incision, or a port access approach. Although cardiopulmonary bypass is required, proponents of the minimally invasive approaches to valve replacement cite the following advantages:

- Less surgical trauma
- Decreased blood loss
- Less mechanical ventilation
- Reduced postoperative pain
- Faster mobility
- Shortened hospital stay
- Reduced perioperative costs
- Improved cosmetic appearance

 Pharmacologic Considerations

- Intravenous antibiotic therapy for 1 to 2 months is considered standard treatment following a prosthetic heart valve replacement to prevent endocarditis from a staphylococcal, streptococcal, or enterococcal infection (Baptiste, 2001).

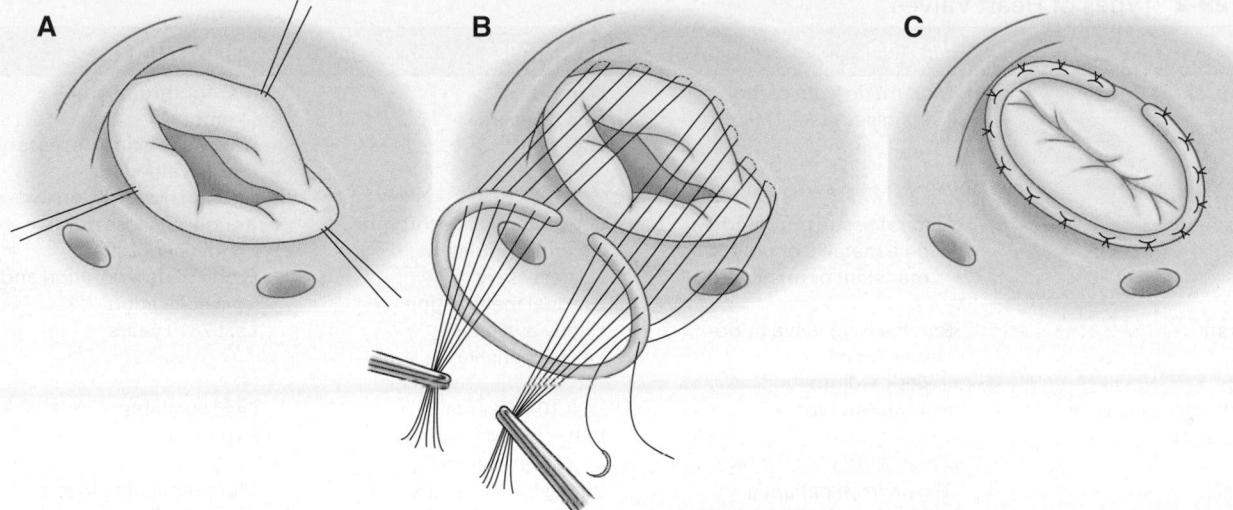

FIGURE 29-6. Annuloplasty ring insertion. (**A**) Mitral valve regurgitation; leaflets do not close. (**B**) Insertion of an annuloplasty ring. (**C**) Completed valvuloplasty; leaflets close.

Repair of Ventricular Aneurysm

An aneurysm of the ventricular wall develops when an infarcted area of myocardium balloons outward. Thrombi commonly form in the crater of the bulging tissue. A ventricular aneurysm is the most lethal complication among clients who survive the acute stage of a myocardial infarction (MI). Because the motion of the myocardium may rupture the aneurysm, an emergency procedure may be performed to suture the weakened area (Fig. 29-8). If waiting is possible, the stretched tissue is excised 4 to 8 weeks after the MI when scar tissue has formed. If surgery is performed too early, it is

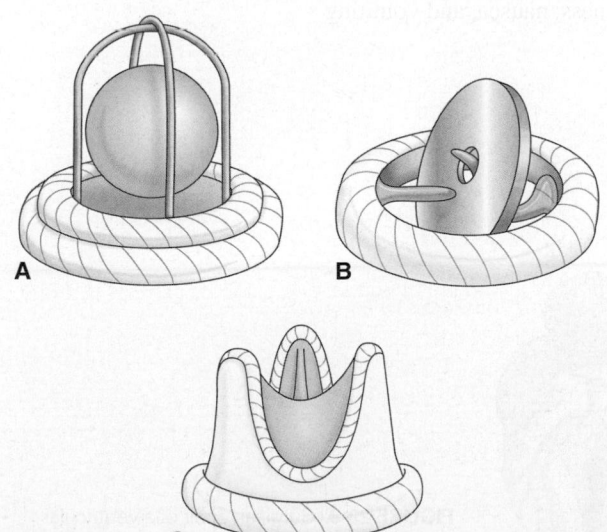

FIGURE 29-7. Common mechanical and biologic valve replacements. (**A**) Caged ball valve (Starr-Edwards, mechanical). (**B**) Tilting-disk valve (Medtronic-Hall, mechanical). (**C**) Porcine heterograft valve (Carpenter-Edwards, biologic).

difficult to differentiate healthy from necrotic tissue, and sutures placed in necrotic tissue usually are not retained.

Removal of Heart Tumors

Primary tumors of the heart, both benign and malignant, are rare. The clinical course and operative procedure depend on the type of tumor and its location in the heart. Benign tumors typically extend from a pedicle or stem, making their removal uncomplicated. Malignant tumors are more difficult to remove, and the prognosis is extremely poor.

Repair of Heart Trauma

A nonpenetrating injury of the chest, such as being crushed against a steering wheel, may cause bruising and bleeding of the heart. Because the pericardium encloses the heart, blood accumulates in the pericardial space, resulting in cardiac tamponade. Sometimes traumatic cardiac tamponade is treated conservatively with bed rest. The inactivity and increased pressure from blood in the pericardium may stop the bleeding. The client may need to have the blood aspirated from the pericardial sac, in which case pericardiocentesis is performed (see Chap. 23). One aspiration is sufficient in most cases, but if bleeding continues, open thoracotomy is indicated to control blood loss.

A penetrating injury, such as a stab wound, also causes blood to leak into the pericardium. A pericardial tear often seals with a clot, whereas a myocardial tear continues to bleed. Large tears necessitate surgery. If the wound is severe enough to cause immediate shock from hemorrhage, the prognosis is poor.

Heart Transplantation

In adults, heart transplantation is indicated for cardiomyopathy (see Chap. 23), end-stage coronary artery disease (see Chap. 25), and end-stage heart failure (see Chap. 28). In newborns and infants, heart transplantation is indicated for a

TABLE 29-2 Types of Heart Valves

TYPE	MATERIAL	ADVANTAGES	DISADVANTAGES
Mechanical	Man-made from carbon, stainless steel, Dacron	Durable Last 20 years Life-long	Risk for thrombi and emboli Anticoagulation necessary Risk for bleeding Sudden malfunction
Bioprosthetic	Natural tissue mounted on a metallic or polymer stent or unstented	Low potential for thrombi No anticoagulation necessary Gradual malfunction	Xenografts less durable than allografts Prone to deterioration and calcification
Xenograft	Porcine (pig) valve or bovine (cow) pericardium	Highly available Less expensive	Last 7–10 years
Allograft (also known as homograft)	Human cadaver	Last 10–15 years Better blood flow characteristics	Less available Expensive
Autograft	Tissue from patient's own pulmonic valve or pulmonary artery	Viable for 20+ years	More difficult to insert surgically

severe congenital cardiac defect. It is performed only when other treatment modalities fail or are unavailable. At any given time, almost 4000 people are waiting for a heart transplant. Approximately 2300 heart transplants are performed per year in the United States (The Cleveland Clinic, 2005).

The National Organ Transplant Act, which Congress passed in 1984, outlaws the sale of human organs. The United Network for Organ Sharing (UNOS) is the organization that maintains a computerized database with which to match organs with recipients (Box 29-2). Once a client is certified as a candidate for transplantation, his or her name and tissue type are placed on a computerized recipient list. Tissue typing is necessary to match the recipient with a donor.

When a donor heart becomes available, it must be removed from the donor and transplanted within 6 hours of being harvested. There are two methods of heart

transplantation. The most common method is an orthotopic heart transplant, in which the recipient's failing heart is removed and the donor heart is sutured onto the native great vessels of the heart (Fig. 29-9).

Many problems are associated with heart transplantation, including the scarcity of donor organs, tissue rejection, postoperative infection, postoperative psychosis, and high cost. To prevent tissue rejection, recipients are given immunosuppressive drugs such as cyclosporine (Sandimmune), azathioprine (Imuran), prednisone (Meticorten), tacrolimus (Prograf), or mycophenolate (CellCept). The client is closely observed for signs of organ rejection, which include the following (Cleveland Clinic Heart Center, 2005):

- Fever over 100.4°F (38°C)
- Flu-like symptoms such as chills, aches, headaches, dizziness, nausea, and vomiting

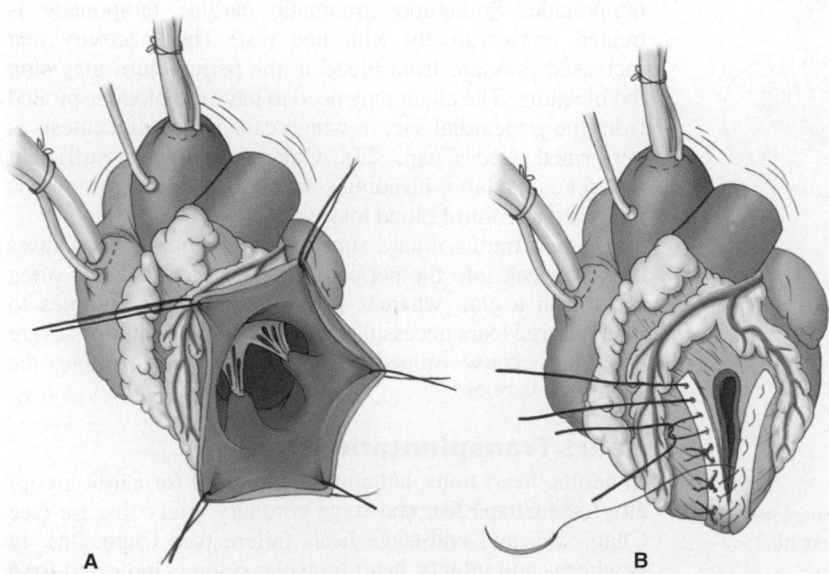

FIGURE 29-8. Surgical repair of a ventricular aneurysm. (**A**) The ventricle is opened and the nonfunctioning tissue from the aneurysm is differentiated from normal myocardium. (**B**) Healthy tissue from the endocardium through the epicardium is approximated.

BOX 29-2 **UNOS Criteria for Thoracic Organ Donation**

Those awaiting heart transplantation are assigned a status code that corresponds to their medical urgency.

Status 1A is a person who has at least one of the following devices or therapies:
- Mechanical circulatory support
- Mechanical circulatory support with a device-related complication
- Continuous mechanical ventilation
- Continuous intravenous infusion of a single high-dose inotropic agent
  or
- Justification of an exceptional case based on recommendation of his or her transplant physician and approval of the Regional Review Board and Thoracic Organ Transplant Committee.

Status 1B must have at least one of the following devices or therapies:
- Left or right implanted ventricular assist device
- Continuous infusion of intravenous inotropes
  or
- Justification of an exceptional case based on recommendation of his or her transplant physician and approval of the Regional Review Board and Thoracic Organ Transplant Committee.

Status 2 is a person who meets neither Status 1A or 1B criteria. Status 7 is a person considered temporarily unsuitable to receive a thoracic organ transplant.

(Adapted from United Network of Organ Sharing [2007]. Policy 3.7 "Allocation of Thoracic Organs." Available at: http://www.unos.org/PoliciesandBylaws2/policies/pdts/policy_9.pdf. Retrieved October 2008.)

- Shortness of breath
- New chest tenderness
- Fatigue and malaise
- Elevated blood pressure

As a result of taking immunosuppressive drugs, clients are at risk for infection. If there are signs and symptoms of infection, which may resemble those of tissue rejection, the client is placed in protective isolation, because an infection can be life threatening. Throughout the client's lifetime, a heart biopsy is performed to detect rejection; cardiac tissue is obtained with an instrument attached to a venous catheter inserted into the heart. When signs of rejection occur, the dose or number of immunosuppressives is increased.

Estimates for the cost of a heart transplant is on average approximately $311,000 for the first year and $40,000 per year thereafter (National Kidney Foundation, 2006). Insurance carriers, Medicare, or Medicaid assume most of this financial burden.

The transplanted heart beats faster than the client's natural heart, averaging about 100 to 110 beats/minute, because nerves that affect heart rate have been severed. The new heart also takes longer to increase the heart rate in response to exercise. CAD is a common problem among heart

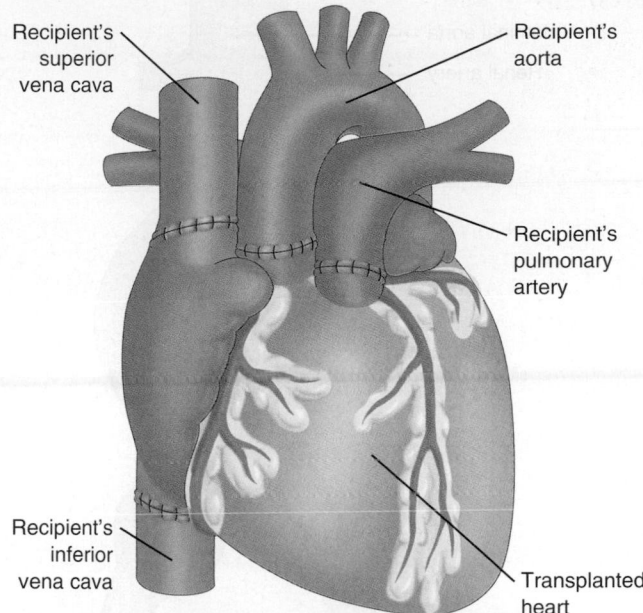

FIGURE 29-9. Orthotopic method of heart transplantation. Note the suture lines indicating the attachment of the donor heart.

transplant recipients; however, they do not experience angina because the transplanted heart's nerve supply is no longer intact. The rate for survival following a heart transplant is 79% for 1 year; 75% for 5 years; and 60% for 10 years. Half of all transplant candidates die within a year if a donor heart is not available (Parks, 2006).

CENTRAL OR PERIPHERAL VASCULAR SURGICAL PROCEDURES

Vascular Grafts

Just as grafts are used to bypass a diseased section of a coronary blood vessel, vascular grafts are used to bypass or replace diseased sections of major systemic blood vessels such as the ascending aorta, descending aorta, femoral, or popliteal arteries. The replacement graft may be made of synthetic fiber, such as Dacron or Teflon, or may be human tissue harvested from cadavers. A clamp is placed above and below the affected area, and the diseased blood vessel is removed. The replacement graft is then sewn in place, and the clamps are removed (Fig. 29-10). Depending on the area involved, cardiopulmonary bypass may be necessary.

Embolectomy and Thrombectomy

When thrombi or emboli occlude a major vessel, a **thrombectomy** (removal of a thrombus) or **embolectomy** (removal of an embolus) is performed. The vessel is opened above the clot, the clot is removed, and the vessel is sutured closed. This type of surgery may be an emergency because complete occlusion results in loss of blood supply to an area.

Endarterectomy

Endarterectomy is the resection and removal of the lining of an artery (see Chap. 38). This type of surgery is performed

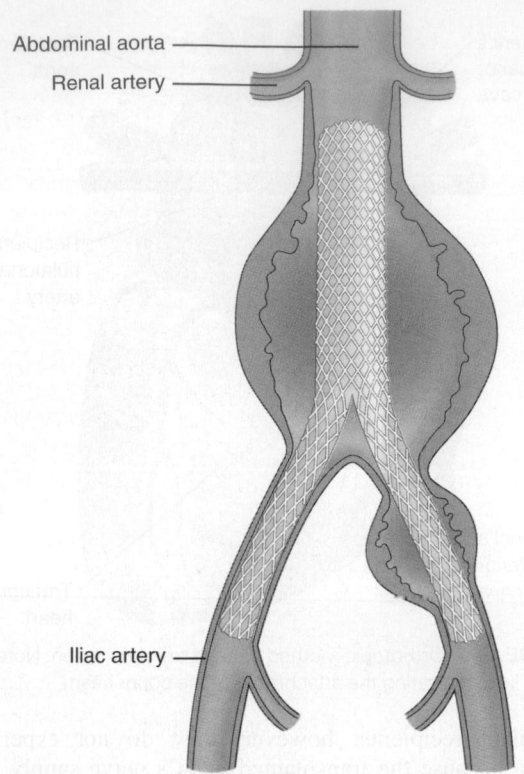

Abdominal aorta

Renal artery

Iliac artery

FIGURE 29-10. Surgical repair of an abdominal aortic aneurysm using a synthetic graft.

to remove obstructive atherosclerotic plaques from the aorta, carotid, femoral, or popliteal arteries (Fig. 29-11).

NURSING MANAGEMENT FOR THE CLIENT UNDERGOING CARDIOVASCULAR SURGERY

The nurse manages the care of the client undergoing cardiovascular surgery throughout the perioperative and rehabilitation phases. Clients who undergo cardiovascular surgery are cared for in an intensive care unit during the immediate postoperative period because of their unstable condition and the need for nurses with expertise in managing complex monitoring equipment.

Hemodynamic Monitoring

Hemodynamic monitoring is used to assess the volume and pressure of blood in the heart and vascular system by means of a surgically inserted catheter. Such monitoring is used to assess cardiac function and circulatory status, detect fluid imbalances, adjust fluid infusion rates, and evaluate the client's response to therapeutic measures, such as drug therapy. Methods for hemodynamic monitoring include direct BP monitoring, central venous pressure (CVP) monitoring, and pulmonary artery pressure monitoring.

Direct Blood Pressure Monitoring

Direct BP monitoring requires the placement of a catheter in a peripheral artery. The artery most commonly used is the radial artery. The brachial and femoral arteries also may be used. The catheter tip contains a sensor that measures and transmits the fluid pressure to a transducer, which electronically converts the data to a visual waveform. A monitor continuously displays the waveform and indicates the client's systolic, diastolic, and mean arterial pressures. This type of equipment eliminates the need to auscultate the BP. Direct BP monitoring may be used in clients with severe and sustained hypertension or hypotension, and during and after cardiac surgery. A three-way stopcock can be attached to the tubing to allow the nurse periodically to draw arterial blood samples for blood gas analysis (Fig. 29-12).

Central Venous Pressure Monitoring

Right atrial pressure, or **central venous pressure** (CVP), is the pressure produced by venous blood in the right atrium. Normal CVP is 2 to 7 mm Hg. This measurement is used to detect an excess or a deficit in venous blood volume.

To monitor CVP, a catheter is inserted into a large vein, usually the jugular or subclavian vein in the neck, and advanced into the superior vena cava. The catheter's proximal end is connected to a three-way stopcock, which controls the direction in which IV fluid flows. The catheter is attached to a transducer that connects to a computer used to analyze hemodynamic data.

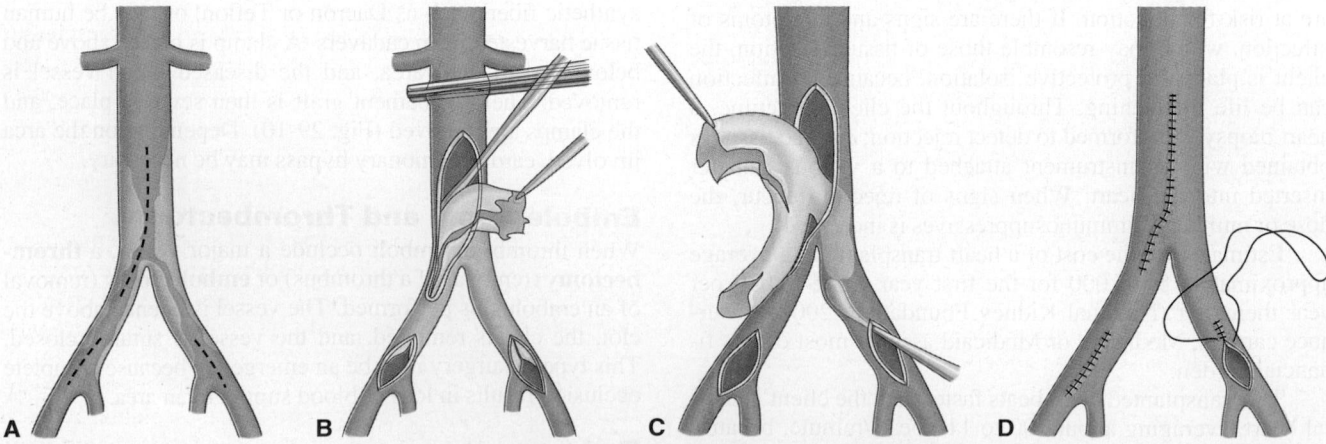

FIGURE 29-11. In an aortoiliac endarterectomy, the vascular surgeon (**A**) identifies the diseased area, (**B**) clamps off blood supply to the vessel, (**C**) removes the plaque, and (**D**) sutures the vessel shut, after which blood flow is restored. (Adapted with permission from Rutherford, R. B. [2005]. *Vascular surgery* [6th ed., Vols. I and II]. Philadelphia: Elsevier.)

A   B   C   D

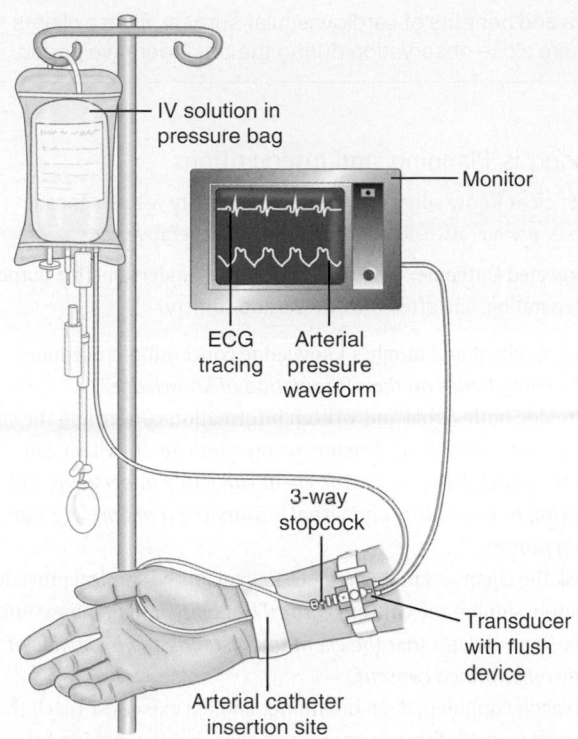

FIGURE 29-12. Example of a direct blood pressure monitoring system. The catheter is inserted in the radial artery. A three-way stopcock is used for drawing arterial blood samples.

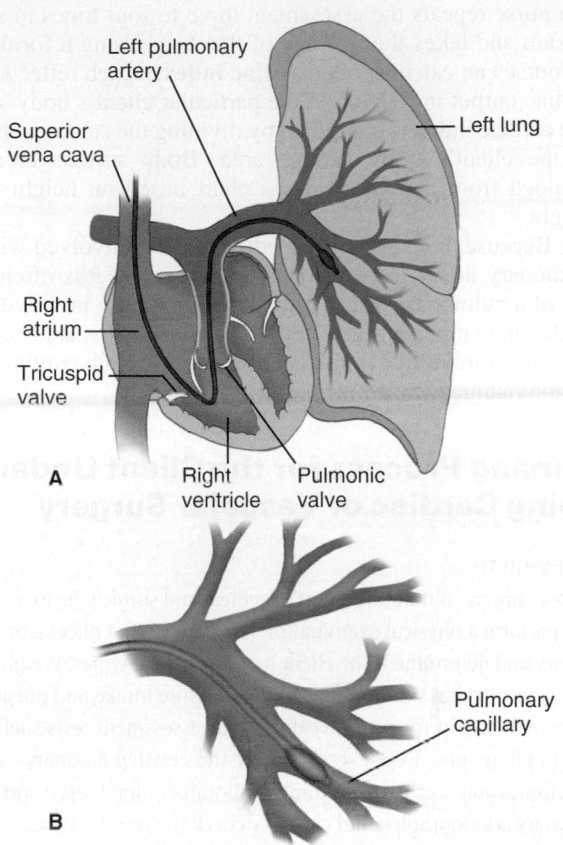

FIGURE 29-13. Fluid status can be monitored with a pulmonary artery catheter. **(A)** Location of the catheter in the heart. The catheter enters the right atrium through the superior vena cava. The balloon is then inflated, allowing the catheter to follow the blood flow through the tricuspid valve, right ventricle, pulmonic valve, and main pulmonary artery. Waveform and pressure readings are noted during insertion to identify the location of the catheter within the heart. The balloon is deflated once the catheter is in the pulmonary artery and properly secured. **(B)** Pulmonary capillary wedge pressure (PCWP). The catheter floats into a distal branch of the pulmonary artery when the balloon is inflated and becomes "wedged." The wedged catheter occludes blood flow from behind, and the tip of the lumen records pressures in front of the catheter. The balloon is then deflated, allowing the catheter to flow back into the main pulmonary artery.

When measuring CVP, the nurse makes sure that the transducer is at the level of the client's right atrium; otherwise, an incorrect reading is obtained. The client is positioned supine or with the head slightly elevated but in exactly the same position as during previous measurements. Between CVP measurements, the head of the bed can be raised or lowered. The physician orders the frequency of CVP measurements; however, the nurse may obtain measurements any time he or she suspects a change in the client's fluid status.

Pulmonary Artery Pressure Monitoring

By inserting a multi-lumen catheter into a peripheral vein with a distal tip in the pulmonary artery, pressures and cardiac output can be measured to assess left ventricular function (see Fig. 17-3 in Chap. 17). When in place, the pulmonary artery catheter can measure both pulmonary artery pressure and right atrial pressure or CVP. Pulmonary artery pressure monitoring aids in the early treatment of fluid imbalances, prevents left-sided heart failure or promotes its early correction, and helps monitor the client's response to treatment.

The pulmonary artery catheter is advanced through the right side of the heart until the distal tip rests in the right or left pulmonary artery. When the small balloon at the tip of the catheter is inflated, the balloon floats forward, eventually wedging in a pulmonary capillary (Fig. 29-13). As the balloon blocks the flow of blood through the capillary, the catheter tip that protrudes from the inflated balloon senses the fluid pressure ahead of it. **Pulmonary capillary wedge pressure** is the retrograde pressure from the fluid on the left side of the heart at the end of left ventricular diastole.

Sometimes this is abbreviated LVEDP, for **left ventricular end-diastolic pressure**. The balloon must be deflated immediately after the pressure is measured to avoid pulmonary infarction from prolonged blockage of capillary blood flow.

To measure cardiac output, a syringe with 5 to 10 mL of 5% dextrose in water solution (D_5W) is pushed through a port of the catheter. In the past, iced injectate was used, but with the newer computers, injectate at room temperature may be used. A computerized probe measures the temperature change as the fluid exits the catheter in the heart. The computer then calculates the rate of temperature change with the speed at which the fluid traveled through the heart. A solution that is quite warm after its instillation indicates impairment of the heart's pump function. If the solution remains close to the instillation temperature, the heart's pump function is working optimally. The computer converts the electronic data into numerical equivalents for cardiac output.

The nurse repeats the assessment three to four times in succession and takes the average of the data. Using a formula, the nurse can calculate the **cardiac index,** which reflects the cardiac output in relation to the particular client's body size. The cardiac index is computed by dividing the cardiac output by the client's body surface area. Body surface area is obtained from a **nomogram,** a chart based on height and weight.

Because there are serious potential risks involved with a pulmonary artery catheter, it is used less and less often. In lieu of a pulmonary artery catheter, a minimally invasive hemodynamic monitoring system may be used. It is attached to a client's arterial line in the radial artery to obtain continuous hemodynamic measurements.

Nursing Process for the Client Undergoing Cardiac or Vascular Surgery

Assessment

Before surgery, obtain the client's medical and surgical history and perform a physical examination (see Chap. 22). Collect a drug history and determine if the client has any drug allergies. Weigh the client, record vital signs regularly, and measure intake and output. Prepare the client for extensive diagnostic assessment tests such as chest radiography, ECG, exercise ECG (stress test), pulmonary function studies, echocardiography, laboratory blood tests, and coronary arteriography, and carefully check the results. Take time to assess the client's understanding of the scheduled procedure.

After open heart surgery, the anesthetist and other members of the operating team send many clients directly from the operating room to the intensive care unit. Obtain a comprehensive surgical report from the anesthetist or anesthesiologist and check all invasive monitoring devices. Systematically assess for signs and symptoms of potential complications, such as hemorrhage and shock, thrombus or embolus formation, cerebral anoxia, cardiac dysrhythmias, fluid overload, electrolyte imbalance, respiratory failure, and cardiac tamponade.

Palpate the peripheral pulses or use a Doppler ultrasound device if the pulses are not palpable. Check for inadequate tissue perfusion, such as a weak or absent pulse, cold or cyanotic extremity, or skin mottling. Assess blood pressures (BP) and pulse rates in both arms after thoracic surgery. Inspect intravenous (IV) sites and monitor the rates of infusing solutions. Calculate urine output and other fluid intake hourly. Perform a neurologic assessment every 30 minutes, including evaluation of level of consciousness, size of pupils and their reaction to light, movement in both arms and legs, verbal response, and status of orientation. Figure 29-14 illustrates postoperative monitoring following cardiovascular surgery.

Gerontologic Considerations

- Many older adults have comorbidities such as diabetes, heart failure, cardiac dysrhythmias, hypertension, and poor renal function, and should carefully consider the potential risks and benefits of cardiovascular surgery. These clients require close observation during the postoperative period.

Diagnosis, Planning, and Interventions

▶ **Deficient Knowledge** related to unfamiliarity with diagnostic tests, preoperative preparations, and postoperative care

▶ **Expected Outcome:** Client and family will understand the purpose, preparation, and aftercare of tests and surgery.

- Assess client and family's knowledge concerning procedures. *Teaching builds on their foundation of knowledge.*
- Provide both verbal and written information concerning the surgical procedure and aftercare, using language the client can understand. *Using terms the client can easily understand and giving both auditory and visual information enhance the learning process.*
- Ask the client or family member to explain the surgical procedure before signing the consent form. *The ability to paraphrase information validates that the client understands and is capable of giving informed consent.*
- Explain coughing, deep breathing, and leg exercises. Teach the use of an incentive spirometer and splinting the incision to cough. *The standard of care for all clients undergoing general anesthesia is to preoperatively teach techniques that prevent postoperative pneumonia and stasis of venous circulation.*
- Promote a relaxed environment conducive to asking questions. *Demonstrating personal interest and encouraging verbal interaction promotes free communication.*
- Clarify misconceptions concerning surgery. *The nurse is obligated to ensure that the client's knowledge and perceptions are accurate.*

▶ **Anxiety** related to fear of surgery

▶ **Expected Outcome:** The client's anxiety will be reduced to a mild level or one the client indicates is tolerable as a result of developing realistic expectations concerning surgery.

- Provide clear information about the surgical procedure and aftercare in short, simple explanations. *Anxiety interferes with the ability to attend to, concentrate on, and process information, especially if it is extensive or complex.*
- Acknowledge emotions and expressions of fear. *Empathetic acceptance of fears decreases anxiety.*
- Demonstrate competence when performing skills. *Sensing that the nurse is knowledgeable and competent relieves the client's insecurity.*

Pharmacologic Considerations

- Narcotic analgesics may be used before surgery to lessen anxiety and sedate the client. Clients who are relaxed and sedated when anesthesia is given require a smaller dose of anesthetic.

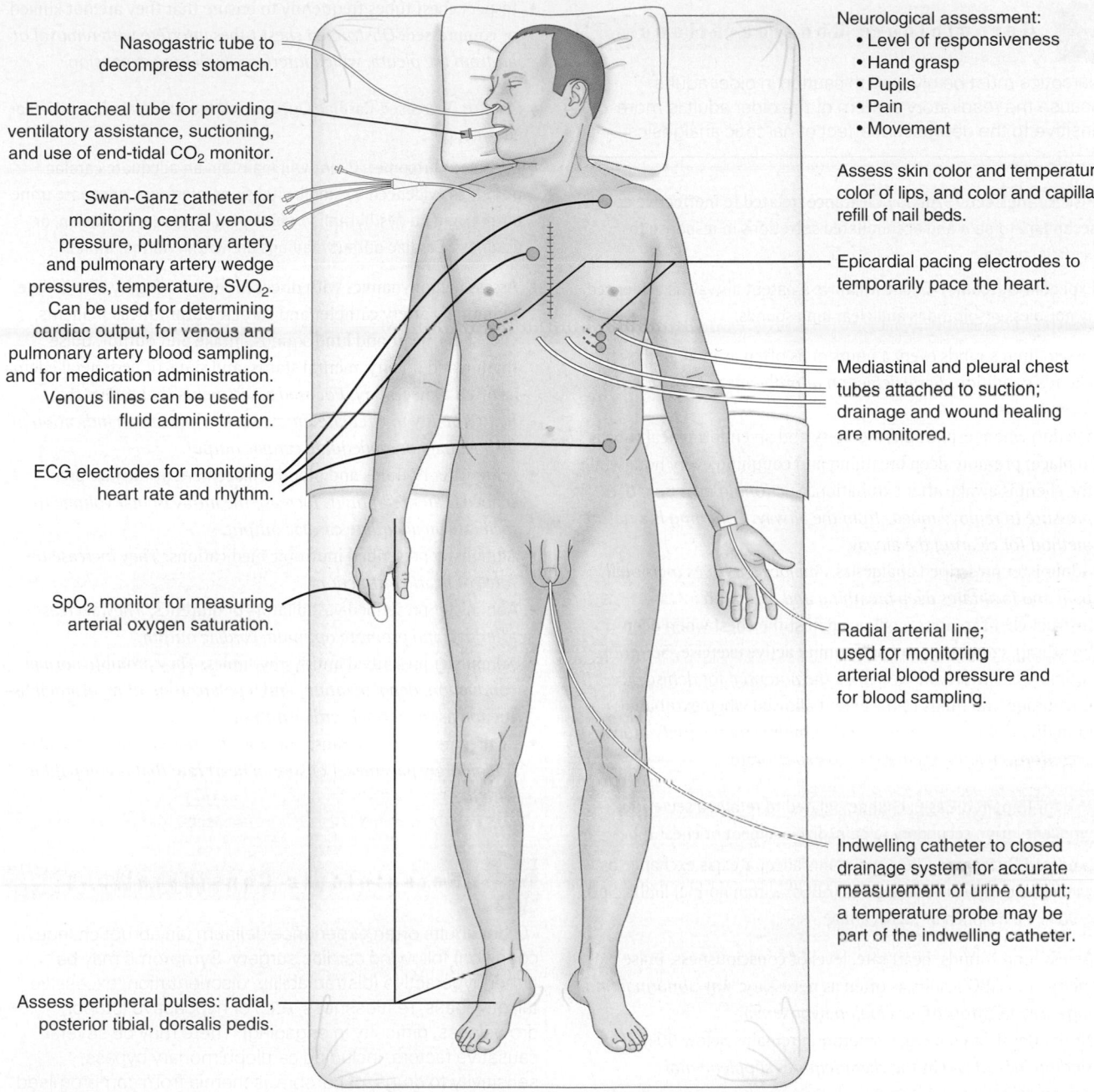

Nasogastric tube to decompress stomach.

Endotracheal tube for providing ventilatory assistance, suctioning, and use of end-tidal CO_2 monitor.

Swan-Ganz catheter for monitoring central venous pressure, pulmonary artery and pulmonary artery wedge pressures, temperature, SVO_2. Can be used for determining cardiac output, for venous and pulmonary artery blood sampling, and for medication administration. Venous lines can be used for fluid administration.

ECG electrodes for monitoring heart rate and rhythm.

SpO_2 monitor for measuring arterial oxygen saturation.

Assess peripheral pulses: radial, posterior tibial, dorsalis pedis.

Neurological assessment:
• Level of responsiveness
• Hand grasp
• Pupils
• Pain
• Movement

Assess skin color and temperature, color of lips, and color and capillary refill of nail beds.

Epicardial pacing electrodes to temporarily pace the heart.

Mediastinal and pleural chest tubes attached to suction; drainage and wound healing are monitored.

Radial arterial line; used for monitoring arterial blood pressure and for blood sampling.

Indwelling catheter to closed drainage system for accurate measurement of urine output; a temperature probe may be part of the indwelling catheter.

FIGURE 29-14. Postoperative monitoring of the client following cardiovascular surgery.

▶ **Acute Pain** related to surgical trauma to skin and operative tissue

▶ **Expected Outcome:** Pain will be reduced to a tolerable level within 30 minutes of a nursing intervention.

• Assess the location, intensity, and quality of pain when assessing vital signs. *Pain assessment is the fifth vital sign. Pain beyond the client's tolerance requires immediate intervention.*

• Demonstrate how to self-administer narcotic analgesia with a patient-controlled analgesia (PCA) pump. *Small, frequent*

self-administrations of an opioid drug control acute pain within consistently tolerable levels.

• Administer narcotic analgesics promptly as prescribed if PCA is not used. *Pain is more easily controlled by giving analgesic medication before the pain becomes severe.*

• Administer non-narcotic analgesics between prescribed doses of narcotic analgesics. *Non-narcotics have a different mechanism of action and are not likely to cause respiratory depression or depressed level of consciousness if given concurrently with narcotics.*

Gerontologic Considerations

- Narcotics must be given with caution in older adults because the respiratory system of the older adult is more sensitive to the depressant effect of narcotic analgesics.

▶ **Risk for Ineffective Airway Clearance** related to ineffective cough secondary to pain and accumulated secretions in response to artificial airway

▶ **Expected Outcome:** Client will have a patent airway as evidenced by noiseless respirations and clear lung sounds.

- Assess lung sounds every 4 hours or as often as indicated by the client's condition. *Early detection of problems allows for swift intervention.*
- Suction when respirations are noisy and an endotracheal tube is in place; promote deep breathing and coughing every hour while the client is awake after extubation. *Suctioning uses negative pressure to remove mucus from the airway. Coughing is a natural method for clearing the airway.*
- Administer prescribed analgesics. *Analgesia relieves incisional pain and facilitates deep breathing and coughing.*
- Instruct client to press a pillow against the chest when deep breathing, coughing, and performing active exercise. *Splinting promotes comfort and decreases the potential for dehiscence.*
- Encourage oral fluids to the extent allowed when extubated; humidify oxygen. *Hydration and humidification liquefy mucous secretions, making them easier to expectorate.*

▶ **Risk for Impaired Gas Exchange** related to retained secretions, hypoventilation secondary to pain, displacement of chest tubes

▶ **Expected Outcome:** Client maintains adequate gas exchange as evidenced by arterial blood gases (ABGs) within normal limits, SpO_2 ≥ 90%, no dyspnea or tachycardia.

- Assess lung sounds, heart rate, level of consciousness, pulse oximetry, and ABG results as often as necessary. *Any abnormal findings are indicators of developing hypoxemia.*
- Notify physician if oxygen saturation remains below 90%. *This finding indicates that the client requires supplemental oxygenation.*
- Administer oxygen as prescribed. *Supplemental oxygen prevents hypoxemia or relieves oxygen deficits.*
- Elevate head of bed as much as possible. *Elevation of the head facilitates maximum chest/lung expansion, promotes comfort, and decreases the work of breathing.*
- Hyperoxygenate with 100% oxygen before suctioning; do not suction for more than 10 to 15 seconds. *Suctioning removes oxygen and can cause hypoxemia, myocardial ischemia, and dysrhythmias. Hyperoxygenation saturates the blood and hemoglobin to compensate for temporary removal during suctioning.*
- Promote rest and administer prescribed sedatives. *Rest reduces oxygen consumption; sedatives promote rest and are sympathetic antagonists.*

- Inspect chest tubes frequently to ensure that they are not kinked or compressed. *Obstructed chest tubes interfere with removal of air from the pleura, which interferes with lung expansion.*

▶ **Risk for Decreased Cardiac Output** related to impaired ventricular contraction.

▶ **Expected Outcome:** Client will maintain an adequate cardiac output as evidenced by stable vital signs, alertness, adequate urine output, and no dysrhythmias, chest pain, dyspnea, confusion, or dizziness. Cardiac output readings are within normal limits.

- Assess hemodynamics with direct BP monitoring by arterial line, pulmonary artery catheter and cardiac output measurements, vital signs, heart and lung sounds, intake and output, pulse rhythm and quality, mental status, and signs of peripheral edema as often as necessary. *Focused assessments that reflect the heart's ability to circulate intravascular fluid are an indication of an adequate or inadequate cardiac output.*
- Administer IV fluids and blood replacement at the rate prescribed. *Parenteral fluids increase the intravascular volume to facilitate an adequate cardiac output.*
- Administer prescribed inotropic medications. *They increase the force of heart contraction.*
- Administer prescribed vasodilators or diuretics. *They decrease afterload and promote optimum cardiac output.*
- Administer prescribed antidysrhythmics. *They promote normal conduction, depolarization, and repolarization of myocardial tissue to ensure normal cardiac output.*
- Be prepared to use a transcutaneous or transvenous pacemaker. *A temporary pacemaker ensures a heart rate that is compatible with life.*

Gerontologic Considerations

- Older adults often experience delirium (an abrupt change in cognition) following cardiac surgery. Symptoms may be either hyperactive (distractability, disorientation, excessive talkativeness, restlessness, etc.) or hypoactive (stupor, drowsiness, difficulty in engaging). There may be several causative factors, including cardiopulmonary bypass, sensitivity to drugs, or cerebral ischemia from compromised blood flow or volume. Identifying and then minimizing or eliminating the causes of delirium after cardiac surgery are critical.

▶ **Risk for Infection** related to impaired skin

▶ **Expected Outcome:** Client will remain free of infection.

- Assess incisions for redness, warmth, swelling, or purulent drainage. *Focused assessments that reflect the inflammatory process signify a possible infection.*
- Practice conscientious hand hygiene. *Hand hygiene is the single most important method for preventing infection.*
- Change moist or loose dressings. Use aseptic technique when changing dressings, IV tubing, bags, or other equipment. *Sterile*

technique prevents the transmission of microorganisms to impaired tissue. Dry, intact dressings are a barrier to microorganisms in the environment.

- Administer prescribed antibiotic therapy. *Antibiotics are administered prophylactically and must be given on time to maintain therapeutic blood levels.*
- Implement infection-control precautions for the immunosuppressed client. *They reduce the potential for exposing such clients to infectious microorganisms.*

▶ **PC: Hemorrhage**

▶ **Expected Outcome:** The nurse will monitor for, manage, and minimize hemorrhage.

- Assess the following as often as necessary: incisional drainage; sites used for cardiopulmonary bypass cannulation; volume and color of chest tube drainage; BP and pulse rate; urinary output; mental status; partial thromboplastin time, prothrombin time, and international normalized ratio; presence of occult blood in stool; bruising; bleeding gums; and hemodynamic measurements. *Abnormal findings of such focused assessments are indicators of bleeding.*
- Report to the physician a cluster of symptoms that suggest significant blood loss. *The nurse works collaboratively to manage complications.*
- Be prepared to administer parenteral fluids, blood replacement, fresh frozen plasma, or antidotes for anticoagulants. *Fluids, blood, and blood products increase blood volume. Fresh frozen plasma replaces clotting factors. Antagonists of anticoagulants restore endogenous clotting mechanisms.*
- Apply direct pressure to bleeding sites. *Pressure promotes stasis of blood.*

▶ **Risk for Ineffective Tissue Perfusion: Peripheral** related to compromised collateral circulation in extremity used to harvest donor vein, cannulation of peripheral artery and vein for cardiopulmonary bypass, venous stasis secondary to inactivity

▶ **Expected Outcome:** Client's donor extremities will be adequately perfused with oxygenated blood; venous blood circulation will be adequate.

- Assess peripheral pulses, dependent edema, capillary refill, skin color and temperature, urinary output, mental status, and Homans' sign as often as necessary. *Focused assessment of these data reflects the status of peripheral blood flow.*
- Position extremity above level of heart. *Gravity promotes venous return to the heart. Reducing edema facilitates potential space for arterial circulation.*
- Encourage leg exercises every hour while awake. *Contraction of skeletal leg muscles propels venous blood toward the heart.*
- Apply elastic stockings or use a mechanical compression device. *Elastic stockings support valves in the leg veins to prevent venous stasis. Mechanical compression devices apply pressure to the tissues of the legs to propel venous blood.*
- Assist the client to ambulate several times a day. *Walking contracts leg muscles that promote venous blood return.*

- Ensure the client avoids prolonged sitting or crossing the legs at the knee. *Gravity and pressure contribute to venous stasis.*
- Encourage oral fluids within prescribed limits. *Adequate fluid volume decreases the potential for hemoconcentration and thrombus formation.*

▶ **PC: Paralytic Ileus** related to intestinal handling during repair of abdominal aortic aneurysm, effects of narcotics and other medications

▶ **Expected Outcome:** The nurse will monitor for, manage, and minimize atony of the bowel.

- Assess bowel sounds, abdominal distention, vomiting or color and amount of nasogastric tube drainage, and bowel elimination pattern as often as necessary. *Such focused assessments help determine the absence of peristalsis in the gastrointestinal tract.*
- Relieve pain with medications other than narcotic analgesics. *Narcotics slow peristalsis.*
- Withhold oral food and fluid. *Keeping the client NPO (nothing by mouth) decreases nausea and vomiting.*
- Ensure that the nasogastric tube remains patent. *A patent nasogastric tube provides an outlet for accumulating secretions and intestinal gas.*

Evaluation of Expected Outcomes

Expected outcomes for the client undergoing cardiovascular surgery are that he or she understands the treatment and recovery regimen and can cope with the fears created by the change in health status and surgical experience. Pain is controlled or eliminated; the airway is patent. The client ventilates adequately to maintain adequate gas diffusion; cardiac output is sufficient to maintain vital signs and renal output within normal ranges. There is no evidence of wound infection, and no significant bleeding develops. The extremities are warm and nonedematous, reflecting adequate arterial and venous circulation; bowel sounds are active.

Client and Family Teaching 29-1 offers discharge instructions after cardiac surgery. ●

▶ ***Stop, Think, and Respond Exercise 29-1***

A client has been in the intensive care unit for the past 4 days after CABG surgery. Normally alert and oriented, the client is very confused, restless, and agitated. What could be possible reasons for this new-onset confusion? What other data will you need to collect? What can you do to help the client right now?

CRITICAL THINKING EXERCISES

1. A client has been told that the physician advises myocardial revascularization. The client tells you that the thought of a long mid-chest incision and leg incision are very frightening. What information would you offer this person?
2. While caring for a client who is recovering from CABG surgery, you gather the following data: the client has leg pain, which the client rates as 8 on a scale of 1 to 10; the

connective tissue. It does not participate in the manufacture of blood cells; however, yellow bone marrow can form blood cells under conditions involving intense stimulation, such as after significant blood loss (hemorrhage). The lymphatic system also plays a role in hematopoiesis.

Blood

Blood consists of cells suspended in a fluid called **plasma** (Fig. 30-1). All blood cells are produced from undifferentiated precursors called **pluripotential stem cells** in the bone marrow (Fig. 30-2). Myeloid stem cells are converted to (1) **erythrocytes**, which are red blood cells (RBCs); (2) several types of **leukocytes**, or white blood cells (WBCs); and (3) **platelets**, also known as *thrombocytes* because they help control bleeding by forming a loose blood clot. Lymphoid stem cells are converted to **lymphocytes**, WBCs with immune functions. Each component of blood has specialized functions (Table 30-1).

Erythrocytes

Erythrocytes (or RBCs) are flexible, anuclear (lacking a nucleus), biconcave disks covered by a thin membrane through which oxygen (O_2) and carbon dioxide (CO_2) pass freely. The flexibility of erythrocytes allows them to change shape as they travel through capillaries. Their major function is to transport O_2 to and remove CO_2 from the tissues.

Production of erythrocytes is called *erythropoiesis*. The rate of erythrocyte production is regulated by **erythropoietin**, a hormone released by the kidneys. Erythrocytes arise from myeloid stem cells, which also require iron and B vitamins such as B_{12}, B_6, and folate to mature properly (Nutrition Notes 30-1). Immature erythrocytes, known collectively as *erythroblasts*, go through several intermediary stages of maturation before being released into the blood. In their immature state, erythroblasts contain a nucleus; the mature erythrocyte has no nucleus.

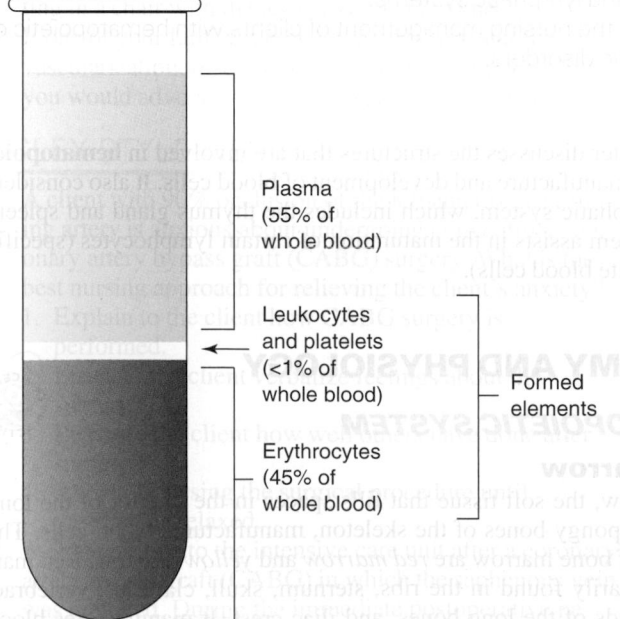

FIGURE 30-1. Components of blood.

Plasma
(55% of
whole blood)

Leukocytes
and platelets
(<1% of
whole blood)

Formed
elements

Erythrocytes
(45% of
whole blood)

The normal number of erythrocytes varies with age, gender, and altitude but ranges between 3.6 and 5.4 million/mm^3. Infants have more erythrocytes than adults; women have fewer erythrocytes than men. People who live at high altitudes or engage in strenuous activity have an increased number of erythrocytes to maximize the transport of oxygen and carbon dioxide.

The red color of blood is caused by **hemoglobin**, an iron-containing pigment attached to erythrocytes. The heme portion of the molecule freely binds with oxygen, forming a substance called *oxyhemoglobin*. Hemoglobin carries oxygen to the cells of the body. In adults, the normal amount of hemoglobin is 12 to 17.4 g/dL. As erythrocytes pass through the lungs, the hemoglobin picks up oxygen and releases CO_2. Oxygenated blood is bright red and carried by arteries, arterioles, and capillaries to all body tissues. After hemoglobin releases oxygen for use by the tissues, the hemoglobin is called *reduced* (or *deoxygenated*) *hemoglobin*. The blood becomes dark red and returns by way of the veins to the heart and lungs, where CO_2 is released and the blood is reoxygenated.

Erythrocytes circulate in the blood for about 120 days, after which the spleen removes them; the liver removes severely damaged erythrocytes. When erythrocytes are destroyed, the iron component of hemoglobin is returned to the red marrow and reused. The residual pigment is stored in the liver as bilirubin and excreted in bile.

Gerontologic Considerations

- The components of blood change only slightly with age. RBCs become slightly less flexible and fewer in number. Lymphocytes also decrease in number, causing a decreased resistance to infection.

Leukocytes

Leukocytes (or WBCs) perform various protective functions such as engulfing invading microorganisms and cellular debris, and manufacturing antibodies (see Chap. 33). They circulate in blood but also migrate from the blood into body tissues to search for and destroy potentially harmful substances.

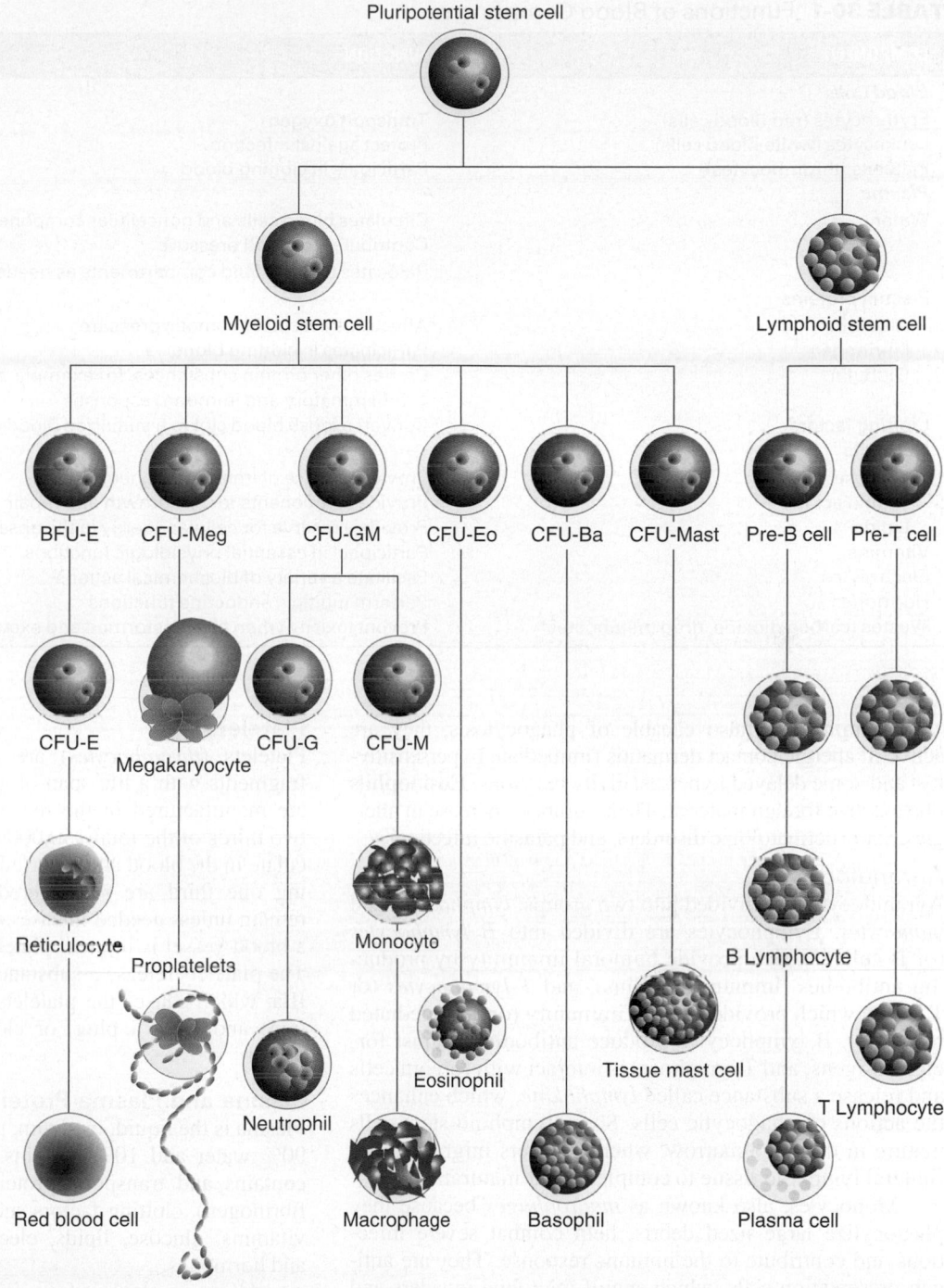

FIGURE 30-2. Hematopoiesis. All blood cells develop from pluripotential stem cells in the bone marrow. (From Smeltzer, S. C., et al. [2008]. *Brunner & Suddarth's textbook of medical–surgical nursing* [11th ed.]. Philadelphia: Lippincott Williams & Wilkins.)

Normal leukocyte count is between 5,000 and 10,000/mm^3. An increased number of leukocytes is called **leukocytosis**; a decreased number is called **leukopenia.** Table 30-2 shows the differential leukocyte count. The life span of leukocytes is only 1 to 2 days; consequently, the demand for the production of WBCs is continuous. The need is even greater with an infection.

Leukocytes are divided into two categories: **granulocytes**, which contain cytoplasmic granules, and **agranulocytes**, which do not contain granules (Fig. 30-3).

Granulocytes

Granulocytes, also called *polymorphonuclear leukocytes*, are divided into three subgroups: neutrophils, basophils, and eosinophils. **Neutrophils** are a major component of the inflammatory response and defense against bacterial infection. Also called *microphages*, they protect the body by **phagocytosis**, the ingestion and digestion of bacteria and foreign substances (Fig. 30-4). Immature neutrophils, called *band cells*, circulate in peripheral blood.

TABLE 30-1 Functions of Blood Components

COMPONENT	FUNCTION
Blood Cells	
Erythrocytes (red blood cells)	Transport oxygen
Leukocytes (white blood cells)	Protect against infection
Platelets (thrombocytes)	Participate in clotting blood
Plasma	
Water	Circulates blood cells and noncellular components
	Contributes to blood pressure
	Relocates to other fluid compartments as needed
Plasma proteins	
Albumin	Affects intravascular osmotic pressure
Fibrinogen	Participates in clotting blood
Globulin	Carries other protein substances, for example, those that are involved in inflammatory and immune responses
Clotting factors	Convert a loose blood clot to a stabilized blood clot
Nutrients	
Glucose	Provides source of immediate energy
Amino acids	Provide components for cell growth and repair
Lipids	Provide a reserve for cellular energy in the absence of glucose
Vitamins	Participate in essential physiologic functions
Electrolytes	Facilitate a variety of biochemical actions
Hormones	Perform multiple endocrine functions
Wastes (carbon dioxide, drug metabolites)	Prevent toxicity when biotransformed and excreted

Basophils are also capable of phagocytosis; they are active in allergic contact dermatitis (immediate hypersensitivity) and some delayed hypersensitivity reactions. **Eosinophils** phagocytize foreign material. Their numbers increase in allergies, some dermatologic disorders, and parasitic infections.

Agranulocytes

Agranulocytes are divided into two groups: *lymphocytes* and *monocytes*. Lymphocytes are divided into *B lymphocytes* (or B cells), which provide humoral immunity by producing antibodies (immunoglobulins), and *T lymphocytes* (or T cells), which provide cellular immunity (or cell-mediated response). B lymphocytes produce antibodies against foreign antigens, and T lymphocytes interact with foreign cells and release a substance called *lymphokine*, which enhances the actions of phagocytic cells. Some lymphoid stem cells mature in the bone marrow, whereas others migrate to peripheral lymphoid tissue to complete their maturation.

Monocytes, also known as *macrophages* because they phagocytize large-sized debris, help combat severe infections and contribute to the immune response. They are antigen-presentation cells, which engulf microbial invaders and display the antigenic surface to T lymphocytes. T lymphocytes then engage B lymphocytes to make the appropriate antibody (see Chap. 34).

TABLE 30-2 Differential White Blood Cell Count

	PERCENT OF TOTAL WBCs	NUMERIC RANGE (mm³)
Neutrophils	60–70	3000–7000
Basophils	1–4	50–400
Eosinophils	0.5–1	25–100
Lymphocytes	20–40	1000–4000
Monocytes	2–6	100–600

Platelets

Platelets (*thrombocytes*) are disklike, non-nucleated cell fragments with a life span of approximately 7.5 days. They are manufactured in the red bone marrow. Approximately two thirds of the total 150,000 to 350,000/mm³ platelets circulate in the blood and contribute to hemostasis. The remaining one third are sequestered in the spleen, where they remain unless needed in cases of significant bleeding. When a blood vessel is injured, platelets migrate to the injury site. The platelets release a substance known as glycoprotein IIb/IIIa, which causes the platelets to adhere (platelet aggregation) and form a plug, or clot, that occludes the injured vessel.

Plasma and Plasma Proteins

Plasma is the liquid, or serum, portion of blood. It consists of 90% water and 10% proteins. Beside blood cells, plasma contains and transports proteins (albumin, globulins, and fibrinogen), clotting factors such as prothrombin, pigments, vitamins, glucose, lipids, electrolytes, minerals, enzymes, and hormones.

Albumin, which is formed in the liver, is the most abundant protein in plasma. Under normal conditions, albumin cannot pass through a capillary wall. Consequently, albumin helps maintain the osmotic pressure that retains fluid in the vascular compartment.

Globulins are divided into three groups: alpha, beta, and gamma. The gamma globulins are also called *immunoglobulins*. Globulins function primarily as immunologic agents; they prevent or modify some types of infectious diseases. Like albumin, they help maintain osmotic pressure in the vascular compartment.

Fibrinogen plays a key role in forming blood clots. It can be transformed from a liquid to fibrin, a solid that controls bleeding.

Granulocytes

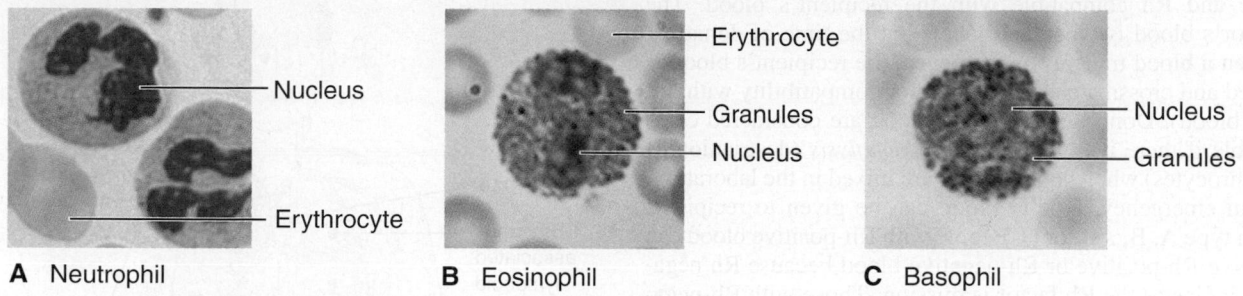

A Neutrophil   **B** Eosinophil   **C** Basophil

Agranulocytes

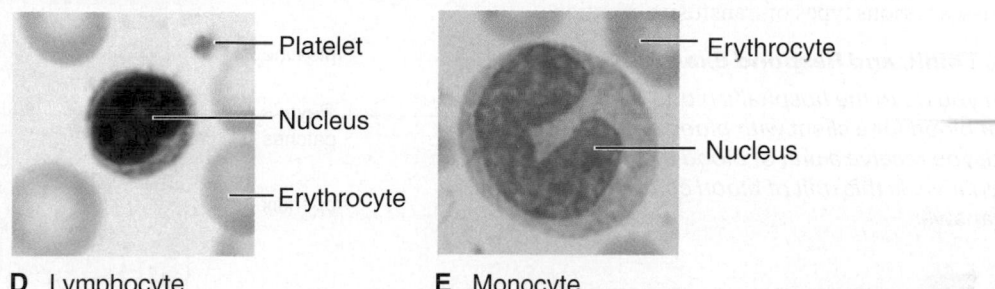

D Lymphocyte   **E** Monocyte

FIGURE 30-3. Categories of leukocytes (or WBCs). *Granulocytes:* (**A**) neutrophil, (**B**) eosinophil, (**C**) basophil. *Agranulocytes:* (**D**) lymphocyte, (**E**) monocyte. (From Cohen, B. J. [2009]. *Memmler's the human body in health and disease.* [11th ed.] Philadelphia: Lippincott Williams & Wilkins.)

Blood Groups

There are four blood groups or types—A, B, AB, and O, which are determined by heredity. Blood type is ascertained by identifying the protein, or *antigen*, on the red cell membranes. Group A has A antigen, group B has B antigen, group AB has A and B antigen, and group O has no antigen. *Antibodies*, immunoglobulins in plasma that inactivate any substance that is nonself, react with incompatible RBC antigens. Therefore, people with type O blood are termed universal donors because they do not have antigens on the red cell membrane. Clients with all other blood types can receive

Type O blood provided the Rh factor is compatible (discussed later). Those with Type O blood, however, can only receive Type O blood. People with type AB blood are considered universal recipients because both A and B antigens are present on the red cell membrane (see Chap. 13 and Table 13-4). Clients with Type AB blood can receive blood from persons with any type of blood, but the Rh factor must be compatible.

The Rh factor is a specific protein on the RBC membrane. If the protein is present, the person is Rh positive. If the protein is absent, the person is Rh negative.

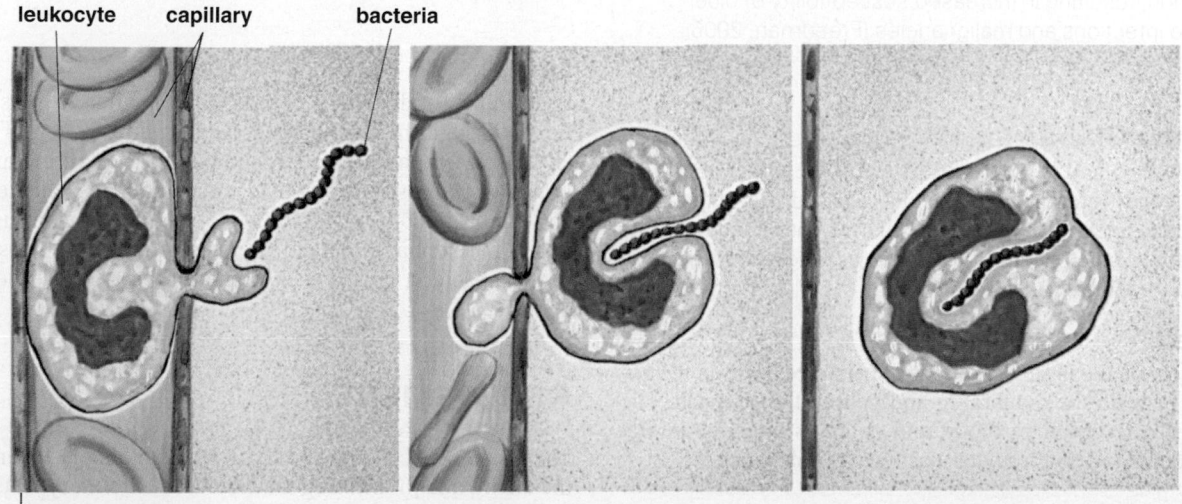

FIGURE 30-4. Phagocytosis. The cell membrane of the neutrophil surrounds and pinches off the bacterium or dead tissue. Enzymes within the cell destroy the foreign material. (From Smeltzer, S. C., et al. [2008]. *Brunner & Suddarth's textbook of medical–surgical nursing* [11th ed.]. Philadelphia: Lippincott Williams & Wilkins.)

When blood is transfused, donor blood must be both type and Rh compatible with the recipient's blood. The donor's blood is typed and labeled at the time of donation. When a blood transfusion is needed, the recipient's blood is typed and crossmatched (matched for compatibility with donor blood). Donor and recipient blood are considered compatible if there is no clumping or *hemolysis* (destruction of erythrocytes) when both samples are mixed in the laboratory. In an emergency, type O blood can be given to recipients with type A, B, AB, or O. People with Rh-positive blood can receive Rh-positive or Rh-negative blood because Rh negative indicates the Rh factor is missing. Those with Rh-negative blood, however, must never receive Rh-positive blood regardless of whether the blood type is compatible. Chapter 13 discusses various types of transfusion reactions.

> ▶ **Stop, Think, and Respond Exercise 30-1**
>
> *When you go to the hospital's blood bank to obtain a unit of blood for a client with blood type A, Rh-positive blood, you receive a unit of blood that is blood type A, Rh negative. Is this unit of blood compatible? Explain your answer.*

LYMPHATIC SYSTEM

The lymphatic system includes the thymus gland, spleen, and a network of lymphatic vessels, lymph nodes, and lymph. This system of **lymphatics** circulates interstitial fluid and carries it to the veins (Fig. 30-5). Along the pathway, the lymphatic system filters and destroys pathogens and removes other potentially harmful substances.

Gerontologic Considerations

- Cellular and humoral immunity are affected by age-related changes in the lymphatic system, including decreases in primary antibody response, T-cell function, and antibody production, resulting in increased susceptibility of older adults to infections and malignancies (Freedman, 2006).

Thymus Gland

The thymus gland is lymphoid tissue in the upper chest that contains undifferentiated stem cells released from bone marrow. Once the undifferentiated cells migrate to the thymus gland, they develop into *T lymphocytes*, so called because they are thymus derived (Fig. 30-6).

Spleen

The spleen is the largest lymphatic structure. It lies in the abdomen beneath the diaphragm and behind the stomach. The spleen is a reservoir of blood and contains phagocytes that engulf damaged erythrocytes and foreign substances.

Lymph Nodes

Lymph nodes, glandular tissue along the lymphatic network, are clustered in the axilla, groin, neck, and large vessels of the thorax and abdomen. Lymphatic ducts, through

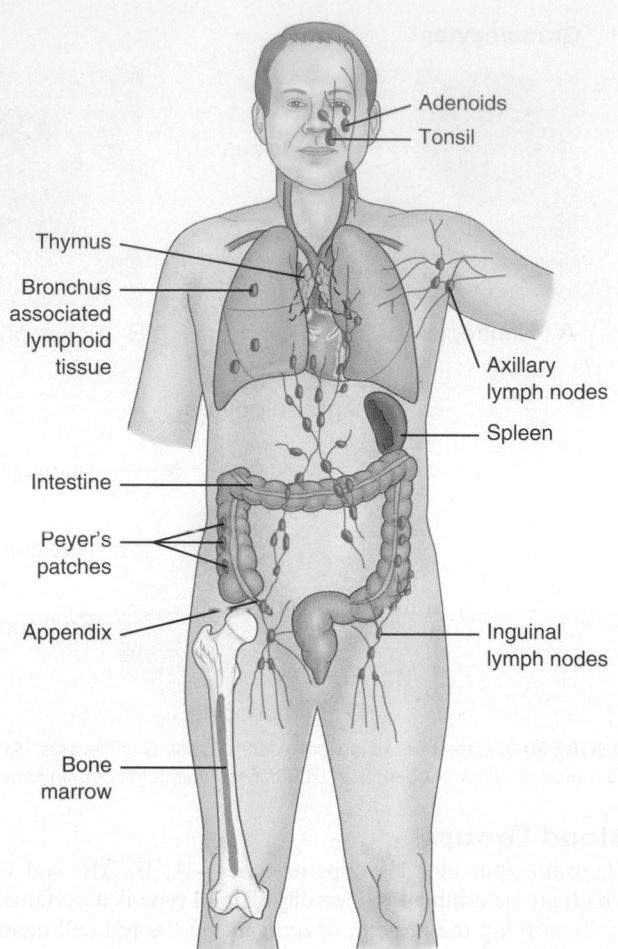

FIGURE 30-5. Central and peripheral lymphoid organs and tissues.

which lymph flows, connect the nodes. The nodes contain both T and B lymphocytes (released from the bone marrow but do not reach the thymus gland) in the smaller nodules of each lymph node.

Lymph

Lymph is fluid with a composition similar to plasma. It flows through the lymphatic system by contraction of skeletal muscles. Lymph enters each node by way of the afferent lymph duct, passes through the node, and leaves by the efferent lymph duct (Fig. 30-7). As lymph passes through the node, macrophages attack and engulf foreign substances such as bacteria and viruses, abnormal body cells, and other debris.

ASSESSMENT

The nurse collects data by taking a health history, examining the client, and monitoring the results of laboratory tests.

History

The health history includes the client's description of signs and symptoms. If abnormalities are present, the nurse

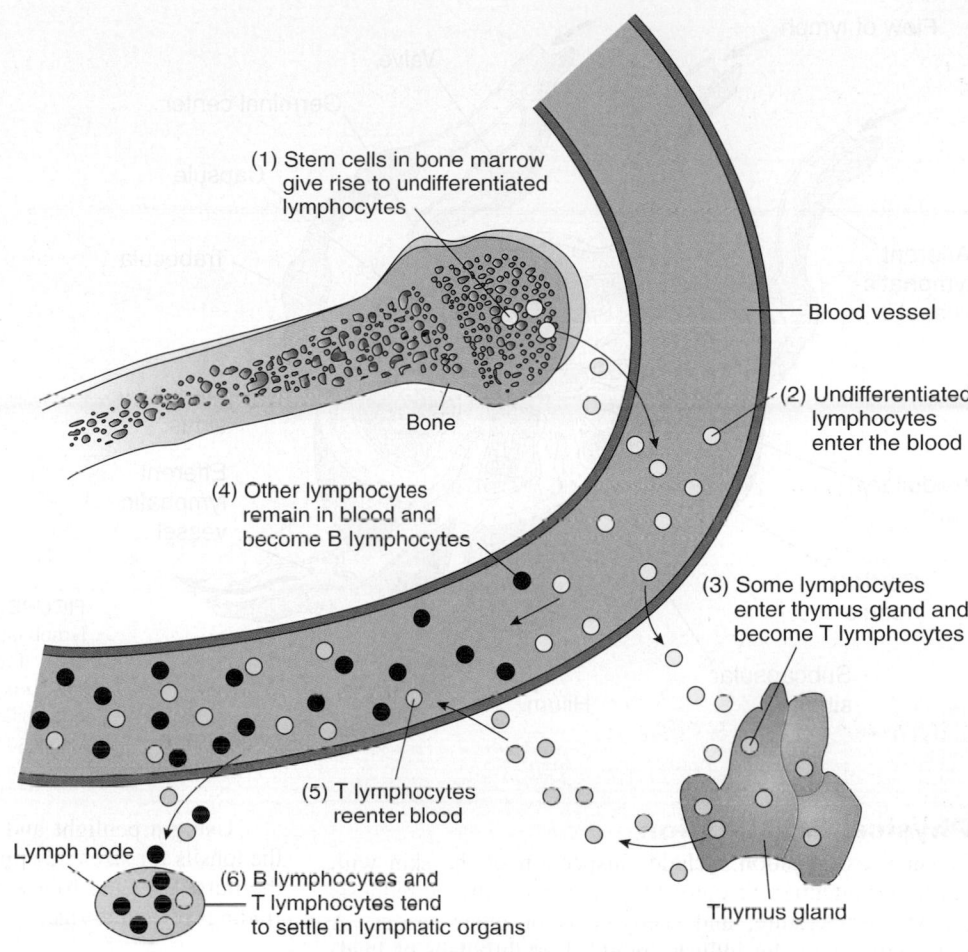

(1) Stem cells in bone marrow give rise to undifferentiated lymphocytes

Bone

Blood vessel

(2) Undifferentiated lymphocytes enter the blood

(4) Other lymphocytes remain in blood and become B lymphocytes

(3) Some lymphocytes enter thymus gland and become T lymphocytes

(5) T lymphocytes reenter blood

Lymph node

(6) B lymphocytes and T lymphocytes tend to settle in lymphatic organs

Thymus gland

FIGURE 30-6. Transformation of T and B lymphocytes.

determines when the signs or symptoms began, their severity, and their frequency. In relation to the hematopoietic and lymphatic systems, it is important to establish if the client:

- Experiences prolonged bleeding from an obvious injury.
- Has unexplained blood loss, as in rectal bleeding, nosebleeds, bleeding gums, or vomiting blood.
- Feels fatigued with normal activities.
- Becomes dizzy or faints.
- Bruises easily.
- Is easily chilled.
- Has frequent infections.
- Feels discomfort in the axilla, groin, or neck.
- Has difficulty swallowing, with localized throat tenderness.
- Has had surgery with lymph node removal or splenectomy, is undergoing treatment for cancer, or has renal failure—all of which may affect blood cell volume or lymphatic circulation.

The nurse obtains a dietary history because compromised nutrition interferes with the production of blood cells and hemoglobin (see Nutrition Notes 30-1).

The nurse takes a drug history of prescription and nonprescription medications. Some antibiotics and cancer drugs contribute to hematopoietic dysfunction. Aspirin and anticoagulants can contribute to bleeding and interfere with clot formation. Because industrial materials, environmental toxins, and household products also can affect blood-forming organs, the nurse explores any exposure to these agents.

 Pharmacologic Considerations

- Many pharmacologic agents affect the hematopoietic system, causing a decrease in various blood components. Closely monitor clients taking medications that depress the hematopoietic system, particularly thrombocytes and leukocytes, for signs of leukopenia (fever, sore throat, chills) and thrombocytopenia (unusual or easy bleeding, oozing from injection sites, bleeding gums, dark, tarry stools).

- The drug epoetin alfa (Epogen, Procrit) can be used to stimulate the production of RBCs. Filgrastim (Neupogen) and pelfigrastim (Neulasta) promote proliferation of neutrophils.

The nurse also asks about foreign travel to countries where malaria or parasitic roundworms are common. The agent that causes malaria following the bite of an infected mosquito invades erythrocytes and causes anemia. Filariasis, also known as elephantiasis, is a consequence of a roundworm infection in which the lymphatic vessels become occluded.

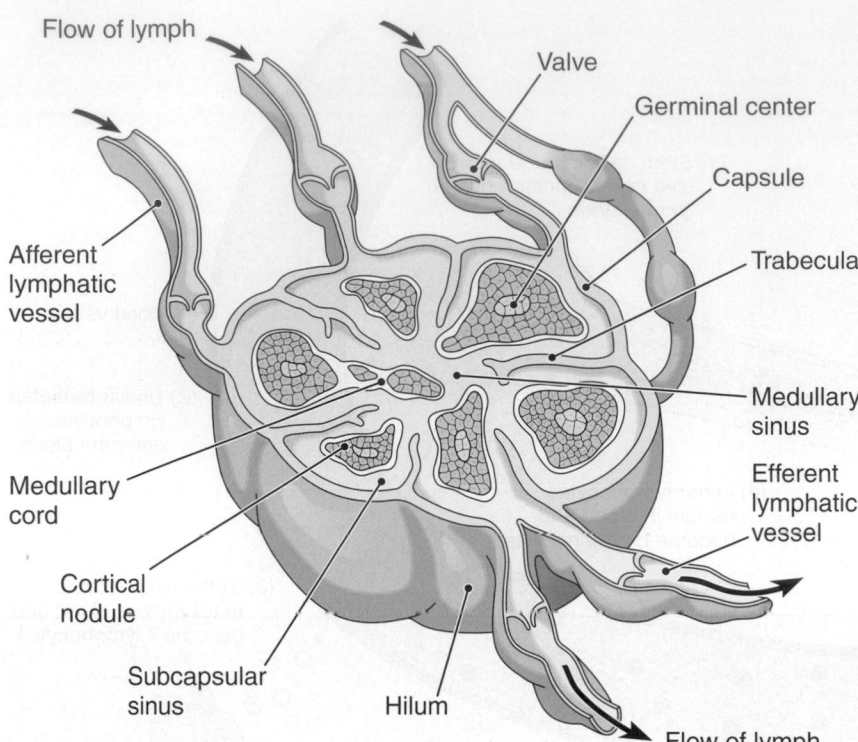

Flow of lymph

Valve

Germinal center

Capsule

Trabecula

Afferent lymphatic vessel

Medullary sinus

Efferent lymphatic vessel

Medullary cord

Cortical nodule

Subcapsular sinus

Hilum

Flow of lymph

FIGURE 30 7. Structure of a lymph node. The lymph filters out bacteria that gain entry to the body. (From Cohen, B. J. [2009]. *Memmler's the human body in health and disease.* [11th ed.] Philadelphia: Lippincott Williams & Wilkins.)

Physical Examination

Physical examination includes inspection of the skin with particular attention to color (e.g., normal, extreme redness, pallor), temperature, and ecchymosis or other lesions. A rapid pulse rate can indicate reduced erythrocytes or inadequate hemoglobin levels.

The nurse palpates the lymph nodes in the neck for tenderness or swelling and notes the size, location, and characteristics of symptomatic lymph nodes (Fig. 30-8). He or she examines the skin adjacent to the node for redness, streaking, and swelling.

Using a penlight and tongue blade, the nurse inspects the tonsils for size and appearance. If the tonsils are present, the nurse uses the following scale to document assessment findings related to size:

- 1 = Tonsils are visible
- 2 = Tonsils extend medially toward the uvula
- 3 = Tonsils touch the uvula
- 4 = Tonsils touch each other

Purulent exudate on the surface of the tonsils suggests tonsillitis.

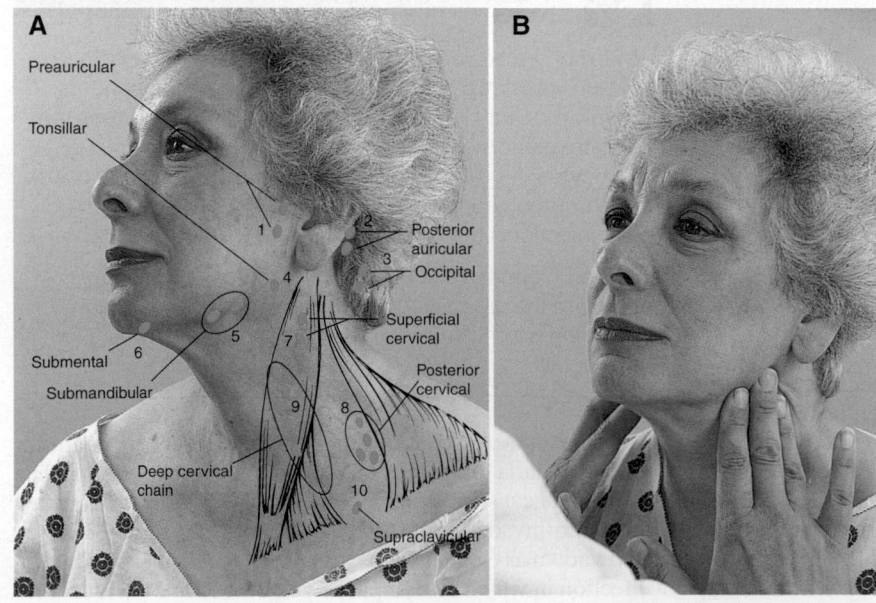

FIGURE 30-8. Assessment of cervical lymph nodes. **(A)** Locations of lymph nodes in the head and neck. **(B)** Palpation of tonsillar lymph nodes. (Photos © B. Proud.)

The nurse examines the extremities to determine if they are of similar size—obstruction of lymphatic circulation can cause unilateral enlargement.

Diagnostic Tests

The nurse obtains a blood sample from a vein, finger, or earlobe. The blood sample is used to perform a complete blood count or to measure the hemoglobin. The physician may order other blood tests that reflect the client's clotting status, such as prothrombin time, fibrinogen level, activated partial thromboplastin time, D-dimer test for fibrin, fibrin degradation products, and factor assays.

A bone marrow aspiration is performed to determine the status of blood cell formation. In this procedure, the physician applies local anesthesia and removes bone marrow from the posterior iliac crest or the sternum. The marrow is examined for the types and percentage of immature and maturing blood cells. The nurse assists the physician, supports the client during the procedure, and monitors the client's status afterward (Nursing Guidelines 30-1).

A Schilling test is used to diagnose pernicious anemia, macrocytic anemia, and malabsorption syndromes. When this test is prescribed, radioactive vitamin B_{12} is given orally, followed in 1 hour by an injection of nonradioactive B_{12}. All urine is collected for 24 to 48 hours after the client receives the nonradioactive B_{12}. Little or no vitamin B_{12} in the urine indicates absence of the intrinsic factor or defective absorption of vitamin B_{12} from the intestinal tract.

Gerontologic Considerations

- The Schilling test may pose a problem in older adults if proper collection of the 24-hour specimen is not possible as a result of cognitive problems or urinary incontinence. The Schilling test is rarely ordered to detect B_{12} deficiencies for older adults because the cause of pernicious anemia in the older population is usually gastric hypoacidity. However, the full Schilling test is indicated if bacterial overgrowth, another cause of B_{12} deficiency, is suspected (Freedman, 2006).

Lymphatic disorders are diagnosed using procedures such as lymph node biopsy, ultrasound of the spleen or selected lymph nodes, and lymphangiography (radiographic examination using contrast media). Additional diagnostic tests include radiography, computed tomography, bone scan, and magnetic resonance imaging. Although they are not specific for hematologic or lymphatic disorders, they are used to rule out other disorders or note changes in organs that have a direct or indirect relationship to a hematologic or lymphatic disorder.

NURSING MANAGEMENT

The nurse collects appropriate data to assist the physician in diagnosing hematologic or lymphatic disorders and the client's response to treatment. Before any diagnostic testing, the nurse determines the client's knowledge of the procedure and offers a description of the test routine, what tasks are necessary to participate in the test, and what discomfort is likely.

The nurse wears gloves when collecting specimens. After collection, he or she checks the specimen for the correct label and immediately takes it to the laboratory. When the test involves a puncture, the nurse assesses the area for excessive bleeding and applies pressure or a pressure dressing to the site as needed. The nurse monitors vital signs to assess the client's recovery, notifies the physician regarding adverse responses, and analyzes and reports test results promptly.

NURSING GUIDELINES 30-1

Assisting With a Bone Marrow Aspiration

- Inform the client of the plan and approximate time for the bone marrow aspiration. Allow time to answer questions.
- Witness the client's signature on a consent form for the procedure as well as for conscious sedation.
- Check the client's medical record for history of allergies, especially to local anesthetics or latex, and the results of coagulation studies that may have been performed.
- Obtain a sterile bone marrow aspiration tray and the type and strength of local anesthetic according to the physician's orders.
- Determine the site from which the physician intends to obtain the sample of bone marrow, for example, iliac crest or sternum.
- Attach a pulse oximeter to the client's finger to monitor oxygenation that may be compromised when conscious sedation is used.
- Position the client on his or her back or side to facilitate access to the aspiration site.
- Cleanse, clip hair, and drape the skin at the test site.
- Suggest distraction techniques to avoid focusing on the pressure or discomfort associated with puncturing the bone that may take approximately 20 minutes.

- Administer analgesia for significant discomfort.
- Be prepared to place samples of the aspirate on slides and allow them to dry.
- Label the biopsy specimen in preservative and ensure its delivery to the laboratory.
- Follow Standard Precautions when there is a potential for contact with blood from the client, equipment, and bedside environment.
- Apply direct pressure followed by a pressure dressing to the site after the needle has been withdrawn.
- Instruct the client to lie on the site for at least 10 minutes or longer.
- Limit the client's activity for approximately 30 minutes after the procedure.
- Monitor the puncture site frequently for continued bleeding; change or reinforce the dressing as needed.
- Report prolonged bleeding, unusual pain at the site that is unrelieved by analgesics, fever, and other signs of an infection such as swelling and purulent drainage.
- Delay bathing or showering for 24 hours.

[TH]INKING EXERCISES

[...]s of blood cell formation.

[...] responsibilities when assisting with [...]tion.

[...]he following blood count values:

Client A — 80,000/mm³ platelets
Client B = 2,400,000/mm³ RBCs
Client C = 24,500/mm³ WBCs

After notifying the physician, what precautions are appropriate to institute?

4. A client reports feeling chronic fatigue and chilled when others feel comfortable. The client has a heart rate of 92 beats/minute at rest and a blood pressure of 110/60 mm Hg. The skin, conjunctiva, and mucous membranes are pale. What additional information is important to obtain? What laboratory or diagnostic tests can the nurse anticipate the physician will order?

NCLEX-STYLE REVIEW QUESTIONS

1. A physician tells a client that her body is not making enough blood cells. After the physician leaves, the client appears very upset and states, "I do not even know how my body is supposed to make blood cells." What is the simplest, yet correct, instruction for the nurse to give the client at this time?
   1. Complex mechanisms within the body make blood cells.
   2. The bone marrow produces blood cells.
   3. Blood cells originate from a healthy immune system.
   4. The lymphatic system produces blood cells.

2. After completion of a bone marrow aspiration, it is essential that the nurse monitor which of the following?
   1. Fluctuations in blood pressure
   2. Bleeding from the puncture site
   3. Changes in the client's pulse
   4. The client's level of consciousness

3. A complete blood count indicates that a client is anemic. Which of the following disorders in the client's health history is most likely contributing to the reduction in red blood cells?
   1. Osteoarthritis
   2. Renal failure
   3. Emphysema
   4. Diabetes mellitus

4. When the nurse reviews a client's complete blood cell count, which of the following is most suggestive that a client is at risk for acquiring an infection?
   1. Low number of platelets
   2. Low number of erythrocytes
   3. Low number of granulocytes
   4. Low number of agranulocytes

5. Which of the following blood types could be transfused into anyone if there is not time to perform a type and crossmatch of the recipient's blood?
   1. AB, Rh positive
   2. AB, Rh negative
   3. O, Rh positive
   4. O, Rh negative

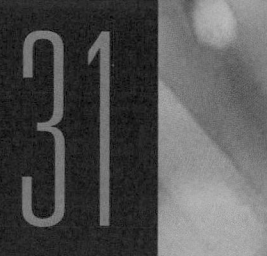

31

Caring for Clients with Disorders of the Hematopoietic System

Words To Know

acute chest syndrome
agranulocytosis
anemia
aplasia
blood dyscrasias
coagulopathies
erythrocytosis
heme
leukocytosis
leukopenia
pancytopenia
sickle cell anemia
thrombocytopenia

Learning Objectives

On completion of this chapter, you will be able to:

1. List seven types of anemia, including examples of inherited types.
2. Identify nutritional deficiencies that can lead to anemia.
3. Discuss clinical problems that clients with any type of anemia experience.
4. Discuss factors that cause sickling of erythrocytes and related adverse effects.
5. List activities a person with sickle cell disease can do to reduce the potential for a sickle cell crisis.
6. Explain the term *erythrocytosis*, give one example of a characteristic disease, and list possible complications.
7. Explain how forms of leukemia are classified.
8. List clinical problems or nursing diagnoses common among clients with leukemia.
9. Explain how the bone marrow dysfunction of multiple myeloma has an effect on the skeletal system.
10. Differentiate agranulocytosis from leukopenia.
11. Explain the term *pancytopenia* and give an example of a disorder that represents this condition.
12. Discuss the meaning of *coagulopathy* and name two coagulopathies.
13. Discuss nursing responsibilities when managing the care of clients with coagulopathies.

This chapter discusses common **blood dyscrasias**, abnormalities in the numbers and types of blood cells, and **coagulopathies**, bleeding disorders that involve platelets or clotting factors. These disorders develop from various pathologic processes, some of which are life-threatening. Despite their differences, many blood disorders have similar symptoms and require similar diagnostic tests.

ANEMIA

Erythrocytes are mature red blood cells (RBCs) to which hemoglobin is attached. Their function is to carry oxygen to cells and transport carbon dioxide (CO_2) to the lungs. **Anemia** is a term that refers to a deficiency of either erythrocytes or hemoglobin. Various terms are used to differentiate the features of erythrocytes and describe pathogenesis related to them (Table 31-1).

Most anemias result from (1) blood loss, (2) inadequate or abnormal erythrocyte production, or (3) destruction of normally formed RBCs. The most common types include hypovolemic anemia, iron deficiency anemia, pernicious anemia, folic acid deficiency anemia, sickle cell anemia, and hemolytic anemias. Although each form of anemia has unique manifestations, all share a common core of symptoms (Box 31-1).

TABLE 31-1 Terms Used to Describe Erythrocytes and Erythrocyte Pathology

DESCRIPTOR	MEANING
Normocytic	Normal cell size
Microcytic	Small cell size
Macrocytic	Large cell size
Megaloblastic	Large immature cell
Normochromic	Normal hemoglobin concentration
Hypochromic	Low hemoglobin concentration
Hyperchromic	High hemoglobin concentration
Aplastic	Decreased cell production
Hemolytic	Premature destruction
Pernicious	Potentially injurious

HYPOVOLEMIC ANEMIA

Hypovolemia is caused by a loss of blood volume, which results in fewer blood cells. Because erythrocytes are the most abundant type of blood cell, one consequence of blood loss is *hypovolemic anemia*.

Pathophysiology and Etiology

A sudden loss of a large volume of blood or a gradual, chronic loss of small amounts of blood causes hypovolemic anemia. An example of the former is trauma, such as a gunshot wound; an example of the latter is gastric bleeding from a peptic ulcer. When blood is lost, the bone marrow responds by increasing production of erythrocytes. As a result, the cells are smaller and contain less **heme**, the pigmented, iron-containing portion of hemoglobin. Consequently, the RBCs are microcytic and hypochromic (see Table 31-1). If the formation of new RBCs cannot compensate for the loss, cellular

BOX 31-1 **Clinical Manifestations of Anemia**

Inadequate RBC Volume
Orthostatic hypotension
Thready pulses
Oliguria
Heart murmur

Compensatory Mechanisms for Lost RBC Function
Tachycardia
Tachypnea
Cool, clammy skin
Amenorrhea

Decreased RBC Function
Dyspnea
Chest discomfort
Acidosis
Headache
Vertigo
Pallor
Constipation
Difficulty concentrating
Decreased bowel sounds

function is compromised from an inadequate oxygen supply and accumulated CO_2.

Assessment Findings

Acute hypovolemic anemia from severe blood loss is evidenced by signs and symptoms of hypovolemic shock: extreme pallor, tachycardia, hypotension, reduced urine output, and altered consciousness (see Chap. 17). Symptoms of chronic hypovolemic anemia include pallor, fatigue, chills, postural hypotension, and rapid heart and respiratory rates.

Laboratory confirmation of acute or chronic hypovolemic anemia is detected through a complete blood count (CBC), which demonstrates decreased erythrocytes, increased *reticulocytes* (erythrocytes in the process of maturation), and low hemoglobin and hematocrit levels (Table 31-2). Mean cell volume is lower than normal as a result of the smaller size of the erythrocytes. The mean cell hemoglobin concentration is below normal, reflecting the reduced hemoglobin level.

Medical Management

Treatment of sudden severe bleeding requires replacement of blood by transfusions. If blood loss is chronic (e.g., from bleeding uterine tumors, peptic ulcer disease, hemorrhoids), the underlying condition is treated. Depending on how much blood is lost, treatment includes blood transfusion or administration of oral, intravenous (IV), or intramuscular (IM) iron to help restore the body's hemoglobin. Oxygen therapy sometimes is necessary if the anemia is severe.

Nursing Process for the Client with Hypovolemic Anemia

Assessment

Question the client to determine possible reasons for the presenting symptoms, obtain vital signs, review laboratory test results, prepare the client for diagnostic tests such as endoscopic examinations, and perform a physical examination to detect sources of bleeding.

Diagnosis, Planning, and Interventions

▶ PC: Hypovolemia

▶ Expected Outcome: The nurse will monitor to detect hypovolemia and manage and minimize blood loss.

• Monitor the results of CBC, especially RBC count and hematocrit and hemoglobin levels. *Lower than normal RBCs and hemoglobin level reflect blood cell loss. The hematocrit level indicates the percentage of RBCs in the volume of whole blood.*

• Assess vital signs every 2 to 4 hours or more often if indicated. *Hypotension and tachycardia are signs of hypovolemia. Changes in vital signs indicate worsening, stabilization, or improvement in the client's condition.*

• Report systolic blood pressure (BP) below 90 mm Hg and heart rate above 100 beats/minute (bpm). *The average adult systolic BP is 120 mm Hg. Decreasing blood pressure reflects hypovolemia and shock. Tachycardia is a heart rate above 100 bpm. A rapid heart rate indicates a compensatory mechanism to oxygenate cells.*

TABLE 31-2 Normal CBC Values

COMPONENT	ADULT MALES	ADULT FEMALES
Red blood cells (erythrocytes)	4.6–6.2 million/mm^3	4.2–5.4 million/mm^3
Hematocrit	40%–54%	38%–47%
Hemoglobin	13.5–18 g/dL	12–16 g/dL
Mean cell volume (MCV)	80–94 μg/m^3	81–99 μg/m^3
Mean cell hemoglobin (MCH)	27–31 picograms/cell	27–31 picograms/cell
Mean cell hemoglobin concentration (MCHC)	32–36 g/dL	32–36 g/dL
Reticulocytes	0.5%–2.0% of RBCs	Slightly higher in females
White blood cells (leukocytes)	5000–13,000/mm^3	5000–10,000/mm^3
Neutrophils	3000–7500/mm^3	3000–7500/mm^3
Eosinophils	50–400/mm^3	50–400/mm^3
Basophils	25–100/mm^3	25–100/mm^3
Monocytes	100–500/mm^3	100–500/mm^3
Lymphocytes	1500–4500/mm^3	1500–4500/mm^3
T lymphocytes	60%–80% of lymphocytes	60%–80% of lymphocytes
B lymphocytes	10%–20% of lymphocytes	10%–20% of lymphocytes
Platelets	150,000–450,000/mm^3	150,000–450,000/mm^3

- Monitor intake and output accurately each shift or every hour. *Urine output is one indication of the circulating blood volume.*
- Report urine output less than 30 to 50 mL/hour. *Low urine volume reflects inadequate renal perfusion. The kidneys must excrete 30 to 50 mL/hour or 500 mL/24 hours to eliminate wastes sufficiently.*
- Use Standard Precautions to examine and test stool and body fluids for evidence of blood. *Blood may be occult (hidden) rather than obvious. Nurses commonly perform tests to detect blood in stool and body fluids.*
- In cases of hemorrhage, apply direct pressure to the bleeding site. Alternatively, apply pressure to a proximal artery. *Compression of blood vessels decreases blood loss.*
- If an IV solution is infusing, increase the rate of flow if the client is bleeding profusely. *A temporary increase in IV fluid administration compensates briefly for rapid blood loss.*
- Place the client in a modified Trendelenburg position if hypovolemic shock develops. *This position facilitates blood flow to the brain.*
- Notify the physician and be prepared to administer blood or blood products. *Crystalloid solutions do not contain blood cells (see Chap. 13). The most definitive management of hypovolemic anemia is to replace lost blood cells.*
- Supplement parenteral fluids with oral fluids, if possible. *Oral fluids contribute to intravascular fluid replacement.*

▶ PC: Hypoxemia

▶ **Expected Outcome:** The nurse will monitor to detect hypoxemia and manage and minimize inadequate oxygenation.

- Monitor oxygen saturation continuously with a pulse oximeter. *It measures the percentage of oxygen bound to hemoglobin.*
- Report a sustained oxygen saturation value below 90%. *Normal oxygen saturation is 95% to 100%; clients become compromised when oxygen saturation falls below 90%.*
- Give oxygen per nasal cannula or simple mask to maintain oxygen saturation at or above 90%. *Supplemental oxygen delivers more than 21% oxygen of room air.*

▶ Activity Intolerance related to reduced cellular capacity to carry oxygen

▶ **Expected Outcomes:** The client will (1) tolerate essential activity as evidenced by a heart rate below 100 bpm and (2) have a respiratory rate less than 28 breaths/minute.

- Limit the client's nonessential activities. *Demands for cellular oxygenation are controlled according to the available supply.*
- Distribute essential tasks over a long period. *Minimizing exertion promotes endurance.*
- Provide periods of rest. *Rest prevents acute hypoxemia.*
- Administer supplemental oxygen during periods of rapid breathing or tachycardia. *Short-term, periodic oxygen administration relieves brief episodes of hypoxemia.*

▶ Risk for Imbalanced Body Temperature related to reduced oxygen for aerobic metabolism

▶ **Expected Outcome:** Temperature will remain at 98.6°F plus or minus 1°F.

- Prevent drafts. *Air circulating over the body promotes heat loss by convection.*
- Provide additional layers of clothing or cover with warmed blankets. *Covering the client in layers of fabric keeps body heat from escaping.*
- Increase the room temperature and add humidity. *Warming the environment decreases heat loss from convection or conduction. The heat index increases when air contains moisture. Increasing environmental humidity reduces heat loss through evaporation.*
- Offer warm oral fluids. *They maintain or promote an increase in core body temperature.*

Evaluation of Expected Outcomes

Blood volume is restored or blood loss is minimized; RBC count and hematocrit level are within normal ranges. The client has 90% or greater saturation of hemoglobin. The client's BP and heart rate are within normal target ranges before, during, and after performing activities of daily living (ADLs). Body temperature is within 97.6°F to 99.6°F. ●

IRON DEFICIENCY ANEMIA
Pathophysiology and Etiology

Iron deficiency anemia develops when iron is insufficient to produce hemoglobin. Examples include when (1) heme cannot be recycled because of blood loss, (2) dietary intake of iron is insufficient, (3) absorption of iron from food is inadequate, and (4) the need for iron exceeds the reserves. Even when a person consumes a healthy diet, he or she absorbs less than 10% of the iron in food. Clients whose nutrition is compromised by unhealthy dieting or who cannot afford to eat a healthy diet, lack knowledge about nutrition, or have malabsorption disorders are at great risk for iron deficiency anemia. The need for iron increases during periods of rapid growth, pregnancy, and the female reproductive years when intermittent blood loss accompanies menses.

Gerontologic Considerations

- Iron deficiency anemia is unusual in older adults. Normally, the body does not eliminate excessive iron, causing total body iron stores to increase with age and necessitating maintenance of hydration. If an older adult is anemic, blood loss from the gastrointestinal or genitourinary tract is suspected. Iron deficiency anemia can develop in older adults because of inadequate intake of iron for many reasons, including living on a fixed income, being unable to shop for food, and lacking energy or motivation to prepare complete meals. These clients require a thorough evaluation of their dietary habits and education in the methods of preventing iron deficiency anemia.

When iron deficiency develops, the iron stores in the body are depleted first, followed by reduced hemoglobin. The result is smaller (microcytic) and fewer RBCs, which leads to manifestations of anemia. Reduced hemoglobin, for whatever reason, compromises the oxygen-carrying capacity of RBCs. Without sufficient oxygen, cells must switch to anaerobic metabolism, which is less efficient than aerobic metabolism at producing energy and sustaining functions at the cellular level.

Assessment Findings

Most clients with iron deficiency anemia have reduced energy, feel cold all the time, and experience fatigue and dyspnea with minor physical exertion. The heart rate usually is rapid even at rest. The CBC and hemoglobin, hematocrit, and serum iron levels are decreased. A blood smear reveals erythrocytes that are *microcytic* (smaller than normal) and *hypochromic* (lighter in color than normal). Other laboratory and diagnostic tests (e.g., stool examination for occult blood) reveal the source of blood loss.

Medical Management

Treatment aims at determining the cause and, when possible, eliminating it. Correction of a faulty diet by adding foods high in iron is an important aspect of treatment. In some instances, an oral supplement or parenteral administration of iron is prescribed. In severe cases, a blood transfusion is necessary, but transfusion is the most expensive and potentially dangerous method for replacing iron.

Pharmacologic Considerations

- To correct iron deficiency anemia, 200 mg ferrous sulfate is given three times per day, 1 hour before meals. Therapeutic response is monitored through periodic hemoglobin and hematocrit counts. If the client cannot swallow tablets, liquid iron preparations are available.

Nursing Management

The nurse focuses on improving the client's nutritional intake of iron. The nurse takes a dietary history and collaborates with the dietitian to resolve dietary deficiencies (Nutrition Notes 31-1). In addition, he or she administers the prescribed oral or parenteral iron supplementation. If a client is taking an oral iron supplement, the nurse instructs as follows:

- Dilute liquid preparations of iron with another liquid such as juice and drink with a straw to avoid staining the teeth.
- Take iron on an empty stomach unless gastric upset occurs; then take with or immediately after meals.
- Avoid taking iron simultaneously with an antacid, which interferes with iron absorption.
- Check with the physician or pharmacist about combining iron with other prescribed or over-the-counter medications to determine appropriate absorption of each.
- Drink orange juice or take other forms of vitamin C with iron to promote its absorption.
- Expect iron to color stool dark green or black.
- Consult the prescribing physician if constipation or diarrhea develops.
- Keep medications containing iron out of the reach of small children, for whom an accidental poisoning may be fatal.

Nutrition Notes 31-1
The Client with Iron Deficiency Anemia

- Heme iron is found in animal foods, such as beef, pork, lamb, egg yolks, oysters, and the dark meat of poultry. It is well absorbed, and its rate of absorption is influenced only by need, not by other dietary factors.
- Adding 3 servings of lean meats per week in the context of a nutrient-rich diet is recommended to help correct iron deficiency anemia.
- Nonheme iron is found in plant foods such as enriched and whole-grain breads, iron-fortified cereals, legumes, and nuts.
- Absorption of nonheme iron is greatly affected by other dietary factors. Vitamin C (citrus fruits and juices, strawberries, red peppers, tomatoes) and foods high in heme iron *enhance* the absorption of nonheme iron when eaten at the same time. Tea, coffee, and wheat bran *inhibit* the absorption of nonheme iron when eaten at the same time.
- To maximize nonheme iron absorption, the client should consume a rich source of vitamin C at every meal and avoid coffee and tea around and during mealtime.

The nurse uses the Z-track technique to administer IM iron (Nursing Guidelines 31-1). For a review of blood transfusion, see Chapter 13. Discharge instructions include pacing activities to minimize fatigue and providing information about oral medications and medical follow-up to determine if the client's hemoglobin level stabilizes within normal limits.

> ▶ **Stop, Think, and Respond Exercise 31-1**
>
> *Why does the nurse use the Z-track technique to administer parenteral iron?*

SICKLE CELL ANEMIA

Sickle cell anemia is so named because erythrocytes become sickle- or crescent-shaped when oxygen supply in the blood is inadequate (Fig. 31-1). This common genetic disorder, found primarily in African Americans but also in people from Mediterranean and Middle Eastern countries, currently affects 1 in every 600 African Americans in the United States (Platt, 2005).

Pathophysiology and Etiology

Hemoglobin A (HbA) normally replaces fetal hemoglobin (HbF) about 6 months after birth. In people with sickle cell anemia, however, an abnormal form of hemoglobin, hemoglobin S (HbS), replaces HbF. HbS causes RBCs to assume a sickled shape under hypoxic conditions.

Sickle cell disease is a hereditary disorder. To manifest this disorder, a person must inherit two defective genes, one from each parent, in which case all the hemoglobin is inherently abnormal. If the person inherits only one gene, he or she carries sickle cell trait. The hemoglobin of those who have sickle cell trait is about 40% affected. Consequently, these people are at less risk for developing signs and symptoms than those who have two defective genes. Many more people have sickle cell trait than have sickle cell disease.

NURSING GUIDELINES 31-1

Administering an Intramuscular Injection by Z-Track Technique

1. Check the medical orders. Read and compare the label on the drug container with the medical order or medication administration record at least three times.
2. Check the client's identity using the identification bracelet.
3. Determine the client's understanding of the purpose and technique for the procedure.
4. Inspect the dorsogluteal site.
5. Obtain the necessary equipment.
6. Wash your hands.
7. Fill the syringe with the prescribed amount of drug and change the needle.
8. Draw up an additional 0.2 mL of air in the syringe.
9. Attach a needle that is at least $1\frac{1}{2}$ to 2 inches long.
10. Don gloves.
11. Position the client on the abdomen or side depending on which injection site you use.
12. Using the side of your hand, pull the tissue laterally about 1 inch (2.5 cm) until it is taut (see Figure A). Swab the site with an alcohol pledget.
13. Insert the needle at a 90° angle while continuing to hold the tissue laterally (see Figure B).
14. Steady the barrel of the syringe with the fingers and use the thumb to manipulate the plunger.
15. Aspirate for a blood return.
16. Instill the medication by depressing the plunger with the thumb.
17. Wait 10 seconds with the needle in place and the skin still held taut.
18. Withdraw the needle and immediately release the taut skin (see Figure C).
19. Apply direct pressure to the injection site with a gauze square, but do not rub it.
20. Cover the injection site with a bandage or gauze square and tape.
21. Discard the syringe without recapping the needle.
22. Remove your gloves and wash your hands.
23. Document the medication administration.

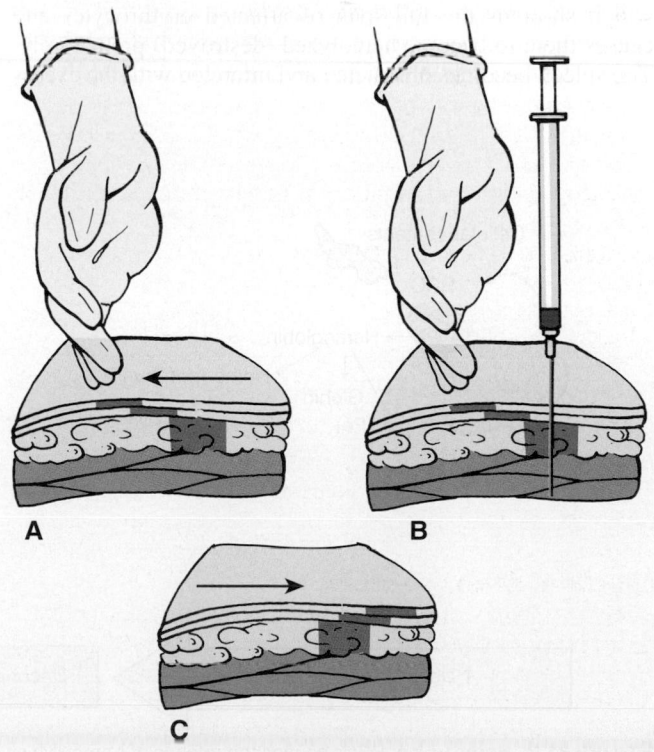

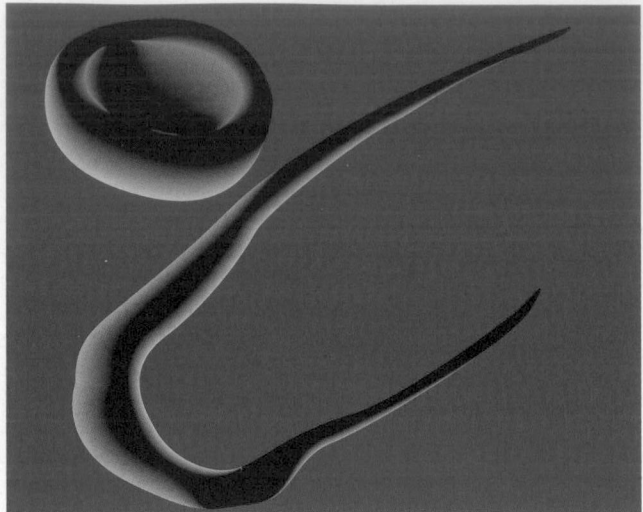

FIGURE 31-1. A normal spherical red blood cell and a sickled cell. (From Smeltzer, S. C. & Bare, B. G. [2008]. *Brunner & Suddarth's textbook of medical–surgical nursing* [11th ed.]. Philadelphia: Lippincott Williams & Wilkins.)

The person with sickle cell anemia suffers from two problems: (1) episodes of *sickle cell crisis* from vascular occlusion, which develops rapidly under hypoxic conditions; and (2) chronic hemolytic anemia. During a sickle cell crisis, the sickle-shaped cells lodge in small blood vessels, where they block the flow of blood and oxygen to the affected tissue. The vascular occlusion induces severe pain in the ischemic tissue. Stroke is a common complication, even in young children.

The anemia results from the defective HbS molecule, which shortens the life span of affected erythrocytes and causes them to become hemolyzed (destroyed) prematurely. The spleen becomes obstructed and infarcted with the excess

dead erythrocytes. The bone marrow enlarges to compensate for the continuous need to produce more erythrocytes. The persistent anemia causes tachycardia, dyspnea, cardiomegaly (enlargement of the heart), and dysrhythmias. Liver dysfunction occurs in about 10% of those affected.

Once the spleen is damaged, risk of infection, especially pneumonia, increases. Hypoperfusion and hypoxia also leave the affected person susceptible to pathogens. One of the unique manifestations of sickle cell disease is **acute chest syndrome**, a type of pneumonia triggered by decreased hemoglobin and infiltrates in the lungs. Acute chest syndrome is characterized by respiratory symptoms such as coughing, wheezing, tachypnea, and chest pain.

Assessment Findings

Signs and Symptoms

Evidence of the accelerated rate of erythrocyte destruction is manifested by jaundice caused by *hyperbilirubinemia* (excess bilirubin pigment in the blood; Fig. 31-2). Secondary consequences include gallstones (see Chap. 47) or a predisposition to infection when the spleen becomes dysfunctional. Anaerobic metabolism compromises growth. Chronic leg ulcers develop from the blockage of the small blood vessels of the legs. Priapism (prolonged erection) occurs from delayed emptying of thick blood from the penis (see Chap. 55). Signs and symptoms of anemia also are present.

The reduced blood flow during sickle cell crisis leads to localized ischemia, severe pain, and possible tissue infarction (necrosis) if the oxygen supply is inadequate. Fever, pain, and swelling of one or more joints are common. Other symptoms depend on the blood vessels involved. Sickle cell crisis can lead to cerebrovascular accident, pulmonary infarction, shock, and renal failure.

Diagnostic Findings

A sickle cell screening test called the *Sickledex test* determines the presence of abnormal HbS. Hemoglobin

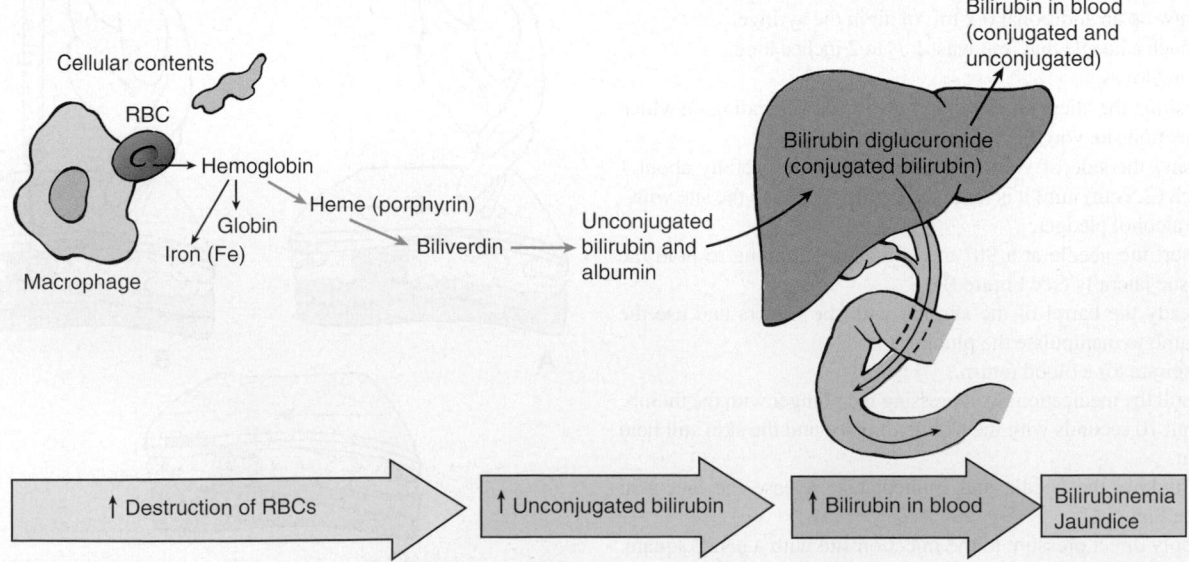

FIGURE 31-2. Hemolysis of RBCs causes the release of heme, which becomes unconjugated bilirubin and must be conjugated in the liver for excretion into the bile. Increased amounts of bilirubin lead to bilirubinemia and jaundice.

electrophoresis determines whether the person has sickle cell disease or carries the sickle cell trait. Hemoglobin levels tend to range between 7 and 10 g/dL in those with sickle cell disease. An increase in secretory phospholipase A is a predictor of acute chest syndrome.

Medical Management

Treatment is supportive rather than curative. Regular blood transfusions decrease the risk of stroke and other complications of infarction. Transfused blood, however, increases blood viscosity (thickness), which can potentially do more harm than good. It also can result in sensitization to minor antigens in donor blood—especially when the source of the donor blood is from someone of different ethnic origin than the recipient. Treatment with hydroxyurea (Hydrea, Droxia), an anticancer agent, shows evidence that it decreases sickling (Anderson, 2006; Porth, 2008). Hydroxyurea is toxic to RBCs with defective hemoglobin. Consequently, the body uses a yet unknown alternative method of hematopoiesis to produce RBCs with HbF (fetal hemoglobin), present during intrauterine development through 6 months of age. Drug-induced formation of HbF, which has a high affinity for oxygen, has several benefits: it induces a milder form of the disease, decreases organ damage, protects against vaso-occlusion, and reduces early mortality (Jones, Davies, & Olujohungbe, 2007).

Pharmacologic Considerations

- Antineoplastic agents, such as hydroxyurea, produce many serious adverse effects. Be thoroughly familiar with the dose, administration, and adverse effects to accurately administer these drugs and competently assess the client for adverse reactions.

Currently, inhaled nitric oxide, a vasodilating agent, is believed to reduce sickling by promoting the binding of oxygen to hemoglobin and is being used on an investigational basis. In the future, clients may abort or relieve pain experienced during sickle cell crises by using handheld inhalers.

Another promising treatment measure is the use of poloxamer 188 (RheothRx), a form of surfactant that is administered by continuous IV infusion for approximately 48 hours at the time of a sickle cell crisis. Poloxamer 188 decreases the viscosity of blood and reduces the clustering of erythrocytes, thus promoting increased vascular blood flow (Gibbs, 2003).

Bone marrow transplantation has cured sickle cell disease in a few people. Researchers continue to investigate the possibility of curing sickle cell disease with gene replacement therapy, but practical application of the technique is remote at this time. Clients with sickle cell disease are subject to potentially life-threatening infections. Continuous antibiotic therapy is prescribed for some; every infection, no matter how minor, is treated promptly with antibiotics. Folic acid is prescribed to facilitate the replacement of hemolyzed erythrocytes.

During sickle cell crisis, clients are given narcotic analgesia on a scheduled basis or can self-administer it using an IV pump. As an alternative to narcotic analgesics, synthetics such as buprenorphine (Buprenex) and nalbuphine (Nubain)

may be prescribed. Oxygen is given to relieve hypoxemia. The client must remain on complete bed rest, be hydrated with IV fluids, and may be given blood transfusions. An iron-chelating agent, such as deferoxamine (Desferal), is used to remove excess iron associated with multiple blood transfusions and erythrocyte destruction.

Pharmacologic Considerations

- Consult the physician if meperidine (Demerol) is prescribed for treating pain in clients with sickle cell crisis. The liver converts meperidine to normeperidine, which is toxic. Grand mal seizures can result.

- If the client had been receiving a narcotic analgesic just prior to changing to a synthetic agent, monitor the client for signs of narcotic withdrawal because the synthetic agents have a similar action to naloxone (Narcan), a narcotic reversing agent (Platt, 2005).

> ### Stop, Think, and Respond Exercise 31-2
> *What is the correlation between sickle cell anemia and stroke (cerebrovascular accident)?*

Nursing Process for the Client with Sickle Cell Anemia

Assessment

Obtain a health history focusing on previous episodes of sickle cell crisis and related complications, which may have had their onset as early as 1 or 2 years of age. Assess vital signs to detect evidence of infection such as fever and tachycardia. During the physical examination, observe the client's appearance, looking for evidence of dehydration, which may have triggered a sickle cell crisis (Smeltzer et al., 2008). Auscultate the lungs and heart to detect abnormal sounds suggestive of pneumonia, acute chest syndrome, and heart failure. Question the client about pain, which may be localized in the joints, bones, or abdomen, and ask the client whether the pain is similar to or different from previous events. Inspect the skin and sclera for jaundice and examine the extremities for ulcerations. Inspect the joints for signs of swelling and collect a urine specimen, which may be concentrated and contain blood cells as a result of renal damage. Assess mental status, verbal ability, and motor strength to detect stroke-related signs and symptoms. Ask the client to identify the therapeutic regimen that the client has used to control or relieve symptoms to determine if the client is experiencing an exacerbation from lack of compliance or drug toxicity if compliance is verified.

Diagnosis, Planning, and Interventions

▶ **Pain** related to obstructed blood flow

▶ **Expected Outcome:** Pain will be reduced or eliminated as evidenced by the client rating the pain at the lower end of a numeric scale.

- Administer prescribed analgesics according to the client's level of pain (i.e., use a non-narcotic analgesic for mild or moderate pain and a narcotic analgesic for severe pain). *Categories of analgesics are efficacious for various levels of pain; the nurse selects the best drug from among those prescribed to manage the client's symptoms.*
- Handle painful joints carefully by supporting the extremity. *Aggressive and unsupported movement escalates pain.*
- Elevate swollen joints. *Elevation relieves edema through increased gravity flow.*
- Provide at least 3000 mL of fluid per day either orally or combined with parenteral solutions. *Hydration dilutes blood cells and promotes blood circulation to ischemic tissues.*
- Keep the skin warm with prewarmed or layered blankets. *Warmth promotes vasodilation.*
- Give oxygen according to the physician's orders. *Supplemental oxygen relieves hypoxemia and reduces the potential for sickling and organ infarction.*
- Use nonpharmacologic methods to relieve pain such as imagery and distraction. *Diverting attention and helping the client concentrate on something pleasant or unrelated to the pain can blunt pain perception.*
- Be prepared to administer whole blood if prescribed. *Donated blood provides RBCs with normal hemoglobin, which improves oxygenation of tissues and relieves ischemic pain.*
- Administer prescribed doses of hydroxyurea. *Hydroxyurea switches production of HbS to HbF.*

▶ **Risk for Infection** related to increased susceptibility to pathogens secondary to dysfunction of the spleen

▶ **Expected Outcome:** Client will be free of infection.

- Perform conscientious hand hygiene. *It is one of the best measures to prevent spread of pathogens.*
- Advise visitors who are ill or have a respiratory infection to delay visiting the client. *Pathogens are transmitted by direct contact, droplets, or air transmission.*
- Recommend influenza and pneumococcal vaccines when the client's health improves. *Immunizations reduce the potential for pulmonary infections.*
- Teach the client aseptic techniques for managing open skin lesions. *Impaired skin provides an opportunity for colonization by infectious microorganisms.*

Evaluation of Expected Outcomes

Pain is absent or controlled within a level that facilitates ADLs. The client's temperature and white blood cell (WBC) count support that the client is free of infection. There is no evidence of cough, respiratory distress, or purulent drainage from skin lesions (see Client and Family Teaching 31-1).

▶ ***Stop, Think, and Respond Exercise 31-3***
What are the differences between HbF, HbA, and HbS?

HEMOLYTIC ANEMIA

The term *hemolytic anemia* refers to the consequence of a widely diverse group of conditions, some acquired, some he-

Client and Family Teaching 31-1
Sickle Cell Anemia

The nurse teaches clients with sickle cell anemia and their families as follows:

- Keep all medical appointments to determine the best drugs and dosages and to detect any developing drug toxicities.
- Never exceed the recommended dosages of analgesics, especially narcotic analgesics, and avoid self-medicating with illegal substances.
- Consume a liberal amount of fluids.
- Dress warmly in cold temperatures.
- Avoid vigorous physical exercise and leg positions or clothing that cause vasoconstriction.
- Stop smoking or other use of nicotine.
- Avoid travel to places with high altitudes.
- Obtain immunizations for pneumococcal pneumonia and influenza caused by *Haemophilus influenzae*.
- See a physician at the first sign of infection.
- Be aware that pregnancy creates risks for maternal and fetal complications. Obtain genetic testing and counseling before conceiving children.

reditary, and some idiopathic, in which there is chronic premature destruction of erythrocytes.

Pathophysiology and Etiology

Some examples of conditions that can produce hemolytic anemia are the use of cardiopulmonary bypass during surgery; arsenic or lead poisoning; invasion of erythrocytes by the malaria parasite; infectious agents; or toxins and exposure to hazardous chemicals. Other causes include the production of antibodies that destroy erythrocytes. Antibodies can be produced against antigens from another person, such as is seen in blood transfusion reactions, as well as against the body's own erythrocytes. As the number of destroyed blood cells increases, the potential for hyperbilirubinemia (excess bilirubin) and jaundice also increases.

Gerontologic Considerations

- Older adults are particularly susceptible to drug-induced hemolytic anemia because they often take more drugs than younger people. Discontinuing the offending drug usually corrects the anemia.

Assessment Findings

Symptoms are similar to those associated with hypovolemic anemia. In more severe forms of hemolytic anemia, the client is jaundiced and the spleen is enlarged. In some cases, hemolysis is so extensive that it causes shock.

Microscopic examination reveals erythrocyte fragments. When an erythrocyte survival study is performed using radioactive chromium, the life span of erythrocytes is 10 days or less. Reaction on a direct Coombs' test (direct antiglobulin test) is positive when the hemolytic anemia results from a transfusion reaction, use of certain drugs, or production of antibodies against the erythrocytes.

Medical and Surgical Management

Treatment includes removing the cause (when possible) and administering corticosteroids. In some cases, the steroid dose can be reduced and then discontinued after several weeks. Blood transfusions often are necessary. Splenectomy is performed if the client fails to respond to medical treatment.

Nursing Management

The nurse obtains a comprehensive health history to help determine the cause of the hemolysis. Until the cause is determined, the nurse provides supportive care to help the client meet basic needs. When the diagnosis is confirmed, he or she implements the medical regimen for treatment and prepares the client for discharge by teaching measures for self-care. The nurse arranges the plan for follow-up evaluations and shares the information with the client.

THALASSEMIAS

Thalassemias are hereditary hemolytic anemias. They are divided into two major groups: alpha-thalassemias and beta-thalassemias. Alpha-thalassemias are found in people from Southeast Asia and Africa; beta-thalassemias are found in people from Mediterranean islands and the Po Valley in Italy.

Assessment Findings

Clients with alpha-thalassemias typically are asymptomatic, as are those with minor forms of beta-thalassemia. Clients with Cooley's anemia, a severe form of beta-thalassemia, exhibit symptoms of severe anemia and a bronzing of the skin caused by hemolysis of erythrocytes. Diagnosis is based on symptoms and the results of hemoglobin electrophoresis.

Medical Management

Treatment of the various forms of thalassemia is symptomatic. Clients usually require frequent transfusions. Those with Cooley's anemia require iron chelation therapy because of the iron deposits in the skin.

Nursing Management

When anemia is severe, the nurse places the client on bed rest and protects him or her from contact with those who have infections. When transfusions are necessary, the nurse closely monitors the rate of administration.

PERNICIOUS ANEMIA

Pernicious anemia develops when a client lacks intrinsic factor, which normally is present in stomach secretions. Intrinsic factor is necessary for absorption of vitamin B_{12}. Vitamin B_{12}, the extrinsic factor in blood, is required for the maturation of erythrocytes.

Pathophysiology and Etiology

The production of intrinsic factor decreases with age and gastric mucosal atrophy. It also decreases secondary to surgical removal of the stomach or small bowel resection, in which the ileum (site for vitamin B_{12} absorption) is removed. Without adequate vitamin B_{12}, erythrocytes remain in an immature form. If the condition is not recognized and treated promptly, degenerative changes in the nervous system develop. Sometimes permanent damage occurs before treatment begins.

 Gerontologic Considerations

- Pernicious anemia accounts for approximately 9% of all anemias in older adults. Pernicious anemia may be accompanied by a dementia with symptoms similar to Alzheimer's disease. Therefore, clients experiencing cognitive changes should be screened, because early detection of pernicious anemia is critical to prevent neurologic damage (Linton & Lach, 2007).

Assessment Findings

Signs and Symptoms

In addition to the usual symptoms of anemia, some clients with pernicious anemia develop stomatitis (inflammation of the mouth) and glossitis (inflammation of the tongue), digestive disturbances, and diarrhea. Anemia may be so severe that dyspnea occurs with minimal exertion. Jaundice, irritability, confusion, and depression are present when the disease is severe. Mental changes usually disappear with treatment. Numbness and tingling in the arms and legs and ataxia are common signs of neurologic involvement. Some affected clients lose vibratory and position senses.

Diagnostic Findings

Diagnosis is established by the client's history, symptoms, and blood and bone marrow studies. The Schilling test is used to confirm the diagnosis. Microscopic examination of a blood smear reveals many large, immature erythrocytes.

Medical Management

Vitamin B_{12} is given intramuscularly in a dose adequate to control the disease. Therapy must continue for life. The typical dose is 100 g IM vitamin B_{12} daily for 2 weeks and then 100 g monthly. No toxic effects have been noted from the use of vitamin B_{12}. Oral vitamin B_{12} seldom is effective, except for short intervals. Iron therapy rarely is needed because mature erythrocytes are manufactured and the hemoglobin level is normal when the condition is corrected. Clients with permanent neurologic deficits benefit from physical therapy.

Nursing Management

If glossitis and stomatitis are present, a soft, bland diet relieves the discomfort associated with eating. Most clients better tolerate small, frequent meals than three large meals. Meticulous oral care after eating is essential to remove particles of food that may irritate the oral mucosal lining and increase soreness.

If a permanent neurologic deficit has occurred, the nurse encourages the client to move about as much as possible to prevent complications associated with immobility, such as contractures and pressure ulcer formation. Assistance with ambulation is necessary because some clients have difficulty walking and are prone to falling. If behavioral changes occur, close supervision is necessary. The nurse emphasizes the importance of lifelong administration of vitamin B$_{12}$. He or she teaches a family member of the client how to administer vitamin B$_{12}$ injections or refers the client to a home health nursing service.

FOLIC ACID DEFICIENCY ANEMIA

Folic acid (vitamin B$_9$) deficiency causes anemia characterized by immature erythrocytes.

Pathophysiology and Etiology

A folic acid deficiency commonly is related to an insufficient dietary intake of foods rich in folic acid (Nutrition Notes 31-2). Older adults and clients with alcoholism, intestinal disorders that affect food absorption, malignant disorders, and chronic illnesses often have a folic acid deficiency because of poor nutrition. Certain drugs, such as anticonvulsants and methotrexate, are folic acid antagonists and interfere with folic acid absorption. Because pregnant women and clients with chronic hemolytic anemias have increased folic acid requirements, they can experience a folic acid deficiency even when they follow a normal diet. Prolonged IV therapy and total parenteral nutrition also can result in a folic acid deficiency. Chronic alcoholism predisposes to folic acid deficiency; affected people tend to obtain most of their calories from alcohol, causing nutritional compromise.

Assessment Findings

Severe fatigue, a sore and beefy-red tongue, dyspnea, nausea, anorexia, headaches, weakness, and lightheadedness occur. Blood test results reveal low hemoglobin and hematocrit levels. The serum folate level is decreased. A Schilling test differentiates pernicious anemia and anemia caused by a folic acid deficiency.

Gerontologic Considerations

- Folic acid deficiency may play a role in depression. Folic acid levels should be measured in older clients who exhibit symptoms of depression (Johnson, 2006).

Nutrition Notes 31-2
The Client with Folic Acid Deficiency Anemia

- *Folate* is the generic term that includes naturally occurring folate (food folate) and synthetic folic acid used in fortified foods and supplements.
- Rich sources of food folate include fortified breads and cereals, green leafy vegetables, orange juice, and dried peas and beans.
- Folic acid can reverse anemia and the gastrointestinal symptoms of vitamin B$_{12}$ deficiency; however, neurologic symptoms continue and, if untreated, can be irreversible. Ascertaining the correct cause of megaloblastic anemia before treatment begins is imperative.

Medical Management

Oral folic acid supplements (1 mg/daily) usually are provided. Parenteral administration of folic acid is required for clients with an intestinal malabsorption disorder. A well-balanced diet that includes foods with a high folate content is also recommended.

Nursing Management

The nurse encourages the client to eat foods high in folate. He or she encourages eating soft, bland foods and performing good oral hygiene. If fatigue is a prominent symptom, the nurse plans adequate rest periods between activities.

ERYTHROCYTOSIS

POLYCYTHEMIA VERA

There are some conditions in which one of the primary characteristics is **erythrocytosis**, an increase in circulating erythrocytes. One of these conditions is *polycythemia vera*, which is characterized by a greater-than-normal number of erythrocytes, leukocytes, and platelets. For people who live at high altitudes, erythrocytosis is a normal phenomenon and usually requires no treatment.

Pathophysiology and Etiology

Polycythemia vera is associated with a rapid proliferation of blood cells produced by the bone marrow. The cause of this accelerated production is unknown. Polycythemia vera usually has an insidious onset and a prolonged course. Despite the abundance of erythrocytes, their life span is shorter. The dead erythrocytes release intracellular potassium, which can cause hyperkalemia, and uric acid, which causes gout-like joint symptoms. The oxygen-combining capacity of the erythrocytes is impaired, which compromises cellular oxygenation. The increased number of erythrocytes makes the blood more viscous than normal and increases the likelihood for the development of thrombi in small blood vessels. Complications include hypertension, congestive heart failure, stroke, tissue and organ infarction, and hemorrhage.

Assessment Findings

Signs and Symptoms

The face and lips are reddish-purple. Fatigue, weakness, headache, pruritus, exertional dyspnea, and dizziness are common. Excessive bleeding after minor injuries, perhaps because of the engorgement of the capillaries and veins, occurs. Hemorrhoids develop. Splenomegaly (enlargement of the spleen) is common. The joints become swollen and painful because of elevated uric acid levels.

Diagnostic Findings

The blood cell count, especially erythrocytes, is elevated, with a similar rise in hemoglobin and hematocrit levels. The platelet and WBC counts are increased. Levels of serum potassium and uric acid are above normal.

Medical Management

Treatment involves measures to reduce the volume of circulating blood, lessen its viscosity, and curb the excessive production of erythrocytes. A phlebotomy (opening a vein to withdraw blood) is done several times a week; 500 mL of blood is removed each time. Anticoagulants are prescribed to reduce the potential for forming clots. Radiophosphorus and radiation therapy can be used to decrease the production of erythrocytes in the bone marrow. Antineoplastic drugs such as mechlorethamine (Mustargen) are given to curb excessive bone marrow activity.

Nursing Management

The nurse observes the client for complications and provides information about drug therapy and techniques to promote circulation and reduce potential thrombi formation. The plan of care includes the following measures:

- Advise drinking 3 quarts (or liters) of fluid per day. *Adequate hydration promotes venous return and ensures sufficient urine production.*
- Teach the client to avoid crossing the legs at the knee and wearing tight clothing. *Restricting blood circulation increases the risk for thrombus formation.*
- Encourage the client to be physically active, change positions frequently, and elevate the lower extremities as much as possible. *Movement and leg elevation promotes the circulation of venous blood.*
- Teach the client how to perform isometric exercises such as contracting and relaxing the quadriceps and gluteal muscles during periods of inactivity. *Contraction of skeletal muscles compresses the walls of veins and increases the circulation of venous blood as it returns to the heart.*
- Help the client apply and use thromboembolic stockings or support hose during waking hours. *Compression of veins promotes venous circulation and prevents the formation of thrombi.*
- Tell the client to rest immediately if chest pain develops. *Chest pain indicates myocardial ischemia. Rest reduces the work of the heart and restores sufficient oxygenated blood flow to overcome the temporary deficiency.*

LEUKOCYTOSIS

Leukocytosis is an increased number of leukocytes above normal limits. Increased leukocytes generally serve as a protective mechanism in response to inflammation and healing, but in some disease conditions such as leukemia, the proliferation of leukocytes is not advantageous.

LEUKEMIA

Leukemia refers to any malignant blood disorder in which proliferation of leukocytes, usually in an immature form, is unregulated. There often is an accompanying decrease in production of erythrocytes and platelets. There are four general types of leukemia, classified according to the bone marrow stem cell line that is dysfunctional (Table 31-3). Acute and chronic lymphocytic leukemias result from bone marrow dysfunction that affects lymphoid stem cells; the primary marrow dysfunction in acute and chronic myelocytic leukemia is in myeloid stem cells (Fig. 31-3).

Pathophysiology and Etiology

The cause of leukemia is unknown, although exposures to toxic chemicals and radiation, viruses, and certain drugs are known to precipitate the disorder. In some cases there is a genetic correlation. Although the increase in leukocytes is rampant, there are many more immature than mature cells. Because of their immaturity, the leukocytes are ineffective at fighting infections. The rapid proliferation of leukocytes results in a decreased production of erythrocytes and platelets. The client eventually develops severe anemia, and the reduction in platelets leads to bleeding. The excessive leukocytes infiltrate the spleen, liver, lymph nodes, and brain if unchecked.

 G e r o n t o l o g i c   C o n s i d e r a t i o n s

- Both acute and chronic leukemias are prevalent in older adults. Approximately 80% of adults with acute leukemia have acute myelogenous leukemia (AML). Older adults with acute lymphoblastic leukemia have a poor prognosis due to the lack of tolerance to pancytopenia that results from prolonged chemotherapy (Freedman, 2006). Rates of both chronic lymphocytic leukemia (CLL) and chronic myelogenous leukemia (CML) increase in adults aged 50 and older (Leukemia and Lymphoma Society, 2008).

TABLE 31-3 Types of Leukemia

TYPE	CELLULAR CHARACTERISTICS	AGE OF ONSET (YR)
Acute lymphocytic (ALL)	Increased immature lymphocytes Normal or decreased granulocytes Decreased erythrocytes Decreased platelets	Younger than 5; uncommon after 15
Chronic lymphocytic (CLL)	Same as above, but erythrocyte and platelet counts may be normal or low	Older than 40; most common type in adults
Acute myelogenous (AML)	Decrease in all myeloid formed cells: monocytes, granulocytes, erythrocytes, and platelets	Occurs in all age ranges
Chronic myelogenous (CML)	Same as above, but greater number of normal cells than in acute form	Older than 20, but incidence increases with age; genetic link in 90% to 95% of cases

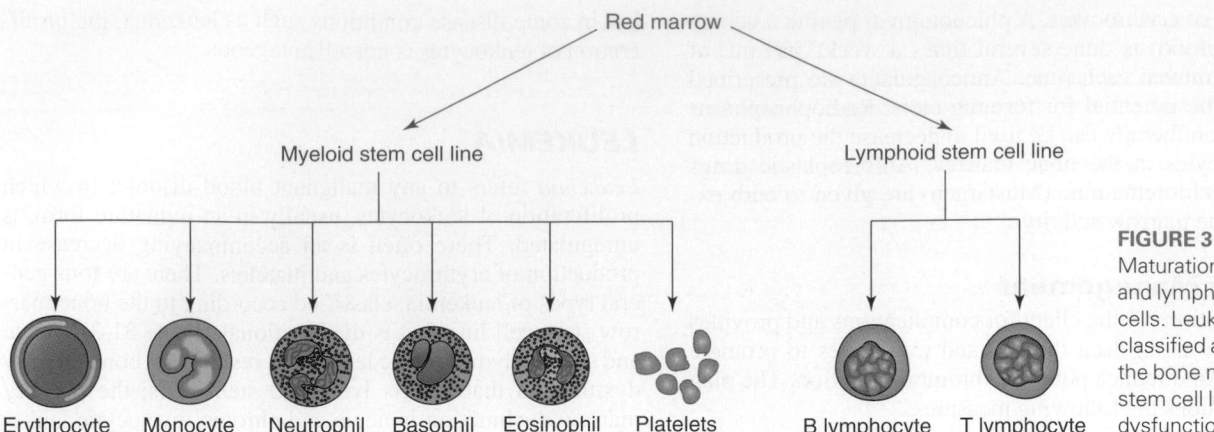

FIGURE 31-3. Maturation of myeloid and lymphoid stem cells. Leukemia is classified according to the bone marrow stem cell line that is dysfunctional.

Assessment Findings

Infections, fatigue from anemia, and easy bruising are hallmarks of leukemia. At the onset of leukemia, particularly in acute lymphocytic leukemia (ALL), a fever is present, the spleen and lymph nodes enlarge, and internal or external bleeding develops. Common sites of bleeding include the nose, mouth, and gastrointestinal tract. The leukocyte count is low, normal, or high, but the number of normal leukocytes is decreased. Consequently, the number of erythrocytes and platelets decreases as well.

Medical Management

Drug therapy is the primary weapon for arresting leukemia. Years of research have led to the development of successful drug protocols using one or combinations of antineoplastic drugs. The type of drug or combination of drugs depends on the form of leukemia. Treatment is most successful in young clients.

Erythrocyte and platelet transfusions are necessary to treat the anemia and decreased platelets. Antibiotics are given when secondary infections develop.

Bone marrow transplantation and stem cell transplantation have increased survival for some clients. The harvesting and use of adult (somatic) stem cells are different from the potential use of harvested embryonic stem cells (Table 31-4). Adult stem cells are classified as either *autologous* (from oneself), *syngeneic* (from an identical twin), or *allogenic* (from another; see Chap. 18). Stem cells are harvested by removing

TABLE 31-4 Comparison of Adult Stem Cells and Embryonic Stem Cells

	ADULT	EMBRYONIC
Source	Bone marrow, peripheral blood, umbilical cord blood	4- to 5-day-old embryo in the blastocyst stage
Donor	Patient, relative, public	Female whose excess ova that have been fertilized in vitro (in a laboratory) are no longer needed for reproductive purposes
Characteristics	Unspecialized and differentiate usually into cells in the tissues where they reside	Unspecialized but have the potential to differentiate into various different body cells
Harvesting Method	Aspiration of bone marrow, *apheresis* (separation of stem cells from differentiated cells) of peripheral blood, collection of blood from the umbilical cord and placenta at birth	Needle aspiration of inner cell mass within the blastocyst
Preservation	Combined with a preservative and frozen until needed	Cultured and *replated* (removal and reculturing) of proliferating cell mass for 6 months or more, then frozen when millions of cells have been grown
Use	Restore the bone marrow's ability to produce blood-forming cells destroyed by high doses of chemotherapy or radiation	Replace various body cells that are diseased or injured (heart muscle following a myocardial infarction, dopamine-producing cells for those with Parkinson's disease, beta cells of those with diabetes mellitus, etc.)
Method of Transplant	IV infusion	Currently restricted to laboratory research on animals to determine how unspecialized cells differentiate
Evidence of Success	*Engraftment* (increased production) of blood cells in 2 to 4 weeks; recovery from disease for at least 5 years to confirm absence of cancer cells	

them from peripheral blood, obtaining cells from bone marrow, or collecting cord blood from a newborn. Malignant stem cells are removed from an autologous specimen before transplantation. Toxic drugs or radiation are administered before transplantation, which renders the client extremely susceptible to infection. The client remains hospitalized for several weeks to observe if normal blood cells are eventually produced, to detect signs of *graft-versus-host disease*, in which the foreign donor cells destroy the recipient's tissues and organs, and to protect the client who is immunosuppressed from acquiring a life-threatening infection (see Chap. 12).

Nursing Process for the Client with Leukemia

Assessment

Begin the initial assessment by obtaining a history of symptoms. Look for a cluster of symptoms that includes weakness and fatigue, frequent infections, nosebleeds or other prolonged bleeding events, and joint pain. Also, look for symptoms associated with leukocyte infiltration of the central nervous system, such as headache and confusion.

Examine the client's body for evidence of bruising. Palpate the abdomen to detect enlargement and tenderness over the liver and spleen. Review laboratory test results, noting the numbers and types of blood cells. Calculate the absolute neutrophil count to determine the client's potential for infection (Box 31-2). In addition, assess the outcome of bone marrow aspiration.

Diagnosis, Planning, and Interventions

▶ **Risk for Infection** related to compromised immunity

▶ **Expected Outcome:** Client will be free of infection as evidenced by normal temperature and no signs of an infectious disorder.

- Implement neutropenic Precautions (Box 31-3). *They reduce exposure to pathogens that are dangerous when immunity is suppressed.*
- Ensure that any staff person, family member, or visitor who is ill temporarily discontinues direct contact with the client. *Eliminating direct contact with others who are infectious reduces the potential for transmitting microorganisms to the client.*

BOX 31-2 Calculating the Absolute Neutrophil Count

Step 1: Use the formula:

$$\text{ANC} = \frac{\%\text{Neutrophils} + \%\text{Bands}}{100} \times \text{Total white blood cell count}$$

Step 2: Interpret results:

ANC of 999 to 500 = risk for infection
ANC of 499 to 100 = high risk for infection
ANC of 99 or less = almost certain development
of infection

BOX 31-3 Neutropenic Precautions

To help prevent infection in clients with neutropenia:
- Place the client in a private room.
- Always wash hands before touching the client; encourage client to remind all staff and visitors to wash hands.
- Tell client to wash his or her hands before and after eating and after using the bathroom.
- Encourage the client to shower daily.
- Place a mask over client's mouth and nose if leaving the room; minimize time client spends in crowded areas.
- Ensure that no raw fruits or vegetables are served.
- Minimize invasive procedures (schedule all blood work to be drawn at one time of the day; discontinue invasive lines as soon as possible).
- Tell client not to handle cut flowers.

- Monitor temperature at least once per shift and continually assess for signs of infection, such as swelling and tenderness, which can appear in any area or organ of the body. *Progressive hyperthermia occurs in some types of infections, and fever (unrelated to drugs or blood products) occurs in most clients with leukemia. Early intervention is essential to prevent sepsis/septicemia in immuno suppressed persons. (Note: Septicemia may occur without fever.)*

▶ **PC: Hemorrhage**

▶ **Expected Outcome:** The nurse will monitor for hemorrhage; if bleeding is detected, the nurse will manage and minimize it.

- Monitor the platelet count. *Suppression of bone marrow and platelet production places the client at risk for spontaneous and uncontrolled bleeding.*
- Inspect the skin for signs of bruising and petechiae; report melena, hematuria, or epistaxis (nosebleeds). *Fragile tissues and altered clotting mechanisms can result in hemorrhage after even minor trauma.*
- Handle client gently when assisting with care and encourage use of electric razors. *Trauma and microabrasions from razors can contribute to anemia from bleeding.*
- Apply prolonged pressure to needle sites or other sources of external bleeding. *Reduced platelet production results in a delayed clotting process.*
- Implement physician orders for transfusions of blood and platelets. *Transfusion restores and normalizes the cell count and oxygen-carrying capacity of RBCs to correct anemia and prevent and treat hemorrhage.*

▶ **Activity Intolerance** related to hypoxia

▶ **Expected Outcomes:** The client will (1) tolerate essential activity as evidenced by a heart rate below 100 bpm and (2) have a respiratory rate less than 28 breaths/minute.

- For interventions, see the discussion that accompanies anemia.

▶ **Risk for Disturbed Body Image** related to hair loss secondary to chemotherapy

▶ **Expected Outcome:** Client will cope with hair loss and changing body image.

- Provide opportunity for client to express feelings about hair loss and changing body image; offer suggestions such as scarves, turbans, baseball caps, or wigs. *Head coverings may increase self-esteem and foster more interactions with others.*

▶ Anxiety and Fear related to unfamiliar experiences and unknown prognosis

▶ **Expected Outcome:** Anxiety and fear will be relieved as evidenced by the client's report of emotional comfort.

- Acknowledge your awareness of the client's anxieties and fears. *Open communication validates and communicates acceptance of the client's feelings.*
- Encourage the client to talk about the disorder and its potential and actual effects. *Vocalizing inner feelings helps identify each client's specific emotional response to the disease and treatment.*
- Explain the plan of care and all treatment procedures. *Explaining the purpose, goal, and plan of care promotes confidence that the healthcare team is dedicated to resolving the illness.*
- Give encouragement and emotional support, and foster hope without implying unrealistic expectations. *A positive attitude sends a message of caring and optimism. Fostering unrealistic hope is not helpful and may significantly decrease the trust that the client places in the healthcare provider.*
- Teach the client and family how to manage their disease and treatment regimen. *Knowledge empowers the client and family and contributes to a sense of control.* (See Client and Family Teaching 31-2.)

Evaluation of Expected Outcomes

Expected outcomes include that the client not acquire an infection and experience no or minimal blood loss. He or she tolerates activity between periods of rest. The client adapts to changes in body image and copes with anxiety and fears. ●

Client and Family Teaching 31-2
Leukemia

If the client is to take medication at home, the nurse explains the dosage schedule because compliance is essential to treat the disease successfully. If untoward effects occur, the healthcare team will make every effort to control the symptoms while continuing chemotherapy. The nurse includes the following points in a teaching plan:

- Have frequent examinations of the blood and sometimes the bone marrow, which are necessary to monitor the results of therapy. (The nurse emphasizes the importance of these examinations to promote wellness rather than focusing on possible complications from drug therapy.)
- Take precautions to avoid physical injury.
- Avoid exposure to people who have infections (e.g., colds).
- Seek medical care promptly if excessive bleeding or bruising or symptoms of illness or infection occur.
- Obtain sufficient rest and eat an adequate diet to prevent secondary infections.
- When feeling well, continue usual activities unless the physician instructs otherwise.
- If sores in the mouth occur, contact the physician as soon as possible. Do not self-treat this problem.
- Contact the physician immediately about any of the following: severe nausea with prolonged vomiting, severe diarrhea, fever, chills, excessive bleeding or bruising, cough, chest pain, cloudy urine, rash, blood in the stool or urine, severe headache, extreme fatigue, increased respiratory rate or difficulty breathing, and rapid pulse rate.
- Follow the physician's recommendations to monitor temperature and weight.
- Keep all clinic or office appointments.

MULTIPLE MYELOMA

Multiple myeloma is a malignancy involving plasma cells, which are B-lymphocyte cells in bone marrow. The overall prognosis is poor but has improved; the median survival rate after diagnosis is 3 to 5 years. Some people have survived for 10 to 20 years or more with aggressive drug therapy or stem cell transplantation (International Myeloma Foundation, 2005).

Pathophysiology and Etiology

The exact triggering mechanism for the disorder is unknown. Multiple myeloma is associated with aging, recurrent infections, drug allergies, and exposure to occupational toxins and radiation (Porth, 2008). Onset before age 40 years is rare. The abnormal plasma cells proliferate in the bone marrow, where they release osteoclast activating factor. This in turn causes osteoclasts to break down bone cells, resulting in increased blood calcium and pathologic fractures. The plasma cells also form single or multiple *osteolytic* (bone-destroying) tumors that produce a "punched-out" or "honeycombed" appearance in bones such as the spine, ribs, skull, pelvis, femurs, clavicles, and scapulae. Weakened vertebrae lead to compression of the spine accompanied by significant pain.

The malignant plasma cells release two types of abnormal proteins. In the process of being excreted by the kidneys, Bence Jones proteins impair renal tubules, causing renal failure. The other protein, called *M-type globulin*, compromises production of functional immunoglobulins (also known as *antibodies*), thus interfering with an optimal immune response (see Chap. 33). The excess production of plasma cells reduces the formation of erythrocytes and platelets, causing anemia and increasing the risk of bleeding. In addition to infection, which may cause death, those with multiple myeloma experience bone pain, pathologic fractures, thrombotic complications such as clot formation in the deep veins of the legs, pulmonary embolism, and stroke caused by increased viscosity of the blood.

Assessment Findings

Signs and Symptoms

The first symptom usually is vague pain in the pelvis, spine, or ribs. As the disease progresses, the pain becomes more severe and localized. The pain intensifies with activity and is relieved by rest. When tumors replace bone marrow, pathologic fractures develop. The client may have an unusually high incidence of infection, especially pneumonia, caused

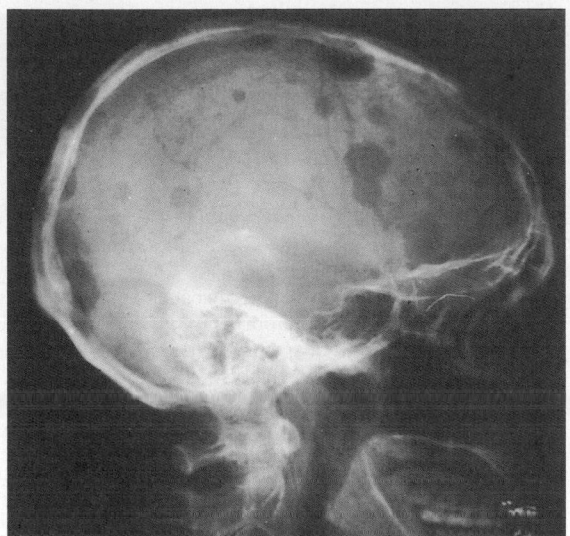

FIGURE 31-4. Multiple myeloma. A radiograph of the skull shows numerous punched out radiolucent areas. (From Rubin, E., & Strayer, D.S. [2008]. *Rubin's pathology: Clinicopathologic foundations of medicine* [5th ed.]. Philadelphia: Lippincott Williams & Wilkins.)

by decreased production of appropriate antibodies. The client may experience symptoms typically associated with anemia: weakness, fatigue, and chills. Bruising and nosebleeds are evidence of decreased platelets. Renal calculi (stones) may develop from hypercalcemia and renal failure.

Diagnostic Findings

Skeletal radiographic studies reveal characteristic bone lesions (Fig. 31-4). Blood cell counts are abnormally low. Serum calcium levels are elevated from bone destruction. Urine samples are positive for Bence Jones protein. Bone marrow aspiration demonstrates increased atypical plasma cells. The uric acid level is elevated from cellular destruction.

Medical Management

Low-dose steroid therapy in combination with anticancer drugs (Drug Therapy Table 31-1) such as bortezomib (Velcade), lenalidomide (Revlimid), and thalidomide (Thalomid) remarkably induce remission, decrease the tumor mass, lessen bone pain, and stimulate killer T-cells of the immune system. Temporary remission occurs in 75% to 87% of clients (International Myeloma Foundation, 2005). Bisphosphonates are prescribed to increase bone density. Analgesics control pain; stronger narcotic analgesics are reserved for the terminal stages of the disease. Allopurinol (Zyloprim) is used to prevent uric acid crystallization and subsequent renal calculus formation. See Chapter 58 for a discussion of the management of renal failure.

Anemia is treated with erythropoietin (Epogen) or blood transfusions. Infections are managed with antibiotics. Back braces are necessary when the spine is involved, and body casts are used when involvement is extensive and causes pathologic fractures.

Autologous bone marrow and peripheral stem cell transplants are now considered standard care for clients with multiple myeloma. However, the choice of drug therapy must be selectively considered if a transplant is anticipated so as not to eliminate this as an option later in the disease process. Another possibility is to harvest stem cells before starting stem cell–damaging drug therapy. Research shows that those who receive a bone marrow or stem cell transplant early in the disease have a mean survival rate of 7 years (University of Arkansas for Medical Sciences, 2007).

Nursing Management

The nurse assesses the client frequently for pain, signs of infection, excessive fatigue, bleeding, thrombus formation, and changes in the quantity or quality of urine production. He or she administers prescribed analgesics for effective pain management. The nurse assists the client with ambulation because immobility can worsen loss of calcium from the bone. He or she provides up to 4000 mL of fluid to prevent renal damage from hypercalcemia and precipitation of protein in the renal tubules. The nurse documents and reports signs suggestive of calculus formation in the kidney, ureters, or bladder (see Chaps. 58 and 59).

Safety is paramount because any injury, no matter how slight, can result in a fracture. When pain is severe, the nurse delays position changes and bathing until an administered analgesic has reached its peak concentration level and the client is experiencing maximum pain relief. The nurse takes measures to reduce the potential for infection.

AGRANULOCYTOSIS

Agranulocytosis refers specifically to a decreased production of granulocytes, including neutrophils, basophils, and eosinophils. This is opposed to **leukopenia**, which is a general reduction in all WBCs. Decreased granulocytes place the client at risk for infection.

Pathophysiology and Etiology

The most common cause of agranulocytosis is toxicity from drugs such as sulfonamides, chloramphenicol (Chloromycetin), antineoplastics, and some psychotropic medications.

Assessment Findings

Fatigue, fever, chills, headache, and opportunistic infections in the mouth, throat, nose, rectum, or vagina can develop.

Medical Management

Treatment includes removal of the cause, such as discontinuing the drug that is producing agranulocytosis. The prognosis is related to the condition's cause and severity. When the cause can be determined and promptly removed, the client usually recovers. Some clients improve after receiving filgrastim (Neupogen) or pegfilgrastim (Neulasta), drugs that supply human granulocyte colony-stimulating factor.

Nursing Management

The nurse determines the names of all drugs (prescription and nonprescription) the client has used in the past 6 to 12 months. Protective isolation is necessary if the leukocyte count is extremely low. Visitors or staff with any type of an

DRUG THERAPY TABLE 31-1 Treatment Options For Multiple Myeloma

Drugs	Advantages	Disadvantages
VAD		
vincristine (Oncovin), doxorubicin (Adriamycin), dexamethasone (Decadron)	Produces remissions in 70% of clients Does not damage stem cells Combination shrinks tumor cells, reduces pressure on nerves, and reduces hypercalcemia	Administered through a central venous catheter Potential for catheter-related complications Vincristine can cause peripheral neuropathy. Adriamycin can cause nausea, vomiting, mucositis, diarrhea, hair loss, cardiac toxicity. Steroid can increase susceptibility to infection, fluid retention, gastric bleeding, hyperglycemia, muscle weakness.
MP		
melphalan (Alkeran), prednisone (Deltasone)	Given orally for 4–7 days and repeated every 4–6 weeks Interferes with replication of cancer cells Produces remission in 60% of clients	Alkylating agent can cause nausea, vomiting, mucositis, pulmonary fibrosis, hair loss, and hyperuricemia. Benefit takes months to achieve. Causes damage to stem cells in bone marrow Contraindicated if stem cell transplant is anticipated
thalidomide (Thalomid)	Inhibits the growth and survival of myeloma cells by altering the production of cytokines needed for their survival Stimulates T cells to attack myeloma cells Used in combination with dexamethasone for initial treatment or singly in clients who relapse after stem cell transplant Taken orally at bedtime Produces remission in 70% of clients	Side effects include sleepiness, peripheral neuropathy, nausea, dizziness, skin rash, headaches, nervousness, depression, mood swings, teratogenesis (absence of limbs) in a fetus if taken even once by the mother during pregnancy. Pregnancy test and effective contraception required throughout drug administration Dose may need reduction if neuropathy develops.
bortezomib (Velcade)	Blocks proteasomes, enzymes that play a role in regulating cell function and growth, thereby destroying cancer cells Given by IV injection twice a week for 2 weeks, followed by a 10-day rest period	Used when clients with multiple myeloma have not responded to at least two other types of drug therapy Considered palliative, not curative Side effects include nausea, vomiting, fatigue, diarrhea, thrombocytopenia, fever, peripheral neuropathy, and pneumonia.
dexamethasone (Decadron)	Synthetic long-acting systemic glucocorticoid with low salt and water retention potential Primary use is to inhibit or help control the inflammatory response by stabilizing the cell membranes of inflammatory cells Given orally or by IV or IM injection	Common adverse effects include but are not limited to potential hypertension related to electrolyte imbalances; nervousness, insomnia, mood swings, ecchymosis, petechiae, facial erythema, poor wound healing, hirsutism, urticaria, muscle weakness, osteoporosis, weight gain.
lenalidomide (Revlimid)	Given orally Stops or slows the growth of cancerous myeloma cells within the bone marrow Used in combination with dexamethasone and is intended for use in clients who have tried one other therapy	Side effects are similar to those of dexamethasone. Potential worsening side effects include blood clots deep venous thrombosis, cytopenias (low blood counts), diarrhea or constipation, rash, muscle cramps, fatigue, insomnia.

infection are restricted from close client contact until the infection has cleared.

PANCYTOPENIA

Pancytopenia refers to conditions such as aplastic anemia in which numbers of all marrow-produced blood cells are reduced.

APLASTIC ANEMIA

Aplastic anemia is more than just a deficiency of erythrocytes, although rarely that is the case. Its name is derived from the word **aplasia**, which means failure to develop. Usually it is manifested by insufficient numbers of erythrocytes, leukocytes, and platelets, collectively described as *pancytopenia.*

Pathophysiology and Etiology

Aplastic anemia is a consequence of inadequate stem cell production in the bone marrow. In some cases, the cause of the disorder is never determined, but it may be autoimmune (self-destroying) in nature (see Chap. 34). In many cases, the bone marrow becomes dysfunctional from exposure to toxic chemicals, radiation, and drug therapy with anticancer drugs and some antibiotics. Clients with aplastic anemia are very ill, and the death rate is high if the bone marrow has been severely damaged.

Assessment Findings

Clients with aplastic anemia experience all the typical characteristics of anemia (weakness and fatigue). In addition, they have frequent opportunistic infections plus coagulation abnormalities that are manifested by unusual bleeding, small skin hemorrhages called *petechiae*, and *ecchymoses* (bruises). The spleen becomes enlarged with an accumulation of the client's blood cells destroyed by lymphocytes that failed to recognize them as normal cells, or with an accumulation of dead transfused blood cells. The blood cell count shows insufficient numbers of blood cells. A bone marrow aspiration confirms that the production of stem cells is suppressed.

Medical Management

In some instances, withdrawal of the causative agent allows the bone marrow to regenerate and assume normal function. Transfusions of whole blood, packed cells, and platelets are given to boost circulating blood cells. Antibiotics are administered to prevent or treat infection. High doses of corticosteroids that suppress the immune system are given in cases of an autoimmune connection. Bone marrow transplantation is considered if a matching donor can be found; otherwise, autologous stem cell transplantation is an alternative (see Chap. 18).

Nursing Management

The nurse assesses for signs of severe anemia, infection, and bleeding tendencies. He or she makes every effort to prevent infection. If the leukocyte count is extremely low, the nurse implements special isolation procedures, such as restricting visitors and using a laminar airflow room.

The nurse includes soft foods in the diet and modifies oral hygiene techniques to prevent bleeding from the gums. He or she collaborates with the physician concerning alternative routes for drugs administered parenterally. If that is not possible, the nurse applies additional pressure to any punctures from injections or sites where IV fluids are administered and discontinued. The nurse monitors the client closely during blood transfusions because the risk of a reaction increases with the repeated introduction of foreign cells from multiple blood donors.

COAGULOPATHIES

The term *coagulopathy* refers to conditions in which a component that is necessary to control bleeding (Fig. 31-5) is missing or inadequate. Two common examples are thrombocytopenia and hemophilia. For information on disseminated intravascular coagulation, a condition in which hypercoagulation (excessive clot formation) is followed by diffuse bleeding as clotting factors are exhausted, refer to texts on trauma and critical care nursing.

THROMBOCYTOPENIA

Thrombocytopenia is a lower-than-normal number of platelets or thrombocytes.

Pathophysiology and Etiology

Thrombocytopenia occurs when platelet manufacture by the bone marrow is decreased or platelet destruction by the spleen is increased. It accompanies leukemia and other malignant blood diseases and is caused by severe infections and certain drugs. Idiopathic thrombocytopenic purpura is thrombocytopenia without a known cause.

Assessment Findings

Thrombocytopenia is evidenced by *purpura*, small hemorrhages in the skin, mucous membranes, or subcutaneous tissues. Bleeding from other parts of the body, such as the nose, oral mucous membrane, and the gastrointestinal tract, also occurs. Internal hemorrhage, which can be severe and even fatal, is possible.

Diagnosis is based on symptoms, a low platelet count, and abnormal bleeding and clotting times. In some instances, bone marrow aspiration is performed. A health history sometimes reveals agents that are associated with drug-induced thrombocytopenia, such as heparin.

Medical and Surgical Management

When possible, the cause is eliminated. Corticosteroids provide symptomatic relief until the platelet count returns to normal. Transfusions of platelets or whole blood are given in a hemorrhagic emergency. If spontaneous recovery does not occur, splenectomy is necessary to stop destruction of platelets in the spleen. Removal of the spleen results in a rise in the platelet count and relief of symptoms.

Clients with idiopathic thrombocytopenia often recover spontaneously. If the cause can be removed or treated, the prognosis is good. Thrombocytopenia in conjunction with illnesses such as leukemia has a poor prognosis.

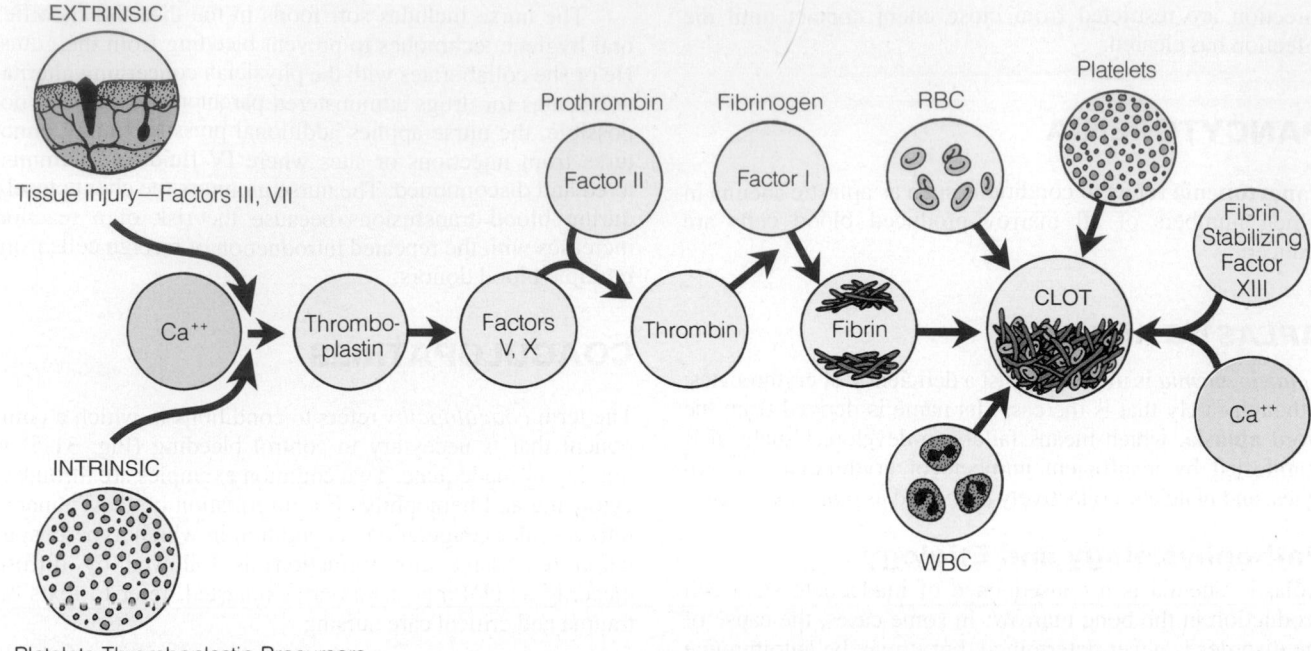

FIGURE 31-5. The normal process of clot formation. Clotting factors are identified by name and Roman numeral or by Roman numeral alone.

Nursing Management

Refer to nursing interventions for managing and minimizing bleeding and hemorrhage discussed with leukemia. If instituting corticosteroid therapy, the nurse observes the client for adverse drug effects. The dose and frequency of steroid medication is tapered before discontinuing it to avoid adrenal insufficiency or crisis (see Chap. 50).

HEMOPHILIA

Hemophilia is a disorder involving an absence or reduction of a clotting factor. The three types of hemophilia are hemophilia A, B, and C. Hemophilia A, the most common type, results from a deficiency of factor VIII. In a less serious form of hemophilia A, *von Willebrand's disease,* the amount and quality of factor VIII is diminished. Hemophilia B, or Christmas disease, is a deficiency of factor IX. Hemophilia C, also known as *Rosenthal's disease* results from a deficiency of Factor XI.

Pathophysiology and Etiology

Hemophilia is inherited from mother to son as a sex-linked recessive characteristic. Daughters can inherit the trait but seldom develop the disease. Women with the trait, however, can transmit the disease to male offspring.

The severity of hemophilia depends on the type inherited. Bleeding typically is noted in infancy and childhood. Milder forms can go unrecognized for years. The disease considerably shortens life expectancy; many clients with hemophilia do not reach adulthood. Those with mild hemophilia may lead full and productive lives despite the illness. Human immunodeficiency virus (HIV) and hepatitis virus have been transmitted to clients with hemophilia

through transfusion of blood and blood products. The testing of donated blood has markedly reduced the risk for acquiring blood-borne pathogens.

Assessment Findings

Persistent oozing and sometimes severe bleeding that occurs spontaneously or after an injury are manifestations of the disease. Bleeding in joints eventually damages the joints and leads to deformity and limitation of motion. Diagnosis is based on the history of symptoms and laboratory tests such as coagulant factor assay, which shows a deficiency of factor VIII, IX, or IX.

Medical Management

Treatment includes transfusions of fresh blood, frozen plasma, factor VIII concentrate, and anti-inhibitor coagulant complex for hemophilia A, factor IX concentrate for hemophilia B, factor XI for hemophilia C, and the application of thrombin or fibrin to the bleeding area. Other measures used to help control bleeding are the administration of fresh frozen plasma, aminocaproic acid (Amicar) that helps to hold a clot in place once it has formed, direct pressure over the bleeding site, and cold compresses or ice packs.

Relatively minor surgical procedures, such as tooth extraction, carry considerable risk and are best performed in a hospital. Transfusions usually are necessary even when minor surgery is performed.

Nursing Management

The nurse obtains a comprehensive health history that includes current symptoms and treatment for the bleeding disorder. He or she questions the client about when the last episode occurred, its location (e.g., mouth, rectum, skin),

Client and Family Teaching 31-3
Hemophilia

The nurse explains the treatment regimen and educates the client and family as follows:

- Eliminate aspirin and nonsteroidal anti-inflammatory drugs (NSAIDs), because these drugs can increase bleeding tendencies.
- Avoid activities that can result in injury.
- Wear a MedicAlert bracelet and inform the dentist and others, when appropriate, of the condition.
- Notify the physician promptly if pain, discomfort, or obvious bleeding from the nose or rectum, in vomitus, or elsewhere occurs. Bleeding in internal organs or structures initially produces only vague symptoms.
- Use a soft toothbrush and rinse the mouth with warm water between and after meals.
- Support painful joints on pillows.

duration, and what treatments, if any, were necessary. The nurse assesses the joints and mobility and inspects the skin for purpura or hemorrhagic areas. Before taking a blood pressure, the nurse asks the client if the use of a blood-pressure cuff has ever produced bleeding under the skin or in the arm joints. The nurse takes the temperature tympanically to avoid oral or rectal injuries. He or she checks the urine and stools for signs of bleeding.

Overall care includes preventing trauma, managing and minimizing bleeding episodes, reducing pain or discomfort, conserving energy, and helping the client learn ways to prevent further bleeding episodes. When the client requires transfusion of products such as whole blood, plasma, or antihemophilic factor for bleeding episodes, the nurse closely observes for signs that bleeding has been controlled. He or she keeps the physician informed of the client's progress because additional treatment modalities often are necessary. Client and Family Teaching 31-3 provides information related to teaching about hemophilia.

CRITICAL THINKING EXERCISES

1. List hematopoietic disorders associated with anemia and an etiology of each.
2. When taking a dietary history from a client with anemia, the frequency and amount of consumption of what foods would be important to ascertain?
3. Discuss the problems that clients with anemia, leukemia, or thrombocytopenia share. What interventions can nurses use regardless of the particular disorder?

4. For what hematopoietic disorders would stem cell transplantation be appropriate?

NCLEX-STYLE REVIEW QUESTIONS

1. A client arrives at the emergency department after a motorcycle accident. Vital signs are T–97.7°F, P–122, R–28, and BP–96/54. The client has suffered profuse blood loss. From the clinical picture, the nurse would be correct in placing this client in which position?
   1. Semi-Fowler's
   2. Modified Trendelenburg ———✓ *legs elevated 45°*
   3. Reverse Trendelenburg
   4. Lithotomy
2. The nurse is assessing a client with anemia possibly resulting from malaria. Which of the following data would be most important to ascertain to assist the physician in making a correct diagnosis?
   1. Recent exposure to radiation
   2. Exercise routine
   3. Foreign travel
   4. Alcohol consumption
3. A client has been diagnosed with pernicious anemia. She exclaims, "I'm worried because my grandmother died of the disease years ago." The nurse is most accurate in giving which of the following explanations?
   1. "We have come a long way in furthering life expectancy."
   2. "We now give vitamin B_{12} to control the disease."
   3. "Regular blood transfusions keep the disease in remission."
   4. "Bone marrow transplant is the only cure for the disease."
4. Which of the following nursing interventions are most appropriate when managing the care of a client with glossitis and stomatitis related to pernicious anemia? Select all that apply.
   1. Give the client a soft, bland diet.
   2. Consult with the physician about initiating iron therapy.
   3. Give the client small, frequent meals rather than three large meals.
   4. Encourage the client to move about as much as possible.
   5. Help the client perform meticulous oral care after meals.
5. A client is being admitted to a medical-surgical floor with a diagnosis of acute lymphocytic leukemia. Which nursing intervention is most important in the acute phase of the disease?
   1. Implement neutropenic precautions.
   2. Monitor blood chemistry results.
   3. Institute standard precautions.
   4. Use a low air flow mattress.

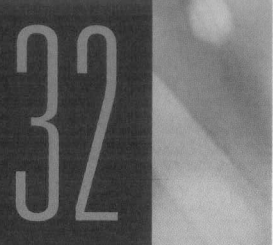

32

Caring for Clients with Disorders of the Lymphatic System

Learning Objectives

On completion of this chapter, you will be able to:

1. Explain the cause and characteristics of lymphedema.
2. Discuss the role of the nurse when managing the care of clients with lymphedema.
3. Describe nursing interventions that promote the resolution of lymphangitis and lymphadenitis.
4. Explain the nature and transmission of infectious mononucleosis.
5. List suggestions the nurse can offer to individuals who acquire infectious mononucleosis.
6. Define the term *lymphoma* and name two types.
7. Name the type of malignant cell diagnostic of Hodgkin's disease.
8. List three forms of treatment used to cure or promote remission of lymphomas.
9. Name at least four problems that nurses address when caring for clients with Hodgkin's disease and non-Hodgkin's lymphoma.

A s described in Chapter 30, the lymphatic system is a network of vessels, known as *lymphatics*, that transport *lymph*, the watery fluid derived from plasma that exits the walls of capillaries and enters interstitial spaces. The lymphatic vessels carry the lymph to and through *lymph nodes*, clusters of bean-sized structures located primarily in the neck, axilla, chest, abdomen, pelvis, and groin. The lymph nodes contain lymphocytes and macrophages, specialized immune defensive cells, that trap, destroy, and remove infectious microorganisms, cellular debris, and cancer cells. The tonsils, thymus gland, and spleen are accessory lymphatic structures.

Most lymphatic fluid circulates with the help of skeletal muscle contraction and is returned to venous circulation through one of two ducts. The *thoracic duct,* located in the posterior abdominal cavity, collects lymph from all body areas except that which circulates above the right diaphragm and deposits the fluid into the left subclavian vein. The *right lymphatic duct* returns lymph from the right side of the head, neck, chest, and right arm and empties it into the right subclavian vein (Fig. 32-1).

Occlusive, inflammatory, infectious, and malignant disorders of the lymphatic system result in fluid distribution problems, tender and painful lymph node enlargement, compromised immune functions, or a combination of these. This chapter discusses such disorders.

OCCLUSIVE, INFLAMMATORY, AND INFECTIOUS DISORDERS

LYMPHEDEMA

Pathophysiology and Etiology

Lymphedema is an accumulation of lymphatic fluid that results from impaired lymph circulation. Primary lymphedema usually is

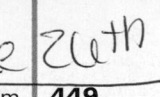

Vessels in purple area drain into right lymphatic duct

Vessels in red area drain into thoracic duct

Right lymphatic duct

Axillary nodes

Mammary vessels

Lumbar nodes

Femoral vessels

Popliteal nodes

Tibial vessels

Thoracic duct

Mesenteric nodes

Cubital nodes

Cisterna chyli

Iliac nodes and vessels

Inguinal nodes

Occipital nodes

Cervical nodes

Parotid nodes

Mandibular nodes

A

Right internal jugular vein

Right lymphatic duct

Right subclavian vein

Right brachiocephalic vein

Left internal jugular vein

Thoracic duct

Left subclavian vein

Superior vena cava

Left brachiocephalic vein

B

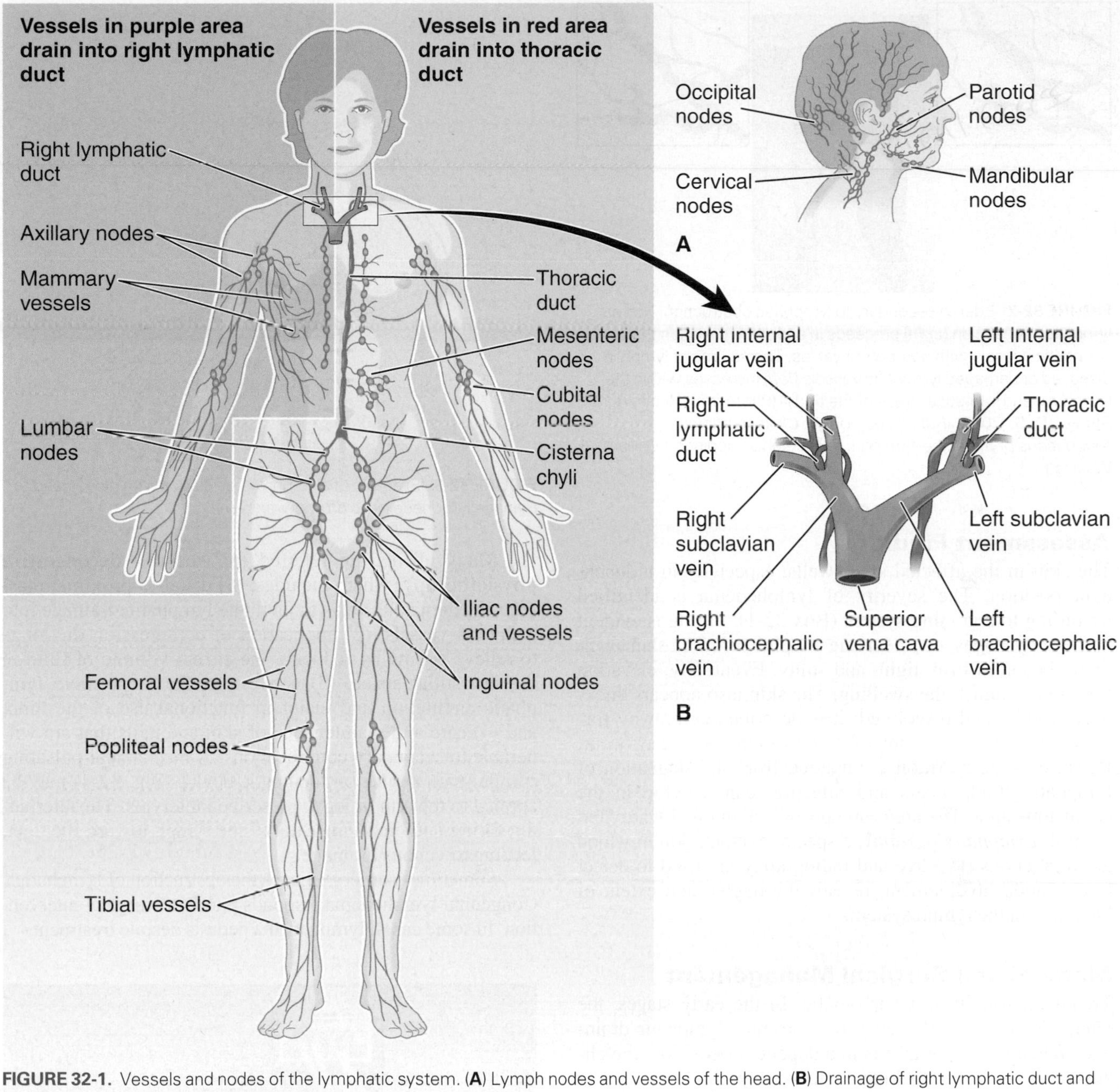

FIGURE 32-1. Vessels and nodes of the lymphatic system. (**A**) Lymph nodes and vessels of the head. (**B**) Drainage of right lymphatic duct and thoracic duct into subclavian veins.

congenitally acquired, although manifestations usually do not appear until adolescence or early adulthood. It affects women more often than men. Secondary lymphedema develops (1) as a complication of other disorders, such as repeated bouts of phlebitis and streptococcal infection, burns, or insect bites; or (2) as a consequence of treatment, such as the removal of multiple lymph nodes at the time of a mastectomy (see Chap. 54) or radiation for cancer. Lymphedema affects more than one fourth of women who have received treatment for breast cancer; this accounts for an appreciable number of the 2 to 3 million Americans affected by this condition (Holcomb, 2006). Worldwide, the most common cause of lymphedema is a parasitic worm; mosquitoes

transmit the parasite, resulting in a condition known as elephantiasis.

The disorder causing lymphedema leads to an accumulation of lymph containing a large percentage of protein within lymphatic vessels. When the volume of the lymph exceeds the capacity of the vessels, the lymph enters the interstitial spaces within soft tissues. The trapped fluid attracts fibroblasts and collagen, eventually causing a non-pitting edema in the late stage that appears different from other types of edema. When massive, the resulting edema leads to chronic deformities in locations such as the arms, legs, and genitalia, with subsequent poor nutrition to tissues (Fig. 32-2).

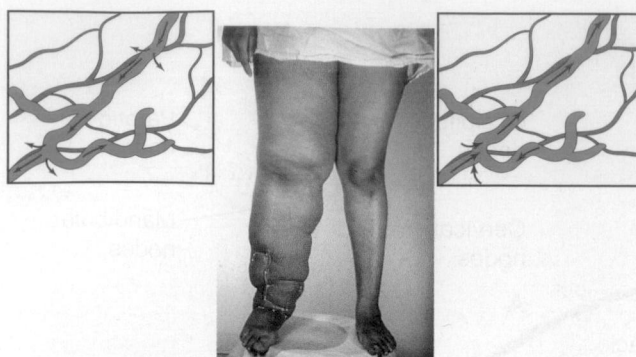

FIGURE 32-2. Edema secondary to lymphatic obstruction. Normal lymphatic circulation (*right*) proceeds in a forward direction through lymphatic vessels with competent valves. The volume of lymph in diseased or damaged lymphatic vessels (*left*) increases within the lymphatic and interstitial areas of the body. (Photo from Rubin, R., & Strayer, D. S. [2008]. *Rubin's pathology: Clinicopathologic foundations of medicine.* [5th ed.]. Philadelphia: Lippincott Williams & Wilkins.)

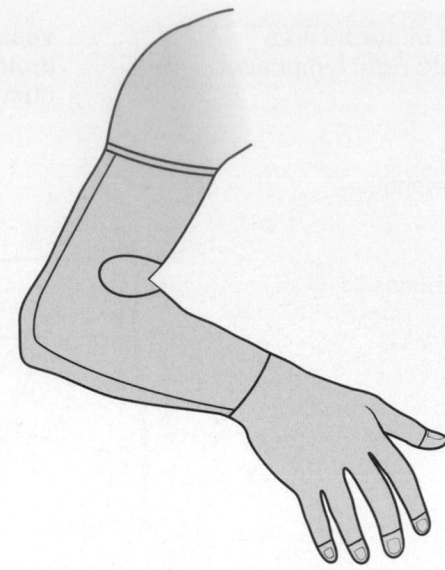

FIGURE 32-3. Example of a compression sleeve with glove used to manage lymphedema in an upper extremity.

Assessment Findings

The skin in the affected area swells, especially in a dependent position. The severity of lymphedema is identified according to a grading system (Box 32-1). Pitting is evident in the early stages, but the tissue remains soft. The skin eventually becomes firm, tight, and shiny. Eventually, elevation does not diminish the swelling. The skin also appears thickened, rough, and discolored; it is described as brawny (orange). Weeping, or oozing of fluid from the skin, may occur. Because tissue nutrition is impaired from the stagnation of lymphatic fluid, ulcers and infection can develop in the edematous area. The area can appear red and feel warm and painful. *Lymphangiography*, a special examination in which an intravenous (IV) dye and radiography are used to detect lymph node involvement, reveals the degree and extent of blockage in the lymph system.

Medical and Surgical Management

Treatment usually is symptomatic. In the early stages, the client elevates the affected part to promote lymphatic drainage. When the leg or arm is in a dependent position, the client wears an elastic stocking or sleeve (Fig. 32-3).

Many clients are referred for **complex decongestive physiotherapy,** which includes: (1) distal-to-proximal massage of edematous areas to facilitate lymphatic drainage into collateral vessels, (2) application of compression dressings to relieve edema by reducing the excess volume of fluid in the interstitial space, (3) active exercise to promote lymphatic circulation and maintain functional use of the limb, and (4) care and maintenance of skin and nails that are vulnerable to secondary complications. A mechanical pulsating compression device or pneumatic device (Fig. 32-4) may be applied to the arm or leg at prescribed intervals. The alternating filling and emptying "milk" the lymph toward the duct, leading to venous drainage.

Sometimes surgery relieves the obstruction of lymphatics. Congenital lymphedema responds poorly to surgical intervention. In some cases, lymphedema persists despite treatment.

BOX 32-1 **Classification of Lymphedema**

Grade I (Mild): Circumference of affected limb is 2 cm, but not more than 4 cm larger than the unaffected limb; client is asymptomatic.

Grade II (Moderate): Circumference of affected limb is 4 cm, but not more than 8 cm larger than the unaffected limb; client experiences symptoms such as heaviness in the limb, pain, and limited movement.

Grade III (Severe): Circumference of affected limb is 8 cm greater than the unaffected limb, involves the entire limb, or is accompanied by infection or cellulitis (inflammation of connective tissue in or close to the skin).

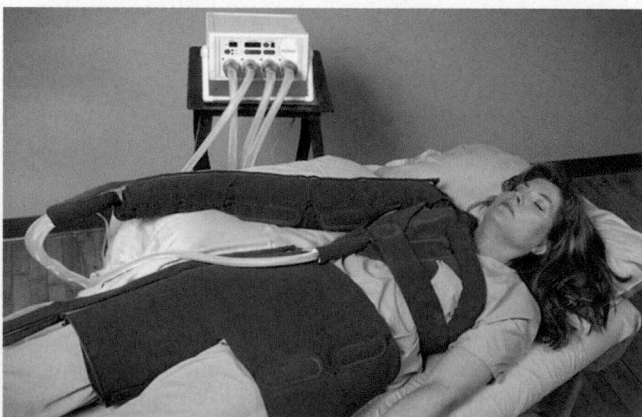

FIGURE 32-4. Example of a pneumatic device that simulates manual lymphatic drainage: the Flexitouch. This device is different than a traditional compression pump; it is a pneumatic device that has a light and variable pressure and works in two phases by treating the trunk first and then the affected extremity based on the principles of manual lymphatic drainage. (Photo courtesy of Tactile Systems Technology, Inc.)

Nursing Management

The nurse inspects and measures the affected area to assess the extent of enlargement and assess the condition of the skin. He or she encourages the client to move and exercise the affected arm or leg to enhance the flow of lymph from the congested area. The nurse instructs the client to elevate the edematous extremities when sitting and teaches how to apply and use elastic garments and mechanical devices.

Extensive emotional support is necessary when the edema is severe. The client's self-esteem often is decreased, which can lead to social withdrawal. The nurse supports the client's self-image by suggesting certain styles of clothing that conceal abnormal enlargement of an arm or leg. For information on client teaching, see the discussion that follows nursing management for clients after a mastectomy in Chapter 54.

▶ **Stop, Think, and Respond Exercise 32-1**

Why is a client at an increased risk for lymphedema after a mastectomy?

LYMPHANGITIS AND LYMPHADENITIS

Lymphangitis is inflammation of lymphatic vessels. When such inflammation affects the lymph nodes near the lymphatics, the condition is called **lymphadenitis.**

Pathophysiology and Etiology

An infectious agent, commonly a streptococcal microorganism, usually causes both lymphangitis and lymphadenitis. The lymph nodes and lymph vessels manifest typical signs of inflammation: redness, swelling, discomfort, and compromised function.

Assessment Findings

Red streaks follow the course of the lymph channels and extend up the arm or leg. Fever also may be present. When lymphadenitis is present, the lymph nodes along the lymphatic channels are enlarged and tender on palpation. Diagnosis is made by visual inspection and palpation.

Medical Management

A broad-spectrum antibiotic commonly is ordered.

Nursing Management

The nurse inspects the area two to three times daily and notes the client's response to antibiotic therapy. He or she gives assistance if the discomfort interferes with activities of daily living. Elevation reduces the swelling. Warmth promotes comfort and enhances circulation. The nurse notifies the physician if the affected area appears to enlarge, additional lymph nodes become involved, or body temperature remains elevated. In severe cases with persistent swelling, the nurse teaches the client how to apply an elastic sleeve or stocking.

INFECTIOUS MONONUCLEOSIS

Infectious mononucleosis is a viral disease that affects lymphoid tissues such as the tonsils and spleen. It can also involve other organs such as the brain, meninges, and liver.

Pathophysiology and Etiology

The **Epstein-Barr virus** causes infectious mononucleosis. This contagious disorder spreads by direct contact with saliva and pharyngeal secretions from an infected person. It is transmitted by kissing; oral spraying during coughing, talking, or sneezing; or sharing food, cigarettes, or other items containing oral secretions. The incubation period can be as long as 30 to 50 days (Box 32-2). The virus most commonly affects young adults, especially those in close living quarters, such as armed services housing and college dormitories.

At the time of infection, macrophages engulf the virus, resulting in a display of the antigen on the cell surface. Active production of T lymphocytes follows. The T lymphocytes trigger the production of B-cell lymphocytes and antibodies. They also infiltrate tissue, particularly the spleen, causing it to enlarge. Force to the abdomen can cause the spleen to rupture when it is enlarged.

The symptoms resolve in approximately 1 to 2 weeks unless complications develop. One episode of infectious mononucleosis produces subsequent immunity; however, the virus remains in the body for the person's lifetime. The Epstein-Barr virus is believed to trigger Hodgkin's lymphoma (discussed later in the chapter) in approximately 40% of people with this disease.

▶ **Stop, Think, and Respond Exercise 32-2**

What factors might make young adults particularly susceptible to acquiring infectious mononucleosis?

Assessment Findings

Signs and Symptoms

Fatigue, fever, sore throat, headache, and cervical lymph node enlargement typically occur. The tonsils ooze white or greenish-gray exudates (Fig. 32-5). Pharyngeal swelling can compromise swallowing and breathing. Some clients develop a faint red rash on their hands or abdomen. The liver and spleen become enlarged. The symptoms persist for several weeks.

Diagnostic Findings

The leukocyte and differential cell counts demonstrate lymphocytosis. A positive slide agglutination test (Monospot, Mono Test, Monosticon) is presumptive evidence that the Epstein-Barr virus is causing the symptoms. A rise in the Epstein-Barr virus antibody titer and a heterophil agglutination

---

BOX 32-2 **Characteristics of Infectious Mononucleosis**

Usual age: 15 to 25 years
Incubation period: 30 to 50 days
Fever: irregular, usually about 2 weeks
Sore throat: marked, whitish-gray exudate
Adenopathy (enlargement of lymph nodes): most commonly anterior and posterior cervical chains; often generalized
Splenomegaly (enlargement of spleen): approximately 50%
Hepatomegaly (enlargement of liver): approximately 10%

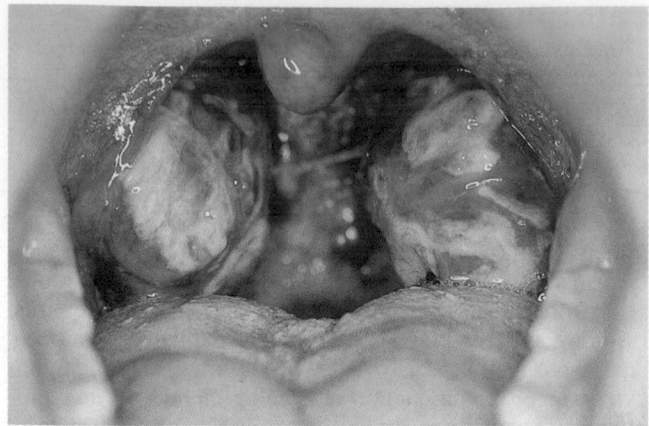

FIGURE 32-5. The throat of a person with infectious mononucleosis is red. The tonsils exude purulent drainage. The appearance can be mistaken for a streptococcal throat infection. (© Dr. P. Marazzi/Science Source/Photo Researchers, Inc.)

test result of 1:224 or greater is conclusive for infectious mononucleosis.

Medical Management

The infection usually is self-limiting. Bed rest, analgesic and antipyretic therapy, and increased fluid intake are recommended. Corticosteroid therapy is prescribed if complications such as hepatic involvement occur. If a bacterial infection such as sinusitis or streptococcal pharyngitis accompanies mononucleosis, an antibiotic is prescribed.

Nursing Management

The nurse inspects the client's throat for the extent of inflammation or edema. He or she gently palpates the lymph nodes to detect swelling and encourages fluids. Soft, bland foods and cool liquids are best for clients with ulcerations of the oral mucosa. The nurse advises the client to rest as much as possible. If the client expresses concern over prolonged time off from work or school, the nurse listens and helps the client cope with the anxiety. He or she advises the client to withhold donating blood for at least 6 months after recovering from the illness.

LYMPHOMAS

The term **lymphoma** applies to a group of cancers that affect the lymphatic system. The types of lymphoma are classified by the microscopic appearance of the malignant cells and how quickly the malignancy spreads. Two of the most common forms of lymphoma are Hodgkin's disease and non-Hodgkin's lymphoma (Table 32-1). Acquired immunodeficiency syndrome–related lymphoma occurs in people who have been infected with the human immunodeficiency virus (HIV).

Gerontologic Considerations

- The risk of lymphoma is increased in older adults, primarily because of the immunologic changes of aging and prolonged exposure to carcinogens.

HODGKIN'S DISEASE

Hodgkin's disease is a malignancy that produces enlargement of lymphoid tissue, the spleen, and the liver, with invasion of other tissues such as the bone marrow and lungs. It may appear in several forms: acute, localized, or latent with relapsing pyrexia (elevated temperature); splenomegaly (enlarged spleen); and as lymphogranulomatosis (multiple granular tumors or growths composed of lymphoid cells).

Pathophysiology and Etiology

Although the exact cause of Hodgkin's disease is unknown, it appears that a virus, particularly the Epstein-Barr virus (the etiologic agent of infectious mononucleosis), causes mutations in some but not all lymphocytes, creating malignant cells known as **Reed-Sternberg cells.** Reed-Sternberg cells are nearly immortal, continue to reproduce prolifically, and, perhaps because of their altered form, are somehow shielded from being destroyed by killer T cells. The virus also is believed to inactivate the immune system's ability to suppress tumor growth. The malignant cells release chemicals known as *cytokines* (see Chap. 33), causing inflammatory symptoms such as pain and fever. Some clients develop generalized itching and a skin rash because of the release of histamine from an atypical allergic/immune response.

The disease is more common in men than in women and most frequently occurs during late adolescence and young adulthood. Some clients survive 10 or more years; others die in 4 to 5 years. A cure is possible when the disease is localized

TABLE 32-1 Comparison of Lymphomas

HODGKIN'S	NON-HODGKIN'S
Four subtypes	Thirty subtypes
Two peaks of onset: ages 15 to 40 and older than age 55 years	Peaks after age 50 years
Reed-Sternberg cells	No Reed-Sternberg cells
Forty percent of affected clients test positive for Epstein-Barr virus	More common in industrial countries; common among clients with immunosuppression
B-cell origin	B- and T-cell origin
Usually starts in lymph nodes above the clavicle, commonly in the neck and chest; 15% are below the diaphragm; spreads downward from initial site	Common in abdomen, tonsils; can develop in areas other than lymph nodes (e.g., brain, nasal passages)
More orderly growth from one node to adjacent nodes	Less predictable growth; spreads to extranodal sites
More curable	Less curable

to one section of the body. Clients who receive treatment usually have remissions that last for months or even years. Death results from respiratory obstruction, cachexia (state of ill health, malnutrition, and wasting), or secondary infections.

Assessment Findings

Signs and Symptoms

Early symptoms of Hodgkin's disease include painless enlargement of one or more lymph nodes. The cervical lymph nodes are the first to be affected. As the nodes enlarge, they press on adjacent structures, such as the esophagus or bronchi. As retroperitoneal nodes enlarge, there is a sense of fullness in the stomach and epigastric pain. Marked weight loss, anorexia, fatigue, and weakness occur. Low-grade fever, pruritus, and night sweats are common. Sometimes marked anemia and thrombocytopenia develop, causing a tendency to bleed. Resistance to infection is poor, and staphylococcal skin infections and respiratory tract infections often complicate the illness.

Diagnostic Findings

A complete blood count demonstrates low red blood cell count, elevated leukocytes, and a paradoxical decrease in lymphocytes. The Reed-Sternberg cells, characterized as giant multinucleated B lymphocytes, are microscopically identifiable in lymph node biopsies. Results of blood chemistry tests such as erythrocyte sedimentation rate are elevated, suggesting a current inflammatory process. Liver enzymes such as alkaline phosphatase are elevated. Lymphangiography, chest radiography, computed tomography, magnetic resonance imaging, or a laparotomy to obtain abdominal nodes for biopsy demonstrate the size of lymph nodes and the spread of the disease in the thorax, abdomen, or pelvis. A bone marrow aspiration and biopsy indicate abnormalities of other blood cells. After diagnosis, the disease is staged from stage I to IV, based on the number of positive lymph nodes and the involvement of other organs (Table 32-2). Staging helps determine treatment.

Stages I, II, III, and IV of adult Hodgkin's disease are subclassified into A and B categories: B for those with defined general symptoms and A for those without B symptoms. The B designation is given to clients with any of the following symptoms:

- Unexplained loss of more than 10% of body weight in the 6 months before diagnosis
- Unexplained fever with temperatures above 100.4°F (38°C)

TABLE 32-2 Stages of Hodgkin's Disease

STAGE	INVOLVEMENT
I	Single lymph node region
II	Two or more lymph node regions on one side of the diaphragm
III	Lymph node regions on both sides of the diaphragm but extension is limited to the spleen
IV	Bilateral lymph nodes affected and extension includes spleen plus one or more of the following: bones, bone marrow, lungs, liver, skin, gastrointestinal structures, or other sites

- Drenching night sweats (Note: The most significant B symptoms are fever and weight loss. Night sweats alone do not confer an adverse prognosis.)

Careful staging and treatment planning by a multidisciplinary team of cancer specialists are required to determine optimal treatment of clients with this disease.

Gerontologic Considerations

- The etiology and presentation of Hodgkin's disease are different in younger adults than in older adults. Older clients may present with Stage IV or the presentation may be impacted by the normal changes of aging (Freedman, 2006).

Medical Management

Treatment of Hodgkin's disease includes localized radiation to affected lymph nodes and chemotherapy with combinations of antineoplastic drugs (Table 32-3). Antibiotics are given to fight secondary infections. Transfusions are prescribed to control anemia. If resistance to treatment develops, autologous bone marrow or peripheral stem cells are harvested, followed by high doses of chemotherapy that destroy the bone marrow (see Chaps. 18 and 31). Normal stem cells are separated from the malignant cells in the harvested specimen, and a transplant is performed.

Pharmacologic Considerations

- Recognizing and treating adverse drug reactions can help optimize response to therapy. Clients with Hodgkin's disease are extremely susceptible to toxic effects of medication and to secondary infection from the combination of treatments (i.e., radiation and chemotherapy) and a weakened immune system from the disease. Supportive measures are necessary for those experiencing toxic effects of chemotherapeutic agents. Bone marrow depression, gastrointestinal disturbances, and alopecia (hair loss) are common adverse effects.

TABLE 32-3 Chemotherapy Regimens For Hodgkin's Disease

REGIMEN	DRUGS
ABVD	Doxorubicin (Adriamycin), bleomycin (Blenoxane), vinblastine (Velban), dacarbazine (DTIC)
MOPP	Mechlorethamine (Mustargen), vincristine (Oncovin), prednisone (Meticorten), procarbazine (Matulane)
MOPP/ABVD	Alternation of drugs from both regimens
For partial remission or relapse within 1 year	
CBV	Cyclophosphamide (Cytoxan), carmustine (BiCNU), etoposide (VePesid)
BEAM	Carmustine (BiCNU), etoposide (VePesid), cytosine arabinoside (Cytosar-U), melphalan (Alkeran)

Gerontologic Considerations

- Because older clients cannot tolerate maximum doses, they respond less well to chemotherapy than younger people. In addition, doxorubicin is not tolerated due to its toxic effects on the kidneys. Although it is necessary to weigh the benefits of chemotherapy against the adverse reactions that may affect older adults, treatment modalities are not based on age alone.

Nursing Process for the Client with Hodgkin's Disease

Assessment

Review the client's past history for infectious mononucleosis or symptoms resembling this disorder. Palpate enlarged lymph nodes and identify their location, size, and other notable characteristics, such as whether they are fixed or mobile. Inquire how long the client has noticed the enlarged lymph nodes and check for the presence and extent of tenderness in the area of lymph node enlargement. Ask if the client experiences fever, chills, or night sweats. Check the client's current weight and deviation from usual weight, enlargement of the liver and spleen, and level of energy and appetite (see Nutrition Notes 32-1). Inspect the appearance of the skin, ask about any itching, and discuss any additional symptoms caused by lymph node enlargement (e.g., coughing, breathlessness, nausea, vomiting).

Diagnosis, Planning, and Interventions

Client and Family Teaching 32-1 describes instructions for nurses to communicate to clients with Hodgkin's disease. Other nursing care includes, but is not limited to, the following:

▶ Risk for Ineffective Airway Clearance and Risk for Impaired Gas Exchange related to compression of trachea secondary to enlarged cervical lymph nodes

▶ Expected Outcome: Breathing will remain adequate to maintain blood oxygen saturation of 90% or greater.

• Assess respiratory status each shift and as needed. Note quality, rate, pattern, depth, flaring of nostrils, dyspnea on exertion, evidence of splinting, use of accessory muscles, and position for

Nutrition Notes 32-1
The Client with Hodgkin's Disease

• Nausea and vomiting often accompany radiation therapy.
• Clients must maintain food and fluid intake.
• Offer clear liquids such as carbonated beverages and water, ice pops, and flavored gelatin until nausea subsides. Thereafter, small, frequent, low-fat meals help prevent nausea.

Client and Family Teaching 32-1
Hodgkin's Disease

The nurse instructs the client as follows:

• Keep appointments for medical follow-up.
• Take prescribed medications as directed. Report side effects to the physician.
• Avoid crowds or people who have infectious diseases.
• Wash hands frequently.
• Avoid oral contact with germ-laden objects.
• Contact the physician if breathing becomes labored.
• Eat small amounts frequently or include a liquid nutritional supplement between meals and at bedtime.
• Reduce work schedule to avoid exhaustion. If that is not possible, rest frequently.
• Consult with an employer about sick-leave considerations or a representative from the Social Security Administration about unemployment benefits and disability payments.
• Obtain a disability sticker to facilitate easy access to public buildings to lessen fatigue.

breathing. *Any deviation from quiet, effortless breathing indicates compromised ventilation.*

• Keep the neck in midline and place the client in high Fowler's position if respiratory distress develops. *This position avoids unnecessary pressure on the trachea and provides for increased lung expansion and improved air exchange.*

• Administer oxygen per physician's orders if blood saturation is consistently less than 90%. *Increasing the percentage of inhaled oxygen beyond 21% in the atmosphere reduces deficits in the blood oxygen level.*

• Place an endotracheal tube, laryngoscope, and bag-valve mask at the bedside for intubation. *Anticipation of the need for airway management ensures that medical intervention and emergency assistance are not delayed.*

▶ Risk for Infection related to immunosuppression secondary to impaired lymphocytes and drug or radiation therapy

▶ Expected Outcome: Client will remain free of infection as evidenced by no fever and no symptoms of secondary infection.

• Restrict visitors or personnel with infections from contact with the client. *Reducing the number of organisms in the environment and restricting visitors and personnel with an infection reduce the transmission of pathogens to the client.*

• Practice conscientious hand hygiene and follow other principles of medical and surgical asepsis. *Cleaning hands and using aseptic techniques reduce the risk of transmitting pathogens from one location to another.*

• Institute infectious disease precautions if normal white blood cells are suppressed to dangerous limits. *Protective isolation techniques provide an environmental barrier against pathogens while a client is highly susceptible to disease.*

▶ **Risk for Impaired Skin Integrity** related to pruritus, inadequate nutrition, and inactivity

▶ **Expected Outcome:** Client's skin will remain intact throughout care.

• Use mild soap for bathing, rinse well, and pat dry. *Mild soap prevents excessive drying of the skin; patting instead of rubbing dry helps prevent friction, which can damage skin.*

• Apply ice to the skin for brief periods, give cool sponge baths, or provide cotton gloves if itching is intolerable. An oral or topical antipruritic medication often is necessary. *Cooling the skin reduces the sensation of itching, and cotton gloves reduce skin trauma from scratching with sharp fingernails. Antipruritic medications block the release of histamine.*

• Trim nails short to avoid scratching when itching occurs. *Trimming fingernails short prevents abrading the skin and providing an entrance for pathogens.*

• Change bedding as soon as possible if night sweats occur. *Wet bedding contributes to skin maceration.*

• Lift rather than pull the client across sheets when changing positions. *Lifting the client prevents shearing forces on the skin.*

• Support and protect bony prominences. *Areas where skin is stretched tautly over bony prominences create ischemia as a result of compressing skin capillaries between a hard surface (mattress) and the bone.*

• Collaborate with the physician to avoid drugs administered by the parenteral route. *Any breaks in skin integrity can provide an open route for the entrance of pathogens.*

▶ **Activity Intolerance and Self-Care Deficit** related to anemia and generalized weakness from disease

▶ **Expected Outcome:** Client will tolerate and perform essential activities as evidenced by heart and respiratory rates within normal limits.

• Divide care into manageable amounts. *Proportioning activities reduces energy expenditures.*

• Provide rest periods between activities. *Rest gives the body time to recover before the next demand for energy.*

• Perform priority activities first. *Client completes most important or necessary activities while energy levels are highest.*

• Assist the client with whatever activities of daily living are independently unmanageable. *Assistance reduces the client's energy expenditure.*

Evaluation of Expected Outcomes

Breathing is noiseless and effortless. The client shows no signs or symptoms of infection, and his or her skin remains intact. He or she can perform essential activities without compromising cardiorespiratory status. ●

NON-HODGKIN'S LYMPHOMAS

Non-Hodgkin's lymphomas are a group of 30 subclassifications of malignant diseases that originate in lymph glands and other lymphoid tissue. Examples include lymphosarcoma, Burkitt's lymphoma, and reticulum cell sarcoma. The incidence of non-Hodgkin's lymphomas is six to seven times that of Hodgkin's disease, and the number of cases continues to rise.

Pathophysiology and Etiology

No single definitive cause for non-Hodgkin's lymphomas has been found, although a genetic link is strongly implicated in some types. An environmental trigger, such as a viral agent, chemical herbicides, pesticides, or hair dye, may induce the disease. The administration of immunosuppressive drugs to prevent transplant rejection also has been correlated with cases of non-Hodgkin's lymphoma.

In non-Hodgkin's lymphoma, chromosomal changes occur in the affected lymphocytes, and lymphoid tissue enlarges to accommodate the proliferative production of malignant cells. Non-Hodgkin's lymphoma is classified as either (1) *indolent,* meaning that the client is relatively asymptomatic at diagnosis and the disorder is relatively responsive to radiation and chemotherapy; or (2) *aggressive,* because the condition has a shorter onset with acute symptoms. Nevertheless, 30% to 60% of aggressive forms of non-Hodgkin's lymphoma are curable with intensive treatment.

Assessment Findings

Symptoms of non-Hodgkin's lymphoma depend on the site of lymph node involvement. Lymph node enlargement, which usually is diffuse rather than localized, occurs in cervical, axillary, and inguinal regions. The diagnosis and differentiation of the subtypes of non-Hodgkin's lymphoma from Hodgkin's disease depend on microscopic examination of lymphoid tissue biopsies. Additional tests are performed to determine the stage of the lymphoma.

Medical Management

Non-Hodgkin's lymphoma is treated with radiation, chemotherapy, or both. The physician may adopt a "watch and wait" approach for clients with indolent forms of non-Hodgkin's lymphoma, choosing to treat the client once the disease accelerates. Immunotherapy with monoclonal antibodies (MABs) and bone marrow transplants (BMTs) also is being used to cure lymphomas or extend the lives of clients with these diseases.

Monoclonal Antibody Therapy

Research continues on the use of biologic therapy (immunotherapy) with MABs to eliminate malignant cells and induce remission. With MABs, human cancer cells are injected into laboratory animals such as mice (see Chap. 18). The mice make lymphocytes that produce antibodies against the cancer cells. The mouse lymphocytes are harvested and fused with a laboratory-grown cell, creating clones called hybridomas that, when administered to a client with cancer, continue to produce tumor-fighting antibodies (Fig. 32-6). The MABs are used alone or are bound to a chemotherapeutic or radioactive agent. The advantage of combining MABs with drugs or radiation is that they target and destroy cancer cells while sparing normal cells. MAB drugs approved for treating non-Hodgkin's lymphoma include rituximab (Rituxan),

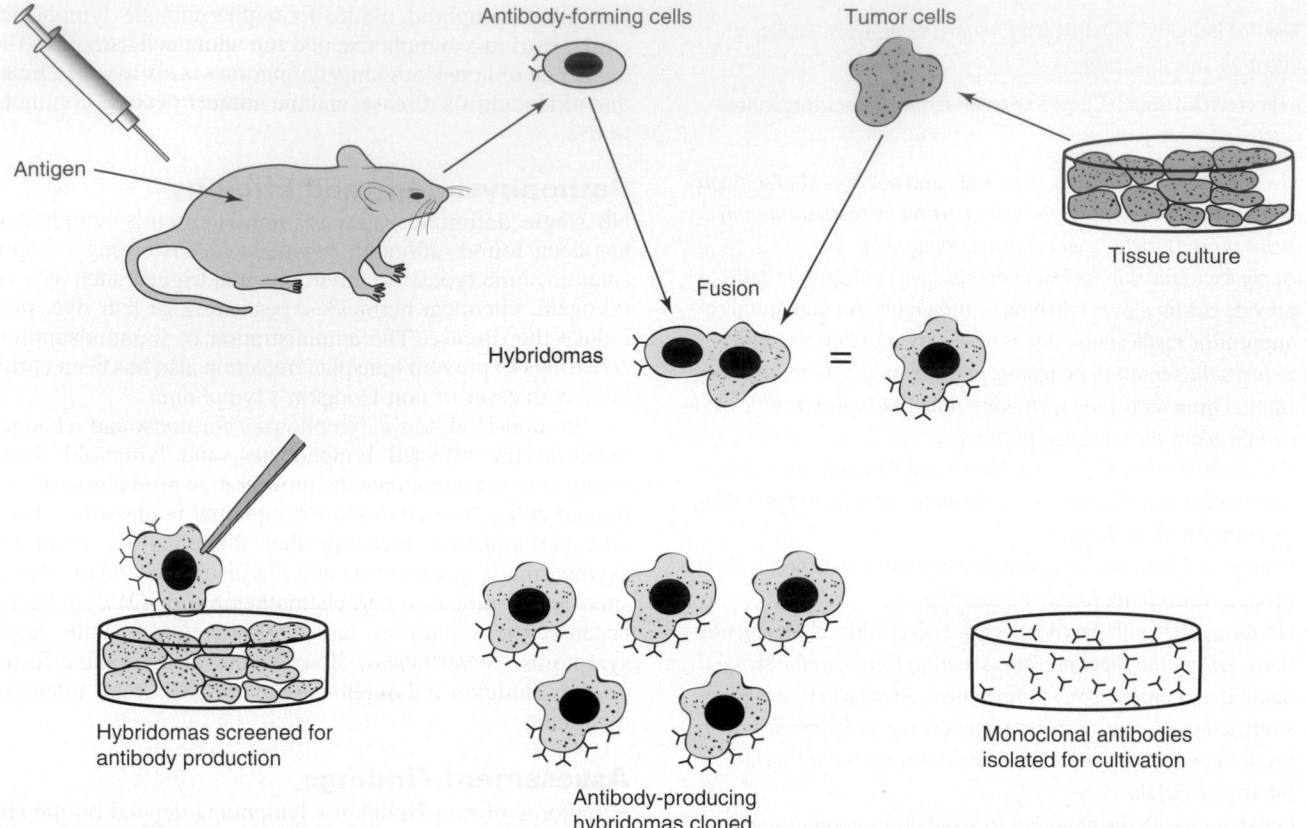

FIGURE 32-6. In monoclonal antibody (MAB) therapy, hybridomas, cloned cells that have been engineered to produce a specific antibody from sensitized mice, attack harmful proteins in the human body such as cancer cells.

ibritumomab and radioactive iodine (Zevalin), tositumomab (Bexxar), and 131I Lym-1 (Oncolym).

Bone Marrow Transplant

Bone marrow and stem cell transplants (see Chaps. 18 and 31) are considered a potential treatment modality when others are ineffective. Autologous (self-donated) bone marrow and peripheral blood stem cells are removed from the client with cancer and frozen. The donor cells are then infused with high doses of drugs and sometimes radiated to destroy all cancer cells. The same is done to the client, thus destroying most remaining bone marrow and stem cells. The frozen marrow and cells are thawed and transplanted into the client's vein, whereupon they recolonize the marrow with normal blood cells.

Instead of autologous transplants, some clients receive allogenic BMTs (i.e., marrow from a human donor), sometimes referred to as *mini-bone marrow transplants* (mini-BMTs). During a mini-BMT, the client is treated with moderate doses of drugs or mild total-body radiation to destroy as many cancer cells as possible and suppress the immune system to reduce the potential for destroying the donor cells. Consequently, when the client undergoes a mini-BMT, the possibility for rejection still exists. The phenomenon is referred to as *graft-versus-host disease* (GVHD) (see Chap. 18). Despite GVHD, allogenic BMTs have two advantages: (1) relapses of lymphoma are less frequent than with autologous transplants, and (2) they induce remissions when a relapse occurs.

Nursing Management

Nursing care is similar for all clients with lymphoma, whether they have non-Hodgkin's lymphoma or Hodgkin's disease. Because chemotherapy and radiation kill many cells, the nurse encourages clients to drink extra fluids ($\geq$2500 mL/day) to facilitate excretion of the cells destroyed by therapy.

 G e r o n t o l o g i c   C o n s i d e r a t i o n s

- Nursing management for older adults with non-Hodgkin's lymphomas must include assessment of the functional status of the cardiopulmonary, renal and central nervous systems to assist the client and family in decision-making regarding risks and benefits of chemotherapy. Advocating for the older client includes planning for end-of-life concerns.

CRITICAL THINKING EXERCISES

1. What are some differences between lymphedema and lymphoma?

2. What teaching is indicated for a person diagnosed with lymphedema?

3. What information can the nurse provide to parents who are concerned about their teenager who has acquired infectious mononucleosis?

4. Explain which lymphoma—Hodgkin's disease or non-Hodgkin's lymphoma—has the better prognosis.

NCLEX-STYLE REVIEW QUESTIONS

1. The nurse is teaching a client with lymphedema how to correctly wear elastic leg stockings. The nurse is correct in instructing that the stockings are to promote which of the following?
1. Circulation in the lower extremities
2. Support of the lower legs during ambulation
3. Lymphatic drainage of the lower extremities
4. Tissue healing of the lower extremities

2. A college student reports to the school health center and is diagnosed with infectious mononucleosis. The student asks the health nurse how the condition was acquired. The best answer by the nurse is that the virus is transmitted by which of the following methods?
1. Contact with microorganisms in the blood
2. Direct contact with an infected person
3. Consuming contaminated food or water
4. The bite of an insect such as a mosquito

3. A client with Hodgkin's disease is admitted to the hospital. In discussing the client's care with the nursing assistant, which nursing explanation is most correct in relation to the chief manifestation of the disease process?
1. Severe itching
2. Tonic-clonic seizure activity
3. Frequent loose stools
4. Enlarged cervical lymph nodes

4. A hospitalized client with Hodgkin's disease is at risk for ineffective airway clearance and impaired gas exchange related to compression of the trachea by enlarged lymph nodes. Which of the following measures would the nurse take first to help ensure that breathing and blood oxygen saturation are remaining adequate?
1. Administer oxygen per the physician's orders.
2. Assess respiratory status during each shift.
3. Place the client in semi- to high-Fowler's position.
4. Restrict visitors and unnecessary personnel.

5. When performing a physical assessment of the client in the early stages of Hodgkin's disease, which is the most likely finding when the nurse palpates the client's lymph nodes?
1. The lymph nodes are fixed and hard.
2. The lymph nodes are enlarged and painless.
3. The lymph nodes are small and firm.
4. The lymph nodes are swollen and tender.

UNIT 8
Caring for Clients with Immune Disorders

33

Introduction to the Immune System

Learning Objectives

On completion of this chapter, you will be able to:

1. Explain the meaning of an immune response.
2. List two general components of the immune system.
3. Discuss the role of T-cell and B-cell lymphocytes.
4. Differentiate between an antigen and an antibody.
5. Name examples of lymphoid tissue.
6. List some cells and chemicals that enhance the function of the immune system.
7. Name three types of immunity, describing how each develops.
8. Discuss techniques for detecting immune disorders.
9. Describe the role of the nurse when caring for a client with an immune disorder.

Although all humans have the same types of cells, each person's cells are unique and different from those of all others. Everyone's body cells are coded with distinct histocompatibility (tissue cell) markers. These markers act as a "fingerprint" that enables the immune system to differentiate self from nonself. When it detects a nonself substance, the immune system protects, defends, and destroys what it perceives as atypical or abnormal. Its primary targets are infectious, foreign, or cancerous cells. The **immune response**, a target-specific system of defense, primarily involves the lymphocytes, which are specialized cells that are located in blood and lymphoid tissue. An immune system that is overly active, as in allergic or autoimmune disorders (see Chap. 34), or one that is functioning poorly, as in acquired immunodeficiency syndrome (AIDS; see Chap. 35), can be life-threatening.

ANATOMY AND PHYSIOLOGY

The immune system is a collection of specialized white blood cells and lymphoid tissues that maintain **immunocompetence**, the ability to cooperatively protect a person from external invaders and the body's own altered cells. The function of these structures is assisted and supported by the activities of natural killer cells, antibodies, and nonantibody proteins such as cytokines and the complement system (Fig. 33-1).

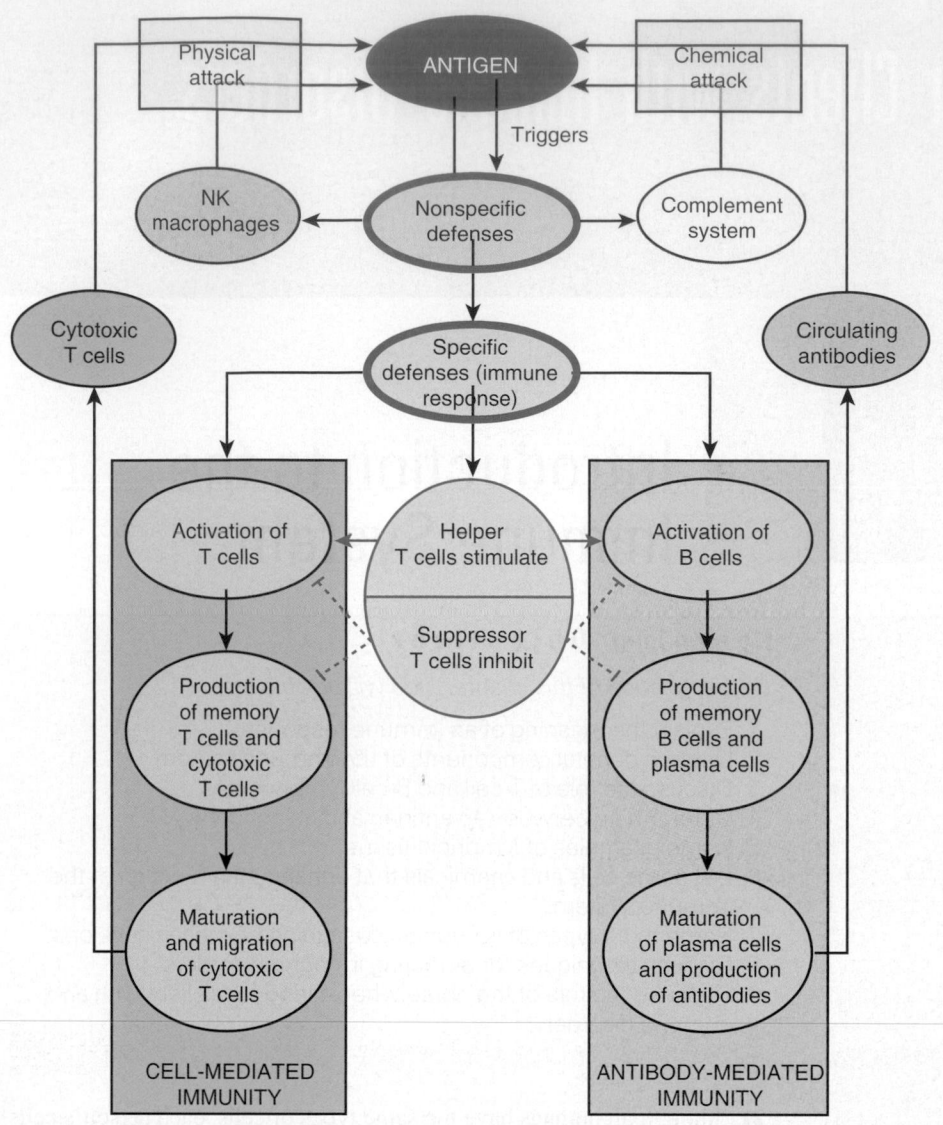

FIGURE 33-1. Schematic representation of the immune response.

White Blood Cells

White blood cells (leukocytes) are produced in the bone marrow. Initially, all blood cells are nonspecific **stem cells** that later differentiate into various types of cells including lymphocytes, neutrophils, and monocytes (see Chap. 30). Figure 33-2 shows the development of various types of blood cells.

Lymphocytes

Lymphocytes, which are either T-cell or B-cell lymphocytes, comprise 20% to 30% of all leukocytes. T-cell and B-cell lymphocytes are the primary participants in the immune response. They distinguish harmful substances and ignore those natural and unique to a person. Table 33-1 identifies various types of lymphocytes and the role they play in the immune response.

T-Cell Lymphocytes

The T-cell lymphocytes are manufactured in the bone marrow and travel to the thymus gland, where they mature to become either regulator T cells or effector T cells. **Regulator T cells** are made up of helper and suppressor cells; **effector**

T cells are killer (cytotoxic) cells. **Helper T cells** are especially important in fighting infection. They recognize **antigens**, which are protein markers on cells, and form additional T-cell clones that stimulate B-cell lymphocytes to produce antibodies against foreign antigens. **Antibodies** are chemical substances that destroy foreign agents such as microorganisms. Helper T cells also are called T4 cells or CD4 cells. **Cytotoxic T cells** bind to invading cells, destroy the targeted invader by altering their cellular membrane and intracellular environment, and stimulate the release of chemicals called lymphokines. **Lymphokines**, a type of cytokine (discussed later in this chapter), attract neutrophils and monocytes to remove the debris. They also promote the maturation of more T cells when they detect antigens and direct B-cell lymphocytes to multiply and mature. **Suppressor T cells** limit or turn off the immune response in the absence of continued antigenic stimulation. The surface molecules of suppressor and cytotoxic (killer) T cells differ from those of helper T cells; cytotoxic T cells sometimes are referred to as T8 or CD8 cells.

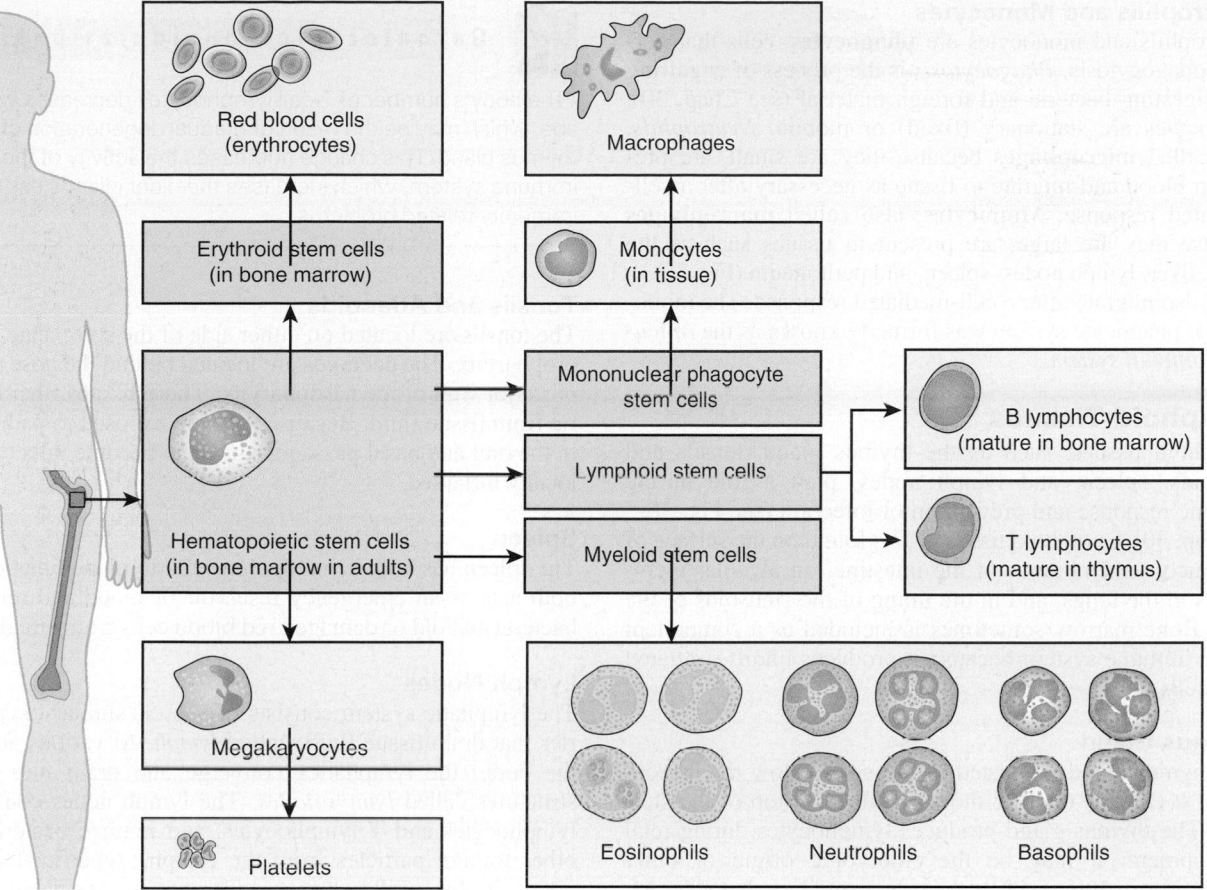

FIGURE 33-2. Origin of blood cells.

The immune response that T-cell lymphocytes perform is called a *cell-mediated response*. A **cell-mediated response** occurs when T cells survey proteins in the body, actively analyze the surface features, and respond to those that differ from the host by directly attacking the invading antigen. An example of a cell-mediated response is one that occurs when an organ is transplanted.

TABLE 33-1 Types and Functions of Lymphocytes

TYPE	FUNCTION
T Cells	
Regulator T cells	
Helper T cells	Recognize antigens; stimulate B cells to produce antibodies
Suppressor T cells	Turn off the immune response
Effector T cells	
Cytotoxic T cells	Bind to and destroy invader cells; stimulate the release of lymphokines
B Cells	
Plasma cells	Produce antibodies
Memory cells	Convert to plasma cells that will produce antibodies when re-exposed to an antigen

 Pharmacologic Considerations

- After organ transplantation, the client's immune system may attack the new organ's cells because it recognizes them as nonself. Therefore, drugs are used to intentionally suppress the immune system. Azathioprine (Imuran), cyclosporine (Sandimmune), and muromonab-CD3 (Orthoclone OKT3) are examples of immunosuppressive drugs.

B-Cell Lymphocytes

The B-cell lymphocytes mature in the bone marrow and migrate to the spleen and other lymphoid tissues such as the lymph nodes. When stimulated by T cells, the B cells become either plasma or memory cells. **Plasma cells** produce antibodies. Formation of antibodies is called a **humoral response**.

Memory cells convert to plasma cells on re-exposure to a specific antigen. When activated, B cells accumulate in lymphoid tissues, which explains the phenomena of swollen and tender lymph nodes that accompany infectious disorders and an enlarged spleen in various immune disorders.

▶ ***Stop, Think, and Respond Exercise 33-1***

Explain the difference between a cell-mediated response and a humoral response.

Neutrophils and Monocytes

Neutrophils and monocytes are **phagocytes**, cells that perform phagocytosis. *Phagocytosis* is the process of engulfing and digesting bacteria and foreign material (see Chap. 30). Phagocytes are stationary (fixed) or mobile. *Neutrophils*, also called **microphages** because they are small, are present in blood and migrate to tissue as necessary after a cell-mediated response. **Monocytes**, also called **macrophages** because they are large, are present in tissues such as the lungs, liver, lymph nodes, spleen, and peritoneum (Fig. 33-3). They also migrate after a cell-mediated response. The mononuclear phagocyte system was formerly known as the *reticuloendothelial system.*

Lymphoid Tissues

Lymphoid tissues, such as the thymus gland, tonsils and adenoids, spleen, and lymph nodes, play a role in the immune response and prevention of infection (see Fig. 30-5 in Chap. 30). Lymphoid tissue also is found on the surface of the mucous membranes of the intestine, on alveolar membranes in the lungs, and in the lining of the sinusoids of the liver. Bone marrow sometimes is included as a component of the immune system because it produces undifferentiated stem cells.

Thymus Gland

The thymus gland is located in the neck below the thyroid gland. It extends into the thorax behind the top of the sternum. The thymus gland produces lymphocytes during fetal development. It may be the embryonic origin of other lymphoid structures such as the spleen and lymph nodes. After birth, the thymus gland programs T lymphocytes to become regulator or effector T cells. The thymus gland becomes smaller during adolescence but retains some activity throughout the life cycle.

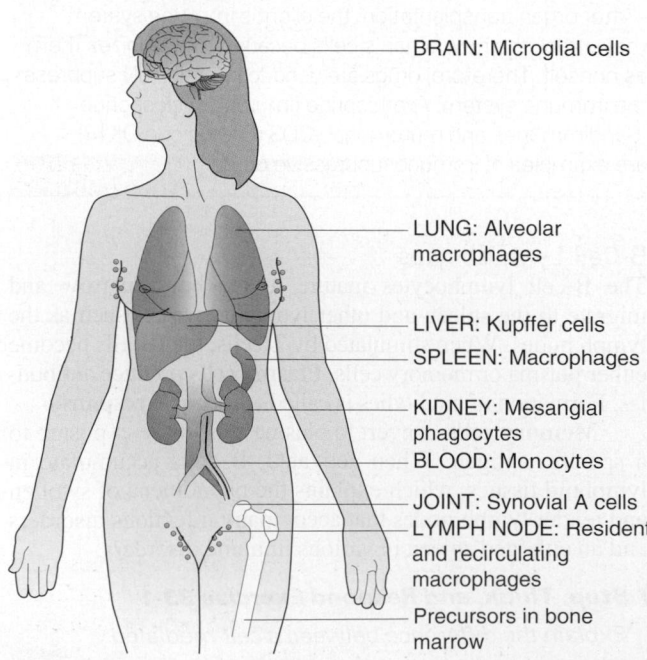

FIGURE 33-3. Location of phagocytes.

BRAIN: Microglial cells

LUNG: Alveolar macrophages

LIVER: Kupffer cells
SPLEEN: Macrophages

KIDNEY: Mesangial phagocytes
BLOOD: Monocytes

JOINT: Synovial A cells
LYMPH NODE: Resident and recirculating macrophages

Precursors in bone marrow

Tonsils and Adenoids

The tonsils are located on either side of the soft palate of the oropharynx. The adenoids are located behind the nose on the posterior wall of the nasopharynx. These tissues filter bacteria from tissue fluid. Because they are exposed to pathogens in the oral and nasal passages, they can become infected and locally inflamed.

Spleen

The spleen has both hematopoietic and immune functions. It both acts as an emergency reservoir of blood and removes bacteria and old or damaged red blood cells from circulation.

Lymph Nodes

The lymphatic system consists of vessels similar to capillaries that drain tissue fluid, called *lymph.* At various areas in the body, the lymphatics converge and drain into larger structures called *lymph nodes.* The lymph nodes contain B lymphocytes and T lymphocytes, and remove bacteria and other foreign particles from the lymph. Superficial lymph nodes in the axilla, groin, and neck are palpable when enlarged.

Natural Killer Cells

Natural killer (NK) cells are lymphocyte-like cells that circulate throughout the body looking for virus-infected cells and cancer cells. NK cells can identify atypical markers on the membranes of these cells without the help of T or B cell lymphocytes. Once identified, NK cells release potent chemicals that lethally alter the target cell's membrane, leading to its demise. Unfortunately, cancer cells can escape NK cell surveillance, which explains how cancer is able to become established and spread beyond its primary site.

Antibodies

Antibodies, proteins produced by B lymphocyte plasma cells, are more correctly referred to as **immunoglobulins** (Ig). There are five types of immunoglobulins: IgA, IgD, IgE, IgG, and IgM. Each immunoglobulin has a separate role in ensuring the maintenance of a healthy state (Table 33-2).

Immunoglobulins bind with antigens and promote the destruction of invading cells in one of two ways. First, immunoglobulins may hinder antigens physically by (1) neutralizing their toxins; (2) linking them together in a process called *agglutination;* and (3) causing them to precipitate, or become solid. Second, antibodies can facilitate the destruction of antigens with other mechanisms—for example, those performed by nonantibody proteins such as the complement system and cytokines.

TABLE 33-2 Types of Immunoglobulins

TYPE	PERCENTAGE OF TOTAL	LOCATION	FUNCTION
IgG	75%	Intravascular and intercellular fluid	Neutralizes bacterial toxins; accelerates phagocytosis
IgA	15%	Body secretions such as saliva, sweat, tears, mucus, bile, colostrum	Interferes with entry of pathogens through exposed structures or pathways
IgM	10%	Intravascular serum	Agglutinates (clusters) antigens and lyses (dissolves) cell walls
IgD	0.2%	Surface of lymphocytes	Binds to antigens; promotes secretion of other immunoglobulins
IgE	0.004%	Surface of basophils and mast (connective tissue) cells	Promotes release of vasoactive chemicals such as histamine and bradykinin in allergic, hypersensitivity, and inflammatory reactions

Nonantibody Proteins

Nonantibody proteins provide additional methods for disabling antigens and further protecting the body. There are two groups of nonantibody proteins. One group is referred to as the *complement system,* and the other is known collectively as *cytokines.*

Complement System

The **complement system** is made up of many different proteins that are activated in a chain reaction when an antibody binds with an antigen. Collectively, the proteins cooperate with antibodies to attract phagocytes, coat antigens to make them more recognizable for phagocytosis (a process known as *opsonization*), and stimulate inflammation through the release of histamine from mast cells and basophils.

Cytokines

Cytokines are chemical messengers released by lymphocytes, monocytes, and macrophages. There are many subgroups of cytokines, including interleukins, interferons, tumor necrosis factor, and colony-stimulating factors.

Interleukins

Interleukins carry messages between leukocytes and tissues that form blood cells. Some interleukins enhance the immune response, whereas others suppress it (Martini & Bartholomew, 2007). Examples of interleukin activity include the following:

- Promotion of inflammation and fever
- Formation of scar tissue by fibroblasts
- Growth and activation of NK cells and additional T cells
- Production of mast cells
- Growth of B cells, formation of plasma cells, and production of antibodies
- Formation of new blood vessels, known as *angiogenesis*
- Stimulation of the anterior pituitary gland to secrete corticotrophin

Pharmacologic Considerations

- Aldesleukin (rIL-2) is a genetically engineered form of human interleukin-2. It is being used as biologic therapy for clients who have not responded to conventional cancer treatments to stimulate the immune system's ability to target cancer cells.

Interferons

Interferons are chemicals that primarily protect cells from viral invasion. They enable cells to resist viral infection and slow viral replication. They have been used as adjunctive therapy in the treatment of AIDS. Interferons also have been used to treat some forms of cancer such as leukemia because they stimulate NK cell activity. Interferon is administered parenterally because digestive enzymes destroy its protein structure.

Tumor Necrosis Factor

When **tumor necrosis factor** (TNF), a type of cytokine, was first discovered, it showed promise as a means of shrinking tumors. Although TNF reduced tumors in laboratory animals, it caused toxic effects in humans. Experiments continue to determine if the antitumor effect can be achieved and the toxic side effects limited by injecting TNF directly into the tumor rather than administering it by a route through which it is systemically absorbed and distributed.

Research has found that TNF helps in cellular repair when administered in small doses. Excess amounts destroy healthy tissue. Consequently, TNF and drugs known as TNF inhibitors are being used to regulate various autoimmune (see Chap. 34) and inflammatory disorders.

Pharmacologic Considerations

- Drugs such as infliximab (Remicade), etanercept (Enbrel), and adalimumab (Humira) are TNF inhibitors. These drugs are being used therapeutically to minimize inflammation. Physicians are administering them to clients with rheumatoid arthritis, ulcerative colitis, and psoriasis. Serious adverse effects have been associated these drugs. Some clients have developed heart failure, infusion reactions, liver dysfunction, and life-threatening infections.

Colony-Stimulating Factors

Colony-stimulating factors (CSFs) are cytokines that prompt the bone marrow to produce, mature, and promote the functions of blood cells. CSFs enable stem cells in bone marrow to differentiate into specific types of cells such as leukocytes, erythrocytes, and platelets. Pharmacologic preparations of CSFs, such as epoetin alfa (Epogen), filgrastim (Neupogen), pegfilgrastim (Neulasta), and sargramostim (Leukine), are used to promote the natural production of blood cells in people whose own hematopoietic functions have become compromised. Consequently, clients with cancer who are receiving antineoplastic drugs may avoid interrupting treatment by reducing their risk of infection, clients who have undergone bone marrow transplantation may recover sooner, and those with chronic renal failure can avoid repeated blood transfusions to compensate for their anemia.

TYPES OF IMMUNITY

The three types of immunity are naturally acquired active immunity, artificially acquired active immunity, and passive immunity (Fig. 33-4). Both forms of active immunity require the person's own production of plasma and memory cells. Passive immunity occurs when ready-made antibodies are provided.

Naturally Acquired Active Immunity

Naturally acquired active immunity occurs as a direct result of infection by a specific microorganism. An example is the immunity to measles that develops after the initial infection. Not all invading microorganisms produce a response that gives lifelong immunity.

Artificially Acquired Active Immunity

Artificially acquired active immunity results from the administration of a killed or weakened microorganism or toxoid (attenuated toxin). The memory cells manufactured by the B lymphocytes "remember" the killed or weakened antigen and recognize it if a future invasion occurs. Recommended immunization schedules are available from the Centers for Disease Control and Prevention, http://www.cdc.gov. Immunizations that are not administered or completed during childhood are recommended for adults. Some immunizations, such as those for tetanus, influenza, and pneumonia require re-administration to maintain adequate immunity.

Gerontologic Considerations

- The amount of antibody produced in response to most foreign antigens decreases with age. Older adults should have an annual influenza vaccine and a pneumococcal vaccine repeated in 5- or 10-year increments. Although vaccination against viral disorders is recommended, vaccines are less effective in older adults than in younger adults, probably because of the decreased immune response that occurs with age.

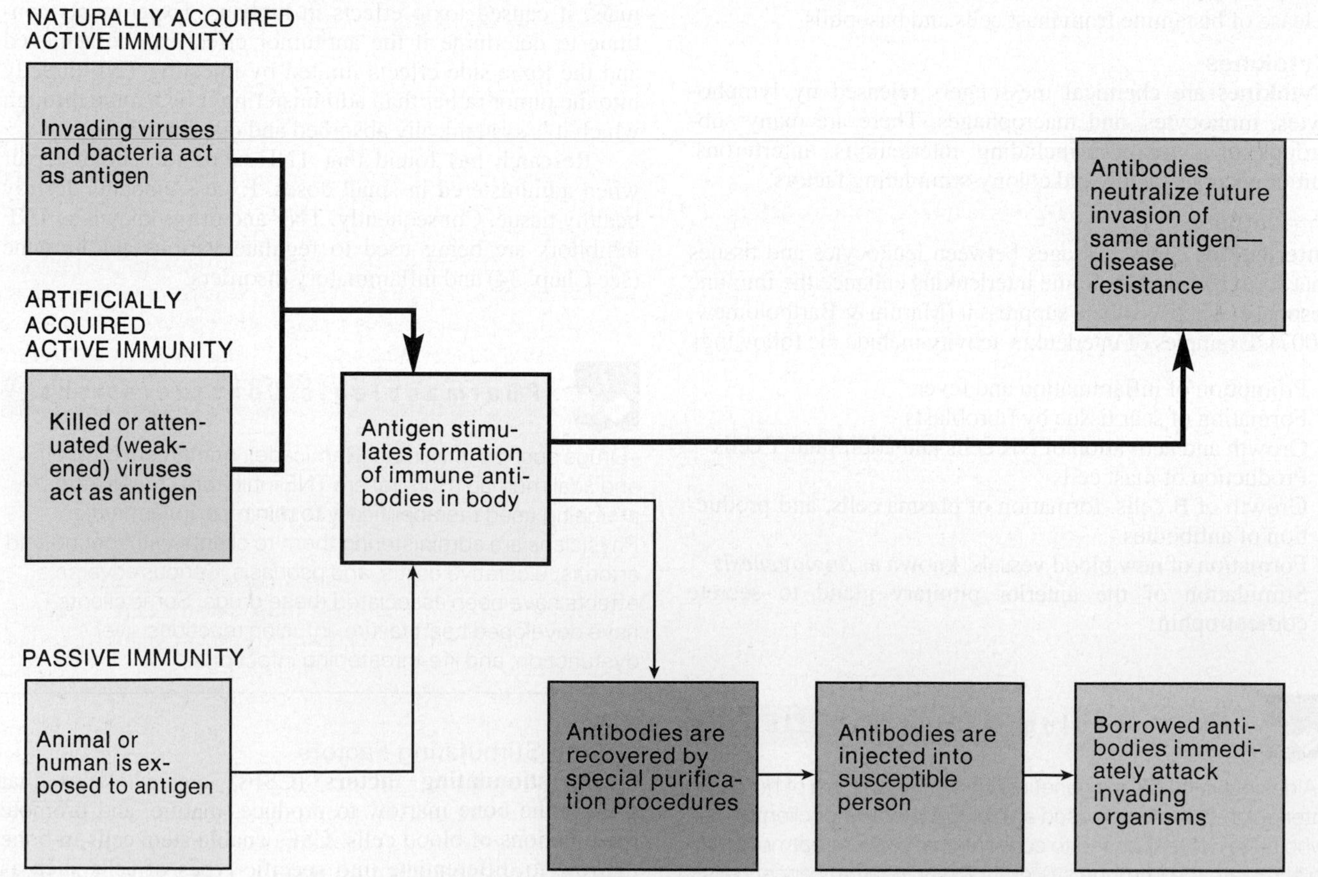

NATURALLY ACQUIRED ACTIVE IMMUNITY

Invading viruses and bacteria act as antigen

ARTIFICIALLY ACQUIRED ACTIVE IMMUNITY

Killed or attenuated (weakened) viruses act as antigen

Antigen stimulates formation of immune antibodies in body

Antibodies neutralize future invasion of same antigen—disease resistance

PASSIVE IMMUNITY

Animal or human is exposed to antigen

Antibodies are recovered by special purification procedures

Antibodies are injected into susceptible person

Borrowed antibodies immediately attack invading organisms

FIGURE 33-4. Active and passive immunity.

Passive Immunity

Passive immunity develops when ready-made antibodies are given to a susceptible person. The antibodies provide immediate but short-lived protection from the invading antigen. No memory cells are produced, and the level of the injected antibodies diminishes over a period of several weeks to a few months.

Ready-made antibodies are obtained from the serum of another organism, either animal or human. Immune serum globulin, also called *gamma globulin* or *immunoglobulin,* is recovered from pooled human plasma. Because the pool comprises plasma from more than one donor, the serum is likely to contain a variety of specific antibodies. Human immune serum is used for passive immunization against measles (rubella), pertussis (whooping cough), hepatitis B, chickenpox (varicella), and tetanus.

Newborns receive passive immunity to some diseases for which their mothers have manufactured antibodies. The circulating maternal antibodies cross the placenta and enter fetal circulation. As with other forms of passive immunity, infants are protected for only a few months after birth.

> ▶ **Stop, Think, and Respond Exercise 33-2**
>
> *Identify the type of immunity that develops from (1) receiving a vaccine for hepatitis B, (2) having chickenpox, and (3) receiving an injection of gamma globulin.*

ASSESSMENT

History

The nurse obtains a history of immunizations, recent and past infectious diseases, and recent exposure to infectious diseases. He or she reviews the client's drug history, because certain drugs (e.g., corticosteroids) suppress the inflammatory and immune responses. The nurse investigates the client's allergy history and questions the client about practices that put him or her at risk for acquired immunodeficiency syndrome (AIDS; see Chap. 35).

Physical Examination

The beginning of the physical examination is a general appraisal of the client's health. The nurse notes whether the client appears healthy, acutely or mildly ill, malnourished, extremely tired, or listless. (Nutrition can affect immune function; see Nutrition Notes 33-1). The nurse records vital signs and weight. The nurse then performs the following:

- Examines the skin for rashes or lesions
- Assesses the abdomen for an enlarged liver or spleen
- Inspects the pharynx for large, red tonsils and purulent drainage
- Palpates the lymph nodes in the neck, axilla, and groin for enlargement and tenderness

Diagnostic Tests

Laboratory tests are used to identify immune system disorders. They usually include a complete blood count with differential. Protein electrophoresis screens for diseases associated with a deficiency or excess of immunoglobulins. T-cell and B-cell assays (or counts) and the enzyme-linked

Nutrition Notes 33-1
Nutrition and Immunocompetence

- Nutrients important in immune system functioning include amino acids such as arginine and glutamine; essential fatty acids and omega-3 fatty acids; the B vitamins, especially vitamin B_6 and folic acid; vitamins A, C, and E; and the minerals copper, iodine, and magnesium.

- Singly or combined, nutrient deficiencies have the potential to affect almost all aspects of immune system functioning. Excesses of certain nutrients, namely, iron, zinc, vitamin E, and polyunsaturated fatty acids, also can impair immune function. The exact amounts and proportions of nutrients needed for optimal immune system function in healthy people, however, are not yet known.

- Until more is known about nutrient interactions, the best dietary advice to maximize immune function in healthy people is to eat a moderate diet that is balanced and varied.

- Several immune-enhancing tube-feeding formulas are available, such as Immune Aid, Impact, Alitraq, Peractive, Crucial, and Vivonex T.E.N. These formulas are enriched with glutamine and/or arginine, omega-3 fatty acids, and nucleotides. These added ingredients enhance the production of T lymphocytes and NK cells, resulting in increased cell-mediated immunity.

immunosorbent assay (see Chap. 35) may be performed. Additional tests are performed when an autoimmune or genetic immune disorder is suspected (see Chap. 34).

Skin tests may be administered. Disease-specific antigens, such as purified protein derivative of the tuberculin toxin, are injected intradermally on the inner aspect of the forearm. The injection area swells if the client has developed antibodies against the antigen (see Chap. 21). The client is not necessarily actively infectious if the test results are positive (see Chap. 21). Skin tests using various common disease antigens such as mumps are administered if anergy is suspected. **Anergy** is the inability to mount an immune response. It is a common finding among clients who have AIDS or are immunosuppressed for other reasons.

NURSING MANAGEMENT

Clear identification of any substances to which the client is allergic is essential. The nurse must consult drug references to verify that prescribed medications do not contain substances to which the client is hypersensitive. He or she explains all diagnostic skin testing procedures to the client and informs the client when to return for interpretation of the results. The nurse ensures that a written consent is obtained before testing for human immunodeficiency virus (HIV) and keeps the results of HIV testing confidential. Standard Precautions (see Chap. 12) are required whenever there is the potential for contact with blood or body fluids. The nurse should follow agency guidelines for controlling infectious diseases or protecting the client who is immunosuppressed. Client teaching includes information about immunizations and instructions regarding drug therapy prescribed for disorders involving the immune system.

CRITICAL THINKING EXERCISES

1. How would you respond to a friend who tells you that her sister has an immune disorder and asks what this means?

2. Discuss the benefit of obtaining immunizations for common childhood diseases.

3. If someone you know has been exposed to hepatitis B, what would you recommend to prevent a subsequent infection?

4. Why are the tonsils and adenoids not being removed as aggressively as they were in the past?

NCLEX-STYLE REVIEW QUESTIONS

1. A client had a splenectomy following a violent motor vehicle accident. The parents ask the nurse if there are any special considerations following the surgical removal of the spleen. Which of the following is the most correct response?

1. The client is susceptible to anemia because the spleen produces red blood cells.
2. The client is susceptible to acidosis because the spleen maintains acid-base balance.
3. The client is susceptible to bleeding because the spleen synthesizes vitamin K.

4. The client is susceptible to infection because the spleen removes bacteria from the blood.

2. A client is suspected of having an immune system disorder. What laboratory test would the nurse expect to be ordered during the initial blood studies?

1. Blood chemistry
2. Complete blood count (CBC)
3. CBC with differential
4. Liver enzyme studies

3. Which of the following types of immunity develops as a result of having an infection with a specific microorganism?

1. Naturally acquired passive immunity
2. Artificially acquired passive immunity
3. Naturally acquired active immunity
4. Artificially acquired active immunity

4. When the nurse examines a client with an immune-related disorder, which of the following are appropriate physical assessments? Select all that apply.

1. The nurse collects a voided urine specimen.
2. The nurse inspects the skin's appearance.
3. The nurse auscultates the abdomen.
4. The nurse palpates the client's neck.
5. The nurse looks at the oral and nasopharynx.

5. When a nurse administers drugs that suppress a client's immune system, which of the following is the client most likely to develop?

1. Allergic reactions
2. Opportunistic infections
3. Malignant cancers
4. Acquired anemia

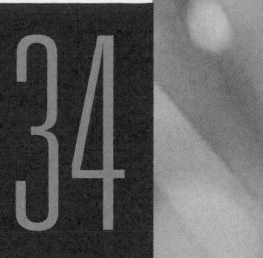

34 Caring for Clients with Immune-Mediated Disorders

Learning Objectives

On completion of this chapter, you will be able to:

1. Describe an allergic disorder.
2. List five examples of allergic signs and symptoms.
3. Name four categories of allergens, and give an example of each.
4. Give four examples of allergic reactions, including two that are potentially life-threatening.
5. Describe diagnostic skin testing.
6. Name three methods for treating allergies.
7. Discuss the nursing management of a client with an allergic disorder.
8. Explain the meaning of autoimmune disorder, and give at least three examples of related diseases.
9. Discuss theories that explain the development of an autoimmune disorder.
10. Name three categories of drugs used in the treatment of autoimmune disorders.
11. Discuss the nursing management of a client with an autoimmune disorder.
12. Give two explanations for how chronic fatigue syndrome develops.
13. List common symptoms experienced by people with chronic fatigue syndrome.
14. Name common nursing diagnoses, desired outcomes, and related nursing interventions for clients who have chronic fatigue syndrome.

The immune system sometimes responds aggressively and destructively to substances that may not always be potentially harmful. Two examples of such a response include allergic and autoimmune disorders. This chapter discusses allergic and autoimmune disorders and the appropriate nursing care for clients who have them. It also explores chronic fatigue syndrome, which is a consequence of an immune-mediated disorder, and nursing management of this condition.

ALLERGIC DISORDERS

An **allergic disorder** is characterized by a hyperimmune response to weak antigens that usually are harmless. The antigens that can cause an allergic response are called **allergens** (Table 34-1). Allergens have a protein component and gain entry to the host from the environment. Allergies can occur at any age, and the pattern of allergic response can vary in the same person during his or her life. For example, a person may suddenly develop an allergic reaction to a substance such as latex, even though he or she has had multiple prior contacts with latex and no past problems. On the other hand, an allergic response to one agent may

TABLE 34-1 Common Allergens

TYPE OF ALLERGEN	EXAMPLES	COMMON REACTION
Ingestants	Food, drugs (especially penicillin)	Gastroenteropathy, dermatitis, asthma, anaphylaxis, urticaria, angioedema, serum sickness
Inhalants	House dust and mites, insect excrement, animal products (dander, saliva, urine), pollens, spores	Allergic asthma, rhinitis, hypersensitivity pneumonitis
Contactants	Plant oils, topical medications, occupational chemicals, cosmetics, metals in jewelry and clothing fasteners, hair dyes, latex	Contact dermatitis, urticaria, or anaphylaxis (rare)
Injectants	Drugs, bee venom	Anaphylaxis, angioedema, acute urticaria

gradually disappear or be replaced by sensitivity to another substance. The reason for these changes is unclear.

Types of Allergies

An allergic disorder is manifested in a variety of ways-depending on the manner in which the allergen gains entry to the body and the intensity of the response. Organs and structures that are primarily involved in allergic reactions include the skin, respiratory passageways, gastrointestinal tract, blood, and vascular system (Table 34-2). Some types of allergic manifestations cause temporary, localized discomfort, whereas others are life-threatening.

▶ **Stop, Think, and Respond Exercise 34-1**

List substances to which you or others you know are allergic and how the symptoms are managed.

Pathophysiology and Etiology

Approximately 10% to 15% of the population develops allergies. The tendency can be inherited. Although members of the same family may have allergies, they may not all be sensitive to the same allergens. Allergy-prone individuals may react to more than one type of antigen. For example, the same person may be sensitive to ragweed pollen and eggs.

The first exposure to an allergen does not produce symptoms; rather, it causes sensitization. **Sensitization** is the process by which cellular and chemical events occur after a second or subsequent exposure to an allergen. Once sensitization occurs, one of four types of hypersensitivity

responses can occur (Fig. 34-1). These may be immediate or delayed, depending on the time it takes for the immune system to mount a response.

Immediate Hypersensitivity Responses: Types I, II, and III

An *immediate hypersensitivity response* is due to antibodies interacting with allergens and occurs rapidly. There are three types of immediate hypersensitivity responses: type I, atopic or anaphylactic, which is mediated by immunoglobulin E (IgE) antibodies; type II, cytotoxic, which is mediated by immunoglobulin M or G (IgM or IgG) antibodies, and type III, immune complex, which is mediated by IgG antibodies. The first two types of responses occur within minutes; type III responses reach a peak within 6 hours after exposure to an allergen.

In type I, the most severe of the three immediate hypersensitivity responses, IgE antibodies attach to basophils or mast cells. **Mast cells** are constituents of connective tissue that contain granules of heparin, serotonin, bradykinin, and histamine (the most potent chemical of this group). With subsequent exposures to the allergen, mast cells and basophils release their vasoactive granules, causing various allergic and inflammatory manifestations.

Anaphylaxis is a rapid and profound type I hypersensitivity response. A massive release of histamine causes vasodilation; increased capillary permeability; **angioneurotic edema** (acute swelling of the face, neck, lips, larynx, hands, feet, genitals, and internal organs); hypotension; and bronchoconstriction.

TABLE 34-2 Types of Allergies

ALLERGY TYPE	SIGNS AND SYMPTOMS	MEDICAL MANAGEMENT
Allergic rhinitis	Sneezing, itching, nasal congestion, watery nasal discharge, itching and redness of the eyes	Antihistamines, nasal decongestants, corticosteroid nasal spray, immunotherapy, allergen avoidance, eye drops
Contact dermatitis	Itching, burning, redness, rash on contact with substance	Allergen avoidance, wearing gloves, topical or oral antihistamines and corticosteroids
Dermatitis medicamentosa	Sudden generalized bright red rash, itching, fever, malaise, headache, arthralgias	Discontinuation of drug, antihistamines and topical corticosteroids
Food allergy	Nausea, vomiting, diarrhea, abdominal cramping, malaise, itching, wheezing, rash, cough	Identification and avoidance of allergenic food Intubation, subcutaneous epinephrine, aminophylline in severe reactions
Urticaria	Itching, swelling, redness, wheals of superficial skin layers	Topical or oral antihistamines and corticosteroids
Angioedema	Itching, swelling, redness of deeper tissues and mucous membranes	Intubation, subcutaneous epinephrine, aminophylline

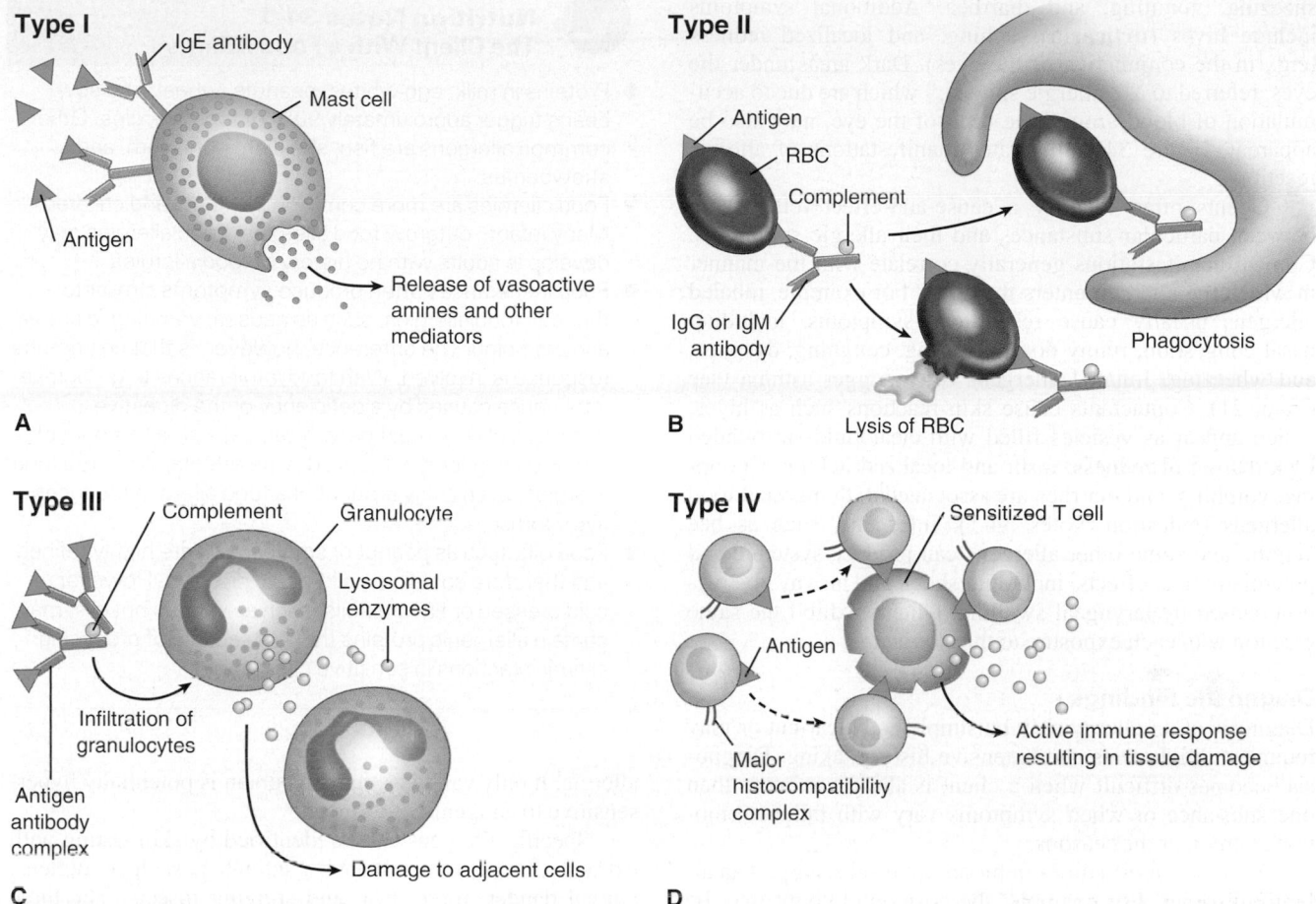

FIGURE 34-1. Types of hypersensitivity responses: (**A**) type I, atopic or anaphylactic; (**B**) type II, cytotoxic; (**C**) type III, immune complex; and (**D**) type IV, delayed.

Delayed Hypersensitivity Response: Type IV

A *delayed hypersensitivity response* is also termed a type IV hypersensitivity response. Antigens are initially phagocytized by macrophages. Sensitized T cells then produce cytokines that cause an inflammatory reaction. Antibody production is not a component of a delayed hypersensitivity response.

A delayed hypersensitivity response may develop over several hours or days, or it may reach maximum severity after repeated exposure. Examples of a delayed hypersensitivity response include a blood-transfusion reaction that occurs days to weeks after blood administration, rejection of transplanted tissues, and reaction to a tuberculin skin test. Delayed hypersensitivity may also explain how people who have been in contact with latex multiple times without showing evidence of an allergy may develop an allergic reaction.

Suppression of the Allergic Response

The body suppresses the allergic response through various mechanisms. One method involves the release of *eosinophil chemotactic factor* (ECF), a chemical mediator, from mast cells. **Chemotaxis** refers to a process of attracting migratory cells to a particular area in the body. ECF attracts eosinophils, whose role is to suppress inflammation by degrading histamine and the other vasoactive chemicals. Epinephrine, a

neurotransmitter, interferes with the release of vasoactive chemicals from mast cells. Corticosteroids, which are anti-inflammatory hormones produced by the adrenal cortex, block the synthesis of prostaglandins and leukotrienes, also known as *slow-reactive substance of anaphylaxis*. Both these substances contribute to vascular permeability and smooth muscle contraction.

> ### Stop, Think, and Respond Exercise 34-2
>
> *Look up the following medications in a drug reference or pharmacology text: diphenhydramine (Benadryl), epinephrine hydrochloride (Adrenalin Chloride), prednisone (Meticorten), montelukast (Singulair), and cromolyn (Intal, Crolom). Correlate their mechanisms of action with events that occur in an allergic reaction.*

Assessment Findings

Signs and Symptoms

Manifestations of anaphylactic reactions include shock (see Chap. 17), laryngeal edema, wheezing, stridor, tachycardia, and generalized itching, as well as hypotension, bronchospasm and angioneurotic edema, as described previously. Less severe localized hypersensitivity responses can include watery eyes, increased nasal and bronchial secretions, sneezing, vomiting, and diarrhea. Additional symptoms include hives (**urticaria**), itching, and localized redness (e.g., in the conjunctiva of the eyes). Dark areas under the eyes, referred to as "allergic shiners," which are due to accumulation of blood around the orbit of the eye, may also be apparent. Figure 34-2 illustrates manifestations of allergic reactions.

Clients often identify a cause-and-effect relationship between particular substances and their allergic symptoms. Clinical manifestations generally correlate with the manner in which the allergen enters the body. For example, inhaled allergens usually cause respiratory symptoms, including nasal congestion, runny nose, sneezing, coughing, dyspnea, and wheezing. Inhaled allergens often trigger asthma (see Chap. 21). Contactants cause skin reactions such as hives, which appear as vesicles filled with clear fluid surrounded by a margin of redness; rash; and localized itching. Cramping, vomiting, and diarrhea are associated with ingested food allergens (Nutrition Notes 34-1). Injectants, such as bee venom, and some other allergens can produce systemic and potentially fatal effects, including shock and airway obstruction caused by laryngeal swelling. Clients exhibit the same reaction with each exposure to the allergen.

Diagnostic Findings

Diagnosis of an allergy may be simple and clear-cut or may require multiple tests and extensive history-taking. Diagnosis becomes difficult when a client is allergic to more than one substance or when symptoms vary with fatigue, emotional stress, or the seasons.

Various abnormalities in blood test results suggest an allergic disorder. For example, the eosinophil count may be elevated. The radioallergosorbent blood test (RAST) measures IgE. On a scale of 0 to 5, a score of 2 or greater is a significant indication for an allergic disorder. The RAST does not identify which, if any, substances to which a person is

Nutrition Notes 34-1
The Client With a Food Allergy

- Proteins in milk, egg whites, peanuts, wheat, and soybeans trigger approximately 90% of food allergies. Other common allergens are fish, shellfish, nuts, corn, and strawberries.
- Food allergies are more common in infants and children. Many infants outgrow food allergies. Food allergies may develop in adults with no history of food allergies.
- Food intolerances often produce symptoms similar to those of food allergies, such as nausea, vomiting, diarrhea, and cramping. The difference, however, is that no immune response is involved. With food intolerances (e.g., lactose intolerance caused by a deficiency of the digestive enzyme lactase), most people can eat a small amount of the offending food without adverse effects. With true food allergies, even a tiny amount of a food allergen produces symptoms.
- Food oils such as peanut or soybean oils are highly refined and therefore contain no allergenic proteins. However, cold pressed or flavored oils, such as various nut oils, may contain allergenic proteins that are capable of producing allergic reactions in sensitive clients.

allergic. It only validates that the person is potentially hypersensitive to antigenic substances.

Specific allergens can be identified by skin testing with extracts of various substances (antigens), such as pollens, animal dander, food, dust, and stinging insects. The three methods of skin testing are the scratch or prick test, the patch test, and the intradermal injection test.

The *scratch* or *prick test* involves scratching the skin and applying a small amount of the liquid test antigen to the scratch. The tester applies one allergen per scratch over the client's forearm, upper arm, or back. The back is more sensitive than the arms. It also provides a larger area for testing because each substance being tested should be distributed at least 3 cm and preferably up to 5 cm (slightly more than 1–2 inches) from one another. Results from a scratch test are identifiable in as little as 20 minutes. If a raised wheal and localized erythema appears, the tester measures its length and width in millimeters. The larger the reaction, the greater the likelihood that the test allergen causes symptoms in the tested person.

The *patch test* is used to identify the offending substance in allergic contact dermatitis. The tester applies a concentrated form of the substance to the skin and covers the area with an occlusive dressing. After 48 hours, the tester removes the dressing and examines the area for erythema, edema, and vesicles.

In the *intradermal injection test*, which usually is performed only when results of a scratch test are negative for allergies, the tester injects a dilute solution of an antigen intradermally. A positive reaction is based on the size of a raised wheal and localized erythema (redness) that forms where the antigen was injected (Fig. 34-3).

To identify food allergens, meticulous record keeping of symptoms and a food diary listing all food and beverages

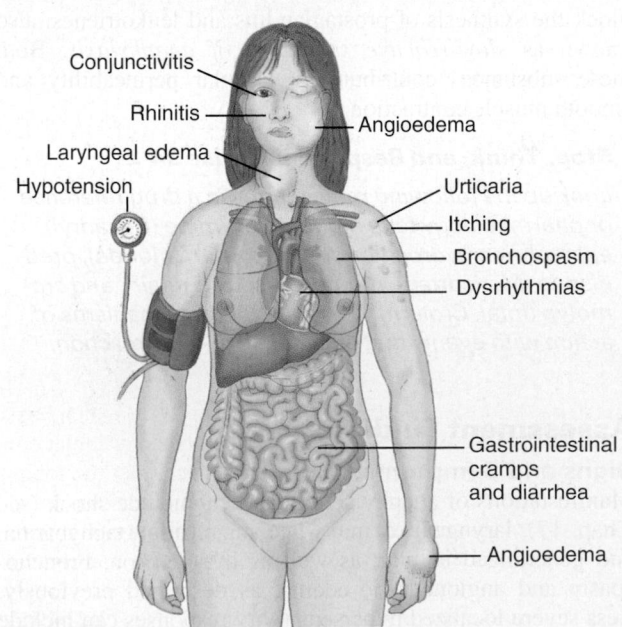

Conjunctivitis
Rhinitis
Laryngeal edema
Hypotension
Angioedema
Urticaria
Itching
Bronchospasm
Dysrhythmias
Gastrointestinal cramps and diarrhea
Angioedema

FIGURE 34-2. Manifestations of allergic reactions.

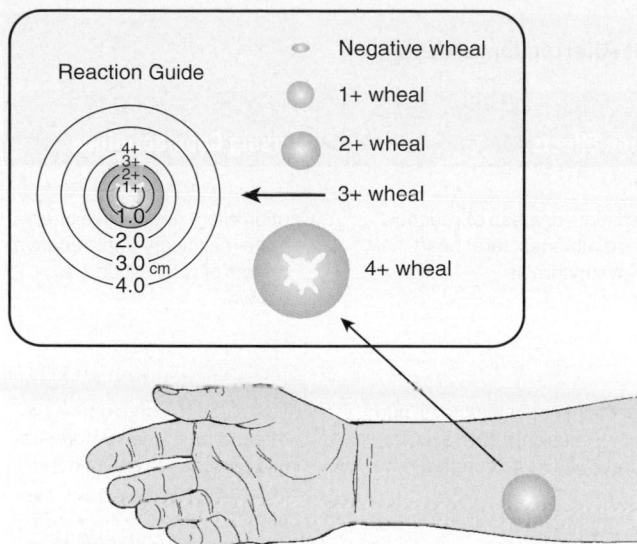

Reaction Guide

- Negative wheal
- 1+ wheal
- 2+ wheal
- ← 3+ wheal
- 4+ wheal

4+
3+
2+
1+
1.0
2.0
3.0 cm
4.0

FIGURE 34-3. The wheal and localized erythema (redness) that appear after an intradermal skin test are measured to interpret the allergic response. The following scale is used: Negative = soft wheal and minimal redness; 1+ = 5–8 mm wheal and redness; 2+ = 7–20 mm wheal and redness; 3+ = 9–15 mm asymmetric wheal and redness; 4+ = >12 mm asymmetric wheal and diffuse redness.

consumed are necessary. Skin testing and a blood test for IgE antibodies provide more objective data. Elimination diets try to establish cause-and-effect relationships: the client completely avoids suspected foods for 1 to 2 weeks and then adds them back to the diet one at a time and in small amounts. That way, if symptoms develop, the offending food can be identified. Because elimination studies are subjective, clients may experience symptoms based on their expectations, not from a true allergy. Clients who have experienced severe allergic reactions should not use elimination diets. Nursing Guidelines 34-1 explains the process of identifying food allergens in more detail.

Complications

Clients with inhalant allergies such as seasonal or allergic rhinitis (also known as *hay fever*) may develop nasal polyps

NURSING GUIDELINES 34-1

Identifying Food Allergens

- Have the client fast for 1 to 2 days, drinking only distilled water.
- Introduce hypoallergenic foods (e.g., rice, tapioca) one at a time.
- Introduce allergenic foods (e.g., wheat, peanuts) one at a time in small quantities.
- Observe client for allergic symptoms after introducing each new food.

from the chronic inflammation. They also are prone to sinus infections related to chronic nasal congestion. Secondary pulmonary infections such as bronchitis also occur. Asthma develops in some clients. The most severe complications among persons with allergies, regardless of type, are anaphylactic shock and angioneurotic edema, which can be lethal without immediate medical interventions.

Medical Management

The treatment used to relieve allergic symptoms depends on the type of allergy. Besides avoiding the allergen if possible, many clients experience symptomatic relief with drug therapy (Drug Therapy Table 34-1).

Pharmacologic Considerations

- To protect against poison ivy, clients can apply bentoquatam 5% (Ivy Block) to the skin before exposure. The cream forms a protective layer on top of the skin. The oral drug pentoxifylline (Trental) may decrease the rash slightly, but clients must take it before exposure.

Desensitization is another option. **Desensitization** is a form of immunotherapy in which a person receives weekly or twice-weekly injections of dilute but increasingly higher concentrations of an allergen without interruption. Repeated exposure to the weak antigen promotes the production of IgG, an antibody that blocks IgE so it cannot stimulate mast cells. When the maximum dose is achieved after 2 to 4 months of treatment, maintenance injections are administered at longer intervals, usually every 2 to 4 weeks. It may take several years before a person treated with desensitization experiences significant relief. After a desensitization injection, the client is observed for 30 minutes to assess for allergic symptoms. Epinephrine (Adrenalin) is administered if a severe reaction occurs. Desensitization for poison ivy, oak, or sumac currently is unavailable.

▶ *Stop, Think, and Respond Exercise 34-3*

List signs and symptoms that suggest a person who is undergoing desensitization needs epinephrine.

Clients with severe allergies to bee venom are advised to carry an emergency kit that contains a premeasured dose of injectable epinephrine (Epipen). The syringe autoinjects the epinephrine when pressed to the skin. The lateral thigh is the site most commonly used for injection (Fig. 34-4).

Recently, *sublingual-swallow immunotherapy (SLIT)* has been used for desensitization against allergens that cause allergic rhinitis. When SLIT is used, a solution or tablet containing grass and pollen allergens is placed under the tongue once a day during allergy season. These allergens do not generally produce a reaction because the sublingual mucosa has very few mast cells. However, cells in the oral mucosa present the antigen to regulatory suppressor T cells that inhibit the inflammatory/allergic response. Consequently, a tolerance to the allergens develops. Repeated SLIT results in

DRUG THERAPY TABLE 34-1 Agents to Treat Allergic Disorders

Drug Category and Examples	Mechanism of Action	Side Effects	Nursing Considerations
Antihistamines diphenhydramine (Benadryl), hydroxyzine (Atarax), fexofenadine (Allegra), astemizole (Hismanal), loratadine (Claritin), cetirizine (Zyrtec)	Block histamine (H₁) receptors	Sedation, dryness of mucous membranes; rare: heart dysrhythmias	Caution client not to drive or operate machinery until sedative effects of medication are known.
Nasal Decongestant Agents flunisolide (Nasalide), oxymetazoline hydrochloride (Afrin)	Vasoconstrict nasal membranes	Headache, transient nasal burning, sneezing, epistaxis, rebound nasal congestion	Advise client to pump spray three to four times before first use and one to two times before each daily use to prime. Caution clients using Afrin to avoid using for longer than 3 to 5 days in a row or rebound nasal congestion may occur.
Nasal Steroid Spray and Inhalant beclomethasone dipropionate (Beconase), fluticasone propionate (Flonase), fluticasone propionate (Flovent)	Anti-inflammatory	Headache, fungal infection of nasal passage or mouth, nasal irritation, cough, flulike illness	Examine nares. Avoid contact with the eyes. Several weeks of therapy may be necessary for full benefit. Report sore throat or signs of oral fungal infection.
Oral Corticosteroids dexamethasone (Decadron), hydrocortisone (Cortef), methylprednisolone (Medrol)	Regulate immune response; control inflammatory response	Euphoria, insomnia, gastrointestinal irritation, increased appetite, weight gain, hyperglycemia	Taper doses when discontinuing; abrupt discontinuation may lead to acute adrenal insufficiency. Give doses in the morning with food. Monitor blood sugar levels. Assess for peripheral edema.
Oral Decongestant Agents pseudoephedrine hydrochloride (Sudafed)	Vasoconstrict nasal membranes (sympathomimetics)	Anxiety, nervousness, palpitations, headache, dizziness, tremors, sleeplessness, hypertension	Use cautiously in clients with severe hypertension, diabetes, glaucoma, hyperthyroidism, prostatic hyperplasia, coronary artery disease, those taking monoamine oxidase inhibitors, and women who are breast-feeding.
Bronchodilators epinephrine (Adrenalin), terbutaline (Brethine)	Dilate airways by stimulating adrenergic receptors located throughout the lungs.	Insomnia, restlessness, anorexia, cardiac stimulation, hyperglycemia, tremor, vascular headache	Avoid taking within 2 hours of bedtime. In pregnant women, Brethine interferes with labor and delivery.

DRUG THERAPY TABLE 34-1 Agents to Treat Allergic Disorders (continued)

Drug Category and Examples	Mechanism of Action	Side Effects	Nursing Considerations
Bronchodilating Inhaled Agents epinephrine (Primatene Mist), metaproterenol (Alupent), ipratropium (Atrovent), ipratropium (Spiriva)	Stimulate adrenergic receptors or block cholinergic receptors	Nervousness, tremor, euphoria, palpitations, hypertension, dysrhythmias, headache	Monitor blood pressure and heart rate. Use caution in those with hypertension, heart disease, diabetes, cirrhosis, or those using digitalis glycosides. Teach proper technique for using inhaler.
Oral or Parenteral Sympathomimetic Agents epinephrine (Adrenalin Chloride), theophylline (Theo-Dur), Elixophyllin), theophylline (Aminophyllin)	Act on alpha and beta receptors	Nausea, anxiety, restlessness, headache, trembling, tachycardia, hypertension, increased urination, increased gastric secretions	Use cautiously in clients with gastritis or peptic ulcer disease, congestive heart failure, hyperthyroidism, or seizure disorders. Monitor vital signs regularly. Give oral drugs with food to decrease gastric irritation.
Leukotriene Antagonists montelukast (Singulair), zileuton (Zyflo)	Block receptors for leukotrienes (slow-reacting substance of anaphylaxis)	Headache, nausea, abdominal upset, flulike symptoms such as fatigue, hepatotoxicity	Avoid if breast-feeding. Monitor for infections. Administer on an empty stomach.

Nursing Management

Throughout the client's care, the nurse observes for signs of an allergic reaction, especially when administering medications, applying substances such as tape or adhesive patches to the skin, or caring for a client receiving contrast media for diagnostic testing. If the nurse suspects a mild allergic reaction, he or she removes or withholds the offending substance and notifies the physician. If a client has an anaphylactic reaction, the nurse acts immediately to stop the client's exposure to the allergen, summons the code team or calls the 911 operator, and provides life support.

Occasionally, the nurse needs to remove a ring from a swollen finger. If applying soap or oil to the finger proves unsuccessful, the nurse may wrap the finger with twine (Fig. 34-5). Once the tissue is compressed, the ring slides off the finger by pulling on the free end of the twine. This technique is preferable to damaging the ring with a metal cutter. If nothing else facilitates ring removal, however, cutting still is a better option than allowing tissue damage from ischemia to develop.

The nurse instructs clients who are scheduled for diagnostic skin testing to avoid taking prescribed or over-the-counter antihistamines or cold preparations for at least 48 to 72 hours before testing. Doing so reduces the potential for false-negative test results. Clients must temporarily discontinue some medications for even longer.

Pharmacologic Considerations

- Some antihistamines are more likely than others to interfere with results of skin testing. Those taking hydroxyzine (Atarax, Vistaril) or cetirizine (Zyrtec) should cease administration for 5 days before skin testing.

The nurse assists the provider who performs diagnostic testing and helps document findings. Once the test is completed, the nurse monitors the client's response until it is safe for the person to return home.

For clients who elect to undergo desensitization, the nurse administers the serial doses and monitors the client for 30 minutes after administration. He or she teaches clients who are being desensitized and those who choose drug therapy for relief of their allergy symptoms how to self-administer prescribed medications, especially those that are delivered by metered-dose or dry-powder inhalers, because many people use these devices incorrectly. The

---

a reduction of symptoms associated with allergic rhinitis and asthma in children with hay fever (Bollinger, 2006). Children tend to prefer SLIT to desensitizing injections.

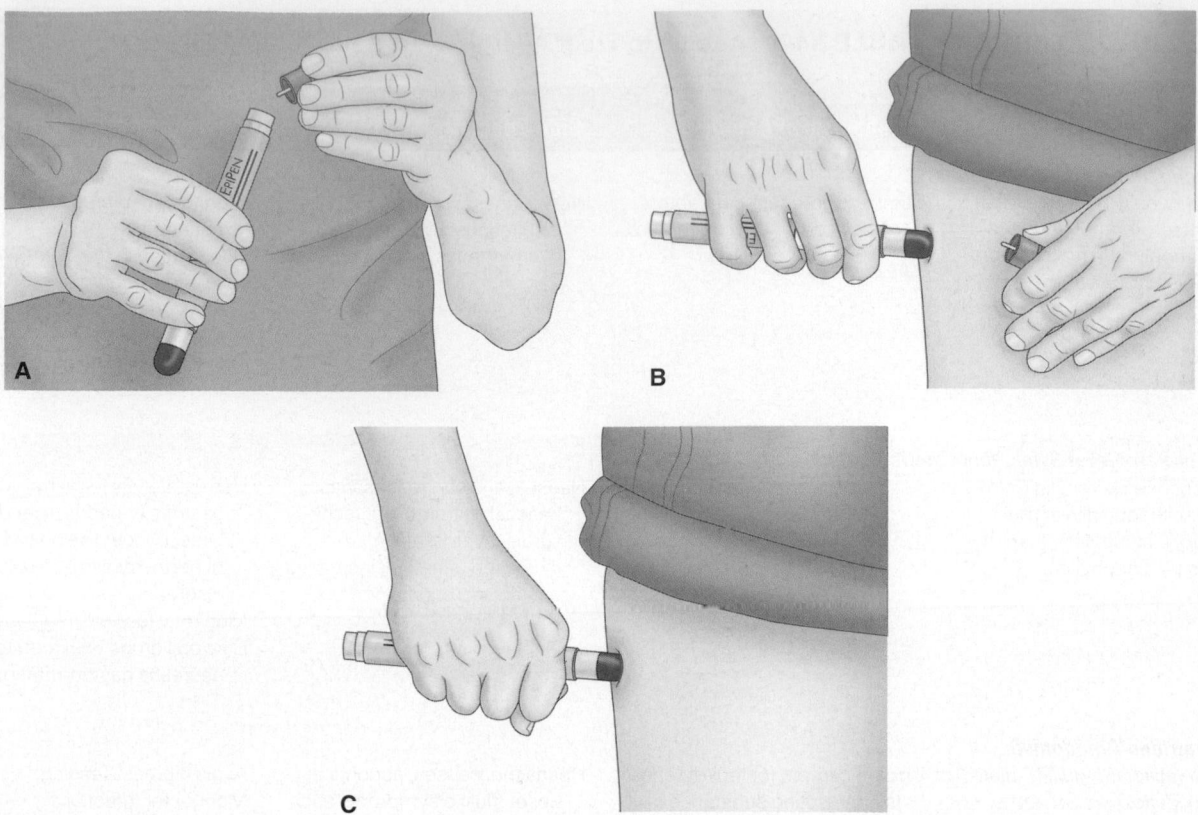

FIGURE 34-4. Self-injection of epinephrine to avoid anaphylactic reaction. (**A**) The client uncaps the Epipen, holding it with the injecting end upright. (**B**) The client positions the device at the middle portion of the thigh. (**C**) The client pushes the device into the thigh as far as possible. The Epipen autoinjects a premeasured dose of epinephrine into the subcutaneous tissue.

nurse must make clients aware of possible side effects and when medical follow-up is necessary.

Techniques for avoiding or reducing exposure in the client's home and work environment are nursing areas for health teaching. Some examples include the following:

- Insist that the environment be smoke free when a person manifests inhalant allergies or respiratory symptoms.
- Keep pets outdoors or at least in one confined area of the home.
- Bathe pets weekly or at frequent intervals.

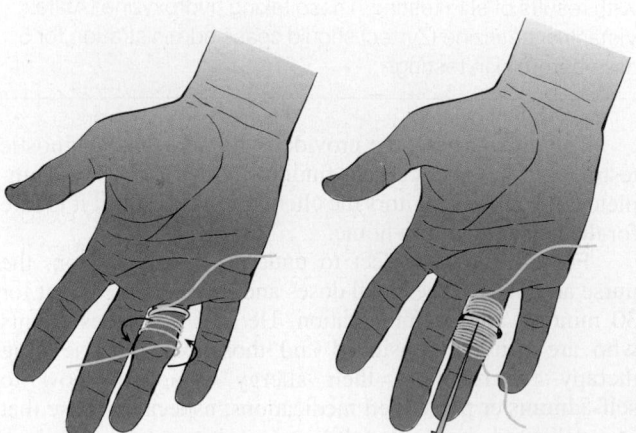

FIGURE 34-5. Technique for ring removal.

- Cover the mattress and box springs with an impervious material to reduce dust mites.
- Eliminate area rugs.
- Contract with an exterminator if cockroaches or other vermin are present.
- Clean humidifiers and heating and cooling ducts to remove mold spores.

For other health teaching information, see Client and Family Teaching 34-1.

▶ **Stop, Think, and Respond Exercise 34-4**
Discuss ways to avoid inhaled and ingested allergens.

Nursing Process for the Client with an Allergic Disorder

Assessment

Obtain a thorough history from the client with an actual or suspected allergic disorder. Gather data about the client's diet history, paying particular attention to foods that cause problems. Determine if others in the family have allergies. Record the client's description of allergic symptoms and the factors that appear to increase or decrease symptoms (e.g., exposures, time of year) in detail. Many clients say they are allergic to substances, but their

Client and Family Teaching 34-1
Allergies

The nurse teaches clients who have allergic disorders and their family members the following guidelines:

● Never begin smoking, or quit if you are currently smoking if your allergy causes respiratory symptoms.
● Understand that treatment for chronic allergic disorders, such as allergic rhinitis and food allergies, may extend over several years.
● Follow the medical regimen as instructed by the physician.
● Do not overuse nose drops or sprays for nasal congestion. Use only prescribed or recommended drugs and only in the dosage suggested by the physician.
● Keep a record of symptoms or lack of symptoms. Bring the record to the physician's office or clinic. The record will help the physician determine therapy.
● Keep a record of symptoms or absence of symptoms each time you add a new food to the diet. Add new foods to the diet slowly and one at a time.
● Avoid environmental substances that cause allergic reactions.
● Seek immediate medical attention if symptoms worsen or new symptoms occur.
● Carry identification, such as a Medic-Alert card or bracelet, to inform medical personnel of allergies, especially if you have a history of anaphylactic reactions.
● Do not miss an immunotherapy appointment; missed appointments may necessitate restarting the series of injections.
● Check prefilled syringes that contain epinephrine for an expiration date. You must refill the prescription and discard the old prescription on or immediately before this date. Keep the directions for use with the product.

BOX 34-1 Products That Contain Latex

Household Products
Carpet backing
Feeding nipples
Pacifiers
Elastic in clothing
Sports equipment
Balloons
Erasers
Toys
Shoe soles
Condoms/diaphragms
Computer mouse pads
Buttons on electronic equipment
Food handled with powdered latex gloves
Handles on racquets, tools, and similar items

Medical Products
Gloves
Face masks
Mattresses
Patient-controlled analgesia
Sports equipment syringes
Ambu bags
Stethoscopes
Blood pressure cuff tubing
Dental devices
Urinary catheters
Tourniquets
Electrode pads
Bulb syringes
Syringe stoppers and medication vial stoppers
Adhesive tape
Bandages
Injection ports
Wound drains

descriptions of manifestations do not always support that conclusion. Identify all prescription and nonprescription drugs that the client takes and has reacted to in the past. Be especially alert to allergic manifestations caused by contact with products that contain latex (Box 34-1). Examine the skin and describe any rashes or eruptions.

Closely observe a client with allergies each time a new drug is added to the therapeutic regimen. This includes drugs given by the nurse and drugs used for diagnostic studies, such as radiopaque dyes. Continue monitoring the client when a second dose of a new drug is given because reactions may follow the first sensitizing dose.

Diagnosis, Planning, and Interventions

▶ **Altered Comfort: Itching** related to histamine release

▶ **Expected Outcome:** The client will have reduced itching and intact skin.

● Remove clothing and wash the skin with soap and flowing water after exposure to contact allergens (e.g., poison ivy, poison oak,

poison sumac). *Reducing the source and duration of contact limits the severity of an allergic skin reaction.*
● Advise the client to limit the frequency of bathing with conventional bar soap and to use superfatted or castile soap. *Conventional bar soap contains lye, which dries the skin and predisposes it to itching and flaking. Superfatted soap uses less lye (sodium hydroxide, caustic soda). Castile soap contains a greater proportion of vegetable (e.g., olive, coconut, soybean, castor) oils.*
● Recommend bathing with tepid rather than hot water when hygiene is necessary and patting the skin dry rather than rubbing a towel vigorously over the skin. *Heat and rubbing intensify itching.*
● Advise the client to avoid scratching the skin. *Scratching releases additional histamine from cells, which leads to a self-stimulating cycle of itching–scratching–more itching.*
● Encourage the client to keep fingernails short or to wear cotton gloves, especially during sleep. *Impaired skin integrity predisposes the client to secondary bacterial infection. Short nails*

prevent skin trauma should the client be unable to resist scratching.

- Apply a skin lubricant or emollient frequently. *Lubricants and emollients act as barriers on the skin that prevent loss of moisture. Moist skin is less vulnerable to trauma and itching.*
- Suggest using distracting techniques such as doing a crossword puzzle or handicraft during periods of itching. *Flooding the brain with alternate stimuli removes the focus from itching.*
- Tell the client to dress in cotton garments rather than those made of rough or synthetic fibers. *Natural fibers facilitate escape of heat from the skin surface, reducing vasodilation and intensification of itching. Rough fabrics irritate the skin, which exacerbates itching.*
- Humidify the environment. *Adding moisture to the environment reduces the potential for dry, itchy skin.*
- Administer prescribed topical, inhaled, oral, or intravenous (IV) drugs. *Antihistamines block histamine receptors, and corticosteroids interfere with release of chemicals from mast cells, thereby relieving itching, redness, rash, and localized swelling.*

Pharmacologic Considerations

- Many antihistamines cause drowsiness, although some newer antihistamines are less likely to do so. Advise the client not to drive a car, operate machinery, or perform tasks that require alertness when taking antihistamines that reduce alertness. Tell clients not to take antihistamines with alcohol or other central nervous system depressants because additive sedative effects can occur. Also, advise clients with disorders of the lower respiratory tract not to take antihistamines. If, for example, these drugs are administered for asthma, a drying effect may occur, making secretions thicker and more difficult to expectorate.

- Suggest that clients avoid the use of nonprescription eye preparations to reduce redness. An ophthalmologist should evaluate and treat itching and redness of the eyes because the symptoms may or may not be caused by an allergy.

Gerontologic Considerations

- Adverse reactions to antihistamines, such as dizziness, sedation, and confusion, are more common in older adults. Careful monitoring of the older adult is necessary. Older men with benign prostatic hypertrophy may experience difficulty voiding while taking antihistamines due to anticholinergic side effects.

▶ **Impaired Home Maintenance** related to an environment that produces moderate to severe allergic symptoms

▶ **Expected Outcome:** The client will modify the home environment, subsequently reducing allergic symptoms.

- Explore ways to avoid the offending allergen. *Preventing contact with the allergen is the first step in avoiding an allergic reaction.*

- Propose using air conditioning during summer months and special furnace filters or electrostatic cleaners for home heating and cooling. *Limiting allergen sources in inhaled air reduces allergic symptoms.*
- Recommend using hypoallergenic products and wearing rubber or vinyl gloves (avoid latex) when using cleaning chemicals. *Hypoallergenic products contain ingredients that do not commonly cause reactions in sensitive people. Gloves act as a barrier between a person's skin and the offending allergen.*

▶ **PC: Anaphylaxis and Angioedema**

▶ **Expected Outcome:** The nurse will manage and minimize manifestations of a severe allergic reaction.

- Closely monitor the client's blood pressure, pulse rate and quality, respiratory effort, and urine output. *Vasodilation and increased capillary permeability affect circulating volume. Hypotension, tachycardia, thready pulse, and oliguria are evidence of reduced circulating volume. Respiratory distress is associated with contraction of smooth muscles in the bronchi or swelling of tissues in the airway.*
- Place the client in semi- or high-Fowler's position if respiratory distress is evident. *An upright position allows greater lung expansion by lowering abdominal organs away from the diaphragm.*
- Maintain an open airway and administer high-flow rates of oxygen. *Cells and organs die when they are deprived of oxygen.*
- Initiate the system for obtaining advanced cardiac life support (ACLS) either through a 911 system in the community or by announcing a "Code Blue" and its location in a healthcare agency. *Implementation of ACLS measures enhances resuscitation efforts.*
- In the healthcare facility, delegate someone to bring the emergency cart to the client's bedside. *When the code team arrives, emergency drugs, an endotracheal tube, a bag-valve mask, and a defibrillator may be needed. Saving time improves the outcome for the client.*
- Administer cardiopulmonary resuscitation with the client on a hard surface if cardiac or respiratory arrest occurs. *Pulmonary resuscitation, preferably with a resuscitation mouthpiece, promotes alveolar capillary diffusion of oxygen. Chest compressions squeeze the heart between the sternum and vertebrae, increasing cardiac output and blood supply to vital organs.*
- Seek the assistance of a registered nurse to insert an IV line as soon as possible if one is not already in place. *Decreased blood pressure reduces the ability to distend and cannulate a vein. Emergency medications usually are administered by the IV route.*
- Report assessment findings as the code team arrives. *Problem-solving and definitive treatment depend on analyzing current data.*
- Assist the code team in delegated activities or intervene in crowd control. *The code team has preassigned responsibilities, but they may need assistance in contacting the laboratory or radiology department for specific requests. Curious spectators or concerned family may interfere with resuscitation efforts.*

Evaluation of Expected Outcomes

The client reports relief of itching. He or she shows no evidence of rash. Skin is smooth and uniform in color. The client makes necessary changes in the home to reduce allergies (e.g., client removes area throw rugs; a friend adopts the family pet; the client contacts a heating-and-cooling specialist to discuss modifications to present system). Vital signs are stable. Breathing is effortless.

AUTOIMMUNE DISORDERS

Autoimmune disorders are those in which killer T cells and autoantibodies attack or destroy natural cells—those cells that are self. **Autoantibodies**, antibodies against self-antigens, are immunoglobulins. They target **histocompatible cells**, cells whose antigens match the individual's own genetic code.

 Gerontologic Considerations

- With age, the body's ability to recognize self from nonself decreases, increasing the risk of autoimmune disorders (e.g., systemic lupus erythematosus). As a person ages, higher levels of autoantibodies may be directed to endocrine glands, so attention to symptoms of hypothyroidism, and hypopituitarism, is important.

Diseases are considered autoimmune disorders when they are characterized by unrelenting, progressive tissue damage without any verifiable etiology. Various specific disorders classified as autoimmune are discussed throughout this text. Refer to Chapter 37 for information on multiple sclerosis, Chapter 58 for discussion of acute glomerulonephritis, and Chapter 63 for coverage of rheumatoid arthritis and systemic lupus erythematosus.

The term **alloimmunity** is used to describe an immune response that is waged against transplanted organs and tissues that carry nonself antigens. See Chapters 29 and 58 for more information.

Pathophysiology and Etiology

Several theories have been proposed to explain the cause of autoimmune disorders (Table 34-3). None appears to explain autoimmunity completely, which suggests that more than one mechanism is responsible.

In many autoimmune disorders, there tends to be a triggering event, such as an infection, trauma, or introduction of a drug that integrates itself into the membranes of the host's cells. One hypothesis is that the triggering event upsets the immune system's tolerance or recognition of self-antigens. A cause-and-effect relationship exists between some viral and bacterial infections (e.g., measles) and the development of a blood disorder called *thrombocytopenic purpura* (see Chap. 31). Another cause-and-effect relationship is found between streptococcal infections and disorders such as rheumatic heart disease (see Chap. 23). Despite such relationships, no scientific evidence has been found to support the hypothesis. It may be that the antigenic surface of the microorganism so closely resembles the person's histocompatible cell markers that the antibodies cannot differentiate between host and invader.

Some believe that certain people are genetically predisposed to autoimmune disorders. Theorists have proposed that the histocompatible cell markers, which are genetically inherited, act as receptors for disease-causing microorganisms, making certain cells more vulnerable than others. Another possibility is that some people inherit a trait for suppressor T-cell dysfunction. The role of suppressor T cells is to mediate immune responses. Without adequate suppressor T-cell function, killer T cells can destroy healthy cells, tissues, and organs without restraint. Consequently, genetic factors may also be a link in explaining why autoimmune disorders have a tendency to occur among blood relatives.

Another interesting phenomenon supports the sequestered antigen theory. Evidence has shown that when a person experiences trauma followed by inflammation to the iris, ciliary body, and choroid layer of one eye, the vision in the untraumatized eye also becomes affected. The term for this phenomenon is *sympathetic uveitis*. The explanation may be related to the fact that during fetal development, the cells and tissues of the eye are not exposed to the lymphatic drainage system. Therefore, the lymphocytes have never learned to

TABLE 34-3 Autoimmunity Theories

THEORY	HYPOTHESIS
Cross-antigen theory	Self-antigens that resemble foreign antigens cause T cells to misidentify natural cells and mount an immune attack.
Tissue injury theory	Infection, trauma, drugs, and radiation alter natural cells. Consequently, they no longer resemble self-antigens.
Viral mutation theory	Viruses alter T-cell receptors that are used to differentiate self from nonself.
Sequestered antigen theory	Some cells, like those of the thyroid, brain, and lens of the eye, are separated from lymphocytes during fetal development. When these cells enter circulation later because of trauma or infection, T cells do not recognize them as "self."
Diminished T-suppressor theory	Reduced numbers of suppressor cells or a shortened life span because of aging and atrophy of the thymus gland alter immunoregulation.
Genetic instruction theory	Genetic coding for antibody production is altered, which explains the familial pattern to some autoimmune disorders.

recognize the histocompatible markers on these ocular cells as self. When trauma occurs and these cells are no longer sequestered, or hidden, from the lymphocytes, the immune system attacks what it perceives to be foreign.

Regardless of whether one or all of these theoretical etiologies is valid, the outcome is clear. The immune system fails to recognize histocompatible cells. Consequently, T and B cells mount a cell-mediated or humoral response (see Chap. 33). The attack may be localized to one organ or type of tissue or it may be systemic (Box 34-2). Cells, tissues, and organs under attack are damaged or destroyed.

Assessment Findings

Signs and Symptoms

Autoimmune disorders produce various signs and symptoms depending on the tissues and organs affected. The symptoms are characteristic of an acute inflammatory response. They develop as antibodies attack normal tissue mistakenly identified as nonself. In some cases, the inflammatory symptoms are episodic. Periods of acute flare-ups (known as **exacerbations**) alternate with periods of **remission** (asymptomatic periods). The duration of these periods is completely unpredictable. During acute exacerbations, clients often experience a low-grade fever, malaise, or fatigue. They also may lose weight.

BOX 34-2	Examples of Autoimmune Disorders

Organ Specific
Blood
  Hemolytic anemia
  Thrombocytopenic purpura
Central nervous system
  Multiple sclerosis
  Guillain-Barré syndrome
Heart
  Endocarditis
Muscles
  Myasthenia gravis
Endocrine
  Hashimoto's thyroiditis
  Type 1 diabetes mellitus
Eye
  Uveitis
Joint
  Ankylosing spondylitis
Gastrointestinal
  Ulcerative colitis
Renal
  Glomerulonephritis

Systemic
Systemic lupus erythematosus
Scleroderma
Rheumatoid arthritis
Sjögren's syndrome

▶ *Stop, Think, and Respond Exercise 34-5*
What could explain why autoimmune disorders have periods of remission and exacerbation?

Diagnostic Findings

Diagnostic testing varies depending on the autoimmune disorder. Overall, elevated circulating antibodies are the hallmark findings for autoimmune disorders. Some examples include elevated erythrocyte sedimentation rate, antistreptolysin O titer, antinuclear antibody titer, and rheumatoid factor.

Medical Management

Autoimmune disorders are rarely cured. The goal of therapy is to induce a remission or slow the immune system's destruction. Drug therapy using anti-inflammatory and immunosuppressive agents is the mainstay for alleviating symptoms (Drug Therapy Table 34-2). Some antineoplastic (cancer) drugs also are used for their immunosuppressant effects. Controlling or limiting side effects of the drugs, one of which is increased susceptibility to infection, is a major concern. Even with remission, most people must continue taking prescribed medications to avoid another acute exacerbation.

 Pharmacologic Considerations

- When taking drugs to suppress the immune system, the client has an increased risk of infection, especially of the respiratory or urinary system. Observe such clients for signs and symptoms of infection such as fever, sore throat, productive cough, and dysuria.

Nursing Process for the Client with an Autoimmune Disorder

Assessment

Obtain a family history during the initial interview with the client and be alert to information about family members who have had chronic diseases with an inflammatory component that involve cardiac, urinary, neurologic, or connective tissues. During acute exacerbations, the client is quite ill; therefore, note elevated vital signs, a finding that suggests an infectious or inflammatory process. Examine the client for signs of localized inflammation and compromised body functions, such as changes in the skin, joints, gait, heart, and renal function. Ask about the client's level of energy, because fatigue is common. Review laboratory test findings for evidence that correlates with an inflammatory process or immunologic changes typical of one of many autoimmune disorders. Teaching points for those with autoimmune disorders are discussed in Client and Family Teaching 34-2.

DRUG THERAPY TABLE 34-2 Immunosuppressive Drugs

Drug Category and Examples	Mechanism of Action	Side Effects	Nursing Considerations
Corticosteroids prednisone (Meticorten), methylprednisolone (Medrol)	Initiates many immunosuppressive and anti-inflammatory cellular responses	Euphoria, initially, depression later, insomnia, gastrointestinal irritation, increased appetite, weight gain	Dose must be tapered. Abrupt withdrawal may cause acute adrenal insufficiency.
Cytotoxic Drugs azathioprine (Imuran)	Suppresses cell-mediated hypersensitivity and alters antibody production	Oral ulceration, nausea, vomiting, pancreatitis, leukopenia, bone marrow suppression, hepatotoxicity, immunosuppression, thrombocytopenia, rash, hair thinning	Follow facility policy on administration of cytotoxic drugs. Instruct clients not to take aspirin. Warn client to report signs of infection and to use effective birth control during treatment and for 4 months after.
cyclophosphamide (Cytoxan)	Interferes with replication of lymphocytes	Cardiotoxicity, anorexia, nausea, vomiting, oral ulceration, hemorrhagic cystitis, leukopenia, thrombocytopenia, anemia, pulmonary fibrosis, reversible alopecia	Advise clients to void every 1 to 2 hours while awake and to drink at least 3 L of fluid per day to reduce risk of cystitis. Do not give drug at bedtime.
methotrexate (Folex-PFS, Mexate-AQ, Rheumatrex)	Inhibits cellular replication	Stomatitis, diarrhea, nausea, vomiting, tubular necrosis, anemia, leukopenia, thrombocytopenia, hepatotoxicity, pulmonary fibrosis, urticaria, photosensitivity, alopecia	Follow facility policy on administration of cytotoxic drugs. Advise client to use birth control while on medication and to report signs of infection immediately.
Immunosuppressives cyclosporine (Sandimmune)	Inhibits lymphocytes; exact mechanism of action unknown	Tremor, gum hyperplasia, nausea, vomiting, diarrhea, nephrotoxicity, leukopenia, thrombocytopenia, hepatotoxicity	Warn client to report signs of infection, take drug at same time every day, take with meals if it causes nausea, avoid pregnancy, and not to stop medication without physician approval. Risk for anaphylaxis is high with injection form. Advise clients to report signs of infection immediately.
tacrolimus (Prograf)	Inhibits T-cell activation; exact mechanism of action unknown	Hypersensitivity, headache, tremor, insomnia, hypertension, diarrhea, nausea, abnormal renal function, anemia, leukocytosis, thrombocytopenia, hyperkalemia, hyperglycemia, hypomagnesemia, pleural effusion, pain, fever, asthenia	Monitor for anaphylaxis for 30 minutes after starting an infusion and frequently thereafter. Have epinephrine (1:1000) and oxygen available at the bedside. Check blood cell counts for suppression. Inform client of an increased risk for cancer. Store diluted solution in glass or polyethylene (not polyvinyl chloride) containers and discard if unused after 24 hours.

Client and Family Teaching 34-2
Autoimmune Disorders

The nurse teaches clients who have autoimmune disorders and their family members the following guidelines:

- Notify a healthcare practitioner of any sign of infection such as cough, fever, severe diarrhea, mouth lesions, or sore throat.
- Notify a healthcare practitioner of any new side effects to prescribed medications.
- Do not stop taking any medications abruptly.
- Avoid crowds or people with infections if you are taking an immunosuppressant drug.
- Limit stress and use stress reduction techniques such as progressive relaxation or breathing exercises.
- Maintain close follow-up with a physician.

Diagnosis, Planning, and Interventions

▶ **Activity Intolerance** related to joint pain secondary to inflammation, malaise, and fatigue

▶ **Expected Outcome:** The client will perform activities of daily living (ADLs) without extreme fatigue or discomfort.

- Encourage rest during periods of severe exacerbation and regular exercise during periods of remission. *Activity levels within a client's level of endurance promote well-being. Endurance is related to the frequency, duration, and intensity of activity (Carpenito-Moyet, 2007).*
- Provide nonpharmacologic and pharmacologic pain management as ordered by the physician. *Nonpainful stimuli (e.g., massage, activity, heat, cold, imagery, pleasant sounds) can reduce or relieve pain. Analgesic anti-inflammatory medications block neurotransmitters that carry pain stimuli to the brain; narcotic analgesics dull the brain, making it less perceptive to pain transmission; corticosteroids suppress the immune response.*

▶ **Risk for Infection** related to immunosuppression secondary to drug therapy for the autoimmune disorder and generally poor physical condition

▶ **Expected Outcome:** The client will be free of infection.

- Instruct the client about signs and symptoms of and the increased risk for infection. *Access to knowledge facilitates an active role in restoring health.*
- Instruct the client to report signs and symptoms of infection (e.g., cough, dyspnea, diarrhea, fever) immediately to the physician. *Early treatment promotes a shorter duration of illness and reduced complications.*
- Tell the client to avoid high-risk activities, such as being in crowds, during periods of immunosuppression. *Risk for infection increases with exposure to others who may have infectious disorders or whose handwashing and hygiene measures are less than adequate.*

▶ Disturbed Personal Identity related to coping with chronic illness and physical changes associated with autoimmune disorders

▶ **Expected Outcome:** The client will maintain a positive self-concept.

- Interact with and frequently show genuine interest in the client. *A person's concept of self is determined to a great extent by the responses of others. The client may interpret lack of interest and avoidance as rejection and being unworthy of attention.*
- Refer the client to community organizations and support groups. *Sharing problems and experiences with others who are similarly affected dispels the idea that a person's symptoms and feelings are unique. A person can more easily resolve and tolerate problems when he or she shares the burden with others.*

Evaluation of Expected Outcomes

The client participates in self-care and ADLs without overwhelming fatigue. There is no evidence of *iatrogenic* (treatment-caused) infection. The client perceives himself or herself realistically, with more positive attributes than negative. ●

CHRONIC FATIGUE SYNDROME

Chronic fatigue syndrome (CFS), also called *chronic fatigue, chronic fatigue immune dysfunction syndrome (CFIDS),* and *myalgic encephalomyelitis (ME),* is a complex of symptoms primarily characterized by profound fatigue with no identifiable cause. The fatigue worsens with physical activity and does not improve with rest. The term *chronic* refers to the fact that the duration of fatigue has been unrelenting for 6 or more months. Some believe that CFS is associated with **fibromyalgia**, pain in fibrous tissues of the body such as muscles, ligaments, and tendons, because both conditions share many symptoms.

From 1989, when the Centers for Disease Control and Prevention (CDC) began to collect surveillance data for CFS, to 2007, the CDC estimates that as many as 1 million people in the United States have symptoms corresponding with CFS, but fewer than 20% have been diagnosed (Centers for Disease Control and Prevention, 2007). Most clients who seek treatment for their symptoms are white women 20 to 50 years of age. CFS also occurs in men as well as in people of other races. Within 5 years after the onset of illness, some people with CFS improve but are not completely symptom-free, while others suffer with their symptoms or feel worse (National Center for Infectious Diseases, 2006). When the duration of symptoms is lengthy, the prognosis is less optimistic.

Pathophysiology and Etiology

No cause for CFS has yet been established. Some believe that the disorder results from immune-system dysregulation, in which the immune system remains activated for an extended period after an infectious triggering event. Although researchers have attempted to find a link between CFS and viral diseases (such as infectious mononucleosis caused by the Epstein-Barr virus, human herpes virus-6

(HHV-6), and enteroviruses), fungal and mycoplasmal infections, or other infections or diseases, no single causal relationship has been found. Some hypothesize that T cells are activated initially in response to a virus and that levels of proinflammatory cytokines, such as various interleukins and tumor necrosis factor, remain elevated (see Chap. 33). It is well documented that cytokines produce achy, flulike symptoms accompanied by fever and malaise during the early stages of infections. People with CFS experience these same symptoms. The difference is that during infections the symptoms are brief, but in CFS they are relentlessly prolonged.

Evidence is mounting that CFS is caused by a combination of immune defects and viral assaults. It has been found that people with CFS produce a defective form of ribonuclease termed RNase L, an enzymatic protein induced by the cytokine interferon that has antiviral activity. The RNase L destroys the RNA in viruses as well as in normal cells. The RNase L attacks the wrong enemy, that is, normal body cells, and leaves the person subject to reactivation of viruses that should remain dormant. Thus, some believe that CFS should be called "chronic viral reactivation syndrome" (Dellwo, 2008).

The fact that serum cortisol levels are low among those with CSF symptoms has led to another hypothesis. Some believe that CSF is a consequence of impaired activation of three neuroendocrine structures: the hypothalamus, pituitary gland, and adrenal glands. Collectively, these structures are sometimes referred to as the *HPA axis*. When the HPA axis functions normally, it is stimulated to release hormones during periods of physical stress, such as an infection, or emotional stress. The hypothalamus secretes corticotropin-releasing hormone, which tells the pituitary to release adrenocorticotropic hormone (ACTH). When ACTH stimulates the adrenal glands, they make corticosterone (cortisol). Cortisol suppresses inflammation and immune activity. Down-regulation of the HPA axis interferes with immune suppression and allows the hyperfunctioning immune processes to continue unabated.

Down-regulation of the HPA axis also helps explain why those with CFS experience **neurally mediated hypotension** (NMH). NMH is a condition in which individuals experience hypotension accompanied by fatigue after standing for more than 10 minutes. Some attribute the symptoms to pooling of blood in the lower limbs, resulting in decreased cerebral oxygenation. Because corticosteroids are associated with fluid retention, reduced cortisol levels may cause the hypotension.

Assessment Findings

Signs and Symptoms

Many clients with CFS report having had a recent illness with flulike symptoms or an upper respiratory infection. Despite having been uncomfortable, most clients do not describe their initial symptoms as being extraordinarily severe. In fact, the opposite is true. Thereafter, however, severe, ongoing fatigue has lasted for at least 6 months without any explanation. Even though the fatigue is constant, it worsens after physical activity. The fatigue is so debilitating that it usually interferes with a person's ability to work in or outside the home.

In addition to fatigue, the client exhibits at least four or more of the following:

- Low-grade fever
- Sore throat
- Tender cervical or axillary lymph nodes
- Muscle weakness
- Myalgia (muscle pain)
- Headaches
- Migrating joint pain without any accompanying swelling or redness
- Unrefreshing sleep
- Neurologic symptoms such as photophobia, defects in the visual field, irritability, forgetfulness, confusion, difficulty concentrating, and depression

▶ **Stop, Think, and Respond Exercise 34-6**

Discuss possible consequences among people who suffer unrelenting fatigue and pain.

Diagnostic Findings

Findings of the medical history and physical examination are unremarkable. Although the client may have other physical or psychological conditions, they are unrelated to the client's presenting symptoms. Results from a battery of blood tests specific for diagnosing diseases associated with fatigue such as alkaline phosphatase; blood urea nitrogen; serum calcium, glucose, and thyroid-stimulating hormone levels; and tests for antinuclear antibodies all fail to reveal an explanation for the client's symptoms. The exhaustive medical workup excludes all diagnoses except CFS. Currently, research is focused on measuring levels of RNase L in CFS. The knowledge that the enzyme is elevated in clients with CFS has not improved diagnosis of the disorder (Centers for Disease Control, 2004).

A **tilt-table test,** one in which the client lies horizontally on a table whose incline is elevated to approximately 70 degrees for 45 minutes, may be done. During the test, the blood pressure and pulse are monitored. The test tends to provoke hypotension in 96% of those eventually diagnosed with CFS (National Center for Infectious Diseases, Chronic Fatigue Syndrome, Information, 2007).

Medical Management

Treatment focuses on relieving the client's symptoms because nothing, as yet, holds promise for a cure. One investigational drug, poly I:polyC12U (Ampligen), is producing modest improvement in some people with CFS. This drug is a synthetic ribonucleic acid that stimulates the production of interferons, which have antiviral functions and modify the immune response. Ampligen has been used in the adjunctive treatment of cancer and acquired immunodeficiency syndrome (AIDS), but results have not been extraordinarily promising. Manufacturers of nicotinamide adenine dinucleotide (NADH), a nutritional supplement known as ENADA, claim it stimulates the production of adenosine triphosphate (ATP), which provides cellular energy. Approximately one third of participants with CFS using Enada in clinical trials report more endurance and less fatigue.

Without any definitive drug treatment, the client is advised to balance activity with rest. An employed client may need to resign from his or her job or negotiate for a less physically demanding position. The physician may prescribe a modest exercise program under the supervision of a physical therapist to avoid muscle atrophy that contributes to weakness. The client is to avoid overexertion at all costs.

Mild pain and fever are treated with aspirin, acetaminophen (Tylenol), or nonsteroidal anti-inflammatory agents such as ibuprofen (Motrin, Advil) or naproxen sodium (Naprosyn, Aleve). Even low doses of tricyclic antidepressants such as amitriptyline (Elavil), doxepin (Sinequan), or nortriptyline (Pamelor) can relieve pain and improve sleep.

Clients who experience hypotension are advised to increase salt and water intake as long as doing so is not contraindicated by cardiac or renal disease. Some clients also experience greater blood pressure stability when fludrocortisone (Florinef), a corticosteroid, is prescribed. An antihypotensive agent such as midodrine (ProAmatine) may be prescribed to increase vascular tone and elevate blood pressure. Several adjunct and alternative therapies are suggested to treat clients with CFS holistically (Nutrition Notes 34-2).

Some clients benefit from cognitive therapy, a form of psychotherapy in which people learn skills to change distorted thoughts about themselves. For example, cognitive therapy may help a person with CFS who believes that he or she is a helpless victim of the disease to perceive himself or herself as capable of dealing with the fatigue. Some promote the use of acupuncture, Eastern exercise and meditation techniques such as yoga and tai chi, and phototherapy (see Chaps. 9 and 13) to contribute to well-being. Until more information is known about CFS, however, clients may fall victim to herbal and dietary claims that promise a cure. As long as the alternative therapy is not dangerous, the client's right to incorporate unproven or unstandardized methods is not challenged.

Nursing Management

The nurse educates the client about his or her disease process and the limitations that it requires (see Client and Family Teaching 34-3 and Nursing Care Plan 34-1).

Gerontologic Considerations

- An older adult who reports CFS should be evaluated for depression.

Client and Family Teaching 34-3
Chronic Fatigue Syndrome

The nurse teaches clients who have CFS and their family members the following guidelines:

● When using over-the-counter analgesics, follow the recommended dosages and frequency for administration. Excess use can lead to increased potential for bleeding, liver, and kidney damage.
● Herbal products also have potential side effects and toxic effects; therefore, consult with the physician and keep him or her informed of any alternative therapeutic approaches you are using.
● Many companies make herbal and health-related supplements, but there is no standard among them for safe, effective dosages. Read and compare labels and ask the physician for his or her opinion on a product's efficacy.
● No scientific evidence has shown that vitamins or minerals alter the course of CFS; however, they are not harmful taken in recommended dosages.
● When searching for a support group, be wary of organizations that

  ● Promise a cure for CFS
  ● Use meetings as an opportunity to criticize specific physicians or treatment programs
  ● Advise abandoning standard treatment regimens
  ● Recommend an untested, unresearched, unscientific approach for managing CFS
  ● Press participants to discuss information of a personal nature
  ● Charge unreasonable fees for membership
  ● Do not tolerate differences of opinion among group participants
  ● Sell health-related items for a profit

● Rely on family and friends. A strong network of family and supportive friends is an important factor in coping with the chronicity of CFS.

Nutrition Notes 34-2
The Client With Chronic Fatigue Syndrome

● Some studies suggest that people with CFS may be marginally deficient in various nutrients, including B vitamins, vitamin C, magnesium, zinc, and essential fatty acids. It is not known, however, whether nutrient deficiencies precede CFS or are a consequence of the disease process. Because the potential benefits outweigh potential risks, a multivitamin and mineral supplement may be prudent.
● An omega-3 fatty acid known as *eicosapentaenoic acid* (EPA) is thought to block the release of cytokines and prostaglandins, and therefore may prevent or reduce inflammation and pain experienced with CFS and other inflammatory autoimmune disorders.
● Fish oils provide the only dietary source of EPA. Fatty fish, such as mackerel, sardines, herring, salmon, and tuna, are the best sources.
● Fish-oil supplements usually are not recommended because no clearly prescribed guidelines on the optimal dose are available. Also, fish-oil supplements have the potential to cause gastrointestinal upset, increased bleeding time, vitamins A and D toxicities, and decreased levels of various immune system components, the significance of which is uncertain.

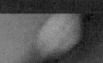

NURSING CARE PLAN 34-1 — The Client with Chronic Fatigue Syndrome

Assessment

- Ask client to rate his or her energy level using a scale of 0 to 10, with 10 being the highest level. Have the client keep an energy diary to track periods during the day when energy levels are highest and lowest to determine any predictable pattern.

- Assess blood pressure and pulse in resting and sitting positions to detect postural changes.
- Have client report his or her estimation of the quality of sleep.
- Determine client's pain level and location of discomfort.

Nursing Diagnosis. Fatigue related to chronic immune response secondary to CFS

Expected Outcome. Client's fatigue will be reduced sufficiently so that he or she can manage ADLs.

Nursing Intervention	Rationale
Have client identify ADLs of high priority.	Setting limits keeps physical and mental stress manageable.
Determine ADLs that the client can delegate.	Delegation ensures completion of ADLs without the client expending personal energy.
Help client perform one or more priority ADLs during a period of peak energy.	Matching periods of activity with peaks in energy minimizes fatigue and avoids overexertion, which contributes to a relapse.
Schedule 5- to 10-minute rest periods every hour or more.	Relaxation can be more restorative than long naps.
Assist client to perform gentle stretching exercises in a chair followed by low-grade active exercises recommended by the physician or physical therapist for 2 to 5 minutes daily.	Stretching exercises promote blood circulation to muscles and ease the response to exercise.
Increase exercise periods by $\frac{1}{2}$ to 1 minute every 2 to 3 weeks according to client's response.	Conditioning increases endurance.

Evaluation of Expected Outcome

Client performs hygiene and essential ADLs between periods of rest.

Nursing Diagnosis. Chronic Pain related to unknown etiology

Expected Outcome. Client's pain will be reduced to a tolerable level.

Nursing Intervention	Rationale
Apply a covered hot or cold pack to joints or muscles for 20 minutes; reapply after allowing the skin some recovery time.	Heat improves circulation and relieves muscle spasm and pain. Cold prevents swelling, numbs sensation, and relieves pain.
Encourage client to float in a pool or tub of tepid water (85°F) for 15 minutes as desired.	Cool temperatures reduce metabolic processes, including the immune response. Submersion in water results in buoyancy, a feeling of weightlessness, and relaxation. Movement and exercise are easier to perform in water.
Massage painful areas gently.	Massage releases endorphins and enkephalins that inhibit neurotransmission of pain.
Administer prescribed analgesics, corticosteroids, and antidepressants.	Medications relieve pain through several physiologic mechanisms.

Evaluation of Expected Outcome

The client's pain is reduced to a level of 5, which is within the client's tolerable range.

Nursing Diagnosis. Risk for Injury related to neurally mediated hypotension

Expected Outcome. The client will remain injury free.

Nursing Intervention	Rationale
Advise client to salt food liberally and to consume at least eight full glasses of fluid per day.	Sodium attracts water. An adequate amount of fluid maintains circulating blood volume, reducing the potential for hypotension.
Keep the signal for assistance within reach, and advise client to use it before attempting to ambulate.	A nursing staff member may support the client in such a way as to break his or her fall and reduce or eliminate injury.
Apply elastic stockings or thigh-high support hose before client lowers legs below the level of the heart.	Elastic fibers compress vein walls and prevent pooling of blood in the extremities.

(care plan continues on page 484)

NURSING CARE PLAN 34-1 **The Client with Chronic Fatigue Syndrome** (Continued)

Nursing Intervention	Rationale
Have client dangle and flex his or her lower limbs before getting out of bed.	Muscle contraction promotes circulation of blood from distal body areas to the heart and brain. Adequate blood flow to the brain reduces hypotensive episodes.
Instruct client to use a shower chair and avoid hot water when performing hygiene.	Remaining seated reduces the potential for injury from a fall. Hot water causes vasodilation and a drop in blood pressure.
Administer prescribed antihypotensive or corticosteroid medications.	Raising vascular tone and promoting sodium and water retention reduce the potential for low blood pressure.

Evaluation of Expected Outcome

Client's blood pressure is within normal limits and no fainting or injuries have occurred.

CRITICAL THINKING EXERCISES

1. A client reports having an allergy to aspirin. What additional information is needed to differentiate a true allergy from the drug's unwanted side effects?
2. A client complains about being delayed from going home for 30 minutes after receiving a desensitizing injection to control his allergies. How would you respond?
3. Explain why allergies, autoimmune diseases, and CFS are classified as immune-mediated disorders.
4. What teaching can you give to a client who seeks relief from symptoms of allergic rhinitis?

NCLEX-STYLE REVIEW QUESTIONS

1. A client who is symptomatic after having been stung by a bee is brought to the emergency department. Which of the following is the initial priority nursing assessment?
   1. Respiratory status
   2. Level of consciousness
   3. Heart rate
   4. Urinary output
2. In a client with an allergy, which of the following findings are likely to be evident when the nurse assesses the pharynx? Select all that apply.
   1. Rashes or lesions
   2. Red tonsils
   3. Excess secretion of lymph
   4. Production of antibodies
   5. Mucoid drainage

3. The nurse is directing care and providing teaching for a client with an autoimmune disorder. Which statement by the client demonstrates a correct understanding of the expected outcome for this client?
   1. "I will be cured of the autoimmune disorder."
   2. "I will need no more pharmacologic therapy."
   3. "I will be asymptomatic by avoiding immunologic triggers."
   4. "I will be in remission or have occasional exacerbations."
4. The nurse is teaching a client with an autoimmune disorder. Which of the following would the nurse stress as most important to avoid?
   1. Crowds during periods of immunosuppression
   2. Regular exercise during periods of remission
   3. Rest during periods of severe exacerbation
   4. Humid environment during periods of remission
5. During an initial physical assessment, an older adult client reports chronic fatigue. When all the assessment findings are normal, it is most appropriate for the nurse to further evaluate the client for which of the following?
   1. Depression
   2. Anxiety
   3. Fear
   4. Confusion

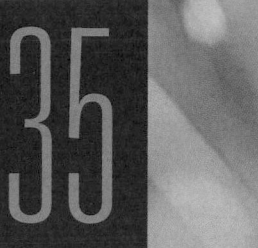

35

Caring for Clients with HIV/AIDS

Learning Objectives

On completion of this chapter, you will be able to:

1. Explain the term *acquired immunodeficiency syndrome (AIDS)*.
2. Identify the virus that causes AIDS.
3. Discuss the characteristics of a retrovirus.
4. Explain how human immunodeficiency virus (HIV) is transmitted.
5. Name at least four methods for preventing transmission of HIV.
6. List three criteria for diagnosing AIDS.
7. Discuss the pathophysiologic process of AIDS.
8. List at least five manifestations characteristic of acute retroviral syndrome.
9. Name two laboratory tests used to screen for HIV antibodies and one that confirms a diagnosis of AIDS.
10. Name two laboratory tests used to measure viral load, and give two purposes for their use.
11. Identify categories of drugs that are used to treat individuals infected with HIV, and give an example of a specific drug in each category.
12. Give the criterion for successful drug therapy for HIV/AIDS.
13. Discuss the nursing management of a client with AIDS, including client teaching.
14. Describe techniques for preventing HIV infection among health care workers who care for infected clients.
15. Discuss two ethical issues that affect healthcare workers in relation to clients with HIV infection.

Acquired immunodeficiency syndrome (AIDS) is an infectious and eventually fatal disorder that profoundly weakens the immune system. A pathogen known as the **human immunodeficiency virus** (HIV) causes AIDS. People can remain well, sometimes up to 10 years or longer, despite being infected with HIV, before the initial infection develops into AIDS. During this asymptomatic period, the infected person can infect others.

 Gerontologic Considerations

- The period between initial infection with HIV and the onset of AIDS-related symptoms is shorter for older adults than for others, and death usually occurs earlier in HIV-infected older people.

The U.S. Public Health Service and the World Health Organization agree that HIV/AIDS is more than an epidemic, a rapidly spreading disease in a particular region. HIV/AIDS is considered a *pandemic*, meaning that it is a disease infecting large numbers of people throughout the world. Based on statistics compiled at the end of 2007 by the Joint

United Nations Programme on HIV/AIDS, an estimated 33.2 million people are infected with HIV worldwide (World Health Organization, 2007). Of that number, 67% live in sub-Saharan Africa, where 60% of the worldwide infected women and 90% of globally infected children reside (Joint United Nations Programme on HIV/AIDS, 2008).

In the early history of HIV/AIDS, HIV occurred more often among homosexual men and intravenous (IV) drug users, but that exclusivity is no longer the case. Increasing numbers of heterosexual women are being infected, which, in turn, leads to transmission of HIV to newborns. To date, nurses are the largest group of healthcare workers to have occupationally acquired HIV infection (CDC, 2003).

 Gerontologic Considerations

- HIV surveillance data indicate that 17% of all new cases of AIDS are in people older than 60 years of age (Bentley, 2006).

Globally, an estimated 2.1 million people died from AIDS in 2007 (World Health Organization, 2007). This figure represents the first decline in the **mortality** or death rate from AIDS since AIDS statistics have been compiled. The decline has been attributed to (1) a change in estimating methods used to calculate statistical data, (2) a decrease in behaviors that contribute to HIV infection, and (3) improved antiretroviral drug therapy.

Despite the decline in the overall rate of HIV infection and death, AIDS continues to be a major public health problem in the United States, especially among African Americans. The rate of HIV infection is 8 times higher in African Americans than in whites (Centers for Disease Control and Prevention [CDC], 2008). In 2003, HIV/AIDS was the second leading cause of death in African American men aged 35 to 44, and the third leading cause of death in African American women in the same age group (CDC, 2003).

HUMAN IMMUNODEFICIENCY VIRUS

It is speculated that HIV is an altered genetic form of simian (monkey) immunodeficiency virus (SIV). It is believed that the transformation allowed the virus to "jump" from chimpanzees to humans in Africa when humans consumed the meat of the chimpanzees.

Subtypes

Two HIV subtypes have been identified: HIV-1 and HIV-2. HIV-1 mutates easily and frequently, producing multiple substrains that are identified by letters from A through O. HIV-2 is less transmittable, and the interval between initial infection with HIV-2 and development of AIDS is longer. HIV-1 is more prevalent in the United States and in the rest of the world. Western Africa is the primary site of infection with HIV-2.

Structural Characteristics

Viruses require a living host cell for survival and duplication. Like all viruses, HIV is genetically incomplete. A

double layer of lipid material surrounds the incomplete HIV, referred to as a **capsid**. Surface-binding proteins, called gp120, project in all directions from the lipid bilayer. Another binding protein, called gp41, which resembles a stalk, attaches the gp120 to the capsid. Inside the capsid are three important enzymes—reverse transcriptase, integrase, and protease—and strands of RNA (Fig. 35-1).

When HIV encounters a helper T-cell lymphocyte, the binding protein gp120 fuses with the T cell's receptor, called a *CD4 receptor*. Another binding protein, gp41, connects the HIV virus to either the T-cell's co-receptors CCR5 or CXCR4 (National Institute of Allergy and Infectious Diseases, 2004). The fusion provides a means by which the capsid can insert its contents into the helper T cell. The discovery of co-receptors has led to the development of a new category of antiretroviral drugs called entry inhibitors (see later discussion).

▶ *Stop, Think, and Respond Exercise 35-1*

What is the role of helper T cells in the immune response?

Replication

To replicate, which means to produce more copies, HIV becomes a parasite of helper T cells (also known as *T4* or *CD4 cells* because of their CD4 receptor; see Chap. 33). HIV alters the helper T cell's genetic code to make more viral particles. To do this, the enzyme **reverse transcriptase** copies the viral RNA into viral DNA, a process called **reverse transcription**. A second viral enzyme, **integrase,** incorporates the reprogrammed viral DNA into the host cell's DNA.

The altered DNA tells the cell how to assemble amino acids to form protein substances, such as the virus. The transformed DNA provides the blueprint or cookbook for making

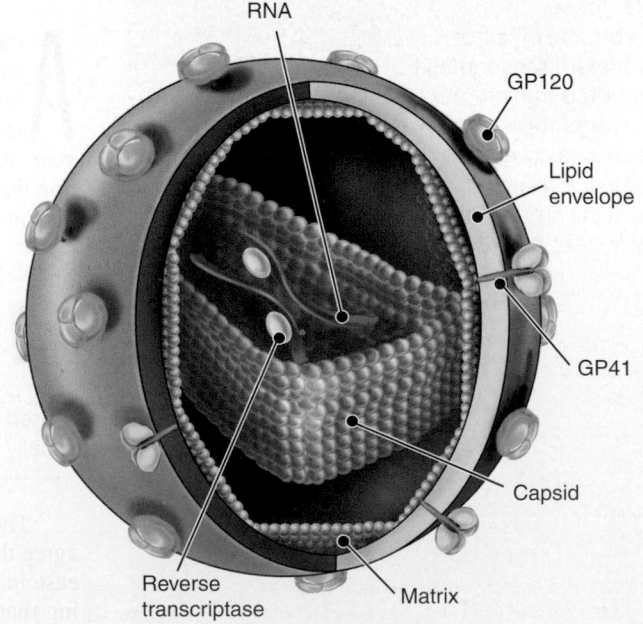

FIGURE 35-1. Structure of HIV, a retrovirus.

clones of HIV along with the enzymes the virus needs to continue reinfecting additional cells.

The T-cell's nucleus follows the DNA's directions and forms long chains of viral particles enclosed within its membrane. **Protease,** the third viral enzyme, cuts the long chains, freeing the replicated viral particles into the cytoplasm of the cell. Some migrate to the cell wall and form buds. When the buds rupture, they release many copies of the virus, which reinfect other helper T cells (Fig. 35-2).

More than 10 billion viral particles are released daily; most, but not all are destroyed. Mutations occur frequently, complicating drug therapy and making production of a vaccine nearly impossible. In February 2005, a new strain of HIV, identified as 3-DCR HIV, was detected in a homosexual man in New York (Medical News Today, 2005). Scientists consider this new strain highly virulent because it converted the man's initial HIV infection to full-blown AIDS in a matter of months; the new strain is highly drug resistant. The infected man also used methamphetamine, which scientists believe can accelerate the replication of the virus, especially in the brain. AIDS activists are warning people to avoid becoming complacent about the potential for acquiring HIV by stressing consistent condom use, avoiding illicit psychostimulants such as methamphetamine that promote disinhibition and hypersexuality, and complying with antiretroviral drug therapy if they have been diagnosed with HIV.

Transmission

HIV is not transmitted by casual contact. There are only four known body fluids through which HIV is transmitted: blood, semen, vaginal secretions, and breast milk. HIV may be present in saliva, tears, and conjunctival secretions, but transmission of HIV through these fluids has not been implicated. HIV is not found in urine, stool, vomit, or sweat.

Stop, Think, and Respond Exercise 35-2

How would you respond to those who avoid drinking from a common cup, such as those used in Christian church services, because they fear acquiring AIDS?

Certain behaviors increase the risk of acquiring HIV from infectious body fluids (Box 35-1). Unprotected sexual intercourse and multiple sexual partners increase the risk of HIV infection and other sexually transmitted diseases. Using a condom is one of the most effective ways to reduce the risk of HIV infection. Condoms are available for both men and women (Client and Family Teaching 35-1).

Gerontologic Considerations

- An accurate sexual history in older adults is important, as sexual activity may continue throughout the lifespan. Heterosexual transmission of HIV in men over age 50 has increased 94% since 1991 (Cichocki, 2007).

Before 1984, blood and blood products were a major source of HIV transmission. Since then, an HIV screening test is performed on donated blood. Although screening donated blood for HIV antibodies reduces the risk of transfusion-related infection with HIV, it is not flawless. Antibody screening cannot identify infected blood from donors who have yet to produce significant antibodies. The window of time between infection (entrance of HIV into the body) and production of antibodies varies from 1 to 6 weeks. Thus, a recently infected person with HIV can donate blood containing the virus, even though the screening test results will be negative for HIV. Other potential methods of transmission include receiving infected semen from a sperm bank or infected organs or tissues for transplantation.

Prevention Strategies

The transmission of HIV is reduced or eliminated by adhering to the following guidelines:

- Abstain from sexual intercourse.
- Have mutually monogamous sex with an uninfected partner.
- Avoid casual sex with multiple partners.
- Use a condom and spermicide that contains nonoxynol-9 during sexual intercourse.

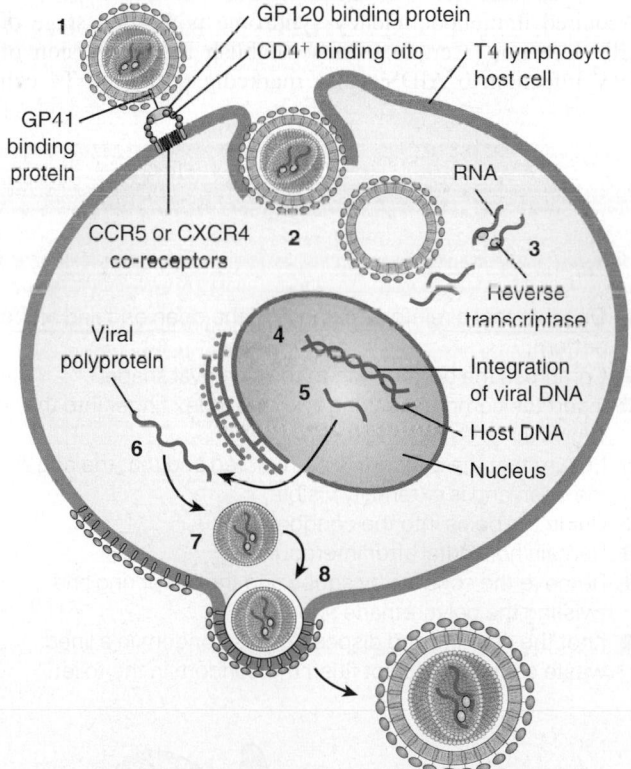

FIGURE 35-2. HIV replication. (1) To enter a T-cell lymphocyte, the HIV must attach to a CD4 receptor and additional co-receptors on the surface of the cell. (2) Internalization and uncoating of the virus with viral RNA and reverse transcriptase. (3) Reverse transcription, which produces a mirror image of the viral RNA and double-stranded DNA molecule. (4) Integration of viral DNA into host DNA. (5) Transcription of inserted viral DNA to produce viral messenger RNA. (6) Conversion of viral messenger RNA to create viral polyprotein. (7) Cleavage of viral polyprotein into viral proteins that make up new virus. (8) Assembly and release of new virus from the host cell.

BOX 35-1 High-Risk Factors for HIV Infection

- Unprotected vaginal, anal, or oral sex
- Contact with blood and infectious body fluids during medical, surgical, dental, or nursing procedures
- Sharing intravenous needles or syringes
- Receiving nonautologous transfusions of blood or blood products

- Receiving plasma or clotting factors that have not been heat treated
- Contact with infected blood on body-piercing, tattoo, and dental equipment
- Transmission from infected mothers to infants during pregnancy, birth, or breast-feeding

- Abstain from using IV drugs, especially psychostimulants, such as methamphetamine, that contribute to disinhibition and hypersexuality.
- Use a new needle and syringe each time IV drugs are injected.
- Refrain from donating blood if engaged in high-risk behaviors.
- Bank **autologous blood** (self-donated) or **directed donor blood** (specified blood donors among relatives and friends) when preparing for nonemergency surgical procedures (Table 35-1).

Some authorities believe that directed donor blood is no safer than blood collected from public donors. Those who support this belief say that directed donors may not reveal their high-risk behaviors that put the potential recipient at risk for blood-borne pathogens such as HIV.

Nurses and other healthcare workers use Standard Precautions (see Chap. 12) when caring for all clients whose infectious status is unknown. Because postexposure protocols can reduce the risk of HIV infection if initiated promptly, nurses must immediately report any needlestick or sharp injury to a supervisor. Infected healthcare workers can continue to practice; however, they usually are restricted from performing procedures in which they may exchange blood with clients.

ACQUIRED IMMUNODEFICIENCY SYNDROME

Acquired immunodeficiency syndrome is the end stage of HIV infection. Certain events establish the conversion of HIV infection to AIDS: (1) a markedly decreased T4 cell

Client and Family Teaching 35-1
Using a Condom

The nurse teaches clients the following points:

Male Condom

- Purchase latex condoms, or vinyl if sensitive to latex.
- Select a strong condom, and use lubricant liberally for anal intercourse.
- Do not store condoms where they are exposed to heat or light.
- Use a new condom each time you engage in sexual intercourse.
- Apply the condom after the penis is erect and before making any sexual contact with a partner.
- Leave a half inch between the tip of the penis and the bottom of the condom.
- Unroll the condom to the base of the penis.
- Expel any air bubbles that have formed.
- On withdrawal, hold the base of the condom and withdraw the penis before it becomes limp.
- When removing the condom, knot the open end, and discard it in a lined waste container.

Female Condom

- Make sure that the purchased condom is labeled for female use; one brand available in the United States is called "Reality."
- Distribute the coated lubricant over the outside by rubbing the outer surface.

- Observe that a reinforced ring is at the open end and at the bottom.
- Compress the bottom ring to form an oval shape.
- Insert the compressed ring with the index finger into the vagina as far as the finger can reach.
- Ensure that the condom is not twisted and that the ring at the open end is externally visible.
- Guide the penis into the condom.
- Remain horizontal after intercourse.
- Remove the condom by squeezing the lower ring and twisting the polyurethane sheath.
- Knot the opening and dispose of the condom in a lined waste container; do not flush the condom in the toilet.

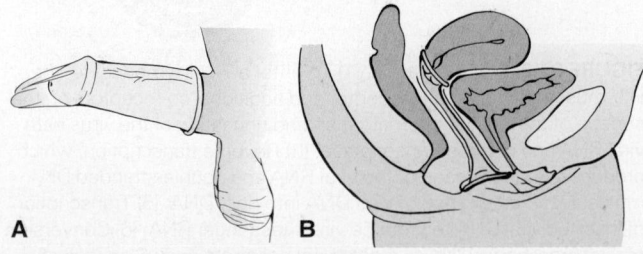

Applied condoms: **(A)** male and **(B)** female.

TABLE 35-1 Guidelines For Autologous and Directed Donor Blood Donation

AUTOLOGOUS DONATION	DIRECTED DONOR DONATION
Donor must weigh 95 lb.	Donor must weigh 110 lb.
Donor must be at least 14 years of age.	Donor must be at least 17 years of age.
Exceptions may be made in medical history.	Donor must meet volunteer donor medical history criteria.
Blood is used only for transfusion to donor.	Client's physician must be informed of directed donation.
	Blood may be transfused to others if not needed by client.
Blood type does not need to be known at time of donation.	Donors should be compatible with blood type of client.
Units that test positive for a disease (other than HIV) will be issued.	Units that test positive for HIV or hepatitis will not be used.
Donation frequency may not be greater than 1 unit every 56 days.	Donation frequency may not be greater than 1 unit every 56 days.
Additional fee to hospital or recipient may be charged for holding blood on reserve.	Additional fees may be charged to the recipient.

count from a normal level of 800 to 1200/mm^3; and (2) the development of certain cancers and **opportunistic infections,** infections that usually do not occur in individuals with a healthy immune system. In 1993, the CDC devised a classification system involving two categories that constitute an AIDS diagnosis: (1) Category 1, 2, or 3, and (2) Category A, B, or C (Table 35-2).

> ▶ **Stop, Think, and Respond Exercise 35-3**
>
> *What classification would be assigned to an HIV-positive person with a T4 cell count of 350/mm^3 who develops Pneumocystis pneumonia?*

Pathophysiology and Etiology

AIDS is transmitted from direct contact with the blood or body fluids of a person infected with HIV or from indirect contact with infected blood or body fluids. When HIV infection occurs, it gradually impairs the ability of infected T4 cells to recognize foreign antigens (e.g., disease pathogens) and stimulate B-cell lymphocytes. While massive numbers of viral particles are being released, infected T4 cells are destroyed by HIV itself and by killer T8-cell lymphocytes that no longer recognize the altered T4 cell's membrane as being self. Although new T4 cells are produced, the process is never as fast as replication of the virus. Eventually, T4 cells become significantly depleted, and immunodeficiency develops (Fig. 35-3). The infected person ultimately dies from an opportunistic infection.

The rate of progression from HIV infection to AIDS is related to the concentration of virus in the blood, the subtype and strain of infecting HIV, and the status of co-receptors on the CD4 cells. For some, the process may take 10 years or more. Although most people infected with HIV die of their disease, a few are long-term survivors. Some explanations for long-term survival include the following:

- The infectious HIV is a weak strain.
- The amount of virus is kept low with stronger-than-normal killer T8 cells.
- Atypical CCR5 or CXCR4 co-receptors hinder the conversion of HIV to AIDS.
- The combination of drugs used for treatment is effective.

Assessment Findings

Signs and Symptoms

At the time of primary HIV infection, one third to more than one half of those infected develop **acute retroviral syndrome** (viremia), which often is mistaken for flu or some other common illness. Some manifestations include fever; swollen and tender lymph nodes; pharyngitis; rash about the face, trunk, palms, and soles; muscle and joint pain; headache; nausea and vomiting; and diarrhea. In addition, there may be enlargement of the liver and spleen, weight loss, and neurologic symptoms such as visual changes or cognitive and motor involvement. However, admission of risk behaviors for HIV narrows the differential diagnosis. Although viral replication is rapid at this time, antibody tests cannot detect the infection.

Eventually, individuals infected with HIV present with a form of cancer that is atypical for the person's age and health history, or an opportunistic infection. For example, **Kaposi's sarcoma,** a type of connective tissue cancer common among those with AIDS, may be noted (Fig. 35-4). Others who acquire *Pneumocystis* pneumonia (discussed later) have a nonproductive cough and shortness of breath. In women, gynecologic problems may be the focus of the chief complaint. Abnormal results of Papanicolaou tests, genital warts, pelvic inflammatory disease, and persistent vaginitis (see Chaps. 53 and 56) also may correlate with HIV infection.

Diagnostic Findings

The **enzyme-linked immunosorbent assay** (ELISA) test, an initial HIV screening test, is positive when there are sufficient HIV antibodies; it also is positive when there are antibodies from other infectious diseases. The test is repeated if results are positive. If results of a second ELISA test are positive, the **Western blot** is performed. A positive result on Western blot confirms the diagnosis; however, false-positive and false-negative results on both tests are possible. Written consent must be obtained before an ELISA or Western blot test is performed. The results of the tests require strict confidentiality.

A total T-cell count, T4 and T8 counts, and T4/T8 ratio determine the status of T lymphocytes. A T4-cell count of less than 500 mm^3 indicates immune suppression; a T4-cell count of 200/mm^3 or less is an indicator of AIDS.

TABLE 35-2 Classification for HIV Infection

CATEGORY 1	CATEGORY 2	CATEGORY 3
T4 cell count ≥500/mm³	T4 cell count 200–499/mm³	T4 cell count <200/mm³
Category A HIV positive with one or more of the following: • Asymptomatic • Persistent generalized **lymphadenopathy** (swollen lymph nodes) • Symptoms formerly known as *AIDS related complex* (ARC), such as anorexia, weight loss, fever, night sweats, rash, fatigue, lowered resistance to infection, diarrhea	**Category B** HIV positive with conditions attributed to or complicated by HIV infection such as: • Bacillary angiomatosis • Candidiasis (oral, vulvovaginal) unresponsive to treatment • Cervical dysplasia or carcinoma • Fever or diarrhea for more than 1 month • Hairy leukoplakia • Herpes zoster (at least two episodes) • Idiopathic thrombocytopenic purpura • Listeriosis • Pelvic inflammatory disease/ tubo-ovarian abscess • Peripheral neuropathy • Toxoplasmosis of the brain • Wasting syndrome	**Category C** HIV positive with one or more of the following: • Candidiasis (bronchial, tracheal, lungs, or esophagus) • Cervical cancer (invasive) • Coccidioidomycosis (disseminated or extrapulmonary) • Cryptococcosis (extrapulmonary) • Cryptosporidiosis for less than 1 month • Cytomegalovirus (other than liver, spleen, or nodes) • Encephalopathy (HIV-related) • Herpes simplex (<1 month) or bronchitis, pneumonitis, esophagitis • Histoplasmosis (disseminated or extrapulmonary) • Isosporiasis (<1 month) • Kaposi's sarcoma • Lymphoma, Burkitt's (or equivalent), immunoblastic (or equivalent), brain (primary) • *Mycobacterium avium* complex or *Mycobacterium kansasii,* disseminated or extrapulmonary • *Mycobacterium tuberculosis,* any site, pulmonary or extrapulmonary • *Mycobacterium,* other species • *Pneumocystis carinii* pneumonia • Pneumonia, recurrent • Progressive multifocal leukoencephalopathy • *Salmonella* septicemia, recurrent

From Centers for Disease Control and Prevention. (1992). 1993 Revised classification system for HIV infection and expanded surveillance case definition for AIDS among adolescents and adults. *Morbidity and Mortality Weekly Report,* 41(51), 961–962.

It now is possible to measure a person's viral load, the number of viral particles in the blood. The **p24 antigen test** and **polymerase chain reaction** test measure viral loads. They are used to guide drug therapy and follow the progression of the disease. Viral load tests and T4-cell counts may be performed every 2 to 3 months once it is determined that a person is HIV positive.

Other general laboratory and diagnostic tests are prescribed when opportunistic infections are involved. In addition, cancer screenings, especially Papanicolaou cervical tests for women (see Chap. 53), are recommended for those infected with HIV. Immunosuppression tends to facilitate the development of cancer and accelerate its progression.

Medical Management

People with HIV and AIDS are treated with antiretroviral drugs, adjunct drug therapy to boost the immune response, and supportive care during opportunistic infections. It usually is recommended that clients infected with HIV receive pneumococcal, hepatitis B, and yearly influenza vaccines. Additional medical management includes treating anorexia, diarrhea, weight loss, and side effects of antiretroviral medications. Research continues on developing an effective AIDS vaccine or reducing the potential for infection with a microbicide (discussed later).

Antiretroviral Drug Therapy

At present, the majority of drugs used to manage clients who are infected with HIV target viral enzymes. When to initiate drug therapy is a subject of debate. The development of **drug resistance,** ineffective response to a prescribed drug because of the survival and replication of exceptionally virulent mutations and noncompliance with drug therapy regimens (Fig. 35-5), and **drug cross-resistance,** diminished drug response to similar HIV drugs, are common. Because drug resistance limits future treatment options, some physicians believe that delaying drug therapy is justified. The current guideline is to initiate treatment if the client develops an

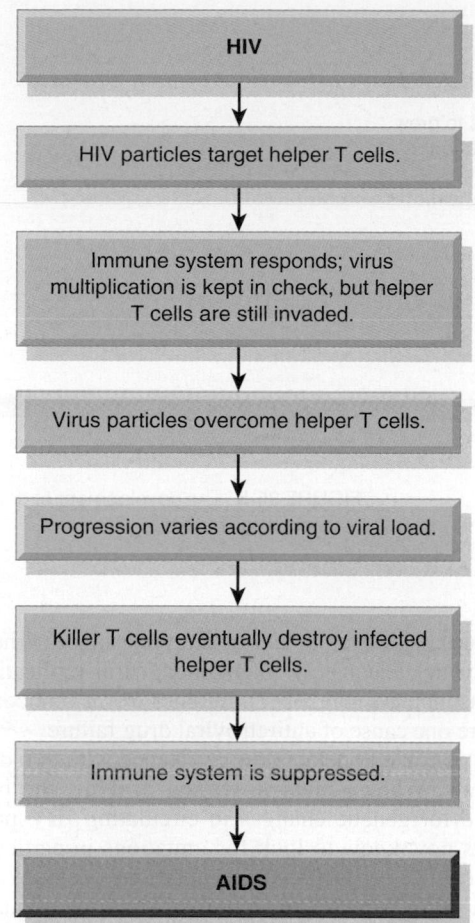

FIGURE 35-3. Progression of HIV infection and development of AIDS.

AIDS-defining illness or has a CD4 T-cell count less than 350 cells/mm³. Antiretroviral drug therapy is also warranted in infected pregnant women, in clients with HIV-associated renal disease, and in clients coinfected with hepatitis B. Treatment may be appropriate for those whose CD4 T-cell count is over 350 cells/mm³ if the benefits of drug therapy

outweigh the risks of initiating treatment earlier than generally recommended (Panel on Antiretroviral Guidelines for Adults and Adolescents, 2008). Therefore, it is critical that clients with HIV comply with regular appointments for laboratory blood tests.

The physician decides when and which antiretroviral drugs to prescribe based on the client's CD4 T-cell and viral load counts, potential compliance, medication side-effect profiles, and drug interactions. Cost is also an issue. Antiretroviral medications are very expensive, as much as $10,000 to $30,000 per year in the United States (Henry J. Kaiser Foundation, 2008). Medicaid pays approximately half the cost of antiretroviral drug therapy; the government-funded **AIDS Drug Assistance Program** (ADAP) covers approximately 30% of their cost. These state-based programs are partially funded by Title II of the Ryan White CARE Act. Some social agencies and pharmaceutical companies have compassionate need programs through which antiretroviral drugs are supplied to people who cannot afford them.

When drug therapy is begun, clients are started on a combination of generally three antiretroviral drugs: two **reverse transcriptase inhibitors,** drugs that interfere with the virus's ability to make a genetic blueprint, and one **protease inhibitor,** a drug that inhibits the ability of virus particles to leave the host cell. Since 2003, a new category of AIDS drugs called **entry inhibitors,** which interfere with the ability of the virus to fuse with and enter the CD4 cell, have become available. Even more recently, **integrase inhibitors**, a class of drugs that prevent the incorporation of viral DNA into the host cell's DNA, have been developed (Fig. 35-6). Because combinations of antiretroviral drugs are more effective, a physician should never prescribe monotherapy (only one drug used for treatment). Some clients take four types of medications (Drug Therapy Table 35-1). Combination therapy, sometimes referred to as a *drug cocktail* or **highly active antiretroviral therapy (HAART),** has several benefits:

- Using different mechanisms, the combination of drugs suppresses replication of the virus.
- The drugs lower the viral load more quickly—sometimes to undetectable levels. Doing so ultimately slows the rate

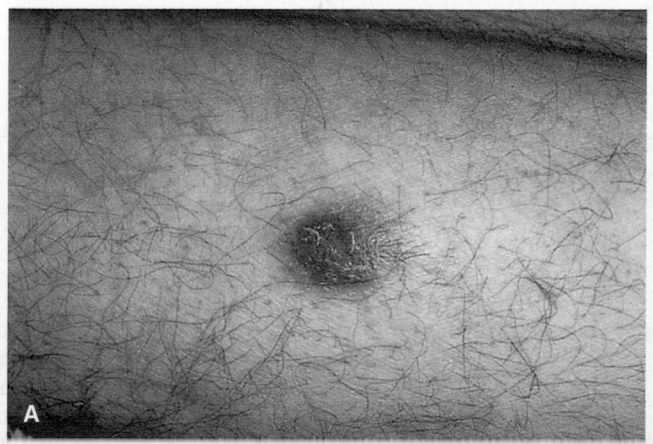
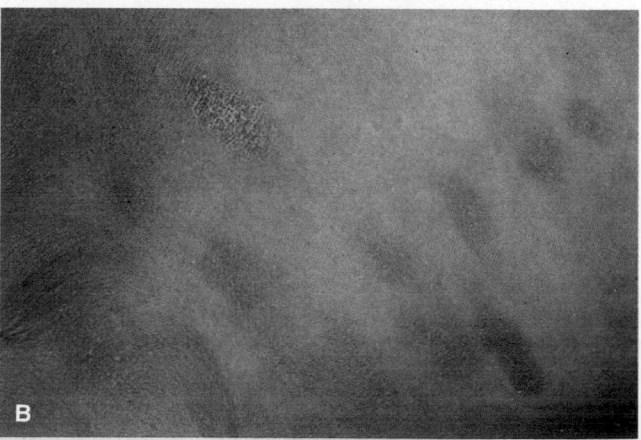

FIGURE 35-4. Kaposi's sarcoma: (**A**) single lesion and (**B**) multiple lesions.

Vir antiretroviral drugs

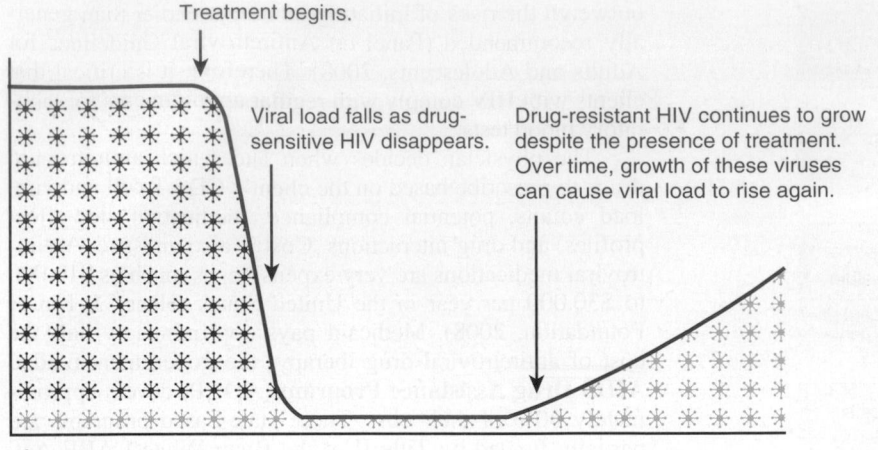

Treatment begins.

Viral load falls as drug-sensitive HIV disappears.

Drug-resistant HIV continues to grow despite the presence of treatment. Over time, growth of these viruses can cause viral load to rise again.

✳ Drug-sensitive HIV

✳ Drug-resistant HIV

FIGURE 35-5. The development of drug-resistant strains of HIV.

of disease progression, prevents opportunistic infections, and, in turn, lengthens survival.

- Combination therapy diminishes the rate of viral mutations and prolongs drug effectiveness.
- Using two or more drugs simultaneously reduces the chance that the virus will develop resistance or cross-resistance.
- Combination of drugs increases the numbers of healthy helper T-cell lymphocytes because it protects many from becoming infected.

The goal of antiretroviral therapy is to keep the CD4 cell count above 350 mm^3 and bring the viral load to a virtually undetectable level. This level is no more than 500 or 50 copies, depending on the sensitivity of the selected viral load test.

Drug Resistance

Clients who neglect to take antiretroviral drugs as prescribed (i.e., every dose, at its designated time, with or without food as directed) risk development of drug resistance. When drug levels are not adequately maintained, viral replication and mutations increase (Fig. 35-7). In other words, noncompliant clients are one cause of antiretroviral drug failure.

It is possible to detect drug resistance with two different blood tests. When **genotype testing** is done, the blood is examined for genetic changes in circulating HIV particles. Scientists now know to look for mutations in particular **codons,** sequences of DNA where mutations occur. With **phenotype testing,** a measured amount of antiviral drug is mixed with the virus until there is a quantity that prevents the virus from reproducing. The higher the dose of drug that eventually inhibits viral growth, the greater is the viral drug resistance.

Reverse Transcriptase Inhibitors

There are three approved categories of reverse transcriptase inhibitors: nucleoside reverse transcriptase inhibitors (NRTIs), non-nucleoside reverse transcriptase inhibitors (NNRTIs), and nucleotide analogues. Nucleosides are

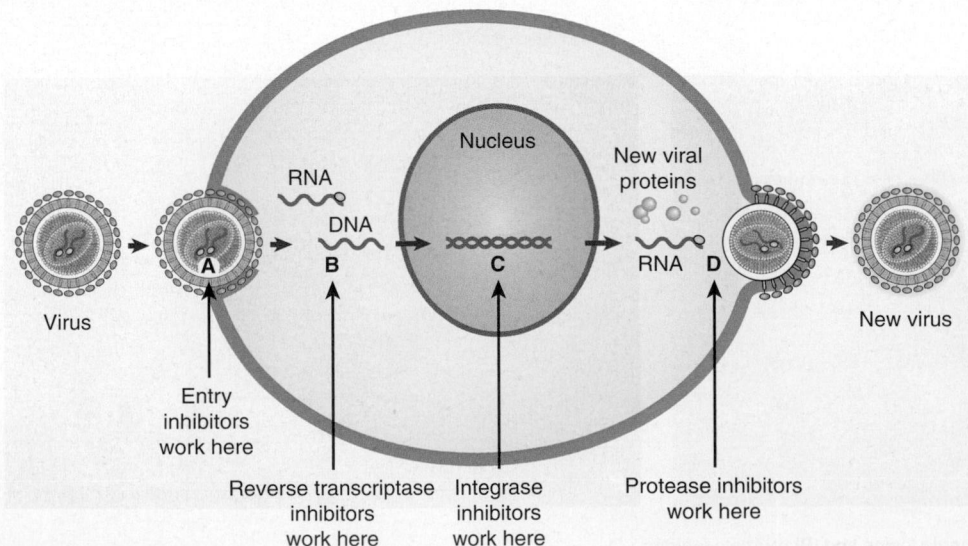

FIGURE 35-6. Current drug therapy interferes with HIV replication by **(A)** blocking the co-receptor on the surface of the T-cell lymphocyte, thus preventing the virus from entering the cell; **(B)** inhibiting the enzyme necessary for converting viral RNA to DNA; **(C)** preventing integration of viral RNA with host cell DNA; and **(D)** preventing virus particles from budding from the infected T cell.

Hydroxurea - sickle cell

DRUG THERAPY TABLE 35-1 Examples of Drugs Used in HIV Therapy

Drug Category and Examples	Side Effects	Nursing Considerations
Entry Inhibitors		
enfuvirtide (Fuzeon)	Injection site reaction such as itching, swelling, redness, pain or tenderness; allergic reactions, increased incidence of pneumonia	Reconstitute 30 to 45 minutes before administration; refrigerate any unused portion, but allow to warm to room temperature before giving. Never shake the reconstituted drug, to avoid foaming. Administer subcutaneously twice daily into the upper arm, thigh, or abdomen. Inject where you can pinch an inch of tissue or insert half the length of the needle. Instill medication slowly and apply gentle pressure after injection. Vigorously massage the site of injection for 3–5 minutes before and after the injection; an electronic vibrator is an option for this purpose. Apply a warm compress to the injection site after the injection. Rotate injection sites.
maraviroc (Selzentry)	Cough, fever, upper respiratory infection, rash, musculoskeletal symptoms, abdominal pain, dizziness	Oral delivery. Recommended dose different when administered with concomitant medications because of potential drug interactions. Must be given in combination with other antiretroviral medications.
Reverse Transcriptase Inhibitors		
Nucleoside Reverse Transcriptase Inhibitors (NRTIs)		
zidovudine (AZT, Retrovir)	Anemia, granulocytopenia, nausea, gastrointestinal pain, diarrhea, myositis, headaches, fever, rash	Monitor T4 cell counts. Administer drug every 4 hours around the clock. Tell client to report extreme fatigue, nausea, vomiting, or rash.
didanosine (ddl, Videx)	Pancreatitis, peripheral neuropathy, nausea, vomiting, abdominal pain, hepatotoxicity, bone marrow suppression, insomnia	Administer on an empty stomach, 1 hour before or 2 hours after eating. Advise client to chew tablets thoroughly or crush tablets and dissolve in at least 1 ounce of water.
Non-Nucleoside Reverse Transcriptase Inhibitors (NNRTIs)		
nevirapine (Viramune, Vistide)	Rash, hepatotoxicity, headache, nausea, vomiting, diarrhea	Use is contraindicated during pregnancy or breast-feeding. Avoid combining with protease inhibitors or oral contraceptives. Monitor hepatic and renal function. Consult physician if severe rash occurs.
efavirenz (Sustiva)	Rash, dizziness, fatigue, unusual dreams, confusion, impaired thinking, amnesia, agitation, hallucinations, hepatotoxicity, false-positive test results for cannabinoids	Control intake of fatty foods, which can elevate drug levels. Assess mental status. Monitor liver function. Warn that drug test results may be falsely positive for marijuana.

(drug table continues on page 494)

DRUG THERAPY TABLE 35-1 Examples of Drugs Used in HIV Therapy (continued)

Drug Category and Examples	Side Effects	Nursing Considerations
Nucleotide Analogues tenofovir (Viread)	Nausea, vomiting, diarrhea, flatulence, lactic acidosis, hepatomegaly, nephrotoxicity, loss of bone density	Administer once a day with a high-fat meal to provide higher blood levels. Monitor renal and hepatic function. Not recommended for women who are pregnant or breast-feeding
Integrase Inhibitors raltegravir (Isentress)	Most common include diarrhea, nausea, headache, pyrexia	Oral tablet must be stored at controlled room temperature of 68°F to 77°F (20°C to 25°C). Dosage is twice daily.
Protease Inhibitors indinavir (Crixivan)	Nephrolithiasis, gastrointestinal intolerance, headache, blurred vision, dizziness, rash, metallic taste, thrombocytopenia, hyperglycemia, lipodystrophy	Monitor for kidney stones. Increase fluid intake to help prevent formation of kidney stones. Wait 1 hour between administration of indinavir and ddl. Give drug 1 hour before or 2 hours after a meal with skim or low-fat milk. Give hard candies to help mask metallic taste. Check blood glucose levels regularly. Observe for signs of bruising or bleeding. Warn that this drug causes a redistribution of body fat.
saquinavir (Invirase, Fortase)	Headache, weakness, muscle aches, nausea, abdominal discomfort, diarrhea, elevated level of creatinine phosphokinase	Administer with or within 2 hours of a full meal. Protect from injury, which may result from weakness. Report alterations in stool or urine color, which may indicate liver dysfunction.

building blocks of DNA and RNA. By binding to viral DNA, NRTIs abort the terminal completion of gene copying.

Non-nucleoside drugs are molecularly similar to nucleoside analogues; however, NNRTIs bind directly to the reverse transcriptase enzyme, thus preventing transcription. They are effective only against HIV-1. The potent combination of drugs from these two classes cripples the virus's ability to copy itself. Unfortunately, drug resistance develops very quickly if the client does not take the NNRTI as prescribed. If drug resistance develops to one NNRTI, cross-resistance usually develops to all others in this same class.

Researchers have developed a third reverse transcriptase inhibitor category, called a nucleotide analogue. Nucleotides are compounds that are part of a chain of substances in nucleic acids (i.e., DNA and RNA). Although nucleotide analogues are technically different from NRTIs and NNRTIs, they act similarly. The essential difference is that nucleotides activate immediately when they enter the CD4 cell. They become incorporated within the viral DNA and cause premature termination of viral DNA synthesis. This group of drugs adds yet another weapon to the arsenal being used to extend the lives of those with AIDS.

Protease Inhibitors

One or two protease inhibitors usually are used in combination with both NRTIs and NNRTIs. Protease inhibitors interfere with the maturation of the viral copies. If viral copies do manage to escape from the host T4 cell, they usually are too immature to invade healthy T4 cells. Because protease inhibitors and reverse transcriptase inhibitors affect separate processes in the viral life cycle, the combination is most likely to control the virus.

Entry Inhibitors

Entry inhibitors, also known as *fusion inhibitors*, are drugs that stop HIV from getting inside a CD4 T-cell by blocking co-receptors on the cell's surface. In 2003, the U.S. Food and Drug Administration (FDA) approved enfuvirtide (Fuzeon), the first drug in this category and maraviroc (Selzentry) in 2007. Enfuvirtide acquired its brand name because it blocks the CXCR4 receptor known as fusin. Maraviroc (Selzentry) blocks the CCR5 receptor. Entry inhbitors are

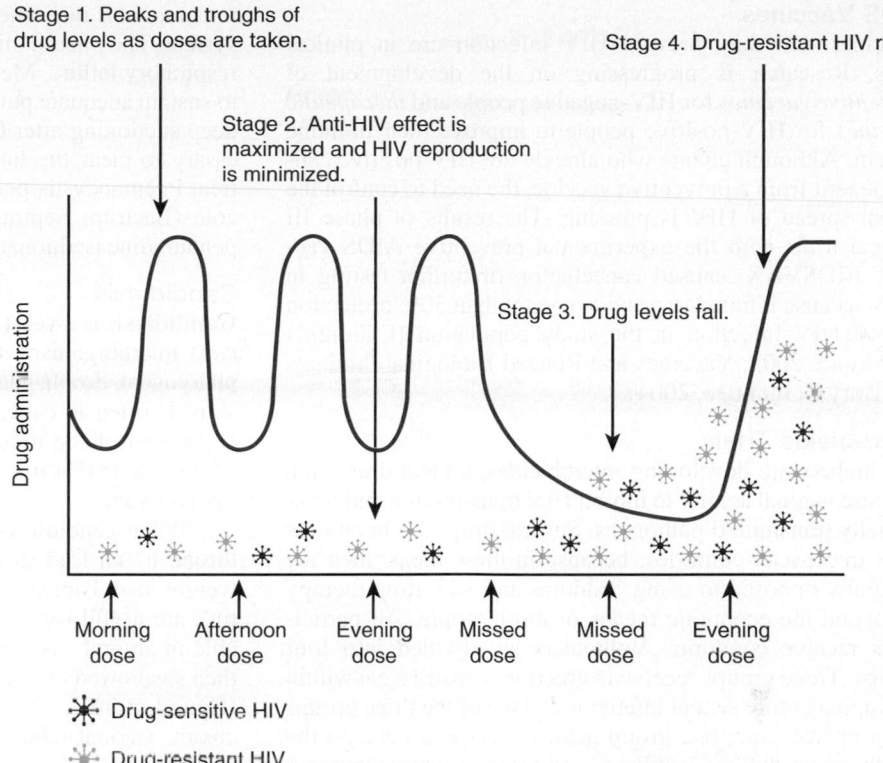

Stage 1. Peaks and troughs of drug levels as doses are taken.

Stage 2. Anti-HIV effect is maximized and HIV reproduction is minimized.

Stage 3. Drug levels fall.

Stage 4. Drug-resistant HIV rises.

Drug administration

Morning dose | Afternoon dose | Evening dose | Missed dose | Missed dose | Evening dose

✳ Drug-sensitive HIV

✳ Drug-resistant HIV

FIGURE 35-7. The effect of noncompliance on drug resistance.

reserved for people who are infected with HIV who are resistant or developing resistance to NRTIs, NNRTIs, and protease inhibitors. People with less advanced HIV/AIDS also may benefit from the inclusion of enfuvirtide in their drug regimen.

Enfuvirtide and maraviroc work best combined with at least one or two other antiretroviral drugs (Body Health Resources, 2003). Potential drug resistance remains a concern. The fear is that once subjected to a specific entry inhibitor, the virus may mutate so as to utilize the other receptor to gain entry. It is not likely that entry inhibitors will develop cross resistance to other categories of antiretroviral drugs. The biggest disadvantage of enfuvirtide is that the medication requires self-injection twice daily, and nearly all users experience some type of reaction at the injection site. The Biojector, a needle-free gas-powered injection system, has been used in Canada to facilitate the ease of injection and decrease the severity of injection site reactions, but it is not available in the United States (HIV and Hepatitis Treatment Advocates, 2007). Use of entry inhibitors requires testing the person with HIV to determine which receptor the virus uses to gain access to the CD4 T-cell (Scondras, 2004).

Integrase Inhibitors

Integrase inhibitors prevent the incorporation of viral DNA into the host cell's DNA by blocking the activity of the integrase enzyme. Preventing integration of viral DNA with host cell DNA interferes with the infected cell's ability to make copies of HIV. Raltegravir (Isentress) is the only currently available integrase inhibitor, although another medication, elvitegravir, is undergoing clinical trials. Raltegravir is combined with other types of anti-HIV drugs to prevent viral mutations. Integrase inhibitors may also be useful in **salvage**

therapy, a treatment option for infected people with significant HIV drug resistance in whom possibilities for effective antiretroviral drug management are limited.

> ### ▶ Stop, Think, and Respond Exercise 35-4
> *Explain the concept of antiretroviral drug resistance and cross-resistance, and techniques for reducing its potential.*

Adjunct Drug Therapy

Other drugs may be used with antiretroviral drug therapy in an overall effort to halt the progression of AIDS. One such drug is hydroxyurea (Hydrea), which usually is used to treat cancer. Hydroxyurea inhibits an enzyme that functions in DNA synthesis, thereby inhibiting or slowing the reproduction of tumor cells. When combined with antiretroviral drugs, hydroxyurea interferes with viral replication, increasing anti-HIV effects.

In addition, administration of endogenous immune substances known as *cytokines,* such as interferons and interleukin-2, may also be helpful (see Chap. 33). Interferons (Roferon-A, Betaseron) activate the cell's own defenses against viruses and are believed to increase blood levels of antiretroviral drugs like zidovudine (Retrovir). Interleukin-2 (IL-2) stimulates the production of lymphocytes. The pharmaceutical counterpart of IL-2 (aldesleukin, Proleukin) is used to increase the numbers of T4 helper and natural killer lymphocytes. Natural killer lymphocytes specifically target virus-infected cells and cancer cells; therefore, the use of IL-2 boosts the body's immune defenses against HIV.

AIDS Vaccines

Vaccines that may prevent HIV infection are in clinical trials. Research is progressing on the development of *preventive vaccines* for HIV-negative people and *therapeutic vaccines* for HIV-positive people to improve their immune system. Although clients who already are HIV positive cannot benefit from a preventive vaccine, the need to control the global spread of HIV is pressing. The results of phase III clinical trials with the experimental preventive AIDS vaccine, AIDSVAX, caused cancellation of further testing in 2003 because it failed to provide greater than 30% protection against HIV infection in the study population (Children's AID Fund, 2005; Vaccines and Related Biological Products Advisory Committee, 2004).

Microbicide Trials

Researchers are developing microbicides, topical drugs that increase vaginal acidity to inhibit HIV transmission and other sexually transmitted pathogens. Several drugs are in clinical trials in African countries, because in these areas, men are culturally opposed to using condoms and HIV drug therapy is beyond the economic means of most people. All participants receive condoms. Volunteers are divided into four groups. Three groups receive instruction to instill a gel within the vagina before sexual intercourse. Two of the three groups test a microbicide; one group instills a placebo gel, and the fourth group did not instill any gel prior to intercourse. All groups have the choice of a condom at the time of intercourse (National Institute of Allergy and Infectious Diseases, 2005).

Researchers are attempting to determine whether drugs used in HIV therapy may be delivered other than via the oral or parenteral route. The impetus to find alternative drug administration routes is related to the following:

1. The oral route requires numerous medications be taken simultaneously around-the-clock, on a schedule that requires near-perfect compliance.
2. The oral route is associated with undesirable gastrointestinal side effects.
3. The parenteral drugs require self-injection, which many people find objectionable.

Although no other alternatives currently exist, some examples under consideration include intradermal preparations that can be absorbed through the skin via creams, gels, or transdermal patches, as well as drugs absorbed through mucous membranes in the form of nasal sprays, buccal patches, or suppositories (Body Health Resources, 2004).

Supportive Care of Opportunistic Infections

Clients with AIDS acquire many infectious disorders, any one of which can cause death. These infectious disorders and their comparative severity are uncommon in populations of relatively healthy people. The management of some common infectious conditions follows.

Pneumocystis Pneumonia

Clients infected with HIV are at particular risk for acquiring **Pneumocystis pneumonia,** a type of pneumonia caused by an organism called *Pneumocystis carinii* which has been renamed *Pneumocystis jiroveci* to distinguish it as the organism that specifically infects humans rather than one that is common to other species of mammals. This form of pneumonia is rare among individuals with an intact immune system. The pneumonia can become so severe as to result in respiratory failure. Mechanical ventilation may be necessary to sustain adequate pulmonary function. Aerosol therapy and deep suctioning after the instillation of saline often are necessary to clear the lungs of thick sputum. To prevent and treat Pneumocystis pneumonia, trimethoprim-sulfamethoxazole (Bactrim, Septra) is prescribed. Monthly aerosolized pentamidine isethionate (NebuPent) also is effective.

Candidiasis

Candidiasis is a yeast infection caused by the *Candida albicans* microorganism. Candidiasis may develop in the oral, pharyngeal, esophageal, or vaginal cavities or in folds of the skin. It often is called *thrush* when located in the mouth. Inspection of the mouth, throat, or vagina reveals areas of white plaque that may bleed when mobilized with a cotton-tipped swab.

When candidiasis affects structures in the mouth and throat, it can lead to problems with eating and subsequent weight loss. Topical antifungals, such as nystatin (Mycostatin), are useful for treating oral candidiasis. They are available in an oral suspension that is swished in the mouth and then swallowed or in an alternate lozenge form. Clotrimazole (Gyne-Lotrimin, Mycelex) and miconazole (Monistat) cream, vaginal tablets, and suppositories are used to treat vaginitis. Sometimes systemic antifungals such as amphotericin B (Fungizone) or fluconazole (Diflucan) are required to control candidiasis.

Cytomegalovirus Infection

Opportunistic infections caused by the cytomegalovirus (CMV) affect immunosuppressed people such as clients with AIDS. CMV can infect the choroid and retinal layers of the eye, leading to blindness. It also can cause ulcers in the esophagus, colitis and diarrhea, pneumonia, and encephalitis. Foscarnet (Foscavir), cidofovir (Vistide), and ganciclovir (Cytovene) are used in combination aggressively to treat acute CMV infections. Maintenance drug therapy follows to reduce the potential for future viral activation.

 Pharmacologic Considerations

- The drug foscarnet is used to treat CMV retinitis and is given by controlled IV infusion. Alterations in renal function, fever, nausea, anemia, numbness in the extremities, and diarrhea are the most common adverse effects.

Cryptosporidiosis

Immunosuppressed clients may develop serious diarrhea as a result of infection with a protozoan called *Cryptosporidium*. The organism is spread by the fecal-oral route from contaminated water, food, or human or animal wastes. Those infected can lose from 10 to 20 L of fluid per day. Losing this magnitude of fluid quickly leads to dehydration and electrolyte imbalances. When diarrhea is accompanied by anorexia, nausea, and vomiting, weight is difficult to maintain.

Definitive diagnosis is made by examining the stool for ova and parasites and other cytologic examinations.

Antibiotic therapy is then implemented. The macrolide family of antibiotics, such as azithromycin (Zithromax) or clarithromycin (Biaxin), or an antiprotozoal agent, such as paromomycin (Humatin), is used.

Management of AIDS-Related Complications

Besides AIDS-related cancers and opportunistic infections, clients may develop **AIDS dementia complex** (ADC). ADC, a neurologic condition, causes degeneration of the brain, especially in areas that affect mood, cognition, and motor functions. Clients exhibit forgetfulness, limited attention span, decreased ability to concentrate, and delusional thinking. Moods range from irritability to euphoria. Possible motor dysfunction is manifested by staggering gait and muscle incoordination, slowing of all movements, or paraplegia, which may be accompanied by incontinence.

Gerontologic Considerations

- The dementia caused by AIDS may be mistaken for other dementias that may affect older adults, and may occur concurrently.

Antiretroviral therapy can delay or prevent ADC. Other drugs, some of which are in clinical trials, may slow the progression of ADC once it manifests. One such drug is memantine (Namenda). It is believed that this medication performs a neuroprotective function. Memantine blocks *N*-methyl-D-aspartate (NMDA) receptors in the brain from being overexcited by a neurotransmitter called *glutamate*. Normal concentrations of glutamate enhance memory and learning; too much glutamate is lethal to brain cells. Research also continues on CPI-1189, an agent that is an antagonist of cytokines such as tumor necrosis factor (see Chap. 33), which are produced during gp120-induced inflammation of brain cells. Until these drugs and others are approved, antiretroviral therapy may be combined with selegiline (Eldepryl), an anti-Parkinson's drug, to treat motor and cognitive impairments of ADC, and with psychiatric drugs to moderate mood and activity levels.

Other clients may develop **distal sensory polyneuropathy** (DSP), which is characterized by abnormal sensations, such as burning and numbness, in the feet and later in the hands. Because neuropathy is a side effect of several antiretroviral drugs, it is difficult to determine if the cause is actually destruction of the sensory peripheral nerves or drug therapy. DSP responds less well to drug therapy than do neuropathics associated with other primary disorders such as diabetes mellitus (see Chap. 51). Nevertheless, an effort is made to preserve and promote nerve function using vitamin B_{12} and thiamine supplementation. Neuropathic pain also may be amenable to treatment with tricyclic antidepressants such as amitriptyline (Elavil) and nortriptyline (Pamelor) or anticonvulsants such as gabapentin (Neurontin) and carbamazepine (Tegretol).

Nursing Management

The role of the nurse involves health teaching and counseling of high-risk populations. Areas of emphasis include HIV prevention strategies such as sexual abstinence and **safer sex practices,** sexual activities in which body fluids are not exchanged. The nurse encourages diagnostic screening for those whose behaviors place them at risk for HIV infection. He or she helps interpret the results of diagnostic tests and monitors the need for continued follow-up in the months after potential exposure.

For clients with an established HIV status, the nurse explains the action of each antiretroviral drug and develops a schedule for the client's self-administration. This includes strong precautions about rigidly adhering to the dosage, time, and frequency of drug administration to avoid development of drug resistance. Describing the side effects of drug therapy is essential, with the admonition to refrain from discontinuing any of the prescribed drugs without first consulting the prescribing physician. The nurse makes appointments for laboratory tests for monitoring the effects of drug therapy.

Referral of HIV-positive clients to support groups and resources for information about new HIV drug development, clinical drug trials, AIDS drug assistance programs, and progress on vaccine development is a very important nursing intervention. Nursing Care Plan 35-1 describes additional nursing management.

Gerontologic Considerations

- HIV education and prevention efforts in the United States are targeted toward young adults, resulting in poor safer sex education for older adults (Cichocki, 2007).

- Older adults with AIDS may lack an adequate support system and feel lonely, anxious, and isolated.

Reducing Occupational Risks

The nurse must observe Standard Precautions whenever there is a risk of exposure to blood and body fluids. He or she must follow the nursing guidelines for safe handling of needles and sharp instruments (Nursing Guidelines 35-1). The Occupational Safety and Health Administration (OSHA) also recommends the following when caring for all clients regardless of their infectious status:

- Transport specimens of body fluids in leak-proof containers.
- Clean and disinfect utility gloves used for cleaning.
- Remove barrier garments (e.g., face shields, glasses) as soon as possible after leaving a client's room.

If exposed to the blood of any client, the nurse should report the incident to the person in charge of employee health immediately. The nurse will be tested for HIV at regular intervals and treated with antiretrovirals, depending on the results of tests or the potential for infection. While awaiting the results of diagnostic tests, the nurse must follow the same sexual precautions as someone who has been diagnosed with AIDS.

Client Teaching

For clients who are healthy enough to continue as outpatients, the nurse develops a teaching plan that includes the following guidelines:

NURSING CARE PLAN 35-1 | **The Client With HIV/AIDS**

Assessment

- *Obtain a thorough history*, including risk factors for HIV infection. List all symptoms, exploring each thoroughly. Determine the client's past and current treatment medications. Inspect the oral mucous membranes and all skin surfaces for rashes, skin breakdown, and opportunistic infections such as her pes lesions. Look for Kaposi's sarcoma, which appear as dark purple lesions that may be painful. Examine the arms and legs for edema. Auscultate the lungs for breath sounds. Question the client about coughing, sputum production, dyspnea, and orthopnea. Palpate the lymph nodes and abdomen for organ enlargement. Gather additional data based on the client's complaints or symptoms. Review results of recent laboratory and diagnostic tests.
- *Obtain vital signs and weight.* Question the client about weight loss and weight before he or she became symptomatic. Explore past and current dietary intake. Ask about factors that interfere with eating, such as difficulty swallowing, diarrhea, and oral discomfort.
- *Assess the client's mental status (see Chap. 67)* and *perform a neurologic assessment (see Chap. 36)*. Look for peripheral neuropathies (sensation changes in extremities), which may be side effects of antiretroviral medications. Ask about any visual changes (e.g., floaters, spots, loss of peripheral vision).
- *Evaluate emotional status*, looking for signs of depression or anxiety.
- *Observe for signs of dehydration.* Examine the skin and mucous membranes for dryness. Evaluate skin turgor. Note additional findings like decreased urine output, hypotension, and slow filling of hand veins. Look for indications of fluid and electrolyte deficit(s) such as excessive thirst, muscle weakness, cramping, nausea, vomiting, cardiac dysrhythmia, shallow respirations, and headache.

Nursing Diagnosis. **Risk for Infection** (opportunistic) related to immunodeficiency

Expected Outcome. Client will experience no secondary infections.

Interventions	Rationales
Follow practices of medical and surgical asepsis.	Aseptic practices break the infection cycle by decreasing or eliminating infectious agents, their reservoirs, and vehicles for transmission.
Place client in protective isolation if T4 cell count is ≤500 mm³.	Keeping the immunosuppressed client in a separate environment and using precautions to limit the introduction of pathogens in that environment reduce the potential for transmission of a nosocomial infection.
Promote hand hygiene especially before meals and after elimination.	The fecal–oral route is a common mechanism for transfer of endogenous microorganisms from one body site to another, where they can become pathogenic. Hand hygiene is the best technique for reducing transmission of microorganisms.
Facilitate adequate sleep and nutrition.	Adequate sleep and nutrition reduce fatigue, stabilize mood, increase protein synthesis, maintain disease-fighting mechanisms of the immune system, promote cellular growth and repair, and improve capacity for learning and memory storage.
Prohibit ill visitors and staff from contact with client.	Microorganisms are transferred by one of three routes: airborne, droplet, and contact.

Evaluation of Expected Outcome

Client is free from secondary infections.

PC: Pneumocystis pneumonia

Expected Outcome. Nurse will manage and minimize pneumonia.

Interventions	Rationales
Auscultate the lungs every 4 hours; monitor oxygen saturation at least once per shift.	Diminished or wet lung sounds and arterial oxygen saturation (SpO_2) ≤90% indicate poor ventilation and oxygen diffusion.
Assist with measures to clear respiratory secretions such as coughing, pharyngeal suctioning, aerosol treatments, and chest percussion.	Clearing the airway promotes gas exchange.
Give oxygen as medically prescribed if SpO_2 is ≤90%.	Keeping SpO_2 above 90% ensures that oxygen in plasma (PaO_2) is between 80 and 100 mm Hg.

NURSING CARE PLAN 35-1 The Client With HIV/AIDS (Continued)

Interventions	Rationales
Provide mechanical ventilation for acute respiratory failure (Paco$_2$ $\leq$50 mm Hg or PaCO$_2$ $\geq$50 mm Hg).	Mechanical ventilation provides a prescribed rate of respiration, tidal volume, and supplemental oxygen when normal breathing is inadequate.
Administer prescribed antimicrobials.	Antimicrobials exert either bactericidal or bacteriostatic functions.

Evaluation of Expected Outcome

Nurse ensures management of pneumonia and control of complications.

Nursing Diagnosis. Risk for Deficient Fluid Volume related to diarrhea secondary to viremia, opportunistic infection, and side effects of medication

Expected Outcome. Client's fluid intake and output will be balanced.

Interventions	Rationales
Keep a record of intake and output, measuring liquid feces.	Measurements provide an objective account of fluid status.
Offer oral fluids every hour while client is awake	Oral intake increases when the nurse encourages it.
Withhold foods, especially caffeine, that are irritating until bowel function improves.	Fibrous foods increase peristalsis and diarrhea; caffeine is a bowel stimulant and diuretic.
Administer prescribed antidiarrheals.	Antidiarrheals slow peristalsis, adsorbing gastrointestinal irritants and water.
Report evidence of dehydration or electrolyte imbalance.	Parenteral fluids and electrolyte additives are alternate ways to restore fluid and electrolyte balance when the oral route is inadequate.

Evaluation of Expected Outcome

Client's fluid intake and output are 1500 mL/24 hours.

Nursing Diagnosis. Risk for Activity Intolerance, Impaired Physical Mobility, and **Deficient Self-Care** related to fatigue, weakness, and neurologic complications

Expected Outcome. Client will tolerate ADLs, maintain mobility, and perform self-care.

Interventions	Rationales
Prevent fatigue by spacing of activities between periods of rest	Aerobic metabolism, which provides greater energy yield than anaerobic metabolism, depends on cellular oxygen.
Assist with ADLs.	Assistance reduces energy expenditure.
Place a commode at the bedside.	Shortening distance between client and toilet conserves energy.
Provide a walker for ambulatory assistance.	Ambulatory aids promote movement and reduce the risk for injury.

Evaluation of Expected Outcome

Client performs ADLs and self-care and maintains mobility.

Nursing Diagnosis. Risk for Impaired Skin Integrity related to impaired capillary blood flow secondary to immobility, skin infection, and rash

Expected Outcome. Client's skin will remain intact.

Interventions	Rationales
Change position every 2 hours.	Relief of pressure ensures that capillary blood flow remains >32 mm Hg to keep tissues oxygenated.
Keep skin clean and dry.	Moist, soiled skin leads to maceration and bacterial growth.
Apply skin moisturizer.	Lubricated skin is more pliable and less likely to break down.
Gently massage intact skin over bony prominences.	Massage increases circulation and delivery of oxygen to tissues.

(care plan continues on page 500)

NURSING CARE PLAN 35-1 **The Client With HIV/AIDS** (Continued)

Interventions	Rationales
Clean and dry perineal area after elimination.	Ammonia from urine and stool debris erode skin. Organisms in stool transmit yeast infections.
Use lubricated wipes or a soft washcloth for cleansing.	Rough textures injure skin.

Evaluation of Expected Outcome

Client's skin is intact

Nursing Diagnosis. **Impaired Oral Mucous Membranes** related to inflammation secondary to opportunistic infections

Expected Outcome. Client's mucous membranes will be pink, moist, and intact.

Interventions	Rationales
Provide meticulous oral care after and between meals.	Oral hygiene removes bacteria and yeast from mouth.
Avoid using mouthwashes that contain alcohol.	Alcohol irritates inflamed tissue.
Use mouth rinses with warm (not hot) plain water, normal saline solution, or water and hydrogen peroxide.	Warmth increases circulation and promotes healing. Water, saline, and dilute peroxide do not irritate oral tissues.
Use a soft toothbrush or foam swabs for oral care.	Soft textures protect gums from injury and infection.

Evaluation of Expected Outcome

Client's mucous membranes are normal.

Nursing Diagnosis. **Powerlessness** and **Hopelessness** related to poor prognosis

Expected Outcome. Client will control his or her time, make other personal choices, and develop a realistic perception of the immediate future.

Interventions	Rationales
Give client choices whenever possible.	Making choices reaffirms a sense of control.
Help client formulate and achieve short-term goals to enjoy more frequent small successes.	Accomplishment of goals enhances hope.
Discourage client from abandoning traditional treatment for therapies that lack any evidence of effectiveness.	Desperate clients may turn to unsubstantiated claims of a cure for AIDS.

Evaluation of Expected Outcome

Client makes personal choices that give a sense of control without further damaging health, and realistically perceives his or her future.

Nursing Diagnosis. **Anticipatory Grieving** related to potential for early death; **Social Isolation** related to rejection by others or death of infected friends; **Interrupted Family Processes** related to abandonment; **Ineffective Coping** related to stress of contending with an incurable disease

Expected Outcome. Client will work through grief, maintain social contacts with family and friends, and cope effectively with crises.

Interventions	Rationales
Be a role model of acceptance for family and friends.	Learning occurs by example.
Make an effort to touch the client.	Touching demonstrates that casual contact does not transmit the disease.
Avoid wearing gloves and other barrier garments unless absolutely necessary.	Unnecessary use of barrier garments implies that the client is unfit to touch.
Refer client to an AIDS support group.	Groups confer acceptance, calm fear, and decrease isolation.

Evaluation of Expected Outcome

Client deals with grief and crises with support of the nurse, family, and friends.

Nutrition Notes 35-1 The Client With HIV/AIDS *high protein, high calorie*

- There are no unanimously agreed upon recommendations for calories or nutrients despite the universal goals of maintaining body weight and lean body mass in clients with HIV/AIDS. Calorie recommendations from the HIV Research of the Nutrition Infection Unit at Tufts University School of Medicine are as follows (the "normal" healthy adult standard commonly used is 30 cal/kg) (Woods et al., 2008):

  - 37 to 45 cal/kg if the client's weight is stable and there are no secondary infections
  - 45 cal/kg if the client has an opportunistic infection
  - 55 cal/kg if the client is losing weight

- A protein intake of 1.2 to 2.0 g/kg is frequently recommended, although there are no data to support this recommendation. This recommendation translates to a rule-of-thumb guideline of 100 to 150 g/day for men and 80 to 100 g/day for women (Woods et al., 2008).

- A Mediterranean diet that is low in saturated fat and refined sugar and high in fruit, vegetables, and whole grains may help improve the common metabolic abnormalities of hypertriglyceridemia and impaired glucose tolerance experienced by many people with HIV/AIDS.

- Low blood levels and inadequate intakes of some vitamins and minerals are associated with faster HIV disease progression and mortality. Nutrient deficiencies may occur from poor intake, malabsorption, infections, or diet–medication interactions. Although food is the preferred source for nutrients, multivitamin and mineral supplements are usually recommended at levels of 100% to 200% of the Daily Reference Intakes. Some evidence suggests that supplements of vitamin A, zinc, and iron can produce adverse outcomes by negatively impacting immune system functioning.

- Nutritional intervention may help alleviate symptoms that interfere with intake or nutrient use:

  - Clients with anorexia should be encouraged to eat small, frequent meals of easily digested food and liquids even when not hungry.
  - Clients with nausea and vomiting may tolerate a low-fat, high-carbohydrate, soft, or liquid diet better than large, high-fat meals.
  - Diarrhea and malabsorption may improve when clients avoid residue, lactose, fat, and caffeine.
  - Liquids should be encouraged to replace fluid and electrolyte losses.
  - Although eating may seem to trigger diarrhea, clients must understand that limiting food intake to control diarrhea only exacerbates wasting.
  - Gravies, sauces, and broth added to soft, nonirritating foods may promote ease of swallowing in clients with oral or esophageal ulcerations. Some clients may require a blenderized or liquid diet. Because temperature extremes (very hot or very cold) can irritate the mucosa, room-temperature foods and liquids are recommended for clients with a sore mouth.

- Clients unable to consume an adequate oral diet may require tube feeding for supplemental or complete nutrition. Because many formulas have the potential to cause diarrhea, closely monitoring the client's tolerance is essential. Advera and Impact are commercial formulas designed for clients with impaired immune function.

- Understand that antiviral drugs do not cure AIDS but may slow its progression.
- Follow the medication schedule religiously; do not omit or increase the dose without physician approval.
- Comply with the timing of antiviral medications around meals.
- Eat small, frequent, well-balanced meals; try to maintain or gain weight (Nutrition Notes 35-1).
- Drink plenty of water.
- Check weight weekly. Report progressive weight loss or loss of appetite to the physician.
- Avoid exposure to people with infections, including colds, sore throats, upper respiratory tract infections, and childhood diseases (e.g., mumps, chickenpox), and people who have recently been vaccinated. Avoid crowds.
- Notify the physician if signs of infection, such as fever, sore throat, diarrhea, respiratory distress, and cough occur, or if signs of a skin, rectal, vaginal, or oral infection appear.
- Wear gloves and a mask when disposing of animal excreta, such as kitty litter, bird cage liners, and hamster shavings; wash hands thoroughly afterward.
- Wash all food before cooking; do not eat raw meat, fish, or vegetables or food that has not been completely cooked.

- Wash bedding and clothes in hot water and separate from the laundry of others, especially if the bedding and clothes are soiled with body secretions.
- Avoid smoking or exposure to secondhand smoke.
- Bathe or shower daily, wash hands before and after preparing food, clean the anal and perineal areas well after each bowel movement, and wash the hands after voiding or defecating. Personal cleanliness is a must.
- When possible, avoid dry and dusty areas, excessive humidity, and extreme heat or cold. Wear clothing appropriate to the weather and temperature.
- Take frequent rest periods, and space activities to prevent fatigue.
- Do not share IV needles, and do not donate blood.
- Inform healthcare personnel of HIV-positive status.

Understanding Financial and Insurance Implications

Despite HIV-specific confidentiality laws, clients infected with AIDS fear that disclosure of their condition will affect employment, health insurance coverage, and even housing. An employer cannot cancel a client's currently active health insurance policy on the basis of AIDS. However, employers

NURSING GUIDELINES 35-1

Safe Handling of Needles and Sharp Instruments

• Do not become distracted when handling needles and sharp instruments. Concentrate on the task being performed.
• Use a clean tray to pass used or contaminated needles and sharp instruments to another person.
• Keep the container for disposal of needles and sharp instruments close by. When necessary, carry the container to the bedside.
• If a client is uncooperative, ask for assistance when obtaining blood specimens, handling body fluids and secretions, giving injections, or starting IV therapy.
• Do not leave uncapped or used needles unattended. Properly dispose of contaminated sharp instruments and needles as soon as they are used.

are more apt to dismiss a worker with a known HIV-positive status from employment to reduce future insurance premiums and death payments. The dismissal often is attributed to some reason not associated with HIV to avoid being charged with discrimination under the Americans With Disabilities Act.

Unemployed persons can apply for a continuation of the employer's health plan for 18 months at self-pay. Thereafter, they can extend their insurance for 11 more months if they meet the Social Security Administration's criteria for being disabled. Eventually, the person infected with HIV may need to obtain private health insurance, which is very expensive. Private insurers often exclude individuals with a pre-existing condition or require a long waiting period before the policy takes effect. An AIDS caseworker often can help an HIV-positive person with health insurance questions.

Discussing Viatical Settlements

A **viatical settlement** is an arrangement in which a terminally ill individual agrees to name a person as beneficiary to his or her life insurance in exchange for immediate cash. It is best to advise a person who is considering this option to work through an attorney or licensed insurance broker who will negotiate the value of the insurance policy with the potential purchaser. Other factors that the client must consider are whether the cash will cancel eligibility for food stamps or other forms of public assistance and that the cash will be considered earned income for tax purposes.

CRITICAL THINKING EXERCISES

1. What advice would you give adolescents to reduce their risk for becoming infected with HIV?
2. People may become complacent about reducing risks for HIV transmission because they believe that if they become infected, they will have a normal life expectancy

with antiretroviral treatment. How would you respond to this statement?
3. A nurse on a medical unit sustains a needlestick injury. What actions should the nurse take? What are the responsibilities of the employing agency?
4. Besides implementing Standard Precautions, what other practices reduce the potential for HIV transmission among healthcare workers?

NCLEX-STYLE REVIEW QUESTIONS

1. A client with AIDS comes into the clinic with a suspected case of candidiasis. Which of the following signs and symptoms would the nurse observe in the client that would likely confirm a diagnosis of candidiasis?
   1. Serious loss of fluids
   2. Inadequate pulmonary function
   3. Red, swollen eyes
   4. White plaque that may bleed when mobilized
2. A nurse is obtaining a client's consent for receiving blood. The client asks if there is any way that HIV can be acquired from the transfusion. The nurse would be most truthful and accurate in answering with which of the following statements?
   1. With any medical procedure there are risks. You must weigh the risks against the benefits.
   2. The blood supply is safe because it is screened for HIV antibodies to ensure quality and safety.
   3. Antibody screening will not detect HIV in blood given by those who have not produced significant antibodies.
   4. Transmission of HIV through screened blood transfusions cannot occur.
3. A nurse's aide attending respite training at an inpatient hospice center asks the nurse what causes the death in a client with end-stage HIV. The nurse is most correct in instructing the nurse's aide that a client infected with HIV ultimately dies from which of the following?
   1. An opportunistic infection
   2. A depleted white blood cell count
   3. Deterioration of the brain tissue
   4. A massive stroke or heart attack
4. The physician orders several laboratory tests for a client suspected of having AIDS. Which laboratory test is most significant for diagnosing antibodies to the human immunodeficiency virus (HIV)?
   1. Venereal disease research laboratory (VDRL) test
   2. Schick test
   3. Dick test
   4. Enzyme-linked immunosorbent assay (ELISA) test
5. A client makes an appointment with a physician because of losing weight and swollen lymph nodes in the axillae and groin. Which situation places the client at highest risk for acquired immunodeficiency syndrome (AIDS)?
   1. The client is an intravenous drug user.
   2. The client drinks excessive amounts of alcohol.
   3. The client had cardiovascular surgery 6 months ago.
   4. The client went to Africa on his vacation.

36

Introduction to the Nervous System

Words To Know

acetylcholine
acetylcholinesterase
arachnoid
axon
brain stem
cauda equina
central nervous system
cerebellum
cerebrum
corpus callosum
decerebrate posturing
decorticate posturing
dendrites
dopamine
dura mater
epinephrine
extrapyramidal
flaccidity
medulla oblongata
meninges
midbrain
myelin
neurilemma
neuron
neurotransmitters
norepinephrine
parasympathetic nervous system
peripheral nervous system
pia mater
pons
pyramidal
subarachnoid space
sympathetic nervous system
synapses
ventricles

Learning Objectives

On completion of this chapter, you will be able to:

1. Name the two anatomic divisions of the nervous system.
2. Name the three parts of the brain.
3. List the four lobes of the cerebrum.
4. Give two functions of the spinal cord.
5. Name and describe the function of the two parts of the autonomic nervous system.
6. Describe methods used to assess motor and sensory function.
7. List six diagnostic procedures performed to detect neurologic disorders.
8. Discuss the nursing management of the client undergoing neurologic diagnostic testing.

The nervous system consists of the brain, spinal cord, and peripheral nerves. It is responsible for coordinating body functions and responding to changes in or stimuli from the internal and external environment. Changes in the functioning of the nervous system can profoundly affect the entire body.

ANATOMY AND PHYSIOLOGY

The nervous system is divided into two anatomic divisions: the **central nervous system (CNS)** and the **peripheral nervous system (PNS)**. The basic structure of the nervous system is the nerve cell or **neuron** (Fig. 36-1). Neurons are either sensory or motor. *Sensory neurons* transmit impulses to the CNS; *motor neurons* transmit impulses from the CNS.

A neuron is composed of a cell body, a nucleus, and threadlike projections or fibers called **dendrites** and axons. Dendrites conduct impulses to the cell body and are called *afferent* ("to" or "toward") nerve fibers. An **axon** is a nerve fiber that projects and conducts impulses away from the cell body. It is therefore called an *efferent* ("away from") nerve fiber. The axon usually is larger than the dendrites.

Neurons are separate units and not directly connected to one another. Impulses travel along neurons, moving from one neuron to the next by means of **synapses**, junctions between the axon of one neuron to the dendrite of another. Substances called **neurotransmitters** (or

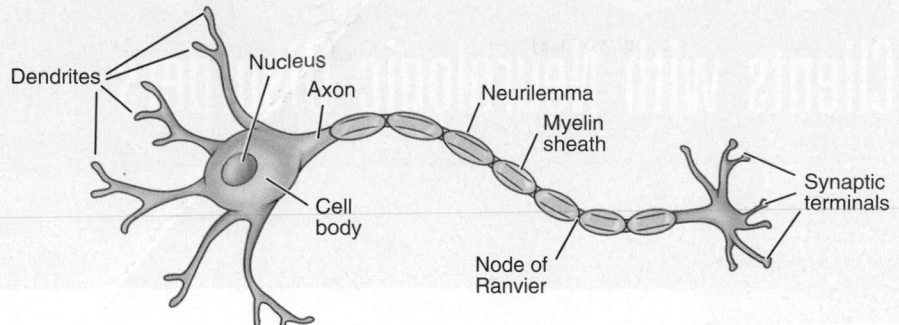

FIGURE 36-1. A neuron, or nerve cell.

neurohormones) accomplish the transmission of an impulse from one neuron to the next (see Chap. 67). Neurotransmitters can either excite or inhibit neurons.

A fatty substance called **myelin** covers some axons in the CNS and PNS. Axons that are covered by myelin are called *myelinated*, white matter, or white nerve fibers. Axons that are not covered with myelin are called *unmyelinated*, gray matter, or gray nerve fibers.

A membranous sheath called the **neurilemma** covers the myelin of axons in peripheral nerves. Myelin serves as an insulating substance for the axon that confines the electrical conduction without allowing it to scatter. However, myelinated nerves are segmented with periodic gaps called the *nodes of Ranvier*. When impulses travel along axons of myelinated nerves, they leap from node to node, a process

called *saltatory conduction*, which is much faster than impulses traveling along axons of unmyelinated nerves.

Central Nervous System

The CNS consists of the brain and spinal cord.

Brain

The brain is divided into three parts: the cerebrum, the cerebellum, and the brain stem. The **cerebrum** consists of two hemispheres connected by the **corpus callosum**, a band of white fibers that acts as a bridge for transmitting impulses between the left and right hemispheres. Each hemisphere has four lobes: frontal, parietal, temporal, and occipital (Fig. 36-2). The cerebral cortex is the surface of the cerebrum. It contains motor neurons, which are responsible for movement, and

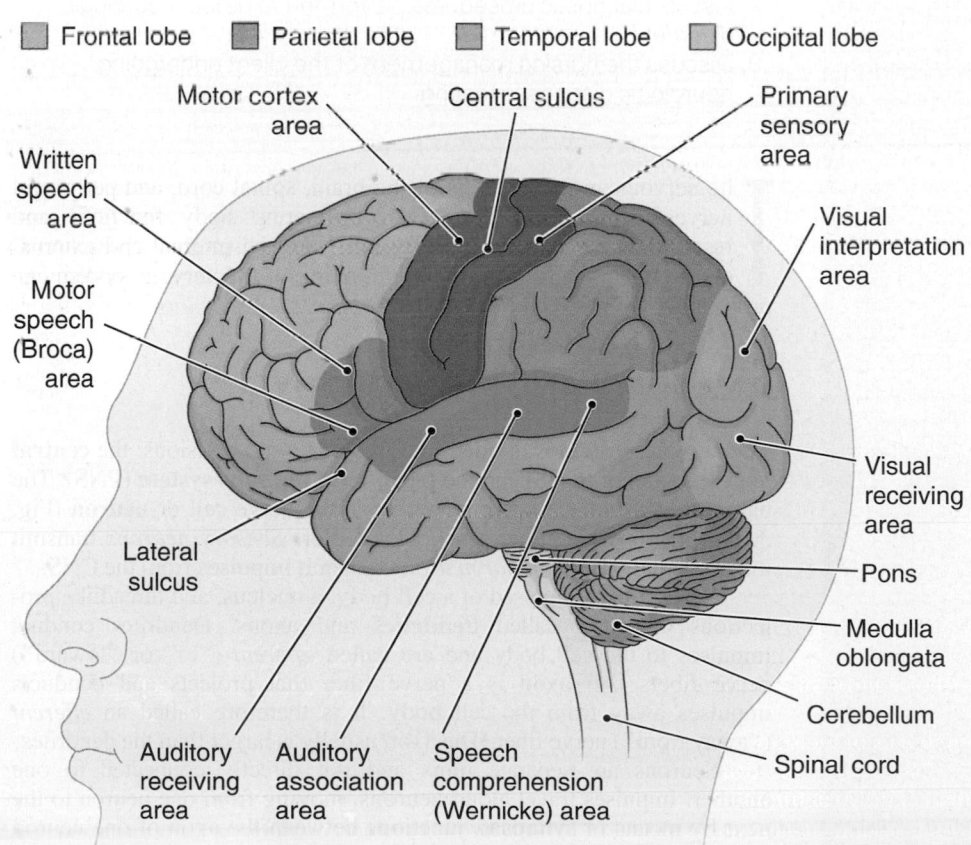

■ Frontal lobe   ■ Parietal lobe   ■ Temporal lobe   ■ Occipital lobe

FIGURE 36-2. Lateral view of the brain showing the four lobes. Shaded areas show the regions of the cerebral cortex that are responsible for different functions.

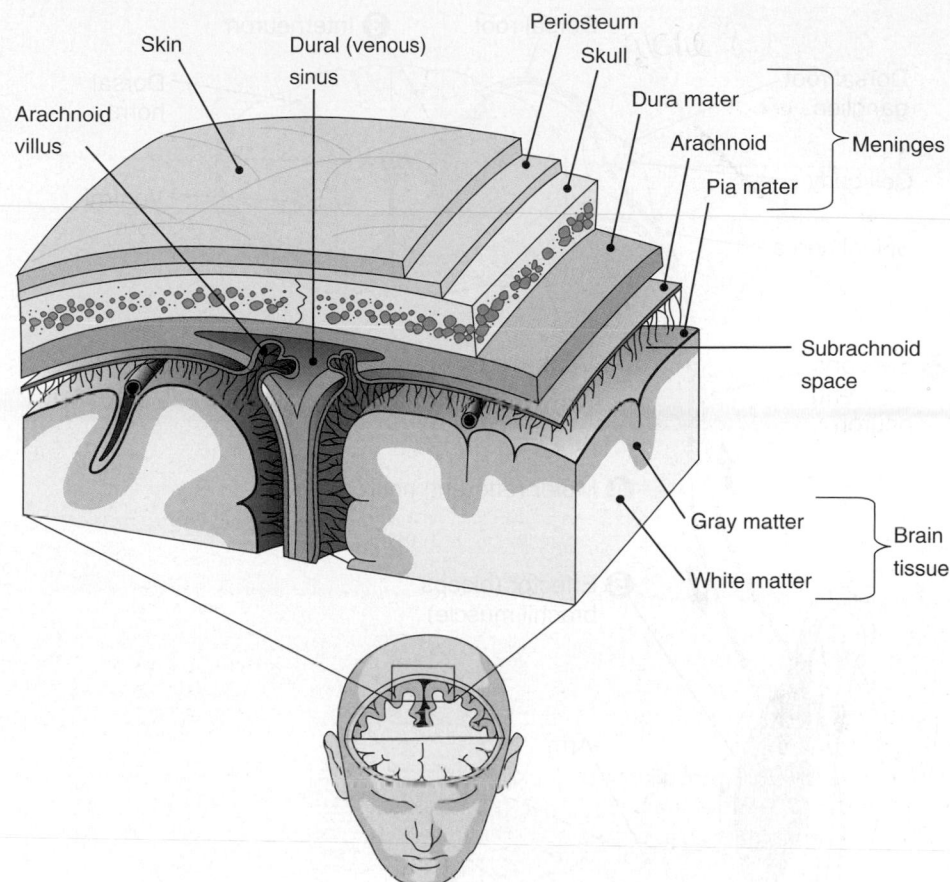

FIGURE 36-3. Frontal section of the top of the head showing the meninges of the central nervous system (pia mater, arachnoid, and dura mater) and related parts. (From Cohen, B. J., & Taylor, J. J. [2009]. *Memmler's structure and function of the human body.* [9th ed.] Philadelphia: Lippincott Williams & Wilkins.)

sensory neurons, which receive impulses from peripheral sensory neurons located throughout the body.

Motor tracts are pyramidal or extrapyramidal. **Pyramidal** motor pathways originate in the motor cortex of the cerebrum, cross over at the level of the medulla, and end in the brain stem and spinal cord. **Extrapyramidal** fibers originate in the motor cortex and project to the cerebellum and basal ganglia. They do not cross over as they connect to motor neurons in the spinal cord.

The **cerebellum**, which is located behind and below the cerebrum, controls and coordinates muscle movement. The **brain stem** consists of the midbrain, pons, and medulla oblongata. The **midbrain** forms the forward part of the brain stem and connects the pons and cerebellum with the two cerebral hemispheres. The **pons** is located between the midbrain and medulla, and connects the two hemispheres of the cerebellum with the brain stem, spinal cord, and cerebrum. The **medulla oblongata** lies below the pons and transmits motor impulses from the brain to the spinal cord and sensory impulses from peripheral sensory neurons to the brain. The medulla contains vital centers concerned with respiration, heartbeat, and vasomotor activity (the control of smooth muscle activity in blood vessel walls).

The brain is protected by the rigid bones of the skull and is covered by three membranes or **meninges:** (1) the **dura mater**, the tough, outermost covering; (2) the **arachnoid**, or middle membrane lying directly below the dura mater; and (3) the **pia mater**, a delicate layer that adheres to the brain

and spinal cord. The **subarachnoid space** lies between the pia mater and the arachnoid membrane (Fig. 36-3).

Within the brain are four hollow structures called **ventricles** (Fig. 36-4). The ventricles manufacture and absorb cerebrospinal fluid (CSF), which constantly circulates in the subarachnoid space of the brain and spinal cord. CSF produced in the ventricles passes down into the subarachnoid space of the spinal cord, then up through the basilar cisterns and over the cerebral hemispheres to the region of the dural sinuses, where most of the absorption occurs. Acting as a

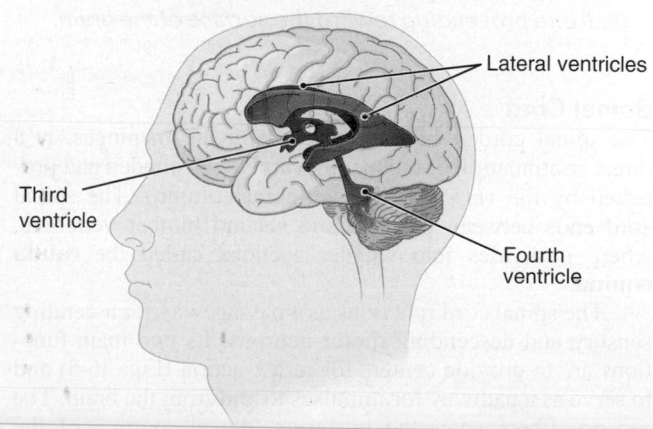

FIGURE 36-4. Ventricles of the brain seen from a lateral view.

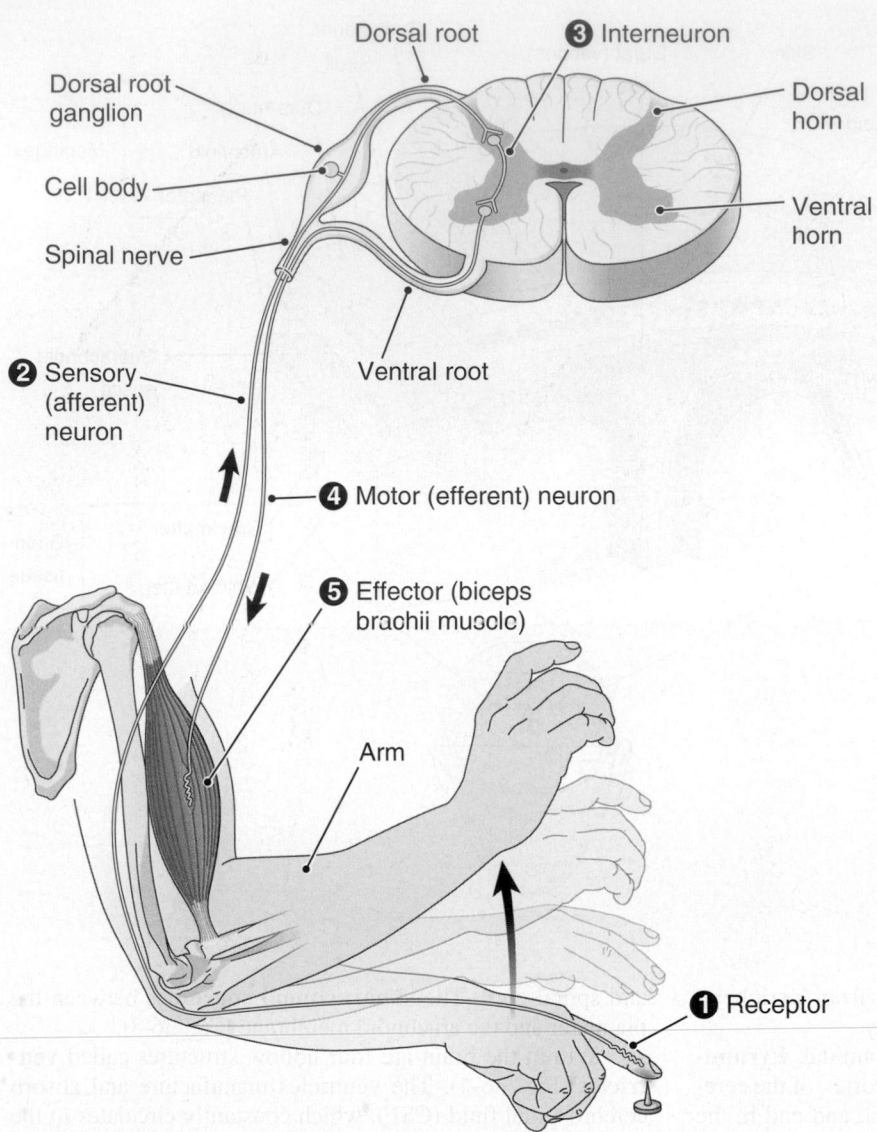

Dorsal root

❸ Interneuron

Dorsal root ganglion

Cell body

Spinal nerve

❷ Sensory (afferent) neuron

Ventral root

Dorsal horn

Ventral horn

❹ Motor (efferent) neuron

❺ Effector (biceps brachii muscle)

Arm

❶ Receptor

FIGURE 36-5. Reflex arc showing the pathway of impulses and cross-section of the spinal cord. Numbers show the sequence of impulses through the spinal cord (solid arrows). (From Cohen, B. J., & Taylor, J. J. [2009]. *Memmler's structure and function of the human body.* [9th ed.] Philadelphia: Lippincott Williams & Wilkins.)

cushion, the CSF protects these structures and helps maintain relatively constant intracranial pressure.

> ▶ *Stop, Think, and Respond Exercise 36-1*
>
> *Name the three layers of meninges, starting below the skull and proceeding toward the surface of the brain.*

Spinal Cord

The spinal cord, which is covered by the meninges, is a direct continuation of the medulla and is surrounded and protected by the *vertebrae* (or vertebral column). The spinal cord ends between the first and second lumbar vertebrae, where it divides into smaller sections called the **cauda equina**.

The spinal cord functions as a passageway for ascending sensory and descending motor neurons. Its two main functions are to provide centers for reflex action (Fig. 36-5) and to serve as a pathway for impulses to and from the brain. The sensory fibers enter the posterior (dorsal) portion of the cord; the nerve fibers that transmit motor impulses run out-

ward to the peripheral nerves from the anterior (ventral) portion of the cord.

Peripheral Nervous System

The PNS consists of all the sensory and motor nerves outside the CNS. The PNS includes the cranial, spinal, and sympathetic and parasympathetic nerves of the autonomic nervous system.

Cranial Nerves

The 12 pairs of cranial nerves, identified by Roman numerals, are as follows:

- *I*: Olfactory nerve: sense of smell
- *II*: Optic nerve: sight
- *III*: Oculomotor nerve: contraction of iris and eye muscles
- *IV*: Trochlear nerve: eye movement
- *V*: Trigeminal nerve: sensory nerve to face, chewing
- *VI*: Abducens nerve: eye movement

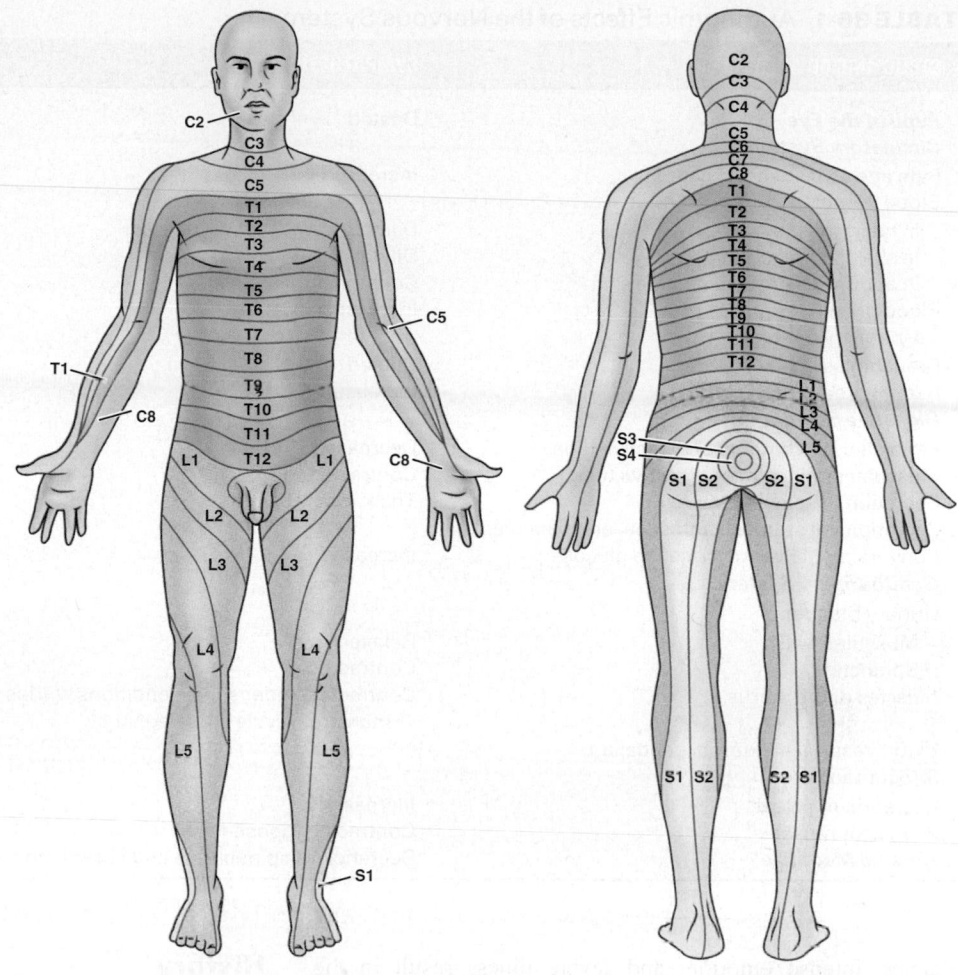

FIGURE 36-6. Dermatome distribution.

- *VII*: Facial nerve: facial expression, taste, secretions of salivary and lacrimal glands
- *VIII*: Vestibulocochlear (or auditory) nerve: hearing, balance
- *IX*: Glossopharyngeal nerve: taste, sensory fibers of pharynx and tongue, swallowing, secretions of parotid gland
- *X*: Vagus nerve: motor fibers to glands producing digestive enzymes, heart rate, muscles of speech, gastrointestinal motility, respiration, swallowing, coughing, vomiting reflex
- *XI*: Accessory (or spinal accessory) nerve: head and shoulder movement
- *XII*: Hypoglossal nerve: movement of the tongue

Spinal Nerves

There are 31 pairs of spinal nerves: 8 cervical, 12 thoracic, 5 lumbar, 5 sacral, and 1 coccygeal. Spinal nerves have two roots: dorsal and ventral. Dorsal nerve fibers are sensory, and ventral nerve fibers are motor. Peripheral sensory nerve fibers in various areas of the body transmit impulses to the spinal nerves, which transmit impulses up the spinal cord to the brain. Motor impulses traveling from the brain and down the spinal cord leave by the ventral root and travel to areas

of the body. Each spinal nerve root innervates a specific area or *dermatome* of the body surface (Fig. 36-6). Knowledge of the distribution of dermatomes is useful for the nurse's assessment and evaluation.

Autonomic Nervous System

The autonomic nervous system consists of the **sympathetic nervous system** and the **parasympathetic nervous system**. It is concerned with functions essential to survival. The two divisions of the autonomic nervous system generally function antagonistically toward each other, yet they maintain homeostasis by stimulating or inhibiting smooth muscles, cardiac muscle, and glands (Table 36-1).

Sympathetic Nervous System

This division of the autonomic nervous system regulates the expenditure of energy. The neurotransmitters of the sympathetic nervous system, collectively known as *catecholamines*, are **epinephrine**, **norepinephrine**, and **dopamine**. The adrenal medulla produces and secretes epinephrine and norepinephrine. Norepinephrine also is produced at sympathetic nerve endings. Dopamine is a precursor (a substance that precedes another) of norepinephrine. Norepinephrine then becomes epinephrine. Stressful situations such as

TABLE 36-1 Autonomic Effects of the Nervous System

STRUCTURE OR ACTIVITY	SYMPATHETIC EFFECTS	PARASYMPATHETIC EFFECTS
Pupil of the Eye	Dilated	Constricted
Circulatory System		
Rate and force of heart beat	Increased	Decreased
Blood vessels		
In heart muscle	Dilated	Constricted
In skeletal muscle	Dilated	*
In abdominal viscera and the skin	Constricted	*
Blood pressure	Increased	Decreased
Respiratory System		
Bronchioles	Dilated	Constricted
Rate of breathing	Increased	Decreased
Digestive System		
Peristaltic movements of digestive tube	Decreased	Increased
Muscular sphincters of digestive tube	Contracted	Relaxed
Secretion of salivary glands	Thick, viscid saliva	Thin, watery saliva
Secretions of stomach, intestine, and pancreas	*	Increased
Conversion of liver glycogen to glucose	Increased	*
Genitourinary System		
Urinary bladder		
Muscular walls	Relaxed	Contracted
Sphincters	Contracted	Relaxed
Muscles of the uterus	Contracted under some conditions; varies with menstrual cycle and pregnancy	Relaxed; variable
Blood vessels of external genitalia	*	Dilated
Integument		
Secretion of sweat	Increased	*
Pilomotor muscles	Contracted (goose-flesh)	*
Adrenal Medullae	Secretion of epinephrine and norepinephrine	*

*No direct effect.

danger, intense emotion, and severe illness result in the release of catecholamines.

Parasympathetic Nervous System

This division of the autonomic nervous system works to conserve body energy and is partly responsible for slowing heart rate, digesting food, and eliminating body wastes. **Acetylcholine** is a neurotransmitter released at the nerve endings of parasympathetic nerve fibers, at some nerve endings in the sympathetic nervous system, and at nerve endings of skeletal muscles. Release of this neurotransmitter allows passage of a nerve impulse from the nerve fiber to the effector organ or structure, where the enzyme **acetylcholinesterase** inactivates acetylcholine.

ASSESSMENT

A neurologic assessment is performed to identify and locate disorders of the nervous system. The scope and extent of the neurologic examination often depend on the symptoms and the probable or actual diagnosis.

 Pharmacologic Considerations

- The use of morphine, heroin, or other narcotic or CNS depressants shortly before a neurologic examination affects the results of a neurologic assessment because these drugs decrease the level of consciousness.

History

A thorough history is essential. The nurse explores all symptoms and asks questions to clarify each symptom. The history must include a record of trauma (no matter how slight) to the head or body within the past 6 to 12 months, a drug history, an allergy history, and a family medical history. The nurse observes the client's speech pattern, mental status, intellectual functioning, reasoning ability, and movement or lack of movement of all extremities.

 Gerontologic Considerations

- When taking the health history of an older adult who has difficulty remembering recent or past events, symptoms, drug and medical history, and other necessary facts, obtain or confirm the information from a family member or friend.

Physical Examination

The physical examination consists of assessment of the cerebral, motor, and sensory areas. The nurse usually assesses intellectual function and speech pattern during the history by noting responses to questions. Additional testing of intellectual function includes asking various questions that require mental tasks (see discussion of Mini-Mental Status Examination, Box 67-2 in Chap. 67).

The nurse evaluates the client's body posture and any abnormal position of the head, neck, trunk, or extremities. If head trauma has occurred, the nurse examines the ears and nose for evidence of bleeding or other drainage. He or she carefully examines the head for bleeding, swelling, or wounds. The nurse does not move or manipulate the client's head during this part of the assessment, especially if there is a recent history of trauma.

Cranial Nerves

The experienced examiner evaluates all or some of the 12 cranial nerves (Table 36-2).

Motor Function

Assessment of motor function includes muscle movement, size, tone, strength, and coordination. The nurse inspects large muscle areas for evidence of atrophy and assesses opposing muscles for equality of size and strength. He or she asks the client to perform tasks such as:

- Pushing the palm or sole against the examiner's palm.
- Picking up small and large objects between the thumb and forefinger.
- Grasping objects firmly.
- Resisting removal of an object from the fist or fingers.

To assess gait, movement, and balance, the nurse asks the client to walk away from the examiner, turn, and walk back. Other tests include climbing a small set of stairs, walking and turning abruptly, and walking heel to toe. In the Romberg test, the client stands with feet close together and eyes closed. If the client sways and tends to fall, this is considered a positive Romberg test, indicating a problem with equilibrium. The examiner stands fairly close to the client during this test in case the client loses balance.

Tests that evaluate motor and cerebral function include doing the finger-to-nose test with eyes closed, writing words, and identifying common objects. The choice of tests depends on the original complaints and the findings of diagnostic tests.

Gerontologic Considerations

- Diseases such as dementia often make it difficult to perform a neurologic assessment. In addition, with age, brain weight and the number of brain cells decrease, and blood flow to the cerebrum is diminished. Although thought processes that involve life experience and judgment may be enhanced with age, older adults often experience short-term memory loss and a slower reaction time. Older adults who have difficulty following directions during a physical examination or diagnostic test need brief instructions given one step at a time during the examination or test. The older person may respond more quickly to mimicking modeling of desired behaviors in addition to verbal instructions.

The nurse evaluates motor response in the comatose or unconscious client by administering a painful stimulus to determine the client's response. An appropriate response is for the client to reach toward or withdraw from the stimulus. Clients with impaired cerebral function manifest abnormal posturing. **Decorticate posturing** (decorticate rigidity) is a position in which the arms are flexed, fists are clenched, and the legs are extended (Fig. 36-7A). **Decerebrate posturing** (decerebrate rigidity) is when the extremities are stiff and rigid (Fig. 36-7B). Decerebrate posturing is more serious

than decorticate posturing. Even more ominous is **flaccidity**, when the client makes no motor response (Fig 36-7C).

> ### Stop, Think, and Respond Exercise 36-2
>
> *Which type of posturing is evidenced by (A) flexion of the arms, (B) extension of the arms, and (C) no movement of any extremities?*

Sensory Function

The nurse evaluates the extremities for sensitivity to heat, cold, touch, and pain. He or she can use various objects such as cotton balls, tubes filled with hot or cold water, and sharp objects (that do not pierce the skin) to check sensation in the extremities.

Level of Consciousness

Depending on the client's symptoms, evaluation of the level of consciousness (LOC) is often necessary. The following classification of LOC applies to altered consciousness from any cause. Differentiating between each level can be difficult; some clients show characteristics of two or more levels:

- *Conscious:* The client responds immediately, fully, and appropriately to visual, auditory, and other stimulation.
- *Somnolent or lethargic:* The client is drowsy or sleepy at inappropriate times but can be aroused, only to fall asleep again. Responses to questions and verbal commands are delayed or inappropriate. Speech is incoherent. Painful stimuli elicit a response.
- *Stuporous:* The client is aroused only by vigorous and continuous stimulation, usually by manipulation or strong auditory or visual stimuli. Stimulation results in one- or two word answers or in motor activity or purposeful behavior directed toward avoiding further stimulation.
- *Semicomatose:* The client is unresponsive except to superficial, relatively mild painful stimuli to which the client makes some purposeful motor response (movement) to evade stimulation. Spontaneous motion is uncommon, but the client may groan or mutter.
- *Comatose:* The client responds only to very painful stimuli by fragmentary, delayed reflex withdrawal; in deeper stages, he or she loses all responsiveness. There is no spontaneous movement, and the respiratory rate is irregular.

Gerontologic Considerations

- The possibility of drug toxicity or abrupt onset of delirium always should be considered when an older person has a change in mental status. The aging brain may develop various compensatory mechanisms. Mental exercises to retain vocabulary, physical exercise to promote circulation, and involvement in social or educational activities can help retain function.

The nurse assesses LOC at frequent intervals after injury to the head or neck, cranial surgery, a cerebrovascular accident (acute phase), a ruptured cerebral aneurysm, and other neurologic disorders. He or she makes this assessment

TABLE 36-2 Cranial Nerve Assessment

CRANIAL NERVE	ASSESSMENT TECHNIQUE	NORMAL FINDINGS
I—Olfactory	Ask client to occlude each nostril separately and close the eyes. Present familiar odors, such as vinegar, lemon, coffee, and ammonia.	Client identifies odors correctly.
II—Optic	Help client cover each eye separately; test visual acuity using a Snellen chart (see Chap. 42) or newspaper, or Jaeger chart.	Client names letters or reads words accurately.
	Client and examiner cover an eye, and examiner moves an object from the periphery toward client's nose from superior, inferior, medial, and lateral positions while both fix their gaze straight ahead. Examiner then tests opposite eye. Inspect optic nerve with an ophthalmoscope.	Client and examiner see object at the same time in the visual field. Optic nerve appears round and lighter than surrounding retina.
III—Oculomotor	In a darkened room, shine a bright light in each pupil; ask client to look at a near and far object (see Chap. 42).	Pupil constricts briskly in response to light and dilates when looking far away.
	Ask client to follow an object you move in horizontal, vertical, and oblique directions (see Chap. 42).	Eye movement is coordinated in all directions.
IV—Trochlear	See assessment for motor function of oculomotor nerve.	Eyes move inferiorly and medially.
V—Trigeminal	Observe for jaw symmetry while client opens mouth.	Appearance is symmetric.
	Instruct client to clamp jaws tightly together.	The muscles contract bilaterally.
	Stroke forehead, cheeks, and jaw with a wisp of cotton, sharp object (e.g., pin), cold and warm objects, and a vibrating tuning fork.	Client shows bilateral sensitivity and correctly identifies sensory experience.
	Touch each cornea with a wisp of cotton.	Client blinks.
	Tap center of chin with a reflex hammer while client slightly opens the mouth.	Jaw closes suddenly and slightly.
VI—Abducens	See assessment for motor function of oculomotor nerve.	Client moves eyes in lateral directions.
VII—Facial	Ask client to wrinkle the forehead, smile, frown, raise eyebrows, look at ceiling, and whistle.	Facial movements are symmetrical.
	Instruct client to close eyelids and resist examiner's efforts to open them.	Both eyes equally resist efforts to open them.
	Apply sweet, sour, salty, and bitter flavors to both sides of the anterior tongue.	Client accurately identifies tastes.
VIII—Vestibulocochlear	Test hearing acuity and perform the Rinne and Weber tests with a tuning fork (see Chap. 43).	Client repeats whispered words correctly; sound is lateralized equally and heard longer by air than by bone conduction.
	Have client stand with both feet close together; note for swaying with eyes open and then shut.	Client maintains balance or sways slightly.
IX—Glossopharyngeal	Touch palate with a tongue blade.	Blade elicits a gag response.
	Ask client to say "ah."	Uvula remains in midline.
X—Vagus	Have client say "la, la, la."	Client speaks clearly and distinctly, with no hoarseness.
XI—Spinal-accessory	Instruct client to shrug the shoulders as you apply resistance.	Client raises shoulders.
XII—Hypoglossal	Tell client to stick out the tongue.	Tongue remains in midline with no lateral deviation.

hourly unless the physician orders otherwise or a change occurs in the client's condition.

The Glasgow Coma Scale (Box 36-1) is a measure of the LOC. The scale consists of three parts: eye opening response, best verbal response, and best motor response. To evaluate responses correctly, several verbal and motor responses are elicited, and the best response is recorded. The eye opening response is determined by talking to the client and calling his or her name. If no response is noted (i.e., the eyes do not open spontaneously), a painful stimulus is introduced and the response noted. The verbal response is evaluated by a verbal reply to questions. The motor response is the ability of the client to follow commands, such as "Wiggle your toes" or "Move your left hand." If there is no response, a painful stimulus is applied and the response noted. The responses are assigned numbers and the numbers are totaled. A normal response is 15. A score of 7 or less is considered coma. The evaluations are recorded on a graphic

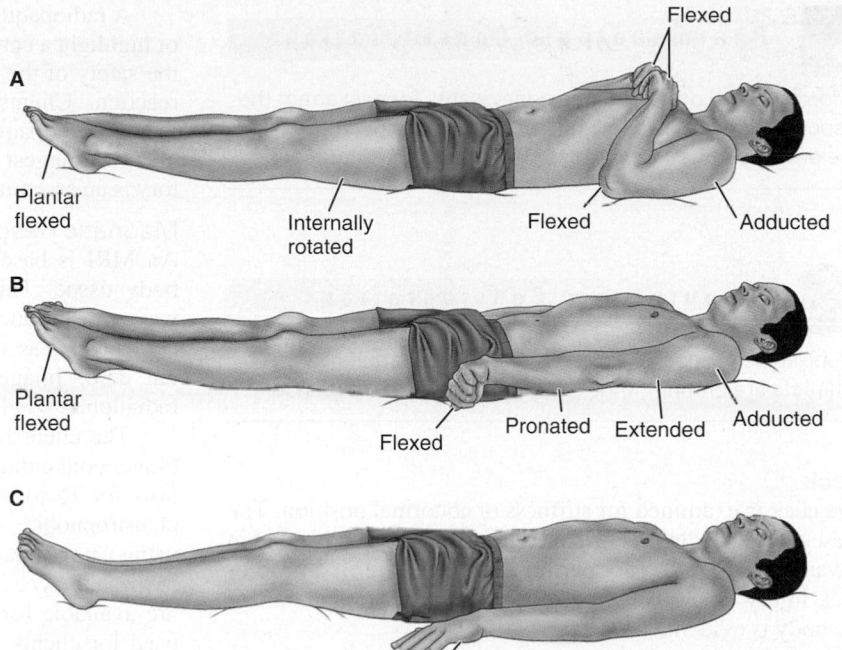

FIGURE 36-7. Abnormal posture response to stimuli: **(A)** decorticate posturing, **(B)** decerebrate posturing. **(C)** Flaccidity is when the client makes no motor response to stimuli.

sheet; connecting lines show an increase or decrease in the LOC.

The Rancho Los Amigos Scale (Box 36-2) is another tool for assessing LOC. Some rehabilitation centers prefer this scale because it is a more flexible assessment tool for identifying the client's status.

Pupils

The size and equality of the pupils and their reaction to light are an assessment of the third cranial (oculomotor) nerve

(see Table 36-2). Pupil size (normal, pinpoint, dilated), equality (equal, unequal in size), and reaction to a bright light (normal, sluggish, no reaction, fixed), are noted (see Chap. 42). When the pupils are examined, any abnormal movement or position of one or both eyes is noted.

Unequal pupils (one pupil larger than the other), dilated or pinpoint pupils, and failure of the pupils to respond quickly to light are, in most instances, abnormal findings. Any sudden change in pupil size, equality, or reaction to light is an important neurologic finding and is reported to the physician at once.

BOX 36-1 Glasgow Coma Scale

The Glasgow Coma Scale is a tool for assessing a client's response to stimuli. A score of 10 or less indicates a need for emergency attention; a score of 7 or less is generally interpreted as coma.

Eye opening response	Spontaneous	4
	To voice	3
	To pain	2
	None	1
Best verbal response	Oriented	5
	Confused	4
	Inappropriate words	3
	Incomprehensible sounds	2
	None	1
Best motor response	Obeys command	6
	Localizes pain	5
	Withdraws (pain)	4
	Flexion (pain)	3
	Extension (pain)	2
	None	1
Total		3 to 15

BOX 36-2 Rancho Los Amigos Scales

Level I: No response to stimuli. Appears in deep sleep.

Level II: Generalized response. First reaction may be to deep pain. Has delayed, inconsistent responses.

Level III: Localized response. Inconsistent responses, but reacts in a more specific manner to stimulus. Might follow simple command "squeeze my hand."

Level IV: Confused. Agitated. Reacts to own inner confusion, fear, disorientation. Excitable behavior, may be abusive.

Level V: Nonagitated. Confused. Inappropriate. Usually disoriented. Follows tasks for 2 to 3 minutes, but easily distracted by environment, frustrated.

Level VI: Confused appropriate. Follows simple directions consistently. Memory and attention increasing. Self-care tasks performed without help.

Level VII: Automatic appropriate. If physically able, can carry out routine activities. Appears normal. Needs supervision for safety.

Level VIII: Purposeful. Alert. Oriented. May have decreased abilities relative to premorbid state.

Pharmacologic Considerations

- Morphine and other narcotic depressants for pain affect the response of the pupils to light, making them pinpoint in size. The drug, not a neurologic disorder, causes the alteration.

Gerontologic Considerations

- Pupillary response is more sluggish in older adults. When cataracts are present, there may be no pupillary response.

Neck

The neck is examined for stiffness or abnormal position. The presence of rigidity is checked by moving the head and chin toward the chest. Do not perform this maneuver if a head or neck injury is suspected or known or trauma to any part of the body is evident.

Gerontologic Considerations

- Range of motion of the neck may be impacted in older adults due to arthritic changes.

Vital Signs

The blood pressure, pulse and respiratory rates, and temperature are closely monitored on all clients with a potential or actual neurologic disorder. The temperature often needs to be monitored every hour because CNS disorders can affect the temperature-regulating ability of the hypothalamus. A sudden increase or decrease in any of the vital signs indicates a change in the neurologic status, and the physician is notified immediately.

Diagnostic Tests

Imaging Procedures

Imaging procedures such as computed tomography (CT), magnetic resonance imaging (MRI), positron emission tomography (PET), and single-photon emission computed tomography (SPECT) are used in the diagnosis of neurologic disorders. Imaging procedures are particularly useful in the diagnosis of neurologic disorders such as brain tumors, Alzheimer's disease, intracranial bleeding or hemorrhage, and cerebral infections.

Computed Tomography

CT scanning uses x-rays and computer analysis to produce three-dimensional views of thin cross-sections, or "slices," of the body. A narrow x-ray beam rotates around the client, and a computer analyzes the results. CT is extremely sensitive to differences in tissue densities, allowing differentiation between intracranial tumors, cysts, edema, and hemorrhage. The client is exposed to the same amount of radiation as in a conventional x-ray.

A radiopaque dye is used during a CT scan to emphasize or highlight a certain area. Use of a radiopaque dye decreases the safety of the procedure, primarily due to risk of allergic reaction. Clients who are allergic to iodine should not receive radiopaque dyes that contain this substance. Seafood allergies suggest an allergy to iodine. A thorough allergy history is an essential part of the neurologic examination.

Magnetic Resonance Imaging

An MRI is based on the magnetic behavior of protons in body tissue. This imaging procedure uses radiofrequency waves to produce images of tissues of high fat and water content such as soft tissue, veins, arteries, the brain, and spinal cord. Images are produced without contrast dye or radiation.

The client lies motionless on a stretcher enclosed in a tunnel containing a powerful magnet. (Fig. 36-8). The MRI lasts for 15 to 90 minutes. For those who may experience claustrophobia, sedation is an option or an "open" MRI using a non-tunneled machine may be performed if the facility has this type of equipment. A call button and an intercom are available for two-way communication. MRI cannot be used for clients with metal implants such as a hip or knee replacement or cardiac pacemaker because metal interferes with the magnetic field.

Positron Emission Tomography

PET uses radioactive substances to examine metabolic activity of body structures. The client either inhales or is injected with a radioactive substance with positively charged particles that combine with negatively charged particles found normally in the body. The energy emitted when these combine is converted into color-coded images indicating metabolic activity of the organ involved. The radioactive substances are short-lived, resulting in minimal radiation exposure. PET is used less frequently than CT or MRI because the equipment is usually available only in major medical centers.

Single-Photon Emission Computed Tomography

SPECT is a relatively new noninvasive imaging tool with the advantage of providing information about the brain's function, whereas CT and MRI only image anatomic

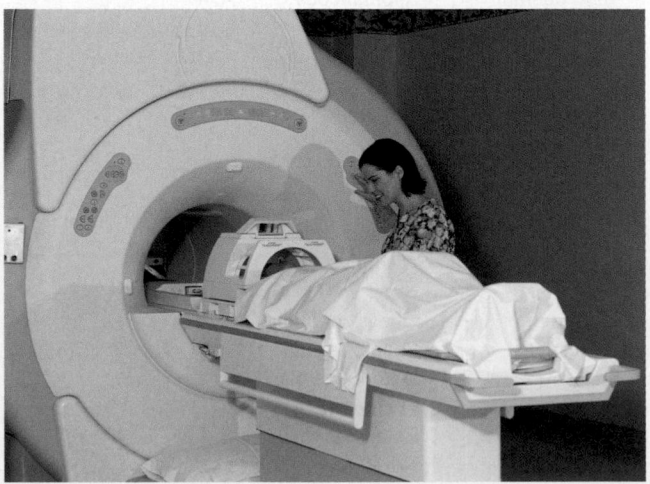

FIGURE 36-8. A technician discusses what the client should expect during magnetic resonance imaging.

structures. SPECT provides information about the brain's cerebral blood flow and the status of receptors for neurotransmitters; it also identifies lesions before they are visible with other imaging techniques (Hinkle, 2002; UTHSC-NRC, 2009). Data from SPECT locate the site causing epileptic seizures, diagnose Alzheimer's and Parkinson's diseases, and detect brain tumors and changes in blood flow that predict the potential or actual area of a stroke and offer prognosis for recovery.

SPECT obtains images of the brain after the client intravenously receives radiopharmaceuticals and radioisotopes approximately 1 hour before the test begins. Once the radioactive substances circulate, there is a scan of the brain. Colored cross-sections of the brain images are evaluated for evidence of pathology. A potential risk of SPECT is the client's allergic reaction to the imaging material.

Lumbar Puncture

Changes in CSF occur in many neurologic disorders. A lumbar puncture (spinal tap) is performed to obtain samples of CSF from the subarachnoid space for laboratory examination and to measure CSF pressure (Fig. 36-9). Bacteriologic tests on specimens of CSF reveal the presence of pathogenic microorganisms. Strict aseptic technique is required during the procedure. The CSF normally is clear and colorless, with a pressure of 80 to 180 mm H_2O; a pressure over 200 mm H_2O is considered abnormal. A lumbar puncture also is performed to inject a drug into the subarachnoid space (intrathecal injection), to administer a spinal anesthetic, to withdraw CSF for the relief of intracranial pressure, or to inject air, gas, or dye for a neurologic diagnostic procedure.

Sometimes a cisternal puncture is performed to remove CSF. The back of the neck is shaved, the skin washed with an antiseptic, and a needle inserted just below the occipital bone of the skull. This procedure is performed more commonly on children. Headache appears to occur less frequently with cisternal puncture than with lumbar puncture.

Contrast Studies

Contrast studies include cerebral angiography, which detects distortion of cerebral arteries and veins, indicating an aneurysm, a tumor, or other vascular abnormality. A radiopaque dye is injected into the right or left carotid artery, the brachial artery, or the femoral artery. A rapid sequence of radiographs is taken as the dye circulates through the cerebral arteries and veins.

For a myelogram, a radiopaque substance is injected into the spinal canal by means of a lumbar puncture. Radiographs are taken to demonstrate abnormalities of the spinal canal such as tumors or a ruptured intervertebral disk.

Electroencephalogram

An electroencephalogram (EEG) records the electrical impulses generated by the brain. Up to 25 electrodes attach to the scalp with a type of skin glue, and electrical activity records on a graph. Techniques such as rapid breathing or looking at a flashing light, known as *photic stimulation*, can induce a seizure during the EEG. In some cases, the physician may request that the client be deprived of sleep before an EEG. Sleep deprivation helps the client fall asleep naturally during the EEG. The electrical activity during sleep provides additional diagnostic information.

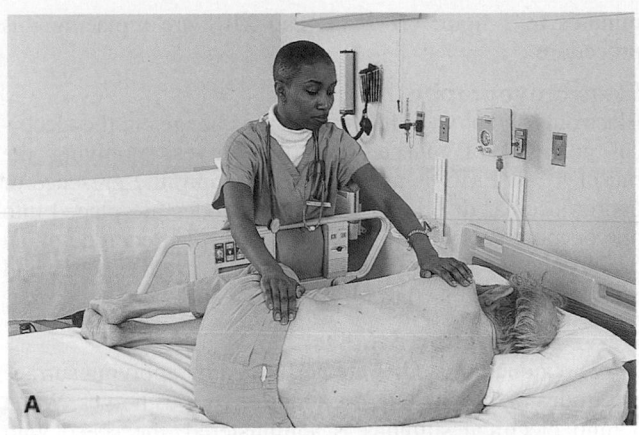

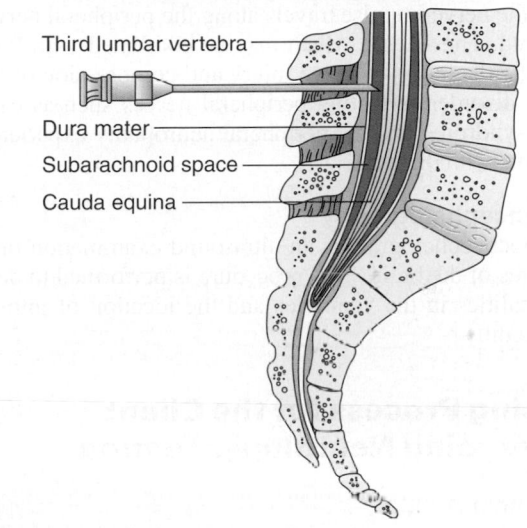

Third lumbar vertebra

Dura mater

Subarachnoid space

Cauda equina

FIGURE 36-9. (**A**) Positioning of the client for lumbar puncture. (**B**) Insertion of the spinal needle into the subarachnoid space.

The nurse is responsible for preparing the client for the EEG as follows:

- Tell the client that he or she will not experience any electrical shock during the test and that the source of the electrical energy is the client's neural activity within the brain.
- Withhold sedatives, coffee, tea, and soft drinks that contain caffeine for at least 8 hours before the test to avoid affecting the diagnostic findings.
- Allow the client to eat; low blood glucose level can alter the EEG.
- Direct the client to shampoo his or her hair to remove oil and hair products. Clean hair facilitates and promotes maintenance of electrode attachment throughout the test.
- Awaken the client around midnight before the EEG to ensure sleep deprivation.

After the EEG is completed, the client who is sleep-deprived can rest and have the hair shampooed to remove the glue used to affix the electrodes to the scalp.

Brain Scan

A brain scan identifies tumors, hematomas in or around the brain, cerebral abscesses, cerebral infarctions, or displaced ventricles. A radioactive material is injected before the procedure. The length of this procedure varies from a few minutes to 1 hour. CT scans and MRI are replacing this procedure.

Electromyography

Electromyography (EMG) studies the changes in the electrical potential of muscles and the nerves supplying the muscles. An EMG is useful in determining the presence of neuromuscular disorders. Needle electrodes are placed into one or more skeletal muscles and the results recorded on an oscilloscope. Pain may occur at needle insertion sites, and muscle soreness may last for some time afterward.

Nerve Conduction Studies

Nerve conduction studies are performed by applying surface electrodes to the skin over locations of various nerves. When a mild electrical stimulus is administered, the speed with which the nerve impulse travels along the peripheral nerve is measured. These tests, which may be combined with EMG, aid in the diagnosis of nerve injury and compression or neurologic disorders affecting peripheral nerves such as carpal tunnel syndrome and the peripheral neuropathy experienced by clients with diabetes.

Echoencephalography

An echoencephalogram is an ultrasound examination of the structures of the brain. This procedure is performed to detect abnormalities in the ventricles and the location of intracranial bleeding.

Nursing Process for the Client Undergoing Neurologic Testing

Assessment

Determine the client's understanding of the diagnostic procedures and answer remaining questions. Check that a consent form has been signed and witnessed. Because some contrast media contain iodine, check the client's history for previous allergic reactions to radiographic dyes, iodine, or seafood. Obtain the client's weight, baseline vital signs, and neurologic data such as LOC, pupil response, and muscle strength in all four extremities. Use the assessment findings for comparison when monitoring the client's condition during and after diagnostic testing. Closely observe the client for any mental or physical deviations from the baseline assessments.

Diagnosis, Planning, and Interventions

Prepare the client for neurologic diagnostic tests following agency policies. If the diagnostic test is performed at the bedside, bring necessary equipment to the room. Assist the physician and support the client during a test performed on the nursing unit. During and after the diagnostic test, monitor for adverse consequences and promote recovery after the test.

Diagnoses, expected outcomes, and interventions include, but are not limited to, the following.

▶ **Deficient Knowledge** related to unfamiliarity with diagnostic testing process

▶ **Expected Outcome:** Client will accurately describe the preparation, procedure, and aftercare that the scheduled diagnostic test involves.

• Clarify the physician's explanation. *Some clients have questions after the physician leaves the nursing unit or healthcare agency.*
• Answer the client's questions. *Clients have the right to information about their plan of care.*
• Describe the procedure to the client as well as what the procedure requires, such as positions to assume or the need to lie still during the procedure. *Specific information decreases anxiety and increases the client's trust and confidence in the nurse.*
• Discuss the preparation for the diagnostic test, which may include temporarily eliminating CNS depressants, such as barbiturates and minor tranquilizers, and CNS stimulants, such as caffeine, for several hours in the case of an EEG. *Drugs that affect neurologic function sometimes are withheld to ensure that factors other than the client's physiology do not affect test results.*
• Explain that hair will be shampooed before an EEG. *Removing scalp and hair oil ensures that electrodes will remain in place until the EEG is completed.*
• Inform the client that he or she will be able to shampoo the hair again after an EEG. *A second shampoo facilitates removing the paste used to secure the electrodes to the scalp.*
• Tell the client to expect some discomfort when undergoing a lumbar puncture, myelogram, EMG, or nerve conduction studies. *Without giving the client information about expected discomfort, the client may assume that he or she is having an adverse reaction.*

▶ **PC: Allergic Reaction** to contrast dye

▶ **Expected Outcome:** The nurse will monitor to detect, manage, and minimize an allergic reaction.

• Report the allergy history to the physician. *Reporting helps the physician decide whether to cancel or modify the diagnostic test by administering a pretest antihistamine or substituting an alternative dye.*
• Identify allergy information prominently on the client's chart. *Documenting allergies on the chart provides a means for communicating the information to all healthcare workers.*
• Attach an allergy band to the client's wrist when that is the agency's policy. *Some healthcare agencies require a second wristband that is a different color than the client identification band to alert personnel that the client has a history of one or more allergies.*
• Administer pretest antihistamines according to the physician's medical order. *Antihistamines block histamine receptors and reduce the manifestations of an allergic reaction.*
• Monitor client for severe hypotension, tachycardia, profuse diaphoresis, sudden change in LOC, dyspnea, and hives or itching. Notify the physician immediately of any such findings. *The most serious allergic reaction is anaphylaxis.*
• Obtain the emergency cart that contains drugs and resuscitation equipment; follow instructions for administering oxygen, intravenous fluids, drugs, and airway management depending on the client's symptoms. *Emergency measures are required to relieve anaphylaxis and other serious allergic reactions.*

● PC: Meningeal Irritation or CNS Changes

● Expected Outcome: The nurse will monitor to detect, manage, and minimize abnormal neurologic changes.

- Observe closely for any neurologic abnormalities such as diminished LOC, weakness, numbness, paralysis in an extremity, unequal or unresponsive pupil reflexes, posturing, and speech disturbance. *Diagnostic tests pose potential risks for neurologic complications, which are characterized by changes in neurologic functions.*

- Assess for changes in vital signs, restlessness, vomiting, and mental changes in orientation and thought processes. *Rising intracranial pressure affects vital signs, stimulates the vomiting center in the brain, and alters the sensorium and cognition.*

- Report the onset of a headache and sudden or severe pain in any area of the body to the physician immediately. *Headache often accompanies increased intracranial pressure; pain of any kind requires further investigation and pain management.*

- Inspect injection sites, especially those made during a lumbar puncture, for signs of a hematoma (collection of blood). *Trauma at an injection site can result in bleeding; bloody drainage also may contain CSF.*

- Position the client flat for at least 3 hours or as directed by the physician after a lumbar puncture or myelogram. *Keeping the client in a recumbent position provides time for CSF to form and replace what has been lost and reduces the potential for a headache.*

- Encourage a liberal fluid intake. *A generous fluid intake helps restore the volume of CSF.*

- Keep the room dark and quiet after a lumbar puncture or myelogram. *Sensory stimulation tends to magnify discomfort.*

- Administer a prescribed analgesic if the client develops a headache. *An analgesic reduces the transmission or perception of pain stimuli.*

Evaluation of Expected Outcomes

Expected outcomes for the client are that he or she understands the preparation and performance involved in the neurologic procedure or diagnostic test and aftercare. Data concerning the client's allergy history are communicated appropriately. Interventions are implemented to control any allergic reaction. Measures to reduce the manifestation of complications are implemented successfully. Interventions to relieve discomfort are carried out. ●

CRITICAL THINKING EXERCISES

1. Discuss appropriate nursing assessments when managing the care of clients with neurologic disorders.

2. A client with a neurologic disorder is being transferred from one nursing unit to another. What information is needed to plan the nursing care of the client?

3. Name two potential complications of neurologic testing procedures. How can the nurse prevent, manage, and minimize them?

4. The nurse providing an end-of-shift [report?] client has a Glasgow Coma Score of [ ] nificance of this score.

NCLEX-STYLE REVIEW QUESTION[S]

1. Following a lumbar puncture, a client asks to am[bulate to] the restroom. Which nursing action is most correct[?]
   1. Explain that the client must lie flat following the [pro]cedure and obtain a bedpan.
   2. Provide a bedside commode and assist the client with its use.
   3. Instruct the client to remain still and insert a urinary catheter.
   4. Assist the client to the restroom and wait outside until finished.

2. A client seen at the neurologist's office reports experiencing chronic dizziness. When the nurse is asked to assist the physician with a diagnostic Romberg text, which nursing intervention is most appropriate to ensure client safety?
   1. Stand close to the client in case the client should begin to sway.
   2. Advise the client to use a handrail while ambulating to avoid falling.
   3. Provide support as the client performs the neurologic test.
   4. Document the results of the testing.

3. An ICU nurse is assessing a client's level of consciousness. Calling the client's name causes the client to awaken but then drift back to sleep when asked questions. When documenting the client's level of consciousness, the nurse would be most correct to document which of the following?
   1. Conscious
   2. Somnolent
   3. Stuporous
   4. Semicomatose

4. A nurse uses the Glasgow Coma Scale to measure the client's level of consciousness. Which of the following methods can the nurse use to evoke and assess the "best verbal response" from the client?
   1. Ask the client to read aloud an interesting item from the newspaper.
   2. Tell the client to pronounce certain difficult technical terms.
   3. Note the client's reaction when the nurse whispers the client's name.
   4. Note the client's responses to general orientation questions.

5. Which of the following post-procedural interventions is appropriate for the nurse to perform when caring for a client who has undergone a lumbar puncture? Select all that apply.
   1. Shampoo the client's hair with warm water.
   2. Administer a prescribed antihistamine.
   3. Position the client flat for several hours.
   4. Stimulate the client to elevate level of consciousness.
   5. Encourage the client to consume a liberal intake of fluid.

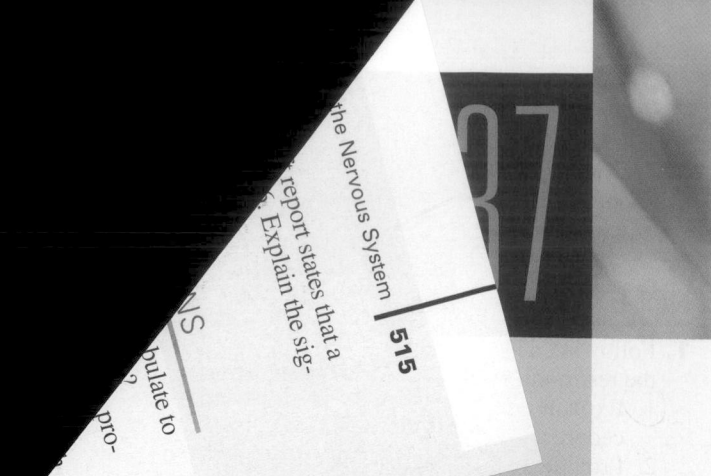

Caring for Clients with Central and Peripheral Nervous System Disorders

Learning Objectives

On completion of this chapter, you will be able to:

1. Discuss at least four signs and symptoms and nursing care of the client with increased intracranial pressure.
2. Name four infectious or inflammatory diseases that affect the central or peripheral nervous system.
3. Discuss three neuromuscular disorders, common related problems, and nursing management.
4. Discuss the nursing management of clients with a cranial nerve disorder.
5. List the signs and symptoms of Parkinson's disease.
6. Discuss the purpose of drug therapy and drugs commonly prescribed for Parkinson's disease.
7. Describe signs and symptoms of Huntington's disease and related nursing management.
8. Discuss the pathophysiology of seizure disorders and different types of seizures.
9. Discuss the nursing management of clients with seizure disorders.
10. Discuss the nursing management of clients with brain tumors.

A cute disorders of the central nervous system (CNS) and peripheral nervous system (PNS) are potentially life-threatening. Chronic neurologic disorders, although not imminently fatal, profoundly affect a person's quality of life. When any part of the CNS or PNS is damaged, removed, or destroyed, a permanent neurologic deficit can occur.

INCREASED INTRACRANIAL PRESSURE

Inside the cranium, there is (1) brain tissue, (2) blood, and (3) cerebrospinal fluid (CSF). The brain represents 84% of the cranial contents; the blood within the cranium contributes 4% of the total; the CSF provides the remaining 12% (Schumacher & Chernecky, 2005). If one or more of these increases significantly without a decrease in either of the other two, intracranial pressure (ICP) becomes elevated.

Pathophysiology and Etiology

Under normal circumstances, autoregulatory mechanisms keep brain tissue perfused with adequate oxygen and glucose. Dilation or constriction of cerebral blood vessels in response to changes in blood pressure, blood oxygen levels, and blood pH maintains constant and consistent tissue perfusion. For example, increased $PaCO_2$ (carbon dioxide level in the blood), decreased blood pH, or decreased PaO_2 (oxygen level in the blood) causes cerebral blood vessels to dilate. Nevertheless, a delicate range of ICP helps maintain autoregulation. Ideally, ICP remains at 15 mm Hg or below to ensure normal cerebral perfusion pressure (CPP) of

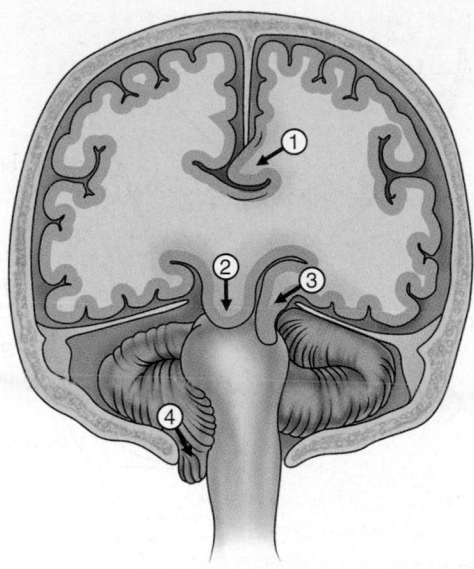

FIGURE 37-1. Major types of intracranial herniations. (1) Cingulate herniation. (2) Central transtentorial herniation. (3) Uncal herniation. (4) Infratentorial herniation of cerebral tonsils.

70 to 100 mm Hg. Many conditions, including brain tumors, swelling or bleeding within the brain from head trauma, and infectious and inflammatory disorders of the brain (e.g., meningitis, encephalitis), cause increased ICP.

When the intracranial volume (and therefore ICP) begins to increase, some initial compensation occurs. CSF production may decrease, or it may displace at a greater rate into venous circulation. However, as ICP continues to rise, vascular autoregulatory mechanisms can become compromised and fail. Hypotension and hypoxia lead to vasodilation, which contributes to increased ICP, compressing blood vessels, and this leads to cerebral ischemia.

If increased ICP continues to be unrecognized or untreated, the contents of the cranium are compressed further. Unrelieved pressure causes brain tissue to herniate or shift from normal locations intracranially and extracranially (Fig. 37-1). The **foramen magnum,** the opening in the lower part of the skull through which the upper part of the spinal cord connects with the brain, provides the only extracranial exit for brain tissue. If the brain stem herniates through the foramen magnum, respiration, heart rate, blood pressure (BP), and the functions of descending and ascending nerve fibers are affected. As increased ICP progresses, the consequences include impaired cellular activity, temporary or permanent neurologic dysfunction, or death.

Assessment Findings

Signs and Symptoms

The signs and symptoms of increased ICP (Box 37-1) can develop rapidly or slowly. When increased ICP develops slowly, subtle changes can be overlooked.

Decreasing level of consciousness (LOC) is one of the earliest signs of increased ICP. Clients may slip from alert and oriented to lethargic, stuporous, semicomatose, and, finally, comatose (see Chap. 36). Confusion, restlessness, and periodic disorientation often accompany decreasing LOC.

Headache is another symptom of increased ICP. Headache, which is more severe in the morning, increases with activities that elevate ICP, such as coughing, sneezing, or straining at stool. Rest or elevation of the head relieves the pain. A constant headache is a grave sign.

Vomiting when associated with a neurologic condition also suggests increasing ICP. Emesis commonly occurs without any forewarning of nausea.

Papilledema (swelling of the optic nerve) is caused by interference with venous drainage from the eye and is observed through examination with an ophthalmoscope. Pressure on the oculomotor nerve usually accompanies increased ICP and affects pupillary response to light. Normal pupillary response to strong light is rapid constriction. In increased ICP, the pupillary response is unequal. One pupil responds more sluggishly than the other or becomes fixed and dilated.

Changes in ICP also influence vital signs. Body temperature may rise or fall depending on the etiology of the increased ICP or because of its effect on the temperature-regulating center. The pulse increases initially but then decreases, systolic BP rises with a widening pulse pressure (the difference between the systolic and diastolic measurements), and the respiratory rate is irregular—three signs

---

B O X 3 7 - 1 **Signs of Increased Intracranial Pressure**	
Early	**Late**
Drowsiness; difficult to awaken	Unresponsive
Restlessness	Glasgow Coma Scale ≤ 12
Confusion	Decreased response to painful stimuli
Irritability	Decorticate or decerebrate posturing
Glasgow Coma Scale ≥ 13	Increased weakness or hemiparesis
Personality changes	Dilated pupil(s)
Sluggish or unequal pupil response	Seizures
Weakness in arms or legs	Cushing's triad: bradycardia, elevated systolic blood pressure
Slow or slurred speech	with wide pulse pressure, irregular breathing
Dull headache, especially upon awakening	Loss of gag and corneal reflexes
Vomiting without nausea	Periods of apnea

called **Cushing's triad.** Cushing's triad occurs late in increased ICP. Later, **Cheyne-Stokes respirations**, consisting of shallow, rapid breathing followed by periods of apnea, occur.

Decorticate or decerebrate posturing (see Chap. 36) develops spontaneously or in response to a painful stimulus when ICP is increased.

Diagnostic Findings

Diagnostic tests that determine the underlying cause of increased ICP include skull radiography, computed tomography (CT), magnetic resonance imaging (MRI), lumbar puncture, and cerebral angiography.

Medical and Surgical Management

Immediate treatment aims at decreasing ICP by relieving the cause if possible. The goals are to maintain BP, prevent hypoxia, and ensure cerebral perfusion. To maintain cerebral tissue perfusion and BP, the physician administers isotonic normal saline, lactated Ringer's, or hypertonic (3%) saline solutions. Hypotonic solutions and solutions containing glucose increase ICP. Providing supplemental oxygen or mechanical ventilation to keep the SaO_2 at 95% and the $PaCO_2$ between 35 and 45 mm Hg prevents hypoxia. The initial practice of hyperventilating the client with increased ICP is avoided because it exacerbates brain injury from cerebral vasoconstriction and cellular necrosis (Lettieri, 2006). The imminent possibility of brain herniation is the only justification for hyperventilation. The client's head is maintained in midline at 30° of elevation to promote venous drainage of blood and CSF. Persistent hyperthermia caused by altered functioning of the hypothalamus may require measures such as administering acetaminophen (Tylenol) or applying a cooling blanket to maintain normothermia. Care must be taken to avoid hypothermia because shivering can increase ICP. The physician can control the client's seizures, which elevate ICP, by administering diazepam (Valium) and fosphenytoin (Cerebyx). Fosphenytoin, a new, parenterally administered anticonvulsant, is a prodrug (i.e., a drug that converts to an active compound when it metabolizes). Fosphenytoin becomes phenytoin (Dilantin) when it metabolizes. It is indicated for short-term parenteral use when oral phenytoin is unavailable or less advantageous. The physician may prescribe a benzodiazepine such as midazolam (Versed) to sedate an agitated client because hyperactivity contributes to transient rises in ICP. Healthcare professionals currently question the use of barbiturate coma therapy because it lowers metabolic brain requirements, and the resultant sedation contributes to hypotension, pneumonia, hypoxia, and respiratory depression.

Pharmacologic Considerations

- Narcotic analgesics depress the respiratory center and raise CSF pressure. Their use is contraindicated in clients with head trauma or increased ICP, unless administration is an absolute necessity.

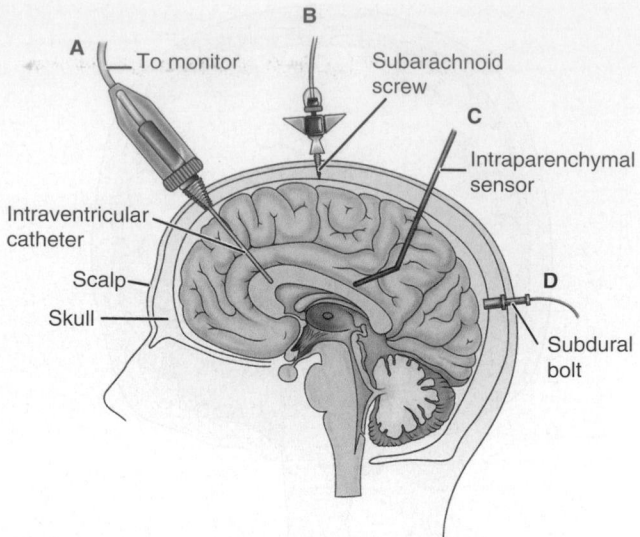

FIGURE 37-2. Techniques for monitoring intracranial pressure (ICP). **(A)** A fiberoptic, transducer-tipped device placed in the ventricle, **(B)** subarachnoid screw, **(C)** intraparenchymal sensor, or **(D)** subdural bolt. These devices connect to a pressure transducer and display system.

Monitoring devices (Fig. 37-2) are inserted to measure ICP and in some cases to withdraw CSF. These devices are connected to a transducer and a monitor that displays the pressure and a waveform to detect the status of ICP. Normal ICP in the ventricles is 1 to 15 mm Hg, moderate elevation values range from 15 to 40 mm Hg, and high levels exceed 40 mm Hg. Although the ICP varies, a rise of 2 mm Hg from a previous measurement is cause for concern. Normal ICP below 20 mm Hg is desirable (Sole et al., 2005).

When the usual measures to reduce ICP are ineffective, osmotic diuretics such as mannitol (Osmitrol) and fluid restriction are used. Care must be taken to avoid precipitating secondary brain injury from hypotension related to hypovolemia. Although corticosteroids, such as dexamethasone (Decadron), have reduced ICP in the past, their use is now restrained. Current thinking is that steroids are not effective in reducing increased ICP with traumatic brain injury (Rangel-Castillo et al., 2008). Among other side effects, steroids may cause upper gastrointestinal bleeding, which can create another complication for a client who is acutely ill.

Depending on the degree and cause of increased ICP, the physician may order the insertion of an indwelling catheter, a nasogastric tube for gastric decompression or provision of tube feedings, a stool softener to prevent straining at stool, and a histamine antagonist such as famotidine (Pepcid) to prevent stress ulcers.

Emergency surgery is done to remove a blood clot if increased ICP results from a head injury with bleeding above or below the dura (see Chap 39). Surgery also is performed to relieve pressure caused by a brain tumor.

Nursing Management

Nursing care of the client with increased ICP is presented in Nursing Care Plan 37-1.

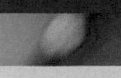

NURSING CARE PLAN 37-1 | **The Client With Increased Intracranial Pressure**

Assessment

- Gather from client or a witness, paramedic, or emergency medical technician the history of circumstances surrounding the altered neurologic state. Also gather past medical history, concurrent health problems being treated, current medications, and allergy history.
- Assess level of consciousness (LOC) and vital signs.
- Assist with a head-to-toe physical examination.

- Perform complete neurologic assessments, including the Glasgow Coma Scale (GCS) or Ranchos Los Amigos Scale (see Chap. 36). Repeat these assessments every 30 to 60 minutes.
- Measure current and daily weights and intake and output measurements.
- Study laboratory findings such as serum electrolyte and arterial blood gas levels.
- Evaluate the presence of bowel sounds and bowel elimination.
- Note evidence of any seizures.

Nursing Diagnosis. Ineffective Tissue Perfusion (cerebral) related to increased ICP as evidenced by decreased LOC, sluggish pupil response, papilledema, and posturing

Expected Outcome. ICP will be between 1 and 15 mm Hg, and the GCS will be 9 or greater.

Interventions	Rationales
Keep head of bed slightly elevated and the head in midline (straight). For clients with a basal skull fracture, keep bed flat.	Head elevation promotes drainage of venous blood and cerebrospinal fluid from the cranium.
Limit movement, space essential nursing tasks, and reduce or eliminate environmental stimuli (e.g., loud noise, bright lights).	Activities that increase BP, use the Valsalva maneuver, impair blood circulation, or decrease oxygenation raise ICP.
Avoid extreme hip flexion.	It compresses femoral blood vessels and interferes with circulation.
Keep client quiet. Change position with assistance and use a turning sheet. Avoid range-of-motion (ROM) exercises until ICP approaches normal unless ordered otherwise by the physician.	Activity increases ICP by raising BP. Increased intracranial pressure (IICP) predisposes to cerebral ischemia and cell damage.
Administer reduced fluid volumes at an even rate for 24 hours. Give diuretics as prescribed; note client's response to therapy.	Reduced fluid volume is one way to decrease the volume in the brain.
Hyperventilate the mechanically ventilated client according to medical orders.	When CO_2 rises in the blood, cerebral blood vessels dilate as an autoregulatory mechanism to prevent cerebral ischemia; however, vasodilation increases volume in an already overloaded cranium. Hyperventilation reduces the intracerebral blood volume, but is only used briefly when the client's condition is severely deteriorating.
Suction the airway only when necessary.	Suctioning stimulates coughing, which raises ICP.
Give 100% oxygen before and after suctioning when it is required.	Preoxygenation reduces the potential for hypoxemia; postoxygenation relieves any oxygen deficit. Keeping blood well oxygenated prevents cerebral ischemia.
Keep suctioning brief, without exceeding 10 to 15 seconds per pass of the catheter.	Prolonged suctioning contributes to hypoxemia and cerebral vasodilation.
Administer a prescribed stool softener.	It increases moisture in stool, making stool easy to pass and reducing the potential for the Valsalva maneuver.
Ensure that a gastric tube used for decompression or nourishment remains patent.	An obstructed gastric tube can contribute to gastric distention and vomiting. Elevated BP and ICP accompany vomiting.
Administer prescribed medications if vomiting or persistent coughing occur.	Suppressing vomiting and coughing reduces the potential for IICP and cerebral ischemia.

Evaluation of Expected Outcome

ICP returns to normal, and cerebral perfusion is restored.

Nursing Diagnoses. Risk for Ineffective Breathing Pattern and **Ineffective Airway Clearance** related to diminished LOC and herniation of the brain stem secondary to increased ICP

Expected Outcomes (1) Respiratory rate will be sufficient to maintain the SpO_2 above 90% and PaO_2 above 80 mm Hg. (2) Airway will be patent.

(care plan continues on page 520)

NURSING CARE PLAN 37-1   The Client with Increased Intracranial Pressure (Continued)

Interventions	Rationales
Attach a pulse oximeter to the finger, earlobe, bridge of the nose, or toe.	A pulse oximeter measures the percentage of oxygen bound to hemoglobin.
Insert an oral airway if client is comatose.	It prevents the tongue from occluding the natural airway.
Administer prescribed oxygen.	Supplemental oxygen provides a greater percentage of oxygen than in room air.
For mechanically ventilated clients, ensure that the ventilator delivers the prescribed tidal volume at the ordered rate.	A mechanical ventilator supplements or controls the client's breathing.
Suction when necessary to clear tracheal secretions or keep endotracheal tube patent.	Artificial airways increase secretions, which reduce the volume of air within the airway.

Evaluation of Expected Outcomes

Respirations are normal, airway is free of secretions, and lungs are clear to auscultation.

Nursing Diagnosis. **Risk for Imbalanced Nutrition: Less than Body Requirements** related to inability to consume food orally secondary to decreased LOC or endotracheal intubation

Expected Outcome. Body weight will remain within 2 lb of preadmission.

Interventions	Rationales
Administer nutritional supplements by gastric tube or total parenteral nutrition (TPN) through a central venous catheter as medically prescribed.	The enteral or parenteral route facilitates a means of providing essential nutrients and fluids.

Evaluation of Expected Outcome

Nutritional needs are met with no evidence of aspiration.

Nursing Diagnosis. **Risk for Infection** related to impaired skin and tissue integrity secondary to surgery, invasive diagnostic or monitoring procedures, or original head injury

Expected Outcome. Client will be free of infection as evidenced by no fever, no purulent drainage from open areas of skin, and white blood cell count within normal limits.

Interventions	Rationales
Keep wounds clean and dry.	Medical asepsis reduces transient pathogens
Use aseptic technique when handling any part of the intracranial monitoring device or changing a dressing applied after surgery.	Surgical asepsis ensures that supplies and equipment are not contaminated with pathogens
Administer antibiotic therapy, if prescribed.	Antibiotics inhibit the growth of or destroy susceptible microorganisms.

Evaluation of Expected Outcome

Temperature is normal with no sign of infection.

PC. **Hyperglycemia** related to administration of TPN

Expected Outcome. The nurse will monitor to detect, manage, and minimize elevated blood glucose level.

Interventions	Rationales
Assess capillary blood glucose levels three times daily and at bedtime.	Capillary blood glucose is a convenient bedside assessment that provides reliable measurements of current blood glucose level.
Follow medical orders for administering insulin according to a sliding scale.	Insulin helps lower blood sugar by facilitating its movement into body cells.

Evaluation of Expected Outcome

Blood glucose level is within normal range or lowered with insulin therapy.

PC. **Stress Ulcer** related to hyperacidity secondary to stress response

Expected Outcome. The nurse will monitor to detect, manage, and minimize the development of a peptic ulcer.

NURSING CARE PLAN 37-1 **The Client with Increased Intracranial Pressure** (Continued)

Interventions	Rationales
Check the pH of gastric secretions per shift.	Obtaining a sample of gastric secretions and using chemical strip for pH provides a quick means for monitoring the acidity of the stomach.
Report a pH of less than 3.	A pH above 3 helps to suppress the release of pepsin, which adds to the gastric pH created by hydrochloric acid.
Administer prescribed drugs that protect the gastric mucosa, reduce histamine secretion, suppress the release of gastric secretions, or neutralize stomach acids.	There are a variety of drugs whose mechanisms of action reduce the potential for developing a peptic ulcer.

Evaluation of Expected Outcome

Gastric mucosa is intact

Nursing Diagnosis. Risk for Impaired Skin Integrity related to low capillary blood flow secondary to pressure and inactivity

Expected Outcome. Skin will remain intact.

Interventions	Rationales
Tilt or turn client from side to side every 2 hours.	Maintaining intracapillary pressure above 32 mm Hg ensures that tissue can exchange oxygen and CO_2 at the cellular level.
Avoid friction by using a lift sheet.	Friction causes abrasions that impair skin integrity.
Use a pressure-relieving mattress or mechanical bed for clients whose position cannot be readily changed.	Specialty mattresses and beds are designed to intermittently reduce pressure on skin throughout the time a client is confined to bed.
Keep skin clean and dry.	Clean, dry skin prevents softening and erosion of epidermal cells.

Evaluation of Expected Outcome

Skin is intact

Nursing Diagnosis. Self-Care Deficit (total or specify type) related to diminished LOC as manifested by inability to follow directions and impaired neuromuscular function

Expected Outcome. Client's basic needs will be met.

Interventions	Rationales
Give client complete care, including bathing, oral care, nutrition, and elimination, until ICP is normal and client can resume these activities independently.	The nurse manages needs that a client cannot perform until neurologic function returns.

Evaluation of Expected Outcome

Basic needs are managed

Nursing Diagnosis. Impaired Verbal Communication related to decreased LOC or endotracheal intubation as evidenced by an inability to speak

Expected Outcome. Client will communicate using body language, pantomime, or writing.

Interventions	Rationales
Look for grimacing or moaning.	Sounds of distress are universal.
Correct problems that may be causing discomfort, such as a wrinkled sheet or an object pressing on the skin.	Astute assessment may determine the cause of discomfort and facilitate prompt intervention.
Provide paper and pencil or a magic slate if client is alert but intubated.	Written communication is an alternative to oral communication.

Evaluation of Expected Outcome

Client communicates needs to others when conscious.
    For additional suggestions for nursing management of a client undergoing surgery or who develops a neurologic deficit, see Chapter 40.

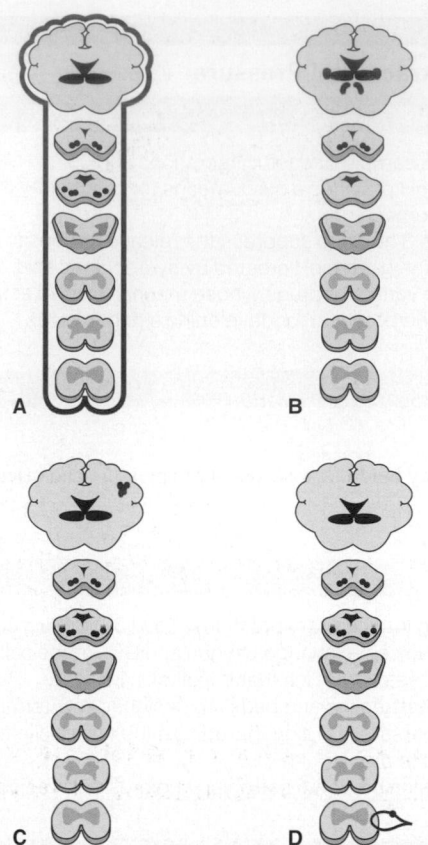

FIGURE 37-3. Sites of infectious and inflammatory disorders. (**A**) Meningitis, (**B**) encephalitis, (**C**) brain abscess, and (**D**) Guillain-Barré syndrome.

> ▶ *Stop, Think, and Respond Exercise 37-1*
>
> *What assessment findings suggest that ICP is increasing beyond the compensatory changes that result from autoregulation?*

INFECTIOUS AND INFLAMMATORY DISORDERS OF THE NERVOUS SYSTEM

Four neurologic conditions have an infectious or inflammatory cause: meningitis, encephalitis, Guillain-Barré syndrome, and brain abscess (Fig. 37-3).

MENINGITIS

Meningitis is an inflammation of the meninges caused by various infectious microorganisms such as bacteria, viruses, fungi, or parasites. The inflammation often extends to the cerebral cortex. Depending on the causative organism, the client's condition may be mild and or it may rapidly become critical. Most adults with bacterial meningitis, the most serious form of meningitis, recover without permanent neurologic damage or dysfunction. When complications do occur, they usually are serious.

Pathophysiology and Etiology

The most highly contagious and potentially lethal form of meningitis is caused by either of two bacteria, meningococci (*Neisseria meningitidis*) and streptococci (*Streptococcus pneumoniae*). Meningococcal meningitis usually affects school-aged children, young adults, and immunosuppressed people. Viruses such as herpes simplex virus, mumps virus, and enteroviruses, which are common intestinal viruses, can cause viral meningitis, a milder form of the disease. Viral meningitis is more common in children and in older adults.

The infecting microorganisms circulate from blood and lymph to cerebral capillaries or by direct extension from infected areas such as the middle ear and the paranasal sinuses. When the pathogens arrive in the cerebral circulation, they travel to the subarachnoid space of the meninges where the inflammatory process begins. In virulent cases, cerebral edema and inappropriate secretion of antidiuretic hormone (ADH), which increases fluid volume, cause increased ICP. *Cerebral vasculitis,* inflammation of blood vessels in the brain, may be present, and cerebral blood flow may be decreased. The client may develop seizures, a brain abscess, neurologic changes, irreversible coma, and death from brain herniation. Neurologic sequelae in survivors include damage to the cranial nerves that facilitate vision and hearing.

Assessment Findings

Signs and Symptoms

Classic symptoms include headache, fever, **nuchal rigidity** (pain and stiffness of the neck, inability to place the chin on the chest). Nausea, vomiting, **photophobia** (aversion to light), restlessness, irritability, and seizures may also develop. Severe irritation of the meninges causes **opisthotonos,** an extreme hyperextension of the head and arching of the back. A positive **Kernig's sign** (inability to extend the leg when the thigh is flexed on the abdomen) and a positive **Brudzinski's sign** (flexion of the neck produces flexion of the knees and hips) are seen (Fig. 37-4).

 Gerontologic Considerations

- Older adults may not exhibit the typical signs and symptoms of meningitis; rather, they may display a change in mental status, slight to no fever, and no nuchal rigidity or headache. Mortality rates are high in older adults with this disease partly because of these atypical signs and symptoms. Contributing factors to death from meningitis are chronic illness and delays in diagnosis.

The client with meningococcal meningitis may have multiple, small to large petechiae that spread over the body, giving the appearance of a rug burn. The petechiae intensify and coalesce (fuse together) to resemble purpura or ecchymoses due to a secondary disturbance in blood coagulation from thrombocytopenia or disseminated intravascular coagulation. Those with viral meningitis develop a nonspecific maculopapular rash.

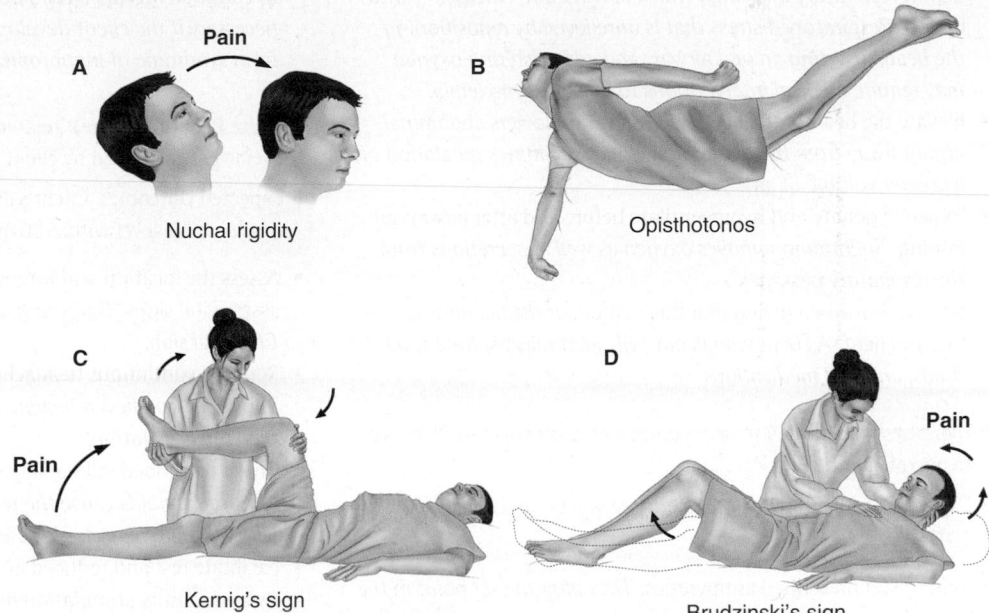

FIGURE 37-4. Signs of meningeal irritation. (**A**) Nuchal rigidity, (**B**) opisthotonos, (**C**) Kernig's sign, and (**D**) Brudzinski's sign.

Diagnostic Findings

A lumbar puncture is performed and samples of CSF are obtained. If the meningitis is bacterial, the CSF appears cloudy. The CSF pressure is elevated, glucose concentration is decreased, protein levels are elevated, and white blood cell (WBC) and red blood cell counts are elevated. Culture and sensitivity studies are performed to identify the specific causative bacteria. If meningitis is viral, the results of culture and sensitivity studies are negative. A CT scan, blood culture, complete blood cell count, and other laboratory tests are used to rule out other possible disorders.

Medical Management

Measures to manage and reduce ICP are used in the acute stage of infection. Taking precautions against diseases and hand hygiene are important in controlling the spread of infection. The local public health department is notified of all cases. Intravenous (IV) fluids and antimicrobial therapy are started immediately when bacterial meningitis is suspected. The appropriate antibiotic, usually penicillin, a cephalosporin, rifampin (Rifadin), vancomycin (Vancocin), or chloramphenicol (Chloromycetin), is determined when the causative microorganism is identified from the results of the sensitivity tests. Drug therapy is continued after the acute phase of the illness to prevent recurrence. Anticonvulsants are necessary if seizures occur. People who have had recent contact with a person with meningococcal meningitis are placed on prophylactic oral rifampin (Rifadin).

Many colleges and universities now recommend immunization for meningococcal meningitis (Menomune). Immunization for *Haemophilus influenzae* type b (Hib), which is part of the series of childhood immunizations, also can reduce the acquisition of bacterial meningitis caused by that pathogen.

Nursing Process for the Client with a Neurologic Infectious or Inflammatory Disorder

Assessment

Obtain a health history. Because the client is acutely ill, interview a family member to obtain information if the client cannot participate in the data-gathering process. Measure vital signs and perform a neurologic examination. After gathering the initial data, initiate an assessment flow sheet for ongoing comparisons. Observe the rate and characteristics of respirations, and auscultate the lungs every 4 to 8 hours. Evaluate the client's abilities to swallow and clear the airway of secretions. Provide for intake and output measurements. Record bowel elimination to ensure that constipation does not develop. Ask the client to indicate the severity of a headache, when present. If a seizure occurs, note its duration, physical manifestations, and whether it involves only one side of the body or starts in one site and spreads elsewhere.

Diagnosis, Planning, and Interventions

▶ **Risk for Impaired Gas Exchange** related to ineffective breathing, ineffective airway clearance, and aspiration

▶ **Expected Outcomes:** (1) Blood gases will be within normal ranges. (2) Breathing will be sufficient to maintain the blood oxygen saturation (SpO_2) above 90%. (3) The airway will be free of oral or gastric secretions.

- Keep an oral airway at the bedside; insert it immediately if respiratory distress develops. *An oral airway holds the tongue forward so it does not occlude the pharynx.*
- Administer oxygen as prescribed. *Supplemental oxygen increases the percentage of oxygen in inhaled gas higher than that in room air.*

- Report respiratory difficulty, which may require emergency intubation. *Respiratory distress that is unrelieved by repositioning the head, inserting an oral airway, and administering oxygen may require medical interventions to prevent hypoxemia.*
- Elevate the head of the bed. *Head elevation lowers abdominal organs away from the diaphragm, which facilitates inhalation of a greater volume of air.*
- Hyperoxygenate and hyperventilate before and after airway suctioning. *Suctioning removes oxygen as well as secretions from the respiratory passages.*
- Use caution when giving oral fluids, food, or medications to a lethargic client. *A client who is not fully alert may aspirate food, fluids, and oral medications.*

▶ **Hyperthermia** related to fever-producing mechanisms secondary to microbial infection

▶ **Expected Outcome:** Body temperature will be controlled below 101°F (38.3°C).

- Administer prescribed antipyretics. *They alter the set point in the hypothalamus.*
- Remove unnecessary clothing and blankets. *Layers of fabric trap body heat and prevent its convection into the environment.*
- Administer tepid sponge baths. *Applying moisture to the body's surface promotes heat loss through evaporation.*
- Apply a cooling blanket beneath the client, but avoid shivering. *It promotes heat loss by conduction. Shivering increases ICP.*
- Maintain adequate hydration. *Adequate fluid volume compensates for fluid loss from perspiration and ensures fluid is available*

to continue this heat-regulating process. *Fluid restriction may be necessary if the client develops cerebral edema and hypervolemia from syndrome of inappropriate antidiuretic hormone (SIADH).*

▶ **Acute Pain (headache)** related to meningeal irritation, cerebral edema as manifested by client's description of head discomfort

▶ **Expected Outcome:** Client's discomfort will be relieved or reduced to a tolerable level within 30 minutes of a nursing measure.

- Assess the location and intensity of discomfort whenever you assess vital signs. *Gathering data about pain is considered the fifth vital sign.*
- Report a continuous headache or one that is unrelieved. *An intense or unrelieved headache suggests rising ICP from acute meningeal irritation.*
- Give a prescribed mild analgesic that does not affect pupil size or reaction. *Opioids cause the pupils to constrict, which interferes with accurate neurologic assessment.*
- Facilitate rest and reduced environmental stimuli. *Reduced activity and sensory stimulation help increase pain tolerance.*

▶ **PC: Seizures** related to meningeal irritation, high fever, or increased ICP

▶ **Expected Outcome:** The nurse will monitor to detect, manage, and minimize seizures.

- Raise and pad side rails with soft material. *Modifying the environment helps reduce the potential for injuries during a seizure (Fig. 37-5).*

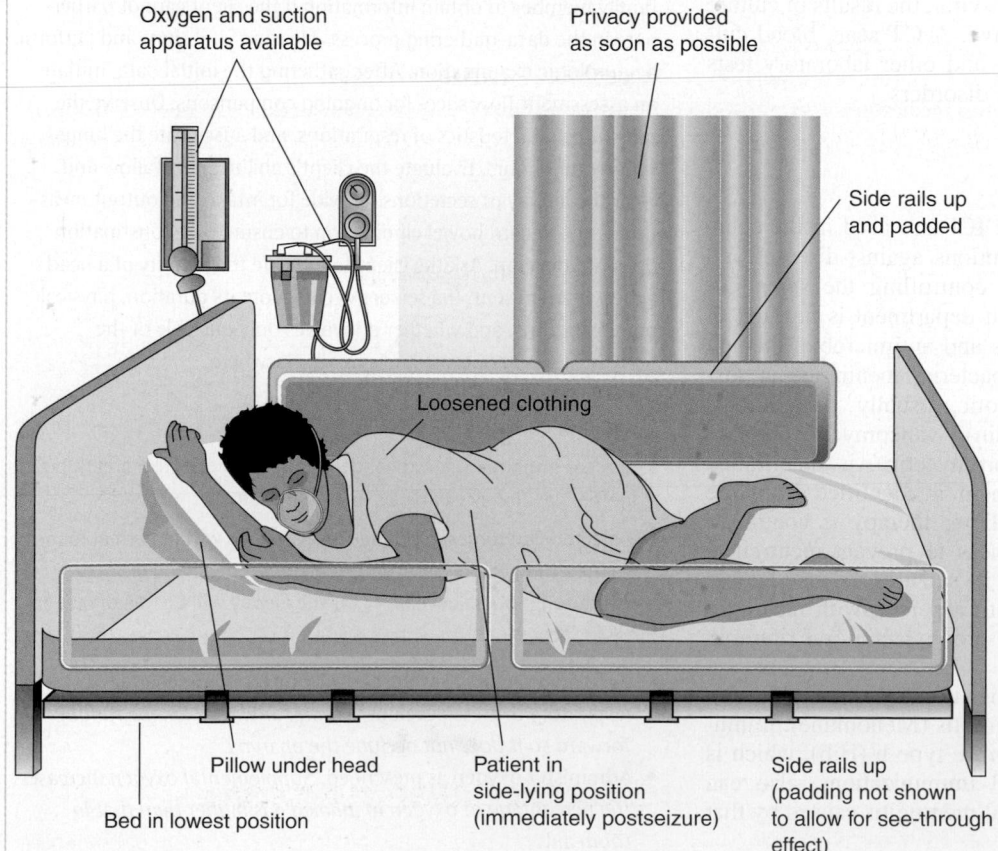

Oxygen and suction apparatus available

Privacy provided as soon as possible

Side rails up and padded

Loosened clothing

Pillow under head

Bed in lowest position

Patient in side-lying position (immediately postseizure)

Side rails up (padding not shown to allow for see-through effect)

FIGURE 37-5. Environmental modifications for seizure precautions.

- Stay with the client if a seizure develops and call for assistance. *A client is defenseless during a seizure. The airway can become obstructed or aspiration can occur if a client is alone during a seizure.*
- Turn client to the side during a seizure. *A lateral position reduces the potential for aspiration of saliva or stomach contents.*
- Do not restrain client's movements. *Doing so during a seizure can cause fractures or other musculoskeletal injuries.*
- Provide privacy. *Privacy protects the client's dignity.*
- Insert a padded tongue blade in the mouth only if the teeth are not tightly shut. *Protecting the tongue and teeth with soft material is dangerous once a seizure begins; if the client experiences an aura before a seizure, there may be time to protect the mouth.*
- Suction client's mouth and pharynx after the seizure. *Suctioning clears accumulated secretions from the airway.*
- Provide oxygen during and after the seizure. *Hypoxemia develops when the client's diaphragm contracts and breathing is irregular throughout the seizure.*
- Reorient client to the surroundings and provide rest after the seizure. *Commonly, clients are sleepy and confused after a seizure.*
- Check for injuries. *A client who experiences a seizure may have oral injuries or contusions to the skin.*
- Administer prescribed anticonvulsants. *They decrease the excitability of neurons in the brain and reduce the potential for additional seizures.*

Evaluation of Expected Outcomes

Oxygenation is adequate throughout care. Temperature is within normal range, and vital signs are stable. The client reports no pain or headache or relief to within a tolerable level. He or she is protected during seizure activity and receives medications that reduce their recurrence. If increased ICP develops, the nurse follows the care described in Nursing Care Plan 37-1.

ENCEPHALITIS

Encephalitis is an inflammatory process affecting the CNS. It is characterized by swelling of the brain and pathologic changes in both the white and gray matter and surrounding meninges.

Pathophysiology and Etiology

Various causes of encephalitis exist, but the most common include vector-borne viral infections, complications from viral infection such as rubeola (measles), or neurotoxic effects associated with childhood vaccination. Viruses that cause encephalitis include the St. Louis, Western equine, Eastern equine, and West Nile viruses. Ticks or mosquitoes can transmit some of these viruses. Infected birds bitten by the common *Culex* mosquito can transmit West Nile and St. Louis viruses. The virus remains in the mosquito's salivary glands, and the mosquito can inject the virus into humans and animals during blood feeding.

In 2007, there were 3630 cases of West Nile Virus in the United States. Less than 1% of those bitten and infected by a mosquito carrying West Nile virus become severely ill (Centers for Disease Control and Prevention, 2008). Susceptible humans become symptomatic hours to weeks following viral transmission (Wisniewski, 2003). Poisoning by drugs and chemicals, such as lead, arsenic, and carbon monoxide, may closely resemble encephalitis clinically.

Severe, diffuse inflammation of the brain occurs. Nerve cell destruction can be extensive. Cerebral edema, neurologic deficits such as paralysis and speech changes, increased ICP, respiratory failure, seizure disorders, and shock can occur.

Assessment Findings

At the onset of viral encephalitis, symptoms include sudden fever, severe headache, stiff neck, vomiting, and drowsiness. During physical assessment, there may be evidence of insect bites. The client may disclose information about immunization or an activity such as recent camping that suggests possible exposure to mosquitoes, other vectors, or a neurotoxic substance. As the infection worsens, the client may develop tremors, seizures, spastic or flaccid paralysis, irritability, and muscle weakness. Lethargy, delirium, or coma develop. Incontinence and visual disturbances such as photophobia, involuntary eye movements, and double or blurred vision occur.

A lumbar puncture is performed. CSF pressure is elevated, but the fluid is clear. In some types of encephalitis, such as West Nile virus infection, blood or CSF shows a rise in IgM antibodies. Electroencephalography (EEG) reveals slow waveforms. The physician may order other diagnostic tests, such as MRI or CT scan, to rule out other etiologies for the symptoms.

Medical Management

Because no specific antiviral measure has been developed, treatment of viral encephalitis is supportive. The client's symptoms are managed with antipyretics, anticonvulsants, anti-inflammatory drugs, and analgesics.

Nursing Management

The nurse monitors vital signs and LOC frequently and compares findings with previous assessments. If urinary retention or urinary incontinence develops, the nurse consults the physician to discuss whether an indwelling urethral catheter is appropriate. The nurse measures fluid intake and output to detect signs of fluid volume deficit and electrolyte imbalances. He or she assesses bowel elimination to determine if the client needs an enema or a stool softener. For additional nursing management, refer to the Nursing Process for the Client With a Neurologic Infectious or Inflammatory Disorder.

Client and Family Teaching 37-1 lists measures such as reducing potential bites from mosquitoes and controlling the mosquito population that prevent the transmission of West Nile virus and St. Louis encephalitis.

GUILLAIN-BARRÉ SYNDROME

Guillain-Barré syndrome (acute postinfectious polyneuropathy, polyradiculoneuritis) affects the peripheral nerves and

Client and Family Teaching 37-1
Measures to Control Exposure to Mosquitoes

● Pay attention to surveillance reports concerning the incidence of birds infected with West Nile virus or St. Louis virus in your community.
● Avoid being outdoors during peak mosquito-biting times, such as early evening.
● Wear clothing that covers as much skin as possible when outdoors.
● Apply insect repellant containing permethrin or DEET to clothing and exposed skin.
● Repair or replace windows and door screens.
● Place netting around strollers and infant carriers.
● Empty outdoor items frequently that may hold standing water, such as pet dishes, birdbaths, flower pots, and pool covers
● Transport discarded tires to a location for waste management.
● Clear gutters of debris that may obstruct the drainage of rain water.

the spinal nerve roots. Most clients begin to show signs of recovery about 1 month after the progression of symptoms ceases. Recovery may be slow and take 1 year or more. Death can occur from complications of immobility, such as pneumonia and infection.

Pathophysiology and Etiology

Although the exact cause of the disorder is unknown, Guillain-Barré syndrome is believed to be an autoimmune reaction (see Chap. 34) that follows a primary disorder, especially one that is infectious. Many clients have a history of a recent viral infection, particularly of the respiratory tract. Others have a history of recent surgery or recent vaccination for a viral disease such as influenza. The syndrome also occurs in clients with malignant diseases and lupus erythematosus.

Antibodies attack the Schwann cells that make up the insulating myelin sheath surrounding the axons on nerves. The affected nerves become inflamed and edematous. As myelin is destroyed, nerve transmission becomes abnormal. Mild to severe ascending muscle weakness, tingling and numbness, or paralysis develops from the legs upward. Overactivity or underactivity of the sympathetic or parasympathetic nervous system is evidenced by changes in BP as well as in heart rate and rhythm. Eventually, the myelin regenerates, function is restored, and recovery begins in reverse sequence from the upper body downward.

Assessment Findings

Although symptoms vary, weakness, numbness, and tingling in the arms and legs that the client may perceive as painful often are the first symptoms. The weakness is progressive and moves to upper areas of the body and affects the muscles

of respiration. Paralysis may follow muscle weakness. If cranial nerve involvement develops, chewing, talking, and swallowing become difficult.

A lumbar puncture reveals elevated CSF protein levels and pressure. The results of electrophysiologic testing show marked slowing in the conduction of nerve impulses. Additional neurologic tests are performed to rule out other possible CNS disorders with similar symptoms.

Medical Management

Plasmapheresis, removal of plasma from the blood and reinfusion of the cellular components with saline, has been shown to shorten the course of the disease if performed within the first 2 weeks. The administering of intravenous immune globulin known as Gamimune N soon after symptoms manifest may enhance improvement. Otherwise, treatment is primarily supportive. For example, the physician may order gabapentin (Neurontin) or a tricyclic antidepressant such as amitriptyline (Elavil) or a narcotic to relieve discomfort (Miller, 2007). If the respiratory muscles are involved, endotracheal intubation and mechanical ventilation become necessary. Difficulty chewing and swallowing necessitate the administration of IV fluids, gastric tube feedings, or total parenteral nutrition (TPN).

Nursing Management

The nurse observes the client closely for signs of respiratory distress. He or she uses a spirometer to evaluate the client's ventilation capacity. To assess for pneumonia, the nurse checks vital signs and lung sounds frequently.

Because immobility incapacitates the client, the nurse provides meticulous skin care and changes the client's position every 2 hours. He or she helps the client perform range-of-motion (ROM) exercises to prevent muscle atrophy. For further aspects of nursing management, see the Nursing Process for the Client With a Neurologic Infectious or Inflammatory Disorder. See also Nutrition Notes 37-1.

▶ *Stop, Think, and Respond Exercise 37-2*

Which of the infectious and inflammatory disorders of the nervous system that have been discussed is the easiest to prevent?

Nutrition Notes 37-1
The Client with a Neurologic Infectious/Inflammatory Disorder

● Infectious disorders often cause anorexia, altered nutrient metabolism, and a negative nitrogen balance, which may further compromise immune system functioning.
● To promote an adequate intake, small frequent meals of nutrient- and calorie-dense foods are encouraged.
● High-protein liquid supplements can deliver a high nutrient load with a minimum amount of effort.

BRAIN ABSCESS

A brain abscess is a collection of purulent material in the brain. If untreated, it can be fatal.

Pathophysiology and Etiology

A brain abscess occurs from an infection in nearby structures such as the middle ear, sinuses, or teeth, or from an infection in other organs. A brain abscess can develop after intracranial surgery or head trauma. It can be secondary to such disorders as bacterial endocarditis, bacteremia, and pulmonary or abdominal infections.

A brain abscess produces neurologic changes according to its location. Because it occupies space in the cranium, increased ICP can develop. Complications include paralysis, mental deterioration, seizure disorder, and visual disturbances.

Assessment Findings

Manifestations of a brain abscess include signs of increased ICP, fever, headache, and neurologic changes such as paralysis, seizures, muscle weakness, and lethargy.

Laboratory tests show an elevated WBC count. Analysis of CSF obtained by lumbar puncture helps confirm the diagnosis, but this procedure has a risk of herniation of the brain stem. A CT scan, MRI, and skull radiographs are safer techniques for diagnosing and locating the abscess.

Medical and Surgical Management

Antimicrobial therapy begins once the diagnosis is confirmed. A craniotomy, discussed later in this chapter, typically is performed to drain the abscess. Cerebral edema and seizures are treated with drug therapy. Additional treatment includes control of fever, mechanical ventilation, IV fluids, and nutritional support.

Nursing Management

The nurse assesses frequently for altered LOC, changes in sensory and motor functions, and signs of increased ICP. He or she monitors vital signs frequently. The nurse measures fluid intake and output because overhydration can lead to cerebral edema. See the Nursing Process for the Client With a Neurologic Infectious or Inflammatory Disorder for more detailed discussion.

NEUROMUSCULAR DISORDERS

A neuromuscular disorder involves the nervous system and indirectly affects the muscles. Some examples include multiple sclerosis (MS), myasthenia gravis, and amyotrophic lateral sclerosis (ALS)—all of which are chronic and progressively debilitating.

MULTIPLE SCLEROSIS

Multiple sclerosis (MS) is a chronic, progressive disease of the peripheral nerves. Its onset is in young adulthood and early middle age. The incidence is greatest between 20 and 40 years of age, and it affects men and women approximately equally. MS is more common in northern temperate zones than in warm climates.

Pathophysiology and Etiology

The cause of MS is unknown, but it is considered an autoimmune disorder that may be triggered by a genetic susceptibility (Bole, 2007). MS is characterized as a **demyelinating disease** because it causes permanent degeneration and destruction of myelin. Myelin acts as an insulator, enabling nerve impulses to pass along a nerve fiber. Loss of myelin and subsequent degeneration and atrophy of nerve axons interrupt transmission of impulses along these fibers (Fig. 37-6).

Many clients experience gradual and continuous worsening of their symptoms. A few have the disease in a mild form and do not experience increased severity of symptoms. For some, the symptoms subside during early phases of the illness (remission), and the client seems healthy for several months or even years. However, with each reappearance (exacerbation), the symptoms become more severe and last longer. Infections and emotional upsets precipitate exacerbations. Some people live a long time with MS, and survival for 20 years after the diagnosis is not unusual.

As the disease progresses, many complications such as pressure ulcers, cachexia, deformities, and contractures develop. Pneumonia, brought about by limited activity, shallow breathing, and general debility, often is the immediate cause of death.

Assessment Findings

Signs and Symptoms

Many clients first dismiss minor symptoms as a result of fatigue or strain. When they no longer can ignore symptoms, clients with MS report blurred vision, **diplopia** (double

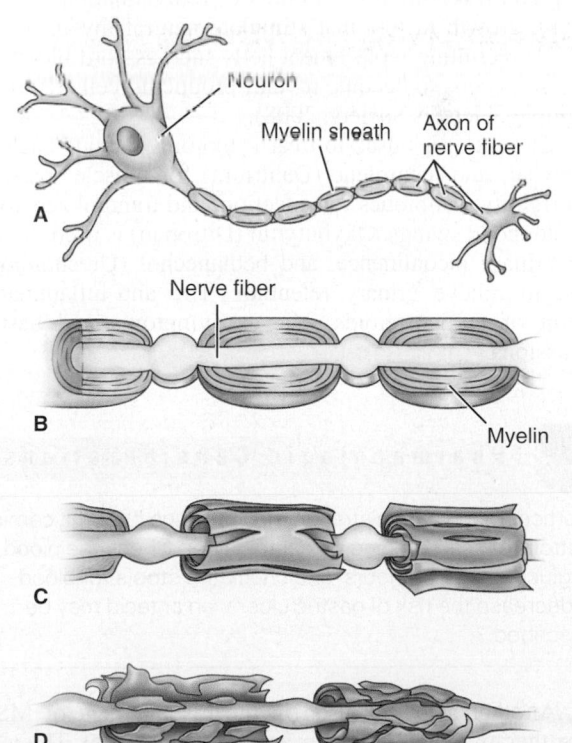

FIGURE 37-6. The process of demyelination. **A** and **B** depict a normal nerve cell and axon with myelin. **C** and **D** show the slow disintegration of myelin, which disrupts axon function.

vision), **nystagmus** (involuntary movement of the eyeball), weakness, clumsiness, and numbness and tingling of an arm or a leg. An intention tremor and slurred, hesitant speech (scanning speech) may develop. Mood swings (emotional lability) are common.

Weakness of an arm or a leg progresses to ataxia (motor incoordination) or paraplegia (paralysis of both legs). Occasional bowel and bladder incontinence leads to total incontinence. Slight visual disturbances end in blindness. The illness impairs intellectual functioning late in its course. Loss of memory, difficulty concentrating, and impaired judgment occur.

Diagnostic Findings

Early diagnosis is difficult because symptoms are vague and in some cases temporary. A lumbar puncture and CSF analysis reveal an increased WBC count. Electrophoresis of the CSF, a technique for electrically separating and identifying proteins, demonstrates abnormal immunoglobulin G bands, described as oligoclonal bands. The bands appear separated rather than homogeneous, which is the normal finding. A CT scan and MRI may or may not disclose lesions in the brain's white matter.

Medical Management

There is no cure for MS, nor is there any single treatment that relieves all symptoms. The primary aim of treatment is to keep the client functional as long as possible. Current research for promoting nerve regeneration exists in four areas: (1) stimulating nearby oligodendrocytes (cells with projections that continue as myelin sheaths) to move to the diseased neurons and replace the damaged myelin, (2) identifying and reversing the inhibitors of remyelination, (3) producing growth factors that stimulate natural myelin repair, and (4) recruiting replacement cells such as cord blood and fetal stem cells to become myelin-producing cells (National Multiple Sclerosis Society, 2008).

Current drugs used to treat symptoms include baclofen (Lioresal) and dantrolene (Dantrium) for muscle spasticity and rigidity, antibiotics for infection, and tranquilizers to alleviate mood swings. Oxybutynin (Ditropan) is used to manage urinary incontinence, and bethanechol (Urecholine) is used to relieve urinary retention. The anti-inflammatory action of corticosteroids relieves symptoms and hastens remissions.

Pharmacologic Considerations

- Corticosteroid administration may produce hyperglycemia, gastrointestinal bleeding, or gastric ulcer. Check the blood for glucose every 4 hours, and check the stools for blood. To decrease the risk of gastric ulcers, an antacid may be prescribed.

Another approach used in the management of MS is drug therapy with glatiramer acetate (Copaxone). This non-interferon/nonsteroidal medication reduces the frequency of exacerbations of MS. Glatiramer changes harmful inflammatory T cells that destroy myelin into protective T cells that suppress myelin depletion. Clients self-administer the drug daily by subcutaneous injection with a prefilled syringe. The drug can produce a brief, mild reaction at the injection site accompanied by flushing, chest tightness, heart palpitations, anxiety, and dyspnea lasting approximately 15 minutes or less.

Nursing Process for the Client with a Neuromuscular Disorder

Assessment

Perform a thorough neurologic assessment. Evaluate pulmonary function, including respiratory rate, depth, and lung sounds, to determine the client's ability to ventilate. To detect early signs of infection, take the client's temperature regularly. Note the client's ability to chew and swallow effectively and observe for drooling, choking when swallowing liquids, and regurgitating fluids through the nose. Assess muscle strength and coordination as well as the client's response to physical activity. Measure intake and output to evaluate fluid status. Monitor the client's elimination patterns. As data accumulate, analyze the trends, using the initial baseline for comparisons. In addition, monitor the client's and caregivers' ability to cope with the progressively debilitating nature of the disorder.

Diagnosis, Planning, and Interventions

▶ **Risk for Ineffective Breathing Pattern** related to weakening of the muscles for respiration

▶ **Expected Outcome:** Ventilation will be sufficient to maintain the SpO$_2$ above 90% and PaO$_2$ above 80 mm Hg.

- Place client in a Fowler's position and support the arms on pillows. *An upright position with the arms supported facilitates maximum chest expansion.*
- Eliminate foods that form intestinal gas or promote the expulsion of gas with a rectal tube. *Intestinal gas rises in the abdomen and places pressure on the diaphragm, which limits the volume of air that the client can inhale.*
- Encourage client to deep breathe several times an hour. *Frequent deep breaths increase tidal volumes, fill alveoli with air, and enhance gas exchange.*
- Notify the physician immediately if the client experiences inadequate ventilation. *Breathing is essential for life; medical interventions may be necessary.*

▶ **Risk for Ineffective Airway Clearance** related to weak or ineffective cough, **Impaired Swallowing**, **Risk for Imbalanced Nutrition: Less than Body Requirements**, and **Risk for Aspiration** related to muscular weakness

▶ **Expected Outcomes:** (1) Airway will be patent. (2) Client will swallow food and fluids without aspiration. (3) Nutritional needs will be met.

- Help client to cough and raise respiratory secretions. *Coughing is a natural protective mechanism for clearing the airway.*
- Suction the oral cavity and airway. *If coughing is ineffective, applying negative pressure with a suction catheter can help clear secretions from the airway.*

Nutrition Notes 37-2
The Client with a Neuromuscular Disorder

● Clients with muscle wasting benefit from an increased protein intake; commercial supplements (e.g., thickened liquids, fortified puddings, fortified gelatins) are tasty and easy options.

● Semisolid foods such as puddings and mashed potatoes are easier to swallow than thin liquids or a regular diet.

● Gastrostomy feedings usually are the best route for clients who require long-term enteral nutritional support.

- Offer liquids frequently in small amounts. *The client may be able to manage small volumes of liquids, but large volumes increase the risk for aspiration.*

- Consult with the dietitian on techniques for modifying the texture and consistency of foods (Nutrition Notes 37-2). *Clients can best swallow smooth foods with texture. Commercial substances are available to thicken liquids to promote swallowing.*

- Provide rest before meals. *The client is more likely to have optimum energy to chew and swallow after rest. Fatigue interferes with attention and coordination.*

- Help client to sit upright when eating. *Sitting is the natural position for eating. It promotes movement of food from the mouth to the esophagus and stomach and reduces the potential for aspiration.*

- Place food in the posterior of the client's mouth. Flex the client's chin toward the chest when swallowing to facilitate passage of food into the esophagus. *Locating food posteriorly facilitates swallowing. Flexing the chin diverts food into the esophagus rather than the airway.*

- Feed client slowly. Wait to place more food in the client's mouth until he or she has swallowed the previous bolus. *Rushing or overloading the client's mouth increases the risk for airway obstruction or aspiration.*

- Consult with the physician about a plan for tube feedings or TPN. *These forms of nourishment may be necessary if oral nutritional intake becomes inadequate or dangerous.*

▶ **Impaired Physical Mobility, Self-Care Deficit** (specify type), and Risk for Impaired Skin Integrity related to diminished muscle strength and inactivity

▶ **Expected Outcomes:** (1) Client will be mobile and use muscles to the maximum extent possible. (2) Basic needs will be met. (3) Skin will remain intact.

- Encourage client to participate in self-care. *Attending to personal needs fosters a positive self-image.*

- Provide rest between bathing, shaving, performing oral care, eating, ambulating, toileting, and participating in diversional activities. *Rest provides time to recover from an activity. It builds stamina and endurance to proceed with additional tasks.*

- Complete whatever tasks the client cannot perform. *The nurse relieves the client of further efforts at self-care when he or she becomes fatigued or weak.*

- Change body position every 2 hours. *Changing position relieves pressure on capillaries that traverse over bony prominences. Relief of pressure reduces the potential for skin breakdown.*

- Perform ROM exercises every 8 hours. *ROM exercises promote joint flexibility and muscle tone. They supplement or complement musculoskeletal activities the client actively performs.*

- Use a foot board and trochanter rolls to promote a neutral body position. *A neutral position keeps the body in good alignment and reduces the potential for contractures.*

- Consult with a physical or occupational therapist on techniques to facilitate client's independence and self-care. *They are experts in maintaining and regaining functional activities.*

- Use pressure-relieving devices when client is in bed or a wheelchair. *Relieving pressure prevents skin breakdown.*

- Keep bed dry and free of wrinkles. *Moisture softens the epidermis, making it vulnerable to breaking down. Wrinkles create pressure that interferes with blood circulation to cells and tissues.*

- Wash and dry the skin well. *Clean, dry skin decreases risk factors that can alter its integrity.*

▶ **Constipation** related to inactivity and abdominal muscle weakness, **Urinary Incontinence** (specify type, such as Total, Functional, or Reflex) related to neuromuscular degeneration

▶ **Expected Outcomes:** (1) Stool will be soft, and bowel elimination will occur at least every 3 days. (2) Urine elimination will be controlled.

- Consult with the physician about a regularly prescribed stool softener, bulk-forming laxative, or suppository. *Medications facilitate bowel elimination through various physical and chemical mechanisms.*

- Include soft fruit or fruit puree in the daily menu. *Fruits are a source of fructose; sugar (fructose) is a natural laxative. Fiber adds bulk to the stool and attracts moisture, making the stool softer and easier to pass.*

- Assist client to move as much as possible. *Activity promotes peristalsis, which propels stool toward the rectum.*

- Place client on a toilet or commode after meals, especially breakfast, or near the time of the client's usual bowel movement. *The gastrocolic reflex is more active after a meal. Most people have a bowel movement at about the same time each day.*

- Help client select clothing that facilitates toileting. *Clients are less likely to be incontinent if they can manipulate clothing to facilitate using a toilet or commode.*

- Assist client to the toilet regularly and frequently. *Clients can maintain continence if they receive some assistance getting to the bathroom and using toilet facilities.*

- Help client use incontinence garments or consult with the physician when client needs an indwelling or external catheter. *When efforts to maintain continence have been exhausted, measures to unobtrusively collect urine can maintain the client's dignity and reduce the potential for skin breakdown.*

▶ **Ineffective Coping** related to feelings of helplessness secondary to chronic illness

▸ **Expected Outcome:** Client will cope effectively with situational stressors.

- Suggest joining a support group of people with a similar disorder or subscribing to the support group's newsletter. *Knowing that others experience similar problems facilitates coping. Clients acquire new coping strategies when others share their problem-solving approaches in person or in written communications.*
- Encourage client to express feelings. *Expressing frustration and other emotions relieves the client's personal emotional burden and fosters support.*
- Provide opportunities in which the client can make choices. *Making choices promotes a feeling of control, which fosters the ability to cope.*
- Facilitate client's network of social support, such as with family, neighbors, coworkers, and church members, through personal visits, telephone conversations, cards, and letters. *A network of supportive others decreases the burden of coping with an illness as an isolated individual.*
- Provide diversional activities that foster feelings of personal accomplishment. *Feeling useful, purposeful, and capable helps a client persevere in coping with adversity.*

▸ **Risk for Caregiver Role Strain** related to unrelenting responsibility for client's care

▸ **Expected Outcome:** Primary caregiver will cope with long-term care of client.

- Listen empathetically while caregiver expresses feelings about caring for the client. *Caregiver is likely to feel less guilty if he or she feels comfortable discussing the stressors involved with someone other than the client or another family member.*
- Help caregiver develop a list of surrogates who may provide regular periods of relief. *The caregiver's dedication will be prolonged if he or she experiences intermittent periods when total responsibility is relieved.*
- Give caregiver permission to meet his or her own needs. *Unless encouraged to do so, caregivers suppress their own needs in deference to those for whom they care.*
- Identify available community resources and offer to facilitate a referral. *The caregiver may be unaware of service organizations whose missions are to provide help and support to clients and caregivers with particular disorders.*

Evaluation of Expected Outcomes

Respirations are of normal rate and depth. The airway is clear, and breathing is effortless. Nutrition is adequate to maintain body weight. The client regains mobility and attends to activities of daily living (ADLs) with minimal or no assistance. Skin is intact with no evidence of breakdown. Bowel elimination is regular; urinary incontinence is minimized or controlled. The client demonstrates effective coping skills. The caregiver continues his or her responsibilities but implements a plan for periodic relief or assistance. •

MYASTHENIA GRAVIS

Myasthenia gravis is a neuromuscular disorder characterized by severe weakness of one or more groups of skeletal muscles. Myasthenia gravis is more common in women, but it can affect both genders. The onset of the illness generally occurs during the young adult years.

Pathophysiology and Etiology

Although its exact cause is unknown, the disease is believed to be autoimmune in nature. It develops when antibodies, perhaps produced by the thymus gland, bind to and degrade acetylcholine receptors on the surface of skeletal muscles (Fig. 37-7). The outcome is extreme muscle weakness during activity. Strength is restored with rest.

Assessment Findings

Muscle weakness varies depending on the muscles affected. The most common manifestations are **ptosis** (drooping) of the eyelids (Fig. 37-8), difficulty chewing and swallowing, diplopia, voice weakness, masklike facial expression, and weakness of the extremities. The respiratory system also is affected. During a myasthenic crisis, the client experiences increased muscle weakness, respiratory distress, decreased tidal volume, and difficulty talking, swallowing, and chewing.

Diagnostic confirmation is made by IV administration of edrophonium (Tensilon), which relieves muscular weakness in a few seconds. The restored muscle strength then dissipates in about 5 minutes. Most manifest an elevated acetylcholine receptor antibody titer. Chest radiography may show an enlargement of the thymus (thymoma). Electromyography measures the electrical potential of muscles.

Medical and Surgical Management

Treatment involves facilitating normal neurotransmission with administration of an anticholinesterase drug, such as

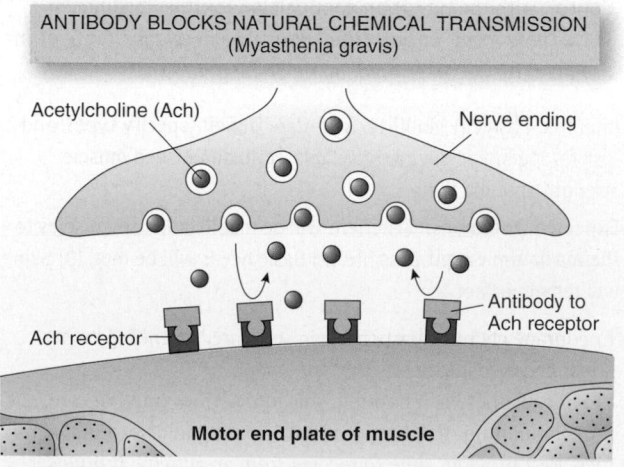

FIGURE 37-7. Inhibition of synaptic transmission of Ach in myasthenia gravis leads to profound muscle weakness. (From Rubin, R., & Strayer, D.S., Eds. [2008]. *Rubin's pathology: Clinicopathologic foundations of medicine.* [5th ed.]. Philadelphia: Lippincott Williams & Wilkins.)

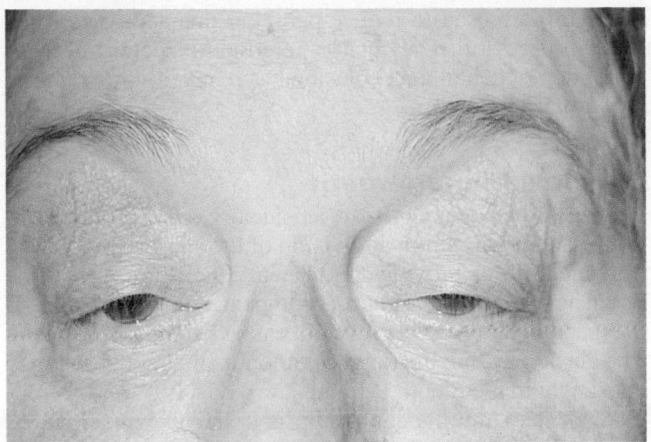

FIGURE 37-8. Ptosis of the eyelids. (From Tasman, W., & Jaeger, E. [2001]. *The Wills Eye Hospital atlas of clinical ophthalmology.* [2nd ed.] Philadelphia: Lippincott Williams & Wilkins.)

pyridostigmine bromide (Mestinon), neostigmine (Prostigmin), or ambenonium chloride (Mytelase). The therapeutic effect prolongs the action of acetylcholine, which sustains muscle contraction. The dose of the drug is adjusted according to the client's response to therapy.

Other treatments include surgical removal of the thymus gland, prednisone or another type of immunosuppressant such as azathioprine (Imuran), and plasmapheresis three times a week for clients who do not respond to other methods of therapy. If myasthenic crisis with severe respiratory distress occurs, the client requires intubation and mechanical ventilation.

Nursing Management

The nurse provides periods of rest for the client to promote restoration of strength. In addition, the nurse supports ventilation by elevating the head of the bed and suctioning secretions that cause difficulty in swallowing for the client. The nurse also makes an effort to understand the client's efforts at communication during periods when the disease compromises intelligible speaking. The nurse demonstrates patience and empathy to help the client deal with his or her change in appearance, function, and life-style. The effects of drug therapy are observed, especially when first initiated or at times of stress. He or she must administer medications at the exact intervals ordered to maintain therapeutic blood levels and prevent symptoms from returning. The nurse observes for signs of drug overdose, such as abdominal cramps, clenched jaws, and muscle rigidity, which indicate that the dose is excessive. For more information, see Nursing Process for the Client With a Neuromuscular Disorder.

AMYOTROPHIC LATERAL SCLEROSIS

Amyotrophic lateral sclerosis (ALS), also known as *Lou Gehrig's disease,* is a progressive and fatal neurologic disorder. The disease is more common in men than in women.

Pathophysiology and Etiology

The cause of ALS is unknown. The disease is characterized by degeneration of the motor neurons of the spinal cord and brain stem, which results in muscle weakness and wasting.

Assessment Findings

Progressive muscle weakness and wasting of the arms, legs, and trunk develop. The client experiences episodes of muscle **fasciculations** (twitching). If ALS affects the brain stem, speaking and swallowing become difficult. The client may display periods of inappropriate laughter and crying. Respiratory failure and total paralysis are seen in the terminal stage.

The disorder is difficult to diagnose in the early stages because no specific diagnostic tests are available for this disease. Electromyography validates weakness in the affected muscles.

Medical Management

There is no specific treatment, and death occurs several years after diagnosis in many cases. The client is encouraged to remain active as long as possible. Death usually results from respiratory arrest or overwhelming respiratory infection. Mechanical ventilation is necessary when ALS affects the muscles of respiration.

A current research study is tracking the effect of the cancer drug tamoxifen on people with ALS. The research commenced after observation that the progression of ALS had slowed in a woman taking tamoxifen for breast cancer. The study hypothesizes that tamoxifen serves as an antagonist of the neurotransmitter glutamate, which is toxic to motor neurons (see the discussion of glutamate and stroke in Chapter 38).

Nursing Management

The nurse performs a comprehensive assessment and develops a plan of care based on the client's identified problems. During the early stages of ALS, the nurse provides assistance with walking, bathing, shaving, and dressing. As ALS progresses, the client becomes totally dependent on the family or healthcare personnel for care. The nurse teaches family members required skills, such as suctioning techniques, how to administer tube feedings, and catheter care. Client and Family Teaching 37-2 provides more information, as does Nursing Process for the Client With a Neuromuscular Disorder. Additional discussion on caring for clients with a neurologic deficit is covered in Chapter 40. Review Chapter 10 for the care of clients in the terminal phase of diseases.

 Client and Family Teaching 37-2
Amyotrophic Lateral Sclerosis

The nurse reviews the following components with the client and family:

● Medication schedule, adverse effects of medications
● Dietary and feeding suggestions
● Agencies that can help with or give home care
● Sources of financial assistance
● Exercises to prevent muscle atrophy
● Positioning and good skin care
● Techniques for preventing skin breakdown

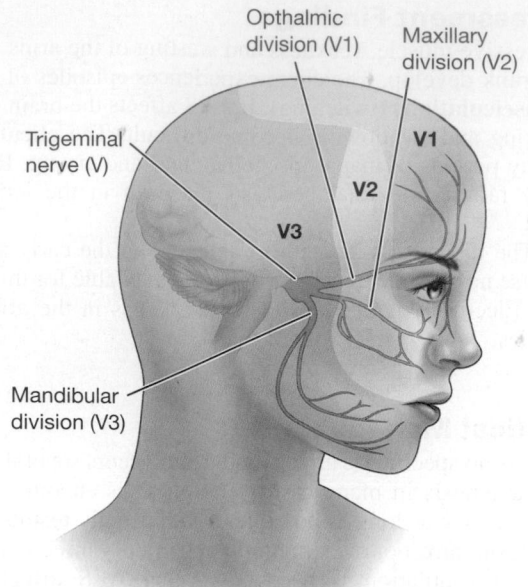

FIGURE 37-9. Areas innervated by the three branches of the trigeminal nerve. These are the areas that become painful in trigeminal neuralgia.

CRANIAL NERVE DISORDERS

TRIGEMINAL NEURALGIA (TIC DOULOUREUX)

Trigeminal neuralgia is a painful condition that involves the fifth (V) cranial nerve (the trigeminal nerve), which has three major branches: mandibular, maxillary, and ophthalmic (Fig. 37-9). This sensory and motor nerve is important to chewing, facial movement, and sensation.

Pathophysiology and Etiology

The cause of the disorder is unknown. It has been suggested that it is related to compression of the trigeminal nerve root. For reasons not fully understood, the client experiences **neuralgia** (nerve pain) in one or more branches of the trigeminal nerve. The slightest stimulus (e.g., vibration of music, passing breeze, temperature change) over trigger points (areas that provoke the pain) can initiate an attack. The forehead over the eyebrow is a common trigger point when the ophthalmic branch of the nerve is affected.

Assessment Findings

The client describes the pain as sudden, severe, and burning. The pain ends as quickly as it begins, usually lasting a few seconds to several minutes. The cycle repeats many times each day. During a spasm, the face twitches and the eyes tear.

Skull radiography, MRI, or CT are performed to rule out other pathologies, such as a brain tumor and intracranial bleeding. Ultimately, the diagnosis is based on the symptoms.

Medical Management

Medical treatment is primarily supportive and symptomatic rather than curative. Narcotic analgesics are necessary. Anticonvulsants such as phenytoin (Dilantin) and carbamazepine (Tegretol) are used to reduce pain, but this approach is not always successful. The client is referred to a dentist because correction of dental malocclusion has relieved some cases of trigeminal neuralgia.

Surgical Management

If medical management is unsatisfactory, surgical intervention is an option. Surgical division of the sensory root of the trigeminal nerve provides permanent relief; however, some permanent loss of sensation accompanies this procedure. If the mandibular branch is severed, eating becomes a problem. The client may bite the tongue without realizing it, food may get caught in the mouth, and the jaw deviates toward the operative side. Until the client adjusts to the altered sensation, swallowing is difficult.

Nursing Process for the Client With Trigeminal Neuralgia

Assessment

Obtain a complete history, and then carefully and gently examine the affected area. Ask the client to identify the location, pattern, and events associated with pain and document the information. Inspect the oral cavity for signs of injury. Weigh the client and assess the client's ability to eat food.

Diagnosis, Planning, and Interventions

▸ Acute Pain related to nerve compression as evidenced by client's description of localized discomfort

▸ Expected Outcome: Pain will be relieved or reduced to a tolerable level.

- Use a scale from 0 to 10 to help client quantify the severity and intensity of pain, both before and after nursing intervention. *Using a scaled range of numbers is the standard for assessing pain. Pain is assessed before and at least 30 minutes after a nursing intervention.*
- Ask at what level the client can tolerate pain. *Pain may not be totally relieved, but asking the client to identify his or her tolerance level provides a realistic goal for achievement.*
- Administer prescribed drugs. *Medications relieve pain by various mechanisms.*
- Observe and record client's response. *If an intervention does not reduce pain to the client's level of tolerance, the nurse pursues additional measures and collaborates with the physician when nursing measures are unsuccessful.*
- Avoid drafts in the room. *Even slight stimulation of the trigeminal nerve can trigger pain.*
- Place a sign on the client's bed stating not to jar the bed or touch client's face in any way. *Sudden, unexpected movement can trigger pain.*
- Advise client to use protective measures such as shielding the face from wind and cold and avoiding shaving and situations or activities that cause pain. *The client can implement life-style changes to reduce or prevent pain from recurring (Client and Family Teaching 37-3).*

Client and Family Teaching 37-3
Trigeminal Neuralgia

The nurse instructs the client as follows:

- Inspect the mouth daily for breaks in the mucous membrane.
- Take small sips or bites of food and concentrate on chewing and swallowing if surgery has been performed.
- Chew on the opposite side.
- Avoid eating hot foods.
- Use mouth rinses after eating.
- Keep regular dental appointments because the warning pain of a cavity, abscess, or other dental problem may be mistaken for neuralgia.

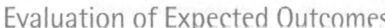

Evaluation of Expected Outcomes

Pain is alleviated or reduced to a level such that the client can continue functioning. The client cooperates with measures to avoid stimuli that trigger episodes of pain.

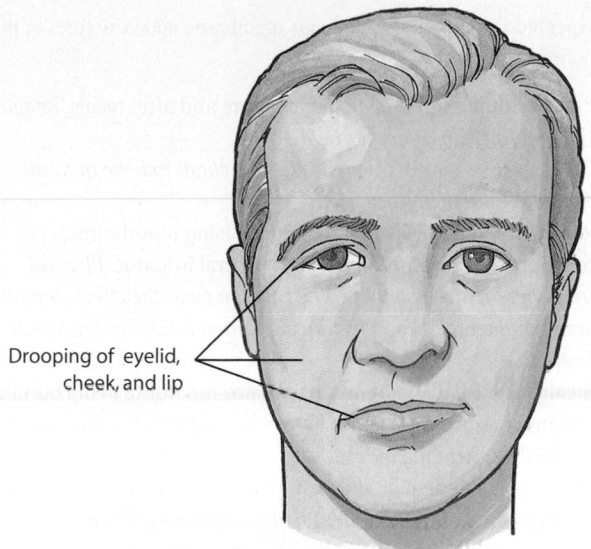

Drooping of eyelid, cheek, and lip

FIGURE 37-10. Weakness or paralysis of facial muscles associated with Bell's palsy results in loss of tone causing the eyelid, cheek, and lip to droop. (From Moore, K.L., & Agur, A. [2006]. *Essential clinical anatomy* [3rd ed.]. Philadelphia: Lippincott Williams & Wilkins.)

BELL'S PALSY

Bell's palsy involves the seventh (VII) cranial nerve, which is responsible for movement of the facial muscles.

Pathophysiology and Etiology

The cause of Bell's palsy is unknown, but a viral link is suspected. Inflammation occurs around the nerve, blocking motor impulses to facial muscles. Inflammation or ischemia resulting from nerve compression leads to impaired nerve function. As a result, there is weakness and paralysis of facial muscles, including the muscles of the eyelids, cheek, and lip on one side of the face (Fig. 37-10). Most clients who recover begin to show improvement in a few weeks. Those whose paralysis is permanent fail to show improvement after 3 months or more.

Assessment Findings

Symptoms develop in a few hours or over 1 to 2 days. Facial pain, pain behind the ear, numbness, diminished blink reflex, ptosis of the eyelid, and tearing on the affected side occur. Speaking and chewing become difficult.

There are no specific diagnostic tests for this disorder; diagnosis is based on symptoms and visual examination of the face. In some instances, it is necessary to rule out other neurologic problems such as brain tumor and stroke, which have comparable symptoms.

Medical Management

Short-term corticosteroid therapy with prednisone (Deltasone, Meticorten) is prescribed to reduce nerve inflammation and edema. Analgesics are prescribed for pain. Electrotherapy or a facial sling helps prevent atrophy of the facial muscles on the affected side. Once the diagnosis is confirmed, the client is assured that a more serious problem (e.g., stroke, tumor) has not occurred.

Nursing Process for the Client with Bell's Palsy

Assessment

Obtain the client's history, noting any recent illness that suggests a viral infection. Perform a physical examination to determine which side of the face is involved and the appearance of affected structures. Note whether the client has any speech impairment and observe the client's ability to chew and swallow food.

Diagnosis, Planning, and Interventions

▶ Risk for (Ophthalmic) Infection related to diminished blink reflex

▶ Expected Outcome: The eye will remain free of infection as evidenced by no redness or purulent drainage.

- Cover the eye with an eye patch. *An eye patch keeps the eyelid closed and protects the eye surface from environmental debris.*
- Apply a protective eye shield at night. *An eye shield ensures that the client does not scratch or injure the eye during sleep.*
- Inspect the eye daily for signs of inflammation and infection. *Early treatment facilitates a quick resolution and minimizes potential impairment of vision.*
- Irrigate the eye with normal saline. *Irrigation flushes debris and microorganisms from the surface and conjunctival folds.*
- Instill prescribed antibiotic ophthalmic ointment. *Antibiotic therapy inhibits the growth of or destroys pathogens.*

▶ Impaired Oral Mucous Membranes related to loss of sensation in the mouth, paralysis of chewing muscles as manifested by trauma to the cheeks, gums, teeth, or tongue

▶ **Expected Outcome:** Oral mucous membrane and structures in the mouth will heal.

• Provide supplies for oral hygiene before and after meals. *Keeping the mouth clean promotes healing.*
• Check client's mouth after eating. *The client may be unaware that oral trauma has occurred.*
• Remove food particles that remain by using mouth rinses, cotton-tipped applicators, or a pulsating oral irrigator. *Physical measures are necessary in some cases to clear the cheek, buccal areas, and teeth of food residue. Retained food interferes with healing.*
• Ensure that food and beverages are not too hot to avoid burning oral mucous membranes. *Extremes in temperatures contribute to thermal injury in the mouth.*
• Encourage biannual dental examinations. *A client with residual paralysis requires regular dental examinations and care to ensure optimum oral health.*

▶ **Impaired Verbal Communication** related to hemiparalysis of facial muscles and pain

▶ **Expected Outcome:** Client will communicate verbally and understandably.

• Instruct client to speak slowly and in short sentences. *Slowing the rate of speech enables the client to coordinate the use of his or her teeth, tongue, and lips while speaking.*
• Provide a pad of paper and a pencil to facilitate communication during severe pain. *Written communication is an acceptable substitute for temporarily impaired oral communication.*

Evaluation of Expected Outcomes

The client understands the techniques for instilling ophthalmic ointment and applying an eye patch and eye shield. The affected eye appears similar to the unaffected eye; there is no redness, swelling of orbital tissue, or drainage that suggests an infection. Vision in the affected eye remains unaffected. The client's mouth is free of retained debris. The soft tissue structures in the mouth are pink, moist, and intact. Teeth are in good repair. The client satisfactorily communicates with spoken words. ●

EXTRAPYRAMIDAL DISORDERS

Extrapyramidal disorders have their origin in the motor cortex and surrounding areas of the cerebellum and basal ganglia. Two common extrapyramidal disorders are Parkinson's disease and Huntington's disease. One of their primary characteristics is abnormal movement.

PARKINSON'S DISEASE

Parkinson's disease usually begins after 50 years of age. It primarily affects the basal ganglia and connections in the substantia nigra and corpus striatum (Fig. 37-11). The term **parkinsonism** is used to describe the cluster of Parkinson's-like symptoms that develop from several etiologies.

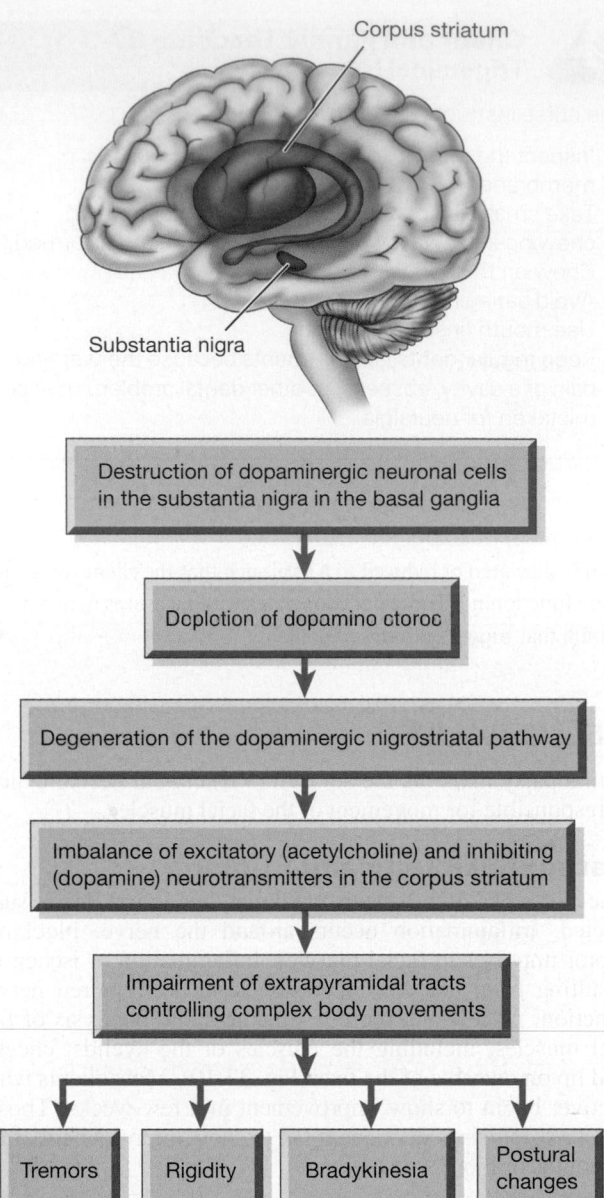

FIGURE 37-11. Nuclei in the substantia nigra protect fibers to the corpus striatum, where the nerve fibers carry dopamine. Loss of dopamine from nerve cells is thought to cause symptoms of Parkinson's disease. (From Smeltzer, S. C., et al. [2008]. *Brunner & Suddarth's textbook of medical–surgical nursing* [11th ed.]. Philadelphia: Lippincott Williams & Wilkins.)

Pathophysiology and Etiology

Parkinson's disease and parkinsonism result from a deficiency of the neurotransmitter dopamine. In the absence of dopamine, another area of the brain, known as the globus pallidus, which responds to acetylcholine, becomes overactive. The imbalance between dopamine and acetylcholine results in a movement disorder that characterizes Parkinson's disease.

In most cases of Parkinson's disease, no cause can be found for dopamine depletion. The symptoms of parkinsonism are associated with exposure to environmental toxins such as insecticides and herbicides and self-administration of an illegal synthetic form of heroin known as MPTP; symptoms also can occur as sequelae of head injuries and encephalitis. Phenothiazine, a category of antipsychotic drugs and other dopamine receptor-blocking antipsychotic drugs used to treat schizophrenia, also produce parkinsonism, but the symptoms are reversible when the drug is discontinued.

Manifestations of the disorder progress so slowly that years may elapse between the first symptom and diagnosis. The symptoms initially are unilateral, but eventually, whether quickly or slowly, become bilateral.

Assessment Findings

Signs and Symptoms

Early signs include stiffness, referred to as *rigidity*, and tremors of one or both hands, described as *pill-rolling* (a rhythmic motion of the thumb against the fingers). The hand tremor is obvious at rest and typically decreases when movement is voluntary, such as picking up an object.

Bradykinesia, slowness in performing spontaneous movements, develops. Clients have a masklike expression, stooped posture, hypophonia (low volume of speech), and difficulty swallowing saliva and food. Weight loss occurs (Nutrition Notes 37-3). A shuffling gait is apparent, and the client has difficulty turning or redirecting forward motion. Arms are rigid while walking (Fig. 37-12).

In late stages, the disease affects the jaw, tongue, and larynx; speech is slurred; and chewing and swallowing become difficult. Rigidity can lead to contractures. Salivation increases, accompanied by drooling. In a small percentage of clients, the eyes roll upward or downward and stay there involuntarily (oculogyric crises) for several hours or even a few days.

Diagnostic Findings

Diagnosis is based on typical symptoms and a neurologic examination. There are no specific tests for this disorder.

Nutrition Notes 37-3
The Client with Parkinson's Disease

● Unintentional weight loss is a common occurrence and may increase the risk for morbidity and mortality. Weight loss may be due to increased energy expenditure related to tremor; impaired intake related to diminished sense of smell, dysphagia, or depression; or from medication side effects such as dry mouth, nausea, anorexia, fatigue, or anxiety. Strategies to prevent or treat unintentional weight loss may include small frequent meals, providing semi-solid foods to facilitate swallowing; and increasing the calorie density of foods served by added sauces, gravies, etc.

● Foods high in fiber, such as crushed bran added to hot cereal and fiber-fortified supplements, help prevent constipation when consumed with adequate fluids. Prunes and prune juice stimulate peristalsis.

● Clients taking levodopa should avoid high intake of protein (meat, fish, poultry, and dairy foods) because protein decreases its effectiveness. However, a high-protein diet may be needed for clients who experience unintentional weight loss.

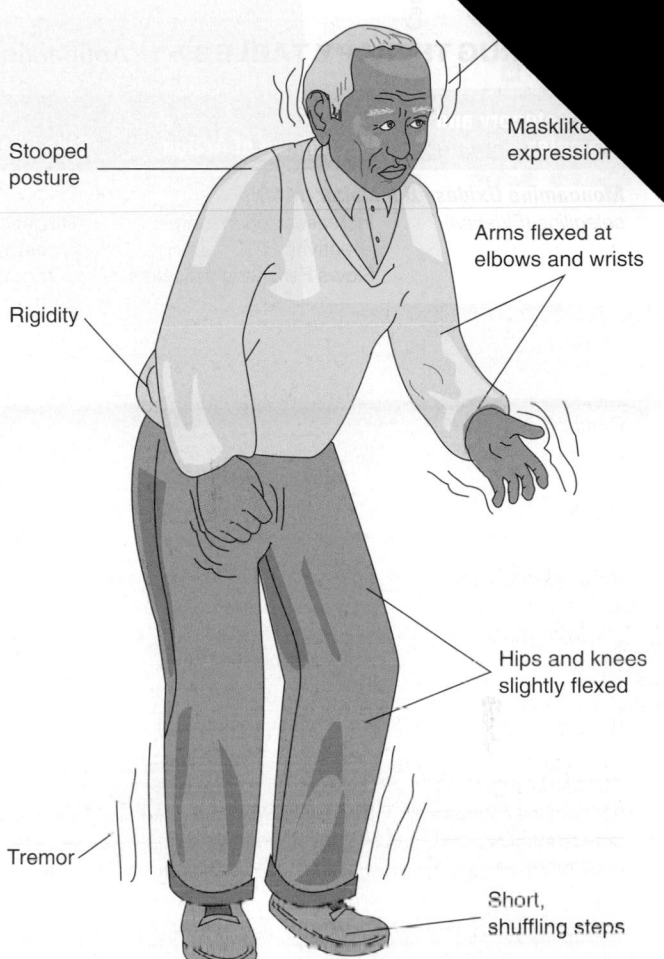

FIGURE 37-12. Typical manifestations of Parkinson's disease.

Medical Management

Treatment aims at prolonging independence. Drugs such as selegiline (Eldepryl), which has neuroprotective properties; dopaminergics such as levodopa (Larodopa) or levodopa-carbidopa (Sinemet); amantadine (Symmetrel); dopamine agonists such as bromocriptine (Parlodel); apomorphine (Apokyn), the newest approved drug; and anticholinergics such as benztropine (Cogentin) are prescribed (Drug Therapy Table 37-1). Their sequence of use is based on the stage of the disorder and the decreasing effectiveness of the medication initially prescribed. Rehabilitation measures, such as physical therapy, occupational therapy, client and family education, and counseling, are used concurrently with drug therapy.

Surgical Management

Stereotaxic pallidotomy is a surgical procedure performed in selected cases (Fig. 37-13). The procedure destroys a part of the globus pallidus to eliminate or reduce tremor, stooped posture, shuffling gait, and stiff movement.

Some clients with Parkinson's disease have obtained relief of symptoms through deep brain stimulation (DBS). DBS involves the implantation of a neurostimulator that works like a pacemaker for the brain (Fig. 37-14). The

TABLE 37-1 Antiparkinson Agents

	Mechanism of Action	Side Effects	Nursing Considerations
(MAOI)	...es dopaminergic ...ty ...arkinson's disease	Dizziness, light-headedness, confusion, nausea, vomiting, diarrhea, dry mouth, palpitations	Never give narcotic analgesics with an MAOI. Administer twice daily with breakfast and lunch. Use ice chips and sugarless candy for dry mouth.
Dopaminergics levodopa (Larodopa, Sinemet)	Dopamine replacement to decrease symptoms	Nausea, vomiting, orthostatic hypotension, dry mouth, constipation, dizziness, cardiac dysrhythmias, sleep disturbance	Do not give with MAOIs. Give with meals. Avoid multivitamins with pyridoxine.
Antiparkinsonism amantadine (Symmetrel)	May increase dopamine release to relieve symptoms	Mood changes, drowsiness, blurred vision, insomnia, nausea, orthostatic hypotension, urinary retention	Do not discontinue abruptly to avoid parkinsonian crisis. Report swelling of fingers, ankles, shortness of breath, difficulty urinating, tremors, slurred speech.
Anticholinergics benztropine (Cogentin), trihexyphenidyl (Artane)	Decrease rigidity, slowed movement (akinesia), tremor, and drooling	Dry mouth, constipation, urinary retention, blurred vision, skin rash, flushing, increased temperature, decreased sweating	Decrease or discontinue dosage if dry mouth interferes with eating. Client must use caution in hot weather. Give with meals. Avoid alcohol and sedatives.
Dopamine Agonists bromocriptine (Parlodel)	Mimics effects of dopamine; may be effective when levodopa has decreased efficacy	Hallucinations, confusion, dizziness, drowsiness, nausea, vomiting, constipation, hypotension, shortness of breath	Give with food. Taper dosage before discontinuing. Monitor mental status.
apomorphine (Apokyn)	Relieves episodes of hypomobility when standard drugs wear off	Nausea, vomiting, hypotension, fainting, hallucinations, excessive sleepiness	Administer by injection with a dosing pen. Must be taken with an antiemetic other than a serotonin antagonist.

neurostimulator sends electrical impulses from a battery implanted under the skin near the clavicle to the globus pallidus, thalamus, or subthalamic nucleus. The electrical stimulus blocks abnormal nerve signals that cause the parkinsonian tremor. DBS eliminates the tremor in approximately 65% of people who have an implanted stimulator. Current research is attempting to produce a similar effect by attaching electrodes to the surface of the brain rather than by implanting a stimulator within the brain.

Many areas of research are being conducted to find additional methods for managing Parkinson's disease. Dopamine-secreting brain cells from pigs have been transplanted into people with Parkinson's disease with some success. However, there is some fear that viruses unique to pigs could jump species and infect humans, similar to the manner in which the human immunodeficiency virus (HIV) transferred from primates to humans. Consequently, this approach to treatment is not actively pursued. Some success has been reported outside the United States with human fetal tissue transplantation, in which brain tissue containing the basal ganglia and dopamine-secreting cells is extracted from an aborted fetus and transplanted into the recipient's brain. This procedure is considered unethical and currently is not approved in the United States. However, the transplantation of retinal pigment epithelial cells shows promise. Preliminary research indicates that these cells have produced and released dopamine, and improved motor symptoms have been sustained for 24 months (Stover et al., 2005). Autotransplantation of cells from a person's own adrenal medulla into the brain also has been used with limited success. There is current interest in transplanting human stem cells as a means of curing Parkinson's disease, but this is only in early experimental stages. Cell transplantation requires craniotomy.

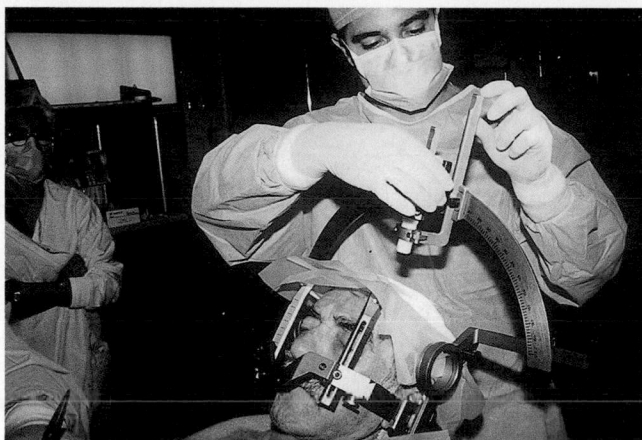

FIGURE 37-13. Client being prepared for pallidotomy. (From Smeltzer, S.C., et al. [2008]. *Brunner & Suddarth's textbook of medical–surgical nursing* [11th ed.]. Philadelphia: Lippincott Williams & Wilkins.)

Gene therapy is still highly experimental. Currently, there are efforts to manipulate a gene for glutamic acid de-carboxylase (GAD). This enzyme is key in the production of the inhibitory neurotransmitter gamma aminobutyric acid (GABA). Researchers think that increasing GABA may inhibit the neurostimulating effects from the globus pallidus similar to the effect achieved with the deep brain stimulator.

Still another research approach for Parkinson's disease is to enhance glial cell–derived neurotrophic factor (GDNF). This substance stimulates growth of dopamine-producing neurons. Finding a technique that improves the delivery of GDNF to the specific target areas in the brain has been the main obstacle of this project.

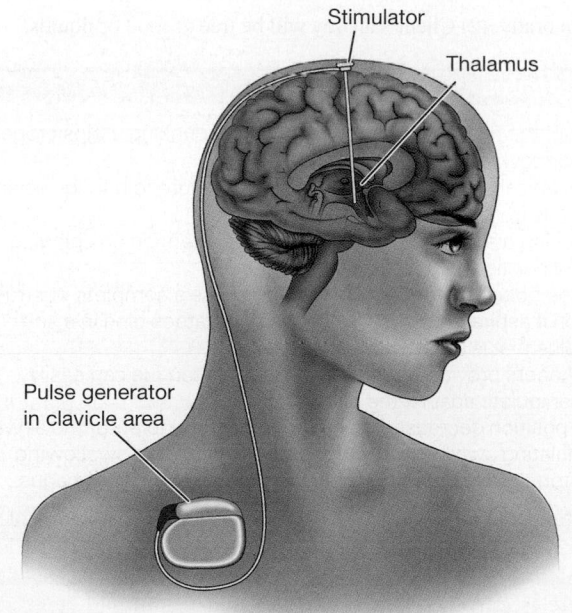

Stimulator

Thalamus

Pulse generator in clavicle area

FIGURE 37-14. Deep brain stimulation with the use of a pulse generator.

Nursing Management

Clients with parkinsonism are admitted to the hospital because of the debilitating effects of the disease. Others are cared for in extended care facilities when they can no longer be managed at home in a chronic state. One of the biggest nursing challenges is managing the client's drug therapy. Levodopa is associated with periods of "breakthrough" or "end-of-dose wearing off" in which symptoms are exacerbated when a consistent level is not maintained. The nurse must administer the drugs closely to the schedule the client previously established at home. Over time, clients may decreasingly respond to their standard drug therapy and have more frequent "off episodes" of hypomobility in which they may be unable to rise from a chair, speak or walk. The drug apomorphine (Apokyn), which was recently approved for these episodes, promises help in relieving this phenomenon. Drugs administered for parkinsonism can cause a wide variety of adverse effects, which requires careful observation of the client. Nursing Care Plan 37-2 provides more discussion of management of the client with an extrapyramidal disorder such as Parkinson's disease or Huntington's disease.

The nurse works with physical and occupational therapists to increase the client's level of activity, optimize his or her gait, improve balance and coordination, and use adaptive equipment to perform activities of daily living.

Gerontologic Considerations

Older adults with Parkinson's disease are more susceptible to the complications of prolonged bed rest and immobility. These clients should be observed closely for such problems as hypostatic pneumonia, pressure ulcers, contractures, and deformities.

- Physical/occupational therapy goals are individualized and may focus on maintaining comfort or function rather than achieving rehabilitation. Techniques can be taught to compensate for embarrassing or disabling symptoms such as shuffling, freezing gait, nuchal rigidity, and lack of control of swallowing to enable the older person maintain self-esteem and social interactions.

HUNTINGTON'S DISEASE

Huntington's disease (Huntington's chorea, hereditary chorea) is a hereditary disorder of the CNS.

Pathophysiology and Etiology

Huntington's chorea is an extrapyramidal disorder that is transmitted genetically and inherited by people of both genders. The basal ganglia and portions of the cerebral cortex degenerate. In the early stages, clients can participate in most physical activities. However, as the disease progresses, hallucinations, delusions, impaired judgment, and increased intensity of abnormal movements develop.

NURSING CARE PLAN 37-2 | The Client with an Extrapyramidal Disorder

Assessment

Determine the following:

- Year of current diagnosis
- Concurrent medical disorders
- Weight and vital signs
- Any unilateral or bilateral hand tremor
- Gait and balance

- Use of assistive ambulatory devices
- Ability to swallow
- Quality of speech
- Bowel and urinary elimination patterns
- Mental and emotional status
- Drug therapy, time and frequency of medication administration

Nursing Diagnoses. Impaired Physical Mobility and **Self-Care Deficit** (specify type) related to muscle rigidity, tremors, choreiform movements, and dementia as evidenced by inability to complete all or some activities of daily living (ADLs)

Expected Outcomes. (1) Client will be physically active. (2) Client will perform self-care to the level at which he or she is capable.

Interventions	Rationales
Assist client with walking and physical activities.	Client is at risk for falls and injuries if activities are not assisted or supervised.
Increase the type and amount of activity gradually.	Client will have more strength and coordination once response to medications has improved.
Minimize fatigue by providing rest periods.	Rest relieves fatigue and restores stamina and endurance.
Promote involvement in self-care activities within the client's individual capacity.	Matching self-care involvement to client's functional level promotes dignity and improves self-image.
Allow ample time to perform ADLs.	Given sufficient time, client is more likely to pace himself or herself to complete ADLs semi-independently.
Modify clothing and self-care supplies to promote independence.	Clothing that is easily put on and taken off and aids for holding a toothbrush, fork, and so forth, facilitate ability to perform self-care.
Assist client, but only when client cannot perform certain tasks.	Too much assistance cultivates dependence on the nurse.

Evaluation of Expected Outcomes

- Client is active in his or her immediate environment and uses assistive devices as necessary.
- Client attends to self-care as much as symptoms allow.

Nursing Diagnoses. Impaired Swallowing and **Risk for Aspiration**

Expected Outcomes. (1) Client will swallow food and liquids taken in orally. (2) Client's airway will be free of food or liquids.

Interventions	Rationales
Place client in a sitting position.	Sitting, the natural position for eating and drinking, helps propel food toward the stomach.
Keep suction equipment at the bedside; use it when the client chokes.	Mechanical suctioning uses negative pressure to pull liquids and solids from the airway.
Decrease environmental distractions.	Reducing distractions helps client focus attention on chewing and swallowing.
Cut food into small pieces. Incorporate mashed potatoes or other pasty foods.	A large bolus of food is more likely to cause a complete obstruction if aspirated. Foods like mashed potatoes bind in a soft bolus that is swallowed more easily.
Thicken liquids with gelatin, cornstarch, applesauce, mashed bananas, ice cream, or a commercial thickener.	Thickeners provide a consistency that the tongue can easily manipulate against the palate.
Position client's chin on the chest during swallowing.	This position decreases the potential for food to enter the airway.
Stroke client's throat as he or she swallows or instruct client to swallow several times in a row.	Stimulating swallowing with stroking or repeated swallowing efforts moves food from the oropharynx to the esophagus.

Evaluation of Expected Outcomes

- Client can swallow food and fluids without choking.
- Client's lungs remain clear of food and liquids.

Nursing Diagnosis. Impaired Verbal Communication related to soft voice or inability to articulate words.

Expected Outcome. Client will communicate needs, feelings, and ideas.

NURSING CARE PLAN 37-2 **The Client With an Extrapyramidal Disorder** (Continued)

Interventions	Rationales
Reduce environmental noise.	A quiet environment helps others hear what the client says.
Listen closely to what the client tries to say.	Attention and patience facilitate understanding.
Ask client to speak slowly.	Altering the rate of speech improves clarity.
Anticipate client's needs.	Doing so reduces client's frustration with having to ask for help.

Evaluation of Expected Outcome

Client's verbalizations are heard and understood.

Nursing Diagnoses. Anxiety and **Ineffective Coping** related to awareness of diminished physical and mental capacities as manifested by periods of agitation, frustration, emotional irritability, and anger

Expected Outcomes. (1) Client will relax and feel secure. (2) Client will accept the gradual loss of physical or mental attributes and will allow others to help without opposition.

Interventions	Rationales
Help client to realistically determine tasks that are feasible and those that are not.	A sense of control reduces anxiety.
Suggest taking a break when the client cannot accomplish an activity.	A break can help the client to regather physical and emotional resources to complete the task successfully.
Offer support and encouragement when client succeeds.	Deserved praise elevates self-esteem and encourages client to persevere.
Help client focus on remaining strengths rather than deficits	Focusing on strengths promotes a more positive attitude
Provide information about support groups whose mission is to provide assistance to clients with similar problems.	Clients are more likely to cope when they have an available network of support.

Evaluation of Expected Outcomes

- Client feels relaxed and in control.
- Client implements strategies that facilitate coping with his or her disability.

Nursing Diagnosis. Risk for Loneliness related to depression and perceived potential for rejection secondary to altered physical appearance or cognitive function

Expected Outcome. Client will maintain social contacts.

Interventions	Rationales
Have client identify persons whose company he or she enjoys and activities they share.	Naming or listing specific people reinforces that the client has a circle of friends.
Encourage client to interact with a few of the designated people for short periods in a place where the client feels secure and comfortable, such as his or her home.	Taking the initiative for contacting friends promotes reestablishing social relationships. Visiting at home shields the client from potential unwanted attention from strangers.
Encourage client to participate in social activities outside the home.	When the client feels more accepted, he or she may extend socialization beyond the home.
Refer client to and encourage joining a support group.	Such groups promote bonding with new acquaintances.

Evaluation of Expected Outcome

Client reestablishes social contacts with previous friends and develops friendships with new acquaintances.

Assessment Findings

Symptoms develop slowly and include mental apathy and emotional disturbances, **choreiform movements** (uncontrollable writhing and twisting of the body), grimacing, difficulty chewing and swallowing, speech difficulty, intellectual decline, and loss of bowel and bladder control. Severe depression is common and can lead to suicide.

Diagnosis is based on symptoms as well as a family history of the disorder. Positron emission tomography (PET)

shows CNS changes, but there is no specific diagnostic test for the disorder. Genetic testing can predict which family members will develop the disease, but not all blood relatives choose to undergo testing.

Medical Management

Treatment is supportive because there is no specific therapy or cure. Tranquilizers and antiparkinson drugs relieve the choreiform movements in some clients. No drugs are available to halt the mental deterioration. Because this disorder is inherited, genetic counseling before a pregnancy is advised.

Nursing Management

Nursing management aims at meeting client and family needs, such as preventing complications as well as encouraging counseling. The stage of the disease determines the scope of nursing care. The client eventually becomes totally dependent on others. Pneumonia, contractures, infections, aspiration of food or fluids, falls, and pressure ulcers are complications. The nurse prevents them by assessing the client frequently and updating the plan of care (see Nursing Care Plan 37-2).

The nurse encourages the client to lead as normal a life as possible. He or she emphasizes the importance of exercise and self-care and explains the medical regimen to the client and family. The nurse demonstrates how to facilitate tasks such as using both hands to hold a drinking glass, using a straw to drink, and wearing slip-on shoes.

SEIZURE DISORDERS

The terms *seizure disorder* and *convulsive disorder* are used interchangeably, but they are not necessarily synonymous. A **seizure** is a brief episode of abnormal electrical activity in the brain. A **convulsion,**, one manifestation of a seizure, is characterized by spasmodic contractions of muscles. **Epilepsy** is a chronic recurrent pattern of seizures.

Pathophysiology and Etiology

Seizure disorders are classified as idiopathic (no known cause) or acquired. Causes of acquired seizures include high fever, electrolyte imbalances, uremia, hypoglycemia, hypoxia, brain tumor, drug abuse, and alcohol withdrawal. Once the cause is removed, the seizures cease. The known causes of epilepsy include brain injury at birth, head injuries, and inborn errors of metabolism. In some clients, the cause of epilepsy is never determined.

Seizures represent abnormal motor, sensory, or psychic neural activity. The abnormal neural activity occurs alone or in combination from discharges in one or more specific areas of the cerebral cortex. Each type of seizure disorder is characterized by a specific pattern of events (Box 37-2).

Types of Seizures

Seizures are divided into two general categories: partial and generalized.

Partial Seizures

Partial, or focal, seizures begin in a specific area of the cerebral cortex. They can progress to generalized seizures. The two subcategories of partial seizures are those with elementary (or simple) symptoms and those with complex symptoms. A client who has a partial seizure with elementary symptoms usually does not lose consciousness, and the seizure lasts less than 1 minute. Partial elementary seizures with motor symptoms are accompanied by uncontrolled jerking movements of a body part, such as a finger, mouth, hand, or foot. Partial elementary seizures with sensory symptoms are

---

BOX 37-2 | **International Classification of Seizures**

I. **Partial (Focal) Seizures**
   A. Partial seizures (no loss of consciousness)
      1. Motor symptoms
      2. Special sensory symptoms
      3. Autonomic symptoms
      4. Psychic symptoms
   B. Complex partial seizures (with loss of consciousness)
      1. Begins as a partial seizure and progresses to complex partial with loss of consciousness.
      2. Loss of consciousness at onset of seizure
II. **Generalized Seizures**
   A. Absence seizures
   B. Myoclonic seizures
   C. Clonic seizures
   D. Tonic seizures
   E. Tonic-clonic seizures
   F. Atonic seizures
III. **Unclassified Seizures**
   All seizures that do not fit into other classifications

---

accompanied by hallucinatory sights, sounds, and odors; mumbling; and the use of nonsense words. The terms *jacksonian, focal motor,* and *focal sensory* describe partial elementary seizures.

A client who has a partial seizure with complex symptoms may have several sensory or motor manifestations, which also last less than 1 minute. After the seizure, the client often is confused. Complex partial seizures are manifested by automatic repetitive movements (**automatisms**) that are not appropriate, such as lip smacking and picking at clothing or objects. The terms *psychomotor* and *psychosensory* are used to describe complex partial seizures.

Generalized Seizures

Generalized seizures involve the entire brain. The client loses consciousness, and the seizure may last from several seconds to several minutes. Types of generalized seizures include absence seizures, myoclonic seizures, and tonic-clonic seizures.

Absence Seizures

Absence seizures, formerly referred to as *petit mal seizures,* are more common in children. They are characterized by a brief loss of consciousness, during which physical activity ceases. The person stares blankly; the eyelids flutter; the lips move; and slight movement of the head, arms, and legs occurs. These seizures typically last for a few seconds, and the person seldom falls to the ground. Because of their brief duration and relative lack of prominent movements, these seizures often go unnoticed. People with absence seizures can have them many times a day.

Myoclonic Seizures

These seizures are characterized by sudden, excessive jerking of the arms, legs, or entire body. In some instances, the muscle activity is so severe that the client falls to the ground. These seizures are brief.

Tonic-Clonic Seizures

Formerly referred to as *grand mal seizures,* tonic-clonic seizures are characterized by a sequence of events that begins with a preictal (or prodromal) phase. The **preictal phase** is the time immediately before a seizure and consists of vague emotional changes, such as depression, anxiety, and nervousness. This phase lasts for minutes or hours and is followed by an **aura,** a sensation that occurs immediately before the seizure. The aura is sensory (i.e., a hallucinatory odor or sound) or a sensation of weakness or numbness. In clients who experience an aura, the aura almost always is the same.

The aura is followed by the epileptic cry, which is caused by spasm of the respiratory muscles and muscles of the throat and glottis. This cry immediately precedes loss of consciousness and the ensuing tonic and clonic phases of the seizure. In the tonic phase, the muscles contract rigidly; in the clonic phase, the muscles alternate between contraction and relaxation, resulting in jerking movements and thrashing of the arms and legs. The skin becomes cyanotic, and breathing is spasmodic. Saliva mixes with air, resulting in frothing at the mouth. The jaws are tightly clenched, and biting of the tongue and inner cheek occurs. Urinary or fecal incontinence is common. The clonic phase lasts for 1 minute or more, gradually subsides, and is followed by the postictal phase. The manifestations of this phase include headache, fatigue, deep sleep, confusion, nausea, and muscle soreness. Many people fall into a deep sleep for several hours.

Status epilepticus is marked by a series of tonic-clonic seizures in which the client does not regain consciousness between seizures. If this extremely dangerous condition is not terminated, death can occur. Status epilepticus occurs spontaneously in acute neurologic disorders or for no known reason; it can be precipitated by the abrupt discontinuation of anticonvulsant medication. Because of this, anticonvulsants must be withdrawn gradually.

Other Seizure Types

Atonic (loss of muscle tone) seizures affect the muscles. The person loses consciousness briefly and falls to the ground. Recovery is rapid. An akinetic (loss of movement) seizure is similar because muscle tone is lost briefly. The client may or may not fall, and recovery is rapid.

Assessment Findings

The client's motor, sensory, and neurologic functions are normal except at the time of a seizure. Identification of seizure activity and type of seizure often depends on a witness's description of the client's actions during the seizure.

A neurologic examination and EEG are performed. Other laboratory or diagnostic studies, such as a CT scan, MRI, serology, and serum electrolyte levels, are used to confirm the diagnosis and to determine the cause of the seizure disorder. When epilepsy is suspected, a series of EEGs is required if the first results are normal.

Medical Management

Once a diagnosis of a seizure disorder is confirmed, one or more anticonvulsant drugs are used to control the seizures. Examples of anticonvulsants are phenytoin (Dilantin), phenobarbital, carbamazepine (Tegretol), ethosuximide (Zarontin), valproic acid (Depakene), felbamate (Felbatol), and fosphenytoin injection (Cerebyx) (Drug Therapy Table 37-2). IV barbiturates or diazepam (Valium) are administered to terminate status epilepticus.

Drug therapy controls the seizures or reduces their frequency or severity. The dose is adjusted over a period of several weeks. The drug is changed or another drug is added to the regimen to obtain optimum control. Blood levels of some anticonvulsant drugs are monitored for accurate dose adjustment and to prevent toxicity (Table 37-1). Serum levels also identify clients who are not taking the drug as ordered.

 Pharmacologic Considerations

- Carbamazepine is taken with meals. The dose is gradually increased until relief is obtained. The effectiveness of carbamazepine may decrease over time.

- Phenytoin requires periodic laboratory evaluation to detect bone marrow depression. This drug also has been implicated in birth defects; therefore, pregnant women or those planning to become pregnant should not take it.

- Clients taking anticonvulsant therapy should carry a MedicAlert bracelet identifying the current medications and disease condition.

Surgical Management

Seizures that are caused by brain tumor, brain abscess, or other disorders often require surgical intervention. Surgery for epilepsy is not considered unless the client does not respond to drug therapy and seizures are frequent and severe. The area of the brain in which abnormal electrical discharges are present is identified (mapped). The surgeon must consider whether removal of the involved area would result in permanent neurologic dysfunction such as paralysis or loss of speech.

Nursing Management

The nurse asks if the client has a history of seizures, the type and pattern of the client's seizure activity, and the current treatment regimen. If the client has no history of seizure, the nurse identifies clients who may be seizure prone. For example, a person who has a high fever, has suffered a recent head injury, is withdrawing from alcohol, or is experiencing hypoglycemia or hypoxia is at risk for having a seizure. The nurse modifies the environment to promote safety if a seizure should occur by placing suction, oral airway, and oxygen equipment at the bedside; padding the side rails and head board; and maintaining the bed in a low position. Prescribed anticonvulsant therapy is administered, and the nurse reinforces the importance of drug compliance following discharge. Nutrition Notes 37-4 provides additional information.

DRUG THERAPY TABLE 37-2 Agents to Control Seizures

Drug Category and Examples	Mechanism of Action	Side Effects	Nursing Considerations
Anticonvulsants phenytoin (Dilantin)	Stabilizes neuronal membranes Limits spread of seizure activity Controls tonic-clonic seizures	Nystagmus, rash, sedation, gingival hyperplasia, liver toxicity, pancytopenia	Evaluate regular serum levels. Evaluate liver function tests, complete blood count and differential. Assess skin daily. Give oral dose with food. Taper dose gradually; never discontinue abruptly. Instruct client to wear MedicAlert bracelet and have regular dental care.
carbamazepine (Tegretol)	Controls partial seizures with complex symptoms, also grand mal seizures	Dizziness, ataxia, nystagmus, rash, nausea, vomiting, liver toxicity, bone marrow suppression	Same as above
ethosuximide (Zarontin)	Reduces frequency of absence (petit mal) seizures	Drowsiness, rash, headache, nausea and vomiting	Same as above
valproic acid (Depakene, Depakote)	Adjunct treatment for multiple seizure types	Nausea and vomiting, drowsiness, diarrhea, liver toxicity	Avoid alcohol intake. Monitor bruising, bleeding gums. See above nursing considerations.
felbamate (Felbatol)	Blocks repetitive firing of neurons and increases the seizure threshold	Anorexia, nausea, vomiting, insomnia, headache, dizziness, mild tremors, hyponatremia and hypokalemia, aplastic anemia, hepatic failure	Monitor electrolytes, liver function tests, and blood cell counts; dosages of phenytoin and carbamazepine may be adjusted if taken concurrently; breast-feeding is contraindicated with drug therapy.
levetiracetam (Keppra)	The precise mechanism(s) of action is unknown; it does not appear to affect GABA neurotransmission like other anticonvulsants.	Weakness, headache, drowsiness, increased incidence of infection, drowsiness, anorexia, cough, double vision	Monitor gait and coordination, be alert to symptoms of infection, if coadministered, phenytoin dose may require adjustment, taper dose when being discontinued, contraindicated while pregnant or breast-feeding
tiagabine (Gabitril)	Allows more GABA to bind to postsynaptic neurons in the brain	Dizziness, nervousness, weakness, tremor, confusion, nausea, vomiting pharyngitis, cough, rash, hair loss, menstrual changes, hypertension, tachycardia, edema	Monitor plasma drug levels; give with food; dose may be incrementally increased; store medication in a closed, light-protected container, dosages of coprescribed anticonvulsants may require adjustment, contraindicated while pregnant or breast feeding.
Barbiturates phenobarbital (Luminal)	Anticonvulsant activity	Sedation, rash, hyperactivity, ataxia, respiratory depression	Take oral dose at bedtime. Monitor vital signs, especially respiratory rate. Administer IM dose in deep muscle mass. Taper dosage before drug is discontinued. Periodic laboratory tests are required.
Benzodiazepines diazepam (Valium)	Skeletal muscle relaxation; adjunct anticonvulsant treatment	Respiratory depression, hypotension, sedation	Monitor BP, pulse, and respiration. Evaluate liver, kidney function, and blood studies. Taper dose before drug is discontinued. Instruct client to wear MedicAlert bracelet.

TABLE 37-1 Anticonvulsant Drug Monitoring

DRUG	THERAPEUTIC LEVEL	TOXIC LEVEL
Carbamazepine	5–12 mcg/mL	>12 mcg/mL
Ethosuximide	40–100 mcg/mL	>100 mcg/mL
Phenobarbital	10–30 mcg/mL	>40 mcg/mL
Phenytoin	10–20 mcg/mL	>30 mcg/mL
Valproic acid	50–100 mcg/mL	>100 mcg/mL

(From Pagana, K. D., & Pagana, T. J. [2008]. *Mosby's diagnostic and laboratory test reference* [9th ed.]. St. Louis: Mosby.)

In the event that a seizure occurs, the nurse positions the client on his or her side and loosens restrictive clothing (see Fig. 37-5). The airway is kept patent; the client is suctioned and oxygen is administered. The mouth is inspected for injuries to the tongue, teeth, and buccal cavity. If the client is incontinent, the nurse cleans the client and changes clothing and bed linen. Documentation includes the situation that preceded the seizure to assist in identifying any precipitating factors or aura, the duration of the seizure, parts of the body involved, vital signs, oxygen saturation, and capillary blood glucose level if indicated.

Nursing Process for the Client with a Seizure Disorder

Assessment

Obtain a complete history, including drug, allergy, and family history. Question the client regarding events or symptoms before and after the seizure. Acquire a description of the client's seizure(s) from an observer. Obtain information about any past head injury, neurologic infection such as meningitis, previous treatment for a seizure disorder, and whether the client takes medication as prescribed.

Nutrition Notes 37-4
The Client with a Seizure Disorder

- Anticonvulsants impair vitamin D metabolism, leading to calcium imbalance, rickets, or osteomalacia if supplemental vitamin D is not given.
- A high-fat diet, known as *ketogenic nutrition therapy,* is used as part of treatment in children whose seizures are not well-controlled on available medications. Fat provides approximately 85% to 90% of the calories in this diet; protein and carbohydrates are severely limited. The high fat content simulates starvation, except that the fat burned for energy comes from food, not stored body fat. Mild dehydration helps concentrate blood ketones; it is not known how or why ketosis affects seizure activity.
- At this time there is little evidence to support the use of ketogenic nutrition therapy in adults.

Note the characteristics of seizures if they occur while under your care. If the client's history is inconclusive and the type of seizure is unknown, it is important to provide a full, detailed description of the seizure (Box 37-3).

Diagnosis, Planning, and Interventions

The newly diagnosed client with seizures needs information about the specific type of disorder, the medications needed to control the seizures, and the precautions, if any, to take. Teach the client as follows:

- Take anticonvulsant medication as prescribed.
- Recognize adverse effects of the medication.
- Keep routine follow-up visits and laboratory appointments for blood level tests.
- Operate a motor vehicle or perform dangerous tasks only when seizures are controlled for at least 6 months.
- Wear a MedicAlert bracelet, tag, or other medical identification.
- Avoid situations known to trigger seizures, such as repetitively flashing or blinking lights, stress, or lack of sleep.

Other nursing care includes, but is not limited to, the following diagnoses, expected outcomes, and interventions.

▶ **Risk for Injury** related to uncontrolled movements and altered consciousness during seizure; **Risk for Impaired Oral Mucous Membranes** related to oral injury during a seizure and side effects of phenytoin drug therapy

▶ **Expected Outcomes:** (1) Client will be free of injuries. (2) Oral mucous membranes and gingiva will remain unaltered.

- Refer to the Nursing Process section on caring for clients with infectious and inflammatory disorders. *Nursing interventions are similar regardless of the cause of a seizure.*
- Use padded head gear on clients with atonic or akinetic seizures. *Loss of consciousness and falls are common with these types of seizures, increasing the potential for head injury.*
- Pad side rails with soft material. *Padding cushions the force on the client's skin and soft tissue when contact with metal side rails occurs during a seizure.*
- Protect client at the onset of the seizure by assisting the client to the floor or moving objects away from the client. *The nurse reduces the risk for serious injuries by modifying the environment and the client's location in the environment.*
- Loosen clothing about the neck. *Tight clothing can impair breathing.*

- Onset—sudden or preceded by an aura
- Duration of seizure
- Behavior immediately before and after
- Type of body movements
- Loss of consciousness, for how long
- Incontinence or not
- Seizure awareness afterward

- Never forcibly restrain the client. *Physically restraining a client during a seizure increases the potential for injuries such as fractures.*
- Inspect the oral cavity and teeth after a generalized seizure. *The nurse assesses the mouth for signs of injury and reports injuries to the physician.*
- Apply ice to bleeding areas; if broken teeth are noted, notify the client's dentist. *Ice constricts blood vessels and reduces bleeding. The client's dentist may be able to reimplant broken teeth or minimize the outcome of the trauma with early interventions.*
- Promote oral hygiene after each meal and recommend dental checkups every 3 to 6 months. *Phenytoin (Dilantin) causes gingival hyperplasia (overgrowth of gum tissue); regular and frequent dental examinations facilitate the maintenance or restoration of teeth and gums.*

▶ **Anxiety** related to unpredictability of seizures and social stigma as evidenced by uneasiness about resuming previous lifestyle activities with social acquaintances

▶ **Expected Outcome:** Anxiety will be reduced as evidenced by a resumption of social interactions.

- Help the client understand the disorder and treatment options. *Knowledge about the disorder and making choices promotes a sense of control.*
- Explain that a variety of drugs are available that can successfully reduce or control seizures. *Drug therapy prevents or reduces seizure activity.*
- Encourage the client to share information about the disorder with others. *Providing accurate information dispels fears and helps eliminate the misconception that people with seizure disorders have subnormal intelligence.*
- Suggest contacting the Epilepsy Foundation. *The Epilepsy Foundation provides counseling, low-cost prescription services, and referrals to agencies for vocational rehabilitation, job opportunities, personal and genetic counseling, and sheltered workshops.*

Evaluation of Expected Outcomes

Expected outcomes for the client are that there are fewer seizures or that they are completely controlled. The client remains safe from injury. The client's mouth and teeth are intact. The client who takes phenytoin understands the importance of regular dental examinations because of the potential for gingival hyperplasia. The client's anxiety is reduced to a tolerable level on a scale of 0 to 10. The client is resolved to maintain social relationships and participate in leisure activities. The client is aware of the services provided by the Epilepsy Foundation and how to contact this organization. ●

BRAIN TUMORS

A brain tumor is a growth of abnormal cells within the cranium. Brain tumors occur in all age groups. Some types are more common in people younger than 20 years of age; others more frequently affect older people.

Gerontologic Considerations

- The overall incidence of brain tumor decreases with age. Headache and papilledema are less common symptoms of a brain tumor in the older adult.

Brain tumors are classified according to whether they are benign or malignant, the type of cells involved, and the site of the tumor. The most common types of adult brain tumors are (1) metastatic tumors from a primary site; (2) gliomas, which involve cells that support structures in the brain, including astrocytes, cells that protect neurons; oligodendrocytes, cells that make myelin, and ependymocytes, cells that line the pathways that carry CSF; and (3) meningiomas, tumors involving the meningeal coverings of the brain and spinal cord. About 50% of all brain tumors are malignant. However, a brain tumor, whether malignant or benign, can result in death.

Pathophysiology and Etiology

The cause of most brain tumors, which occur in various areas of the brain (Fig. 37-15), remains unknown. A small percentage are congenital, such as hemangioblastomas. Genetic factors are associated with two types of brain tumors, *astrocytoma,* a gliomal tumor in the frontal lobe, and *neurofibromatosis.* Other causative factors include viral infection, exposure to radiation, head trauma, and immunosuppression. The brain also is the site of metastatic lesions from primary tumors, especially those of the lung and breast.

Tumors that arise from cerebral tissue, such as malignant gliomas and glioblastomas, and angiomas that involve cerebral blood vessels, expand in the confines of the skull and encroach on brain tissue that is vital for life. Extracerebral tumors, such as meningiomas, press on the brain tissue from without.

Assessment Findings

Signs and Symptoms

Because tumors take up space and block the flow and absorption of CSF, symptoms associated with increased ICP occur. The classic triad of headache, vomiting, and papilledema is common. Headache is most common early in the morning. It becomes increasingly severe and occurs more frequently as the tumor grows. Vomiting occurs without nausea or warning. Seizures also develop. Symptoms of disturbed neurologic function, such as speech difficulty, paralysis, and double vision, may be manifested, depending on the tumor's location.

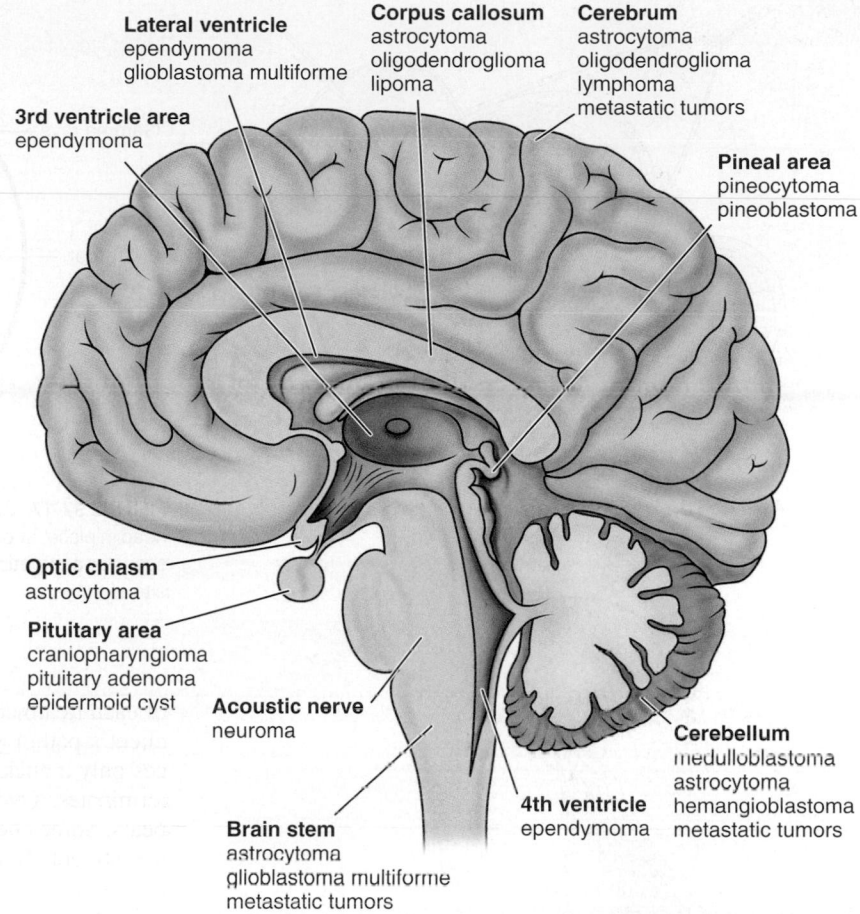

Lateral ventricle
ependymoma
glioblastoma multiforme

3rd ventricle area
ependymoma

Corpus callosum
astrocytoma
oligodendroglioma
lipoma

Cerebrum
astrocytoma
oligodendroglioma
lymphoma
metastatic tumors

Pineal area
pineocytoma
pineoblastoma

Optic chiasm
astrocytoma

Pituitary area
craniopharyngioma
pituitary adenoma
epidermoid cyst

Acoustic nerve
neuroma

Brain stem
astrocytoma
glioblastoma multiforme
metastatic tumors

4th ventricle
ependymoma

Cerebellum
medulloblastoma
astrocytoma
hemangioblastoma
metastatic tumors

FIGURE 37-15. Common sites for a brain tumor.

When the ICP is greatly increased, areas of the brain can herniate. If the brain stem is forced through the foramen magnum, the client is in grave danger because the vital centers that control respiration and heart rate are compressed. Respirations become deeper, labored, and noisy and then slow to only periodic. Unless the condition is relieved, the client dies of respiratory failure and cardiac arrest. Hyperthermia occurs as the temperature-regulating center in the brain is affected. Coma progressively deepens.

Diagnostic Findings
Diagnosis is confirmed with CT scan, MRI, brain scan, and cerebral angiography, which reveal the tumor's size and location.

Medical Management
Treatment depends on several factors, including the tumor's location and type (primary or metastatic) and the client's age and physical condition. Brain tumors are treated by surgery, radiation therapy, chemotherapy, or a combination of these methods.

Metastatic tumors and some primary tumors are inoperable, and radiation therapy and chemotherapy are the only treatment choices. Clients who cannot withstand surgery, chemotherapy, or radiation therapy are kept as comfortable and free from pain as possible. Intra-arterial or intrathecal administration of antineoplastic drugs is used to destroy the tumor or slow tumor growth. Symptomatic drug therapy includes corticosteroids and osmotic diuretics to reduce cerebral edema, analgesics, anticonvulsants, and antibiotics.

Complications, such as increased ICP, paralysis, mental changes, infection, seizures, and prolonged immobility, are treated symptomatically.

Surgical Management
Surgery for an operable brain tumor involves a craniotomy (incision through the skull) or craniectomy (excision of part of the skull). A section of bone (bone flap) is removed to reach the brain (Fig. 37-16). After the tumor is removed, the dura is reapproximated (the cut edges are lined up and sewn together), the bone flap replaced, and the skin sutured. The bone flap is not reinserted when increasing ICP or tumor growth is expected.

The client's postoperative symptoms are determined by the location and function of any damaged or removed brain tissue. Brain tissue does not regenerate.

Another method of removing brain tumors uses a laser beam directed at the tumor site. This surgical technique enables the physician to reach tumors that previously were considered inoperable. Radioisotopes also are surgically

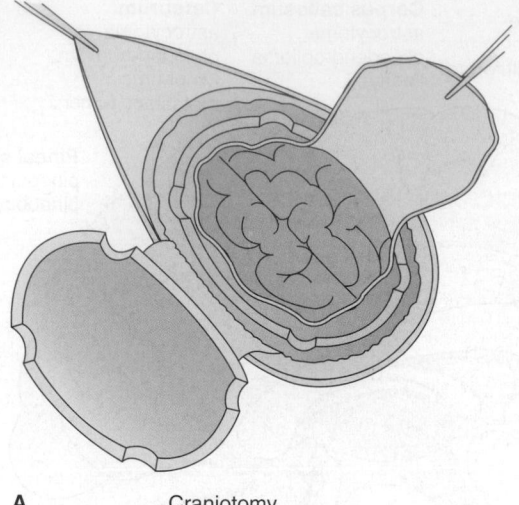

A Craniotomy

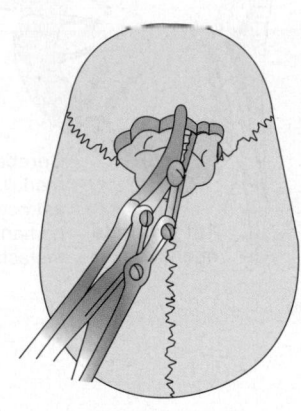

B Craniectomy

FIGURE 37-16. Neurosurgical techniques: (**A**) craniotomy; (**B**) craniectomy.

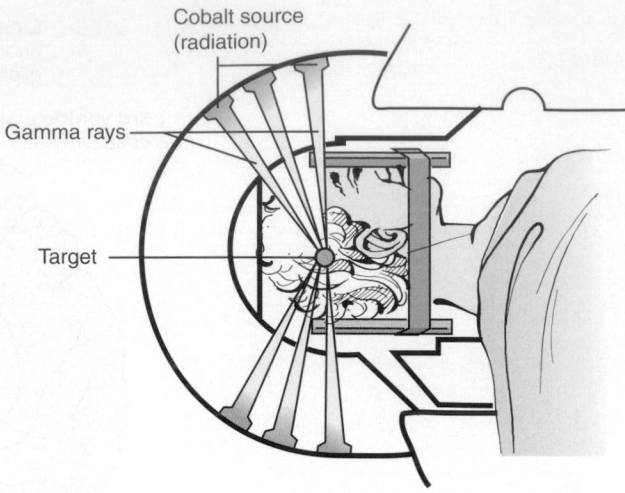

FIGURE 37-17. Gamma-knife radiosurgery. A head frame holds the head in place, and a plastic localizer is used during the pretreatment scans as a targeting landmark. Gamma rays converge on the targeted site of the tumor.

inserted into the tumor. However, the cure rate for this procedure is about the same as for external radiation therapy.

Gamma-Knife Radiosurgery
Gamma-knife radiosurgery is a noninvasive alternative for treating tumors deep within the brain or that conventional surgery can only partially remove. Removing these types of tumors through conventional surgery is difficult or generally impossible and can create the potential for damaging healthy brain tissue.

The gamma knife targets the lesion without making an incision, thus eliminating the risk for surgical complications and dangers of prolonged general anesthesia. The gamma knife directs gamma radiation from many computer-calculated directions so that all converge at a precise target area. Radiation is then delivered through holes in a helmet applied to the client's head. A box-shaped head frame attached to the scalp with screws holds the helmet in place and ensures that there is no head movement. (Fig. 37-17). Treatment, done on an outpatient basis or as a 24-hour inpatient stay, involves more than one procedure. The duration

of each treatment varies from 2 to 4 hours, depending on the client's pathology. The client remains awake and experiences only a clicking sound, as the procedure commences and terminates. Over time, the brain tumor shrinks and disappears. Some clients develop headache and minor nausea after a treatment. Temporary hair loss may occur if the radiated tumor is close to the surface of the skull.

Nursing Management
Nursing management depends on the area of the brain affected, tumor type, treatment approach, and the client's signs and symptoms. If the tumor is inoperable or has expanded despite treatment, increased ICP is a major threat (see Nursing Care Plan 37-1). See Chapter 39 for the care of the client undergoing intracranial surgery. Clients who receive chemotherapy and radiation are supported through the adverse effects associated with antineoplastic drug administration and effects of radiation (see Chap. 18). The nurse clarifies the client's and family's questions concerning treatment modalities. He or she directs the client to appropriate professionals to discuss treatment alternatives. The nurse explains hospice care and services to clients with brain tumors that no longer are at a stage where they can be cured.

Before the client is discharged, the nurse evaluates the client's and family's immediate and long-term needs. The nurse develops an individualized teaching plan that addresses the following components:

- Medication regimen
- Appointments for chemotherapy or radiation therapy
- Adverse effects of chemotherapy or radiation and techniques for managing them
- Nutritional support
- Home care considerations
- Rehabilitation (exercises, physical therapy)
- Referrals to support services for physical, emotional, and financial assistance

Nursing Process for the Client with a Brain Tumor

Assessment

Identify affected areas after a thorough history and neurologic examination. Perform a physical assessment and record the abnormal findings.

Diagnosis, Planning, and Interventions

Depending on the stage of the disease and the selected method(s) of treatment, the nurse's role includes but is not limited to the following.

▶ Acute Pain related to increased ICP secondary to expansion of the tumor or a sequela of surgery

▶ Expected Outcome: Pain will be controlled within client's level of tolerance.

- Assess and monitor characteristics of pain every time you measure vital signs. *Pain assessment is the fifth vital sign.*
- Administer prescribed analgesia and monitor for respiratory depression. *Narcotic analgesics relieve pain, but tolerance develops. High doses of narcotic analgesics depress the respiratory center in the brain.*
- Give analgesia on a scheduled rather than an as-needed basis. *Regular administration of analgesia is most effective at controlling pain.*
- Advocate for patient-controlled analgesia or transdermal analgesic patch. *Methods that facilitate frequent administration of small doses of IV analgesia or continuous absorption through the skin provide more continuous pain relief.*

▶ Imbalanced Nutrition: Less than Body Requirements related to nausea and vomiting or altered LOC

▶ Expected Outcome: Nutritional and fluid needs are met as evidenced by maintenance of weight and intake above 2000 mL.

- Administer prescribed antiemetics before meals. *A client is likely to consume adequate food without nausea or vomiting.*
- Determine client's food preferences and supply them. *Catering to likes and dislikes promotes a greater intake of food.*
- Give small, frequent servings of food or nourishing beverages. *Large servings tend to overwhelm a client. He or she may consume more food overall if smaller amounts are served several times a day. Liquid nutritional supplements provide extra calories and nutrients in an easily consumed form.*
- Collaborate with the physician concerning gastric tube feedings or TPN. *Enteral and parenteral routes for nutrition may be used when the oral route is no longer adequate.*

▶ Impaired Oral Mucous Membranes related to fluid volume deficit, tissue damage secondary to chemotherapy or radiation as manifested by xerostomia (oral lesions)

▶ Expected Outcome: Oral mucous membranes will be pink, moist, and intact.

- Relieve discomfort with a prescribed topical anesthetic. *It blocks sensory nerves and relieves local discomfort.*
- Provide meticulous mouth care. *The mouth contains many microorganisms that thrive on particles of food and sugar clinging to teeth. Increased microbial growth fosters the potential for dental decay and impaired tissue.*
- Offer mouth rinses of tap water or medicated solutions frequently. *Liquids keep the mouth moist and flush debris from the oral cavity.*

▶ Anticipatory Grieving related to uncertain future, physical and social losses

▶ Expected Outcome: Client will express feelings and deal with potential losses while working through acceptance of the diagnosis.

- Give the opportunity to express feelings privately. *A person is more likely to be open and frank in an environment where others will not overhear intimate feelings.*
- Remain with client when emotions are overwhelming. *A supportive other helps client endure emotional pain and cope more effectively.*
- Help clarify any and all questions the client may have. *Honest and accurate information facilitates the client's right to self-determination.*
- Reassure client that he or she will not be abandoned and that comfort and preservation of dignity are priorities of nursing care. *Most clients fear that they will be left alone when dying and will experience extreme pain or discomfort.*
- Assist client to complete unfinished business however he or she defines it. *Taking care of tasks, accomplishing specific goals, or communicating feelings to significant others helps clients die more peacefully.*
- Refer client and family to the local hospice organization if the client is in the terminal stage. *Hospice organizations help client and family meet their physical and emotional needs.*

Evaluation of Expected Outcomes

The client reports that pain is relieved or resolved to a tolerable level. Nutritional intake is sufficient to maintain body weight. Oral mucosa is intact. The client and family progress through the grieving process and implement a plan for postdischarge care. ●

CRITICAL THINKING EXERCISES

1. When caring for a client with a seizure disorder, what nursing interventions are indicated?
2. What information can the nurse provide to a person who recently has been diagnosed with multiple sclerosis?
3. What discharge teaching is appropriate when discussing home care with the spouse of a client in the late stage of Parkinson's disease?
4. An older female adult client with myasthenia gravis is concerned about the cost of medications under her Medicare prescription drug plan. She questions the necessity of neostigmine (Prostigmin) and pyridostigmine

(Mestinon). What information is important to provide this client to promote drug compliance following discharge?

NCLEX-STYLE REVIEW QUESTIONS

1. Understanding that older adults often do not exhibit the typical signs and symptoms of meningitis, the nurse would be especially vigilant for which of the following signs and symptoms in older clients with suspected meningitis? Select all that apply.
   1. No nuchal rigidity or headache
   2. Pressure ulcers
   3. Hypostatic pneumonia
   4. Papilledema
   5. Change in mental status
2. A client diagnosed with Guillain-Barré syndrome is being placed on a medical floor. When selecting the equipment to place in the client's room, the nurse is most correct to include items that facilitate which of the following?
   1. Supplemental oxygen
   2. Cardiac monitoring
   3. Nasogastric suction
   4. Intravenous therapy
3. To ensure the safety of a client with Parkinson's disease using a wheeled walker, it is best for the nurse to remind the client to do which of the following?
   1. Maintain a constant pace of walking.
   2. Keep the walker a full arm's length in front.
   3. Pick up the walker when taking a step.
   4. Stand straight with the head up.
4. Which of the following nursing interventions is most appropriate for managing and minimizing seizures when caring for a client with a neurologic infectious disorder?
   1. Restrain client's movements.
   2. Suction client's mouth and pharynx during the seizure.
   3. Place client in supine position during the seizure.
   4. Provide oxygen during and after the seizure.
5. A client with Parkinson's disease has difficulty swallowing. To promote adequate nutrition and reduce the risk for aspiration, which of the following nursing measures are appropriate? Select all that apply.
   1. Modify the texture and consistency of food.
   2. Have the client flex the chin when swallowing.
   3. Encourage frequent sips of liquid while eating.
   4. Position the client in a sitting position.
   5. Allow ample time for consuming meals.

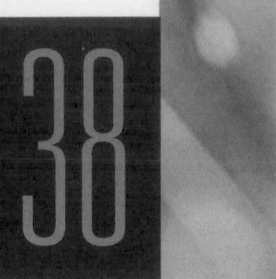

38

Caring for Clients with Cerebrovascular Disorders

Words To Know
aneurysm
bruit
cephalalgia
cerebral infarction
cerebrovascular accident
collateral circulation
endarterectomy
expressive aphasia
hemianopia
hemiplegia
receptive aphasia
transient ischemic attack

Learning Objectives

On completion of this chapter, you will be able to:

1. Identify three common types of headaches and their characteristics.
2. List nursing techniques that supplement drug therapy in reducing or relieving headaches.
3. Explain the cause and significance of a transient ischemic attack.
4. Discuss medical and surgical techniques used to reduce the potential for a cerebrovascular accident.
5. Differentiate between ischemic and hemorrhagic strokes.
6. Identify five manifestations of a cerebrovascular accident; discuss those that are unique to right-sided and left-sided infarctions.
7. Identify at least five nursing diagnoses common to the care of a client with a cerebrovascular accident and interventions for them.
8. Describe a cerebral aneurysm and the danger it presents.
9. Discuss appropriate nursing interventions when caring for a client with a cerebral aneurysm.

Cerebrovascular disorders are major medical problems that affect adults. Some, such as headaches, can disrupt a client's life-style, causing tremendous discomfort and anxiety. Others, such as cerebrovascular accident and transient ischemic attacks, are life-threatening.

HEADACHE

Aching in the head is referred to as **cephalalgia**. This symptom accompanies many disorders such as meningitis, increased intracranial pressure (ICP), brain tumors, and sinusitis. When the duration is relatively brief, a headache is considered transient and benign. Although there are many types of headaches, *tension*, *migraine*, and *cluster* headaches are the most common (Table 38-1). Tension headaches, the most common of the three, occur when a person contracts the neck and facial muscles for a prolonged period of time. Migraine headaches, which are recurrent and severe and last for a day or more, have a vascular origin. Cluster headaches may be a variant of migraine headaches; they are episodic, reccurring over 6 to 8 weeks, with only brief periods of recovery between multiple daily attacks.

Pathophysiology and Etiology

Neither the skull nor the brain itself contains sensory nerves. A vast network of sensory and motor nerves, however, is distributed throughout the scalp and facial muscles. During stressful conditions, people tend to contract muscles about the neck, face, and scalp, and a tension headache may develop. A tension headache also can develop when a person

TABLE 38-1 Features of Common Headaches

FEATURE	CLUSTER HEADACHE	MIGRAINE HEADACHE	TENSION HEADACHE
Client gender	Usually male	Usually female	Equally male/female
Age at onset	20–50 yr	10–40 yr	Any age
Frequency of attacks	1–8/day	1–8/month	Almost daily
Duration of attacks	30 min–4 hr	4–72 hr	Gradual onset, steady
Intensity of pain	Excruciatingly relentless	Moderate to severe	Constant dull ache
Location of pain	Strictly unilateral	Unilateral or bilateral	Bilateral
Nasal congestion	70%	None	None
Droopy, teary eye	Common	Uncommon	Uncommon
Incidence of associated nausea and vomiting	Rare	Common	Rare
Incidence of attacks awakening client from sleep	Common	Rare	Rare
Characteristic behavior	Client cannot remain still during severe attack	Client prefers hibernation	Client prefers hibernation
Family history	7%	90%	Associated with stress
Treatment	Refer to physician	Refer to physician	Refer to physician

contracts the neck and facial muscles for a prolonged period. When the tensed muscles sensitize *nociceptors,* pain-relaying nerves in the head, the nociceptors transmit neurochemicals such as prostaglandin and substance P to the brain, which registers the presence and location of discomfort (see Chap. 11).

Researchers are getting closer to finding what causes migraine headaches. They have targeted three sequential contributing cofactors: (1) changes in particular serotonin receptors that promote (2) dilation of cerebral blood vessels, and pain intensification from (3) neurochemicals released from the trigeminal nerve (Fig. 38-1). It also has been suggested that fluctuations in reproductive hormones, chemicals in certain foods, a food-related allergy, or drugs can trigger migraines (Box 38-1).

The cause of cluster headaches is unknown. Cluster headaches can be triggered by vasodilating agents such as nitroglycerin, histamine, and alcoholic beverages. Some suggest that lower than normal levels of the neurotransmitter serotonin occurs, which may explain the mechanism by which serotonin-enhancing drugs provide relief. Acetylcholine, a parasympathetic neurotransmitter, also may play a role in cluster headaches.

Assessment Findings

Symptoms vary from a mild ache to severe, disabling pain. Clients may describe a tension headache as pressure or steady constriction on both sides of the head. Some people correlate the onset of the headache with anxiety or emotional conflict.

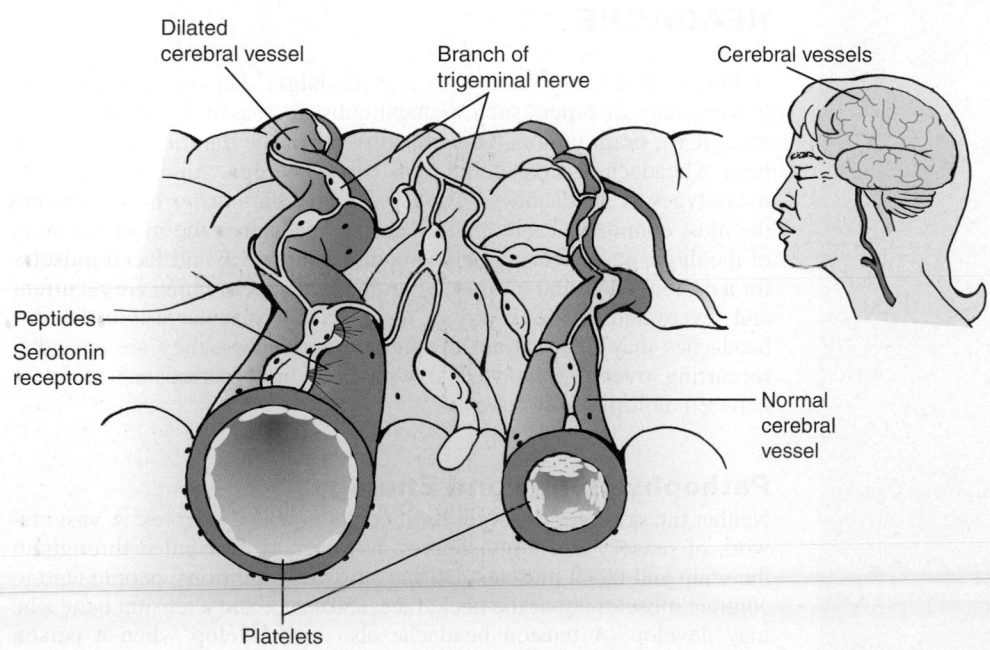

FIGURE 38-1. Chemical developments in migraine headaches. Cerebral blood vessels dilate in response to serotonin from platelets. Peptides released from the trigeminal nerve intensify pain.

BOX 38-1 Substances That Trigger Migraine Headaches

Foods
Aged cheese
Alcohol
Bananas, figs, raisins
Caffeine
Citrus fruits
Chocolate
Dairy products
Fermented or pickled food
Nuts
Onions
Pea or lima bean pods
Processed foods containing nitrites, sulfites, or monosodium glutamate (MSG)
Saccharin or aspartame
Yeast-containing products

Drugs
Analgesic overuse
Benzodiazepine withdrawal
Cimetidine
Decongestant overuse
Estrogen replacement
Fenfluramine
Indomethacin
Nifedipine
Nitrates
Oral contraceptives
Reserpine
Theophylline

Events
Stress
Menstruation; menopause
Sleep changes; excess or loss
Overexertion
Hunger or fasting
Odors, smoke, or perfume
Strong glare or flashing lights

Diagnosis is based on the pattern of headaches accompanying signs and symptoms. Persistent heada... require tests such as computed tomography (CT) scan, bra... scan, head and neck radiographs, and angiography to rule out other neurologic disorders such as a brain tumor or intracerebral hemorrhage.

Medical Management

Transient tension headaches usually are relieved by rest, a mild analgesic, and stress management techniques such as relaxation or imaging (see Chap. 67). For severe, recurrent tension headaches, counseling and psychotherapy may help clients deal with emotional stressors in healthier ways. Antidepressants also help some clients.

Mild analgesics usually are ineffective for migraine headaches. Drug therapy with methysergide (Sansert) may be prescribed to prevent migraines, or drugs such as sumatriptan (Imitrex) may be prescribed to interrupt migraines that have already developed (Drug Therapy Table 38-1). Prophylactic drug therapy may be necessary if migraine headaches occur several times a month and produce severe impairment, or if acute attacks are not adequately relieved. Although this may not prevent all migraines, it may reduce the frequency, intensity, and duration of attacks. Antiemetics may control nausea and vomiting that accompany an acute attack. Some clients learn to shorten or abort migraines with biofeedback techniques (see Chap. 67).

PharmacologicConsiderations

- Once prophylactic drug therapy eliminates or reduces migraine headaches, the physician may gradually reduce or discontinue the dose. Drugs used to abort a migraine in progress can still be used even if the client is receiving prophylactic migraine drug therapy.

- Some clients have experienced reduced frequency of migraines by taking an herbal form of feverfew (*Chrysanthemum parthenium*). Clients should consult or inform their physician about therapy with herbs because many herbs interact with medications.

Clients who have "classic" migraines experience an *aura,* a sensory phenomenon that precedes the headache like seeing flashing lights or wavy lines for about 10 to 30 minutes. For others with the more "common" form of migraine, the prodromal period before the headache is marked by a change in mood, difficulty concentrating, or unusual fatigue. The client with a migraine describes the pain as "throbbing" or "bursting." Nausea and vomiting, vertigo, sensitivity to light, irritability, and fatigue accompany the headache.

A person with a cluster headache has pain on one side of the head, usually behind the eye, accompanied by nasal congestion, *rhinorrhea* (watery discharge from the nose), and tearing and redness of the eye. The pain is so severe that the person is not likely to lie still; rather he or she paces or thrashes about.

Symptoms of cluster headaches are controlled with various drugs, including an ergotamine derivative such as dihydroergotamine (Migranal) or methysergide (Sansert). Some clients respond to corticosteroids such as triamcinolone (Aristocort) and prednisone (Deltasone), lithium carbonate (Eskalith), vasoconstricting drugs in the "triptan" group such as sumatriptan (Imitrex) and zolmitriptan (Zomig), anticonvulsants such as gabapentin (Neurontin) and divalproex (Depakote), and beta-adrenergic blockers such as atenolol (Tenormin) and propranolol (Inderal). Inhaled or injected drugs are preferred because they are absorbed more rapidly than those administered by the oral route (see Drug Therapy Table 38-1). Oxygen may be used during a headache to reduce the vasodilating compensatory response occurring in the brain. For clients who do not respond to pharmacologic interventions, neurosurgical

Anti hypertensive effects

Check BP & heartrate

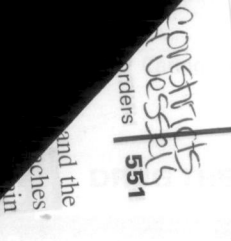

RAPY TABLE 38-1 Drugs For Managing Headaches

	Mechanism of Action	Side Effects	Nursing Considerations
Migraine Prophylaxis			
Neuronal stabilizers			
topiramate (Topamax)	Potentiates the action of gamma aminobutyric acid (GABA), an inhibitory neurotransmitter	Drowsiness, pain, agitation, anxiety, tremor, flulike symptoms, rash, weight loss or gain, may decrease effectiveness of oral contraceptives, kidney stones	Increase dose gradually, advise caution regarding driving or hazardous activities, contraindicated if breast-feeding, do not crush tablets because of bitter taste, provide a liberal fluid intake
lamotrigine (Lamictal)	Thought to inhibit the release of glutamate, an excitatory neurotransmitter	Drowsiness, dizziness, nausea, double and blurred vision, rash, rhinitis	Do not discontinue abruptly, monitor drug levels, contraindicated if breast-feeding
Beta-adrenergic blockers			
atenolol (Tenormin)	Block the beta receptors for norepinephrine and epinephrine, thereby preventing cerebral vasoconstriction	Hypotension, bradycardia, impotence, peripheral edema, depression, fatigue	Monitor pulse and blood pressure, withhold drug if pulse is < 60 bpm, teach to change positions slowly, contraindicated if breast-feeding
Tricyclic antidepressants			
amitriptyline (Elavil)	Sustains levels of the neurotransmitters serotonin and norepinephrine	Nervousness, drowsiness, orthostatic hypotension, dry mouth, blurred vision, constipation, urinary retention, weight gain	Therapeutic effect may be delayed for 1–6 weeks, take measures to prevent falls, monitor elimination patterns
Ergotamine derivative			
methysergide (Sansert)	Displaces serotonin on cranial artery receptors, promotes vasoconstriction	Insomnia, postural hypotension, nausea, vomiting, heartburn, abdominal pain, diarrhea, flushing, rash, edema	Requires 1–2 days of administration to provide migraine prophylaxis; drug should be discontinued over 2–3 weeks, use measures to prevent falls, contraindicated if breast-feeding, weigh daily, limit sodium if edema develops
Aborting Acute Migraine Attacks			
Ergot alkaloids			
ergotamine (Cafergot)	Blocks alpha-adrenergic receptors promoting cerebral vasoconstriction	Weakness, paresthesias, cool skin, confusion, nausea, vomiting, diarrhea, rapid irregular heart rate, chest pain, renal failure	Begin drug therapy as soon as possible after migraine begins; have the client lie down for 2–3 hours after drug administration; high doses can increase the frequency of headaches; notify physician if migraines occur more frequently or are unrelieved; contraindicated if breast-feeding
Serotonin agonists			
zolmitriptan (Zomig)	Reverses vasodilation of cranial blood vessels and reduces the pain pathways associated with a migraine	Weakness, paresthesias, drowsiness, dizziness, coronary artery vasospasm, dry mouth, nausea, vomiting, flushing, dyspnea	Administer immediately after migraine aura passes; repeat q2h up to 10 mg in 24 hrs if headache returns; do not administer with an ergot alkaloid; report chest pain immediately; discard opened and unused tablets
sumatriptan (Imitrex)	Causes vasoconstriction of cranial carotid arteries; relieves photophobia, sensitivity to sound, nausea and vomiting associated with migraine attacks	Coronary artery vasospasm, tingling, numbness, warm sensation, dizziness, pain on injection	Available by oral, intranasal spray, or subcutaneous injection; give any time after symptoms develop; oral dose can be repeated in 2 hours, a second injection can be repeated in 1 hour if headache is unrelieved or reccurs
Nonsteroidal anti-inflammatory drugs			
acetaminophen/aspirin/ caffeine (Excedrin Migraine)	Blocks transmission of pain over nociceptors; caffeine causes vasoconstriction	GI distress, allergic reactions if sensitive to aspirin, nervousness, tachycardia, insomnia, can cause rebound headache if taken too frequently	Limit administration to no more than 2 tablets in 24 hours, avoid caffeine and alcohol, give for relief of mild-to-moderate symptoms; not for pediatric use or those who may have an ulcer or bleeding disorder

techniques such as rhizotomy may be the only hope for relief (see Chap 11).

Nursing Process for the Client with a Headache

Assessment

Ask the client questions about the location, type of pain, and past history of the same type of headache, because another disorder or problem may be occurring. Determine whether the pain is in one area or over the entire head; factors that appear to bring on, worsen, or relieve the headache; how long the pain lasts; and symptoms such as tearing, nasal congestion, nausea or vomiting, or sensitivity to light.

When assessing clients with chronic headaches or headaches that cause various symptoms, obtain a complete medical, allergy, and family history, as well as a record of frequency and description of the pain, including its numeric intensity during an attack. Record vital signs to use as a baseline for comparison.

Diagnosis, Planning, and Interventions

The nurse reinforces the drug therapy regimen and instructs the client on self-administration of medications. The nurse teaches the client with migraines to take medication as soon as symptoms begin and to minimize noise and other pain-provoking stimuli (Client and Family Teaching 38-1). In addition, the following nursing interventions are appropriate for clients with headache.

▶ Pain related to muscle tension, changes in cerebral blood flow, or unknown etiology

▶ Expected Outcome: Headache will be reduced or eliminated within 30 minutes of nursing intervention.

- Eliminate environmental factors that intensify pain, such as bright light and noise. *Sensory stimuli decrease pain tolerance.*
- Administer prescribed medications as early as possible and note their effect. *Medications that relieve headaches are in many different categories with various mechanisms of action. If the medication is ineffective, collaborate with the physician to modify the method of treatment.*

Client and Family Teaching 38-1
Migraine Headaches

The nurse includes the following instructions:

- Follow the indications and dosage regimen for medication, and notify the physician of any adverse drug effects.
- Identify and avoid factors that precipitate or intensify an attack. Keeping a food diary may help identify foods that trigger attacks.
- Keep a record of the attacks, including activities before the attack, and environmental or emotional circumstances that appear to bring on the attack.
- Lie down in a darkened room, and avoid noise and movement when an attack occurs, if that is possible.

- Offer a back massage to promote muscle relaxation. *Massage relaxes tense muscles, causes local dilation of blood vessels, relieves headache. This approach is not likely to help a client with migraine or cluster headache.*
- Apply warm (or cool) cloths to the forehead or back of the neck. *Warmth promotes vasodilation; cool stimuli reduce blood flow.*
- Provide distraction with soft, soothing music, or suggest using a relaxation tape or one that provides guided imagery. *Reduced anxiety can relieve a tension headache; clients with migraine or cluster headaches are not receptive to this approach.*

Evaluation of Expected Outcome

Head pain is reduced or eliminated. The client demonstrates understanding of the medication regimen and possible side effects. He or she identifies ways to modify behavior to minimize pain. ●

TRANSIENT ISCHEMIC ATTACKS

A **transient ischemic attack** (TIA) is a sudden, brief attack of neurologic impairment caused by a temporary interruption in cerebral blood flow. Symptoms may disappear within 1 hour; some continue for as long as 1 day. When the symptoms terminate, the client resumes his or her presymptomatic state. A TIA is a warning that a cerebrovascular accident (CVA, also known as *stroke*) can occur in the near future; one third of people who experience TIA subsequently develop a stroke.

Pathophysiology and Etiology

TIAs result from impaired blood circulation in the brain, which can be caused by atherosclerosis and arteriosclerosis, cardiac disease, or diabetes (see Chaps. 25, 27, and 51). Circulation is impaired by atherosclerosis (buildup of fatty plaque) in cerebral blood vessels and the formation of thrombi and microemboli. The inelastic arterial system affected by arteriosclerosis restricts the volume of blood circulating through blood vessels. Dysrhythmias and ineffective heart contraction are the catalysts for thrombi that can travel to cerebral vessels. Hypertension, which is associated with some of the previously mentioned etiologies, reduces the blood traveling to the brain and increases the potential for ruptured cerebral vessels from the elevated pressure. Smoking and other forms of tobacco use aggravate hypertension. Some medications, such as estrogens used for hormone replacement therapy and oral contraceptives, are thrombogenic. During the ischemic period, motor, sensory, and cognitive functions are temporarily affected.

Assessment Findings

Symptoms of a TIA include temporary light-headedness, confusion, speech disturbances, loss of vision, diplopia, variable changes in consciousness, and numbness, weakness, impaired muscle coordination, or paralysis on one side. The symptoms are short-lived.

A neurologic examination during an attack reveals neurologic deficits. Auscultation of the carotid artery may reveal a **bruit** (abnormal sound caused by blood flowing over the

DRUG THERAPY TABLE 38-2 Drugs to Prevent or Treat Cerebrovascular Disorders

	Mechanism of Action	Side Effects	Nursing Considerations
...(Plavix)	Decreases clot production by interfering with platelet aggregation	Dizziness, diarrhea, nausea, abdominal pain, neutropenia, bleeding, rash	Administer with food or meals; monitor white blood cell count, and assess for excessive bleeding; explain need for regular, follow-up laboratory tests
Glycoprotein IIb/IIIa inhibitors eptifibatide (integrilin), tirofiban (aggrastat)	Block platelet binding receptors; more potent than aspirin and heparin alone.	Most common undesirable effect of therapy is internal, intracranial, and superficial bleeding; may have hypersensitivity, anaphylactoid reactions, nausea, vomiting, hypotension	Must have baseline assessment data and lab data; if platelet counts fall below 90,000/mm^3, notify the provider
Thrombolytics alteplase (Activase); recombinant tissue plasminogen activator (r-TPA)	Reestablishes blood flow to ischemic areas by dissolving thrombi, contraindicated in clients with history of cerebrovascular accident or bleeding tendencies	Cardiac dysrhythmias, hypotension, bleeding at venous or arterial access sites, nausea, vomiting	Use caution when administering with heparin because of increased risk for hemorrhage; monitor PT and PTT; apply pressure to control superficial bleeding
Anticoagulants heparin sodium (Hepalean)	Inhibits thrombus and clot formation by blocking conversion of prothrombin to thrombin and fibrinogen to fibrin	Hemorrhage, bruising, thrombocytopenia, alopecia, chills, fever	Monitor closely for bleeding or hemorrhage when combined with oral anticoagulants; give subcutaneously (usually in the abdomen) or IV; rotate injection sites; avoid areas within 2 inches of umbilicus; apply pressure to all IM injection sites; monitor for epistaxis and other bleeding; ensure protamine sulfate is available in case of overdose
warfarin sodium (Coumadin)	Prevents thrombi; prolongs clotting times by interfering with vitamin K–dependent clotting factors	Increased bleeding, nausea, leukopenia, alopecia, dermatitis, fever, rash	Monitor complete blood counts, PT, and INR frequently; advise client to wear a MedicAlert tag; instruct client to report any unusual or excessive bleeding; advise client to avoid excessive intake of vitamin K-rich foods, such as collard greens, spinach, other salad greens, broccoli, cabbage, soybean and canola oils

Vitamin K for overdose (handwritten note)

rough surface of one or both carotid arteries). Ultrasound examination of the carotid artery shows an irregular shape to the artery lining caused by atherosclerotic plaques. A carotid arteriogram shows narrowing of the carotid artery. A CT scan or magnetic resonance imaging (MRI) is used to rule out other neurologic disorders with similar manifestations, such as a brain tumor.

Gerontologic Considerations

- Older adults may ignore the symptoms of a TIA, attributing them to part of the normal aging process.

Medical and Surgical Management

Therapy for clients who have had a TIA and others who have a high potential for experiencing a CVA (stroke) is complex. Clients must control their blood pressure with or without medications (see Chap 27), lose excess weight, and stop tobacco and alcohol abuse. To manage atherosclerosis and the consequences of cardiac dysrhythmias, especially atrial fibrillation (see Chap 26), cholesterol-lowering drugs (see Chap. 25) and prophylactic anticoagulant or antiplatelet therapy are prescribed. Specific antiplatelet or anticoagulant medicines include daily aspirin, clopidogrel (Plavix), ticlopidine (Ticlid), warfarin (Coumadin), and dipyridamole (Persantine) (Drug Therapy Table 38-2). Clients with diabetes are educated in techniques to control blood sugar

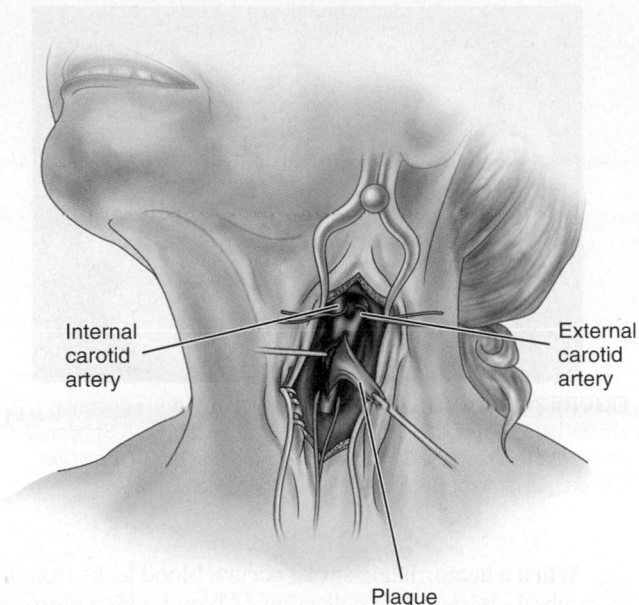

Internal carotid artery

External carotid artery

Plaque

FIGURE 38-2. In endarterectomy, plaque—a potential source of emboli in TIAs and CVAs—is surgically removed from the carotid artery.

within normal ranges with diet, exercise, and medications (see Chap 51).

Pharmacologic Considerations

Aspirin (1.0 to 1.3 g/day orally) is given prophylactically because it inhibits platelet aggregation and therefore prevents blood clots from forming within arteries. If gastric upset occurs, aspirin may be given with food, with an antacid, or in an enterically coated form.

- If the client is receiving an oral anticoagulant to prevent thromboembolic disorders, the dose is adjusted according to laboratory findings. Optimum therapeutic results are obtained when prothrombin levels are 1.5 to 2.5 times the normal control value, or the international normalized ratio value is 2.0 to 3.0.

If narrowing of the carotid artery by atherosclerotic plaques is the cause of the TIAs, a carotid **endarterectomy** (surgical removal of atherosclerotic plaque) is a treatment option (Fig. 38-2). A percutaneous transluminal coronary angioplasty (PTCA), also called a balloon angioplasty (see Chap. 25), is performed to dilate the carotid artery and increase blood flow to the brain.

▶ *Stop, Think, and Respond Exercise 38-1*

For a client who has had a TIA, what client teaching related to reducing risk factors for stroke is appropriate?

Nursing Management

The nurse obtains a complete history of symptoms and medical, drug, and allergy histories. He or she weighs the client,

because obesity, hyperlipidemia, and atherosclerosis are related to cerebrovascular disease. The nurse checks the client's capillary blood sugar to help identify hyperglycemia associated with undiagnosed or uncontrolled diabetes mellitus. He or she measures vital signs and notes if blood pressure (BP) is 140/90 mm Hg or greater. The nurse asks the client about smoking habits. Although symptoms of a TIA usually are not permanent, the nurse performs a neurologic examination to identify the client's current status and establish a baseline for future comparisons. He or she documents and reports even subtle changes.

If the client undergoes carotid artery surgery, the nurse performs frequent neurologic checks to detect paralysis, confusion, facial asymmetry, or aphasia. He or she monitors the heart rhythm because dysrhythmias (see Chap. 26) can alter blood flow to the brain as well. Because it is possible for the neck to swell after surgery, the nurse observes the client closely for difficulty breathing or swallowing and hoarseness. The nurse places an airway at the bedside and is prepared for endotracheal intubation if an airway obstruction occurs.

The nurse teaches the client to:

- Maintain hydration by drinking the equivalent of eight glasses of fluid a day, unless contraindicated.
- Follow directions for drug therapy, including medications for controlling hypertension and diabetes.
- Monitor for signs of bruising or bleeding if antiplatelet or anticoagulant drugs are prescribed.
- Keep appointments for laboratory tests and medical follow-up to monitor the effectiveness of therapy.
- Report any future instances of sensory or motor impairment, or call 911 for emergency assistance.

Pharmacologic Considerations

- For clients taking an antiplatelet or anticoagulant drug, bleeding can occur at any time, even when the prothrombin level appears to be within safe limits. Observe the client for evidence of unusual bleeding, such as easy bruising, nosebleeds, excessive bleeding from small cuts, and blood in the urine or stool. Keep parenteral vitamin K, the antidote for oral anticoagulants, available.

CEREBROVASCULAR ACCIDENT (STROKE)

A **cerebrovascular accident,** or stroke, is a prolonged interruption in the flow of blood through one of the arteries supplying the brain. Stroke is the third leading cause of death among adult Americans. Each year, approximately 780,000 Americans have a new or recurrent stroke (American Heart Association/American Stroke Association, 2008).

Brain and cerebral nerve cells are extremely sensitive to a lack of oxygen; if the brain is deprived of oxygenated blood for 3 to 7 minutes during stroke, both the brain and

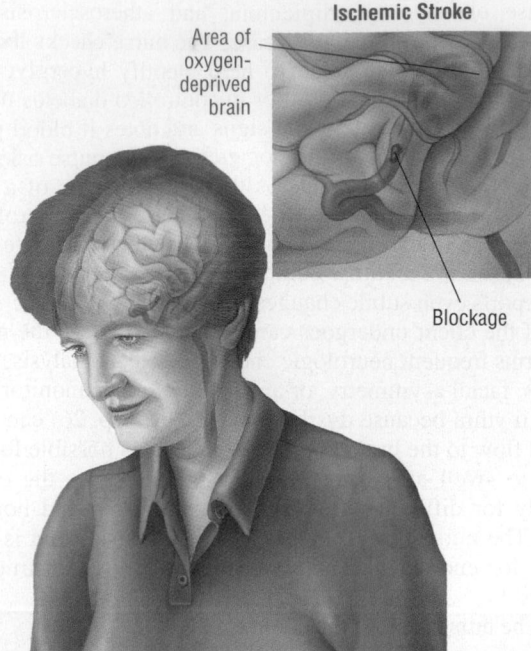

Ischemic Stroke

Area of oxygen-deprived brain

Blockage

FIGURE 38-3. In ischemic stroke, arterial blood flow to part of the brain is blocked by a clot that forms in a cerebral artery (*thrombotic stroke*) or by a clot that travels to and lodges in a cerebral artery from another location (*embolic stroke*). (From the Anatomical Chart Company.)

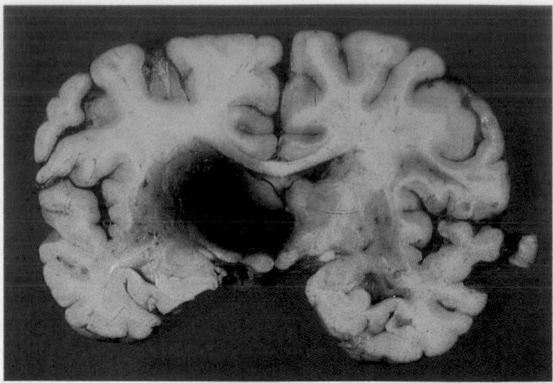

FIGURE 38-4. Cerebral hemorrhage. A postmortem specimen shows bleeding into the basal ganglia. (From Rubin, R., & Strayer, D. S., eds. [2008]. *Pathology: Clinicopathologic foundations of medicine* [5th ed.]. Baltimore: Lippincott Williams & Wilkins.)

nerve cells begin to die. Once these cells are destroyed, the outcome is irreversible. Although the site of the cellular damage is located in the brain, the consequences are widespread. About one third of stroke victims die; most survivors have permanent disabilities. Permanent neurologic deficits have a profound physical, emotional, and financial effect on the client and the family.

Pathophysiology and Etiology

There are two main types of stroke: *ischemic strokes* and *hemorrhagic strokes*. Ischemic strokes occur when a thrombus or embolus obstructs an artery carrying blood to the brain (Fig. 38-3); about 80% of strokes are the ischemic variety. Hemorrhagic strokes occur when a cerebral blood vessel ruptures and blood is released in brain tissue (Fig. 38-4).

When ischemic strokes occur, glucose and oxygen to brain cells are reduced. The reduced glucose quickly depletes the stores of adenosine triphosphate (ATP), resulting in anaerobic cellular metabolism and the accumulation of toxic by-products such as lactic acid. Although some brain cells die from anoxia, the lack of oxygen destroys additional brain cells by a secondary mechanism. Oxygen depletion triggers the release of glutamate, an excitatory neurotransmitter that activates neuronal receptors known as *N*-methyl-D-aspartate (NMDA) receptors (see Chap 11). The receptors allow large amounts of calcium followed by glutamate to enter the cells. Once glutamate is inside the brain cells, it literally overexcites them, causing disordered enzyme activities that release toxic free radicals, which destroy the cells (Fig. 38-5). This secondary assault extends the zone of **cerebral infarction** (death of brain tissue).

When a hemorrhagic stroke occurs, blood leaks from intracerebral arteries. The collection of blood adds volume to the intracranial contents, resulting in elevated pressure (see Chap. 37). Hemorrhagic strokes are more common in particular areas of the brain such as the cerebellum, the structure that facilitates balance and coordination, and brain stem, which controls breathing, BP, and heart rate.

Various factors increase the risk for a CVA. Some are controllable and some are uncontrollable (Box 38-2). Atherosclerosis and arteriosclerosis are major contributors to the formation of thromboemboli and subsequent CVAs. Common causes of cerebral hemorrhage are rupture of cerebral vessels (discussed later in this chapter), hemorrhagic disorders such as leukemia and aplastic anemia, severe hypertension, and brain tumors.

Gerontologic Considerations

- A major risk factor for stroke is hypertension. The older adult with hypertension living on a limited income may not adhere to the medication regimen because of financial constraints, increasing the risk of CVA. Client education is important to provide risk-benefit information. The symptoms of decreased alertness, drowsiness, weakness, or falling may be attributed to other health concerns common in older persons.

Assessment Findings

Signs and Symptoms

In some instances, clients experience one or more TIAs days, weeks, or years before a CVA, or there may be no warning and the symptoms develop suddenly. Signs of an impending stroke include the following:

- Numbness or weakness of one side of the face, an arm, or leg
- Mental confusion
- Difficulty speaking or understanding
- Impaired walking or coordination
- Severe headache

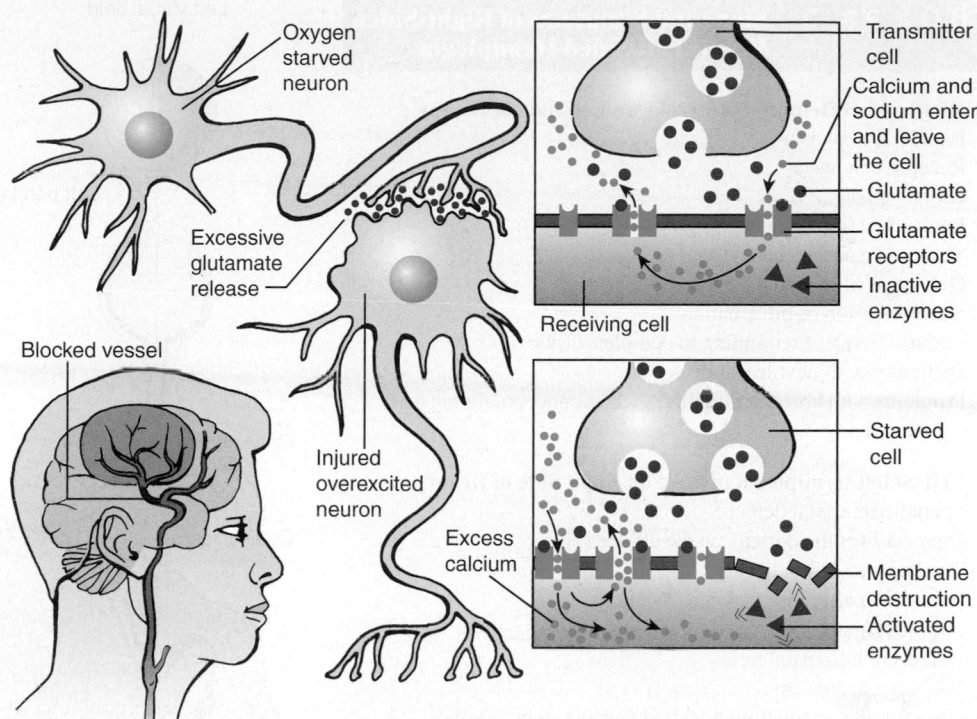

FIGURE 38-5. During a stroke, oxygen is depleted, which causes release of glutamate. Glutamate activates NMDA receptors and overexcites brain cells, leading to the release of toxic free radicals, which destroy the cells.

Immediately after a large cerebral hemorrhage, the client is unconscious. Breathing is noisy and labored. The cheek on the side of the CVA blows out on exhalation. The eyes deviate toward the affected side of the brain. The pulse is slow, full, and bounding. Initially, BP is elevated. Temperature is elevated during the acute phase and persists for several days. The level of consciousness (LOC) ranges from lethargy and mental confusion to deep coma, which can persist for days or even weeks. The longer the coma, the poorer the prognosis and the less likely that consciousness will return.

Clinical manifestations following a stroke are highly variable and depend on the area of the cerebral cortex and the affected hemisphere (Box 38-3), the degree of blockage (total, partial), and the presence or absence of adequate **collateral circulation**, circulation formed by smaller blood vessels branching off from or near larger occluded vessels.

BOX 38-2 | **Risk Factors for Cerebrovascular Accident**

Uncontrollable
- *Age*: Risk of CVA increases with each decade beyond age 55 years.
- *Sex*: Men have a slightly higher risk than women.
- *Race*: African Americans experience more CVAs than do other groups.
- *Genetics*: Those whose blood relatives have had a CVA are at increased risk.

Controllable
- *Hypertension*: 40% to 90% of clients with CVA have previous hypertension.
- *Atrial fibrillation*: 15% of those with atrial fibrillation, a dysrhythmia associated with thromboembolic complications, develop a CVA.
- *Hyperlipidemia*: High blood cholesterol and low-density lipo-protein (LDL) levels increase the risk for atherosclerosis and CVA.

- *Diabetes*: Elevated blood glucose level increases triglycerides and accelerates their conversion to LDLs.
- *History of TIA or CVA*: 35% of clients who already have had a TIA will have a CVA within 5 years; after one CVA, 42% of men and 24% of women have another.
- *Smoking*: Nicotine is a vasoconstrictor.
- *Obesity*: It contributes to hypertension, hyperlipidemia, and diabetes.
- *Thrombogenic substances*: Stimulants such as herbal products derived from *ephedra* plants, estrogens, and oral contraceptives increase risk.
- *Valvular disease or replacement*: Thrombi and emboli form and break free from vegetations or valve replacements.

BOX 38-3 Signs and Symptoms of Right-Sided Versus Left-Sided Hemiplegia

Right-Sided Hemiplegia (Stroke on Left Side of Brain)
Expressive aphasia
Receptive aphasia
Global aphasia
Intellectual impairment
Slow and cautious behavior
Defects in right visual fields
Short retention of information
Require frequent reminding to complete tasks
Difficulty with new learning
Problems with abstract thinking, such as conceptualizing and generalizing

Left-Sided Hemiplegia (Stroke on Right Side of Brain)
Spatial-perceptual defects
Disregard for the deficits on the affected side
Tendency to distractibility
Impulsive behavior; unaware of deficits
Poor judgment
Defects in left visual fields
Misjudge distances
Difficulty distinguishing upside-down and right-side-up
Impairment of short-term memory
Neglect left side of body; objects and people on left side

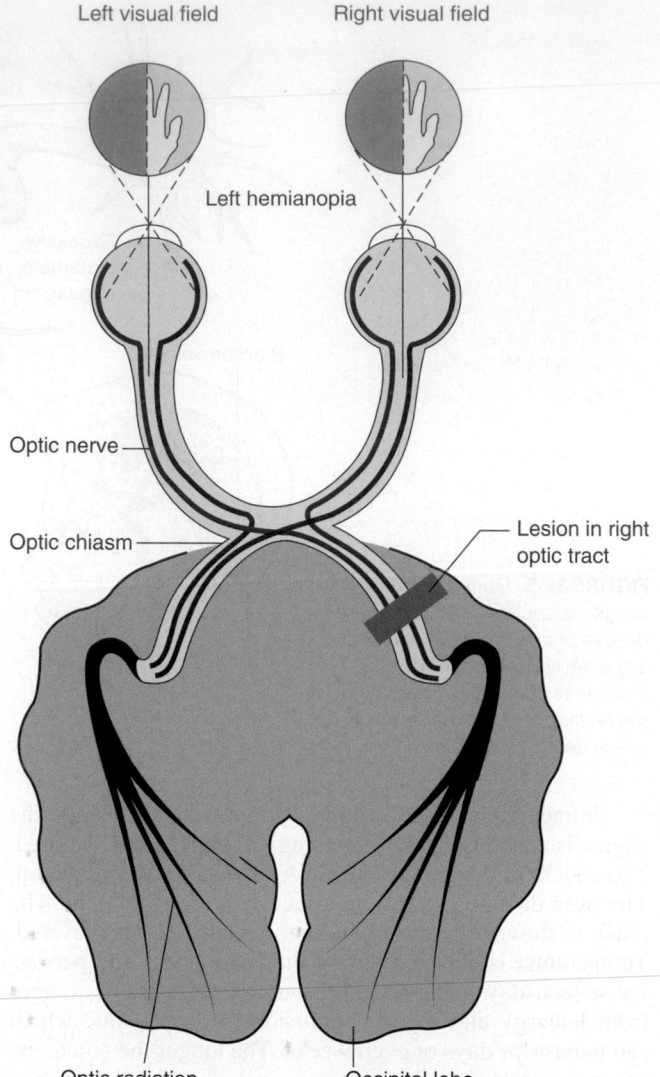

FIGURE 38-6. Hemianopia is a visual-field defect in which a person experiences an inability to see the left or right half of an image. It develops when a stroke involves the visual pathway.

A common neurologic result of a CVA in the motor area of the cerebrum is **hemiplegia** (paralysis on one side of the body). Hemiplegia occurs on the side opposite the area of the brain that is affected because motor nerves cross over (decussate) at the level of the neck. For example, when the motor area on the right side of the brain incurs a CVA, hemiplegia develops on the left side of the body: There is left-sided hemiplegia when the CVA occurs in the right hemisphere of the brain. Immediately after the CVA, the affected side is flaccid. This progresses to spastic limbs. The arm typically is more severely affected than the leg.

Expressive aphasia, the inability to speak, or **receptive aphasia**, the inability to understand spoken and written language, can result, depending on where the client's speech center is located in the brain. For most, the speech center is in the dominant hemisphere (i.e., if a person is right handed, the speech center is in the left hemisphere). A right-handed person who has a CVA in the left brain usually develops aphasia, and vice versa for a left-handed person.

Confusion and emotional lability are characteristic symptoms of a CVA. Hemianopia on the affected side is another potential consequence. **Hemianopia** is the ability to see only half of the normal visual field (Fig. 38-6). When looking straight ahead, the client cannot see to the right (in left-sided stroke) or left (in right-sided stroke) with either eye. This condition is caused by damage to the visual area of the cerebral cortex or its connections to the brain stem (optic radiations).

Neurologic deficits that result from a CVA may subside completely, partially, or not at all.

Diagnostic Findings

A CT scan or MRI differentiates a CVA from other disorders, such as a brain tumor or cerebral edema, and shows the size and location of the infarcted area. Transcranial Doppler ultrasonography determines the size of intracranial vessels and the direction of blood flow, and locates the obstructed cerebral vessel. Single-photon emission computed tomography (SPECT) also determines cerebral blood flow. An electroencephalogram reveals reduced electrical activity in the involved area, but is not a specific diagnostic test for a CVA. A lumbar puncture often is performed. If subarachnoid bleeding has occurred, the cerebrospinal fluid will be bloody. Cerebral angiography shows displacement or blockage of cerebral vessels.

Medical and Surgical Management

A CVA is a medical emergency. Treatment varies and is directed toward relieving the cause, if known. Tissue plasminogen activator (TPA), a thrombolytic agent, has been

BOX 38-4 Inclusion and Exclusion Criteria for Therapy with Tissue Plasminogen Activator (TPA)

Inclusion Criteria
- Clinical evidence of an ischemic attack
- Age >18 years
- Signed consent, if possible
- Onset of stroke within 3 hours of initiation of therapy (or from time client was last seen as "normal")
- Normal prothrombin and partial thromboplastin times

Exclusion Criteria
- Stroke or serious head trauma in past 3 months
- Major surgery or invasive procedure within past 14 days
- Gastrointestinal or urinary bleeding within past 21 days
- Puncture of noncompressible artery or biopsy of internal organ within past 7 days
- Seizure preceding or during stroke
- History of intracranial hemorrhage or known history of cerebral vascular malformations
- Pericarditis, endocarditis, septic emboli, recent pregnancy, or active inflammatory bowel disease

found to limit neurologic deficits when given within 3 hours after the onset of an ischemic CVA (Box 38-4). It is contraindicated in hemorrhagic CVAs, as is anticoagulant therapy. Several neuroprotective agents, such as NMDA receptor blockers, calcium and glutamate antagonists, and antioxidants, are nearing completion in clinical trials. Hypothermia also is being used to protect damaged cells by reducing their metabolic need for oxygen.

If atherosclerosis of the carotid artery is the cause, a carotid endarterectomy is considered. A ruptured cerebral aneurysm is treated surgically.

In many cases, treatment is supportive because medical or surgical interventions cannot repair damaged brain tissue. The best treatment available involves an intensive medical program aimed at rehabilitation and the prevention of future CVAs.

Nursing Management

Detailed nursing management for the client with a CVA is discussed in Nursing Care Plan 38-1. Client and family teaching also is essential and focuses on the following points:

- Administer medications as directed and understand the potential side and adverse effects.
- Implement eating and swallowing techniques that reduce the potential for aspiration (Nutrition Notes 38-1).
- Perform the Heimlich maneuver to clear the airway if the client cannot speak or breathe after swallowing food (see Chap. 20).
- Continue follow-up care with the speech pathologist and dietitian.
- Contact community resources such as medical supply companies that rent or sell special care devices such as a hospital bed, bedside commode, walker, or tripod cane.

- Remove throw rugs, clutter, and electrical cords from the client's home environment to reduce the potential for falls.
- Perform regular exercises, change the client's position frequently, and apply braces or splints designed to maintain extremities in proper anatomic position.

 Gerontologic Considerations

- The older adult is more susceptible to the complications of prolonged bed rest and inactivity such as hypostatic pneumonia, pressure ulcers, and contractures that may be involved in the rehabilitation period after a CVA.

- Healthcare providers should avoid stereotypes that suggest older persons may lack motivation or the ability to participate in rehabilitation efforts, or that the outcomes will not be positive. The healthcare provider may need to encourage family or friends to overcome these beliefs to prevent dampening motivation.

- Rehabilitation of the older client with a CVA is subject to more complications than rehabilitation of a younger adult. The nurse must work closely with the family and social service agencies to help the family assume the care of the client to the extent possible or to facilitate a transfer to a rehabilitation center or long-term care facility.

 Nutrition Notes 38-1
The Client With a Cerebrovascular Accident

- When the client can resume oral intake after a CVA, individualize the diet according to his or her ability to chew and swallow. Semisolid and medium-consistency foods such as pudding, scrambled eggs, cooked cereals, and thickened liquids are easiest to swallow. Cold foods stimulate swallowing. The client should avoid tepid foods, because they are more difficult to locate in the mouth, and extremely hot foods, which can cause overreaction. The client should also avoid foods most likely to cause choking: peanut butter, bread, tart foods, dry or crisp foods, and chewy meats. Progress the texture as swallowing ability improves.
- Clients with decreased salivation benefit from added gravies and sauces. Thinking of a specific food before eating stimulates salivation, as do eating dill pickles and sucking on lemon slices.
- To minimize the volume of food needed, provide nutritionally dense foods such as thickened commercial beverages, fortified puddings, fortified cooked cereals, and scrambled eggs.
- When a normal diet is resumed, encourage the client to eat "heart healthy"—less saturated and trans fats and more fruits, vegetables, and whole grains. Encourage overweight clients to lose weight to reduce cardiac workload. Sodium restriction is appropriate for clients with hypertension.

NURSING CARE PLAN 38-1 | The Client With a Cerebrovascular Accident

Assessment

Determine the following:

- Time symptoms began
- Medical, drug, and allergy history from the family (or client if he or she can report)
- Vital signs and LOC
- Size and response of pupils to light

- Any musculoskeletal weakness or paralysis
- Capacity to speak or understand spoken language
- Changes in visual field
- Ability to swallow
- Any alteration in bladder or bowel control
- Integrity of the skin; evidence of soft tissue injury as a consequence of falling

Nursing Diagnoses: Impaired Swallowing related to hemiplegia; **Risk for Aspiration** related to impaired swallowing; **Risk for Deficient Fluid Volume** related to impaired swallowing; **Risk for Imbalanced Nutrition: Less than Body Requirements** related to impaired swallowing

Expected Outcomes: (1) Client will swallow without aspiration. (2) Fluid intake will be at least 2000 mL/24 hours. (3) Client will consume sufficient calories to maintain admission weight.

Interventions	Rationales
Elevate client's head for eating or drinking; position client on his or her side at other times.	Sitting and facing food or liquids raises client's awareness and attention; a side-lying position prevents aspiration if vomiting occurs or saliva accumulates in the mouth.
Keep a suction machine at the bedside.	Mechanical suctioning facilitates clearing the airway of saliva, food, and fluids.
Limit distractions (e.g., turn off the television when the client eats or drinks).	The client can better concentrate and follow nursing instructions when distracting stimuli are reduced.
Use a thickening agent for watery substances; request viscous or pureed food from the dietary department.	The tongue can more easily manipulate thickened liquids against the palate and oral pharynx.
Request small, frequent nourishment from the dietary department rather than three large meals.	Eating small amounts is less tiring, and the client may consume more on a daily basis.
Offer or remind client to load the fork or spoon with a small amount of food.	A small amount is easier to manage in the mouth and less likely to cause a complete airway obstruction.
Place thickened liquids or pureed food on the unaffected side of the mouth.	The client can feel and use the unaffected side of the mouth for chewing and swallowing.
Lower client's chin to his or her chest when swallowing.	Lowering the chin helps close the laryngopharynx and reduces the potential for aspiration.
Encourage client to swallow several times.	Several efforts at swallowing may be necessary to move food to the esophagus.
Check the mouth for pocketed food before offering more.	The client may be unaware of food that remains unswallowed
Instruct client to use the tongue to relocate pocketed food or apply gentle pressure on the cheek to reposition food. Collaborate with the physician concerning gastric or enteral tube feedings if oral intake is inadequate.	Physical manipulation helps reposition trapped food.

Evaluation of Expected Outcomes

The airway remains patent, and lungs are clear to auscultation. There is an adequate intake of food and fluids.

Nursing Diagnoses: Total Urinary Incontinence; Bowel Incontinence or **Risk for Constipation** related to diminished LOC, confusion, and immobility

Expected Outcome: Urinary and bowel elimination will be controlled independently or with minimal assistance.

Interventions	Rationales
Maintain a record of bowel elimination.	It provides data that can indicate if the client requires a stool softener, laxative, suppository, or enema.
Place an elevated seat over the toilet.	An elevated seat reduces the work of transferring to the toilet seat and back to a wheelchair.
Assist client to the toilet every 2 hours while he or she is awake and after each meal.	Positioning and environmental cues may help stimulate the client to eliminate. The gastrocolic reflex that promotes bowel evacuation is stronger soon after eating.
Dress client in unrestricted clothing that facilitates elimination needs.	Clothing that is easy to undo or lower reduces the potential for incontinence.

NURSING CARE PLAN 38-1 **The Client With a Cerebrovascular Accident** (Continued)

Interventions	Rationales
Avoid negative comments if incontinence occurs; acknowledge client's success when he or she eliminates while on the toilet or commode.	Criticism lowers self-confidence and self-esteem; praise encourages client to continue efforts at controlling elimination.
Apply incontinence garments or place absorbent pads beneath client.	Concealment of urine or stool preserves client's dignity.
Collaborate with the physician concerning the insertion of an external or indwelling catheter.	An external catheter is less likely to predispose to a urinary tract infection; a catheter helps keep the skin dry and reduces embarrassment of incontinence.
Administer a prescribed suppository or low-volume enema when necessary.	Chemical or mechanical stimulation increases intestinal contraction, which helps to evacuate the bowel.

Evaluation of Expected Outcome

Bowel and urinary elimination are managed at the highest level the client can achieve.

Nursing Diagnoses: Self-Care Deficit related to hemiplegia; **Unilateral Neglect** related to hemianopia; **Impaired Mobility: Physical** related to hemiplegia

Expected Outcomes: (1) Client will resume independent activities of daily living (ADLs). (2) Client will identify and care for paralyzed body parts. (3) Client will use assistive devices to achieve mobility.

Interventions	Rationales
Approach and place objects within client's field of vision.	Client is likely to ignore objects and people that are located in areas where the visual field is impaired.
Help reintegrate the weak side by reminding the client to look at it.	Calling attention to the neglected side of the body helps the client recognize and accept that it exists.
Set realistic goals for self-care.	Unrealistic goals lead to frustration and discouragement.
Consult with an occupational therapist (OT) or physical therapist (PT) regarding modifications in clothing, utensils, and assistive devices.	Therapists have expertise in measures to accommodate for neurologic deficits.
Attach a trapeze above the bed.	Client can use a trapeze with one hand to independently facilitate position changes.
Perform range-of-motion (ROM) exercises at least once each shift.	ROM exercises maintain joint mobility and muscle tone.
Support the affected arm in a sling when the client is upright.	An arm sling improves posture and reduces musculoskeletal changes in the shoulder joint.
Position client to avoid contractures (e.g., use a foot board, trochanter roll at the hip, rolled cloth in the paralyzed hand).	Skeletal muscles tend to become permanently shortened unless efforts are made to maintain normal anatomic position.
Consult the PT about devices to assist ambulation, such as a log brace and walker.	A brace promotes stability when standing and walking. A walker supports the client and facilitates ambulation.

Evaluation of Expected Outcomes

Client performs ADLs alone or with assistance and learns to use assistive devices.

Nursing Diagnosis: Risk for Impaired Skin Integrity related to pressure over bony prominences secondary to immobility

Expected Outcome: Skin will remain intact.

Interventions	Rationales
Keep skin clean and dry.	Cleaning the skin removes transient bacteria. Drying the skin prevents maceration, a process in which skin is softened and easily eroded.
Use a turning sheet and get assistance when changing client's position.	A turning sheet prevents shearing, the movement of a layer of tissue in one direction as another moves in opposition.
Massage skin areas that blanch when pressure is relieved.	Massage improves blood flow to tissue, but it is contraindicated if tissue is already damaged as evidenced by a sustained lack of color when pressure is relieved.
Use pressure-relieving devices or a therapeutic bed that alternately distributes the client's body weight.	Tissue damage occurs unless intracapillary pressure is maintained at 32 mm Hg or more; relief of pressure at least every 2 hours reduces tissue hypoxia.

(care plan continues on page 562)

NURSING CARE PLAN 38-1 **The Client With a Cerebrovascular Accident** (Continued)

Evaluation of Expected Outcome

Skin is intact; there is no evidence of pressure sores.

Nursing Diagnosis: Impaired Verbal Communication related to expressive aphasia

Expected Outcome: Client will make needs understood either verbally or nonverbally.

Interventions	Rationales
Ask questions requiring a "yes" or "no," and suggest the client respond by nodding the head.	Nodding the head is a form of body language that communicates agreement or disagreement.
Instruct client to speak slowly when attempting to communicate orally.	If unpressured to quickly respond, the client may be able to formulate words and sentences more easily.
Have client point to or write key words or phrases.	Some clients retain the ability to read written language although they may not be able to express themselves orally.
Support and practice techniques used in speech therapy.	Practicing new techniques helps to promote mastery.

Evaluation of Expected Outcome

Client can communicate either orally, in writing, or with techniques that facilitate nonverbal communication.

Nursing Diagnoses: Risk for Ineffective Coping and **Risk for Compromised Family Coping** related to diminished psychosocial resources to deal with multiple stressors

Expected Outcome: Client and family will cope with illness and changes in life-style.

Interventions	Rationales
Listen and try to identify clues to client's or family's future concerns.	Identifying problems that require actions facilitates coping.
Acknowledge personal strengths.	Recognition of strengths promotes confidence in the ability to overcome current problems.
Encourage individuals in the client's social network to collaborate on problem-solving.	Successful outcomes are more likely when there is a team effort.
Refer client and family to a discharge planner, social worker, or community social services for arranging extended care, home care, and respite care.	The health team includes persons with expertise in assisting clients and their families with postdischarge issues.

Evaluation of Expected Outcome

- Client and family cope with the client's neurologic deficits; referrals are made to services or facilities that can assist with long-term recovery.
- The family pursues a plan for postdischarge management.

▶ *Stop, Think, and Respond Exercise 38-2*

When a client with an evolving CVA arrives in the emergency department, her speech is difficult to understand, the left side of her face has a drooped appearance, and she cannot move her left arm and leg. Before this client becomes a candidate for TPA, what other information is important to gather?

CEREBRAL ANEURYSMS

An **aneurysm** is a weakening in the wall of a blood vessel. Most aneurysms occur in arteries, where blood flow is under high pressure. Cerebral aneurysms usually occur in the circle of Willis, a ring of arteries that supply the brain (Fig. 38-7).

Pathophysiology and Etiology

Aneurysms develop at a weakened area in the blood vessel wall. The defect is congenital or secondary to hypertension and atherosclerosis.

An aneurysm can affect cranial nerve function (see Chap. 36) as the aneurysm presses on these structures. For many, there is no prior warning that an aneurysm exists. Berry aneurysms, a type of congenital cerebral aneurysm, can rupture at any time without prior symptoms. The sudden cerebral hemorrhage causes immediate neurologic changes from increased ICP, interruption of oxygenated blood flow to the surrounding cells and tissues, and blood collecting in the subarachnoid space. Occasionally, there is a slow leakage of blood from an aneurysm, in which case symptoms are less severe.

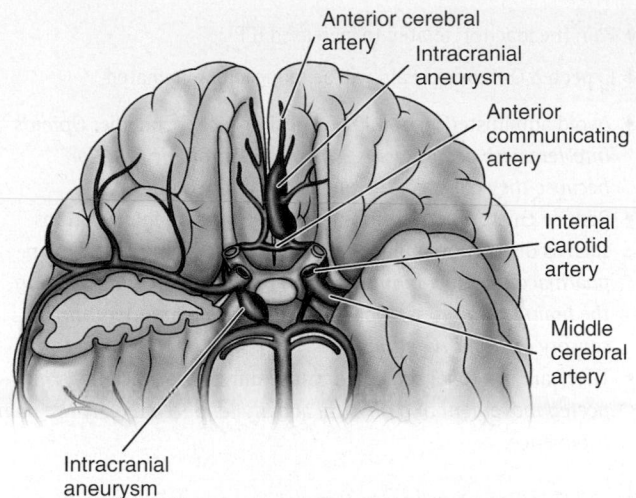

FIGURE 38-7. An intracranial aneurysm may occur in any of the cerebral arteries that make up the circle of Willis.

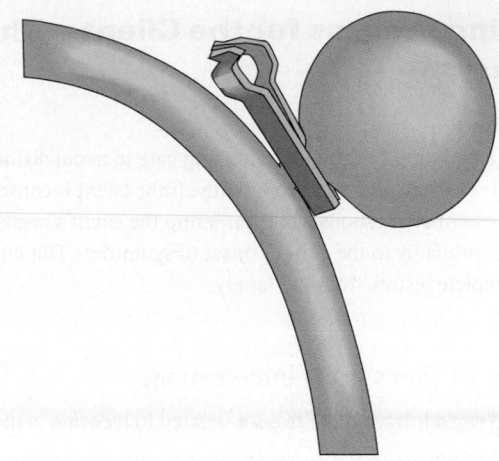

FIGURE 38-8. An aneurysm is clamped to prevent rupture. Wrapping the aneurysm with supportive material is another alternative.

Assessment Findings

Symptoms include sudden and severe headache, dizziness, nausea, and vomiting, usually followed by a rapid loss of consciousness. If the ruptured aneurysm produces a slow leak, a stiff neck, headache, visual disturbances, and intermittent nausea develop.

Cerebral angiography can reveal an unruptured aneurysm. The procedure is performed with caution because the added fluid pressure can increase the risk of rupturing the blood vessel, dislodge plaque-formed emboli, and cause ischemia from vasospasm. A CT scan and MRI are safer for locating the site of the aneurysm and determining the amount of blood in the subarachnoid space. A lumbar puncture reveals grossly bloody cerebrospinal fluid when an aneurysm ruptures. The physician may identify the status and prognosis of the client based on criteria in the Hunt-Hess classification system (Table 38-2). As the grade increases, the prognosis becomes less optimistic.

Medical Management

Conservative management is attempted until a decision is made regarding surgical repair of the aneurysm. Some aneurysms are considered inoperable because of anatomic location, and only medical treatment is possible.

Complete bed rest, the prevention of rebleeding at the rupture site, and treatment of complications are primary goals. Absolute bed rest in a quiet area, preferably a private room, is essential. Visitors are restricted except for family members. The head of the bed is elevated to reduce ICP and cerebral edema. Hypertension is treated with antihypertensive agents.

Anticonvulsants are given to prevent seizures. Tranquilizers or barbiturates are used to keep the conscious client relaxed and quiet. Increased ICP is managed with osmotic diuretics and corticosteroids (see Chap. 37).

Mechanical ventilation is necessary to support respirations and provide oxygenation if the client is unconscious. Aminocaproic acid (Amicar) is used to delay lysis (breaking up) of the blood clot because lysis results in rebleeding.

Surgical Management

Surgical repair is attempted after the initial hemorrhage because the danger of further hemorrhage from the weakened aneurysm is great. The operation is not without hazard; manipulation of the small cerebral vessels can result in increased vasospasm or thrombosis and cerebral infarction. The risks of surgery are less serious than the dangers of recurrent hemorrhage from the aneurysm. Surgical approaches with a craniotomy include wrapping or clipping the aneurysm in an attempt to control further bleeding (Fig. 38-8).

An alternative to direct repair of the aneurysm by a craniotomy approach is ligation of or application of a clamp to one of the carotid arteries. This is an extracranial (outside the cranium) procedure because the surgical approach is below the jaw. The purpose of this approach is to obstruct blood flow to the vessel that has an aneurysm, thus reducing the pressure in the aneurysm and preventing rupture or further bleeding. Collateral circulation in the cerebral vessels must be adequate for success.

TABLE 38-2 The Hunt-Hess Scale for Grading a Client with a Cerebral Aneurysm

CLASSIFICATION	CLINICAL CRITERIA
Grade I	Alert, oriented, asymptomatic
Grade II	Alert, oriented, headache, stiff neck
Grade III	Lethargic or confused, minor focal deficits such as hemiparesis (weakness on one side)
Grade IV	Stupor, moderate to severe focal deficits such as hemiplegia
Grade V	Comatose, severe neurologic deficits such as posturing (see Chap. 39)

(Adapted from Hickey, J. V. [2008]. *The clinical practice of neurological and neurosurgical nursing* [6th ed.]. Philadelphia: Lippincott Williams & Wilkins.)

Nursing Process for the Client with an Aneurysm

Assessment

Perform a neurologic examination, taking care to avoid disturbing the client. Measure vital signs frequently. If the client is conscious, ask only essential questions while gathering the client's history, limiting it primarily to the current onset of symptoms. Obtain a more complete history from the family.

Diagnosis, Planning, and Interventions

▶ **PC: Increased Intracranial Pressure** related to bleeding in the brain

▶ **Expected Outcome:** The nurse will monitor for, manage, and minimize ICP.

- Use the Glasgow Coma Scale (GCS) to assess neurologic status at least every hour (see Chap. 36). *The GCS is a systematic assessment tool for documenting neurologic function and identifying early clinical changes.*
- Report neurologic changes as soon as a trend indicates worsening of the client's condition. *Early collaboration with the physician facilitates implementing medically prescribed interventions that will reduce or eliminate more serious complications.*
- Keep client calm and physically still. *Activity or emotional distress elevates BP and ICP, which could cause or contribute to more bleeding.*
- Avoid any activities that cause a Valsalva maneuver such as coughing, straining at stool, and rough position changes. *Bearing down raises BP and increases the potential for rupture of the aneurysm or increased bleeding if the aneurysm has already ruptured.*
- Follow the physician's orders for fluid restrictions and drug therapy for reducing hypertension, potential seizures, restlessness, and anxiety. *Interventions that reduce BP, large motor movements, and emotional stress help to reduce ICP.*
- Elevate client's head or follow the physician's directive for body position (some prefer that the client remain flat). *Head elevation helps venous blood and cerebrospinal fluid drain from cerebral areas and reduces the volume in the cranium.*
- Limit visitors to the immediate family; suggest they take turns and stay briefly. *Although visitors' and family members' desires to interact with the client are well intentioned, the stimulation can increase ICP or trigger a seizure.*

▶ **PC: Seizures** related to increased ICP

▶ **Expected Outcome:** The nurse will monitor to detect, manage, and minimize seizures.

- Institute seizure precautions (see Chap. 37). *Seizure precautions are used to prevent or minimize seizure-related injuries.*
- Implement anticonvulsant drug therapy as prescribed. *Anticonvulsants reduce excitation of neurons in the brain that result in seizure activity.*

▶ Pain (headache) related to increased ICP

▶ **Expected Outcome:** Pain will be reduced or eliminated.

- Avoid administering opioid analgesics, except codeine. *Opioids interfere with accurate assessment of neurologic function because they constrict the pupils and depress LOC.*
- Reduce environmental stimuli, and use nursing interventions such as distraction, guided imagery, and soothing music. *Non-pharmacologic techniques for pain relief are based on blocking the brain's awareness of pain by substituting another form of sensory or cognitive stimulus.*
- Take care not to jar the bed or cause unnecessary activity. *Unexpected movement and physical activity tend to intensify the pain experience.*

▶ **Self-Care Deficit** related to imposed rest and decreased LOC

▶ **Expected Outcome:** Client's basic needs will be met.

- Perform only those activities of daily living for the client that are absolutely necessary. *Keeping the client quiet, which reduces the risk for life-threatening complications, takes greater precedence over bathing, ambulating, and the like.*
- Provide rest between necessary nursing tasks. *Limiting tasks to brief moments prevents overstimulating the client.*
- Feed client calorie-dense foods in small amounts at frequent intervals. *In this way, the client's hunger is managed without requiring a large intake of food at any one time.*

▶ **Risk for Ineffective Peripheral Tissue Perfusion and Risk for Impaired Skin Integrity** related to imposed inactivity

▶ **Expected Outcomes:** (1) Peripheral circulation will be maintained. (2) Skin will remain intact.

- Apply elastic stockings to lower extremities or use a pneumatic compression device. *Intermittent compression passively moves venous blood toward the heart in a way similar to active skeletal muscle contraction. Elastic stockings support the valves of veins in the lower extremities to prevent venous stasis.*
- Use pressure-relieving pads or a similar type of mattress. *Relieving pressure promotes the circulation of oxygenated blood through capillaries to peripheral cells and tissues and facilitates venous blood return.*

Evaluation of Expected Outcomes

The ICP is maintained within a safe range. The client does not manifest seizures. His or her level of discomfort is tolerable. Essential needs for nutrition, hydration, ventilation, and elimination are met. Peripheral circulation is adequate; there are no signs of skin breakdown. For the client who undergoes a craniotomy, refer to Chapter 37.

Discharge teaching depends on the method of treatment and the recommendations of the physician. Usually, the nurse instructs clients to avoid heavy lifting, straining at stool, extreme emotional situations, and other work-related activities that could raise BP and increase ICP.

When the client must restrict his or her life-style, the changes are likely to cause financial, physical, and social hardships for the client and family. Referrals to a social service worker, counselor, or social service agency are appropriate.

CRITICAL THINKING EXERCISES

1. What suggestions could you give to someone who has migraine headaches to help reduce their severity?

2. A client is brought to the emergency department after being found unconscious at home. A CVA is the tentative diagnosis. The family is advocating for the administration of a thrombolytic agent. What factors may be contraindications to this form of treatment?

3. The family of a client who has had a stroke is concerned about postdischarge care. The client has left-sided paralysis, is incontinent, and has expressive aphasia. What help can you offer the family?

4. When assigned to care for a client with a leaking cerebral aneurysm, what nursing interventions are appropriate for reducing the potential for a serious intracranial bleed?

NCLEX-STYLE REVIEW QUESTIONS

1. A client arrives at the headache center for an initial evaluation. The client describes flashing lights before the headache begins. The nurse is most correct in documenting the presence of which of the following?
1. A premonition of a migraine headache
2. An aura prior to a migraine headache
3. A papillary response creating the headache
4. Intense photophobia prior to the headache onset

2. When a nurse assesses a client, which finding suggests that the client is having transient ischemic attacks (TIAs)?
1. Brief periods of photosensitivity
2. Brief periods of mental depression
3. Brief periods of unilateral weakness
4. Brief periods of stabbing head pain

3. When providing a dietary tray to a client with hemianopia, it is best for the nurse to do which of following?
1. Place the tray most convenient for staff, as the cl will need to be assisted.
2. Place the tray on the right side of the client to allow for self-feeding.
3. Place the tray on the left side of the client to allow for self-feeding.
4. Place the tray directly in front of the client to allow for self-feeding.

4. What nursing intervention is most appropriate to decrease the frustration experienced by a client with expressive aphasia?
1. Use a picture or alphabet board with frequently needed topics.
2. Ask the client to shake head yes or no to different options.
3. Offer emotional support by telling the client you know how frustrating this must be.
4. Arrange for family to be present when attempting to communicate with the client.

5. A client with a leaking cerebral aneurysm is being treated conservatively with complete rest, anticonvulsants, and sedatives. If the nurse observed the following when caring for the client with a cerebral aneurysm, for which one is it most important to intervene?
1. The client is not sleeping well.
2. The client is constipated.
3. The client has a diminished appetite.
4. The client has a sore throat.

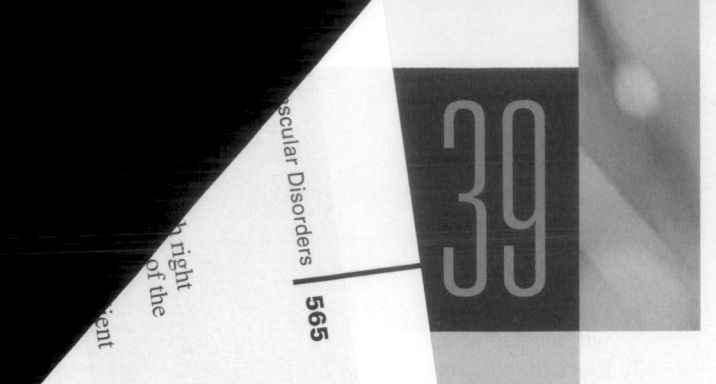

39 Caring for Clients with Head and Spinal Cord Trauma

Words To Know

autonomic dysreflexia
autoregulation
Battle's sign
cerebral hematoma
chemonucleolysis
closed head injury
concussion
contrecoup injury
contusion
coup injury
craniectomy
cranioplasty
craniotomy
diskectomy
epidural hematoma
extramedullary
functional electrical stimulation
halo sign
infratentorial
intracerebral hematoma
intramedullary
laminectomy
open head injury
otorrhea
paraplegia
paresthesia
periorbital ecchymosis
poikilothermia
rhinorrhea
spinal fusion
spinal shock
subdural hematoma
supratentorial
tentorium
tetraplegia
uncal herniation

Learning Objectives

On completion of this chapter, you will be able to:

1. Differentiate a concussion from a contusion.
2. Explain the differences between epidural, subdural, and intracerebral hematomas.
3. Discuss the nursing management of a client with a head injury.
4. Discuss the nursing management of a client undergoing intracranial surgery.
5. Explain spinal shock, listing four symptoms.
6. Discuss autonomic dysreflexia and at least five manifestations.
7. List possible long-term complications of spinal cord injury.
8. Describe the nursing management of a client with a spinal cord injury.
9. Identify the anatomic difference between intramedullary and extramedullary spinal nerve root compression.

H ead and spinal cord trauma can result in permanent disability and dysfunction. This chapter discusses head injuries, which include lacerations, skull fractures, and bleeding and swelling within the brain and surrounding tissues. It also discusses spinal disorders caused by trauma and mechanical injury.

HEAD INJURIES

Injury to the head can cause concussions, contusions, hematomas, or skull fracture.

CONCUSSION

Pathophysiology and Etiology

A **concussion** results from a blow to the head that jars the brain. It usually is a consequence of falling, striking the head against a hard surface such as a windshield, colliding with another person (e.g., between athletes), battering during boxing, or being a victim of violence. A concussion results in diffuse and microscopic injury to the brain. The force of the blow causes temporary neurologic impairment but no serious damage to cerebral tissue. There is generally complete recovery within a short time. However, in older adults, recovery may take longer.

Assessment Findings

The client may experience a brief lapse of consciousness, with temporary disorientation, headache, blurred or double vision, emotional irritability, and dizziness. Skull radiography, computed tomography (CT) scan, and magnetic resonance imaging (MRI) rule out a more serious head injury (e.g., skull fracture, intracranial bleeding).

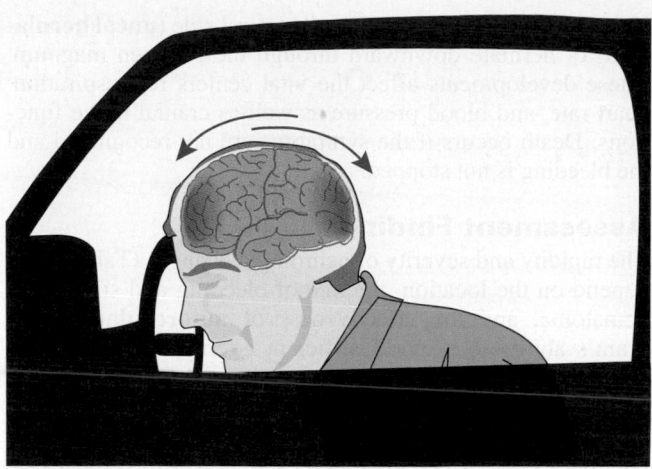

FIGURE 39-1. Coup injuries occur at the point of contact, and contrecoup injuries occur when the brain rebounds and hits the opposite side of the skull.

Medical Management

The client's activity is temporarily halted until the seriousness of the injury is determined. Mild analgesia (usually acetaminophen) relieves the headache. The client is observed for neurologic complications.

Nursing Management

The nurse performs a neurologic assessment (see Chap. 36). If findings are normal and the client does not require hospitalization, the nurse instructs the family to watch the client closely for signs of increased intracranial pressure (ICP). Common signs of increased ICP include behavioral alterations, sleepiness, personality changes, vomiting, and speech or gait disturbances (see Chap. 37). The nurse instructs the client and family to contact a physician or return to the emergency department (ED) if any of these symptoms occur.

CONTUSION

A **contusion** is more serious than a concussion and leads to gross structural injury to the brain.

Pathophysiology and Etiology

Contusions result in bruising and, sometimes, hemorrhage of superficial cerebral tissue. When the head is struck directly, the injury to the brain is called a **coup injury**. Dual bruising can result if the force is strong enough to send the brain ricocheting to the opposite side of the skull, which is called a **contrecoup injury** (Fig. 39-1). Edema develops at the site of or in areas opposite to the injury. A skull fracture can accompany a contusion.

Assessment Findings

Signs and symptoms vary depending on the severity of the blow and the degree of head velocity. Clients exhibit hypotension, rapid and weak pulse, shallow respirations, loss of consciousness, and pale, clammy skin. While unconscious, they usually respond to strong stimuli, such as pressure applied to base of the nail (Fig. 39-2). On awakening, clients often have temporary *amnesia* (loss of memory) for recent events. Permanent brain damage can impair intellect and gait and cause speech difficulty, seizures, and paralysis.

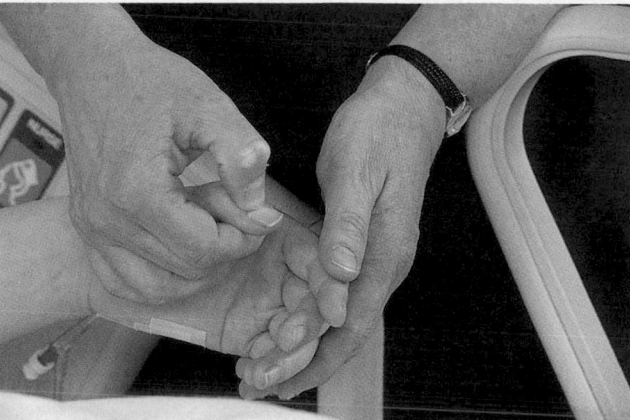

FIGURE 39-2. The nurse tests the client's motor response by assessing response to a painful stimulus. (Photo © B. Proud.)

Skull radiography is performed to rule out or confirm skull fracture. CT or MRI detects bleeding or small hemorrhages in brain tissue, a shift in brain tissue, and edema at the injury site.

Medical Management

The unstable client's vital functions are supported with drug therapy and mechanical ventilation if necessary.

Nursing Management

The nurse observes the client closely for changes in level of consciousness (LOC), signs of increased ICP (see Chap. 37), neurologic changes, respiratory distress, and changes in vital signs every 1 to 2 hours. If symptoms develop, the nurse reports them to the physician.

Prevention of health problems is a major component of nursing care. To reduce the potential for both minor and life-threatening head injuries, the nurse stresses the importance of:

- Using seatbelts for all passengers in automobiles
- Restraining infants in approved car seats located in the rear seats of automobiles
- Wearing protective head gear while riding, skiing, bicycles or motorcycles and when participating in contact sports such as hockey, baseball, or softball
- Raising neck restraints on the backs of car seats
- Not driving under the influence of alcohol or drugs

CEREBRAL HEMATOMAS

A **cerebral hematoma** is bleeding within the skull. The accumulation of blood forms an expanding lesion. People at high risk for cerebral hematomas are those receiving anticoagulant therapy or those with an underlying bleeding disorder, such as hemophilia, thrombocytopenia, leukemia, and aplastic anemia (see Chap. 31).

Pathophysiology and Etiology

Most hematomas result from head trauma or cerebral vascular disorders. The types are epidural hematoma, subdural hematoma, and intracerebral hematoma (Fig. 39-3).

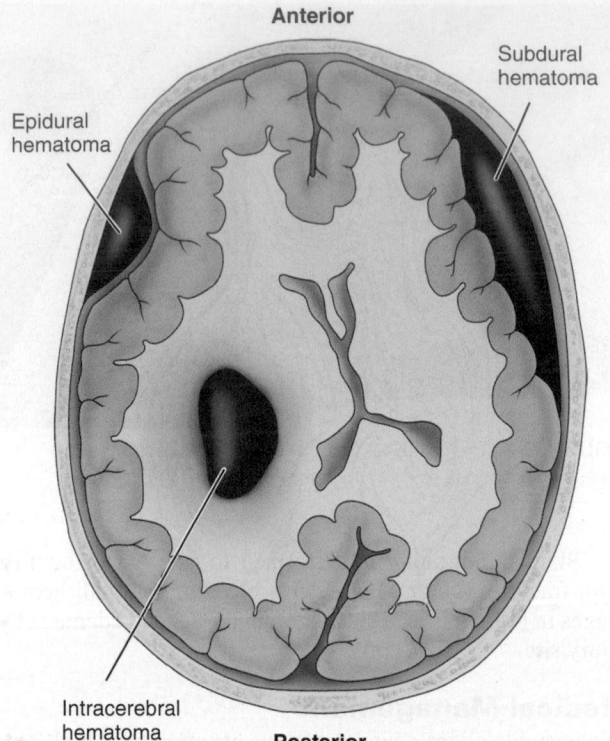

FIGURE 39-3. Location of epidural, subdural, and intracerebral hematomas.

An **epidural hematoma** stems from arterial bleeding, usually from the middle meningeal artery, and blood accumulation above the dura. It is characterized by rapidly progressive neurologic deterioration. A **subdural hematoma** results from venous bleeding, with blood gradually accumulating in the space below the dura. Subdural hematomas are classified as acute, subacute, and chronic according to the rate of neurologic changes. Symptoms progressively worsen in a client with an acute subdural hematoma within the first 24 hours of the head injury. Clients with subacute and chronic subdural hematomas become symptomatic after 24 hours and up to 1 week later. An **intracerebral hematoma** is bleeding within the brain that results from an open or closed head injury or from a cerebrovascular condition such as a ruptured cerebral aneurysm (see Chap. 38).

Bleeding increases the volume of brain contents and ICP, which disrupts blood flow and causes the brain to become ischemic and hypoxic. Unrelieved increased ICP also causes the brain to shift to the lateral side (**uncal herniation**) or herniate downward through the foramen magnum. These developments affect the vital centers for respiration, heart rate, and blood pressure as well as cranial nerve functions. Death occurs if the symptoms are not recognized and the bleeding is not stopped.

Assessment Findings

The rapidity and severity of neurologic changes (Table 39-1) depend on the location, the rate of bleeding and size of the hematoma, and the effectiveness of **autoregulation**, the brain's ability to provide sufficient arterial blood flow despite rising ICP. MRI and CT scan show densities that indicate the location of the hematoma and shifts in cerebral tissue. ICP monitoring (see Chap. 37) provides direct and continuous data for evaluating the extent to which the lesion is expanding or responding to treatment.

Medical Management

In some cases, the body walls off and absorbs a subdural hematoma with no treatment. However, a rapid change in LOC and signs of uncontrolled increased ICP indicate a surgical emergency.

Surgical Management

Surgery consists of drilling holes (*burr holes*) in the skull to relieve pressure (Fig. 39-4), removing the clot, and stopping the bleeding. If the source of bleeding cannot be located by means of burr holes, more invasive surgery is performed. Epidural hematomas require more prompt intervention because the rate of bleeding is greater from an arterial bleed than from a venous bleed.

Intracranial surgery consists of three possible procedures: craniotomy, craniectomy, and cranioplasty. A **craniotomy** is a surgical opening of the skull to gain access to structures beneath the cranial bones. It is performed to remove a blood clot or tumor, stop intracranial bleeding, or repair damaged brain tissues or blood vessels. A **craniectomy** is removal of a portion of a cranial bone. **Cranioplasty** is the repair of a defect in a cranial bone (see Chap. 37). A metal or plastic plate or wire mesh is used to replace the removed bone or to reinforce a defect in a cranial bone.

One of two surgical approaches is used to enter the brain above or below the **tentorium**, a double fold of dura mater that separates the cerebrum from the cerebellum. A **supratentorial** (above the tentorium) approach is made through a

TABLE 39-1 Differences in Cerebral Hematomas

TYPE	LOCATION	SIGNS AND SYMPTOMS
Epidural	Arterial blood collects between the skull and dura.	Client may be alert after initial unconsciousness, but then becomes increasingly lethargic before lapsing into coma. Common symptoms are headache, ipsilateral (same side as injury) pupil changes, and contralateral (opposite side to injury) hemiparesis (weakness or paralysis).
Subdural	Venous blood collects between the dura and subarachnoid layers.	Deterioration in LOC is progressive. There are ipsilateral pupil changes, decreased extraocular muscle movement, and contralateral hemiparesis, with periodic episodes of memory lapse, confusion, drowsiness, and personality changes.
Intracerebral	Blood collects within the brain.	Client shows classic signs of increased ICP: headache, vomiting, seizures, posturing, hyperthermia, irregular breathing.

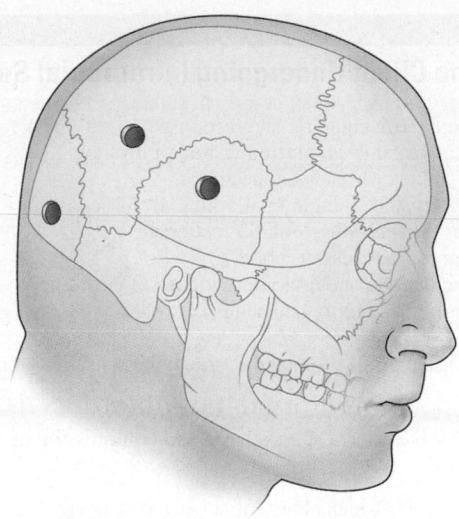

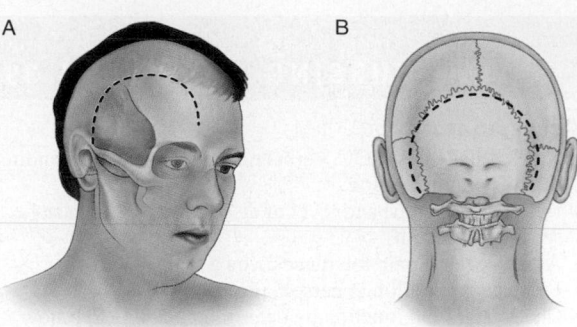

A   B

FIGURE 39-5. (**A**) A supratentorial incision is made behind the hairline on the side of pathology. (**B**) An infratentorial incision is a horseshoe-shaped incision around the occipital lobe.

FIGURE 39-4. Neurosurgical procedures may require the use of burr holes to make a bone flap in the skull, aspirate a brain abscess, or evacuate a hematoma.

scalp incision at the site where a particular cerebral lobe requires surgical access. The **infratentorial** (below the tentorium) approach provides an opening to the midbrain and structures of the brain stem. The incision is made at the back of the head with the client in a sitting position (Fig. 39-5).

In cranial surgery, after several burr holes are made in the skull, a saw is used to cut a section of bone (bone flap). The bone flap is removed to provide a visual field for surgery. After surgery is completed, the bone flap usually is replaced. In some instances, such as with an inoperable tumor, the bone flap is not replaced, allowing the tumor to expand, and thus reducing the rate at which ICP rises. Complications associated with intracranial surgery include cerebral edema, infection, neurogenic shock (see Chap. 17), fluid and electrolyte imbalances, venous thrombosis (especially in the arms and legs), increased ICP, seizures, leakage of cerebrospinal fluid (CSF), and stress ulcers and hemorrhage.

Pharmacologic Considerations

- An osmotic diuretic such as mannitol may be prescribed to reduce ICP after intracranial surgery. Inspect the mannitol vial before use. If the solution contains crystals, warm the vial in hot water and shake it vigorously. Do not administer the drug if crystals are in the solution.

Nursing Management

The nurse regards a head injury, no matter how mild it appears, as an emergency. He or she obtains a history of the injury and performs a neurologic examination, paying particular attention to vital signs, LOC, presence or absence of movement in the arms and legs, and pupil size, equality, and reaction to light. If trauma caused the head injury, the nurse examines the head for bleeding, abrasions, and lacerations. He or she evaluates respiratory status, paying particular

attention to the client's ability to maintain adequate oxygenation. The nurse reports neurologic changes immediately. See Chapter 37 for nursing care of a client with increased ICP who is treated medically.

Preoperative Nursing Care

Once the physician determines that operative intervention is necessary, the nurse prepares the client for surgery. He or she uses electric hair clippers to remove hair where burr holes will be drilled or an incision will be made (sometimes this is deferred until the client is in the operating room). The nurse takes vital signs and maintains a record of continuing neurologic assessment findings. He or she administers prescribed medications, such as the anticonvulsant phenytoin (Dilantin) to reduce the risk of seizures before and after surgery, an osmotic diuretic, and corticosteroids. Preoperative sedation usually is omitted. Before surgery, the nurse restricts fluids to avoid intraoperative complications, reduce cerebral edema, and prevent postoperative vomiting. If indicated, the nurse inserts an indwelling urethral catheter and intravenous (IV) line. To prevent thrombophlebitis and deep vein thrombosis, which may develop from prolonged inactivity during neurosurgery, the nurse applies antiembolism stockings.

Postoperative Nursing Care

After surgery, the nurse places the client in either a supine position with the head slightly elevated or a side-lying position on the unaffected side. He or she performs postoperative and neurologic assessments every 15 to 30 minutes. The nurse maintains a neurologic flow sheet to compare trends in assessment findings. Edema around the eyes (periorbital edema) may make examination of the pupils difficult during the immediate postoperative period. Ecchymosis also can be present. The nurse removes antiembolism stockings briefly every 8 hours and reapplies them to reduce the risk of thrombus or embolus.

It is important to monitor the client's body temperature closely, because hyperthermia increases brain metabolism, increasing the potential for brain damage. Therefore, elevated temperature must be relieved with an antipyretic and other measures.

The nurse observes the client closely for increased ICP. He or she restricts fluids to control cerebral edema and to increase cerebral perfusion. The nurse also administers corticosteroids when prescribed. Nursing Care Plan 39-1 and Client and Family Teaching 39-1 provide more information.

NURSING CARE PLAN 39-1 — Care of the Client Undergoing Intracranial Surgery

Assessment

- Assess vital signs, LOC, verbal response, and understanding of oral communication.
- Determine the type and level of discomfort (e.g., headache, sensitivity to light).
- Assess level of pain tolerance using a scale of 0 to 10.
- Evaluate orientation to person, place, and time.
- Check cognitive function by determining ability to follow simple instructions or perform basic mathematical calculations.
- Check pupil size, equality, and response to light. Look for changes in visual field, blurred vision, or diplopia.
- Assess symmetry in facial appearance.
- Test mobility and strength in all four extremities.
- If client is unconscious, look for restlessness.
- Check appropriateness of mood.
- Ask about nausea, and look for evidence of vomiting.
- Monitor seizure activity and status of corneal blink and gag reflexes.
- Monitor urine production, and evaluate the sensation of thirst.

Nursing Diagnosis: Risk for Ineffective Breathing Pattern related to depressive effects of anesthesia and compression of medulla secondary to edema of the brain

Expected Outcome: Breathing will be sufficient to maintain an SpO_2 of at least 90% and a PaO_2 of at least 80 mm Hg.

Interventions	Rationales
Monitor SpO_2 with a pulse oximeter.	SpO_2 of at least 90% indicates PaO_2 is at least 80 mm Hg.
Maintain a patent airway by keeping the head erect and in midline, inserting an oral or nasopharyngeal airway if necessary, and suctioning secretions.	Neck flexion or rotation can compromise the diameter of the natural airway; an oral or pharyngeal airway prevents the tongue from obstructing the airway; suction removes secretions that reduce air exchange.
Encourage client to deep breathe at least 10 times each hour or to use a bedside spirometer.	Gas exchange depends on moving atmospheric air to the level of the alveoli and exhaling to remove CO_2.
Avoid administering narcotic analgesia.	Narcotics depress respirations.
Elevate the head of the bed.	Elevating the head lowers abdominal organs away from the diaphragm, which helps improve inspired volume and reduce intracranial swelling.
Report signs of hypoxemia; be prepared to administer supplemental oxygen or provide mechanical ventilation.	Delivering oxygen at a greater concentration than room air increases oxygenation of blood; mechanical ventilation assists breathing.

Evaluation of Expected Outcome

Client's airway is patent, and respirations are normal.

Nursing Diagnosis: Risk for Ineffective Tissue Perfusion (Cerebral) related to cerebral edema and bleeding within the cranium

Expected Outcome: ICP will be adequate to perfuse the brain as evidenced by normal neurologic signs and symptoms.

Refer to Nursing Care Plan: The Client With Increased Intracranial Pressure in Chapter 37 for interventions.

Evaluation of Expected Outcome

Client shows neurologic stability.

Nursing Diagnosis: Pain related to chemicals released from traumatized tissue, swelling of cerebral tissue, irritation of meninges

Expected Outcome: Pain will be reduced to client's preidentified level of tolerance within 30 minutes of intervention.

Interventions	Rationales
Assess presence, type, and level of pain whenever you assess vital signs and as needed.	Pain assessment is the fifth vital sign.
Reduce bright lights and noise.	Annoying and disturbing sensory stimuli lower the pain threshold.
Minimize activity when pain is acute.	Movement and disturbed rest intensify pain.
Administer prescribed analgesia.	Non-narcotic analgesia is preferred because it does not interfere with neurologic assessment findings.

Evaluation of Expected Outcome

Client reports no pain or a tolerable level of pain.

PC: Seizures

Expected Outcome: The nurse will monitor to detect, manage, and minimize seizure activity.

NURSING CARE PLAN 39-1 **Care of the Client Undergoing Intracranial Surgery** (Continued)

Interventions	Rationales
Observe client for changes in consciousness and involuntary muscle contraction.	Seizures are categorized as generalized or partial; manifestations vary (see Chap. 43).
Pad side rails; keep the bed in low position.	Padding reduces the potential for trauma.
	Serious injury is less likely if a client falls from a bed in low position.
Stay with the client if a seizure occurs; protect him or her from injury, suction secretions, and promote adequate ventilation.	During a seizure, a client cannot protect himself or herself. Secretions accumulate, increasing the risk for aspiration. Contraction of the diaphragm and intercostal muscles can lead to hypoxia.
Administer prescribed anticonvulsants.	They decrease excitation of brain neurons.

Evaluation of Expected Outcome

The nurse detects seizures and implements interventions to minimize their consequences.

Nursing Diagnosis: Risk for Infection related to impaired skin integrity and suppressed inflammatory response.

Expected Outcome: Client will remain free of infection

Interventions	Rationales
Assess temperature, pulse rate, lung sounds, and characteristics of urine. Note the presence of a cough.	Body temperature and pulse rate rise in response to infection. Pneumonia and urinary tract infections are common after surgery because of retained pulmonary secretions, urine stasis, or bacteria entering the urinary tract from the anus.
Inspect the dressing and wound for evidence of purulent drainage.	Impaired skin provides an entrance for microorganisms. Purulent drainage is characteristic of infection
Follow principles of asepsis when assessing the incision and changing the dressing.	Asepsis reduces or eliminates pathogens.
Administer prescribed antibiotics.	They interfere with the growth and reproduction of pathogens.

Evaluation of Expected Outcome

The surgical site remains free of infection; no other evidence of infection develops

Nursing Diagnosis: Risk for Hyperthermia related to hypothalamic dysfunction or infection

Expected Outcome: Client will maintain body temperature within normal range.

Interventions	Rationales
Measure body temperature every 4 hours.	Routine assessment of body temperature provides early indications of changes in client's thermoregulation
Help client maintain an adequate oral fluid intake.	Perspiration assists with heat loss through evaporation.
Remove heavy blankets if client develops a fever. Place client on an electrical cooling blanket to reduce fever.	Blankets trap body heat and interfere with convection. A cooling blanket reduces body temperature through conduction.
Administer a prescribed antipyretic when fever does not respond to heat reduction methods.	Antipyretics lower the set-point for body temperature in the hypothalamus.

Evaluation of Expected Outcome

Temperature does not exceed 99.8°F.

Nursing Diagnosis: Disturbed Thought Processes related to cognitive deficits secondary to structural changes in brain tissue and physiology

Expected Outcomes: Client will be oriented to person, place, and time.

Interventions	Rationales
Orient client at frequent intervals.	Until cognition and sensorium return to normal, client may not recall his or her location and the reasons for medical care.
Provide environmental clues such as a calendar with large numbers.	An easy-to-read calendar within client's vision helps reorient the client to time.
Investigate contributing causes of disorientation and restlessness (e.g., full bladder, pain) and intervene as appropriate.	Clients may sense that they are uncomfortable but be unable to identify specifics of their distress.
Share current events, and turn on newsworthy television or radio programs.	Sensory stimulation and communication tend to elevate cognitive functions.
Repeat explanations or answers to questions as needed.	Repetition reinforces information and promotes storage of memory.

(care plan continues on page 572)

NURSING CARE PLAN 39-1 Care of the Client Undergoing Intracranial Surgery (Continued)

Evaluation of Expected Outcome

Client is oriented to person, place, and time.

Nursing Diagnosis: Risk for Injury related to confusion and poor judgment

Expected Outcome: Client will remain free of injuries.

Interventions	Rationales
Locate client near nursing station.	Placing the client in an optimal site for nursing observation increases the nurses' ability to assist the client when necessary.
Place a signal cord within the client's reach; remind client to use it when he or she needs assistance.	The signal cord can help prevent injuries if the client cannot make his or her needs known.
Place a bed/chair alarm that sounds if the client attempts to get out of bed without assistance.	Such an alarm calls attention to the need for assessment and assistance.

Evaluation of Expected Outcome

No injuries occur

Nursing Diagnosis: Risk for Ineffective Coping related to multiple stressors involving physical losses, lengthy rehabilitation, and compromised finances

Expected Outcome: Client and family will cope with neurologic deficits, participate fully in rehabilitation, and seek assistance from social agencies.

Interventions	Rationales
Consult with the physician about the client's prognosis.	Giving false reassurance is nontherapeutic; offering encouragement promotes motivation.
Concur with physician's explanations if client or family raises questions.	Giving consistent responses reinforces that the client has received the same information as other members of the healthcare team.
Keep client and family informed of progress or changes as they occur.	It is easier to cope with and adapt to small changes.
	Problem-solving is more effective when client and family are provided with facts.
Accept client's and family's behavior under stress in a nonjudgmental manner.	Responses to stress vary. Intolerance of a person's response interferes with a therapeutic alliance between the nurse, client, and family.
Encourage problem-solving techniques and acknowledge positive outcomes.	Unity and cohesiveness develop when client and family resolve problems collaboratively.
Refer client and family to a social worker, discharge planner, or home health agency.	Such providers can assist client and family with the transition from the hospital to other options for care.

Evaluation of Expected Outcomes

Client and family effectively cope with the stress of surgery and possibility of long-term disability.

Pharmacologic Considerations

- Codeine may be prescribed for postoperative pain after intracranial surgery because respiratory depressant effects are less likely with this drug than with other narcotic analgesics.

▶ Stop, Think, and Respond Exercise 39-1

You are caring for two clients with head injuries. Client A lost consciousness at the time of his head injury. He was alert and oriented on arrival in the ED, but 2 hours later he does not respond even when you press on his nailbeds. Client B has been hospitalized for 1 day. He has not been fully alert since admission and continues to be lethargic. He requires more and more stimulation to give a response. Which client's condition is more serious? Explain your choice.

SKULL FRACTURES

A skull fracture is a break in the continuity of the cranium. The most common types are simple, depressed, or comminuted fractures (Table 39-2).

Client and Family Teaching 39-1
Care After Intracranial Surgery

If the client is discharged directly home, the nurse must explain the purposes for prescribed medications (e.g., anticonvulsants, anti-inflammatory drugs, drugs to control gastric acidity), schedule for administration, and side effects to report. In addition, the nurse must provide the following verbal and written instructions:

● Watch for signs of intracranial bleeding and infection (expect swelling around the eye and below the incision).
● Expect sensory changes such as hearing a "clicking" sound around the bone flap, which will disappear as healing takes place. Understand that headaches also are common, but notify the surgeon if a mild analgesic such as acetaminophen (Tylenol) fails to relieve them.
● Care for the surgical site as directed by the physician. Some recommendations include keeping the incision clean, avoiding scrubbing the incision, securing remaining hair away from the incision, resuming shampooing the hair when the staples or sutures are removed, and wearing a hat when outside to avoid sunburn until hair growth resumes.
● Maintain safety precautions at home, including ambulating only with assistance and ensuring well-lit and clutter-free rooms. Do not drive until the risk of seizures has been eliminated.
● Engage in exercises that promote strength and endurance.
● Use techniques to ensure bowel and bladder elimination (see Chap. 40).
● Follow feeding or nutritional suggestions
● Keep follow up appointments for measuring anticonvulsant blood levels, electroencephalograms, and continued medical care and evaluation.

Pathophysiology and Etiology

A skull fracture results from a blow to the head. It can be associated with an **open head injury**, in which the scalp, bony cranium, and dura mater (the outer meningeal layer) are exposed, or it may be a **closed head injury**, in which an intact layer of scalp covers the fractured skull.

Open head injuries create a potential for infection because they expose internal brain structures to the environment. They are less likely to produce rapid increased ICP because the opening gives the brain some room to expand as pressure increases.

TABLE 39-2 Types of Skull Fractures

TYPE	DESCRIPTION
Simple	Linear crack without any displacement of the pieces
Depressed	Broken bone pushed inward toward the brain
Comminuted	Bone splintered into fragments

Basilar skull fractures are located at the base of the skull. Trauma in this location is especially dangerous because it can cause edema of the brain near the origin of the spinal cord (*foramen magnum*), interfere with circulation of CSF, injure nerves that pass into the spinal cord, or create a pathway for infection between the brain and middle ear (Fig. 39-6), which can result in meningitis.

Assessment Findings

Signs and Symptoms

Simple skull fractures produce few, if any, symptoms and heal without complications. The client may complain of a localized headache. A bump, bruise, or laceration may be visible on the scalp.

Symptoms depend on the area of the brain that has been injured. For example, a large bone fragment that is pressing on the motor area can cause hemiparesis. In any type of skull fracture, shock can develop from injury to the skull or some other area of the body.

Because basilar skull fractures tend to tear the dura, **rhinorrhea**, leaking of CSF from the nose, or **otorrhea**, leakage of CSF from the ear, may occur. In some cases, **periorbital ecchymosis**, referred to as *raccoon eyes*, or bruising of the mastoid process behind the ear, called **Battle's sign**, can be present (Fig. 39-7). Conjunctival hemorrhages can occur as well. Injury to the brain tissue may result in seizures. Epilepsy can develop as a sequela of head injury.

Diagnostic Findings

Skull radiographs, CT scan, or MRI show brain tissue injuries such as a fracture line or embedded skull fragments (compound skull fracture), cerebral edema, or a subdural or epidural hematoma.

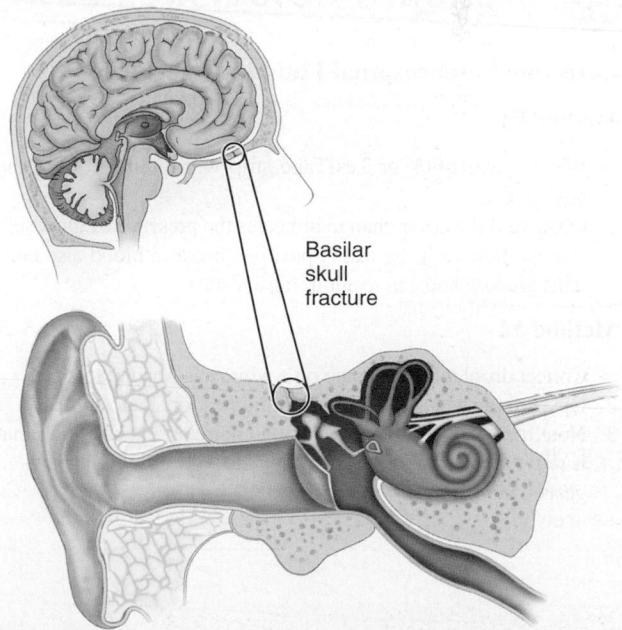

FIGURE 39-6. Basilar fractures allow cerebrospinal fluid to leak from the nose and ears. (Adapted from Hickey, J. V. [2008]. *The clinical practice of neurological and neurosurgical nursing* [6th ed.]. Philadelphia: Lippincott Williams & Wilkins.)

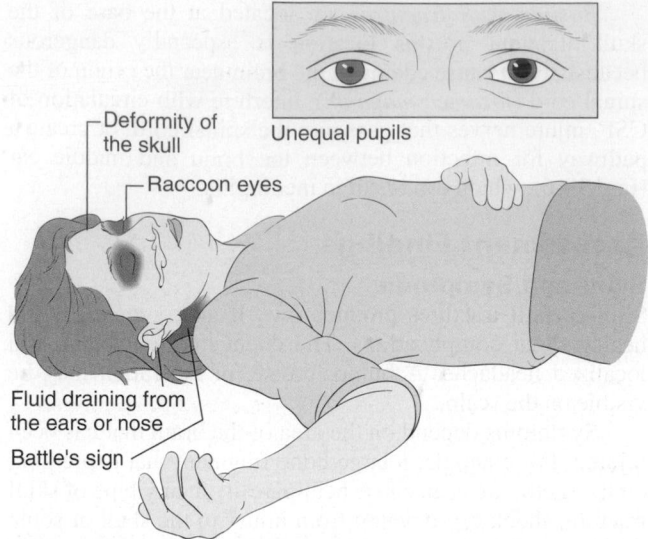

Deformity of the skull

Unequal pupils

Raccoon eyes

Fluid draining from the ears or nose

Battle's sign

FIGURE 39-7. Signs of a skull fracture may include skull deformity, unequal pupils, periorbital ecchymosis (*raccoon eyes*), fluid from the ears or nose, and periauricular ecchymosis (*Battle's sign*). (LifeART image © Lippincott Williams & Wilkins.)

Medical and Surgical Management

Simple skull fractures require bed rest and close observation for signs of increased ICP. If the scalp is lacerated, the wound is cleaned, debrided, and sutured.

Depressed skull fractures require a craniotomy to remove bone fragments and control bleeding, elevation of the depressed fracture, and repair of damaged tissues. A piece of mesh is inserted to replace the bone fragments that are removed. Additional treatment includes antibiotics to control infection, an osmotic diuretic to prevent or treat cerebral edema, and an anticonvulsant to prevent or treat seizures. Use of corticosteroids following head injuries and neurosurgery occurs less and less because research studies are showing a higher incidence of deaths associated with such use as compared with those not treated with corticosteroids (Brain Trauma Foundation, American Association of Neurological Surgeons, Congress of Neurological Surgeons, 2007).

Nursing Management

Most clients are hospitalized for at least 24 hours after a significant head injury. The nurse examines the client to identify signs of head trauma and tests drainage from the nose or ear (Nursing Guidelines 39-1). To detect any CSF drainage, the nurse looks for a **halo sign**, which is a blood stain surrounded by a clear or yellowish stain. If drainage is present, the nurse allows it to flow freely onto porous gauze and avoids tightly plugging the orifice.

The nurse performs neurologic assessments, which include an hourly evaluation of LOC and of pupil, motor, and sensory status, even if the injury appears mild. It is possible for a hematoma to accompany a skull fracture. The nurse obtains vital signs every 15 to 30 minutes and prepares for the possibility of seizures. See Chapter 37 for additional nursing care.

 Gerontologic Considerations

- Nurses should assess older adults for risk of falls and implement appropriate preventative interventions. However, if a fall occurs, the older adult should be assessed for skull fracture.

 NURSING GUIDELINES 39-1

Detecting Cerebrospinal Fluid in Drainage

Method #1

1. Wet a Dextrostick or Tes-Tape strip with drainage from the nose or ear.
2. Observe if the color change indicates the presence of glucose.
3. Use method #2 if the test is positive, because blood also contains glucose and can result in false results.

Method #2

1. Collect droplets of drainage on a white absorbent pad.
2. Observe the wet area after a few minutes for a halo sign.
3. Note if a pale yellow or clear ring encircles a central ring that is red: the red ring indicates blood; the pale yellow ring suggests CSF.

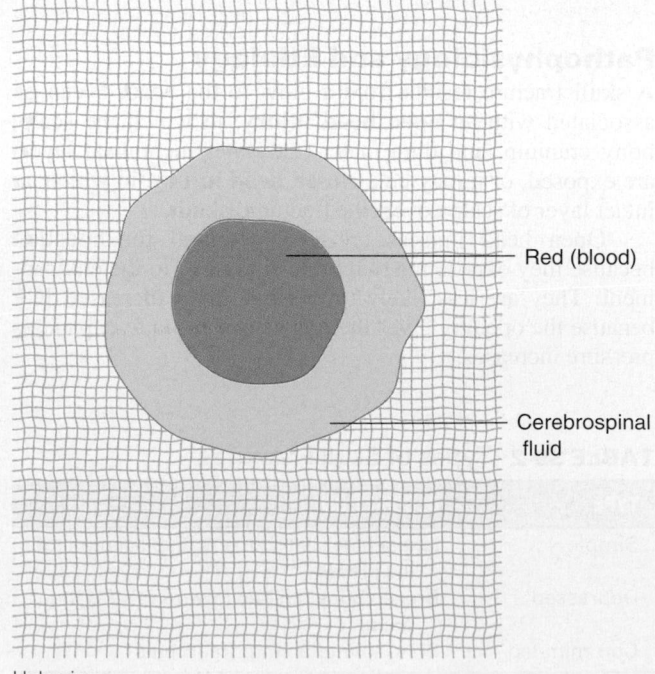

Red (blood)

Cerebrospinal fluid

Halo sign.

SPINAL CORD INJURIES

Spinal cord trauma is serious and sometimes fatal. The cervical and lumbar vertebrae are the most common sites of injury. Correct emergency management at the time of injury is crucial because moving the client incorrectly can permanently damage the spinal cord.

Pathophysiology and Etiology

Common causes of spinal cord injury include accidents and violence. Vehicular accidents are the leading cause, followed by violence, falls, sports, and miscellaneous injuries.

Trauma to the back can fracture or collapse one or more vertebrae, causing a portion of bone to injure the spinal cord and interfere with the transmission of nerve impulses (Fig. 39-8). Even with no fracture, edema may lead to cord compression, which may permanently damage the cord.

Spinal cord injury also can lead to bleeding within the cord. Because the blood has no place to drain, it forms a hematoma that occupies space and compresses the nerve roots. Injury to the cord also can completely or partially sever spinal cord nerve fibers. With such an injury, the client experiences various consequences of motor and sensory dysfunction below the site of the injury that affect functional abilities (Table 39-3).

Tetraplegia (a term that replaces *quadriplegia*), refers to weakness, paralysis and sensory impairment of all extremities and the trunk when there is a spinal injury at or above the first thoracic (T1) vertebrae. **Paraplegia**, weakness or paralysis and compromised sensory functions of both legs and lower pelvis, occurs with spinal injuries below the T1 level. When the tracts of the spinal nerves are completely severed, no effective nerve regeneration occurs. Muscle spasms occur spontaneously, but they are not evidence that the client is regaining motor function. Many paraplegics return home, live independently, and, in some instances, resume work. Tetraplegics may return home but require extensive physical care.

Complications

Respiratory arrest and spinal shock are immediate complications of spinal cord injury. Long-term complications include autonomic dysreflexia, pressure ulcers, respiratory infections, urinary and fecal impairment, spasticity and contractures, weight gain or loss, calcium depletion, urinary calculi, sexual dysfunction, and pain.

Spinal Shock (Areflexia)

Spinal shock is a loss of sympathetic reflex activity below the level of injury within 30 to 60 minutes of a spinal injury. It is characterized by immediate loss of all cord functions below the point of injury. In addition to paralysis, manifestations include pronounced hypotension, bradycardia, and warm, dry skin. If the level of injury is in the cervical or upper thoracic region, respiratory failure can occur. Bowel and bladder distention develops. The client does not perspire below the level of injury, which impairs temperature control. The client manifests **poikilothermia**, body temperature of the environment. Spinal shock may persist for 1 week to months until the body adjusts to the damage imposed by the injury. Until then, vital functions require medical support.

Autonomic Dysreflexia (Hyperreflexia)

Autonomic dysreflexia is an exaggerated sympathetic nervous system response in people with spinal cord injuries above T6. It can occur suddenly at any time after spinal shock subsides. Box 39-1 lists factors that precipitate autonomic dysreflexia. Characteristics of this acute emergency are as follows:

- Severe hypertension
- Slow heart rate
- Pounding headache
- Nausea
- Blurred vision
- Flushed skin
- Sweating
- Goosebumps (erection of pilomotor muscles in the skin)
- Nasal stuffiness
- Anxiety

Uncontrolled autonomic dysreflexia can lead to seizures, stroke, and death. Prevention is the best treatment, but additional measures such as administering antihypertensive drug therapy with nifedipine (Procardia), nitroglycerin ointment, phentolamine (Regitine), hydralazine (Apresoline), or diazoxide (Hyperstat); raising the client's head; and relieving the precipitating cause are necessary once it develops.

Pressure Ulcers

Pressure ulcers develop in 20% to 80% of people with spinal cord injuries (Regan, Teasell, & Mortenson, 2006). Risk factors include immobility, muscle atrophy, skin shear due to

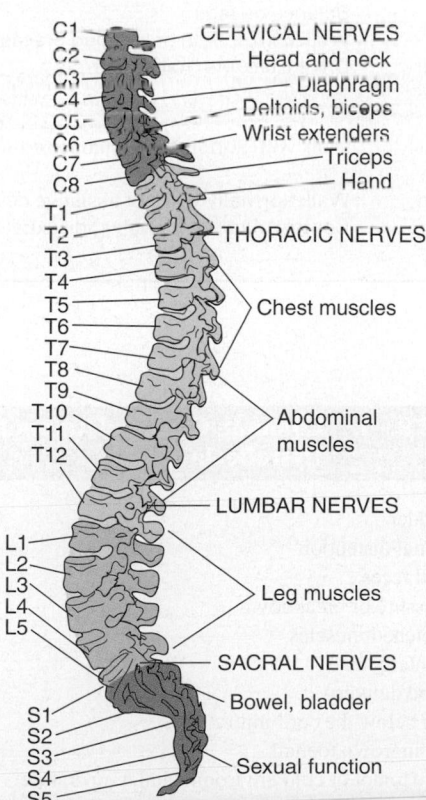

C1 — CERVICAL NERVES
C2 — Head and neck
C3 — Diaphragm
C4 — Deltoids, biceps
C5
C6 — Wrist extenders
C7 — Triceps
C8 — Hand
T1
T2 — THORACIC NERVES
T3
T4
T5 — Chest muscles
T6
T7
T8
T9
T10
T11 — Abdominal muscles
T12
— LUMBAR NERVES
L1
L2
L3 — Leg muscles
L4
L5
— SACRAL NERVES
S1
S2 — Bowel, bladder
S3
S4 — Sexual function
S5

FIGURE 39-8. Structures affected by spinal nerves.

TABLE 39-3 Consequences of Spinal Cord Injuries

LEVEL OF INJURY	COMMON MOTOR EFFECTS	COMMON SENSORY EFFECTS	FUNCTIONAL ABILITIES
C1–C3	Paralysis below neck; impaired breathing; bowel and bladder incontinence; sexual dysfunction	No sensation below neck	Breathe with assistance of ventilator Swallow and speak Use a power wheelchair with movement of head and neck control Operate computer or appliances, such as TV or lights, using voice-activation device or mouth stick
C4, C5	Shoulder elevation possible; ventilation support required	No sensation below clavicle	Breathe with ventilator assistance or possibly independently Use a power wheelchair with sip-and-puff or hand control Drink independently using a long straw and bottle
C6–C8	Some elbow, upper arm, and wrist movement; can do diaphragmatic breathing	Some sensation in arms and thumb; sensation in chest impaired	Eat, groom, bathe, and attain bed mobility with assistive devices Transfer from bed to chair using a slide board Perform self-catheterization (males); more difficult for females Use manual wheelchair in flat environment Drive with hand controls
T1–T6	Paralysis below waist; control of hands; abdominal breathing	No sensation below midchest	Perform personal care and household activities independently Use manual wheelchair, including up and down curbs Stand between bars with leg splints
T7–T12	Varying degrees of trunk and abdominal control	Varying degrees of sensation below waist	Transfer from bed to wheelchair independently Propel wheelchair over uneven surfaces and rough terrain Care for bowel and bladder independently Perform light housekeeping and meal preparation Balance on legs Walk with splints or long leg braces
L1–L2	Hip adduction impaired	No sensation below lower abdomen; some sensation in inner thighs	Drive a car with hand controls
L3–L5	Knee and ankle movement impaired	No sensation below upper thighs	Walk with support of walker or crutches
S1–S5	Varying degrees of bowel/bladder control and sexual function	No sensation in perineum	Walk normally without assistive devices Control bladder, bowel, and sexual functions

C, cervical; T, thoracic; L, lumbar; S, sacral.

spasticity and traumatic transfer techniques, skin contact with urine and feces, loss of sensation, and altered nutrition.

Respiratory Infections

Clients with spinal cord injuries may not be able to breathe normally and cough to clear secretions. The spinal nerves that transmit impulses to the diaphragm, intercostal muscles, neck, and abdominal muscles may no longer function. Consequently, the risk of inadequate ventilation and pneumonia is high.

Urinary and Fecal Impairment

Although the kidneys continue to produce urine, the muscles of the bladder and urinary sphincter may no longer be controlled voluntarily. This may result either in reflexive emptying when the bladder fills with urine, or failure to empty,

BOX 39-1 | **Common Causes of Autonomic Dysreflexia**

- Full bladder
- Abdominal distention
- Impacted feces
- Skin pressure or breakdown
- Overstretched muscles
- Sexual intercourse
- Labor and delivery
- Sunburn below the cord injury
- Infected ingrown toenail
- Exposure to hot or cold environmental temperature
- Taking over-the-counter decongestants

which causes urine to reverse-fill the ureters and kidney pelvis as the bladder becomes overly distended. Bacteria are likely to colonize the bladder because clients may not completely empty it.

In addition, clients may have no urge to defecate and may be prone to fecal accumulation within the bowel. The connection between the spinal cord nerves and muscles needed for bowel elimination may be severed, or the rectal sphincter may not dilate to allow the passage of stool. In either case, there is a risk of fecal impaction.

Spasticity and Contractures

Clients with spinal cord injuries experience intermittent spasticity, uncontrolled jerking movements, muscle stiffness, and rigidity. Spasticity occurs because nerve signals between the brain and nerves below the level of injury are interrupted. Instead of a coordinated effort, an unregulated spinal reflex may cause an overly active muscle response. Muscle spasms pull the joints into a shortened position, increasing the potential for skin impairment and contractures.

Pharmacologic Considerations

- Various medications may be prescribed as muscle relaxants for clients who experience spasticity. Examples include benzodiazepines such as clonazepam (Klonopin); skeletal muscle relaxants such as baclofen (Lioresal) and dantrolene (Dantrium); and alpha-2 adrenergic agonists such as tizanidine (Zanaflex), a drug that increases inhibition of motor neurons. Botulinum toxin type A (Botox) is also injected into spastic muscles to loosen and relax them. Injections are repeated every 3 to 6 months.

Contractures result from the inability to move a joint freely because of an imbalance between opposing muscle groups; a strong muscle overpowers a weaker one. After spinal cord injury, this may be a consequence of muscle spasticity. Contractures such as flexed elbows, wrists, hips, or knees; clenched fists; and thumb-in-palm may develop any time after the injury (Fig. 39-9).

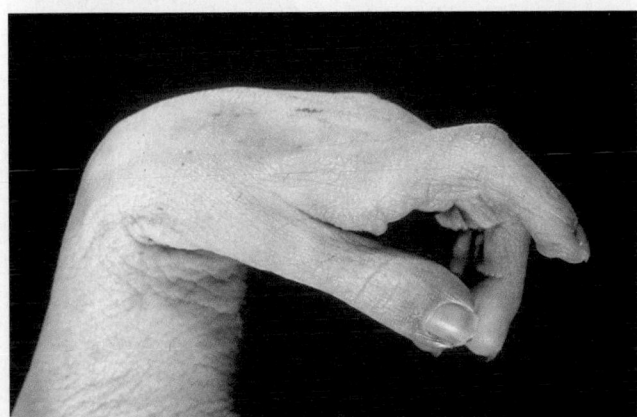

FIGURE 39-9. Contractures can occur when a joint is not exercised regularly. Use of the joint can be permanently lost. (© Siebert/ Custom Medical Stock Photo.)

Weight Change

After spinal cord injury, clients tend to lose weight initially but gain weight after weeks, months, and years of inactivity. Clients must be taught how to make healthy food choices by selecting foods that are both relatively low in calories as well as nutritious.

Calcium Depletion

Following a spinal cord injury, clients experience demineralization of their bones because physical activity is one mechanism for maintaining bone density. Within the first 4 to 6 months, spinal cord injury clients lose 25% of their bone mass and 33% after 1 ½ years (University of Washington, 2002). This places clients at high risk for fractures from falls or even activities of daily living. Preventive methods include administering calcium and vitamin D supplements, and ossification agents such as bisphosphonates, calcitonin, and selective estrogen receptor modulators (see Chap 63). Functional electrical stimulation, which is discussed later, may be helpful to increase bone density.

Urinary Calculi

Clients with spinal cord injury are at risk for forming calculi (stones) in the kidneys or bladder at a higher rate than the general population. The etiology of stone formation is discussed in Chapters 58 and 59. It is assumed that crystallization is associated with urinary retention and immobility. Bladder calculi tend to occur soon after injury, whereas renal calculi can develop both soon after the injury and years later (Hansen, Sorensen, & Kristensen, 2007).

Sexual Dysfunction

Sexuality is affected differently in males and females who sustain spinal cord injuries. In most males whose S2 to S4 spinal nerves are undamaged, involuntary *reflex erections* occur as a result of touching the penis or stimulating other erotically sensitive areas of the body such as the nipples, ears, or neck. *Psychogenic erections* occur depending on the level and extent of spinal cord injury when males experience an arousing thought, triggering nerve stimulating impulses from the brain to the nerves of the spinal cord at the T10 to L2 levels. Drugs for erectile dysfunction such as tadalafil (Cialis) and others may help promote a reflex erection. Other alternatives for treatment of sexual dysfunction include penile injection therapy, application of a vacuum pump, or penile implant (see Chap. 55). Achieving an erection facilitates intercourse, but it may not ensure fertility. Men often have impaired ejaculation with decreased motility of sperm, reducing their ability to biologically father a child. Alternative fertility measures may facilitate pregnancy.

Women with spinal cord injuries can conceive and bear children. However, they experience decreased vaginal lubrication, impaired clitoral and vaginal sensations, and an inability to contract the pubococcygeal muscles of the pelvic floor. Although using a vibrator may help women with an injury below the T6 level achieve an orgasm, it may be unperceived or feel different than it did before the injury (Spinal Cord Injury Info Sheet, 2007).

Pain

Clients with spinal cord injuries may experience one or more types of pain (see Chap 11). Neuropathic pain, which is caused by trauma to structures of the nervous system, develops in approximately 40% of clients (Jeffrey, 2006). It is described as being sharp, shooting, or burning. Nociceptive pain, which originates in musculoskeletal structures such as those associated with muscle spasms, and visceral pain, which emanates from within the abdomen, may also occur. Pain relief involves medications such as opioid and nonopioid analgesics, antidepressants such as duloxetine (Cymbalta) that are known to relieve pain, anticonvulsants such as pregabalin (Lyrica), and topical lidocaine (patch) (Dworkin et al., 2007).

Assessment Findings

The degree and location of the spinal cord injury determine the immediate symptoms. There is pain in the affected area, difficulty breathing, numbness, and paralysis. If the injury is high in the cervical region, respiratory failure and death occur because the diaphragm is paralyzed. If the cord is completely severed, permanent loss of function below the level of the injury occurs. If damage to the cord is minimal, some function is maintained.

A neurologic examination reveals the level of spinal cord injury. Radiography, myelography, MRI, and CT scan show evidence of fracture or compression of one or more vertebrae, edema, or a hematoma.

Medical and Surgical Management

Initial Treatment

Initially, the head and back are immobilized mechanically with a cervical collar and back support. An IV line is inserted to provide access to a vein if shock develops. Vital signs are stabilized. Corticosteroids are given to reduce spinal cord edema, thereby decreasing potential damage to injured nerves. Riluzole (Rilutek), a neuroprotective drug that blocks the neurotoxic effects of glutamate, may be administered. BA-210 (Cethrin), an FDA-approved orphan drug that is currently in phase II clinical trials, is being investigated with hopes that it will promote regrowth of neurons and reduce neuronal death after acute spinal cord injury.

Pharmacologic Considerations

- Riluzole affects the body's ability to fight infection, so white blood cell counts should be measured periodically while taking this drug. Also, riluzole should be taken on an empty stomach. Clients should avoid eating or drinking caffeine-containing products and charcoal-broiled foods.

After the client is stabilized, the injured portion of the spine is further immobilized using a cast or brace or surgical intervention. Traction with weights and pulleys is applied to provide correct vertebral alignment and to increase the space between the vertebrae. Additional weight is added over the next few days to increase the space between the vertebrae and to move them into correct alignment. A turning frame is used to change the client's position without altering the alignment of the spine (Fig. 39-10).

Depending on the extent of the injury, surgery may be necessary to remove bone fragments, repair dislocated

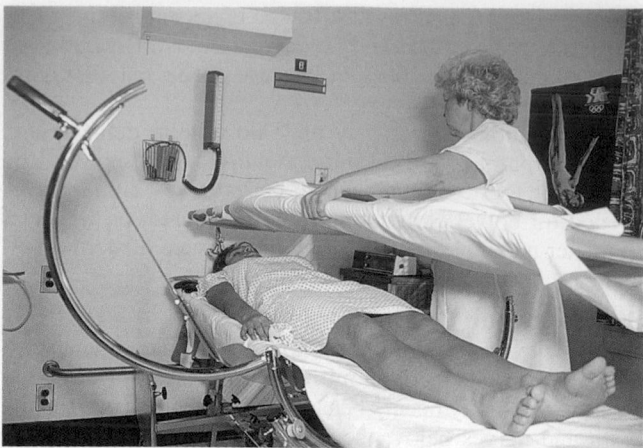

FIGURE 39-10. The nurse frequently turns a client on a mechanical turning frame to relieve pressure.

vertebrae, and stabilize the spine. The vertebrae are fused with bone obtained from the iliac crest or stabilized with a steel rod. External immobilization with a brace or cast often is necessary.

Long-Term Management

After the initial period of therapeutic care, the focus of treatment turns to rehabilitative and restorative measures.

Functional Electrical Stimulation

While the client is undergoing physical and occupational therapy, **functional electrical stimulation (FES)** may be used to activate paralyzed muscles and prevent muscle atrophy. FES is used in a variety of ways. Surface or implanted electrodes attached to the quadriceps, hamstring, and gluteal muscles help paralyzed legs pedal a stationary bicycle, stand, or walk (Fig. 39-11). Electrodes attached to the forearm and

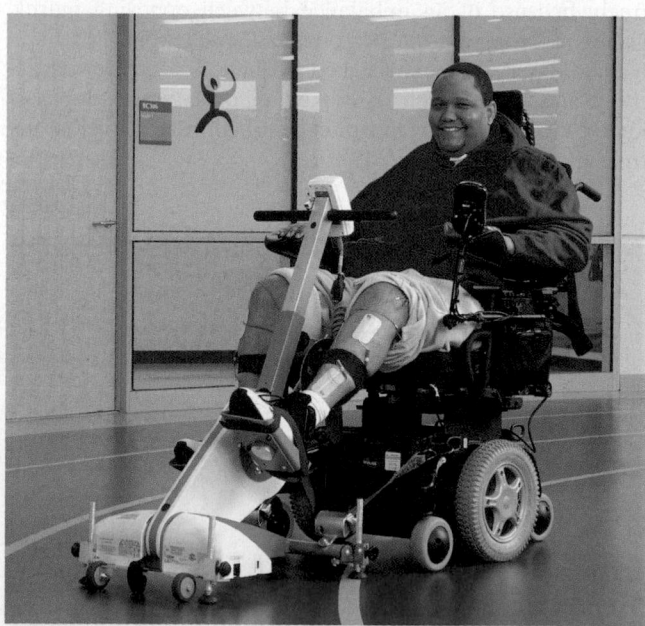

FIGURE 39-11. Functional electrical stimulation (FES) facilitates the movement of paralyzed muscles to pedal a modified bicycle. (Photo courtesy of the Center for SCI Recovery at Rehabilitation Institute of Michigan.)

flexors and extensors of the hand help the hand open and close to allow grasping of objects, reduce stiffness, maintain or increase range of motion, and increase circulation. FES is also being used to restore bladder continence by stimulating the sacral nerves, causing contraction of the detrusor muscle necessary for bladder emptying. In addition, FES improves breathing; when the electrodes are implanted in respiratory muscles, they reduce the need for mechanical ventilation.

Treadmill Training

Treadmill training, which is also known as weight-supported ambulation, is suitable only for those clients with an incomplete spinal cord injury (i.e., some remaining connections between the spinal cord and brain). Treadmill training increases the function within the remaining connections. The client is suspended in a harness above the treadmill, and therapists move the person's legs in a walking fashion (Fig 39-12).

Tendon Transfer Surgery

Clients with injuries from vertebrae C5 through T1 have weak or nonfunctioning wrists and hands and may benefit from tendon transfer surgery. Tendon transfer is a surgical procedure that repositions tendons from a working muscle to a paralyzed one. The goal of the surgery is to restore a pinching motion with the thumb and flexion of the wrist. The presurgical preparation and postsurgical rehabilitation are both demanding for clients; strengthening and range-of-motion exercises and physical therapy are required.

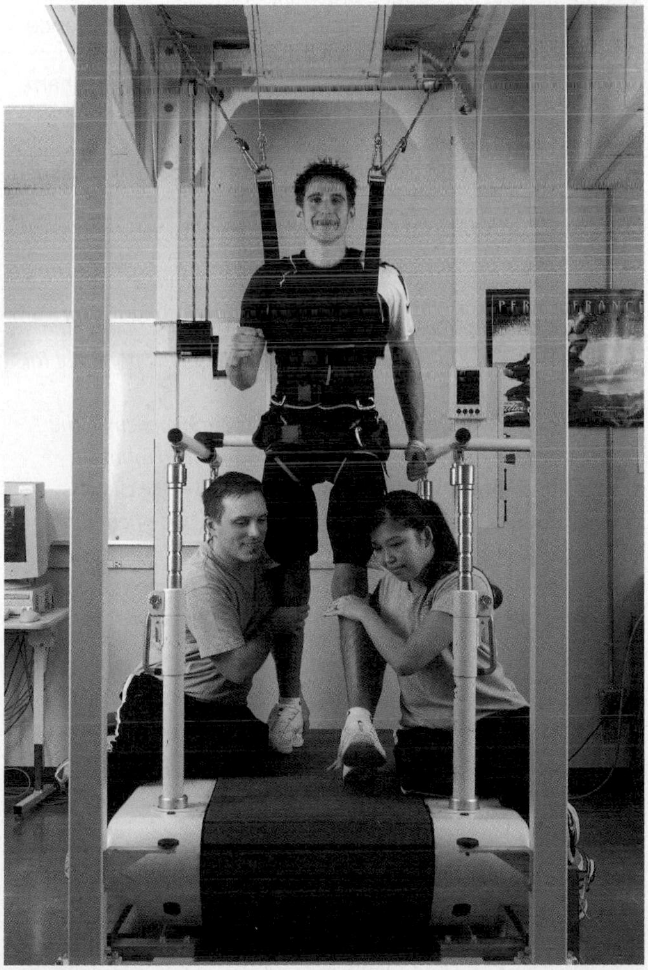

Cell Transplantation

Nerve cells in the central nervous system, which includes the spinal cord, lose the ability to regenerate when injured. Consequently, there is a focus on finding cells that, when transplanted, can replace the nerve cells that have been damaged. Stem cells are *pluripotent,* that is, they can differentiate into a variety of cell types, including spinal nerves (see Chap 18). However, use of embryonic stem cells is currently politically and ethically controversial. Autologous stem cells from bone marrow have been collected from clients and reimplanted in the area surrounding the injured spinal cord with promising results (Yoon et al., 2007).

Other researchers are investigating the therapeutic effectiveness of using host stem-like Schwann cells and olfactory ensheathing cells harvested from the mucosa of nasal tissue for promoting nerve regeneration and growth of axons and restoring function when implanted into the injured spinal cord (Lavdas, et al., 2008; Lima et al., 2006; Raisman, 2005).

FIGURE 39-12. Walking is simulated by supporting body weight in a harness above a treadmill. (Photo courtesy of the Center for SCI Recovery at Rehabilitation Institute of Michigan.)

Nursing Process for the Initial Care of the Client with Spinal Trauma

The nurse provides immediate supportive care after the spinal cord injury and plans or administers rehabilitative measures to prevent long-term complications.

Assessment

On the client's arrival in the ED, obtain information about the injury and treatment given at the scene from family, witnesses, or those who transported the client to the hospital. After gathering such facts, perform a neurologic assessment, taking care to document findings on a flow sheet to provide a database for future comparison. Assess vital signs, paying particular attention to respiratory status. During the acute phase, repeat neurologic assessments frequently. Determine if the client has movement and sensation below the level of injury, look to see if neurologic damage is worsening, and observe for signs of respiratory distress and spinal shock.

Diagnosis, Planning, and Interventions

Keep the client's body and head aligned and limit all movement. If directed by the physician, insert a urinary retention catheter. Assist with immobilization of the injured spine (Fig. 39-13). Burr holes in the skull are required for inserting the pointed ends of traction tongs or the halo traction apparatus. When applying traction, check that the weights hang free. Instruct others on the nursing team never to lift or remove the weights or increase or decrease the amount of prescribed weight. The use of external stabilizing devices such as the halo vest facilitates early discharge from the acute care facility. Teach the client in a halo vest measures to ensure the client's safety and prevent complications (Client and Family Teaching 39-2).

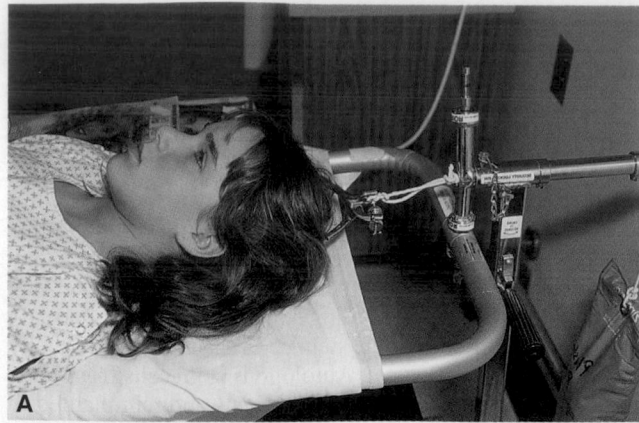

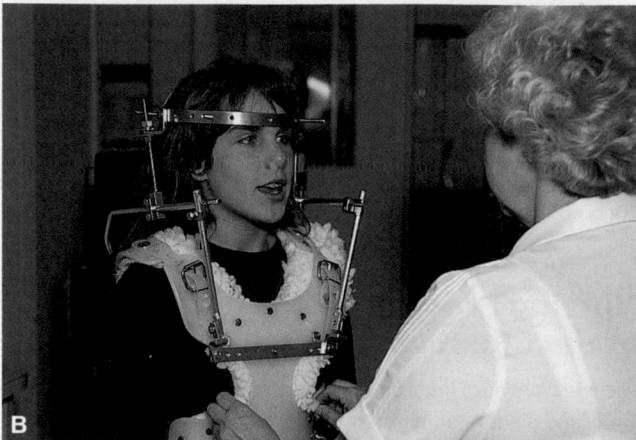

FIGURE 39-13. (**A**) Traction for cervical fractures may be applied with tongs. (**B**) A halo vest may be used to maintain alignment in cervical injuries. (From Smeltzer, S. C., et al. [2008]. *Brunner & Suddarth's textbook of medical–surgical nursing* [11th ed.]. Philadelphia: Lippincott Williams & Wilkins.)

 Client and Family Teaching 39-2
Halo Vest Management

The nurse teaches the client as follows:

● Turn your whole body rather than trying to turn your head; you will not be able to look down.
● Do not drive a car.
● Walk only on level surfaces until you become accustomed to the vest; avoid stairs, curbs, and uneven terrain unless assistance is available.
● Take care getting in and out of vehicles to avoid bumping the halo and loosening the pins.
● Use a mirror to inspect the pin sites and as a guide while cleaning them.
● Clean the pin sites two to three times a day with cotton-tipped applicators saturated with hydrogen peroxide; remove loose crusts.
● Use a clean applicator after making a full circle around the pin site.
● Clip the hair that grows around the pin sites.
● Report pain, redness, drainage from pin sites, fever, or neck tingling or pain to the physician.
● Never independently adjust the vest if it becomes tight or loose; consult the physician.
● Pad the vest if it causes pressure or friction.
● Take sponge baths to maintain hygiene; seek assistance for areas you cannot reach such as around the anus.
● Use a dry shampoo or consult physician on how to shampoo hair without wetting the vest.
● Use pillows for support and comfort when sleeping.
● Wear loose-fitting clothing with wide necklines for ease in dressing.
● Wear shoes with flat heels that are easy to slip on and off.

Besides monitoring for and intervening in cases of spinal shock and autonomic dysreflexia, the nurse's role may include the following.

▶ **Ineffective Breathing Pattern, Ineffective Airway Clearance, and Risk for Impaired Gas Exchange** related to paralysis of respiratory, chest, and abdominal muscles

▶ **Expected Outcomes:** (1) Client will breathe independently at a rate of 16 to 20 breaths/minute. (2) The airway will be free of secretions. (3) The client's blood oxygen saturation (SpO$_2$) will be 90% or higher.

● Maintain a patent airway. *A patent airway maximizes passage of air in and out of the lungs.*
● Be prepared for endotracheal intubation and mechanical ventilation if respiratory failure occurs. *An endotracheal tube provides an airway from the nose or mouth to an area above the mainstem bronchi. Mechanical ventilation provides a means to regulate respiratory rate, volume of air, and percentage of oxygen when a client cannot breathe independently.*
● Suction the airway to remove secretions. *A client with spinal trauma may not be able to cough effectively. An artificial airway increases the production of respiratory secretions. Suctioning helps ensure adequate ventilation and reduces the potential for pneumonia.*
● Administer oxygen as prescribed. *To prevent hypoxemia, the client may require more oxygen than available in room air.*
● Help the client use a spirometer as prescribed if the client is ventilator free. *This helps prevent atelectasis and pneumonia.*
● Encourage obtaining a pneumococcal pneumonia and yearly influenza immunization. *Prophylaxis of common community acquired respiratory infections reduces the potential for pulmonary complications.*

▶ **PC: Neuropathic Pain** related to irritated nerve root and soft tissue injury

▶ **Expected Outcome:** The nurse will monitor to detect, manage, and minimize neuropathic pain.

● Administer prescribed analgesia intravenously. *IV administration of an analgesic avoids administration of injections into tissues where absorption is compromised.*
● Assist the physician with nerve block procedures if analgesia is ineffective. *A nerve block is a form of regional anesthesia in which an anesthetic agent is injected close to the nerve that is transmitting pain impulses.*

‣ Impaired Physical Mobility and Risk for Disuse Syndrome related to loss of motor function

‣ **Expected Outcomes:** (1) Client's ability to be mobile will be maintained. (2) Client will use assistive devices to move and perform activities of daily living. (3) Client will not experience complications associated with inactivity and immobility.

- Position client to avoid joint contractures and foot drop. *Mobility depends on preventing permanent changes to the musculo-skeletal system. Inactivity causes joints to assume a position of flexion.*
- Help client perform exercises identified by the physical therapist. *Active and passive exercise maintains joint flexibility and reduces muscle atrophy and atony. For exercises to be effective, clients must perform them several times a day.*
- Apply leg braces when ambulation is possible. *Braces support joints, allowing the client to ambulate independently or with a walker or crutches.*
- Maintain skin integrity by changing client's position at least every 2 hours, using pressure-relieving devices, massaging bony prominences, using a mechanical lift for bed-to-chair transfers, and keeping skin clean and dry. *Position changes and pressure-relieving devices ensure that capillary pressure stays above 32 mm Hg, thus providing oxygenated blood to cells for their continued survival. Massage increases blood flow to temporarily deprived areas. Using a mechanical lift prevents injuries to the client as well as the nurse. Keeping skin clean and dry prevents maceration and decreases the potential for bacterial growth.*
- Facilitate urine elimination. Teach the client to perform intermittent catheterization every 3 to 4 hours if capable. If a leg bag is used, attach the catheter to the bag and empty and clean the device regularly. *Urinary retention and stasis may contribute to autonomic dysreflexia and formation of renal calculi.*
- Keep the bowel evacuated. If necessary, manually remove stool. *Infrequent bowel evacuation leads to constipation and impaction. A high-fiber diet and a bowel program using a suppository or enema every 3 days approximately 30 minutes after a meal normalize bowel movements.*
- Keep client hydrated. *Adequate hydration reduces potential for formation of thrombi and renal calculi.*
- Provide oral or enteral nutrition. *A well-balanced diet provides nutrients and elements necessary for energy and to sustain cellular growth and repair (Nutrition Notes 39-1).*

‣ Anxiety and Risk for Ineffective Coping related to prognosis of neurologic deficits

‣ **Expected Outcome:** (1) Anxiety will be relieved. (2) Client will cope effectively with stressors.

- Discuss information about prognosis with the physician. *Communication facilitates mutual understanding of client's potential for recovery and rehabilitation.*
- Tell client and family that determining the severity of deficits immediately after a spinal cord injury is difficult. Explain that the outcome varies depending on the specific injury and client's response to rehabilitation. *Until the initial trauma and swelling*

Nutrition Notes 39-1
The Client With a Spinal Cord Injury

- Clients have varying nutritional needs, depending on the nerves injured and the resulting complications.
- Tetraplegic and paraplegic clients have lower caloric requirements because their energy expenditure is reduced, and their caloric intake should be adjusted to avoid excessive weight gain. Nutrient needs, however, are stable or higher, depending on complications. For example, prolonged immobility promotes nitrogen excretion, causing an increased protein requirement.
- Clients with skin breakdown have increased requirements for protein (meat, milk, supplements), vitamin C (citrus fruit and juices, strawberries, "greens," tomatoes), and zinc (meat, seafood, milk, egg yolks, legumes, whole grains), which are needed to promote healing.
- Extended immobility accelerates calcium loss from bone, leading to hypercalcemia and hypercalciuria. A high fluid intake (up to 3 L/day) helps dilute urine, thus preventing the precipitation of calcium renal stones.

---

have resolved, any assumptions about the client's outcome are premature. Successful rehabilitation depends on the level of the cord injury, development of complications, client's motivation and perseverance, and intervention of the healthcare team.

- Be a good listener and offer encouragement as the client makes progress. *Such encouragement can contribute to the client's resolve to put forth continued effort.*

Evaluation of Expected Outcomes

Breathing is adequate to maintain oxygenation. Pain is relieved or reduced to a tolerable level. The client regains mobility using minimal assistive devices. Complications from inactivity are prevented or reduced. The client's level of anxiety is mild, and he or she begins to cope with the effects of the injury and the challenge of rehabilitation. The client and family demonstrate understanding of post-discharge home care. ●

‣ ***Stop, Think, and Respond Exercise 39-2***

When providing hygiene to the client with a spinal cord injury, a red area that does not blanch is noted at the base of the coccyx. What actions are appropriate?

SPINAL NERVE ROOT COMPRESSION

There are two basic types of spinal nerve root compression: **intramedullary** lesions that involve the spinal cord and **extramedullary** lesions that involve the tissues surrounding the spinal cord. The most common site of nerve root compression is at the level of the three lower lumbar disks; however, nerve root compression also occurs in the cervical spine.

Pathophysiology and Etiology

Pressure on spinal nerve roots results from trauma, herniated (ruptured) intervertebral disks, and tumors of the spinal cord and surrounding structures (Fig. 39-14). Stress caused by poor body mechanics, age, or disease weakens an area in the vertebra, causing the spongy center of the vertebrae, the *nucleus pulposus,* to swell and herniate. This condition is commonly called a *slipped disk;* the displacement puts pressure on the nearby nerves.

Pain along the distribution of the nerve root is common. Actions that increase pressure intensify the pain. Weakness and changes in sensation occur. The symptoms intensify with increasing nerve root compression.

Assessment Findings

Symptoms vary depending on the cause of compression and level involved. They usually include weakness, paralysis, pain, and **paresthesia** (numbness, tingling). When a herniated disk in the lumbar region compresses the sciatic nerve, the client describes feeling pain down the buttocks and into the posterior thigh and leg. Physical examination reveals weakness or paralysis of the extremity innervated by the compressed nerve. If a nerve in the lumbar or sacral area is affected, the client experiences pain when lying supine and lifting the leg without bending the knee. The pain increases when straining, coughing, or lifting a heavy object. Walking and sitting become difficult. Spinal radiography, CT, MRI, myelography, and EMG show displacement or herniation of an intervertebral disk, tumor, or bleeding around the nerve root.

Medical Management

When a client has a herniated intervertebral disk, conservative therapy is tried first. Metastatic spinal cord tumors also are treated conservatively because removal is not feasible.

A herniated cervical disk is treated by immobilizing the cervical spine with a cervical collar or brace. Later, as inflammation subsides, the client wears the collar or brace intermittently when walking or sitting. Bed rest with a firm mattress and bed board is used for clients with a lumbar herniated disk.

Skin traction, which can be applied in the home, is used to decrease severe muscle spasm as well as increase the distance between adjacent vertebrae, keep the vertebrae correctly aligned, and, in many instances, relieve pain. Treatment relieves symptoms for an extended period.

Hot moist packs are used to treat muscle spasm. Skeletal muscle relaxants, such as carisoprodol (Rela) and chlorzoxazone (Paraflex), help clients with a herniated intervertebral disk. Diazepam (Valium), a tranquilizer with skeletal muscle-relaxing action, is used for its twofold effect: to reduce anxiety associated with the pain of a herniated disk and to relax the skeletal muscle. Drugs such as aspirin, phenylbutazone (Butazolidin), and corticosteroids are used to treat inflammation. Reducing inflammation and muscle spasm helps ease pain, but additional analgesics are given to control pain. Clients with an inoperable spinal cord tumor are given analgesics to maintain comfort.

Pharmacologic Considerations

- Clients who take a skeletal muscle relaxant or tranquilizer for a herniated intervertebral disk, back strain, or spasms of the back muscles may experience drowsiness and dizziness. They require assistance with ambulatory activities and should not drive or operate equipment.

Surgical Management

If conservative therapy fails to relieve symptoms of a herniated disk with spinal nerve root compression, surgery is considered. Procedures for relieving spinal nerve root compression include the following:

- **Diskectomy**—removal of the ruptured disk
- **Laminectomy**—removal of the posterior arch of a vertebra to expose the spinal cord. The surgeon can remove whatever lesion is causing compression: a herniated disk, tumor, blood clot, bone spur, or broken bone fragment.

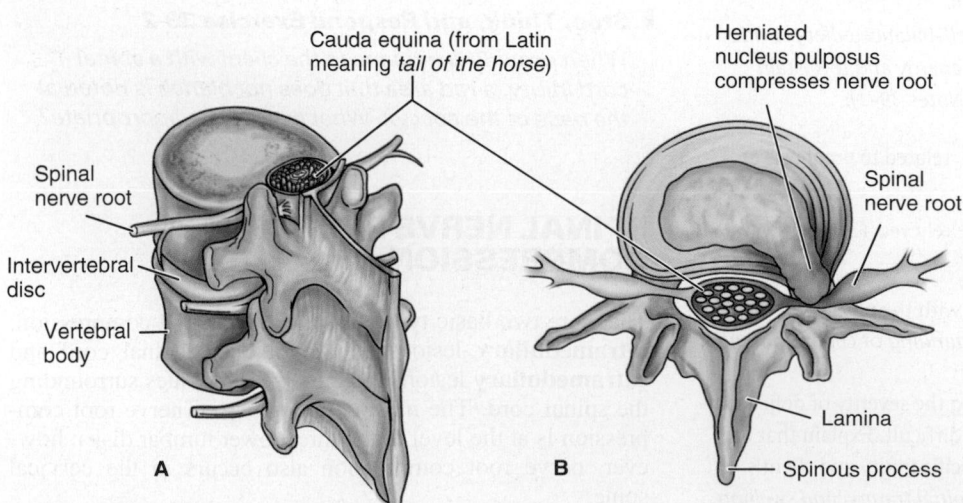

Cauda equina (from Latin meaning *tail of the horse*)

Herniated nucleus pulposus compresses nerve root

Spinal nerve root

Intervertebral disc

Vertebral body

Spinal nerve root

Lamina

Spinous process

A

B

FIGURE 39-14. (**A**) Normal lumbar spine vertebrae, intervertebral disks, and spinal nerve root. (**B**) Ruptured vertebral disk.

NURSING GUIDELINES 39-2

Nursing Care After Specific Spinal Surgeries

Postcervical Diskectomy

- Keep a cervical collar in place at all times; do not remove without a physician's order.
- Instruct client to keep the neck straight in midline position until healing occurs.
- Support client's head, neck, and upper shoulders when moving from a lying to sitting to standing position or when getting into and out of a chair.
- Observe for Horner's syndrome, a complication following anterior cervical diskectomy from cervical sympathetic nerve damage. Manifestations are lid ptosis (drooping), constricted pupil, regression of eye in the orbit, and lack of perspiration on one side of the face.

Postlumbar Laminectomy or Diskectomy with Spinal Fusion

- Logroll when turning client every 2 hours; maintain alignment at all times.

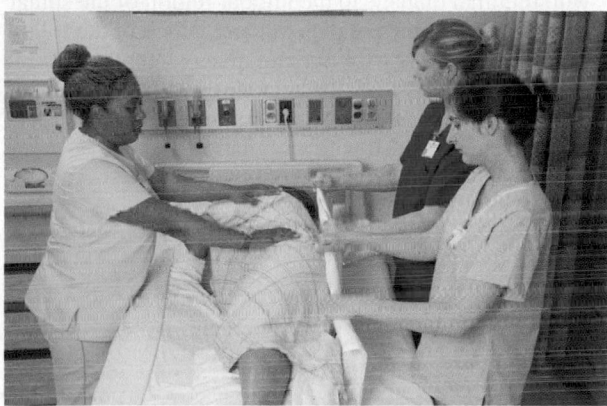

Roll client in a coordinated movement.

- Caution client to avoid turning self.
- Teach client to avoid twisting or jerking the back; sitting during the first week and prolonged sitting thereafter (client should use a straight-backed chair and not slump); bending from the waist (client should bend from the knees and hips).

- Diskectomy with **spinal fusion**—removal of the ruptured disk followed by grafting a piece of bone taken from another area, such as the iliac crest, onto the vertebra to fuse the vertebral spinous process. Bone also may be obtained from a bone bank.
- **Chemonucleolysis**—injection of the enzyme chymopapain into the nucleus pulposus to shrink or dissolve the disc, which then relieves pressure on spinal nerve roots

Spinal fusion stabilizes the vertebrae weakened by degenerative joint changes, such as osteoarthritis, and by laminectomy. It results in a firm union; the client loses mobility and must become accustomed to a permanent area of stiff-

ness. When a portion of the lumbar spine is fused, the client usually does not feel the stiffness after a short time because motion increases in the joints above the fusion. Motion is more limited when the area of fusion is in the cervical spine. Spinal fusion also is performed for spinal cord tumors, fractures and dislocations of the spine, and Pott's disease (tuberculosis of the spine).

Nursing Management

The nurse performs a neurologic examination and notes any limitation of motion and the type of movement that causes pain. Nursing Guidelines 39-2 outlines nursing responsibilities unique to various types of spinal surgery. For clients being treated conservatively, the nurse uses a firm mattress or applies a bedboard because a firm surface supports the spine and promotes alignment. He or she maintains the client on bed rest, placing him or her in semi-Fowler' position, with the knees and head slightly elevated to relieve lumbosacral pain. The nurse applies halo vest traction. For intermittent pelvic or cervical skin traction, he or she attaches the skin device to the client, supports the weights, and lowers them gently to avoid a sudden and strong pull (Box 39-2). The nurse reminds the client to roll from side to side without twisting the spine. When the client gets out of bed, the nurse reinforces the use of proper body mechanics. He or she advises clients with cervical nerve root compression to avoid extreme hyperextension of the neck and side-to-side rotation of the head. The nurse administers prescribed muscle relaxants and analgesics. He or she applies moist heat for no longer than 20 minutes, but repeats several times a day.

The nurse periodically evaluates the client's response to conservative therapy. It is important to note the activities and positions that increase pain and the gain or loss in motion or sensation since the previous observation. Comparison of current symptoms with those first exhibited provides an evaluation of response to therapy. It is important to note a change in symptoms when the client is removed from traction.

Nursing interventions after spinal surgery are as follows:

- Monitor vital signs.
- Assist client to perform hourly deep-breathing exercises while awake but avoid forced coughing because it increases pressure within the spinal canal.
- Examine the dressing for CSF leakage or bleeding.
- Assess neurovascular status (color, temperature, mobility, sensation) in extremities below the area of surgery, which may result from edema or hemorrhage at the operative site.
- Report an inability to void or an output of less than 240 mL in 8 hours.
- Use a fracture bed pan.

BOX 39-2 Maintaining Traction

For proper application and use of traction:
- The prescribed amount of weight must be used.
- Traction weights must hang above the floor.
- Ropes must move freely through the pulley grooves.
- The client's position must be in line with the pull of the traction apparatus.

CRITICAL THINKING EXERCISES

1. A man involved in a motor vehicle accident is brought to the ED. You are told that he was not wearing a seat belt and struck his head on the steering wheel. What neurologic assessments would you make? Why?

2. You are caring for a paraplegic client. What signs and symptoms suggest that the client is experiencing autonomic dysreflexia? What nursing measures are appropriate?

3. The family of a tetraplegic client in an extended care facility wants to assume home care of the client, whose condition is stable. What recommendations would be appropriate at this time?

4. What health teaching is essential to provide a client who is recovering from back spasms associated with a herniated (ruptured) vertebral disk?

NCLEX-STYLE REVIEW QUESTIONS

1. A nurse on a medical flight crew is assessing an alert but lethargic client with a possible closed head injury. The nurse is correct in giving priority attention to which of the following for data relating to the client's neurologic status?
1. Temperature and blood pressure
2. Respiratory rate and breathing effort
3. Level of consciousness and pupillary responses
4. Peripheral vision and cranial nerve function

2. The nurse is obtaining a history from the wife of a client who has just arrived in the ED. Which statement by the wife characterizes the progression of disease symptoms associated with an epidural hematoma?
1. "My husband had a headache all day. He rested in bed with the lights out."
2. "I noticed that he was confused and then collapsed in the kitchen. It happened so fast."
3. "I have noticed that he has become increasingly more forgetful over the past week."
4. "His coordination was poor this morning, but he still drove to the hospital."

3. A client is undergoing intracranial surgery. Which of the following interventions is most important to prevent the complications of thrombophlebitis and deep vein thrombosis?
1. Restrict the intake of fluids
2. Discourage preoperative sedation
3. Apply elastic support stockings
4. Administer prescribed corticosteroids

4. Which of the following is the most important reason for the nurse to monitor a client's body temperature closely after intracranial surgery?
1. Hyperthermia increases the risk for tetraplegia.
2. Hyperthermia increases the risk for cerebral edema.
3. Hyperthermia increases the risk for immobility.
4. Hyperthermia increases the risk for brain damage.

5. A nurse in a rehabilitation setting is caring for a client with minimal damage to the lumbar region of the spinal cord. In developing the plan of care, which of the following will be a priority for nursing management?
1. Total paralysis from the neck down
2. Symptoms of autonomic dysreflexia
3. Assistance needed with ambulation
4. Assistance needed with feeding

40

Caring f
Neurolo

586 | UNIT 9 Caring for Clients

Medical and Surgi

The focus of managem
lize the client and
client with a CVA
or hypotension
or spinal cord
mechanica
the inju
forei
cli

Words To Know

Credé's maneuver
cutaneous triggering
neurologic deficit
reflex incontinence

Learning Obje

On completion of this chap......

1. Define neurologic deficit.
2. Describe the three phases of a neurologic deficit.
3. Give the primary aims of medical treatment of a neurologic deficit.
4. Name six members of the healthcare team involved with the management of a client with a neurologic deficit.
5. Describe nursing management of a client with a neurologic deficit.

This chapter discusses the management of a client with a **neurologic deficit**, a condition in which one or more functions of the central and peripheral nervous systems are decreased, impaired, or absent. Examples include paralysis, muscle weakness, impaired speech, inability to recognize objects, abnormal gait or difficulty walking, impaired memory, impaired swallowing, or abnormal bowel and bladder elimination. The client with a neurologic deficit faces many problems. Often, the deficit affects more than one body system. The client may be unable to walk, talk, perform simple tasks such as feeding and bathing, or recognize family members.

Many members of the healthcare team are involved in the complex management of the client with a temporary or permanent neurologic deficit: the physician, nurse, nursing assistant, social worker, physical therapist, occupational therapist, speech therapist, prosthetist, psychotherapist, dietitian, pharmacist, and vocational counselor. With intensive therapy and a coordinated approach by all team members, many clients have the potential to regain normal or near-normal function or successfully adapt to the changes in function.

PHASES OF A NEUROLOGIC DEFICIT

Neurologic deficits are divided into three phases: acute, recovery, and chronic. Not all clients with a neurologic deficit experience all three phases. Some clients have deficits that begin with an acute phase and move into a recovery phase or into a lifelong chronic phase.

ACUTE PHASE

The acute phase follows a sudden neurologic event, such as a cerebrovascular accident (CVA) or a head or spinal cord injury. During the acute phase, the client usually is critically ill, with many signs and symptoms, such as altered level of consciousness (LOC), hypertension or hypotension, fever, difficulty breathing, or paralysis.

cal Management

...ent during the acute phase is to stabi-
...revent further neurologic damage. The
... may require management of hypertension
... through drug therapy. The client with a head
... injury may require respiratory support through
... ventilation or surgical intervention to stabilize
...ed area or remove bone fragments, blood clots, or
...n objects. Sometimes, surgery is postponed until the
...nt is stabilized and the acute phase has passed. In other
instances, surgery is performed during the acute phase as a
lifesaving measure.

Nursing Management

The nurse performs frequent and thorough neurologic
assessments to evaluate the client's status, need for additional medical or surgical interventions, and response to
treatment. He or she uses the Glasgow Coma Scale (see
Chap. 36) or other neurologic assessment tools such as the
Mini-Mental Status Examination (see Chap. 67). When significant changes occur, the nurse immediately reports them
to the physician. The nurse assesses vital signs as often as
necessary and maintains the blood pressure (BP) to ensure
adequate cerebral oxygenation. He or she measures intake
and output and observes for signs of electrolyte imbalances
and dehydration. The nurse reports a urinary output of less
than 500 mL/day or urinary or bowel incontinence.

Beginning basic rehabilitation during the acute phase is
an important nursing function. Measures such as position
changes and prevention of skin breakdown and contractures
are essential aspects of care during the early phase of rehabilitation. The nursing goal is to prevent complications that
may interfere with the client's potential to recover function.
(See Nursing Process section for additional nursing
management.)

RECOVERY PHASE

The recovery phase begins when the client's condition is stabilized. It starts several days or weeks after the initial event
and lasts weeks or months.

Medical and Surgical Management

Medical management during the recovery phase aims at
keeping the client stable and preventing or treating complications, such as pneumonia, and further neurologic
impairment.

Nursing Management

During recovery, the nurse works with team members to plan
a rehabilitation program in several domains according to the
client's abilities and limitations (Table 40-1). Various
assessment tools can help identify a client's level of functioning and potential for improvement with a rehabilitation
program, including:

- The National Institute for Health Stroke Scale
  (http://www.ninds.nih.gov/doctors/NIH_Stroke_Scale_
  Booklet.pdf)

TABLE 40-1 Domains of Neurologic Impairment

DOMAIN	DESCRIPTION
Motor	A single deficit, or combination of deficits, involving the face, arms, and legs, which affects speech, swallowing, muscle tone and strength, gait, coordination, and ability to use objects for their intended purpose
Sensory	Altered sensation (e.g., numbness, tingling, exaggerated sensation), or altered perception (e.g., inability to identify objects by touch, loss of writing ability)
Vision	Loss of vision in one eye or in the temporal or nasal fields; blindness
Language	Disturbances in comprehension, naming, repeating, clarity of speech, reading
Cognition	Changes in memory, attention, orientation, calculation, and construction
Affect	Altered mood, lability of mood

- The American Heart Association's Stroke Outcome Classification (http://stroke.ahajournals.org/cgi/content/full/
  29/6/1274)
- The Barthel Index (Table 40-2)

Rehabilitation is designed to meet the client's immediate and long-term needs. Environmental changes may be
necessary to help the client adapt to the disability and fully
regain any remaining functions. Even though deficits can be
temporary, a prolonged period and enrollment in a rehabilitation program often are necessary before recovery of partial
or full function can occur. A successful rehabilitation
program includes not only nurses and physicians, but also
several other providers, such as physical therapists, occupational therapists, speech therapists, and enterostomal therapists, all of whom recommend devices or procedures to
prevent complications and enhance the client's remaining
abilities.

With continuous assessment and identification of the
client's needs, the nurse plays an important role in rehabilitation. Devices that help a client walk, eat, groom, and perform
other motor skills are recommended or devised to suit particular needs. Flotation pads for wheelchairs, walkers, padded
ankle-foot boots to prevent foot drop, and range-of-motion
(ROM) exercises are examples of the many appliances and
procedures used in rehabilitation. (See Nursing Process section for additional nursing management.)

CHRONIC PHASE

For some clients (e.g., those with multiple sclerosis or Alzheimer's disease), neurologic deficit results in a prolonged
or lifelong chronic phase. In this phase, the client shows little
or no improvement, remains stationary, or progressively
worsens. Physical and psychological rehabilitation continues
in the chronic phase to prevent complications such as pressure ulcers and muscle contractures.

TABLE 40-2 Modified Barthel Index

ITEM	UNABLE TO PERFORM TASK	SUBSTANTIAL HELP REQUIRED	MODERATE HELP REQUIRED	MINIMAL HELP REQUIRED	FULLY INDEPENDENT
Personal hygiene	0	1	3	4	5
Bathing self	0	1	3	4	5
Feeding	0	2	5	8	10
Toilet	0	2	5	8	10
Stair climbing	0	2	5	8	10
Dressing	0	2	5	8	10
Bowel control	0	2	5	8	10
Bladder control	0	2	5	8	10
Ambulation	0	3	8	12	15
or wheelchair*	0	1	3	4	5
Chair/bed transfer	0	3	8	12	15

*Score only if client is unable to ambulate and is trained in wheelchair management.

DEPENDENCY NEEDS			
CATEGORIES	MBI TOTAL SCORES	DEPENDENCY LEVEL	HOURS OF HELP REQUIRED PER WEEK (MAXIMUM)
1	0–24	Total	27.0
2	25–49	Severe	23.5
3	50–74	Moderate	20.0
4	75–90	Mild	13.0
5	91–99	Minimal	<10.0

Medical and Surgical Management

Medical management continues throughout the chronic phase and uses a wide range of therapies and treatments, such as control of BP, physical therapy, dietary management, and treatment of complications related to disuse and immobility. In some cases, surgery is performed to correct deformities or problems that have developed. Examples include muscle and skin grafts to close a pressure ulcer, surgery to correct a contracture deformity, or removal of a kidney stone (a complication of prolonged immobility).

> ▶ *Stop, Think, and Respond Exercise 40-1*
>
> *You have been caring for a client with a head injury who is being transferred to an extended care facility for rehabilitation. What information is important to include to help nurses at the new facility plan the client's care?*

Nursing Management

Clients in the chronic phase often are admitted to a hospital for treatment of complications. They also are transferred to a skilled nursing facility or long-term care facility when family members no longer can manage their care, or when the disease has progressively worsened so that skilled care is mandatory. Nursing management focuses on preventing physical and psychological complications. Therapy in a rehabilitation center may include retraining in skills such as using the telephone, handling money, shopping, using public transportation, maintaining a household, and vocational training.

PSYCHOSOCIAL ISSUES AND HOME MANAGEMENT

Overview

Leaving the inpatient setting, where the daily, intensive support of the healthcare team is readily available, and returning home with life-altering changes can be tremendously frightening. The client and family need additional support to adapt to a new life-style. Although many clients recover sufficiently to assume responsibility for some aspects of their own care, others do not. The burden of care often falls on the spouse, who may have physical problems as well, or the adult children, who may not be available or willing to share this responsibility.

Financial resources are strained during a lengthy hospitalization, and may continue after discharge. Adapting the home to accommodate a wheelchair or special bed can be costly. Wide doorways, ramps instead of stairs, and special fixtures in the bathroom for bathing and toileting are examples of changes that often are necessary. The client may have been the major wage earner. Some clients can enter training programs that allow them to find employment outside the home, whereas others can learn skills that enable them to be employed at home. Others, because of age or extreme physical disability, cannot be gainfully employed.

Nursing Management

The nurse listens and is alert to subtle hints about the client's and family's adaptation to the client's change in functional status. The nurse asks direct questions to identify problems and needs. He or she evaluates the client's ability to perform self-care, resume his or her role in the family, and call on a support system. The nurse takes appropriate steps to help the client and family attain and maintain a home life as near normal as possible. For example, the nurse assesses available facilities, the family support system, physical aids required (e.g., a wheelchair, cane, walker), and the amount of assistance the client requires with activities of daily living. He or she encourages the family to help plan for the client's return home, to ask questions about care, and to seek assistance from those agencies that can provide emotional, physical, and financial support.

Coping

The nurse addresses each client individually. He or she offers reassurance and emotional support and displays empathetic understanding of the multiple problems the client is facing. Many clients have difficulty coping with their disability. Crises such as being unable to move; having limited movement; being unable to attend to one's most basic needs; and having to totally depend on others for housing, clothing, mobility, and food generate strong emotional responses. Some clients eventually accept their disability; others do not. The nurse provides encouragement and praise throughout rehabilitation and shows personal interest and pleasure in each accomplishment, no matter how small, to help clients accept what they cannot or never will be able to do.

The nurse gives clients time to talk about their problems, fears, and concerns. Once needs are identified, he or she encourages the client to set attainable goals, which may help maintain independence as long as possible. The nurse works with the client and family to develop solutions and possible alternatives. This helps the client and family meet each problem as it arises, understand the limitations, establish goals, and work toward a solution.

With rehabilitation comes the client's awareness of progress or lack thereof. At times, improvement is slow and barely noticeable. A client often has difficulty coping. Discouragement, depression, withdrawal, and anger are not unusual. The nurse suggests available support groups for those with neurologic deficits for emotional, physical, and social support.

Gerontologic Considerations

- The slower response to stimuli that may accompany aging can lead to increased frustration, irritability, or depression. Teach caregivers and clients to allow extra time if needed to formulate answers to questions or perform activities. Encourage family caregivers to use respite care services or seek resources to prevent exhaustion.

Socialization

As soon as clients can respond to those around them, the nurse encourages socialization with others. At first, socialization can be limited to healthcare team members and family. The nurse encourages the family to talk to the client, discuss current events, and motivate the client to respond. Those with speech difficulties tend to become withdrawn and depressed. The nurse encourages visitors to talk to the client, include the client in their conversations, and ask the

client questions. The nurse suggests that family members use patience when trying to understand what a client with aphasia is trying to communicate.

Occupational and recreational therapies are part of the rehabilitation program and require a team effort. In the beginning, occupational therapy is designed to help strengthen muscles that are under voluntary control. Later, certain tasks are learned or relearned to help the client interact with others. Participation in these therapies increases socialization time and helps the client interact with others.

Gerontologic Considerations

- Older adults with a neurologic deficit may lack an adequate support system once they are discharged from the hospital. Involve social service and other agencies to assist these clients and their caregivers with rehabilitation and to prevent social isolation.

Family Processes

The nurse recognizes that the family faces many disruptions because of the permanent disability of a family member. Life-styles are altered, financial resources are strained, conflicts arise, and people must accept new responsibilities. The nurse allows the family time to deal with and accept these changes. The nurse provides the family with opportunities to talk and openly express their anger, fears, guilt, and helplessness. Although no single perfect solution to any problem exists, the following suggestions may help the family adjust to present and future changes:

- Include the family in the client's rehabilitation.
- Give encouragement and praise when a family member is able to help with a part of home care or shows interest in becoming involved in the client's care.
- Explain the purpose of each segment of rehabilitation (e.g., ROM exercises, positioning).
- When the family expresses a desire to assume responsibility for certain procedures to be performed at home, teach each procedure or task slowly and give the family time to practice under supervision.
- Prepare a list of public or private agencies that may assist with home care, transportation, and financial and emotional support.

Client and Family Teaching

The nurse develops a teaching plan for home care management that incorporates the therapies prescribed by the physician and other members of the team. The client and family usually have many questions. The nurse must begin teaching long before discharge so that the client and family have sufficient time to learn and understand home care management. The individualized teaching plan includes discussion of the topics presented in Client and Family Teaching 40-1.

Pharmacologic Considerations

- Clients with impaired swallowing often have difficulty taking pills or capsules; liquid medications are preferred. If a client

Client and Family Teaching 40-1
Home Care for the Client with a Neurologic Deficit

The nurse addresses the following key areas and points when teaching the client and family.

Skin Care

● Know how to inspect and care for the skin. A pressure ulcer that is beginning to develop may not cause discomfort.
● Change position at least every 2 hours to relieve pressure on bony prominences.
● Contact a healthcare provider immediately if the skin is reddened, warm, or disrupted.

Body Alignment

● Understand that good body alignment is important.
● Be able to demonstrate how to put joints through a full ROM. Perform ROM exercises several times per day or as ordered by the physician or physical therapist.
● Know how to use various devices, such as rolled blankets or pillows, to support or align areas of the body, such as the back, hips, and legs. Be able to explain the use of a footboard or other device to prevent footdrop.

Nutrition and Fluids

● Be sure to take fluids frequently. A high fluid intake is important to prevent urinary tract complications.
● Consume a balanced diet; this is important in maintaining optimal health.
● It may be easier to tolerate small meals and between-meal snacks than three large meals.
● Take time to chew food and drink fluids.

Bowel and Bladder

● Continue a bowel and bladder training program.

● Include adequate dietary fiber to facilitate regular bowel elimination.
● Use a clean technique for irrigating, changing, or inserting catheters at home (as demonstrated by the nurse).
● Inspect the urine for cloudiness (which may indicate a urinary tract infection).
● Contact a physician if chills and fever occur or if the urine is bloody, cloudy, or has an offensive odor.
● Know how to perform skin care of the genitalia and perineum, including the special care that must be given to the anal area and the genitalia after defecation. (A male client with an external urinary sheath should be able to demonstrate its application and know how to clean the penis daily to remove urine and dried secretions.)

Activity

● Make use of social contacts, hobbies, and changes in the daily routine to relieve boredom.
● Avoid fatigue and exposure to infection.
● Take deep breaths every 1 or 2 hours while awake and to cough to raise secretions.

Therapies, Community Services, and Equipment

● Work with therapists and follow their advice about performance or practice of the therapies.
● When needed, use services available for home care.
● Contact agencies or retail stores from which home care equipment may be purchased, rented, or borrowed.
● If necessary, consult with a social service worker for information regarding financial assistance or the availability of loan closets that allow people who need certain types of equipment to borrow these materials.

---

must take solid medications at home, advise family members to check with their physician or pharmacist before crushing or breaking tablets or opening capsules; some medications must not be crushed or opened.

Nursing Process for the Client with a Neurologic Deficit

Assessment

Obtain a thorough history (including drugs and allergies) from the client or family. Assess vital signs and level of comfort. Weigh the client for future comparisons. Perform a general neurologic assessment and use a standardized assessment tool (see Table 40-2) to note the extent of neurologic deficits related to swallowing, vision, weakness or paralysis of extremities, speech, and language compre-

hension. Ask about any seizures and for a description of those that have occurred. Evaluate airway, breathing, circulation, and LOC. Inspect the skin, auscultate the abdomen for bowel sounds, palpate the bladder for distention, and determine the client's ability to control bowel and bladder. Explore the client's emotional and mental status, such as stability of mood, evidence of depression, and motivation for rehabilitation.

Diagnosis, Planning, and Interventions

In addition to the diagnoses discussed in the following section, many nursing diagnoses may apply for the client and family facing a neurologic deficit (Box 40-1).

▶ Risk for Impaired Skin or Tissue Integrity related to immobility, incontinence, or other factors (specify)

▶ Expected Outcome: Skin will remain intact and free from infection.

Additional Nursing Diagnoses for the Client and Family Facing a Neurologic Deficit

Diagnoses for the Client

- **Deficient Knowledge** (specify) related to cognitive limitation, lack of recall, misinterpretation of information
- **Impaired Memory** related to neurologic disturbances
- **Relocation Stress Syndrome** related to losses involved in decision to move, feeling of powerlessness
- **Ineffective Role Performance** related to change in ability to resume role
- **Chronic Confusion** related to cognitive changes
- **Powerlessness** related to inability to control situation, dependence on others
- **Hopelessness** related to feeling overwhelmed by prognosis
- **Ineffective Coping** related to chronic stress
- **Deficient Diversional Activity** related to immobility, depression, withdrawal, inability to participate in social activities, monotonous environment
- **Ineffective Therapeutic Regimen Management** related to insufficient knowledge of tests, treatments, home care management, other (specify)
- **Impaired Home Maintenance** related to inability to care for self, inadequacies such as housing, care, financial resources (specify)
- **Impaired Adjustment** related to inability to accept the physical changes and impaired cognition
- **Impaired Social Interaction** related to aphasia, immobility
- **Social Isolation** related to immobility, lack of transportation, other (specify)

Diagnoses for the Family

- **Caregiver Role Strain** related to complexity or amount of care needed
- **Interrupted Family Processes** related to changes in health status, disability of family member
- **Compromised Family Coping** related to exhaustion of supportive capacity

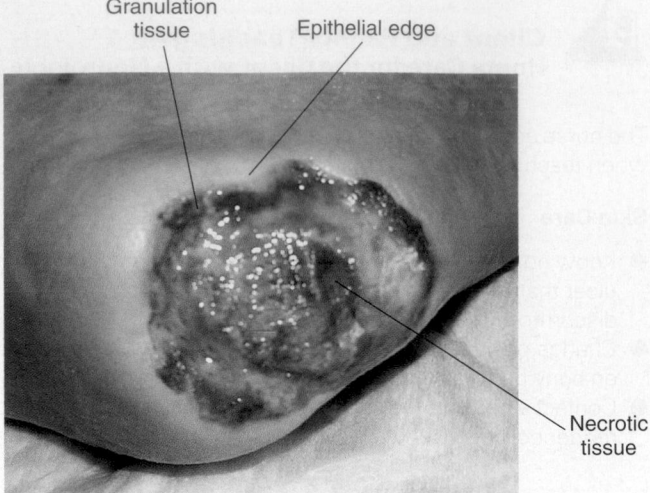

FIGURE 40-1. Pressure ulcer of the elbow in a client with a CVA cared for at home. This client was admitted to the hospital for treatment of multiple pressure ulcers.

▶ Risk for Disuse Syndrome related to musculoskeletal inactivity and neuromuscular impairment

▶ Expected Outcome: Client will maintain ROM in all joints.

- Keep extremities aligned with pillows, trochanter rolls, and splints. *A neutral position facilitates functional use of the limbs.*
- Perform passive ROM exercises with the weak or paralyzed extremity (Fig. 40-2). *ROM maintains joint flexibility and prevents permanent contractures.*

- Inspect all pressure points daily; keep skin clean and dry at all times. *Assessment enables identification of problems. Clean, dry skin reduces bacteria and the moisture that promotes their reproduction.*
- Massage bony prominences that blanch when pressure is relieved. *Massage increases circulation to the tissues, bringing oxygen and removing carbon dioxide and cellular wastes. Massage is contraindicated if the skin is already impaired, as evidenced by areas that remain reddened with relief of pressure.*
- Use a flotation mattress and other devices to relieve pressure when client is lying and sitting. *The integument becomes impaired when capillary pressure falls below 32 mm Hg (Fig. 40-1).*
- Encourage adequate nutrition and provide supplements as ordered. *Protein, vitamin C, and zinc are important for healing/ maintaining skin integrity. Supplements may be necessary to meet increased need for vitamin C and zinc.*
- Change client's position every 2 hours. *Doing so relieves pressure over bony prominences and maintains sufficient capillary pressure to keep integument intact.*

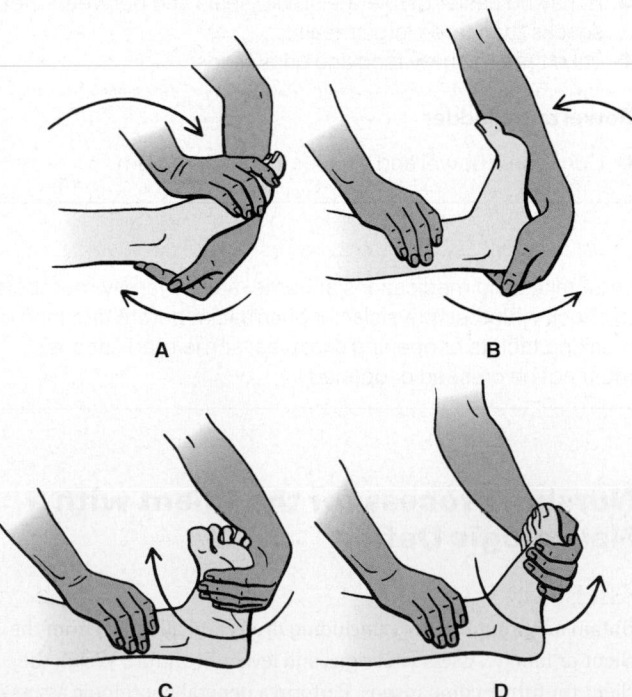

FIGURE 40-2. Passive ROM exercises for the affected foot in hemiplegia. The motions should be conducted slowly and smoothly, with a momentary pause when spasticity causes resistance. As soon as the client exhibits movement, these exercises can be done actively rather than passively.

NURSING GUIDELINES 40-1

Implementing a Bowel Training Program

Some clients can achieve self-controlled emptying of the bowel provided they and those who care for them exert the persistent effort required. Bowel control typically is easier to achieve than bladder control.

For a bowel training program:

- Keep a record of bowel movements over several weeks. Doing so helps determine the time of day the client is most likely to have a bowel movement.
- Encourage liquids throughout the day. Include foods that produce bulk, such as fresh fruits and vegetables, in the diet. Eliminate foods that cause loose stools.
- Assist client to the bathroom at a certain time each day. The physical activity involved in getting out of bed often increases peristalsis and encourages defecation.
- Administer a low-volume enema or suppository each day at the same time to stimulate a bowel movement. Later, bowel

function will become regulated so that the client can have a bowel movement at this time without these aids.

Steps for administering a suppository or enema:

1. Tape the paralyzed client's buttocks together to keep a suppository in place. Remove the tape at the time the suppository is expected to work.
2. Give enemas slowly, about 1 to 2 oz, followed by a waiting period, to clients with tetraplegia or paraplegia who can retain sufficient enema solution.
3. Check the temperature of the enema solution immediately before administration. Insert the rectal tube gently, especially for clients who cannot feel, because they are vulnerable to trauma.
4. Allow the client privacy and sufficient time to have a bowel movement.

- Prevent footdrop with a footboard. *A footboard positions the foot and ankle in such a way as to prevent plantar flexion.*
- Remove and reapply elastic stockings at least twice a day. *Elastic stockings support vein walls, reduce hemostasis, and decrease the potential for thrombophlebitis.*

▶ Constipation or Diarrhea (specify) related to prolonged immobility, tube feedings, decreased fluid intake, effect of disease or injury on the spinal cord nerves

▶ Expected Outcome: Client will have regular bowel movements at least every 3 days.

- Keep a daily record of all bowel movements. *A database helps identify problems.*
- Administer a prescribed stool softener daily. *Stool softeners moisturize the feces, which facilitates passage of stool without straining.*
- Increase client's daily fluid intake. *Oral fluids contribute to moisture in stool.*
- Institute a bowel training program (Nursing Guidelines 40-1). *Bowel training promotes bowel continence.*
- Perform a digital examination of the rectum if there is no bowel elimination in 3 days or if client passes liquid stools. *A digital examination helps determine if hard stool is in the rectum; passage of liquid stool may accompany fecal impaction.*
- Add high-fiber foods to the diet. *Fiber increases fecal bulk and pulls water into the feces, promoting regular bowel elimination.*
- Discuss persistent diarrhea with physician. *Bacterial growth in warm enteral formula, contamination of tube feeding equipment, and low-fiber formulas can cause enteritis and diarrhea.*

the lower rectum, and bisacodyl (Dulcolax), which stimulates peristalsis in the terminal section of the colon. Enemas used in a bowel training program may be plain water, glycerin, and Fleet brand enema.

▶ Total Urinary Incontinence or Urinary Retention related to effects of disease or injury to the nervous system or spinal cord nerves, loss of bladder tone

▶ Expected Outcome: Client will void, the bladder will empty with no urinary retention, or both.

- Use an indwelling catheter or intermittent catheterization. *Some neurologic deficits are permanent; urinary elimination and continence may require a catheter.*
- Measure intake and output when client has an indwelling urethral catheter and takes fluids poorly, and when first removing an indwelling urethral catheter. *Measuring intake and output helps identify whether fluid volume is within normal expectations.*
- Palpate the lower abdomen for bladder distention; notify the physician if client cannot void. *The bladder is not palpable unless it becomes distended. The urge to void occurs when the bladder contains 150 to 300 mL; urination needs to occur several times a day to avoid overdistention.*
- Ensure client uses incontinence pads or absorbent underwear. *Disposable, porous pads and underwear wick urine away and keep bedding dry.*
- Institute a bladder training program as soon as possible (Nursing Guidelines 40-2). *Bladder training promotes urinary continence.*

Pharmacologic Considerations

- Examples of suppositories used for a bowel training program are glycerin suppositories, which soften the stool in

Gerontologic Considerations

- A behavioral or cognitive change such as irritability may be the only sign of urinary retention in older adults with a neurologic deficit.

NURSING GUIDELINES 40-2

Implementing a Bladder Training Program

- Record the times the client voids over several weeks to help establish voiding patterns.
- Plan a voiding schedule that is similar to the assessed voiding patterns.
- Encourage increased fluid intake; clients who remain relatively immobile for the rest of their lives are subject to bladder infections and calculus (stone) formation in the urinary tract.
- Advise client to note any sensation (chilliness, lower abdominal discomfort, restlessness) that precedes voiding. Doing so helps the client identify when he or she needs to void.
- Encourage client to void every 30 minutes to 2 hours while awake. If the client can use the bedpan or urinal, keep these

readily available, and answer the call light promptly when the client requires assistance.
- Instruct client to bend at the waist or press inward and downward over the bladder, a technique referred to as **Credé's maneuver**. It increases abdominal pressure and facilitates emptying the bladder.
- Use other measures to stimulate voiding, such as running water and placing a hand in a basin of water.
- Propose that paralyzed clients with **reflex incontinence**, which occurs spontaneously when the bladder is full, lightly massage or tap the skin above the pubic area, a method known as **cutaneous triggering** that stimulates relaxation of the urinary sphincter

---

- Functional problems and diminished muscular strength that accompany aging may complicate recovery for a client with a neurologic deficit. For example, an age-related delay in the relaxation of the internal bladder sphincter can make bladder training more difficult.

▶ **Impaired Physical Mobility** related to muscle weakness and paralysis

▶ **Expected Outcome:** Client will tolerate increased physical mobility as demonstrated by use of devices for mobility and remain free of contractures.

- Perform active or passive ROM exercises on the affected and unaffected extremities, or encourage client to perform ROM exercises independently (Fig. 40-3). *ROM exercises prevent contractures and muscle atrophy.*
- Regularly position clients with paraplegia or tetraplegia in an upright posture. *An upright posture helps the client take in the immediate environment and helps promote circulation through regulation of baroreceptors.*
- Apply an abdominal binder and elastic stockings before the client gets up. *An abdominal binder and elastic stockings decrease pooling of blood in distal areas, thereby preventing dizziness and faintness.*
- Suggest using parallel bars or a walker (Fig. 40-4). *Before ambulating independently, clients can learn to support body weight and move forward with a variety of ambulatory aids.*

▶ **Risk for Sexual Dysfunction** related to disturbance or loss of nerve function to genitalia

▶ **Expected Outcome:** Client will explore sexual alternatives.

- Be alert to subtle references to sexual dysfunction or problems. *Most clients are hesitant to discuss sexuality openly and frankly.*
- Allow client time to talk or ask questions. *Most clients refrain from sexual discussions if they sense the nurse is unreceptive or pressed for time.*

- Convey acceptance; recommend that the client and sexual partner speak with a physician or sexual therapist. *Medical and behavioral approaches may provide alternatives to former sexual activities.*
- Explain to paralyzed men that spontaneous erections may occur when the bladder is full. *Spontaneous erections are unpredictable and sometimes circumstantially inconvenient.*
- Offer information about penile implants (see Chap. 55). *A penile implant provides temporary or permanent penile erection, which facilitates vaginal penetration during intercourse.*

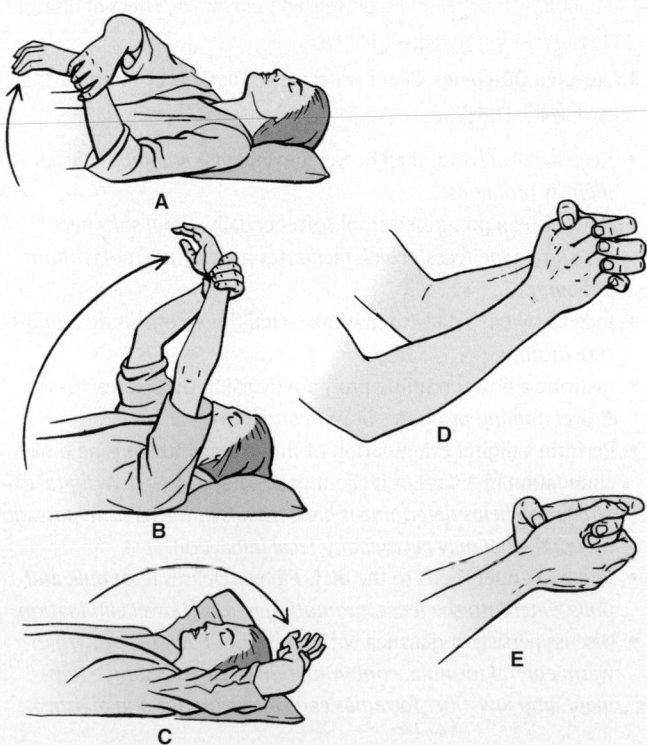

FIGURE 40-3. Range-of-motion exercises of the affected hand and arm that hemiplegic clients can learn to do themselves. (**A–C**) The client uses the unaffected hand to grasp the affected arm at the wrist and raise it over the head. (**D** and **E**) The client grasps the paralyzed hand and extends each affected finger slowly in turn.

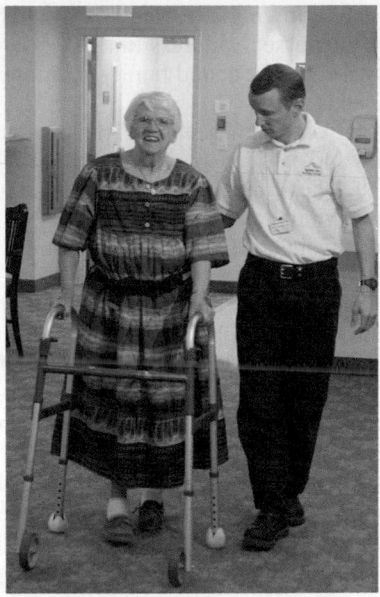

FIGURE 40-4. Ambulatory training in the physical therapy department starts as soon as the client can stand.

- Inform paralyzed men that ejaculation is rare and sperm motility is diminished, which reduces the potential for fathering children. *Clients with paraplegia or tetraplegia have the right to information about their potential for fertility.*
- Suggest that having intercourse on a water bed may facilitate sexual activity. *The buoyancy of a water bed promotes pelvic movement.*
- Share that some couples use mutual masturbation or electronic vibrators during sexual activity. *Orgasmic arousal can be achieved using alternatives.*
- Instruct female clients that they are still fertile and may need contraception if a pregnancy is undesired. *Motor paralysis does not affect ovulation.*

▶ **Risk for Injury** related to muscle weakness, paralysis, seizure disorder, loss of calcium from bone, other (specify)

▶ **Expected Outcome:** Client remains free from injury.

- Use caution when moving and lifting a client who has been immobile. *Prolonged immobility results in calcium loss from bones and increased susceptibility to fractures.*
- Use a mechanical lift to safely transfer client (Fig. 40-5). *It uses principles of physics to raise, lift, and lower clients with minimal exertion on the part of caregivers.*
- Implement seizure precautions for clients with head injuries or brain tumors (see Chap. 37, Nursing Process for the Client With a Seizure Disorder, for specific interventions). *The client is at risk for injury during a seizure because he or she cannot implement self-protective interventions.*

▶ **Risk for Situational Low Self-Esteem** related to effects of disability on perception of self-worth

▶ **Expected Outcome:** Client will maintain positive self-regard, accept changes in body function, express feelings about the disability, and participate in rehabilitation.

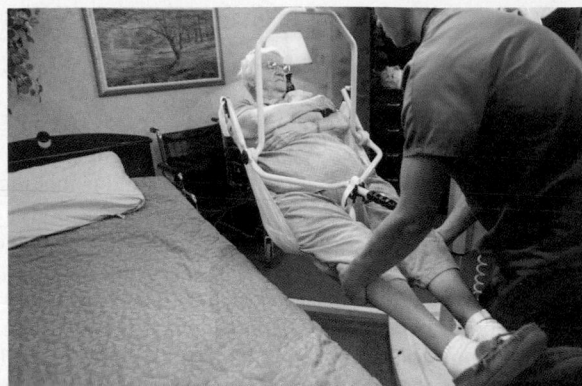

FIGURE 40-5. A mechanical lift may be used to transfer a client to and from the bed, wheelchair, or shower.

- Assess for signs of negative responses, such as refusal to discuss loss, lack of participation in care, and increased isolation. *Nonverbal cues provide more reliable feedback about self-regard than do verbalizations.*
- Convey respect and hope; encourage verbalization of feelings. *Remaining nonjudgmental and giving the client an opportunity to express feelings help relieve stressors.*
- Help client identify his or her positive attributes and strengths from past experiences. *Focusing on successes rather than failures helps decrease feelings of helplessness and hopelessness.*
- Identify ways to support client's independence and role in the family. *Helping the client maintain his or her previous level of functioning maintains self-esteem.*

▶ **Risk for Dysfunctional Grieving** related to loss of body function

▶ **Expected Outcome:** Client will adaptively progress through various stages of grieving.

- Convey support and acceptance of client's feelings. *Grief is a normal response to loss; suppressing grief delays emotional healing.*
- Explain that grieving involves a sequence of emotions. *The grief process is a universal experience that begins with shock and progresses through denial, anger, depression, bargaining, and eventually acceptance.*
- Support grief work: explain denial; promote hope during depression; encourage adaptive outlets for anger; encourage decision-making in all aspects of self-care; focus on present and future goals. *Grief work promotes acceptance of losses.*

Evaluation of Expected Outcomes

Expected outcomes vary, depending on the original goals and nursing diagnoses. The client has no evidence of skin breakdown. Complications associated with inactivity and immobility do not develop. The client works through the grieving process and accepts altered abilities. Defecation and urinary elimination are managed. The client is physically active, as demonstrated by use of trapeze, wheelchair, and other methods for mobility. The client continues sexual activities or learns about sexual alternatives. No injuries occur. The client participates in decision-making regarding daily activities, social outlets, vocational options, and applicable therapies.

CRITICAL THINKING EXERCISES

1. Discuss methods to help clients achieve success in a bowel and bladder training program.
2. A client had a CVA 6 months ago and is paralyzed on his right side. He cannot speak and shows signs of mental changes. He now appears agitated and is making motions with his left hand to various areas of his body, mainly his abdomen. What assessments could you make to determine the possible cause of his agitation?
3. A family is planning to care for a client who has had a CVA at home. Ideally, discharge planning begins at the time of admission. What equipment and supplies would you recommend that the family obtain?
4. A client had a spinal cord injury at T11 and is paraplegic. During a conference, team members mention his depression and withdrawal. What other members of the healthcare team and services may be helpful in this client's care?

NCLEX-STYLE REVIEW QUESTIONS

1. A client is in the skilled rehabilitation setting during the early phase of rehabilitation. When developing the client's nursing plan of care, which long-term goal would be most appropriate?
   1. The client will maintain adequate nutritional status.
   2. The client will exhibit no skin breakdown or contractures.
   3. The client will exhibit no signs of clinical depression.
   4. The client will function using all extremities.
2. A home care nurse is helping client and cope with a recent disability. They have identified several needs.

Which of the following interventions would be most important for the nurse to address first?
   1. Identify for the client and family solutions to their stated needs.
   2. Encourage outside assistance from community agencies and resources.
   3. Assist the client and family to identify solutions and attainable goals.
   4. Call the physician and ask for suggestions on solving the needs.
3. When the nurse is assisting a neurologically impaired client with activities of daily living (ADLs), which approach is best?
   1. Complete all ADLs as quickly as possible.
   2. Eliminate whatever the client cannot perform.
   3. Let the client rest between activities.
   4. Perform all ADLs without involving the client.
4. When planning strategies for managing bowel elimination for the client with paraplegia due to a spinal cord injury, which nursing intervention is most appropriate to include?
   1. Administer a tap-water enema just before bedtime
   2. Encourage a high-fiber diet to increase stool bulk
   3. Change disposable absorbent undergarments when soiled
   4. Pad the rim of the bedpan to prevent skin breakdown
5. The nurse initiates a teaching plan for the family and client with neurologic deficits due to Parkinson's disease. Which nursing instruction is the highest priority?
   1. Encourage social interactions.
   2. Reduce home safety hazards.
   3. Enhance the immune system.
   4. Maintain a balanced diet.

UNIT 10
Caring for Clients with Sensory Disorders

41

Introduction to the Sensory System

Words To Know

accommodation
audiometry
caloric stimulation test
central vision
conductive hearing loss
conjunctivitis
decibels
electronystagmography
near point
nystagmus
ophthalmoscopy
otoscope
proptosis
ptosis
refraction
Rinne test
Romberg test
sensorineural hearing loss
tonometry
tuning fork
visual acuity
visual field examination
Weber test

Learning Objectives

On completion of this chapter, you will be able to:

1. Describe the anatomy and physiology of the eyes.
2. Discuss tests that are used for visual screening.
3. Identify questions to ask during an eye assessment.
4. Describe diagnostic studies for eye function
5. Explain the anatomy and physiology of the ears.
6. Describe methods for assessing the ear and hearing acuity.
7. Describe specific diagnostic tests for ear function.

The special senses of vision and hearing allow humans to view their world, hear what is in their environment, communicate with others, and maintain their balance. Eye and ear disorders occur throughout the life cycle. Many of the disorders can result in changes in visual acuity or hearing loss, as well as problems with balance and communication. Nurses can be instrumental in early identification of eye and ear problems, and they may play an important role in reducing the severity and/or long-term effects of eye and ear disorders. This chapter focuses on the structure and function of the eyes and ears and the diagnostic tests used to evaluate their function.

THE EYES

ANATOMY AND PHYSIOLOGY

The *eyeballs* are globes located in a protective bony cavity or *orbit* of the skull. The frontal, maxillary, zygomatic, sphenoid, ethmoid, lacrimal, and palatine bones form the walls of the orbit. Fat and muscle protect the posterior, superior, inferior, and lateral aspects of each eyeball.

The muscles that permit movement include the superior and inferior rectus (move eye up and down), the medial and lateral rectus (move eye toward the nose and the temple), and the superior and inferior oblique muscles (move eye to the left and right). Six cranial nerves innervate the eye, ocular muscles, and lacrimal apparatus: the optic, oculomotor, trochlear, trigeminal, abducens, and facial cranial nerves.

Extraocular Structures

The eyelids, eyelashes, and tears protect the anterior or exposed surface of the eye. The upper and lower eyelids are folds of skin that meet at an angle referred to as the *canthus*. The outer or lateral canthus is the outer angle, and the inner or medial canthus is at the inner aspect of the eye. The line between the lateral and medial canthus usually is horizontal. Children with Down syndrome have a line that slants upward and outward. People of Asian descent have an epicanthal fold, which is a fold of skin that covers the inner canthus.

The eyelids protect against foreign bodies and adjust the amount of light that enters the eye. The eyelashes trap foreign debris. Periodic blinking clears dust and particles from the surface of the eyes. The eyelids also spread tears over the surface of the eye. The eyelids have multiple glands, including sebaceous, sweat, and accessory lacrimal glands. They are lined with a sensitive, transparent mucous membrane called *conjunctiva*. This membrane extends from the lid margins and meets the *cornea* (the transparent domelike structure that covers most of the anterior portion of the eyeball) at the *limbus*, which is the outermost edge of the iris. The lacrimal *caruncle* is a small, reddish elevation on the conjunctiva located at the inner canthus.

Tears, composed of water, sodium chloride, and lysozyme, an antibacterial enzyme, are produced by *lacrimal (tear) glands* found beneath the bony orbital ridge. The *lacrimal apparatus* includes the lacrimal glands, *punctum, lacrimal canals, lacrimal sac,* and *nasolacrimal ducts*. Tears flow across the eyes, continually bathing and lubricating the surface. The tears drain through the punctum into the lacrimal canals and lacrimal sac to the nasolacrimal ducts, tiny openings at the junction of the upper and lower lids, and then into the nose (Fig. 41-1).

Intraocular Structures

Three layers form the intraocular structures. The first layer is the *sclera*, commonly referred to as the "white of the eye." It is composed of tough connective tissue. The sclera protects structures in the eye. It connects directly to the cornea, anterior chamber, iris, and pupil.

The middle layer is the *uvea*, or vascular coat of the eye, located immediately under the sclera. The uvea includes the *choroid* (contains blood vessels and darkly pigmented cells that prevent light from scattering inside the eye) and the *iris* (the highly vascular, pigmented portion of the eye surrounding the pupil). The *pupil* is an opening that dilates and constricts in response to light. The choroid gives rise to the *ciliary body,* composed of *ciliary processes* and the *ciliary muscle*. The ciliary processes produce *aqueous humor*, a nutrient-rich liquid that nourishes eye structures. The ciliary muscle helps change the shape of the lens when adjusting to near or far vision. The *anterior chamber*, behind the cornea, is filled with clear aqueous humor, which provides nourishment to the cornea. The lens lies behind the pupil and iris.

The *posterior chamber* is a small space behind the lens. Aqueous fluid, produced in the posterior chamber by the ciliary processes, flows from the posterior chamber to the anterior chamber. It then drains into the *canal of Schlemm*.

Vitreous humor is thick, gelatinous material that maintains the spherical shape of the eyeball. It also maintains the

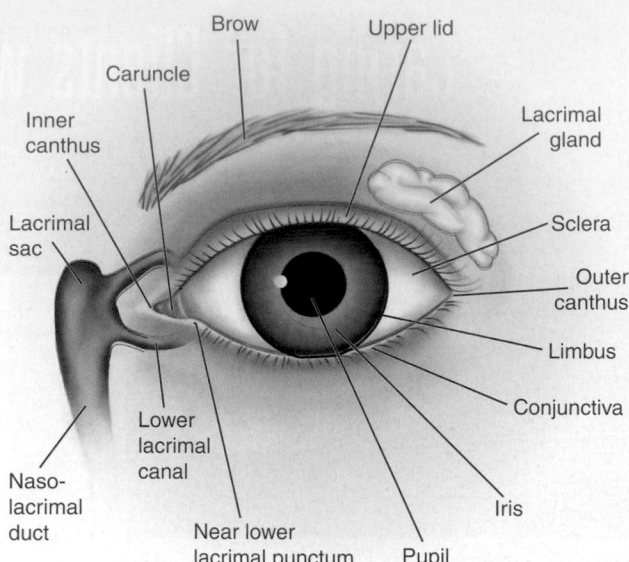

FIGURE 41-1. External structures of the eye and position of the lacrimal structures.

placement of the retina (Fig. 41-2). The *retina*, the innermost layer of the eye, is composed of a pigmented outer layer and an inner neurosensory layer. Light stimulates this neurosensory layer, which contains nerve cells called *rods* and *cones*. Rods function in night or dim light and assist in distinguishing black and white. Cones function in bright light and are sensitive to color. The nerve cells of the retina extend from the optic nerve.

The *macula lutea*, or the "yellow spot," is composed entirely of cones and allows for detailed vision. It lies in the center of the retina. The *fovea centralis* or *foveola* is at the center of the macula. The blood vessels are displaced from the fovea centralis, allowing light to pass to the cones. The density of the cones decreases away from the fovea centralis, as the number of rods increases in the periphery of the retina. The *optic disc*, the anterior surface of the optic nerve, is easily distinguished from the macula because of the vasculature that radiates from the optic disc. No blood vessels radiate directly from the macula (Fig. 41-3). The macula is the area of the eye that provides **central vision**, the ability to discriminate letters, words, and the details of any image. If the macula degenerates or is damaged, only the ability to see movement and gross objects in the peripheral fields of vision remains.

Visual Function

The function of the eyeball is to convert light energy into nerve signals that are transmitted to and interpreted in the cerebral cortex. Every object reflects light. For a person to see it clearly, the reflected light must pass through the intraocular structures—the cornea, anterior chamber, pupil, lens, and vitreous humor. These structures cause **refraction**, which means that the light rays bend and change speed. The lens focuses the light into an upside-down and reversed image on the retina. The rods and cones in the retina send nerve impulses by way of the optic nerve and optic tract to the visual cortex of the occipital lobe. This is where the image is interpreted.

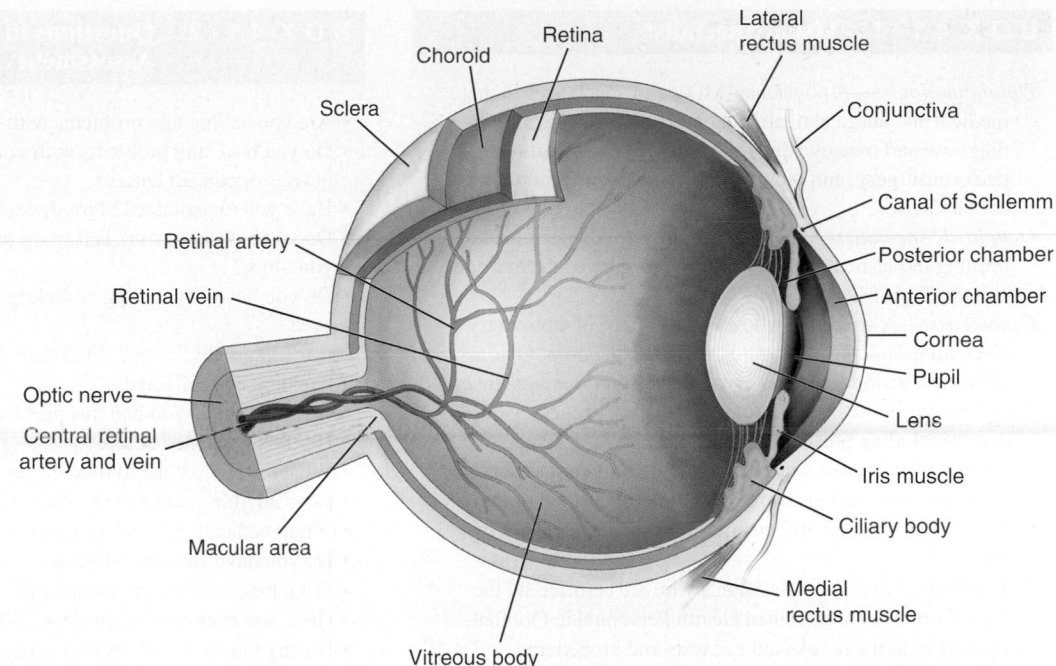

Retina
Choroid
Sclera
Retinal artery
Retinal vein
Optic nerve
Central retinal
artery and vein
Macular area
Vitreous body
Lateral
rectus muscle
Conjunctiva
Canal of Schlemm
Posterior chamber
Anterior chamber
Cornea
Pupil
Lens
Iris muscle
Ciliary body
Medial
rectus muscle

FIGURE 41-2. Three-dimensional cross-section of the eye.

The lens is more convex on the posterior side and can change shape, a process known as **accommodation**. The ciliary muscles contract or relax to focus an image onto the retina, which allows the person to clearly see distant or near objects. For viewing distant objects, the ciliary muscles relax and the lens flattens. The opposite occurs to view objects that are closer. The closest point a person can clearly focus on an object is called the **near point**. Aging results in loss of lens elasticity and makes the use of reading glasses for near vision necessary. When the lens becomes opaque, as when a cataract forms, light is blocked from reaching the macula and the visual image becomes blurred or cloudy.

 Gerontologic Considerations

- Teaching aids with black print at font size 22 or larger on ivory background minimizes glare and should be used for clients experiencing age-associated lens changes. Indirect lighting (over the shoulder) also minimizes glare. Color perception may be altered in older adults experiencing yellowing of the lens.

ASSESSMENT

The ophthalmic assessment provides information about a client's eye health. Nurses usually examine the client's external eye appearance, pupil responses, and eye movements, as well as obtain information about the client's ophthalmic condition. For more complex examinations, nurses need additional education or training. Ongoing eye examinations and treatment require the care of specialists. Box 41-1 provides a list of specialists and technicians who provide eye care and treatment.

Clients often ask nurses when to have an eye examination. The American Academy of Ophthalmology (2008)

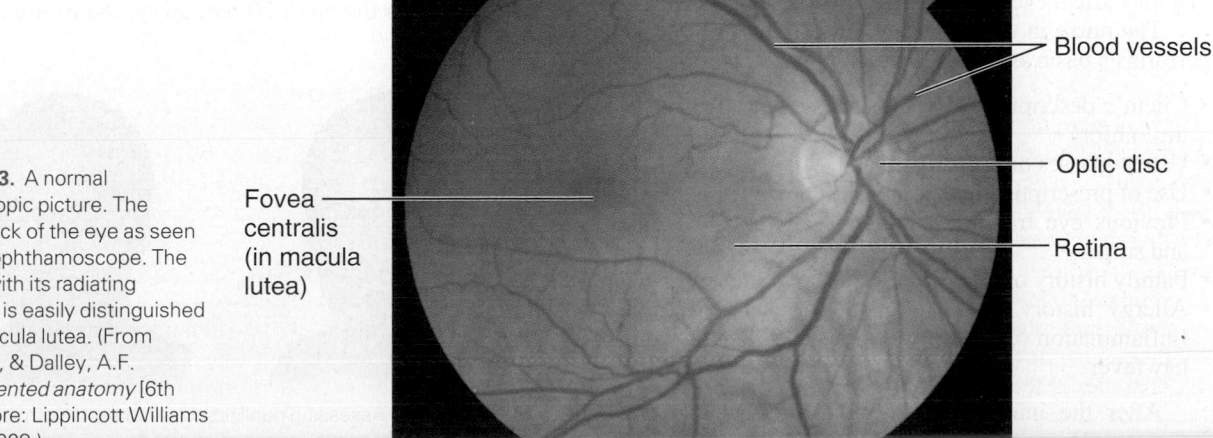

Fovea centralis (in macula lutea)

Blood vessels
Optic disc
Retina

FIGURE 41-3. A normal opthalmoscopic picture. The fundus or back of the eye as seen through an ophthamoscope. The optic disc, with its radiating vasculature, is easily distinguished from the macula lutea. (From Moore, K. L., & Dalley, A.F. *Clinically oriented anatomy* [6th ed.]. Baltimore: Lippincott Williams & Wilkins, 2009.)

recommends that adults who do not have any signs of eye disease or risk of any eye disorders have a thorough screening at age 40, because signs of disease and visual changes begin to occur at this time. Adults with a personal or family history of eye disease, diabetes, or hypertension should see an ophthalmologist to determine how frequently they need an eye examination. Symptoms that require attention include bulging of the eyes; dark spot in the center of the client's field of vision; difficulty focusing; blurred, cloudy, double, or hazy vision; loss of peripheral vision; or sudden loss of vision. Chapter 42 provides more information on eye disorders.

Nursing Assessment

The nurse obtains a history to identify any specific problems that the client is experiencing and possible causes. Box 41-2 lists questions that nurses may ask when taking an ocular history. The nurse gathers information related to eye problems: past and current ability to see; any discomfort, pain, or other symptoms; how long the client has experienced problems; any treatments and medications; and other illnesses that may affect eye health.

The nurse in the acute care, outpatient, or home setting performs a basic assessment of ocular health by obtaining:

- Client's description of vision changes, any visual or eye discomfort
- Use of glasses or contacts
- Use of prescription and nonprescription eye medication
- Previous eye trauma, ophthalmic and medical diseases, and surgery
- Family history of inherited eye diseases such as glaucoma
- Allergy history associated with seasonal **conjunctivitis** (inflammation of the conjunctiva) that often accompanies hay fever

After the interview, the nurse inspects the eyes for symmetry. He or she also observes the lid margins for signs of inflammation, exudate, or loss of eyelashes. The nurse determines the pupil size, and their change and response to light. Normal pupils are round, of equal size, and constrict simultaneously when stimulated (Fig. 41-4). The nurse checks the extraocular muscles by asking the client to keep his or her head still while following an object moved up, down, left, and right (Fig. 41-5). Other observations include looking for:

- **Ptosis**—drooping upper eyelid
- **Proptosis**—an extended or protruded upper eyelid that delays closing or remains partially open
- **Nystagmus**—uncontrolled oscillating movement of the eyeball

In addition, the nurse can examine the client for age-related changes in the eye. Table 41-1 reviews these changes.

Visual Screening Tests

The *Snellen eye chart* (Fig. 41-6) is a simple screening tool for determining **visual acuity**, the ability to see far images clearly. With the chart 20 feet away, the examiner asks the

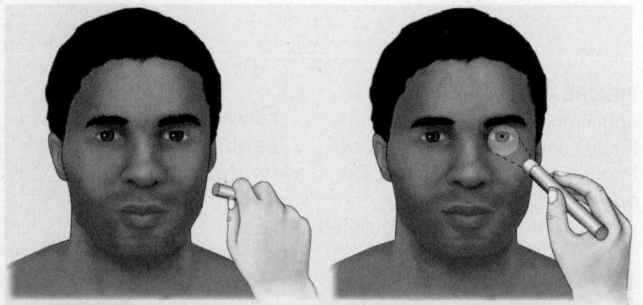

FIGURE 41-4. Assessing pupil response to light. Normal pupils constrict simultaneously when stimulated.

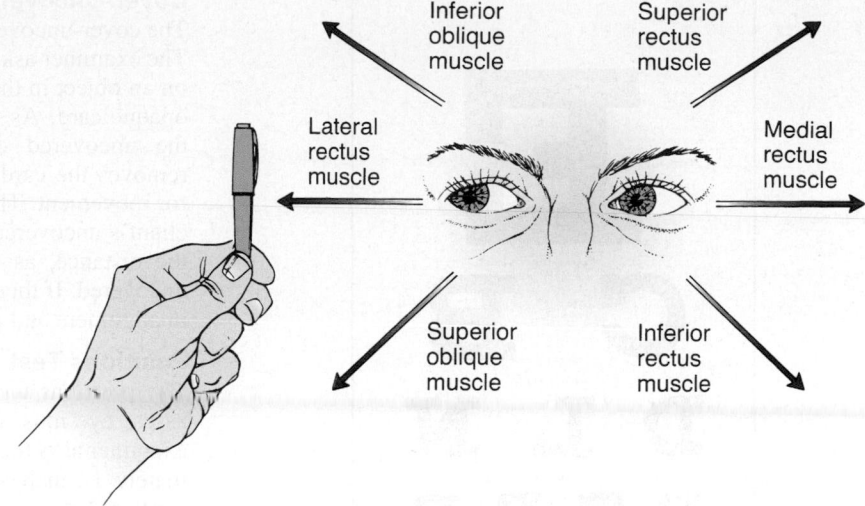

FIGURE 41-5. Assessing extraocular movements.

client to cover one eye and identify letters of decreasing size. Results for each eye are expressed as a fraction that compares the client's vision with standard norms. If a client has 20/20 vision (normal vision), it means that he or she sees letters at 20 feet that others see clearly and accurately at 20 feet; a client with 20/40 vision sees letters at 20 feet that most others can read at 40 feet, and so on. If the client cannot identify even the largest letters on the chart, the examiner asks him or her to count the number of fingers that the examiner

holds up. If the finger count is inaccurate, the examiner tests the client's ability to distinguish light from dark. Visual acuity also is measured with a computerized refractor that records the strength and type of lenses necessary to correct the client's visual problem.

The *Jaeger chart* and *Rosenbaum Pocket Vision Screener* evaluate near vision. These charts contain words, numbers, and letters in various print sizes. The examiner instructs the client to cover one eye and then hold

TABLE 41-1 Age-Related Changes in the Eye

	STRUCTURAL CHANGE	FUNCTIONAL CHANGE	FINDINGS
Eyelids and lacrimal structures	Loss of skin elasticity and orbital fat; decreased muscle tone; development of wrinkles	Turned-in lid margins (entropion) and turned-out lid margins (ectropion) cause irritation to cornea and conjunctiva or to the eyelids themselves	Client reports burning and sensation of object in eye; increased tearing; inflammation; ulceration may occur
Refractive changes; presbyopia	Lens cannot readily accommodate with aging (see Chap. 42)	Client holds reading materials at increasing distance to focus	Client reports needing increased light; needs reading glasses or bifocals
Cataract	Lens develops opacities	Interference with focus of a sharp image on the retina	Client reports increased glare, decreased vision, and changes in color perception
Conjunctiva	The conjunctiva (white portion of the eye) becomes slack and more susceptible to chronic inflammations with age	Part of the conjunctiva may become caught between the lids during blinking. Harmless degenerative plaques may appear on the conjunctiva; tear glands and the conjunctiva may lose the ability to lubricate the eye	Client reports dry eyes and may have to use artificial tears
Cornea	Arcus senilis, a harmless white circle that may appear on the margin of the cornea, is a common occurrence in older adults	Composed of cholesterol and its derivatives, its presence does not necessarily indicate an overall increased cholesterol level	No complaints
Posterior vitreous detachment	Liquefaction and shrinkage of vitreous body	May lead to retinal tears and detachment	Client reports light flashes, cobwebs, and floaters
Age-related macular degeneration	Yellowish aging spots in the retina (drusen) appear and coalesce in the macula	Affects central vision. (see Chap. 42).	Affects reading vision

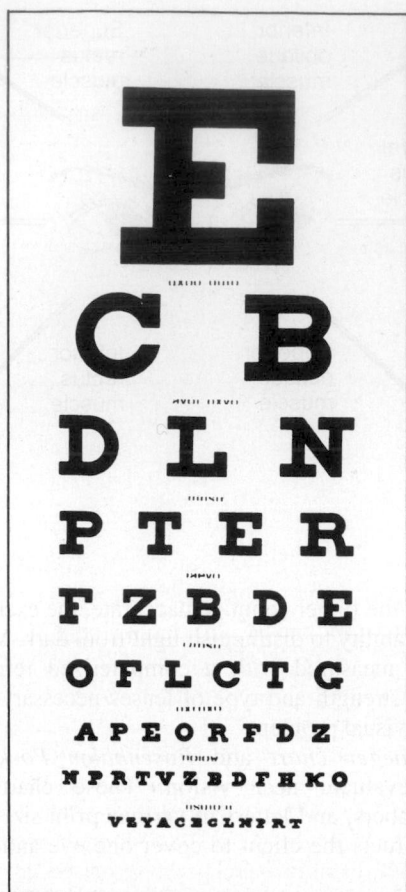

FIGURE 41-6. The Snellen chart is used to assess visual acuity, or far vision.

the chart approximately 14 inches away and read the smallest print that he or she can see comfortably. The size of the print the client reads indicates the quality of his or her near vision.

Color vision is assessed with *Ishihara polychromatic plates.* The client receives a series of cards on which the pattern of a number is embedded in a circle of colored dots. The numbers are in colors that color-blind individuals commonly cannot see. Clients with normal vision readily identify the numbers.

▶ ***Stop, Think, and Respond Exercise 41-1***

A client asks you what 20/200 visual acuity means. What is the best explanation?

Extraocular Muscle Function Tests

Corneal Light Reflex Test

The *corneal light reflex test* assesses the alignment of the eyes. The examiner holds a penlight approximately 12 inches from the client's face and asks the patient to stare straight ahead. The reflection of light should be in the same spot on each eye, indicating parallel alignment. If the light reflex is uneven, it indicates deviated alignment of the eyes, possibly due to muscle weakness or paralysis.

Cover-Uncover Test

The cover-uncover test assesses extraocular muscle function. The examiner asks the client to stare straight ahead and focus on an object in the distance, while covering one eye with an opaque card. As the eye is covered, the examiner observes the uncovered eye for movement. The examiner then removes the card and observes the previously covered eye for movement. The test is repeated on the opposite eye. The client's uncovered eye should remain fixed on the object in the distance, as should the eye that is covered and then uncovered. If there is movement, it may indicate a deviation in alignment and muscle weakness.

Positions Test

The positions test or cardinal positions of gaze is done to assess eye muscle strength and cranial nerve function. The examiner asks the client to focus on an object that is approximately 12 inches away and moves this object through six cardinal positions in a clockwise direction. As the object is moved, the examiner observes the client's eye movements, which should be smooth and symmetrical in all six directions. If asymmetrical movements are noted, it indicates weakness in the extraocular muscles or dysfunction of the cranial nerve that innervates that muscle.

Diagnostic Studies

Ophthalmoscopy

Direct **ophthalmoscopy** is examination of the fundus or interior of the eye. This examination is done with a direct ophthalmoscope, an instrument that illuminates the internal surface of the eyes and allows the examiner to see the lens, retina, retinal blood vessels, and the optic disc under magnification (Fig. 41-7).

Indirect ophthalmoscopy uses an instrument that produces a bright, intense light. The ophthalmologist uses this

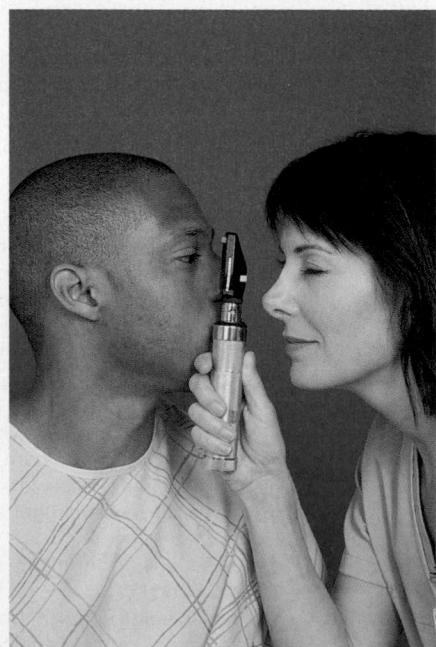

FIGURE 41-7. The examiner looks at the interior of the eye with a direct ophthalmoscope.

instrument in conjunction with an ophthalmoscope to see larger areas of the retina, although no magnification is involved.

Retinoscopy

Use of a *retinoscope* and trial lenses determines the focusing power of each eye. A retinoscope is a hand-held instrument that produces a line of light. The light appears distorted in the eyes of clients with refractive errors. Trial lenses of varying refractive powers are then placed in front of the eye until the light streak does not deviate in any direction.

Tonometry

Tonometry measures intraocular pressure (IOP). It is done by using a tonometer to indent or flatten (applanate) the surface of the eye. The principle is that a soft eye indents more easily than a hard eye. The force that produces indentation is measured and converted to a pressure reading. Normal IOP is 10 to 21 mm Hg. High readings indicate high IOP; low readings indicate low IOP (Smeltzer et al., 2008).

There are various methods for performing tonometry. *Applanation tonometry* provides the greatest accuracy, but the *indentation* method may be used because it is smaller and more portable. Before either is used, a topical anesthetic solution is instilled in the lower conjunctival sac. Anesthesia begins almost immediately and lasts a few minutes. The client does not feel the tonometer while the eye is anesthetized. A *noncontact* tonometer, although less accurate, blows a puff of air against the cornea, and no local anesthetic is required.

Visual Field Examination

A **visual field examination** or perimetry test measures peripheral vision and detects gaps in the visual field. The client fixes his or her gaze on a stationary point straight ahead. A light or white object is moved from a point on the side, where it cannot be seen, toward the center. The client indicates the point at which he or she sees the stimulus without directly looking at it. Certain disorders, such as glaucoma, stroke, brain tumor, or retinal detachment, are associated with changes in the visual field.

Color Vision Testing

Assessing a client's ability to differentiate color is essential for determining a person's ability to function within an environment dictated by color codes. For example, traffic lights or work equipment mandate that people be able to distinguish different colors. Ishihara polychromatic plates are the most common test for color vision. Different plates, bound in a book, have dots of primary colors embedded in a background of secondary colors. Clients must identify the hidden shape. Clients with diminished color vision are not able to do this successfully.

Amsler Grid

Clients with macular problems are tested with an Amsler grid. It is made up of a geometric grid of identical squares with a central fixation point. The examiner instructs the client to stare at the central fixation point on the grid and report if they see any distortion of the squares. Clients with macular problems may say some of the squares are faded or wavy.

Slit-Lamp Examination

A *slit lamp* is a binocular microscope that magnifies the surface of the eye. A beam of light, narrowed to a slit, is directed at the cornea, facilitating an examination of structures and fluid in the anterior segment of the eye. This examination is used to identify disorders such as corneal abrasions, iritis, conjunctivitis, and cataracts.

Retinal Angiography

Retinal angiography or *fluorescein angiography* is used to detect vascular changes and blood flow through the retinal vessels. Sodium fluorescein, a water-soluble dye, is injected into a peripheral vein. The examiner uses a special camera to photograph the appearance and distribution of the dye in the retinal arteries, capillaries, and veins at 1-second intervals. The photographs provide a record of vascular filling and emptying defects. Many conditions affect retinal circulation, such as diabetes mellitus, hypertension, drug toxicity, tumors, and acquired immunodeficiency syndrome. Intravenous fluorescein causes skin to yellow slightly for 6 to 8 hours. The urine also turns bright yellow, but the color becomes less noticeable over the following 24 to 36 hours as the dye is excreted.

Ultrasonography

Ultrasonography is used when pathologic changes such as an opaque lens, cloudy cornea, or bloody vitreous make it difficult to look directly at the posterior of the eye. Using sound waves, the contour and shape of contents in the eye are imaged and recorded. After instillation of anesthetic ophthalmic drops, an ultrasound probe is placed on the cornea and a recording is made on an oscilloscope. This technique is helpful in detecting eye lesions and measuring for an intraocular lens implant before extracting a cataract.

Retinal Imaging

A new ophthalmologic screening tool uses a *retinal imaging* system to produce a high-resolution image of almost the entire retina without having to dilate the pupil. The Panoramic200 Scanning Laser Ophthalmoscope (Optos, Dunfermline, Scotland) can detect retinal disorders such as diabetic retinopathy, and provides an excellent baseline screening test.

NURSING MANAGEMENT

Although nurses may not be directly involved in caring for clients who are undergoing eye examinations and tests, it is essential that they engage in assuring that clients receive eye care to preserve their eye function and/or prevent further visual loss. Careful assessment of the function and structure of the eyes provides the nurse with a baseline and assists with determining if further action is warranted.

THE EARS

ANATOMY AND PHYSIOLOGY

The ear is divided into three areas: the outer, middle, and inner sections (Fig. 41-8). Sound is perceived because of a chain reaction involving all three areas of the ear. The inner ear also helps maintain balance.

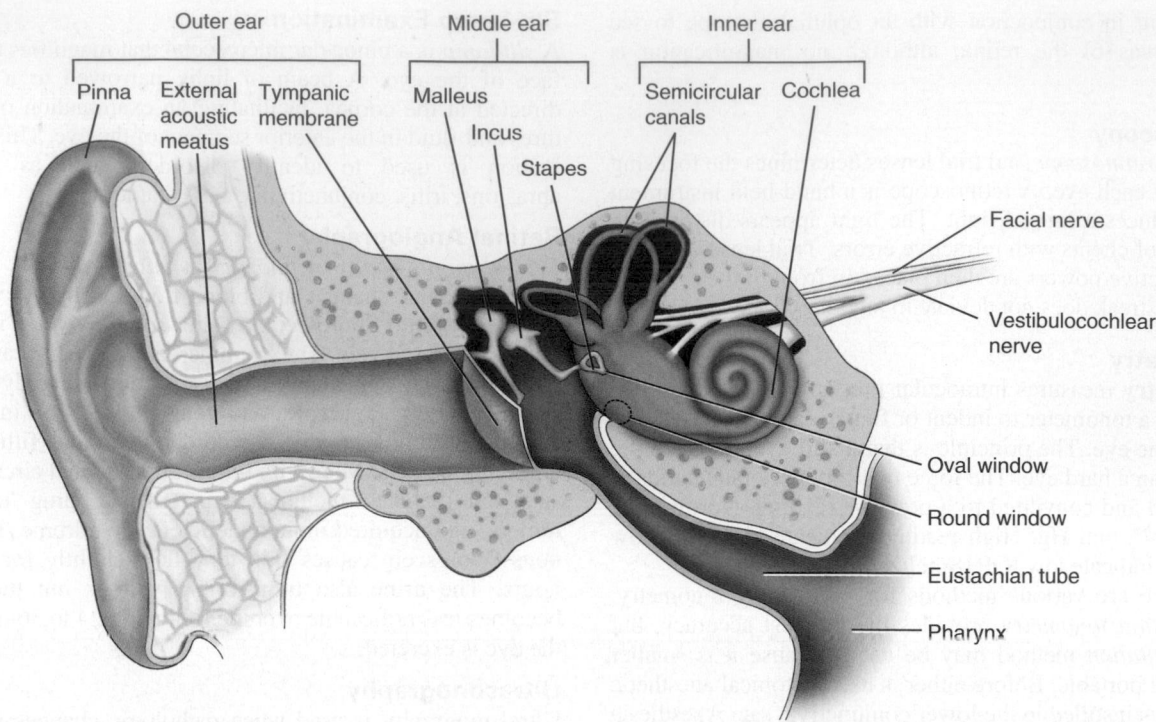

FIGURE 41-8. Anatomy of the ear. The outer, middle, and inner subdivisions are shown.

Outer Ear

The outer ear, or *auricle*, consists of the *pinna*, the fleshy external projection of the ear, and the *external acoustic meatus*, a 1-inch canal that extends to the *tympanic membrane*, or eardrum. The outer ear collects sound waves and directs them inward. The external acoustic meatus contains the glands that produce *cerumen*, a waxy substance that lubricates the ear canal, protects the eardrum, and helps prevent external ear infections. Chewing and talking help to move cerumen to the outer area of the external acoustic meatus, where it is easily washed away.

Gerontologic Considerations

- Older clients form drier cerumen and experience an increased incidence of impaction in the external acoustic meatus. Nonprescription preparations are available for softening hardened cerumen. Refer the client to a healthcare provider if hearing remains diminished.

Middle Ear

The middle ear is a small, air-filled cavity in the temporal bone. The *eustachian tube* extends from the floor of the middle ear to the pharynx and is lined with mucous membrane. It equalizes air pressure in the middle ear. A chain of three small bones, the *malleus*, the *incus*, and the *stapes*, stretches across the middle-ear cavity from the tympanic membrane to the *oval window*. They move when struck by sound waves transmitted from the outer ear. When these bones are set in motion, the footplate of the stapes, which is very flexible, strikes the oval window, agitating the fluid in the inner ear.

Inner Ear

The inner ear, or *labyrinth*, consists of a series of cavities and canals that contain fluid. It contains the *cochlea*, which provides for hearing, the *semicircular canals*, which promote balance, and the *vestibulocochlear nerve (cranial nerve VIII)*.

The fluid motion created by the vibrating stapes excites the nerve endings in the sensitive sound receptors of the *organ of Corti* located in the cochlea. The impulses are then converted to nerve impulses and transmitted along the cochlear nerve to the brain, where sound is perceived.

Nerve receptors for balance are found in both the vestibule and semicircular canals. They transmit information about motion through the vestibular nerve, which joins with the cochlear nerve to form the eighth cranial nerve, the vestibulocochlear nerve (formally called the *auditory* or *acoustic nerve*).

ASSESSMENT

The screening of hearing in adults is generally voluntary. The American Speech-Language-Hearing Association

BOX 41-3	Nursing Assessment of the Ear and Basic Hearing Acuity

- Obtain client's appraisal of his or her hearing, including whether the client experiences tinnitus.
- Observe for actions that suggest a hearing problem such as leaning forward, turning the head, or cupping a hand to the ear to hear better.
- Document the use of a hearing aid.
- Ask client about allergies, a history of upper respiratory and middle ear infections, high fevers, or exposure to loud sounds, because all these can cause hearing loss.
- Inspect external ear for signs of infection, such as swelling, redness, drainage, or evidence of trauma.
- Shine a penlight into the ear to grossly inspect the ear canal; straighten the ear canal by gently pulling the ear up and back for an adult and downward and backward for small children.
- Palpate the areas in front of and behind the ear lobe for tenderness and swelling.
- Perform a basic hearing acuity test.

(ASHA, 2008) recommends that adults be screened at least every decade through the age of 50 and every 3 years after that. Although family practice physicians assess and treat many ear disorders, they refer some clients to *otolaryngologists*, physicians who specialize in the diagnosis and treatment of ear, nose, and throat disorders. An *audiologist* is a paraprofessional with special training in performing hearing tests, measuring hearing loss, and recommending methods for improving the perception of sound. Box 41-3 outlines the nursing assessment.

Pharmacologic Considerations

- Many commonly administered medications are potentially ototoxic, such as furosemide (Lasix), cisplatin, salicylates (aspirin), and many antibiotics. Nurses need to be aware of these potential effects. It is necessary to make sure the client is taking the prescribed dosages and monitor for signs of impaired hearing.

Basic Auditory Acuity Tests

One general method is used to assess a client's gross auditory acuity. The method is referred to as the *whisper test*. For this test, the examiner covers the untested ear with his or her palm and stands 1 to 2 feet from the client's uncovered ear. He or she whispers a number or a phrase and asks the client to repeat it. The examiner provides several numbers to ensure valid test results. Another technique is to sit beside the client and bring a ticking watch toward the ear. The client should perceive the sound at the same time as the nurse, who is assumed to have normal hearing.

Otoscopic Examination

An otoscopic examination involves inspecting the external acoustic canal and tympanic membrane using an **otoscope**, a hand-held instrument with a light, lens, and optional speculum for inserting into the client's ear (Fig. 41-9). If normal, the canal appears smooth and empty. The normal tympanic membrane is intact, looks pearly gray, and transmits light. Excessive cerumen interferes with inspection.

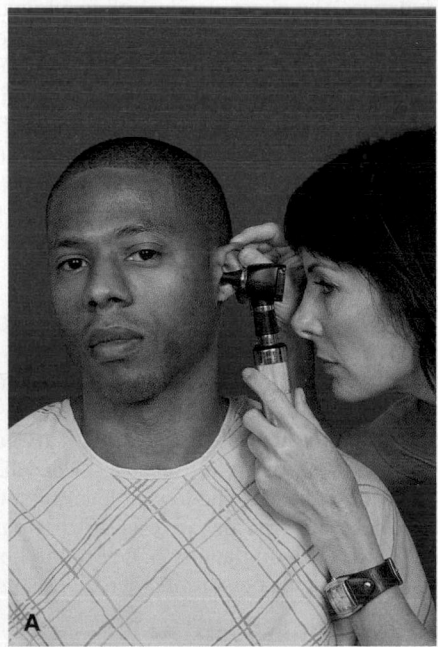

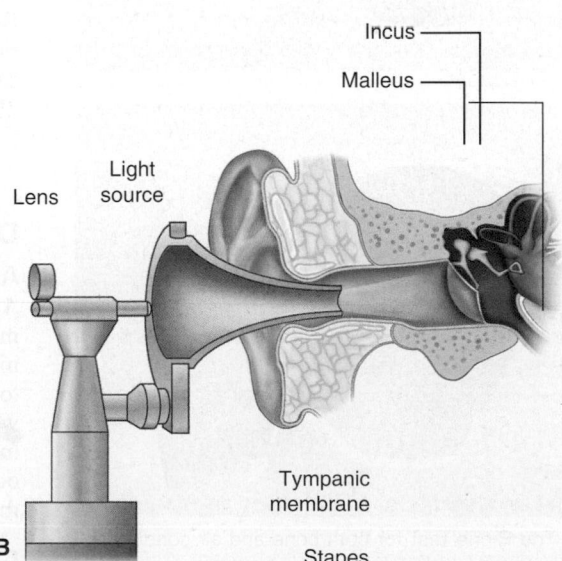

Incus
Malleus
Light source
Lens
Tympanic membrane
Stapes

FIGURE 41-9. Technique for using the otoscope. **(A)** The examiner pulls the adult client's pinna up and back before inserting the otoscope. **(B)** Position of the otoscope in the ear.

Tuning Fork Tests

A **tuning fork** is an instrument that produces sound in the same range as human speech. It is used to screen for conductive or sensorineural hearing loss. A **conductive hearing loss** involves interference in the transmission of sound waves to the inner ear. **Sensorineural hearing loss** is the result of nerve impairment.

The Rinne test and Weber test identify types of hearing loss. For the **Rinne test** (Fig. 41-10), the tuning fork is struck, placed on the mastoid process behind the ear, and held there until the client indicates the sound is no longer heard. Immediately after that, the still-vibrating tuning fork is held beside the ear, and the client again says when the sound is no longer heard. Normally, air conduction beside the ear measures twice as long as by bone conduction through the mastoid.

The **Weber test** is performed by striking the tuning fork and placing its stem in the midline of the client's skull or center of the forehead (Fig. 41-11). A person with normal hearing perceives the sound equally well in both ears. If the sound seems lateralized to one ear, it suggests a conduction hearing loss in that ear or a sensorineural loss in the opposite ear.

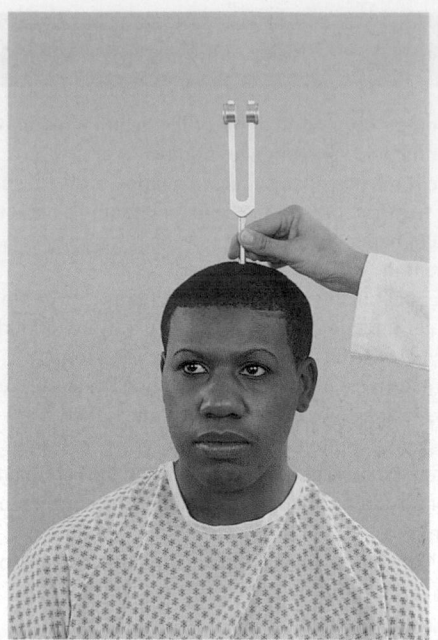

FIGURE 41-11. The Weber test for bone conduction of sound.

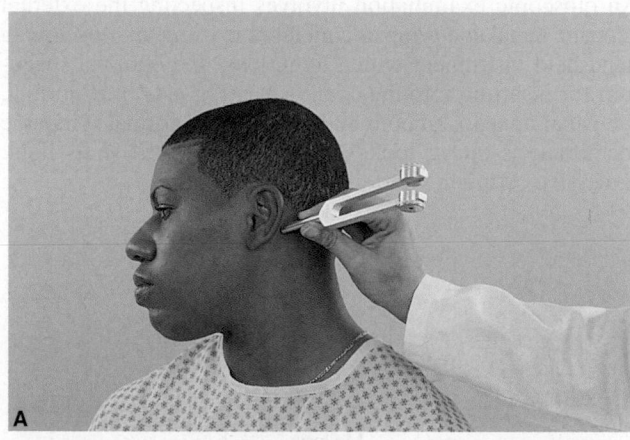

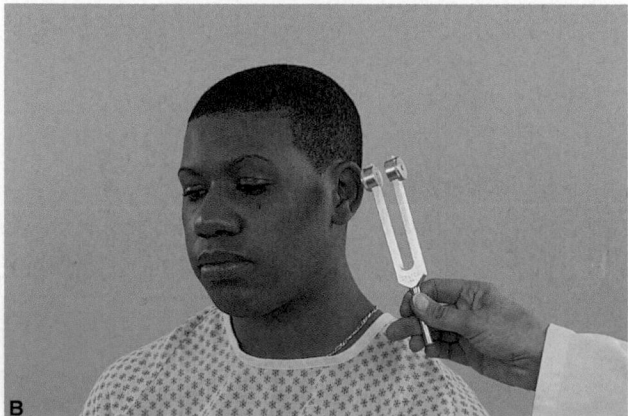

FIGURE 41-10. The Rinne test for both bone and air conduction of sound. **(A)** The tuning fork is first placed on the mastoid process behind the ear. **(B)** The tuning fork is then held beside the ear.

 Gerontologic Considerations

- Careful documentation of conduction times assessed using the Rinne and Weber tests is important. This information enables early identification of hearing changes and may impact selection of assistive hearing devices (see Chap. 43).

Romberg Test

The **Romberg test** is used to evaluate a person's ability to sustain balance. The client stands with feet together and both arms extended. The client closes his or her eyes. Swaying, losing balance, or arm drifting are abnormal responses. Because central nervous system lesions cause similar abnormal results, additional testing is needed to confirm an inner ear dysfunction. For clients who are unsteady, this test may not be appropriate. For all clients, the examiner needs to be close by to prevent the client from completely losing his or her balance and falling.

Diagnostic Studies

Audiometry

Audiometry is done by an audiologist. Audiometric testing measures hearing acuity precisely. During the test, controlled intensities of sound, measured in **decibels** (dB), are projected to one ear at a time through a headset. The client indicates when the sound is heard. The lowest level of sound that normal individuals can first perceive is 20 dB; painful sounds occur at 120 dB. Hearing acuity is determined by measuring the intensity at which a person first perceives sound.

Caloric Stimulation Test

A **caloric stimulation test** assesses vestibular reflexes of the inner ear that control balance. Warm (40°C) or cool (25°C) water or air is instilled into the external meatus of each ear separately. The fluid alters the temperature of the temporal bone and creates convection currents in the fluid of the inner ear that simulate movement of the head. Nystagmus, a quivering movement of the eyes, is the expected response. Slight dizziness also may be experienced. A diminished response in one eye is significant for an inner ear disorder such as Ménière's disease (discussed in Chap. 43).

Electronystagmography

Electronystagmography is a more precise method for evaluating vestibular function, the mechanisms that facilitate maintaining balance. It is performed in conjunction with caloric stimulation. When the fluid is instilled within the ear, a machine records the duration and velocity of the eye movements with electrodes attached superiorly, inferiorly, and laterally about the eyes.

▶ **Stop, Think, and Respond Exercise 41-2**

A client is having an assessment of balance. The physician tells you that the Romberg test is appropriate and will be performed. What is an important action for the nurse?

NURSING MANAGEMENT

Often, testing and care of ear function are done in outpatient settings. Assessment of ear structure and hearing function is done as screening in most healthcare settings, providing a foundation for further testing and referrals.

CRITICAL THINKING EXERCISES

1. If a client reports having difficulty seeing, what additional data are important to obtain?
2. A 60-year-old client tells you that he has not had his eyes examined in 5 years. What should you advise him?
3. What cues can a nurse observe in an older client with possible hearing loss?
4. A client tells you that her hearing has diminished over the years. She has seen an online advertisement for a hearing aid that gave the ordering information. What is your response?

NCLEX-STYLE REVIEW QUESTIONS

1. What advice would the nurse give to a client who has just undergone fluorescein angiography? Select all that apply.
   1. Expect hives or rashes within 4 hours.
   2. Expect mild headaches for 24 to 36 hours.
   3. Expect red and swollen eyes for 6 to 9 hours.
   4. Expect skin to appear slightly yellow for 6 to 8 hours.
   5. Expect urine to appear bright yellow for 24 to 36 hours.
2. A 65-year-old client asks the nurse why his vision is not as sharp as it once was. The nurse's best response is:
   1. "It is not unusual for older clients to have dry eyes."
   2. "Older adults are more prone to eye infections."
   3. "The lenses in an older adults's eyes accommodate more slowly."
   4. "Vision in older adults gradually worsens with age."
3. To test a client's ability to read small print, a nurse in a clinic asks the client to hold a Jaeger chart and instructs her to do which of the following?
   1. Cover one eye while reading the smallest print with the other
   2. Hold the chart at arm's length while reading the chart with one eye
   3. Read the bottom line of the chart from right to left with both eyes
   4. Read the smallest print on the chart that can easily be read with both eyes
4. A client who states that he was walking in a densely wooded area and was struck in the eye with a pine tree branch arrives in the eye clinic. He tells you that his right eye feels like it is scratched because it is burning and very irritated. As the LVN, you prepare the client for which of the following examinations?
   1. Retinoscopy
   2. Slit-lamp examination
   3. Tonometry
   4. Visual field examination
5. A client is being seen in a physician's office for an annual check-up. The client tells the nurse that he has been experiencing constant itchiness in his right eye. What specific questions about this problem should the nurse ask to obtain more information about the client's complaint? Select all that apply.
   1. Has this happened before?
   2. How long have you had this problem?
   3. Is the other eye ever itchy?
   4. Is there any drainage?
   5. Do any family members have eye conditions?

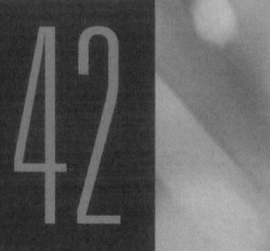

42

Caring for Clients with Eye Disorders

Words To Know
astigmatism
cataract
corneal transplantation
corneal trephine
diplopia
emmetropia
endophthalmitis
enucleation
glaucoma
hordeolum
hyperopia
intraocular lens implant
iridectomy
keratitis
keratoplasty
macular degeneration
myopia
photophobia
presbyopia
retinal detachment
trabeculoplasty
uveitis
visually impaired

Learning Objectives

On completion of this chapter, you will be able to:

1. Explain the different types of refractive errors.
2. Differentiate the terms *blindness* and *visually impaired*.
3. Identify appropriate nursing interventions for a blind client.
4. Discuss the nursing management of clients with eye trauma.
5. Describe the technique for instilling ophthalmic medications.
6. Explain how different infectious and inflammatory eye disorders are acquired.
7. Specify the visual changes that result from delayed or unsuccessful treatment of macular degeneration.
8. Differentiate between open-angle and angle-closure glaucoma.
9. Distinguish categories and mechanisms of actions of medications used to control intraocular pressure.
10. Identify a category of drugs contraindicated in clients with glaucoma.
11. Name activities clients with glaucoma should avoid because they elevate intraocular pressure.
12. Describe methods for improving vision after a cataract is removed.
13. Discuss postoperative measures that help prevent complications after a cataract extraction.
14. Give classic symptoms associated with a retinal detachment.
15. Discuss the care and cleaning of an eye prosthesis.

One in three Americans has some form of vision-impairing eye disease by 65 years of age (EyeCareAmerica, 2008). Approximately 18 million people in the United States have some degree of visual impairment, and this includes the more than 1 million who are legally blind (American Foundation for the Blind, 2008). This chapter discusses common disorders that can affect the eyes, as well as the accompanying treatment and nursing care measures.

IMPAIRED VISION

REFRACTIVE ERRORS

Emmetropia, or normal vision, means that light rays are bent to focus images precisely on the retina. In refractive errors, vision is impaired because light rays are not sharply focused on the retina. Refractive errors include myopia, hyperopia, presbyopia, and astigmatism.

Myopia is nearsightedness. People who are myopic hold things close to their eyes to see them well. **Hyperopia** is farsightedness. People who are hyperopic see objects that are far away better than objects that are close. **Presbyopia** is associated with aging and results in difficulty with near vision. People with presbyopia hold reading material or handwork at a distance to see it more clearly. **Astigmatism** is visual

Emmetropia (normal refraction): Parallel light rays are focused, on the retina, Nearby vision requires contraction of ciliary muscle to bring object into focus. Vision defects are present if light rays converge in front of or behind the retina or if the eyeball is shaped abnormally.

Myopia (nearsightedness): Parallel light rays are focused in front of the retina as a result of increased anteroposterior diameter of the eyeball. Myopic persons cannot focus sharply on a distant object. As the individual moves closer to the object, the rays become more focused, and the focal point finally falls on the retina.

Hyperopia (farsightedness): The eyeball is abnormally short. Parallel light rays are focused beyond the retina. Focus on distant objects occurs through accommodation. As objects move closer to the eye, accommodation can no longer compensate, and images become blurred. The near point is abnormally distant.

Astigmatism (defect of the curvature of the cornea and lens producing refractive errors): Parallel rays are imperfectly focused on the retina. Light striking peripheral areas is bent at different angles and not focused on a single point on the retina.

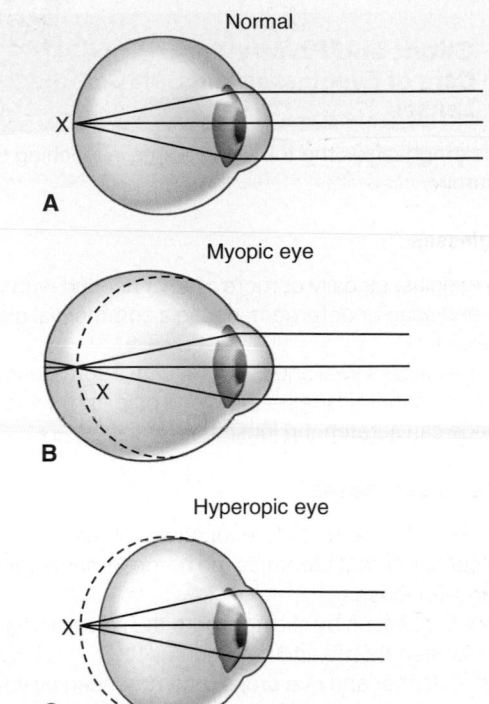

FIGURE 42-1. Eyeball shape affects visual acuity in some refractive errors. Ocular focusing of parallel light rays is shown in **(A)** normal, **(B)** myopic, and **(C)** hyperopic eyes.

distortion caused by an irregularly shaped cornea. Many people have both astigmatism and myopia or hyperopia. Box 42-1 presents a summary of refractive errors.

Pathophysiology and Etiology

Refractive errors are inherited or occur as a result of surgical treatment of disorders of the cornea or lens. Myopia occurs in people with elongated eyeballs. Because of the excessive length of the eye, light rays focus in the vitreous body before they reach the retina. Hyperopia results when the eyeball is shorter than normal, causing the light rays to focus at a theoretical point behind the retina (Fig. 42-1). Presbyopia occurs because of degenerative changes. Presbyopia is caused by the gradual loss of elasticity of the lens, which leads to decreased ability to accommodate, or focus, for near vision. The loss of accommodation progresses gradually. Astigmatism results from unequal curvatures in the shape of the cornea.

Assessment Findings

People with refractive errors experience blurred vision. Some seek help for recurrent headaches caused by straining to see clearly.

Refractive errors are detected with the Snellen and Jaeger charts. During retinoscopy, the vision of myopes improves when concave trial lenses correct the focusing power of the eyes. Hyperopes experience improvement when convex lenses are used. The amount of power needed to improve visual acuity indicates the degree of refractive error. The refractive error is not always the same in both eyes.

Medical Management

Refractive errors usually are corrected with eyeglasses or contact lenses. The lenses bend light rays to compensate for the refractive error. Not everyone can wear contact lenses; people with a history of recurrent eye infections, low tear production, or severe allergic reactions are more likely to have trouble with them.

Surgical Management

A number of procedures are used to correct refractive errors. These include:

- *Incisional radial keratotomy (RK)*—Under local anesthesia, the eye surgeon reshapes the cornea by making incisions. It is made flatter for clients with myopia and more cone-shaped for clients with hyperopia, enabling light rays to converge directly at the back of the retina. This procedure is not always successful. Some clients report a worsening of their vision. When RK is successful, clients no longer need to wear corrective lenses.

- *Laser-assisted in situ keratomileusis (LASIK)*—The eye surgeon uses a laser called a femtosecond laser or a surgical blade to create a thin corneal flap, which is gently folded back to expose the inner cornea. A cool-beam laser then resculpts the cornea. The flap is returned to its original position, and sutures are not required. Eyedrops and/or ointments are used to promote healing. Vision is regained very quickly with little or no discomfort.

- *Photorefractive keratectomy (PRK)*—This procedure involves the removal of the epithelial layer (top surface) of the cornea. A laser sculpts the cornea to correct refractive errors. A bandage-type contact lens promotes epithelial healing. There is some discomfort with PRK. Although LASIK is the preferred, because of more rapid recovery

Client and Family Teaching 42-1
Care of Eyeglasses and Soft Contact Lenses

The nurse emphasizes the following points in teaching the client and family:

For Eyeglasses

● Clean eyeglasses daily or more often if needed with warm water and soap or detergent, or use a commercial glass cleaner.
● Rinse the glasses well and dry them with a soft, clean cloth.
● Do not use paper tissues—the wood pulp from which they are made can scratch the lenses.

For Soft Contact Lenses

● Wash and rinse hands before touching lenses.
● Use a container that identifies the compartments for the right and left lenses.
● Remove a soft lens by sliding it onto the sclera and grasping it between thumb and forefinger.
● Use lens cleaner and eye drops recommended by your eye doctor. Follow directions for their use.
● Clean, rinse, and dry the lens case each time lenses are removed. It is recommended that lens cases be replaced every six months.
● Take out the lenses and call the eye doctor right away if any of the following symptoms develop:
  ● Significant vision changes
  ● Red eyes
  ● Eyes that hurt or feel itchy
  ● Excessive tearing
● Do not use saliva to clean the lenses.
● Do not use solutions for cleaning lenses other than those that have been recommended.

---

and lack of discomfort, PRK may still be used for clients with thin corneas

• *Intrastromal corneal ring segments (ICRS)*—The eye surgeon implants these semicircular pieces of plastic through a small incision in the cornea to correct mild myopia. The implant changes the shape of the cornea. If necessary, ICRS can be reversed, with the cornea resuming its original shape within a few weeks.
• *Phakic intraocular lenses (IOLs)*—Clients who do not have cataracts can have phakic IOLs surgically implanted in front of their natural lenses. Because this procedure involves surgical incision into the eyeball, there is a higher risk of complications. This procedure is an option for clients who cannot safely have LASIK. It corrects more severe myopia or hyperopia but preserves the client's ability to focus for near vision.
• *Conductive keratoplasty (CK)*—This procedure, used only for clients with presbyopia, involves the application of heat to the periphery of the cornea to make it tighter and steeper. Clients generally experience immediate improvement without discomfort. Retreatment may be necessary.

Client and Family Teaching 42-2
Postoperative Instructions for LASIK or PRK

LASIK

● Understand that stitches are not needed—the corneal flap remains in place through natural eye pressure.
● Use antibiotic eyedrops as ordered for up to 1 week to prevent infection.
● Resume normal activity within 3 days but avoid strenuous exercise for 1 week.
● Avoid rubbing eyes for about 1 week.
● Realize that healing occurs within 1 week but that it may take 1 to 3 months for vision to fully stabilize.
● Expect that discomfort may occur for 5 to 6 hours after the procedure. If necessary, use nonsteroidal anti-inflammatory drugs (NSAIDs) for relief.

PRK

● Use antibiotic and anti-inflammatory eye medications as ordered for 2 to 5 days after surgery.
● Understand that clear contact lenses are placed on each eye for 2 to 5 days to prevent infection.
● Understand that the epithelial layer begins to regenerate in 2 to 5 days, but realize that complete healing takes 3 to 4 months.
● Avoid rubbing eyes for at least several weeks.
● Avoid strenuous exercise for 1 week.
● Use pain medication for 1 to 2 days after surgery if necessary. Pain fibers are located on the surface of the cornea.

Any procedure potentially provides complete correction of refractive error but can result in overcorrection or undercorrection. Other complications include decentered ablation, dry eye syndrome, epithelial abrasion, or infection. With RK, increased glare from microscarring of the cornea may occur. With LASIK, the most common procedure, complications include wrinkles in the flap, debris under the flap, a displaced flap, or infection or inflammation of the flap.

Nursing Management

Nurses, especially those in pediatric offices, industrial sites, community school systems, and public health clinics, perform screening examinations and refer clients to eye specialists. They are instrumental in teaching clients how to care for their corrective lenses and remove and clean contact lenses (Client and Family Teaching 42-1). In addition, nurses provide preoperative and postoperative care and teach clients about postoperative care at home. Client and Family Teaching 42-2 provides some postoperative teaching points for clients having LASIK or PRK.

BLINDNESS

Definitions related to low vision refer to the *best corrected visual acuity* (BCVA). As indicated in Chapter 41, 20/20 is considered to be normal visual acuity. To pass a driving test, visual acuity of 20/40 in at least one eye is commonly required. *Blindness* is a legal term for a BCVA of 20/200 or less even with corrective lenses. The term **visually impaired** is used to describe a BCVA between 20/70 and 20/200 in the better eye with the use of glasses. Many people who are considered blind perceive light and motion. People with severe loss of visual field also are referred to as blind and are not able to perceive light. The BCVA is defined as 20/400 to no light perception. Blindness can be congenital or caused by injury, a high fever that damages the optic nerve, or disorders such as cataracts, glaucoma, retinal detachment, macular degeneration, and tumors.

Medical Management

Vision is improved to its maximum extent with corrective lenses. Clients who are severely visually impaired or blind are referred to a rehabilitation center or other resource for supportive services. Blind or nearly blind clients are taught skills for independent living, how to use a cane for mobility, and how to read and write Braille, a system that uses raised dots to form letters of the alphabet and numbers. Some individuals use trained guide dogs.

Nursing Process for the Client Who Is Blind

Assessment

In addition to assessing the degree of the client's impairment, ask questions about how the client is coping with his or her visual problems. Grief is a normal response to being newly blind or having severely compromised vision. Anger and sadness are typical reactions as clients face their disability. Help and support clients during depression. It is therapeutic to acknowledge the grief rather than attempt to cheer clients. Another helpful approach is to express confidence that the client has the inner resources to deal with the adversity.

Gerontologic Considerations

- Visual impairment curtails activities that older adults may have been able to enjoy previously, such as reading, watching television, and engaging in hobbies or other forms of recreation. Nursing interventions such as referring clients to resources for visual assistive devices can help prevent depression and withdrawal.

Diagnosis, Planning, and Interventions

One of the nurse's most important roles is to help the visually impaired client achieve independence. Whether the condition is temporary, because both eyes are patched, or permanent, the following measures are appropriate:

- Introduce yourself each time you enter the room because many voices sound similar.
- Call the client by name during group conversations because the blind client cannot see to whom questions or comments are directed.

- Speak before touching the client.
- Tell the client when you are leaving the room.

In addition, the care of a client who is blind or whose vision is severely impaired includes, but is not limited to, the following:

▶ **Disturbed Sensory Perception: Visual** related to impaired vision

▶ **Expected Outcome:** Client will independently complete activities of daily living (ADLs).

- Ask client's preference for where to store hygiene articles and other objects needed for self-care. *Involving the client promotes his or her control over the environment.*
- Keep personal care items in the same location at all times. *Doing so provides client with the ability to locate toiletries easily.*
- Move food items from the tray to a larger surface area. *Doing so facilitates locating food and eating utensils without accidental spilling or dropping.*
- At mealtimes, describe where food is on the plate using the positions on the face of a clock. *This measure assists the client to identify the location of food.*
- Offer to open containers, butter bread, and so forth. *Allowing the client a choice facilitates independence.*

▶ **Risk for Injury** related to compromised vision

▶ **Expected Outcome:** The client will remain free of trauma.

- Orient client to the physical environment. *Orientation assists the client to remain familiar with the environment and to avoid injury.*
- Indicate the location of the signal cord for obtaining nursing assistance. *Doing so facilitates the client's ability to get help.*
- Keep doors fully open rather than ajar. *This measure helps maintain a safe environment.*
- Help client to feel where the door to the bathroom is located. *This intervention promotes independence and prevents injury.*
- Remove chairs or objects that are in the client's walking pathway. *Doing so maintains a safe environment.*
- Instruct client to grasp your elbow and walk slightly behind and to the side when ambulating. *This positioning helps the client to feel secure and ensures safety.*

Gerontologic Considerations

- A nightlight should be used to promote visibility and thus enhance safety for older adults requiring nocturnal voiding. Objects, chairs, electrical cords, rugs, and footstools are placed away from areas where the client walks, and assistance is given whenever the client is out of bed.

▶ **Risk for Impaired Home Maintenance** related to decreased vision.

▶ **Expected Outcome:** The client will resume independent living.

- Discuss client's network of support that can help with shopping, banking, and transportation. *This discussion assists the client to plan for meeting needs outside the home.*

- Offer a home health nursing referral for the purpose of assessing the client's needs for a home aide. *Home care nurses can provide assistance with household tasks.*

▶ Situational Low Self-Esteem related to impaired adjustment to loss of vision

▶ Expected Outcome: The client will redevelop a positive self-image.

- Call attention to tasks the client successfully performs without assistance if the client focuses on self-pity. *Encouragement promotes positive feelings about ability to care for self.*
- Help client clarify those activities that are essential and then develop a plan for mastering each one. *A plan reduces frustration and systematically helps client achieve short-term goals.*
- Review progress to nurture self-confidence, self-reliance, and improved self-image. *Reminding the client of progress promotes a positive self-image.*

▶ Interrupted Family Processes related to conflict in reversed roles

▶ Expected Outcome: The family will remain cohesive and supportive.

- Encourage client and family members to verbalize their feelings. *Acknowledging feelings provides them with validation for what they are feeling and experiencing.*
- Promote a discussion of other life changes that were difficult but to which they eventually adjusted. *This discussion provides information that can help to form a plan of care.*
- Have each person share a list of inner strengths of the other to promote insight that, regardless of roles, what each brings to the relationship remains unchanged. *Listing strengths gives information that family members can refer to for positive feedback.*

▶ Deficient Diversional Activity related to transition from sighted to nonsighted

▶ Expected Outcome: The client will develop interests in activities that contribute to the enjoyment and enrichment of life.

- Refer the partially sighted client to the public library where large-print editions of books and magazines are available, as well as recordings of printed books ("talking books"). *Diversional activities must be tailored to the client's abilities.*
- Suggest that the partially sighted client use a magnifying lens to read. *This measure enables the client to enhance his or her sight.*
- Contact or refer clients who can read Braille to special agencies for books, Braille typewriters, and other visual assistive devices. *Appropriate referrals assist the client to reach maximum potential.*
- Inform client about the availability of optical scanners that use synthesized voice. *Scanners make it possible for the client to "read" printed materials.*
- Tell client that telephone companies exempt visually impaired customers from directory assistance charges and offer a "talking" yellow pages information service. *Providing clients with information about available resources assists them to achieve more independence.*

- Instruct client that laws prohibit the exclusion of patrons with guide dogs from public restaurants, public transportation, schools, and places for entertainment. *Possessing accurate knowledge assists clients to make informed decisions.*

Evaluation of Expected Outcomes

The client can perform self-care activities. He or she remains free of injury and demonstrates an ability to arrange for outside support to meet needs. The client expresses more positive feelings about ability to meet needs independently. The family provides positive support, as evidenced by sharing, planning activities, and relying on one another. The client begins to access resources that provide diversional activities and support. ●

EYE TRAUMA

Trauma or injury to the eye and surrounding structures can result in decreased or total loss of vision.

Pathophysiology and Etiology

Children and adults are subject to eye injuries from wind, sun, chemical sprays, direct blows to the eye, lacerations, and penetrating objects, such as fish hooks and bits of metal or wood. Cell and tissue injury causes an inflammatory response. Secondary infections may follow the initial injury. When trauma involves the cornea, scar tissue may affect the refraction of light. If the capsule that contains the lens is damaged, aqueous fluid and vitreous penetrate the lens, causing it to become an opaque cataract. Penetrating trauma can lead to **endophthalmitis**, a condition in which all three layers of the eye and the vitreous are inflamed; removal of the eye may be necessary.

Assessment Findings

Signs and Symptoms

The injured eye is painful or described as feeling "gritty." There is tearing, and the client usually tries to relieve discomfort by squeezing the eyelids closed. The effort helps control eye movement and reduces the light entering the eye. Vision may be blurred. If the bony orbit is fractured, the eyes may appear asymmetrical and the client has **diplopia** (double vision).

Blows to or near the eye usually result in swelling and bleeding into soft tissues with ultimate discoloration (black eye) of the area. On inspection, hemorrhage may be observed in the subconjunctival tissue. The eye may appear to recede into the orbit, and there may be a change in the normal size or shape of the iris or pupil. Adjacent lid structures may be lacerated, bloody, and swollen. Shining a penlight obliquely across the eye detects an obvious or obscured foreign body. Sometimes the upper lid must be everted to detect an object trapped beneath (Fig. 42-2). If treatment has been delayed, there may be purulent drainage in the conjunctival sac. A rust ring is seen in retained foreign bodies that contain iron.

Diagnostic Findings

Staining the surface with fluorescein dye identifies a minute foreign body or abrasion to the cornea. A slit-lamp

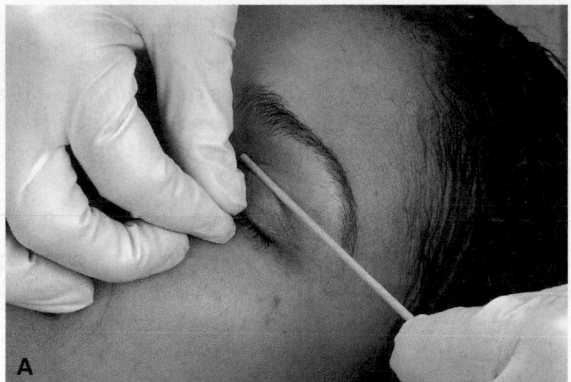 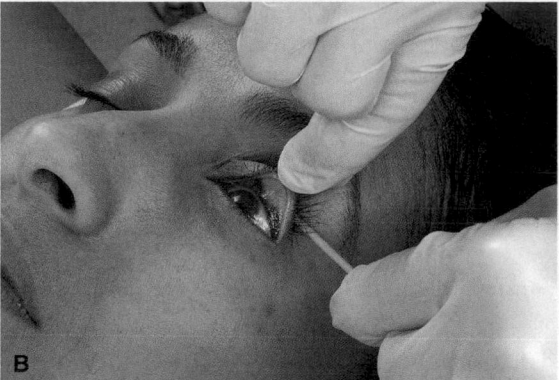

FIGURE 42-2. To evert the eyelid, (**A**) the examiner gently grasps the upper eyelashes and pulls downward, then places an applicator midway on the upper lid. (**B**) The examiner uses slight pressure to evert the lid over the applicator. The eyelid resumes its normal position when the client looks upward or the eyelash is pulled gently forward.

examination provides magnification and light to visualize structures in the anterior and posterior segments. Radiography and computed tomography help find a penetrating foreign body. A radiograph confirms an orbital fracture.

Medical and Surgical Management

After emergency first aid is performed, the eye is anesthetized to ease examination. Antibiotic ointment or drops are instilled, and the eye is patched. Clients with blunt trauma are hospitalized to reduce the danger of intraocular complications. To repair a laceration of the eyelid, the physician injects a local anesthetic and the lid margins are approximated with sutures. A cut on the eyeball, especially the cornea, is serious and requires immediate treatment. Surgery is performed if internal eye structures are damaged.

Nursing Process for the Client With Eye Trauma

Assessment

If the trauma does not involve gross injury, gently inspect the eye. Darken the room and direct a penlight at the eye to inspect for the presence of a foreign body. If none is visible, evert the lower lid and instruct the client to look up. Inspect the inferior conjunctival sac using direct vision or magnification. If this fails to locate a foreign body, evert the upper lid and direct the client to look down (see Fig. 42-2). If possible, perform a gross vision assessment.

Diagnosis, Planning, and Interventions

Recommend the use of glasses with shatter-resistant lenses or safety goggles to prevent eye trauma while working with substances that can injure the eyes. When eye trauma occurs, obtain a brief history of the type or cause of injury from the client or a family member. If eye pain is severe, or if the client cannot or is unwilling to permit an initial examination, loosely patch both eyes and refer the client immediately for medical treatment. If a foreign body is present, pressure on the eye may push the object into the tissues of the eyeball. Provide instructions for home care and instilling eye medications if needed (Client and Family Teaching 42-3).

The care of a client with eye trauma includes, but is not limited to, the following:

▶ Acute Pain related to trauma of the eye or surrounding structures

▶ Expected Outcome: The client's eye discomfort will be reduced to a tolerable level.

- Implement emergency measures, such as irrigating the eye, dimming bright lights, and closing and patching both eyes. *Measures neutralize chemical burns and reduce pain from glare and movement.*

Client and Family Teaching 42-3
Instilling Eye Medications at Home

The nurse provides the following instructions for the client to instill eye medications at home:

- Wash hands thoroughly.
- Wipe the lids and lashes in a direction away from the nose with a moistened, soft gauze pad, paper tissue, or cotton ball. Use a separate item for each wipe.
- Pull the tissue near the cheek downward, forming a sac in the lower lid.
- Tilt the head slightly backward and toward the eye in which the medication is to be instilled.
- Do not allow the tip of the container to touch the eye.
- Instill the prescribed number of drops into the conjunctival pocket, or apply a thin ribbon of ointment directly into the conjunctival pocket, beginning at the inner corner and moving outward.
- Close the eye gently.
- Wipe away excess medication that falls onto the skin.
- Secure dressing to the face with tape and use an eye shield for additional protection, especially at night.
- Do not rub the eye, and visit an ophthalmologist or return to the emergency department if the eye is not completely comfortable within a short time.
- Keep all follow-up visits to check the condition of the eye and surrounding structures.

- Instill anesthetic eyedrops under the direction or standing orders of a physician. *Anesthetic eyedrops reduce pain. They must not be given repeatedly after corneal injury because of the risk for masking injury, delaying healing, and causing corneal scarring (Smeltzer et al., 2008).*
- Apply cool compresses or an ice pack for the first 24 hours, followed thereafter by warm compresses. *Cold reduces swelling.*

▶ **Impaired Tissue Integrity** related to physical or chemical injury to the epithelium

▶ **Expected Outcome:** The tissue of the eye will not be permanently damaged.

- For a chemical splash, take the client to the nearest sink or water fountain, instruct him or her to hold the eyes open, and flush the eyes with running water. *Running water removes chemicals and reduces the potential for chemical burn.*
- Tilt client's head to the side, and direct the flow of solution from the nasal area outward of the affected eye. *Doing so prevents the solution from flowing into the other eye and causing damage.*
- Continue flushing the eye(s) for 10 to 15 minutes. *Flushing removes the chemical, neutralizes the effects of the chemical, and prevents tissue ulceration.*
- After irrigation, instill an antibiotic if prescribed. *Antibiotics prevent infection.*
- Apply an eye pad after irrigation. Instruct the client to close the eye while the eye pad is applied over the lid, and secure the pad with tape. *These measures prevent further injury and reduce eyelid movement.*

▶ **Risk for Infection** related to disruption of corneal and conjunctival tissue

▶ **Expected Outcome:** The client will not acquire a secondary ophthalmic infection.

- Wash hands before examining the eyes or performing any procedures about the face. *Handwashing prevents infection.*
- Use sterile solutions to irrigate the eye in nonemergency situations. *Sterile solutions reduce the introduction of microbes.*
- Instill antibiotic ointment or drops as prescribed. *Antibiotics prevent infection.*
- Do not use a container of ophthalmic medication for anyone other than the client. *This measure prevents cross-contamination.*
- Avoid contaminating the medication dropper or tube by holding the tip above the eye and adjacent tissue. *This position reduces the risk of infection.*
- Change gauze eye dressings on a regular basis using aseptic technique. *Maintaining asepsis prevents the introduction and transmission of infection.*

Evaluation of Expected Outcomes
Pain is reduced or eliminated. Trauma is minimized by immediate first-aid measures. No purulent exudate is noted. ●

▶ *Stop, Think, and Respond Exercise 42-1*
You are accompanying a group of 10-year-old children on a field trip. One of the boys runs into a tree branch and immediately starts crying and holding his eye, stating that something is stuck in it. What action should you take?

INFECTIOUS AND INFLAMMATORY EYE DISORDERS

CONJUNCTIVITIS

Conjunctivitis is an inflammation of the conjunctiva. It commonly is called *pinkeye* because of hemorrhage of the subconjunctival blood vessels, which cause the pink appearance. Some forms are highly contagious.

Pathophysiology and Etiology
Conjunctivitis results from a bacterial, viral, or rickettsial infection. The microorganisms most often are introduced by air transmission, direct contact with sources on the fingers, a contaminated face towel or washcloth, or transmission from infected lesions near the eye. Allergic reactions, trauma from chemicals, or foreign bodies in the eye also cause conjunctivitis. A local inflammatory response follows damage to the tissue. Untreated conjunctivitis, especially when caused by *Neisseria gonorrhoeae* and *Chlamydia trachomatis,* can lead to blindness.

Assessment Findings
Symptoms include redness, excessive tearing, swelling, pain, burning or itching, and, possibly, purulent drainage from one or both eyes. In infections with the herpes simplex virus, lesions appear on or near the lid margins. In severe cases, lymph nodes in the neck or throat area are enlarged.
    Although cultures identify the causative microorganism, more often than not, the disorder is diagnosed by visual inspection and a history of exposure to someone with similar symptoms.

Medical Management
Treatment includes antibiotic or antiviral ointment or drops. Warm soaks or sterile saline irrigations are used to remove purulent drainage, reduce swelling, and relieve pain or itching. If an allergen causes the conjunctivitis, antihistamines and decongestants are prescribed.

Nursing Management
The nurse cleans the eye and instills or applies the prescribed medication. He or she provides health teaching so that the client can assume the necessary care independently. Because many forms of this condition are infectious, the nurse identifies methods for preventing its spread, including instructing the client to:

- Remain at home and apart from other people as much as possible while contagious.
- Use separate towels, linens, and other personal items.
- Wash hands often and thoroughly with soap and water.

- Use new tissue each time when wiping discharge from eye.
- Discard eye make-up items and do not use new make-up until conjunctivitis clears.
- Return to physician if discharge becomes thick and yellowish.

UVEITIS

Uveitis is an inflammation of the uveal tract, which consists of the iris, ciliary body, and choroid.

Pathophysiology and Etiology

The cause of uveitis is unknown, but it definitely produces inflammatory changes. Pathogens seldom are identified. Although the disorder occurs randomly, it is detected with some frequency among clients with juvenile rheumatoid arthritis, ankylosing spondylitis, tuberculosis, toxoplasmosis, histoplasmosis, and herpes zoster infection. Because some of these diseases are autoimmune disorders, uveitis may be an atypical antigen-antibody phenomenon (see Chap. 33). Complications such as glaucoma, cataracts, and retinal detachment are known to occur secondary to uveitis.

Assessment Findings

Symptoms include blurred vision and **photophobia**, a sensitivity to light. Eye pain is experienced in varying degrees. The eye appears red and congested, and the pupil reacts poorly to light.

Uveitis is confirmed by its clinical appearance during slit-lamp examination. Skin tests for primary disorders, such as tuberculosis, are performed to confirm or rule out this etiology.

Medical Management

Treatment includes oral and topical corticosteroids, mydriatic (dilating) eyedrops such as atropine, and antibiotic eyedrops. Analgesics are prescribed for pain. Sunglasses reduce the discomfort of photophobia.

Nursing Management

The nurse instructs the client on the medication regimen and drug-administration technique and stresses compliance with therapy. Failure to follow the medication regimen can result in serious complications. The nurse also emphasizes the importance of close follow-up during treatment.

KERATITIS AND CORNEAL ULCER

Keratitis is an inflammation of the cornea. A corneal ulcer is an erosion in the corneal tissue.

Pathophysiology and Etiology

Trauma to the cornea (e.g., wearing hard contact lenses for an extended period) and infectious agents (e.g., bacteria, fungi, viruses) cause keratitis. Secondary infections are common once the epithelium is damaged. Most clients experience severe pain because of the abundance of nerve endings in the cornea. Inflammation and disruption of the tissue interfere with the transparency and smoothness of the cor-

nea, temporarily impairing vision. When and if scar tissue forms, visual impairment is permanent. The degree of visual change depends on the size and density of the corneal scar tissue.

Assessment Findings

Keratitis is associated with localized pain or the sensation that a foreign body is present. Blinking increases the discomfort. Photophobia, blurred vision, tearing, purulent discharge, and redness develop.

In addition to flashlight illumination and slit-lamp examination, fluorescein drops or strips provide evidence of corneal tissue erosion.

Medical and Surgical Management

Treatment is begun promptly to avoid permanent loss of vision. Keratitis is treated with topical anesthetics, mydriatics (drugs that dilate the pupil), and local and systemic antibiotics. Dark glasses are recommended to relieve photophobia. Treatment in the early stages of a corneal ulcer is the same as for keratitis. Once corneal scar tissue has formed, the only treatment is **corneal transplantation (keratoplasty)**.

Nursing Management

The nurse removes exudate that harbors microbes and instills antibiotic eye medication. He or she follows aseptic principles to avoid transferring microorganisms to the injured corneal tissues. The nurse advises the client who wears contact lenses to stop wearing them temporarily.

BLEPHARITIS

Blepharitis is an inflammation of the lid margins.

Pathophysiology and Etiology

One form of blepharitis is associated with hypersecretion from sebaceous glands, which causes greasy scales to form. This type often occurs in conjunction with dandruff of the scalp or seborrheic dermatitis found about the ears and eyebrows. Infectious agents such as staphylococci cause other cases. Some cases are combinations of both. Blepharitis can coexist with conjunctivitis and lead to the development of hordeola and chalazia, which are discussed later.

Assessment Findings

The lid margins appear inflamed. Patchy flakes cling to the eyelashes and are readily visible about the lids. Eyelashes may be missing. Purulent drainage may be present.

The condition is definitively diagnosed by scraping the lid margins and examining the scales microscopically, although that usually is not necessary.

Medical Management

A topical antibiotic ointment is prescribed. The condition also improves with cleaning of the eyelids once or twice daily. Because seborrhea (excessive oiliness of the skin) of the face and scalp is associated with blepharitis, frequent washing of the face and hair is recommended.

Nursing Management

The nurse reinforces the instructions for conscientious performance of hygiene measures. Many clients become discouraged because the condition takes some time to improve. Noncompliance contributes to the chronicity of the condition.

HORDEOLUM (STY)

A **hordeolum** or sty is an inflammation and infection of the Zeis or Moll glands, types of oil glands at the edge of the eyelid.

Pathophysiology and Etiology

Staphylococcus aureus is the most common causative pathogen. The microorganisms multiply in the oil gland, which initiates an inflammatory response. A collection of purulent exudate accompanies the inflammation in the channel of the gland. As debris accumulates, it causes swelling and localized discomfort. Sties are common in clients with diabetes mellitus because their glucose-rich blood readily supports microbial growth.

Assessment Findings

A sty appears as a tender, swollen, red pustule in the internal or external tissue of the eyelid. A culture of the exudate, although seldom performed, identifies bacterial pathogens.

Medical and Surgical Management

Treatment of a sty includes warm soaks of the area and a topical antibiotic. Severe cases require incision and drainage.

Nursing Management

The nurse assures the client that treatment provides relief from pain and discomfort. He or she explains how to avoid transferring microorganisms from the sty to areas of the body by cleaning the unaffected eye first and changing the washcloth, towel, and water after contact with the affected eye. The nurse also instructs the client to use separate fresh tissues, cotton balls, or gauze for each wiping stroke when cleaning exudate from the eye.

CHALAZION

A *chalazion* is a cyst of one or more meibomian glands, a type of sebaceous gland in the inner surface of the eyelid at the junction of the conjunctiva and lid margin.

Pathophysiology and Etiology

A chalazion forms when the meibomian gland becomes obstructed and the release of sebaceous secretions is blocked. Consequently, the meibomian gland becomes inflamed and enlarged.

Assessment Findings

A chalazion appears similar to a sty, but the swelling in the upper or lower eyelid is not tender. As the chalazion matures, it feels hard. The enlargement within the eyelid causes clients to feel self-conscious about their appearance and affects their visual acuity.

If a chalazion grows large enough to obscure the pupil or compress corneal tissue, the distortion of vision is similar to that caused by astigmatism.

Medical and Surgical Management

Treatment of a chalazion is not necessary if the cyst is small and does not interfere with vision. Warm soaks and massage of the surrounding area are prescribed to promote spontaneous drainage. If the cyst is firm, becomes infected, or interferes with closure of the eyelid, it is surgically excised.

Nursing Management

The nurse prepares the client for examination and treatment by a physician. He or she gives instructions on methods for carrying out the treatment measures. Some points to include when teaching clients with infectious and inflammatory eye disorders are as follows:

- Comply with the full course of prescribed drugs to achieve satisfactory results.
- Wash hands thoroughly before cleaning the eyelids, instilling eyedrops, or applying eye ointment.
- Do not rub the eyes, and keep hands away from the eyes.
- Use a separate washcloth or towel if the disorder is infectious.
- Do not use nonprescription eye products during or after treatment unless approved by the physician.
- Eliminate the use of eye cosmetics or use hypoallergenic products and replace them frequently to avoid harboring microorganisms.
- Keep all follow-up appointments.

MACULAR DEGENERATION

Macular degeneration is the breakdown of or damage to the macula, the point on the retina where light rays converge for the most acute visual perception. The disorder usually occurs in both eyes, but the vision in one eye tends to deteriorate more rapidly.

Pathophysiology and Etiology

Macular degeneration, which tends to affect older adults, is usually referred to as age-related macular degeneration (AMD). AMD is the leading cause of vision loss in clients older than 60 years of age (National Eye Institute, 2006). Risk factors for developing AMD include race (it is more common among Caucasians), smoking, and heredity.

The two main types of AMD are referred to as the dry type and the wet type. In the dry type, the outer layers of the retina break down over a long period of time and characteristic small yellowish spots (drusen) are apparent under the retina. When drusen form within the macula, the client gradually experiences blurred vision. This type of macular degeneration does not have any treatment or cure.

The wet type has been further classified. The first is called classic choroidal neovascularization. It has a more abrupt onset and is characterized by enlarged drusen. The underlying problem stems from an opening between one of the membranous layers of the retina and the choroid. Serous fluid seeps into the separation and elevates an area of the

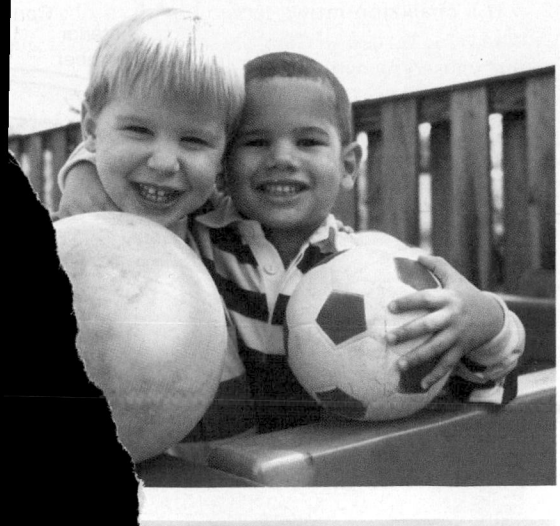

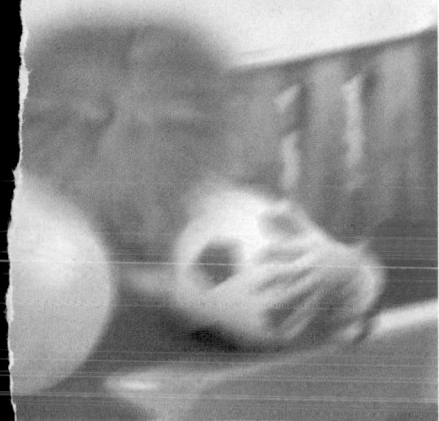

...ss associated with macular degeneration.
...sion. **(B)** View with age-related macular
... of the National Eye Institute, National

One or more blood vessels grow into the
...a subretinal hemorrhage. After the bleed,
...he damage almost always is confined to
...nd vision loss can be severe. The second
...lt choroidal neovascularization; it differs
...m in that the new vessel growth and leak-
...unced, resulting in vision loss that is less

Findings

...generation, blurred vision is the first symp-
...ich becomes more noticeable when clients
...ose work. In wet macular degeneration, cli-
...listortion of vision, such as straight lines
...r letters in words looking broken. A client's
...r may also be diminished. When the macula
...ly damaged, clients compare their vision to
... the bull's-eye area of the image is absent
...peripheral field, or side vision, is unaffected;
...ot see images by looking at them directly.
...angiography shows pooling of the dye in
...Optical coherence tomography uses fiberop-
...ages of the ocular tissue structure.

Medical Management

One of two procedures may be performed. *Laser photocoagulation* seals the serous leak and destroys the encroachment of blood vessels in the area. It must be performed early to prevent progression of the disorder. For many clients, the diagnosis is made too late, and laser treatment no longer is an option. Dangers of this procedure include destruction of healthy tissue and loss of vision. *Photodynamic therapy* uses an intravenous injection of a photosensitizing drug and a nonthermal laser application to reduce proliferation of abnormal blood vessels and eliminate the risk to the retina.

Research on the use of medications that are directly injected into the vitreous (intravitreal injection) is showing great promise in the treatment of wet AMD. Ranibizumab (Lucentis) and pegaptanib (Macugen) bind and inhibit vascular endothelial growth factor, a protein that is involved with angiogenesis (formation of new vessels). Both medications slow the progression of choroidal neovascularization and actually improve vision in many clients. A transient loss of vision related to increased intraocular pressure (IOP), burning sensation, eye pain, and floaters may occur. Bevacizumab (Avastin), a drug originally developed for treatment of colorectal cancer, is the focus of a recent trial in which it is being compared with ranibizumab. Bevacizumab works in a similar fashion to ranibizumab; however, it is at least as effective, has fewer side effects, and is more cost effective.

Macular translocation is a new surgical procedure for wet AMD. A retinal detachment is created, moving the retina so that the macula is a slight distance from the area of choroidal neovascularization. Laser treatments can then be used without as much risk to the macula. More research to refine this procedure is being conducted.

Diet and vitamins are also used to slow the progression of all types of AMD. Studies are in progress to demonstrate whether supplements with zinc and lutein as well as zeaxanthin and other antioxidants are effective for clients diagnosed with AMD. Clients are also instructed to eat a healthy diet that includes two to three servings of cold-water fish (e.g., salmon) per week, and daily servings of leafy green vegetables and a variety of fruits and other vegetables (Nutrition Notes 42-1).

The client may be provided with suggestions for coping with the visual impairment. Aids, such as magnifying glasses, may be of value, and high-intensity reading lamps

Nutrition Notes 42-1
The Client with Macular Degeneration

- Several studies suggest that carotenoids other than beta-carotene, namely lutein and zeaxanthin, form the yellow pigment in the macula and may protect the eye against damage by filtering out visible blue light. Sources of these phytochemicals include dark green leafy vegetables, broccoli, peas, kiwi, red grapes, oranges, corn, mangoes, and honeydew melon.
- One study showed that the risk of macular degeneration was half as great in people who ate spinach or collard greens two to four times per week than in people who ate these vegetables less than once per month.

have helped some people. The ophthalmologist may refer the client to a specialized center for evaluation and selection of assistive devices.

Nursing Management

The nurse helps the client cope with loss of vision. For additional nursing management of the client with permanent visual impairment, review the information that accompanies the previous discussion of blindness.

GLAUCOMA

Glaucoma, a major cause of blindness in the United States, is a group of eye disorders caused by an imbalance between the production and drainage of aqueous fluid. When the drainage system is obstructed, the anterior chamber becomes congested with fluid and IOP rises. Optic nerve damage can occur as a result of the increased IOP.

Glaucoma is classified as either open-angle or angle-closure. *Open-angle glaucoma,* formerly called *chronic* or *simple glaucoma,* is the most common form. Its onset is slow, and the client may not experience noticeable symptoms for several years. *Angle-closure glaucoma* is less common, but immediate recognition and treatment are required to prevent blindness.

Pathophysiology and Etiology

Glaucoma occurs congenitally; secondary to other eye disorders such as ocular trauma, ophthalmic infections, and cataract surgery; or as a primary disease among adults older than 40 years of age. It is more prevalent among those who have a family history of the disorder. The incidence is higher among African Americans, who are four to eight times more likely to develop blindness from glaucoma than are other ethnic groups.

Open-angle glaucoma occurs when structures in the drainage system (i.e., trabecular meshwork and canal of Schlemm) degenerate and the exit channels for aqueous fluid become blocked. As the IOP rises, it causes edema of the cornea, atrophy of nerve fibers in the peripheral areas of the retina, and degeneration of the optic nerve.

Angle-closure glaucoma occurs in people who have an anatomically narrow angle at the junction where the iris meets the cornea (Fig. 42-4). This deviation makes them vulnerable to angle closure when nearby structures protrude into the anterior chamber and occlude the drainage pathway. For example, an attack can be precipitated when the iris thickens in response to a mydriatic drug, by pupil dilation while sitting in the dark, or when the lens enlarges with age and bulges forward. A delay in treatment may result in partial or total loss of vision in the affected eye.

Assessment Findings

Signs and Symptoms

Clients with open-angle glaucoma may be asymptomatic, and the condition may not be discovered until the client has a routine ophthalmologic examination. When symptoms do occur, they often are ignored because they are not dramatic. Clients may complain of eye discomfort, occasional and

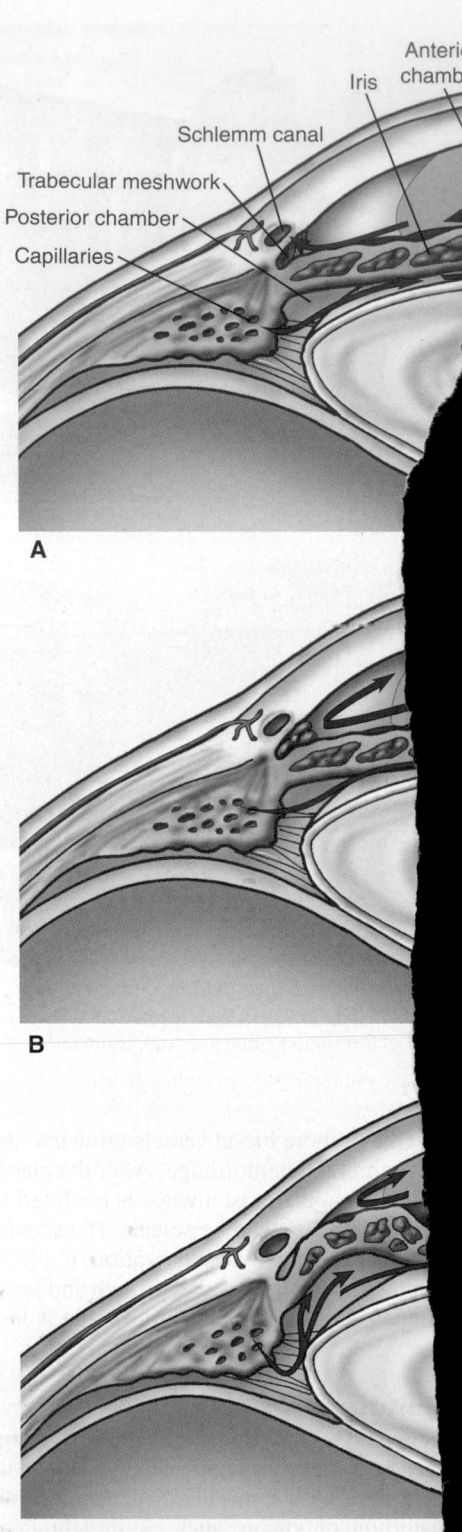

A

B

C

FIGURE 42-4. (A) In the normal eye, the pathway to flow to the canal of Schlemm is wide and unob... open-angle glaucoma, the flow is obstructed at th... meshwork. **(C)** In angle-closure glaucoma, the mo... impaired because increased pressure in the poste... produces a forward bowing of the iris, which narro... the canal of Schlemm.

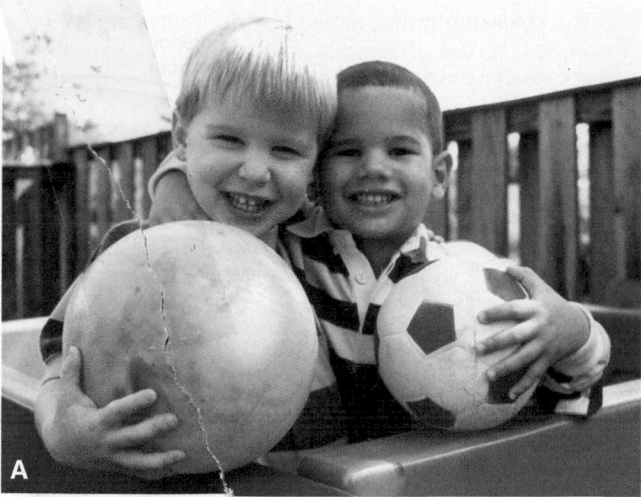

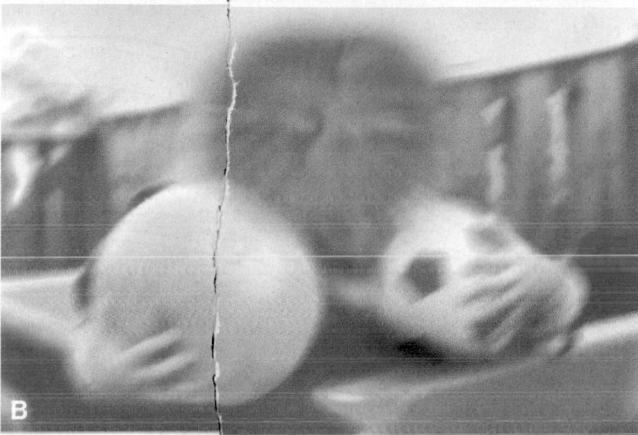

FIGURE 42-3. Visual loss associated with macular degeneration. **(A)** View with normal vision. **(B)** View with age-related macular degeneration. (Courtesy of the National Eye Institute, National Institutes of Health.)

retina, like a blister. One or more blood vessels grow into the defect and produce a subretinal hemorrhage. After the bleed, scar tissue forms. The damage almost always is confined to the macular area, and vision loss can be severe. The second form is termed occult choroidal neovascularization; it differs from the classic form in that the new vessel growth and leakage are less pronounced, resulting in vision loss that is less severe.

Assessment Findings

In dry macular degeneration, blurred vision is the first symptom of disease, which becomes more noticeable when clients try to read or do close work. In wet macular degeneration, clients experience distortion of vision, such as straight lines appearing wavy or letters in words looking broken. A client's perception of color may also be diminished. When the macula becomes irreparably damaged, clients compare their vision to a target in which the bull's-eye area of the image is absent (Fig. 42-3). The peripheral field, or side vision, is unaffected, but the client cannot see images by looking at them directly.

Fluorescein angiography shows pooling of the dye in the blister area. Optical coherence tomography uses fiberoptics to provide images of the ocular tissue structure.

Medical Management

One of two procedures may be performed. *Laser photocoagulation* seals the serous leak and destroys the encroachment of blood vessels in the area. It must be performed early to prevent progression of the disorder. For many clients, the diagnosis is made too late, and laser treatment no longer is an option. Dangers of this procedure include destruction of healthy tissue and loss of vision. *Photodynamic therapy* uses an intravenous injection of a photosensitizing drug and a nonthermal laser application to reduce proliferation of abnormal blood vessels and eliminate the risk to the retina.

Research on the use of medications that are directly injected into the vitreous (intravitreal injection) is showing great promise in the treatment of wet AMD. Ranibizumab (Lucentis) and pegaptanib (Macugen) bind and inhibit vascular endothelial growth factor, a protein that is involved with angiogenesis (formation of new vessels). Both medications slow the progression of choroidal neovascularization and actually improve vision in many clients. A transient loss of vision related to increased intraocular pressure (IOP), burning sensation, eye pain, and floaters may occur. Bevacizumab (Avastin), a drug originally developed for treatment of colorectal cancer, is the focus of a recent trial in which it is being compared with ranibizumab. Bevacizumab works in a similar fashion to ranibizumab; however, it is at least as effective, has fewer side effects, and is more cost effective.

Macular translocation is a new surgical procedure for wet AMD. A retinal detachment is created, moving the retina so that the macula is a slight distance from the area of choroidal neovascularization. Laser treatments can then be used without as much risk to the macula. More research to refine this procedure is being conducted.

Diet and vitamins are also used to slow the progression of all types of AMD. Studies are in progress to demonstrate whether supplements with zinc and lutein as well as zeaxanthin and other antioxidants are effective for clients diagnosed with AMD. Clients are also instructed to eat a healthy diet that includes two to three servings of cold-water fish (e.g., salmon) per week, and daily servings of leafy green vegetables and a variety of fruits and other vegetables (Nutrition Notes 42-1).

The client may be provided with suggestions for coping with the visual impairment. Aids, such as magnifying glasses, may be of value, and high-intensity reading lamps

Nutrition Notes 42-1
The Client with Macular Degeneration

- Several studies suggest that carotenoids other than beta-carotene, namely lutein and zeaxanthin, form the yellow pigment in the macula and may protect the eye against damage by filtering out visible blue light. Sources of these phytochemicals include dark green leafy vegetables, broccoli, peas, kiwi, red grapes, oranges, corn, mangoes, and honeydew melon.

- One study showed that the risk of macular degeneration was half as great in people who ate spinach or collard greens two to four times per week than in people who ate these vegetables less than once per month.

have helped some people. The ophthalmologist may refer the client to a specialized center for evaluation and selection of assistive devices.

Nursing Management

The nurse helps the client cope with loss of vision. For additional nursing management of the client with permanent visual impairment, review the information that accompanies the previous discussion of blindness.

GLAUCOMA

Glaucoma, a major cause of blindness in the United States, is a group of eye disorders caused by an imbalance between the production and drainage of aqueous fluid. When the drainage system is obstructed, the anterior chamber becomes congested with fluid and IOP rises. Optic nerve damage can occur as a result of the increased IOP.

Glaucoma is classified as either open-angle or angle-closure. *Open-angle glaucoma,* formerly called *chronic* or *simple glaucoma,* is the most common form. Its onset is slow, and the client may not experience noticeable symptoms for several years. *Angle-closure glaucoma* is less common, but immediate recognition and treatment are required to prevent blindness.

Pathophysiology and Etiology

Glaucoma occurs congenitally; secondary to other eye disorders such as ocular trauma, ophthalmic infections, and cataract surgery; or as a primary disease among adults older than 40 years of age. It is more prevalent among those who have a family history of the disorder. The incidence is higher among African Americans, who are four to eight times more likely to develop blindness from glaucoma than are other ethnic groups.

Open-angle glaucoma occurs when structures in the drainage system (i.e., trabecular meshwork and canal of Schlemm) degenerate and the exit channels for aqueous fluid become blocked. As the IOP rises, it causes edema of the cornea, atrophy of nerve fibers in the peripheral areas of the retina, and degeneration of the optic nerve.

Angle-closure glaucoma occurs in people who have an anatomically narrow angle at the junction where the iris meets the cornea (Fig. 42-4). This deviation makes them vulnerable to angle closure when nearby structures protrude into the anterior chamber and occlude the drainage pathway. For example, an attack can be precipitated when the iris thickens in response to a mydriatic drug, by pupil dilation while sitting in the dark, or when the lens enlarges with age and bulges forward. A delay in treatment may result in partial or total loss of vision in the affected eye.

Assessment Findings

Signs and Symptoms

Clients with open-angle glaucoma may be asymptomatic, and the condition may not be discovered until the client has a routine ophthalmologic examination. When symptoms do occur, they often are ignored because they are not dramatic. Clients may complain of eye discomfort, occasional and

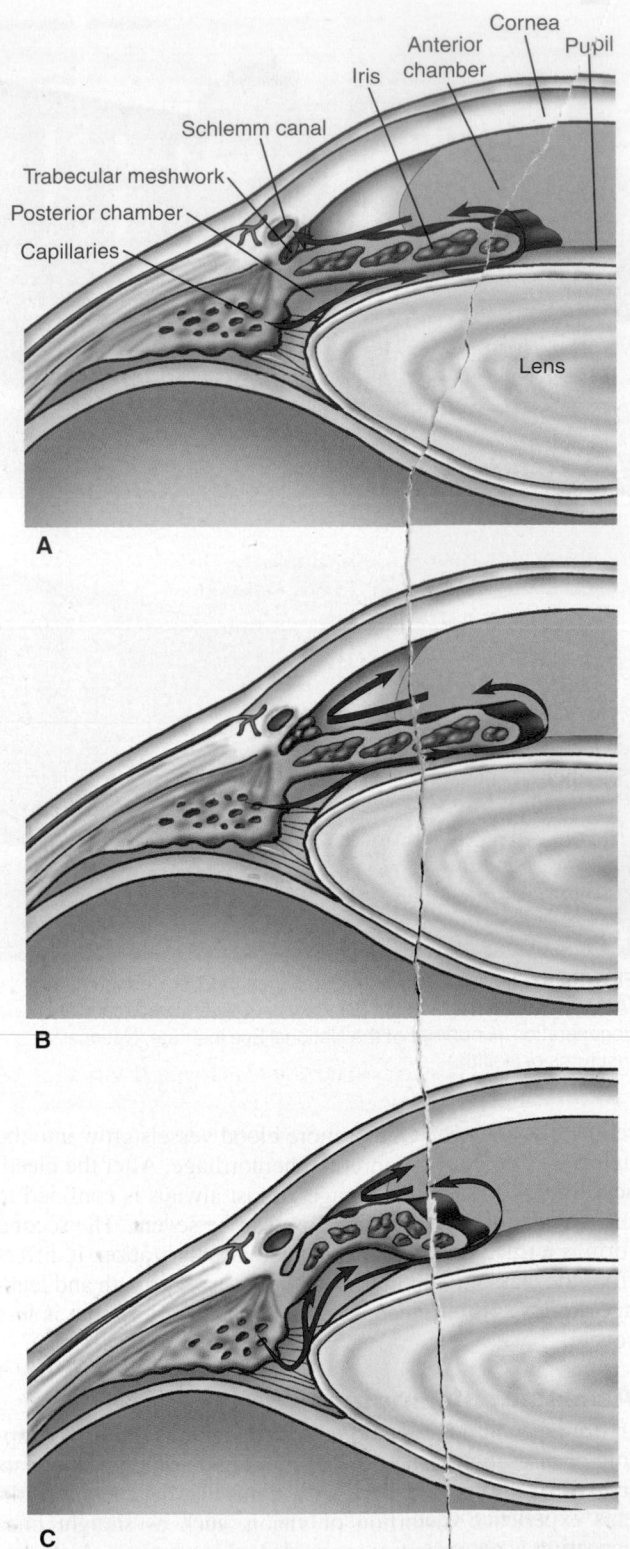

FIGURE 42-4. (A) In the normal eye, the pathway for aqueous humor to flow to the canal of Schlemm is wide and unobstructed. **(B)** In open-angle glaucoma, the flow is obstructed at the trabecular meshwork. **(C)** In angle-closure glaucoma, the movement of fluid is impaired because increased pressure in the posterior chamber produces a forward bowing of the iris, which narrows the approach to the canal of Schlemm.

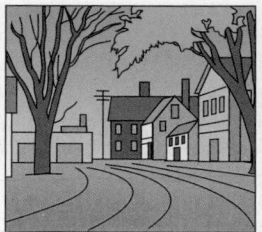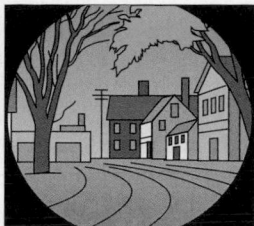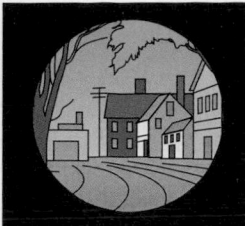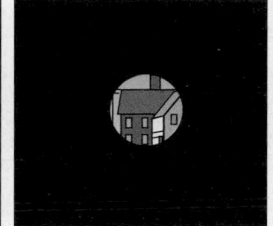

FIGURE 42-5. Gradual loss of vision from glaucoma.

temporary blurred vision, the appearance of halos around lights, reduced peripheral vision, and the feeling that their eyeglass prescription needs to be changed (Fig. 42-5).

In contrast, clients with acute angle-closure glaucoma become symptomatic quite suddenly. The eyes become rock hard, painful, and sightless. Nausea and vomiting may occur. The conjunctiva is red; the cornea becomes cloudy and commonly is described as appearing "steamy." The attack is self-limiting, but with each subsequent attack, vision becomes more impaired.

Diagnostic Findings

The optic disc, when visualized directly with an ophthalmoscope or with retinal angiographic photographs, shows a cupping effect (widening and deepening). When the anterior chamber of the eye of a client with angle-closure glaucoma is inspected with a penlight or slit lamp, the angle between the iris and cornea is narrow. Tonometry reveals elevated IOP and reduced aqueous outflow. The visual field examination demonstrates a loss of peripheral vision; nasal and superior areas usually are impaired first.

Other tests used to monitor glaucoma, particularly the optic nerve and internal structures, include scanning laser polarimetry and optical coherence tomography. Ultrasound biomicroscopy evaluates how fluids flow through the eye angles. Gonioscopy uses special lenses to better visualize the eye structures. These methods not only establish a baseline but also determine whether the glaucoma has progressed.

Medical Management

Initially, glaucoma may be treated with medications. Clients with open-angle glaucoma use topical beta-blockers, such as timolol (Timoptic) (Drug Therapy Table 42-1). Beta-blockers decrease the flow rate of aqueous humor into the eye. Other medications to control IOP may be given; as many as four topical medications may be used at a time. Miotics such as carbachol (Miostat) and pilocarpine (Pilocar) constrict the pupil. These medications pull the iris away from the drainage channels so that the aqueous fluid can escape. Other eye medications that are used for lowering IOP include echothiophate iodide (Phospholine Iodide), epinephrine, and dipivefrin (Propine). Acetazolamide (Diamox) and methazolamide (Neptazane), which are carbonic anhydrase inhibitors, slow the production of aqueous fluid. Oral medications, including carbonic anhydrase inhibitors such as acetazolamide (Diamox) and dichlorphenamide (Daranide), may be used to supplement or replace topical medications. However, side effects are more problematic with the oral preparations.

In an acute attack of angle-closure glaucoma, analgesics are given to relieve pain, and the client is kept at complete rest. Laser surgery (see Surgical Management) is usually performed before medications are prescribed, but clients frequently require medications after surgery.

Surgical Management

When compliance is poor (e.g., client fails to instill eyedrops as directed) or drug therapy no longer is effective (i.e., IOP fails to decrease sufficiently), or if the client develops severe adverse reactions to the medication, more aggressive treatment becomes necessary to preserve vision. One of several procedures that create accessory drainage channels can be performed. These procedures include laser or surgical **iridectomy**, laser **trabeculoplasty**, and **corneal trephine**.

Laser iridectomy, in which holes are burned into the iris to increase areas for drainage, is performed first. If this procedure is unsuccessful, it is followed by a standard surgical iridectomy, in which a section of the iris is removed. Either a peripheral or sector iridectomy is used. In a peripheral iridectomy, a small section of iris is removed at the outer margin of the iris. In a sector or keyhole iridectomy, a larger segment of the iris is removed in the direction of the pupil (Fig. 42-6). A laser trabeculoplasty is an alternative to a surgical iridectomy. In this procedure, the laser beam is directed at the trabecular network, which lies near the canal of Schlemm, creating multiple openings for drainage. A corneal trephine is similar to a trabeculoplasty in that it produces a small hole at the junction of the cornea and sclera to provide an outlet for aqueous fluid. The opening is then covered by a flap of the conjunctiva.

Nursing Management

The nurse determines the client's history of symptoms, the medications that have been prescribed, and whether the client is adhering to the prescribed medication schedule (or taking any other medications). It is also is important to ask when the client was first diagnosed with glaucoma.

Acute angle-closure glaucoma is an emergency. The nurse refers the client for medical treatment immediately because vision can be permanently lost in 1 to 2 days. Severe pain requires analgesics. To promote the maximum effect from analgesic drug therapy, it is essential to limit sensory stimulation, such as loud noise, activity, and movement. The nurse informs the physician immediately if the client states that the pain has worsened despite treatment. While clients are incapacitated by their pain or if the disease results in loss of vision, the nurse assists with meeting basic needs. Mydriatics (drugs that dilate the pupil) must never be administered to clients with glaucoma. The nurse consults the physician if

DRUG THERAPY TABLE 42-1 Drugs Used in Managing Glaucoma

Drug Category and Examples	Mechanism of Action	Side Effects	Nursing Considerations
Cholinergics (Miotics) pilocarpine (Pilocar), carbachol (Miostat)	Increase aqueous fluid outflow by contracting the ciliary muscle and causing miosis (constriction of the pupil) and opening of trabecular meshwork	Periorbital pain, blurry vision, difficulty seeing in the dark	Warn clients about diminished vision in dimly lit areas.
Adrenergic Agonists dipivefrin (Propine)	Reduce production of aqueous humor and increase outflow	Eye redness and burning; can have systemic effects, including palpitations, elevated blood pressure, tremor, headaches, and anxiety	Teach clients punctal occlusion to limit systemic effects.
Beta-Adrenergic Blockers betaxolol (Betoptic), timolol (Timoptic)	Decrease aqueous humor production and decrease intraocular pressure	Can have systemic effects, including bradycardia, exacerbation of pulmonary disease, and hypotension; common ocular side effects are burning/stinging, discomfort, dry eyes, and eyelid erythema	Contraindicated in clients with asthma, chronic obstructive pulmonary disease, second- or third-degree heart block, bradycardia, or cardiac failure; teach clients punctal occlusion to limit systemic effects. Because it may cause blurred vision, advise driving with caution.
Alpha-Adrenergic Agonists apraclonidine (Iopidine), brimonidine (Alphagan)	Decrease aqueous humor production	Eye redness, dry mouth and nasal passages	Teach clients punctal occlusion to limit systemic effects.
Carbonic Anhydrase Inhibitors acetazolamide (Diamox), methazolamide (Neptazane), dorzolamide (Trusopt)	Decrease aqueous humor production	Oral medications (acetazolamide and methazolamide) associated with serious side effects, including anaphylactic reactions, electrolyte loss, depression, lethargy, gastrointestinal upset, impotence, and weight loss; topical form (dorzolamide) side effects include topical allergy	Do not administer to clients with sulfa allergies; monitor electrolyte levels.
Prostaglandin Analogs latanoprost (Xalatan)	Increase uveoscleral outflow	Darkening of the iris, conjunctival redness, possible rash	Instruct clients to report any side effects.

drugs with anticholinergic properties, such as atropine sulfate, are prescribed, because dilation of the pupil can further obstruct drainage of aqueous fluid, raise IOP, and damage whatever vision remains.

Because glaucoma tends to run in families, the nurse advises adults to be examined regularly. Early diagnosis and treatment are essential for preventing loss of vision. Clients who already are diagnosed with glaucoma are encouraged to maintain close follow-up and comply with the medication regimen. The nurse explains drug-instillation techniques. Besides eyedrops, some clients insert an ocular therapeutic system under the upper lid. An *ocular therapeutic system* is a small, thin film that contains eye medication. The film, which is replaced weekly, continuously releases the medication and eliminates the need for frequent eyedrop instillation.

If a client has difficulty remembering when to take the medication, the nurse recommends a watch with a timer. For the client who does not understand the chronic and progressive nature of the disease, it is important to stress that glaucoma has no cure but can be controlled and that blindness caused by glaucoma usually is preventable.

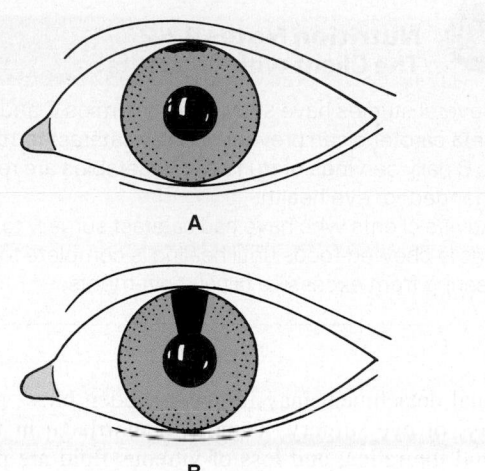

FIGURE 42-6. (**A**) Appearance of the eye after peripheral iridectomy. (**B**) Appearance of eye after keyhole (sector) iridectomy.

Other general instructions include the following:

- Obtain assistance from a family member, relative, or friend if you have trouble instilling eyedrops.
- Avoid all drugs that contain atropine. Check with physician or pharmacist before using any nonprescription drug; preparations for cold or allergy symptoms may contain an atropine-like drug.
- Maintain regular bowel habits; straining at stool can raise IOP.
- Avoid heavy lifting and emotional upsets (especially crying) because they increase IOP.
- Limit activities that strain or tire the eyes.
- Keep an extra supply of prescribed drugs on hand for vacations, holidays, or in case some is lost or spilled.
- Seek medical attention immediately if pain or a visual disturbance occurs.
- Tell all physicians that you have this disorder and the treatment prescribed by the ophthalmologist. Carry identification stating that you have glaucoma in case of illness or injury.

▶ **Stop, Think, and Respond Exercise 42-2**

What is appropriate advice for a person with a family history of glaucoma?

CATARACTS

A **cataract** is a condition in which the lens of the eye becomes opaque. One or both eyes may be affected.

Pathophysiology and Etiology

Cataracts occur as a result of the aging process or are congenitally acquired, caused by injury to the lens, or secondary to other eye diseases. When cataracts occur in response to injury, they usually develop quickly. Most cataracts result from degenerative changes associated with aging and develop slowly. A high incidence of cataracts occurs among people with diabetes and those with a family history. Prolonged exposure to ultraviolet rays (e.g., sunlight, tanning

lamps), radiation, or certain drugs (e.g., corticosteroids) has been associated with cataract formation. In all cases, vision decreases because light no longer has a transparent pathway to the retina.

Assessment Findings

One of the earliest symptoms is seeing a halo around lights. Other symptoms include difficulty reading, changes in color vision (colors that look faded or yellow), glaring of objects in bright light, distortion of objects, blurred vision, poor night vision, and double vision in one eye. As the cataract worsens, visual acuity is so severely reduced that the client can only read the largest letter on a Snellen chart, count fingers, and distinguish movement. On inspection, a white or gray spot is visible behind the pupil (Fig. 42-7).

Under ophthalmoscopic and slit-lamp examination, the lens appears in varying stages of opacity. Some lenses are so cloudy that the examiner cannot see through the cataract to the posterior of the eye. Tonometry determines whether the cataract is increasing the IOP.

Surgical Management

Cataracts cannot be treated medically and are surgically removed. Surgery often is performed under local anesthesia. A tranquilizer is given before and during surgery to relax the client. Occasionally general anesthesia is used and has certain advantages, especially with an apprehensive client. The lens is removed by *intracapsular extraction* (removal of the lens within its capsule) or *extracapsular extraction* (removal of the lens, leaving the posterior portion of its capsule in position). *Phacoemulsification,* which uses ultrasound to break the lens into minute particles that are then removed by aspiration, is a technique that may accompany the extracapsular method. When phacoemulsification is used, a smaller incision is required and most clients return to full activity sooner than after the other methods.

After surgery, vision is restored with one of three methods: corrective eyeglasses, a contact lens, or an **intraocular lens** (IOL) **implant.** When cataract eyeglasses are prescribed, the correcting lens for the *aphakic eye* (the eye without a lens) causes the client to see objects about one-third larger than normal. These lenses also distort peripheral vision, and the client

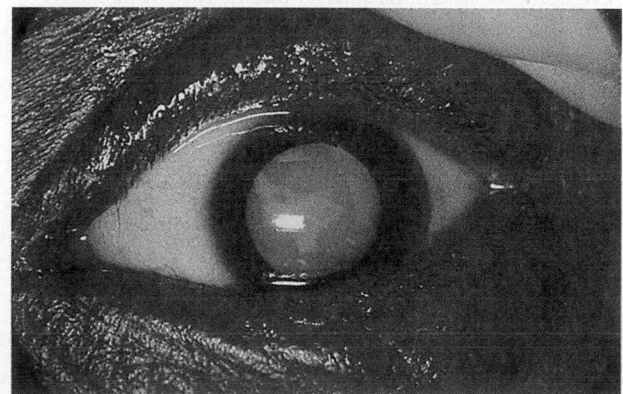

FIGURE 42-7. A cataract is a cloudy or opaque lens that appears gray or milky. (From Rubin, R., & Strayer, D. S., eds. [2008]. *Rubin's pathology: Clinicopathologic foundations of disease* [5th ed.]. Philadelphia. Lippincott Williams & Wilkins.)

must learn to turn his or her head to see objects that are not in the center of vision. If only one lens is removed, the client must use one eye or the other to avoid seeing a distorted image. A coating usually is applied to the eyeglasses so that only the aphakic eye with a corrective lens is used.

A contact lens also can restore vision after cataract extraction. Advantages of the contact lens are that peripheral vision is not lost and objects appear about their actual size. A disadvantage is that the lens must be removed at night, cleaned, and reinserted daily, which can be difficult for an older client who has poor manual dexterity or a cataract in the other eye.

Insertion of an IOL at the time of cataract surgery is the most often used method for improving vision. Most commonly, IOLs are inserted behind the iris. Ultrasonography is performed before surgery to determine the size and prescription of the IOL. A monofocal (single-vision) or multifocal lens is implanted to correct presbyopia.

Clients may experience cloudy vision at some point after cataract surgery involving an IOL. The IOL is positioned on the posterior capsule or membrane, which is the back surface of the client's natural lens. This membrane may become cloudy, interfering with visual acuity. To restore the client's vision, a simple laser procedure is performed to open the membrane. Other complications of cataract surgery include infection, loss of vitreous, intraocular hemorrhage, retinal detachment, and displacement of the IOL implant. Loss of vitreous is serious because the vitreous body does not regenerate. Its loss, as well as hemorrhage, seriously damages the eye.

Nursing Management

Cataract surgery is usually performed in an outpatient setting. The client wears a protective eye shield for 24 hours after the procedure and then at night and during naps for about a week. Clients need to wear sunglasses when in bright light for at least one week. Eyedrops, used several times a day, are prescribed for at least one week to prevent infection. The nurse is responsible for providing preoperative and postoperative care of the surgical client as well as discharge instructions (Nursing Care Plan 42-1). In addition, the nurse instructs the client that for at least one week he or she must avoid the following:

- Engaging in strenuous activity and heavy lifting
- Bending and stooping and other exercise that potentially increases IOP
- Immersing the eyes in water
- Any activity that potentially could cause dust or other particles to lodge in the eye

Nutrition Notes 42-2 provides additional information.

RETINAL DETACHMENT

In **retinal detachment**, the sensory layer becomes separated from the pigmented layer of the retina (Fig. 42-8).

Pathophysiology and Etiology

In general, retinal separation is associated with a hole or tear in the retina caused by stretching or degenerative changes.

Nutrition Notes 42-2
The Client with Cataracts

- Several studies have shown that vitamins C and E and beta carotene can prevent or delay cataract formation. Five to 9 daily servings of fruits and vegetables are recommended for eye health.
- Advise clients who have had cataract surgery to eat soft, easily chewed foods until healing is complete to avoid tearing from excessive facial movements.

Retinal detachment may follow a sudden blow, penetrating injury, or eye surgery. Tumors, hemorrhage in front of or behind the retina, and loss of vitreous fluid are particularly likely to lead to retinal detachment. This condition may also be a complication of other disorders, such as advanced diabetic changes in the retina. In many instances, the cause of retinal detachment is unknown. Retinal separation is more common after 40 years of age.

The separation of the two layers of the retina deprives the sensory layer of its blood supply. Vision is lost in the affected area because the sensory layer no longer can receive visual stimuli. Vitreous fluid moves between the separated layers of the retina, holding the layers apart and causing further separation.

Three types of retinal detachment have been identified:

- *Rhegmatogenous*—Fluid moves under the retina through a tear and separates it from the pigmented layer; this is the most common form
- *Tractional*—The retina separates from the pigmented layer secondary to scar tissue on the retina's surface
- *Exudative*—Fluid moves under the retina secondary to inflammatory disorders or injury to the eye; there are no tears in the retina

Assessment Findings

Many clients notice definite gaps in their vision or blind spots. They describe the sensation that a curtain is being drawn over their field of vision, and they often see flashes of light. Seeing spots or moving particles, called *floaters,* is common. Complete loss of vision may occur in the affected eye. The condition is not painful, but clients usually are extremely apprehensive. When the retina is inspected with an ophthalmoscope, the tissue appears gray in the detached area.

Surgical Management

Surgical interventions for retinal reattachment include laser surgery, cryopexy, diathermy, retinopexy, and scleral buckling. The method chosen depends on the extent of detachment.

Several procedures are used for small tears or holes. *Laser surgery* involves making of small burns around the tear to attach the retina back in place. The exudate that forms between the retina and choroid results in adhesion of the retina to the choroid. *Cryopexy* involves the application of a supercooled probe to the tear, assisting the retina to reattach. *Diathermy* uses electric current to heat the tissue around the tear.

Pneumatic retinopexy is a less invasive method used to repair larger retinal tears. Methods described previously are

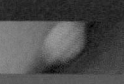

NURSING CARE PLAN 42-1 | **Postoperative Management of the Client Undergoing Eye Surgery**

Assessment

Clients having eye surgery require the usual preoperative care. Frequently, they have surgery in ambulatory care settings, so preoperative assessments may be done before the day of surgery. Obtain preoperative vital signs to have a baseline for postoperative monitoring.

Depending on the type of surgery, it is important to ask the client about medications. Check to ensure that instructions about withholding any medications before surgery were followed. Examples include the following:

- Anticoagulation therapy withheld as ordered. For example, if the client takes warfarin (Coumadin), a prothrombin time of 1.5 is the desired level before surgery.
- Aspirin withheld for 5 to 7 days
- Nonsteroidal anti-inflammatory drugs (NSAIDs) withheld for 3 to 5 days

In addition, check the preoperative orders and administer eyedrops as ordered.

PC. Ophthalmic Hemorrhage or **Increased Intraocular Pressure** (IOP)

Expected Outcome. Bleeding and IOP will be managed and minimized.

Interventions	Rationales
Report sudden or intense pain immediately.	Pain may indicate hemorrhage or increased IOP, which may require emergency surgery.
Instruct client to avoid coughing, vomiting, straining at stool, bending forward, or lifting anything heavier than 5 lb.	Avoiding these activities prevents the IOP from rising.

Evaluation of Expected Outcome

Client experiences no complications.

Nursing Diagnosis. Pain related to surgery.

Expected Outcome. Client will experience little or no pain or discomfort.

Interventions	Rationales
Acknowledge client's discomfort and administer prescribed analgesic that is appropriate for the level of pain.	Acknowledging and treating the client's pain provide validation and pain relief.
Keep room lights dim. Provide dark glasses if light causes discomfort.	These measures reduce eye sensitivity to light.
If allowed, instruct client to gently use a clean, moist washcloth to remove eye discharge.	This measure promotes increased comfort.

Evaluation of Expected Outcome

Client reports little or no pain.

Nursing Diagnosis. Risk for Infection related to impaired tissue integrity.

Expected Outcome. The incised tissue will heal without evidence of infection.

Interventions	Rationales
Perform conscientious handwashing before an eye assessment or treatment procedure.	Consistent and meticulous handwashing remains the primary method to reduce or prevent the transmission of microorganisms.
Follow principles of asepsis when cleaning the eye or applying a new dressing.	Asepsis prevents infection of operative site.
Keep the tips of all medication applicators clean.	Doing so prevents contamination of equipment and prevents infection of the operative site.

Evaluation of Expected Outcome

The incision heals without evidence of redness, swelling, or unusual drainage.

Nursing Diagnosis. Risk for Injury related to compromised vision

Expected Outcome. Client's safety will be maintained.

(care plan continues on page 622)

NURSING CARE PLAN 10-1 Postoperative Management of the Client Undergoing Eye Surgery (Continued)

Interventions	Rationales
While client is hospitalized, raise side rails and identify the location of the signal device.	These measures provide client with security and orient the client as to how to get needed assistance.
Encourage client to use a dim light or night light in the room after sundown.	Total darkness presents safety challenges to the visually compromised client. Minimal light provides a light source and prevents injury.
Reorient the confused client. Ask a family member to sit at the bedside if confusion persists.	These measures provide the client with a sense of where he or she is and where things are. Visual compromise can cause confusion. Having someone stay promotes safety.
Apply a shield over the patched eye.	The shield provides additional protection and prevents client from rubbing or accidentally poking the eye.
Assist client to ambulate; ensure the pathway is clear.	Doing so maintains client's safety.

Evaluation of Expected Outcome

Client remains free of injury.

---

used to seal the tear. A gas bubble is then injected within the vitreous to push the detached retina against the sclera. The gas bubble expands at first but then disappears within 2 to 6 weeks. A disadvantage of this procedure is that the client may have to position himself/herself in a face down position for a certain period of time each day for 7 to 10 days following the procedure. However, it is simpler and less expensive than other surgical procedures.

Scleral buckling is a surgical procedure in which a tiny synthetic band is attached outside the eyeball to lightly push the wall of the eye against the detached retina (Fig. 42-9). Sometimes a vitrectomy, in which the vitreous is removed and replaced by gas to help reattach the retina, is also performed. As healing occurs, the eye produces fluid that fills the eye and takes the place of the gas. With both scleral buckling and vitrectomy, the use of laser or cryopexy "welds" the retina back in place.

Nursing Management

Anyone with sudden loss of vision is referred immediately for examination by a physician. Clients are kept on flat bed rest, and sometimes positioned on their side, with the affected eye in dependent position (e.g., if the tear is on the left side the client will lie on his or her left side), until surgery is performed. Sedation may be ordered. The eyes are patched and covered with an eye shield. Mydriatic eyedrops are instilled as ordered to dilate the pupil and facilitate further examination of the retina.

If surgery is performed, the client is kept on complete bed rest with position restrictions for several days. The head may be immobilized. The client is not turned or moved without orders. If an air bubble is instilled to promote contact between the retina and sclera, the client is positioned with the face parallel to the floor so that the bubble floats to the posterior of the eye. If floaters are still seen after the eye heals, the nurse can tell the client that they eventually become absorbed or settle to the inferior floor of the eye, out of the line of vision. For additional postoperative nursing management, see Nursing Care Plan 42-1.

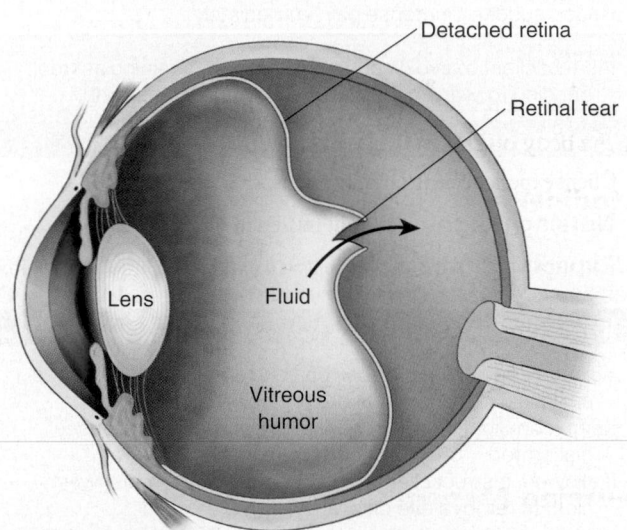

FIGURE 42-8. Retinal detachment.

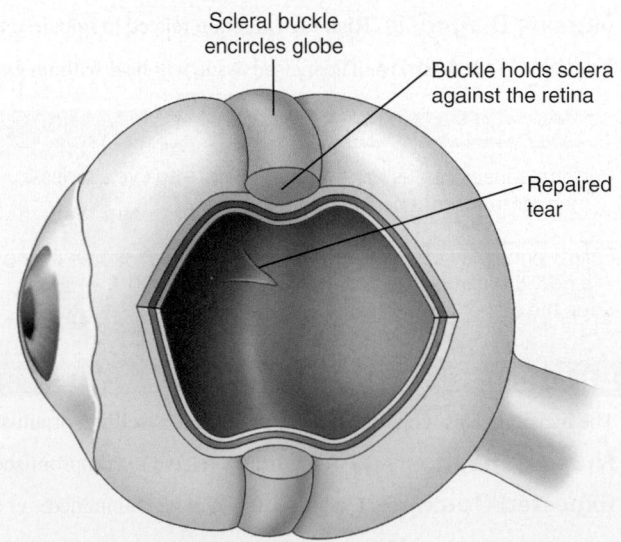

FIGURE 42-9. Scleral buckle.

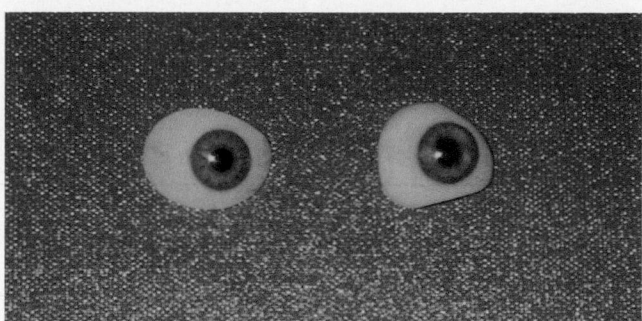

FIGURE 42-10. Eye prostheses. (*Left*) Anophthalmic ocular prosthesis. (*Right*) Scleral shell. (From Smeltzer, S. C., et al. [2008]. *Brunner & Suddarth's textbook of medical–surgical nursing* [11th ed.]. Philadelphia: Lippincott Williams & Wilkins.)

ENUCLEATION

Enucleation is the surgical removal of an eye. It is necessary when the eye is destroyed by injury or disease, when a malignant tumor develops (rare), or to relieve pain if the eye is severely damaged and sightless. Sometimes only the contents of the eyeball are removed and the sclera is left in place. Other times, the entire eyeball is removed as well as tissues in the bony orbit.

Medical and Surgical Management

When enucleation is performed, a metal or plastic ball is buried in the capsule of connective tissue from which the eyeball is removed. A pressure dressing is applied to control hemorrhage, a complication of enucleation. After the tissues have healed, a shell-shaped prosthesis is placed over the buried ball (Fig. 42-10). The shell is painted to match the client's remaining eye. The shell is the only portion that is removed for cleaning.

Nursing Management

The nurse observes the client after surgery for signs and symptoms of bleeding or infection. The client usually is allowed out of bed the day after surgery. When healing is complete, in about 2 to 4 weeks, the nurse teaches the client how to insert and remove the prosthetic shell. The prosthesis typically is removed before going to bed and inserted the next morning. The nurse instructs the client to hold the head over a soft surface, such as a bed or padded table, when removing or inserting the prosthesis to avoid damage if he or she drops the prosthetic eye. The client should clean the shell after removal and keep it in a safe place where it will not become scratched or broken.

CRITICAL THINKING EXERCISES

1. Discuss preventive measures for transmitting an infectious eye disorder.

2. Explain the preoperative and postoperative management for a client undergoing a cataract extraction.

3. A client has a family history of glaucoma and is concerned that she will suddenly go blind, like her grandmother. What should you tell her would be reasons to seek immediate medical attention?

4. You are a new LPN/LVN working in a physician's office that has a large percentage of older clients. Many of them use eyedrops. After reviewing the procedure for administration of eyedrops, outline what instructions you will provide to your clients.

NCLEX-STYLE REVIEW QUESTIONS

1. The nurse is assessing a client with a history of cataracts. Which of the following findings would indicate that the client is experiencing a recurrence?
   1. The client notices definite gaps in vision or blind spots.
   2. The client reports that the visual image is blurred or cloudy.
   3. Tears flow incessantly throughout the examination.
   4. The client's eyes are red and swollen.

2. The nurse is providing teaching for a client with blepharitis. Which of the following would the nurse be most likely to recommend?
   1. Avoid outdoor activities.
   2. Frequently wash the face and hair.
   3. Avoid use of soap on the face.
   4. Use dark glasses at all times.

3. A client has glaucoma that has not been treated. Which of the following symptoms caused by chronic progression of the disease is the client most likely to report to the nurse?
   1. Bulging eyes
   2. Double vision
   3. Tunnel vision
   4. Bloodshot eyes

4. A client has angle-closure glaucoma. Once the intraocular pressure has been temporarily reduced, an iridectomy is performed. When the nurse assesses the operative eye following surgery, which finding is most expected?
   1. The pupil appears cloudy and gray.
   2. The pupil is a fixed size and shape.
   3. There is absence of colored area of the iris.
   4. A section of the iris appears black.

5. The client with a detached retina undergoes a scleral buckling procedure. Postoperatively, which client problem should be the nurse's highest priority?
   1. Pain
   2. Vomiting
   3. Anxiety
   4. Boredom

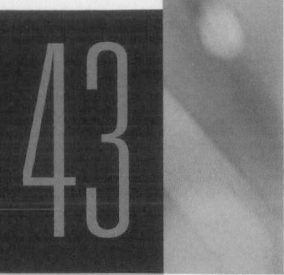

43

Caring for Clients with Ear Disorders

Words To Know

acoustic neuroma
cochlear implant
labyrinthitis
mastoidectomy
mastoiditis
Ménière's disease
myringoplasty
myringotomy
otalgia
otitis externa
otitis media
otosclerosis
ototoxicity
presbycusis
sign language
speech reading
stapedectomy
tinnitus
tympanotomy

Learning Objectives

On completion of this chapter, you will be able to:

1. List types of hearing impairment and the acuity levels for each.
2. Name techniques that clients with impaired hearing use to communicate with others.
3. Give examples of support services available for the hearing impaired.
4. Discuss the role of the nurse in caring for clients with a hearing loss.
5. Name conditions that involve the external ear.
6. Explain the technique for straightening the ear canal of adults to facilitate inspection and the administration of medication.
7. Discuss methods for preventing or treating disorders of the external ear.
8. Name conditions that affect the middle ear.
9. Describe nursing interventions appropriate for managing the care of a client with ear surgery.
10. Explain the pathophysiology of Ménière's disease, and name some consequences of this inner-ear disorder.
11. Discuss the nursing management of clients with Ménière's disease.

E ar disorders occur throughout the life cycle. Many ear disorders result in hearing loss, a common sensory deficit among older adults. Hearing aids can compensate for some but not all forms of hearing loss. Nurses play a pivotal role in preventing hearing loss by reducing the severity and frequency of ear infections among children and advocating for measures that reduce exposure to loud noise.

HEARING IMPAIRMENT

Hearing impairment is described as mild, moderate, severe, or profound, depending on the intensity of sound required for a person to hear it (Table 43-1). Diminished hearing results from a conductive loss, sensorineural loss, or both. Conductive hearing loss occurs from conditions such as an accumulation of cerumen in the external acoustic meatus or failure of the tiny ear bones to vibrate. Sensorineural hearing loss includes such etiologies as atherosclerosis, a tumor of the vestibulocochlear nerve, infections, and drug toxicity. **Presbycusis** is hearing impairment that is associated with old age. Clients with a hearing impairment often have **tinnitus**, in which the client hears buzzing, whistling, or ringing noises in one or both ears. Box 43-1 elaborates on causes of conductive and sensorineural hearing loss. Hearing loss also can result from repeated exposure to excessive noise, such as live concerts, high volumes from stereos or headphones, or a loud work environment (machinery or jackhammers).

TABLE 43-1 Hearing Acuity

HEARING RANGE	DECIBELS (DB)	WITHOUT A HEARING AID	WITH A HEARING AID
Normal	20–120	Can hear faint to painful sounds	Unnecessary
Mild impairment	40–120	Cannot hear unvoiced consonants such as "s" and "f"	Helpful, but not necessarily worth the expense
Moderate impairment	60–120	Cannot hear conversational volume unless others talk loudly	Beneficial for restoring ability to hear normal conversations
Severe impairment	70–120	Misses most conversational content	Amplifies 40 dB sounds to 75 dB, but also amplifies nonspeech and background noise
Profound impairment	90–120	Depends heavily on speech reading	Helps hearing vowels, but amplified speech and background noise are painful
Total deafness	120	Hears only painfully loud sounds or vibrations created by loud sounds	Not useful for understanding speech

Hearing loss seriously impairs the ability to protect oneself and communicate with others. The age at which hearing loss occurs plus the severity of the impairment have extensive consequences. For example, hearing loss during the first 3 years of life, the most critical period for learning to make sounds, affects language acquisition at the word, phrase, and sentence levels. If uncorrected, hearing deficits can lead to depression and social isolation.

BOX 43-1 Common Causes of Conductive and Sensorineural Hearing Loss

Conductive Hearing Loss
- External ear conditions
  - Impacted ear wax or foreign body
  - Otitis externa
- Middle ear conditions
  - Trauma
  - Otitis media
  - Otosclerosis
  - Tumors

Sensorineural Hearing Loss
- Trauma
  - Head injury
  - Noise
- Central nervous system infections (e.g., meningitis)
- Degenerative conditions
  - Presbycusis
- Vascular conditions
  - Atherosclerosis
- Ototoxic drugs
- Tumors
- Ménière's disease

Mixed Conductive and Sensorineural Hearing Loss
- Middle ear conditions
- Temporal bone fractures

Adapted from Porth, C. M. (2007). *Essentials of pathophysiology: Concepts of altered health states* [2nd ed.], p. 889. Philadelphia: Lippincott Williams & Wilkins.

Medical Management

Besides treating the cause of the hearing loss, medical management includes a recommendation for a hearing aid, a battery-operated device that fits behind the ear, in the ear, or in the ear canal and amplifies sound. Clients with a conductive hearing loss benefit more from the use of a hearing aid because the structures that convert sound into energy and facilitate perception of sound in the brain continue to function. Clients who use hearing aids are challenged with some related problems. Some experience a whistling noise because of a poor fit or improper function. Others may not have the appropriate hearing aid for their hearing loss. It is important that clients seek assistance when they have hearing aid problems. Client and Family Teaching 43-1 provides tips for hearing aid care.

Some clients with hearing deficits learn **sign language**, a method for communication that uses a hand-spelled alphabet and word symbols (see Fig. 7-6 in Chap. 7). Clients also learn **speech reading**, also called *lip reading*.

Many technological devices have been developed to promote communication. Some television programs are transmitted using closed-caption inserts in which the dialogue is printed on the bottom of the screen or a person who simultaneously signs is displayed in a corner of the screen. Some theaters provide headsets that amplify actors' voices for individual patrons. Theaters are also increasingly offering closed captioning for patrons. Telephones can be adapted with a hearing amplifier that increases sound from incoming callers. Text-based telecommunications equipment, such as the telecommunication device for the deaf (TDD), teletype (TTY), and text telephone (TT), were designed for people with severe hearing impairments. These devices are a combination of a special typewriter keyboard and telephone used to call someone else with a similar machine. For people who use TDDs or similar devices, a business directory is available, or the users can call a relay center and the center will communicate for them. Computer modems also facilitate communication.

Many other products allow the hearing impaired to perceive (rather than hear) sound. For example, light-activated alarms in smoke detectors, alarm clocks, doorbells, and telephones flash when sound is produced. Hearing dogs, such as guide dogs for the blind, are specially trained to warn their owners when certain sounds occur.

Client and Family Teaching 43-1
Tips for Hearing Aid Care

The nurse emphasizes the following points when teaching the client:

Cleaning

● Wash only the ear mold with soap and water, daily or frequently.
● Clean cannula with a small pipe-cleaner–like device.
● Make sure ear mold is dry before snapping onto receiver.

Malfunctioning

● Inadequate amplification, a whistling noise, or pain from the ear mold may be signs of malfunctioning.
● If a hearing aid malfunctions:
    ● Ensure that the switch is on.
    ● Check that batteries are charged and in position.
    ● Contact hearing aid dealer if the above does not fix the problem.

Recognizing Complications

● The external auditory canal is prone to increased moistness secondary to occlusion from the hearing aid.
● Seek medical treatment if symptoms related to otitis externa or pressure ulcers in the external auditory canal or meatus occur.

Adapted from Smeltzer, S. C., et al. (2008). *Brunner & Suddarth's textbook of medical–surgical nursing* [11th ed.], p. 2122. Philadelphia: Lippincott Williams & Wilkins.

Surgical Management

Sensorineural hearing loss usually is irreversible. For the client who is profoundly deaf or has severe hearing loss and for whom a hearing aid is ineffective, a **cochlear implant** may be beneficial. This device has an external microphone that captures incoming sounds, as well as an external sound processor implanted behind the ear that captures the sound, converts it to digital signals, and sends them to an internal implant. This internal processor converts the signals into electrical energy and stimulates the auditory nerve. The brain then perceives this as sound (Fig. 43-1). A cochlear implant does not restore normal hearing, and what a person hears through a cochlear implant is not the same things as the amplified sounds he or she hears through a hearing aid. However, the cochlear implant does provide a means for clients to learn or relearn sounds in the environment and to understand speech.

Nursing Management

The nurse observes for signs of hearing impairment such as leaning forward, turning and cupping the ear to hear better, and asking that words be repeated (Box 43-2). He or she assesses gross hearing using the techniques described earlier (as described in Chap. 41). The nurse also determines the clarity of the client's speech. He or she refers a client for the diagnosis and subsequent treatment of a hearing impairment, as well as speech therapy. Many people reject the idea that their hearing is impaired. Some consider it a sign of aging and deterioration. If the client fears that wearing a hearing aid is a stigma, the nurse describes the various types of hearing aids that are available, some of which fit almost unnoticeably in the ear (Fig. 43-2). The nurse also stresses the importance of avoiding the purchase of a hearing aid from a mail-order catalogue or a company salesperson.

Gerontologic Considerations

- Unfamiliar environments may contribute to disorientation or confusion in the hearing impaired older adult. Nursing interventions should include speaking clearly in a low tone of normal volume during frequent reorientations and teaching related to assistive hearing devices. The client's ability to care for the assistive device will influence selection of a hearing aid from various styles available.

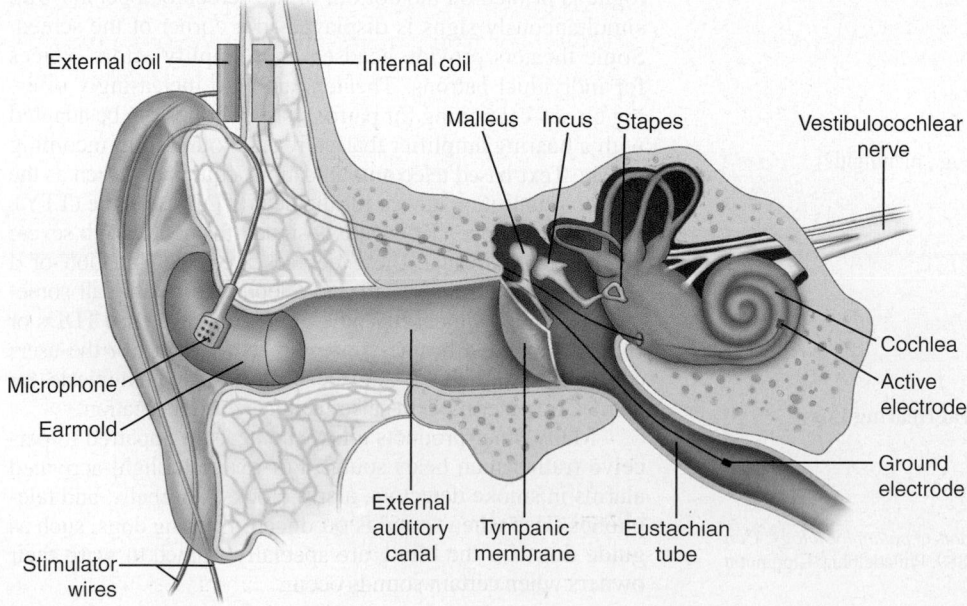

FIGURE 43-1. With a cochlear implant, sound is passed from the external transmitter to the inner coil by magnetic conduction and is then carried over an electrode to the cochlea.

Speech deterioration: slurring or dropping ends of words
Fatigue: result of straining to hear
Indifference: related to depression, isolation, or disinterest
Social withdrawal: afraid to participate in social activities
Insecurity: lack of self-confidence
Indecision and procrastination: fear of making mistakes
Suspiciousness: fear that people are talking about him or her because of inability to hear the whole conversation
False pride: attempts to hide hearing loss
Loneliness and unhappiness: boredom, isolation, and fear
Tendency to dominate the conversation: able to control the conversation

Adapted from Smeltzer, S.C., et al. (2008). *Brunner & Suddarth's textbook of medical–surgical nursing* (11th ed.), p. 2102. Philadelphia: Lippincott Williams & Wilkins.

If a hearing impairment exists, the nurse obtains information about its severity and the methods used to understand the speech of others. When a client hears poorly, the nurse determines the communication method the client prefers: speech reading, signing, writing, or typing. Suggestions for

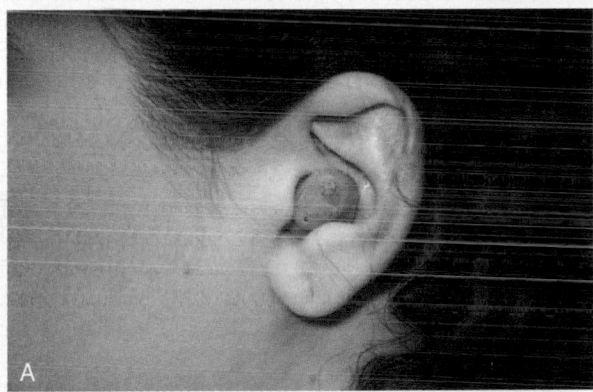

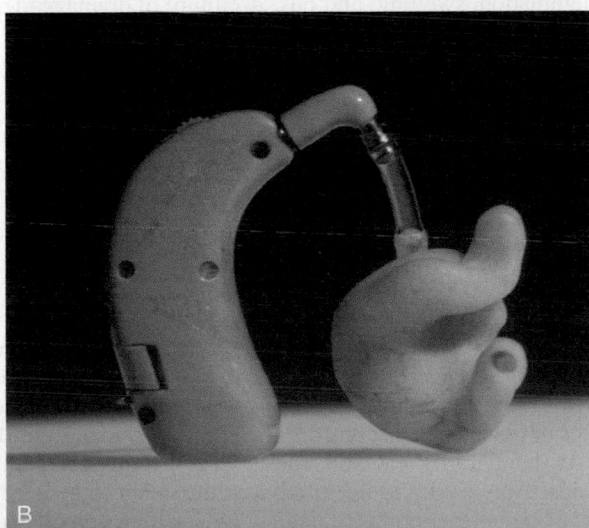

FIGURE 43-2. Examples of hearing aids. (**A**) in the ear, (**B**) behind-the-ear. (© Custom Medical Stock Photo.)

oral communication are listed in Nursing Guidelines 43-1. If the client uses a hearing aid, the nurse safeguards the instrument, assists the client with its insertion, and helps maintain its function.

To protect their self-esteem, some clients with a hearing impairment nod their heads as if they are following the conversation or laugh along with others to conceal the fact that they do not understand what has been said. The nurse encourages clients with a hearing loss to be forthright and inform others about the hearing deficit. In addition, he or she identifies assistive hearing devices and aids for communication discussed earlier. The nurse advises clients to maintain previously established relationships because a physical impairment is unlikely to affect genuine friendships.

The nurse uses illustrations, pamphlets, and written directions to aid teaching and includes a family member. He or she asks the client to repeat information and demonstrate technical skills. The nurse initiates a referral to a community agency to evaluate if and how well the client is performing self-care after discharge.

▶ *Stop, Think, and Respond Exercise 43-1*

What recommendations can you make for someone to prevent injury to the ears or hearing loss?

DISORDERS OF THE EXTERNAL EAR

Various disorders such as impacted cerumen, injury from foreign objects, or otitis externa affect the external acoustic meatus. If these disorders are not treated carefully and adequately, they may spread to the middle ear.

IMPACTED CERUMEN

Impacted cerumen is accumulated ear wax that obstructs the external acoustic meatus.

Pathophysiology and Etiology

Impacted cerumen is more common among people who have excessive thick or dry cerumen. Both qualities interfere with drainage toward the proximal end of the meatus, where cerumen normally leaves the ear during regular shampooing and showering. The trapped cerumen interferes with the transmission of sounds carried on air waves.

Assessment Findings

The client reports having a sense of fullness or pain in the ears, referred to as **otalgia**, and diminished hearing. The client asks that words be repeated, misinterprets questions, or raises the volume on the television or radio. Visual inspection with an otoscope shows an orange-brown accumulation of cerumen in the distal end of the external acoustic meatus. Audiometric, Rinne, and Weber tests reveal conductive hearing loss.

Medical Management

Dried cerumen is hydrated by instilling 1 or 2 drops of half-strength peroxide, warm glycerin, or mineral oil, or it is

NURSING GUIDELINES 43-1

Communicating With People Who Have a Hearing Loss

- Eliminate background noise as much as possible.
- Stand or sit on the side of the client's better ear.
- Ensure that there is adequate natural or artificial light.
- Get the client's attention.
- Face the client.
- Speak clearly and at a normal pace without exaggerating pronunciations.
- Do not shout, but avoid dropping conversational volume at the end of a sentence.

- Promote a clear image of your mouth; do not chew gum or cover your mouth.
- Use gestures and facial expressions to enhance what is being said orally.
- Rephrase whatever the client does not understand.
- Remain patient, positive, and relaxed.
- Provide paper and pencil if the client communicates by sign language or has speech that is difficult to understand.
- Use a support person who can communicate by signing.

softened with commercial agents, such as carbamide peroxide (Debrox) and triethanolamine (Cerumenex). Cerumen is removed mechanically by irrigating the ear if the eardrum is intact or using an instrument called a *cerumen spoon*.

Nursing Management

The nurse inspects the ears and implements measures to remove excessive cerumen. Ear drops can be warmed by holding the container in the hand for a few moments or placing it in warm water. If irrigation or instillation of liquids is ordered, the nurse warms the liquid to body temperature. Cold or hot liquids cause dizziness, and the potential for injury exists if the liquid is hot. The nurse avoids inserting the irrigating syringe too deeply so as to close off the auditory canal. He or she directs the flow toward the roof of the canal rather than the eardrum.

FOREIGN OBJECTS

Pathophysiology and Etiology

Foreign objects find their way into the ear either by accident or by deliberate insertion. Sharp objects can scratch the skin or cause blunt penetration of the eardrum. Insect stings cause local inflammation of the tissue.

Assessment Findings

The client describes discomfort, diminished hearing, feeling movement, or hearing a buzzing sound. On gross inspection, there is evidence of abrasion from trauma, or an insect or an object is seen. Inspection with a penlight or otoscope reveals swelling and redness in the auditory canal.

Medical Management

Mineral oil is instilled into the ear to smother an insect. Solid objects are removed with small forceps.

Nursing Management

The nurse instructs clients to clean the ears with a face cloth rather than inserting objects into the ears. A hat with earflaps or a scarf is recommended when venturing into the woods or other areas with a high insect population.

OTITIS EXTERNA

Otitis externa is an inflammation of the tissue in the outer ear.

Pathophysiology and Etiology

Inflammation usually is caused by an overgrowth of pathogens. The microorganisms tend to follow trauma to the lining of the ear, or their growth is supported by retained moisture from swimming. Another possibility is that a hair follicle becomes infected, causing a furuncle or an abscess to develop.

Assessment Findings

The tissue in the external ear looks red. Sometimes it is difficult to see the tympanic membrane because of swelling. Clients describe discomfort that increases with manipulation during the examination. Hearing is reduced because of swelling. In severe infections, a fever develops and the lymph nodes behind the ear enlarge.

Otoscopic examination reveals diffuse or confined inflammation, swelling, and pus. A culture of drainage identifies the specific pathogen.

Medical Management

Treatment includes warm soaks, analgesics, and antibiotic ear medication, often with corticosteroid medication, such as neomycin/polymyxin/hydrocortisone otic solution (Cortisporin, Otocort).

Nursing Management

The nurse instructs the client to carry out the medical treatment and provides health teaching to prevent recurrence. For example, he or she advises swimmers to wear soft plastic ear plugs to prevent trapping water in the ear. If chewing produces or potentiates discomfort, the nurse encourages the client to temporarily eat soft foods or consume nourishing liquids. Above all, the nurse advises the client to avoid the use of nonprescription remedies unless they have been approved by the physician and to contact the physician if symptoms are not relieved in a few days.

DISORDERS OF THE MIDDLE EAR

OTITIS MEDIA

Otitis media is an acute inflammation or infection in the middle ear. Clients may have acute or chronic forms of either serous otitis media, also known as secretory or nonsuppurative otitis media, or the purulent or suppurative type. Although otitis media is more common among young children, adults can and do develop middle ear infections.

Pathophysiology and Etiology

Serous otitis media, a collection of pathogen-free fluid behind the tympanic membrane, results from irritation associated with respiratory allergies and enlarged adenoids. Purulent otitis media usually results from the spread of microorganisms from the eustachian tube to the middle ear during upper respiratory infections.

When fluid or pus collects in the middle ear, pressure increases, which causes the eardrum to bulge and spontaneously rupture in some cases. Rupture results in a jagged tear of tissue that heals slowly and sometimes incompletely. Scarring interferes with the vibration of the eardrum, causing diminished hearing. Clients with perforated eardrums are prone to repeated infections.

Other potentially serious complications can occur. Because the middle ear connects with the mastoid process, a part of the temporal bone, pathogens that are unresponsive to antibiotic therapy can spread, causing **mastoiditis**, or they can travel deeper in the inner ear, causing **labyrinthitis**. Infection also may extend to the meninges, causing meningitis, or brain abscess may result from its extension to the brain. If septicemia occurs, the infection can spread to the large veins at the base of the brain and cause lateral sinus thrombosis. Facial nerve damage and facial paralysis may result from the infection. With prompt and adequate treatment, complications are rare.

Assessment Findings

The client often describes a history of having had a recent upper respiratory infection or seasonal allergies. Signs and symptoms vary widely depending on the type and severity of the inflammation but may include a fever, tinnitus, malaise, severe earache, and diminished hearing. Tenderness behind the ear indicates mastoiditis. The eardrum looks red and bulging. Pressure in the middle ear or dysfunction of inner ear structures can cause nausea, vomiting, and dizziness. If the tympanic membrane perforates, fluid drains into the external acoustic canal and pain is relieved.

The white blood cell count shows an elevated number of neutrophils and eosinophils. If the eardrum has ruptured and drainage is present, the cultured drainage reveals a specific infectious microorganism.

Medical and Surgical Management

Prompt treatment usually prevents rupture of the eardrum. In some cases, the fluid is aspirated by needle. Antibiotics are given to control the infection. The overuse of antibiotics, however, has created another problem: microorganisms are becoming resistant and, for some infections, the available antibiotics are of limited benefit.

To reduce the consequences of spontaneous rupture of the eardrum, subsequent scarring, and hearing loss, the physician performs a **myringotomy** or **tympanotomy**, an incisional opening of the tympanic membrane. The incised opening facilitates drainage of the purulent material, eases the pressure, and relieves the throbbing pain. The incision heals readily, with little scarring.

Plastic surgery (**myringoplasty**) usually is successful in repairing the perforated eardrum. In one technique, the edges of the perforation are cauterized and a patch of blood-soaked absorbable gelatin sponge (Gelfoam) is used as a scaffolding over which new tissue grows until it has filled in the defect. Chronic infections are prevented if the eardrum is repaired. In the case of mastoiditis, a **mastoidectomy** is performed to remove the diseased tissue. With early and effective antibiotic therapy, mastoiditis is rare.

Nursing Management

After myringotomy, the discharge from the ear is bloody and then purulent. To remove the drainage, the nurse wipes the external ear repeatedly with a dry sterile cotton applicator. An alternative is to insert a loose (not tightly packed) cotton pledget in the external ear to collect drainage. The nurse changes the cotton when it becomes moist.

OTOSCLEROSIS

Otosclerosis is the result of a bony overgrowth of the stapes and a common cause of hearing impairment among adults. Fixation of the stapes occurs gradually over many years.

Pathophysiology and Etiology

The underlying cause of otosclerosis is unknown. The condition, which is more common in women than in men, usually becomes apparent in the second and third decades of life. It seems to be accelerated during pregnancy. Most clients have a family history of the disease, which indicates a possible hereditary relationship.

Otosclerosis interferes with the vibration of the stapes and the transmission of sound to the inner ear. Although hearing loss in otosclerosis is of the conductive type, when and if progression of the disease involving the cochlea of the inner ear occurs, a mixed type of hearing loss develops.

Assessment Findings

Signs and Symptoms

A progressive, bilateral loss of hearing is the most characteristic symptom. The client notices the hearing loss when it begins to interfere with the ability to follow conversation. There is particular difficulty hearing others when they speak in soft, low tones, but hearing is adequate when the sound is loud enough. Tinnitus appears as the loss of hearing progresses. It is especially noticeable at night, when surroundings are quiet, and can be quite distressing to the client.

The eardrum appears pinkish-orange from structural changes in the middle ear. When the Rinne test is performed, the sound is heard best when the tuning fork is applied behind the ear. The sound lateralizes to the more affected ear when the Weber test is performed.

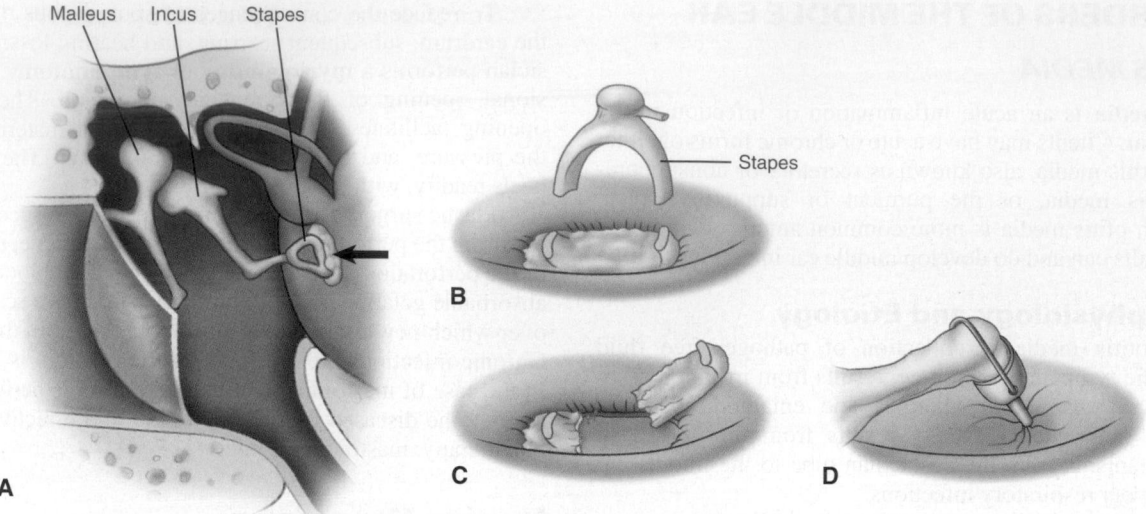

FIGURE 43-3. Stapedectomy for otosclerosis. (**A**) Arrow points to the diseased area at the foot of the stapes in the middle ear. (**B**) Stapes broken away surgically from its diseased base. (**C**) The footplate is removed from its base. Tissue is placed over any remaining otosclerotic tissue. (**D**) A metal prosthetic stapes in position bridges the gap between the incus and inner ear, improving sound conduction.

Diagnostic Findings

Audiometric tests reveal the type and severity of hearing loss. A computed tomography (CT) scan demonstrates the location and extent of excessive bone growth.

Medical and Surgical Management

Although otosclerosis has no cure, a hearing aid helps. The level of restored hearing depends greatly on the severity of the sensorineural involvement. The outcome is best when the hearing loss is purely conductive. If the surgical treatment is selected, a **stapedectomy** is performed on the ear most affected. In this procedure, all or part of the stapes is removed and a prosthesis is inserted that can vibrate the oval window (Fig. 43-3). Once the stapes is freed or replaced, the client experiences an immediate, dramatic improvement in hearing. Hearing temporarily diminishes after surgery because of swelling, but eventually returns. Complications include dislodgment of the prosthesis and continued hearing loss, infection, dizziness, and facial nerve damage. Depending on the outcome of surgery, the procedure may be repeated for the opposite ear.

Nursing Management

The nurse uses selected alternatives for communicating with the client as identified earlier in Nursing Guidelines 43-1. It is important to give the preoperative client an explanation of what to expect in the immediate postoperative period. The nurse tells the client that activity is restricted for 24 hours or more after surgery and that hearing may be temporarily the same as or worse than before surgery.

After surgery, the nurse positions the client on the nonoperative side. He or she takes care to prevent dislodgment of the prosthesis as a result of coughing, sneezing, or vomiting. Nausea and dizziness are common problems. The nurse assesses facial nerve function by checking symmetry when the client smiles or frowns.

Nursing Process for the Client Recovering From Stapedectomy

Assessment

After the client returns from surgery, take vital signs as well as monitor for complications, drainage from the affected ear, and level of discomfort. It is important to report any elevation in temperature.

Diagnosis, Planning, and Interventions

▶ Impaired Comfort (pain, nausea, vertigo) related to tissue disruption (Carpenito-Moyet, 2008, p. 118)

▶ Expected Outcome: Client will experience relief of discomfort to at least a tolerable level.

- Administer prescribed analgesic and assess again in 30 minutes. *Ongoing assessment determines effectiveness of pain medication. Response to pain and pain medication is unique for each client.*
- Give an antiemetic for nausea or vomiting. *Antiemetics promote relief of nausea.*
- Validate client's feelings of discomfort. *This measure promotes the nurse–client relationship and reassures the client that his or her needs are important.*
- Provide small, frequent sips of fluid or light food. *Doing so prevents nausea.*
- Limit head movement and avoid jarring the bed. *Movement aggravates vertigo. Limiting movement minimizes pain, dizziness, and nausea.*

▶ Risk for Infection related to impaired tissue integrity secondary to the surgical incision

▶ Expected Outcome: Client will remain free of a secondary infection.

- Adhere strictly to aseptic principles when changing a dressing or cleaning the ear. *Using aseptic technique reduces the introduction and transmission of microorganisms and protects the client from exposure to pathogens.*
- Administer prescribed antibiotics. *Appropriate and timely administration of antibiotics promotes a consistent blood level needed to treat or prevent infection.*
- Instruct client to keep his or her hands away from the dressing or packing. *Doing so maintains integrity of the dressings and prevents contamination from opportunistic infections.*
- Keep external ear and surrounding skin meticulously clean and free of purulent drainage. *This measure promotes healing and prevents infection through reduction of microorganisms.*

▶ **Risk for Injury** related to vertigo

▶ **Expected Outcome:** Client will be free of injury.

- Encourage client to use the side rails and handrails for support when preparing to ambulate. *Side and hand rails prevent client from falling or causing injury to the affected ear. Basic safety measures prevent injury.*
- Walk with the client who is dizzy. *Assistance promotes the client's safety and reduces the chance for injury.*

Evaluation of Expected Outcomes

The client remains comfortable, as evidenced by minimal complaints of pain, and no complaints of nausea or vertigo. He or she has no signs or symptoms of infection. The client experiences mild vertigo but maintains safety. The prescribed medical regimen and restrictions are discussed with the client or a family member. Client and Family Teaching 43-2 reviews other teaching points important to include in a discharge plan. ●

 Client and Family Teaching 43-2
The Client With a Stapedectomy

The nurse teaches the client and family members to:

- Refrain from blowing the nose because this action can dislodge the prosthesis.
- Avoid high altitudes or flying.
- Refrain from lifting heavy objects, straining when defecating, or bending over at the waist; these activities increase pressure in the middle ear.
- Prevent water from getting in the ear. Avoid swimming, showering, and washing the hair until approved by the physician.
- Follow the physician's instructions for keeping the ear clean.
- Stay away from people with respiratory infections. If a head cold occurs, contact the physician immediately.
- Notify the physician immediately if severe pain, excessive drainage, a sudden loss of hearing, or fever occurs.
- Adhere to the restriction of activities recommended by the physician until told otherwise.

DISORDERS OF THE INNER EAR

MÉNIÈRE'S DISEASE

Ménière's disease is a term given to the episodic symptoms created by fluctuations in the production or reabsorption of fluid in the inner ear. This ear disease is analogous to glaucoma of the eye in that there is too much circulating fluid (Smeltzer et al., 2008).

Pathophysiology and Etiology

Acute attacks of Ménière's disease appear to be associated with changes in fluid volume within the labyrinth of the inner ear, which consists of bony and membranous parts. This structure is needed for both hearing and balance. The bony labyrinth protects the delicate membranous inner ear, and the membranous labyrinth is filled with a fluid called endolymph. When a person moves his or her head, the endolymph also moves, and nerve receptors within the membranous labyrinth send signals to the brain about the movement. In Ménière's disease, an increase in endolymph causes the membranous labyrinth to dilate like a balloon; this is referred to as endolymphatic hydrops. The drainage system or endolymphatic duct becomes blocked. The blockage sometimes results from scar tissue or congenital narrowing of the duct. Eventually, hair cells in the inner ear are destroyed, which leads to functional deafness. In addition, the inner ear structures are disrupted and distorted, leading to chronic problems with imbalance and unsteadiness even when clients are not experiencing attacks.

The cause of Ménière's disease is not known. Generally, physicians attribute the disease to viral infections of the inner ear, a head injury, hereditary factors, or allergic reactions. More recent theories about its etiology center on autoimmune factors.

Ménière's disease typically is unilateral, appears during middle age, and occurs equally in men and women. It causes a triad of hearing loss, vertigo, and tinnitus. When the fluid accumulates, it dilates the cochlear duct, which diminishes hearing. It also affects equilibrium as the vestibular system becomes damaged, and tinnitus occurs. At times, the client is symptom free except for permanent, residual hearing loss as the number of attacks increase. Occasionally, clients recover spontaneously.

Assessment Findings

Onset of Ménière's disease may be sudden, and symptoms may occur daily or infrequently. Vertigo is the most incapacitating symptom; clients report whirling dizziness and the need to lie down. Severe vertigo causes nausea and vomiting. Typically, clients also experience tinnitus and hearing loss that lasts for several hours as well as headaches and abdominal discomfort. Nystagmus of the eyes may result from an imbalance in vestibular control of eye movements. Generally, hearing returns between attacks but gradually becomes worse with repeated attacks.

An attack lasts from a few minutes to weeks. Because episodes can be unexpected, some clients are reluctant to leave their homes for fear they will have an attack in public. Continued employment becomes impossible for some clients.

In addition to a thorough medical history and physical examination, clients should have hearing and balance tests. A caloric stimulation test and electronystagmography (ENG) demonstrate a difference in eye movement response. A CT scan or magnetic resonance imaging (MRI) rules out other possible causes of the symptoms, such as a tumor that involves the vestibulocochlear nerve. Audiometry identifies the type and magnitude of the hearing deficit. Electro-cochleography, which records the electrical activity of the inner ear in response to sound, helps confirm the diagnosis.

Medical and Surgical Management

Treatment aims at reducing fluid production in the inner ear, facilitating its drainage, and treating the symptoms that accompany the attack. A low-sodium or sodium-free diet lessens edema. Smoking is contraindicated to prevent vaso-constriction, which interferes with fluid drainage. Treatment of the allergy or avoidance of the allergen is recommended. Bed rest may be necessary during acute attacks. Specific drug therapy may include the following:

- Meclizine (Antivert)—an antihistamine often prescribed because it suppresses the vestibular system
- Diazepam (Valium) or other tranquilizers—may be or-dered for acute episodes to help control vertigo; used only for short-term therapy because of the addictive potential
- Promethazine (Phenergan)—an antiemetic to help control the nausea and vomiting; has an antihistamine effect
- Hydrochlorothiazide or other diuretics—may decrease the fluid in the endolymphatic system and relieve symptoms

If clients become extremely incapacitated, surgery becomes an option. Surgeries range from decompression of the endolymphatic sac to insertion of intraotologic catheters to vestibular nerve section. Box 43-3 presents a brief description of specific surgical procedures.

Nursing Management

The nurse obtains a history of symptoms, their duration, and complete medical, drug, and allergy histories. He or she assesses gross hearing and performs the Rinne and Weber tests. It also is important to determine the extent and effect of the client's disability.

The client with Ménière's disease requires a great deal of emotional support because of the unpredictability of the attacks and the resulting impairments. During an attack, the nurse administers prescribed drugs, limits movement, and promotes the client's safety. He or she assists the client with activities of daily living because the least amount of motion can produce severe vertigo.

The nurse is available, empathic, and responsive to the client. Trust and confidence develop when the client does not feel abandoned or required to convince caregivers of the necessity for attention. Clients are comforted when the nurse acknowledges that dealing with temporary or permanent hearing loss is a challenge.

If a low-sodium or salt-free diet is recommended, the di-etitian provides a list of foods to avoid or a specific diet to follow. If an allergy is suspected as the cause of the disorder, the nurse advises the client to take the prescribed antihist-amines as directed and to avoid known allergens. If a hearing aid is recommended, the nurse refers the client to an audiolo-gist for instructions on its use and care.

> ### Stop, Think, and Respond Exercise 43-2
>
> *A nurse admits a client with Ménière's disease who is having an acute episode. After assessing the client, the nurse selects Risk for Deficient Fluid Volume as the best nursing diagnosis. Complete the diagnostic state-ment with expected outcomes.*

OTOTOXICITY

Ototoxicity describes the detrimental effect of certain medi-cations on the eighth cranial nerve or hearing structures. Signs and symptoms of ototoxicity include tinnitus and sen-sorineural hearing loss. Vestibular toxicity includes signs and symptoms of light-headedness, vertigo, nausea, and vomiting. Drugs associated with ototoxicity include salicy-lates, loop diuretics, quinidine, quinine, and aminoglycosides. Box 43-4 lists selected ototoxic substances. It is important that nurses be knowledgeable about the ototoxic effects of certain medications. Nurses must carefully monitor the dosage and frequency of administration as well as assess the client for changes in hearing.

BOX 43-3 | **Surgical Procedures for Ménière's Disease**

- *Endolymphatic sac decompression*: A shunting procedure that involves the insertion of a shunt or drain in the endo-lymphatic sac to equalize pressure in the endolymphatic space. This procedure is safe and usually is the first choice. It is done as an outpatient procedure.
- *Middle and inner ear perfusion*: Antibiotics, such as genta-micin or streptomycin (considered to be ototoxic), are infused into the middle and inner ear. This procedure decreases vestibular function and vertigo, but holds a high risk for significant hearing loss. Clients usually stay over-night. Clients may experience a period of imbalance for sev-eral weeks.
- *Intraotologic catheters*: A catheter is inserted in the external ear canal through or around the tympanic membrane to the round window, for the purpose of instilling medications. Potential treatments are for sudden hearing loss, vertigo, tin-nitus, and slowly progressive sensorineural hearing loss.
- *Labyrinthectomy*: Excision of the labyrinth through the transcanal or transmastoid route assists in eliminating ver-tigo. Auditory function of the inner ear is destroyed, and potential complications include facial nerve injury and total hearing loss.
- *Vestibular nerve section*: This procedure has the highest success rate in eliminating vertigo and is used for clients who are incapacitated by Ménière's disease and already have significant hearing loss. Cutting the nerve prevents the brain from receiving input from the semicircular canals. The procedure requires a brief hospital stay.

(Adapted from Smeltzer, S. C., et al. [2008]. *Brunner & Suddarth's textbook of medical–surgical nursing* [11th ed.]. Philadelphia: Lippincott Williams & Wilkins, p. 2113.)

BOX 43-4 Selected Ototoxic Substances

Loop Diuretics
Bumetanide (Bumex)
Furosemide (Lasix)   *will help reduce excess fluid*
Acetazolamide

Chemotherapeutic Agents
Cisplatin
Carboplatin

Antimalarials
Quinine
Chloroquine

Anti-inflammatory Agents
Salicylates (aspirin)
Indomethacin

Chemicals
Alcohol
Arsenic

Aminoglycoside Antibiotics
Amikacin
Gentamicin
Kanamycin
Netilmicin
Neomycin
Streptomycin
Tobramycin

Other Antibiotics
Erythromycin
Minocycline
Polymyxin B
Vancomycin

Metals
Gold
Mercury
Lead

ACOUSTIC NEUROMA

An **acoustic neuroma**, also known as a vestibular schwannoma, is a benign Schwann cell tumor that progressively enlarges and adversely affects cranial nerve VIII (which consists of the vestibular and cochlear nerves). Most acoustic tumors arise in the auditory canal and extend into the cerebellar region, pressing on the brain stem.

Pathophysiology and Etiology

Acoustic neuromas are rare, occurring in 1 in 100,000 people. Men and women are affected equally, and diagnosis is usually made between the 30 and 60 years of age. The cause of acoustic neuroma is unknown. The tumor usually is unilateral. Hearing loss occurs secondary to compression of the cochlear nerve or interference with the blood supply to the nerve and cochlea.

Assessment Findings

Signs and symptoms vary according to the size and location of the tumor. The client may exhibit or experience any or all of the following signs and symptoms—usually unilateral:

- Hearing loss (usually gradual)
- Impaired facial movement
- Altered facial sensation, including numbness and tingling
- Tinnitus in the affected ear
- Vertigo with or without balance disturbance

Initial audiometric studies reveal significant differences in hearing and presence of tinnitus and vertigo. MRI or CT scans with contrast agents is done to determine the location and extent of the tumor. ENG may demonstrate nystagmus, which is related to inner ear problems. Cerebrospinal fluid (CSF) studies demonstrate increased pressure and the presence of proteins.

Medical and Surgical Management

Treatment depends on how fast the tumor is growing. In some instances, if the acoustic neuroma is small or growing slowly, or if the client is not experiencing symptoms, the physician may elect to monitor the client with regular assessments and tests. A form of radiation therapy called gamma-knife radiosurgery, which allows the physician to apply radiation beams without surgery, may also be useful (see Chap. 37). Imaging scans help the physician locate and direct the beams. Local anesthesia is generally given, and the client's head is in a lightweight frame to stabilize it. Generally the client will only have one treatment. It may take weeks, months, or even years before the effects of the radiosurgery are evident. The physician monitors the client with imaging and hearing studies. Clients may experience neck soreness and pain where the frame is attached to the head, but they usually resume activities within 24 hours of treatment.

Surgical removal of the tumor remains the preferred treatment. The challenge for the physician is to remove the tumor and retain facial nerve function. Usually hearing loss already has occurred, so destruction of the hearing mechanism that occurs with the surgical approach is not a consideration. If the client has little or no hearing loss, however, the suboccipital or middle cranial fossa approach is used, with close monitoring of cranial nerve VIII function.

Complications of acoustic neuroma excision include the following:

- Facial nerve paralysis
- CSF leak
- Meningitis
- Cerebral edema
- Increased intracranial pressure

Nursing Management

The assessment of a client with acoustic neuroma includes evaluating hearing function, observing the client's facial movements, and testing for facial sensation. If the client has hearing deficits, the nurse can use the communication measures outlined in Nursing Guidelines 43-1. For clients with vertigo, the nurse takes measures to protect the client from injury.

After surgery, the nurse implements the aforementioned measures as well as monitoring the client for signs of increased intracranial pressure, including restlessness, confusion, or unresponsiveness, pupillary changes, bradycardia, hypertension, and respiratory changes. It also is important that the nurse maintain strict asepsis to prevent transmission of microorganisms. Clients are at risk for wound infection and meningitis.

CRITICAL THINKING EXERCISES

1. A client with a history of Ménière's disease arrives at the clinic complaining of severe vertigo and nausea. What precautions are important to take while the client is at the clinic?
2. A male refugee from Somalia is scheduled for a mastoidectomy because of severe and untreated ear infections that affected the mastoid. Identify two goals for this client after he returns from surgery.
3. A young woman comes in the clinic complaining of severe pain of her left ear; it hurts to touch it. She says that she swims at least 3 days a week. She is diagnosed with otitis externa. The nurse practitioner prescribes analgesics and application of heat to the affected ear and also tells the client to avoid swimming for 2 weeks. Because this client swims regularly for exercise, what further instructions can the nurse provide to prevent future problems?
4. A client is diagnosed with an acoustic neuroma. The client asks the nurse why this is a problem because it is not cancerous?

NCLEX-STYLE REVIEW QUESTIONS

1. What actions would the nurse perform while administering ear drops to remove excessive cerumen? Select all that apply.
   1. Avoid inserting the irrigating syringe too deeply.
   2. Boil the solution once.
   3. Direct the flow of the ear drops toward the eardrum.
   4. Direct the flow of the ear drops toward the roof of the canal.
   5. Shake the ear drops container vigorously.
   6. Warm the ear drops by holding the container in the hand for a few minutes.
2. A client arrives at the emergency department after an insect has entered the ear. Which of the following solutions would the nurse instill into the client's ear to smother the insect?
   1. Carbamide peroxide
   2. Hot water
   3. Mineral oil
   4. Triethanolamine
3. For a client with Ménière's disease, which medication is most appropriate to administer during an acute attack?
   1. acetaminophen (Tylenol)
   2. meclizine (Antivert)
   3. meperidine (Demerol)
   4. triazolam (Halcion)
4. Which is the best evidence that the antibiotic the nurse is administering for the treatment of acute otitis media is having a therapeutic effect?
   1. Ear discomfort is relieved.
   2. Ear drainage is thin and watery.
   3. Ringing sounds within the ear stop.
   4. The ear feels less warm to the touch.
5. The nurse helps the team leader plan interventions to promote effective communication with the client with otosclerosis. Which is the most appropriate nursing order to include in the care plan of this client?
   1. Drop voice at the end of each sentence.
   2. Face the client when speaking to him or her.
   3. Raise pitch of voice one octave higher.
   4. Speak directly into the client's ear.

44

Introduction to the Gastrointestinal System and Accessory Structures

Words To Know
barium enema
barium swallow
cholangiography
cholecystography
colonoscopy
enteroclysis
esophagogastroduodenoscopy
flexible sigmoidoscopy
gallbladder series
lower gastrointestinal series
panendoscopy
percutaneous liver biopsy
peristalsis
proctosigmoidoscopy
radionuclide imaging
ultrasonography
upper gastrointestinal series
virtual colonoscopy

Learning Objectives

On completion of this chapter, you will be able to:

1. Identify major organs and structures of the gastrointestinal system.
2. Discuss important information to ascertain about gastrointestinal health.
3. Identify facts in the client's history that provide pertinent data about the present illness.
4. Discuss physical assessments that provide information about the functioning of the gastrointestinal tract and accessory organs.
5. Describe common diagnostic tests performed on clients with gastrointestinal disorders.
6. Describe nursing measures after liver biopsy.
7. Explain nursing management of clients undergoing diagnostic testing for a gastrointestinal disorder.

The gastrointestinal (GI) system (Fig. 44-1) may be divided into two sections: the upper GI tract and the lower GI tract. The upper GI tract begins at the mouth and ends at the jejunum. The lower GI tract begins at the ileum and ends at the anus. Accessory structures include the peritoneum, liver, gallbladder, and pancreas. The primary functions of the GI tract are digestion (Table 44-1) and distribution of food.

ANATOMY AND PHYSIOLOGY

Mouth
Food normally enters the GI system at the mouth, where it is chewed (masticated) before being swallowed. Food that contains starch undergoes partial digestion when it mixes with the enzyme *salivary amylase,* which the *salivary glands* secrete. Table 44-2 outlines how oral structures participate in digestion.

Esophagus
The *esophagus* begins at the base of the pharynx and ends at the opening to the stomach. Layers of muscle tissue surround the esophagus. They consist of striated muscle tissue in the proximal esophagus, striated and smooth muscle in the mid-esophagus, and smooth muscle in the lower esophagus. Coordinated movement of these muscle layers propels food into the stomach. These wavelike contractions are known as **peristalsis**.

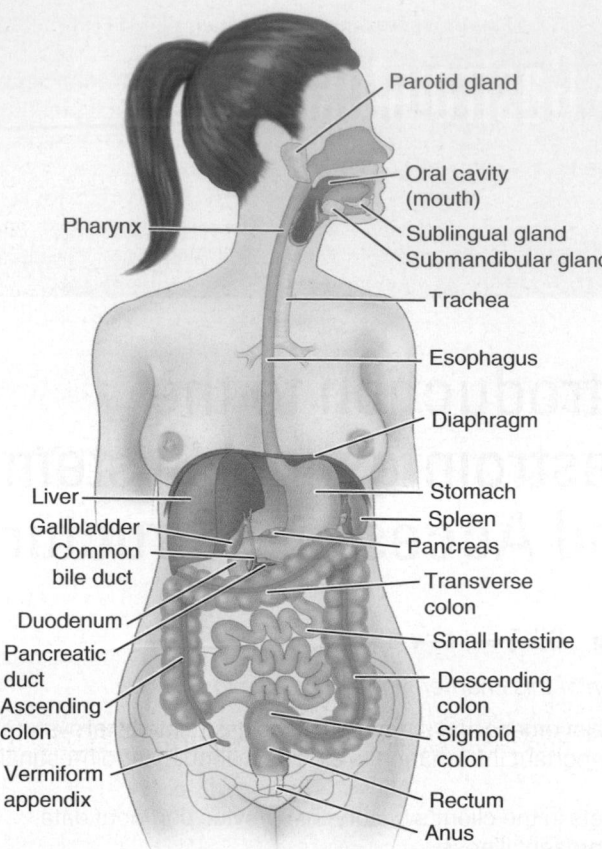

FIGURE 44-1 Organs of the gastrointestinal tract.

An *upper esophageal sphincter* or *hypopharyngeal sphincter* prevents food or fluids from re-entering the pharynx.

Stomach

The stomach temporarily holds ingested food and prepares it by mechanical and chemical action to pass in semiliquid form into the small intestine. The opening between the esophagus and stomach is called the *lower esophageal sphincter* or *cardiac sphincter*. The opening between the stomach and duodenum is called the *pyloric sphincter*. Both sphincters are circular bands of muscle fibers. When contracted, these sphincters keep stomach contents enclosed (or confined). When the pyloric sphincter relaxes, stomach contents flow to the duodenum.

Gastric secretions that contain digestive enzymes are released continuously but increase when food is eaten. Gastric secretions are acidic because they contain hydrochloric acid (HCl). The contractions of the stomach mix the food with the gastric secretions and move the mixture of semiliquid food, called *chyme*, to the small intestine by peristalsis. The time required for the stomach to empty depends on the amount and composition of food. Fats, for example, delay stomach emptying.

Small Intestine

The small intestine is divided into three portions: duodenum, jejunum, and ileum. The *duodenum*, which is approximately 10 inches long, is the first region of the small intestine and the site where bile and pancreatic enzymes enter. These secretions continue to promote the chemical breakdown of food and transform chyme to an alkaline state. Peristalsis mechanically propels the mixture, which is semiliquid at this point, into the jejunum and ileum, which have a combined length of approximately 23 feet.

The primary function of the small intestine is to absorb nutrients from the chyme. Absorption of different nutrients occurs at different sites in the small intestine (Table 44-3). When a part of the small intestine is diseased or removed surgically, absorption in that area is diminished or lost altogether.

The *ileocecal valve* lies at the distal end of the small intestine and regulates the flow of intestinal contents, which are liquid at this point, into the large intestine. It also prevents the reflux of bacteria from the large intestine, preserving the relative sterility of the small intestine.

Large Intestine

The large intestine, approximately 4 to 5 feet long and 2 inches in diameter, receives waste from the small intestine and propels waste toward the *anus,* the opening from the body for elimination. The large intestine absorbs water, some electrolytes, and bile acids. The cecum, colon, rectum, and anal canal make up the structures of the large intestine through which fecal material passes.

The *cecum* is a pouchlike structure at the beginning of the large intestine. The *appendix,* a narrow blind tube at the tip of the cecum, has no known function in humans.

TABLE 44-1 Selected Digestive Enzymes/Secretions

LOCATION	ENZYME	SUBSTANCE THE ENZYME ACTS ON	PRODUCTS OF ENZYMATIC ACTION
Salivary glands	Salivary amylase	Starch	Smaller carbohydrates
Stomach	Pepsin	Proteins	Polypeptides (process activated by HCl)
	Gastric lipase	Triglycerides (lipids)	Glycerides and fatty acids
	HCl	Proteins	Smaller polypeptides
Pancreas	Trypsin	Proteins and polypeptides	Smaller polypeptides, amino acids
	Nucleases	Nucleic acids	Nucleotides (base + sugar + phosphate)
	Pancreatic amylase	Starch	Smaller carbohydrates
	Pancreatic lipase	Lipids, especially triglycerides	Glycerides, free fatty acids, glycerol
Small intestine	Peptidases	Peptides	Amino acids
	Lactase, maltase, sucrase	Disaccharides	Monosaccharides
	Intestinal lipase	Fats	Glycerides, fatty acids, glycerol
Liver	Bile	Fats	Glycerides, fatty acids, glycerol

HCl, hydrochloric acid.

TABLE 44-2 How Oral Structures Participate in Digestion

STRUCTURE	CONTRIBUTION TO THE DIGESTIVE PROCESS
Teeth	Reduce food to sizes appropriate for swallowing; break down dense particles
Tongue	Place food in proper position for swallowing; mixes secretions to moisten food
Salivary glands	Moisten and lubricate foods in the mouth; add ptyalin enzyme for digestion of starches
Muscles of mastication	Provide movement for the grinding of food into smaller particles; provide more surface area for the digestive enzymes to act

(From Bullock, B A & Henze, R.L. [2000]. *Focus on Pathophysiology*, p. 722. Philadelphia: Lippincott Williams &Wilkins.)

The colon is divided into the *ascending, transverse, descending,* and *sigmoid* colons and *rectum.* In the colon, the unabsorbed material becomes fecal matter, which is composed of water, food residue, microorganisms, digestive secretions, and mucus. Water is reabsorbed by means of diffusion across the intestinal membrane as the mixture moves through the colon. By the time the mixture reaches the descending and sigmoid colon, the portion of the bowel adjacent to the rectum, it is a formed mass. The rectum holds and retains fecal matter through the contraction of the internal and external anal sphincters. As fecal mass accumulates, it distends the rectal wall, creating the urge to defecate. When the external anal sphincter relaxes, the fecal matter is expelled through the anus.

Gerontologic Considerations

- Although the older adult may have less control of the rectal sphincter because of age-related changes in innervation, diminished awareness of the filling reflex, and decreased muscle tone, changes in patterns of defecation should always be assessed.

TABLE 44-3 Sites of and Requirements for Absorption of Dietary Constituents and Manifestations of Malabsorption

DIETARY CONSTITUENT	SITE OF ABSORPTION	REQUIREMENTS	MANIFESTATIONS
Water and electrolytes	Mainly small bowel	Osmotic gradient	Diarrhea Dehydration Cramps
Fat	Upper jejunum	Pancreatic lipase Bile salts Functioning lymphatic channels	Weight loss Steatorrhea Fat-soluble vitamin deficiency
Carbohydrates			
Starch	Small intestine	Amylase Maltase Isomaltase α-dextrins	Diarrhea Flatulence Abdominal discomfort
Sucrose	Small intestine	Sucrase	
Lactose	Small intestine	Lactase	
Maltose	Small intestine	Maltase	
Fructose	Small intestine		
Protein	Small intestine	Pancreatic enzymes (e.g., trypsin, chymotrypsin, elastin)	Loss of muscle mass Weakness Edema
Vitamins			
A	Upper jejunum	Bile salts	Night blindness Dry eyes Corneal irritation
Folic acid	Duodenum and jejunum	Absorptive; may be impaired by some drugs (i.e., anticonvulsants)	Cheilosis Glossitis Megaloblastic anemia
B$_{12}$	Ileum	Intrinsic factor	Glossitis Neuropathy Megaloblastic anemia
D	Upper jejunum	Bile salts	Bone pain Fractures Tetany
E	Upper jejunum	Bile salts	Uncertain
K	Upper jejunum	Bile salts	Easy bruising and bleeding
Calcium	Duodenum	Vitamin D and parathyroid hormone	Bone pain Fractures Tetany
Iron	Duodenum and jejunum	Normal pH (hydrochloric acid secretion)	Iron-deficiency anemia Glossitis

(From Porth, C.M. [2007]. *Essentials of Pathophysiology: Concepts of altered health states* (2nd ed.), p. 625. Philadelphia: Lippincott Williams & Wilkins.)

If any portion of the large intestine becomes diseased or is surgically removed, its absorptive function is diminished or lost. This may result in the passage of loose stools and potential fluid and electrolyte imbalance. Passage of liquid stool, which contains many bile salts, makes the client especially vulnerable to skin breakdown in the perianal area. If stool remains in the large intestine too long, constipation results. The client may then strain to evacuate hard, solid stool, which can disrupt skin integrity.

Accessory Structures

The three accessory digestive organs are the liver, gallbladder, and pancreas. Although not an accessory structure itself, the peritoneum encloses the abdominal organs.

Peritoneum

The *peritoneum,* a membrane that lines the inner abdomen, encloses the viscera and the serous fluid that it secretes. It allows the abdominal organs to move about without creating friction. The walls of the digestive organs normally prevent the gastric and intestinal contents from escaping into the peritoneal cavity. Any perforation that allows material to seep out of the digestive tract is serious because the microorganisms and enzymes can cause a severe inflammation and infection of the surrounding tissue. This condition is known as *peritonitis.*

Liver

The *liver,* the largest glandular organ in the body, weighs between 1 and 1.5 kg (2 and 3 lb). It is located in the right upper abdomen just under the diaphragm, which separates the liver from the right lung. The liver is involved in many vital, complex metabolic activities. It forms and releases bile; processes vitamins, proteins, fats, and carbohydrates; stores glycogen; contributes to blood coagulation; metabolizes and biotransforms many chemicals (including drugs), bacteria, and foreign matter; and forms antibodies and immunizing substances (gamma globulin). See Chapter 47 for more information.

Gallbladder

The *gallbladder* is attached to the midportion of the undersurface of the liver. It normally has a thin wall and holds approximately 60 mL of bile. The liver forms approximately 1 L of bile each day. When the bile reaches the gallbladder from the common hepatic duct, water and minerals are absorbed from the bile to form a more concentrated product. Gallbladder contraction, triggered by ingested food (especially fats), causes bile to be released first through the cystic duct and then the common bile duct into the duodenum, where it aids in the absorption of fats, fat-soluble vitamins, iron, and calcium. Bile also activates the pancreas to release its digestive enzymes and an alkaline fluid that neutralizes stomach acids that reach the duodenum.

Pancreas

The *pancreas* is both an *exocrine gland,* one that releases secretions into a duct or channel, and an *endocrine gland,* one that releases substances directly into the bloodstream. As an endocrine organ, it produces the hormones insulin and glucagon (see Chap. 51). As an exocrine organ, it produces various protein-, fat-, and carbohydrate-digesting enzymes. At the appropriate time for digestion, the pancreatic enzymes are released in inactive forms and transported to the duodenum, where they are activated.

ASSESSMENT

Many conditions can disrupt the normal function of the GI system. In addition to disorders of the GI tract and accessory organs, many disorders involving other organ systems can affect GI function. As a result, the client with a GI disorder may experience a wide variety of health problems that involve disturbances of ingestion, digestion, absorption, and elimination. Accurate recording of the client's health history and physical assessment findings helps the healthcare team to diagnose and treat GI disorders.

History

The objective of the history is to identify the client's specific problem and its possible cause. The history includes the chief complaint; a focus assessment of current nutritional, metabolic, and elimination patterns; and past history.

The nurse gathers as much data as possible about why the client has sought treatment and current symptoms. This includes how long the symptoms have been present and what appears to cause or be related to them. Pertinent information to elicit includes which types of food produce distress and when symptoms are most likely to occur. The nurse also determines what measures, if any, the client uses to relieve the symptoms and the effects of these measures.

During GI assessment, the focus is on nutritional, metabolic, and elimination patterns, including quality of the client's appetite; problems associated with chewing or swallowing; what and how much the client eats each day; discomfort before, during, or after food consumption; nutritional supplements, if any, that the client uses (e.g., vitamins, herbs, home remedies); weight gain or loss; and bowel elimination patterns (usual consistency and color of stools, visible blood, stool frequency, effort or pain with passage of stool). After obtaining a current health history, the nurse obtains a history of all past medical and surgical disorders and their treatment. He or she compiles a family history of illnesses and causes of death. A family history of digestive disorders is especially important because several, such as colorectal cancer, have a hereditary link. The nurse also explores the client's work history to evaluate the possibility of exposure to environmental toxic wastes or radioactive materials.

The nurse obtains a complete allergy history, including adverse reactions to foods, because food allergies can cause various GI symptoms. The medication history includes prescription and nonprescription drugs, especially those affecting GI function. For each drug, the nurse lists the name, dose, frequency, and reason for taking.

▶ **Stop, Think, and Respond Exercise 44-1**

A client says that she has been experiencing nausea and occasional vomiting for several days. What questions should you ask to gain more information?

Physical Examination

General Appearance

The nurse assesses the client's overall physical condition and measures weight, height, and vital signs. He or she evaluates general appearance with regard to age and body size, and assesses hygiene, energy, breathing pattern, emotional attitude, and mental status to the degree that they may affect the client's general appearance.

Skin

Using natural sunlight or bright artificial light, the nurse inspects the skin for any abnormal color, such as a yellowish tint indicating jaundice. In very dark-skinned clients, he or she inspects the hard palate, gums, conjunctiva, and surrounding tissues for discoloration. If the skin appears jaundiced, the nurse inspects the sclera to see if it is yellow. Inspection of the skin of the face and abdomen is necessary to look for other abnormalities, such as *spider angiomas* (superficial red discolorations consisting of blood vessels that assume a spider-shaped pattern), distended abdominal veins (*caput medusae*), and scars. The nurse also assesses for dryness of the oral mucosa and skin turgor. Mucous membranes may be dry and skin turgor may be poor in clients who are dehydrated as a result of fluid losses from the GI tract.

Mouth

The nurse examines the lips for sores, cracks, lesions, or other abnormalities. Using a tongue blade and a flashlight, he or she inspects the mouth for inflammation, sores, swellings, or discolorations. Assessment of the quality of oral care is essential and includes evaluating for missing teeth and partial plates, bridges, or dentures. If the client has dentures, the nurse asks if they fit well and whether the client can eat regular food. If the client can eat only soft foods, the nurse communicates this information to the physician and dietary department.

Abdomen

The nurse continues the physical assessment by having the client lie supine, with the knees flexed, for the abdominal examination. (This position assists in relaxing the abdominal muscles.) Abdominal areas typically are described in quadrants (right upper, right lower, left upper, and left lower), with the umbilicus as the center point for both horizontal and vertical divisions (Fig. 44-2). The nurse then observes the abdomen's contour, noting whether it is flat, round, concave, or distended, as well as the effort associated with breathing. Distention may cause dyspnea as a result of upward pressure on the diaphragm (see Chap. 21).

Abdominal auscultation is done before palpation because palpation disrupts normal bowel sounds. Using a stethoscope, the nurse listens over each quadrant for bowel sounds, which sound like gurgles. He or she describes the location, pitch quality, and frequency, which usually is every 5 to 30 seconds. Listening for a full 5 minutes over each quadrant is important to confirm absence of bowel sounds. Generally, bowel sounds are described as absent, normal, hypoactive, or hyperactive. Measurement of abdominal girth is done at the widest point (usually at the umbilicus). Using a pen, the nurse marks the measurement location on the abdomen to ensure that additional examiners use the same reference point.

In the next part of the examination, the nurse percusses the abdomen to elicit changes in sounds from dullness over an area with a solid mass, such as the liver, to resonance over less dense structures or those filled with air.

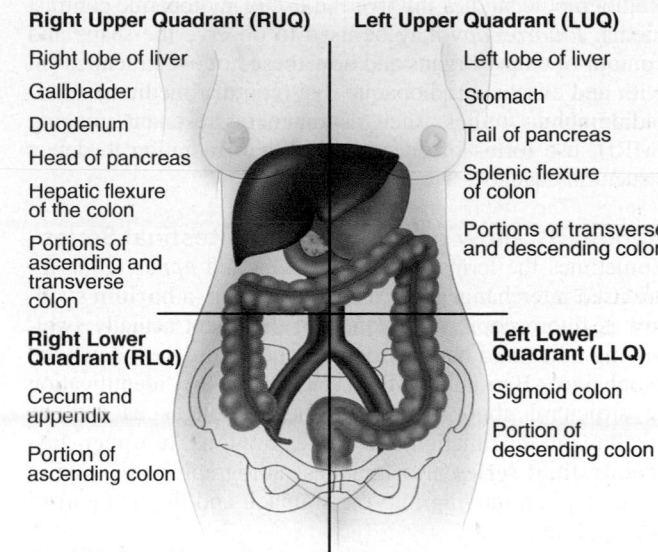

Right Upper Quadrant (RUQ)
Right lobe of liver
Gallbladder
Duodenum
Head of pancreas
Hepatic flexure of the colon
Portions of ascending and transverse colon

Left Upper Quadrant (LUQ)
Left lobe of liver
Stomach
Tail of pancreas
Splenic flexure of colon
Portions of transverse and descending colon

Right Lower Quadrant (RLQ)
Cecum and appendix
Portion of ascending colon

Left Lower Quadrant (LLQ)
Sigmoid colon
Portion of descending colon

FIGURE 44-2 Abdominal quadrants.

The nurse next palpates the abdomen to determine whether it is soft or firm and to detect masses and areas of pain or tenderness. If the client reports tenderness, the nurse probes the lower liver margin. He or she may feel an enlarged liver below the right lower rib cage. Pain or discomfort in this area may suggest a liver disorder, gallbladder or intestinal disease, or a pancreatic disorder.

Anus

The nurse examines the anal area for external hemorrhoids, skin tags, or fissures (small tears in the anal opening). He or she inspects the skin surrounding the anus for breaks, lesions, rash, inflammation, and drainage. If and when stool passes, the nurse examines its characteristics. The shape, color, and consistency of stool usually are helpful in the differential diagnosis of GI disorders. Foods and medications can alter the color of stool (Table 44-4).

Diagnostic Tests

Various studies, both radiographic and nonradiographic, are used to identify the location and structural appearance of organs or other space-occupying masses (air, fluid, tumors, foreign objects) in the abdomen, chest, or GI system.

TABLE 44-4 Foods and Medications That Alter Stool Color

ALTERING SUBSTANCE	COLOR
Meat protein	Dark brown
Spinach	Green
Carrots and beets	Red
Cocoa	Dark red or brown
Senna	Yellow
Bismuth, iron, licorice, and charcoal	Black
Barium	Milky white

From Smeltzer, S. C., et al. (2008). *Brunner & Suddarth's textbook of medical–surgical nursing* (11th ed.), p. 1127. Philadelphia. Lippincott Williams & Wilkins.

Radiographic studies involve the use of radiopaque contrast media. *Fluoroscopy* may be used to observe the shape and contour of empty organs and how these hollow structures fill with and evacuate radiopaque dye (contrast medium). Nonradiographic studies, such as magnetic resonant imaging (MRI), use forms of energy other than radiation to detect structural changes.

Barium Swallow or Upper Gastrointestinal Series

Sometimes the terms *barium swallow* and *upper GI series* are used interchangeably. Strictly speaking, a **barium swallow** is fluoroscopic observation of the client actually swallowing a flavored barium solution and its progress down the esophagus. Barium swallow facilitates the identification of structural abnormalities of the esophagus as well as swallowing dysfunction and oral aspiration. An **upper gastrointestinal series** also includes radiographic observation of the barium moving into the stomach and the first part of the small intestine.

Structural abnormalities in the esophagus include tumors, strictures, varices, and hiatal hernia. Structural abnormalities below the esophagus include gastric tumors, peptic ulcers, and numerous gastric disorders (see Chap. 48). If only a barium swallow is performed, the examination may take as little as 20 minutes. If stomach filling and emptying need to be observed, the test may take approximately 1 hour.

For several days before the procedure, the client is on a low-residue diet. Usually, he or she takes nothing by mouth (NPO) for 8 to 12 hours before the test (Nutrition Notes 44-1). A laxative may be given to clean out the GI tract. Smoking stimulates gastric motility, so the client is asked not to smoke the day of the procedure. With rare exceptions (e.g., anticonvulsants, insulin), all medications are withheld.

Barium is very constipating. Once any test using barium is over, the nurse encourages the client to drink fluids liberally to dilute the barium and promote its elimination from the GI tract. He or she advises the client that stools will appear white, streaky, or clay colored from the barium. The nurse must wait to obtain stool specimens until the client has fully excreted the barium. In some cases, a laxative may help with evacuation. In all cases, failure to have a bowel

movement within a reasonable time must be reported to the physician, because the retained barium may cause a blockage.

Small Bowel Series

A small bowel series is fluoroscopy of the small intestine after the ingestion of a contrast medium. It is used to identify tumors, inflammation, or obstruction in the jejunum or ileum. It is performed like an upper GI series, but the client must swallow more barium for the small intestine to be well visualized. If the healthcare provider suspects an obstruction or *fistula* (a leaking channel between two structures), he or she substitutes a water-soluble contrast medium such as methylglucamine diatrizoate (Gastrografin) for the barium. The test takes 5 to 6 hours, which is when the contrast medium reaches the lower portion of the small intestine. When a small bowel series fails to detect subtle small bowel disease, enteroclysis may be indicated.

Enteroclysis

Also known as a *small bowel enema,* **enteroclysis** requires nasal or oral placement of a flexible feeding tube, the tip of which is positioned in the proximal jejunum. This study uses two contrast media. First, 750 to 1000 mL of a thin barium suspension is infused through the tube, followed by 750 to 1000 mL of methylcellulose. The two contrast media fill in and pass through the intestinal loops. The examiner observes the intestine continuously by fluoroscopy and takes periodic radiographs of the various sections of the small intestine. Even with normal motility, this process can take up to 6 hours. If sedation is administered to ensure the client's comfort, he or she requires monitoring accordingly. The risk that the contrast media may be aspirated is increased if the client vomits while under sedation. Therefore, positioning of the client on his or her side and availability of a suction apparatus are critical.

Barium Enema or Lower Gastrointestinal Series

A **barium enema** or **lower gastrointestinal series** is used to identify polyps, tumors, inflammation, strictures, and other abnormalities of the colon. It is performed in the radiology department. The radiographic technologist rectally instills 1000 to 1500 mL of barium solution. He or she observes the rectum, sigmoid colon, and descending colon fluoroscopically during filling. To facilitate this process, the examiner directs the client to make multiple position changes. The client must retain the barium during this test, which may take up to 30 minutes.

During the test, the client may experience abdominal cramping and a strong urge to defecate. The nurse reassures the client that most people can retain the instilled barium throughout the test. Radiographs are taken again after the client expels the barium. In some cases, air is instilled to compress the barium residue against the wall of the lower intestine to aid in detecting mucosal defects. Stool specimens are not collected until the barium has been expelled completely.

To reduce the formation of stool and remove any residual stool, the client follows prescribed restrictions and procedures 24 to 48 hours before the barium enema:

- Low-residue diet 1 to 2 days before the test
- Clear liquid diet the evening before the test

Nutrition Notes 44-1
The Client Undergoing Diagnostic Gastrointestinal Testing

- Many GI tests require at least an 8-hour fast beforehand. Repeated or multiple tests performed over several days can compound potential or existing nutritional problems.
- Encourage adequate fluid intake to promote dilution and elimination of dyes and other test substances.
- Observe for subsequent signs and symptoms of intolerance in clients whose test requires ingesting a special solution, such as a carbohydrate solution. For instance, clients tested for lactose intolerance may experience cramping, abdominal distention, and diarrhea after ingestion of the substrate used for testing.

- A laxative the evening before the test
- NPO after midnight
- Cleansing enemas the morning of the test (if not contraindicated by inflammation or active bleeding)

The amount of fluids is not restricted, and the client usually does not have to withhold oral medications. The client may have up to three cleansing enemas (or until the evacuated solution appears clear) before the procedure. After the examination is complete, the client may resume eating. The nurse encourages the client to rest and to drink fluids liberally. He or she also monitors the passage of stool and informs the client that feces will appear white until the barium is completely eliminated.

Oral Cholecystography or Gallbladder Series

Oral **cholecystography** or **gallbladder series** identifies stones in the gallbladder or common bile duct, and tumors or other obstructions. The test also determines the ability of the gallbladder to concentrate and store a dyelike, iodine-based, radiopaque contrast medium. After the dye is absorbed, it goes to the liver, is excreted into the bile, and passes into the gallbladder, making it radiographically visible. Radiography of the gallbladder should be performed before other GI examinations in which barium is used because residual barium tends to obscure the image of the gallbladder and its ducts.

Instructions prior to the procedure vary, but generally a client is asked to eat a fat-free meal the night before the test. It is important to ask the client whether he or she is allergic to iodine. Under the direction of a physician, the client swallows six iodine-containing contrast tablets—one every 5 minutes after the evening meal the night before the procedure with a total of 250 mL of water or more. After the client ingests the contrast agent, he or she needs to be NPO after midnight and may not eat or drink until after the test is complete. If the contrast dye causes nausea and vomiting, the client or nurse needs to notify the physician so that more tablets can be ordered or the test rescheduled. Once the initial radiographs are obtained, a fatty test meal or fatty synthetic substance may be given to stimulate gallbladder contraction and emptying. Additional radiographs are taken to determine the gallbladder's ability to empty.

Cholangiography

Performed in the radiology department or during surgery, **cholangiography** determines the patency of the ducts from the liver and gallbladder. It is used when the gallbladder is not distinctly visualized with an oral cholecystogram, vomiting interferes with the retention of the oral dye, or the status of the ductal system needs to be determined during or after surgery. There are four specific types of cholangiography:

- *Endoscopic retrograde cholangiopancreatography (ERCP)*— With the use of endoscopy, dye is injected through a catheter into the common bile duct and the pancreatic duct.
- *Intraoperative cholangiography*—The contrast agent is injected directly into the bile duct during gallbladder surgery.
- *Magnetic resonance cholangiopancreatography (MRCP)*— This newer technique for visualizing the bile ducts, the pancreatic duct, and the gallbladder does not use contrast dye but rather magnetic resonance imaging (MRI), thus

obtaining computerized images. These images provide clear and detailed views.
- *Percutaneous transhepatic cholangiography (PTC)*— Ultrasound is used to guide a needle into the bile ducts so that dye can be directly injected.

If a contrast agent is used, no matter how it is introduced, it spreads into the biliary system. Radiographs are then taken to show narrowing or blockages within the biliary system.

The client must sign a consent form. If a contrast agent is going to be used, the nurse asks the client if he or she is allergic to iodine or shellfish. The nurse checks physician orders to determine if the client needs a cleansing enema. It may also be necessary to restrict food and fluids for several hours before the procedure. The nurse informs the client that he or she may experience a warm sensation and nausea when the dye is instilled. After the procedure, the client may eat and drink. To promote dye excretion, the nurse encourages the client to drink liberally.

Radionuclide Imaging

Radionuclide imaging detects lesions of the liver or pancreas and assists in evaluating gastric emptying. A radionuclide is a radioactive natural or synthetic element, such as technetium. Once the radionuclide is injected intravenously or ingested orally, the radiologist may examine a body organ by passing the radionuclide imaging scanner over the structure. This test is helpful in demonstrating the size of the organ, as well as defects or lesions such as tumors. Specialized radionuclide studies are done to identify sites of bleeding or inflammation in the GI tract. Radionuclides have rather short half-lives, lasting a few hours to days, during which they emit radiation, which usually is less than with diagnostic radiography.

Pretest measures include weighing the client to calculate the radionuclide dose and determining pregnancy and lactation. Breast milk may be pumped and discarded so that the nursing child remains safe from radioactivity. The test is contraindicated in pregnant women.

Computed Tomography

Computed tomography (CT) scanning may be performed to detect structural abnormalities of the GI tract. These tests help detect metastatic lesions that might not be apparent on regular GI radiographs. Oral barium sulfate or IV calcium phosphate may be given to provide contrast for the hollow GI organs examined by CT scan. The client is NPO for 6 to 8 hours before the CT test. Before the test, the bowel may be cleaned to reduce stool and gas. Drugs may be administered to decrease peristalsis or improve gastric motility.

Continuous-motion (helical or spherical), three-dimensional CT scans enable examiners to have detailed pictures of GI organs and vessels. This procedure is referred to as *colonography*. Clients are prepared as above. A small tube is inserted into the colon, air is introduced to inflate the colon, and computer images are produced.

Magnetic Resonance Imaging

Magnetic resonance imaging (MRI) uses magnetic energy rather than radiation to visualize soft tissue structures. It is used to examine GI structures when CT scanning is inadequate. Oral contrast agents are used to enhance the evaluation of GI disorders, such as abscesses or bleeding.

The client is NPO for 6 to 8 hours before the MRI. He or she must remove any metal objects, credit cards, wristwatch, jewelry, and the like. Clients with pacemakers may need a cardiology consult prior to the MRI to determine if there are any risks or contraindications. IV fluids, if required, must be infused by gravity during MRI because the changes in electrical charges during the test can affect mechanical infusers or pumps. The nurse informs clients that the scanner, a narrow, tunnel-like machine that will enclose them during the test, makes loud repetitive noises while the test is in progress. Clients who are claustrophobic (fear enclosed spaces) may need sedation, because it is imperative that they lie still and not panic during the test.

Magnetic Resonance Elastrography

Magnetic resonance elastrography (MRE), a new noninvasive methodology developed by physicians at the Mayo Clinic (2008), combines MRI with low-frequency sound waves (referred to as shear waves). The resulting images enable physicians to ascertain the firmness of the liver, thus allowing them to better predict clients who are at risk for developing fibrosis (scar tissue) and eventually cirrhosis (hardening of the liver). If detected early, treatment of the underlying cause can be initiated before the client develops cirrhosis, which is an irreversible and eventually fatal condition. Physicians previously could only rely on palpation, which is inconclusive, or a liver biopsy, which is diagnostic for only a small portion of the liver, and very invasive, with risks of bleeding. MRE shows great promise for other parts of the body, such as breasts, muscles, and brain tissue.

Ultrasonography

In **ultrasonography** (also called *ultrasound*), high-frequency sound waves are directed through the body, where they bounce off nearby structures, such as the liver and pancreas. The returning sound waves are then interpreted and recorded electronically. Ultrasonography, which shows the size and location of organs and outlines structures and abnormalities, helps detect cholecystitis, cholelithiasis, pyloric stenosis, and some disorders of the biliary system. It may be useful in detecting changes caused by appendicitis. Although the client can drink water before ultrasonography, the nurse discourages drinking through a straw, smoking, or chewing gum. In these activities, the client may swallow air and thereby distort sound wave transmission.

Endoscopic ultrasonography uses a fiberoptic scope with a small high-frequency ultrasonic transducer to obtain direct images of specific areas along the GI tract. The images have higher resolution and help in staging tumors and evaluating changes in the intestinal walls.

Percutaneous Liver Biopsy

In a procedure called **percutaneous liver biopsy,** the physician obtains a small core of liver tissue by placing a needle through the client's lateral abdominal wall directly into the liver. The tissue is then examined microscopically to detect abnormalities, which may include malignant changes, infectious or inflammatory processes, liver damage (cirrhosis), and signs of rejection in clients who have received a liver transplant.

Although the procedure is most often performed in the hospital operating room, it may be done in a physician's office or other outpatient site or in a radiology department. The client must have coagulation studies before the procedure, since a major complication after a liver biopsy is bleeding. Ultrasound or CT scanning is performed before or during the biopsy to identify an appropriate site for placement of the biopsy needle. The client usually receives a sedative and anesthetic to promote comfort and cooperation.

Pharmacologic Considerations

- Before biopsy procedures, clients at risk for serious bleeding may receive precautionary vitamin K, which promotes blood clotting.

- If sedatives, IV medications or dyes, or general anesthetics are administered, the client must be monitored appropriately.

When assisting with a percutaneous liver biopsy, the nurse ensures that the biopsy equipment is assembled and in order. He or she helps the client assume a supine position with a rolled towel beneath the right lower ribs. Before the physician inserts the needle, the nurse instructs the client to take a deep breath and hold it to keep the liver as near to the abdominal wall as possible. After specimen cells are obtained, they are placed in a preservative. The nurse makes sure that the specimen container is labeled and delivered to the laboratory (Nursing Guidelines 44-1).

Gastrointestinal Endoscopy

Gastrointestinal endoscopy is the direct visual examination of the lumen of the GI tract. It facilitates evaluation of the appearance and integrity of the GI mucosa and detects lesions. It provides access for therapeutic procedures. GI endoscopy is performed using a flexible fiberoptic endoscope. Diagnostic uses include obtaining biopsies of the mucosa, obtaining samples of fluids found in the GI tract, and injecting dyes for radiographic purposes. Therapeutic uses include inserting tubes and drains, electrocautery, and injecting medications. Among the variations of GI endoscopy (Box 44-1) are **proctosigmoidoscopy, esophagogastroduodenoscopy** (EGD) (Fig. 44-3), small bowel enteroscopy, peritoneoscopy, **colonoscopy, virtual colonoscopy, flexible sigmoidoscopy,** and **panendoscopy.**

Before an endoscopic procedure, the client follows dietary and fluid restrictions and bowel preparation procedures if the examination involves the lower GI structures. For the client undergoing an EGD, it is necessary for the client to spray or gargle with a local anesthetic. For an EGD and a colonoscopy, the client receives an anxiolytic agent such as midazolam (Versed) before the procedure to provide sedation and relieve anxiety.

Pharmacologic Considerations

- For certain diagnostic tests of the GI tract, clients may take oral preparations to cleanse the bowel in order to promote clear visualization of internal structures. These preparations include polyethylene glycol/electrolytes (GoLYTELY,

NURSING GUIDELINES 44-1

Assisting With a Percutaneous Liver Biopsy

- Explain that the purpose of the procedure is to obtain a small sample of liver tissue for a differential diagnosis of liver disease or to evaluate the extent of liver disease.
- Check the results of coagulation studies (PTT, APPT, PT, and platelet count).
- Check that the informed consent form has been signed.
- Instruct the client to lie supine with the right arm behind the head.
- Tell the client that the site will be cleansed and then draped with a sterile barrier.
- The physician will instruct the client to take a deep breath and hold it while the needle is introduced, sample obtained, and needle withdrawn; this takes only a few seconds.
- Monitor vital signs throughout the procedure.
- Place a pressure dressing over the biopsy site.
- Assist the client to lie on the right side after the procedure and place a small pillow under the costal margin.
- Instruct client to remain in this position for at least two hours to prevent the release of blood, bile, or both.
- Instruct the client that she or he should remain in bed for 8-12 hours, except to go to the bathroom. The client should avoid coughing or straining during this time.

- Continue to monitor vital signs according to agency policy. Changes in vital signs may indicate bleeding.
- Monitor the biopsy site frequently for bleeding, swelling, or hematoma.
- Assess breath sounds regularly. Report diminished breath sounds immediately.
- Assess the abdomen for distention or rigidity. Report if the client is experiencing abdominal pain.
- Instruct the client to avoid heavy lifting and strenuous activity for 5 to 7 days after the procedure.
- Instruct the client to follow physician orders for blood-thinning medications.
- Instruct the client to call if he or she experiences the following symptoms:
  - Severe pain at the biopsy site
  - Shortness of breath
  - Chest pain
  - Bleeding from the biopsy site
  - Fever
  - Abdominal pain
  - Weakness or diaphoresis
  - Heart palpitations

NuLYTELY, Colyte). The solution is reconstituted with water and the client instructed to drink 240 mL every 10 minutes until 4 L is consumed or fecal returns are clear. Clients can only drink clear liquids when administration of the solution begins. This polyethylene glycol/electrolyte solution produces watery stools, but usually is not associated with increased risk of fluid and electrolyte imbalance.

- Other bowel preparation medications include ones that contain a large amount of phosphorus (e.g., Phospho-soda, Visicol). These medications work by creating an osmotic diarrhea, which can result in risk of fluid and electrolyte imbalance. Instruct clients to drink adequate amounts of clear liquids during the bowel cleansing process.

During an endoscopic procedure, the nurse monitors respirations and vital signs. Assessing the client's level of pain and discomfort during the procedure is important, as is medicating the client as indicated. After the test, the nurse assesses the client's vital signs, respiratory status, level of consciousness, and abdominal symptoms. The nurse monitors the client for complications, especially signs of perforation. These include fever, abdominal distention, abdominal or chest pain, vomiting blood, or bright red rectal bleeding. The nurse offers the client light food and fluids, unless the procedure was an EGD.

After an EGD, the client may not have food or fluids until the gag reflex returns. Once the gag reflex is present, the nurse may introduce clear fluids and advance the diet to regular foods and fluids according to the client's tolerance. Occasionally, the client may complain of a sore throat after

EGD. If the client's gag reflex has returned, the nurse may offer saline gargles, ice chips, or cool drinks.

Client and Family Teaching 44-1 outlines discharge instructions following a colonoscopy.

Laboratory Tests

Depending on the suspected or confirmed diagnosis, various blood and urine tests may be ordered. Laboratory tests may include a complete blood count, urinalysis, serum bilirubin, cholesterol, serum ammonia level, prothrombin time, protein electrophoresis, and enzymes, such as amylase, lipase, aspartate aminotransferase, and lactic acid dehydrogenase. Common tumor marker blood studies include carcinoembryonic antigen and alpha-fetoprotein. Tests specific to the GI system are described in the following sections.

Gastric Analysis

Analysis of gastric fluids assists in determining problems with the secretory activity of the gastric mucosa. It also helps evaluate gastric retention in clients who may have partial or complete pyloric or duodenal obstruction. For 8 to 12 hours before the test, the client is NPO. A small nasogastric tube is inserted into the stomach. Gastric contents are aspirated every 15 minutes for at least 1 hour and analyzed for acidity (pH), volume, and cytology if indicated.

Helicobacter pylori Tests

Helicobacter pylori, a bacterium, is believed to be responsible for the majority of peptic ulcers. Blood tests are used to determine whether there are antibodies to *H. pylori* in the blood. These tests cannot be used to determine whether treatment is effective, because the results remain positive even after the bacteria are eliminated.

BOX 44-1 Common Gastrointestinal Endoscopic Procedures

Esophagogastroduodenoscopy (EGD)
Examination of the esophagus, stomach, and duodenum through an endoscope advanced orally to inspect, treat, or obtain specimens from any one or all of the upper GI structures.

Colonoscopy
Examination of the entire large intestine with a flexible fiberoptic colonoscope. Clients are sedated briefly (and monitored accordingly) with IV medication during the procedure. The colonoscope is advanced anally from the rectum to the cecum, allowing visualization of the rectum, sigmoid, and descending colon. The distal portion of the small intestine, the terminal ileum, may be inspected as well. Air may be instilled to promote visualization within the folds of the intestinal mucosa. Physicians may remove polyps or perform biopsies as indicated.

Virtual Colonoscopy or Computed Tomography (CT) Colonography
A noninvasive procedure requiring the same preparation as a colonoscopy. Sedation is not required. A small flexible rubber catheter is inserted in the rectum, and air or carbon dioxide is pumped through the tube to distend the colon. With the use of a CT scanner, images are taken with the client in a supine and prone position. Any other procedures cannot be done (e.g. removal of polyps and/or biopsies).

Although there are some concerns that the level of detail is not as great as with colonoscopy, it is a good diagnostic method. There is less risk of bowel perforation, and clients do not require sedation or pain relievers for this procedure. For clients on blood thinner medications, virtual colonoscopy is a good alternative. Unfortunately, many insurance companies do not cover this procedure unless there are associated symptoms.

Proctosigmoidoscopy
Examination of the rectum and sigmoid colon using a rigid endoscope inserted anally about 10 inches. To facilitate examination, the client must lie in a knee-chest position. The test is brief and no sedation is needed.

Peritoneoscopy
Examination of GI structures through an endoscope inserted percutaneously through a small incision in the abdominal wall with the client receiving a local, spinal, or general anesthetic. Also called *laparoscopy*.

Small Bowel Enteroscopy
Endoscopic examination and visualization of the lumen of the small bowel.

Panendoscopy
Examination of both the upper and lower GI tracts.

Urea breath tests are also used to test for the presence of *H. pylori*. In addition, they can determine whether treatment has been effective. The client either drinks a urea solution or swallows a urea capsule. Breath tests are then conducted by having the client blow up a small balloon (Fig. 44-4) or by blowing bubbles in a small container of breath-collection liquid. If *H. pylori* bacteria are present, they break down the urea, releasing carbon. The blood carries the air to the lungs, where it is exhaled, and the air is analyzed.

In addition, fecal matter can be tested for *H. pylori*. The test, called the *Helicobacter pylori* stool antigen (HpSA) test, is also an accurate diagnostic tool. If bacteria are present in the stool, then the stomach is infected. Like the urea breath test, the stool test can also be used to determine whether treatment is effective.

More invasive tissue tests may be done with endoscopy and tissue biopsy. There are three types:

- The rapid urease test, which detects urease, an enzyme produced by *H. pylori*.

Client and Family Teaching 44-1
Discharge Instructions Following Colonoscopy

When the client is alert and managing fluids and small amounts of food, he or she may be discharged. The nurse provides the following instructions:

- Mild cramping and flatulence are expected; these symptoms will resolve within 24 hours.
- If you had a small growth or polyp removed, you may experience a slight amount of bleeding that resolves on its own.
- Avoid eating high-fat or high-fiber foods for at least 24 hours following the procedure.
- Biopsy results will be available in 5 to 7 days.
- Report the following problems that, if present, may indicate bowel perforation, hemorrhage, or infection:
  - Nausea
  - Vomiting
  - Fever
  - Excessive bleeding
- Resume your usual medication regimen unless instructed otherwise.

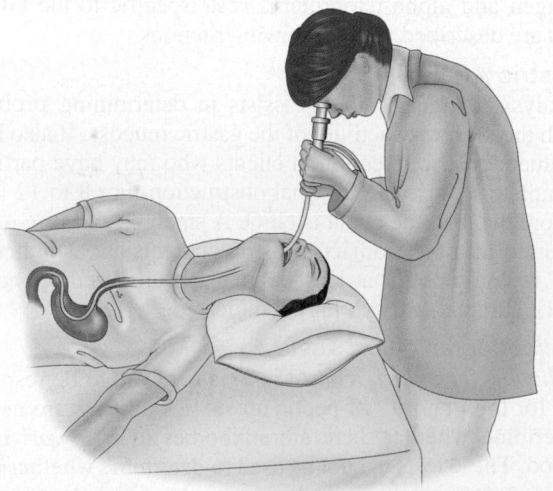

FIGURE 44-3 Esophagogastroduodenoscopy.

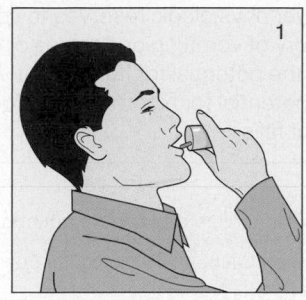 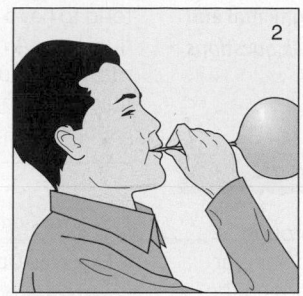 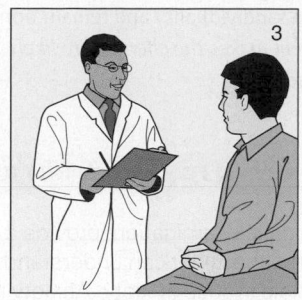

FIGURE 44-4 The breath test indicating *Helicobacter pylori* is performed in three easy steps: (**1**) the client takes a ^{14}C-urea capsule and waits about 10 minutes. (**2**) The client blows up a balloon. (**3**) The client waits while the air in the balloon is analyzed for gastric urease.

- A histology test that allows the physician to find and examine the actual bacteria.
- A culture test that involves growing *H. pylori* in a tissue sample.

Hydrogen Breath Testing

This test involves collecting a breath sample before and at intervals after ingestion of a carbohydrate solution. The two major gases in expired air are hydrogen and carbon dioxide. Elevated hydrogen levels in the expired breath sample indicate carbohydrate malabsorption. The type of solution used for the test depends on the suspected type of malabsorption. Lactose malabsorption (lactose intolerance) is a common disorder investigated using this technique.

Stool Analysis

Stool specimens are collected to identify white blood cells (indicating inflammation), red blood cells (indicating GI blood loss), and fat (indicating malabsorption). They also are collected to identify infection. Only a small amount of stool needs to be collected; samples should always be placed in a covered container. To examine for microorganisms, specimens should be fresh and warm. Routine cultures may reveal bacterial infections (e.g., *Salmonella, Shigella, Campylobacter*). Placement of the specimen in a specific preservative to detect parasites and their ova allows diagnosis of parasitic infections (e.g., *Giardia, Cryptosporidium*).

A simple test that determines the presence of occult blood in the stool is the Hemoccult test. A positive result indicates that the client is bleeding or has recently bled from somewhere in the GI tract. Substances that may cause false-positive results include red meat, iodine-containing antiseptic preparations, aspirin (greater than 325 mg per day) and other nonsteroidal anti-inflammatory agents, and excessive alcohol. Substances that may cause false-negative results include ascorbic acid (vitamin C greater than 250 mg per day) and iron supplements.

Nursing Process for the Client Undergoing Diagnostic Testing for a Gastrointestinal Disorder

Assessment

Interview the client to determine past familiarity with the test or similar procedure. Ask the client to discuss previous experiences or current expectations. If the client is responsible for self preparation before the test, explore those preparations. Review the client's history and explore any data on prior hypersensitivity or allergy to test preparations. In particular, ask about reactions to radionuclide or iodine-based contrast medium (dye), signaled by allergy to seafood. In some situations, label an allergic client's chart and apply a special band or tag to the client's identification bracelet.

 Pharmacologic Considerations

- Some, all, or none of the client's medications may be withheld before and during testing, depending on the test procedure, the client's medication regimen, and physician's orders.

Take vital signs and weigh the client if required before the procedure. Encourage the client to empty the bladder before some tests. It is important to record other essential baseline data for later comparison and identification of serious reportable changes or complications (e.g., rectal bleeding). In addition, record the client's informed consent.

Diagnosis, Planning, and Interventions

▶ Anxiety related to lack of knowledge of test procedure or possible test findings

▶ **Expected Outcomes:** (1) Client will demonstrate knowledge of the test procedure. (2) Client will express feelings of relief from anxiety.

- Explain the test's purpose and procedure and what to expect afterwards. *Providing such information reassures the client about what will occur, thus relieving anxiety.*
- Review test preparations. *Such review ensures that the client understands and carries out preparations as required.*
- Provide printed directions. *Printed directions reinforce verbal instructions.*
- Encourage client to express fears. *Expressing feelings assists in alleviating fear and clarifying misconceptions.*
- Discuss the client's perceptions and expectations of the test. *Having knowledge of the client's understanding provides an opportunity to reinforce the knowledge and to clarify expectations for the test.*

- Respect the client's individuality and remain nonjudgmental and supportive. *Respect makes the client more likely to ask questions without fear of ridicule.*

Gerontologic Considerations

- Before any diagnostic examination, provide a thorough explanation in terms the client can understand and answer any questions to help reduce anxiety. Anxiety regarding the diagnostic examination may be due to pain from positioning or being rushed.

▶ **Acute Pain** related to test procedure

▶ **Expected Outcome:** Client will state no or minimal discomfort.

- Use pillows or blankets for positioning to relieve discomfort if the client has physical problems that cause pain (e.g., arthritis). *Supportive positioning alleviates and relieves pain.*
- Medicate the client with opioid analgesic or sedative if ordered before the procedure. *Analgesia or conscious sedation reduces pain and discomfort during the procedure.*
- Tell the client to inform test personnel if he or she experiences pressure or cramping during the instillation of test fluids. *Test personnel can slow the instillation or take other measures to relieve discomfort.*
- Teach the client to expel gas and test fluids from the bowel when he or she experiences the urge. *Ignoring the urge to expel bowel contents increases pain and discomfort.*

▶ **Risk for Deficient Fluid Volume** related to fluid restriction or loss associated with diarrhea or vomiting

▶ **Expected Outcome:** Client will maintain fluid volume balance as evidenced by normal findings on intake and output records.

- Weigh client and monitor the color and amount of urine. *These data provide a baseline for the client's response to tests, fluid loss related to diarrhea or vomiting, or both.*
- Monitor pulse rate and blood pressure. *Changes may indicate dehydration.*
- Report dizziness and confusion. *Such findings may indicate dehydration.*
- Administer oral fluids as soon as possible. *These fluids replace fluid loss.*
- When testing is complete, monitor intake and output and encourage liberal intake. *These measures ensure that client is taking in adequate fluids.*

Gerontologic Considerations

- Fluid restrictions and the multiple enemas or laxatives required for GI tests may greatly impact fluid balance and electrolyte levels in the older adult. Older adults are at higher risk for dehydration than are younger people because they tend to have fewer physiologic reserves to compensate for fluid loss. A history of vomiting or diarrhea or diuretic therapy may compound the potential for fluid deficit. Additionally, any fluid deficit has potential for blood pressure decrease and associated risk of falls.

▶ **Risk for Constipation** related to barium retention

▶ **Expected Outcome:** Client achieves regular bowel elimination pattern within 2 to 3 days.

- Encourage client to drink at least 2000 mL of fluid per 24 hours after tests using barium. *This amount provides sufficient fluid to facilitate evacuation of stool.*
- Administer post-test laxative or enema if ordered. *A laxative or an enema promotes quicker evacuation of barium.*
- Monitor stool passage, observing the stool for barium. *Stools with barium appear light-colored or white-streaked.*
- Report diminished or hyperactive bowel sounds. *Such sounds may indicate barium retention.*

Evaluation of Expected Outcomes

The client reports minimal anxiety and pain, maintains adequate fluid balance, and evacuates all barium. Normal bowel elimination resumes, as evidenced by statement from client.   ●

Gerontologic Considerations

- After the diagnostic test, the older adult may experience dizziness or confusion secondary to prolonged time without food or fluids. Provide nourishment as soon as possible after the examination and give assistance with ambulation when necessary.

- Inform older clients and their families that diminished intestinal and sphincter muscle tone may contribute to constipation, diarrhea, or fecal incontinence following a diagnostic test; appropriate early nursing interventions should be implemented.

CRITICAL THINKING EXERCISES

1. A client is preparing for an esophagogastroduodenoscopy (EGD). This includes withholding food and fluids for 6 to 12 hours and receiving a sedative before the test. In addition, the nurse will spray the client's throat with a local anesthetic or the client will gargle with the local anesthetic. What precautions does the nurse take before the client goes for the EGD?
2. When the client returns from the EGD, what is important for the nurse to assess?
3. A client is complaining of epigastric pain. What areas of the abdomen should be included in the nurse's assessment?
4. A client has a potential diagnosis of colon cancer. Which tests do you anticipate the physician will order for the client?

NCLEX-STYLE REVIEW QUESTIONS

1. A client is scheduled for a barium enema. Which of the following statements indicates that the client understands the pre-procedure instructions?
   1. "I can eat whatever I want before the test."
   2. "I can only have clear liquids the day before the test."
   3. "I cannot eat any spicy foods for 7 days before the barium enema."
   4. "I have to abstain from all food and fluids for 24 hours before the test."

2. The client with epigastric pain is scheduled for a radiograph of the upper gastrointestinal tract. After the nurse explains the procedure, which statement best indicates that the client understands what the procedure involves?
   1. "A flexible tube will be inserted into my stomach."
   2. "Dye will be infused into my vein before the test."
   3. "I will have to swallow a large amount of barium."
   4. "My body will be placed within an imaging chamber."

3. The nurse needs to assess a client's abdomen. To best accomplish this, the nurse directs the client to lie in which of the following positions?
   1. In a semi-Fowler's position
   2. On the right side with knees straight
   3. Prone with knees slightly bent
   4. Supine with knees flexed

4. The client with possible cholecystitis is scheduled for an oral cholecystography, a radiograph of the gallbladder. The night before the test, the client orally takes several tablets that will facilitate a sharper radiographic image. Before administering the contrast substance, which question is essential for the nurse to ask?
   1. Can the client tolerate holding still?
   2. Does the client want any anesthesia?
   3. How many radiographs has the client had?
   4. Is the client allergic to iodine?

5. After a liver biopsy is done on a client with cirrhosis, which nursing action is most appropriate?
   1. Ambulating the client twice each shift
   2. Elevating the client's legs on two pillows
   3. Keeping the client in high Fowler's position
   4. Positioning the client on the right side

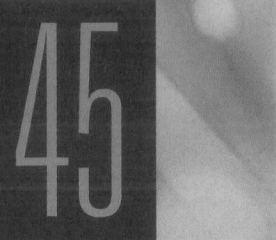

45

Caring for Clients with Disorders of the Upper Gastrointestinal Tract

Words To Know
anorexia
bariatric surgery
diverticulum
dumping syndrome
dyspepsia
esophagitis
fundoplication
gastrectomy
gastric decompression
gastritis
gastroesophageal reflux disease
gastrostomy
hiatal hernia (diaphragmatic hernia)
jejunostomy
morbid obesity
nasoenteric intubation
nasogastric intubation
odynophagia
orogastric intubation
peptic ulcer
percutaneous endoscopic gastrostomy (PEG)
pyrosis

Learning Objectives

On completion of this chapter, you will be able to:

1. Discuss assessment findings and treatment of eating disorders, esophageal disorders, and gastric disorders.
2. Describe the nursing management of a client with a nasogastric or gastrointestinal tube or gastrostomy.
3. Identify strategies for relieving upper gastrointestinal discomfort.
4. Discuss the nursing management of clients undergoing gastric surgery.

Digestion begins in the mouth and continues in the stomach and small intestine, with food traveling through the esophagus in between. The nurse is responsible for managing the care of clients with disorders affecting the upper gastrointestinal (GI) tract (see Fig. 44-1).

DISORDERS THAT AFFECT EATING

ANOREXIA

Simple **anorexia**, or lack of appetite, is a common symptom of many diseases. Prolonged anorexia may lead to serious consequences, such as malnutrition.

Pathophysiology and Etiology

The appetite center, which stimulates or suppresses the appetite, is located in the hypothalamus. Pleasant or noxious food odors, effects of drugs, emotional stress, fear, psychological problems, or illnesses may affect appetite.

Brief periods of anorexia are not life-threatening but can cause temporary malnutrition. During periods of reduced food consumption, most people have a sufficient reserve of stored glycogen, which provides energy through the process of *glycogenolysis,* the conversion of glycogen to glucose. Hormones such as glucagon, glucocorticoid hormones from the adrenal cortex, and thyroid hormones stimulate the liver to carry out *gluconeogenesis.* Selective reabsorption by the kidneys can temporarily maintain electrolyte balance.

 Gerontologic Considerations

- With age, the salivary glands become less active and the numbers of taste buds are reduced, contributing to anorexia in the older adult. Anorexia and weight loss in the older adult can also result from ill-fitting dentures or dysphagia or may be a manifestation of depression. Decreased appetite may result from diminished oxygenation to the

NURSING GUIDELINES 45-1

Managing the Care of Clients With Anorexia

- Provide foods that the client likes during meals.
- Offer nourishing beverages (egg nog, milk shakes, and commercial concentrates such as Ensure or Instant Breakfast) as between-meal snacks.
- If the client is hospitalized or in another healthcare facility, encourage family members to bring favorite foods that can be refrigerated or reheated.
- Conduct a daily caloric count if necessary to determine total proteins and carbohydrates in the client's diet.
- Keep serving sizes and containers small to avoid overwhelming the client.
- Serve and keep hot foods hot and cold foods cold.
- Encourage eating in the company of others.
- Formulate a nutritional plan with the client and dietitian that promotes weight gain (approximately 600 calories per meal).
- If necessary, arrange for supplementation based on documented deficiencies in the client's intake.
- Consult the physician and dietitian in cases of prolonged anorexia.

appetite centers in the brain caused by atherosclerosis or decreased cardiac stroke volume.

Assessment Findings

Signs and Symptoms

Hunger usually is absent, and clients describe having no desire for food. Some clients state that they feel nauseous when they smell food or even think about eating. Some eat a small amount only because they feel they should or others coerce them to do so. Amounts of weight loss vary, depending on how long the anorexia and reduced food intake have lasted. Eventually, the client may show signs of *hypovitaminosis* (vitamin deficiency). The body does not store any water-soluble vitamins (B vitamins, including folic acid and vitamin C) except for vitamin B_{12}. Therefore, deficiencies in these vitamins may be seen in more acute phases of illness. The body does store fat-soluble vitamins (A, D, E, and K) but requires fat absorption to do so. Chronic illnesses and those that directly affect fat absorption (e.g., cystic fibrosis, pancreatitis, liver disease) result in deficiency of the fat-soluble vitamins.

Diagnostic Findings

Depending on the chronicity of the anorexia, hemoglobin level and blood cell counts may be reduced. Red blood cells (RBCs) may become abnormally enlarged. Serum albumin, electrolyte, and protein levels may be low, with accompanying cardiac dysrhythmias. For example, an elevated U wave on the electrocardiogram may indicate potassium deficiency.

Medical and Surgical Management

Management depends on the cause. Short-term anorexia (less than 1 week) usually requires no medical intervention. Persistent anorexia may require various approaches, such as a high-calorie diet, high-calorie supplemental feedings, tube feedings, and total parenteral nutrition (TPN). Psychological support, psychiatric treatment, or both may be essential for the client whose anorexia is linked with *anorexia nervosa,* a psychiatric disorder, instead of a defined organic disease (see Chap. 70).

Nursing Management

To maintain sufficient nutrition and sustain normal body weight, the client must eat an adequate quantity of food. In assisting the client to meet this goal, the nurse monitors weight daily. He or she also obtains a complete medical and allergy (drugs and food) history from the client or a family member and compiles a dietary history, including a description of the client's eating patterns and food preferences. For more information, see Nursing Guidelines 45-1.

Additional nursing measures depend on any consequences of anorexia. In the case of altered bowel patterns (diarrhea or constipation) from reduced bulk secondary to liquid supplements, potential interventions include the following:

- Keep a record of the client's bowel movements.
- If the client experiences diarrhea, consult with the physician and dietitian about changing the type of supplement.
- If the client is constipated, change formula to one that contains fiber to add bulk to stools.
- Dilute the formula temporarily until the client adjusts to the concentrated contents.
- Assist the client and dietitian to increase dietary fiber.
- Administer a prescribed stool softener to promote ease and frequency of bowel elimination.

NAUSEA AND VOMITING

Nausea and vomiting are common and often coexisting problems. If these symptoms are prolonged, weakness, weight loss, nutritional deficiency, dehydration, and electrolyte and acid-base imbalances may result.

Pathophysiology and Etiology

Some of the more common causes of nausea and vomiting include drugs, infections and inflammatory conditions of the GI tract, intestinal obstruction, systemic infections, lesions of the central nervous system, food poisoning, emotional stress, early pregnancy, and uremia. Nausea generally precedes vomiting and usually results from distention of the duodenum. Increased salivation and peripheral vasoconstriction, which causes cold, clammy skin and tachycardia, accompany nausea. The vomiting center, located in the medulla, is particularly sensitive to parasympathetic neurotransmitters released in response to gastric irritation. The Valsalva maneuver, which accompanies the forceful expulsion of stomach contents, causes dizziness, hypotension, and bradycardia.

Assessment Findings

Signs and Symptoms

The client describes an unpleasant feeling, identified as nausea, which usually is associated with loss of appetite and refusal to eat. When a client vomits, others may observe him or her retching while he or she evacuates the stomach contents. The process occurs once or several times in succession.

The client who experiences excessive fluid loss (dehydration) with vomiting may complain of excessive thirst and report decreased or no urine production. Eyes and oral mucosa appear dry or dull, and poor skin turgor reflects fluid loss (see Chap. 16).

Gerontologic Considerations

- Severe and prolonged episodes of vomiting can be especially serious for older adults whose nutritional and fluid intake is marginal; more profound electrolyte imbalances and severe dehydration can result.

- Teach older adults about potential bradycardia, hypotension, or dizziness that accompany the Valsalva maneuver, and the safety precaution of calling for assistance or remaining seated until the symptoms pass to decrease the risk of falling (see Chap. 65).

The client's history may include ingestion of noxious substances, such as excessive amounts of alcohol, presumably contaminated food, or drugs that commonly cause GI side effects. Exposure to other people with similar symptoms suggests a bacterial or viral cause. When vomiting is secondary to intestinal obstruction, the abdomen is distended, tender, and firm to the touch. Bowel sounds may be absent or hypoactive.

Diagnostic Findings

Prolonged vomiting may lead to low levels of serum sodium and chloride. Bicarbonate levels may rise to compensate for the loss of chloride and accumulation of metabolic acids. The hematocrit value, if high, is secondary to the hemoconcentration that accompanies dehydration.

Medical and Surgical Management

Sometimes nausea and vomiting are short-lived and do not require medical intervention. In some instances, intravenous (IV) fluids, electrolyte replacement, and drug therapy are necessary. Elimination of the cause necessitates various interventions, ranging from stopping a drug to surgical intervention for intestinal obstruction. Symptomatic relief may be achieved by administering an antiemetic agent (Drug Therapy Table 45-1), providing IV fluid and electrolyte replacement, and temporarily restricting food intake until the cause of vomiting is eliminated (Nutrition Notes 45-1).

Nutrition Notes 45-1
The Client with Nausea

● The client should eat small meals and eat and drink slowly.
● Dry, salty foods, such as crackers and pretzels, may relieve nausea.
● Fried food, spicy food, and foods with strong odors should be avoided.
● Cold foods may be preferable to hot foods.

Pharmacologic Considerations

- Consult the physician for changes in drug orders if a client cannot retain oral medications.

Nursing Process for the Client with Nausea and Vomiting

Assessment

Obtain a complete medical, dietary, drug, and allergy history. In addition, compile a list of symptoms that occurred before and along with the nausea and vomiting, how long the problem has existed, and the frequency, color, and amount of vomited material. Because the cause may be unknown, list the foods and where the client has eaten in the past 24 hours. In addition, assess general appearance, weight, and vital signs. Documenting intake and output and monitoring for signs of fluid volume deficit are additional essential assessment requirements (see Chap. 16).

Diagnosis, Planning, and Interventions

▶ **Deficient Fluid Volume** related to prolonged vomiting and decreased intake of oral fluids

▶ **Expected Outcome:** Fluid balance will be restored as evidenced by intake of 1500 to 3000 mL/day with similar fluid loss.

● Offer clear fluids in small amounts. *Slow introduction of fluids allows client to develop tolerance and determine if he or she can advance the diet.*
● Recommend commercial over-the-counter beverages such as Gatorade. *Gatorade replaces fluids and electrolytes.*
● Inform physician if urine output is below 500 mL/day or serum electrolyte levels are abnormal. *Such findings indicate severe dehydration and the need for IV replacement fluids.*
● Monitor weight daily. *Daily monitoring helps to determine trends in weight loss or gain.*
● Assess skin turgor and mucous membranes. *Decreased skin turgor and dry mucous membranes indicate dehydration.*

▶ **Imbalanced Nutrition: Less than Body Requirements** related to nausea and vomiting

DRUG THERAPY TABLE 45-1 Antiemetic Medications

Drug Category and Examples	Mechanism of Action	Side Effects	Nursing Considerations
Serotonin Receptor Antagonist ondansetron (Zofran)	Blocks receptors for $5HT_3$, which affects the neural pathways involved in nausea and vomiting	Headache, dizziness (low blood pressure), myalgia (muscle aches and pains), malaise, fatigue, drowsiness	Review client's allergy history before administering medication. Provide oral drug form q8h around the clock for 1 to 2 days after chemotherapy or radiation to prevent nausea and vomiting. Caution client about side effects that may make activities such as driving a car or operating other machinery hazardous.
Phenothiazine prochlorperazine (Compazine)	Inhibits the CTZ and vomiting center in the brain	Drowsiness, hypotension, changes in heart rhythms, photophobia, blurred vision, dry mouth, discolored urine	Tell client that this drug is for short-term control of nausea and vomiting and should be used exactly as directed. Explain side effects and advise client not to save any medicine for a later date or give any to anyone else. Monitor older clients because effects of this drug may lead more rapidly to dehydration than in younger clients.
Antihistamines hydroxyzine (Atarax, Vistaril)	Blocks H_1 receptors, decreasing stimulation of the CTZ and vomiting center	Drowsiness, tremor, dry mouth, hypersensitivity reaction (includes difficulty breathing), tremors, loss of coordination, sore muscles, or muscle spasms	Take full health history to help determine underlying cause of nausea and vomiting. Give by deep intramuscular injection in volume prescribed to control vomiting. Report breathing problems, tremors, muscle problems and incoordination.
promethazine (Anergan, Phenergan)	Blocks H_1 receptors, decreasing stimulation of the CTZ and vomiting center	Dizziness, drowsiness, poor coordination, confusion, restlessness, excitation, epigastric distress, thickened bronchial secretions, urinary frequency, dysuria	Take drug and health history. Because this drug interacts with several others, review potential for drug interactions; for example, do not administer medication if client is taking an monoamine oxidase inhibitor (MAOI). Do not give to a client with a lower respiratory tract disorder. Advise client to avoid drinking alcohol when taking this medication.
dimenhydrinate (Dramamine)	Inhibits vestibular stimulation in the ear, thereby relieving motion sickness	Drowsiness, confusion, nervousness, restlessness, headache, dizziness, vertigo, tingling, heaviness and weakness of hands, epigastric discomfort, low blood pressure, nasal stuffiness, chest tightness, rash, photosensitivity	Advise client not to take if pregnant or lactating. Review client history for glaucoma, peptic ulcer, bronchial asthma, heart problems because drug may pose a danger. Urge client to avoid alcohol because serious sedation could result. Advise client to report breathing problems, tremors, loss of coordination, visual disturbances or hallucinations, and irregular heartbeat.

Handwritten notes:
- *When pt. undergoes chemo* (next to ondansetron)
- *IM* (next to hydroxyzine)
- *Suppository or pill form* (next to promethazine)

▶ **Expected Outcome:** Client's nutritional status will be adequate as evidenced by maintenance of weight and normal electrolyte and blood values.

- When client tolerates clear fluids, advance diet to full liquids, then to soft, bland foods, such as creamed soups, crackers, or toast. *Advancing diet slowly helps client develop tolerance for fluids and food.*
- Collaborate with the dietitian to provide nutritional foods. *The dietitian can help create a plan that assists client to increase caloric intake with foods that he or she can tolerate.*
- Discourage caffeinated or carbonated beverages. *Such drinks may decrease appetite and lead to early satiety.*

CANCER OF THE ORAL CAVITY

Cancer cells undergo changes in structure and appearance. They multiply, eventually forming a colony of abnormal and dysfunctional cells (see Chap. 18). When cancer affects the oral cavity, cells in the lips, mouth, or pharynx undergo malignant changes. When cancers of the oral cavity are detected early, the rate of cure is fairly good.

Pathophysiology and Etiology

Development of oral cancers is linked with smoking, chewing tobacco, and drinking alcohol in excess. Lip cancer is associated with pipe smoking and prolonged exposure to wind and sun. As cancer cells in the oral cavity increase, the mass may distort a client's appearance; exert pressure on surrounding tissue, making it difficult to masticate (chew); cause local pain; or produce *dysphagia* (difficulty swallowing).

The most common oral cancer is squamous cell carcinoma. Malignant growths can be found anywhere in the oral cavity, but cancers usually occur on the lips, sides of the tongue, or floor of the mouth. Untreated, cancerous growths may extend into nearby tissue, such as the middle ear or nasal sinuses; infiltrate regional lymph nodes; or invade large blood vessels, such as the carotid arteries, that are near the oral cavity. Serious hemorrhage (carotid blowout) and death may result when cancer cells invade an artery that becomes ulcerated or when necrosis follows radiation therapy.

Assessment Findings

The early stage of oral cancer is characteristically asymptomatic. At first, the client may notice a lesion, lump, or other abnormality of the lips or mouth. Other changes, such as pain, soreness, and bleeding follow. If a lesion is on the tongue, the client commonly experiences difficulty eating or tasting food. Pain and numbness also follow. Dentists and oral hygienists may be the first to notice changes in mouth tissues, such as *leukoplakia,* a white patch on the tongue or inner cheek that may become cancerous. A biopsy of the lesion discloses malignant cells, which confirms the diagnosis of oral cancer.

Medical and Surgical Management

Treatment depends on the location and type of tumor, extent (or stage) of involvement, and the client's physical condition. In cases of hemorrhage, transfusions are given to replace lost blood. Ligation of the bleeding vessel usually is necessary. Drugs such as antianxiety agents are prescribed to relieve the client's apprehension.

Surgical treatment of most oral cancers includes tumor excision alone or with follow-up radiation therapy and chemotherapy. The radiation therapy may include a combination of external beam radiation and surgical implantation of radioactive interstitial implants. Surgical excision may result in complete cure, provided that it is performed early.

A neck dissection is performed if the cancer has spread to the lymph nodes near the jaw or below the ears. Cancer of the tongue usually involves radical surgery to remove part or all of the tongue. Excision of the tumor from parts of the jaw or palate is disfiguring.

For clients with advanced disease, treatment is palliative only. Chemotherapy or radiation therapy is used to relieve pain and temporarily decrease tumor size. A tracheostomy and tube feedings are instituted to maintain an adequate airway and provide nourishment.

Nursing Management

General nursing management of the client with oral cancer is much the same as for any client with cancer (see Chap. 18). The focus of attention, however, is on maintaining a patent airway, promoting adequate fluid and food intake, and supporting communication that the tumor or treatment may have impaired. To review care of the client needing airway management, refer to Chapter 20 and the discussion of endotracheal intubation and tracheostomy care.

Nurses collaborate with speech pathologists to address communication problems. They must be patient when the client chooses to communicate by speaking and clarify or repeat what he or she says if speech is not understandable. Nurses may substitute written forms for communicating if speech is impaired. They also offer the client pencil and paper, a Magic Slate, or an alphabet board, or they suggest that the client use hand signals.

When the client returns from the operating room after oral surgery, he or she should be positioned flat, either on the abdomen or side, with the head turned to the side to facilitate drainage from the mouth. After recovery from the anesthetic, the client is positioned with the head of the bed elevated, which makes it easier for the client to breathe deeply and cough up secretions. It also controls edema in the operative area.

After oral surgery, there should be equipment for suctioning, administration of oxygen, and tracheostomy at the client's bedside. If the client does not have a tracheostomy, a tracheostomy tray must be nearby for emergency use because respiratory distress or airway obstruction requires immediate attention. If the client has a tracheostomy, the nurse suctions secretions from the cannula and cleans it on a regular basis.

The nurse should not irrigate the client's mouth until the client is awake and alert. When and if mouth irrigation is carried out, the nurse should turn the client's head to the side to allow the solution to run in gently and flow out into an emesis basin. The nurse instills only a small amount of solution and then waits for the fluid to drain before administering more. In addition, he or she suctions the mouth as necessary to remove secretions, blood, or irrigating solution.

The client must not receive oral liquids or foods until a written order exists. The nurse observes the client's ability to swallow small amounts of liquid. In cases of coughing or other difficulty, the nurse must suction the liquid from the mouth immediately.

The client may receive prescribed antiemetics if he or she experiences nausea or vomiting. If the client has a gastric tube, the nurse checks it for patency. Clients should not use a straw because it causes the client to swallow air, which can distend the stomach.

The client's emotional response to radical oral surgery is a real and difficult problem. Extensive surgery of the mouth and adjacent structures is not only disfiguring but incapacitating. It interferes with communication, eating, and control of saliva. Although healthcare providers explain the extent of surgery before the operation, many clients and families cannot grasp all the ensuing effects. The first time family members or clients see the effects of surgery, the experience usually is traumatic. The nurse needs to promote effective coping and therapeutic grieving at this time. Responses may range from crying or extreme sadness and avoiding contact with others to refusing to talk about the surgery or changes in appearance. Allowing the client time to mourn, accept, and adjust to losses is essential. To facilitate adaptation, the client needs opportunities to express feelings. Nurses must observe severely depressed clients closely. Clients who are suicidal need psychological evaluation and counseling. In addition, the nurse provides time for family members to express fears, ask questions, and grieve. It may help to refer clients and family members to support groups and counselors.

Nutritional management is a particular challenge when caring for clients with oral cancer. If the client can take oral nourishment, a nutritional consultation may be necessary to modify the diet according to the client's ability to chew and swallow. Because oral tissues are sensitive, the client should avoid hot and cold liquids and spicy foods. The nurse can consult with the physician about prescribing a topical anesthetic mouthwash containing lidocaine (Xylocaine), which numbs the tissues, or a systemic analgesic to relieve pain. Providing nourishment by a route other than the mouth may be necessary.

▶ *Stop, Think, and Respond Exercise 45-1*

A client comes to the clinic complaining of difficulty chewing and swallowing. What questions should you ask?

Gastrointestinal Intubation for Feedings or Medications

At some time during the care of the client with oral cancer, as well as when caring for others with GI disorders, the nurse may have to perform gastrointestinal (GI) intubation, which is the insertion and management of GI tubes. GI intubation is performed to provide nutrition, medications, or both; to carry out **gastric decompression**, which is removal of gas and fluids from the stomach; to lavage the stomach to remove ingested toxins; to diagnose GI disorders, a process that may include aspiration of gastric contents for analysis; to treat GI obstruction; or to apply pressure to a GI bleed.

GI tubes are advanced to the upper GI tract by way of the mouth or nose or introduced directly into the stomach or small intestine through the abdominal wall. The nasal route is the preferred route for passing a tube when the client's nose is intact and free from injury. Examples of different types of GI intubation include **nasogastric intubation** (tube passes through nose into stomach via esophagus), **orogastric intubation** (tube passes through mouth into the stomach), **nasoenteric intubation** (tube passes through the nose, esophagus, and stomach to the small intestine), **gastrostomy** (tube enters the stomach through a surgically created opening into the abdominal wall), and **jejunostomy** (tube enters jejunum or small intestine through a surgically created opening into the abdominal wall). See Table 45-1. A gastric tube lies in the stomach; an intestinal tube extends past the pylorus.

The type of tube selected depends on the reason for placing the tube. In general, smaller (narrower), more flexible tubes are used for feeding because they tend to be more easily tolerated by clients; larger tubes are used for decompression because they allow for evacuation of large pieces of debris or blood clots from the upper GI tract. Tubes used for feeding are longer and end in the upper,

TABLE 45-1 Nasogastric, Nasoenteric, and Feeding Tubes

TUBE TYPE	LENGTH	SIZE (FRENCH)	LUMEN	OTHER CHARACTERISTICS
Nasogastric Tubes				
Levin (plastic or rubber)	125 cm	14–18	Single	Circular markings serve as guidelines for insertion.
Gastric sump Salem (plastic)	120 cm	12–18	Double	Smaller lumen acts as a vent.
Moss	90 cm	12–16	Triple	Tube contains both a gastric decompression lumen and a duodenal lumen for postoperative feedings.
Sengstaken-Blakemore (rubber)	100 cm	12–16	Triple	Two lumens are used to inflate the gastric and esophageal balloons; one lumen attached to suction to aspirate gastric contents.
Minnesota	100 cm	12–16	Quadruple	As above, but fourth lumen is attached to suction esophageal contents.
Nasoenteric Decompression Tubes				
Andersen (like Miller-Abbott; rubber)	2.44 m	16	Double	Used for temporary management of early mechanical obstruction. One lumen is Tungsten weighted; other is used as a vent.
Nasoenteric Feeding Tubes				
Dobbhoff or Keofeed II (polyurethane or silicone rubber)	160–175 cm	8–12	Single	Tip is tungsten weighted, radiopaque.

small intestine; instilling the feeding formula below the pylorus reduces the potential for vomiting and aspiration. The disadvantage of the long tubes is that the distal location is difficult to assess without a chest or abdominal radiograph.

Nursing Process for the Client Receiving Tube Feedings

Assessment

Before beginning a tube feeding, determine why the client requires it—such as to improve nutritional and hydration status for chronic illness. It is essential to evaluate renal function and check for any digestive issues, just as it is important to assess previous stool patterns, present weight, and any vomiting.

Diagnosis, Planning, and Interventions

When a client is receiving tube feedings, medications, or both (Table 45-2), ensure that the lungs remain free of liquid substances, infection does not develop, and intake and output are appropriate for the client's age and size. Additional objectives include providing adequate nutrition, promoting appropriate stool patterns (amount, consistency, and frequency), and preserving intact skin and nasal mucosa. Keep mucous membranes moist because they tend to dry from mouth breathing and restricted oral fluids. Provide frequent mouth care to relieve discomfort from dryness and unpleasant tastes and odors. Ice chips and analgesic throat lozenges, gargles, or sprays may help if the client's mouth and throat become sore. Provide mouth care after removal of the tube and inform the client that a sore throat (an aftereffect of intubation) may persist for several days.

The client is at risk not only for dry mouth but also fluid-volume deficit resulting from insufficient fluid intake. Be aware of the client's normal fluid needs and whether the formula alone can meet them. Observe for signs and symptoms of dehydration. For example, if urine output is less than 500 mL/day, administer formula and additional water as ordered.

While ensuring adequate hydration, protect the client from infections that stem from microbes in the tube-feeding formula. Signs and symptoms of infection include diarrhea, fever, or abnormal white blood cell count. To prevent infection, wash hands before handling equipment; keep the feeding formula refrigerated or unopened until it is ready for use; warm the bolus, intermittent, or cyclic feeding formula (Box 45-1) to room temperature just before

---

BOX 45-1 Tube Feeding Methods

Liquid nourishment is administered by bolus, intermittent, cyclic, or continuous methods. Intermittent cyclic and bolus tube feedings are physiologically preferable to continuous feedings for long-term use because they resemble a more normal pattern of intake, allowing hormone and enzyme levels to rise and fall rather than being constantly stimulated. Continuous feedings, however, may be preferred to decrease the risk of aspiration.

Depending on institutional policy and individual feeding orders, the feeding tube is flushed with water at various intervals to ensure patency. Many tube feeding formulas are available to suit a client's different nutritional needs. Nursing observation of tolerance of the feeding is essential to determine which tube and formula are best for the client.

Bolus Tube Feedings
- Allow introduction of 250 to 400 mL formula through the tube in a short period (usually 15–30 minutes)
- Administered by syringe or gravity flow system attached to the distal end of the feeding tube

Intermittent Tube Feedings
- Allow delivery of between 250 and 400 mL formula over 30–60 minutes
- Delivered by gravity flow system or an electronic feeding pump

Continuous Tube Feedings
- Allow formula to be administered at lower rates— usually 1.5 mL/minute over a longer time (usually 12–24 hours)
- Delivered by gravity flow system or an electronic feeding pump

Cyclic Tube Feedings
- Allow formula to be administered continuously for 8–12 hours during sleep followed by a 12- to 16-hour pause
- Ensure adequate nutrition during weaning from tube to oral feeding
- Alternate with oral food intake until client can take most nutrition orally

---

administering; hang continuous formula-feeding containers with only the volume necessary for 4 to 6 hours; flush the tubing with water before adding more formula and after giving a bolus or intermittent feeding or medications; discard any premixed formula after

---

TABLE 45-2 Medication Administration by Way of Feeding Tube

TYPE	PREPARATION
Liquid	None
Simple compressed tablets	Crushed and dissolved in water
Buccal or sublingual tablets	Give as intended
Enteric-coated tablets	Cannot be crushed; change in form required
Time-release tablets	Some can be opened; cannot be crushed because doing so may release too much drug too quickly (overdose); check with pharmacist

24 hours; thoroughly clean and dry all equipment used for bolus feedings (i.e., syringe, feeding adapters, tubing, containers) after each use; and replace the infusion container and tubing used for a continuous tube feeding every 24 hours or as directed by agency policy.

    The plan of care contains the following diagnoses, outcomes, and interventions.

▶ **Imbalanced Nutrition: Less than Body Requirements** related to inadequate dietary intake

▶ **Expected Outcome:** Nutrition will be adequate as evidenced by stable body weight.

- Maintain feeding schedule, drip rate, and amount administered by gravity drip, bolus feeding, or continuous controlled pump. *Feeding at set rate and amount ensures the client will receive the appropriate amount, calories, and nutrients, and assists client to digest the feeding without discomfort.*
- Aspirate and measure residual content before each intermittent feeding or every 4 to 8 hours for continuous feedings. Delay feeding if residual content measures more than 100 mL or 10% to 20% of the hourly amount of a continuous feeding. Readminister the residual amount. *Measuring the residual content ensures that the client digests feedings and will not be overfed. Readministering residual amounts ensures that the client does not lose nutrients and digestive enzymes.*
- Maintain tube function by:
  - Administering 15 to 30 mL of water before and after medications and feedings (every 4 to 6 hours with continuous feedings). *This measure ensures tube patency and decreases the risk of bacterial infection and crusting or blockage of the tube.*
  - Changing tube feeding container and tubing per agency policy. *Regular changes prevent blockage and infection.*
- Monitor weight daily. *Daily monitoring checks for trends in weight loss or gain.*
- Consult with physician and dietitian if client experiences any problems with tube feeding, such as nausea, bloating, diarrhea, or cramping. *Such problems may indicate poor tolerance of feeding, wrong formula for client, or other issues.*

▶ **PC: Aspiration**

▶ **Expected Outcome:** The nurse will manage tube feedings to reduce risk for aspiration during feedings or vomiting episodes.

- Check tube placement and gastric residual before feedings. *Checking prevents improper infusion and assists in preventing vomiting.*
- Place client in semi-Fowler's position during and 30 to 60 minutes after an intermittent feeding, and at all times for a continuous feeding. *Proper positioning prevents regurgitation.*
- Stop feeding if client vomits or aspiration is suspected. *In these cases, cessation prevents further problems and allows for treatment of the immediate problem.*

Gerontologic Considerations

- A diminished gag reflex that may occur with aging increases the risk for aspiration.

▶ **Risk for Diarrhea** related to hypertonic feeding solutions, lack of dietary fiber, high carbohydrate and electrolyte content, or other factors (e.g., gastroenteritis, deficient fluid volume)

▶ **Expected Outcome:** Client will have normal bowel patterns with formed stool.

- Consult with physician about decreasing the infusion rate. *A decreased infusion rate provides time for carbohydrates and electrolytes to be diluted, preventing increased fluid from the vascular system going to the jejunum.*
- Administer feedings at room temperature. *Cold or warm feedings stimulate peristalsis.*
- If possible, administer feedings continuously. *Bolus or intermittent feedings cause sudden distention of the small intestine.*
- Instruct client to remain in semi-Fowler's position during and after feedings (as discussed previously). *This position slows movement of feeding into the intestine.*
- Consult with physician and dietitian if diarrhea persists. *Client may require a different formula if all other possible causes for diarrhea are ruled out.*

Evaluation of Expected Outcomes

The client maintains his or her weight. Lungs are clear to auscultation, and the client has not vomited. Bowel patterns are normal with formed stool. ●

Gastrointestinal Intubation for Decompression

The larger GI tube is used to relieve abdominal distention caused by problems after surgery, episodes of acute upper GI bleeding, or symptoms associated with intestinal obstruction, or for diagnostic purposes. It is inserted by following the same procedure as is used for insertion of a feeding tube (Fig. 45-1).

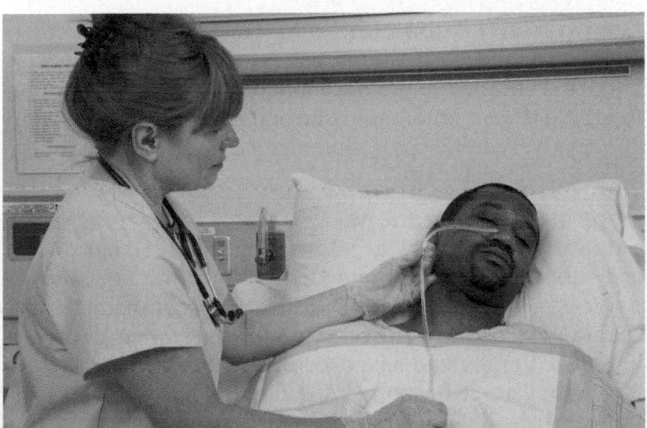

FIGURE 45-1. The nurse determines the length of nasogastric tubing for a client by measuring from the tip of nose to the tip of earlobe, and then to the tip of the xiphoid process.

NURSING GUIDELINES 45–2

Managing the Care of a Client Needing GI Suction and Decompression

- Locate the suction source, usually a wall outlet or portable machine.
- Adjust the suction level on the wall outlet or portable machine to provide the amount and frequency of suction specified by the physician.
- Select intermittent high, low, or continuous suction when using a Salem sump tube; select low intermittent suction when using a Levin tube because the single lumen may adhere to the lining of the stomach during continuous suction. (If the tube is used only to obtain specimens for diagnostic purposes, manual suction may be achieved by attaching a syringe to the end of the tube and drawing back on the plunger.)
- Insert the gastric decompression tube in accord with accepted standards and connect it to the suction.

Maintain Safe Suction

- Observe the amount and quality of the gastric contents being suctioned and the client's response.
- Monitor the procedure frequently because abdominal or gastric distention caused by suction failure may have serious consequences, such as strain on surgical sutures or vomiting around the tube.

- Check equipment frequently to make sure it is operating properly. If the suction is not operating satisfactorily, obtain another suction machine.

Maintain Tube Patency

- If the decompression tube is occluded, irrigate or replace it.
- First review the client's chart. The physician may order irrigation on an as-needed basis.
- When irrigating the tube, use normal saline solution to prevent disturbance of electrolyte balance. Also use a large syringe to instill the irrigant into the distal end of the tube.
- After the fluid is instilled, remove it by gently pulling back on the plunger.
- Document the amount of solution used and the amount of fluid returned on the client's intake and output.

Ensure Client Comfort

- Provide ice chips sparingly because water pulls electrolytes into the gastric secretions, which are then removed by suction, increasing the risk for an electrolyte disturbance.

Some tubes, such as a gastric sump tube, have a double lumen, one of which serves as a vent, allowing a small amount of air to be drawn in when the tube is connected to suction. Sump tubes decrease the possibility of the stomach wall adhering to and obstructing the tube openings during gastric decompression. A common problem associated with vented tubes is leakage from the vent lumen. The nurse may prevent this by keeping the vent above the level of the client's stomach. Newer gastric sump tubes have a one-way antireflux valve that allows air to enter but prevents gastric contents from escaping. In many cases, decompression tubes are connected to a source of suction (Nursing Guidelines 45-2).

Gastrostomy Tubes for Long-Term Feeding

A client with a gastrostomy has a transabdominal opening into the stomach that provides long-term access for administering fluids and liquid nourishment. Creating a gastrostomy is a relatively minor procedure that can be performed surgically or endoscopically.

General Considerations

Surgical placement of a gastrostomy involves laparotomy and surgical creation of an external stoma through which a gastrostomy tube is placed. When a **percutaneous endoscopic gastrostomy** (PEG) is performed, an endoscope is introduced orally and advanced into the stomach so that the physician can see the correct location for the tube. This location also is identified on the external abdominal surface before an incision is made. Two physicians or one physician and a specially trained nurse usually perform the PEG, which can be done either in the endoscopy suite or at the bedside

with the client needing minimal sedation (Fig. 45-2). Because of the reduced risks, endoscopic placement is preferred to surgical laparotomy unless the client has ascites, is morbidly obese, or has had previous gastric surgery. If the client's condition eventually improves, the gastrostomy tube is removed and the opening closes over time. Rarely, the gastrostomy opening may require surgical closure.

Gastric feedings are administered by bolus, intermittent, cyclic, or continuous feeding methods, using the same techniques described previously. Bolus feedings are not given

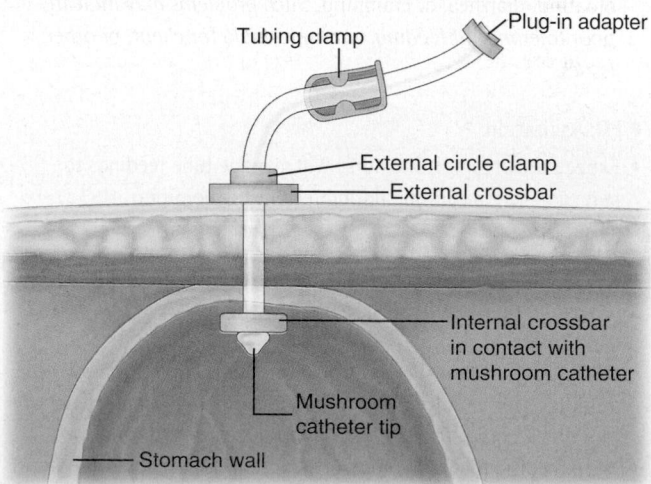

FIGURE 45-2. Detail of abdomen and percutaneous endoscopic gastrostomy (PEG) tube, showing catheter fixation.

BOX 45-2 Prevention of Complications Related to PEG Tubes

- PEG tubes are most often stabilized with internal and external bumpers. The internal bumper prevents the tube from being dislodged from the stomach or intestine. The external bumper secures the tube to the abdominal wall and prevents the tube from migrating.
- Bumpers that are too tight may cause:
  - Pressure ulcer on the abdomen.
  - "Buried bumper syndrome," in which the internal bumper becomes buried in the abdominal wall, possibly leading to GI bleeding, perforation, or peritonitis.
- Bumpers that are too loose may cause:
  - Free movement of the tube, leading to irritation, ulceration of the tract, or both.
  - Dislodgment.
- A new PEG tube insertion site may have a slight amount of bleeding, mucus, or both; report any prolonged drainage or other problems.
- The tube insertion site should be inspected for signs of irritation, infection, drainage, or gastric leakage.
- New PEG tubes are usually taped or sutured until the tract heals.
- Once the tract heals, there is less risk for trauma to the abdominal wall. The PEG tube is more easily replaced in a healed tract.

(Adapted from Clinical Query [2004]. How does a PEG tube stay in? *Nursing 2004, 34*[6], 21.)

through tubes inserted below the pylorus because such placement causes abdominal cramping and diarrhea. Intermittent, cyclic, or continuous feedings simulate the normal passage of food into the small intestine and usually are well tolerated.

Gastrostomy feeding devices may be skin-level devices (known as *buttons*) or tubes. Some tubes have a double lumen to allow infusion of two different fluids at once, such as administration of medications and delivery of feeding formula without interruption. For stabilization, most gastrostomy tubes have an external bumper and a firm internal bumper or an inflatable balloon. The advantage of the firm internal bumper is that it is difficult to dislodge accidentally; the disadvantage is that it may be difficult or painful to remove when replacement is desired. The advantage of the balloon-style internal bumper is that it is relatively painless and easy to replace; disadvantages include relative ease of accidental dislodgment and gradual loss of fluid from the inflated balloon, resulting in leakage. The volume of fluid placed in the balloon is measured regularly and replaced as necessary. Box 45-2 provides further information about preventing complications for clients with a PEG tube.

Nursing Management

Before insertion of a PEG tube, the nurse weighs the client, assesses vital signs, auscultates bowel sounds, and offers an opportunity to empty the bladder. Other activities include determining the client's perception of the procedure, clarifying information, and checking that proper consent forms are signed and in order. The nurse prepares the client's skin and conducts other ordered preprocedural activities, such as inserting an IV line and administering sedatives.

The nurse monitors vital signs (i.e., respiratory rate, oxygen saturation, heart rate and rhythm) throughout the procedure according to institutional protocol. He or she monitors and documents the client's tolerance of the procedure. Monitoring of vital signs and response to the procedure continues in the postprocedural period. The nurse observes the stoma and surrounding skin for signs of infection and checks dressings frequently for evidence of bleeding and drainage.

The nurse must examine the appearance and volume of the drainage from the gastrostomy tube during the first 24 hours when the tube may be temporarily attached to gravity drainage. He or she auscultates bowel sounds and palpates the abdomen lightly for signs of distention and tenderness. He or she inspects the oral mucosa for excessive dryness. In addition, the nurse notes the client's tolerance of the instilled formula when tube feeding is initiated, promptly reporting abdominal distention, vomiting, fever, and severe pain to the physician. Another important nursing intervention is to monitor the characteristics and pattern of bowel elimination and trends in daily weight.

Accidental removal of the gastrostomy device necessitates immediate replacement. Clients who have recently placed gastrostomy devices (less than 2 weeks) do not have a well-established tract and are at high risk for inadvertent replacement into the peritoneum instead of the stomach. If fluids are administered into this device, the resulting peritonitis may be life-threatening. For this reason, the nurse notifies the physician immediately and takes steps to ensure proper placement of the replacement device. For clients with well-established tracts, the nurse can maintain patency of the tract by inserting a clean catheter (i.e., Foley) and inflating the balloon to hold the catheter in place. The diameter of the replacement device should be the same as that of the device that was removed. The nurse notifies the physician so a new feeding device can be inserted. It is safe to administer gastric feedings through a catheter until it is replaced.

 Pharmacologic Considerations

- Never crush and administer an enteric-coated drug through any type of enteral feeding tube (nasogastric, nasoenteric, or gastrostomy).

DISORDERS OF THE ESOPHAGUS

Various disorders can affect the esophagus. Examples include gastroesophageal reflux disease, esophageal diverticulum, hiatal hernia, and cancer. Esophageal varices, which result from hypertension in the portal venous system, are discussed in Chapter 47.

GASTROESOPHAGEAL REFLUX DISEASE

Gastroesophageal reflux disease (GERD) is a common disorder that develops when gastric contents flow upward into the esophagus. All adults and children normally have some degree of reflux, especially after eating. Gastroesophageal reflux is considered a disease process only when it is excessive or causes undesirable symptoms, such as pain or respiratory distress.

Pathophysiology and Etiology

GERD results from an inability of the lower esophageal sphincter (LES; also called the *cardiac sphincter*) to close fully, allowing the stomach contents to flow freely into the esophagus. Obesity and pregnancy increase susceptibility to GERD because of the upward pressure that increased abdominal girth associated with these conditions places on the diaphragm.

Assessment Findings

Signs and Symptoms

The most common symptoms associated with GERD are epigastric pain or discomfort (**dyspepsia**), burning sensation in the esophagus (**pyrosis**), and regurgitation. Other symptoms include difficulty swallowing (dysphagia), painful swallowing (**odynophagia**), inflammation of the lining of the esophagus (**esophagitis**), aspiration pneumonia, and respiratory distress. Clients with esophagitis related to GERD may experience bleeding from the lining of the esophagus, manifested by vomited blood (*hematemesis*) or tarry stools (*melena*). Sometimes *occult* (hidden) *bleeding* for long periods produces iron-deficiency anemia. Because the esophagus is anatomically close to the heart, clients with epigastric pain may think they are having a heart attack. Until a myocardial infarction is ruled out as a cause for the discomfort, it is considered a potential diagnosis. Prolonged or severe esophagitis can lead to scarring and stricture formation. In these events, the client may report a sensation of feeling food "stick" in the esophagus for varying periods.

Diagnostic Findings

Barium-swallow findings show inflammation or stricture formation from chronic esophagitis. Upper endoscopy with biopsy confirms esophagitis. Tests of stool may show positive findings of blood. Ambulatory 24-hour esophageal pH monitoring allows for observation of the frequency of reflux episodes and their associated symptoms. Another method of pH monitoring uses radiotelemetry technology, in which a pH-measuring capsule is attached endoscopically to the lining of the esophagus. The client, who does not need a catheter, wears a recording device around the waist that records acid and non-acid reflux data. This device may be worn longer than 24 hours (Holmes, 2006). Bronchoscopy with analysis of fluids found in the lungs and nuclear medicine scans may be used to test for aspiration. Esophageal motility testing is used to evaluate the muscles of the esophagus by assessing pressures with a catheter and sensor. It usually is performed in clients who do not respond to treatment for GERD to determine what surgery might be needed. A gastric emptying study may also be done to evaluate the effectiveness of the stomach to empty its contents into the duodenum. Ineffective gastric emptying may lead to gastroesophageal reflux and aspiration. The gastric emptying study may help determine what medications and/or surgery are needed.

Medical and Surgical Management

Treating GERD begins with conservative measures first, depending on the symptoms and presence of erosive esophagitis. Education and lifestyle changes may include weight loss, maintaining an upright position following meals, elevating the head of the bed when sleeping, avoiding food and fluids 2 to 3 hours before bedtime, and avoiding foods that intensify symptoms.

Medications may also be effective. Antacids, whether aluminum, magnesium, or calcium-based, continue to be a primary treatment, because they neutralize stomach acids. A newer foam antacid tablet, composed of alginic acid and sodium bicarbonate, is used with other drugs. The tablet disintegrates as it reaches the stomach and turns into a foam that forms a barrier to the reflux of liquid. It reduces the number of reflux incidents and is particularly useful after the client has eaten a meal and when he or she is lying down. Other medications used to control esophageal reflux are discussed in Drug Therapy Table 45-2. Generally, histamine$_2$-receptor (H$_2$) antagonists, proton-pump inhibitors, or both are used for 2 to 3 months if GI bleeding or other symptoms are present. H$_2$ antagonists, such as ranitidine, cimetidine, or famotidine, are used for the short-term treatment of duodenal and gastric ulcers for managing GERD. Prokinetic or promotility drugs may be used for mild to moderate GERD caused by incompetence of the LES or delayed gastric emptying. Drugs such as metoclopramide (Reglan) increase LES pressure and promote movement of food through the stomach.

Pharmacologic Considerations

- Antacids may be given two to four times per day or as frequently as every 1 to 2 hours. They are not administered within 1 hour of H$_2$ antagonists or many other oral medications because they may decrease absorption of the other drug.

- Most antacids contain a combination of magnesium hydroxide and aluminum hydroxide. The magnesium component may tend to cause diarrhea in some clients. In such cases, switching to an aluminum-only antacid (e.g., AlternaGel) or a calcium-containing antacid (e.g., Tums) may be helpful.

The most common surgical procedure performed for GERD is **fundoplication**, a procedure that tightens the LES by wrapping the gastric fundus around the lower esophagus and suturing it into place. Fundoplication may be performed using laparoscopic technique, endoscopic technique, or open laparotomy. Esophageal strictures may be managed by endoscopic dilatation. Recurrent strictures may require repeat dilatation. In some cases, clients are taught self-dilatation using a tapered flexible dilator in the

DRUG THERAPY TABLE 45-2 Medications Used To Treat Problems In The Upper GI Tract

Drug Category and Examples	Mechanism of Action	Side Effects	Nursing Considerations
Antacids			
calcium carbonate (Tums)	Neutralize gastric acid to relieve heartburn and sour stomach	Constipation, hypercalcemia, hypophosphatemia	Avoid using in large amounts for a prolonged time. These drugs may be used as calcium supplements.
aluminum hydroxide (AlternaGel, Gaviscon)		Constipation, indigestion	Do not administer to clients on a sodium-restricted diet. Do not administer with tetracycline.
aluminum hydroxide with magnesium hydroxide (Maalox, Mylanta)		Hypermagnesemia, hypophosphatemia	Observe for central nervous system depression and other symptoms of hypermagnesemia, especially in clients with renal failure.
Histamine$_2$-receptor (H$_2$) Antagonists			
cimetidine (Tagamet)	Suppress gastric acid by blocking H$_2$ receptors	Blood abnormalities (agranulocytosis, neutropenia, thrombocytopenia), diarrhea, dizziness, sleepiness, headache, confusion, increased plasma creatinine level, cardiac rhythm disturbances, erectile dysfunction (reversible), rash	Give drug with meals and at bedtime. Urge client to report sore throat, fever, unusual bruising/ bleeding, or dizziness.
ranitidine (Zantac)		Headache, GI disturbance, insomnia, nausea/vomiting, rash, blood abnormalities, erectile dysfunction	Give drug with meals and at bedtime. Encourage regular checkups. Urge client to report sore throat, fever, unusual bruising/ bleeding, dizziness, severe headache, or muscle/joint pain.
famotidine (Pepcid)		Headache, dizziness, diarrhea, constipation, muscle cramps, erectile dysfunction	Give drug with meals and at bedtime. Encourage regular checkups. Advise client to report sore throat, fever, unusual bruising/ bleeding, dizziness, severe headache, or muscle/joint pain.
Anti-ulcer/Cytoprotective Agents			
sucralfate (Carafate)	Protect ulcers from acid and pepsin	Dizziness, insomnia, vertigo, constipation, GI discomfort, dry mouth, rash, back pain	Give drug to client with an empty stomach 1 hour before or 2 hours after meals and at bedtime. Do not administer concurrently with an antacid or H$_2$ antagonist. Advise client to report severe gastric pain.
Proton Pump Inhibitors			
omeprazole (Prilosec)	Suppress gastric acid by blocking enzymes associated with the final step of acid production	Headache, fatigue, dizziness, depression, abdominal pain, cramps, gas, nausea, diarrhea, flulike symptoms, rash, arthralgia	Give before meals to prevent upset stomach. Instruct client to swallow capsule whole without breaking, opening, or crushing contents. Caution client not to drive car or operate machinery if side effects are severe.
lansoprazole (Prevacid)		Diarrhea, abdominal pain, nausea/vomiting, constipation, dry mouth, headache, dizziness, vertigo, insomnia, upper respiratory symptoms (reversible), rash	Give drug before meals. Arrange for client to be medically monitored while taking drug. Advise client to report worsening symptoms, severe headache, fever, or chills.
GI Motility Agents			
metoclopramide (Reglan)	Stimulate upper GI tract and gastric emptying without stimulating release of gastric acid	Restlessness, drowsiness, fatigue, extrapyramidal symptoms, parkinson-like reactions, nausea, diarrhea	Instruct client not to use alcohol or sleeping pills because resulting sedation may be dangerous. Advise client to report severe depression, diarrhea, and involuntary tremors or tics of the face, eyes, arms, and legs.

(drug table continues on page 660)

DRUG THERAPY TABLE 45-2 Medications Used To Treat Problems In The Upper GI Tract *(continued)*

Drug Category and Examples	Mechanism of Action	Side Effects	Nursing Considerations
cisapride (Propulsid)		Headache, abdominal pain, diarrhea, constipation, nausea/vomiting, serious cardiac dysrhythmias from potential drug interactions, runny nose	Assess medication history and for gallbladder disease, GI bleeding or obstruction, pregnancy, or lactation. Give 15 minutes before each meal and at bedtime.
bethanechol (Urecholine)		Abdominal discomfort, salivation, nausea/vomiting, sweating, flushing	Instruct client not to use alcohol or sleeping pills because resulting sedation may be dangerous. Administer on an empty stomach. Monitor bowel function, especially in older adults.
Anticholinergics			
atropine sulfate (Atropine)	Relax smooth muscles of GI tract and inhibit gastric secretions	Blurred vision, dilated pupils, cycloplegia, dizziness, nervousness, insomnia, dry mouth, increased intraocular pressure, palpitations, heart rhythm changes, life-threatening paralytic ileus, urinary retention, intolerance to heat	Assess for health conditions that may contraindicate therapy. Give 30 minutes before meals. Be sure client has adequate fluid intake. Keep room temperature cool but comfortable. Tell client to report eye pain, abnormal heartbeats, difficulty swallowing, or breathing problems.
dicyclomine HCl (Bentyl)		Constipation, dry mouth, blurred vision, sensitivity to light, difficulty urinating, irregular heartbeat, intolerance to heat	Ensure adequate fluids. Keep room temperature stable to prevent problems resulting from heat intolerance. Tell client to report eye pain, abnormal heartbeats, difficulty swallowing, breathing problems, and so forth. Assess for health conditions that contraindicate therapy (glaucoma, bronchial asthma).
propantheline bromide (Pro-Banthine [Can])		Constipation, dry mouth, blurred vision, sensitivity to light, difficulty urinating, irregular heartbeat, intolerance to heat	
Combination Drugs for PUD			
bismuth subsalicylate (BSS), metronidazole (MTZ), and tetracycline hydrochloride (TCN) (Helidac)	Combination medication of anti-ulcer and antibiotic to treat PUD and remove *H. pylori* infection.	Most common side effects are nausea, diarrhea, abdominal pain, melena, upper respiratory infection, constipation, anorexia	One dose contains 4 pills; follow directions for administration. Each dose should be taken with a full glass (8 oz.) of water. If a dose is missed, do not double the dose.

home setting. Newer devices to treat GERD (Holmes, 2006) are listed below:

- The Stretta system uses electrodes to create tiny lesions on the LES. As the lesions heal, the tissue tightens, increasing the muscle mass of the LES and preventing reflux.
- The Bard EndoCinch suturing system creates small tucks in the LES with sutures to strengthen the muscle.
- The Enteryx implant injects a solution in the LES. The liquid becomes spongy and reinforces the LES, preventing reflux.

These minimally invasive procedures take approximately 45 minutes and may be performed using conscious sedation. Recovery time for clients is short—generally 1 to 2 days.

Because these procedures are new, the long-term effects are unknown.

Nursing Management

The nurse educates the client with GERD about diet and lifestyle changes needed to reduce reflux symptoms. Dietary management consists of avoiding foods and beverages that increase gastric acidity (e.g., black and red pepper, regular and decaffeinated coffee, alcohol) and avoiding items that lower pressure in the LES (e.g., alcohol, chocolate, peppermint, licorice, citrus fruits, caffeine, high-fat foods). Additional measures include losing weight, avoiding tight-fitting garments, elevating the head of the bed, stopping smoking, and avoiding food and drink for several hours before bedtime. Nurses must advise pregnant clients that symptoms of GERD usually resolve after delivery. The nurse teaches the client how to self-administer medications to control reflux. He or she emphasizes strict compliance with drug therapy to reduce symptoms. The nurse also teaches the client about the importance of controlling severe GERD to prevent possible complications, such as esophageal stricture formation and esophageal cancer. He or she closely observes the client having fundoplication for postoperative abdominal distention and nausea, because many clients cannot belch or vomit after undergoing this procedure.

▶ *Stop, Think, and Respond Exercise 45-2*

You are assigned to care for a client with GERD. After lunch, the client tells you that he needs to take a nap. What should you advise?

ESOPHAGEAL DIVERTICULUM

A **diverticulum** is a sac or pouch in one or more layers of the wall of an organ or structure. Esophageal diverticula (plural) are found at the junction of the pharynx and the esophagus or in the middle or lower portion of the esophagus.

Pathophysiology and Etiology

The most common esophageal diverticulum, known as *Zenker's diverticulum*, occurs at the pharyngeal–esophageal juncture. Men are more likely than women to have this condition. Diverticula result from a congenital or an acquired weakness of the esophageal wall. They trap food and secretions, which then narrow the lumen, interfere with the passage of food into the stomach, and exert pressure on the trachea. The trapped food decomposes in the esophagus, causing esophagitis or mucosal ulceration.

Assessment Findings

The client has foul breath and experiences difficulty or pain when swallowing, belching, regurgitating, or coughing. Auscultation of the middle to upper chest may reveal gurgling sounds. A barium swallow determines the structural abnormalities in the esophagus. Esophagoscopy usually is contraindicated secondary to the risk of esophageal perforation.

Medical and Surgical Management

For mild symptoms, treatment usually includes a bland, soft, semisoft, or liquid diet to facilitate passage of food. Eating four to six small meals a day is recommended.

Clients with more severe symptoms may require surgical excision of the diverticulum. If the diverticulum is at the lower esophagus, it is repaired through a thoracic (chest) approach. The surgical approach for an esophageal diverticulum at the junction of the pharynx and esophagus usually is above the clavicle (collarbone).

Nursing Management

The nurse explains that oral hygiene will not alleviate the foul breath. He or she provides instructions for dietary modifications or arranges a consultation with a dietitian. See the section on Nursing Management of Hiatal Hernia and Nursing Care Plan 45-1 as well.

HIATAL HERNIA

A **hiatal or** diaphragmatic hernia is a protrusion of part of the stomach into the lower portion of the thorax. There are two types of hiatal hernias:

- *Axial or sliding*—The junction of the stomach and esophagus and part of the stomach slide in and out through the weakened portion of the diaphragm (Fig. 45-3A).
- *Paraesophageal*—The fundus is displaced upward, with greater curvature of the stomach going through the diaphragm next to the gastroesophageal junction (Fig. 45-3B).

Pathophysiology and Etiology

A hiatal hernia results from a defect in the diaphragm at the point where the esophagus passes through it. It is particularly common in women. There is congenital muscle weakness or weakness resulting from trauma. Factors that increase intraabdominal pressure also contribute to the potential for hiatal hernia and include multiple pregnancies, obesity, and loss of muscle strength and tone that occurs with aging. Hiatal hernia develops in approximately 60% of people older than 70 years of age. When the upper portion of the stomach slips from its usual position and becomes trapped, gastroesophageal reflux occurs.

Assessment Findings

The client describes having heartburn, belching, nausea, and a feeling of substernal or epigastric pressure or pain after eating and when lying down. He or she may report increased symptoms when bending at the waist. If scars form, swallowing becomes difficult. As food distends the esophagus, the client may vomit. Reflux does not usually accompany gastroesophageal hernias, because the gastroesophageal sphincter remains intact. Sliding hernias, however, are often associated with reflux. A barium swallow confirms the diagnosis by outlining the abnormal positioning of the stomach. An esophagoscopy shows the extent of irritation and scarring in the esophagus.

Medical and Surgical Management

Medical management of hiatal hernia is the same as that of GERD. The narrowed esophagus is stretched endoscopically, but the procedure may need to be repeated often. Clients who do not respond to a rigid medical regimen are treated surgically, which involves restoring the stomach to its proper position and repairing the diaphragmatic defect.

Nursing Process for the Client With an Esophageal Disorder

Assessment

Ask the client about his or her appetite, particularly changes, difficulty swallowing, and problems after meals, such as discomfort, bloating, regurgitation, and belching. If the client indicates that he or she has pain after meals, ask if the pain follows every meal or certain foods, if other things (e.g., a particular position) seem to aggravate it, and if the pain is a burning sensation or associated with stomach fullness or pressure. In addition, determine if the client has experienced any weight loss. Finding out if the client has tried

NURSING CARE PLAN 45-1 | The Client Undergoing Gastrointestinal Surgery

Preoperative Assessment

In addition to performing assessments for the client with a GI disorder:

- Obtain a complete health, drug, tobacco, and allergy history.
- Ask approximately how long symptoms have lasted, whether eating is normal, and how much weight, if any, the client has lost.

- Assess bowel sounds for presence and quality.
- Ask about food intolerance and current dietary management.
- Determine bowel elimination patterns and stool characteristics.
- Assess understanding of diagnostic tests, scheduled surgery, and preparations for surgery.

Nursing Diagnosis: Anxiety related to test results, diagnosis, and surgical procedure.

Expected Outcome: Anxiety will be mild as evidenced by a calm demeanor, appropriate questions, and expressions of fear.

Interventions	Rationales
Provide time for client to verbalize fears and express needs related to diagnosis and surgery.	Being present and supportive encourages communication.
Allow client to express his or her personal reaction to the threat to well-being.	Expressing feelings without being judged can help reduce fears.
Explain tests, procedures, and surgery, using nonmedical speech and allowing time for questions.	Education helps to increase coping skills.
Keep client informed of progress and explain delays or changes in plans.	Adequate explanations make clients feel more secure and less anxious.
If surgery is emergent (such as in GI hemorrhage), provide explanations to family member and anticipate questions and concerns that client will have after surgery.	Family members will have decreased anxiety and be less anxious and better able to provide support when seeing client after surgery.

Evaluation of Expected Outcome

Client is less anxious, expressing fears and questions about diagnosis and surgery.

Nursing Diagnosis: Deficient Knowledge related to preoperative preparation.

Expected Outcome: Client will demonstrate exercises satisfactorily and acknowledge the purpose of equipment and procedures that may be used after surgery.

Interventions	Rationales
Using nonmedical language, instruct client about common postoperative equipment: intravenous (IV) line, infusion pump, nasogastric suction, oxygen, urinary catheter, wound drain, cardiac monitor, and pulse oximeter.	Providing understandable explanations helps client learn information effectively.
Prepare client by explaining reasons for postoperative treatments and procedures, such as frequent assessment of vital signs and performance of breathing exercises.	Such explanation promotes postoperative compliance with needed treatments and procedures.
Explain postoperative administration of analgesics to reduce and manage pain.	Client fear pain—understanding that pain will be managed will reduce fear.
Evaluate client's learning through return demonstrations of deep breathing, coughing, moving legs, and turning, as well as verbalization of instructions.	Having client provide explanations and demonstrations reinforces instructions and helps nurse determine if client needs further teaching.

Evaluation of Expected Outcome

Client can discuss the surgical procedure and demonstrate how to turn, deep breathe, cough, and splint incision.

Postoperative Assessment

Refer to Standards for Postoperative Care in Chapter 14. When the client returns from surgery:

- Assess vital signs.
- Review the record about the type of surgery performed and the client's progress during surgery and in the postanesthesia recovery unit.
- Inspect the surgical dressing for drainage and tubes or catheters for placement, patency, and type of drainage.

- Carefully observe nasogastric tube drainage for evidence of bleeding. Although the nasogastric tube may contain a small amount of dark blood when the client first returns from the operating room, the drainage should promptly return to the yellow-green of normal gastric secretions.
- Inspect the IV site and note the current rate and progress of fluid infusion.
- Document fluid intake and output as well as level of consciousness and comfort.

NURSING CARE PLAN 45-1 **The Client Undergoing Gastrointestinal Surgery** (Continued)

- Closely monitor the client for change in vital signs, especially fluctuations in blood pressure (BP may increase initially in response to shock), increased pulse rate, and elevated temperature; extreme restlessness; difficulty breathing (increased respiratory rate, cyanosis); severe pain, especially after an analgesic has been given or in an area other than the operative site; abdominal distention or rigidity; excessive or absent nansogastric output; urinary output less than 35mL/hour if catheterized or failure to void within 8 hours of surgery; failure to pass flatus or stool more than 48 hours after surgery; profuse diaphoresis; excessive bloody drainage from the nasogastric tube, surgical drains, or surgical dressing; separation of the surgical wound edges; and unusual color or odor of drainage.

Nursing Diagnosis: Imbalanced Nutrition, Less than Body Requirements related to poor nutritional intake before surgery and changed GI system after surgery.

Expected Outcome: Client will achieve optimal caloric intake to maintain weight.

Interventions	Rationales
Assess client for changes in physiologic status that will interfere with nutrition.	Malnutrition contributes to poor recovery from surgery.
Administer total parenteral nutrition (TPN) as ordered (see Chap. 13).	TPN provides adequate calories, nutrition, and fluid replacement and supports metabolic needs.
Administer nasogastric feedings as ordered (see section in this chapter).	Nasogastric feedings provide adequate calories, nutrition, and fluid replacement and support metabolic needs.
When bowel sounds return, advance oral diet as ordered and tolerated. Encourage small, frequent meals.	An advanced diet provides opportunity for client to eat and adjust. Small, frequent meals prevent fullness and nausea.
Monitor food intake.	Such monitoring helps identify trends in client's nutritional status.
Weigh client twice a week.	Weighing determines weight loss, gain, or maintenance.
Report laboratory values such as low blood cell and hemoglobin counts and decreased iron, serum protein, transferrin, or ferritin level.	Such findings may indicate malnutrition.

Evaluation of Expected Outcome

Client attains optimal nutrition as evidenced by reasonable weight and tolerance of six small meals of soft foods and liquids.

PC: Dumping Syndrome

Expected Outcome The nurse will minimize and manage problems associated with dumping syndrome.

Interventions	Rationales
Offer small, frequent feedings low in simple sugars.	Small frequent feedings delay entry of foods into the jejunum, allowing time for dilution and absorption.
Withhold oral fluids at meals. Provide fluids 1 hour after meals	These measures avoid rapid emptying of food from the stomach.
Encourage client to lie down for about 30 minutes after a meal.	Lying down for 30 minutes helps food to remain longer in the stomach.
Maintain bed rest if dizziness and weakness occur.	Bed rest decreases other symptoms, such as nausea, vomiting, and palpitations.

Evaluation of Expected Outcome

Client does not have any signs or symptoms of dumping syndrome and follows dietary restrictions.

---

antacids or other over-the-counter medications to relieve symptoms is also important. Weigh the client and check for signs of malnutrition and dehydration. When completing the history, ask about past infections, exposure to irritants, and alcohol and tobacco use.

Diagnosis, Planning, and Interventions

For clients who undergo thoracic surgery to repair a hiatal hernia, nursing care is the same as for clients who have chest surgery (see Chap. 20). Regardless of the surgical approach, postoperative care will likely involve intubation for gastric decompression to prevent stomach distention and avoid pressure on the surgical repair (see Nursing Guidelines 45-2). When managing nonsurgical care of clients with hiatal hernia or other esophageal disorders, the care plan includes, but is not limited to, the following.

▶ **Imbalanced Nutrition: Less than Body Requirements** related to difficulty swallowing

▶ **Expected Outcome:** Client will consume adequate nutrients to gain or maintain weight.

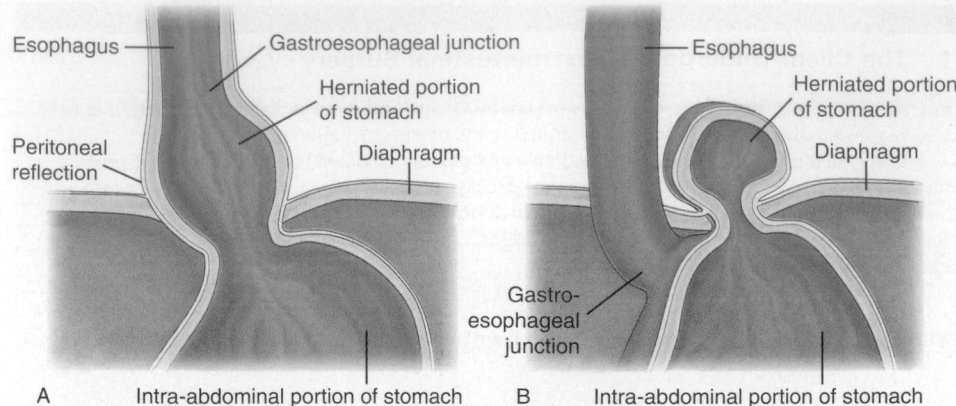

FIGURE 45-3. (**A**) Sliding hiatal hernia. (**B**) Paraesophageal hiatal hernia.

- Encourage client to eat frequent, small, well-balanced meals. *This meal plan provides adequate nutrition without overloading the upper GI system.*
- Instruct client to eat slowly and to chew food thoroughly. *Slow eating and thorough chewing promote easy passage of food to the stomach through the esophagus.*
- Suggest that the client avoid foods and beverages that cause discomfort. *Clients with GERD should avoid foods and beverages that decrease LES pressure and stimulate gastric acid secretion (e.g., caffeine, chocolate).*
- Record daily weights. *A daily record reveals trends in weight gain or loss.*
- Instruct client to avoid alcohol or tobacco products. *They may suppress the appetite and can irritate the digestive tract.*

▶ **Acute Pain** related to pressure, reflux of gastric secretions, or difficulty swallowing

▶ **Expected Outcome:** Client will experience relief from epigastric discomfort.

- Tell client to avoid very hot or cold fluids or spicy foods. *These foods stimulate esophageal spasm and secretion of hydrochloric acid in the stomach.*
- Inform client to remain upright for at least 2 hours after meals. *An upright position helps prevent reflux.*
- Discourage client from eating before bedtime. Raise the head of the bed on blocks 4 to 8 inches. *These measures help to prevent reflux.*
- Tell client to avoid activities that may involve the Valsalva maneuver (e.g., lifting heavy objects, straining for bowel movements). *The Valsalva maneuver increases intra-abdominal pressure and may cause the stomach to wedge above the diaphragm.*
- Instruct client to take medications as prescribed. *Excessive antacids may cause rebound stomach acidity. Prescribed medications reduce acidity effectively, prevent esophageal irritation, and relieve pain.*

Evaluation of Expected Outcomes

The client consumes adequate nutrients as evidenced by maintenance of weight and adherence to small, frequent meals. He or she states relief from epigastric pain.

CANCER OF THE ESOPHAGUS

Esophageal cancer is a serious condition. Clients usually do not experience symptoms until the disease has progressed to interfere with swallowing and passage of food, leading to weight loss.

Pathophysiology and Etiology

Esophageal cancer affects men more often than women. Clients usually are diagnosed in the fifth or sixth decade of life. There are two types of esophageal cancer. The most common is squamous cell carcinoma, which begins in the cells lining the esophagus. It generally occurs in the middle to upper part of the esophagus. The other type is adenocarcinoma, which begins in the glandular tissue of the lower part of the esophagus. As the cancer advances, the mass occupies space and interferes with swallowing. If the tumor grows unchecked, it may obstruct passage of food into the stomach, promoting the possibility of aspiration, or the tumor may ulcerate, leading to occult or frank blood loss.

In general, the major cause of esophageal cancer is chronic irritation of the esophagus from any source. Esophageal cancer is strongly correlated with alcohol abuse and cigarette smoking. Clients with GERD are at higher risk for adenocarcinoma of the esophagus. Other risk factors include habitual ingestion of hot liquids or foods, poor or inadequate oral hygiene, and nutritional deficiencies (Smeltzer et al., 2008).

Assessment Findings

Symptoms usually develop slowly. Beginning symptoms are mild, with vague discomfort and difficulty swallowing some foods. Weight loss accompanies progressive dysphagia. As the disease continues, solid foods become almost impossible to swallow, and the client resorts to consuming liquids only. He or she may experience regurgitation of food and liquids. The tumor also may hemorrhage, resulting in hemoptysis. By the time swallowing difficulty is pronounced, the cancer may have invaded surrounding tissues and lymphatics. Expansion of the tumor causes back pain and respiratory distress. Pain is a late symptom. The client also exhibits weight loss and weakness.

A barium swallow demonstrates a filling defect caused by a space-occupying mass. A biopsy of tissue removed during esophagoscopy or an esophagogastroduodenoscopy

(EGD) reveals malignant cells. A bronchoscopy may determine whether the cancer cells have affected the trachea. An endoscopic ultrasound or mediastinoscopy may evaluate for cancer in the surrounding lymph nodes or other mediastinal structures. Computed tomography (CT) of the chest and abdomen and positron emission tomography (PET) also determine whether metastasis has occurred.

Medical and Surgical Management

If esophageal cancer is diagnosed in early stages, treatment is directed at a cure and includes surgery, chemotherapy, and/or radiation. The surgery is a complete resection of the esophagus (esophagectomy), which involves removing the tumor and a wide margin of tumor-free tissue as well as surrounding lymph nodes. If the tumor is in the upper two thirds of the esophagus, the surgeon removes the affected area and replaces that portion of esophagus with a section of jejunum or colon. The surgery is very risky, particularly if the tumor is high in this part of the esophagus, because of pulmonary complications as well as problems with the anastomosis and the transplant to replace the cancerous esophageal tissue (Smeltzer et al., 2008). If the tumor is in the lower one third of the esophagus, the surgeon removes the affected area and attaches the remaining esophageal tissue to the stomach.

Clients who are not candidates for surgery are treated with palliative measures and, possibly, endoscopic laser surgery to destroy some of the tumor. Esophageal dilatation may be used to enlarge the obstructed area. A prosthesis (stent placement) may be inserted at the tumor site to widen the narrowed area or when a fistula forms at the tumor site. Radiation, chemotherapy, laser therapy, and/or photodynamic therapy may also be used as palliative measures. Laser therapy may be used to destroy the cancerous tissue and relieve obstruction when surgery is not effective or cannot be used. Photodynamic therapy combines chemotherapy with special light to eliminate cancer cells and relieve symptoms such as difficulty swallowing.

Nursing Management

The nurse must consult with the dietitian before instituting measures for weight reduction or gain as ordered. A major nursing goal is adequate or improved nutrition and eventually stable weight. The nurse encourages small, frequent meals. If the client has difficulty swallowing, the nurse ensures that the client receives soft foods or high-calorie, high-protein semi-liquid foods. The client needs to refrain from consuming foods that contain significant air or gas, such as soufflés and carbonated drinks. To reduce bloating, the client should avoid drinking from straws or narrow-necked bottles to reduce the volume of air trapped in the esophagus or stomach. The client should receive liquid supplements between meals.

The nutritional needs of the client with inoperable cancer of the esophagus are met with nasogastric or gastrostomy tube feedings or TPN. In such cases, essential nursing management involves caring for the skin at the tube insertion site, preventing infection, administering nourishment, maintaining tube patency, and preparing the client or family for self-care or home care after discharge. (See the earlier sections on GI Intubation and gastrostomy.)

Clients who return from esophageal or gastric surgery need to be turned and to perform deep breathing and coughing every 2 hours. They also must know how to support the surgical incision for coughing and deep breathing. The nurse may use an incentive spirometer to motivate the client and provide immediate feedback on respiratory efficiency. The client must ambulate to mobilize secretions, increase depth of respiration, and promote expulsion of intestinal gas.

To avoid gastric distention, the client should not have oral nourishment until bowel sounds resume and are active. The nurse provides oral liquids, when allowed, to thin secretions. To minimize dyspnea, the nurse gives frequent, small meals and does not allow the client to lie down immediately after eating.

The nurse explains the rationale underlying the prescribed treatment and instructs the client and family to adhere to the therapeutic regimen, follow the necessary dietary modifications, and attend medical follow-up appointments regularly. He or she emphasizes that the client should inform the physician immediately of worsening symptoms, steady weight loss, difficulty swallowing soft foods, abnormal bleeding, or other new problems.

GASTRIC DISORDERS

GASTRITIS

Gastritis is inflammation of the stomach lining (gastric mucosa). It may be acute or chronic.

Pathophysiology and Etiology

The causes of gastritis include dietary indiscretions; reflux of duodenal contents; use of aspirin, steroids, nonsteroidal anti-inflammatory drugs (NSAIDs), alcohol, or caffeine; cigarette smoking; ingestion of poisons or corrosive substances; food allergies; infection; and gastric ischemia secondary to vasoconstriction caused by a stress response. The bacterium *Helicobacter pylori* may contribute to chronic gastritis.

Gastric secretions are highly acidic. *Parietal cells* in the stomach increase acid production (hydrochloric acid) in response to seeing, smelling, and eating food. The parasympathetic vagus nerve releases histamine and acetylcholine, chemicals that also stimulate the parietal cells. An increasing level of acid triggers the conversion of pepsinogen to pepsin, creating a chemical mixture strong enough to digest the stomach wall. However, because mucus protectively coats the stomach lining, pepsin normally has little effect on the stomach wall.

Prostaglandin E, a lipid compound secreted in the stomach, apparently promotes the production of mucus, which contains buffering substances and mechanically bars penetration by stomach acids. The submucosal layers of the stomach can become inflamed, however, when irritating substances reduce or penetrate the mucous layer. Consequently, the client experiences epigastric discomfort, often described as *heartburn*. The mucus-producing cells usually heal and regenerate in 3 to 5 days. Chronic irritation leads to ulceration.

- Changes of aging include thinning of the gastric mucosa, predisposing older adults to superficial gastritis and gastric ulcers.

- Common chronic conditions in older adults such as osteoarthritis, vascular, or cardiac problems may require medications such as aspirin, NSAIDs, or anticoagulants, which increase the risk for gastritis, gastric bleeding, and gastric ulcers.

Assessment Findings

Usually the client complains of epigastric fullness, pressure, pain, anorexia, nausea, and vomiting. When a bacterial or viral infection causes the gastritis, the client may experience vomiting, diarrhea, fever, and abdominal pain. Drugs, poisons, toxic substances, and corrosives can cause gastric bleeding. Clients may describe seeing blood in emesis or note a darkening of their stool color. Chronic gastritis may give rise to no symptoms or symptoms similar to mild indigestion.

A complete blood count may reveal anemia from chronic blood loss. Stool testing for occult blood often detects RBCs. In difficult cases, gastroscopy may be performed to visualize the mucosa and obtain specimens, which are examined for pathogens or cellular abnormalities. Clients may also be tested for *H. pylori.*

Medical and Surgical Management

Treatment depends on the cause and symptoms. Ingestion of poisons requires emergency treatment. In acute cases, eating is restricted and IV fluids are given to correct dehydration and electrolyte imbalances, particularly if vomiting is severe. Antiemetics are prescribed to control nausea and vomiting, and antibiotics may be prescribed to inhibit or destroy infection.

The usual treatment of chronic gastritis is the avoidance of irritating substances, such as alcohol and NSAIDs. Some clients may wish to avoid spicy foods, high-fat foods, and caffeine, depending on the degree to which these items aggravate their symptoms. Various drugs, such as antacids, H_2-receptor antagonists, and proton pump inhibitors may be prescribed. A combination of drugs may be used to treat *H. pylori* (see the section on Medical and Surgical Management of peptic ulcer disease).

Nursing Management

The nurse monitors the client's symptoms. Evaluating the client's response to dietary modifications and prescribed medications is important. The nurse observes the color and characteristics of any vomitus or stool that the client passes. In addition, he or she teaches about diet, drug therapy, and the need for continued medical follow-up. For complications such as ulcer formation, refer to the section on Nursing Management of peptic ulcer disease.

PEPTIC ULCER DISEASE

A **peptic ulcer** is a circumscribed loss of tissue in an area of the GI tract that is in contact with hydrochloric acid and pep-

sin. Most peptic ulcers occur in the duodenum; however, they may develop at the lower end of the esophagus, in the stomach, or in the jejunum after the client has had surgery at the spot where the stomach and the jejunum were sutured. Gastric ulcers are more likely to recur and have the highest incidence for undergoing malignant changes. Men are affected more frequently by peptic ulcer disease (PUD) than women are. The highest incidence occurs during middle life, but the condition can occur at any age.

Pathophysiology and Etiology

PUD occurs when the normal balance between factors that promote mucosal injury (gastric acid, pepsin, bile acid, ingested substances) and factors that protect the mucosa (intact epithelium, mucus, and bicarbonate secretion) is disrupted. The single greatest risk factor for the development of PUD is infection with the gram-negative bacterium *H pylori.* Transmission of the bacterium is thought to be by fecal–oral or oral–oral pathways. *H. pylori* is present in the gastric or duodenal mucosa of 80% to 90% of clients with PUD. The bacteria, which shelter themselves in the bicarbonate-rich mucus, are a factor in chronic gastritis and PUD. The mechanism by which this microorganism makes the mucosa more susceptible to erosion is not yet completely understood. It appears that *H. pylori* secretes an enzyme that theoretically depletes gastric mucus, making it more vulnerable to injury.

Family history is thought to be an additional risk factor for the development of PUD. A genetic component may exist, as demonstrated by the high incidence among first-degree relatives. Another explanation is the clustering of infection with *H. pylori* in families. Other risk factors include chronic use of NSAIDs, cigarette smoking, and physiologic stress. PUD resulting from physiologic stress is seen most often in the intensive care unit and may accompany increased intracranial pressure (Curling's ulcer), burns (Cushing's ulcer), and sepsis.

Ulcers develop when there is prolonged hyperacidity or chronic reduction in mucus. Once gastric acid has penetrated the mucosal layer, the acid begins to digest the stomach wall (Fig. 45-4). Histamine, released from the injured cells, aggravates the condition by triggering hypersecretion of more hydrochloric acid and pepsin. The body responds with

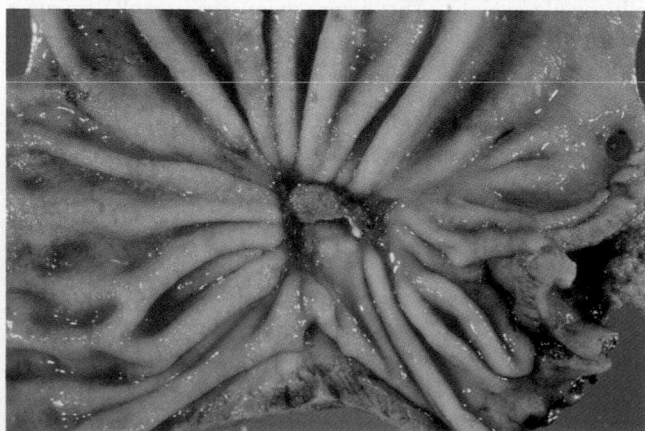

FIGURE 45-4. Gastric ulcer. (From Rubin, R., & Strayer, D. S., eds. [2008]. *Rubin's pathology: Clinicopathologic foundations of medicine* [5th ed.]. Philadelphia: Lippincott Williams & Wilkins.)

the inflammatory process. Capillary permeability is increased; the mucosa swells and bleeds easily.

Because food dilutes stomach acid, clients with PUD experience more discomfort when the stomach is empty than after eating food. Unless the process is controlled, the erosion can lead to an obstruction from scar formation or penetrate the entire thickness of the stomach wall, spilling gastric contents into the peritoneal cavity, a process that may be accompanied by hemorrhage.

Aging and chronic stomach inflammation, such as in recurrent gastric ulcers, cancer of the stomach, or a long history of alcoholism, lead to atrophy of the glandular epithelium of the stomach. The chronic gastric inflammation causes the parietal cells to secrete less hydrochloric acid, resulting in hypochlorhydria (reduced gastric acidity) or achlorhydria (absence of hydrochloric acid). In addition, the gastric mucosa produces intrinsic factor, which the body requires for the absorption of vitamin B_{12}. Chronic gastric inflammation inhibits the production of intrinsic factor, leading to poor absorption of this essential nutrient. As a result, the client is at high risk for pernicious anemia.

Gerontologic Considerations

- Physical changes that occur with aging include degeneration of the gastric mucosa, resulting in a loss of parietal cells. The loss of parietal cells decreases the production of the intrinsic factor and hence decreases the absorption of vitamin B_{12}, leading to pernicious anemia.

Assessment Findings

Signs and Symptoms

Most clients with PUD have abdominal pain, which usually is confined to the epigastrium and does not radiate. Clients most often describe it as having a "burning" quality. They usually complain of pain that occurs 1 to several hours after meals and disturbs sleep. Eating food may relieve the pain. Back pain suggests that the ulcer is irritating the pancreas. Approximately 20% of clients may have bleeding as the first sign of the ulcer. Hemorrhage, hematemesis, or melena may occur. Protracted vomiting secondary to scarring and resultant obstruction also are seen among those who have ignored earlier symptoms. Some clients also have unexplained weight loss.

Diagnostic Findings

The diagnosis is suggested by the history and confirmed by results of an upper GI series or EGD. To differentiate between benign and malignant ulcers, a gastric washing or biopsy for cytologic analysis may be performed. Typically, the hemoglobin level and RBC count are low from chronic blood loss. Vomiting alters electrolyte levels. In addition, tests for *H. pylori* are performed.

Medical and Surgical Management

Most clients with PUD have *H. pylori*. Thus, the goals of treatment are to (1) eradicate the bacteria and (2) reduce the acid levels in the digestive system to relieve pain and

promote healing. Use of only one antibiotic is inadequate to kill the bacterium; eradication therapy includes a combination of antibiotics for at least 2 weeks. Drugs are also prescribed to reduce acid, relieve pain, and promote healing, including H_2 antagonists, antacids, proton pump inhibitors, and cytoprotective agents. These drugs may be prescribed for longer than 2 weeks. The following list provides examples of drugs used to treat PUD:

- *Antibiotics:* Commonly prescribed antibiotics are amoxicillin (Amoxil) and clarithromycin (Biaxin), which exert bactericidal effects to eradicate *H. pylori*.
- *Amebicides:* Metronidazole (Flagyl) assists in the eradication of *H. pylori*.
- *Histamine$_2$-receptor (H_2) antagonists:* Cimetidine (Tagamet), famotidine (Pepcid), nizatidine (Axid), and ranitidine (Zantac) block H_2 receptors and decrease hydrochloric acid secretion in the stomach, relieving pain and promoting healing.
- *Antacids:* These drugs initially are used to neutralize existing stomach acid and provide quick pain relief. They are not absorbed from the GI tract and therefore do not produce alkalosis, even when given in large doses.
- *Proton pump inhibitors:* Omeprazole (Prilosec), lansoprazole (Prevacid), esomeprazole (Nexium), rabeprazole (AcipHex), and pantoprazole (Protonix) block the final step in acid production at the surface of parietal cells. These medications also promote healing and appear to inhibit the growth of *H. pylori*.
- *Cytoprotective agents:* Sucralfate (Carafate) forms a seal over the ulcer, protecting it from irritation. Misoprostol (Cytotec), a synthetic prostaglandin, is used to sustain the mucosal layer especially among clients who require large doses or long-term treatment with aspirin or NSAIDs. Bismuth salts such as bismuth subsalicylate (Pepto-Bismol) suppress *H. pylori*, assist in healing mucosal lesions, and protect the lining of the stomach and intestines.
- *Combination drugs:* Some drug companies provide medication combinations for the treatment of PUD, which include two antibiotics with an H_2 antagonist or cytoprotective agent. Examples include Prevpac and Helidac.

Pharmacologic Considerations

- Sucralfate is administered 2 hours after an H_2 antagonist to ensure the absorption of the H_2 antagonist. It may be given for 4 to 6 weeks.

Clients with PUD may experience obstruction resulting from edema and inflammation. Gastric intubation is necessary, along with treatment for the ulcer. Treatment of hemorrhage includes complete rest for the GI tract, blood transfusions, and gastric lavage with saline solution. IV fluids are administered until the bleeding has stopped. If more conservative measures are unsuccessful, endoscopic laser therapy or endoscopic injections of epinephrine or anhydrous alcohol into the ulcer bed may be used to control bleeding.

Ulcers that persist (referred to as refractory ulcers) despite medical interventions, repeatedly recur, cause severe hemorrhage, create unrelieved obstruction, cause perforation, or are predisposed to malignant changes justify surgical interventions as described in Table 45-3. If a total **gastrectomy** (removal of the stomach) is performed, the client receives vitamin B_{12} injections or intranasal vitamin B_{12} for life because, without the stomach, the intrinsic factor necessary for absorption of vitamin B_{12} no longer is produced. vitamin B_{12} therapy usually is not necessary for 1 or 2 years after surgery because the body uses very small amounts of this vitamin and body reserves usually are sufficient for several years.

Clients with a gastrojejunostomy are at risk for developing dumping syndrome when they begin to take solid food. **Dumping syndrome**, which produces weakness, dizziness, sweating, palpitations, abdominal cramps, and diarrhea, results from the rapid emptying (dumping) of large amounts of hypertonic chyme (a liquid mass of partly digested food) into the jejunum. This concentrated solution in the gut draws fluid from the circulating blood into the intestine, causing hypovolemia. The drop in blood pressure can produce syncope. As the syndrome progresses, the sudden appearance of carbohydrates in the jejunum stimulates the pancreas to secrete excessive amounts of insulin, which in turn causes hypoglycemia.

Nursing Management

The nurse must explore each symptom of PUD in depth. For example, if pain occurs, the nurse determines its type, onset in relation to eating food, location, and duration. A dietary history must include relevant questions pertaining to foods that cause distress, the amount of food eaten at each meal, and whether eating food relieves pain.

For a client to continue eating, it may be necessary to modify ingredients, temperature, or consistency of foods, as well as to use smaller portions on smaller plates. Clients need nutritional supplements. If the client is receiving tube feedings, reinstilling the gastric residual is necessary because it contains partially digested nutrients and essential electrolytes.

In addition, the nurse notes the client's bowel patterns and stool characteristics. He or she also evaluates the client's emotional status and response to activity. The nurse monitors the nonsurgical client closely for medical complications, which includes assessing vital signs and fluid status. Nursing Guidelines 45-3 describes assessment of gastric pH. For a discussion of appropriate nursing management of a surgical client, refer to the Nursing Management section that accompanies the discussion of cancer of the stomach.

Nursing Process for the Client With a Gastric Disorder

Assessment

Ask about current symptoms, looking for specific information about such symptoms as indigestion, fullness, heartburn, nausea,

vomiting. How long has the client had these symptoms? When do they occur? For example, does the client experience problems before or after eating or with certain foods? Do situations such as stress make the problems worse? Does anything relieve the problem? Having the client provide a record of dietary intake for the last 72 hours may be useful. Also, ask about previous gastric problems and treatments/surgery. Assess for signs of abdominal discomfort/pain, malnutrition, and dehydration.

Diagnosis, Planning, and Interventions

▶ **Risk for Deficient Fluid Volume** related to vomiting, diarrhea, and/or bleeding

▶ **Expected Outcome:** Client will maintain adequate fluid balance.

- Assist client to set a goal for minimum oral liquid intake during waking hours. *Involving the client in planning helps meet his or her needs.*
- Provide fluids with calories and electrolytes hourly. Offer different choices. *Frequent fluid intake maintains fluid balance. Various choices prevent monotony.*
- Monitor fluid intake and output. *This record helps indicate trends in fluid balance and early signs of dehydration.*

▶ **Deficient Knowledge** about dietary management and gastric disorder

▶ **Expected Outcome:** Client will demonstrate knowledge of dietary management as evidenced by appropriate choices of foods and fluids.

- Review client's fluid and nutritional needs. *Understanding of fluid and nutritional needs promotes better compliance and intake.*
- Provide a list of foods and substances to avoid. *Doing so may help prevent gastric irritation.*
- Review medications with client, including reasons for medications, schedule, and side effects and their management. *Such review promotes better compliance and outcomes.*

Evaluation of Expected Outcomes

Fluid intake is 2000 mL/24 hours, with a urine output of 1850 mL/24 hours. Nutritional intake is adequate as evidenced by maintenance of pre-illness weight. The client adheres to medical regimen as evidenced by appropriate choice of foods and fluids and compliance with medication schedule.

CANCER OF THE STOMACH

Pathophysiology and Etiology

Cancer of the stomach is a malignancy characterized by either an enlarged mass or ulcerating lesion that expands or penetrates several tissue layers. Stomach malignancies are most common among natives of Japan, as well as in African Americans and Latinos. Although a single etiology has not been identified, factors that are linked to stomach cancer

TABLE 45-3 Surgical Procedures to Treat Peptic Ulcer Disease

PROCEDURE	DESCRIPTION	ILLUSTRATION
Vagotomy	A branch of the vagus nerve is cut to reduce gastric acid secretion.	
Pyloroplasty	The pylorus is repaired or reconstructed to expand the stomach outlet narrowed by scarring or improve gastric motility and emptying.	
Antrectomy	The antrum (lower portion of the stomach, including the pylorus) is removed to eliminate a benign ulcer in the lesser curvature of the stomach if the ulcer has not healed after 12 weeks of medical treatment or is recurring.	
Gastroduodenostomy (Billroth I)	Part of the stomach is removed, while the remaining portion is connected to the duodenum. Usually, a vagotomy also is performed. This procedure is done to remove an ulcerated area in the stomach that is prone to hemorrhage, perforation, and obstruction.	
Gastrojejunostomy (Billroth II)	Same as Billroth I, except the remaining portion is connected to the jejunum in cases of extensive duodenal inflammation or perforation.	
Total gastrectomy	The entire stomach is removed and the esophagus is joined to the jejunum to remove an ulcer high in the stomach near the gastroesophageal junction. It is performed to treat a gastric malignancy.	

NURSING GUIDELINES 45-3

Assessing the pH of Aspirated Fluid

Purpose: To evaluate the effectiveness of antacid or H_2 antagonist therapy in peptic ulcer disease by aspirating stomach fluid and testing gastric pH. Desired pH range is 4.0 to 6.0.

- Obtain a pH test kit.
- Put on gloves.
- Verify that the distal tip of the client's nasogastric tube is in the stomach and has not migrated to the intestine.
- Use a separate syringe for withdrawing the test specimen because antacid residue or irrigating solution in the nasogastric tube will falsely raise the gastric pH.
- Connect the syringe to the tube.
- Instill a small amount of air to clear fluid from the gastric tube just before aspirating.
- Aspirate a small amount of fluid.
- Drop a sample of the gastric fluid onto a pH color indicator strip.
- Compare the color on the test strip with the color guide supplied in the test kit.
- Record the findings.

Client and Family Teaching 45-1
Discharge Instructions for the Client with Stomach Cancer

The type and extent of teaching depends on the surgery that is performed. If tube or gastrostomy feedings, tracheostomy care, and suction techniques will continue after discharge, the nurse involves the client and a family member in practicing these procedures while the client is still hospitalized. He or she identifies where medical supplies can be purchased and offers a referral for home care from a local community agency. Other points to instruct the client and family about in the discharge teaching plan include the following:

- Adhere to the diet (e.g., foods to eat or avoid) recommended by the physician.
- Also adhere to the dietary, fluid, and positional modifications to avoid the dumping syndrome.
- Take medications exactly as prescribed. Follow the directions on the label, paying particular attention to when you should take the drug (e.g., before, after, or with food or meals).
- Monitor weight weekly. Report any significant weight loss to the physician.
- Keep appointments for periodic medical follow-up.

---

include (1) heredity; (2) chronic inflammation; (3) *achlorhydria* (absence of free hydrochloric acid in the stomach), which may promote bacterial growth; (4) chronic ingestion of highly salted, smoked, or pickled foods; (5) nitrates and nitrites, nitrogen-based chemical additives in cured meats, which combine with other nitrogen-containing substances in the stomach to produce nitrosamines—known carcinogens; and (6) tobacco and alcohol abuse. The most common type of stomach cancer is adenocarcinoma, which arises from the glandular cells in the inner layer of the stomach. Stomach cancer often spreads to the lymph nodes and metastasizes to the liver, pancreas, esophagus, or duodenum.

Assessment Findings

Early symptoms are vague. As the tumor enlarges, symptoms include a prolonged feeling of fullness after eating, anorexia, weight loss, and anemia. Stool usually contains occult blood. Pain is a late symptom. A barium swallow or CT scan and a tissue biopsy obtained by gastroscopy or open laparotomy help confirm the diagnosis. Gastric analysis may disclose no free hydrochloric acid. CT scanning or ultrasonography helps determine the depth of the cancer.

Medical and Surgical Management

A subtotal (partial) or total gastrectomy is the only curative approach. The type and extent of surgery usually depend on tumor location, symptoms, and any metastasis. A subtotal gastrectomy preserves more normal digestion. Even though surgery may not achieve a complete cure, it still may be performed to control bleeding or relieve obstruction at the cardiac or pyloric junction.

Chemotherapy with drugs such as 5-fluorouracil (5-FU) or doxorubicin (Adriamycin) and palliative radiation also may be used. For some clients with a specific genetic mutation in their cancer cells, a drug called imatinib mesylate (Gleevec), used in the treatment of leukemia, may be taken orally every day in capsule form. It targets the specific mutation, preventing cell growth without harming healthy tissue. Its use is limited, and surgery remains the treatment of choice.

Nursing Management

The nurse's role in management of gastric cancer includes teaching the public, especially susceptible ethnic groups or clients with a family history of stomach cancer, how to change their dietary habits to reduce the predisposition for this disease. The nurse also may instruct high-risk groups, such as those who have undergone vagotomy or must take medications to reduce hydrochloric acid formation, on the early warning signs of cancer and the value of frequent health assessments. Nursing roles in managing clients undergoing surgery for gastric cancer are extensive. See Nursing Care Plan 45-1 and Client and Family Teaching 45-1.

MORBID OBESITY

Morbid obesity is defined as a body mass index (BMI) of 40 or higher (Box 45-3) or a body weight of more than 20% of ideal.

BOX 45-3	**Calculating Body Mass Index (BMI)**

To calculate BMI, divide weight in pounds by height in inches squared, and then multiply by 703:

$$BMI = \frac{Weight \; (pounds)}{[Height \; (inches)]^2} \times 703$$

- Underweight = < 18.5
- Normal weight = 18.5 to 24.9
- Overweight = 25 to 29.9
- Obesity = ≥ 30
- Morbid obesity = ≥ 40

Pathophysiology and Etiology

Obesity has now reached epidemic levels in the United States, with one third of the population categorized as obese (having a BMI of 30 or higher) (CDC, 2008). The etiology of obesity involves several factors. Genetic predisposition to obesity is a factor, but it is sometimes difficult to separate hereditary factors from learned diet and lifestyle habits. It is clear that obesity results from excessive caloric intake, ready access to an abundance of food, and a sedentary lifestyle. A low resting metabolic rate may also be a factor. Clients with morbid obesity are at greater risk for diabetes, heart disease, hypertension, stroke, osteoarthritis, gallbladder disease, and some forms of cancer, including colorectal and kidney cancer.

Assessment Findings

Clients with morbid obesity often weigh 100 pounds more than their ideal body weight. They may already have hypertension, heart disease, and type 2 diabetes. Many clients are unable to engage in physical activity without getting severely short of breath, and they cannot participate easily in normal activities of daily living, such as bathing and other self-care activities. In addition, they may have poor self-esteem and suffer from depression.

Medical and Surgical Management

Several prescription medications are currently approved for the treatment of obesity. Sibutramine (Meridia) is prescribed for clients who are at least 30 pounds overweight. It inhibits the reuptake of serotonin and norepinephrine (see Chapter 70), which control mood and appetite, thus acting as an antidepressant and suppressing appetite. Sibutramine is used cautiously in clients with hypertension because it can elevate blood pressure. Orlistat (Xenical) works to bind to gastric and pancreatic lipase to prevent the digestion of 30% of ingested fat, thereby decreasing caloric intake. Undigested fat is excreted in stool. Clients with gallbladder problems or those with chronic problems related to absorption of food cannot take orlistat. Clients taking this medication may experience an increased number of bowel movements, increased flatus and oily discharge from the rectum, and decreased absorption of fat-soluble vitamins. To compensate for this problem, clients are advised to take a multivitamin.

Bariatric surgery, or gastric bypass surgery, is a procedure designed to help clients reduce their weight through surgical changes to the upper GI digestive system. It is performed only after other methods for weight reduction have failed. Selected clients should be morbidly obese and motivated to lose weight, and they should accept the surgery-related risks and the lifestyle changes necessary for weight management. In addition, they can have no associated physiologic reasons for the obesity, such as endocrine problems, or any psychopathology that interferes with understanding of the risks involved, such as bipolar disorder or schizophrenia (Beauchamp-Johnson, 2006).

There are three types of bariatric surgery:

- *Restrictive*—This procedure limits food intake into the stomach by creating a small pouch from the top of the stomach and narrowing the passage into the lower part of the stomach. It reduces the amount of food the stomach can hold and slows passage of food through the stomach. The two types widely used for restrictive purposes are called vertical banded gastroplasty (VBG) and laparoscopic gastric banding (Lap-Band).
- *Malabsorptive*—This procedure bypasses the major portion of the small intestine so that it no longer functions as part of the digestive system. In this way, fewer calories and nutrients are absorbed. This procedure is rarely used because of the high risk of nutritional deficiencies. One type is called jejunoileal bypass.
- *Combination*—This procedure combines the restrictive and malabsorptive methods to reduce stomach capacity and partially bypass the small intestine. The Roux-en-Y gastric bypass (RYGB) procedure creates a small stomach pouch by stapling the stomach and then dividing the upper jejunum, rerouting the upper half (called the Roux limb) and attaching it to the stomach pouch. The other end of the jejunum is attached to the Roux limb at a lower point. The end effect is that food moves through the esophagus into the small gastric pouch, passes through the pouch into the Roux limb, and then passes into the remaining small intestine, bypassing the lower stomach and duodenum (Smith, 2006). The RYBG procedure can be performed laparoscopically.

As with any surgical procedure, there are risks. Postoperative bleeding, blood clots, bowel obstruction, and infection may occur (Smeltzer et al., 2008). Other problems may involve nausea and/or distention in the stomach pouch related to overeating or poor chewing of food, dumping syndrome, diarrhea or constipation, and nutritional deficiencies. Long-term goals for this surgery are resolution of chronic health problems, such as type 2 diabetes, hypertension, increased cholesterol and triglycerides, and obstructive sleep apnea. It is hoped that clients will gain increased mobility and greater quality of life.

Nursing Management

The nurse manages the care of clients having bariatric surgery as he or she would for clients having any other type of gastric surgery. However, clients have greater risk of complications related to their morbid obesity. For example, obstructive sleep apnea may be a problem. The client may require continuous positive airway pressure (CPAP) or bilevel positive airway pressure (BIPAP) (see Chapter 20). The obesity can also contribute to poor wound healing, infection, and wound dehiscence. Pain is another possible complication, and effective management is needed so that clients better comply with breathing and mobility exercises.

Discharge teaching must emphasize the preoperative instruction related to lifestyle changes and need for medical follow-up. During the first 3 to 6 months following this surgery, clients may experience flu-like symptoms such as body aches, fatigue, chills, as well as dry skin, thinning and/or hair loss, and mood changes (Mayo Clinic, 2007). Postoperative dietary guidelines for clients having a RYGB are presented in Client and Family Teaching 45-2.

Client and Family Teaching 45-2
Dietary Guidelines After Roux-en-Y Gastric Bypass Surgery

Postoperatively, clients who have had Roux-en-Y gastric bypass (RYGB) surgery have a stomach about the size of an egg. Although it will stretch some, it will never be more than the size of a cup. As time passes, some dietary restrictions will ease. When teaching the client about avoiding discomfort and complications, the nurse emphasizes the following points:

- Gradually progress to 5 or 6 small meals daily, with each feeding providing protein, fat, and complex carbohydrate. Restrict total amount to less than 1 cup.
- Plan to take an hour to eat, chewing food slowly and thoroughly.
- Do not drink fluids with meals. Withhold fluids for 15 minutes before eating to 90 minutes after eating. Take fluids in sips. Drink adequate amounts of water. Avoid liquid calories, such as juice and sodas.
- Choose breads, cereals, and grains that provide less than 2 g of fiber per serving.
- Avoid commonly problematic foods such as tough, fibrous, or overcooked meats; doughy breads, pasta, rice, skins and seeds of fruits and vegetables, nuts, and popcorn.
- Avoid all sweets.
- Avoid any foods that cause discomfort. Maintain a food diary to track what causes discomfort.
- Stop eating when you feel full.

CRITICAL THINKING EXERCISES

1. An older adult is admitted to a healthcare facility because of unexplained weight loss. What assessments are appropriate?
2. A man is diagnosed with a peptic ulcer. He tells you that he had an ulcer many years ago and that he watched his diet carefully and used antacids, and eventually the symptoms subsided. He asks if he should start doing this again. What should you advise him?
3. Clients having upper abdominal surgery are more prone to pulmonary complications. What are some reasons for this?
4. A few days after a client had a gastrectomy, he ate a small meal of rice with cooked vegetables, bread, vanilla pudding, and 8 ounces of juice. Shortly afterward, he complained of feeling weak, dizzy, sweaty, and very crampy. The nurse suspects dumping syndrome. What actions should the nurse take?

NCLEX-STYLE REVIEW QUESTIONS

1. The physician prescribes sucralfate (Carafate) for a client with peptic ulcer disease. When the client asks the nurse to explain the action of the medication, which of the following is the most accurate response?
   1. Sucralfate blocks histamine receptors in the stomach.
   2. Sucralfate covers the ulcer with a protective barrier.
   3. Sucralfate inhibits gastric acid production.
   4. Sucralfate makes gastric secretions less acidic.
2. A client experiences persistent indigestion, feeling of gastric fullness, and unexplained weight loss. The nurse reviews the results of the client's diagnostic tests. Which finding best suggests that the client's symptoms are related to cancer of the stomach?
   1. An elevated level of gastrin is found in the blood
   2. Gastric irritation is noted during a gastroscopy
   3. Gastric analysis shows absence of hydrochloric acid
   4. Hemoglobin and hematocrit are decreased
3. The nurse implements the teaching plan on dumping syndrome for the client who has recently undergone a gastrojejunostomy. After the nurse provides information about restricting carbohydrates, which additional information should the nurse plan to teach this client to help reduce the potential for experiencing the symptoms of dumping syndrome?
   1. Lie down for a short time after eating
   2. Meditate or relax just prior to eating
   3. Sleep with the head of the bed elevated
   4. Walk several times a day between meals
4. During a routine home visit, a client describes what the nurse believes may be symptoms related to a hiatal hernia. Which modification in the client's bed is most appropriate to recommend at this time?
   1. Consider sleeping in a waterbed temporarily
   2. Elevate the legs on pillows when retiring at night
   3. Place a bed board between the mattress and springs
   4. Raise the head of the bed on 4-inch blocks

5. A client has been experiencing difficulty swallowing, and undergoes esophagoscopy, which reveals that the client has a stricture near the end of the client's esophagus. To help improve the client's ability to swallow, the best recommendation the nurse can make is to instruct the client to do which of the following?

1. Avoid drinking beverages while eating a meal
2. Chew everything very thoroughly
3. Eat a variety of foods containing a thickener
4. Refrain from consuming milk and dairy products

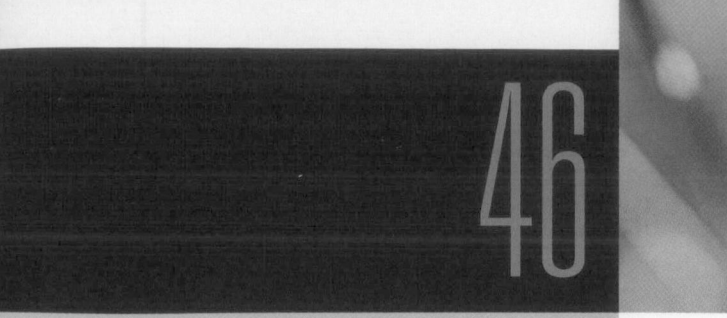

46

Caring for Clients with Disorders of the Lower Gastrointestinal Tract

Learning Objectives

On completion of this chapter, you will be able to:

1. List factors that contribute to constipation and diarrhea and describe nursing management for clients with these problems.
2. Explain the symptoms of irritable bowel syndrome.
3. Contrast Crohn's disease and ulcerative colitis.
4. Describe the features of appendicitis and peritonitis.
5. Describe nursing management for a client with acute abdominal inflammatory disorders.
6. Describe the nurse's role as related to care measures for the client with intestinal obstruction.
7. Differentiate diverticulosis and diverticulitis.
8. Identify factors that contribute to the formation of an abdominal hernia.
9. Discuss nursing management for a client requiring surgical repair of a hernia.
10. Describe warning signs of colorectal cancer.
11. List common problems that accompany anorectal disorders.

The lower gastrointestinal (GI) tract includes the small and large intestines from the duodenum to anus (see Fig. 44-1). The material that moves down the lower GI tract consists of food residues, microorganisms, digestive secretions, and mucus. The mixture of these substances composes feces. Disorders of the lower GI tract usually affect movement of feces toward the anus, absorption of water and electrolytes, and elimination of dietary wastes.

ALTERED BOWEL ELIMINATION

People differ greatly in their bowel habits. Normal bowel patterns range from three bowel movements per day to three bowel movements per week. In differentiating normal from abnormal, the consistency of stools and the comfort with which a person passes them are more reliable indicators than is the frequency of bowel elimination. The type and amount of food a person consumes greatly affect stool consistency. High-fiber diets, such as those containing whole grains, fresh fruits, and uncooked vegetables, form an increased residual of cellulose, an insoluble, indigestible product, in the bowel. Cellulose absorbs water. The combination of cellulose and water increases and softens fecal volume, which speeds the passage of feces through the lower GI tract.

Diseases or disorders of the lower GI system usually manifest themselves as changes in bowel elimination. The most common problems are constipation and diarrhea. Irritable bowel syndrome is a motility problem in which constipation and diarrhea are alternately present.

CONSTIPATION

Pathophysiology and Etiology

Constipation is a condition in which stool becomes dry, compact, and difficult and painful to pass. Normally, fecal matter collects in the rectum and presses on the internal anal sphincter, creating an urge to defecate (eliminate stool). Peristalsis and distention of the colon facilitate the signal to release stool. The gastrocolic reflex facilitates stool passage by accelerating peristalsis. This reflex is most active after eating, particularly after the first meal of the day.

A diet low in fiber predisposes people to constipation because the stools produced are small in volume and dry. The lower GI tract propels low-volume stools more slowly. Whenever stool remains stationary in the large intestine, moisture continues to be absorbed from the residue. Consequently, retention of stool, for any number of reasons, causes stool to become dry and hard.

Constipation may result from insufficient dietary fiber and water, ignoring or resisting the urge to defecate, emotional stress, use of drugs that tend to slow intestinal motility, or inactivity. It may stem from several disorders, either in the GI tract or systemically. Anatomic disorders of the colon, rectum, and anus, which predispose a person to constipation, include strictures (e.g., secondary to disease or intestinal resection), anal stenosis, and anterior displacement of the anus.

Impaired GI motility also may lead to chronic constipation. Motility may be impaired in the absence of other disorders (intestinal pseudo-obstruction) or as a result of visceral myopathies, musculoskeletal disorders, neuropathy, or spinal cord lesions. Systemic disorders that predispose clients to constipation include hypothyroidism, diabetes, pheochromocytoma, porphyria, and hypercalcemia (resulting from hyperparathyroidism and excessive production of vitamin D). Constipation may also result from chronic use of laxatives ("cathartic colon") because such use can cause a loss of normal colonic motility and intestinal tone. Laxatives also dull the gastrocolic reflex. Chronic lead poisoning or concurrent medications such as opioids, tranquilizers, antidepressants, and antihypertensives may also result in constipation.

Gerontologic Considerations

- Constipation is a common problem in older adults and often results from inadequate intake of dietary fiber, lack of exercise, and decreased fluid intake. The risk for constipation is also increased by an age-related decrease in the peristaltic action of the GI tract. Constipation can also occur in older adults who feel rushed when defecating or cannot get to the toilet in time.

Assessment Findings

Signs and Symptoms

Bowel elimination is infrequent or irregular. Clients describe feeling bloated. The abdomen may be tympanic or distended, and bowel sounds may be hypoactive. The client experiences rectal fullness, pressure, and pain when he or she attempts to eliminate stool. What he or she passes usually is hard and dry. Rectal bleeding may result as the tissue stretches and tears while the person tries to pass the hard, dry stool. When a practitioner inserts a gloved and lubricated finger in the rectum, the stool may feel like small rocks, a condition referred to as *scybala*.

Sometimes, if he or she has been constipated for a long time, the client may begin passing liquid stool around an obstructive stool mass (**encopresis**), a phenomenon sometimes misinterpreted as diarrhea. The liquid stool results from dry stool stimulating nerve endings in the lower colon and rectum, which increases peristalsis. The increased peristalsis sends watery feces from higher in the bowel than the retained stool. This symptom is most common in residents of nursing homes and school-aged children who have a long-standing history of constipation, stool-withholding behavior, or both. It may be necessary to check for a fecal impaction.

Diagnostic Findings

A thorough history and physical examination are necessary to determine the underlying cause and need for further diagnostic testing. Frequently, treatment is based on findings of the history and physical examination, precluding the need for a more aggressive approach. Abdominal radiography helps determine the extent of the constipation. A barium enema is performed if a structural abnormality is suspected. In *defecography*, a thick barium paste is inserted into the rectum. Radiographs are taken as the client expels the barium to determine whether there are any anatomic abnormalities or problems with the muscles surrounding the anal sphincter. Anorectal motility and/or colonic motility studies may be performed to confirm a motility disorder. These studies use flexible catheters with sensors that measure the pressure of muscle contractions. Colonic transit or marker studies are used to determine how long it takes for food to travel through the intestines. For one or more days, clients swallow capsules that contain radiographically visible plastic particles. After 5 to 7 days, radiographs are taken to determine whether any particles are left and if so, where they are. The location of the particles can help determine whether there is colonic inertia related to muscle and/or nerve impairment or pelvic floor dysfunction.

Medical and Surgical Management

Treating the cause provides the best relief. For quick symptomatic relief, the physician prescribes an enema or a laxative in oral or suppository form, followed by prophylactic administration of a stool softener. Drug Therapy Table 46-1 provides information about types of laxatives that may be used to treat constipation. Dietary management also is promoted.

Nursing Process for the Client With Constipation

Assessment

Complete the assessments performed on any client with a GI disorder (see Chap. 44). Obtain a complete history as well as a drug history, including the frequency with which the client uses laxatives or enemas. In discussing bowel elimination, determine the client's

DRUG THERAPY TABLE 46-1 Agents Used to Treat Constipation

Drug Category and Examples	Mechanism of Action	Nursing Considerations
Chemical Stimulants bisacodyl (*Dulcolax*) cascara (generic) castor oil (*Neoloid*) senna (*Senokot*)	Directly stimulate the nerve plexus in the intestinal wall, causing increased movement and stimulation of local reflexes. Lead to intestinal evacuation.	Prior to administration assess client's abdomen for tenderness, rigidity, and bowel sounds. Ask when client had last bowel movement. Repeated use in the older adult may cause orthostatic hypotension and weakness from electrolyte loss. Encourage client to maintain adequate fluid intake. After administration assess client for: • Bowel activity and stool consistency • Bowel sounds • Serum electrolytes for clients with repeated use
Bulk Forming Agents magnesium sulfate (*Epsom salts*) magnesium citrate (*Citrate of Magnesium*) magnesium hydroxide (*Milk of Magnesia*) polycarbophil (*FiberCon*) psyllium (*Metamucil*)	Increase intestinal motility by increasing fluids in intestinal contents. This in turn enlarges bulk, stimulates local stretch receptors, and activates bowel reflex activity.	Prior to administration assess client's abdomen for tenderness, rigidity, and bowel sounds. Ask when client had last bowel movement. Magnesium products may cause ECG changes with prolonged use. After administration assess the client for: • Amount, color, and consistency of stool • Daily pattern of bowel activity • Bowel sounds • BUN, serum creatinine, and magnesium levels for clients with repeated or chronic use
Hyperosmotic Agents lactulose (*Chronulac*) polyethylene glycol (PEG) glycerin (Fleet Babylax)	Similar action as bulk-forming agents; pulling water into intestine results in distention and peristalsis, leading to evacuation. The action of these drugs is limited to only the large intestine.	Assess for chronic constipation. After use, assess for abdominal bloating and potential electrolyte imbalance. Possible rectal irritation if given by the PR route.
Emollients and Lubricants docusate (*Colace*) glycerin (*Sani-Supp*) mineral oil (*Agoral Plain*)	Lubricants ease defecation without stimulating movement in the GI tract. Products form a slippery coat on intestinal contents, decreasing the loss of water out of the contents and preventing the contents from becoming hard or impacted. Clients with lower GI surgery such as hemorrhoidectomy or those for whom straining could be harmful (such as in heart dysrhythmias) benefit from lubricants.	Prior to administration assess client's abdomen for tenderness, rigidity, and bowel sounds. Ask when client had last bowel movement. Encourage client to maintain adequate fluid intake. Monitor bowel function to evaluate drug effectiveness.

definition of constipation. Some clients are unaware that a daily bowel movement is not necessarily a rigid standard for proper bowel function.

Obtain a description of the bowel elimination pattern, asking about frequency, overall appearance and consistency of stool, blood in the stool, pain, and effort necessary to pass stool. Ask the client to keep a record of bowel elimination. In addition, assess dietary habits, fluid intake, and activity level. Physical examination includes the anal area, looking for fissures, redness, and hemorrhoids. Auscultate the abdomen for bowel sounds and palpate for distention and masses. Finally, inspect the stool or gently insert a lubricated, gloved finger in the anal canal to assess the characteristics of the unpassed stool.

Diagnosis, Planning, and Interventions

Major goals of nursing management are restoring normal bowel function, relieving rectal discomfort and anxiety, and helping the client understand how to maintain normal bowel function. To make these goals measurable, the nurse must add specific criteria.

When constipation is related to dietary habits, decreased fluid intake, stress, lack of exercise, or other factors, suggest a high-fiber diet that includes plenty of raw fruits and vegetables, whole-grain breads, and coarse brans and cereals (Nutrition Notes 46-1). Teach clients to drink eight or more full glasses of water and fruit juice daily to promote regularity, because fructose is a natural laxative. In addition, urge the client to schedule time to exercise each day because such activity promotes intestinal motility.

The client must respond quickly to the urge to defecate and allow sufficient time to evacuate the bowel. Encourage the client to use the toilet at regular intervals even without the urge to defecate, particularly after meals, when the gastrocolic reflex is most active. Help the client and family understand the need for privacy during bathroom times. Instruct the client to avoid excessive straining to have a bowel movement.

Discourage self-treatment with daily or frequent enemas or laxatives. Chronic use of such products causes natural bowel function to be sluggish. In addition, laxatives containing stimulants can be habit forming, requiring continued use in increasing doses. Teach the client about the use of fiber supplements, such as those containing psyllium. Agents considered "natural" sometimes contain ingredients that lead to chronic laxative dependence. The client must discuss any medication he or she uses for control of chronic constipation with the physician or nurse practitioner. If long-term treatment with stool softeners is indicated, the nurse provides a list of safe medications, such as those containing mineral oil, magnesium, or nonabsorbable sugar (i.e., sorbitol, lactulose).

Nutrition Notes 46-1
The Client With Constipation

A *high-fiber diet* is a vague term that does not quantify or qualify fiber content. Individual tolerance and "need" for fiber vary. To achieve a high fiber intake, most daily grain choices should be whole grains (e.g., 100% whole wheat bread, whole wheat or bran cereal, oats, brown rice, whole wheat pasta). Clients should look for whole grain breads that provide at least 2 g of fiber per serving and whole grain cereals that provide at least 5 g fiber per serving. An adequate fluid intake is essential. In addition, encourage clients to:

● Consume approximately one-half cup of dried peas or beans (legumes) daily. These vegetable proteins are low-fat, high-fiber alternatives to meat. Legumes include split peas; black-eyed peas; pinto, kidney, and navy beans; and red and yellow lentils.
● Consume plenty of fruits and vegetables daily; actual amounts recommended vary with total calories consumed. Because the skin and seeds of fruit are especially rich in insoluble fiber, whole fruits are recommended over canned fruit or fruit juice. Likewise, minimal peeling and scraping of vegetables is encouraged. Most fruits and vegetables provide 1 to 3 g of fiber per serving.
● Consider slowly adding coarse, unprocessed wheat bran, a natural laxative, to the diet. Start with 1 teaspoon daily and work up to 2 to 3 tablespoons daily to decrease the likelihood of flatus, distention, cramping, and diarrhea. Mix wheat bran with juice or milk; add it to muffins, quick bread, or casseroles; or sprinkle it over cereal, applesauce, or other foods.
● Seeds and nuts (sesame, sunflower, and poppy seeds, crunchy peanut butter, popcorn) are also sources of fiber.

Pharmacologic Considerations

- Narcotics and sedatives decrease peristalsis and can result in constipation. Assess bowel function daily. The client may require a stool softener to minimize the constipating effects of these drugs.

Diagnoses, outcomes, and interventions are as follows.

▶ Constipation related to immobility or inadequate fluid intake as evidenced by infrequent passage of stool and abdominal distention

▶ **Expected Outcomes:** Client attains a normal pattern of elimination, and stools are soft and easily passed.

● Review usual pattern of elimination. *Constipation has many possible reasons; assessing usual pattern is the first step in identifying the cause.*
● Review current medications. *Many medications affect bowel elimination.*
● Encourage client to slowly increase dietary fiber intake to 25 g/day. Bran cereals, fresh fruits and vegetables, and beans are excellent sources of insoluble fiber, which promotes normal bowel function. Remind client to add these foods gradually. *Fiber absorbs water in the colon and forms a gel, adding bulk and easing defecation. Adding fiber gradually helps to avoid bloating, gas, and diarrhea.*
● Instruct client to increase fluids to six to eight glasses per day. *This intake prevents hard, dry stools.*
● Encourage client to be out of bed, increase activity, or develop a regular exercise program. *Activity increases peristalsis and promotes bowel elimination.*
● Administer laxatives, suppositories, and enemas as ordered. *Treatments should be used only as ordered to avoid cathartic bowel.*

▶ **Acute Pain** related to rectal distention, difficulty passing stool, or anal tears

▶ **Expected Outcome:** Client will state reduced or no rectal discomfort.

- Apply lubricant in rectum and around anus with glove. *Lubricant provides emollient action for passage of stool and healing of anal tears.*
- Assist client to soak rectal area in tub of warm water. *Soaking in a warm tub relieves pain, helps to heal anal tears, and soothes rectal distention.*

Evaluation of Expected Outcomes

The client has soft, formed stool every 2 days. He or she reports feeling more comfortable after warm soaks and application of lubricant. ●

DIARRHEA

Pathophysiology and Etiology

Diarrhea is the frequent passage of larger-than-normal amounts of liquid or semiliquid stool (more than three bowel movements per day). It results from increased peristalsis, which moves fecal matter through the GI tract much more rapidly than normal. The swift velocity causes intestinal cramping and decreases the time available for water to be absorbed from stool in the large intestine. Consequently, the stool is either very soft or liquid.

Three major problems associated with severe or prolonged diarrhea include dehydration, electrolyte imbalances, and vitamin deficiencies. When diarrhea results from a disease that causes malabsorption, the client is at risk for a nutritional deficiency. The sudden onset of acute abdominal pain or a rise in temperature may indicate perforation of the bowel.

Diarrhea may be related to bacterial or viral infections affecting the intestine; lactose intolerance; food allergies or intolerance; uremia; intestinal disease such as diverticulitis, ulcerative colitis, malabsorption, or intestinal obstruction; rapid addition of fiber to the diet; consumption of highly spiced or seasoned food; overuse of laxatives; and adverse effects of drugs, especially antibiotics or concentrated tube-feeding formulas. The most common cause is infection by bacterial, parasitic, or viral agents. The client may give a history of contacts with ill people in his or her household, foreign travel, or use of water from an impure source (e.g., lakes, streams). The client also may mention long-standing abdominal pain or diarrhea or a family history of metabolic or inflammatory disorders.

Diarrhea also may result from several metabolic disorders and diseases such as cystic fibrosis, pancreatic insufficiency, or inflammatory bowel disease. It may be caused by surgical resection of large portions of the small bowel (short bowel syndrome). Other causes include immunoglobulin A deficiency, overeating, concurrent medication (especially antibiotics), and irritable bowel syndrome.

Assessment Findings

Signs and Symptoms

Stools are watery and frequent. In severe cases, blood and mucus pass with the stool. The client usually experiences urgency (**tenesmus**) and abdominal discomfort. Bowel sounds are hyperactive. Skin around the anus may become excoriated from contact with fecal matter and products of the digestive process (e.g., gastric acid, bile salts). Fever may be present. Infectious diarrhea typically has a sudden onset, with accompanying generalized malaise.

Diagnostic Findings

Routine stool cultures are obtained to identify bacterial infections as the cause for infectious diarrhea. They do not identify parasites, however, which necessitate the use of other measures. Stool specimens obtained to identify parasites and their ova are placed in special preservatives and analyzed separately by the microbiology department. Several samples may be needed because parasites are not typically shed with each stool. Routine ova and parasite analysis may identify amebic infections; however, such infections may require serologic (blood) tests.

Blood in the stool may be common with certain infections and disease processes. Nurses typically test stool specimens, collecting a specimen from the client (e.g., Hemoccult testing). A proctosigmoidoscopy or colonoscopy may be performed to identify chronic inflammation or alteration in the mucosal layer of the large intestine. These studies often are carried out to identify the cause of chronic inflammation. An upper GI series with small-bowel follow-through allows for radiologic examination of the small bowel and identification of inflammation. Upper GI endoscopy allows for identification of malabsorptive disorders such as celiac disease.

Medical and Surgical Management

Treatment of diarrhea that is mild or of short duration, such as that caused by dietary changes or acute illness, involves resting the bowel by limiting intake to clear liquids for one or two meals and gradually advancing to a regular diet. When diarrhea persists and stools are frequent and large, or if the person is very young, elderly, or debilitated, medical treatment may include one or more of the following measures:

- Administration of an antidiarrheal agent, such as diphenoxylate hydrochloride with atropine sulfate (Lomotil), loperamide hydrochloride (Imodium), or a combination product such as kaolin and pectin (Kaopectate)
- Fluid and electrolyte replacement by either the oral or intravenous (IV) route
- Dietary adjustments, which may involve eliminating foods that cause diarrhea
- Total parenteral nutrition (TPN) if diarrhea is severe and prolonged and if the introduction of oral fluid and food results in another episode of diarrhea

Chronic diarrhea depletes the bowel of helpful organisms and allows yeasts and fungi to thrive unchecked. To recolonize the bowel, capsules or granules containing *Lactobacillus acidophilus* (Bacid or Lactinex) are prescribed. These agents are referred to as *probiotics.*

Nursing Process for the Client with Diarrhea

Assessment

Conduct the assessments performed on the client with a GI disorder (see Chap. 44). In addition, obtain a complete health, dietary, allergy, and drug history. It is important to include a history of newly prescribed drugs, such as antibiotics, as well as the pattern of laxative and enema use. Ask about any recent incidence of constipation, because diarrhea can result from an impacted fecal mass. Observe emotional status, because anxiety affects bowel motility. To help determine a cause-and-effect relationship, ask about the onset of diarrhea in relation to the possibility of eating tainted foods. Learning that others who ate the same food have similar symptoms may support the possibility of food-related diarrhea. Ask the client about recent foreign travel. Drinking unsanitary water or consuming uncooked food washed with contaminated water may transmit some intestinal pathogens.

Depending on the severity and duration of the diarrhea, it may be necessary to examine the anal area for redness or other tissue changes. Abdominal auscultation helps identify characteristics of bowel sounds. Palpate for distention and masses, monitor the frequency and characteristics of stools, and measure the volume of liquid stools to assess fluid loss. Also assess for signs of dehydration, electrolyte imbalance, and metabolic acidosis (see Chap. 16). Baseline data collection includes recording daily weights and taking vital signs. Report the sudden onset of acute abdominal pain to the physician immediately.

Diagnosis, Planning, and Interventions

Provide a list of foods and beverages to avoid. Temporary dietary changes may be necessary to reduce the number of stools and to rest the bowel (Nutrition Notes 46-2). If medication is prescribed,

Nutrition Notes 46-2
The Client With Diarrhea

- Reintroducing food after a bout of diarrhea usually calls for a diet low in insoluble fiber to reduce the volume of stool. Insoluble fiber is found mostly in whole grains, high-fiber cereals, raw vegetables, corn, nuts, seeds, and the skins and seeds of fruit.
- Foods high in soluble fiber help slow GI motility; examples include oatmeal, ripe bananas, and applesauce.
- Foods such as mashed potatoes, pasta, bread made with white flour, white rice, and low-fiber cereals are easy to tolerate.
- Yogurt is usually well tolerated and contains probiotics that promote the growth of healthy GI bacteria. Milk should be avoided for a few days because lactose intolerance may occur during periods of acute diarrhea.
- The diet is advanced as tolerated.
- Encourage potassium-rich foods as tolerated. Examples include bananas, canned apricots and peaches, apricot nectar, orange juice, grapefruit juice, tomato juice, fish, potatoes, and meat.

explain its purpose and routine for use and identify common side effects. Caution the client to avoid self-treatment of diarrhea and to consult the physician if the diarrhea does not respond to dietary restrictions and antidiarrheal medications. Advise the client with an underlying GI disorder (e.g., Crohn's disease, ulcerative colitis) to consult the physician or nurse practitioner before using drugs that affect motility (e.g., loperamide, diphenoxylate hydrochloride). Use of these drugs in diseases that affect bowel mucosa may cause dangerous complications. Also advise the client to contact the physician if diarrhea is prolonged or accompanied by severe abdominal pain, blood or mucus passes with stool, fever develops, or urine output decreases. The care plan may include the following.

▶ **Diarrhea** related to an enteric infection, as manifested by frequent liquid stools and abdominal cramping

▶ **Expected Outcome:** Client will develop a normal bowel elimination pattern of one soft, formed stool every 1 to 3 days and will not experience pain or cramping.

- Encourage client to withhold foods until the acute attack subsides. *Withholding food rests the bowel and slows peristalsis.*
- Give clear liquids as tolerated, but limit high-sugar drinks. *Drinking clear liquids prevents dehydration; high-sugar drinks have high osmolality, which may aggravate diarrhea.*
- Advance oral intake as tolerated, initially offering foods high in soluble fiber such as oatmeal, ripe bananas, and applesauce. *Soluble fiber helps slow GI motility.*
- Teach client to avoid foods high in insoluble fiber, such as whole grain bread and cereals, bran cereals, and raw vegetables. Caffeinated and carbonated beverages should also be avoided. *Such items stimulate GI motility.*
- Encourage the intake of yogurt. *Yogurt contains probiotics that help promote the growth of healthy GI bacteria.*
- Administer antidiarrheal medications as ordered for prolonged diarrhea. *These medications slow intestinal motility and inhibit peristalsis.*
- Encourage client to rest in a comfortable position with legs bent toward the abdomen. *This position relaxes abdominal muscles and reduces discomfort.*
- Advise client to avoid carbonated beverages or drinking with a straw. *These increase volume of swallowed air, which in turn increases gas and cramping.*

▶ **Risk for Deficient Fluid Volume** related to frequent passage of watery stools and inadequate fluid intake

▶ **Expected Outcome:** Client's output will not exceed fluid intake.

- Assess hydration status by monitoring intake and output, skin turgor, and moisture of mucous membranes. *Assessment provides a baseline.*
- If diarrhea is severe, offer water, electrolyte solutions (e.g., Gatorade), and clear liquids as allowed and tolerated. *These substances replace fluids and electrolytes and prevent dehydration.*
- Report urine output of less than 240 mL in 4 hours. *Such a finding indicates dehydration.*

- Monitor the number and consistency of stools. *A record documents stool output and provides a baseline to guide fluid replacement.*
- Observe for symptoms of sodium and potassium loss, such as weakness, abdominal or leg cramping, or dysrhythmias. Note results of blood chemistry testing. *Excessive diarrhea causes severe loss of electrolytes.*

▶ **Risk for Imbalanced Nutrition: Less than Body Requirements** related to anorexia and malabsorption secondary to rapid passage of stool through the GI tract

▶ **Expected Outcome:** Client maintains adequate nutritional intake and maintains body weight.

- Notify physician if client cannot tolerate resuming a progressive diet. *This client may require other medical interventions.*
- Instruct client to limit foods that aggravate diarrhea, such as fatty foods and foods high in insoluble fiber. *These foods stimulate GI motility.*
- Advise the client to avoid caffeine (e.g., coffee, chocolate, tea) and milk. *Caffeine stimulates peristalsis; milk intolerance may occur during periods of acute diarrhea.*
- Weigh client as indicated. *A record provides a baseline for monitoring weight loss, particularly for clients with prolonged diarrhea.*

▶ **Risk for Impaired Skin Integrity** related to mechanical and chemical trauma to the rectum

▶ **Expected Outcome:** Client's perianal tissue will remain intact.

- Assist with or administer perianal care after each bowel movement. Provide or use premoistened, nonirritating, non–alcohol-based wipes rather than toilet paper for the anal area. *These measures prevent perianal excoriation.*
- Apply a medicated ointment, such as one containing vitamins A and D or zinc oxide, if perianal area is reddened. *The ointment minimizes excoriation of the perianal skin.*
- If perianal skin becomes excoriated or desquamated, apply a wound hydrogel. *Moisture-barrier ointments protect against further excoriation and promote healing.*

Evaluation of Expected Outcomes

The client's bowel elimination pattern is normal, as evidenced by one to two soft, formed stools every 2 days. The client states that he or she has no pain or cramping. Urine output does not exceed fluid intake. Weight remains stable. Skin remains intact with no signs of redness or excoriation. ●

IRRITABLE BOWEL SYNDROME

Irritable bowel syndrome (IBS) is a functional motility disorder primarily affecting the colon. It refers to a cluster of symptoms that occur despite the absence of an identifiable disease process. People with IBS experience abdominal pain and cramping, bloating and flatus, as well as diarrhea and/or constipation, with or without the presence of mucus. Often, either diarrhea or constipation predominates. IBS does not cause inflammation of the bowel or changes in bowel tissue, and it does not increase the risk of colorectal cancer.

It is estimated that one in five people in the United States have IBS (Mayo Clinic, 2008). Women are affected more often than men, which suggests a hormonal influence.

Pathophysiology and Etiology

Fluctuating intestinal motility tends to be an underlying factor that causes symptoms. Changes in motility may result from a neuroendocrine dysregulation involving the autonomic nervous system. This affects motor function in the GI tract through neuron stimulation and inhibition, influencing bowel motility. When a parasympathetic neurotransmitter (e.g., acetylcholine) is released, intestinal motility increases and diarrhea results. An opposite effect occurs when the smooth muscle of the gut responds to sympathetic neurotransmission. Other factors may also be involved, such as infection or irritation, as well as disturbances in vasculature of the bowel or metabolism (Smeltzer et al., 2008).

Assessment Findings

Signs and Symptoms

Most clients with IBS describe having chronic constipation with sporadic bouts of diarrhea. Some report the opposite pattern, although less commonly. Most clients experience various degrees of abdominal pain that defecation may relieve. Many clients suffer with belching and flatulence (intestinal gas). In general, symptoms do not awaken people from sleep. Some clients with IBS report anxiety, insecurity, depression, or anger.

Weight usually remains stable, indicating that when diarrhea occurs, malabsorption of nutrients does not accompany it. When loose stools are inspected, although passed frequently, they usually are of low volume and may contain mucus. Blood usually is not found in the stool because the bowel is not locally inflamed.

Diagnostic Findings

Radiographic and endoscopic tests rule out other disorders with similar symptoms, such as peptic ulcer disease, colorectal cancer, diverticulitis, or inflammatory bowel disease. Specifically, a barium enema and colonoscopy may show the spasms, distention, and mucus accumulations associated with IBS (Smeltzer et al., 2008) (Fig. 46-1).

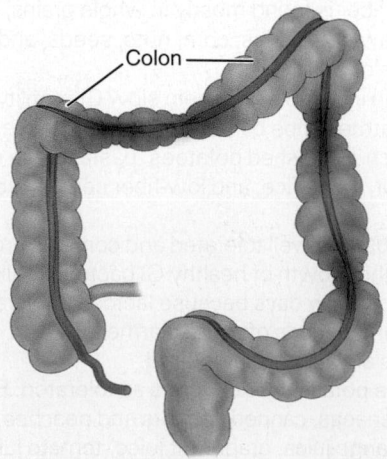

Colon

FIGURE 46-1. In irritable bowel syndrome, the spastic contractions of the bowel are visible in x-ray contrast studies.

Medical and Surgical Management

Dietary changes reduce flatulence and abdominal discomfort. By trial and error, the client eliminates common food sources that cause discomfort or intestinal gas, such as beans or cabbage. At the same time, a high-fiber diet or a bulk-forming agent, such as products containing psyllium (e.g., Metamucil), is prescribed to regulate bowel elimination. The fiber draws water into constipated stool and adds bulk to watery stool. An anticholinergic, such as dicyclomine (Bentyl), has an antispasmodic effect if taken before meals. Either a prescription or nonprescription antidiarrheal is used for temporary relief from diarrhea.

Nursing Management

Most clients with IBS are not hospitalized. Nurses become involved in their care during diagnostic testing, follow-up visits, or hospitalization for a concurrent problem. During these encounters, the nurse gathers a comprehensive database of symptoms, helps manage the problems associated with constipation and diarrhea, explains therapeutic treatments, evaluates the client's understanding of the regimen for self-care, and monitors the response to therapy. By keeping a diary in which they record daily food consumption and symptoms, clients can determine what foods cause problems. Avoiding problem foods helps alleviate symptoms. Eating at regular intervals helps many clients. For clients with diarrhea, eating frequent small meals may be effective. For more specific nursing interventions, refer to the preceding discussions of clients with constipation and diarrhea.

▶ *Stop, Think, and Respond Exercise 46-1*

A neighbor confides that she has IBS. She wonders if you can provide her with any tips about managing her condition. What is your best response?

INFLAMMATORY BOWEL DISEASE

Inflammatory bowel disease (IBD) is a chronic illness characterized by exacerbations and remissions. The term IBD refers to several chronic digestive disorders believed to result from the immune system's attacking the bowel. **Crohn's disease** and **ulcerative colitis** are the most common inflammatory diseases that include IBD. These two distinct disorders are grouped together because of their similar symptoms and treatments (Table 46-1). Because of the similarity in presenting symptoms and results of diagnostic procedures, differential diagnosis may be difficult. Unlike IBS, IBD does not resolve without medical intervention.

CROHN'S DISEASE

Crohn's disease is also called *granulomatous colitis, ileitis,* and *regional enteritis.* This chronic inflammatory condition can occur in any portion of the GI tract but predominantly affects the bowel in the terminal portion of the ileum. In general, this disease begins in young adulthood, although it can occur in older adults. Clients who are more prone to this disorder include those with a family history of the disease, those who are white with a European and/or Jewish ancestry, and those who smoke.

Pathophysiology and Etiology

The inflammation in Crohn's disease extends transmurally through all the layers of the bowel, but the submucosal layer is most involved. Hyperemia (increased blood supply), edema, and ulcerations characterize affected areas. Endoscopic examination shows inflamed areas alternating with healthy tissue. The inflamed areas occur randomly, a phenomenon described as **skip lesions.** The bowel is described as having a "cobblestone" appearance because of the deep ulcerations that form among the edematous tissue (Fig. 46-2).

Because Crohn's disease is a transmural inflammatory process, inflammation can extend beyond the lining of the bowel. As a result, inflammatory channels containing blood, mucus, pus, or stool may develop. Such an inflammatory channel is called a **fistula**; two or more are referred to as *fistulae.* Fistulae may form a channel between the bowel and the skin surface (enterocutaneous fistulae). Common sites for enterocutaneous fistulae are perianal and perilabial sites. Inflammation also may extend between the bowel and other pelvic organs (e.g., vagina), between the bowel and bladder, or between loops of bowel (enterovaginal, enterovesical, and enteroenteric fistulae, respectively). Fistulae also may form between the rectum and vagina in women, as evidenced by passage of stool from the vagina. Chronic inflammation in Crohn's disease also may lead to scarring and stricture formation and eventual obstruction of the lumen.

The cause of Crohn's disease is unknown. Because incidence is increased among family members, a genetic predisposition is presumed. Other possible contributing factors include allergic and autoimmune responses triggered by diet or infectious microbial antigens. Recurrent attacks on the tissue are believed to result from an exaggerated immune response, which explains the chronic nature of the disease. The role of stress in the development of symptoms and subsequent exacerbations has not been defined. As with any chronic illness, stress may influence the client's ability to cope with symptoms. This issue is certainly confused by the fact that many clients with IBD also may have IBS. Diarrhea as a response to anxiety may be confused with exacerbation of the disease.

Assessment Findings

Signs and Symptoms

Usually, onset is insidious, and the course of the disease varies. Usually, most clients have abdominal pain, distention, and tenderness in the lower abdominal quadrants, especially on the right side. Pain may be associated with eating. The client may have a history of chronic diarrhea and fatigue. Growth failure is a common early symptom in children and adolescents. Fever may be present. As Crohn's disease progresses, anorexia, weight loss, dehydration, and signs of nutritional deficiencies occur. Symptoms gradually increase in some clients, whereas acute exacerbations alternate with remissions in other clients. The symptoms may go into remission spontaneously.

The systemic nature of this disease is evidenced by symptoms outside the GI tract, referred to as *extraintestinal manifestations of IBD.* They include arthritis, arthralgias, skin lesions (erythema nodosum and pyoderma gangrenosum), inflammation in the eyes (uveitis, conjunctivitis, and iritis), and disorders of the liver and gallbladder. Usually,

TABLE 46-1 Comparison of Crohn's Disease and Ulcerative Colitis

FACTOR	CROHN'S DISEASE	ULCERATIVE COLITIS
Course	Prolonged, variable	Exacerbations, remissions
Pathology		
Early	Transmural thickening	Mucosal ulceration
Late	Deep, penetrating granulomas	Mucosal minute ulceration
Clinical Manifestations		
Location	Ileum, right colon (usually)	Rectum, left colon
Bleeding	Usually not, but may occur	Common—severe
Perianal involvement	Common	Rare—mild
Fistulae	Common	Rare
Rectal involvement	About 20%	Almost 100%
Diarrhea	Less severe	Severe
Diagnostic Study Findings		
Radiography	Regional, discontinuous lesions	Diffuse involvement
	Narrowing of colon	No narrowing of colon
	Thickening of bowel wall	No mucosal edema
	Mucosal edema	Stenosis rare
	Stenosis, fistulae	Shortening of colon
Sigmoidoscopy	May be unremarkable unless accompanied by perianal fistulae	Abnormal inflamed mucosa
Colonoscopy	Distinct ulcerations separated by relatively normal mucosa in right colon	Friable mucosa with pseudo-polyps or ulcers in left colon
Therapeutic Management	Corticosteroids, sulfonmides (sulfasalazine [Azulfidine])	Corticosteroids, sulfonamides; sulfasalazine useful in preventing recurrence
	Antibiotics	Bulk hydrophilic agents
	Parenteral nutrition	Antibiotics
	Partial or complete colectomy, with ileostomy or anastomosis	Proctocolectomy, with ileostomy
	Rectum can be preserved in some patients	Rectum can be preserved in only a few patients "cured" by colectomy
	Recurrence common	
Systemic Complications	Small bowel obstruction	Toxic megacolon
	Right–sided hydronephrosis	Perforation
	Nephrolithiasis	Hemorrhage
	Cholelithiasis	Malignant neoplasms
	Arthritis	Pyelonephritis
	Retinitis, iritis	Nephrolithiasis
	Erythema nodosum	Cholangiocarcinoma
		Arthritis
		Retinitis, iritis
		Erythema nodosum

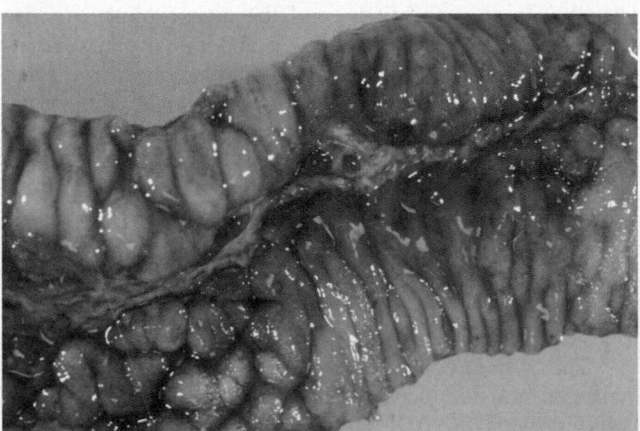

FIGURE 46-2. Crohn's disease. (From Rubin, R., & Strayer, D. S., eds. [2008]. *Rubin's pathology: Clinicopathologic foundations of medicine* [5th ed.]. Philadelphia: Lippincott Williams & Wilkins.)

extraintestinal manifestations become quiescent when the bowel disease is under control.

During the physical examination, palpation may reveal an abdominal mass. Inspection of the perineum and perianal areas may reveal scars from previous fissures, skin tags, or evidence of fistulae or perianal abscesses.

Diagnostic Findings

Stool cultures fail to reveal an etiologic microorganism or parasite, but occult blood and white blood cells (WBCs) often are found in the stool. Results of blood studies indicate anemia from chronic blood loss and nutritional deficiencies. The WBC count and erythrocyte sedimentation rate may be elevated, confirming an inflammatory disorder. Serum protein and albumin levels may be low because of malnutrition. Low serum levels of the fat-soluble vitamins also reflect the client's malnourished state.

All these laboratory findings do not confirm IBD because they can be associated with several other disorders, especially acute infections. Abnormal serum electrolyte levels and a disturbed acid-base balance may accompany severe diarrhea. Serologic tests for IBD may be helpful in some cases. These tests allow for the identification of certain antibodies common to those with Crohn's disease (anti-*Saccharomyces*antibodies, or ASCAs) and those with ulcerative colitis (antineutrophil cytoplasmic antibodies, or ANCAs). These tests do not confirm IBD because clients with IBD may not test positive for the antibodies, and some clients who do not have IBD may test positive. These tests may, however, serve as an important adjunct to other diagnostic tests.

Barium enema findings may show inflammation in the large intestine, but confirmation of the diagnosis requires endoscopic examination (colonoscopy or sigmoidoscopy). Endoscopic evaluation allows for identification of mucosal abnormalities (e.g., skip lesions, ulcerations, cobblestone appearance, bowel wall thickening, and presence of fistula tracts). Biopsies taken during colonoscopy or sigmoidoscopy are examined under the microscope for evidence of chronic inflammation and possible granuloma. A granuloma is an aggregate of inflammatory cells and, when identified on biopsy, confirms the diagnosis of Crohn's disease. The absence of a granuloma does not rule out the diagnosis of Crohn's disease.

Clients with Crohn's disease are vulnerable to intestinal perforation during barium enema and endoscopy because of poor integrity of the bowel wall. They are monitored accordingly. Esophagogastroduodenoscopy (EGD) with biopsy is indicated when inflammation is suspected in the upper GI tract. An upper GI series with small-bowel follow-through allows for radiographic examination of the small intestine and identification of inflammation that endoscopy cannot evaluate.

Medical Management

Treatment is supportive. The dietary approach varies. A high-fiber diet may be indicated when it is desirable to add bulk to loose stools. A low-fiber diet may be indicated in cases of severe inflammation or stricture. A high-calorie and high-protein diet helps replace nutritional losses from chronic diarrhea. The client may need nutritional supplements, depending on the area of the bowel affected. When the small intestine is inflamed, some clients experience lactose intolerance, requiring avoidance of lactose-rich foods.

Some clients need an elemental diet formula, such as Tolerex, Vivonex, or Peptamen, that reduces proteins, fats, and carbohydrates to an easily absorbed form. Elemental diets effectively induce remission in Crohn's disease without medications. Unfortunately, clients are not allowed to eat or drink normally while on the elemental diet, making this treatment modality unacceptable for many. In addition, elemental formulas are not very palatable. Some may need to be administered through a nasogastric tube. Success with elemental diet therapy requires extensive education and client motivation. Newly introduced polymeric diets (Modulen, Nestle, U.S.A.) may provide the benefit of inducing remission and are more palatable. TPN may become necessary to provide intestinal rest. IV fluids, electrolytes, and whole blood are given to correct anemia and restore fluid and electrolyte balance.

Drug therapy involves supplementary vitamins, iron, antidiarrheal and antiperistaltic drugs to reduce peristalsis and rest the bowel, anti-inflammatory corticosteroids and

5-aminosalicylic acid (5-ASA) medications, immune modulating agents, and antibiotics (Drug Therapy Table 46-2). Vitamin and iron supplements are used for known deficiencies and malabsorption. Antidiarrheal agents, such as diphenoxylate (Lomotil) and loperamide (Imodium), usually are used sparingly and only when clients do not have an infection. Decreasing motility in cases of infection predisposes clients with IBD to **toxic megacolon**, a complication that is discussed in the section on ulcerative colitis.

Considered first-line treatment for IBD, 5-ASA drugs contain salicylate, which is bonded to a carrying agent that allows the drug to be absorbed in the intestine. These drugs work by decreasing the inflammatory response. The 5-ASA medications include sulfasalazine (Azulfidine), olsalazine (Dipentum), and mesalamine (Asacol, Pentasa). Mesalamine also is available in enema or suppository form (Rowasa) and may be used to treat distal disease. Folic acid usually is recommended for clients taking sulfasalazine, which interferes with absorption of this nutrient. Corticosteroids (prednisone) are used during acute exacerbations of symptoms and when 5-ASA drugs cannot control the symptoms. Hydrocortisone is available in enema form (Cortenema) and is effective in controlling distal disease without posing a high risk of systemic side effects. Long-term corticosteroid use is undesirable because of the potentially severe side effects; the dose usually is tapered and discontinued when the symptoms are in remission.

Failure to maintain remission necessitates the use of an immune-modulating agent such as mercaptopurine (6-MP) or azathioprine (Imuran). These agents often allow clients to discontinue corticosteroids without exacerbating symptoms. Other immune modulators are cyclosporine (Sandimmune), tacrolimus (Prograf), and methotrexate (MTX). Antibiotics such as metronidazole (Flagyl) and ciprofloxacin (Cipro) are effective adjuncts to treating Crohn's disease, especially related fistulae.

Treatment of moderate to severely active and fistulizing Crohn's disease includes infliximab (Remicade), which has proved safe and effective in achieving and maintaining remission in many clients with Crohn's disease. Infliximab is an antibody that interferes with the inflammatory process early in the immune response by inhibiting tumor necrosis factor (TNF). Adalimumab (Humira) is a similar medication used in clients for whom infliximab has not been effective. Clients learn to self-administer adalimumab by subcutaneous injection every other week. The potentially serious risk of infection, including tuberculosis, is associated with its use. Certolizumab also pegol (Cimzia), a drug approved in 2008, also inhibits TNF. Injections are given every other week initially and then monthly if the medication is effective. Certolizumab poses a risk of infection because of its effect on the immune system.

Surgical Management

Surgical treatment is reserved for complications such as intestinal obstruction, perforation, or fistula formation. The need for surgical intervention is common in Crohn's disease. In fact, more than 75% of clients with Crohn's disease require surgery within 20 years of the onset of symptoms, and 90% require surgery within 30 years. Unlike surgical treatment for ulcerative colitis, removing the inflamed portion of the intestine does not alter disease progression or

DRUG THERAPY TABLE 46-2 Agents for Disorders of the Lower GI Tract

Drug Category and Examples	Mechanism of Action	Side Effects	Nursing Considerations
Antidiarrheals			
Absorbent Antidiarrheals	Act by coating the walls of the GI tract and absorbing substances.		
bismuth subsalicylate (Pepto-Bismol)		Constipation, dark discoloration of oral mucous membranes and stools	Do not administer to clients who are allergic to aspirin or salicylates.
kaolin and pectin (Kaopectate)		Constipation, abdominal pain	This drug may interfere with absorption of nutrients and other drugs.
Opiate-related Antidiarrheals	Act by slowing overall GI motility.		
diphenoxylate with atropine sulfate (Lomotil)		Sedation, dizziness, dry mouth, paralytic ileus, constipation	Monitor closely for proper bowel function. Advise client not to drive or operate dangerous machinery while taking this drug.
loperamide (Imodium)		CNS depression, abdominal pain and distention, nausea, vomiting, constipation	If necessary and prescribed, administer naloxone to counteract CNS depression from overdosage. Avoid prolonged use.
Laxatives, Cathartics, and Bulk-Forming Agents			
bisacodyl (Dulcolax)	See Drug Therapy Table 46-1.	Abdominal cramps, nausea, vomiting, rectal irritation (from suppository form)	Advise client that prolonged use creates dependence. Do not administer within 1 hour of milk or antacids.
magnesium preparations (milk of magnesia, magnesium citrate, magnesium oxide)		Abdominal cramps, diarrhea, nausea, vomiting	Monitor serum magnesium levels and avoid prolonged use. Explain that these drugs may interfere with absorption of histamine$_2$-receptor antagonists, phenytoin, steroids, and some antibiotics.
mineral oil		Leakage of oil from rectum, diarrhea, abdominal cramps	Mineral oil may cause lipid pneumonitis if aspirated. Do not administer to clients who are vomiting and therefore at risk for aspiration. Prolonged use in high doses may result in poor absorption of fat-soluble vitamins. Monitor serum levels of these vitamins.
polyethylene glycol (GoLYTELY, Colyte)		Nausea, vomiting, abdominal distention and cramps	Administer for bowel evacuation prior to GI testing. Explain that large amounts may be administered. Compliance may be difficult.
psyllium (Metamucil, Citrucel)		Nausea, vomiting, diarrhea, intestinal gas, abdominal cramps	Do not give if client has intestinal obstruction or fecal impaction. Some forms require reconstitution with water.
Anti-inflammatory 5-Acetylsalicylic Acid Medications			
sulfasalazine (Azulfidine), olsalazine (Dipentum), mesalamine (Pentasa, Asacol, Rowasa)	Act in response to inflammation; anti-inflammatory properties of some drugs in this class are not fully understood.	Headache, diarrhea, abdominal pain and cramps, malaise, hair loss, rash, harmless orange discoloration of urine, bone marrow suppression, photosensitivity, decreased sperm motility (sulfasalazine)	These drugs are contraindicated in clients allergic to salicylates. Continued GI symptoms may indicate an exacerbation of the disease and should be reported to the physician. Routine blood tests to monitor for bone marrow suppression are indicated.

DRUG THERAPY TABLE 46-2   Agents for Disorders of the Lower GI Tract (Continued)

Drug Category and Examples	Mechanism of Action	Side Effects	Nursing Considerations
			Encourage application of sunscreen to prevent skin damage (sulfasalazine). Decreased sperm motility is reversible with discontinuing sulfasalazine. Clients taking Asacol may report passing the tablets whole in the stool, which is not harmful. They should notify the physician if this occurs repeatedly.
Anti-inflammatory Corticosteroids prednisone, methylprednisolone (Medrol)	Modify enzyme activity in the body and inhibit inflammatory immune response.	Cushingoid appearance, hypertension, acne, water retention, weight gain, hair loss, increased appetite, hypokalemia, gastric irritation, ulcer formation, adrenal suppression, decreased resistance to infection, complications associated with prolonged use (osteoporosis, development of cataracts, growth retardation, peptic ulceration, hyperglycemia)	Monitor closely for side effects, especially with long-term use. Administer with food to decrease gastric irritation. Encourage low-sodium diet to minimize water retention. Clients with diabetes may have increased insulin needs; monitor blood glucose levels. Abrupt withdrawal may precipitate addisonian crisis, which may be fatal. Caution clients that drug should be weaned. Monitor blood pressure. Monitor linear growth in children. Instruct clients taking prednisone to wear a bracelet or necklace that states they are taking prednisone and may need additional corticosteroids during a medical crisis. Clients taking corticosteroids may not have a normal immune response to infection. Monitor closely for signs of infection, prevent exposure through universal precautions, and encourage consultation with physician regarding routine immunizations. Encourage regular physical examinations to monitor for long-term side effects. Clients should consider a calcium supplement to help prevent osteoporosis. Encourage client to undergo routine blood tests used to screen for bone marrow suppression and hepatic dysfunction.
Immune-Modulating Agents mercaptopurine, 6-MP (Purinethol), azathioprine (Imuran)	Inhibit the synthesis and function of RNA and DNA, impacting immune suppression.	Bone marrow suppression, increased vulnerability to infection, rash, arthralgias, hepatic dysfunction, nausea, vomiting, diarrhea, pancreatitis, hair loss, development of neoplasms	Clients taking these agents may not have a normal immune response to infection. Monitor closely for signs of infection, prevent exposure through universal precautions, and encourage client to consult the physician before routine immunizations.

(drug table continues on page 686)

DRUG THERAPY TABLE 46-2 Agents for Disorders of the Lower GI Tract (*Continued*)

Drug Category and Examples	Mechanism of Action	Side Effects	Nursing Considerations
			Drugs may be teratogenic: women of childbearing age should consult their physician before considering pregnancy. Sexually active females should use appropriate birth control. Drugs may be toxic to infants when transmitted through breast milk.
Biologic Agents infliximab (Remicade)	Works through the monoclonal antibodies and is specific for certain tumor necrosis factors.	Infusion-related reactions: pruritus, rash, chest pain, hypotension, hypertension, dyspnea; other potential side effects: headache, nausea, vomiting, fatigue, fever, autoantibody, lupus-like syndrome, lymphoproliferative disorders, increased susceptibility to infection	Drug is currently approved for a single dose in moderate to severely active Crohn's disease and is being investigated for multidose use to maintain remission in both Crohn's disease and ulcerative colitis. Clients often are given acetaminophen (Tylenol) and diphenhydramine (Benadryl) before the infusion to minimize side effects. Clients with a history of previous infusion reaction may be pretreated with prednisone. Drug is administered intravenously over 2 hours: monitor client for infusion reaction every 1/2 hour during the infusion. Should a reaction develop, discontinue the infusion and notify the ordering physician. Instruct client to continue routine medications unless otherwise directed by physician. Encourage client to undergo routine medical follow-up care. Clients taking this medication may not have a normal immune response to infection. Monitor closely for signs of infection, prevent exposure through universal precautions, and encourage client to consult physician before routine immunizations. Safety during pregnancy and breastfeeding has not been established.

recurrence. Many clients who undergo surgery for Crohn's disease require additional surgery within a few years. An intestinal transplant, a new approach to surgical intervention for clients with severe Crohn's disease, may be performed on clients who have lost intestinal function. The procedure does not provide a cure but does improve the client's quality of life (Smeltzer et al., 2008).

Surgical removal of a large amount of intestine results in the loss of absorptive surface, called **short bowel syndrome**. Massive bowel resection results in dependence on TPN, possibly for life. Removal of the colon requires a permanent ileostomy because the disease tends to recur in any rectal pouch. Ileostomy is discussed in Chapter 48.

Nursing Management

A health history assists in determining the onset, duration, and nature of the client's GI problems. Medical, drug, allergy, and diet histories also are important. Nursing care focuses on monitoring the client for complications, managing fluid and nutrition replacement, supporting the client emotionally, and teaching about diet and medications.

The nurse determines the average number of stools the client passes each day and their appearance. Providing regular skin care to avoid breakdown is essential (see Nursing Process for the Client With Diarrhea). In addition, the nurse asks the client about weight loss and whether any foods increase the frequency of bowel movements or cause discomfort. The client requires assistance to maintain adequate nutritional intake. The nurse monitors the client's intake and collaborates with the dietitian to replace uneaten food with something more acceptable.

Physical examination includes auscultating and lightly palpating the abdomen and inspecting the rectal area. The nurse takes vital signs, weighs the client, and measures and documents intake and output. Advising the client to report whenever a bowel movement occurs is important so it can be inspected and a sample sent to the laboratory for occult blood and other analyses.

ULCERATIVE COLITIS

In ulcerative colitis, the chronic inflammation usually is limited to the mucosal and submucosal layers of the colon and rectum. The disease is most common in young and middle-aged adults but can occur at any age. Some clients experience prolonged remission, whereas others experience mild to severe (and potentially life-threatening) exacerbations of symptoms.

Pathophysiology and Etiology

Although the exact cause is unknown, some believe that multiple factors trigger ulcerative colitis, including genetic predisposition, infection, allergy, and abnormal immune response. The connection between the disease and a malfunction of the immune system is supported by the fact that clients with ulcerative colitis often have other coexisting immune-related disorders such as ankylosing spondylitis and other extraintestinal manifestations.

Inflammation usually begins in the rectum and extends proximally and continuously. As a rule, no healthy tissue appears between inflamed areas, as in Crohn's disease. When inflammation remains confined to the most distal area of the large intestine, the client has **ulcerative proctitis**. When inflammation extends beyond the sigmoid colon, the client has ulcerative colitis. **Pancolitis** occurs when a client's entire colon is affected with ulcerative colitis, and he or she experiences severe bouts of bloody diarrhea, pain, cramps, fatigue, and weight loss. **Fulminant colitis**, also affecting the entire colon, is a progression of severity of the ulcerations, with severe pain, copious diarrhea, and potential dehydration and shock.

The lining of the colon tends to bleed easily in ulcerative colitis. Ulceration may extend to the muscular layer of the bowel wall. Superficial abscesses form in depressions in the mucosa. Poor integrity of the bowel wall may lead to *toxic megacolon,* a complication in which the colon dilates and becomes atonic (lacks motility). The thin bowel wall is vulnerable to perforation under these conditions, leading to peritonitis, septicemia, and the need for emergency surgical repair.

Assessment Findings

Signs and Symptoms

The onset of the disease usually is abrupt. Clients experience severe diarrhea and expel blood and mucus along with fecal matter. Cramps and abdominal pain in the lower left quadrant (LLQ) accompany diarrhea. Eating precipitates cramping and diarrhea, resulting in anorexia, dehydration, and fatigue. Clients usually experience weight loss. The urge to defecate may come so suddenly and with such urgency that the client is incontinent. Some clients experience such incontinence during sleep. Despite intense tenesmus, clients may expel very little stool, or they may have 10 to 20 stools per day. This disease is usually marked by exacerbations and remissions.

Diagnostic Findings

Laboratory findings are similar to those described in the section on Crohn's disease. Barium enema reveals evidence of inflammation. Definitive diagnosis requires proctosigmoidoscopy or colonoscopy with biopsy. Endoscopic examination and biopsy of the lining of the colon reveals characteristic inflammatory lesions. Biopsies of the intestinal mucosa reveal evidence of chronic inflammation. These diagnostic studies usually are withheld in cases of toxic megacolon because of the high risk of perforation. Typical preparation for these procedures often is modified because clients cannot tolerate cathartics, which can lead to exacerbation of the ulcerative colitis. Instead, clients have a clear liquid diet before the procedure and a gentle tap-water enema on the day of the examination.

Medical and Surgical Management

Medical treatment aims toward achieving and maintaining remission. The diet is kept as normal as possible but modified to increase caloric and nutritional content. The client is instructed temporarily to refrain from eating foods associated with discomfort. If all foods cause discomfort, the symptoms are likely from the disease itself and not food. The client may be given TPN and intermittent lipid infusions to rest the bowel completely. The use of an elemental diet, as described with Crohn's disease, has not proved effective in ulcerative colitis.

Blood transfusions and iron are given to correct anemia. The client also may need parenteral fluids and electrolytes. Because frequent bowel movements interfere with absorption of nutrients, supplementary vitamins are prescribed.

Medications used to treat Crohn's disease also are used to treat ulcerative colitis (see section on Crohn's Disease and Drug Therapy Table 46-2). Corticosteroids, given orally, intravenously, or rectally, are used if the disease does not respond to other measures. Because of unacceptable side effects associated with long-term use of corticosteroids, the dose is tapered and discontinued according to the client's response. When tapering corticosteroids without exacerbating the disease becomes impossible, immunomodulating agents (azathioprine, 6-mercaptopurine) are used to decrease the immune response and allow tapering. The goals of therapy are to induce and retain remission, allowing the client to be as healthy as possible when contemplating elective surgery, or both.

Surgery is necessary when the disease does not respond to medical treatment or with complications such as dysplastic tissue (a precancerous condition), perforated colon, or hemorrhage. Removal of the colon under elective, nonemergent circumstances offers the client the best possible outcome and is the definitive cure. The current standard treatment is ileoanal pull-through and anastomosis (see Chap. 48). This procedure typically is performed in two stages, several weeks apart. In the first stage, the colon is removed, and a rectal "pouch" is created from a section of the ileum. The rectal mucosa is removed to create a temporary ileostomy. In the second stage, the surgeon closes the ileostomy and connects the intestine to the rectum, allowing the client to defecate normally. When an emergency colectomy is performed (i.e., for toxic megacolon or perforation), an anastomosis (rejoining of the bowel) may be impossible, necessitating creation of a permanent ileostomy.

Nursing Management

The nurse obtains a health history to identify the nature of the abdominal pain, number and frequency of stools, anorexia, and weight loss. He or she asks the client about dietary patterns, including daily amounts of alcohol and caffeine. The nurse auscultates the abdomen for bowel sounds and their characteristics and palpates the abdomen to determine any pain or tenderness.

The nurse compiles a comprehensive database and conducts frequent focused assessments to identify early changes in the symptoms, which may herald rapidly progressing complications. Until the disease is confirmed, preparing clients for diagnostic tests is necessary. The nurse needs to question radiographic and endoscopic protocols for harsh laxatives and cleansing enemas when the client is experiencing severe diarrhea, because bowel irritation and stimulation tend to aggravate the client's symptoms.

Once the diagnosis is confirmed, the physician orders drug and fluid therapy. If antispasmodics and opiates are pre-

---

Client and Family Teaching 46-1
Inflammatory Bowel Disease

The nurse should include the following topics when teaching the client and family about IBD:

- Comply with special dietary modifications and understand that compliance with these is important.
- Know the name, purpose, dosage, and adverse effects of prescribed drugs.
- Use medications to control symptoms rather than cure the disease.
- Keep all follow-up physician and laboratory appointments so that potentially dangerous complications of disease and side effects of medications can be monitored.
- Use proper techniques for rectal hygiene and skin care.
- Know signs to report immediately to the physician such as more frequent bowel movements, extreme fatigue, severe abdominal pain, visible blood in the stool, adverse drug effects, or weight loss.
- Have regular medical checkups, even when symptoms subside, because clients with ulcerative colitis have an increased risk for the development of colon cancer.

---

scribed, the nurse must exercise great caution when administering them because they may trigger the development of toxic megacolon. The nurse reports any sudden onset of abdominal distention, severe pain, or fever in a client with acute ulcerative colitis. In addition, he or she observes the client receiving steroids for subtle changes because these drugs mask inflammatory symptoms accompanying complications. The dosage and frequency of steroids gradually are tapered when clients no longer need them. The nurse teaches the client about the disease and measures for self-care as soon as he or she is well enough to learn (Client and Family Teaching 46-1).

Clients who are discharged and need high levels of care, such as enteral feedings or TPN, require extensive teaching specific to their home care needs. Central venous catheter care and maintenance of TPN are a few examples of these special learning needs. The nurse thoroughly covers all technical procedures for the client or significant other to perform and allows time for the client or caregiver to perform them with nursing supervision before discharge. The nurse makes a referral to a home care agency to provide continuity of care and to ease the transition from acute care to home care.

ACUTE ABDOMINAL INFLAMMATORY DISORDERS

Appendicitis and peritonitis are among disorders known as *acute abdominal inflammatory disorders.*

APPENDICITIS

Appendicitis is inflammation of a narrow, blind protrusion called the *vermiform appendix* located at the tip of the cecum in the right lower quadrant (RLQ) of the abdomen. Appendicitis can occur at any age but is most common in adolescents and young adults. It is difficult to diagnose at its onset because the initial symptoms resemble a host of other disorders such as gastroenteritis, Crohn's disease, ovarian cyst, tubal pregnancy, and inflammation of the kidney or ureter.

Pathophysiology and Etiology

Like other parts of the bowel, the appendix fills with food and empties digested material regularly. Its location and shape contribute to the inefficiency of this process. The inflammation begins when the opening of the appendix narrows or becomes obstructed (Fig. 46-3). The obstruction may result from a hard mass of feces, called a *fecalith,* a foreign body, local edema, or a tumor. The blockage interferes with drainage of secretions from the appendix, and they accumulate in the confined space. The appendix enlarges and distends, and the swelling compresses surrounding blood vessels. The locally damaged cells are then easily infected with bacteria from within the intestinal lumen. Unless the inflammation resolves, the appendix can become gangrenous or it ruptures, spilling bacteria throughout the peritoneal cavity.

Assessment Findings

An attack of abdominal pain is the most frequent symptom. At first, the pain is generalized throughout the abdomen or

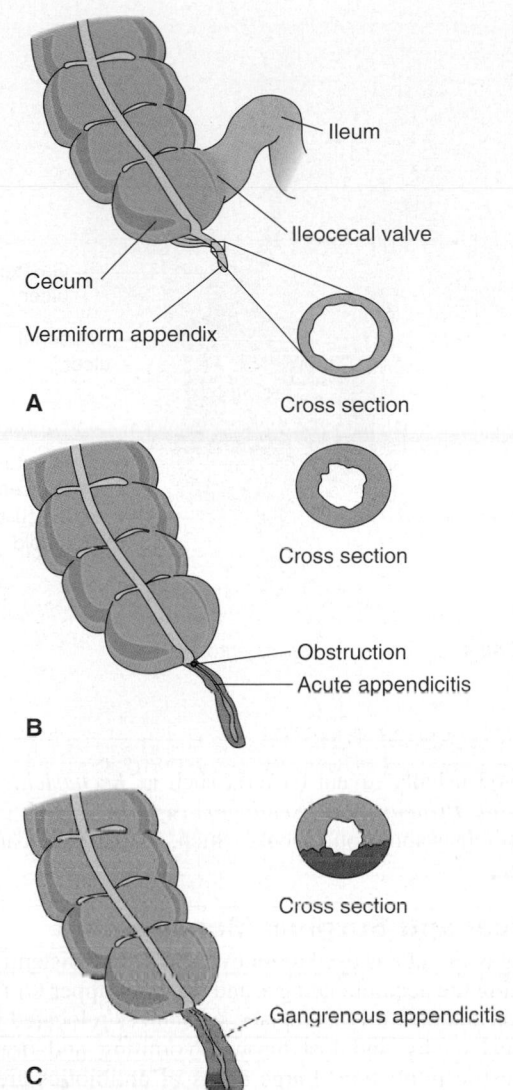

Ileum

Ileocecal valve

Cecum

Vermiform appendix

A Cross section

Cross section

Cross section

Obstruction

Acute appendicitis

B

Cross section

Gangrenous appendicitis

C

FIGURE 46-3. (**A**) Normal appendix. (**B**) Acute appendicitis resulting from obstruction (note the narrowing in the cross section). (**C**) Appendicitis and gangrene.

around the umbilicus. Later, the pain localizes in the RLQ at McBurney's point, an area midway between the umbilicus and the right iliac crest. Often, the pain is worse when manual pressure near the region is suddenly released, a condition called *rebound tenderness*. When an examiner deeply palpates the left lower abdominal quadrant, and the client feels pain in the RLQ, this is referred to as a positive Rovsing's sign and suggests acute appendicitis. Fever, nausea, and vomiting may be present. The abdomen is tense, and the client usually flexes the right hip to relieve the discomfort. The location of the appendix may influence the type of pain. For example, if the tip of the appendix is against the rectum, the client may experience pain with defecation. If the tip is near the bladder or against a ureter, the client may experience pain with urination (Smeltzer et al., 2008). Box 46-1 describes precautions to follow when a client may have appendicitis.

If the appendix perforates, clients experience more diffuse abdominal pain. The abdomen appears distended secondary to a **paralytic ileus** (intestine lacks peristalsis). Perforation generally occurs 24 hours following the onset of

BOX 46-1 | **Precautions When Assessing a Client for Appendicitis**

- Avoid multiple or frequent palpation of the abdomen—there is danger of causing the appendix to rupture.
- Perform the test for rebound tenderness at the end of the examination. A positive response causes pain and muscle spasm and makes it difficult to complete the rest of the assessment.
- Do not administer laxatives or enemas to a client who is experiencing fever, nausea, and abdominal pain, even though the client may complain of feeling constipated. Laxatives and cathartics may cause the appendix to rupture.

abdominal pain. Clients have a fever of 37.7°C (100°F) or higher and are very ill.

Gerontologic Considerations

- Older adults with appendicitis may not display the type of acute pain that younger adults with the condition experience. Severe pain may be absent, minimal, or referred in the older adult, causing a delay in diagnosis and a greater incidence of complications. Additionally, the temperature may not be elevated in the older adult with an infection.

A WBC count reveals moderate leukocytosis. When a differential count of leukocytes is performed, it shows an ever-increasing number of immature neutrophils, indicating a progressive worsening of the inflammatory condition. A computed tomography (CT) scan or abdominal ultrasound shows enlargement at the cecum.

Medical and Surgical Management

Antibiotics are given, and the client is restricted from eating or drinking while a decision is made about surgery. IV fluids are prescribed to meet the client's fluid needs. Analgesics may be withheld initially to avoid masking symptoms that may affect the diagnosis. If symptoms worsen, the surgeon performs an **appendectomy** to remove the appendix before it spontaneously ruptures. The appendix has no known function in the body. Its removal results in cure with no physiologic changes. If the appendix perforates or ruptures, an abscess or peritonitis can develop.

Nursing Management

The nurse assesses vital signs and the client's pain to detect early changes in the symptoms. If ordered, the nurse administers IV fluid therapy and observes the client's response to antibiotics. When analgesics are withheld, the nurse is empathetic and facilitates comfort with positioning, imagery, and distraction.

When surgery is indicated, preparing the client quickly is important to avoid delay that may cause surgical complications. Soon after surgery, if no complications occur, the client ambulates and tries light nourishment. Convalescence may be rapid, although postoperative progress depends on the client's age, general physical condition, and extent of complications. A healthy young adult usually can return to normal activities soon. Clients need to avoid heavy lifting or unusual exertion, however, for several months. For more specific nursing interventions when caring for a client undergoing surgery, see Chapter 14.

> ▶ **Stop, Think, and Respond Exercise 46-2**
>
> *An older adult client presents with vague symptoms of lower abdominal pain, nausea, and one episode of vomiting. In the initial assessment, what is an important question to ask?*

PERITONITIS

Pathophysiology and Etiology

In **peritonitis,** the peritoneum, a serous sac lining the abdominal cavity, becomes inflamed. Peritonitis may be caused by perforation of a peptic ulcer, the bowel, or the appendix; abdominal trauma, such as gunshot or knife wounds; IBD; ruptured ectopic pregnancy; or infection introduced during peritoneal dialysis, a procedure used to treat kidney failure. Figure 46-4 illustrates common causes of peritonitis.

Spillage of chemical contents and bacteria inflames the peritoneum, which leads to localized abscess formation or generalized inflammation. The intestinal tract initially responds with hypermotility, but, eventually, *paralytic ileus* ensues, with air and fluid trapped in the bowel. The proliferation of bacteria leads to tissue edema and leakage of fluid. Fluid in the abdominal cavity has increasing amounts of bacteria, protein, blood, cellular debris, and white blood cells. As generalized peritonitis occurs, vascular fluid shifts to the abdomen, lowering blood pressure and producing hypovolemic shock or septic shock. If the condition is not treated promptly or adequately, death may follow.

Assessment Findings

Signs and Symptoms

Symptoms include severe abdominal pain, distention, tenderness, nausea, and vomiting. Fever may be absent initially, but the temperature rises as infection becomes established. The client avoids moving the abdomen when breathing because movement increases pain. He or she may draw the knees up toward the abdomen to lessen the pain. Lack of bowel motility typically accompanies peritonitis. The abdomen feels rigid and boardlike as it distends with gas and intestinal contents. Bowel sounds typically are absent. The pulse rate is elevated, and respirations are rapid and shallow. If the peritonitis is unresolved, severe weakness, hypotension, and a drop in body temperature occur as the client nears death.

Diagnostic Findings

The results of a WBC count show marked leukocytosis. Abdominal radiographs reveal free air and fluid in the peritoneum. A CT scan or ultrasonography identifies structural changes in abdominal organs. Cultures of peritoneal fluid

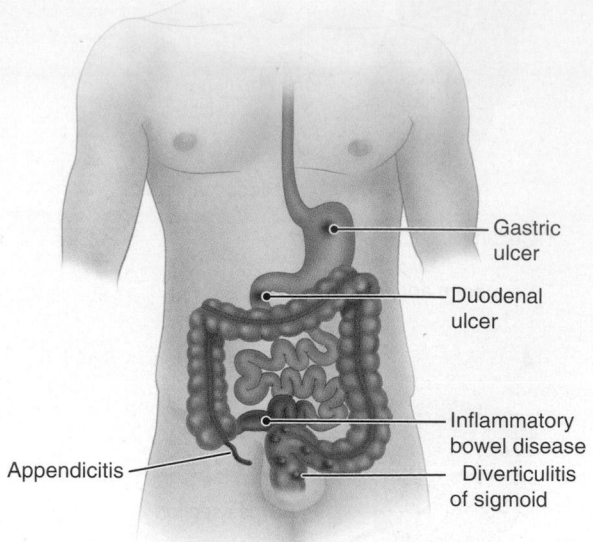

FIGURE 46-4. Common causes of peritonitis.

and blood usually reveal bacteria such as *Escherichia coli, Klebsiella, Proteus,* and *Pseudomonas.* If untreated, clients develop sepsis and septic shock, which, if untreated, can lead to death.

Medical and Surgical Management

A nasogastric tube is used to relieve abdominal distention by suctioning the accumulated gas and stagnant upper GI fluids. IV fluids and electrolytes replace substances relocated in the peritoneal cavity and lost through vomiting and drainage from gastric intubation. Large doses of antibiotics are prescribed to combat infection. Analgesics such as meperidine (Demerol) or IV morphine sulfate are ordered to relieve pain and promote rest. Antiemetics are prescribed for nausea and vomiting. The perforation is surgically closed so that intestinal contents can no longer escape.

Nursing Management

The nurse monitors the acutely ill client while completing preparations for diagnostic tests or surgery. He or she administers analgesics and infuses IV fluids with secondary administrations of antibiotics. If ordered, a nurse passes a nasogastric tube and connects it to suction (see Chap. 45). The client may need a urinary retention catheter. The nurse assesses the circulatory status by taking vital signs frequently and monitoring central venous and pulmonary artery pressures.

For the client who has had surgery, the nurse assesses the client's vital signs, fluid balance, incision, dressing, and drains. Assessing the client's pain level is important, as is medicating according to the medical orders. For clients who have prolonged recovery time, TPN may be initiated.

Clients are fearful of the emergent nature of the peritonitis and subsequent surgery. The nurse provides frequent explanations and emotional support. Clients also need monitoring for continued abdominal infection. If the client experiences abdominal distention, fever, changes in level of consciousness, or deviations in vital signs, the nurse must notify the physician quickly. Refer to Chapter 14 for further management of the postoperative client.

INTESTINAL OBSTRUCTION

Intestinal obstruction occurs when a blockage interferes with the normal progression of intestinal contents through the intestinal tract. Obstruction is more common in the small intestine than in other parts of the tract. Obstruction in the large intestine generally occurs in the sigmoid colon. The causes are classified as mechanical or functional (adynamic, or lacking peristalsis; also called *paralytic ileus*), and as partial or complete. The severity depends on the region of the bowel affected, degree to which the lumen is obstructed, and degree to which blood circulation to the intestine is impeded (Smeltzer et al., 2008). An intestinal obstruction is extremely dangerous and may be fatal if not treated promptly.

Pathophysiology and Etiology

Mechanical obstructions result from a narrowing of the bowel lumen with or without a space-occupying mass. A mass may include a tumor, *adhesions* (fibrous bands that constrict tissue), incarcerated or strangulated hernias, **volvulus** (kinking of a portion of intestine), **intussusception** (telescoping of one part of the intestine into an adjacent part), or impacted feces or barium (Table 46-2).

In functional obstruction, the intestine can become adynamic from an absence of normal nerve stimulation to intestinal muscle fibers. Paralytic ileus is common 12 to 36 hours after abdominal surgery. It also can result from inflammatory conditions (e.g., peritonitis), electrolyte disturbances (e.g., hypokalemia), or adverse drug effects (e.g., narcotics, cholinergic blockers). Even a vascular embolus or low blood flow during shock can interfere with the neuromuscular function of the bowel.

When the intestinal contents cannot move freely, the portion above the obstruction distends, whereas the portion below the obstruction is empty. If the obstruction is complete, no gases or feces are expelled rectally. Both forward and reverse peristalsis becomes forceful in an attempt to clear the obstruction. Stasis of the accumulating volume and the violent muscular peristaltic contractions potentiate the risk for intestinal rupture.

Locally, the increased pressure pushes electrolyte-rich fluid from the intestine and capillaries into the peritoneal cavity. Failure of the mucosa to reabsorb the secretions contributes to water and electrolyte imbalances and shock. Increasing pressure on the bowel from severe distention and edema impairs circulation and leads to necrosis and eventually gangrene of a portion of the bowel. Perforation of the gangrenous bowel, which results from pressure against weakened tissue, causes the intestinal contents to seep into the peritoneal cavity, resulting in peritonitis.

Small bowel obstruction and large bowel obstruction are similar in terms of development and resulting pathophysiology. Dehydration occurs more slowly with large intestine

TABLE 46-2 Mechanical Causes of Obstruction

CAUSE AND COURSE OF EVENTS	APPEARANCE
Adhesions—Loops of intestine adhere to areas that heal slowly or scar after abdominal surgery. The adhesions cause the intestinal loop to kink 3 to 4 days later.	
Intussusception—One part of the intestine slips into another lower part (like a telescope shortening). The intestinal lumen narrows	
Volvulus—The bowel twists and turns on itself, obstructing the intestinal lumen. Gas and fluid accumulate in the trapped bowel.	
Hernia—The intestine protrudes through a weakened area in the abdominal muscle or wall. Intestinal flow and blood flow to the area may be completely obstructed.	
Tumor—A tumor in the intestinal wall extends into the intestinal lumen; or a tumor outside the intestine causes pressure on the intestinal wall. The lumen becomes partially obstructed; if the tumor is not removed, complete obstruction results.	

obstruction, however, because the colon can absorb the fluid contents and distend to a considerably greater size.

Assessment Findings

Signs and Symptoms

Nausea and abdominal distention are common. When an obstruction occurs high in the GI tract, the client usually vomits whatever contents are in the stomach and small intestine. The emesis appears to contain bile or fecal material. If the obstruction is lower in the GI tract, vomiting may occur later or not at all. The client may have one or two bowel movements soon after the intestine has been obstructed because he or she is expelling material already past the obstruction. The client may experience severe intermittent cramps. Sudden, sustained pain, abdominal distention, and fever are symptoms of perforation.

In a functional obstruction, peristalsis is absent; therefore, bowel sounds are not heard. In a mechanical obstruction, the bowel sounds usually are high-pitched above the obstructed area. Pulse and respiratory rates are elevated. Blood pressure falls, and urine output decreases if shock develops.

Clinical symptoms associated with large bowel obstruction occur more slowly. Constipation may be the only symptom for many days. Eventually the client experiences abdominal distention. It is possible to see loops of bowel outlined through the abdominal wall, and the client complains of lower abdominal cramps and pain. Fecal vomiting also may occur. The client can have symptoms of shock.

Diagnostic Findings

A radiographic study of the abdomen shows air and fluid collecting in a segment of the intestine. A barium enema (used when the risk of perforation is low) pinpoints the location of the obstruction. Tests of serum electrolytes may indicate low levels of sodium, potassium, and chloride. Metabolic alkalosis is evidenced by arterial blood gas results. A complete blood count (CBC) shows an increased WBC count in instances of infection. The hematocrit level is elevated if dehydration develops.

Medical and Surgical Management

While diagnostic tests are performed to determine the cause and appropriate treatment for the client's obstruction, the client receives medical support. The client receives nothing by mouth (NPO). IV fluids with electrolytes are administered to correct fluid and electrolyte imbalances, and antibiotics are ordered to treat infection.

To relieve intestinal distention, cramping, and vomiting, and to reduce the potential for intestinal rupture with peritonitis, intestinal decompression is begun. Intestinal decompression is accomplished by suctioning large amounts of accumulated secretions and gas through a nasogastric tube or longer intestinal tube, which may or may not be weighted. Nasogastric tubes are used when the obstruction is partial or located high in the small intestine.

Before surgery, decompression alone may be sufficient to relieve a functional obstruction or symptoms in clients who are undergoing surgery for mechanical obstruction. In some cases, mechanical obstructions are treated during colonoscopy by removing obstructing polyps or destroying benign tumors with laser therapy or electrocautery. Most mechanical obstructions, however, require surgery. Usually, a section of the obstructed bowel is removed and then the proximal and distal sections are reconnected (bowel resection and anastomosis). In some cases, a temporary or permanent ostomy (see Chap. 48) may be performed.

Nursing Management

In addition to the assessments performed on the client with a GI disorder, the nurse obtains complete medical, drug, and allergy histories, assesses fluid intake and output, and takes vital signs. Documenting all symptoms and obtaining detailed information about each is important. For example, if vomiting has occurred, the nurse gathers information regarding its onset, amount, and color. If an intestinal tube has been inserted, the nurse monitors its progress (Nursing Guidelines 46-1).

The care of a client with an intestinal obstruction involves managing pain, maintaining fluid balance to prevent deficits related to fluid shifts and losses from vomiting, and helping the client deal with fear related to severe, possibly life-threatening symptoms and an unstable condition. The nurse also manages pain by maintaining the patency of the decompression tube and administering a prescribed narcotic analgesic as long as blood pressure and respiratory rate indicate that doing so is safe. The nurse maintains uninterrupted infusion of IV fluids and shortens the siege of vomiting by maintaining intestinal decompression, even though intestinal fluid is lost in the suctioning. It is crucial to monitor urinary output hourly and to report output below 50 mL/hour, a finding that may indicate that the client is going into shock.

DIVERTICULAR DISORDERS

Diverticula are sacs or pouches caused by herniation of the mucosa through a weakened portion of the muscular coat of the intestine or other structure (Fig. 46-5). They can appear anywhere in the GI tract (see Chap. 45), but they appear most commonly in the colon, especially the sigmoid area, in people older than 50 years of age.

DIVERTICULOSIS AND DIVERTICULITIS

Asymptomatic diverticula are called **diverticulosis**. When the diverticula become inflamed, the term **diverticulitis** is used.

Pathophysiology and Etiology

The incidence of diverticula is higher in people who have a low intake of dietary fiber. There also may be a congenital predisposition. It is thought that most diverticula result from weakness in the muscular coat associated with aging.

Diverticula become inflamed when fecal material is trapped in one or more blind pouches. The inflammation causes swelling of the tissue in the area. If the localized swelling involves several diverticula in one area, the edema may be severe enough to cause an intestinal obstruction. Abscesses form when the inflamed tissue becomes infected with intestinal bacteria present in the bowel. The swollen tissue has the potential to rupture into the peritoneal cavity or form a fistular connection with an adjacent organ such as the bladder.

Assessment Findings

Constipation alternating with diarrhea, flatulence, pain and tenderness in the LLQ, fever, and rectal bleeding may occur. A palpable mass may be felt in the lower abdomen. When the diverticula bleed, the stools appear maroon and are sometimes described as resembling "currant jelly."

A barium enema shows an irregular mucosal wall. A colonoscopy helps visualize the areas of inflammation. A CT scan generally is used first as an alternative to a barium enema or colonoscopy because both require an aggressive bowel preparation that may be contraindicated when the large intestine is acutely inflamed. Risk of perforation is increased. A CBC shows leukocytosis. A stool specimen may reveal occult blood.

NURSING GUIDELINES 46-1

Managing the Care of Client With an Intestinal Tube

Preparations

- Auscultate and examine the abdomen for bowel sounds, distention, and tenderness.
- To provide a baseline for reference, measure abdominal girth, placing a measuring tape about the largest diameter of the abdomen.
- Mark the measuring location on the skin (with an indelible marker) to facilitate consistency when obtaining future comparison measurements.
- Assemble all the equipment the physician will need. If a weighted double-lumen tube is selected, label the tip of the adapter leading to the lumen through which tungsten gel is instilled to avoid confusing which lumen to use for suction.

Tube Advancement

- After the physician inserts the tube, ambulate the client, if possible, to facilitate tube passage through the pylorus. When a radiographic image indicates that tube has advanced beyond the stomach, position the client as follows:
  - On the right side for 2 hours, then
  - On the back in a Fowler's position for 2 hours, then
  - On the left side for 2 hours.
- Observe the lines or numbers on the tube periodically to evaluate the tube's progressive movement and approximate anatomic location.
- Advance the tube several inches at specified intervals as directed to avoid tension as it descends into the intestine.

- Stabilize or tape the tube to the nose after a radiographic image verifies that the tube has reached the obstruction. Coil the excess length, securing it to the client's hospital gown.
- Attach the proximal end to suction.
- Prepare for radiography to be performed daily to evaluate progress toward relieving the obstruction.

Removal

- Remove the tube once the obstruction is relieved or another treatment replaces intubation.
- Disconnect the tube from suction.
- If removing a weighted tube, withdraw the tungsten gel by aspirating it with a 10-mL syringe. Remove the tungsten gel in the other types of tubes after the tube is withdrawn.
- Withdraw 6 to 10 inches of the tube between 10-minute pauses. When the tube is in the esophagus, as determined by 18 inches of length remaining in the client, flush the tube with a small amount of air to remove debris.
- Clamp the tube to prevent secretions from being deposited in the client's upper airway and instruct the client to hold the breath while the tube exits the esophagus.
- If removing a Cantor-like or Harris-like tube, grasp the bag of tungsten gel with a forceps and withdraw it from the client's mouth when it reaches the oropharynx.
- Once the tungsten gel is removed from the bag, remove the tube from the client's nose. Provide nasal and oral hygiene immediately afterward.

Medical and Surgical Management

Diverticula noted during routine examination require no treatment if they do not cause symptoms. Avoiding foods that contain seeds of any kind is recommended, although there is no scientific evidence to support this practice. A high-fiber diet supplemented with bran or prescription of a bulk-forming agent (e.g., Metamucil) helps avoid constipation.

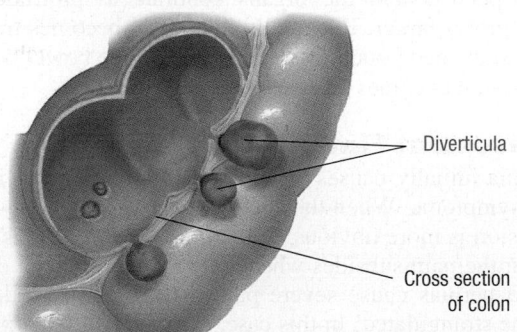

Diverticula

Cross section
of colon

FIGURE 46-5. Intestinal diverticula, particularly common in the sigmoid colon of older adults, usually do not cause symptoms except for occasional rectal bleeding. They may become inflamed and infected from fecal matter that becomes lodged in the pouchlike herniations. (From Anatomical Chart Company. [2006]. *Atlas of pathophysiology* [2nd ed.]. Philadelphia: Lippincott Williams & Wilkins.)

When symptoms occur, the diet is temporarily adjusted to low-residue foods. If the inflammation is severe and accompanied by pain and local tenderness, the client is maintained on IV fluids for several days with no oral intake. As the inflammation subsides with antibiotic therapy, oral fluids and food are reintroduced.

If diverticulitis does not respond to medical treatment, or if complications such as perforation, intestinal obstruction, or severe bleeding occur, surgery becomes necessary. The portion of colon that contains the diverticula is removed, and the continuity of the bowel is reestablished by joining the remaining portions of the colon. Depending on the location and extent of the disease and whether there is intestinal obstruction, a temporary colostomy may be necessary (see Chap. 48). The continuity of the bowel is restored, and the colostomy is closed 3 to 6 weeks later.

Nursing Management

In addition to the assessments performed on the client with a GI disorder, the nurse obtains a history of symptoms, diet, drug use, and allergies and asks questions regarding pain, bowel elimination, and diet habits. He or she takes vital signs to establish a baseline and to determine if the client is febrile. The nurse examines the abdomen for pain, tenderness, and masses.

Explaining the underlying pathology and rationale for treatment is important. Because dietary compliance reduces the potential for recurrences, consulting the dietitian for teaching is useful. If surgery becomes necessary, the nurse prepares the client before surgery and manages the postoperative care. A dietary consult or a list of foods to eat or avoid is necessary. The nurse also includes the following points in the teaching plan:

- Follow the diet recommended by the physician, which will probably reduce pain and discomfort.
- Bran adds bulk to the diet. Unprocessed bran can be sprinkled over cereal or added to fruit juice.
- Avoid the use of laxatives or enemas except when recommended by the physician.
- Avoid constipation. Do not suppress the urge to defecate.
- Drink at least 8 to 10 large glasses of fluid each day.
- Take prescribed medications as directed, even if symptoms improve.
- Exercise regularly if the current lifestyle is somewhat inactive.
- If severe pain or blood in the stool occurs, see a physician immediately.

ABDOMINAL HERNIA

Although **hernia** refers to the protrusion of any organ from the cavity that normally confines it, the term most commonly is used to describe the protrusion of the intestine through a defect in the abdominal wall. Certain areas in the abdominal wall are weaker than other areas and more vulnerable to the development of a hernia. These areas include the inguinal ring, the point on the abdominal wall where the inguinal canal begins; the femoral ring at the abdominal opening of the femoral canal; and the umbilicus.

If the protruding structures can be replaced in the abdominal cavity, it is a *reducible hernia*. Placing the client in a supine position and applying manual pressure over the area may reduce the hernia. An *irreducible* or *incarcerated hernia* is one in which the intestine cannot be replaced in the abdominal cavity because of edema of the protruding segment and constriction of the muscle opening through which it has emerged. If the process continues without treatment, the blood supply to the trapped segment of bowel can be cut off, leading to gangrene. This development is referred to as a *strangulated hernia*.

Pathophysiology and Etiology

The most common abdominal hernias are *inguinal, umbilical, femoral,* and *incisional* (Box 46-2), with inguinal hernias the most common type. Inguinal hernias are more prevalent in men than women. Umbilical and femoral hernias are more frequent in women than men.

A hernia develops when intra-abdominal pressure increases, such as while straining to lift something heavy, having a bowel movement, or coughing or sneezing forcefully. When abdominal pressure increases, a segment of the intestine moves through a weak area of abdominal muscle. In the areas that are naturally predisposed to weakness, the abdominal wall may be thin or stretched from an inadequate amount of collagen. Such a condition may be present at birth or develop as a result of aging, abdominal surgery, or obesity.

BOX 46-2 **Types of Hernias**

Inguinal: Protrusion of the hernial sac contains the intestine at the inguinal opening.
  Direct: Hernia extends through inguinal ring; it follows spermatic cord in males and round ligament in females.
  Indirect: Protrusion follows the posterior inguinal wall; it often descends into the scrotum in males.
Umbilical: Hernia occurs in the umbilical region, through which the hernial sac protrudes. This type occurs in children when the umbilical orifice fails to close shortly after birth. It may occur in obese adults who have prolonged abdominal distention.
Femoral: Intestines descend through the femoral ring where the femoral artery passes into the femoral canal, below the inguinal ligament. Incidence of strangulation is high.
Incisional: This type occurs through the scar of a surgical incision when healing is impaired. Careful surgical technique, particularly prevention of wound infection, can prevent incisional hernias. Obese, older, or malnourished clients are prone to the development of incisional hernias.

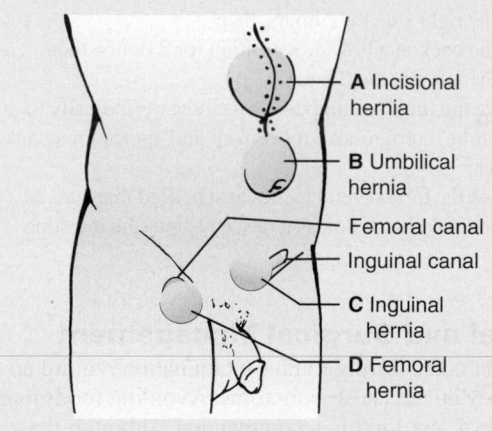

A Incisional hernia
B Umbilical hernia
Femoral canal
Inguinal canal
C Inguinal hernia
D Femoral hernia

At first, the defect in the abdominal wall is small. As the hernia persists and the organs continue to protrude, the defect grows larger. Eventually the bowel becomes trapped in the weakened pouch. If blood supply to the bowel is compromised, it becomes gangrenous.

Assessment Findings

A hernia initially causes swelling on the abdomen with no other symptoms. When the client coughs or bears down, the protrusion is more obvious. Sometimes the swelling is painful, but the pain subsides when the hernia is reduced. Incarcerated hernias cause severe pain and, if not treated, may become strangulated. In this case, the client suffers extreme abdominal pain. The severe pressure on the loop of intestine protruding outside the abdominal cavity causes intestinal obstruction.

Medical and Surgical Management

When a hernia forms, it tends to enlarge, leading to serious complications. Surgery is the only method of eliminating a hernia. Some clients, either because they are unwilling to have or are not candidates for surgery, may wear a truss, an apparatus that presses over the hernia and prevents protrusion of the bowel. The client also may lie supine while manual pressure is applied over the protruding area to reduce the hernia periodically. Some clients learn to do this themselves.

A **herniorrhaphy**, the surgical repair of a hernia, is the recommended treatment. When a herniorrhaphy is performed, the protruding intestine is repositioned in the abdominal cavity and the defect in the abdominal wall is repaired. Herniorrhaphy is performed under local, spinal, or general anesthesia. Some types of hernias can be treated using a laparoscopic approach. When a hernia is neglected for many years, the tissues in the area weaken, and postoperative healing may be impaired. Obese people who have put off surgical repair for a prolonged period are especially prone to recurrence of the hernia, despite surgical repair. For these cases, the surgeon also may perform a **hernioplasty**. The weakened area is reinforced with wire, fascia, or mesh. The obese client usually is advised to lose weight before the surgery to lessen the possibility of recurrence.

Strangulation is an acute emergency. Unless surgery is performed promptly, blood flow to the intestine is impaired. If necrosis occurs, the gangrenous part of the intestine must be excised and portions of the intestine reconnected.

Nursing Management

If the client is managing herniation with a truss and not undergoing surgery, nursing care centers primarily on teaching. The nurse educates the client about ways to avoid constipation, control a cough, and perform proper body mechanics. The client needs to know the signs of incarceration and strangulation of the hernia. The nurse teaches the client how to wear a truss and observe for and treat skin irritation from friction caused by continuous rubbing. Advising the client to keep the skin clean and dry or to use cornstarch to absorb moisture is an important intervention. The nurse also explains that compression from a truss may produce localized edema from interference with lymphatic and venous blood flow.

When surgery is scheduled, the nurse prepares the client and manages postoperative care (see Chap. 14). The assessment of clients undergoing surgery includes obtaining a complete medical and drug history because malnutrition, diabetes, or concurrent use of corticosteroids or antimetabolite cancer drugs can affect wound healing. The nurse also obtains the client's allergy history, especially to seasonal inhalants (i.e., ragweed pollen), and smoking history because sneezing and coughing can increase intra-abdominal pressure after surgery and place the client at risk for weakening the surgical repair. Before surgery, the nurse takes vital signs, auscultates the lungs to identify infectious or respiratory risk factors, and documents the client's weight and duration of the hernia. These factors influence the potential for postoperative healing complications. The client's previous surgical experience may affect how the client feels about this surgery. The nurse also assesses the client's urinary and bowel patterns to determine if the client has any preexisting problems affecting elimination. After surgery, the nurse inspects the scrotum of male clients because it is common for edema to follow surgical repair.

Hernia repairs are performed mainly on an outpatient basis. Therefore, the nurse teaches measures to the client and significant others who will provide care after discharge. The nurse needs to reinforce verbal instructions with written instructions about signs and symptoms of possible complications (i.e., bleeding, infection) and the need to report these symptoms to the physician. The instructions include techniques for avoiding constipation and straining to have a bowel movement. The nurse also includes instructions to avoid strenuous exertion and heavy lifting until the physician determines that the client can safely undertake such activities. For clients who perform heavy physical labor, it is essential to explore how they may modify the manner in which they perform their jobs, take an extended sick leave, or apply for a temporary leave of absence. The nurse explains to those whose work is sedentary or light that they usually can return to full employment with few activity restrictions within a few weeks.

CANCERS OF THE COLON AND RECTUM

Intestinal malignancies may develop anywhere in the lower GI tract. Colorectal cancer ranks as the third most common cancer among men and women in the United States, and second among causes of cancer deaths. The incidence of the disease increases with age. For colorectal screening, fecal occult blood testing is recommended every 1 to 2 years and colonoscopy every 5 to 10 years in clients older than 50 years of age. This screening may be performed in younger clients with risk factors, such as a family history of colorectal cancer or ulcerative colitis.

Gerontologic Considerations

- Regular health examination and screenings for colorectal cancer should be encouraged because of increased incidence of cancer in the older adult.

Pathophysiology and Etiology

Many malignant colorectal tumors develop from benign adenomas in the mucosal and submucosal intestinal layers. Adenocarcinoma accounts for nearly 95% of cases of colorectal cancer. A benign polyp may become malignant and then invade the surrounding tissues and structures. Cancer cells break away and spread to other body parts, most commonly the liver and the lungs. It is believed that genetic, environmental, and lifestyle factors spark the transformation from a benign to a cancerous state. Catalysts seem to include chronic bowel inflammation, as in ulcerative colitis, and a lifetime pattern of eating low-fiber, high-fat foods.

Having a blood relative with this disease is a high-risk factor. Genetic testing may be done to identify some types of familial colon cancer. At some point, the normal cells undergo mutation, which affects their proliferation and growth pattern. Some believe that an *oncogene*, a genetic messenger that stimulates tumor growth, is not adequately

BOX 46-3 Symptoms of Colorectal Cancer Related to Location of the Lesion

Right-Sided Lesions
Dull abdominal pain
Melena (black, tarry stools)

Left-Sided Lesions
Abdominal pain and cramping
Narrowing of stools
Constipation
Abdominal distention
Bright red blood in stool

Rectal Lesions
Tenesmus (ineffective painful straining with defecation attempts)
Rectal pain
Feeling of incomplete evacuation after a bowel movement
Alternating constipation and diarrhea
Bloody stools

(From Smeltzer, S. C., et al. [2008] *Brunner & Suddarth's textbook of medical–surgical nursing* [11th ed.]. Philadelphia: Lippincott Williams & Wilkins.)

suppressed. Without growth inhibition, the neoplastic cells reproduce rapidly and later proceed to invade the muscle wall. Other research suggests that a gene mutation interferes with the ability of colon cells to copy their DNA molecule correctly.

Although the malignant growth remains in situ (confined to its site of origin), it may change the shape of the stool, compressing it or making it appear pencil-like as it passes by the protruding mass. Untreated, the cancer extends to other organs by way of the mesentery lymph nodes or portal vein leading to the liver.

Assessment Findings

The chief characteristic of cancer of the colon is a change in bowel habits, such as alternating constipation and diarrhea. Occult or frank blood may be present in the stool. Sometimes a client may feel dull, vague abdominal discomfort. Pain is a late sign of cancer. On physical assessment, the abdomen feels distended, and a mass may be palpated in the abdomen or rectum. Box 46-3 lists symptoms associated with colorectal cancer based on the location of the cancer.

A number of diagnostic tests are performed for colorectal cancer, including fecal occult blood test; sigmoidoscopy; barium enema; colonoscopy; and digital rectal examination. (Note that the last two are recommended screening tests.) Newer diagnostic tests include virtual colonoscopy (see Chap. 44) and DNA testing of stools, which involves looking for cellular genetic changes that can be a sign of cancer. Genetic screening may detect chromosomal markers for particular types of colon cancer. An elevated carcinoembryonic antigen (CEA) test result suggests a tumor. Unfortunately, a CEA test is not effective in identifying colorectal cancer in its earliest, most treatable stages. Unless malignant growths are elevated from the mucosal wall, a barium enema may not provide conclusive evidence either. A tissue sample taken during a proctosigmoidoscopy or colonoscopy may detect malignant cells in the area of the biopsy. A CBC may show a low erythrocyte count from chronic blood loss.

Medical and Surgical Management

When polyps are discovered during endoscopic examination, they are removed and examined. Even if the polyps are benign, the client continues to undergo periodic radiographic and endoscopic examinations to identify recurrent polyps for early malignant changes. An exception to this rule is the finding of juvenile polyps in young children. These benign growths do not tend to recur. The primary treatment of colorectal cancer is surgical, but sometimes treatment involves a combination of surgery, radiation therapy, and chemotherapy.

An encapsulated colorectal tumor may be removed without taking away surrounding healthy tissue. This type of tumor, however, may call for partial or complete surgical removal of the colon (**colectomy**). Occasionally, the tumor causes a partial or complete bowel obstruction. If the tumor is in the colon and upper third of the rectum, a **segmental resection** is performed. In this procedure, the surgeon removes the cancerous portion of the colon and rejoins the remaining portions of the GI tract to restore normal intestinal continuity.

Cancers in the lower third of the rectum are treated with an **abdominoperineal resection**—wide excision of the rectum and creation of a sigmoid colostomy. The surgical procedures used to treat cancers in the middle third of the rectum vary. A low resection with a temporary colostomy usually is attempted to preserve the anal sphincter. Radiation therapy is indicated in many cases of colon cancer, whereas chemotherapy usually is reserved for those with evidence of lymphatic infiltration or metastasis. If the cancer metastasizes, a colostomy may be performed to relieve an intestinal obstruction. In some cases, the obstruction is relieved or bleeding is controlled with laser surgery.

Nursing Management

The nurse advises and prepares clients for routine colorectal screening. He or she follows standard guidelines for collecting stool specimens and sending them to the laboratory for analysis. The nurse instructs the client how to collect specimens at home, if applicable (Client and Family Teaching 46-2). The nurse advises anyone who is asymptomatic but whose stool test results are positive for blood to undergo a colonoscopy, the next step in cancer detection. Nursing management of the client with a colostomy is discussed in Chapter 48.

ANORECTAL DISORDERS

Clients with anorectal disorders usually experience localized pain and bleeding, and thus seek medical attention. They also may have problems with perianal itching, tenderness,

Client and Family Teaching 46-2
Fecal Occult Blood Testing (FOBT)

The nurse should include the following points when instructing a client about the procedure for FOBT, which the client may perform at home:

Seven to 10 Days Before and Throughout the Test
- Do not drink alcohol or take aspirin, NSAIDs, vitamin C, or iron preparations
- Check with physician if anticoagulants, steroids, colchicines (used to treat gout), or cimetidine (for peptic ulcer treatment) have been prescribed

Two Days Before and Throughout the Test
- Consume a high-fiber diet and avoid red meat, substituting with poultry and fish
- Avoid turnips, cauliflower, broccoli, cantaloupe, horseradish, and parsnips

During the Test
- Collect stool within a toilet liner or bedpan
- Use an applicator stick and remove a sample from the center of the stool
- Apply a thin smear of stool onto the test area supplied with the screening kit
- Take care to cover the entire space
- Place two drops of developer solution onto the test area
- Wait precisely 60 seconds
- Observe for a blue color, indicating a positive reaction (for more valid results, test samples from several stools over 3 to 6 days)

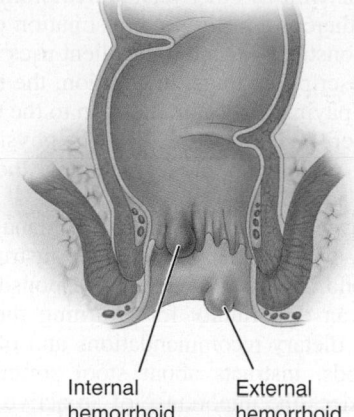

FIGURE 46-6. Internal and external hemorrhoids.

and swelling. They may delay defecation secondary to pain and other discomfort.

HEMORRHOIDS

Hemorrhoids are dilated veins outside or inside the anal sphincter (Fig. 46-6). Thrombosed hemorrhoids are veins that contain clots.

Pathophysiology and Etiology

Chronic straining to have a bowel movement or frequent defecation with chronic diarrhea likely weakens the tissue supporting the veins. Clients whose work requires prolonged sitting are at increased risk for the development of hemorrhoids. Pregnancy, prolonged labor, portal hypertension, or other intra-abdominal conditions that interfere with venous blood return can cause or aggravate the condition. The veins near the anal sphincter probably are displaced downward from their natural location as the result of a loss of supporting tissue. Without adequate connective tissue and smooth muscle support, the veins dilate and fill with blood. Dry stool passes by the engorged hemorrhoids, which stretches and irritates the mucosa, giving rise to the local symptoms of burning, itching, and pain. Passing dry, hard stool causes the hemorrhoids to bleed.

Assessment Findings

External hemorrhoids may cause few symptoms, or they can produce pain, itching, and soreness of the anal area. They appear as small, reddish-blue lumps at the edge of the anus. Thrombosed external hemorrhoids are painful but seldom cause bleeding.

Internal hemorrhoids cause bleeding but are less likely to cause pain, unless they protrude through the anus. The amount of bleeding varies from an occasional drop or two of blood on toilet tissue or underwear to chronic loss of blood, leading to anemia. Internal hemorrhoids usually protrude each time the client defecates but retract after defecation. As the masses enlarge, they remain outside the sphincter.

An anoscope, an instrument for examining the anal canal, or a proctosigmoidoscope, allows visualization of internal hemorrhoids. A colonoscopy rules out colorectal cancer, which has similar symptoms.

Medical Management

Small external hemorrhoids may disappear without treatment, or the client may obtain relief through symptomatic treatment. The physician may recommend warm soaks, an ointment that contains a local anesthetic for the relief of pain and itching, topical astringent pads to relieve swelling, a diet that corrects or prevents constipation, and a stool softener. In some cases the hemorrhoid is ligated (tied off) with a rubber band. Infrared photocoagulation, in which the protein and water in hemorrhoidal tissue are destroyed, is an alternative to traditional surgery.

Surgical Management

A **hemorrhoidectomy**, the surgical removal of hemorrhoids, may be necessary in chronic and severe cases. The procedure is performed using conventional surgery or laser surgery; the client receives a local anesthetic or regional nerve block. Internal packing of lubricated gauze, external gauze dressing, or a perineal pad is applied to absorb blood. A T-binder holds the absorbent material in place.

Nursing Management

The nurse gathers a complete history, including drug and allergy histories. Because bleeding accompanies many colorectal disorders, it is important to ask the client to describe the bleeding as well as other related symptoms. The nurse determines if there is a history of constipation or alternating diarrhea and constipation, and if the client uses any prescription or nonprescription drugs. In addition, the nurse obtains a diet history, paying particular attention to the type of foods (especially fiber) included in the diet. The physical examination involves putting on gloves, draping the client, and inspecting the anus.

Health teaching is focused on self-management. The nurse reviews the physician's home care instructions, demonstrates wound care to the client or responsible caregiver and provides an opportunity for returning the demonstration, provides dietary recommendations and offers a list of high-fiber foods, instructs about stool softeners as indicated, emphasizes the importance of an active lifestyle and increased fluid intake, and cautions against the prolonged use of laxatives.

ANORECTAL ABSCESS

An anorectal abscess is an infection with a collection of pus in an area between the internal and external sphincters.

Pathophysiology and Etiology

The original source of the infection may be microorganisms harbored in the intestine itself. An anorectal abscess is common in clients with Crohn's disease. Anorectal infections, however, also are transmitted from others through anal intercourse or insertion of foreign bodies into the rectum.

Usually, infectious microorganisms invade anal crypts, small tubular cavities in the anal skin and rectal mucosa. A purulent exudate collects, and the pressure causes pain and swelling. The abscess eventually may develop into a fistulous tract.

Assessment Findings

Clients with an anorectal abscess experience pain that is aggravated by walking and sitting or other activities that increase intra-abdominal pressure such as coughing, sneezing, and straining to have a bowel movement. A swollen mass is evident in the anus. Fever and abdominal pain develop if the abscess has extended into deeper tissues. Foul-smelling drainage may leak from the anus if the abscess spontaneously ruptures. A culture of anal drainage reveals the infectious microorganism.

Medical and Surgical Management

Analgesics and sitz baths are prescribed to relieve symptoms. Antibiotic therapy is used to treat gonorrheal, staphylococcal, streptococcal, or other drug-sensitive bacteria. An incision and drainage to remove the infected material may be necessary. If a fistula has formed, deeper excision and removal of the fistulous tract are necessary. Because fistula formation frequently is associated with Crohn's disease, additional diagnostic testing may be necessary to determine the presence of this condition.

Nursing Management

To limit the spread of infectious microorganisms, the nurse instructs the client to practice scrupulous handwashing after each bowel movement, to use separate hygiene articles, to cleanse the bathtub after each use, and to use a condom if having anal intercourse. Refer to the nursing management of a client with an anorectal disorder for specific nursing interventions.

ANAL FISSURE

An anal **fissure** (fissure in ano) is a linear tear in the anal canal tissue.

Pathophysiology and Etiology

Constipation is the leading cause of anal fissures. Other factors that may lead to formation of a slitlike tear include eversion of the anus during vaginal delivery and trauma to the anus, such as during anal intercourse or through the insertion of foreign bodies or medical instruments. When the anal canal is excessively stretched, the skin rips apart, exposing the underlying tissue.

Assessment Findings

Severe pain and bleeding on defecation are common. If constipation was not an original problem, it becomes one. Most clients with an anal fissure are reluctant to defecate because of the associated pain. The torn area may be visible when the anus is visually inspected, and the irregular surface of the fissure may be felt during a digital examination. Anoscopy provides evidence of the altered integrity of the anal mucosa.

Medical and Surgical Management

Treatment includes applying anesthetic creams, ointments, or suppositories; taking sitz baths and analgesics; and preventing constipation. Surgical excision of the area may be necessary.

Nursing Management

The nurse includes the following in the plan of care:

- Teach the client how to insert a suppository.
- Instruct the client in how to take a sitz bath.
- Discuss strategies to relieve constipation.

Refer to Nursing Care Plan 46-1 for more information.

ANAL FISTULA

An anal fistula (fistula in ano) is a tract that forms in the anal canal.

Pathophysiology and Etiology

When healing of an anorectal abscess is inadequate, an inflamed tunnel develops, connecting the area of the original abscess with perianal skin (Fig. 46-7). Purulent material drains from the opening.

Assessment Findings

The client reports pain on defecation. The opening of the fistula appears red, and pus leaks from the external opening of the fistula or can be expressed if the area is compressed. If

NURSING CARE PLAN 46-1 | The Client With an Anorectal Condition

Assessmemt

Include the following questions in the health history:

- Do you have any burning, itching, or pain in the anorectal area? If so, when do these symptoms occur— with defecation? How long do they last? Do you have any other discomfort, such as abdominal cramps?
- Is any blood in the stool or on the toilet tissue when you wipe the rectum? How much? Is the blood bright or dark red?

- Is there mucus or pus from the rectal area?
- What is your stool pattern?
- Do you use laxatives? If so, how often?
- What is your typical diet?
- Do you exercise regularly? If so what is the exercise?
- Do you sit or stand for long periods?

Nursing Diagnosis: Risk for Constipation related to fear of painful elimination

Expected Outcome: Client identifies measures that prevent or treat constipation.

Interventions	Rationales
Instruct client, unless contraindicated, to increase intake of water to 2 L/day.	Such fluid intake prevents hard, dry stools and eases defecation.
Provide a list of high-fiber foods.	A high-fiber diet promotes bulk of stool and prevents constipation.
Instruct client in the use of laxatives or stool softeners as ordered.	Prolonged use of these measures is not encouraged; they should be used only as indicated.
Teach the client to heed the urge to have a bowel movement.	This measure prevents constipation.

Evaluation of Expected Outcome

Client practices measures that prevent constipation, as evidenced by increased fluid and fiber intake and the passage of soft, formed stools.

Nursing Diagnosis: Acute Pain related to surgical procedure.

Expected Outcome Client will report that pain management regimen relieves his or her pain.

Interventions	Rationales
Administer pain medications as ordered.	Medications promote ongoing pain relief.
Encourage client to rest in a comfortable position that removes pressure from surgical site, or to use a flotation device.	These measures relieve pressure and decrease pain at the surgical site.
Apply ice and analgesic ointments as indicated.	These measures promote pain relief.
Use warm compresses or sitz baths three to four times daily as indicated.	Warmth through compresses or baths relaxes the rectal sphincter spasm and soothes irritated tissues.

Evaluation of Expected Outcome

Client states that positioning and use of sitz baths relieve pain.

Nursing Diagnosis: Risk for Ineffective Therapeutic Regimen Management related to knowledge deficit

Expected Outcome: Client will demonstrate ability to manage therapeutic regimens.

Interventions	Rationales
Instruct client to cleanse perianal area with warm water and to dry with cotton wipes.	These measures prevent infection and irritation.
Teach client how to do sitz baths at home, using warm water, three to four times each day.	Sitz baths promote healing, decrease skin irritation, and relieve rectal spasms.
Instruct client to take a sitz bath after each bowel movement.	Sitz baths also help keep the perianal area clean.
Encourage client to follow diet and medication instructions.	Encouragement promotes compliance with therapeutic regimen and prevents complications.
Encourage moderate exercise.	Activity promotes healing and normal stool patterns.

Evaluation of Expected Outcomes

(1) Incision heals without complications. (2) Client has no signs of infection and eats a diet high in fiber.(3) Vital signs are normal. (4) Stools are soft-formed and regular.

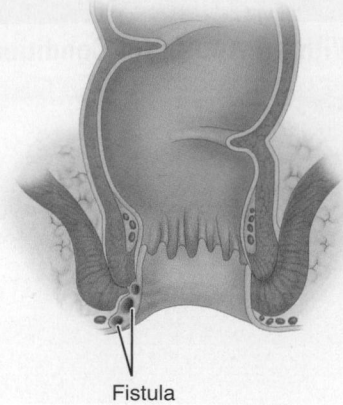

FIGURE 46-7. Anal fistula.

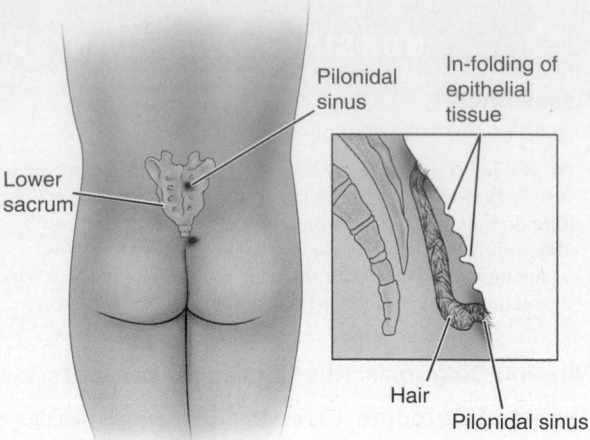

FIGURE 46-8. Pilonidal sinus on lower sacrum about 5 cm (2 in) above the anus in the intergluteal cleft. Hair particles emerge from the sinus tract, and localized indentations (pits) can appear on the skin near the sinus openings.

the fistula is superficial, it feels cordlike on palpation. A proctosigmoidoscopy or colonoscopy may identify Crohn's disease, which predisposes the client to an anorectal abscess or anal fistula.

Medical and Surgical Management

Antibiotics are prescribed to treat infection. Treatment of underlying Crohn's disease often allows for resolution of the fistula without surgical intervention. Most simple low-lying fistulae can be managed by **fistulotomy**. This procedure involves incising the fistula along with partial sphincter division and is reserved for those fistulae that arise from relatively normal surrounding tissue. Another surgical procedure, referred to as **fistulectomy**, involves an excision of the fistulous tract. This type usually is the recommended surgery.

If a sphincter division compromises fecal continence, a noncutting seton may be placed into the fistula to allow for drainage of the fistula and to minimize the risk for future abscesses. A *seton* is a nonabsorbable suture or drain that is passed from the cutaneous opening of the fistula into the lumen of the anal canal and then back out onto the skin, where it is tied to itself. The seton can be gradually tightened to cut through the sphincter or left in place as a drain.

Nursing Management

The nurse teaches the client to self-administer medications, keep the anal region clean, and avoid transferring microorganisms to other hygiene articles that they share with family members (e.g., bar soap). For surgical nursing care, refer to Nursing Care Plan 46-1.

PILONIDAL SINUS

Pilonidal means "a nest of hair." A **pilonidal sinus** is an infection in the hair follicles in the sacrococcygeal area above the anus (Fig. 46-8). Other local infections, such as osteomyelitis and furuncles of the skin, also have common presenting signs and symptoms and must be ruled out. The terms *pilonidal sinus* and *pilonidal cyst* are both used to describe the condition.

Pathophysiology and Etiology

The condition typically occurs after puberty. People who have a deep intergluteal cleft and those who have abundant hair in the perianal and lower back regions are predisposed to the condition. Inadequate personal hygiene, obesity, and trauma to the area also contribute to its development.

A sinus or cyst begins to form when the skin deep in the cleft softens as a result of being chronically moist. Stiff hairs then irritate and pierce the soft, macerated skin, becoming embedded in it. The irritation inflames the tissues. Infection readily follows because the break in the skin allows microorganisms to enter. Several channels may lead from the sinus to the skin.

Assessment Findings

Pain and swelling at the base of the spine and purulent drainage occur. On inspection, the sinus opening may be located in the gluteal fold. Dilated pits of the hair follicles in the sinus are a unique characteristic.

Medical and Surgical Management

The abscess is drained, and the tissue is incised. The sinus and all its connecting channels are laid open, and purulent material and hair are removed. Packing is inserted into the cavity, and the wound heals by secondary intention. In some cases, the wound edges are approximated. Healing by primary intention, however, sometimes allows the purulent material to reform and collect, causing another abscess. Because the infection is localized, systemic antibiotics usually are not prescribed.

Nursing Management

The nurse teaches the client how to minimize discomfort and facilitates postoperative bowel elimination. As appropriate, the nurse instructs a family member in the procedures of removing the packing, cleaning the incised tissue, and redressing the area. See Nursing Care Plan 46-1 for additional nursing management.

CRITICAL THINKING EXERCISES

1. The admitting department notifies the nursing unit to expect a client with ulcerative colitis. Based on the characteristics of the disease process, what assessments are essential to obtain at the time of admission?

2. As you assist an older adult with using a bedpan, you notice blood on the toilet tissue. What other data are appropriate to gather at this time?

3. A 65-year-old client recently diagnosed with diverticulosis tells you that she is very concerned about having acute problems with diverticulitis like her mother. What information could you provide that can most help her prevent diverticulitis?

4. A 45-year-old friend tells you that his physician has scheduled him for a colonoscopy. The friend asks you why he needs to have one, because he feels fine and is not having any bowel problems. What is most important to ask?

NCLEX-STYLE REVIEW QUESTIONS

1. A client with appendicitis is awaiting treatment. Which of the following instructions would the nurse give the client while a decision is being made about surgery?
1. Drink plenty of fluids.
2. Use over-the-counter analgesics.
3. Refrain from eating.
4. Gently massage the abdomen.

2. Which of the following signs would the nurse expect when assessing a client with suspected peritonitis? Select all that apply.

1. The abdomen feels rigid.
2. The stools appear maroon.
3. Respirations are slow and labored.
4. The pulse rate is elevated.
5. Rectal bleeding is present.

3. A client being treated for intestinal obstruction is vomiting profusely. Which of the following actions would the nurse take first to control the vomiting?
1. Maintain uninterrupted infusion of intravenous fluids.
2. Provide prescribed narcotic analgesics.
3. Check if intestinal decompression is working.
4. Elevate the upper part of the client's body.

4. A client with a long history of ulcerative colitis is admitted to the hospital for a colectomy. The nursing team identifies the nursing diagnosis of Bowel Incontinence related to sudden urgency for defecation on the care plan. Which intervention is most appropriate when managing this nursing diagnosis?
1. Keeping the bedside commode nearby
2. Answering the client's signal for help promptly
3. Putting a disposable diaper on the client
4. Assisting the client to the bathroom frequently

5. The nurse assesses the client with diarrhea for signs of fluid volume deficit. Which assessment finding best indicates that the client is becoming dehydrated?
1. The client's blood pressure is elevated.
2. The client's heart rate is irregular.
3. The client's mucous membranes are pink.
4. The client's urine is dark yellow.

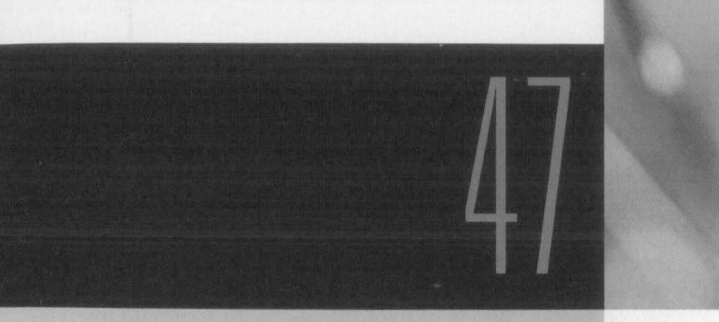

47

Caring for Clients with Disorders of the Liver, Gallbladder, or Pancreas

Words To Know

alpha fetoprotein
ascites
balloon tamponade
biliary colic
caput medusae
cholecystitis
choledocholithiasis
cholelithiasis
cholestasis
cirrhosis
esophageal varices
fetor hepaticus
hepatic encephalopathy
hepatic lobectomy
hepatitis
hepatorenal syndrome
injection sclerotherapy
laparoscopic cholecystectomy
lithotripsy
open cholecystectomy
pancreatectomy (partial, total)
pancreatitis
portal hypertension
radical pancreatoduodenectomy (Whipple procedure)
steatorrhea
T-tube

Learning Objectives

On completion of this chapter, you will be able to:

1. Explain possible causes of jaundice.
2. List common findings manifested by clients with cirrhosis.
3. Discuss common complications of cirrhosis.
4. Identify the modes of transmission of viral hepatitis.
5. Discuss nursing management for clients with a medically or surgically treated liver disorder.
6. Identify factors that contribute to, signs and symptoms of, and medical treatments for cholecystitis.
7. Name techniques for gallbladder removal.
8. Summarize the nursing management of clients undergoing medical or surgical treatment of a gallbladder disorder.
9. Describe the treatment and nursing management of pancreatitis.
10. Describe the treatment of pancreatic carcinoma.
11. Explain the nursing management of clients undergoing pancreatic surgery.

The liver, gallbladder, and pancreas play important roles in digestion. They also are responsible for many other physiologic activities (see Chap. 44). Their poor function impairs the digestive process and the client's overall nutritional status.

DISORDERS OF THE LIVER

The liver has four lobes. Each lobe is surrounded by connective tissue that extends in the lobe itself and divides the liver into smaller units referred to as lobules. The liver is supported by intra-abdominal pressure and various attachments called *mesenteries,* which connect the liver to the adjacent intestines, abdominal wall, and diaphragm. Unless it is abnormally enlarged, the liver usually is not palpable. Figure 47-1 illustrates the liver and the surrounding structures.

The liver has various functions (Box 47-1) and a rich blood supply. It receives arterial blood from the hepatic artery, an indirect branch of the aorta. The portal vein transports blood from the intestinal tract to the liver. After blood has traversed vascular pathways inside the liver, the hepatic veins collect the blood and transport it to the inferior vena cava and then back to the heart (Fig. 47-2).

Microscopically, the liver's internal structure includes smaller branches of the hepatic artery, the hepatic and portal veins, the lymphatics, and the bile ducts. The cellular constituents of the liver are the hepatic parenchymal cells (hepatocytes), which perform most of the liver's metabolic functions, and the Kupffer cells, which engage in the liver's immunologic, detoxifying, and blood-filtering actions. The smallest bile ducts, *canaliculi,* are between the lobules of the liver. They receive secretions from the hepatocytes, carrying them to larger bile

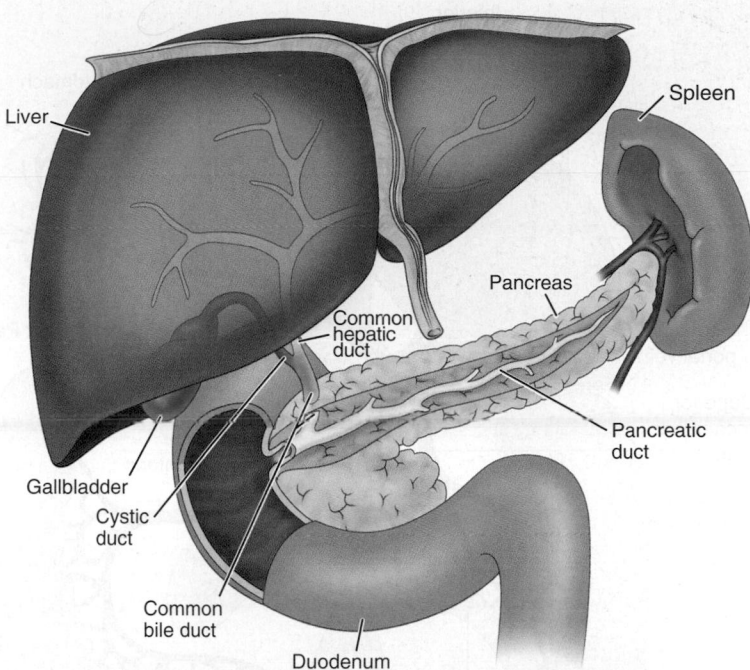

FIGURE 47-1. The liver and biliary system.

ducts and, eventually, the hepatic duct. This duct joins with the cystic duct from the gallbladder to form the common bile duct, which empties into the small intestine. The sphincter of Oddi controls the amount of bile that enters the duodenum from the common bile duct.

Gerontologic Considerations

- Changes in the liver that accompany the aging process include decreases in organ weight, blood flow, and size and number of hepatocytes; increase in fibrous tissue; and changes in metabolism of medications. However, liver function is not significantly affected unless disease is present.

JAUNDICE (ICTERUS)

Jaundice, also called *icterus,* is a greenish-yellow discoloration of tissue. It is a sign of disease, but it is not itself a unique disease. Jaundice accompanies many diseases that directly or indirectly affect the liver and is probably the most common sign of a liver disorder.

Jaundice results from an abnormally high concentration of the pigment *bilirubin* in the blood. Normally, total bilirubin concentration ranges from 0.2 to 1.3 mg/dL. If the serum bilirubin level exceeds 2.5 mg/dL (43 mcmol/L), jaundice is visible, notably on the skin, oral mucous membranes, and (especially) sclera.

To understand the scope and significance of jaundice, it is important to know how bile is formed and excreted. Bilirubin is produced in the liver, spleen, and bone marrow. It also results from hemoglobin metabolism and is a by-product of hemolysis (red blood cell [RBC] destruction). The

reticuloendothelial system also produces bilirubin. The liver removes bilirubin from the body, excreting it in *bile,* of which bilirubin is the major pigment. Thus, serum contains a normal amount of bilirubin. Serum bilirubin levels increase when (1) there is excessive destruction of RBCs or (2) the liver cannot excrete bilirubin normally.

There are two forms of bilirubin. *Indirect* or *unconjugated bilirubin* binds with protein as it circulates in the blood. This form normally circulates in the blood; when its level is elevated, the usual cause is increased hemolysis. The other form of bilirubin is *direct* or *conjugated bilirubin,* which circulates freely in the blood until reaching the liver. The liver conjugates direct bilirubin with glucuronide. The conjugated bilirubin is excreted in the bile. As the bile enters

BOX 47-1 Functions of the Liver

- Metabolizes glucose
- Regulates blood glucose concentration
- Converts glucose to glycogen to glucose to maintain normal glucose levels
- Synthesizes amino acids from the breakdown of protein or from lactate that muscles produce during exercise to form glucose (*gluconeogenesis*)
- Converts ammonia (by-product of gluconeogenesis) into urea
- Metabolizes proteins and fats
- Stores vitamins A, B$_{12}$, D, and some B-complex vitamins, as well as iron and copper
- Metabolizes drugs, chemicals, bacteria, and other foreign elements
- Forms and excretes bile
- Excretes bilirubin
- Synthesizes factors needed for blood coagulation (e.g., prothrombin, fibrinogen)

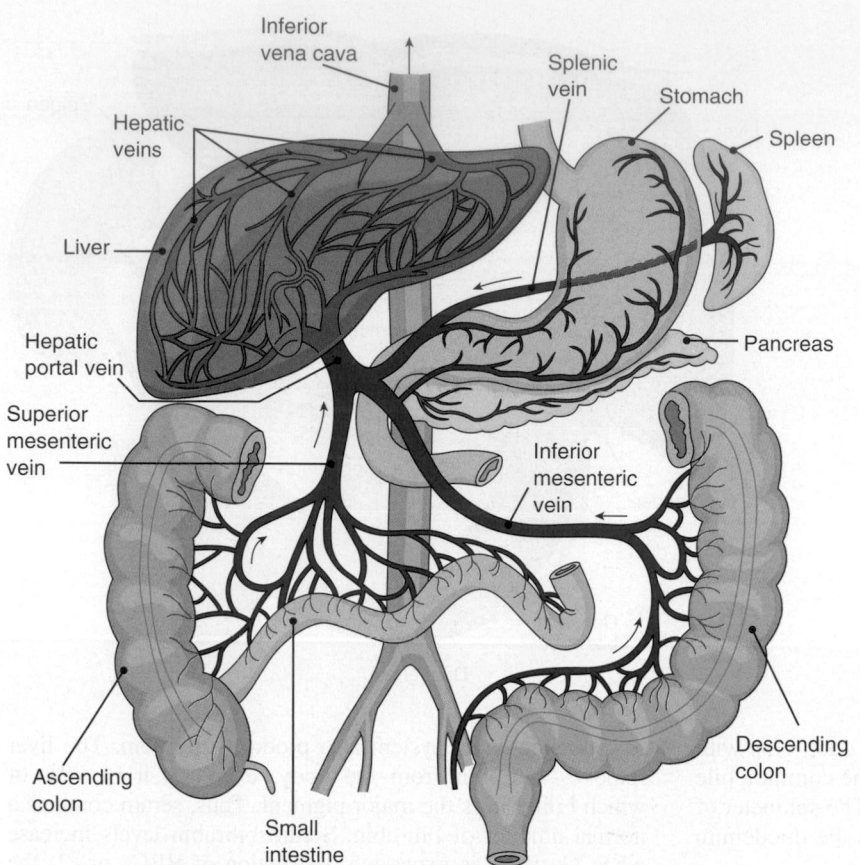

FIGURE 47-2. Hepatic portal system. Veins from the abdominal organs carry blood to the hepatic portal vein leading to the liver. After blood travels through vascular pathways inside the liver, the hepatic veins carry it to the inferior vena cava and back to the heart.

the bile ducts and moves into the intestine, bacterial enzymes transform the direct bilirubin into *urobilinogen*. Some urobilinogen is changed into *urobilin*, the brown pigment of stool; some is excreted in the urine; and some is carried back to the liver by the bloodstream for re-excretion in the bile (Fig. 47-3).

There is no direct test for indirect bilirubin levels. They are calculated by subtracting direct bilirubin levels from total bilirubin levels. For example, if the total bilirubin level is 1.0 mg/dL and the conjugated bilirubin level is 0.1 mg/dL, then the indirect bilirubin level is 0.9 mg/dL.

There are three forms of jaundice: (1) *hemolytic jaundice,* caused by excess destruction of RBCs (see Chap. 31); (2) *hepatocellular jaundice,* caused by liver disease (damaged liver cells cannot clear normal amounts of bilirubin from the blood); and (3) *obstructive jaundice,* caused by a block in the passage of bile between the liver and intestinal tract (Table 47-1). Because unconjugated and conjugated bilirubin are distinct and can be differentiated, they are important in the differential diagnosis of diseases that produce jaundice.

CIRRHOSIS

Cirrhosis is a degenerative liver disorder caused by generalized cellular damage.

Pathophysiology and Etiology

Once liver cells are irreversibly damaged, nonfunctional fibrous connective scar tissue replaces them, which leads to

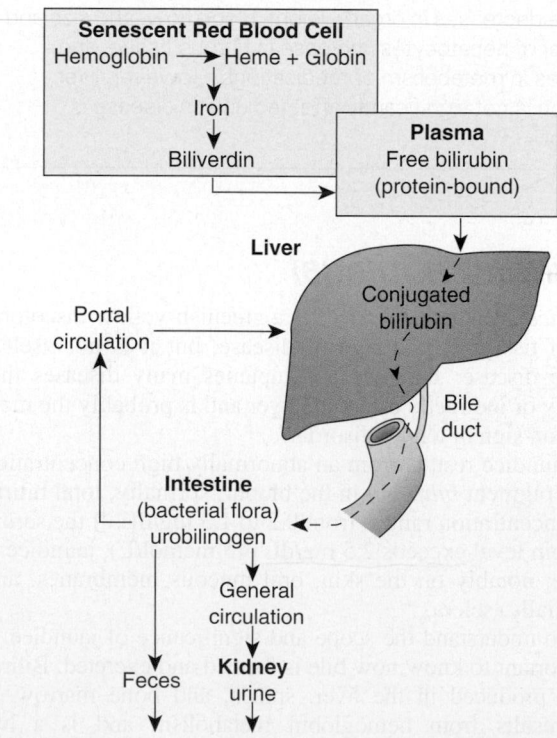

FIGURE 47-3. Formation, circulation, and elimination of bilirubin.

TABLE 47-1 Types of Jaundice

TYPE	DESCRIPTION	CHANGES IN BILIRUBIN LEVELS
Hemolytic	Hemolytic processes (e.g., multiple blood transfusions, pernicious anemia, sickle cell anemia) cause an over-production of bilirubin.	Elevated unconjugated bilirubin levels
Hepatocellular	Liver cells damaged by viral infections, medications, or chemical toxicity cannot clear bilirubin from the blood.	Elevated conjugated and unconjugated bilirubin levels
Obstructive	Gallstones, inflammation, or tumors obstruct the bile duct, causing reabsorption of bile into the blood.	Elevated conjugated bilirubin levels

considerable anatomic distortion and partial or complete occlusion of blood channels in the liver. The liver becomes increasingly unable to carry out its many functions. This leads to disturbances in digestion and metabolism, defects in blood coagulation, fluid and electrolyte imbalances, and impaired ability to metabolize hormones and detoxify chemicals. Because bile begins to drain into the intestine, the client experiences fat malabsorption and an inability to absorb fat-soluble vitamins (A, D, E, and K). Portal hypertension, esophageal varices, ascites, and hepatic encephalopathy are complications of advanced cirrhosis (see later discussion).

There are several types of cirrhosis: Laënnec's, postnecrotic, and cardiac. *Alcoholic* or *Laënnec's cirrhosis,* the most common type, results from chronic alcohol intake and is frequently associated with poor nutrition. It also can follow chronic poisoning with certain chemicals (e.g., carbon tetrachloride, a cleaning agent) or ingestion of hepatotoxic drugs (e.g., acetaminophen). Alcoholic cirrhosis is characterized by necrotic liver cells, which gradually are replaced by scar tissue. Eventually the amount of scar tissue exceeds functional liver tissue. The liver takes on a characteristic "hobnail" appearance, in which there are islands of normal tissue, regenerating tissue, and scar tissue. The disease develops over a long period of 30 years or more.

Postnecrotic cirrhosis results from destruction of liver cells secondary to infection (e.g., hepatitis), metabolic liver disease, or exposure to hepatotoxins or industrial chemicals.

In *biliary cirrhosis,* scarring occurs around the bile ducts in the liver. The cause usually is related to chronic biliary obstruction and infection. Primary biliary cirrhosis refers to a progressive autoimmune disease of the liver. Chronic inflammation causes destruction to the small intrahepatic biliary ducts, preventing the flow of bile into the small intestine. Eventually, cirrhosis and liver failure result.

The prognosis for clients with cirrhosis is based on bilirubin and albumin levels, presence of ascites (accumulation of serous fluid in the peritoneal cavity), neurologic involvement, and nutritional status. Table 47-2 provides information on classification of severity of the disease.

Assessment Findings

Signs and Symptoms

Signs and symptoms of cirrhosis increase in severity as the disease progresses and are categorized as compensated or decompensated (Box 47-2). *Compensated cirrhosis* is less severe, and signs and symptoms are more vague. As the disease progresses, it is referred to as *decompensated cirrhosis.* Signs and symptoms of decompensated cirrhosis are very pronounced and indicate liver failure.

The client's history often correlates with factors that predispose to cirrhosis, such as chronic alcohol use, hepatitis, and exposure to toxins. The client typically experiences chronic fatigue, anorexia, dyspepsia, nausea, vomiting, and diarrhea or constipation, with accompanying weight loss. Many clients report passing clay-colored or whitish stools as a result of no bile in the gastrointestinal (GI) tract. They also may report dark or "tea-colored" urine from increased concentrations of urobilin. Abdominal discomfort and shortness of breath are common complaints as a result of organ compression from the enlarged liver. Many clients mention nosebleeds, bleeding from the gums, or easy bruising. Skin may itch (pruritus) from accumulated bile salts.

A client with cirrhosis has an enlarged liver and sometimes an enlarged spleen, causing the abdomen to appear

TABLE 47-2 Child-Pugh Classification of Severity of Liver Disease

PARAMETER	POINTS ASSIGNED*		
	1	2	3
Ascites	Absent	Slight	Moderate
Bilirubin (mg/dL)	<2	2–3	>3
Albumin (g/dL)	>3.5	2.8–3.5	>2.8
Prothrombin time			
Seconds over control	<4	4–6	>6
INR	<1.7	1.7–2.3	>2.3
Encephalopathy	None	Grade 1–2	Grade 3–4

*A total score of 5–6 is considered grade A (well-compensated disease); 7–9 is grade B (significant functional compromise); and 10–15 is grade C (decompensated disease). INR, international normalized ratio. (From Child-Pugh Classification of Severity of Liver Disease, medicalCRITERIA.com, http://www.medicalcriteria.com/criteria/gas_liver.htm. Accessed on December 28, 2008. Reprinted with permission.)

BOX 47-2 Clinical Manifestations of Cirrhosis

Compensated
Intermittent mild fever
Vascular spiders
Palmar erythema (reddened palms)
Unexplained epistaxis
Ankle edema
Vague morning indigestion
Flatulent dyspepsia
Abdominal pain
Firm, enlarged liver
Splenomegaly

Decompensated
Ascites
Jaundice
Weakness
Muscle wasting
Weight loss
Continuous mild fever
Clubbing of fingers
Purpura (due to decreased platelet count)
Spontaneous bruising
Epistaxis
Hypotension
Sparse body hair
White nails
Gonadal atrophy

BOX 47-3 Common Blood Test Findings in Cirrhosis

Blood studies of clients with cirrhosis are likely to show:
- Increased unconjugated and conjugated bilirubin levels
- Increased enzyme levels of AST (SGOT), ALT (SGPT), and GGT
- Low RBC count—cells appear large
- Decreased leukocytes and thrombocytes
- Low fibrinogen level
- Prolonged PT
- Decreased platelet count
- Low serum albumin level
- Increased globulin level
- Hypokalemia

ALT, alanine transaminase; AST, aspartate phosphatase; GGT, gamma glutamyltransferase; PT, prothrombin time; RBC, red blood cell; SGOT, serum glutamic-oxaloacetic transaminase; SGPT, serum glutamic-pyruvic transaminase.

distended. The skin, sclera, or oral mucous membranes are jaundiced. Edema may be present in the legs and feet. Veins over the abdomen may be dilated (**caput medusae**). Because the dysfunctional liver cannot fully metabolize estrogen, men may present with *gynecomastia* (enlarged breasts) and testicular atrophy. *Palmar erythema* (bright pink palms) and *cutaneous spider angiomata* (tiny, spider-like blood vessels) may be visible. These findings also are related to an inability to inactivate estrogen.

 Gerontologic Considerations

- Older adults need to be carefully assessed for alcohol abuse using standardized screening instruments. Some older adults may self-medicate with alcohol and not be aware of the potential for addiction or risk for organ damage.

Diagnostic Findings

A liver biopsy, which reveals hepatic fibrosis, is the most conclusive diagnostic procedure. The biopsy is obtained percutaneously with mild sedation (see Nursing Guidelines 44-1) or through a surgical incision. It also can be performed in the radiology department with ultrasound or computed tomography (CT) to identify appropriate placement of the trochar or biopsy needle.

Certain blood tests provide information about liver function (Box 47-3). Prolonged prothrombin time (PT) and low platelet count place the client at high risk for hemorrhage. The client may receive intravenous (IV) administration of vitamin K or infusions of platelets before liver biopsy to reduce the risk of bleeding. Other tests used to examine the liver include CT, magnetic resonance imaging (MRI), and radioisotope liver scan, all of which may demonstrate the liver's enlarged size, nodular configuration, and distorted blood flow.

Medical and Surgical Management

No specific cure for cirrhosis exists. The principal aim of therapy is to prevent further deterioration by abolishing underlying causes and preserving what liver function remains. Various approaches are used to relieve associated symptoms. An optimal diet and vitamin and nutritional supplements promote healing of liver cells (Nutrition Notes 47-1). Improved nutritional status helps the client feel better. Malnutrition may be treated with enteral or parenteral feedings. Because absorption of the fat-soluble vitamins is impaired, special attention is given to their supplementation (see Table 44-1). Vitamin K also is used to correct coagulopathy, which results from prolonged PT and partial thromboplastin time (PTT). Vitamin B complex, vitamin C, and iron also may be prescribed. IV albumin may be given if hypoproteinemia is severe. The client *must not* consume alcohol.

Altered ammonia metabolism may be responsible for precipitating hepatic encephalopathy (see Complications of Cirrhosis). Lactulose is administered to detoxify ammonium and to act as an osmotic agent, drawing water into the bowel, which causes diarrhea in some clients. Antacids may be used to reduce gastric disturbances and decrease the potential for GI bleeding. Potassium-sparing antidiuretics such as spironolactone are used to treat ascites (see Complications of Cirrhosis).

Transfusions of platelets may be necessary to correct thrombocytopenia (low platelet count). Packed RBCs may be administered in cases of anemia or blood loss.

Nutrition Notes 47-1
The Client With Cirrhosis

- Nutrition therapy for clients with cirrhosis is individualized according to symptoms and tolerance.
- Dietary restrictions are used only when they can be expected to improve symptoms. Fat is restricted for clients with fat malabsorption (steatorrhea). Medium-chain triglyceride oil may be given for calories when fat intake is limited. Sodium is restricted to 2–3 g per day when ascites is present. Fluid restriction is imposed in clients with hyponatremia.
- A high-calorie diet is recommended for clients with malnutrition, weight loss, or infection. Adequate calories are essential to ensure protein sparing.
- A high-protein diet is used to prevent muscle wasting. A protein-restricted diet is no longer recommended for most people with hepatic encephalopathy because it may worsen malnutrition and muscle wasting, and protein intolerance is much less common than previously thought.
- A carbohydrate controlled diet is used for clients with diabetes or insulin resistance.
- Small frequent meals and the use of nutritional supplements may help boost intake in clients who have nausea, vomiting, or fatigue.

BOX 47-4 Liver Transplants and Organ Donation

The United Network for Organ Sharing (UNOS) administers the Organ Procurement and Transplantation Network. Through this network, the organization adds clients who need transplants to a national waiting list and generates a list of potential recipients when a donor organ becomes available. The UNOS bases its list of potential recipients on such factors as genetic similarity, organ size, medical urgency, and time on the waiting list.

Many transplanted livers are from cadaver donors. Some centers, however, now have "living related donor" programs, in which portions of livers for transplantation come from living donors. In either type of transplant, recipients need life-long immunosuppressant therapy to suppress the immune system and prevent rejection of the transplanted organ.

The organs available are nowhere close to the number needed. Many potential recipients succumb to liver failure while waiting for donor organs. Transplantation costs are high, and the condition of potential recipients is fragile, jeopardizing the chances for successful transplantation. The decision to do a liver transplantation is based on careful scrutiny and assessment of the client, with consideration of the potential for success and improved quality of life.

Cholestyramine may be prescribed to bind bile salts and relieve pruritus. Additional measures to relieve pruritus include skin care and routine cleansing with a nondrying agent. Skin is patted dry, and moisturizing lotion is applied immediately after bathing. Ursodeoxycholic acid (Actigall) may be used to promote bile flow from the liver. Sodium intake is carefully regulated and often restricted because of the potential for water retention, which can lead to edema, circulatory congestion, and heart failure. Fluid intake also may be restricted. Liver transplantation is an option for treating liver failure as well as chronic liver disease (Box 47-4).

Nursing Management

If the client has active alcoholism, the nurse monitors vital signs closely. A rise in blood pressure (BP), pulse, and temperature correlates with alcohol withdrawal; the nurse must recognize and treat these appropriately along with the other presenting symptoms (see Chap. 71).

The nurse weighs the client daily and keeps an accurate record of intake and output. If the abdomen appears enlarged, the nurse measures it according to a set routine (Fig. 47-4). Because of the anorexia that accompanies severe cirrhosis, the client may better tolerate frequent, small, semisolid or liquid meals rather than three full meals a day.

Careful evaluation of the client's response to drug therapy is important because the liver cannot metabolize many substances. The nurse reports any change in mental status or signs of GI bleeding immediately because they indicate secondary complications.

The nurse provides educational information specific to the liver disorder. He or she can refer the client to the American Liver Foundation (or a similar organization) for information about available support groups. The nurse emphasizes the need for abstinence from alcohol and all nonprescription drugs unless approved by the physician. In addition, he or she contacts social services about referrals to alcohol or drug cessation programs. Additional teaching depends on the type and cause of the disorder and the physician's prescribed or recommended home care (Client and Family Teaching 47-1). Nursing Care Plan 47-1 describes additional nursing management.

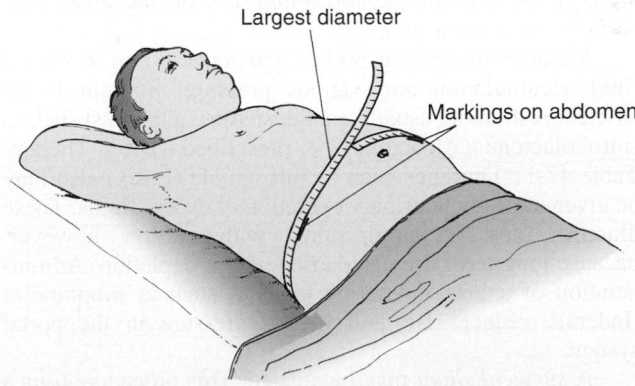

FIGURE 47-4. To measure abdominal girth, place a tape measure around the largest diameter of the abdomen. Make guide marks on the skin so that future measurements are obtained from the same site.

Client and Family Teaching 47–1
Cirrhosis

The following topics are appropriate for a teaching plan:

- Follow the diet recommended by the physician.
- Consult a dietitian if you require a special diet (i.e., a low-sodium diet to prevent edema and ascites). Many metabolic liver disorders require highly specialized diets and necessitate extensive teaching from nursing and nutritional staff. Some diets require routine monitoring and home care.
- Avoid situations that could further damage the liver, such as drinking alcohol, taking tranquilizers, or inhaling chemicals such as benzene or vinyl chloride, which are toxic.
- Rest frequently, especially if activity causes fatigue.
- Avoid exposure to people with known infections.
- Continue skin care.
- Avoid nonprescription drugs (especially aspirin and products that contain it because they contribute to bleeding problems) unless approved by the physician.
- Be prepared for rejection as a blood donor because of liver disease.
- Contact the physician immediately about vomiting of blood, tarry stools, extreme fatigue, yellow skin, light-colored stools, or dark urine.

Complications of Cirrhosis

Portal Hypertension

The portal system consists of gastric veins from the stomach, the mesenteric vein from the intestines, the splenic vein from the spleen and pancreas, and the portal vein. All these veins drain into and through the liver and out the hepatic veins into the inferior vena cava.

In the scarred cirrhotic liver, intrahepatic veins may be compressed. Consequently, blood backs up into the portal system, which is the venous pathway through the liver. This congestion and increased fluid pressure in the portal system are called **portal hypertension**. As the normal pathway for blood is obstructed, the collateral veins become distended and engorged with blood (Fig. 47-5). These distended collateral vessels develop primarily in the esophagus (esophageal varices) and rectum (hemorrhoids) and on the abdominal surface (caput medusae).

Methods of treating portal hypertension aim to reduce fluid accumulation and venous pressure. Sodium is restricted. A diuretic, usually an aldosterone antagonist such as spironolactone (Aldactone), is prescribed (Drug Therapy Table 47-1). Diuretics such as furosemide (Lasix) also may be given to promote urinary excretion of excess fluids. These diuretics must be administered with caution, however, because long-term use can cause sodium depletion. Administration of a beta-adrenergic blocker, such as propranolol (Inderal), reduces BP and lowers pressure in the portal system.

A *surgical shunt* may be created. This procedure uses a graft to decompress the portal system by diverting blood flow into the systemic circulation. It is not frequently performed, however, because of the high incidence of complications and shunt failure. An alternative, nonsurgical method of shunt placement is a *transjugular intrahepatic portosystemic shunt (TIPS)*. This invasive radiologic procedure involves the creation of a tract from the hepatic to the portal vein. In TIPS, a cannula with an expandable stent is inserted into the portovenous system through the jugular vein. The stent serves as the intrahepatic shunt between the hepatic vein and portal circulation to relieve portal hypertension. TIPS may be carried out using conscious sedation or anesthesia (see Chap. 14).

Esophageal Varices

Dilated, bulging esophageal veins are referred to as **esophageal varices**. A single dilated, bulging esophageal vein is called a *varix*. Esophageal varices overfill as a result of portal hypertension. They are especially vulnerable to bleeding because they lie superficially in the mucosa, contain little protective elastic tissue, and are easily traumatized by rough food or chemical irritation. Figure 47-6 depicts the pathogenesis of esophageal varices.

Esophageal bleeding is a cardinal sign of esophageal varices. It may be slight but chronic, or massive and rapid. Massive bleeding from esophageal varices is a life-threatening medical emergency requiring immediate intervention. Once bleeding begins, clotting disorders common to liver damage occur. Barium swallow or esophagoscopy confirm the diagnosis of esophageal varices.

Measures to treat portal hypertension reduce the potential for bleeding varices. In addition, a soft diet and elimination of alcohol, aspirin, and other locally irritating substances may prevent varices. Antitussives and stool softeners are prescribed when the client is symptomatic, to reduce coughing or straining, which increases vascular pressure.

Esophageal varices also are treated with injection sclerotherapy or variceal banding. In **injection sclerotherapy** (also referred to as *endoscopic sclerotherapy*), the physician passes an endoscope orally to locate the varix. He or she then passes a thin needle through the endoscope into the varix and then directly injects a sclerosing agent (sodium tetradecyl, sodium morrhuate). The sclerosing agent solidifies and stops circulation to the varix.

In *variceal banding* (*variceal band ligation*), another endoscopic procedure, the physician uses a device with small rubber bands at the end of the endoscope. After locating the varix, the physician places a rubber band over it. The band restricts blood flow to the varix, which sloughs off after a few days. Persistent portal hypertension allows varices to form again, making it necessary to repeat sclerotherapy or banding procedures regularly.

Another procedure involves placing a distal splenorenal shunt (DSRS). The splenic vein is detached from the portal vein and reattached to the left renal vein. This procedure helps reduce pressure in the varices and control bleeding.

Acute hemorrhage from esophageal varices is life-threatening. Resuscitative measures include administration of IV fluids and blood products. IV octreotide (Sandostatin) is started as soon as possible. Octreotide reduces pressure in the portal venous system and is preferred to the previously used agents, vasopressin or terlipressin. Urgent endoscopy is indicated to allow for treatment with sclerotherapy or

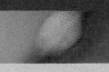

| NURSING CARE PLAN 47-1 | The Client With a Liver Disorder |

Assessment

- Obtain complete diet, drug, and allergy histories and a history of symptoms from client or family. Depending on the circumstances, in depth questioning may be necessary. Contributing factors may include exposure to toxic chemicals, history of hepatitis, or long-term alcohol abuse.

- Pay special attention to ventilation, abdominal size, weight, and any jaundice or other symptoms of liver disease.
- Analyze food intake and fluid records.
- Review laboratory and diagnostic studies and the physician's progress notes daily to assess client's response to therapy.

Nursing Diagnosis: Fatigue related to malnutrition and liver disease.

Expected Outcome: Client will report improved energy and adhere to conserve energy.

Interventions	Rationales
Assess client's ability to perform activities of daily living and pattern of fatigue.	Data provide a baseline for comparison and help nurse and client to target ways to conserve energy.
Assist client to set small, short-term goals that will be easy to achieve.	Such goals help the client accomplish tasks without being overwhelmed or exhausted.
Encourage client to separate essential and nonessential tasks and to delegate.	Doing so creates a realistic picture of what must be done and who should do it.
Encourage the client to limit demands on his or her time.	Doing so helps the client set priorities and balance demands with available energy.
Teach strategies for energy conservation such as sitting instead of standing in the shower, storing items within easy reach, and breaking large tasks into smaller ones.	These strategies enhance energy and give a client more control over activities.
Offer a high-protein (if client does not have severe liver disease) and high-calorie diet.	Inadequate nutrition contributes to fatigue.
Encourage client to rest frequently.	Inadequate sleep contributes to fatigue.

Evaluation of Expected Outcome

Client participates in appropriate activities, gradually increases activities, and reports feeling stronger and more energetic.

Nursing Diagnosis: Imbalanced Nutrition: Less than Body Requirements related to loss of appetite, nausea, and vomiting.

Expected Outcome: Client will identify nutritional requirements and consume adequate nutrition.

Interventions	Rationales
Encourage client to eat six small meals a day.	Small, frequent meals reduce the sensation of fullness and the stimulus for vomiting.
Consult the dietitian for ways to provide nutritional meals that complement the prescribed diet.	Such meals will provide foods that the client is likely to eat within dietary restrictions.
Provide high-carbohydrate snacks or supplements to meals.	Doing so provides additional calories.
Offer highest-calorie meal when the client's appetite is greatest.	Clients with liver disease usually are hungriest at breakfast, so providing the highest-calorie meal at the beginning of the day would be most logical.
If vomiting is a problem, administer antiemetics before meals.	Antiemetics prevent nausea and vomiting.
Monitor food intake and ask dietitian to calculate caloric intake.	Tracking nutritional intake provides a record of foods the client best tolerates at different times of day.
Ask family members to assist with meal planning and preparation, adapting to the client's cultural preferences.	These measures enhance the client's ability to eat preferred foods and meet nutritional requirements within dietary restrictions.

Evaluation of Expected Outcome

Client reports improved appetite, identifies appropriate foods that meet dietary requirements, and demonstrates appropriate weight gain.

Nursing Diagnosis: Ineffective Breathing Pattern related to ascites and liver enlargement

Expected Outcome: Client will breathe without effort.

(care plan continues on page 710)

NURSING CARE PLAN 47-1 **The Client With a Liver Disorder** (Continued)

Interventions	Rationales
Assess respiratory pattern, noting what causes and relieves dyspnea.	Assessing the cause of dyspnea helps the nurse provide relief measures and improve client's ventilatory efforts.
Place client in an upright or semi-Fowler's position.	These positions facilitate lung expansion by reducing pressure on the diaphragm.
Schedule rest periods after activity.	Rest reduces metabolic and oxygen requirements.
Provide supplemental oxygen if client becomes short of breath.	Oxygen therapy decreases dyspnea by reducing the central drive mediated by chemoreceptors in the carotid bodies.

Evaluation of Expected Outcome

Client reports decreased shortness of breath and improved comfort with breathing.

Nursing Diagnosis: **Excess Fluid Volume** related to peripheral edema, ascites, and sodium retention

Expected Outcome: Client will maintain fluid balance.

Interventions	Rationales
Assess location and extent of edema.	These measures help locate changes in peripheral edema and ascites.
Measure and record abdominal girth daily.	
Monitor weight daily.	Abdominal girth and weight reflect changes in body fluid volume.
Restrict sodium and fluid intake as ordered.	Such restrictions reduce peripheral edema and ascites.
Administer prescribed diuretics and potassium.	These measures promote fluid excretion through the kidneys to maintain fluid and electrolyte balance.
Monitor serum albumin levels. Administer protein supplements as ordered.	Low albumin levels can cause severe peripheral edema because they lead to impaired movement of fluid from interstitial spaces to intravascular spaces.
Maintain IV infusion rates carefully.	Doing so prevents inadvertent infusion of excess fluid volumes.
Encourage client to turn at least every 2 hours when in bed.	Edematous tissue is vulnerable to ischemia and pressure ulcers.

Evaluation of Expected Outcome

Client maintains fluid balance, as evidenced by stable BP, adequate urine output, and decreased peripheral edema and ascites.

Nursing Diagnosis: **Ineffective Protection** related to risk for impaired blood coagulation, bleeding from portal hypertension, and infection.

Expected Outcome: Client will not demonstrate evidence of new bleeding or infection.

Interventions	Rationales
Carefully monitor vital signs.	Changes may indicate the onset of bleeding or infection.
Notify physician promptly when client has signs of infection: fever, chills, or drainage.	Prompt treatment reduces the risk of morbidity and mortality.
Monitor bleeding times, clotting studies, and platelet counts.	Abnormal results indicate increased risk for bleeding.
Teach client to avoid aspirin or nonsteroidal anti-inflammatory drugs and to use electric razors and toothbrushes.	These drugs can cause GI bleeding, and aspirin interferes with platelet function. Electric razors and soft toothbrushes can minimize unnecessary trauma.
Practice aseptic measures and teach family members to do so	Asepsis reduces the risk of infection.
Observe stools for color and consistency.	Tests detect blood in stool and may indicate issues with GI bleeding.
Test stool for occult blood.	
Note any complaints of anxiety, epigastric fullness, weakness, and restlessness.	These findings may indicate bleeding and early shock
Monitor for ecchymosis, epistaxis, petechiae, and bleeding from gums.	These findings indicate altered clotting mechanisms.
Monitor client carefully during blood transfusions.	Doing so can help detect a transfusion reaction.
Administer vitamin K as ordered.	Vitamin K promotes clotting

Evaluation of Expected Outcome

Client does not exhibit any new signs of bleeding or infection. Vital signs are stable, and laboratory values are normal.

Nursing Diagnosis: **Impaired Skin Integrity** related to pruritus, jaundice, bleeding tendencies, and edema.

Expected Outcome: Skin will remain intact.

NURSING CARE PLAN 47-1   The Client With a Liver Disorder (Continued)

Interventions	Rationales
Provide frequent skin care, avoiding drying soaps and alcohol based lotions.	Skin care remove waste products deposited in skin and prevents drying.
Encourage client to keep fingernails short and smooth.	Doing so prevents excoriation and infection from scratches.
Turn client at least every 2 hours, massaging bony prominences with emollients.	Turning and massage mobilize edema and improve circulation.
Use nonallergenic bed linens; instruct family to avoid harsh detergents.	These measures decrease skin irritation.

Evaluation of Expected Outcome

Skin remains intact with no evidence of pressure ulcers.

Nursing Diagnosis: Chronic Pain related to liver enlargement and ascites.

Expected Outcome: Client will report increased level of comfort.

Interventions	Rationales
Encourage client to remain on bed rest when experiencing abdominal discomfort, changing position frequently.	These measures relieve pressure and promote comfort.
Administer prescribed analgesics.	These drugs relieve chronic pain.
Explain the pain management regimen.	Adequate explanations help the client understand implementation of the pain-control plan.
For client receiving opioids, monitor sedation and respiratory status when dose is increased.	Usually, clients receiving long-term opioids develop a tolerance to the respiratory depressant effects. They still require monitoring for sedation and respiratory problems.
Instruct client in nonpharmacologic techniques to relieve pain.	Other interventions supplement pain medications and improve comfort level.

Evaluation of Expected Outcome

Client reports that pain medication is effective and that comfort is improved

PC: Hepatic Encephalopathy

Expected Outcome: The nurse will minimize and manage problems associated with hepatic encephalopathy.

Interventions	Rationales
Assess cognitive and neurologic status at least every 8 hours.	Baseline data provide a means by which to determine change.
Restrict dietary protein as ordered.	Protein is a source of ammonia, which contributes to encephalopathy.
Give small and frequent feedings high in carbohydrates.	Carbohydrates provide energy and space protein breakdown.
Restrict medications that increase encephalopathy.	Sedatives, hypnotics, and opioids may precipitate hepatic encephalopathy and increase confusion.
Monitor laboratory results, especially ammonia levels.	Increased ammonia levels indicate hepatic encephalopathy, which can lead to coma.
Administer medications that reduce serum ammonia levels, such as lactulose.	Reduced serum ammonia levels are a key goal.
Identify potentially dangerous items and modify the environment.	Doing so promotes the client's safety.
Report any new or sudden increase in mental confustion.	Confusion indicates increased hepatic encephalopathy and possible coma. It requires immediate medical intervention.
Orient client to name, place, time, and date as needed.	Doing so reinforces reality and provides the client with cues about the world.
If hepatic coma develops, monitor respiratory status and initiate measures to prevent complications.	Clients in hepatic coma are at increased risk for pneumonia and infection.
Implement measures to prevent skin breakdown and pressure.	These clients are at increased risk for skin breakdown and pressure ulcers.

Evaluation of Expected Outcome

Client remains free from injury.

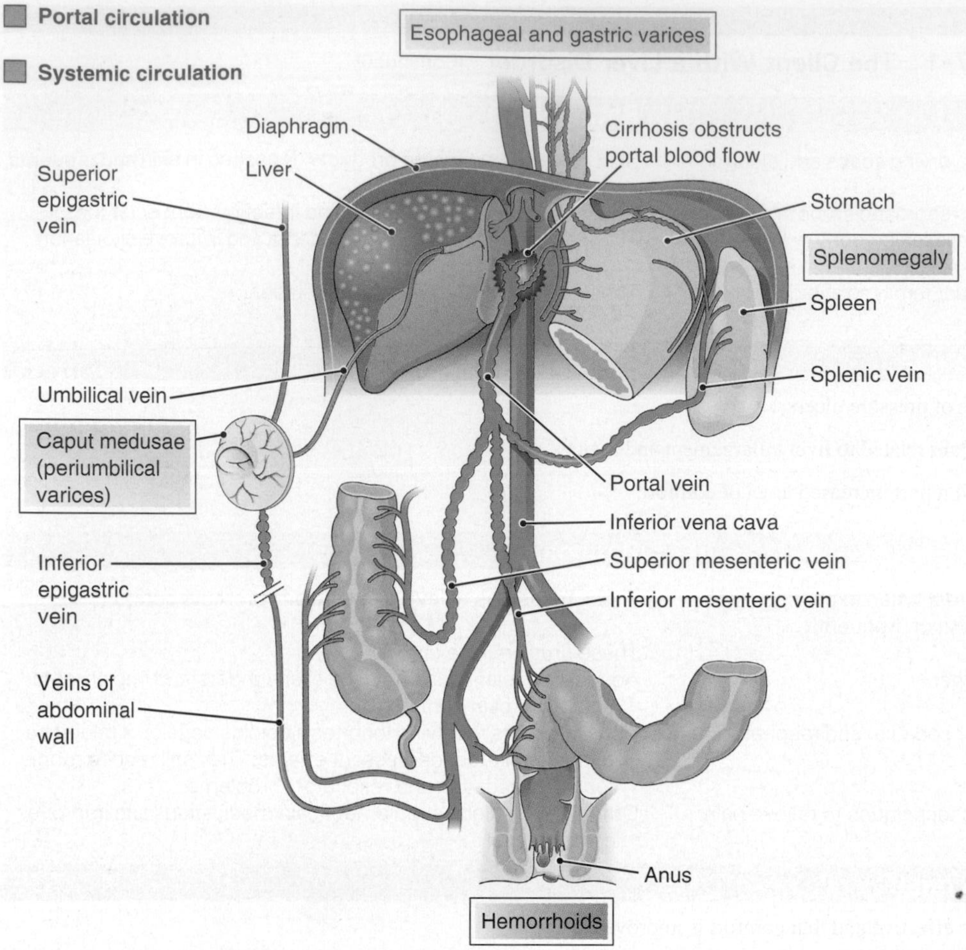

■ Portal circulation

■ Systemic circulation

Esophageal and gastric varices

Diaphragm

Cirrhosis obstructs portal blood flow

Superior epigastric vein

Liver

Stomach

Splenomegaly

Spleen

Splenic vein

Umbilical vein

Caput medusae (periumbilical varices)

Portal vein

Inferior vena cava

Superior mesenteric vein

Inferior epigastric vein

Inferior mesenteric vein

Veins of abdominal wall

Anus

Hemorrhoids

FIGURE 47-5. Portal hypertension results from obstruction of blood in the portal circulation in cirrhosis and other disorders. With the increased pressure, collateral vessels become distended, primarily in the esophagus, rectum, and abdominal surface.

banding. If a skilled endoscopist is not available or bleeding is too rapid to permit endoscopy, **balloon tamponade** with a Sengstaken-Blakemore tube may be useful in compressing the varices and stemming the flow of blood (Fig. 47-7). Unfortunately, this method usually allows only temporary relief from hemorrhage, necessitating endoscopy with sclerotherapy or banding after the client's condition is stabilized.

Ascites

Ascites is collection of fluid in the peritoneal cavity. Undoubtedly, portal hypertension is a major underlying factor in the development of ascites. It leads to a cascade of events, referred to as the **hepatorenal syndrome**, that ultimately alter fluid distribution and interfere with fluid excretion.

Increased pressure in the portal system forces serum proteins into the peritoneal cavity. The proteins draw plasma from the circulating blood by osmosis. The kidneys respond to decreases in blood volume and renal BP by initiating the renin-angiotensin-aldosterone system (see Chap. 27). In response, the body conserves sodium ions, which further contributes to fluid retention. Low renal blood volume also may suppress antidiuretic hormone, causing water to be reabsorbed rather than eliminated as urine. These combined factors promote fluid accumulation in the abdomen. Ascites is visible as extensive and massive abdominal swelling.

Abdominal paracentesis may be performed to remove ascitic fluid. Abdominal fluid is rapidly removed by careful

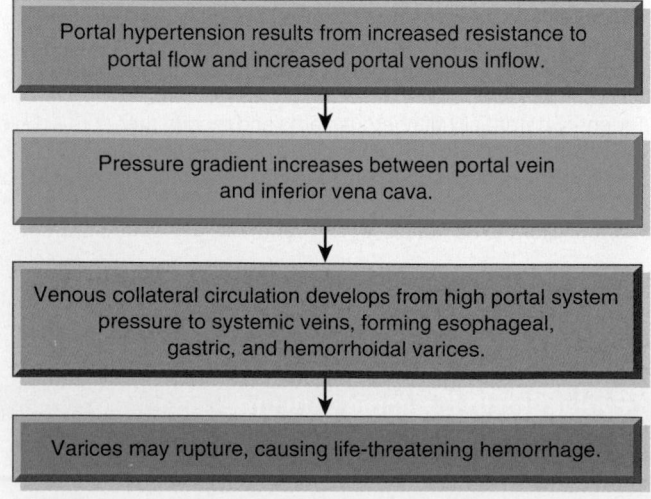

Portal hypertension results from increased resistance to portal flow and increased portal venous inflow.

↓

Pressure gradient increases between portal vein and inferior vena cava.

↓

Venous collateral circulation develops from high portal system pressure to systemic veins, forming esophageal, gastric, and hemorrhoidal varices.

↓

Varices may rupture, causing life-threatening hemorrhage.

FIGURE 47-6. Pathogenesis of esophageal varices.

DRUG THERAPY TABLE 47-1 Selected Medications Used for Liver, Gallbladder, and Pancreatic Disorders

Drug Category and Examples	Mechanism of Action	Side Effects	Nursing Considerations
Drugs For Liver Disorders **Procoagulant** vitamin K (AquaMEPHY-TON, Mephyton, Konakion)	Promotes blood coagulation in bleeding conditions resulting from liver disease	Dizziness, transient hypotension, rapid and weak pulse, diaphoresis, flushing, skin rash, anaphylaxis	Instruct client not to take additional vitamin supplements unless specifically directed to do so by the physician. Assess adequacy of therapy by measuring prothrombin time.
Aminoglycoside antibiotic kanamycin (Kantrex)	Decreases intestinal bacteria, thereby decreasing serum ammonia level	Diarrhea, cramping, ototoxicity, nephrotoxicity	Administer orally to decrease intestinal bacteria and serum ammonia levels. Note that discoloration does not indicate the loss of potency. Assess adequacy of therapy by measuring serum ammonia levels.
Laxative and ammonia reduction agent lactulose (Cephulac, Chronulac, Constilac, Duphalac, Heptalac, Portalac)	Degrades intestinal bacteria	Diarrhea, cramping, abdominal distention, flatulence, nausea, vomiting, belching, hypernatremia	Because acidic stools excoriate the perianal area, perform careful cleansing after bowel movements to maintain skin integrity. Monitor serum sodium level for hypernatremia. Assess adequacy of therapy by measuring serum ammonia levels.
Bile acid sequestrant cholestyramine (Questran)	Reduces pruritus by binding bile salts for excretion in feces	Headache, anxiety, vertigo, dizziness, insomnia, fatigue, tinnitus, constipation, hematuria, dysuria, skin rash, muscle and joint pain	Give all other drugs at least 1 hour before or 4 hours after cholestyramine because drug interferes with absorption of fat-soluble vitamins (A, D, E, and K), as well as many other drugs. Mix powder with liquid. Taking the medication in its dry form causes esophageal irritation and severe constipation.
Potassium-sparing diuretic spironolactone (Aldactone, Spirotone)	Promotes excretion of sodium and water, particularly in cases of ascites	Headache, drowsiness, lethargy, confusion, ataxia, diarrhea, gastric bleeding, cramping, vomiting, urticaria, skin eruptions, hyperkalemia, dehydration, hirsutism, agranulocytosis	To enhance absorption, give with meals. Protect drug from light. Monitor serum electrolytes, intake and output, weight. Administer in the morning to prevent nocturia. Avoid potassium supplements and salt substitutes.
Immune agents interferon alfa-2b, recombinant (Intron A)	Promotes virus-fighting capacities	Dizziness, confusion, paresthesia, lethargy, depression, insomnia, anxiety, fatigue, amnesia, malaise, hypotension, chest pain, anorexia, nausea, diarrhea, abdominal pain, dyspepsia, constipation, stomatitis, gingivitis, transient impotence, gynecomastia, leukopenia, anemia, thrombocytopenia, dyspnea, cough, rash, pruritus, alopecia, dermatitis, flulike symptoms (fever, fatigue, chills, headache, muscle aches), back pain, diaphoresis	Administer intramuscularly or subcutaneously for chronic hepatitis. Administer at bedtime to minimize daytime drowsiness. Monitor for flulike symptoms. Monitor blood studies for hematologic side effects. Explain to the client the increased risk of infection when taking this drug. Advise avoiding contact with those who have an acute illness and those who have recently received oral polio vaccine. The client should not receive vaccines prepared with live virus, unless specifically instructed to do so by the physician.

(drug table continues on page 714)

DRUG THERAPY TABLE 47-1 Selected Medications Used for Liver, Gallbladder, and Pancreatic Disorders (*Continued*)

Drug Category and Examples	Mechanism of Action	Side Effects	Nursing Considerations
Immunosuppressives cyclosporine (Sandimmune)	Prevent rejection of transplanted organ	Tremor, headache, seizures, confusion, paresthesia, hypertension, gum hyperplasia, nausea, vomiting, diarrhea, nephrotoxicity, hepatotoxicity, anemia, leukopenia, thrombocytopenia, hemolytic anemia, acne, flushing, infection, hirsutism, anaphylaxis, gynecomastia	Administer from a glass container or dropper to minimize adherence of the drug to container walls. Monitor cyclosporine blood levels to ensure that the client's level is within therapeutic range. Monitor renal function, blood urea nitrogen (BUN) and creatinine levels. Monitor liver enzyme levels for hepatotoxicity. Because the client is at increased risk of infection when taking this drug, advise against contact with those who have an acute illness and those who have recently received oral polio vaccine. The client should not receive vaccines prepared with live viruses, unless specifically instructed to do so by the physician.
tacrolimus (Prograf, FK-506)	Prevent rejection of transplanted organ	Headache, tremor, insomnia, paresthesia, hypertension, peripheral edema, diarrhea, nausea, constipation, abnormal liver function test, anorexia, abdominal pain, abnormal renal function, elevated creatinine or BUN levels, oliguria, hyperkalemia, hypokalemia, hyperglycemia, hypomagnesemia, anemia, leukocytosis, thrombocytopenia, pleural effusion, dyspnea, atelectasis, pruritus, rash, back pain, ascites, anaphylaxis	Monitor for neurotoxicity and nephrotoxicity, especially in clients who receive high doses, or who have renal dysfunction. Monitor serum magnesium and electrolyte levels and blood glucose levels. Monitor liver enzymes. Inform client of an increased risk of infection when taking this drug. The client should avoid contact with those who have an acute illness and those who have recently received oral polio vaccine. The client should not receive vaccines prepared with live viruses, unless specifically instructed to do so by the physician.
For Gallbladder Disease **Gallstone-dissolving agents** chenodiol—also called chenodeoxycholic acid (Chenix)	Suppresses hepatic synthesis of cholesterol and cholic acid	Diarrhea, cramping, heartburn, constipation, nausea, anorexia, epigastric distress, elevated liver enzymes, possible hepatotoxicity	Administer orally to dissolve gallstones; may require long-term therapy for effectiveness. Monitor the client's liver enzyme levels. Avoid administering during pregnancy.
ursodiol (Actigall)	Suppresses hepatic synthesis of cholesterol and inhibits intestinal absorption of cholesterol	Headache, fatigue, anxiety, depression, sleep disorders, rhinitis, nausea, vomiting, dyspepsia, metallic taste, abdominal pain, biliary pain, diarrhea, constipation, flatulence, cough, pruritus, rash, dry skin, urticaria, alopecia, myalgia, back pain	Administer orally to dissolve cholesterol-related gallstones; may require long-term therapy for effectiveness and may be helpful in promoting bile flow in liver disease. Monitor the client's liver enzyme levels.
For Pancreatic Disorders **Pancreatic enzymes** pancreatin (Creon, Bioglan, Panazyme, Donnazyme, Entozyme) pancrelipase (Pancrease, Cotazym, Creon 10 and Creon 20, Protilase, Ultrase, Viokase, Zymase)	Promote digestion and fat, protein, and carbohydrate absorption	Anorexia, nausea, diarrhea, allergic reactions, perianal irritation	Administer with meals and snacks. Monitor stool consistency. Open capsules and sprinkle onto a small quantity of soft food. Do not crush or chew enteric-coated preparations. Expect dosage to vary with degree of malabsorption, amount of fat in diet, size of the meal and enzyme activity of individual preparations (300 mg pancrelipase/17 g dietary fat). Cautious use in clients with a history of allergy to pork products or enzymes.

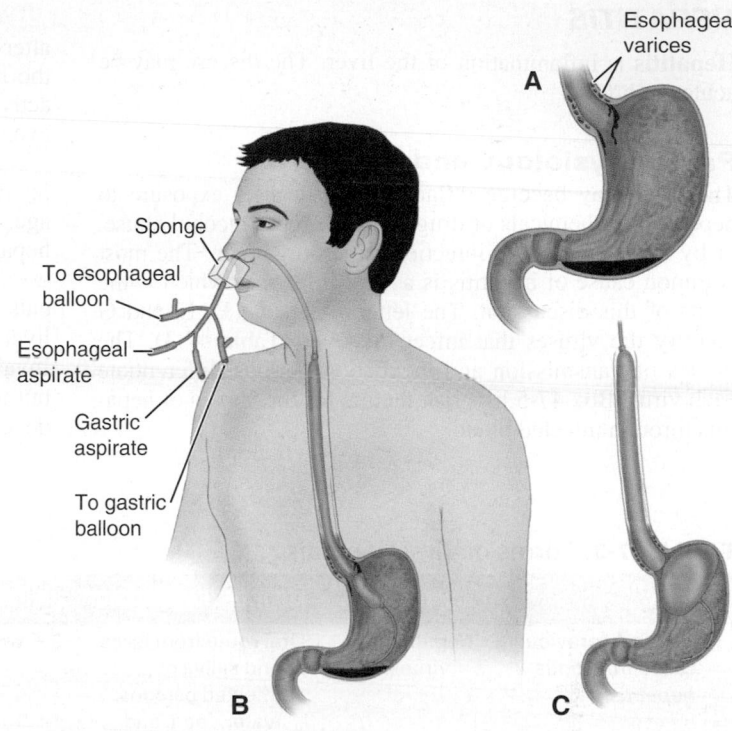

FIGURE 47-7. Balloon tamponade to treat esophageal varices. **(A)** Dilated, bleeding esophageal veins (varices). **(B)** A Sengstaken-Blakemore tube in place with uninflated balloons in the esophagus and stomach. The tube has four separate openings: two are used to inflate the two balloons, and two allow for aspiration of esophageal and gastric secretions. **(C)** Inflated balloons compress bleeding esophageal varices.

introduction of a needle through the abdominal wall, allowing the fluid to drain. This usually eases severe discomfort caused by distention and relieves breathing difficulty secondary to a high volume of abdominal fluid pressing on the diaphragm and lungs. Up to 6 to 8 L of fluid may be removed over 60 to 90 minutes. A total of 15 L may be removed over a longer period, depending on the need. IV albumin is simultaneously infused to pull fluid back into the vascular space. Monitoring of BP and urine output is crucial to evaluate the effects of the fluid shifts. Diuretic therapy is prescribed if the circulatory volume becomes excessive.

Additional treatment includes maintenance diuretic therapy and a sodium-restricted diet. The potassium-sparing diuretic spironolactone (Aldactone) may be chosen because it specifically antagonizes the hormone aldosterone. Reversing the effects of aldosterone causes the excretion of sodium and water, retention of potassium, and reduction of ascitic fluid.

If ascites repeatedly develops despite conservative treatment, the physician may surgically insert an internal catheter to redirect the ascitic fluid back into the vascular space. See the section on portal hypertension for more information.

Hepatic Encephalopathy

Hepatic encephalopathy is a central nervous system (CNS) manifestation of liver failure that often leads to coma and death. This neurologic complication is related to an increased serum ammonia level, but not singularly. Ammonia forms in the intestine by bacterial action on ingested proteins. The liver normally detoxifies ammonia by converting it to urea, which the kidneys then excrete in urine. A failing liver, as in advanced cirrhosis, can no longer break down ammonia, causing it to accumulate in the blood. Ammonia can cross the blood-brain barrier and enter brain cells, where it interferes with brain metabolism, cell membrane pump mechanisms, and neurotransmission.

Indications of CNS effects include disorientation, confusion, personality changes, memory loss, a flapping tremor called *asterixis,* a positive Babinski reflex, sulfurous breath odor (referred to as **fetor hepaticus**), and lethargy to deep coma. Symptoms usually worsen after the client eats a high-protein meal or has active GI bleeding, because both dietary protein and digested blood cells increase ammonia volume in the intestine. In addition to an elevated serum ammonia level, electroencephalography may show abnormal waveforms.

Treatment includes eliminating dietary protein, removing residual protein (such as blood if the client had a recent GI hemorrhage), and depleting intestinal microorganisms with drugs, laxatives, and enema therapy. Antibiotics, such as neomycin or kanamycin (Kantrex), which are poorly absorbed from the GI tract, are prescribed to destroy intestinal microorganisms and thereby decrease ammonia production. The administration of lactulose (Cephulac) reduces the serum ammonia concentration. In the colon, lactulose splits into lactic acid and acetic acid, attracts ammonia from the blood, and forms a compound that can be eliminated in the feces. Levodopa (L-dopa) is a precursor of dopamine that restores normal neurotransmission in the brain. Supportive measures include administering IV fluids containing electrolytes and multivitamins or total parenteral nutrition (TPN).

The prognosis for clients with hepatic encephalopathy is grim. Only a few survive without a liver transplant.

HEPATITIS

Hepatitis is inflammation of the liver. The disease may be acute or chronic.

Pathophysiology and Etiology

The liver may become inflamed shortly after exposure to hepatotoxic chemicals or drugs, after lengthy alcohol abuse, or by invasion with an infectious microorganism. The most common cause of hepatitis is a viral infection, which is the focus of this discussion. The letters A, B, C, D, E, and G identify the viruses that infect the liver (Table 47-3). The modes of transmission and incubation periods differentiate each virus. Box 47-5 lists risk factors for the spread of hepatitis through infected blood.

Once the virus invades the *hepatocytes* (liver cells), it alters their structure. An immune reaction ensues, in which the infected cells become inflamed and dysfunctional. The active disease process affects the uptake, conjugation, and excretion of bilirubin.

Most people recover from acute infection, but a few suffer from chronic active hepatitis and subsequent liver damage. In chronic persistent hepatitis (most common with hepatitis B, C, and D), liver damage does not worsen, but it does not improve, and the liver remains enlarged. Some clients may develop cirrhosis. Others deteriorate rapidly with liver failure and die unless liver transplantation is performed. Invasion of the transplanted liver by the virus is common, but it usually takes years before the newly transplanted liver develops cirrhosis.

TABLE 47-3 Forms of Viral Hepatitis

TYPE	CAUSE	MODE OF TRANSMISSION	INCUBATION	SIGNS AND SYMPTOMS	OUTCOME
Hepatitis A (previously called *infectious hepatitis*)	Hepatitis A virus (HAV)	Oral route from feces and saliva of infected persons; water, food, and equipment contaminated with HAV	3–5 weeks	May occur with or without symptoms; flulike illness Preicteric phase: headache, malaise, fatigue, anorexia, fever Icteric phase: dark urine, jaundice, tender liver	Usually mild with full recovery; fatality rate <1%; no carrier state or increased risk of chronic hepatitis, cirrhosis, or hepatic cancer
Hepatitis B (previously called *serum hepatitis*)	Hepatitis B virus (HBV)	Infected blood or plasma; needles, syringes, surgical or dental equipment contaminated with infected blood; also sexually transmitted through vaginal secretions and semen of carriers or those actively infected	2–5 months	Arthralgias, rash; may occur without symptoms	May be severe; fatality rate 1% to 10%; carrier state possible; increased risk of chronic hepatitis, cirrhosis, and hepatic cancer; some infected people become carriers
Hepatitis C (previously called *non-A, non-B hepatitis—NANB*)	Hepatitis C virus (HCV); may be more than one virus	Infected blood or blood products; sexual contact	2–20 weeks	Similar to HBV, although less severe and without jaundice	Frequent occurrence of chronic carrier state and chronic liver disease; increased risk of hepatic cancer
Hepatitis D (also called *delta hepatitis*)	Hepatitis D virus (HDV)	Same as HBV; cannot infect alone; occurs as dual infection with HBV	2–5 months	Similar to HBV	Similar to HBV with greater likelihood of carrier state, chronic active hepatitis, and cirrhosis
Hepatitis E	Hepatitis E virus (HEV)	Fecal–oral routes; low risk of person–person contact; found more in countries with poor sanitation and water quality	2–9 weeks	Similar to HAV—very severe in pregnant women	Similar to HAV—very severe in pregnant women
Hepatitis G	Hepatitis G virus (HGV, GB virus-C, or GBV-C)	Infected blood or blood products	14-145 days	Similar to HCV	Causes persistent infection; does not affect clinical course or cause chronic liver disease

---

BOX 47-5 **Risk Factors for Acquiring Blood-borne Hepatitis**

- History of illicit IV drug use
- Occupational exposure through sharps injuries (needlesticks)
- Perinatal exposure (child born to woman who has hepatitis)
- Blood transfusion
- Organ transplant
- Exposure to contaminated equipment that penetrates the skin (includes tattoos and body piercings)
- Sexual contact with infected person
- Hemodialysis
- Impaired immune response

Hepatitis A is usually transmitted via the oral–fecal route (eating or drinking something contaminated by the feces of an infected person). If food or drinking water is contaminated because of inadequate handwashing or poor sanitation, the virus can spread rapidly. Hepatitis A can also occur as a result of eating raw or undercooked shellfish from water contaminated by sewage. Occasionally, hepatitis A is transmitted via blood transfusions. Hepatitis A rarely leads to chronic illness, but clients may need to be hospitalized.

Gerontologic Considerations

- Although hepatitis A commonly is found in younger people, older adults may contract hepatitis through contact with younger people who have the disease, such as grandchildren, wait staff, or supermarket or nursing home employees.

Hepatitis B and C are transmitted through the blood or sexual contact. Hepatitis B and C commonly are associated with hepatocellular carcinoma. Therefore, routine monitoring (e.g., blood test for alpha fetoprotein and ultrasound) should be carried out for clients with chronic forms of these diseases.

Hepatitis G is considered to be non-A, non-B, and non-C disease. It occurs 14 to 145 days after a blood transfusion. It cannot be identified as can the other types, and thus it is designated type G. Hepatitis G is similar to hepatitis C.

Other types of hepatitis include:

- *Autoimmune hepatitis*—results from an abnormal immune system response. Treatment of this uncommon form consists of the administration of corticosteroids and immune-modulating agents (azathioprine or 6-mercaptopurine) (see Drug Therapy Table 46-1). Without treatment, many of these clients will die or require a liver transplant.
- *Toxic hepatitis*—develops when certain chemicals toxic to the liver (e.g., chloroform, phosphorus, carbon tetrachloride) cause liver necrosis. Treatment includes removing the toxin and treating symptoms. If liver damage is severe and

prolonged, the prognosis is not good without a liver transplant.
- *Drug-induced hepatitis*—occurs when a drug reaction damages the liver. This form of hepatitis can be severe and fatal. Examples of drugs that may cause a severe reaction are anesthetic agents, antidepressants, or anticonvulsants. High-dose corticosteroids are administered to treat the reaction. Liver transplantation may be necessary.

Pharmacologic Considerations

- Many drugs are potentially hepatotoxic. Liver impairment may occur in some persons with normal, short-term doses, prolonged use, or high doses of hepatotoxic drugs. Examples of drugs capable of causing hepatotoxicity are the penicillins, acetaminophen (Tylenol), methotrexate, and allopurinol (Zyloprim). Oral bile acids given to dissolve gallstones also can be hepatotoxic; frequent monitoring of liver function is necessary. In clients with liver disease, barbiturates, narcotics, and any drug metabolized or detoxified by the liver are contraindicated or used with caution.

Assessment Findings

Signs and Symptoms

The signs and symptoms of the various forms of hepatitis sometimes are indistinguishable. The phases of all forms of hepatitis are as follows:

1. *Incubation phase:* the virus replicates within the liver; the client is asymptomatic. Late in this phase the virus can be found in blood, bile, and stools (for hepatitis A). At this point, the client is considered infectious.
2. *Preicteric or prodromal phase:* nausea; vomiting; anorexia; fever; malaise; arthralgia; headache; right upper quadrant (RUQ) discomfort; enlargement of the spleen, liver, and lymph nodes; weight loss; rash; and urticaria.
3. *Icteric phase:* jaundice, pruritus, clay-colored or light stools, dark urine, fatigue, anorexia, and RUQ discomfort; symptoms of the preicteric phase may continue.
4. *Posticteric phase:* liver enlargement, malaise, and fatigue; other symptoms subside; liver function tests begin to return to normal.

Not all clients with hepatitis experience all the listed symptoms, and the severity of any one symptom may vary. Even though the symptoms are categorized, not all clients with hepatitis necessarily develop jaundice.

Gerontologic Considerations

- Although recurrent severe pain is the predominant symptom of chronic hepatitis in young to middle-aged adults, older adults report the pain with chronic hepatitis as being mild or absent.

Diagnostic Findings

Serologic analysis can detect specific viral antibodies. Ribonucleic acid (RNA) testing may be performed to identify the virus itself. Test results may take up to 1 week. The white blood cell count may be elevated. Evidence of **cholestasis** (ineffective bile drainage) is seen with elevated bilirubin levels. Hepatic aminotransferase (alanine aminotransferase [ALT] and aspartate aminotransferase [AST]) levels rise during the incubation period and begin to fall once symptoms appear. Chronic disease may result in persistent elevation of the transaminases. A prolonged PT or PTT reflects poor synthetic liver function. Additional indicators of poor synthetic function include low blood glucose and serum albumin levels. Liver biopsy and histologic examination of the specimen allow for evaluation of the severity of the disease by identifying inflammation, fibrosis, and cirrhosis.

Medical and Surgical Management

Treatment is symptomatic and includes bed rest, a balanced diet of small feedings at intervals, and IV fluid administration if the client is extremely ill or has a low oral fluid intake. Supplementation of vitamins, especially the fat-soluble vitamins, is necessary regardless of oral intake because these vitamins are poorly absorbed. In some cases, antiemetics are given to relieve vomiting, but usually drug therapy is avoided until the liver recovers.

Recombinant interferon alfa-2b (Intron A, Roferon-A) may be given to clients with chronic hepatitis B, C, and D to force the virus into remission. It frequently is administered in combination with ribavirin (Rebetol), a synthetic antiviral also used to treat respiratory syncytial virus infection. The combination therapy increases the likelihood of a sustained virus-free response (more than 6 months). Ribavirin may cause birth defects, so clients of childbearing age need to be counseled about using strict birth-control methods while taking this drug.

For clients with chronic disease who do not respond to medical treatment, a liver transplantation may be performed (see Box 47-4). This involves total removal of the diseased liver and transplantation of a healthy liver in the same location. Immunosuppression must be done for transplantation to succeed. Immunosuppressant agents include cyclosporine, tacrolimus, sirolimus, corticosteroids, and azathioprine. The goal is to find immunosuppressive agents that effectively reduce rejection of transplanted organs and cause the fewest side effects.

Nursing Management

The nurse practices preventive techniques to control the spread of hepatitis viruses and teaches the family and general public how to reduce the risk of infection (Box 47-6). Nursing care in the early stages focuses on maintaining physical rest, supporting nutritional intake (Nutrition Notes 47-2),

---

BOX 47-6 Measures For Preventing Viral Hepatitis Transmission

Preventing Hepatitis A[*]
- Receive hepatitis A virus (HAV) vaccine, especially when considered at high risk (healthcare workers, day-care workers, food preparers, foreign travel).
- Obtain immune globulin (IG) injection if exposed (in household or sexual contacts with infected individuals) to hepatitis without previous immunization.
- Observe Standard Precautions. Wear gloves if hands come into contact with body fluids; wear gown and face shield if body fluids may be splashed.
- Require child care staff to wear gloves during diaper changes and to perform adequate handwashing.
- Perform conscientious handwashing, even after removing gloves.
- Screen food handlers.
- Avoid eating from public salad bars and buffets that do not have sneeze guards or other hygienic devices and practices to prevent food contamination.
- Use liquid soap dispensers and hand dryers in public restrooms rather than bar soap and cloth towels.
- Avoid placing fingers and hand-held objects in mouth.
- Do not share cigarettes, eating utensils, or beverage containers.
- Avoid eating raw seafood or seafood harvested from possibly polluted water.
- Use a pocket mask when giving pulmonary resuscitation.

- Drink bottled water in developing countries. Avoid ice unless it was made from bottled water.

Preventing Hepatitis B[†]
- Receive hepatitis B virus (HBV) vaccine, especially if in a high-risk category (dialysis, blood dyscrasias, IV drug abuser, homosexual, healthcare worker, school teacher).[**]
- Adhere to American Academy of Pediatrics guidelines for immunization.
- Obtain hepatitis B immune globulin (HBIG) if exposed to HBV and not previously vaccinated within 24 hours but no later than 7 days after blood contact.
- Observe Standard Precautions (wear gloves if hands may come into contact with body fluids; wear gown and face shield if body fluids may be splashed).
- Do not recap needles.
- Dispose of needles and other sharp objects in a puncture-resistant container.
- Use a condom when engaging in sexual intercourse.
- Do not share razors, fingernail tools, toothbrushes, or any personal care item that may come into contact with blood or body fluids.
- If contemplating surgery, investigate the possibility of donating and storing your own blood for later use.
- Wear a mouth shield when giving mouth-to-mouth resuscitation.

[*]Prevention of hepatitis A also prevents hepatitis E; no vaccine or postexposure treatment is available for hepatitis E.
[†]Prevention of hepatitis B also prevents hepatitis C, D, and G; no vaccine or postexposure treatment is available for hepatitis C, D, or G.
[**]Hepatitis B vaccination is not routinely given to older adults. In general, older adults should receive the vaccine only if they are traveling to areas where they may be exposed to the disease. Immunogenicity is somewhat reduced in older adults.

Nutrition Notes 47-2
The Client With Hepatitis

● Nutrition therapy for clients with hepatitis is based on symptoms and tolerance. Some clients may not require any nutrition intervention; others may need a high-calorie, high-protein diet to replenish losses and small frequent meals to maximize intake.

● A high-protein diet of 1.5 to 2.0 g/kg is used to promote liver cell regeneration in clients with hepatitis.

---

and preventing complications. Before discharge, the nurse teaches self-care measures to promote health and avoid transmitting the infection to others. The client must avoid alcohol and drugs that can further damage the liver. For clients who develop chronic active or persistent hepatitis and require liver transplants, see Nursing Process for the Client Having Surgery for a Liver Disorder.

▶ *Stop, Think, and Respond Exercise 47-1*

You are assigned to a client who is recovering from abdominal surgery. She tells you that the client in the next room has chronic hepatitis and that she is afraid she will catch it. Which answer would best help this client?

- *"Don't worry. That kind of hepatitis can only be transmitted sexually."*
- *"There are many kinds of hepatitis—do you know which kind she has?"*
- *"Hospital staff always use precautions to prevent any possibility of transmission of infectious diseases to other clients."*
- *"There is no problem—that client is not a carrier of the disease."*

TUMORS OF THE LIVER

A tumor of the liver is an abnormal mass of cells in the liver. Liver tumors may be benign or malignant (see Chap. 18). If malignant, the tumor may be a primary lesion (classified as a *hepatoma*) or a metastasis.

Pathophysiology and Etiology

Primary malignancies (hepatomas) are rare but appear to have an increased incidence in people with previous hepatitis B or D virus infections or cirrhosis, especially those with the postnecrotic form. The most common liver malignancy is a metastatic lesion from the breast, lung, or GI tract. Causes of benign liver tumors are tuberculosis and fungal and parasitic infections. Oral contraceptives and anabolic steroids also have been implicated in the development of benign hepatic lesions.

Tumor cells grow at an accelerated rate. They function in a disorganized manner and eventually impair the liver's physiologic activities. They may obstruct bile flow,

leading to jaundice, liver failure, portal hypertension, and ascites.

Assessment Findings

Symptoms can be vague and confused with those of cirrhosis. Jaundice is common. Once the tumor is sufficiently large, the client may report pain in the RUQ. Weight loss and debilitation are common. The client usually experiences bleeding tendencies. Eventually, the abdomen becomes distended from liver enlargement and related ascites.

Alpha fetoprotein, a serum protein normally produced during fetal development, is a marker that, if elevated, can indicate a primary malignant liver tumor. Total bilirubin and serum enzyme (ALT, AST, alkaline phosphatase) levels are elevated. A liver scan, ultrasonography, MRI, or CT scan identifies the tumor and its location. A biopsy, performed to identify the specific type of tumor cells, also can define and disclose damage to adjacent liver tissue.

Medical and Surgical Management

If the tumor is confined to a single lobe of the liver, a **hepatic lobectomy** may be attempted to remove primary malignant or benign tumors. Metastatic tumors usually are considered inoperable because they often are scattered throughout the liver. The frequency of metastasis and poor survival rate usually eliminate liver transplantation as a therapeutic option. Sometimes biliary ducts obstructed by disease are bypassed with percutaneous biliary or trans-hepatic drainage. A catheter is inserted under fluoroscopy through the abdominal wall, past the obstruction, into the duodenum. This procedure relieves the pressure and pain caused by bile buildup and decreases jaundice and pruritus. In some cases *cryosurgery* or *cryoablation* is used. This technique uses liquid nitrogen at –196°C to destroy tumors. Two or three freeze-and-thaw cycles are administered through probes inserted with open laparotomy. The effectiveness of this procedure is still being evaluated (Smeltzer et al., 2008).

For malignant tumors, short-term improvement may be achieved using IV chemotherapy or infusions directly into the hepatic artery or in the peritoneum. Doxorubicin hydrochloride (Adriamycin) and 5-fluorouracil (5-FU) are common choices for drug therapy. Unfortunately, results from chemotherapy tend to be transient. Radiation therapy may be administered to reduce pain and discomfort.

Nursing Management

In the terminal stages of the disease, the nurse keeps the client as comfortable as possible by administering analgesics, supporting ventilation compromised by ascites, and reducing discomfort from pruritus. When the liver fails and coma develops, the nurse institutes safety measures and continues performing total care. While the client is alert, the nurse provides support for the client and family as both begin grieving their potential losses. As appropriate, he or she makes referrals for hospice care. Additional nursing management depends on symptoms and treatment. Client and Family Teaching 47-2 provides information regarding tumors of the liver.

Client and Family Teaching 47-2
Tumors of the Liver

The nurse emphasizes the following points when teaching the client and family:

- Follow diet recommended by physician.
- Plan rest periods during the day.
- Avoid heavy lifting.
- Take medications exactly as prescribed. Follow directions on the label, particularly with regard to taking the drug before, after, or with food or meals.
- Record weight weekly or as recommended by the physician. Report any significant weight gain or loss to the physician.
- Contact physician about significant increase in abdominal size, fever, nausea, vomiting, vomiting of blood (bright red, coffee grounds), tarry stools, difficulty with concentration or changes in level of consciousness, jaundice, or swelling of the ankles.
- Make and keep appointments for periodic follow-up office visits.

Nursing Process for the Client Having Surgery for a Liver Disorder

Assessment

Determine whether the client will be undergoing a lobectomy or a liver transplantation (see Chap. 14 for perioperative nursing management). Postoperative assessments include checking vital signs and the function of drains and tubes. Observe carefully for potential complications (hemorrhage, shock, infection, rejection in cases of transplant, electrolyte imbalances, and hepatic coma). In addition, observe the client with cirrhosis for signs of alcohol withdrawal. Standard postsurgical assessments include evaluating breathing pattern, airway patency, and pain.

Diagnosis, Planning, and Interventions

▶ **Risk for Deficient Fluid Volume** related to hemorrhage from surgical site and fluid loss from drainage, tubes, or both

▶ **Expected Outcome:** Client will maintain fluid balance as evidenced by adequate urine output and normal BP and pulse.

- Monitor intake and output at least every 8 hours. *Urine output less than 30 mL is inadequate for renal function and indicates hypovolemia.*
- Monitor vital signs at least every 4 hours; do so more frequently if client is hypovolemic. *Hypovolemia causes hypotension and decreased oxygenation.*
- Monitor IV infusion replacement solutions and rates. *Fluids replace intravascular volume and promote kidney function.*
- Monitor serum and urine osmolality, serum sodium, blood urea nitrogen (BUN), creatinine, and hematocrit levels. *Decreased intravascular volume will elevate these fluid volume levels.*

▶ Hyperthermia related to infection, rejection, or both

▶ **Expected Outcome:** Body temperature will be below 101°F.

- Monitor temperature frequently. Report elevation above 101°F immediately. *This finding may indicate wound infection and require cultures. It also can indicate a need to change immunosuppressant drugs if rejection is suspected after liver transplantation.*
- If client is diaphoretic, assist with bathing and changing into dry clothes. *These measures increase comfort and minimize shivering caused by water evaporation from the skin.*
- If client is shivering, cover with light blanket. If client is not shivering, cover with a sheet only. *Shivering increases body temperature. A light blanket will prevent shivering. A sheet should be sufficient to keep a client who is not shivering covered but not too warm.*
- Administer antipyretics as ordered. *They help reduce fever, which enhances the immune response.*
- Notify physician if client's mental status changes. *This finding can indicate septic shock.*
- Place client on hypothermia blanket as ordered. *Cooling blankets are used if temperature rises to 105°F to control fever.*

▶ **Imbalanced Nutrition: Less than Body Requirements** related to anorexia, impaired use of proteins and carbohydrates, and nausea, vomiting, and sluggish peristalsis

▶ **Expected Outcome:** Weight will remain stable, and the client will tolerate oral feedings.

- Initially administer nutrition by IV access. *Client will not tolerate oral liquids until bowel sounds resume and he or she passes flatus or stool.*
- After removal of the nasogastric tube, give small sips of clear liquids. *Small sips prevent nausea and vomiting.*
- Progress diet to full liquids and then soft foods. *Advancing the diet as tolerated prevents nausea, vomiting, or gastric discomfort.*

Evaluation of Expected Outcomes

Fluid balance is adequate as evidenced by moist mucous membranes, good skin turgor, intake of 2400 mL and output of 2300 mL, BP of 136/88 mm Hg, and pulse rate of 84 beats/minute. Body temperature remains below 101°F. The client tolerates food, nourishment meets metabolic needs, and the client's weight stabilizes. ●

DISORDERS OF THE GALLBLADDER

Several disorders affect the *biliary system*, which refers to the *gallbladder* and *bile ducts*, which carry bile (Fig. 47-8). These disorders impair the drainage of bile into the duodenum. Box 47-7 defines terms related to the biliary system.

CHOLELITHIASIS AND CHOLECYSTITIS

Cholelithiasis denotes stones that form in the gallbladder. Gallstone formation represents the most common abnormality of the biliary system. If the stones are located in the

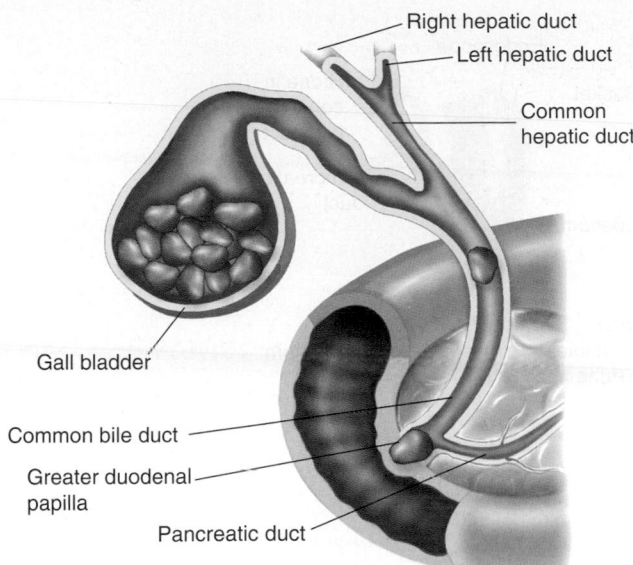

FIGURE 47-8. Gallstones may form in many locations within the biliary tree.

common bile duct, the condition is referred to as **choledo-cholithiasis**. The formation of stones often leads to **chole-cystitis**, an inflammation or infection of the gallbladder. Cholecystitis may be chronic or acute.

Pathophysiology and Etiology

Cholelithiasis and cholecystitis are intimately related and almost always coexist. Their incidence increases progressively with age. Gallstones are more frequent in women than in men, particularly women who are middle-aged or have a history of multiple pregnancies, diabetes, and obesity or frequent weight changes. The cause of cholelithiasis remains unestablished, but bile stasis, dietary factors, and infection are suspected. The formation of pigmented stones is associated with hemolytic anemia, which increases free

---

BOX 47-7 Terms Related to the Biliary System

Cholecystitis: inflammation of the gallbladder
Cholelithiasis: the presence of calculi in the gallbladder
Cholecystectomy: removal of the gallbladder
Cholecystostomy: opening and drainage of the gallbladder
Choledochotomy: opening into the common duct
Choledocholithiasis: stones in the common duct
Choledocholithotomy: incision of common bile duct for removal of stones
Choledochoduodenostomy: anastomosis of common duct to duodenum
Choledochojejunostomy: anastomosis of common duct to jejunum
Lithotripsy: disintegration of gallstones by shock waves
Laparoscopic cholecystectomy: removal of gallbladder through endoscopic procedure
Laser cholecystectomy: removal of gallbladder using laser rather than scalpel and traditional surgical instruments

---

bilirubin (see Chap. 31). Cholesterol-type stones are linked to a high-fat diet or predisposition to hypercholesterolemia.

Symptoms tend to develop when one or more gallstones partially or totally impair the passage of bile, causing the gallbladder to become inflamed, swollen, and distended with bile. Each time the person eats fatty foods, *cholecystokinin*, a hormone secreted by the small intestine, stimulates the gallbladder to send bile for its digestion. The gallbladder responds by contracting forcefully. Discomfort results from a combination of the inflammation and contractile spasms. Digestion problems result from the reduced or absent bile. If the swelling and distended volume remain unrelieved, the gallbladder can become necrotic or rupture, leading to peritonitis.

Assessment Findings

Signs and Symptoms

Initially, clients experience belching, nausea, and RUQ discomfort, with pain or cramps after high-fat meals. Symptoms become acute when a stone blocks bile flow from the gallbladder. With acute cholecystitis, clients usually are very sick with fever, vomiting, tenderness over the liver, and severe pain called **biliary colic**. The pain may radiate to the back and shoulders. The gallbladder may be so swollen that it becomes palpable. Slight jaundice may be noted. The urine appears dark brown; the stools may be light-colored.

Diagnostic Findings

Various tests are performed to rule out other disorders with similar symptoms. Eventually, the stones and structural changes in the gallbladder are imaged by means of *cholecystography* (gallbladder imaging), ultrasonography, CT scan, or radionuclide imaging. Percutaneous transhepatic cholangiography distinguishes jaundice caused by liver disease from jaundice caused by gallbladder disease. Endoscopic retrograde cholangiopancreatography (ERCP) locates stones that have collected in the common bile duct. Magnetic resonance cholangiopancreatography is a noninvasive technique that uses MRI to detect gallstones and gallbladder disorders.

Clients with jaundice have elevated bilirubin levels. Leukocytosis findings correlate with inflammation. In addition, serum liver enzymes may be elevated. The PT may be prolonged as a result of interference with absorption of vitamin K.

Medical and Surgical Management

When the gallbladder is acutely inflamed, the client takes nothing by mouth. Instead, a nasogastric tube is inserted, and antibiotics and parenteral fluids are prescribed until the inflammation subsides. Treatment of mild or chronic cholecystitis involves a low-fat diet. To relieve pain and discomfort, analgesics, anticholinergics, and even nitroglycerin are prescribed. Fat-soluble vitamins may be ordered to compensate for their reduced absorption. A bile-binding resin, such as cholestyramine (Questran), is prescribed to relieve pruritus.

Clients who are a surgical risk and whose gallstones appear radiolucent on diagnostic studies receive oral bile acids, either chenodeoxycholic acid (CDCA, chenodiol, Chenix) or ursodeoxycholic acid (UDCA, ursodiol, Actigall), in an attempt to dissolve the gallstones. These drugs, which may take at least 6 to 12 months to be effective, are

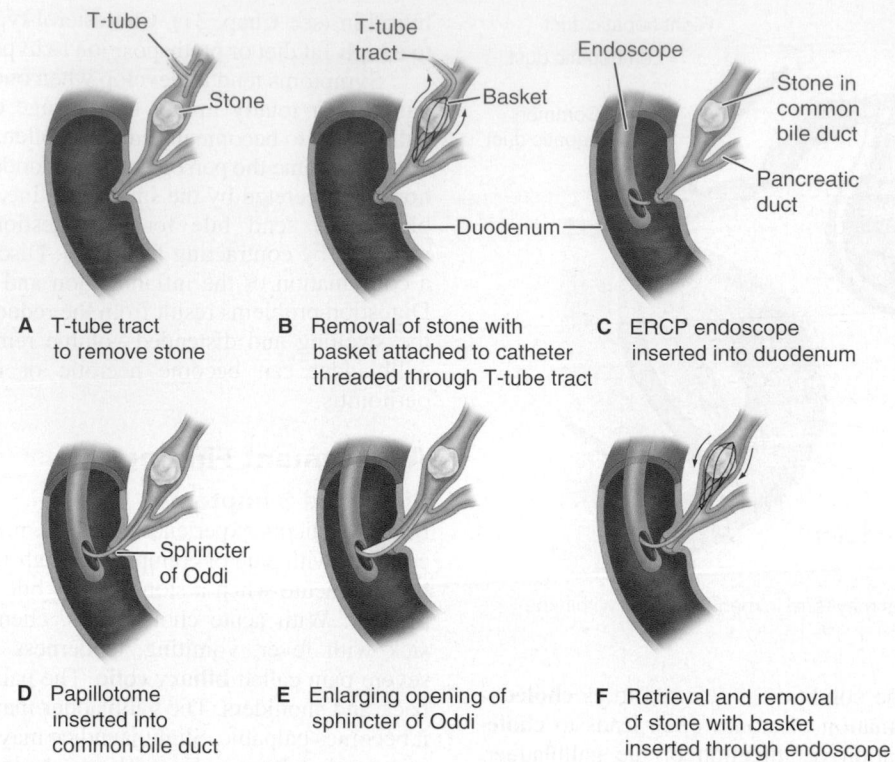

A T-tube tract to remove stone

B Removal of stone with basket attached to catheter threaded through T-tube tract

C ERCP endoscope inserted into duodenum

D Papillotome inserted into common bile duct

E Enlarging opening of sphincter of Oddi

F Retrieval and removal of stone with basket inserted through endoscope

FIGURE 47-9. Nonsurgical techniques for removing gallstones.

only moderately successful. The success rate is greatest when the stones are small, but the rate of recurrence within 5 years is high.

 Pharmacologic Considerations

- When chenodiol (Chenix) is prescribed to dissolve gallstones, therapy may last for 2 years or more.

Dissolving the stones by direct contact may be attempted by instilling a solvent, methyl-tert-butyl ether, into the gallbladder or common bile duct through a percutaneously placed catheter. If successful, the stones clear in hours or a few days. The rate of recurrence is unknown at this time.

Lithotripsy, a nonsurgical procedure using shock waves generated by a machine called a *lithotriptor*, may be tried to break up some types of gallstones. The shock waves are directed at the gallbladder while the anesthetized client lies in a specially designed water tank. After the shock waves fragment the gallstones, endoscopy or direct contact dissolution removes the fragments.

Stones in the common bile duct can be removed by performing a *sphincterotomy* (opening of the sphincter of Oddi where the common bile duct joins the duodenum) using an endoscope. The stone is snared or retrieved using a basket-like attachment on the endoscope. Other nonsurgical techniques for removing gallstones are depicted in Figure 47-9.

Laparoscopic cholecystectomy is the preferred surgical procedure for gallbladder removal. It is the treatment of choice for about 80% of clients with gallbladder disease.

The procedure requires general anesthesia, but the surgery is performed with an endoscope inserted in one of three or four small puncture sites in the abdomen (Fig. 47-10). After inflating the abdomen with carbon dioxide to displace abdominal structures and provide a better view, the surgeon drains the gallbladder, dissects the vessels and ducts, and then grasps and removes the gallbladder. Next, the surgeon

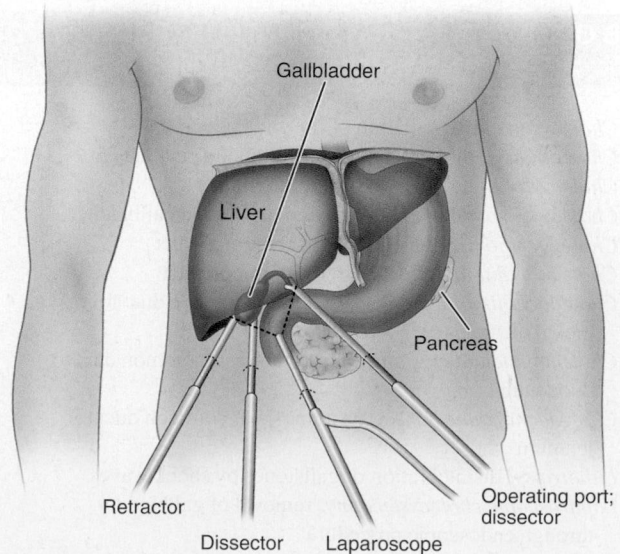

FIGURE 47-10. In laparoscopic cholecystectomy, the abdominal organs are viewed on a television monitor while the gallbladder is removed.

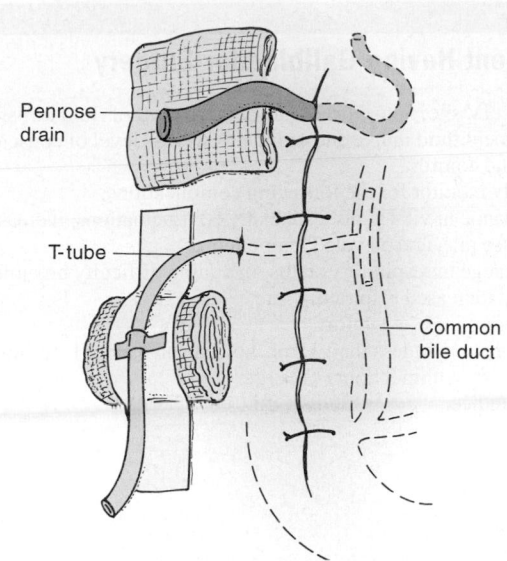

FIGURE 47-11. After an open cholecystectomy, a wound drain removes exudates from the area formerly occupied by the gallbladder and a T-tube diverts bile, which the liver is still forming.

staples the puncture sites closed and covers the incisions with a light dressing.

Most clients return home in the evening or the morning after the procedure. Although a nasogastric tube may have been inserted during surgery, it is removed before the client is awake and alert. Mild analgesics are administered to relieve minor discomfort. The client may eat food once the effects of the anesthetic subside. A prolonged recovery period usually is unnecessary. Most clients resume normal activities within 1 week.

For some clients, laparoscopic removal is inappropriate. When the gallbladder is extremely distended and fragile from inflammation and infection or contains unusually large or multiple stones, its removal through a small abdominal opening may be impossible or dangerous. In these cases, the surgeon performs an **open cholecystectomy**. This procedure involves a laparotomy (abdominal incision). A *Penrose drain,* a wide, flat rubber tube, or a *vacuum drain,* a plastic tube connected to a bulb or other collecting device, is inserted in the wound to remove serosanguineous fluid. After surgery, clients experience a lengthy period of gastric decompression and acute postoperative pain. Hospitalization lasts about 1 week, and a 6-week recovery period follows discharge.

During cholecystectomy, a *choledochotomy,* surgical opening and exploration of the common bile duct, may be performed. A **T-tube** (a tube used to drain bile) usually is inserted while the surgical wound heals (Fig. 47-11). The T-tube is brought through the abdomen near the incision and connected to gravity drainage. Bile salts such as dehydrocholic acid (Decholin) may be prescribed to promote drainage.

Nursing Management

During an attack of biliary colic, the nurse ensures that the client rests, monitors the client's tolerance to eating and adminis-

ters prescribed antispasmodics or analgesics. Nutrition Notes 47-3 outlines other dietary considerations. If gastric decompression is required, the nurse inserts a nasogastric tube and connects it to suction (see Chap. 45). If lithotripsy or another procedure is initiated to remove the stones, close observation of the client after the procedure for increased pain, shock, or signs of internal bleeding is important.

Same-Day Surgery

When outpatient or laparoscopic surgery is scheduled, the nurse instructs the client about presurgical procedures, laboratory testing, and the consent form. On the day of surgery, the nurse completes preoperative skin preparation, inserts an IV line, and administers sedation. After the client recovers from anesthesia and before discharge, the nurse provides intensive instruction to the client and the accompanying caregiver regarding self-care. Giving written instructions for reference is useful. In accordance with agency policy, the nurse performs follow-up measures, such as telephoning the client the day after surgery to inquire about recovery progress.

Cholecystectomy

The nurse asks the client to describe symptoms experienced before admission such as the type and location of pain or discomfort. He or she asks whether any foods cause pain or discomfort and discusses other problems, such as nausea, vomiting, or abdominal cramping. The nurse inspects the skin and sclera for jaundice and palpates the abdomen for tenderness. Routine presurgical and postsurgical assessments are necessary when the client returns from surgery (Nursing Care Plan 47-2). If a T-tube is in place after an open cholecystectomy, the nurse monitors and records the drainage and maintains tube patency by keeping the collector below the level of the incision. This prevents bile from flowing back into the duct. A physician's order is necessary to clamp a T-tube. As healing occurs, the physician may direct that the T-tube be clamped temporarily before a meal and reopened later after eating.

The nurse measures bile drainage every 8 hours or according to agency policy. If more than 500 mL of bile drains within 24 hours or if drainage is significantly reduced, the nurse notifies the physician. Preventing tension on the tubing is important because it may become dislodged internally. A return of normal color to stool and urine indicates that bile is being deposited normally in the GI tract. Client and Family Teaching 47-3 provides more information related to teaching a postoperative cholecystectomy client about his or her care.

Nutrition Notes 47-3
The Client With Gallbladder Disease

- A low-fat diet is commonly recommended prior to gallbladder surgery, even though its efficacy has not been established.
- After gallbladder surgery, there is no need for a fat-restricted diet. A regular diet is resumed.

NURSING CARE PLAN 47-2 | The Client Having Gallbladder Surgery

Postoperative Assessment

See Chapter 14 for perioperative management. When the client returns from surgery:

- Assess vital signs.
- Review chart for type of surgery and client's progress during surgery and in the postanesthesia recovery unit.
- Inspect surgical dressing for drainage and tubes or catheters for placement, patency, and type of drainage.
- Carefully observe nasogastric tube for type and amount of drainage. If there is a T-tube, monitor drainage for amount. If there is a Penrose drain, observe and change dressing as needed.
- Inspect IV site; note current rate and progress of fluid infusion.
- Document fluid intake and output, as well as level of consciousness and comfort.
- Closely monitor for the following complications:
  - Change in vital signs, especially BP fluctuations, increased pulse rate, and elevated temperature.
  - Change in respiratory status, including difficulty breathing and increased respiratory rate.
  - Abdominal discomfort.
  - Urine output less than 35mL/hour if catheterized, or failure to void within 8 hours of surgery.
  - Jaundice.

Nursing Diagnosis: Acute Pain related to surgical incision.

Expected Outcome: Client will report that analgesics relieve pain.

Interventions	Rationales
Administer analgesics as ordered.	Timely administration provides maximum and effective pain control.
Teach client to splint incision when moving or coughing.	Splinting reduces pain and discomfort.
Maintain patency of nasogastric and T-tubes if present.	Doing so maintain drainage flow, preventing pressure of accumulated fluids and reducing pain.

Evaluation of Expected Outcome

Client reports decreased abdominal pain and demonstrates good splinting technique when moving or coughing.

Nursing Diagnosis: Risk for Ineffective Breathing Pattern related to proximity of incision (if an open cholecystectomy) to lungs, inhibiting deep breathing.

Expected Outcome: Client will report comfort with breathing and exhibit unlabored breathing and effective respirations.

Interventions	Rationales
Place client in upright or semi-Fowler's position.	These positions facilitate lung expansion.
Encourage client to deep breathe, cough, and splint incision at least every 2 hours.	These measures provide for lung expansion and mobilize secretions.
If client has shallow breaths, instruct him or her to use incentive spirometer.	It promotes deeper breathing and more lung expansion.
Ambulate client as soon as possible four times a day, increasing distance each time. Encourage client to sit at least twice a day.	Ambulation and sitting prevent pulmonary complications and promote lung expansion.
Auscultate lung sounds at least every 8 hours.	Auscultation detects retained secretions and atelectasis early, helping prevent respiratory complications.

Evaluation of Expected Outcome

Client demonstrates adequate lung function, as evidenced by ability to take deep breaths and cough and no signs of respiratory complications.

Nursing Diagnosis: Impaired Skin Integrity related to altered biliary drainage after surgery and insertion of T-tube, Penrose drain, or both.

Expected Outcome: Incision and skin around T-tube and drain will remain intact and not be irritated.

Interventions	Rationales
Inspect all drainage tubes to ensure they are connected to drainage bags, appropriately covered with sterile dressings, and fastened to client's clothing to prevent dislodgment or kinking.	Doing so prevents bile from leaking onto skin.
Keep drainage collector for T-tube below incision and maintain connection to gravity drainage.	These measures promote drainage of bile through T-tube.

NURSING CARE PLAN 47-2 **The Client Having Gallbladder Surgery** (Continued)

Interventions	Rationales
Change dressings frequently as needed. Apply protectants such as zinc oxide or petrolatum to skin around drainage tubes.	These measures prevent skin irritation.
Observe sclerae for jaundice. Report abdominal pain, nausea, vomiting, bile drainage around T-tube, or clay-colored stools.	These findings may indicate obstruction of bile drainage.

Evaluation of Expected Outcome

Skin around drainage tubes remains intact and free of irritation.

Nursing Diagnosis: Imbalanced Nutrition: Less than Body Requirements related to high metabolic needs and decreased ability to digest fatty foods.

Expected Outcome: Client will maintain weight and optimal nutritional status.

Interventions	Rationales
Offer a diet low in fats and high in carbohydrates and proteins. Instruct client that fats are restricted for 4 to 6 weeks after surgery.	Initially bile is drained and unavailable for fat digestion. As the biliary ducts dilate to accommodate the bile volume once held by the gallbladder, sufficient bile will be released into the GI tract to emulsify fats and allow for digestion.
Administer vitamins A,D,E, and K as indicated.	These fat-soluble vitamins are needed for adequate nutritional intake.
Consult with dietitian if client is having difficulty meeting nutritional needs.	Doing so provides client with a resource for nutritional information and alternatives to dietary restrictions.
Instruct client to weigh himself or herself weekly.	This provides a record of weight maintenance, loss, or gain.
Encourage client to increase activity.	Increased activity promotes appetite.
Instruct client to maintain a record of nutritional intake and any problems with GI symptoms during or after meals.	This method helps client to track and avoid foods that causes GI symptoms.

Evaluation of Expected Outcome

Client reports that weight remains stable and that he or she is tolerating the diet very well.

Nursing Diagnosis: Risk for Ineffective Therapeutic Regimen Management related to insufficient knowledge for self-care.

Expected Outcome: Client will demonstrate knowledge of discharge instructions as evidenced by adequate wound care and repetition of dietary and medication instructions.

Interventions	Rationales
Reinforce diet instructions as above, with rationales as to why client must restrict fat.	Knowledge improves understanding of and compliance with dietary restrictions.
Provide verbal and written information that the client can understand about any prescriptions.	Clients learn in various ways. Presenting understandable information promotes learning.
Demonstrate and have client or family member return demonstration of wound care, dressing changes, and care of T-tube and drainage collector.	Return demonstrations allow the nurse to determine the client or family member's ability and knowledge, reinforce instructions, and correct misconceptions.
Instruct client or family member to notify the physician if the wound appears red or swollen or has purulent drainage, or if T-tube output increases.	Such findings indicate infection or obstruction below the T-tube, which needs intervention.
Explain that initially stools may be loose and frequent.	Bile will initially trickle continuously into the digestive system because the gallbladder no longer stores bile.
Instruct client to notify physician of clay-colored stools, dark brown urine, or jaundice.	These findings indicate obstruction and require early intervention.
Recommend that the client avoid lifting anything over 5 lb for at least 1 month.	This will prevent incisional hernia formation.

Evaluation of Expected Outcome

Clients manages self-care at home as evidenced by proper wound healing, compliance with dietary and medication regimen, and no complications.

**Client and Family Teaching 47-3
Postoperative Teaching Following a
Cholecystectomy**

The nurse emphasizes the following points when teaching
the client and family:

● Meet with a dietitian to review foods that should be
avoided.
● Read labels on food products to determine their fat
content.
● If applicable, explain the purpose of drug therapy, the
schedule to follow for administration, and the potential
side effects.
● Continue taking medication as long as prescribed, even if
symptoms disappear.
● Understand that frequent monitoring of the effect of drug
therapy may be necessary.
● Notify the physician immediately of severe pain, jaundice,
fever, or if the color of the stools or urine changes.

Gerontologic Considerations

- The incidence of gallstones is common in older adults. Older
adults may recover more slowly from surgery of the
gallbladder. They also are more prone to develop
postoperative complications, such as pneumonia and
thrombophlebitis, due to decreased movement in bed,
inadequate performance of deep-breathing exercises, and
lack of ambulation shortly after surgery.

DISORDERS OF THE PANCREAS

The pancreas is in the upper abdomen. Disorders of the pancreas can affect both exocrine and endocrine functions.

ACUTE PANCREATITIS

Pancreatitis, inflammation of the pancreas, may be acute or
chronic with a long history of relapse and recurrences. Acute
pancreatitis ranges from mild to severe and can be fatal.
Characteristics of the mild form are inflammation and edema
of the pancreas. Although the client is very ill, pancreatic
function usually returns to normal within 6 months. In the
severe form, more generalized and complete enzymatic digestion of the pancreas occurs. The tissue becomes necrotic, and
the client develops many local and systemic complications.

Pathophysiology and Etiology

Primarily, the pancreas becomes inflamed when the organ's
own enzymes—especially trypsin—cause the pancreas to
digest itself (*autodigestion*). Autodigestion develops when
there is reflux of bile and duodenal contents into the pancreatic duct, which activates the exocrine enzymes that the pancreas produces. Swelling of the opening to the pancreatic

duct impairs or even obstructs the release of bicarbonate,
which neutralizes chyme as it enters the small intestine. It
also obstructs the release of the enzymes trypsin, which
digests proteins; amylase, which digests carbohydrates; and
lipase, which digests fats. As the enzymes accumulate in the
gland, they begin to digest the pancreatic tissue itself. Eventually, destruction of the pancreas leads to impairment of endocrine functions.

The causes of acute pancreatitis vary widely. Known
causes include structural abnormalities, abdominal trauma,
infections, metabolic disorders (e.g., hyperlipidemia, hypercalcemia), vascular abnormalities, inflammatory bowel disease, hereditary factors, ingestion of alcohol or certain other
drugs, or refeeding after prolonged fasting or anorexia. Sometimes, however, acute pancreatitis develops without any of
these predisposing factors or other identifiable causes.

Complications from severe acute pancreatitis are serious
and sometimes fatal. Hyperglycemia results from an imbalance of glucagon, insulin, and somatostatin. Necrosis and
hemorrhage of the gland, peritonitis, severe fluid and electrolyte imbalance, shock, pleural effusion, acute respiratory distress syndrome, and blood coagulation problems ensue.
When lipase digests the fatty tissue around the pancreas, calcium binds with the released fatty acids. In rare cases, this
reduces the level of circulating calcium to a dangerous
degree, resulting in tetany and convulsions. Pancreatic cysts
and abscesses also can develop.

Assessment Findings

Signs and Symptoms

The most common complaint of clients with pancreatitis is
severe mid- to upper-abdominal pain, radiating to both sides
and straight to the back. Nausea, vomiting, and flatulence
usually are present. The client may describe the stools as
being frothy and foul-smelling, a sign of **steatorrhea**,
increased fat in the stool, from poor fat digestion. The symptoms, which worsen after the client eats fatty foods or drinks
alcohol, are relieved when the client sits up and leans forward or curls into a fetal position.

Physical examination may reveal jaundice. Bowel
sounds are diminished or absent with accompanying distention, and the abdomen is tender to palpation. The client may
be hypotensive, indicating hypovolemia and shock caused
by the release of large amounts of protein-rich fluid into the
tissues and peritoneal cavity. The client may be feverish and
tachycardic. Breathing is shallow from severe pain. Severe
pancreatitis may result in bruising around the umbilicus or
on the flanks.

Diagnostic Findings

Elevated serum and urine amylase, lipase, and liver enzyme
levels accompany significant pancreatitis. If the common
bile duct is obstructed, the bilirubin level is above normal.
Blood glucose levels and white blood cell counts can be elevated. Serum electrolyte levels (calcium, potassium, and
magnesium) are low. Pancreatic edema and necrosis appear
on CT scan with vascular enhancement. Various endoscopic
examinations and ultrasound may be performed to assist the
differential diagnosis and to determine the presence of pancreatic cysts, abscesses, and pseudocysts (fibrous capsules
filled with fluid, blood, enzymes, pus, and tissue debris).

Medical and Surgical Management

Medical treatment concentrates on relieving pain, reducing pancreatic secretions, restoring fluid and electrolyte losses, and preventing or treating systemic complications such as respiratory distress syndrome, acute (renal) tubular necrosis, and bleeding abnormalities. The client usually receives nothing by mouth, and a nasogastric tube may be inserted and connected to suction if the client is experiencing problems with nausea and vomiting. This relieves nausea, distention, and vomiting and reduces stimulation of the pancreas by gastric contents that otherwise may enter the duodenum. Along with general fluid therapy for hydration purposes, IV albumin may be given to pull fluid trapped in the peritoneum back into the circulation. Parenteral nutrition may be administered if the client is weak and debilitated to reduce the metabolic stress associated with acute pancreatitis (Smeltzer et al., 2008). Diuretics are given if circulating fluid is excessive.

Atropine or other anticholinergics are given to reduce the activity of the vagus nerve, which stimulates the pancreas. Histamine$_2$-receptor (H$_2$) antagonists such as famotidine (Pepcid) or proton pump inhibitors such as omeprazole (Prilosec) may be administered to suppress gastric acid and decrease pancreatic activity. IV antibiotic therapy is prescribed to prevent localized abscesses or to treat systemic sepsis. If pseudocysts develop, they may be located by CT scan and drained by percutaneous needle aspiration. Improvement, if it is forthcoming, usually occurs in about 1 week. A clear liquid diet is prescribed initially, with a slow progression to a low-fat diet. Alcohol, caffeine, and pepper, which are digestive stimulants, are withheld. If pancreatic exocrine function is impaired, pancreatic enzyme replacement therapy is administered with meals to promote digestion.

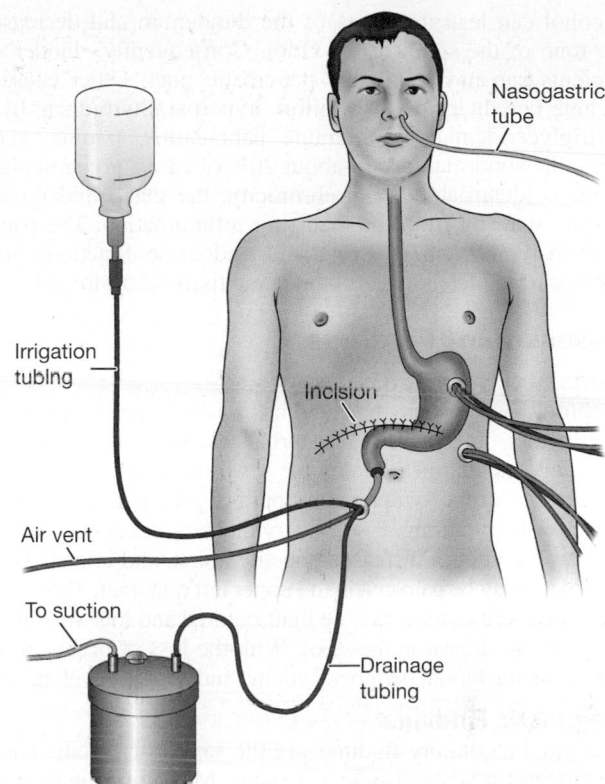

FIGURE 47-12. Multiple sump tubes are used after pancreatic surgery. Triple-lumen tubes consist of ports that provide tubing for irrigation, air venting, and drainage.

Pharmacologic Considerations

- If motility and absorption are not impaired, malnourished clients may be given nasojejunal feedings of an elemental formula during an acute attack of pancreatitis; their extremely low fat content causes only minimal pancreatic stimulation. TPN is used cautiously; some clients with pancreatitis cannot tolerate a high-glucose concentration even with insulin coverage. IV lipids are used sparingly when pancreatitis is related to hyperlipidemia.

In severe cases, surgical management involves opening the abdomen to debride necrotic tissue. Every 2 to 3 days, the process is repeated to prevent the spread of infection. Multiple sump drains, inserted into the cavity to remove debris, are attached to continuous irrigation (Fig. 47-12). If acute cholecystitis or obstruction of the common duct is thought to be a coincidental or inciting factor, drainage and simple stone removal may be necessary.

Nursing Management

Nursing management involves monitoring the client for life-threatening changes and alcohol withdrawal if substance abuse is part of the client history. It also entails performing the prescribed treatment measures. The nurse is responsible for inserting a nasogastric tube, maintaining its patency, and infusing IV fluids. If gastric decompression is prolonged, the client can receive jejunal feedings of a low-fat formula or TPN. The nurse must monitor blood glucose levels closely. Clients with acute pancreatitis require frequent administrations of analgesics. Most clients with acute pancreatitis are severely ill. The nurse must continuously monitor intake and output, especially urine volume. If the physician inserts a pulmonary artery or central venous catheter, the nurse monitors pressure measurements. Cardiac monitoring is continuous because electrolyte imbalances can produce dysrhythmias. The nurse continues to perform other assessments, including vital signs, lung sounds, serum electrolyte values, and observes for bleeding tendencies. If the client develops severe respiratory problems, he or she may require intubation and mechanical ventilation. The nurse must report any sudden change in the client's general condition or symptoms (i.e., pain or abdominal distention) to the physician immediately.

When surgery is performed, the nurse infuses irrigation solution and ensures that suction is functioning effectively. He or she also provides skin care if pancreatic drainage leaks from the sump drain sites.

CHRONIC PANCREATITIS

Pathophysiology and Etiology

Chronic pancreatitis is prolonged and progressive inflammation of the pancreas. In most cases, alcohol is the cause.

Alcohol can lead to edema of the duodenum and decrease the tone of the sphincter of Oddi. Consequently, duodenal contents can move into the pancreatic duct. Other causes include hereditary predisposition, hyperparathyroidism, hypertriglyceridemia, autoimmune pancreatitis, trauma, and anatomic abnormalities. In about 20% of cases, no particular cause is identifiable. With chronicity, the gland undergoes fibrotic scarring from the recurring inflammation. The pancreas hardens, and exocrine and endocrine functions are partly or completely lost as pancreatic tissue is destroyed.

Assessment Findings

Signs and Symptoms

In chronic pancreatitis, the client has severe to persistent pain, weight loss, and digestive disturbances, such as flatulence, vomiting, and diarrhea. If pseudocysts form, they contribute to the severity of the symptoms by putting pressure on adjacent organs or by rupturing. If secondary diabetes develops, the client may experience increased appetite, thirst, and urination. A firm mass may be palpated in the upper left quadrant. The urine may be dark; the stools may be light-colored and foul-smelling. Fatty streaks appear in the stool. With the loss of plasma proteins from the blood, peripheral edema and ascites develop.

Diagnostic Findings

Abnormal laboratory findings are the same for chronic pancreatitis as for acute disease. CT scans, MRI, ultrasound, and ERCP studies of the pancreas show diagnostic results similar to those in clients with acute pancreatitis. Results of a glucose tolerance test show an impaired ability to metabolize carbohydrates because of malfunctioning endocrine cells in the islets of Langerhans.

Medical and Surgical Management

Treatment depends on the cause and whether the pancreatic duct is obstructed. If the duct is not obstructed, treatment consists of abstinence from alcohol, a clear liquid to bland, fat-free diet, and correction of associated biliary tract disease or hyperparathyroidism. The client who adheres to treatment may have good results.

Drug therapy with meperidine (Demerol) is ordered in deference to morphine sulfate (morphine causes spasm of the sphincter of Oddi). Narcotics are prescribed cautiously. The focus is on management of pain using nonopioid methods. Treatment for insulin and digestive enzyme deficiencies includes diet, insulin, and pancreatic enzyme replacement therapy. Such therapy uses pancreatic enzymes, such as pancreatin (Creon, Bioglan, Panazyme, Donnazyme, Entozyme) or pancrelipase (Pancrease, Cotazym, Creon 10 and Creon 20, Protilase, Ultrase, Viokase, Zymase, Pancrecarb, Ilozyme), which help digest and absorb fats, proteins, and carbohydrates.

Pharmacologic Considerations

- The effectiveness of a conventional pancreatic enzyme such as pancrelipase (Ilozyme) is increased when the gastric pH is 4 or above; but enteric-coated preparations such as pancreatin (Panteric) require a pH of under 4 to 5 to avoid being broken down in the stomach.

When surgery is part of treatment, some or all of the pancreas (**partial or total pancreatectomy**) may be removed. If there is scarring, with stricture and stenosis of portions of the pancreatic duct, various surgical measures can be performed to attempt reconstitution of the duct. A pancreaticojejunostomy (joining of the pancreatic duct to the jejunum) can relieve ductal obstruction. Pancreatic autotransplantation is a recent surgical development. It involves excision and relocation of the pancreas. During this procedure, innervation is severed, effectively treating pain symptoms. Although exocrine function is lost, necessitating enzyme replacement, endocrine function and normal insulin production are preserved.

Nursing Process for the Client with Pancreatitis

Assessment

Initial assessment includes a history of symptoms the client experienced before admission as well as a complete medical history. Ask about the frequency and amount of alcohol ingestion and determine when the client had his or her last drink as a method of evaluating if or how soon withdrawal symptoms may occur. For reliability, involve family members in compiling assessment data (if possible), especially if the client's condition is serious. During the interview, obtain a description of pain with respect to location, type, severity, and circumstances that aggravate or relieve it. The physical examination includes gentle palpation of the abdomen, especially the epigastric area, for pain, tenderness, distention, or rigidity.

Include an immediate evaluation of vital signs, because shock often is an outstanding symptom of acute pancreatitis. A description of the client's general appearance is important. Periodic weights provide a comparison for when more serious symptoms occur. Instruct the client to save stool for inspection or laboratory testing. Initiate blood glucose testing as indicated.

Diagnosis, Planning, and Interventions

Administer prescribed analgesics. The client may exhibit or develop tolerance as a result of cross-addiction to alcohol or chronic use of analgesics. Monitor for signs of alcohol withdrawal, which may develop within the first 24 hours of admission. Implement measures to manage nutrition and blood glucose levels and administer insulin as indicated. The client requires therapeutic skin care to prevent breakdown from frequent, loose stools. If surgery is planned, manage preoperative and postoperative care. Diabetic and diet teaching begin before the client is discharged from the hospital (Client and Family Teaching 47-4). Provide referrals to a community substance abuse rehabilitation program if appropriate.

Other care can include the following nursing diagnoses, expected outcomes, and interventions.

▶ **Chronic Pain** related to distention, edema, and irritation of the inflamed pancreas

▶ **Expected Outcome:** Client will report reduced pain.

Client and Family Teaching 47-4
Pancreatitis

Most clients with pancreatitis require a prolonged recovery period. The following instructions are usual:

- Follow the written instructions for a bland, low-fat, calorie-controlled diet.
- Eat four or more small meals daily.
- Take prescribed medications, including enzyme replacements, as directed.
- If alcohol abuse is known to cause acute or chronic pancreatitis, avoid all alcoholic beverages. Strongly consider self-referral to Alcoholics Anonymous or a medical treatment center. Urge the family to attend Al-Anon meetings. (If insulin administration is necessary because of diabetes mellitus, see Chap. 51.)

- Administer analgesics as ordered. *Prompt administration of analgesics provides a therapeutic level of analgesia and promotes pain relief.*
- Withhold oral feedings. *Doing so limits the reflux of bile and duodenal contents into the pancreatic duct, preventing activation of the exocrine enzymes produced by the pancreas.*
- Instruct client to remain on bed rest. *Bed rest reduces metabolic rate and thus decreases secretion of pancreatic and gastric enzymes.*
- Report unrelieved pain or sudden increased intensity of pain. *Increased pain stimulates secretion of pancreatic enzymes. Sudden increased pain may indicate pancreatic rupture.*
- Administer anticholinergic medications as ordered. *They reduce gastric and pancreatic secretions.*
- Maintain continuous nasogastric drainage. *Drainage removes gastric contents and prevents gastric secretions from entering the duodenum.*

▶ **Ineffective Breathing Pattern** related to severe pain and pancreatic distention, edema, and inflammation

▶ **Expected Outcome:** Client will maintain adequate lung function as evidenced by improved breathing patterns and clear lungs.

- Position client with head of bed elevated or in semi-Fowler's position. *These measures reduce pressure on the diaphragm from abdominal distention and promote lung expansion.*
- Reposition client at least every 2 hours. *Repositioning prevents atelectasis and pooling of respiratory secretions.*
- Monitor pulse oximetry. Report episodes of desaturation to physician. *Pulse oximetry helps show changes in respiratory status and promotes early interventions.*
- Encourage client to deep breathe and cough every 2 hours. *Deep breathing and coughing clear the airway and reduce atelectasis.*

▶ **Deficient Fluid Volume** related to vomiting, decreased fluid intake, fever, diaphoresis, and fluid shifts

▶ **Expected Outcome:** Client will be adequately hydrated as evidenced by sufficient urine output and normal BP and skin turgor.

- Monitor intake and output at least every 8 hours. *This record can show if fluid loss is excessive.*
- Monitor serum electrolytes and BUN levels. *Findings might indicate a need for fluid and electrolyte replacements.*
- Administer IV fluids and electrolytes as ordered. *Replacing fluids and electrolytes restores fluid balance.*
- Administer plasma, albumin, and blood products as ordered. *Clients with severe pancreatitis lose large amounts of blood and plasma, which decreases effective circulating blood volume.*

▶ **Diarrhea** related to impaired fat and protein digestion

▶ **Expected Outcome:** Client experiences decreased diarrhea.

- Monitor number and characteristics of stools. *Such monitoring provides a baseline for determining fluid and electrolyte loss from stools.*
- Maintain low-fat diet if client is allowed food. *Decreased fat intake reduces the amount that the client cannot properly digest.*
- Administer antidiarrheal medications if ordered. *They assist in decreasing diarrhea and, in turn, reduce fluid and electrolyte losses.*

▶ **Risk for Injury** related to alcohol withdrawal

▶ **Expected Outcome:** Client remains uninjured with stable vital signs and no seizures.

- Monitor client for signs of CNS stimulation, such as agitation or belligerence. Observe for signs of hand tremors and emotional lability. *Such findings may indicate that the depressant effects of alcohol are wearing off.*
- Report if client's heart rate is over 100 beats/minute, diastolic BP is greater than 100 mm Hg, or temperature is above 100°F (36.6°C). *Such findings may indicate signs of alcohol withdrawal and the need for medical intervention.*
- Minimize environmental stimuli. *Extraneous lights and noise can increase agitation and possibly cause confusion.*
- Administer prescribed sedatives. *They provide appropriate sedation as the client withdraws from the effects of alcohol.*
- Provide a safe environment for the client if he or she is extremely agitated or at risk for seizures. Place client near nurses' station if he or she requires close observation. *Anticipating safety needs prevents harm to the client. If the client is near the nurses' station, the nurses can more closely monitor his or her activities.*
- Pad side rails and keep oral suction available. *If the client has a seizure or becomes extremely agitated, padded side rails, other safety measures, and immediate availability of suction can prevent further injury.*
- If a seizure occurs, initiate seizure precautions by protecting, but not restraining, the client. Observe the client throughout the seizure. After the seizure, ensure that the airway is clear and administer oxygen briefly according to agency policy. *Restraining a client during a seizure can cause more injury. Staying with the client during and after the seizure provides protection for the client and ensures that his or her airway is patent.*

Evaluation of Expected Outcomes

The client reports relief of pain, with an increased ability to sleep and rest more comfortably. He or she breathes deeply at a rate of

12 to 20 breaths/minute and maintains adequate pulmonary ventilation, as evidenced by clear lungs and 95% saturation by pulse oximetry. Fluid intake and output are balanced as evidenced by urine output of at least 50 mL/hour and normal BP and skin turgor. The client reports fewer stools and that stools have more form. Alcohol withdrawal occurs without hypertension or seizures. ●

CARCINOMA OF THE PANCREAS

Carcinoma of the pancreas may occur in the gland's head, body, or tail. Some tumors are primary lesions, whereas others are metastases from other locations. Because tumors of the head of the pancreas tend to cause obstructive jaundice, they usually are diagnosed earlier. Nevertheless, most are discovered late in the disease and invariably have a lethal prognosis.

Pathophysiology and Etiology

When sufficient malignant cells accumulate, they block the pancreatic duct, producing symptoms similar to chronic pancreatitis. There is some question as to whether the pancreatitis is a precursor or consequence of tumor development. Tumors in the body or tail of the pancreas can press on the portal vein and lead to the formation of varices and bleeding. Once a tumor develops, it tends to grow rapidly. By the time symptoms are serious enough for the client to seek medical assistance, the tumor may have spread to adjacent structures, such as the liver or spleen.

Besides pancreatitis, factors that correlate with pancreatic cancer include diabetes mellitus, a high-fat diet, and chronic exposure to carcinogenic substances (i.e., petrochemicals). Although data are inconclusive, a relationship may exist between cigarette smoking and high coffee consumption (especially decaffeinated coffee) and the development of pancreatic carcinoma.

Assessment Findings

Signs and Symptoms

Symptoms may not appear until the disease is far advanced. The most common symptoms are left upper abdominal pain that may be referred to the back, jaundice, anorexia, and weight loss. The client may describe light-colored stools but dark urine, typical symptoms of obstructive jaundice. Pruritus may accompany jaundice.

A mass may be palpated in the left upper quadrant. The mass may be a tumor or an enlarged gallbladder, which tends to expand as a result of obstructed passage of bile. Ascites may be present in late stages of the disease. Some clients develop thrombophlebitis from pancreatic tumor products, which increase the blood's coagulability.

Diagnostic Findings

Abdominal ultrasonography or CT scan demonstrates pancreatic enlargement but does not indicate the underlying cause. A biopsy obtained by ERCP or percutaneous needle aspiration provides evidence of malignant cells.

Elevated serum amylase, alkaline phosphatase, and bilirubin levels support the evidence that the pancreas is diseased, but they do not confirm carcinoma. The level of carcinoembryonic antigen is elevated, but this elevation is a less specific tumor marker than is CA 19–9.

Medical and Surgical Management

The prognosis is poor. In some cases, resection of a tumor at the head of the pancreas is possible by **radical pancreatoduodenectomy (Whipple procedure)** (Fig. 47-13). This surgical procedure involves removing the head of the pancreas, resecting the duodenum and stomach, and redirecting the flow of secretions from the stomach, gallbladder, and pancreas into the jejunum. The tumor may be irradiated during surgery, or radioactive seeds may be implanted. Because metastasis to the spleen is so common, some surgeons also may perform a splenectomy. Rather than do an extensive resection, others are inclined to do a total pancreatectomy. This radical surgery then creates a malabsorption syndrome and historically brittle diabetes, which must be treated after surgery. Some complications associated with this surgery include bleeding tendencies caused by a vitamin K deficiency and liver and kidney failure.

Pharmacologic Considerations

- Clients with carcinoma of the head of the pancreas usually require vitamin K before surgery to correct a prothrombin deficiency.

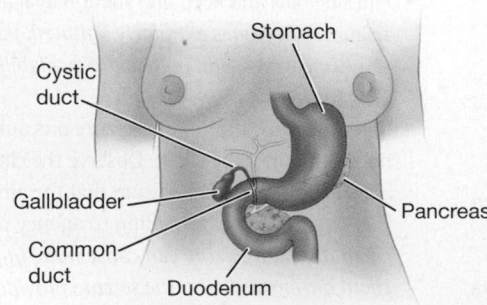

Before surgery

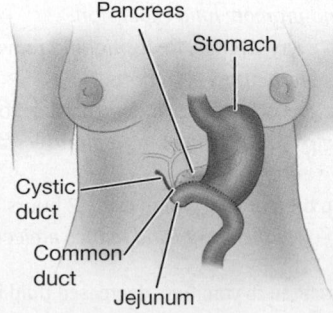

After surgery

FIGURE 47-13. Radical pancreatoduodenectomy (Whipple procedure). The head of the pancreas is removed, as well as the gallbladder. The common duct is sutured to the end of the jejunum, and the remaining portion of the pancreas and the end of the stomach are sutured to the side of the jejunum.

A cholecystojejunostomy, a rerouting of pancreatic and biliary drainage, may be done to relieve obstructive jaundice. This measure is considered palliative only. For inoperable tumors, radiation therapy or chemotherapy with 5-fluorouracil (5-FU) or mitomycin (Mutamycin) may be tried. These treatments do not cure the disease. Despite surgery, chemotherapy, or radiation therapy, most clients die within 3 to 12 months after the onset of symptoms.

Nursing Management

Nursing management for those treated medically is the same as for any client with a terminal malignant disorder (see Chap. 18). Clients undergoing palliative surgery require care similar to that of clients having general abdominal surgery. If clients have severe anorexia and weight loss, they are poor risks for immediate surgery. These clients may receive preoperative IV fluids, TPN, or a special diet to improve nutritional status and correct any fluid or electrolyte imbalances. Most surgical clients have a nasogastric tube inserted. Once the biliary obstruction is relieved, the color of the skin, stools, and urine returns to near normal. Clients undergoing the Whipple procedure or one of its variations require more intensive nursing management because of the profoundly invasive nature of the procedure.

Initially, the nurse evaluates the client's general physical condition and obtains a history of all symptoms present before admission. He or she asks about the onset of symptoms, weight loss, bleeding tendencies, and the type of pain or abdominal discomfort. Physical examination includes inspection for jaundice, a visual examination of stools and urine, and palpation of the abdomen for tenderness and distention. Laboratory tests include blood or urine samples for analysis and detection of glucose. The nurse records vital signs and weight and assesses nutritional status.

The nurse observes the client after surgery for complications such as shock, pancreatic abscess formation, and hemorrhage. See Chapter 14 for postoperative nursing management measures for pain control, anxiety, and impaired skin integrity. Immediate postoperative assessments include vital signs and a review of the chart for the type and extent of surgery. The nurse also checks the surgical dressing and all drains and tubes for patency, as well as noting the amount and color of drainage throughout the entire postoperative course.

Close observation for signs of bleeding, such as easy bruising, blood in the urine or stool, or bleeding from the incision, drains, or tubes, is important. The nurse also monitors for signs of infection (elevated temperature, increased pain, abdominal distention, abdominal tenderness, and purulent drainage from the incisional site).

The surgery for carcinoma of the pancreas is very serious, with potentially major complications and poor outcomes. Nursing diagnoses can include the following:

- **Acute Pain** related to surgical procedure
- **Deficient Fluid Volume** related to hemorrhage and loss of fluids
- **Ineffective Breathing Pattern** related to abdominal discomfort and drainage tubes

- **Risk for Infection** related to invasive procedure and poor physical condition
- **Risk for Imbalanced Nutrition: Less than Body Requirements** related to high metabolic requirements and decreased ability to digest food
- **Risk for Injury** related to failure to consume adequate calories or get enough insulin
- **Anticipatory Grieving** related to shortened life span and poor prognosis

Clients who have surgery for pancreatic carcinoma and their significant others require diligent and caring attention. The nurse providing care focuses on:

- Assessing pain with a rating scale from 0 to 10
- Administering medications as prescribed
- Emptying drainage collection devices before they become full, taking care to avoid contaminating the drainage port
- Replacing fluids as ordered
- Monitoring serum electrolyte levels
- Auscultating lung sounds
- Instructing client to splint abdomen when turning or moving
- Encouraging client to deep breathe and cough at least every 2 hours
- Using aseptic technique to change or reinforce dressings when they become moist
- Following agency policy for changing IV sites, tubing, and infusing solutions
- Reassigning staff with potentially infectious symptoms to assignments that do not require direct client care or advising them to take sick leave
- Discouraging family or friends who may be ill from visiting until they are well
- Monitoring blood glucose levels several times each day
- Administering IV solutions, TPN, or both per orders
- Monitoring oral and IV caloric intake
- Teaching client about pancreatic enzyme replacement and a low-fat diet
- Providing support to client and family members as they begin to cope with the prognosis
- Helping client and family gain access to support services, hospice, and other organizations for palliative care and support

Care for clients with pancreatic tumors also must consider the psychological and emotional outcomes. If the client is discharged home, he or she and the family members require extensive teaching and home health services. The teaching plan should address schedules and techniques for administering prescribed medications, how to check the blood glucose level, recommended diet, importance of drinking fluids and eating, skin care (particularly around the incision), and the future schedule for follow-up visits, radiation therapy, or chemotherapy. The nurse also must review with the client and family symptoms to report to the physician: jaundice, dark urine, bleeding tendencies, vomiting, tarry stools, increased pain, swelling of the extremities, abdominal enlargement, decreased urine output, weight loss, and calf pain.

CRITICAL THINKING EXERCISES

1. A client has jaundice. What questions can you ask to help determine the cause?

2. How would you reassure someone who is interested in becoming a nurse, yet has reservations because of potentially acquiring a blood-borne disease, such as hepatitis B?

3. A clinic nurse hears a male client with hepatitis telling the medical assistant that he is taking cough syrup for his bad cold and cough. Does the nurse need to follow up?

4. A client with acute pancreatitis is admitted to the medical-surgical unit. She has poor skin turgor and tachycardia, and she complains of nausea and is having dry heaves. In addition, she rates her abdominal pain as 8 on a 0 to 10 scale. An IV line is running, and the client is taking nothing by mouth. After about 2 hours, the client is more comfortable. Signaling with her call light, she asks for something to drink. How do you respond?

NCLEX-STYLE REVIEW QUESTIONS

1. A client has had surgery for pancreatic carcinoma. Which of the following interventions should the nurse consider when caring for this client? Select all that apply.
1. Empty drainage collection devices regularly.
2. Instruct the client to avoid splinting the abdomen when turning.
3. Monitor blood glucose levels several times each day.
4. Instruct the client to avoid deep breathing and coughing.
5. Discourage visitors who are ill from visiting until they are well.

2. After a liver biopsy on the client with cirrhosis, which nursing order is most appropriate to add to the plan of care?
1. Elevate the client's legs on two pillows.
2. Ambulate the client twice each shift.
3. Keep the client in high Fowler's position.
4. Position the client on his right side.

3. After taking nothing by mouth for several days, a client with pancreatitis has a nasogastric tube removed and is placed on a bland, low-fat diet. Which food item, if found on the client's breakfast tray, should be removed?
1. Whole wheat toast
2. Scrambled eggs
3. Skim milk
4. Stewed prunes

4. A college student is diagnosed with hepatitis A. An infection control nurse is consulted on measures for reducing the potential transmission of the hepatitis A virus to others. Based on the routes of transmission for this disease, which infection control measure is essential to include in the plan for care?
1. Wear gloves whenever entering the client's room.
2. Don a mask and gown when providing direct care.
3. Maintain the client in a private room at all times.
4. Perform vigorous handwashing after leaving the room.

5. A client has suspected cholecystitis. When the client describes discomfort to the nurse, the client is most likely to indicate that the pain becomes worse at which of the following times?
1. Before arising in the morning
2. After periods of activity
3. Especially on an empty stomach
4. Shortly after eating food

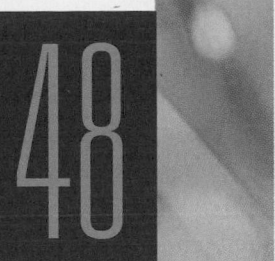

48

Caring for Clients with Ostomies

Words To Know

abdominoperineal resection
anastomosis
appliance
colostomy
continent ileostomy (Kock pouch)
double-barrel colostomy
effluent
enterostomal therapist
ileoanal reservoir (anastomosis)
ileostomy
loop colostomy
ostomate
ostomy
segmental resection
single-barrel colostomy
stoma
wound, ostomy, and continence nurses
  (WOCNs)

Learning Objectives

On completion of this chapter, you will be able to:

1. Differentiate between ileostomy and colostomy.
2. Discuss preoperative nursing care of a client undergoing ostomy surgery.
3. List complications associated with ostomy surgery.
4. Discuss postoperative nursing management of a client with an ileostomy.
5. Describe the components used to apply and collect stool from an intestinal ostomy.
6. Cite reasons for changing an ostomy appliance.
7. Summarize how to change an ostomy appliance.
8. Explain how stool is released from a continent ileostomy.
9. Describe the two-part procedure needed to create an ileoanal reservoir.
10. Discuss various types of colostomies.
11. Explain ways that clients with descending or sigmoid colostomies may regulate bowel elimination.

The term **ostomy** refers to an opening between an internal body structure and the skin. The most common intestinal ostomies are the **ileostomy**, an opening from the distal small intestine, and the **colostomy**, an opening from the colon (Table 48-1). Fecal material exits through a **stoma**, an opening on the exterior abdominal surface. Most ostomies are created in response to an inflammatory bowel disorder that fails to respond to medical treatment or complications such as rupture of a portion of intestine, irreversible obstruction, compromised blood supply to the intestine, or cancerous tumor. Whether an ostomy is temporary or permanent, each client requires an individually adapted plan of care that incorporates preparation for surgery, recovery from surgery, and knowledge required for ongoing self-care.

ILEOSTOMY

In the usual surgical procedure for a conventional ileostomy, the entire colon and rectum are removed (total colectomy). The terminal end of the ileum is brought out through a separate area on the right lower quadrant of the abdomen slightly below the umbilicus, near the outer border of the rectus muscle (Fig. 48-1). The cut end is everted and sutured to the skin, a process referred to as creating a *matured* stoma. When an ileostomy is performed, the stoma continually releases stool and gas. The fecal material discharged from an ileostomy is liquid or mushy and contains digestive enzymes.

TABLE 48-1 Types of Intestinal Ostomies

TYPE	STOMA LOCATION	FECAL CONSISTENCY	FECAL CONTROL
Conventional ileostomy	Lower abdomen	Liquid	Never
Continent ileostomy	Lower abdomen	Liquid	By siphoning
Ascending colostomy	Middle right abdomen	Semiliquid	Never
Transverse colostomy	Center of the abdomen below the belt line	Semiliquid	Never
Descending colostomy	Middle left abdomen	Soft	Sometimes
Sigmoid colostomy	Lower left abdomen	Formed	Usually

THE OSTOMY APPLIANCE

The matured stoma promotes healing and provides a smooth peristomal area that permits the immediate postoperative application of an **appliance**, the collection device worn over a stoma. Clients with an ileostomy always wear an appliance, which requires frequent emptying. Ostomy suppliers provide various appliances to meet the individual needs of the **ostomate** (client with an ostomy). All appliances consist of one-piece or two-piece devices with a pouch for collecting feces and a faceplate, or disk, which is attached to the abdomen with an opening through which the stoma protrudes (Fig. 48-2). The faceplate adheres to the skin either with self-adhesive backing or another bonding substance such as an adhesive powder, paste, or wafer. Karaya gum, which becomes gelatinous when in contact with moisture, is commonly used in place of an adhesive. Karaya gum protects the skin and promotes adhesion of the ostomy appliance. Karaya gum rings are used around the stoma. They are pulled or pushed into any shape and are ideal for correcting problems created by an ill-fitting appliance. Unlike rings made of rigid material, a karaya gum ring fits snugly around the stoma without injuring it.

A disposable, or temporary, appliance is preferred in the immediate postoperative phase because the size of the stoma changes over time as a result of swelling from the procedure itself. The size of the stoma may change rapidly and differ from one appliance change to the next. After the stoma heals and reaches its final size and shape, a permanent (reusable) appliance is fitted.

Reusable equipment consists of a sturdier pouch with a custom-sized faceplate and "O" ring. The pouch is designed to fasten into position when pressed over the ring, much like snapping a lid on a plastic margarine tub. The pouch has a clamp at the bottom, which can be released when the pouch needs to be emptied. The pouch may be fastened to a belt for more security. The belt supports the weight of the liquid fecal material and prevents the faceplate from being pulled away from the abdominal skin. Foam rubber, gauze, or flannel padding is placed under a belt if the belt cuts into the flesh. The client requires two sets of permanent appliances so that one can be cleaned periodically. Disposable equipment may be appropriate for some clients. Disposable bags, faceplates, and attachment rings are replaced with new ones with each change of the ostomy appliance (usually daily with bathing).

Pharmacologic Considerations

- Some medications, especially vitamins, antibiotics, and antituberculosis drugs, cause particularly strong odors that cling to the appliance. The client can obtain a list of drugs that may leave an odor on an ostomy appliance from an ostomy association or ostomy appliance manufacturers.

- Clients with an ileostomy should avoid enteric-coated products and some modified-release drugs, such as slow-release beads and layered tablets. These products may pass through without being absorbed. When changing the

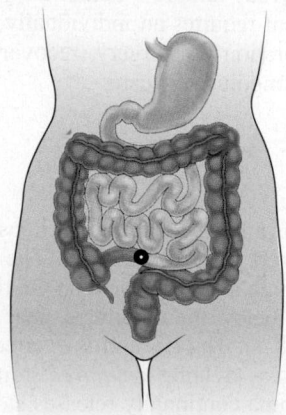

FIGURE 48-1. Total colectomy is removal of the entire colon and rectum. The terminal end of the ileum is brought out through the abdomen to form an ileostomy. (Shaded portion represents the section that has been removed.)

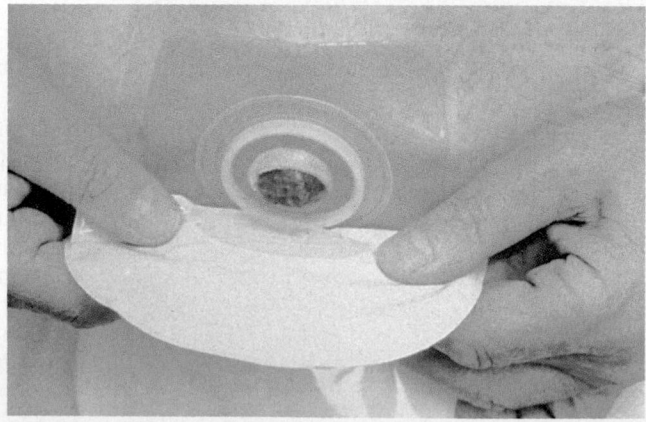

FIGURE 48-2. The ostomy appliance. (Courtesy of Convatec, a Bristol-Myers Squibb Company.)

ileostomy appliance, check for undissolved—and therefore unabsorbed—capsules. Such findings mean that the client has not received the desired effect of the medication; contact the physician.

- Some preparations such as Slow-K (potassium chloride) leave a "ghost" of the wax matrix coating, but that does not indicate the drug has been unabsorbed. Clients with an ileostomy may need monthly vitamin B_{12} injections or intranasal vitamin B_{12} because the terminal ileum may be compromised to such an extent as to interfere with dietary absorption of the vitamin.

PREOPERATIVE PERIOD
Surgical Management

Before surgery, the physician explains the purpose for the surgical procedure along with its benefits and risks. He or she describes the appearance and function of the stoma, where it will be placed, and its required care. The physician carefully marks the site to ensure that it is away from bony prominences, skin creases, and scars; is within the rectus abdominis muscle; is unobstructed; and is visible to the client. Clients benefit from preoperative interactions with a specially certified nurse, referred to as an enterostomal therapy nurse, **enterostomal therapist**, or **wound, ostomy and continent nurse (WOCN)**. This nurse assists with marking placement of the stoma and collaborates with the surgeon regarding placement and the client's educational needs.

The physician identifies potential risks from the total colectomy, such as possible bladder and sexual dysfunction secondary to parasympathetic nerve injury. Sexual dysfunction in men after a total colectomy is unusual but sometimes occurs. If such dysfunction persists after a colectomy, operative and nonoperative options are available to facilitate erection. Young male clients may wish to collect and store sperm for later use if they plan to have children. A colectomy may slightly diminish fertility in women; however, this procedure does not preclude the ability to achieve a full-term pregnancy with a normal vaginal delivery.

Cleansing of the bowel before surgery is carried out using dietary restrictions in combination with laxative or lavage agents (e.g., GoLYTELY, NuLYTELY, Colyte), depending on the client's condition (i.e., presence or absence of obstruction) and according to the surgeon's preference. Opinions vary regarding the need for antibiotic prophylaxis. Many surgeons order a combination of intravenous (IV) antibiotics (i.e., a third-generation cephalosporin and metronidazole) before surgery and continue administration after surgery.

Whenever possible, prednisone should be tapered and discontinued before surgery to avoid negative effects of the drug on tissue healing. A preoperative "stress dose" of IV steroid (i.e., hydrocortisone) is given to clients who have been on prednisone within the previous 6 months to prevent adrenal crisis. Adrenal crisis is potentially life-threatening and can result from the abrupt withdrawal of corticosteroids or significant stress after the client has been treated with corticosteroids. See Chapter 50 for additional information on adrenal crisis.

Immunosuppressive agents such as azathioprine, 6-mercaptopurine, and cyclosporine should be discontinued 3 to 4 weeks before surgery to prevent negative effects on tissue healing. Aspirin-containing compounds are discontinued at least 1 week before surgery to minimize the risk of bleeding. Blood samples are taken before surgery, and the client's blood is typed and cross-matched for replacement of losses that occur during surgery.

Nursing Process for the Client Before Ileostomy Surgery

Assessment

Obtain complete medical, allergy, diet, and drug histories. Ask the client if he or she has been taking corticosteroids. If so, monitor the client closely for signs and symptoms of adrenal insufficiency such as weakness, lethargy, hypotension, nausea, and vomiting as the dosage is tapered. Perform a physical assessment, paying particular attention to inspecting the skin over the abdomen, auscultating bowel sounds, and obtaining the client's vital signs and weight. In addition, check the preoperative laboratory test results to determine if blood cell counts and serum electrolyte levels are within normal ranges. Obtain a description of preoperative measures the client may have been asked to take, such as dietary modifications and antibiotic therapy. Implement medical orders for cleansing the bowel, inserting a nasogastric tube, and preparing the client for surgery.

Referral to community and professional resources before surgery may positively affect the client's postoperative quality of life. Resources for education and support include the medical and surgical teams and the lay public (e.g., Crohn's & Colitis Foundation of America, United Ostomy Associations of America).

Healthcare teams hold several views about beginning ostomy instructions before surgery. Some believe that such teaching helps clients to accept the ostomy. Others believe that this type of teaching creates premature stress and anxiety. Often, an enterostomal therapist provides ostomy instruction, whether before or after surgery. He or she is certified to care for ostomates and manage their unique problems. The enterostomal therapist also is an excellent resource for nurses providing direct care to ostomates. If the client expresses a readiness to learn or asks questions about ostomy care, provide information about ostomy equipment and general principles of ostomy management. Also, if the client so desires, arrange a preoperative visit with the enterostomal therapy nurse.

Diagnosis, Planning, and Interventions

- Anxiety related to change in health status and fear of the unknown

- Expected Outcome: Client will experience reduced anxiety.

- Provide an overview of preoperative procedures, using explanations the client understands. *Explanations enable the client to know what to expect.*
- Allow time for the client to ask questions and express fears. *Adequate time and support promote communication and assist the client to verbalize anxiety.*

- Assess previous positive coping skills and assist client to access them again. *Past successful coping methods are likely to be effective now.*

▶ Disturbed Body Image related to the stoma and altered bowel elimination

▶ Expected Outcome: Client verbalizes what the changes will be and the benefits to future health.

- Encourage the client to discuss feelings about the stoma. *Such discussion enables the client to express concerns and fears about the fecal diversion.*
- Inform the client that an assigned staff nurse will be there when the client first views and touches the stoma. *Such information gives reassurance that a familiar nurse will be available to answer questions and give support.*
- If the client expresses interest, provide a list of appropriate community resources. *Knowing that others have experienced the same surgery and can share their experience and offer advice and support may help the client.*

Evaluation of Expected Outcomes
The client verbalizes fears and demonstrates positive coping skills. He or she discusses what physical changes to expect. ●

POSTOPERATIVE PERIOD
Surgical Management
The rectum is packed with gauze during surgery to absorb drainage and promote gradual healing. The rectal pack usually is removed in 5 to 7 days. Afterward, irrigations may be ordered to promote healing. A nasogastric tube is used for gastrointestinal (GI) decompression until normal bowel motility resumes. Fluid, electrolyte, and nutritional balances are maintained with IV fluids until oral nourishment is possible. Within several days, the nasogastric tube is removed and oral feedings begin. Antibiotic therapy continues. Analgesics are prescribed for pain relief. Wound healing is monitored, and complications that develop are managed.

Possible postoperative complications include intestinal obstruction; bleeding; and impaired blood supply to, stenosis of, or prolapse or excessive protrusion of the stoma. Intestinal obstruction, a serious complication, may result from a twisted, strangulated, or incarcerated segment of the remaining intestine or a bolus of poorly chewed or inadequately digested food. When a collection of food causes obstruction, the physician may irrigate the stoma in an attempt to correct the problem. If the bowel is twisted or strangulated, surgical intervention is necessary.

Prolapse or protrusion of the ileostomy is fairly common. If it is moderate (1 or 2 inches), no treatment is required. A severe prolapse of the stoma is a serious complication, however. If edema occurs, it may cause an obstruction and restrict stomal blood supply. Stomal necrosis results if the prolapse is not promptly and skillfully managed. Once the stoma prolapses, recurrence is likely.

Nursing Process for the Client Recovering From Ileostomy Surgery

Assessment
Review the medical record for information regarding the type of surgery and any problems during or immediately after surgery. Obtain vital signs; inspect the dressing and stoma for bleeding and signs of infection (Table 48-2); monitor the rate and progress of fluid and blood infusions; check the function of the gastric suction; measure intake and output; and inspect the collection appliance, special drains, packing, or tubes. Record all immediate postoperative findings to provide a database.

Diagnosis, Planning, and Interventions
Nursing Guidelines 48-1 provides instructions for replacing an ostomy appliance. In logical steps and at a pace that promotes comprehension, teach the client and another family member about managing the ostomy, adopting dietary modifications, recognizing how drug therapy affects bowel elimination, and adjusting to various surgery-related changes, such as possible sexual dysfunction. Client and Family Teaching 48-1 lists additional topics to include in the teaching plan.

TABLE 48-2 Characteristics of Healthy and Unhealthy Stomas

CHARACTERISTICS	HEALTHY STOMA	UNHEALTHY STOMA
Color	Bright pink or red	Dusky blue or black
Size	Comparable in diameter with the intestine from which it has been formed; may be somewhat large after surgery because of edema	Larger or smaller in comparison to size after resolution of postoperative edema
Opening	Patent, unobstructed	Tight or narrow
Surface	Moist, shiny with an overlying layer of mucus; may bleed slightly when being cleansed	Dull, dry; excessive bleeding
Length	Protrudes from or is just flush with the skin	Protrudes beyond 2 inches from the skin or retracts beneath it
Sensation	Painless	Peristomal burning
Function	Regular passage of feces	Sparse or absent elimination of feces

NURSING GUIDELINES 48-1

Changing an Ostomy Appliance

Assemble clean gloves, scissors, ostomy belt, stoma gauge, faceplate, pouch, adhesive or protectant (e.g., karaya gum), and cleaning materials such as gauze pads, water, or adhesive solvent.

- Wash hands and put on gloves.
- Empty pouch when it is one-third full.
- Change the faceplate only when needed, that is, if it becomes loose or tight or client experiences discomfort. If the faceplate is changed too frequently, skin around stoma may become raw and excoriated secondary to removal of protective layers of epithelium with the faceplate.
- If the ostomy appliance is being replaced routinely, schedule the change when the gastrocolic reflex is less active. For many clients, this time is early in the morning, before eating, or 2 or 3 hours after mealtime.
- Gently ease the faceplate from the skin. If the faceplate was applied with adhesive, roll the adhesive from the skin and appliance. If it does not roll off, use a small amount of solvent, which chemically loosens the adhesive bond. Because some solvents irritate the skin, apply solvent sparingly between the body and faceplate using a sprayer, medicine dropper, or gauze pad. Avoid rubbing, which may further irritate skin. Clean the area with soap and water and pat dry after a solvent has been used.
- Inform the client that the most common causes of discomfort are reactions to the adhesive or solvent used to remove it or irritation from leaking fecal drainage. In such cases, the client may experience stinging, tingling, or itching immediately after an appliance change. These sensations should quickly subside. If a sensation is prolonged or intensified, remove the appliance regardless of whether it has been on for 1 hour or several days. When using a new adhesive product, remember to patch test it first on nonirritated skin at the inner aspect of the client's forearm.
- After removing the faceplate and pouch, protect the peristomal area from drainage by placing a tissue cuff around the stoma or using a receptacle such as a small paper cup to collect the drainage. Use a soapy washcloth to clean the skin around the stoma and wipe the soap from the skin. Pat the area or allow it to air dry.
- Inspect the stoma and skin carefully. If excoriation is observed, use a temporary appliance or hydrocolloid dressing, such as DuoDERM or Tegasorb, to cover the excoriated skin to promote moist healing.
- Create an even surface for reapplying the pouch by filling irregular hollows in the peristomal skin with karaya paste before replacing the faceplate.
- Measure the circumference of the stoma and cut a comparable hole in the faceplate, allowing 18-inch margin to account for potential swelling in a new stoma.
- Secure the pouch to the faceplate. Be sure to smooth out ridges or openings in the closure. Also be sure to seal the pouch.
- Peel the backing from the faceplate.
- Affix the faceplate to the skin.

Client and Family Teaching 48-1
Postoperative Ileostomy Care

The nurse discusses the following issues with the client and his or her family:

- Restrict oral intake only with medical supervision.
- Eat slowly and chew food well with the mouth closed to help lessen the development of gas.
- Avoid food that cause discomfort, excessive gas, or loose stools.
- Drink extra fluids, especially in warm weather.
- Dilate the stoma if the volume of stool decreases for some unexplained reason. To do this, cut the nail on the index or little finger, cover the finger with a finger cot, lubricate it thoroughly, and then insert the finger gently into the stoma for a few minutes.
- Clean the pouch thoroughly to prevent odors.
- Use an internal odor-absorbing substance or one that can be added to the pouch to control lingering or stubborn odors.
- Use an old or disposable pouch when medications or offending foods that cause disagreeable odors are excreted.
- Slip a plastic cover over the pouch to act as a second barrier against escaping odors.
- Check with a physician before self-administering any drug, especially a laxative or antidiarrheal agent.

In addition to the measures discussed in the following, postoperative care includes standard pain management (see Chap. 11) and postoperative interventions (see Chap. 14).

▶ **Risk for Impaired Skin Integrity** related to effects of fecal material and adhesives on the skin

▶ **Expected Outcome:** Client will maintain intact peristomal skin.

- Demonstrate safe, gentle removal of the pouch. *This type of removal prevents skin irritation.*
- Gently cleanse the peristomal area with warm water and mild soap. *Gentle cleansing minimizes skin irritation and abrasions.*
- Teach the client to apply a skin barrier, such as a wafer, gel, paste, or powder. *The skin barrier protects the peristomal skin from digestive enzymes and bacteria.*

▶ **Risk for Infection** related to fecal contamination of the surgical wound

▶ **Expected Outcome:** Client's wound is free from infection.

- Apply dressing securely, covering the surgical wound completely. *The dressing protects the incision from contact with fecal material.*
- Change the ostomy pouch when it is loose and leaking. *Changing at the appropriate time minimizes the risk of fecal drainage entering the incision.*

- When drainage leaks near the incision, wipe it away from the incision and change the dressing if soiled at all. *These measures keep fecal drainage away from incision, ensuring that the dressing always is clean.*
- Observe for signs of wound infection: wound drainage, abdominal pain, and elevated temperature. *These signs indicate possible wound infection.*

▶ **Bowel Incontinence** related to loss of sphincter control and change in intestinal motility

▶ **Expected Outcome:** Client will have no or minimal leaking from the appliance or soiling with fecal material.

- Instruct the client how to prepare the drainage pouch for a secure fit around the stoma, leaving an extra 1/8 inch in the appliance opening. (Use a gauge for measuring, provided by the manufacturer.) *Accurate preparation provides room for stoma clearance and potential swelling.*
- Press the adhesive faceplate around the stoma for about 30 seconds. *This measure ensures secure attachment of the pouch to the peristomal skin.*
- Demonstrate frequent emptying of the pouch. *Frequent emptying prevents tension on the pouch and skin from the weight of the drainage.*
- Use the following measures to prevent leakage:
  - Press the adhesive faceplate from the stomal edge outward. *This technique prevents the formation of wrinkles.*
  - Ask the client to remain inactive for 5 minutes. *This period allows time for body heat to strengthen the adhesive bond.*
  - Allow a small amount of air to be trapped in the pouch. *Liquid feces will then drain to the bottom of the pouch, placing less tension on it.*
  - Make several pinhole-sized punctures at the upper edge of the pouch. *Punctures allow excess gas to escape and decrease tension on the pouch.*

▶ **Risk for Deficient Fluid Volume** related to decreased appetite, vomiting, or increased loss of fluids and electrolytes from ileostomy

▶ **Expected Outcome:** Client maintains adequate fluid and electrolyte balance.

- Assess fluid balance. *This evaluation determines any deficits.*
- Examine serum and urine test results for sodium and potassium levels. *Review may indicate imbalances and other potential problems (e.g., acidosis, cardiac dysrhythmias).*
- Observe skin turgor and appearance of the tongue. *Poor skin turgor and dry tongue indicate fluid deficits.*

▶ **Risk for Sexual Dysfunction** related to altered body image

▶ **Expected Outcome:** Client will plan modifications for maintaining sexual fulfillment.

- Encourage the client and partner to verbalize fears and concerns about intimacy. *Discussion allows client and partner to express feelings and explore needs.*

Client and Family Teaching 48-2
Sexual Modifications for Ostomates

The nurse offers the following suggestions to clients with ostomies:

- Always practice good hygiene. Bathe and apply a fresh pouch before having sex.
- Disguise the pouch by enclosing it within a purse-string cloth cover.
- When anticipating sexual activity, avoid eating or drinking substances that activate the bowel or create a lot of gas.
- Fashion a cummerbund with a pocket or fold into which the pouch can be held.
- Remove the belt and temporarily secure the pouch to the skin with tape.
- If accidents happen, cultivate a sense of humor, which may relieve the anxiety of the sexual partner as well.
- Consult with members of a local ostomy group who also may provide support and counseling regarding sexual matters.

- Reassure the client who is not experiencing sexual dysfunction that intercourse will not harm the healed ostomy. *Fear can interfere with sexual relations; reassurance assists clients to reestablish sexual relationships.*
- Recommend alternative sexual positions and modifications (Client and Family Teaching 48-2). *Different positions and other modifications may enable the client to avoid embarrassment about the stomal appearance until he or she is more comfortable.*
- Refer clients who experience sexual dysfunction to a sexual therapist, enterostomal therapist, or advanced practice nurse. *Clients and partners may need assistance to determine problems and solutions, including alternative methods to achieve sexual satisfaction.*

▶ **Ineffective Coping** related to disturbed body image and altered bowel function

▶ **Expected Outcome:** Client will cope effectively with body changes.

- Ensure privacy when teaching and providing ileostomy care. *Privacy allows client to get used to changes without fear of embarrassment in front of others.*
- Help the client to set realistic goals and identify personal skills and knowledge. *Participation in the care plan allows the client to make decisions and move toward independence.*
- Use empathetic communication, allowing time for client to express fears and concerns. *A supportive environment promotes coping.*
- Refer the client to support networks, such as ostomy groups or other ostomates. *Resources help client to problem solve and increase coping skills.*

Evaluation of Expected Outcomes

Peristomal skin is not reddened, there is no evidence of edema or drainage, and the client does not complain of burning sensations. The incision heals without infection. Stool is contained in the ostomy pouch. The client maintains adequate fluid balance as evidenced by balanced intake and output, good skin turgor, moist tongue and mucous membranes, and normal serum and urine sodium and potassium levels. The client reports that he or she has attained satisfactory sexual performance. He or she also demonstrates coping skills as evidenced by interest in self-care, ability to seek assistance, and ability to maintain relationships. ●

Gerontologic Considerations

- Older adults with ostomies who also experience chronic disorders such as poor vision and arthritis may encounter difficulty in changing the appliance, performing skin care, irrigating the colostomy stoma, and caring for the permanent appliance. Consult with an enterostomal therapist about which equipment may best meet the client's needs.

- Healthcare professionals must assess the older adult's ability to provide long-term self-care for the ostomy, or identify available resources such as a family member, visiting nurse, or home healthcare nurse. In some instances, a skilled nursing facility or nursing home may be necessary.

CONTINENT ILEOSTOMY (KOCK POUCH)

A **continent ileostomy (Kock pouch)** is the creation of an internal reservoir for the storage of GI **effluent** (discharged fecal material or liquid feces). The reservoir stores this effluent for several hours until the client removes it with a catheter. Doing so eliminates the need for an external appliance.

Surgical Management

After removing the diseased portion of the ileum, the surgeon forms a reservoir with a portion of the terminal ileum and creates a nipple valve by telescoping (*intussusception*) the distal ileal segment into the reservoir. The surgeon then forms a permanent external stoma and anchors it to the abdominal wall (Fig. 48-3).

During the operation, the surgeon inserts a temporary catheter through the nipple valve and sutures the catheter in place so that its end protrudes from the external stoma. Then the surgeon packs the perineal area from which the lower intestine was removed with gauze. The packing remains in place for about 1 week.

Nursing Management

The nurse reinforces the perineal packing, as needed, during the postoperative period. In addition, the nurse checks the abdominal dressing for drainage and connects the stomal catheter, if ordered, to low, intermittent suction that empties the reservoir continuously, thereby preventing tension on

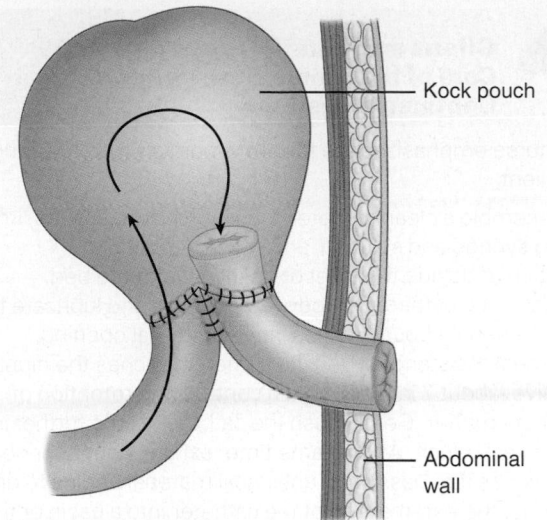

FIGURE 48-3. Continent ileostomy.

healing suture lines. He or she checks the ileal catheter frequently for the following signs of obstruction: lack of fecal drainage, the client's complaint of feeling full in the area of the ileal pouch, or leakage of liquid stool around the catheter. The nurse notes the color and amount of drainage, observes the size and color of the stoma, and administers either routine or as-needed irrigations of the ileal catheter, using small amounts of normal saline solution if the catheter appears to be obstructed, according to physician's orders. He or she keeps the skin clean around the stoma, changes the gauze dressing over the stoma when it becomes wet with mucus or serosanguineous drainage, and changes the dressing every 6 to 8 hours as drainage decreases.

The nurse also monitors ileal output carefully during the entire postoperative period. As GI function resumes, the initial amount of ileal drainage usually is high. If excessive fluids and electrolytes are lost, parenteral fluid and electrolyte replacement is necessary. When ileal drainage stabilizes, about 10 to 14 days after surgery, the physician removes the ileal catheter. The reservoir then holds the accumulating effluent until the nurse or client siphons it. Initially the reservoir is emptied every 2 to 4 hours. As the capacity of the reservoir increases, usually in about 6 months, the client or caregiver performs the procedure three or four times daily.

The nurse includes the information presented in Client and Family Teaching 48-3 in his or her teaching plan. For additional nursing management, refer to the discussion that addresses similar problems experienced by a client with ileoanal reservoir.

ILEOANAL RESERVOIR

The **ileoanal reservoir**, also called an ileoanal **anastomosis** (a surgical connection between two structures, Fig. 48-4), is a procedure that maintains bowel continence. It is performed on selected clients who have chronic ulcerative colitis or whose disease does not affect the anorectal sphincter. Besides allowing the client to control bowel elimination, this procedure, as opposed to a conventional

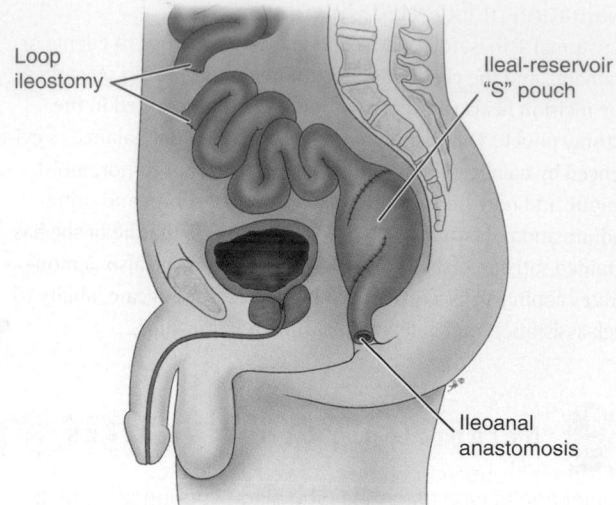

FIGURE 48-4. An ileoanal anastomosis joins a section of ileum to create an ileal reservoir. The distal end of the ileum is sutured above the anus. Intestinal effluent is temporarily discharged through the proximal stoma of a loop ileostomy until the second stage of surgery is performed.

Client and Family Teaching 48-3
Care of the Stoma and Catheter After a Continent Ileostomy

The nurse emphasizes the following points when teaching the client:

● Assemble a clean catheter, lubricant, basin, tissues, irrigating syringe and solution, and gauze dressing.
● Sit on or beside the toilet or on the side of the bed.
● Warm the catheter to body temperature and lubricate the tip. Insert it about 2 inches into the stomal opening.
● Expect resistance when the catheter reaches the nipple valve (about 2 inches), which controls the retention of waste matter. Gently push the catheter a little further into the ileal pouch. At the same time, exhale, cough, or bear down as if to pass stool until fecal material begins to drain.
● Direct the external end of the catheter into a basin or the toilet about 12 inches below the stoma.
● If the catheter is obstructed, try the following measures:
  ● Bear down as if to have a bowel movement.
  ● Rotate the catheter tip inside the stoma.
  ● Milk the catheter.
  ● If these are not successful, remove the catheter, rinse it, and try again.
  ● Notify the physician if efforts to unblock the catheter do not result in any drainage.
  ● Never wait longer than 6 hours without obtaining drainage.
● Allow 5 to 10 minutes for drainage to cease; then remove the catheter, clean it with soapy water, and store it in a sealable plastic bag until needed again.
● Wash the area around the stoma and pat the skin dry.
● Place an absorbent pad or dressing over the stoma.

---

ileostomy with total colectomy, preserves innervation to the male genitalia. Subsequently, the male client is unlikely to experience bladder dysfunction, erectile dysfunction, or infertility.

Surgical Management

An ileoanal anastomosis is performed in two stages. In the first stage, the surgeon creates a temporary ileostomy, removes a large length of diseased colon down to the terminal section of the rectum above the anal sphincter, joins several distal loops of healthy ileum to form a pouch for holding stool, and connects the ileal reservoir to the anal cuff. After the first stage of surgery, clients experience an almost continuous discharge of mucus from the anus and a frequent discharge of fecal material from the ileostomy. Initially, clients cannot control the frequent watery discharge.

The second stage is performed 2 or 3 months later. At this time, the surgeon closes the temporary ileostomy and reunites the two sections of ileum. The area where the two sections of bowel are joined is called an *anastomosis.* The anastomosis establishes a normal flow of fecal material through the ileum to the reservoir. The fecal material, which is stored in the ileal reservoir, is then expelled from the anus.

Control is achieved as edema subsides and the anal sphincter becomes stronger.

Nursing Management

The preoperative assessment of a client having an ileoanal reservoir (both stages) is essentially the same as for the client with an ileostomy. The postoperative assessment after the first stage of ileoanal reservoir surgery includes making the same observations and assessments as those for an ileostomy. In addition, the nurse inspects the anal area for drainage and checks the drain or drainage tube in the presacral area if there is one. After the second stage, when the ileostomy is closed and the ileum is connected to the anal reservoir, the nurse inspects the anal area and the operative sites for drainage.

The postoperative plan of nursing care involves measures pertaining to general surgery and related client problems, such as risk for fluid volume deficit, risk for bowel incontinence, and impaired perianal skin integrity (refer to Nursing Process for the Client Recovering From Ileostomy Surgery). To reduce the risk for bowel incontinence, the nurse instructs the client to perform perineal exercises to reestablish anal sphincter control and enlarge the ileoanal reservoir. These exercises involve tightening the anus as if trying to prevent a bowel movement and holding the contraction for a count of 10 before relaxing. The nurse should urge the client to do 10 repetitions of this exercise four to six times a day.

Keeping the perianal area clean is especially important. After first-stage ileoanal surgery, the nurse teaches the client to use a squirt bottle to clean the perianal area and avoid skin irritation. After the second-stage repair, the nurse instructs the client to cleanse the anus with warm, soapy water to remove mucus, stool, or both. The client also must dry the area well. Refer to Client and Family Teaching 48-4 for information that the nurse teaches the client and family.

Client and Family Teaching 48-4
Postoperative Ileoanal Reservoir Care

The nurse discusses the following issues with the client and his or her family:

● Continue performing perineal strengthening exercises daily.
● Apply protective ointments or creams as recommended by the physician.
● Inspect the anal area daily using a hand-held mirror.
● Contact physician if the anal area becomes sore or skin changes (e.g., ulceration, bleeding) are apparent.
● Use a thin sanitary shield or disposable, lined underwear to absorb fecal drainage until anal sphincter control is achieved.

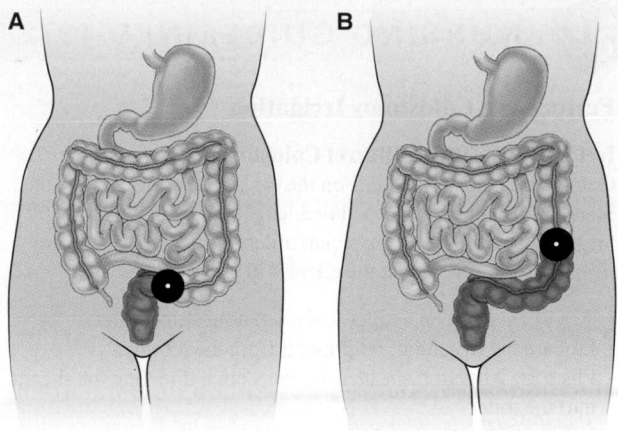

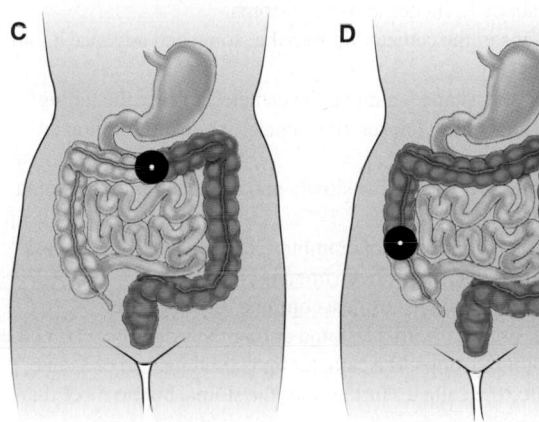

FIGURE 48-5. Placement of colostomies, with shaded areas representing the sections of the bowel that have been removed or are currently inactive: (**A**) Sigmoid colostomy—feces are solid. (**B**) Descending colostomy—feces are semi-mushy. (**C**) Transverse colostomy—feces are mushy. (**D**) Ascending colostomy—feces are fluid.

COLOSTOMY

A colostomy is an opening in the large bowel created by bringing a section of the large intestine out to the abdomen and fashioning a stoma. A cancerous lesion, an ulcerative inflammatory process, multiple polyposis (condition of numerous polyps), and traumatic injury to the bowel are indications for a colostomy.

Types of colostomies are described according to their placement. A temporary or permanent colostomy may be created in the sigmoid, descending, transverse, or ascending areas of the colon (Fig. 48-5). The consistency of the fecal material ranges from semiliquid to formed depending on the intestinal area from which the colostomy is formed (see Table 48-1). Regular irrigations may control a sigmoid colostomy, and sometimes a descending colostomy, thus eliminating the need for the client to constantly wear an appliance (Nursing Guidelines 48-2).

The stoma may be found anywhere from the lower right, center, to middle or lower left positions on the abdomen. The terms *single-barrel, double-barrel,* and *loop* are used to describe the appearance of the colostomy.

Surgical Management

Single-Barrel Colostomy

The term **single-barrel colostomy** indicates that the ostomy has a single stoma through which fecal matter passes. The colon is cut above the diseased area, and the healthy end is brought through the abdominal wall to form the matured stoma. The diseased portion of the bowel is removed, with the remaining distal end closed for later reconnection (**segmental resection**). For tumors in the lower third of the sigmoid, that portion, the rectum, and anus may be surgically removed through a perineal incision in a procedure referred to as an **abdominoperineal resection**. After performing an abdominoperineal resection, the surgeon leaves a drain or pack in the perineal area for about 1 week, after which it is removed and irrigations of the perineal wound may be ordered.

Double-Barrel Colostomy

A **double-barrel colostomy**, which is performed most often in the transverse section of the large intestine, contains both a proximal and distal stoma. Each stoma is everted and sutured in place. The proximal stoma expels the fecal material. The distal stoma leads from the lower portion of the cut bowel to the anus. Because fecal drainage has been diverted, the distal portion of the bowel does not pass feces. The distal stoma and the anus may expel mucus. When a double-barrel colostomy has been performed, the physician is asked to identify the distal and proximal stomas. A diagram is provided in the medical record, and the nurse may duplicate it on the nursing care plan. This information is essential when assessing bowel function and whether irrigations are required. Irrigation may be ordered for both the proximal and distal portions of the bowel or for the proximal portion only.

A double-barrel colostomy often is temporary and usually performed to rest a portion of the bowel to treat a disorder such as acute diverticulitis, chronic constipation, or inflammatory bowel disease. The interval before reestablishing the continuity of the bowel may be 16 months or longer. When the diseased portion of the bowel is removed or

NURSING GUIDELINES 48-2

Performing Colostomy Irrigation

Irrigation for Single-Barrel Colostomy

Colostomy irrigation begins on the 4th or 5th postoperative day. Standard irrigation is a scheduled irrigation, using 500 to 1500 mL tepid water. Check physician orders. Try to use colostomy irrigation equipment that the client will use at home.

- Ask client to sit on a toilet seat or chair near the toilet.
- Prepare the irrigation, purging air from the tubing.
- Place the irrigation sheath over the stoma, directing the sheath into the toilet.
- Lubricate the distal end of the catheter.
- Hang the container of irrigant so that the bottom of the solution bag is about 12 inches above the stoma.
- Gently insert the catheter tip into the stoma and advance it 2 to 3 inches (Fig. A).
- If there is resistance, remove the catheter, release the tubing clamp, and gently reinsert the catheter while the solution is flowing.
- Allow the irrigant to flow slowly and gradually into the stoma (Fig. B).
- If the client complains of cramping, clamp the tubing and ask the client to take a few deep breaths.
- Once the cramping subsides, continue the irrigation.
- If water escapes from the stoma during the irrigation, clamp the tubing until it stops. If a catheter tip is used instead of a cone, introduce the catheter further into the stoma, but no more than 6 inches.
- When the prescribed amount of solution is instilled, remove the catheter. The client may remain sitting or walk around (clamp the distal end of the irrigation sheath). Complete drainage usually takes 30 minutes.
- If the irrigant fails to return properly, gently massage the lower abdomen or have the client take several deep breaths and relax or reposition his or her body. Notify the physician if these measures do not work.
- Document the procedure, including the amount of irrigant used, appearance of returns, and client's response.

Irrigation for Double-Barrel Colostomy

If the client has a double-barrel colostomy, irrigate the proximal stoma in the same manner as a single-barrel colostomy. To irrigate the distal stoma, try the following:

- Have the client sit on a toilet or a bedpan, because the irrigation fluid and a small amount of mucus will leave by way of the anus. During the immediate postoperative period, necrotic tissue also may be expelled.
- Use a bulb syringe (Fig. C), short catheter, container of solution, plastic sheath or apron, and an emesis basin as another technique for irrigation. This method calls for several instillations of 250 to 500 mL solution at a time, sometimes twice a day. Some clients have found this method effective for controlling spillage for 24 hours or more. It may be used as an alternate choice when the standard method cannot be used.

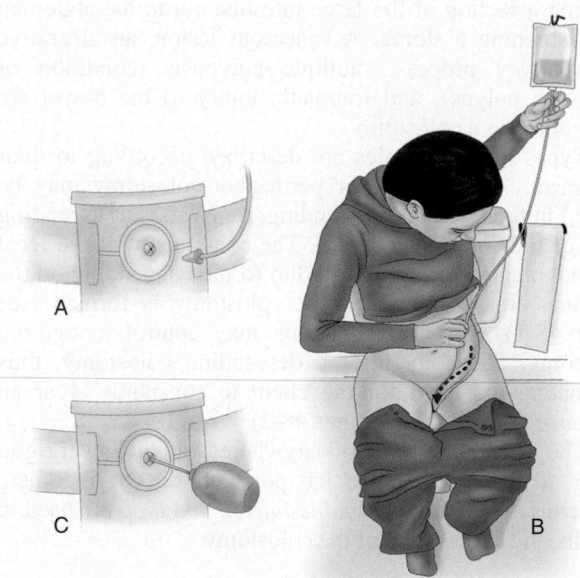

(**A**) Irrigating catheter has a cone attachment to prevent injury to stomal tissue. (**B**) Irrigating fluid is instilled with sleeve in place; drainage empties into toilet. (**C**) A bulb syringe method may be used to stimulate fecal drainage.

---

healed, the bowel is reconnected and functions normally. In the meantime, the stoma may need irrigation or alternative methods for regulating bowel elimination (Box 48-1).

> ### ▶ Stop, Think, and Respond Exercise 48-1
>
> *A client calls the physician's office 4 months after a double-barrel colostomy. He tells the triage nurse that the stool is more liquid than usual and that he is emptying the pouch every 4 hours. What questions does the triage nurse need to ask?*

Loop Colostomy

A **loop colostomy** indicates that a loop of bowel has been lifted through the abdomen and is supported in place with a glass rod or plastic butterfly device. About 24 to 72 hours after surgery, the anterior wall of the loop is opened at the client's bedside or in a treatment room, either by incising the bowel or using a cautery machine to form the stoma. The posterior wall of the bowel is left intact, which results in a proximal and distal opening to the bowel.

By delaying the opening of the intestinal loop, the initial healing of the incision occurs without danger of

BOX 48-1   Regulating Bowel Elimination Without Irrigating

Some ostomates learn to regulate bowel elimination without irrigating frequently. The following tips may be encouraging to new ostomates, who may be able to establish regular elimination patterns.

- Insert a suppository, such as glycerin or bisacodyl (Dulcolax), into the stoma. The suppository should be recommended by the physician. Up to 7 days or more of daily use may be needed before a regular elimination pattern is established. Initially movements may occur three or four times daily, but each day movements should decrease until only one or two movements occur daily.

Other methods to stimulate bowel elimination and a regular schedule include:

- Drinking prune or fruit juice.
- Eating fiber-rich foods and dried fruits and performing mild exercise.
- Using a stool softener, mineral oil, or milk of magnesia if recommended by the physician

Nutrition Notes 48-1
The Client With an Ostomy

For both colostomy and ileostomy clients:

- Fiber is restricted after ostomy surgery to prevent irritation and slow transit time until healing is complete. Thereafter, small amounts of foods containing fiber are added individually to the diet so that the client's tolerance can be evaluated. Foods not tolerated initially may be reintroduced weeks or months later. Most clients resume a normal diet within 6 weeks after surgery.
- The primary nutrition concerns are fluids and electrolytes. Eight to 10 cups of fluid are recommended daily. Reassure the client that extra fluids do not contribute to watery stools but are excreted as urine. Fluid restriction should not be used to control liquid feces. Sodium and potassium requirements may increase because of increased losses.
- Eating small, frequent meals at regular times is recommended. Eating a large meal in the middle of the day instead of in the evening may help decrease stool output at night.
- Clients should take small bites of food and chew food thoroughly.
- Foods that may help decrease odor include buttermilk, parsley, yogurt, kefir, and cranberry juice. Odor-causing foods include dried peas and beans, fish, eggs, onion, garlic, vegetables from the cabbage family, asparagus, beer, and other alcoholic beverages.
- Banana flakes, applesauce, pasta, potatoes, smooth peanut butter, and cheese may help thicken stools.
- Because they may cause obstruction, nuts, corn, cabbage, coconut, dried fruit, unpeeled apples, and grapes should be avoided.

For colostomy clients:

- Eventually, a high-fiber diet may improve stool consistency and regularity in clients with a colostomy. Increase fiber gradually.

For clients with an ileostomy:

- Lactose intolerance may occur.
- Limit liquids with meals if output is high.
- Oral rehydration formulas, such as Gatorade, may help maintain fluid and electrolyte balance.

---

contamination. Opening the bowel does not cause any discomfort because the bowel lacks pain receptors. When a loop colostomy is opened, the bed and client's clothing are well protected. Preparing the client for the pungent odor of cauterized tissue, which subsides shortly, and the initial gush of fecal material is important. A temporary ostomy pouch initially is used to receive the flow of liquid feces.

Nursing Management

Preoperative nursing management is similar to that for clients having an ileostomy. Because a colostomy may be performed for cancer of the colon or rectum, however, the client may be more anxious about the procedure. Postoperative cancer treatment options also may serve to increase the client's anxiety. Nurses and/or dieticians will review postoperative dietary restrictions and expectations (Nutrition Notes 48-1).

Nursing Process for the Client Following Colostomy Surgery

Assessment

After the client returns from surgery, assessments include taking vital signs, checking dressings, and monitoring nasogastric tubes and IV infusions. Review the client's chart for the type of colostomy and the location of the stoma(s). If an abdominoperineal resection was performed, check the drain or packing in the perineal area and note the characteristics of the drainage.

Monitor vital signs every 4 hours or as ordered. Take the client's temperature by a route other than rectal. Report a sudden elevation in temperature over 101°F (38.3°C) or an increase in pain and abdominal tenderness or distention to the physician immediately. Also, check the surgical dressing frequently in the early postoperative period and observe the characteristics of the stoma. Monitor urine output and the volume of suctioned gastric secre-

tions. If urine output is markedly decreased or less than 500 mL/day, inform the physician immediately.

Diagnosis, Planning, and Interventions

Perform standard postsurgical measures to maintain the airway and relieve pain and anxiety. Also, perform nasogastric decompression (see Chap. 45) and monitor fluid and electrolyte status. It may be necessary to measure fluids lost through decompression and replace them with additional IV fluids. An indwelling catheter may be used to relieve abdominal pressure and prevent urine retention during the first few days after surgery.

Client and Family Teaching 48-5 Postoperative Colostomy Care

The nurse emphasizes the following points when teaching the client and his or her family:

- Inspect the stoma for changes in appearance. Changes in the size and color of the stoma vary with activity and emotional status. Anger or extreme annoyance may cause the stoma to turn red or purple. Small beads of blood may ooze from the surface. Fright may cause the stoma to blanch. These reactions are normal and insignificant as long as the tissues revert to their normal state when the cause is alleviated.
- Eat a regular diet, but avoid gas-forming foods to control intestinal gas.
- If experiencing problems with constipation, increase fiber in the diet and drink extra water—these measures generally correct the problem.
- Eliminate food items that result in diarrhea. This may help to control the problem because diarrhea may be related to diet. Characteristics of diarrhea include both increased stool output and liquid nature of the stool. One or two loose stools per day do not necessarily indicate a problem. If diarrhea persists for more than 2 days, contact the physician.
- Eat slowly with the mouth closed and chew food well to decrease gas that results chiefly from swallowing air rather than from digestion.

- With the exception of tight clothing, do not alter preferences in clothing. If you require firm support (e.g., wear girdles or braces, have back problems), find a stoma shield that is helpful in preventing irritation or undue pressure on the stoma.
- Check body weight weekly. Contact physician if there is a sudden weight loss or gain.
- Perform irrigations at approximately the same time each day. The best time to irrigate is after a meal because food in the digestive tract stimulates peristalsis and defecation.
- The physician may recommend that the schedule for irrigations gradually progress to every other day, every third day, or even twice a week. If constipation occurs, contact physician regarding a change in the irrigation schedule.
- Do not restrict travel or activities outside the home. Changes in stool pattern may be normal when daily routines change. Preassembled kits that contain all materials needed for irrigation and changes of the colostomy appliance are available. If traveling by air, take ostomy supplies in carry-on luggage to prevent their loss if luggage is misdirected or lost. Necessary items also may be assembled individually and placed in waterproof containers.

Teach how to care for the colostomy by demonstrating the irrigating procedure and, if possible, outlining nonirrigation methods for keeping the ostomy patent and establishing a regular pattern of bowel elimination. The time between the use of these methods and eventual regularity is unique to each client. Natural methods are the least predictable for regulating the bowel, but many clients learn to recognize subtle clues that the bowel will be moving. They then have sufficient time to reach a bathroom and eliminate in private.

In addition, demonstrate skin and stoma care and appliance application and removal. To provide ample learning time, divide material that the client must learn into small units. After demonstrating one aspect of care, have the client return the demonstration. When the client feels self-confident, add additional material. Reinforce verbal information and demonstrated skills with printed material that may be available from ostomy associations or the enterostomal therapy nurse. Finally, arrange a dietary consultation to discuss nutrition and food modifications. Client and Family Teaching 48-5 outlines important teaching for the client with a colostomy.

▶ **Risk for Bowel Incontinence** related to unpredictable bowel elimination pattern

▶ **Expected Outcome:** Client will not experience accidental soiling.

- Instruct the client how to keep the ostomy appliance intact. *Proper application prevents accidental soiling.*
- Schedule colostomy irrigation or suppository insertion for a descending or sigmoid colostomy. *These measures assist with maintaining predictable bowel elimination.*

▶ **Risk for Diarrhea or Constipation** related to changes in bowel motility

▶ **Expected Outcome:** Client will maintain expected consistency of feces according to location of the colostomy.

Diarrhea

- Instruct client to keep a record of food intake, noting time of problems with loose stools or diarrhea. *A food record helps identify specific foods that irritate the GI tract.*
- Inform client about the need to reduce or eliminate offending foods. *Such information helps prevent diarrhea.*
- Teach client to report prolonged problems with increased stool volume, watery stool consistency, nausea, vomiting, or abdominal pain to the physician. *Ostomates can experience gastroenteritis.*

Constipation

- Gently dilate the stoma with a lubricated-gloved finger. *Dilation assists with expelling stool.*
- Advise client to increase fluid intake. *Increased intake will add fluid to stool, making it easier to pass.*
- Encourage client to eat regular meals. *Dieting or fasting can decrease stool volume and slow elimination.*
- Provide high-fiber, nonirritating foods. *Such foods increase stool bulk and moisture.*
- Offer foods such as coffee or stewed prunes. *These foods promote elimination.*
- Consult with physician if preceding measures fail. *Client may benefit from irrigation, suppository, or laxative.*

Evaluation of Expected Outcomes

The client reports a predictable stool pattern and no problems with soiling. Stool consistency is as expected, and the client has not had constipation or diarrhea.   ●

CRITICAL THINKING EXERCISES

1. In what ways does the care of a 20-year-old client with an ileostomy differ from that of a 60-year-old client with a colostomy?

2. A client with an ileostomy is disturbed by having to empty liquid stool from his appliance frequently. He intends to reduce his intake of fluids. What information is important to give this client?

3. What recommendations are appropriate for the client with a colostomy who has been experiencing an unusual amount of intestinal gas?

4. Discharge is planned for a client with a new colostomy. He tells the nurse that when he gets home he will just drink liquids and avoid solid food until the colostomy is working more normally. What should the nurse teach this client?

NCLEX-STYLE REVIEW QUESTIONS

1. Why should a nurse ensure that a client with an ostomy discontinues immunosuppressive agents 3 to 4 weeks before surgery?
  1. To minimize the risk of bleeding during surgery
  2. To control effects on tissue healing after surgery
  3. To prevent adrenal insufficiency after surgery
  4. To avoid cleansing of the bowel during surgery

2. Which of the following nursing interventions would be most likely to initially help a client with an ileostomy cope effectively with body changes?

  1. Provide detailed written instructions about ileostomy care.
  2. Involve family members when providing ileostomy teaching.
  3. Set realistic goals with client to approach the ileostomy.
  4. Reassure the client that the changes are common and temporary.

3. The care plan for the client with the colectomy includes providing measures for caring for the ileostomy that was created at the time of surgery. When implementing the plan of care, the best time of day to perform stomal care and change the appliance is after the client does which of the following?
  1. Awakens in the morning
  2. Has showered after breakfast
  3. Has been ambulating in the hall
  4. Finishes the evening meal

4. A client with bowel obstruction is scheduled for a laparotomy, possible colon resection, and temporary colostomy. A few days after surgery, the physician orders daily colostomy irrigations. Which position is best to place the client when irrigating the colostomy?
  1. Kneeling in the bathtub
  2. Lying on the left side
  3. Sitting on the toilet
  4. Standing at the sink

5. During a conversation concerning the client's feelings about a colostomy, the client says to the nurse, "How will I ever adjust to this colostomy?" Which nursing response is most appropriate at this time?
  1. Say nothing, but quote her statement in the chart
  2. Encourage the client to express her concerns
  3. Reassure her that adjustment will come with time
  4. Recommend she investigate care in a nursing home

UNIT 12
Caring for Clients with Endocrine Disorders

49

Introduction to the Endocrine System

Words To Know

adenohypophysis
adrenal cortex
adrenal glands
adrenal medulla
adrenocorticotropic hormone
antidiuretic hormone
calcitonin
corticosteroids
estrogen
feedback loop
follicle-stimulating hormone
glucagon
glycogenolysis
hormones
hypophysis
hypothalamus
insulin
islets of Langerhans
luteinizing hormone
melatonin
neurohypophysis
nuclear scan
ovaries
oxytocin
pancreas
parathormone
parathyroid glands
pineal gland
pituitary gland
progesterone
prolactin
radioimmunoassay
radionuclide
somatostatin
somatotropin
testes
testosterone
tetraiodothyronine
thymopoietin

Learning Objectives

On completion of this chapter, you will be able to:

1. Identify the chief function of the endocrine glands.
2. Describe the general function of hormones.
3. Explain the relationship between the hypothalamus and the pituitary gland.
4. Discuss the regulation of levels of hormones.
5. List endocrine glands and the hormones they secrete.
6. Name other organs that are not classified as endocrine glands but secrete hormones.
7. Outline information to include when taking the health history of a client with an endocrine disorder.
8. Describe physical assessment findings that suggest an endocrine disorder.
9. List examples of laboratory and diagnostic tests that identify endocrine disorders.
10. Discuss the nursing management of clients undergoing diagnostic tests to detect endocrine dysfunction.

The endocrine glands (Fig. 49-1) secrete **hormones,** chemicals that accelerate or slow physiologic processes, directly into the bloodstream. This characteristic distinguishes endocrine glands from exocrine glands, which release secretions into a duct. Hormones circulate in the blood until they reach receptors in target cells or other endocrine glands. They play a vital role in regulating homeostatic processes such as:

- Metabolism
- Growth
- Fluid and electrolyte balance
- Reproductive processes
- Sleep and wake cycles

Table 49-1 presents an overview of the hormones involved in the endocrine system.

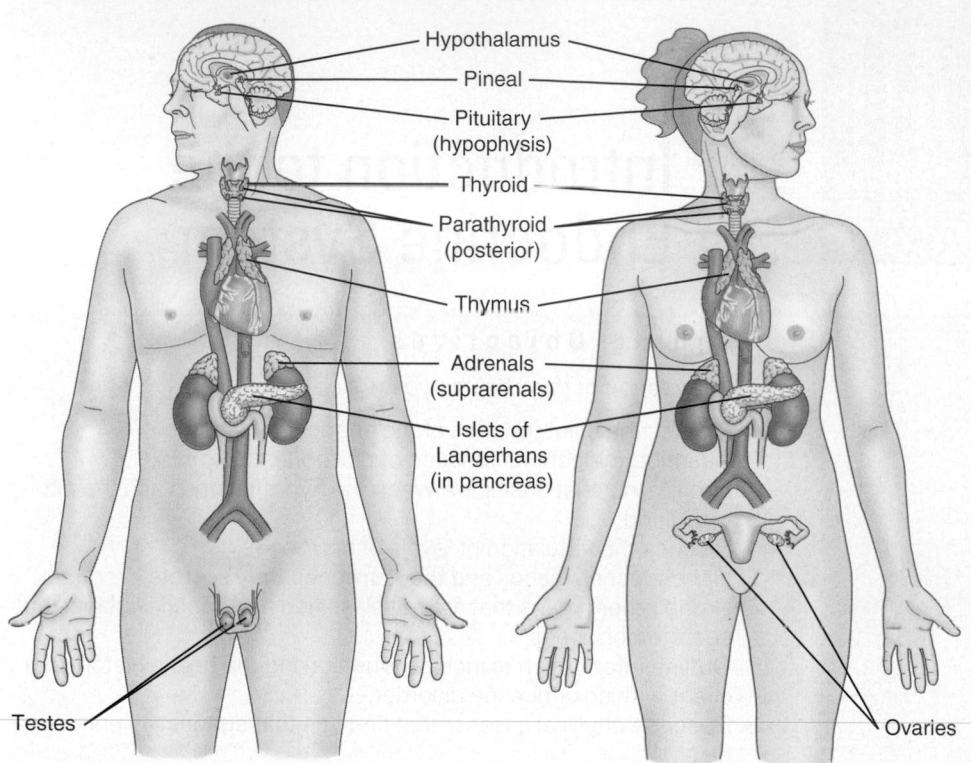

FIGURE 49-1. The glands of the endocrine system.

Labels: Hypothalamus, Pineal, Pituitary (hypophysis), Thyroid, Parathyroid (posterior), Thymus, Adrenals (suprarenals), Islets of Langerhans (in pancreas), Testes, Ovaries

---

▶ **Stop, Think, and Respond Exercise 49-1**

Give examples of hormones that affect metabolism, growth, fluid and electrolyte balance, reproductive processes, and sleep and wake cycles.

ANATOMY AND PHYSIOLOGY

Pituitary Gland

Many endocrine glands respond to stimulation from the **pituitary gland** (or **hypophysis**), which is connected by a stalk to the **hypothalamus** in the brain (Fig. 49-2). The pituitary is divided into three lobes: the anterior lobe (**adenohypophysis**), intermediate lobe (pars intermedia), and posterior lobe (**neurohypophysis**). The pituitary gland is called the *master gland* because it regulates the function of other endocrine glands. The term is somewhat misleading, however, because the hypothalamus influences the pituitary gland.

Hypothalamus

The hypothalamus, a portion of the brain between the cerebrum and the brain stem, projects down toward the pituitary gland. This creates a pathway for neurohormones, also known as releasing hormones or factors, that stimulate and inhibit secretions from the anterior and posterior lobes of the pituitary gland. Under the influence of the hypothalamus, the lobes of the pituitary gland secrete various hormones (Fig. 49-3).

So far, six hypothalamic hormones have been identified:

- Thyrotropin-releasing hormone (TRH), which stimulates the release of **thyroid-stimulating hormone** (TSH) from the anterior pituitary gland
- Corticotropin-releasing hormone (CRH), which causes the anterior pituitary gland to secrete **adrenocorticotropic hormone** (ACTH)
- Gonadotropin-releasing hormone (GnRH), which triggers sexual development at the onset of puberty and continues to cause the anterior pituitary gland to secrete **luteinizing hormone** (LH) and **follicle-stimulating hormone** (FSH)

TABLE 49-1 Endocrine Hormones

GLAND	HORMONE RELEASED	HORMONE FUNCTION	HORMONE REGULATOR
Posterior pituitary	Antidiuretic hormone (ADH)	Increases water absorption from kidneys; raises blood pressure	Hypothalamic secretions, blood osmolarity
	Oxytocin	Stimulates contraction of pregnant uterus and release of breast milk after childbirth	Hypothalamic secretions, uterine stretch, suckling
Anterior pituitary	Somatotropin (growth hormone)	Stimulates bone and muscle growth; promotes protein synthesis and fat mobilization	Hypothalamic secretions
	Prolactin	Promotes production and secretion of milk after childbirth	Hypothalamic hormones
	Thyroid-stimulating hormone (TSH)	Stimulates production and secretion of thyroid hormones	Blood thyroxine levels; hypothalamic secretions
	Adrenocorticotropic hormone (ACTH)	Stimulates adrenal cortex to secrete cortisol and other steroids	Corticotropin-releasing hormone (CRH) from the hypothalamus; blood cortisol levels
	Luteinizing hormone (LH) in females and interstitial cell–stimulating hormone (ICSH) in males	Initiates ovulation and the secretion of sex hormones in both genders	Hypothalamic secretions, estrogen and testosterone levels
	Follicle-stimulating hormone (FSH)	Stimulates development of ovum in ovaries and sperm in testes	Hypothalamic secretions, progesterone
Thyroid	Tetraiodothyronine (thyroxine or T_4) and triiodothyronine or (T_3)	Increases oxygen consumption and heat production; stimulates, increases, and maintains metabolic processes	TSH regulated by thyrotropin-releasing hormone (TRH) from the hypothalamus
	Calcitonin	Inhibits calcium release from bone, thus lowering blood calcium levels	Blood calcium concentrations
Parathyroids	Parathyroid hormone (PTH)	Increases blood calcium by stimulating calcium release from bone; decreases blood phosphate level	Calcium concentrations in blood
Thymus	Several thymosin and thymopoietin hormones; thymic humoral factor; thymostimulin; factor thymic serum	Stimulates T-cell development in thymus and maintenance in other lymph tissue; involved in some B cells developing into antibody-producing plasma cells	Not known
Pineal gland	Melatonin	Involved in circadian rhythms; antigonadotropic effect induces sleep	Exposure to light-dark cycles; darkness stimulates release and light diminishes release
Adrenal medulla	Epinephrine (adrenaline)	Constricts blood vessels in skin, kidneys, and gut, which increases blood supply to heart, brain, and skeletal muscles, leads to increased heart rate and blood pressure; stimulates smooth muscle contraction; raises blood glucose levels	Sympathetic nervous system
	Norepinephrine	Constricts blood vessels; increases heart rate and contraction of cardiac muscles; increases metabolic rate	Sympathetic nervous system
Adrenal cortex	Corticosteroids:		
	Glucocorticoids	Regulates blood glucose by affecting carbohydrate metabolism; affects growth; decreases effects of stress and anti-inflammatory agents	ACTH; stress and serum electrolyte concentrations
	Mineralocorticoids (mainly aldosterone)	Regulate sodium, water, and potassium excretion by the kidneys	Renin and angiotensin
	Gonadocorticoids (mainly androgens—male sex hormones)	Contribute to secondary sex characteristics (greater androgenic effect in women after menopause)	ACTH
Pancreas (islets of Langerhans)	Insulin	Lowers blood sugar; increases glycogen storage in liver; stimulates protein synthesis	Blood glucose concentrations

(table continues on page 750)

TABLE 49-1 Endocrine Hormones (continued)

GLAND	HORMONE RELEASED	HORMONE FUNCTION	HORMONE REGULATOR
	Glucagon	Stimulates glycogen breakdown in liver; increases blood sugar (glucose) concentration	Blood glucose and amino acid concentration
Ovary follicle	Estrogens	Develop and maintain female sex organs and characteristics; initiates building of uterine lining	FSH and LH
Ovary (corpus luteum)	Progesterone and estrogens	Influences breast development and menstrual cycles; promotes growth and differentiation of uterine lining; maintains pregnancy	FSH
Testes	Androgens (mainly testosterone)	Develop and maintain male sex organs and characteristics; aid sperm production.	FSH and ICSH

Adapted from Campbell, N. A., & Reece, J. B. (2008). *Biology* (8th ed.). Redwood City, CA: Benjamin Cummings.

- Growth hormone–releasing hormone (GHRH), which results in the release of **somatotropin** (growth hormone [GH]) from the anterior pituitary gland. GHRH secretion is controlled by another hypothalamic hormone, **somatostatin**, which is also secreted by other tissues outside the hypothalamus such as the pancreas.
- Somatostatin, which inhibits GHRH and TSH and also blocks the secretion of several gastrointestinal hormones, including gastrin, cholecystokinin, and secretin; lowers the blood flow within the intestine; suppresses the release of insulin and glucagon from the pancreas; and suppresses the release of exocrine enzymes from the pancreas.
- Hypothalamic dopamine, which inhibits the release of **prolactin** from the anterior pituitary gland. (Dopamine, of which there are five variants, is produced in several structures within the brain, one of which is the hypothalamus.)

Pharmacologic Considerations

- Somatostatin and octreotide (Sandostatin), a drug that mimics the actions of somatostatin, have been used to reduce gastrointestinal bleeding. Clients treated with this form of drug therapy require fewer blood transfusions compared with those managed with other drugs affecting gastrointestinal function (Tomagno et al., 2004).

- Following delivery of a newborn, a dopamine antagonist such as metoclopramide (Reglan) may be prescribed to the mother to stimulate the production of breast milk.

Hormone Regulation

A feedback loop controls hormone levels. A **feedback loop** is a mechanism that turns hormone production off and on to keep concentrations of hormones within a stable range at all times (Fig. 49-4). Feedback can be either negative or positive. Most hormones are secreted in response to negative feedback; a decrease in levels stimulates the releasing gland; in positive feedback, the opposite occurs. Most endocrine disorders result from overproduction or underproduction of specific hormones.

Thyroid Gland

The **thyroid gland** is located in the lower neck anterior to the trachea (Fig. 49-5). It is divided into two lateral lobes joined by a band of tissue called the *isthmus*. The thyroid concentrates iodine from food and uses it to synthesize **tetraiodothyronine** (thyroxine or T_4) and **triiodothyronine** (T_3). These two hormones regulate the body's metabolic rate. **Calcitonin**, another thyroid hormone, inhibits the release of calcium from bone into the extracellular fluid. A rise in the serum calcium level stimulates the release of calcitonin from the thyroid gland.

Parathyroid Glands

The **parathyroid glands** are four (some people have more than four) small, bean-shaped bodies, each surrounded by a capsule of connective tissue and embedded within the lateral lobes of the thyroid (Fig. 49-6). The upper parathyroids are found posteriorly at the junction of the upper and middle thirds of the thyroid. The lower parathyroids typically lie among the branches of the inferior thyroid artery. They secrete **parathormone**, which increases the level of calcium in the blood when there is a decrease in the serum level. Parathormone does so by (1) causing calcium and phosphorus to be released from bones; (2) interfering with the urinary excretion of calcium, but promoting the urinary excretion of

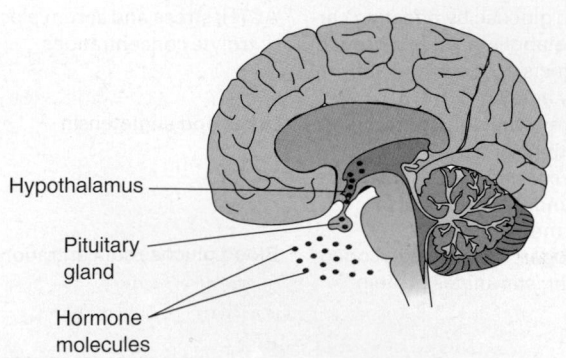

FIGURE 49-2. The hypothalamus regulates pituitary activity.

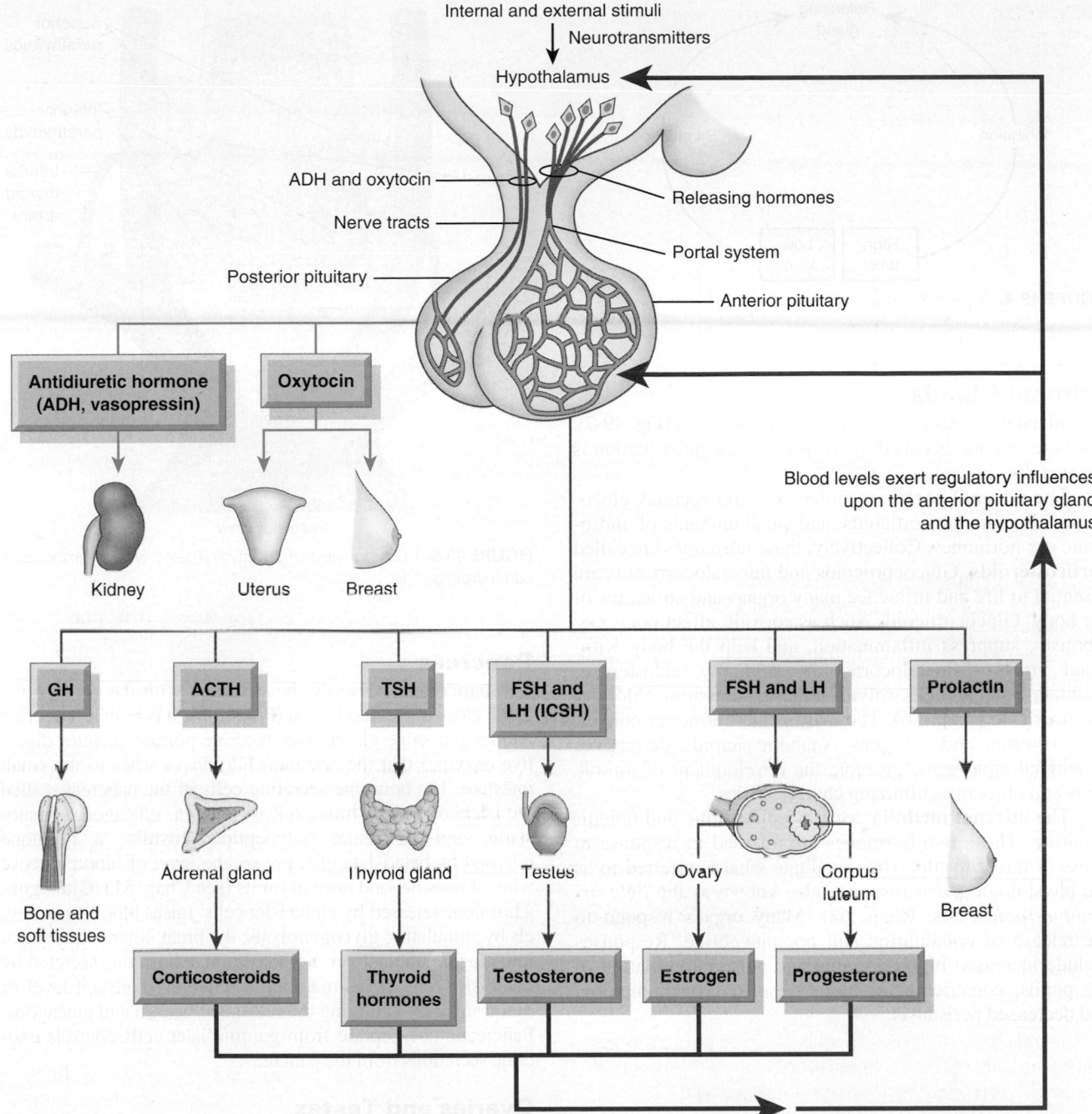

Internal and external stimuli

Neurotransmitters

Hypothalamus

ADH and oxytocin

Nerve tracts

Releasing hormones

Portal system

Posterior pituitary

Anterior pituitary

Blood levels exert regulatory influences
upon the anterior pituitary gland
and the hypothalamus

**Antidiuretic hormone
(ADH, vasopressin)**

Oxytocin

Kidney

Uterus

Breast

GH

ACTH

TSH

**FSH and
LH (ICSH)**

FSH and LH

Prolactin

Bone and
soft tissues

Adrenal gland

Thyroid gland

Testes

Ovary

Corpus
luteum

Breast

Corticosteroids

**Thyroid
hormones**

Testosterone

Estrogen

Progesterone

FIGURE 49-3. The pituitary gland, the relationship of the brain to pituitary action, and the hormones secreted by the anterior and posterior pituitary.

phosphorus; and (3) activating vitamin D, which causes an increase in calcium absorption within the intestine.

Thymus Gland

The **thymus gland** is located in the upper part of the chest above or near the heart. It secretes **thymosin** and **thymopoietin**, which aid in developing T lymphocytes, a type of white blood cell involved in immunity (see Chap. 33). The thymus gland is large during childhood but usually shrinks by adulthood. Despite its reduced size, the thymus gland

continues to support the production of T lymphocytes, but the rate of production decreases with age. Functional disorders of the gland are rare.

Pineal Gland

The **pineal gland** is attached to the thalamus in the brain. It secretes **melatonin**, which aids in regulating sleep cycles and mood (see Chap. 69). Melatonin is believed to play a role in hypothalamic-pituitary interaction.

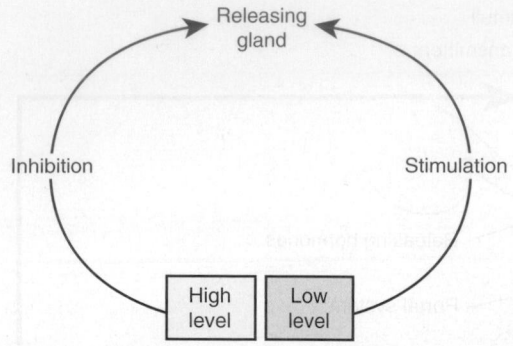

FIGURE 49-4. A feedback loop regulates hormone levels.

Adrenal Glands

The **adrenal glands** are located above the kidneys (Fig. 49-7). The outer portion is called the *cortex,* and the inner portion is the *medulla.*

The **adrenal cortex** manufactures and secretes gluco-corticoids, mineralocorticoids, and small amounts of andro-genic sex hormones. Collectively, these hormones are called **corticosteroids.** Glucocorticoids and mineralocorticoids are essential to life and influence many organs and structures of the body. Glucocorticoids, such as cortisol, affect body me-tabolism, suppress inflammation, and help the body with-stand stress. Mineralocorticoids, primarily aldosterone, maintain water and electrolyte (sodium, potassium, chloride) balances (see Chap. 16). The androgenic hormones convert to testosterone and estrogens. Anabolic steroids, derivatives of adrenal androgens, promote the development of muscle mass and other masculinizing characteristics.

The **adrenal medulla** secretes epinephrine and norepi-nephrine. These two hormones are released in response to stress or threat to life. They facilitate what is referred to as the physiologic stress response also known as the *fight-or-flight response* (see Chap. 67). Many organs respond to the release of epinephrine and norepinephrine. Responses include increased blood pressure and pulse rate, dilation of the pupils, constriction of blood vessels, bronchodilation, and decreased peristalsis.

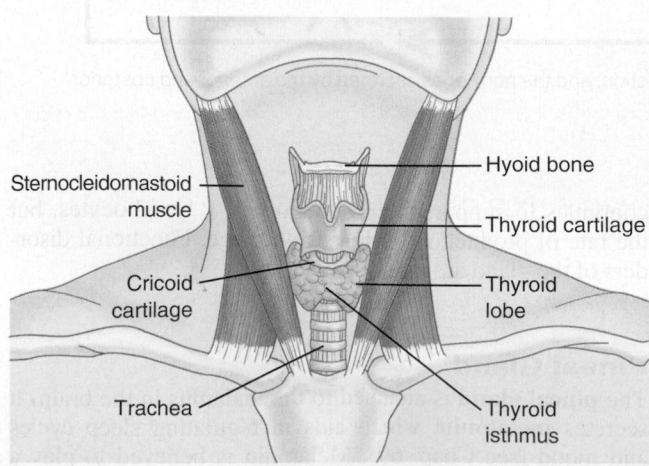

FIGURE 49-5. The thyroid gland and surrounding structures.

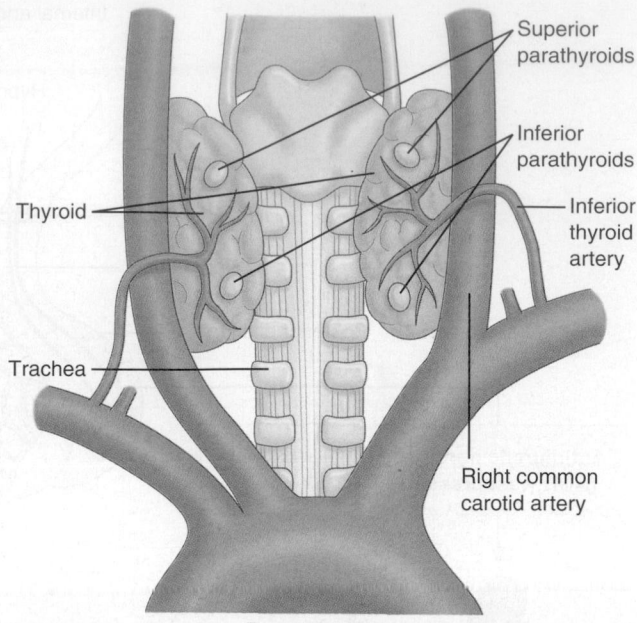

Posterior view

FIGURE 49-6. Posterior view of the thyroid gland with the imbedded parathyroid glands.

Pancreas

The **pancreas** lies below the stomach, with the head of the gland close to the duodenum (Fig. 49-8). It is both an exocrine and an endocrine gland. The exocrine portion secretes diges-tive enzymes that the common bile duct carries to the small intestine. The hormone-secreting cells of the pancreas, called the **islets of Langerhans,** release insulin, glucagon, somato-statin, and pancreatic polypeptide. **Insulin,** a hormone released by beta islet cells, lowers the level of blood glucose when it rises beyond normal limits (see Chap. 51). **Glucagon,** a hormone released by alpha islet cells, raises blood sugar lev-els by stimulating **glycogenolysis,** the breakdown of glycogen into glucose, in the liver. Somatostatin, a hormone secreted by delta islet cells, helps maintain a relatively constant level of blood sugar by inhibiting the release of insulin and glucagons. Pancreatic polypeptide from gamma islet cells controls exo-crine secretions from the pancreas.

Ovaries and Testes

The sex glands, the female **ovaries** and the male **testes,** are important in the development of secondary sex characteris-tics, manufacture of hormones, and development of the ovum (female) and sperm (male).

The ovaries produce **estrogen** and **progesterone.** The testes are the major source of the hormone **testosterone,** which is involved with the development and maintenance of male secondary sex characteristics, such as facial hair and a deep voice. The functions and roles of these hormones are discussed in Chapters 52, 53, and 55.

Additional Hormone-Releasing Organs

Other organs are not typically considered endocrine glands, yet they secrete one or more hormones among the other major functions that they perform. For example, the atria of

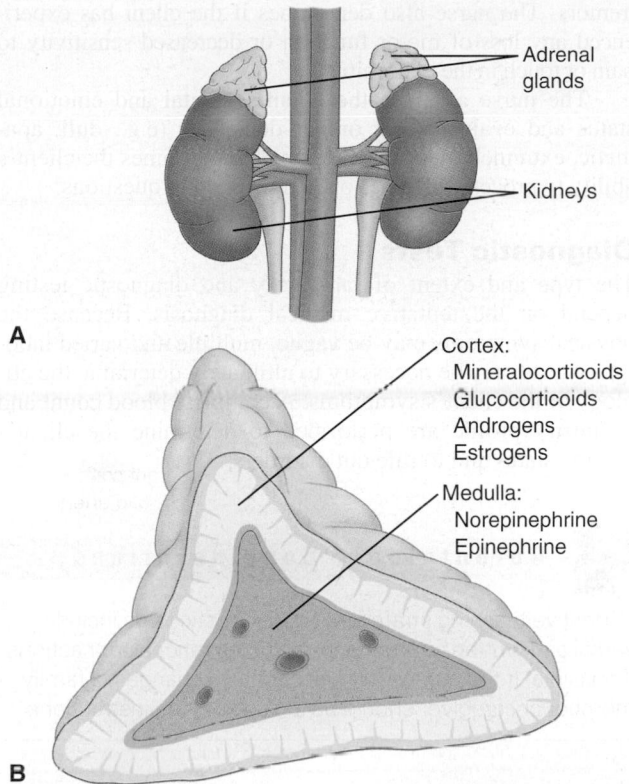

A

B

FIGURE 49-7. (**A**) The adrenal glands sit on top of each kidney. (**B**) Cross-section of one adrenal gland; each gland is composed of the outer cortex and the inner medulla, both of which secrete specific hormones.

Adrenal glands

Kidneys

Cortex:
Mineralocorticoids
Glucocorticoids
Androgens
Estrogens

Medulla:
Norepinephrine
Epinephrine

the heart secrete *atrial natriuretic peptide* (ANP), a hormone that helps reduce blood volume by promoting urinary excretion of sodium (see Chap. 16). Conversely, the kidneys release *renin,* a hormone that initiates the production of

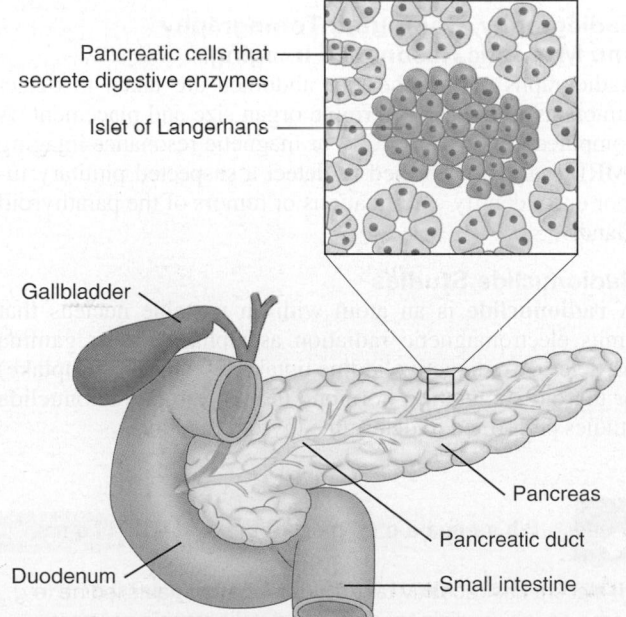

Pancreatic cells that secrete digestive enzymes

Islet of Langerhans

Gallbladder

Pancreas

Pancreatic duct

Duodenum

Small intestine

FIGURE 49-8. The pancreas secretes hormones from the islets of Langerhans. Digestive enzymes are released from the common bile duct.

angiotensin and aldosterone to increase blood pressure and blood volume. The kidneys also secrete *erythropoietin,* a substance that promotes the maturation of red blood cells.

During pregnancy, the placenta provides maternal circulation to the developing fetus, but it also secretes hormones such as estrogen; progesterone; corticotrophin-releasing hormone (CRH), which determines the length of gestation and the onset of labor; and human chorionic gonadotropin (Marieb & Hoehn, 2007). When exposed to sunlight, epidermal skin cells form a precursor of vitamin D; the liver continues the conversion, and the kidneys complete the activation process. And lastly, hormone-secreting cells within the gastrointestinal tract aid in the regulation of digestion. For example, gastrin is released within the stomach to increase the production of hydrochloric acid. Cholecystokinin released from cells in the small intestine stimulates contraction of the gallbladder to release bile when dietary fat is ingested.

ASSESSMENT

History

The health history becomes important in the diagnosis of many endocrine disorders. Some endocrine disorders are inherited or have a tendency to occur in families; therefore, a complete family history is essential. The nurse also obtains diet and drug histories.

The nurse documents an allergy to iodine, a component of contrast dyes, or seafood, and informs the physician. He or she also reports whether the client has had a diagnostic test that used iodine (e.g., intravenous pyelography, gallbladder series) within the past 3 months. This information is essential before initiating a thyroid test. The nurse identifies the current symptoms. Sometimes the symptoms of endocrine disorders are vague or resemble other physical or mental disorders. Examples are fatigue, personality changes, inability to sleep, and frequent urination. At other times, symptoms are dramatic, such as a change in mental acuity or sudden weight loss.

Gerontologic Considerations

- Obtaining a drug history is essential before a diagnostic examination for an older adult because side effects or interactions may contribute to changes in endocrine function. If the older adult is cognitively impaired, a family member or the caregiver should provide information regarding medications and dosage history.

Physical Examination

The nurse obtains the client's height, weight, and vital signs and notes his or her general physical appearance. The nurse examines body structures to detect evidence of hypersecretion or hyposecretion of hormones (see Chaps. 50 and 51 for assessment findings unique to specific endocrine glands). He or she inspects the skin for excessive oiliness or dryness,

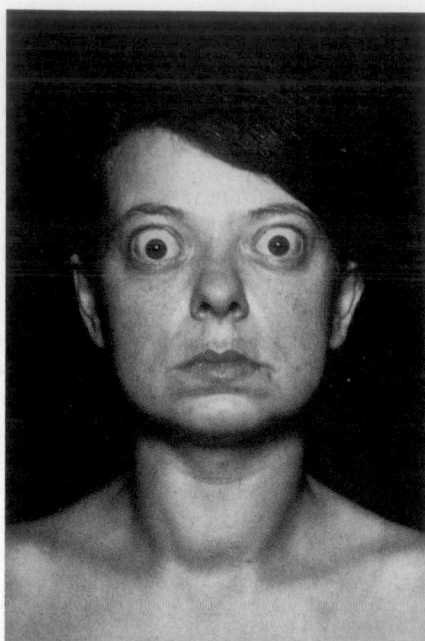

FIGURE 49-9. Exophthalmos in a person with hyperthyroidism. (From Rubin, R., & Strayer, D. S., eds. [2008]. *Rubin's pathology: Clinicopathologic foundations of medicine* [5th ed.]. Philadelphia: Lippincott Williams & Wilkins.)

excessive or absent areas of pigmentation, excessive hair growth or loss, and skin breaks that heal poorly. The nurse examines the shape and color of the nails and determines whether they are thin, thick, or brittle. He or she examines the eyes for *exophthalmos*, abnormal bulging or protrusion of the eyes (Fig. 49-9), and periorbital swelling. The nurse observes the client's facial expression and general features. He or she visually inspects the neck for thyroid enlargement and gently palpates the thyroid gland (Fig. 49-10). Repeated or forceful palpation of the thyroid in the case of thyroid hyperactivity can result in a sudden release of a large amount of thyroid hormones, which can have serious implications. The nurse notes the pulse rate and rhythm. He or she examines the extremities for edema and changes in pigmentation, auscultates the lungs for abnormal sounds, and examines outstretched hands for

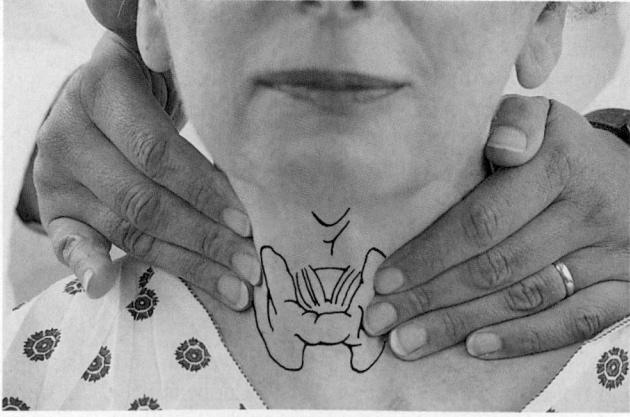

FIGURE 49-10. With the client's head slightly tilted to the side, the examiner displaces the thyroid laterally with his or her fingers and palpates the thyroid as the client swallows. The examination is repeated on the opposite side.

tremors. The nurse also determines if the client has experienced any loss of motor function or decreased sensitivity to pain or touch in the extremities.

The nurse assesses the client's mental and emotional status and evaluates his or her demeanor (e.g., dull, apathetic, extremely nervous). He or she determines the client's ability to process information and respond to questions.

Diagnostic Tests

The type and extent of laboratory and diagnostic testing depend on the tentative medical diagnosis. Because the physical symptoms may be vague, multiple and varied laboratory tests may be necessary to ultimately determine the etiology of the client's symptoms. A complete blood count and chemistry profile are performed to determine the client's general status and to rule out disorders.

Gerontologic Considerations

- Effective teaching strategies for diagnostic tests include verbal and written instructions, including rationale for actions if possible. If the older adult has cognitive changes, a family member or caregiver should be included in the instructions.

Hormone Levels

Measuring blood hormone levels helps evaluate the functioning of some endocrine glands. These tests include cortisol levels (morning and evening) to determine adrenal hyperfunction or hypofunction, antidiuretic hormone (ADH) levels to determine the presence or absence of ADH, testosterone levels to detect increased or decreased total testosterone levels, and a thyroid panel that measures TSH, T_3, and T_4 levels to identify diseases associated with increased or decreased thyroid hormones.

Radiography, Computed Tomography and Magnetic Resonance Imaging

Radiographs of the chest or abdomen are taken to detect tumors as well as to determine organ size and placement. A computed tomography (CT) or magnetic resonance imaging (MRI) scan is performed to detect a suspected pituitary tumor or to identify calcifications or tumors of the parathyroid glands.

Radionuclide Studies

A **radionuclide** is an atom with an unstable nucleus that emits electromagnetic radiation as alpha, beta, or gamma particles. A radioactive iodine uptake test (RAI, ^{131}I uptake) or thyroid-stimulating hormone (TSH) test are radionuclide studies performed to determine thyroid function.

Pharmacologic Considerations

- If a client has recently taken a drug that contains iodine (e.g., some cough medicines) or has had radiographic contrast studies that used iodine, thyroid test results may be inaccurate. Other drugs (e.g., salicylates, corticosteroids) also affect the results of thyroid tests. Be sure to enter on the laboratory request slip all drugs the client is taking or has taken within the past 3 months.

A **radioimmunoassay** determines the concentration of a substance in plasma. Venous blood samples are required for radioimmunoassay tests. A radioactively labeled substance (e.g., hormone, protein, antibodies, antigens) is combined in the laboratory with a blood sample to determine the quantity of the substance to be identified. For example, a T_3 determination by radioimmunoassay evaluates thyroid function.

A **nuclear scan** uses a radioactive substance that is taken orally or injected intravenously. The dose of the radioactive substance is larger than the dose used for radionuclide studies. Certain endocrine organs are visualized or their activity determined by means of special equipment. Examples of scans include thyroid scan, adrenergic tumor scan, and parathyroid scan.

NURSING MANAGEMENT

The nurse prepares the client for laboratory and diagnostic testing. He or she explains the general purpose of the test, type of test, and how it will be performed. The nurse encourages the client and family to ask questions and discuss the results with the physician.

Nurses must consult the institution's procedure manual and the physician's orders for the required preparation for each diagnostic procedure. Some tests, such as a CT scan, require no special preparation other than a general explanation. Some tests require fasting; others require temporary elimination of certain foods from the diet.

The nurse explains to the client how to participate in the test. For example, some tests require the client to save all voided urine during a particular time frame or to return for additional testing.

If a client is anxious about the use of radioactive materials for tests, the nurse offers assurance that these substances are safe and ordinarily pose no danger to the client or others.

CRITICAL THINKING EXERCISES

1. Explain why the pituitary gland is considered the master gland. Give some examples that support the terminology.
2. Discuss the meaning and purpose of a feedback loop.
3. Based on the principle of the feedback loop, if a client's T_3 and T_4 hormone levels are low, what hormone level(s) is/(are) most likely elevated?
4. When examining a client, the nurse notes that the client's eyes bulge and protrude from the bony orbits. What is the term for this condition, and what hormonal disorder may be the cause? What diagnostic test would be ordered to confirm or rule out a hormonal cause for the condition?

NCLEX-STYLE REVIEW QUESTIONS

1. A client diagnosed with parathormone deficiency is admitted to the hospital. As the nurse initiates the care plan, which body system should be the focus of care?
   1. Skeletal
   2. Urinary
   3. Respiratory
   4. Integumentary
2. The nurse takes vital signs for a client scheduled for open heart surgery in the next few minutes and notes that the client's pulse, respirations, and blood pressure are elevated. The nurse explains to the client that the elevations are a normal response to stress and anxiety and are due to the release of which hormone?
   1. Insulin
   2. Epinephrine
   3. Thyroxine
   4. Aldosterone
3. The nurse gently palpates the neck of a client diagnosed with a thyroid disorder. The client asks why the nurse's touch is so gentle. Which response by the nurse is most appropriate?
   1. "Forceful palpation can result in excessive release of thyroid hormone."
   2. "This type of palpation is the way my instructor in nursing school taught me to do it."
   3. "Gentle palpation prevents closing off the trachea, which would cause you to gasp for air."
   4. "Forceful palpation causes pain in an area that is already enlarged and tender to touch."
4. A client is to undergo radioimmunoassay tests. Which of the following is a prerequisite for the test?
   1. Venous blood samples
   2. A radioactive substance injected intravenously
   3. A computed tomography (CT) scan
   4. Radiographs of the chest
5. A nurse is explaining the rationale for a nuclear scan test to a client with a thyroid disorder. Which of the following would be the *best* explanation?
   1. The test determines the concentration of a substance in plasma.
   2. The test visualizes certain endocrine organs and their activities.
   3. The test detects tumors of the parathyroid glands.
   4. The test evaluates for suspected pituitary tumors.

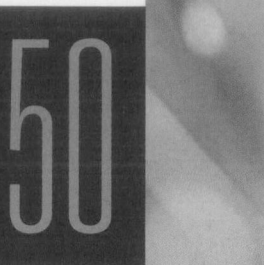

50 Caring for Clients with Disorders of the Endocrine System

Words To Know

acromegaly
addisonian crisis
adrenalectomy
adrenal insufficiency
carpopedal spasm
cushingoid syndrome
Cushing's syndrome
diabetes insipidus
goiter
hyperparathyroidism
hyperplasia
hyperthyroidism
hypoparathyroidism
hypophysectomy
hypothyroidism
myxedema
pheochromocytoma
Simmonds' disease
syndrome of inappropriate antidiuretic
    hormone secretion
tetany
thyroiditis
thyrotoxic crisis

Learning Objectives

On completion of this chapter, you will be able to:

1. Describe the physiologic effects of hyposecretion and hyperse-cretion of the pituitary, thyroid, parathyroid, and adrenal glands.
2. Describe the nursing management of clients with pituitary disorders
3. Describe thyroid disorders and nursing management of clients with these disorders.
4. Compare the differences in physiologic effects, assessment find-ings, and management of disorders affecting the parathyroid glands.
5. Identify disorders of the adrenal glands and describe nursing management of clients with these disorders.
6. Identify symptoms of emergency conditions resulting from endo-crine disorders.

A disorder of any endocrine gland can profoundly affect the other en-docrine glands, as well as many major body systems. This chapter discusses the care of clients with various endocrine disorders and considers the ways in which these disorders affect systemic physi-ology. The chapter's focus is on disorders affecting the pituitary, thy-roid, parathyroid, and adrenal glands. Diabetes mellitus is presented separately in Chapter 51. Disorders of the ovaries and testes are dis-cussed in Chapters 53 and 55, respectively.

DISORDERS OF THE PITUITARY GLAND

Pituitary disorders usually result from excessive or deficient production and secretion of a specific hormone. When oversecretion of growth hor-mone (GH) occurs before puberty (when the ends [epiphyses] of the long bones are not yet fully united), *gigantism* results. When secretion of GH during childhood is insufficient, *dwarfism* occurs. Refer to a pe-diatric text for further discussion of gigantism and dwarfism.

Oversecretion of GH during adulthood results in *acromegaly*. Con-versely, an absence of pituitary hormonal activity causes panhypopitui-tarism, or *Simmonds' disease*.

ACROMEGALY (HYPERPITUITARISM)

Pathophysiology and Etiology

Acromegaly is a condition in which GH is oversecreted after the epiphy-ses of the long bones have sealed. GH is overproduced when the pituitary gland is insensitive to feedback inhibiting hormones such as *somatostatin*, a hypothalamic hormone, and *insulin-like growth factor 1* (IGF-1). IGF-1, a hormone released by the liver, stimulates the growth of bones and tis-sue (National Institute of Diabetes & Digestive & Kidney Diseases,

2008). Unchecked GH allows sustained production of IGF-1, leading to lengthening and widening of bones, organ enlargement, increased blood glucose levels, and hyperlipidemia. Hypersecretion results from **hyperplasia** (increased numbers of cells), which in the majority of cases is caused by an *adenoma,* a benign tumor. As with other cranial tumors, a benign pituitary tumor becomes a space-occupying lesion and can affect other cerebral structures (see Chap. 37).

Assessment Findings

Signs and Symptoms

A client with acromegaly has coarse features, a huge lower jaw, thick lips, a thickened tongue, a bulging forehead, a bulbous nose, and large hands and feet (Fig. 50-1). When the overgrowth is from a tumor, headaches caused by pressure on the sella turcica, a bony depression in which the pituitary gland rests, are common. Partial blindness may result from pressure on the optic nerve. The heart, liver, and spleen may be enlarged. Despite enlarged tissues, muscle weakness is common, and hypertrophied joints become painful and stiff. Osteoporosis of the spine and joint pain develop. Many men experience erectile dysfunction, and women may have amenorrhea (absence of menstruation), increased facial hair, and deepened voices that result from compression of areas of the pituitary responsible for producing gender-related hormones (Fig. 50-2). Some people develop diabetes mellitus.

Diagnostic Findings

Skull radiography, magnetic resonance imaging (MRI), and computed tomography (CT) reveal pituitary enlargement. Bone radiographs show thickened long bones and skull bones. A glucose tolerance test in combination with a GH measurement is the most reliable method of confirming acromegaly. Ingestion of a bolus of glucose should lower GH levels, but GH levels remain elevated in persons with acromegaly (National Institute of Diabetes, Digestive & Kidney Disease, 2008). Increased blood levels of IGF-1 can also indicate acromegaly in nonpregnant women; they typically

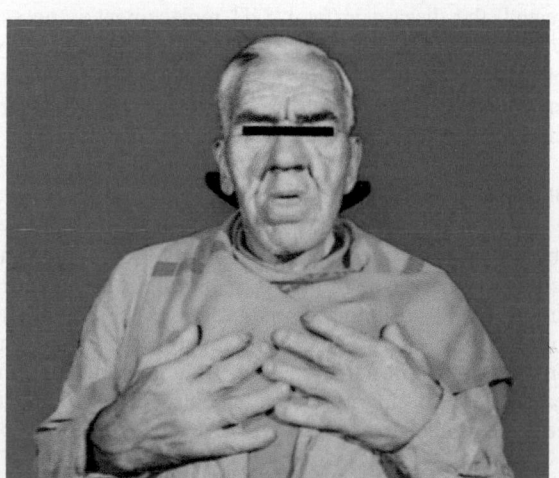

FIGURE 50-1. Acromegaly is characterized by enlargement of the facial features, hands, and feet. (From Willis MC, CMA-AC. [2002]. *Medical terminology: A programmed learning approach to the language of health care.* Baltimore: Lippincott Williams & Wilkins.)

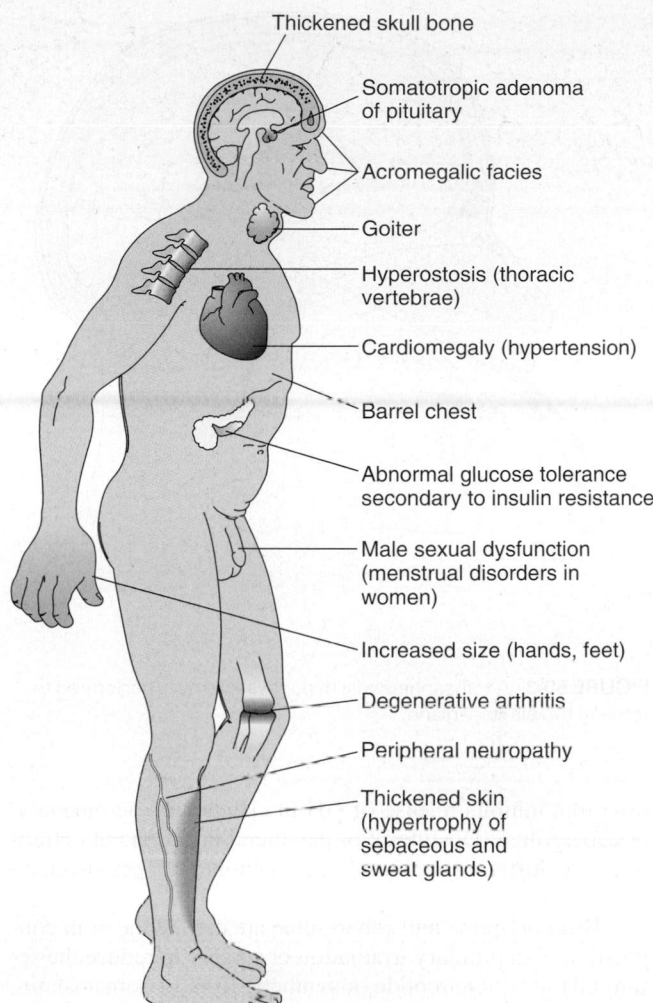

Thickened skull bone

Somatotropic adenoma of pituitary

Acromegalic facies

Goiter

Hyperostosis (thoracic vertebrae)

Cardiomegaly (hypertension)

Barrel chest

Abnormal glucose tolerance secondary to insulin resistance

Male sexual dysfunction (menstrual disorders in women)

Increased size (hands, feet)

Degenerative arthritis

Peripheral neuropathy

Thickened skin (hypertrophy of sebaceous and sweat glands)

FIGURE 50-2. Clinical manifestations of acromegaly. (From Rubin, R., & Strayer, D. S. [2008]. *Rubin's pathology: Clinicopathologic foundations of medicine* [5th ed.]. Philadelphia: Lippincott Williams & Wilkins.)

have IGF-1 levels two to three times higher than normal in pregnant women.

Medical and Surgical Management

The treatment of choice is surgical removal of the pituitary gland (transsphenoidal **hypophysectomy**) through a nasal approach (Fig. 50-3). The surgeon may substitute an endoscopic technique using microsurgical instruments to reduce surgical trauma. The client who is a surgical risk may undergo a primary method of treatment that includes a series of radiation treatments over 4 to 6 weeks, to remove tumor fragments that remain after surgery. Clients undergo frequent monitoring for evidence of tumor recurrence. Even if the disease is arrested successfully, physical changes are irreversible. If surgery or radiation therapy removes or destroys normal pituitary tissue, replacement therapy with thyroid hormone, corticosteroids, antidiuretic hormone (ADH), and sex hormones is necessary.

Medical treatment includes either oral administrations of bromocriptine mesylate (Parlodel), an oral antiparkinsonism

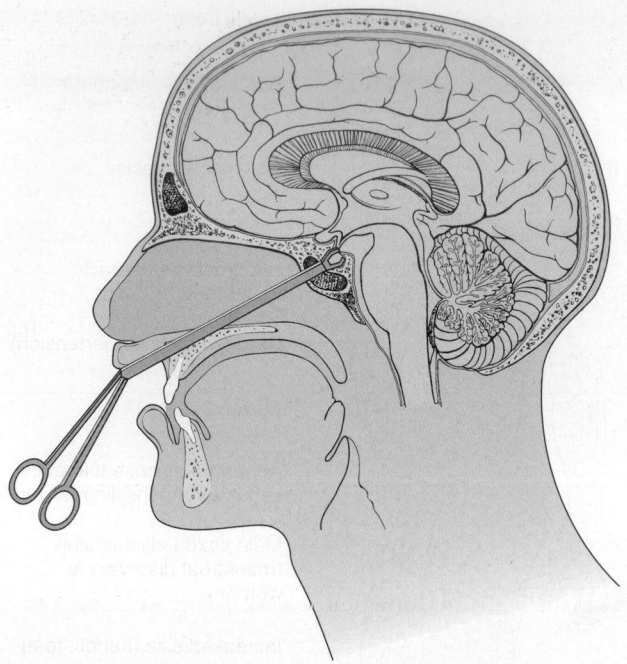

FIGURE 50-3. A transsphenoidal hypophysectomy is performed to remove the pituitary gland.

drug that inhibits release of GH in clients with acromegaly, or cabergoline (Dostinex); or parenteral injections of octreotide (Sandostatin), lanreotide (Somatuline), or pegvisomant (Somavert).

Bromocriptine and cabergoline are used alone or in conjunction with pituitary irradiation or surgery to reduce the serum GH level. Octreotide, a synthetic form of somatostatin, stops the production of GH and IGF-1 and effectively relieves symptoms for a short time. One form of octreotide is injected subcutaneously every 8 hours; a longer-acting form, Sandostatin LAR Depot, is injected intramuscularly every month. Both forms may cause gastrointestinal (GI) side effects, gallstones, and diabetes. Pegvisomant, a GH receptor antagonist, is the newest and most effective drug for treating acromegaly. Injected subcutaneously once a day, it normalizes the IGF-1 level in 93% to 97% of cases by blocking the GH stimulation of IGF-1 produced by the liver (van der Lely & Kopchick, 2006). Pegvisomant may be combined with octreotide or lanreotide. Clients who take pegvisomant must be monitored for liver damage.

Nursing Management

Until the client has surgery or receives radiation treatment, nursing priorities include helping the client cope with changes in physical appearance, pacing activities to accommodate the client's fatigue, and relieving discomfort from headaches, abdominal distention resulting from organ enlargement, and skeletal pain. The nurse evaluates the client's pain, discerning type and location, gives analgesics as prescribed, and notes whether the client reports relief from pain. The nurse encourages self-care and activities when the client's strength and endurance permit.

The client may experience severe psychological stress because of the prominent physical changes, sexual dysfunc-

tion, and decreased libido. The nurse discusses such issues to help the client cope with changes. If the client expresses concern over sexual dysfunction, the nurse brings it to the physician's attention. Referral to a sex therapist could be indicated.

Postoperatively, the client undergoes frequent neurologic assessments (see Chap. 36) to detect signs of increased intracranial pressure and meningitis. If the client has nasal packing, the nurse monitors drainage from the nose and postnasal drainage for the presence of cerebrospinal fluid. The nurse modifies oral and facial hygiene to promote cleanliness without contributing to trauma near the operative site. The nurse also reminds the client to avoid drinking from a straw, sneezing, coughing, and bending over to prevent dislodging the graft that seals the operative area between the cranium and nose.

SIMMONDS' DISEASE (PANHYPOPITUITARISM)

Pathophysiology and Etiology

Simmonds' disease is a rare disorder caused by destruction of the pituitary gland followed by cessation of pituitary hormonal activity. Events such as postpartum emboli or hemorrhage, surgery, tumor, and tuberculosis can destroy pituitary function. This disease affects all hormones of the anterior pituitary.

Assessment Findings

The gonads and genitalia atrophy. Because of the impaired pituitary stimulus, the thyroid and adrenals fail to secrete adequate hormones. Signs and symptoms of hypothyroidism, hypoglycemia, and adrenal insufficiency (Addison's disease—see later discussion) are apparent. The client ages prematurely and becomes extremely cachectic. Results of laboratory tests show decreased hormone levels (e.g., thyroid, corticosteroid, reproductive hormones).

Medical Management

Treatment includes administration of replacement hormones for the glands that depend on the pituitary for stimulation. If untreated, the disease is fatal. GH replacement is necessary only for children. Deficiency of TSH requires replacement with levothyroxine (Synthroid) or liothyronine (Cytomel) for the client's lifetime. Male clients receive testosterone and female clients receive estrogen; both sexes receive FSH and LH.

Nursing Management

The nurse administers all hormone replacements as prescribed. Teaching the client to adhere to the medication schedule and never to omit a dose is important. The nurse monitors blood hormone levels and assesses mental status, emotional state, energy level, and appetite. He or she is alert to any alterations in nutrition. Most clients with Simmonds' disease tolerate four to six small meals per day better than three regular meals.

DIABETES INSIPIDUS

Diabetes insipidus (DI) is a disorder characterized by the excretion of extremely large volumes of urine. *Neurogenic* or *central diabetes insipidus* develops when there is insufficient ADH (also known as *vasopressin)* from the posterior pituitary gland. A second type is called *nephrogenic diabetes insipidus.* Both have identical symptoms. The difference is that in nephrogenic diabetes insipidus, the secretion of ADH is normal, but the receptors in the renal tubules partially or completely fail to respond to the hormone.

Pathophysiology and Etiology

ADH, secreted by the posterior pituitary, regulates the reabsorption of water in the kidney tubules. Its function is to increase fluid volume. ADH is released in response to thirst and fluid losses such as hemorrhage, which lowers blood pressure. ADH also raises blood pressure by signaling the peripheral arterioles to constrict; hence, its alternative name, vasopressin (Marieb & Hoehn, 2007). Lack of ADH secretion or an ineffective response to it causes the client to produce large volumes of dilute urine. If the client fails to drink a compensatory volume of fluid, dehydration with concentrated levels of electrolytes occurs.

Neurogenic diabetes insipidus can result from head trauma that damages the pituitary or from primary or metastatic brain tumors. In some congenital incidences, symptoms occur shortly after birth. Neurogenic diabetes insipidus also can occur after *hypophysectomy,* surgical removal of the pituitary.

Nephrogenic diabetes insipidus is less common than neurogenic diabetes insipidus. The client generally acquires nephrogenic diabetes insipidus as a side effect from drugs such as lithium (Eskalith), a drug used for managing bipolar disorder (see Chap 69); demeclocycline (Declomycin), an antibiotic in the tetracycline family, and amphotericin B (Amphocin), an antifungal antibiotic. Nephrogenic diabetes insipidus also is associated with elevated levels of prostaglandin E_2, which has been shown to interfere with the action of vasopressin (Wilden, 2006).

Assessment Findings

Signs and Symptoms

Urine output may be as high as 20 L/24 hours. Urine is dilute, with a specific gravity of 1.002 or less. Limiting fluid intake does not control urine excretion. Thirst is excessive and constant. Activities are limited by the frequent need to drink and void. Weakness, dehydration, and weight loss develop.

Diagnostic Findings

A fluid deprivation test can diagnose DI and differentiate neurogenic DI from nephrogenic DI. The protocol for a fluid deprivation test involves withholding fluid from the client for 5 to 6 hours while concurrently measuring his or her urine volume, urine specific gravity, and serum osmolality (osmotic pressure of the serum compared with water). In both types of DI, the excreted urine volume continues to be excessive, with a low specific gravity almost equal to that of water; the serum osmolality is high because of the client's dehydration from the water restriction. At the completion of the fasting phase of the test, the client receives an infusion of desmopressin acetate (DDAVP), a synthetic analog of vasopressin. If the urine becomes more concentrated following the infusion, the symptoms result from insufficient ADH (i.e., neurogenic DI). If the urine continues to be dilute, with

low specific gravity, the symptoms result from a failure of the renal tubules to respond to ADH, and the diagnosis is nephrogenic DI.

Medical Management

Desmopressin (DDAVP) nasal solution and lypressin (Diapid) nasal spray are synthetic drugs with ADH activity that reduce urine output to 2 to 3 L/24 hours (Client and Family Teaching 50-1). If the client cannot take oral fluids to meet the excessive fluid volume loss, intravenous (IV) fluids are necessary.

The management of nephrogenic DI is different. Beside ensuring that the client has a sufficient intake of fluid, the physician also wants to reduce the client's urine output by reducing the amount of sodium excreted by the renal tubules. Therefore, the physician restricts the client's use of dietary sodium. The physician prescribes a thiazide diuretic, such as hydrochlorothiazide (HydroDIURIL). The thiazide acts at the proximal convoluted tubule, leaving less fluid for excretion in the distal convoluted tubules, the portion affected by nephrogenic DI. Consequently, the client excretes water, but the total volume is less than in an untreated state. Sometimes the physician prescribes the thiazide diuretic combined with spironolactone (Aldactone) or amiloride (Midamor), potassium-sparing diuretics to help prevent hypokalemia. In addition, the physician prescribes indomethacin (Indocin), an anti-inflammatory drug that acts as a prostaglandin inhibitor, to reduce the level of prostaglandin E_2. Lastly, the physician restricts the client's intake of dietary protein to reduce the work of the kidney to excrete protein nitrogenous wastes.

Nursing Management

Nursing measures include correcting fluid volume deficit. The nurse closely monitors the rate of IV infusions to ensure that the prescribed amount is given over the required period and measures fluid intake and output. If the client is acutely ill or extremely dehydrated, fails to take oral fluids, or is beginning to receive medical treatment, the nurse measures urine output every 30 minutes while administering prescribed fluid and drug therapy. He or she weighs the client daily to identify weight gain or loss and observes for signs of

**Client and Family Teaching 50-1
Self-Administration of Lypressin Nasal Spray**

The nurse teaches the client the following administration steps:

1. Hold container upright.
2. Place nozzle in nostril while in sitting position.
3. Spray prescribed number of times in each nostril.
4. Avoid exceeding the number of sprays per self-administration; the excess is not absorbed and therefore wastes the volume of prescribed drug.
5. Do not inhale medication.
6. Report nasal irritation to the physician.
7. Monitor urine output and level of thirst.

fluid excess or deficit. The nurse notifies the physician of sudden or steady weight gain or loss.

The nurse teaches the client to consume sufficient fluid to control thirst and to compensate for urine loss. In addition, the nurse explains other methods for reducing fluid loss such as remaining in air-conditioned areas during hot and humid weather and avoiding strenuous physical activity. The nurse stresses compliance with drug (and diet) therapy and reassures the client that treatment can control symptoms.

SYNDROME OF INAPPROPRIATE ANTIDIURETIC HORMONE SECRETION

The **syndrome of inappropriate antidiuretic hormone secretion** (SIADH) is characterized by renal reabsorption of water rather than its normal excretion.

Pathophysiology and Etiology

Causes of SIADH include lung tumors, central nervous system (CNS) disorders, brain tumors, cerebrovascular accident, head trauma, and drugs such as vasopressin, general anesthetic agents, oral hypoglycemics, and tricyclic antidepressants. The continued release of ADH increases fluid volume and causes *hyponatremia* (decreased serum sodium level).

Assessment Findings

Water retention, headache, muscle cramps, and anorexia develop. As the condition worsens, the client experiences nausea, vomiting, muscle twitching, and changes in level of consciousness (LOC). Diagnosis is based on symptoms and a history of a disorder associated with SIADH. Serum sodium levels and serum osmolarity are decreased. Urine sodium levels and osmolarity are high.

Medical Management

When possible, treatment aims at eliminating the underlying cause. Osmotic diuretics, such as mannitol (Osmitrol), and loop diuretics, including furosemide (Lasix), help correct water retention. Severe hyponatremia is treated with IV administration of a 3% hypertonic sodium chloride solution.

Nursing Management

The nurse closely monitors fluid intake and output and vital signs. He or she carefully assesses LOC and immediately reports any changes to the physician. The nurse checks closely for signs of fluid overload (confusion, dyspnea, pulmonary congestion, hypertension) and hyponatremia (weakness, muscle cramps, anorexia, nausea, diarrhea, irritability, headache, weight gain without edema).

The nurse gives the client and family extensive information about the medication schedule and adverse effects of drug therapy, especially if several medications are prescribed. He or she stresses the importance of adhering to the medication schedule and not omitting a dose.

DISORDERS OF THE THYROID GLAND

Thyroid disorders are difficult to detect because symptoms are vague until the disease advances to a severe level.

Treatment often is long term, and the client requires periodic follow-up to monitor response. Thyroid disorders include hyperthyroidism, thyrotoxic crisis, hypothyroidism, thyroid tumors, and endemic and multinodular goiters.

HYPERTHYROIDISM

Hyperthyroidism also is called *Graves' disease, Basedow's disease, thyrotoxicosis,* or *exophthalmic goiter.*

Pathophysiology and Etiology

There is no one etiologic factor for hyperthyroidism. Researchers have suggested that it may be autoimmune or inherited. Hypersecretion of thyroid hormones accompanies thyroid tumors, pituitary tumors, and hypothalamic malignancies. It also may result from stress or infection. The metabolic rate increases because of the oversecretion of the thyroid hormones thyroxine (T_4) and triiodothyronine (T_3). Both T_4 and T_3 increase the metabolic rate. Hyperthyroidism is more common in women than in men.

Assessment Findings
Signs and Symptoms

Symptoms vary from mild to severe. Clients with hyperthyroidism characteristically are restless despite feeling fatigued and weak, highly excitable, and constantly agitated. Fine tremors of the hands occur, causing unusual clumsiness (Fig. 50-4). The client cannot tolerate heat and has an increased appetite but loses weight. Diarrhea also occurs. Visual changes, such as blurred or double vision, can develop. *Exophthalmos*, seen in clients with severe hyperthyroidism, results from enlarged muscle and fatty tissue surrounding the

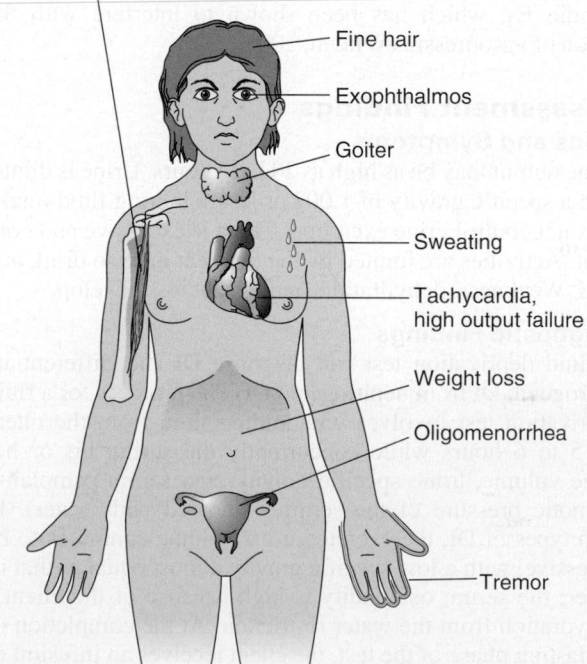

Muscle wasting

Fine hair

Exophthalmos

Goiter

Sweating

Tachycardia, high output failure

Weight loss

Oligomenorrhea

Tremor

FIGURE 50-4. Clinical manifestations of hyperthyroidism (From Rubin, R., & Strayer, D.S. [2008]. Rubin's pathology: Clinico-pathologic foundations of medicine [5th ed.]. Philadelphia: Lippincott Williams & Wilkins.)

TABLE 50-1 Symptoms of Thyroid Dysfunction

BODY SYSTEM OR FUNCTION	HYPERTHYROIDISM	HYPOTHYROIDISM
Metabolism	Increased, with symptoms of increased appetite, intolerance to heat, elevated body temperature, weight loss despite increased appetite	Decreased, with symptoms of anorexia, intolerance to cold, low body temperature, weight gain despite anorexia
Cardiovascular system	Tachycardia, moderate hypertension	Bradycardia, moderate hypotension
Central nervous system	Nervousness, anxiety, insomnia, tremors	Lethargy, sleepiness
Skin and skin structures	Flushed, warm, moist	Pale, cool, dry; face appears puffy, hair coarse; nails thick and hard
Ovarian function	Irregular or scant menses	Heavy menses, may be unable to conceive, loss of fetus also possible
Testicular function		Low sperm count

rear and sides of the eyeball (see Fig. 49-10). Neck swelling caused by the enlarged thyroid gland often is visible. Table 50-1 compares the signs and symptoms of hyperthyroidism and hypothyroidism.

Gerontologic Considerations

- Older adults have an increased incidence of nodules and small goiters on the thyroid gland. Symptoms of thyroid disease in older adults often are atypical or minor and easily attributed to normal aging or other chronic conditions. For example, older adults may not experience restlessness or hyperactivity and may not appear nervous. Symptoms seen most often in older adults include anorexia, weight loss, palpitations, angina, and atrial fibrillation.

Diagnostic Findings

The protein-bound iodine; free thyroxine (FT$_4$), a thyroxine that is not bound to protein; thyroglobulin; and serum T$_3$ and T$_4$ levels are elevated. The TSH level is decreased. Thyroid ultrasonography shows an enlarged thyroid gland. A thyroid scan indicates an increased uptake of radioactive iodine (RAI; ^{131}I and ^{123}I) throughout the gland or confined to a single nodule. The isotope of iodine that is used for diagnostic purposes does not destroy the thyroid gland.

Gerontologic Considerations

- Changes in hormone levels may accompany aging. Although levels of T$_4$ tend to remain constant, levels of T$_3$ may decrease with age. The most reliable thyroid function test to diagnose hyperthyroidism in an older adult is a serum T$_4$ level.

Medical and Surgical Management

Antithyroid drugs, such as propylthiouracil (PTU, Propyl-Thyracil) and methimazole (Tapazole), are given to block the production of thyroid hormone preoperatively or for long-term treatment for clients who are not candidates for surgery or radiation treatment. If clients receive antithyroid drugs as the only treatment and do not comply with prescription therapy early in its management, the disorder may reactivate. About 40% to 70% of those who comply with antithyroid drug therapy for 1 to 2 years experience remission, but they need to continue with follow-up care to detect any sign of recurrence (Mathur, 2008).

The physician may prescribe potassium iodide (Lugol's solution) in combination with an antithyroid drug such as propylthiouracil. Potassium iodide creates a negative feedback effect on the hypothalamus. When the hypothalamus senses the high level of iodine, it suppresses the secretion of thyroid-releasing hormone, and thyroid hormone levels are reduced.

The combination of potassium iodide solution and an antithyroid drug can curb thyroid activity before surgery to reduce the postoperative potential for bleeding and thyrotoxicosis (discussed later). Antithyroid medications, however, are avoided during pregnancy because they can induce hypothyroidism, or cretinism, in the fetus. Drug Therapy Table 50-1 discusses these and other drugs used to treat thyroid disorders.

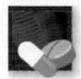

Pharmacologic Considerations

- Potassium iodide should not be administered to anyone who is allergic to seafood, which is also high in iodine. (This agent can also be used to protect the thyroid gland from the effects of a radiation exposure after release of radiation in a nuclear power plant accident or nuclear bomb; see Chapter 15.)

- Antithyroid drugs such as methimazole (Tapazole) are administered every 8 hours around the clock, unless directed otherwise by the physician.

- The most serious adverse effect of antithyroid drugs is agranulocytosis, which occurs most often in the first 2 months of therapy and necessitates discontinuing the drug. Instruct the client to report sore throat, fever, chills, headache, malaise, weakness, or unusual bleeding or bruising.

DRUG THERAPY TABLE 50-1 Agents to Treat Thyroid Disorders

Drug Category and Examples	Mechanism of Action	Side Effects	Nursing Considerations
Antithyroid Agents methimazole (Tapazole), propylthiouracil (PTU)	Inhibits synthesis of thyroid hormones	Paresthesias, nausea, agranulocytosis, bleeding, rash, diarrhea, vomiting	Caution clients to avoid use during pregnancy. Monitor results of blood tests for bone marrow depression. Administer in three equal doses every 8 hours. Alert client to notify the physician of fever, sore throat, unusual bleeding or bruising, or malaise.
Iodides strong iodine solution (Lugol's solution)	Inhibits synthesis and release of T_3 and T_4	Iodism: metallic taste, burning mouth, sore teeth and gums, nausea, abdominal pain, diarrhea, rash	Monitor for symptoms of acute iodine toxicity: vomiting, abdominal pain, diarrhea, circulatory collapse. Dilute with fruit juice or water. Advise client to drink solution with a straw to avoid staining teeth.
Radioactive Iodine sodium iodine ^{131}I and ^{123}I	Used in diagnostic scans; destroys thyroid tissue in hyperthyroidism and thyroid malignancies	Allergy to iodine, nausea, vomiting	Follow precautions for body fluids for 24 hours after diagnostic testing. Monitor for signs of hypothyroidism.
Beta-Adrenergic Blockers propranolol (Inderal)	Reduces symptoms of hyperthyroidism—tachycardia, tremors, nervousness	Nausea, vomiting, diarrhea, constipation, bradycardia, congestive heart failure, dysrhythmias, hyperglycemia	Monitor cardiac function. Administer with meals. Instruct client not to discontinue abruptly. Assess blood glucose level regularly for clients with diabetes.
Thyroid Hormone Replacement Drugs *Synthetic source of T_4:* levothyroxine (Synthroid) *Natural (animal source) of T_3/T_4:* dessicated thyroid (Armour thyroid, S-P-T, Thyrar, Thyroid Strong) *Synthetic source of T_3:* liothyronine (T3, Cytomel, Triostat) *Synthetic source of T_3/T_4:* liotrix (Thyrolar); combination of levothroxine and lyothyronine	Increases metabolic rate of body tissues	Hyperthyroidism: tachycardia, tremors, headache, nervousness, insomnia, diarrhea, weight loss, heat intolerance	Monitor response closely. Monitor thyroid function tests. Advise client that drug usually is required for lifetime. Administer drug as a single daily dose before breakfast. Thyroid preparations interact with digitalis, estrogen, beta blockers, glucagon, and anticoagulants. Once therapy is begun, one drug should not be substituted for another.

^{131}I is used to destroy hyperplastic thyroid tissue by radiation. The thyroid is quick to remove iodine, including RAI, from the bloodstream. Antithyroid drugs are given for 6 months or more before administration of ^{131}I. If symptoms do not improve, a second and perhaps a third dose of ^{131}I is given. About 6 to 8 weeks after the initial dose of ^{131}I, most clients notice some remission of symptoms. The extended time lag before relief of symptoms is a disadvantage of this treatment method. A more common and unfortunate result of treatment is hypothyroidism, because accurately determining the precise amount of thyroid tissue that radiation will destroy is very difficult. This complication may not develop until long after the administration of ^{131}I, and clients must remain under medical supervision for many years.

Subtotal thyroidectomy (partial removal of the thyroid gland) or a *partial thyroid lobectomy* (removal of the upper or lower portion of one lobe) is an effective treatment for a confined area or nodule within the thyroid that is increasing production of thyroid hormones. Occasionally, an entire lobe with or without the isthmus is removed. *Total thyroidectomy* (removal of the entire thyroid gland) is performed if a cancerous tumor is present or the hyperthyroidism is in an advanced stage and involves all of the glandular tissue. Clients commonly receive antithyroid drug therapy for several weeks before surgery to prevent a dramatic release of thyroid hormones into the bloodstream during surgery. Single thyroid nodules less than 3 cm in diameter can be removed by minimally invasive endoscopic techniques in which the surgeon makes three to four small incisions in the neck rather than the typical single incision, which is several inches long.

Complications of thyroidectomy include the following:

- Accidental removal of or alteration in the blood supply to the parathyroid glands, which are embedded in thyroid tissue, resulting in hypocalcemia. One or more parathyroid glands may be reimplanted into nearby muscular tissue where they will eventually attach, grow, and function normally (http://www.endocrineweb.com/surthyroid.html).
- Hemorrhage caused by the vascularity of the thyroid and surrounding tissue
- Thyrotoxicosis (or thyroid storm) as a result of excessive secretion of thyroid hormones during surgical excision
- Damage to the recurrent laryngeal nerve, which affects the function of the vocal cords. If the recurrent laryngeal nerve is damaged either temporarily or partially, breathing may be impaired because the vocal cords cannot open properly during inspiration; the voice may sound weak, hoarse, or breathy; and aspiration and pneumonia may occur if the vocal cords do not close completely during swallowing.

Nursing Management

The nurse monitors heart rate and blood pressure (BP) regularly. He or she records the client's sleep pattern and daily weights. The nurse promotes rest and helps the client avoid excess physical stimulation. Increased caloric intake can compensate for increased metabolism (Nutrition Notes 50-1).

The nurse informs the client that effects of antithyroid therapy usually are not apparent until the thyroid gland has secreted the excess thyroid hormone into the bloodstream. This process may take several weeks or more. If RAI is used to destroy thyroid tissue, the nurse tells the client that it does

Nutrition Notes 50-1
The Client With Hyperthyroidism

- Calorie needs increase between 10% and 50% above normal to replenish glycogen stores and correct weight loss. A high protein intake helps replenish losses from muscle catabolism.
- Clients experiencing steady weight loss despite eating large amounts of food often are frustrated and discouraged. Encourage frequent meals and the intake of nutritionally dense foods (fortified milkshakes, foods fortified with skim milk powder, eggs, cheese, butter, or milk).
- After treatment restores normal metabolism, calories are adjusted downward to avoid excess weight gain.

not seriously affect other tissues. Possible transient effects after use of ^{131}I and ^{123}I are nausea, vomiting, malaise, fever, and gland tenderness.

Nursing Care Plan 50-1 discusses care of the client undergoing thyroid surgery.

THYROTOXIC CRISIS

Pathophysiology and Etiology

Thyrotoxic crisis (also known as thyroid storm and thyrotoxicosis), an abrupt and life-threatening form of hyperthyroidism, is thought to be triggered by extreme stress, infection, diabetic ketoacidosis, trauma, toxemia of pregnancy, or manipulation of a hyperactive thyroid gland during surgery or physical examination. Although rare, this condition may occur in clients with undiagnosed or inadequately treated hyperthyroidism.

The oversecretion of T_3 and T_4 is followed by a release of epinephrine. Metabolism is markedly increased. The adrenal glands produce excess corticosteroids in response to the stress created by this hypermetabolic state.

Assessment Findings

The temperature may be as high as 106°F (41°C). The pulse rate is rapid, and cardiac dysrhythmias are common. The client may experience persistent vomiting, extreme restlessness with delirium, chest pain, and dyspnea.

The diagnosis is based on the symptoms and a recent medical history that indicates symptoms of severe hyperthyroidism. Laboratory tests, such as serum T_3 and T_4 determinations, may be used to confirm the diagnosis. In thyrotoxic crisis, serum thyroid determinations are markedly elevated.

Medical Management

Immediate treatment is necessary. Antithyroid drugs (e.g., propylthiouracil, methimazole) are used to block the synthesis of thyroid hormones. An IV corticosteroid may be given to replace depletion that results from overstimulation of the adrenals during the hypermetabolic state. IV sodium iodide prevents the thyroid gland from releasing thyroid hormones. Propranolol (Inderal), a beta blocker, reduces the effect of thyroid hormones on the cardiovascular system. Supportive therapy includes IV fluids, antipyretic measures, and oxygen therapy.

NURSING CARE PLAN 50-1 | The Client Undergoing Thyroid Surgery

Assessment

- Obtain complete medical, drug, and allergy histories.
- Check and compare present weight with preillness weight.
- Measure vital signs each shift and more often if findings are abnormal.

- Perform a physical examination, but avoid palpating the thyroid gland (manipulation releases excess thyroid hormones).
- Determine client's preoperative compliance with antithyroid drug therapy.
- Explore client's knowledge of the operative procedure and perioperative care.

Nursing Diagnosis: Anxiety related to perception of pending surgery

Expected Outcome: Anxiety will be reduced to a tolerable level as evidenced by a rating below 5 on a scale from 0 to 10, uninterrupted sleep, no restlessness or purposeless activity, and moderate emotional responses.

Interventions	Rationales
Be calm and confident during interactions with client.	A nurse who conveys expertise helps reduce anxiety and builds a sense of security.
Interact with client frequently and respond promptly to requests for assistance.	Trust develops when a client obtains attention and support in a reasonable amount of time.
Give client opportunities to talk and ask questions about the surgery and subsequent health management issues.	If a nurse is receptive to questions, the client is more likely to verbalize concerns about the impending procedure.
Encourage the presence of those who give the client emotional support.	Significant others with whom the client has emotional bonds potentiate security.

Evaluation of Expected Outcomes

Client reports decreased anxiety.

Nursing Diagnosis: Deficient Knowledge related to unfamiliarity with perioperative measures that reduce potential postoperative complications

Expected Outcome: Client will demonstrate breathing and leg exercises and the technique for postoperative head support.

Interventions	Rationales
Provide routine instructions for deep breathing and leg exercises (see Chap. 14).	These measures decrease the potential for pneumonia, thrombi, and other complications.
Show client how to support the neck with the hands when rising to sit (Fig. 50-5).	Supporting the head avoids straining neck muscles or the surgical incision.

Evaluation of Expected Outcomes

Client performs exercises and supports the head as taught before surgery.

Nursing Diagnosis: Risk for Ineffective Breathing Pattern related to compression of the trachea from edema of the glottis, accumulated blood in the operative area, recurrent laryngeal nerve damage, or retained secretions

Expected Outcome: Breathing will be regular, noiseless, and effortless with an SpO_2 of at least 90%.

Interventions	Rationales
Elevate the head of the bed 30° or more.	Head elevation reduces edema.
Apply an ice bag to the neck if prescribed.	Cold promotes vasoconstriction, thereby reducing edema and bleeding.
Place a tracheostomy set in client's room.	Having a means for establishing a patent airway is an emergency life-saving measure.
Assemble oral/pharyngeal suction equipment at client's bedside and suction client if he or she cannot raise respiratory secretions.	Suctioning clears the airway of substances that compromise movement of gases into and out of the lungs.
Observe for dyspnea and restlessness.	Increased breathing effort is evidence of a compromised airway.
Report signs of respiratory distress to the nurse in charge and the physician.	Sharing information aids in collaborative efforts to prevent complications.

Evaluation of Expected Outcomes

Client maintains normal ventilation with no airway obstruction.

PC: Hemorrhage

Expected Outcome: The nurse monitors to detect, manage, and minimize signs of hemorrhage.

NURSING CARE PLAN 50-1   The Client Undergoing Thyroid Surgery (Continued)

Interventions	Rationales
Monitor vital signs every 1 to 4 hours.	Tachycardia and hypotension suggest cellular hypoxia and fluid volume deficit secondary to bleeding.
Inspect the surgical dressing frequently for bleeding. Check the back of the neck for bloody drainage.	Gauze dressing material wicks blood from the surgical incision. Gravity causes blood to drain posteriorly, which interferes with its visibility on the surface of the surgical dressing.
Attend to client's complaints of fullness in or around the surgical incision.	Blood may accumulate beneath the sutured incision rather than drain externally.
Place suture or staple removal equipment in client's room or stock equipment in a clean utility room.	The incision may need to be opened to remove clotted blood or ligate blood vessels that continue to bleed.

Evaluation of Expected Outcomes

There is no evidence of excessive bleeding in or around the operative site.

Nursing Diagnosis: Impaired Verbal Communication related to hoarseness secondary to recurrent laryngeal nerve damage

Expected Outcome: Client will regain normal volume and quality of speech.

Interventions	Rationales
Minimize unnecessary vocalizations for client.	Resting the voice reduces strain on the vocal cords.
Deliver bedside humidification.	Inhalation of moist air helps relieve hoarseness.
Provide an alternate means (pad of paper, magic slate, alphabet board) for the client to ask questions or make needs known.	Written communication provides a substitute for verbal interactions.
Ensure that client has access to a signal cord or bell with which to summon a caregiver.	A light or bell signals a need for assistance and is essential when a client cannot call for help.
Assess the quality of client's voice periodically every 2 to 4 waking hours for the first 2 postoperative days.	The nurse must report a weakening of the voice or loss of the ability to project sounds.

Evaluation of Expected Outcomes

Speech is at the presurgical volume.

Nursing Diagnosis: Risk for Aspiration related to recurrent laryngeal nerve damage

Expected Outcome: Lungs will be free of food or liquids.

Interventions	Rationales
Prepare oral/pharyngeal suction equipment.	Suctioning provides a way to clear the airway.
Have client sit upright.	An upright position promotes the mechanics of swallowing and a more forceful cough if substances enter the airway.
Provide thickened substances initially.	Watery food and beverages are more difficult to swallow.
Encourage client to place a very small amount in his or her mouth at any one time.	Controlling ingested substances increases the potential success for swallowing the mass.

Evaluation of Expected Outcomes

Client does not experience respiratory distress, and lungs are clear on auscultation.

Nursing Diagnosis: Pain related to tissue trauma secondary to operative procedure

Expected Outcome: Client will report an increased comfort level within 30 minutes of a pain-relieving intervention.

Interventions	Rationales
Administer analgesics as prescribed.	They interfere with pain transmission and perception.
Place pillows under the head, neck, and shoulders.	Pillows support the operative area, preventing excessive muscular pulling and possible separation of the incision.
Maintain head support when client's position is changed.	Head support reduces muscle contraction and tension on the surgical incision.

(care plan continues on page 766)

NURSING CARE PLAN 50-1   The Client Undergoing Thyroid Surgery (Continued)

Evaluation of Expected Outcomes

Client is comfortable or pain free.

PC: Tetany

Expected Outcome: The nurse will monitor to detect, manage, and minimize tetany.

Interventions	Rationales
Observe for spontaneous spasm of the fingers or toes, mouth twitching or jaw tightening when you tap the cheek anteriorly to the earlobe (Chvostek's sign), and spasm of the fingers toward the wrist when you inflate a BP cuff midway between systolic and diastolic pressures for 3 minutes (Trousseau's sign) (see Chap. 16).	Tetany develops when the parathyroid glands, which regulate blood calcium levels, are accidentally removed during a thyroidectomy. Hypocalcemia results in neuromuscular hyperexcitability.
Note crowing respirations and dyspnea.	Manifestations of hypocalcemia include symptoms caused by laryngeal spasm.
Be prepared to implement seizure precautions.	Seizures may occur when the blood calcium level falls below normal.
Have calcium gluconate for IV administration available if prescribed by the physician.	Calcium replacement controls symptoms of tetany.

Evaluation of Expected Outcomes

No complications develop.

PC: Thyrotoxic Crisis

Expected Outcome: The nurse will monitor to detect, manage, and minimize thyrotoxic crisis.

Interventions	Rationales
Assess for hyperthermia, tachycardia, chest pain, cardiac dysrhythmias, and altered level of consciousness.	Excess levels of thyroid hormones raise body temperature and accelerate cardiac activity by increasing the rate of metabolism.
Notify the physician if symptoms of thyrotoxic crisis develop.	Collaborative measures are necessary to control symptoms and their consequences.
Implement measures to reduce body temperature such as administering antipyretics or placing client on an aquathermia pad.	Measures to reduce body temperature help prevent complications such as seizures and brain damage.
Follow medical orders for measures to reduce heart rate and dysrhythmias.	Tachycardia increases myocardial demands for oxygen; unless managed, it can lead to myocardial infarction, acute heart failure, or cardiac arrest.

Evaluation of Expected Outcomes

No complications develop.

Nursing Management

The client with thyrotoxic crisis is acutely ill. The nurse monitors vital signs, especially the temperature, frequently. Failure to respond to an antipyretic drug requires other measures, such as a cooling blanket or ice application. A cool room also may help reduce body temperature. The nurse gives all therapeutic treatment measures as ordered because the situation must be corrected as soon as possible.

HYPOTHYROIDISM

Hypothyroidism occurs when the thyroid gland fails to secrete adequate thyroid hormones.

Pathophysiology and Etiology

This condition may originate in the thyroid (primary hypothyroidism) or in the pituitary, in which case insufficient TSH is secreted. Regardless of the cause, the result of inadequate thyroid hormone secretion is a slowing of all metabolic processes (see Table 50-1). Severe hypothyroidism is called **myxedema**. Advanced, untreated myxedema can progress to myxedemic coma. Signs of this life-threatening event are hypothermia, hypotension, and hypoventilation. A client with hypothyroidism experiencing infection, trauma, or excessive chills, or taking narcotics, sedatives, or tranquilizers, can lapse into a myxedemic coma.

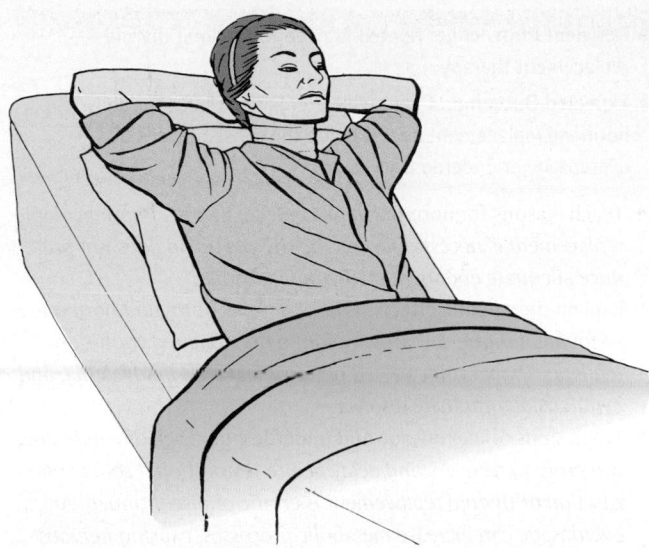

FIGURE 50-5. After a thyroidectomy, the client uses the hands to support the head while rising to a sitting position. This type of support helps avoid strain to the neck muscles and surgical incision.

Assessment Findings

Signs and Symptoms

Signs and symptoms are opposite those of hyperthyroidism in many respects. Metabolic rate and physical and mental activity slow down. The client is lethargic, lacks energy, dozes frequently during the day, is forgetful, and has chronic headaches. The face takes on a masklike, unemotional expression, yet the client often is irritable. The tongue may be enlarged and the lips swollen, and there may be edema of the eyelids. Temperature and pulse rate are decreased; the client is intolerant to cold. Weight increases despite a low caloric intake. The skin is dry, and hair characteristically is coarse and sparse and tends to fall out. Menstrual disorders are common. Constipation may be severe. The voice is low pitched and hoarse, and speech is slow. Hearing may be impaired. The client may experience numbness or tingling in the arms or legs that is unrelieved by position change.

Gerontologic Considerations

- Hypothyroidism is difficult to identify in older adults because symptoms closely resemble normal aging—for example, anorexia, constipation, weight loss, muscular weakness and pain, joint stiffness, apathy, and depression.

Hypothyroidism may lead to an enlarged heart caused by pericardial effusion and an increased tendency toward atherosclerosis and excessive effort by the heart to pump blood. Anemia also may be present. Early recognition of hypothyroidism is difficult because many of the symptoms are nonspecific and may not be sufficiently dramatic to bring the client to the physician. This condition can go untreated for years.

Diagnostic Findings

In primary hypothyroidism, levels of TSH are increased because of the negative feedback to the pituitary gland; that is, the low levels of thyroid hormones cause the pituitary gland to increase secretion of TSH (see Chap. 49). The level of FT_4 is decreased. The RAI uptake may be decreased. The T_3 and T_4 levels show no response in primary untreated hypothyroidism but may show a response if hypothyroidism results from failure of the pituitary to secrete TSH.

Medical Management

Hypothyroidism is treated with thyroid replacement therapy (see Drug Therapy Table 50-1). Thyroid hormone in the form of desiccated thyroid extract, or with one of the synthetic products, such as levothyroxine sodium (Synthroid) or liothyronine sodium (Cytomel), are oral thyroid preparations. A low dose of thyroid hormone is given initially and then increased or decreased until the optimal dose is achieved.

Pharmacologic Considerations

- During initial therapy with a thyroid replacement, the most common adverse reaction is signs of hyperthyroidism (which would indicate drug overdosage). Other adverse reactions are rare.

- Early effects of thyroid replacement therapy may be observed within 48 hours of the initial dose. However, a complete therapeutic response to thyroid hormone replacement therapy may not be evident until the client has concluded several weeks of therapy.

Gerontologic Considerations

- Dosages of thyroid replacement drugs are lower in older adults, and drug therapy is initiated slowly and increased cautiously. Older adults receiving thyroid replacement therapy are at increased risk for adverse reactions associated with cardiac function.

- Untreated hypothyroidism becomes a risk factor for coronary artery disease, indicating a need for cardiac stress testing and lipid level monitoring. Metabolic changes of hypothyroidism can be corrected with proper treatment. Older adults and family members should be advised that T_4 replacement with levothyroxine sodium must be maintained for life, with at least annual follow-up visits.

Nursing Process for the Client with Hypothyroidism

Assessment

Obtain medical, drug, and allergy histories as well as a thorough description of symptoms. Check vital signs and weight. During the physical examination, observe for symptoms of hypothyroidism:

lethargy, fatigue, anorexia, weight gain, hair loss, brittle nails, and cold intolerance.

Once a definitive diagnosis is made, observe for adverse effects of thyroid replacement therapy. Note the following signs of hyperthyroidism: dyspnea, rapid pulse rate, palpitations, precordial pain, hyperactivity, insomnia, dizziness, and GI disorders if the dose of thyroid hormone is too high. Once replacement therapy has begun, expect a dramatic change in a few weeks.

Diagnosis, Planning, and Interventions

▶ **Activity Intolerance** related to fatigue and depressed cognitive processes

▶ **Expected Outcome:** Client will demonstrate increased activity tolerance.

- Assess activity tolerance. *Altered metabolism from reduced secretion of thyroid hormone compromises client's ability to perform physical activities.*
- Allow adequate rest between activities. *Conserving energy increases endurance.*
- Assist with hygiene and other self-care activities as needed. *Such assistance extends the client's tolerance until he or she can progress to independent self-care.*

▶ **Constipation** related to decreased bowel function

▶ **Expected Outcome:** Stools will be moist and easily and regularly passed.

- Assess bowel elimination patterns and stool characteristics. *A record of bowel elimination and stool characteristics helps determine the need for measures to promote defecation.*
- Provide high-fiber foods. *Fiber increases stool bulk and promotes additional water in the intestinal mass. Bulky stool creates pressure in the rectum, which causes the stimulus to defecate.*
- Encourage adequate fluid intake. *Moist stool is expelled more easily than dry stool.*
- Encourage increased physical activity (e.g., short walks) within the client's tolerance. *Physical activity promotes the movement of intestinal contents toward the rectum and anus.*

▶ **Risk for Imbalanced Body Temperature** related to hyposecretion of thyroid hormones

▶ **Expected Outcome:** Body temperature will be maintained.

- Assess body temperature; report deviations from usual values. *Decreased metabolism lowers body temperature; reduced muscle contraction from inactivity interferes with the generation of body heat.*
- Provide extra warmth with blankets or clothing. *Layers of fabric that trap and hold warm air next to the body surface conserve or increase body heat.*
- Protect the client from exposure to cold or drafts. *Body heat is lost through convection as air currents pass over the warmer areas of exposed skin.*

▶ **Deficient Knowledge** related to need for lifelong thyroid replacement therapy

▶ **Expected Outcome:** Client will verbalize the need for daily hormone replacement and describe the consequences of overdosage or underdosage.

- Teach reasons for hormone replacement therapy. *Pharmacologic replacement is necessary when the thyroid gland does not produce adequate endogenous thyroid hormone.*
- Explain therapeutic effects. *When the level of thyroid hormone is adequate, fatigue, lethargy, weight gain, impaired cognition, tendency to feel cold, altered physical features, bradycardia, and hypotension gradually resolve.*
- Teach signs of overdosage and underdosage. *Lack of compliance can prolong recovery and delay health restoration if self-administration of thyroid replacement is erratic or discontinued. An overdosage can increase metabolic processes, causing nervousness, tremor, tachycardia, hypertension, and insomnia.*
- Assist the client to develop a schedule for taking medication each day. *Such a schedule helps the client avoid missing one or more doses.*
- Explain the need for continued follow-up to monitor hormone status. *Response to thyroid replacement therapy is evaluated through laboratory tests that measure TSH, T_3, and T_4 levels and regular medical examinations by the prescribing physician.*
- Recommend that the client obtain and wear a MedicAlert tag at all times. *It helps healthcare personnel to assess an unconscious client more readily if they are aware of a pre-existing health problem.*

PC: Myxedema and Myxedemic Coma

▶ **Expected Outcome:** The nurse will monitor to detect myxedema or myxedemic coma and will manage and minimize these conditions should they develop.

- Assess for decreased pulse, respirations, BP, and temperature. *Changes in vital signs accompany decreased metabolism.*
- Cover the client with warm blankets if temperature is below normal. *The heat from warmed cotton blankets is conducted to the skin and superficial blood vessels.*
- Assess for changes in LOC, difficulty waking, or increasing confusion. *Profound hypothyroidism slows all body functions, including the ability to remain awake and alert.*
- Monitor oxygenation status using a pulse oximeter. *A stuporous or comatose client may be unable to protect his or her airway, causing the blood oxygen saturation (SpO_2) to fall below 90%.*
- Administer oxygen as prescribed to maintain SpO_2 at or above 90%. *Maintaining SpO_2 at 90% ensures that the arterial oxygen pressure (PaO_2) is between 80 and 100 mm Hg.*
- Maintain a patent airway using an oral or pharyngeal airway. *An artificial airway keeps the tongue from obstructing the upper airway.*
- Consult with the physician or respiratory therapist if the client requires endotracheal intubation and mechanical ventilation. *An endotracheal tube maintains an airway and provides a means to oxygenate a client who does not breathe adequately.*

- Implement medical directives for IV fluids and administration of vasopressors and thyroid replacement hormone. *Clients with myxedema or myxedemic coma are treated with IV administration of levothyroxine and vasopressors.*
- Carefully administer analgesics; avoid administering sedatives or hypnotics. *CNS depressants interfere with the client's neurologic status and subsequent assessment of it.*

Evaluation of Expected Outcomes/Teaching Plan

Client reports feeling rested and meets self-care needs. He or she has regular stools without discomfort. The client reports feeling comfortable, not cold, in a normal temperature setting. He or she describes the medication regimen, possible side effects, and precautions. The client does not develop myxedema or myxedemic coma, or if it develops, the nurse collaborates with the physician to restore a normal physiologic state.

Symptoms associated with hyperthyroidism and hypothyroidism often affect learning and retention ability. The nurse carefully explains the treatment regimen, including the dose of the medications and possible adverse effects. If a special diet has been recommended, the nurse obtains a dietary consultation and reviews sample diets with the client.

A teaching plan includes the following:

- Weigh self weekly; keep a record of symptoms and weight in case the medication dose needs adjustment.
- Avoid stressful situations.
- Maintain good nutrition (Nutrition Notes 50-2).
- Notify the physician if symptoms worsen or adverse drug effects occur.

THYROID TUMORS

Tumors of the thyroid can cause hyperthyroidism. They are more commonly benign, but all nodules must be evaluated.

Pathophysiology and Etiology

A *follicular adenoma* is the most common benign thyroid lesion. In adult women, a thyroid nodule is most likely this type, but as it enlarges, surgical excision and pathologic examination are necessary to be certain. *Papillary carcinoma* is the most common malignant lesion; it usually occurs in clients who received radiation treatments to the head or neck region in the past. It tends to spread only to nearby lymph nodes and rarely to other parts of the body. The cure rate of thyroid cancer depends on the type of tumor present.

Assessment Findings

Symptoms are vague, and the client may be unaware of the lesion. Often a routine physical examination reveals a nodular thyroid. As the tumor enlarges, the client often notices a swelling in the neck. Benign tumors cause symptoms of hyperthyroidism in some clients. Malignant tumors can cause voice changes, hoarseness, and difficulty swallowing.

Biopsy of the lesion confirms the diagnosis. Thyroid cancer is suspected when the gland is firm and palpable and when results of RAI studies show poor concentration in the suspect area.

Medical and Surgical Management

If there are no symptoms of hyperthyroidism with a benign nodule, treatment usually is not needed. The nodule is examined yearly. If the enlargement causes such symptoms as difficulty swallowing and noticeable neck swelling, surgical removal of the lesion is considered. Although treatment of malignant lesions varies, a thyroidectomy (total or subtotal) typically is performed. A modified radical neck dissection is indicated if there is metastasis. After a thyroidectomy, thyroid hormone replacement therapy is given to restore thyroid function and to suppress pituitary TSH so that it no longer stimulates growth of residual thyroid tissue. ^{131}I is administered to destroy remaining thyroid tissue as well as to treat lymph node metastasis, if present.

Nursing Management

If the thyroid tumor is malignant, the physician explains the planned treatment and expected outcome. The nurse provides emotional support, especially if the tumor has metastasized and radical surgery is necessary. When RAI is used after surgery, the client is isolated and placed on radiation precautions (see Chap. 18). The nurse handles body fluids carefully to prevent spread of contamination.

ENDEMIC AND MULTINODULAR GOITERS

The word **goiter** refers to an enlarged thyroid gland.

Pathophysiology and Etiology

An *endemic goiter* is caused by a deficiency of iodine in the diet, by the inability of the thyroid to use iodine, or by relative iodine deficiency caused by increasing body demands for thyroid hormones. *Nontoxic goiter* (also called *simple* or *colloid goiter*) is an enlarged thyroid, usually with no symptoms of thyroid dysfunction. The gland may enlarge as a result of consuming excessive goitrogenic foods such as soybeans and peanuts or taking certain drugs such as lithium that may cause hyperplasia of the gland (Understanding Goiter, 2001). *Nodular goiters* contain one or more areas of hyperplasia. This type of goiter appears to develop for essentially the same reasons as an endemic goiter (Fig. 50-6).

Nutrition Notes 50-2
The Client With Hypothyroidism

- Until normal metabolism is restored, clients experience weight gain even if calorie intake is low.
- After hormone replacement therapy begins, the client may still need to follow a low-calorie diet to attain or maintain normal weight. A high-fiber diet promotes satiety and regularity.
- Additional modifications, such as low-fat, low-cholesterol, and low-sodium diets, are necessary if the client has cardiovascular complications.

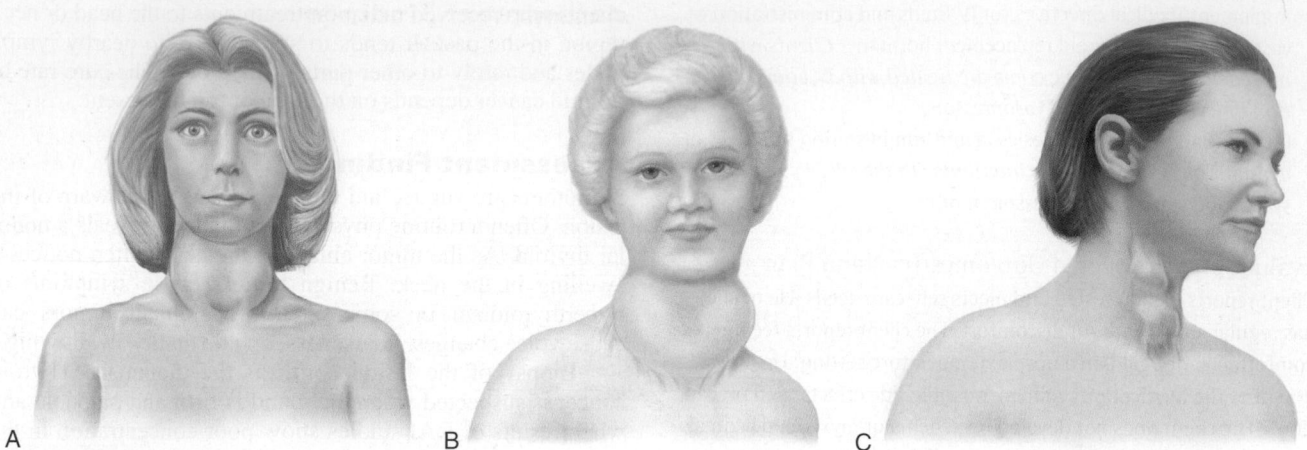

FIGURE 50-6. Thyroid abnormalities. (**A**) Toxic goiter (Graves' disease) with exophthalmos. (**B**) Nontoxic goiter. (**C**) Nodular goiter. (Provided by Anatomical Chart Co.)

Assessment Findings

The thyroid gland enlarges. The client has a sense of fullness in the neck area. Continued gland enlargement eventually results in difficulty swallowing and breathing as the thyroid presses on the trachea and esophagus. When the gland has enlarged, it is visible as a swelling in the neck. Nodular goiters also produce enlargement, but the gland has an irregular surface on palpation.

A thyroid scan shows an enlarged gland and a decreased uptake of ^{131}I. Tests of thyroid function are performed, but results may or may not be abnormal and, thus, are inconclusive.

Medical Management

Treatment depends on the cause. If the diet is deficient in iodine, foods high in iodine, such as seafood or iodized salt, are recommended. Potassium iodide to supplement iodine intake may be given. In some instances, a thyroidectomy is recommended, especially when the gland is grossly enlarged.

Nursing Management

If the client has respiratory distress because of the enlarged thyroid, the nurse closely observes respiratory status and elevates the head of the bed to relieve respiratory symptoms. He or she provides a diet high in iodine and iodized salt. Natural iodine content is highest in seafood; it is also found in varying amounts in bread, milk, eggs, meat, and spinach. A soft diet may be necessary if the client has difficulty swallowing.

THYROIDITIS

Thyroiditis, inflammation of the thyroid gland, can be acute, subacute, or chronic.

Pathophysiology and Etiology

There are multiple etiologies and, consequently, subtypes of thyroiditis that involve inflammation of the gland, release of higher than normal levels of hormone, and changes in thyroid function from hyperactivity to hypoactivity. Inflammation causes the gland to enlarge and become tender in some cases. Excess thyroid hormone released from stores within the thyroid gland rather than from stimulation from the pituitary produces a hypermetabolic state. As the stores of thyroid hormone deplete, a hypometabolic state ensues. In some cases, the thyroid gland recovers; in other cases, the hypothyroidism becomes permanent.

Acute thyroiditis, most common in children, appears to result from bacterial infection of the gland. Acute thyroiditis is fairly rare due to the efficacy of antibiotic therapy. One type of *subacute thyroiditis* can follow an upper respiratory viral infection while another, which is most likely autoimmune in nature, accompanies the postpartum period. The most common type is *Hashimoto's thyroiditis,* a chronic form of thyroiditis, believed to be an autoimmune disorder.

Assessment Findings

Signs and Symptoms

Signs and symptoms of acute thyroiditis include high fever, malaise, and tenderness and swelling of the thyroid gland. Subacute thyroiditis produces symptoms of a swollen and painful or painless gland. Chills, fever, and malaise approximately 2 weeks after infection accompany thyroiditis of a viral etiology. When signs of hyperthyroidism develop, the client experiences tachycardia, tremors, intolerance of heat, weight loss, and emotional irritability. Once the gland is destroyed, symptoms of hypothyroidism such as lethargy, weight gain, weakness, constipation, and dry hair develop.

Diagnostic Findings

In acute thyroiditis, laboratory test results show an elevated white blood cell (WBC) count. During a thyroid scan, inflamed and damaged thyroid cells fail to concentrate radioactive iodine. During the hypermetabolic phase of the disease, thyroid function tests elevate. In Hashimoto's thyroiditis, high titers of antimicrosomal and antithyroglobulin antibodies are evident, reflecting the autoimmune nature of the disease.

Medical and Surgical Management

Acute thyroiditis requires administration of appropriate antibiotics. The treatment of subacute thyroiditis is symptomatic and includes analgesics for pain and discomfort. Corticosteroids also may be prescribed to reduce inflammation. The treatment of Hashimoto's thyroiditis includes thyroid hormone replacement therapy. Surgery is required if the gland becomes excessively large.

Nursing Management

Management depends on the type of thyroiditis and severity of symptoms. The nurse gives antipyretics for fever. He or she elevates the head of the bed if the client has difficulty breathing. The nurse offers a soft diet if the gland is markedly enlarged and the client has difficulty swallowing.

If a client has undergone surgery (see Nursing Care Plan 50-1), the nurse instructs the client before discharge in the care of the surgical wound and to avoid excessive strain on the wound until it is healed. Because the incision is made in a neck crease, the healed scar is barely visible. If a client appears concerned about scarring, the nurse may suggest that the client wear clothing that covers the neck until the scar is almost invisible.

The nurse discusses the symptoms of hypothyroidism, hyperthyroidism, and hypoparathyroidism, with instructions to notify the physician immediately if they occur. If medication is prescribed, the nurse reviews the dosage and adverse effects of each drug. A teaching plan includes techniques for wound care, the need to take thyroid replacement medication in the morning at the same time each day to avoid insomnia and CNS stimulation, and side effects that require notification of the physician (chest pain, tachycardia, and dyspnea).

▶ *Stop, Think, and Respond Exercise 50-1*
When reviewing a client's medical record, you read that the physician has detected an enlarged thyroid gland. What are some possible causes?

DISORDERS OF THE PARATHYROID GLANDS

When the parathyroid gland dysfunctions, hyperparathyroidism or hypoparathyroidism develops. Calcium and phosphorus levels are affected.

HYPERPARATHYROIDISM

Hyperparathyroidism can be a primary or secondary condition.

Pathophysiology and Etiology

The most common cause of *primary hyperparathyroidism* is an adenoma of one of the parathyroid glands. In primary hyperparathyroidism, excessive secretion of parathyroid hormone (parathormone) results in increased urinary excretion of phosphorus and loss of calcium from the bones. The bones become demineralized as the calcium leaves and enters the bloodstream. Renal stones may develop as calcium becomes concentrated in the urine.

In *secondary hyperparathyroidism,* the parathyroid glands secrete excessive parathormone in response to hypocalcemia (low serum calcium level), which may result from vitamin D deficiency, chronic renal failure, large doses of thiazide diuretics, and excessive use of laxatives and calcium supplements.

Assessment Findings
Signs and Symptoms

Excessive calcium in the blood depresses the responsiveness of the peripheral nerves, accounting for fatigue and muscle weakness. The muscles become hypotonic (loss of or decrease in muscle tone). Cardiac dysrhythmias may develop. Because the bones have lost calcium, there is skeletal tenderness and pain on bearing weight; the bones may become so demineralized that they break with little or no trauma (pathologic fractures). Other possible effects include nausea, vomiting, and constipation. Large amounts of calcium and phosphorus passing through the kidneys predispose the client to the formation of stones in the urinary tract, pyelonephritis, and uremia.

Diagnostic Findings

The diagnosis is based on elevated serum calcium and decreased serum phosphorus levels without other causes of hypercalcemia. The results of a 24-hour urine test show increased urine calcium levels. Skeletal radiographs show calcium loss from bones. An MRI or CT scan identifies a parathyroid adenoma if it is present. Parathormone levels are elevated in hyperparathyroidism.

Medical and Surgical Management

Secondary hyperparathyroidism is managed by correcting the cause (e.g., vitamin D therapy for a vitamin D deficiency, correction of renal failure, calcium-restricted diet). Sodium and phosphorus replacements often are ordered. Hormone replacement with synthetic calcitonin (Calcimar) is avoided because it is associated with allergic reactions and drug resistance. The latter is caused by antibodies that neutralize the hormone.

The only treatment for primary hyperparathyroidism is surgical removal of hypertrophied glandular tissue or of an individual tumor of one of the parathyroid glands. Before surgery, the physician determines the number of the four glands to be removed, based on the cause of hyperparathyroidism and laboratory and diagnostic test results. One or more of the parathyroids is left in place because they are necessary for calcium and phosphorus metabolism.

Nursing Management

The nurse closely measures the client's intake and output. He or she observes for signs of urinary calculi from hypercalcemia, flank pain, and decreasing urine output (see Chap. 58). The nurse encourages a large volume of fluid to keep the urine dilute (Nutrition Notes 50-3). He or she assesses the client's ability to perform self-care, provides a safe environment to prevent falls and other injury, encourages frequent rest periods, and monitors fatigue level.

The primary nursing responsibility is teaching the client about the effects of the disease, the planned medical management, and the importance of following the prescribed treatment. If the client undergoes surgery, the nursing management is similar to that for thyroid surgery. In addition, the nurse observes the client for symptoms of hypoparathyroidism.

HYPOPARATHYROIDISM

Hypoparathyroidism is a deficiency of parathormone that results in hypocalcemia.

Pathophysiology and Etiology

Parathormone regulates calcium balance by increasing calcium absorption from the GI tract and bone resorption of calcium. Hypocalcemia affects neuromuscular functions. It causes hyperexcitability, resulting in spastic muscle contractions and *paresthesias* (abnormal sensations).

The most common causes of hypoparathyroidism are trauma to the glands and inadvertent removal of all or nearly all these structures during thyroidectomy or parathyroidectomy. The idiopathic form of this disorder is rare but may be autoimmune in origin or caused by the congenital absence of the parathyroids.

Assessment Findings

Signs and Symptoms

The main symptom of acute and sudden hypoparathyroidism is **tetany**. The client may report numbness and tingling in the fingers or toes or around the lips. A voluntary movement may be followed by an involuntary, jerking spasm. Muscle cramping may be present. Tonic (continuous contraction) flexion of an arm or a finger may occur. If a nurse taps the client's facial nerve (which lies under the tissue in front of the ear), the client's mouth twitches and the jaw tightens. The response is identified as a positive *Chvostek's sign* (see Chap. 16). The nurse may elicit a positive *Trousseau's sign* by placing a BP cuff on the upper arm, inflating it between the systolic and diastolic BP, and waiting 3 minutes. The nurse observes the client for spasm of the hand (**carpopedal spasm**), which is evidenced by the hand flexing inward (see Chap. 16).

Laryngeal spasm can occur, causing dyspnea, with long, crowing respirations as air passes around the constriction. Cyanosis may be present, and the client is in danger of asphyxia and cardiac dysrhythmias. Nausea, vomiting, abdominal pain, and seizures can develop.

In chronic hypoparathyroidism, the client experiences neuromuscular irritability, constipation or diarrhea, numbness and tingling of the arms and legs, loss of tooth enamel, and muscle pain. Positive Chvostek's and Trousseau's signs may or may not be elicited, depending on the degree of hypocalcemia.

Diagnostic Findings

The serum calcium level is decreased, the serum phosphorus level is increased, and the urine levels of both are decreased. In chronic hypoparathyroidism, radiographs show increased bone density.

Medical Management

Tetany and severe hypoparathyroidism are treated immediately by the administration of an IV calcium salt, such as calcium gluconate. Endotracheal intubation and mechanical ventilation may be necessary if acute respiratory distress occurs. Bronchodilators also are used. Parathyroid replacement therapy is not the usual treatment because of its associated incidence of allergic reactions. If it is used, drug resistance develops in approximately 2 weeks.

Long-term treatment after trauma to or inadvertent removal of the parathyroids includes administration of oral calcium, vitamin D, or vitamin D_2 (calciferol), which increases the serum calcium level. The dose is related to the degree of hypocalcemia, which is determined by frequent monitoring of serum and urine calcium levels. A diet high in calcium and low in phosphorus usually is recommended (see Nutrition Notes 50-3).

Nursing Management

The nurse is alert for signs of tetany and assesses for Chvostek's and Trousseau's signs. He or she monitors the client with chronic hypoparathyroidism for increasing severity of symptoms. The nurse is prepared to administer IV calcium salt and observes the client during such administration for adverse effects, such as flushing, cardiac dysrhythmia (usually a bradycardia), tingling in the arms and legs, and a metallic taste. Local tissue necrosis may occur if the IV fluid escapes into surrounding tissues. The nurse monitors serum calcium levels to determine the effectiveness of therapy.

If the client has chronic hypoparathyroidism, the nurse obtains complete medical, drug, and allergy histories. He or she examines the client for symptoms of the disorder, primarily for the effect of hypocalcemia on the CNS. The nurse assesses the arms and legs for evidence of muscle spasm. He or she auscultates the lungs because the client may have dyspnea or other respiratory difficulty. During assessment of vital signs, attention to heart rate and rhythm is particularly important.

The nurse keeps an emergency tracheostomy tray, mechanical ventilation equipment, artificial airway, and endotracheal intubation equipment at the client's bedside if hypocalcemia is severe. He or she inserts an IV line for the emergency administration of calcium. The nurse observes frequently for respiratory distress and notifies the physician immediately if this problem occurs.

Until hypocalcemia is corrected, the nurse must assist the client with activities of daily living (ADLs). Movement, noise, and other environmental disturbances can trigger muscle contractions or convulsions. Thus, minimizing all forms of stress is essential until serum calcium levels approach normal and symptoms are relieved.

Clients who require lifetime treatment of the disorder need careful review of the prescribed treatment. Because normal calcium levels depend on drug and diet therapy, the nurse

Nutrition Notes 50-3
The Client With a Parathyroid Disorder

- Clients with hyperparathyroidism should use a low-calcium diet (fewer dairy products) and drink at least 3 to 4 L of fluid daily to dilute the urine and prevent renal stones from forming. It is especially important that the client drink fluids before going to bed and periodically throughout the night to avoid concentrated urine.
- Clients with hypoparathyroidism need more calcium and vitamin D than can be provided through food alone, yet they should be encouraged to eat foods rich in calcium, such as milk, yogurt, green leafy vegetables, and fortified orange juice. Carbonated beverages should be avoided because they are high in phosphorus (phosphoric acid).

Client and Family Teaching 50-2
Hypoparathyroidism

The nurse develops a teaching plan that includes the following points:

- Take drugs at the doses and intervals prescribed.
- Never increase, decrease, or omit drug doses unless advised by the physician. Increasing the dose can cause symptoms of hypercalcemia; decreasing or omitting the dose can cause the original symptoms to return.
- If nausea, vomiting, or severe diarrhea develops, contact the physician.
- Read food labels carefully so that you include foods that are part of the diet and avoid those that are not. Adherence to the recommended diet is necessary.

---

must stress the importance of these two aspects of treatment. Consultation with a dietitian may be necessary to provide a list of foods to include or to avoid in the prescribed diet. The nurse gives the client a list of the symptoms of hypercalcemia and hypocalcemia, either of which can occur if the dose of the prescribed drug is too high or too low or if the drug is omitted. He or she emphasizes the need to contact the physician immediately about any symptoms. The nurse reminds the client that the physician may need periodically to adjust the dose of the drug; therefore, recognizing the symptoms associated with hypercalcemia and hypocalcemia is essential. Client and Family Teaching 50-2 outlines more teaching points

DISORDERS OF THE ADRENAL GLANDS

Adrenal dysfunction includes pathology of the outer portion of the adrenal gland, the *cortex,* which synthesizes and secretes the hormones known as *corticosteroids:* mineralocorticoids, glucocorticoids, and gonadocorticoids, or sex hormones, sometimes referred to as androgens. The sex hormones are secreted in small amounts by the adrenal glands in comparison with that which is secreted by the testes and ovaries. Androgenic gonadocorticoids, one source of testosterone, cause masculinizing effects in women after menopause, when ovarian estrogen levels decline. Disorders of the adrenal glands also involve the *medulla,* the inner portion, which secretes the catecholamines norepinephrine (noradrenaline) and epinephrine (adrenaline). Proper secretion of these hormones is essential to life.

ADRENAL INSUFFICIENCY (ADDISON'S DISEASE)

Adrenal insufficiency is classified as either primary or secondary.

Pathophysiology and Etiology
Primary adrenal insufficiency (Addison's disease) results from destruction of the adrenal cortex by diseases such as

tuberculosis. It also may be an autoimmune disorder, in which antibodies formed by the client's immune system destroy adrenal tissue. In many instances, the cause is unknown.

The consequences of decreased adrenal cortical function include decreased available glucose and hypoglycemia. The glomerular filtration rate of the kidneys slows dramatically, causing decreased urea nitrogen excretion.

Secondary adrenal insufficiency is the result of surgical removal of both adrenal glands (*bilateral adrenalectomy*), hemorrhagic infarction of the glands, hypopituitarism (caused by pituitary failure or surgical removal of the pituitary), or suppression of adrenal function by the administration of corticosteroids. Clients with secondary adrenal insufficiency after bilateral adrenalectomy or surgical removal of the pituitary gland do not experience true adrenal insufficiency because corticosteroids are administered to replace the hormones no longer secreted by the adrenals.

Assessment Findings
Signs and Symptoms
Decreased or absent adrenocortical hormones lead to symptoms of adrenal insufficiency, which are the same in primary and secondary adrenal insufficiency (Box 50-1). Clients with primary adrenal insufficiency usually experience symptoms gradually. Clients with secondary adrenal insufficiency develop symptoms suddenly or over several days to weeks.

Diagnostic Findings
A dose of synthetic ACTH, cosyntropin (Cortrosyn), is administered intramuscularly as a screening test for adrenal function. In primary adrenal insufficiency, an absent or a low cortisol response indicates adrenal insufficiency. In secondary insufficiency, the decrease in serum cortisol levels is less significant.

The serum cortisol level is decreased. Serum sodium and fasting blood glucose levels are low, and serum potassium, calcium, and blood urea nitrogen levels are increased. The WBC count often is elevated. A glucose tolerance test shows evidence of hypoglycemia. In Addison's disease, the glucose

| BOX 50-1 | Signs and Symptoms of Adrenal Insufficiency |

- Increased urinary excretion of sodium and retention of potassium followed by dehydration and reduced blood plasma volume
- Weakness, fatigue, dizziness, hypotension, postural hypotension, hypothermia
- Vascular collapse because of poor myocardial tone, decreased cardiac output, weak and irregular pulse
- Weight loss, anemia, anorexia, gastrointestinal symptoms
- Nervousness, periods of depression
- Hypoglycemia from a deficiency of the hormones that facilitate the conversion of protein into glucose; episodes of hypoglycemia may occur 5 to 6 hours after eating—the period before breakfast is especially dangerous
- Abnormally dark pigmentation, especially of exposed areas of the skin and mucous membranes, and decreased hair growth (primary adrenal insufficiency)

level in the bloodstream does not rise as high as normal and returns to its fasting level more quickly than it would under normal conditions. The fasting blood glucose level may be low. Radiographs of the adrenals show calcification. An abdominal CT scan reveals atrophy of the adrenal glands.

Medical Management

Clients with primary adrenal insufficiency require daily corticosteroid replacement therapy for the rest of their lives. Fludrocortisone (Florinef), a synthetic corticosteroid preparation that possesses mineralocorticoid and some glucocorticoid properties, frequently is selected for replacement therapy. An additional glucocorticoid may be necessary, depending on the client's response to therapy.

Pharmacologic Considerations

- The more common adverse reactions to Florinef include frontal and occipital headache, arthralgia, edema, and hypertension. Dosage increases may be necessary during stressful periods to prevent drug-induced adrenal insufficiency.

Treatment for secondary adrenal insufficiency caused by bilateral adrenalectomy or pituitary failure is the same as treatment for primary adrenal insufficiency. Treatment of secondary adrenal insufficiency resulting from discontinuation of corticosteroid therapy or hemorrhagic infarction of the gland varies and depends on the ability of the adrenals to return to normal function.

If the client is not given or does not take the medication, acute adrenal crisis can develop (see next section). This also applies to clients on long-term corticosteroid therapy for the treatment of disorders such as allergies, rheumatoid arthritis, and collagen diseases who abruptly discontinue taking their prescribed steroid. If the drug is to be discontinued, the dose must be tapered over time. Client and Family Teaching 50-3 discusses important information to teach clients receiving corticosteroid therapy.

Nursing Process for the Client With Addison's Disease

Assessment

Obtain a complete health history that includes presence or absence of weight loss, salt craving, nausea and vomiting, abdominal cramps, diarrhea, muscle weakness, and decreased stress tolerance. Take vital signs frequently. Monitor blood sugar levels; hypoglycemia may occur in clients with primary adrenal insufficiency. These clients must never receive insulin by error because insulin lowers the blood glucose to a critically low level that could result in brain damage, coma, or death.

Diagnosis, Planning, and Interventions

Nursing management of the client with primary adrenal insufficiency is essentially the same as that of the client with secondary

Client and Family Teaching 50-3
Corticosteroid Therapy for Adrenal Insufficiency

The nurse explains adrenal insufficiency and the importance of lifetime corticosteroid replacement. A teaching plan includes the following points:

- Never omit, increase, or decrease a dose. Lifetime corticosteroid replacement therapy is necessary. If the prescribed drug is not taken, adrenal insufficiency, which is life-threatening, will occur.
- Seek medical attention for dosage readjustment whenever there is stress. The body has limited ability to handle stress of any kind. Examples of stress include an infection, a motor vehicle accident (even if not noticeably hurt), a family crisis, and a heavy work load.
- Avoid exposure to infections and excessive fatigue.
- If an infection (e.g., sore throat, upper respiratory tract infection) or other type of illness occurs, contact the physician immediately. An increased medication dose may be necessary.
- Seek immediate medical attention if vomiting, diarrhea, or any other condition prevents the medication from being taken orally or interferes with proper drug absorption. Parenteral administration will be necessary. (The physician instructs the client on the procedures to follow if the medication cannot be taken orally.)
- Wear identification, such as a MedicAlert tag or bracelet, stating that the wearer has adrenal insufficiency. If an accident or other problem occurs, medical personnel must be made aware of the need for corticosteroids.
- Follow the diet recommended by the physician.

---

adrenal insufficiency because the major problem in both types is a lack of adrenal cortical hormones. The client with secondary adrenal insufficiency because of surgery (bilateral adrenalectomy, surgical removal of the pituitary) has a controlled deficiency that hormone replacement therapy corrects.

▶ Risk for Deficient Fluid Volume related to inadequate fluid intake, fluid loss secondary to inadequate adrenal hormone secretion

▶ Expected Outcome: Fluid intake will be 1500 to 3000 mL/day.

- Keep careful records of fluid intake and urine output. *Data collection is necessary to determine if a problem is developing.*
- Weigh the client daily on the same scale, at a similar time, with similar clothing. *Consistency in data collection helps the nurse accurately compare assessment findings.*
- Notify the physician if dehydration, signs of hyponatremia, or progressive weight loss occurs. *The physician and nurse collaborate to manage a client's problem.*
- Encourage the client to drink fluids and eat the prescribed diet to maintain fluid and electrolyte balance (Nutrition Notes 50-4). *Fluid and nutritional needs are easier to meet orally than parenterally.*

Nutrition Notes 50-4
The Client With Addison's Disease

- A high-protein, moderate-carbohydrate diet that is low in refined carbohydrates is recommended to reduce the risk of hypoglycemia from excess insulin secretion. The risk of hypoglycemia is also lessened by consuming frequent meals and snacks, especially a substantial bedtime snack.
- A high sodium intake is necessary unless fludrocortisone (Florinef) (a sodium-retaining hormone) is used.
- Unless otherwise contraindicated, 2 to 3 L of fluid per day is recommended.
- Potassium requirements are determined on an individual basis.

- If serum sodium levels are decreased, instruct the client to add salt to food. If excessive perspiration occurs, increase fluid and salt intake. *Salt is sodium chloride. Sodium is an electrolyte that attracts water and reduces its excretion. Increasing oral fluid intake compensates for unusual loss of body fluid.*

▶ PC: Hypoglycemia

▶ **Expected Outcome:** The nurse will monitor to detect, manage, and minimize episodes of low blood glucose.

- Minimize any reason for fasting, such as before a diagnostic test. *Eating carbohydrates regularly maintains the blood glucose level.*
- Observe for symptoms of hypoglycemia: hunger, headache, sweating, weakness, trembling, emotional instability, visual disturbances, and, finally, disorientation and loss of consciousness. *Physiologic and emotional changes accompany a low blood glucose level.*
- Check the client's blood glucose level with a glucometer 30 minutes before each meal, at bedtime, and whenever the client is symptomatic. *Checking capillary blood glucose provides a numeric assessment of the blood glucose level.*
- Follow agency protocol for raising the client's blood glucose level, which may include offering the client the equivalent of 15 g of carbohydrate such as 1/2 c of grape juice or administering 3 to 4 glucose tablets if the level is below 70 mg/dL and rechecking the level in 15 minutes. If the blood glucose level continues to be low, repeat the method for increasing blood sugar. *Glucose, a monosaccharide found in various carbohydrate food sources and commercially available in glucose tablets that contain 4 or 5 g of glucose per tablet, should raise the blood glucose level within 15 minutes of consumption.*
- Give the client milk and graham crackers or provide the next meal when the blood glucose level recovers to a level above 70 mg/dL. *Milk and graham crackers contain forms of carbohydrate that take longer to absorb and tend to maintain the blood glucose level for an extended period.*
- Contact the physician if the client continues to be symptomatic and the blood glucose level is below 80 mg/dL. *Regulation of blood glucose level may require parenteral administration of glucose, which the nurse cannot implement independently.*

- Instruct the client to remain in bed. *Dizziness and fainting may accompany the low blood glucose level; maintaining bed rest protects the client from injuries from a fall.*
- Offer five or six small meals per day rather than three regular meals to control hypoglycemic episodes; if client is eating three meals per day, give between-meal snacks of milk and crackers. *Eating carbohydrates frequently and regularly helps stabilize blood glucose levels within a normal range.*

▶ Fatigue related to fluid, electrolyte, and glucose imbalances

▶ **Expected Outcome:** Client will demonstrate endurance to meet self-care needs independently.

- Assist with bathing and grooming as needed. *The nurse helps the client until the client can resume total self-care.*
- Provide rest between activities. *Rest replenishes energy.*
- Control environmental stimuli to promote rest. *Stimulation interferes with client's ability to relax physically and become refreshed.*

▶ Risk for Injury related to hypotension, muscle weakness

▶ **Expected Outcome:** Client will experience no injuries or falls.

- Tell the client to lie down if he or she becomes dizzy when rising or changing position. *Blood tends to pool temporarily in dependent areas, causing a deficit in the brain when assuming an upright position.*
- Take the client's BP if symptoms such as weakness and faintness occur. *Measuring BP provides objective data for assessing hemodynamic changes.*
- Keep side rails raised. *They remind the client that he or she should not ambulate independently.*
- Instruct the client to ask for assistance getting out of bed. *Assistance can support and reposition the client if syncope develops.*
- Emphasize the importance of getting out of bed slowly. *Moving quickly aggravates symptoms of hypotension and potentiates the risk for fainting and falling.*

Evaluation of Expected Outcomes

Fluid intake approximates output; electrolytes remain within normal limits. The client has sufficient energy for ADLs. No injuries occur.

ACUTE ADRENAL CRISIS (ADDISONIAN CRISIS)

Clients with either primary or secondary adrenal insufficiency are at risk for **addisonian crisis**, a life-threatening endocrine emergency.

Pathophysiology and Etiology

Acute adrenal crisis occurs when the adrenal glands suddenly fail. Because the hormones of the adrenal cortex are prominent in facilitating the body's adaptive reactions to stress, clients with Addison's disease may develop acute adrenal crisis when faced with extreme stress. Even uncomplicated surgery requires more physiologic adaptive ability than a client with Addison's disease usually possesses. Salt deprivation, infection, trauma, exposure to cold, overexertion, or any abnormal stress can cause adrenal crisis. Acute adrenal crisis can occur when corticosteroid therapy is suddenly discontinued. If the condition is untreated, coma and death result.

Assessment Findings

Adrenal crisis may be sudden or gradual. It may begin with anorexia, nausea, vomiting, diarrhea, abdominal pain, profound weakness, headache, intensification of hypotension, restlessness, or fever. Unless the corticosteroid dose is increased to meet the demand, the client progresses to acute adrenal crisis. The BP markedly decreases and shock develops.

Diagnosis is based on symptoms and history. Case finding can show an omission of daily corticosteroid therapy. (See section on Diagnostic Findings for adrenal insufficiency.)

Medical Management

Adrenal crisis is an emergency; death may occur from hypotension and vasomotor collapse. Corticosteroids are given IV in solutions of normal saline and glucose. Antibiotics are administered because of an extremely low resistance to infection.

Nursing Management

Two important nursing tasks are the recognition of signs and symptoms of adrenal crisis and the accurate administration of corticosteroid drugs. A client with a diagnosis of adrenal insufficiency is a candidate for acute adrenal crisis; therefore, the nurse constantly observes such clients for this problem. He or she administers the correct dose of corticosteroid therapy at the correct time. Doses must never be omitted or abruptly discontinued, because this can result in adrenal crisis. Once the condition is recognized, the nurse takes vital signs frequently, paying special attention to heart rate and rhythm. He or she observes for signs of hyponatremia and hyperkalemia. The nurse keeps the client warm and as quiet as possible until treatment is initiated and the condition is stabilized.

PHEOCHROMOCYTOMA

Pheochromocytoma is a tumor of the adrenal medulla that causes hyperfunction.

Pathophysiology and Etiology

A pheochromocytoma usually is a benign tumor. Hyperfunction causes the adrenal medulla to secrete the catecholamines epinephrine and norepinephrine excessively. Exercise, emotional distress, trauma such as surgery, manipulation of the tumor, and postural changes can trigger episodic symptoms. Excessive secretion of epinephrine leads to hypertension and increases the potential for cerebrovascular accident, palpitations, and tachycardia. People who should be assessed for pheochromocytoma include those who (1) have hypertension that is difficult to control, (2) take more than four medications to control their blood pressure, or (3) develop hypertension before 35 years of age.

Assessment Findings

Symptoms include elevated BP (intermittent or, more frequently, persistent), tremors, nervousness, sweating, headache, nausea, vomiting, hyperglycemia, polyuria, and vertigo. The level of vanillylmandelic acid in a 24-hour urine specimen is markedly increased. Urinary catecholamine determination on the same or a different specimen may be elevated. CT, MRI, ultrasonography, aortography, and retrograde pyelography reveal the tumor. A drop in BP after a test injection of the alpha-adrenergic blocker phentolamine (Regitine) supports the presence of a pheochromocytoma; when compared with baseline measurements, the systolic BP falls more than 35 mm Hg and the diastolic BP falls more than 25 mm Hg.

Medical and Surgical Management

Treatment involves surgical or minimally invasive laparoscopic removal of the tumor by means of *unilateral adrenalectomy* (removal of one adrenal gland). Phentolamine is given before and during surgery to control hypertension. Alpha-adrenergic blockers, such as phenoxybenzamine (Dibenzyline), are used to control hypertension before surgery or when surgery is contraindicated, or to treat a malignant pheochromocytoma. Medical treatment includes metyrosine (Demser), an enzyme inhibitor that reduces synthesis of catecholamines to decrease hypertensive attacks.

Nursing Management

The nurse monitors the BP closely when initiating drug therapy or during dose changes. He or she notifies the physician of a sudden decrease in BP. If the client undergoes adrenalectomy, the nurse assesses for signs and symptoms of acute adrenal insufficiency (see earlier discussion).

CUSHING'S SYNDROME (ADRENOCORTICAL HYPERFUNCTION)

Cushing's syndrome is an endocrine disorder that results from excessive secretion of hormones by the adrenal cortex.

Pathophysiology and Etiology

An overproduction of adrenocortical hormones results from (1) overproduction of ACTH by the pituitary gland, with resultant hyperplasia of the adrenal cortex and excessive production and secretion of glucocorticoids, mineralocorticoids, and gonadocorticoids; (2) benign or malignant tumors of the pituitary gland or adrenal cortex; or (3) prolonged administration of high doses of corticosteroids. Those clients who take corticosteroids are advised to remain compliant and avoid discontinuing their administration abruptly to avoid addisonian or adrenal crisis. When these types of medications are no longer necessary, they are discontinued gradually (see section on Adrenalectomy later in this chapter).

Hyperadrenalism affects most body systems and causes many changes in appearance and physiology. The term **cushingoid syndrome** refers to the physical changes that accompany this disorder (Fig. 50-7). Examples of physiologic alterations include suppression of the inflammatory response, hyperglycemia, hypokalemia, hypernatremia with subsequent weight gain and elevated BP, peptic ulcer,

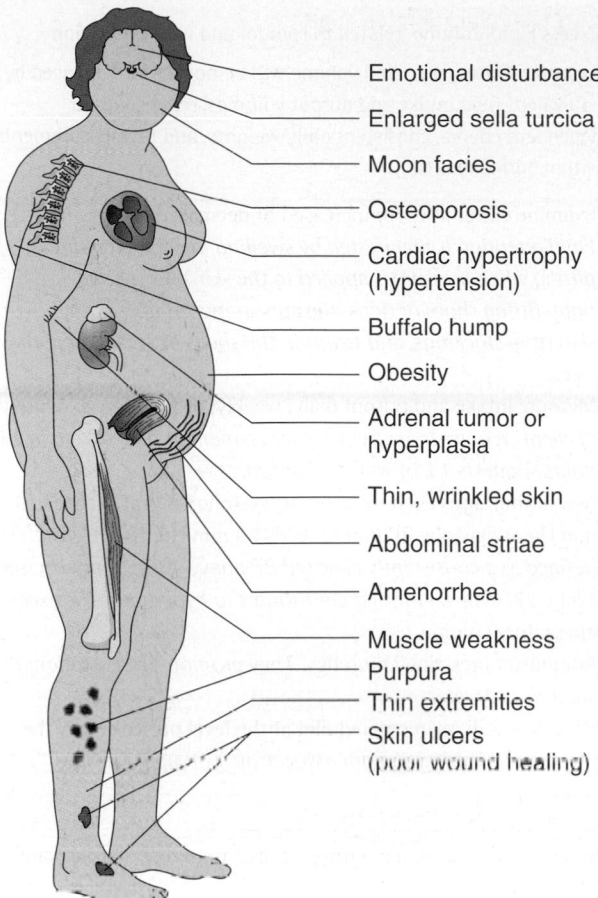

- Emotional disturbance
- Enlarged sella turcica
- Moon facies
- Osteoporosis
- Cardiac hypertrophy (hypertension)
- Buffalo hump
- Obesity
- Adrenal tumor or hyperplasia
- Thin, wrinkled skin
- Abdominal striae
- Amenorrhea
- Muscle weakness
- Purpura
- Thin extremities
- Skin ulcers (poor wound healing)

FIGURE 50-7. Clinical manifestations of Cushing's syndrome. (From Rubin, R., & Strayer, D. S. [2008]. *Rubin's pathology: Clinicopathologic foundations of medicine* [5th ed.]. Philadelphia: Lippincott Williams & Wilkins.)

demineralization of bones, and muscle weakness. Increased levels of androgenic gonadocorticoid hormone cause women to acquire male secondary sex characteristics. People of both sexes experience decreased sexual drive. Many clients suffer from depression, and the endocrine imbalance may cause psychosis.

Assessment Findings

Signs and Symptoms

Physical examination reveals muscle wasting and weakness resulting from extensive protein depletion. Carbohydrate tolerance is lowered, and signs and symptoms of diabetes mellitus develop (see Chap. 51). Fat is redistributed, leading to facial fullness and the characteristic moon face and buffalo hump. The skin is thin, and the face is ruddy. The client has increased susceptibility to wounds, and healing is prolonged; however, the immunosuppressive effects of the disorder usually mask symptoms of infection.

Because the blood vessels are fragile, the client bruises easily, and striae often form over extensive skin areas. The bones become so demineralized that the client may have backache, kyphosis, and collapse of the vertebrae. He or she retains sodium and water, and peripheral edema and hypertension develop. The client reports mood changes and

difficulty coping with stressors that were manageable in the past. The family may report serious mental changes. In women, Cushing's syndrome produces masculinization with hirsutism and amenorrhea. These sexual changes and alterations in appearance are reversible when adrenocortical hormone levels return to normal (Fig. 50-8).

Diagnostic Findings

Diagnosis is tentatively based on the physical changes. Urine levels of 17-hydroxycorticosteroids (17-OHCS) and 17-ketosteroids (17-KS) almost always are increased. Plasma and urine cortisol levels are elevated. An overnight dexamethasone suppression test is used as an initial screening. The client takes 1 mg oral dexamethasone; the next morning plasma cortisol levels are obtained. If these results are above normal (5 mg/dL), 0.5 mg dexamethasone is given every 6 hours, and 24-hour urine collections are tested for 2 consecutive days. Clients without the disorder have decreased 17-OHCS and 17-KS levels; these levels remain elevated in those with Cushing's syndrome.

To determine whether the symptoms of Cushing's syndrome are the result of pituitary stimulation, plasma ACTH is measured in conjunction with the administration of dexamethasone. If ACTH levels subsequently are found to be low or normal and the cortisol level is elevated, it suggests that the adrenal gland alone is hyperfunctioning. If both the ACTH and cortisol levels are elevated, a pituitary or hypothalamic etiology is more likely.

Laboratory blood test results also reveal increased serum sodium, decreased serum potassium, and increased blood glucose levels. Abdominal radiographs, CT, or MRI may show adrenal enlargement, and an IV pyelogram may show changes in the renal shadow caused by an abnormally large adrenal gland.

Medical and Surgical Management

Treatment depends on whether a tumor or adrenal hyperplasia causes the disorder. It is directed toward removing the cause and lowering plasma cortisol levels. Radiation therapy

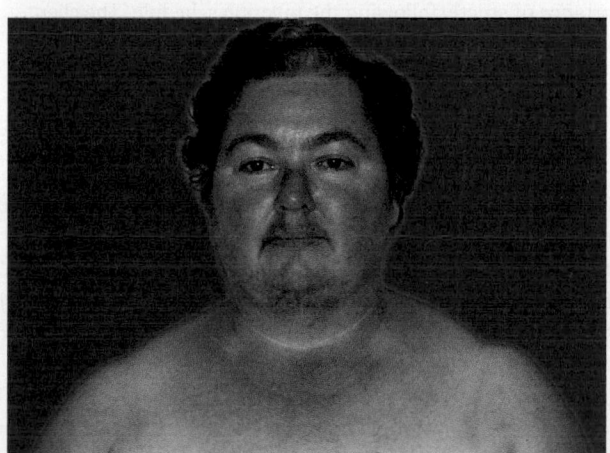

FIGURE 50-8. This woman with Cushing's syndrome exhibits a moon face, buffalo hump, increased facial hair, and thinning of the scalp hair. (From Rubin, R., & Strayer, D. S. [2008]. *Rubin's pathology: Clinicopathologic foundations of medicine* [5th ed.]. Philadelphia: Lippincott Williams & Wilkins.)

or removal of the pituitary may be used for adrenal hyperplasia. Bilateral adrenalectomy may be preferred if both adrenals are involved.

Drug therapy includes diuretics for edema as well as an antihypertensive agent. A diet low in sodium and carbohydrates controls edema and blood glucose level. Antibiotics are used to treat infection.

If cushingoid syndrome results from exogenous administration of a corticosteroid preparation, the drug is slowly withdrawn by tapering the dose over days or weeks. In some instances, as in the treatment of a disorder such as leukemia, or to prevent rejection of transplanted organs, the syndrome is allowed to persist.

Nursing Process for the Client With Cushing's Syndrome

Assessment

Obtain thorough medical, drug, and allergy histories, and observe for symptoms of an adrenal disorder: altered skin pigmentation and integrity, decreased energy level, mental changes, sexual dysfunction, and changes in mood, appetite, weight, and bowel patterns. Monitor vital signs every 4 hours and test the blood or urine (or both) for glucose three or four times per day. If the urine tests positive for glucose or the blood glucose level is elevated, report the information to the physician.

Because the client is at risk for the development of peptic ulcers, observe the color of each stool and test the stool for occult blood. If the client reports epigastric pain or discomfort or the stool has a black appearance or tests positive for blood, make the physician aware of the assessment findings.

Diagnosis, Planning, and Interventions

If corticosteroid therapy has caused a cushingoid appearance and the dose is to be tapered over time, give the client and family a detailed explanation of the tapering schedule. Review the directions printed on the prescription container and emphasize the importance of strictly following the tapering schedule. The client may find it helpful to use a calendar to enter the dosage for each day. Another option to ensure compliance is to write the entire tapering schedule on a card and instruct the client to cross off each day.

Depending on many factors, such as age and severity of the disorder, clients with Cushing's syndrome may or may not be scheduled for adrenalectomy or irradiation of the pituitary. Until such time as further treatment is scheduled, emphasize the importance of continued medical supervision. Highlight important points, such as avoiding trauma to the skin; contacting the physician if sores or cuts do not heal or become infected, if easy bruising occurs, or if stools are dark or black; following the recommended diet; reading food labels carefully; avoiding exposure to infection; avoiding nonprescription drugs (unless approved by the physician); weighing self weekly; and reporting marked weight gain or edema to the physician.

Diagnoses, expected outcomes, and interventions include, but are not limited to, the following.

▶ **Excess Fluid Volume** related to sodium and water retention

▶ **Expected Outcome:** Fluid volume will be normal as evidenced by equivalent fluid intake and output volumes, reduced or no dependent edema, consistent daily weights, and BP measurements within normal limits.

- Examine extremities for increased or decreased edema. *Fluid retention is manifested by swelling in dependent areas, pitting when pressure is applied to the skin over a bone, tight-fitting shoes or rings, the appearance of lines in the skin from stockings, and seams in the shoes or areas where they lace.*
- Measure intake and output daily, weekly, or as ordered. *Acutely ill clients require more frequent assessment. A gain of 2 lb in 24 hours suggests 1 L of water retention.*
- Assess vital signs each shift; report systolic BP that exceeds 139 mm Hg or diastolic BP that exceeds 89 mm Hg. *Hypertension is defined as a consistently elevated BP above 139/89 mm Hg (see Chap. 27). One factor that contributes to hypertension is excess circulatory volume.*
- Administer prescribed diuretics. *They promote the excretion of sodium and water.*
- Provide a sodium-restricted diet at the level prescribed by the physician. *Limiting sodium reduces the potential for fluid retention.*

▶ **Risk for Impaired Skin Integrity** related to thinning of skin and edema

▶ **Expected Outcome:** Skin will remain intact.

- Inspect the skin daily, especially over bony prominences, for open lesions or ulcers. *The skin is thin and fragile and prone to breaking down with minimal trauma.*
- Encourage the client to change positions frequently. *Relieving pressure on capillaries helps maintain a supply of oxygenated blood to cells and tissues. Cells deprived of oxygenated blood are prone to cellular death.*
- Handle the client gently; use interventions that relieve pressure on the skin. *Gentleness reduces the potential for skin abrasions, and interventions that cushion the weight and force of gravity against body surfaces help prevent the development of pressure ulcers.*
- Exercise care when performing tasks that may damage the skin, such as removing tape when discontinuing an IV infusion. *The skin's fragility increases its potential for injury.*

▶ **Fatigue** related to muscle wasting and protein depletion

▶ **Expected Outcome:** Client will demonstrate energy to complete ADLs.

- Provide frequent rest periods between activities. *Rest restores energy and improves endurance.*
- Assist the client with activities when muscle wasting or pain secondary to osteoporosis is severe. *The nurse relieves client of responsibilities until the client can safely and comfortably manage self-care.*

▶ Risk for Infection related to suppressed inflammatory response and immune function

▶ **Expected Outcome:** Client will be free from infection.

- Observe for signs and symptoms that indicate infection: a skin injury that does not heal, increased temperature, sore throat, or cough. *Signs of infection or inflammation are less dramatic in these clients than in others. What may appear to be a minor problem could be masking a more serious problem.*
- Make every effort to prevent exposing the client to infectious microorganisms. *Microorganisms are spread by direct and indirect contact. A client with suppressed defenses is more likely to succumb to an infection.*
- Immediately notify the physician if an infection is suspected. *The nurse collaborates with the physician on medical interventions.*

▶ Risk for Injury related to demineralization of bones

▶ **Expected Outcome:** Client will be safe from injury such as bone fracture.

- Protect the client from falls by applying supportive slippers and keeping the environment free of clutter and water spills. *The force of a fall is more likely to cause a fracture when the bones are porous. Environmental safety reduces the potential for injury.*
- Use side rails and instruct the client to seek assistance when getting out of bed. *Assistance reduces the incidence and consequences of a fall.*

▶ Risk for Self-Directed Violence related to mood changes and depression

▶ **Expected Outcome:** Client's mood will stabilize with no depressive symptoms.

- Assess mental status, including suicidal ideation, regularly. *A depressed client is likely to appear sad, be tearful, have difficulty sleeping or sleep more than expected, neglect hygiene, have a poor appetite and reduced energy, and lack interest in the future. Clients who entertain thoughts of suicide usually admit to their despair when openly questioned.*
- Explain that a depressed mood is a common symptom of the disorder or side effect of corticosteroid therapy. *Depressed clients may blame themselves for their inability to cope with stressors. Providing information as to the cause of the depressed mood may help the client to persevere with the treatment regimen.*
- Maintain safety by removing items that could be used for suicide, checking on the client frequently, transferring the client to a room close to the nursing station, and offering to stay with the client when he or she is feeling self-destructive. *Eliminating the opportunity or methods by which the client can harm himself or herself may prevent a suicide attempt.*
- Collaborate with the physician about a referral to a mental health practitioner or agency. *Counseling, drug therapy, and psychotherapy after discharge provide long-term measures for keeping a client safe from self-harm.*

▶ Disturbed Body Image related to changes in appearance

▶ **Expected Outcome:** Client will express a positive self-image.

- Offer the client opportunities to express feelings over physical changes. *Verbalizing feelings with a supportive person increases the client's ability to cope with stress.*
- Explain that when the cause of the disorder is eliminated, some physical changes gradually improve, but others, such as striae and kyphosis, are permanent. *Being honest and sharing accurate information promotes the client's trust and confidence.*
- Offer suggestions such as wearing loose clothing, a hat, or cap, to help disguise physical changes that the client finds difficult to tolerate. *Although the client's perception of physical changes probably is more exaggerated than others', he or she may feel more confident in social situations with techniques that minimize changes in appearance.*

Evaluation of Expected Outcomes

Fluid volume is normal, with no evidence of edema, hypertension, or weight gain. The client meets self-care needs without fatigue. Temperature and WBC count are within normal limits. Skin is intact. The client is free from injury, such as pathologic fractures. He or she demonstrates normal range of moods and denies suicidal ideation. The client copes effectively with physical changes. ●

HYPERALDOSTERONISM

The secretion of aldosterone, a mineralocorticoid, is regulated by serum levels of potassium and sodium, the renin-angiotensin system, and ACTH. The hypersecretion of aldosterone creates extreme electrolyte imbalances.

Pathophysiology and Etiology

The cause of primary hyperaldosteronism may be a benign aldosterone-secreting adenoma of one of the adrenals, an adrenal malignant tumor, or unknown. Pregnancy, congestive heart failure, narrowing of the renal artery, and cirrhosis can cause secondary hyperaldosteronism.

Excessive secretion of aldosterone results in increased reabsorption of sodium and water and excretion of potassium by the kidneys. Figure 50-9 presents an overview of the renin-angiotensin-aldosterone system.

Assessment Findings

Headache, muscle weakness, increased urine output, fatigue, hypertension, and cardiac dysrhythmias are seen. Serum potassium levels are decreased and serum sodium levels are increased in the absence of other causes, such as diuretic therapy or diarrhea. The serum bicarbonate, serum aldosterone, and plasma renin levels are increased. CT or MRI may rule out or locate an adrenal tumor. Adrenal venography may identify small tumors that CT scanning fails to reveal.

Medical and Surgical Management

If the cause is an adrenal tumor, unilateral adrenalectomy may be performed. Medical management may include administration of spironolactone, a potassium-sparing

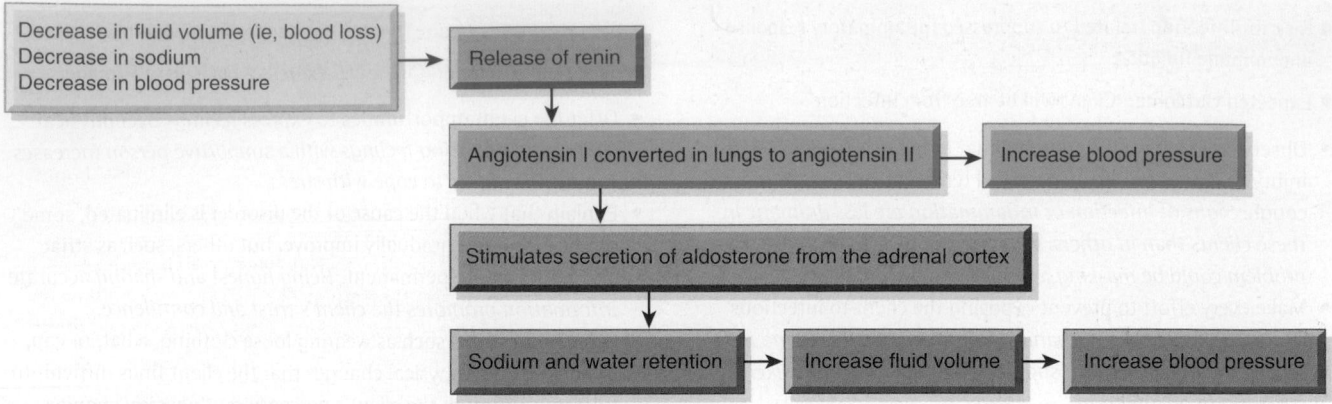

FIGURE 50-9. The renin-angiotensin-aldosterone system.

diuretic, and an antihypertensive agent to control BP. A sodium-restricted diet may be necessary.

Nursing Management

The nurse monitors vital signs every 4 hours or as ordered. He or she reports marked elevations to the physician. The nurse measures fluid intake and output and weighs the client every 2 to 7 days. Daily examination of the extremities for edema is essential. The nurse observes for signs of hypokalemia and hypernatremia (see Chap. 16).

OPEN ADRENALECTOMY

An open **adrenalectomy** is a surgical removal of the adrenal gland(s). It is usually performed to remove a cancerous tumor. Surgeons prefer an open adrenalectomy to a laparoscopic approach when malignancy is present or the gland is 4 or more inches in diameter. In some instances, removal of the ovaries, testes, and both adrenal glands (which secrete male and female hormones), is considered to control cancers of the breast and prostate, which depend on hormones for growth.

The adrenals are surgically approached by means of an abdominal incision or a flank incision under and following the position of the 12th rib. The abdominal incision usually is long because adequate exposure is needed to access the adrenals, which lie posteriorly. The flank incision is the same surgical approach used for kidney surgery.

Nursing Management
Preoperative Period

Major goals include reduced anxiety and an understanding of preparations for surgery and possible postoperative events. The nurse keeps the client on bed rest and minimizes anxiety. The client who requires surgery to halt progression of a metastatic disease may be anxious as well as depressed and needs time to discuss the surgery and anticipated results. If the client has a pheochromocytoma, the nurse monitors BP frequently before surgery. When bilateral adrenalectomy is scheduled, the nurse may start IV administration of a solution containing a corticosteroid preparation the morning of surgery. Some surgeons prefer to initiate corticosteroid administration during removal of the adrenals. Additional preparations are the same as for the client having general surgery (see Chap. 14).

Postoperative Period

When the client returns from surgery, the nurse reviews the surgical record because postoperative observations and management depend on whether one or both adrenal glands were removed. In addition to the complications associated with general anesthesia, the nurse observes for such problems as hemorrhage, atelectasis, and pneumothorax because the adrenals are located close to the diaphragm and inferior vena cava. He or she monitors vital signs frequently and closely observes for signs of adrenal insufficiency (addisonian crisis, adrenal crisis), which may occur when:

- The prescribed dose of a corticosteroid preparation is inadequate to meet the client's needs (bilateral adrenalectomy).
- The remaining adrenal gland does not produce sufficient hormone to meet the client's needs (unilateral adrenalectomy).
- The prescribed dose of a corticosteroid preparation is not given.

If symptoms of adrenal insufficiency occur, the nurse notifies the physician immediately. He or she should never omit administering a prescribed corticosteroid because corticosteroid replacement is essential to life. Acute adrenal insufficiency is managed with infusions of IV solutions, glucose, and cortisol. Client and Family Teaching 50-4 provides detailed instructions for postdischarge management of the client who has undergone bilateral adrenalectomy.

Nursing Process for the Client Undergoing an Adrenalectomy

Assessment

Check vital signs as soon as the client returns to the unit to establish a baseline. Conduct other routine postoperative assessments, such as examining the dressing over the incision and the patency and characteristics of fluid from incisional drains, noting LOC, checking infusion of IV fluids, auscultating the lungs and abdomen, observing breathing patterns, identifying level of pain, measuring intake and output, and monitoring whether the client is performing leg exercises. Closely observe for acute adrenal crisis evidenced by

Client and Family Teaching 50-4
Discharge Instructions After Adrenalectomy

The nurse emphasizes the following points when teaching the client:

- The functions of the adrenal glands include providing a physiologic response to stress, suppressing inflammation, raising blood sugar levels, conserving sodium to maintain blood volume and blood pressure, and contributing hormones that affect sexual characteristics.
- Follow the prescribed treatment regimen.
- Care for the surgical wound as directed until it has healed.
- Adhere to the prescribed medication schedule.
- Obtain sufficient sleep and rest to prevent fatigue and support activities of daily living.
- Eat a well-balanced diet.
- Keep appointments for scheduled blood tests and health-care appointments.
- Avoid infections and stressful situations.
- Carry identification indicating that the adrenal glands have been surgically removed.
- Seek immediate medical help if it is not possible to take the prescribed corticosteroid drug or if symptoms of adrenal insufficiency and adrenal crisis develop.

hypotension and shock, nausea, vomiting, dehydration, muscle weakness, and hypoglycemia. Monitor blood studies for electrolyte imbalances and assess closely for any signs of infection. Throughout the postoperative period, continue to monitor pulse, BP, temperature, breath sounds, blood glucose levels, and urinary output.

Diagnosis, Planning, and Interventions
Pain related to tissue trauma

▶ **Expected Outcome:** Pain will be eliminated or reduced to a tolerable level within 30 minutes of a nursing intervention.

- Assess pain whenever assessing vital signs. *Pain assessment is the fifth vital sign; assess pain whenever you take vital signs and more often if indicated.*
- Give an analgesic promptly before pain increases. *Giving an analgesic before pain becomes intolerable more easily relieves and controls pain.*
- Assess and note the client's response to the analgesic. *The nurse is obligated to manage the client's pain; the client may require additional measures if the analgesic is ineffective.*
- Offer comfort measures such as massage, skin care, and emotional support. *Nonpharmacologic approaches complement and supplement pain-relieving medications.*

▶ **Ineffective Airway Clearance** related to inadequate coughing secondary to incisional pain

▶ **Expected Outcome:** The airway will be clear as evidenced by normal breath sounds and respiratory rate and effort.

- Support the incision firmly when turning or changing the client's position. *Movement of the skin and tissue underlying the incision stimulates nociceptors that transmit pain impulses to the CNS. Limiting pain facilitates movement, circulation, and breathing.*
- Apply firm support over the incision when the client deep breathes and coughs. *Pressing on the incision with a pillow or folded bath blanket promotes fuller lung expansion and more effort when coughing, both of which help to maintain a patent airway.*
- Change the client's position every 2 hours. *Movement helps prevent stasis of respiratory secretions.*
- Encourage deep breathing and coughing every 2 hours. *Deep breathing and coughing open and clear respiratory passages.*
- Encourage adequate (2000 mL) intake of oral fluids. *When oral fluids are absorbed, they contribute to the volume in all fluid compartments. Adequate oral intake thins mucus.*
- Consult with the physician about the need for suctioning or aerosolized respiratory treatments if the lungs sound congested or sputum is thick and difficult to raise. *Suctioning is a mechanical means to remove retained secretions; it is useful if the client's natural cough is ineffective. Respiratory treatments provide medications that dilate the bronchi and thin mucoid secretions so they are more easily expelled.*

▶ **Risk for Infection** related to decreased cortisol secretion or immunosuppression secondary to steroid therapy replacement

▶ **Expected Outcome:** The wound is clean and dry with no signs of infection.

- Observe strict aseptic technique for all procedures, such as changing the dressing on the surgical wound. *Medical asepsis reduces microorganisms; surgical asepsis uses techniques in which microorganisms are absent or destroyed before contact with a susceptible host.*
- Notify the physician if vital signs change, purulent drainage is on the dressing, or analgesics do not control pain. *The nurse reports findings that may require medical interventions.*
- Inspect the wound during each dressing change. Notify the physician about excessive redness, swelling of the suture line, or purulent drainage. *Impaired skin from an incision increases the potential for infection. Nurses must report abnormal wound characteristics immediately.*

▶ **Risk for Injury** related to postural hypotension and weakness secondary to adrenal insufficiency

▶ **Expected Outcome:** Client will be free from injury.

- Assist with ambulatory activities and observe for weakness and dizziness. *Until the client's condition is stable and BP is normal, he or she requires assistance.*

- Notify the physician of continued hypotension or weakness. *Persistent symptoms may represent an impending adrenal crisis, which requires more definitive medical treatment.*

Evaluation of Expected Outcomes

Client reports pain relief and improved comfort. Lungs are clear to auscultation; client coughs and breathes effectively. There is no evidence of infection. Safety is maintained; the client is injury free. ●

CRITICAL THINKING EXERCISES

1. When caring for a client receiving fludrocortisone (Florinef) orally after bilateral adrenalectomy, nurses have a team conference to review the client's potential for acute adrenal insufficiency. What information is appropriate to discuss?

2. A nurse is assigned to a client recently admitted because of unexplained weight loss, insomnia, and fullness in the throat. The attending physician, several medical students, and a physician's assistant subsequently palpate this enlargement. Later, the client becomes restless and disoriented. The heart rate increases to 165 beats per minute, respirations are rapid, and the temperature is recorded at 103.8°F (39.8°C). What is a possible explanation for the changes in the client's condition and what methods would be used to manage them?

3. A client had a thyroidectomy this morning. It is now 8:00 PM, and the client complains of difficulty swallowing clear liquids and pressure in the area of the throat incision. The BP is normal, but the pulse rate is elevated. You see no drainage on the surface of the dressing. What actions would you take at this time?

4. How do the clustered terms "sugar, salt, and sex" relate to hormones produced by the adrenal cortex?

NCLEX-STYLE REVIEW QUESTIONS

1. A client diagnosed with hypothyroidism is taking a thyroid replacement. Prior to discharge from the hospital, the nurse instructs the client to report to the physician any side effects of the drug, including chest pain, insomnia, and hyperactivity. What is the best explanation for the nurse's instruction?
  1. The side effects indicate that the dosage is too low and needs to be increased.
  2. The side effects determine whether the medication should be changed.
  3. The side effects of thyroid replacement often mimic those of hyperthyroidism.
  4. The side effects indicate that an adverse drug reaction is occurring.

2. A client who is diagnosed with Cushing's syndrome asks the nurse about the cause of the disorder. Which response by the nurse is most accurate?
  1. "Cushing's syndrome results from decreased iodine in the diet."
  2. "Cushing's syndrome results from overproduction of ACTH by the pituitary."
  3. "Cushing's syndrome is caused by a reduction of calcium from the bone."
  4. "Cushing's syndrome is caused by an elevation in blood glucose."

3. The nurse weighs a client hospitalized with cushingoid syndrome daily. Which of the following statements is best for explaining the nurse's action?
  1. In clients with cushingoid syndrome, excess fluid volume results from sodium and water retention, which causes weight gain.
  2. In clients with cushingoid syndrome, fat is frequently redistributed, causing weight gain.
  3. In clients with cushingoid syndrome, sodium fluctuates, causing excess urine output and weight loss.
  4. In clients with cushingoid syndrome, excessive urine output results in fluid volume deficit and weight loss.

4. A nurse is performing client teaching for newly prescribed antithyroid drugs. The nurse emphasizes that the client should report which of the following findings to the physician?
  1. The client's activity tolerance improves.
  2. The client experiences a sore throat.
  3. The client shows weight gain.
  4. The client feels more relaxed.

5. A client is prescribed antithyroid therapy to treat hyperthyroidism. The client asks the nurse when a desired effect can be expected. Which of the following information would be accurate for the nurse to tell the client about the effects of antithyroid drug therapy?
  1. The effects can be experienced after several weeks or more.
  2. The effects can be experienced after completing at least 2 years of medication.
  3. The effects are usually experienced by clients younger than 30 years of age.
  4. The effects may or may not be experienced by all clients.

51

Caring for Clients with Diabetes Mellitus

Words To Know

diabetes mellitus
diabetic ketoacidosis
diabetic nephropathy
diabetic retinopathy
fasting blood glucose
glycemic index
glycosuria
glycosylated hemoglobin
hyperglycemia
hyperosmolar hyperglycemic nonketotic
  syndrome
hypoglycemia
insulin independence
insulin resistance
ketoacidosis
ketonemia
ketones
Kussmaul respirations
lipoatrophy
lipohypertrophy
lipolysis
metabolic syndrome
oral glucose tolerance test
polydipsia
polyphagia
polyuria
postprandial glucose
pre-diabetes
random blood glucose
renal threshold
rule of 15
tight glucose control

Learning Objectives

On completion of this chapter, you will be able to:

1. Define and distinguish the two types of diabetes mellitus.
2. Identify the three classic symptoms of diabetes mellitus.
3. Name three laboratory methods used to diagnose diabetes mellitus.
4. Describe the methods used to treat diabetes mellitus.
5. Discuss the nursing management of the client with diabetes mellitus.
6. Explain the source of ketones and cause of diabetic ketoacidosis.
7. List three main goals in the treatment of diabetic ketoacidosis.
8. Identify two physiologic signs of hyperosmolar hyperglycemic nonketotic syndrome.
9. Describe the treatment of hyperosmolar hyperglycemic nonketotic syndrome.
10. Explain the cause and treatment of hypoglycemia.
11. Differentiate between the symptoms of hypoglycemia and hyperglycemia.
12. Describe common chronic complications of diabetes mellitus.

Diabetes mellitus, a metabolic disorder of the pancreas, affects carbohydrate, fat, and protein metabolism. This disease is reaching epidemic proportions in the United States. Some experts believe that diabetes in adults is one consequence of **metabolic syndrome**, which includes obesity, especially in the abdominal area; high blood pressure; elevated triglyceride, low-density lipoprotein (LDL), and blood glucose levels; and a low high-density lipoprotein (HDL) level (see Chap. 25).

Although no age group is exempt from diabetes, the American Diabetes Association (2007) indicates that 90% to 95% of affected people acquire the disease as adults. For 2007, estimates were that 23.6 million people in the United States have diabetes, with 5.7 million being undiagnosed (Centers for Disease Control and Prevention [CDC], 2008). Incidence is increased among African Americans, Latinos, Native Americans, and Asian Americans (including Pacific Islanders). The World Health Organization predicts that, as a result of longer life expectancies, diabetes will affect 366 million people worldwide by 2030 (WHO, 2004). At present, diabetes is the seventh cause of death in the United States (U.S. National Center for Health Statistics, 2005). Because of the chronic nature of diabetes, affected people experience many debilitating and life-threatening complications before death. Research is providing exciting discoveries, however, that may eventually cure this disease.

DIABETES MELLITUS

The Expert Committee on the Diagnosis and Classification of Diabetes Mellitus (2002) has identified and described the two major forms of diabetes mellitus:

- *Type 1*, formerly called insulin-dependent diabetes mellitus (IDDM), is characterized by no insulin production by the beta cells in the islets of Langerhans of the pancreas (Fig. 51-1). The onset of type 1 diabetes is more likely in childhood and adolescence, but the disease can occur at any age (American Diabetes Association, 2008). Type 1 diabetes accounts for approximately 5% to 10% of all diagnosed cases of diabetes (National Institute of Diabetes and Digestive and Kidney Diseases [NIDDK], 2008).
- *Type 2*, formerly known as non–insulin-dependent diabetes mellitus (NIDDM), is characterized by insulin resistance or insufficient insulin production. Type 2 diabetes is more common in aging adults. However, in 2007, slightly more than 50% of people with newly diagnosed disease were in the 40- to 59-year age group (CDC, 2008), and type 2 diabetes also is being detected in obese children. The incidence of this form of diabetes now accounts for 20% of all newly diagnosed cases (Kimball, 2008).

Pre-Diabetes Mellitus

The NIDDK (2008) has developed criteria that identify people with pre-diabetes, which can lead to type 2 diabetes, heart disease, and stroke. People with **pre-diabetes** may have either *impaired fasting glucose* (IFG) or *impaired glucose tolerance* (IGT), or both. A person with IFG has a fasting blood glucose level of 100 to 125 mg/dL after an overnight fast (see discussion of Diagnostic Findings). In IGT, a person has a blood glucose level of 140 to 199 mg/dL after a glucose tolerance test lasting 2 hours. The NIDDK (2008) estimates that 57 million Americans have pre-diabetes. A significant number of those with pre-diabetes will develop the disease; however, many can delay or avoid type 2 diabetes with weight loss and increased physical activity.

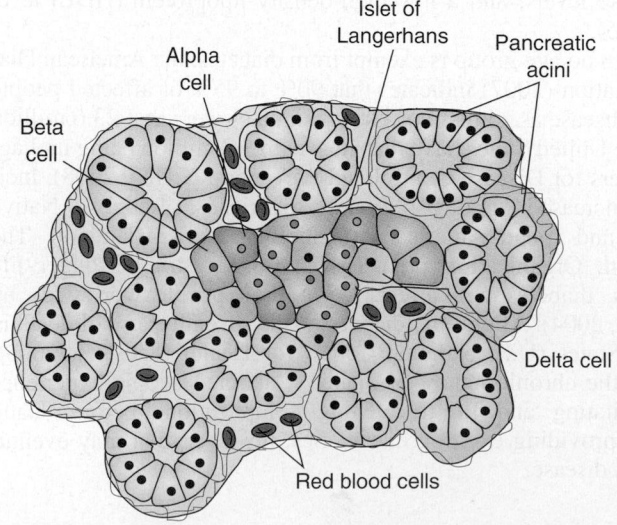

FIGURE 51-1. Islet of Langerhans in the pancreas. (From Guyton, A. C., & Hall, J. E. [2006]. *Textbook of medical physiology* [11th ed.]. Philadelphia: W. B. Saunders.)

Hyperglycemia

Hyperglycemia, an elevated blood glucose level, is associated with other disorders or their management. For example, pancreatitis (see Chap. 47) causes both exocrine and endocrine disturbances. When production of adrenocortical hormones is excessive, as in Cushing's syndrome (see Chap. 50), or with the administration of glucocorticoid drugs for immunosuppressive purposes, secondary diabetes develops. Impaired glucose metabolism and hyperglycemia also are associated with drugs such as loop and thiazide diuretics, levodopa, and oral contraceptives, and with the administration of total parenteral nutrition. A normal blood glucose level is restored once these diabetogenic regimens are discontinued.

Pathophysiology and Etiology
Type 1 Diabetes Mellitus

Insulin has three functions: (1) it carries glucose into body cells as their preferred source of energy, (2) it promotes the liver's storage of glucose as glycogen, and (3) it inhibits the breakdown of glycogen back into glucose. In type 1 diabetes, the islet cells, or endocrine portion of the pancreas, cease to produce insulin. Without insulin, the blood glucose level rises beyond its normal range—sometimes to 300 to 1000 mg/dL, and the body breaks down fat and protein as alternative sources of cellular energy (Porth, 2008). The breakdown of fat, known as **lipolysis**, results in the accumulation of fatty acids and **ketones**, metabolic byproducts of fat metabolism. When ketones accumulate in the blood, clients with diabetes are prone to developing a form of metabolic acidosis known as **ketoacidosis**. In type 1 diabetes, ketoacidosis develops quite suddenly because of the total cessation of insulin production.

Type 1 diabetes is considered an autoimmune disorder. Faustman and colleagues (2005) have shown that a genetic mutation causes killer (CD8) T-cell lymphocytes to attack and destroy the insulin-producing islet cells. The hypothesis is that people with type 1 diabetes lack a protein marker, known as major histocompatibility complex, or MHC, that helps the T cells identify natural cells as "self." Consequently, the T cells misidentify islet cells as unnatural and subsequently destroy them. This same research has now found a way to destroy the islet-attacking T cells using tumor necrosis factor-alpha (TNF-alpha) and stimulate the growth of new islet cells with the bacillus Calmette-Guérin (BCG) vaccine. A human trial began in January 2008. If successful, this discovery may eventually mean that type 1 diabetes can be cured rather than controlled with daily injections of insulin. Faustman's research also may help in curing other autoimmune diseases (Massachusetts General Hospital, 2005; Children with Diabetes, 2008).

There is additional good news of a possible cure for type 1 and insulin-dependent type 2 diabetes. Scientists have gone forward with a U.S. Food and Drug Administration (FDA)–approved human trial with insulin-deficient research participants. The clinical trial involves the administration of a recombinantly produced gene known as INGAP, which in animal studies stimulated new growth of pancreatic islet cells, progressively reduced blood glucose concentration, and reversed diabetes 30% to 40% of the time (McGill University Health Center, 2008; Reuters World News, 2008).

Type 2 Diabetes Mellitus

Diabetes mellitus, especially type 2, runs in families, although a specific gene for diabetes has not been isolated. The consensus is that type 2 diabetes mellitus is an inherited disease and that obesity, especially intra-abdominal obesity, is likely a cofactor that triggers its onset. In research conducted on mice, scientists possibly have found the link between obesity and type 2 diabetes (Dongsheng et al., 2005). Their findings show that obesity causes low-grade inflammation that then causes changes in liver function accompanied by hyperglycemia and **insulin resistance**, a decreased sensitivity to insulin at the tissue level.

When type 2 diabetes is manifested, the beta cells of the islets of Langerhans secrete increased levels of insulin into the bloodstream to offset hyperglycemia, but the blood glucose level remains higher than normal because there is a deficiency of *transmembrane glucose tranporters* on the surface of cells. Transmembrane glucose transporters form channels that facilitate diffusion of glucose into cells, and they may function only at 20% efficiency in people with type 2 diabetes. This contributes to hyperglycemia. Exercise increases transmembrane glucose transporter levels in skeletal muscles, which explains how exercise helps reduce blood sugar (Kimball, 2008). Eventually, the overstimulated beta cells become exhausted, resulting in a decline in insulin production, and the client with type 2 diabetes may also become insulin deficient, like those with type 1 diabetes. The correlation of obesity, sedentary lifestyle, and insulin resistance helps explain how dieting, exercise, and weight loss control type 2 diabetes and delay, reduce, or eliminate the need for medication to treat the disease.

An excessive level of glucose in the blood leads to **glycosuria**, glucose in the urine, and urinary excretion. Glycosuria appears when the blood glucose level rises above 180 mg/dL. At this level, the kidneys' **renal threshold**, the ability to reabsorb glucose and return it to the bloodstream, is impaired. The hypertonicity from concentrated amounts of glucose in the blood pulls fluid into the vascular system, resulting in **polyuria**, excessive urine production. The client experiences urinary frequency accompanied by increased excreted urine. Because so much water is lost, **polydipsia**, excessive thirst, develops.

While the needed glucose is being wasted, the body's requirement for fuel continues. The person with diabetes feels hungry and eats more (**polyphagia**). Despite eating more, he or she loses weight as the body uses fat and protein to substitute for glucose. Ketones, chemical intermediate products in fat metabolism, such as beta-hydroxybutyric acid, acetoacetic acid, and acetone, cause ketoacidosis when they accumulate.

The bicarbonate buffer system buffers ketones. Thus, **ketonemia** (increased ketones in the blood) causes a decreased alkali (base) reserve, leading to acidosis. **Kussmaul respirations** (fast, deep, labored breathing) are common in ketoacidosis (Fig. 51-2). Acetone, which is volatile, can be detected on the breath by its characteristic fruity odor. If treatment is not initiated, the outcome of ketoacidosis is circulatory collapse, renal shutdown, and death. Ketoacidosis is more common in people with diabetes who no longer produce insulin, such as those with type 1 diabetes. People with type 2 diabetes are more likely to develop hyperosmolar hyperglycemic nonketotic syndrome (HHNKS; see later discussion), because with limited insulin, they can use enough glucose to prevent ketosis but not enough to maintain a normal blood glucose level.

Infection, failure to eat, vomiting, and stress invite ketosis because they increase the demand for insulin, which the pancreas cannot accommodate in diabetes. In addition, people with diabetes mellitus are at increased risk for vascular disorders such as atherosclerosis, cerebrovascular accidents, myocardial infarction, peripheral vascular disease with decreased ability to heal, renal failure, blindness, and neuropathy. Women are prone to complications during pregnancy; men are prone to erectile dysfunction (see Chap. 55).

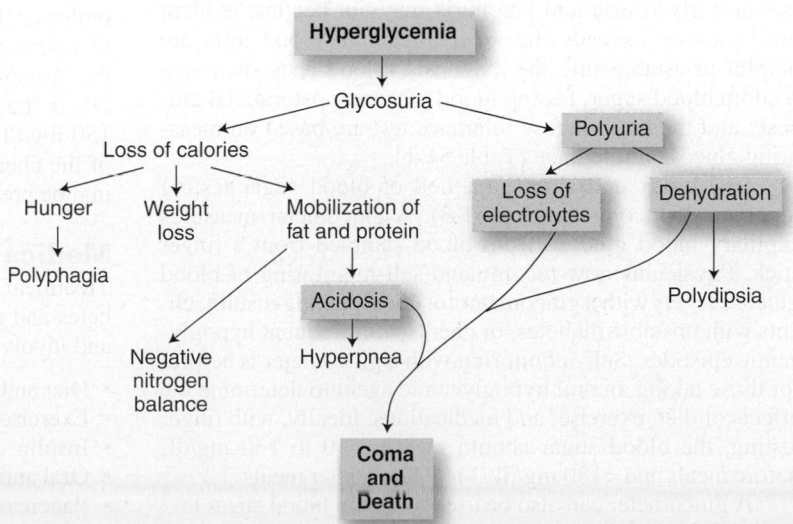

FIGURE 51-2. Signs and symptoms of uncontrolled hyperglycemia in diabetes mellitus. (From Rubin, R., & Strayer, D.S. [2008]. *Rubin's pathology: Clinicopathologic foundations of medicine*, 5th ed. Philadelphia: Lippincott Williams & Wilkins.)

▶ *Stop, Think, and Respond Exercise 51-1*
Identify some differences between type 1 and type 2 diabetes mellitus.

Assessment Findings

Signs and Symptoms

The three classic symptoms of both types of diabetes mellitus are polyuria, polydipsia, and polyphagia. Additional symptoms include weight loss, weakness, thirst, fatigue, and dehydration. These signs and symptoms have an abrupt onset in clients with type 1 diabetes. Clients with type 2 diabetes have a gradual onset of symptoms. Some develop skin, urinary tract, and vaginal infections, possibly because the elevated level of blood glucose supports bacterial growth. There may be changes in visual acuity manifested by blurred vision because the hypertonicity of body fluid affects the cells in the lens and retina (Porth, 2008).

Gerontologic Considerations

- Symptoms of hyperglycemia in older adults may include depression, cognitive changes, lethargy, unexplained weight loss, urinary incontinence, falls, or nonketotic hyperosmolar syndrome. High glucose levels over an extended time period, hypertension, and dyslipidemia contribute to complications in older adults with diabetes (Barzilai, 2006).

Diagnostic Findings

Although diabetes mellitus is a highly complex disease, screening for its detection is relatively simple. Normally, urine contains no detectable glucose or ketones; in diabetes, one or both may be present. Because the body fails to use glucose adequately, it excretes glucose in the urine. If the body metabolizes fats faster than it can use the ketones, ketones also appear in the urine. The relative ease of these urinary tests facilitates early detection of diabetes (Nursing Guidelines 51-1).

Blood Sugar Testing

Because glycosuria and ketonuria may not become evident until glucose exceeds the renal threshold, blood tests are helpful in establishing the diagnosis. Blood tests such as a random blood sugar, fasting blood glucose, postprandial glucose, and the oral glucose tolerance test are based on measuring glucose intolerance (Table 51-1).

One quick and simple method of blood sugar testing involves a glucometer (Fig. 51-3). A glucometer measures capillary blood glucose from blood sampled from a finger stick. Physicians now recommend self-monitoring of blood glucose levels with a glucometer for clients taking insulin, clients with unstable diabetes, or clients with frequent hypoglycemic episodes. Self-monitoring with a glucometer is helpful for those taking an oral hypoglycemic agent to determine the effects of diet, exercise, and medications. Ideally, with finger testing, the blood sugar should measure 90 to 130 mg/dL before meals and <180 mg/dL 1 to 2 hours after meals.

A glucometer can also be used to obtain blood sugar levels from alternate sites such as the upper arm, forearm, thigh,

NURSING GUIDELINES 51-1

Performing Urine Glucose Testing

Method: Test-Tape and Diastix

- Have the client empty his or her bladder to eliminate glucose and ketones that have been stored in the bladder for hours; save this specimen in case the client cannot void later.
- Encourage the client to drink water; ask the client to void in 30 minutes.
- For the client with an indwelling catheter, clamp the catheter for 30 minutes and take the specimen directly from the catheter, not the drainage bag.
- Test the second voided specimen to detect current concentration of glucose and ketones.
- Dip the testing strip into the urine and wait for the recommended time.
- Observe the color change and document the results.

or calf. These tests are described as less painful or even painless, because the fingertips have a higher number of nerve endings. However, alternate sites are regarded as lagging test sites because they actually provide a measurement of blood glucose as it was 20 to 35 minutes prior to the test (Becton, Dickinson and Company, 2009). Consequently, alternate sites are only an option for people whose glucose levels are relatively stable and are not an option for people who require tight glucose control. **Tight glucose control** involves maintaining near-normal blood glucose levels by taking short-acting insulin throughout the day and intermediate-acting insulin at bedtime. Controlling blood glucose levels can delay the onset of complications associated with diabetes.

Glycosylated Hemoglobin

Once a client with diabetes receives a treatment regimen to follow, the physician can assess the effectiveness of treatment and the client's compliance by obtaining a glycosylated hemoglobin, or hemoglobin A1c, test. The results of this test reflect the amount of glucose that is stored in the hemoglobin molecule during its life span of 120 days. Normally, the level of glycosylated hemoglobin is less than 7%. According to the American Diabetes Association, a hemoglobin A1c of 7% is the equivalent of an average blood glucose level of 150 mg/dL. Amounts of 8% or greater indicate that control of the client's blood glucose level has been inadequate during the previous 2 to 3 months.

Medical Management

Treatment depends on many factors, such as the type of diabetes and the ability of the pancreas to manufacture insulin, and involves combinations of the following:

- Diet and weight loss
- Exercise
- Insulin
- Oral antidiabetic agents
- Pancreas transplantation
- Islet cell transplantation

TABLE 51-1 Diagnostic Tests For Detecting Glucose Intolerance

TEST	IMPLEMENTATION	DIAGNOSTIC RESULT
Random blood glucose	Blood specimen is drawn without preplanning.	≥200 mg/dL in the presence of symptoms is suggestive of diabetes mellitus.
Fasting blood glucose	Blood specimen is obtained after 8 hours of fasting.	In the nondiabetic client the glucose level will be between 70 and 110 mg/dL. In the diabetic client glucose is ≥ 110 mg/dL but <126 mg/dL.
Postprandial glucose	Blood sample is taken 2 hours after a high-carbohydrate meal.	In the nondiabetic client, the glucose level will be between 70 and 110 mg/dL. In the client with diabetes mellitus, the result is ≥140 mg/dL but <200 mg/dL.
Oral glucose tolerance test	Diet high in carbohydrates is eaten for 3 days. Client then fasts for 8 hours. A baseline blood sample is drawn and a urine specimen is collected. An oral glucose solution is given and time of ingestion recorded. Blood is drawn at 30 minutes and 1, 2, and 3 hours after the ingestion of glucose solution. Urine is collected simultaneously. Drinking water is encouraged to promote urine excretion.	In the nondiabetic client, the glucose returns to normal in 2 to 3 hours and urine is negative for glucose. In the diabetic client, blood glucose level returns to normal slowly; urine is positive for glucose.
Glycosylated hemoglobin or hemoglobin A1c	Single sample of venous blood is withdrawn.	The amount of glucose stored by the hemoglobin is elevated above 7.0% in the newly diagnosed client with diabetes mellitus, in one who is noncompliant, or in one who is inadequately treated.

Gerontologic Considerations

- Cognitive problems such as depression, dementia, or episodes of delirium can interfere with the older adult's management of diabetes. The family or caregiver should be included in teaching about treatments and monitoring.

- Older adults should be treated aggressively. However, client preferences, functional and cognitive abilities, or concurrent comorbidities may dictate treatment modifications. Complications may occur more frequently in clients taking multiple medications.

Diet and Weight Loss

Diet is a major component of treatment for every person with diabetes. Formulation of a diabetic diet depends on the client's sex, age, height and weight, activity level, occupation, state of health, former dietary habits, and cultural background (Nutrition Notes 51-1). When dietary allowances (calories, percentages of carbohydrates, fats, and proteins) are prescribed, the client is given a diet prescription and a list of substitutions and exchanges to vary the diet. For example, the physician determines that the client with diabetes may have 1500 calories per day. The calories are then distributed according to the percentage of carbohydrates, fats, and proteins that equal the total prescribed caloric amount. A dietitian provides the client with a list of foods in six different categories—starch/bread, meat, vegetable, fruit, milk, and fat—and indicates how many items from each category the client can consume for breakfast, lunch, dinner, and snacks (Fig. 51-4). The dietitian gives the client a list of foods in

each category and their equivalent amounts. The client can then exchange or substitute one food for another in the specified amount for variety (Box 51-1).

Carbohydrate counting is a flexible alternative to using the exchange system. This method of dietary management involves an individualized meal pattern that specifies the number of carbohydrate "choices" (1 choice = 15 g carbohydrate) for each meal and snack. Most adults are allowed 3 to 5 carbohydrate choices per meal and 1 to 2 for each snack, depending on their calorie needs. Clients are generally advised to add 4 to 6 ounces of lean meat or meat substitute, some healthy fats, and little to no saturated or trans fats to complete their daily intake (Dudek, 2010). Carbohydrate choice lists, similar to the exchange lists, can help clients with identifying sources of carbohydrates and the

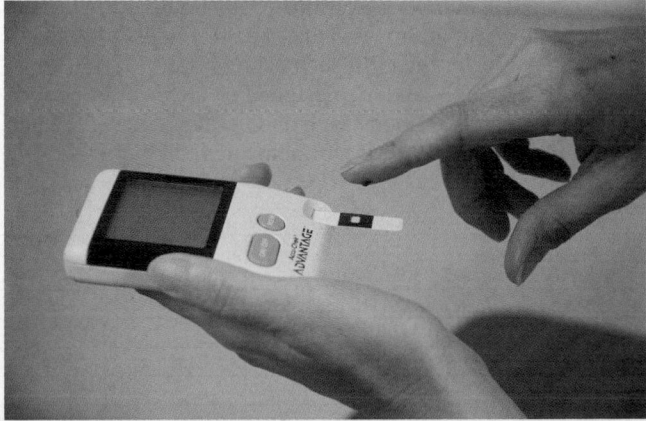

FIGURE 51-3. Example of a blood glucose monitor that uses blood sampled from a finger stick.

Nutrition Notes 51-1
The Client with Diabetes Mellitus

● Nutritional therapy is the cornerstone of treatment for all clients with diabetes, regardless of weight, blood glucose levels, or use of medication. There no longer is one diabetic diet that is appropriate for all clients; meal plans are individualized according to the assessment data and treatment goals.

● For all people with diabetes, saturated fat, trans fat, and cholesterol are limited to help decrease the risk of cardiovascular complications. Two or more servings of fish per week are recommended for their omega-3 fatty acid content. The recommendations regarding other dietary components, such as fiber, protein, total carbohydrate, vitamins, and minerals, are unchanged from those of the general population.

● Because most clients with type 1 diabetes are of normal weight, calorie allowances are calculated for weight maintenance.

● For clients with type 2 diabetes, weight loss is the focus of nutritional intervention. A low-calorie diet may immediately improve clinical symptoms. A 1/2- to 1-lb loss per week is recommended, but even a mild to moderate weight loss (e.g., total of 10 to 20 lb) can lower blood glucose levels and improve insulin action.

---

appropriate portion sizes. Clients also need to know how to read the Nutrition Facts label in order to count carbohydrates accurately.

For some clients, dietary modifications alone can control type 2 diabetes. These clients have a mild form of diabetes, with the pancreas producing some insulin. The client with diabetes who is overweight is placed on a weight-reduction diet because diabetes is less easily controlled in the presence of obesity. Even a moderate weight loss improves the body's use of insulin.

Clients may also use the **glycemic index**, a measure of how fast a carbohydrate food is likely to raise blood sugar, to help maintain normal blood sugar levels. The glycemic index assigns a number to various foods relative to glucose, which is given an arbitrary value of 100. Foods with glycemic indices greater than 70, such as a waffle (76), raise low blood sugar quickly and are designed to cover brief periods of intense exercise. Foods with indices less than 55, such as low-fat yogurt (14), slowly help prevent hypoglycemia

during the night or when a person exercises for long periods (Brand-Miller et al., 2007).

Exercise

Exercise helps metabolize carbohydrates and control blood glucose levels because glucose-transporting receptors within skeletal muscles allow the muscles to take in glucose from the blood *independent* of insulin. This provides energy during exercise and lowers blood sugar. Exercise, therefore, reduces the need for insulin because blood sugar can be lowered without it, an advantage for those with diabetes. It also explains why hypoglycemia can accompany exercise.

Exercise also improves circulation of blood, which is compromised in the client with diabetes. Exercise also lowers cholesterol and triglyceride levels and improves muscle tone. An exercise program for the client with diabetes specifies the type of exercise and the length of time to perform it. The program is tailored according to the client's needs and life-style. Most importantly, the client needs to exercise consistently each day. Sporadic periods of exercise are discouraged because wide fluctuations in blood glucose levels can occur. It is necessary to regulate food and insulin requirements during times of increased activities.

Insulin

All clients with type 1 diabetes must rely on insulin therapy. The goal of pancreas and islet cell transplantation (see later discussion), which is performed only for clients with type 1 diabetes, is that the client will acquire **insulin independence**—that is, the client's own naturally produced insulin will regulate blood glucose levels within consistently normal ranges. Better yet, the use of techniques to reverse autoimmunity or to stimulate islet cell regeneration with gene therapy (discussed earlier) may eventually cure clients with type 1 diabetes. Additional possibilities for eliminating the need for exogenous insulin include transplantation of stem cells. Until then, clients with type 1 diabetes continue to require daily, multiple, or continuous injections of insulin. Clients with type 2 diabetes eventually may become dependent on insulin therapy when the beta cells cease to function and antidiabetic agents are no longer effective.

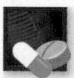

Pharmacologic Considerations

- The three important properties of insulin are *onset*, when the insulin first begins to act in the body; *peak*, the time when insulin is exerting maximum action; and, *duration*, the time the insulin remains in effect.

	1 Starch/Bread	2 Meat	3 Vegetable	4 Fruit	5 Milk	6 Fat
Breakfast	2			1	1	1
Snack time						
Lunch	2	1	1	1		1
Snack time				1		
Dinner	2	2	1	1		2
Snack time	1			1	1	

FIGURE 51-4. A sample diabetic meal plan for 1500 calories.

BOX 51-1 Sample Starch/Bread Category Foods and Equivalent Amounts

Bran cereals, flaked (Bran Buds, All Bran)	1/2 cup
Bread	1 oz
Bulgur, cooked	1/2 cup
Cooked cereals	1/2 cup
Grits, cooked	1/2 cup
Pasta, cooked	1/3 cup
Rice (white or brown), cooked	1/3 cup
Shredded wheat	1/2 cup
Unsweetened cereals	3/4 cup
Wheat germ	3 Tbsp
Lentils, cooked	1/2 cup
Baked beans	1/3 cup
Beans and peas, cooked (kidney, split)	1/2 cup
Corn	1/2 cup
Corn on cob	1/2 large cob (5 oz)
Lima beans	1/2 cup
Peas, green (canned or frozen)	1/2 cup
Plantain	1/3 cup
Potato, baked (3 oz)	1/4 large
Potato, mashed	1/2 cup
Squash, winter (acorn, butternut)	1 cup
Tortilla, corn or flour	1 6-inch
Yam, sweet potato, plain	1/2 cup

Source: American Diabetes Association, American Dietetic Association. 2008. *Choose your foods: Exchanges lists for diabetes.*

- The measurement of insulin must be accurate because clients may be sensitive to minute dose changes. Observe the client for signs of hypoglycemia at the expected onset and again at the peak of action.

Table 51-2 includes commonly used insulin preparations, which are divided into four categories: rapid acting, short acting, intermediate acting, and long acting. Some clients with type 2 diabetes maintain glycemic control with a once-daily injection of an intermediate-acting insulin, combination of intermediate-acting and short-acting insulin in a 70:30 or 50:50 proportion, or long-acting insulin. Clients with type 1 diabetes may self-administer three to four injections or more throughout the day unless they use an insulin pump (discussed later).

Human Insulin

Human forms of insulin are gradually replacing purified insulin extracts from beef and pork pancreas. Beef and pork insulin is essentially a "foreign" substance, and the human immune system produces antibodies that blunt their effect, requiring higher doses of insulin (Kimball, 2008). Human insulin also appears to cause fewer allergic reactions than insulin obtained from animal sources; however, clients who switch from animal to synthesized human insulin must be monitored for low blood glucose levels initially because the human form of insulin is used more effectively.

Several methods are used to produce human insulin through genetic engineering. First, the conversion of pork insulin to human insulin results from changing one amino acid. Second, insertion of the human gene for insulin into strains of the bacteria *Escherichia coli* produces Humulin insulin; use of yeast organisms instead of *E. coli* yields Novolin insulin. Third, further modification of human insulin to work faster than Humulin has led to the development of lispro (Humalog) and aspart (NovoLog); conversely, glargine (Lantus) insulin is human insulin that has been modified to work more slowly than other human insulins (Kimball, 2008).

Gastrointestinal enzymes inactivate insulin; therefore, insulin must be injected. In the United States, Exubera, an inhaled form of insulin, has been discontinued for a variety of reasons: it is twice as expensive as injectable insulins, it is bulky and complicated to use, and it affects lung function. In Australia, a pharmaceutical company has developed a transdermal method for delivering insulin, which has been successful in preclinical trials on pigs (Barnes, 2006).

TABLE 51-2 Insulin Preparations

INSULIN	ONSET	PEAK	DURATION
Rapid Acting			
Insulin lispro (Humalog)	5–15 min	1–2 hr	3–4 hr
Aspart (NovoLog)	15 min	1 hr	3–4 hr
Short Acting			
Regular insulin (Humulin R, Novolin R, Iletin II Regular)	30 min–1 hr	1–3 hr	6–8 hr
Intermediate Acting			
Isophane insulin suspension (NPH, Humulin N, Novolin N)	1–1.5 hr	4–12 hr	24 hr
Insulin zinc suspension (Lente)	1–2.5 hr	7–15 hr	24 hr
Long Acting			
Extended insulin zinc suspension (Ultralente, Humulin U)	4–8 hr	8–10 hr	18–30 hr
Glargine (Lantus)	2–4 hr	No peak	≥24 hr
Insulin Mixtures			
Humulin 50/50	15 min	2–4 hr	20–22 hr
Humulin 70/30	30 min	7–12 hr	16–24 hr
Novolin 70/30	30 min	0 8 hr	10–16 hr
Humalog 75/25	15 min	2 hr	20–22 hr

▸ *Stop, Think, and Respond Exercise 51-2*

Identify which of the following insulins is rapid acting, short acting, intermediate acting, and long acting: glargine (Lantus), Lente, lispro (Humalog), Novolin R.

Administration of Insulin

Insulin is prescribed in units. U100 means that 1 mL contains 100 units of insulin. The physician specifies both the dosage and the type of insulin to be used. When combining two types of insulin in the same syringe, the short-acting regular insulin is withdrawn into the syringe *first* and the intermediate-acting insulin is added next, a practice referred to as "clear to cloudy." The mixture is administered within 15 minutes to ensure that the onset, peak, and duration of each separate insulin remains intact. Glargine (Lantus) insulin cannot be mixed with other types of insulin in the same syringe. Combination mixtures of insulin, such as Humulin 70/30, Novolin 70/30, and Humulin 50/50, eliminate the need for mixing insulins from two separate vials

Regular insulin can be administered intravenously and subcutaneously. The intravenous (IV) route is used to (1) treat severe hyperglycemia or (2) prevent or control elevated blood sugar by adding it to a total parenteral nutrition solution that contains a high concentration of glucose. The subcutaneous route is used most commonly for administering insulin (Fig. 51-5); insulin is absorbed more rapidly when injected in the abdomen than in the arms or thighs. Clients with diabetes are taught to use the abdomen as the preferred site for self-administration. Subcutaneous injection sites require rotation to avoid **lipoatrophy**, breakdown of subcutaneous fat at the site of repeated injections, and **lipohypertrophy**, buildup of subcutaneous fat at the site of repeated injections, either of which eventually interferes with insulin absorption in the tissue. Because insulin is an anabolic hormone, it also causes weight gain.

Other techniques for injecting insulin subcutaneously include an insulin pen, jet injector, or insulin pump.

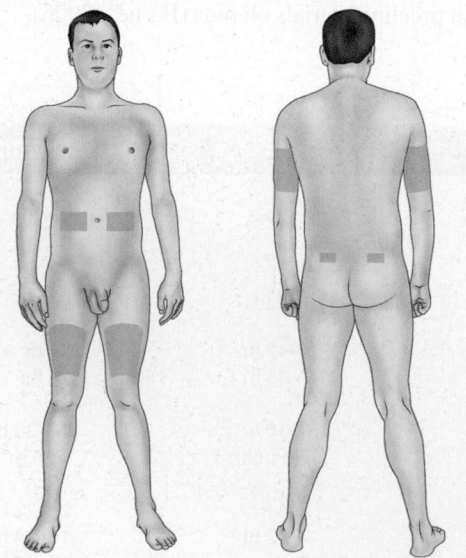

FIGURE 51-5. Subcutaneous injection sites used for administering insulin.

Gerontologic Considerations

- Changes in taste sensation (sweet and salty) that accompany aging may contribute to older adults' unintentional consumption of foods higher in sugar content, resulting in the risk for hyperglycemia. Teaching plans should emphasize blood glucose testing prior to insulin administration.

- Some older clients experience difficulty in administering insulin because of problems such as decreased visual acuity or arthritis. Assess the client's ability and resources for self-administration of insulin before developing a teaching program. Appropriate aids, such as a magnifier that fits over the syringe, pre-filled syringe, or insulin pens are available.

Insulin Pen. An insulin pen is a device in which a cartridge containing 150 to 300 units of insulin is loaded into an injecting pen with a disposable needle attached. Each time the insulin is injected, a new needle is attached. Once the device is loaded, the client (1) selects the number of units for injection by dialing in the dose in 1- to 2-unit increments, (2) cleans and pierces the skin, and (3) injects the programmed amount (Fig. 51-6).

Jet Injector. A jet injector uses high pressure and rapid speed, rather than a needle, to instill insulin through the skin. The pressure transforms the liquid into a fine mist that is distributed over a wide area of tissue, resulting in faster absorption (Fig. 51-7). Although a jet injector offers several advantages, such as reducing pain at the site and eliminating the use of needles and their appropriate disposal, the cost tends to make this form of administration less practical.

Insulin Pump. An insulin pump provides a means for delivering insulin by continuous infusion. The device has three components: pump, tubing, and needle (Fig. 51-8). The pump itself contains a reservoir for rapid-acting or short-acting insulin, a battery-operated infuser, and a computer chip that enables a person to regulate basal (continuous) and premeal bolus doses in 0.05- to 0.1-unit increments. The pump, which is worn in a pouch or belt holder, is attached to tubing with a needle. The needle is inserted in the subcutaneous tissue of the abdomen and can remain in the same site for up to 3 days. Clients who are interested in controlling their diabetes with an insulin pump need to consider both its advantages and disadvantages (Box 51-2).

Oral Antidiabetic Agents

Oral antidiabetic drugs are prescribed for clients with type 2 diabetes who meet the following criteria:

- Fasting blood glucose level less than 200 mg/dL
- Insulin requirement of less than 40 units/day
- No ketoacidosis
- No renal or hepatic disease

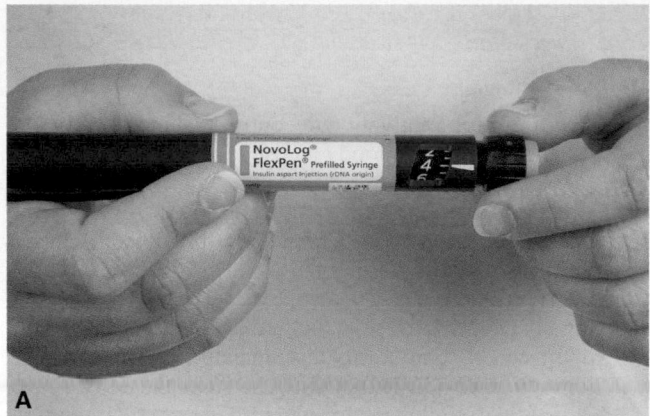

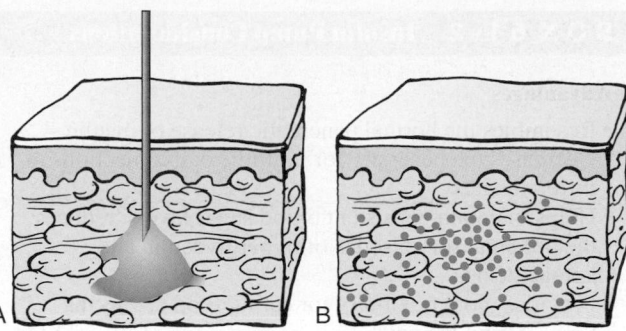

FIGURE 51-7. (**A**) Needle produces a pool of insulin beneath the skin, which is slowly absorbed. (**B**) Jet injector produces an insulin mist beneath the skin, which is absorbed more quickly.

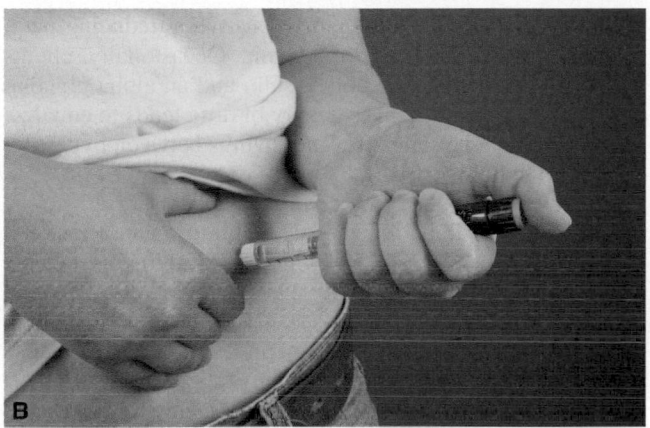

FIGURE 51-6. To use an insulin pen, the person (**A**) dials in the dose and (**B**) injects the needle into the cleaned site, pressing the button to deliver insulin.

 Gerontologic Considerations

- Older adults may take several medications for chronic comorbidities. Both prescription and nonprescription drugs should be assessed for any interactions with oral antidiabetic agents.

Sulfonylureas and Meglitinides

Sulfonylureas such as glyburide (DiaBeta, Glynase, Micronase) and glipizide (Glucotrol) were modified from sulfa-containing antibiotics when it was found that they reduced the blood glucose level. The sulfonylureas, which have evolved through several generations, and the meglitinides, nonsulfonylureas such as repaglinide (Prandin), are described as being "insulin releasers" because they stimulate the pancreas to secrete more insulin. Although they are effective

Before 1995, only one category of drugs, the sulfonylureas, was used to lower the blood glucose level. Since then, many new drugs have been developed that help control type 2 diabetes by various mechanisms. Recently developed drug categories include biguanides, alpha-glucosidase inhibitors, thiazolidinediones, and meglitinides. Drug Therapy Table 51-1 lists examples of oral hypoglycemic drugs.

Pharmacologic Considerations

- Oral antidiabetic drugs may be used in conjunction with insulin therapy in some clients with insulin-dependent diabetes; this reduces the insulin requirements and decreases the incidence of hypoglycemic reactions.

- Observe the client receiving an oral antidiabetic agent for signs of hypoglycemia. The time when hypoglycemia may occur is not predictable.

- Use of alcohol with some oral hypoglycemic drugs may result in abdominal cramps, nausea, flushing, headache, and hypoglycemia.

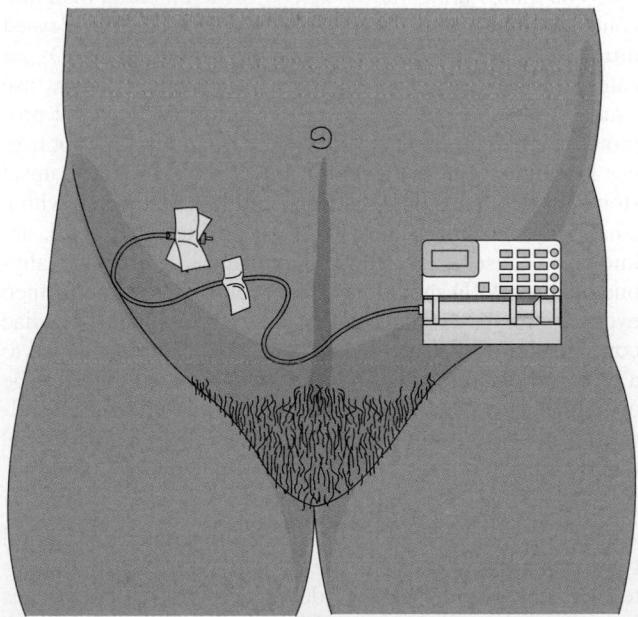

FIGURE 51-8. An insulin pump contains a syringe preloaded with insulin that is delivered to a client through tubing and needle in the abdomen. (From Pillitteri, A. [2007]. *Maternal and child health nursing* [5th ed.]. Philadelphia: Lippincott Williams & Wilkins.)

B O X 5 1 - 2 **Insulin Pump Considerations**

Advantages

- Resembles the normal pancreatic release of insulin
- Decreases the necessity for multiple daily injections in different sites
- Helps maintain consistent blood sugar levels; reduces the potential for episodes of hyperglycemia and ketoacidosis
- Provides more flexibility for eating food at varying times during the day
- Facilitates the instillation of smaller doses than those of insulin syringes

Disadvantages

- Requires high motivation to control diabetes by frequently checking blood glucose levels and adjusting the infusion
- Creates a potential for hyperglycemia if the pump fails, the tubing becomes kinked or obstructed, or the needle is displaced
- Interferes or creates a nuisance factor when participating in active sports, sexual intercourse, or bathing; the pump can be temporarily disconnected without removing the needle, but doing so stops the delivery of insulin until it is reconnected

---

drugs, they tend to cause weight gain, hypoglycemic reactions, and *secondary failure,* a phenomenon in which the pancreas cannot continue making sufficient insulin, perhaps as a result of the gland's overstimulation. Repaglinide has a short duration of action, making hypoglycemia less common than with sulfonylureas, but must be taken with each meal.

 Pharmacologic Considerations

- The sulfonylureas may interact with other drugs such as diuretics, antihypertensives, and thyroid preparations, which, depending on the specific drug, may increase or decrease the effects of the sulfonylurea.

Biguanides and Thiazolidinediones

Metformin (Glucophage) is the only biguanide approved for use. The thiazolidinediones (TZDs), which include rosiglitazone (Avandia) and pioglitazone (Actos), are the newest drugs used for type 2 diabetes. The biguanides and TZDs are categorized as "insulin sensitizers"—they help tissues use available insulin more efficiently. Metformin does not promote weight gain like the sulfonylureas, and it does not trigger low blood glucose levels. It may, however, cause upset stomach, flatulence, and diarrhea, and it is associated with a small risk of lactic acidosis. TZDs, on the other hand, are known to cause weight gain, edema, and liver damage; anyone taking a TZD should have liver function tests performed every 2 months during the first year of treatment. Cardiac complications associated with the use of rosiglitazone led to a proposal that this drug be withdrawn, but it continues to be available. However, troglitazone (Rezulin), the first developed TZD, was withdrawn from the market after its initial approval because several deaths were related to its use.

Alpha-Glucosidase Inhibitors

Alpha-glucosidase inhibitors include drugs such as miglitol (Glyset) and acarbose (Precose). Alpha-glucosidase is an intestinal enzyme that breaks down complex carbohydrates into glucose, a simple sugar. When this enzyme is inhibited, the process of forming glucose is slowed and glucose is absorbed more slowly from the small intestine. Consequently, blood glucose is balanced with the body's available insulin. Drugs in this category must be taken 15 minutes

before each meal. They are most effective in reducing postprandial (after a meal) hyperglycemia. Occasionally, clients with type 1 diabetes take both insulin and an alpha-glucosidase inhibitor because this category of drug tends to equalize blood glucose levels and prevents swings between hyperglycemia and hypoglycemia.

Unfortunately, a person who develops hypoglycemia while taking an alpha-glucosidase inhibitor cannot respond to the first line of treatment, which is drinking fruit juice, because the drug interferes with the conversion of fructose in the juice to glucose. In this case, the better treatment is to give glucose either in tablets or by injection because glucose requires no further breakdown for absorption.

Adjuvant Drugs

Pramlintide (Symlin) and exenatide (Byetta) are new drugs based on hormones with glucose-regulating functions. They are used along with traditional drugs for managing diabetes. Pramlintide is similar to *amylin,* a hormone that is secreted by the beta cells of the pancreas. Amylin lowers blood sugar after meals and causes a sense of satiety that controls overeating. Exenatide mimics *incretin,* a hormone released from cells that line the ileum and colon. Incretin promotes the secretion of insulin and improves the metabolism of carbohydrates. When combined with other diabetic agents, both pramlintide and exenatide regulate blood sugar more effectively and result in weight loss, an advantage over medications that affect only insulin levels. The disadvantage of these adjuvant drugs is that they require multiple daily injections. A long-acting injection is being developed.

Sitagliptin (Januvia) is an oral medication that works similarly to pramlintide; however, instead of promoting the action of amylin, it blocks its breakdown. It is classified as a dipeptidyl peptidase-4 (DPP-4) inhibitor. Januvia should be combined with other hypoglycemic agents and not used as a single agent. The FDA recently approved Janumet, a combination of sitagliptin and metformin in one pill.

 Pharmacologic Considerations

- Make certain that the client understands that insulin and the oral antidiabetic drugs are used to control hyperglycemia, but do not cure diabetes.

DRUG THERAPY TABLE 51-1 Oral Hypoglycemic Agents

Drug Category and Examples	Mechanism of Action	Side Effects	Nursing Considerations
Second-Generation Sulfonylureas glimepiride (Amaryl), glipizide (Glucotrol), glyburide (DiaBeta, Glynase PresTab, Micronase)	Stimulates insulin release; are more potent than first-generation sulfonylureas	Increased risk of cardiovascular mortality, anorexia, nausea, vomiting, heartburn, diarrhea, hypoglycemia, allergic skin reactions, insulin "burn out"	Give before breakfast. Monitor urine and serum glucose levels. Avoid administering to pregnant women. Caution client to avoid alcohol. Teach client appropriate diet, exercise, signs and symptoms of hypoglycemia and hyperglycemia, avoidance of infection. Do not abruptly discontinue medication.
Alpha-Glucosidase Inhibitors acarbose (Precose), miglitol (Glyset)	Delays digestion of carbohydrates Effects are additive to sulfonylureas in type 2 diabetes	Abdominal pain, flatulence, diarrhea, hypoglycemia	Give three times a day 15 min before each meal. Monitor urine and serum glucose levels. Inform client of gastrointestinal side effects.
Biguanide Compound metformin (Glucophage)	Improves use of insulin in type 2 diabetes	Anorexia, nausea, heartburn, diarrhea, lactic acidosis, hypoglycemia, allergic skin reactions, flatulence	Monitor urine and serum glucose levels. Avoid administering to pregnant women. Caution client to avoid use of alcohol. Instruct client not to discontinue medication.
Thiazolidinediones (TZDs) rosiglitazone (Avandia), pioglitazone (Actos)	Increases effects of circulating insulin	Headache, pain, liver injury, hypoglycemia, hyperglycemia, infections, fatigue, risk for heart attack and heart failure	Give once daily in morning. Monitor liver function periodically. Report weight gain and edema which may indicate a predisposition for heart failure.
Meglitinides repaglinide (Prandin)	Stimulates insulin release	Upper respiratory infections, hypoglycemia, hyperglycemia, headache	Monitor urine and serum glucose levels. Teach client appropriate diet, exercise, signs and symptoms of hypoglycemia and hyperglycemia, avoidance of infection.
Dipeptidyl peptidase IV (DPP-4) Inhibitor sitagliptin (Januvia)	Increases effects of incretin; prolongs the release of insulin and reduces production of glucose by the liver	Upper respiratory tract infection; nasopharyngitis and headache.	Assess blood sugar levels to evaluate response to therapy Do not use in clients with type 1 diabetes. Assess renal function before beginning drug therapy; contraindicated in renal dysfunction
Adjuvant Drugs exenatide (Byetta)	Mimics incretin	Heartburn, headache, nausea, vomiting, diarrhea, weight loss, dizziness, pancreatitis	Refrigerate unused prefilled pen; Inject 1 hour before morning and evening meals in upper thighs or arms Administer antibiotic or oral contraceptive one hour before exenatide

(drug table continues on page 794)

DRUG THERAPY TABLE 51-1 Oral Hypoglycemic Agents (*Continued*)

Drug Category and Examples	Mechanism of Action	Side Effects	Nursing Considerations
pramlintide (Symlin)	Mimics amylin; lowers blood sugar especially after meals; slows move-of food from stomach	Injection site reactions, anorexia, nausea, vomiting, stomach pain, indigestion, fatigue, dizziness, hypoglycemia	Bring drug to room temperature before injecting Administer subcutaneously in the abdomen or thighs prior to a meal or consumption of >30 g of carbohydrate Use with insulin, but give separate injections at least 2 inches from the insulin injection site Do not use if cloudy Check blood sugar before and after meals and at bedtime Contraindicated with other medications that slow gastric emptying
Combination Drugs metformin and sitagliptin (Janumet)	Combination product for use as adjunct to diet and exercise to improve glycemic control in adults with type 2 diabetes when mono-therapy is not controlling levels.	Lactic acidosis can occur based on the metformin component; diarrhea; upper respiratory infection; headache.	Baseline blood levels (hematologic assessment) and minimal monitoring of hematologic assessment Report all suspected adverse reactions to the FDA. Assess and educate clients on the signs of lactic acidosis: malaise, myalgias, respiratory distress, increasing somnolence, nonspecific abdominal distress.

Gerontologic Considerations

- The eating and sleeping habits of older adults often differ from those of young or middle-aged persons. This should be taken into consideration when planning meals and scheduling the dosage of insulin or an oral hypoglycemic agent.

▶ **Stop, Think, and Respond Exercise 51-3**

Name at least one oral antidiabetic agent in each of the following categories: (1) promotes release of insulin, (2) enhances response to insulin (insulin sensitizer), and (3) slows the breakdown of complex carbohydrates.

Pancreas Transplantation

Replacing the pancreas involves a whole or partial organ transplant. The usual candidate is a client with type 1 diabetes who has renal failure and will benefit from a combined kidney and pancreas transplant. Clients with type 2 diabetes are not offered the option of a pancreas transplant because usually their problem is insulin resistance, which does not improve with a transplant.

Because the pancreas is both an exocrine and endocrine gland, transplanting it requires a means for exocrine enzymatic drainage and venous absorption of insulin. Exocrine drainage is accomplished by establishing a duodenal or urinary bladder connection with the transplanted pancreas. Insulin is released into the portal vein, which carries blood to the liver. Although bladder connections have a lower incidence of organ rejection, they also tend to cause urologic complications and are used less often than originally.

As with any transplant, lifelong immunosuppressive drug therapy is required because without it, the new organ is destroyed. Because type 1 diabetes can be managed with insulin, many experts believe that the risks involved with immunosuppression outweigh the benefit that can be achieved with a pancreas transplant, unless a kidney transplant also is necessary.

Islet Cell Transplantation

Some clients with type 1 diabetes are recipients of islet cell transplants, the insulin-producing components of the pancreas, rather than a transplant of the entire organ or part of the organ. Two human pancreases are necessary to obtain sufficient numbers of islet cells for transplantation. The fragile islet cells must be transplanted within 12 hours of harvesting (NIDDK, 2007).

After the pancreas is harvested, the islet cells are separated from the tissue and injected through the abdominal wall into the client's portal vein, where they migrate to the liver and begin to release insulin. Presently, islet cell transplantation surgeons use a combination of tacrolimus (Prograf), sirolimus (Rapamune), and dacliximab (Zenapax) to prevent rejection. The current practice is to avoid using a steroid with other immunosuppressive drugs because steroids raise the blood glucose to levels the new islet cells have difficulty overcoming.

Transplanted islet cells tend to lose their ability to function over time, and approximately 70% of recipients resume insulin administration within 2 years. However, the amount of insulin and the frequency of its administration are reduced because of improved control of blood glucose levels (NIDDK, 2007).

Nursing Management

The nurse obtains a complete medical, drug, and allergy history, including a list of all symptoms and their duration. He or she determines when the client was diagnosed with diabetes and if others in the family also are diabetic. If the client is a diagnosed diabetic, the nurse asks the client to identify his or her prescribed treatment regimen and when he or she last consumed food and self-administered medications. The nurse weighs the client and performs a complete head-to-toe physical examination because diabetes affects many systems. The nurse looks for physical changes associated with diabetes:

* Changes in the skin over insulin injection sites, impaired skin areas that appear to be healing poorly, ulcerations or evidence of skin or soft-tissue infection
* Vital signs, peripheral pulses, temperature of the extremities, inspection of the extremities for edema or changes in color
* Decreased visual acuity and visual changes such as blurred vision
* Muscle atrophy, weakness, or loss of sensation

See Nursing Care Plan 51-1 for managing the care of a client with diabetes mellitus. The nurse monitors the client's blood glucose level before meals and at bedtime. It is also necessary to monitor postprandial blood sugar for the client on tight glucose control. The nurse tests the urine for ketones if the blood glucose level is high. He or she administers prescribed medications and evaluates the client's response to their effects. If hypoglycemia develops, the nurse uses the **rule of 15**: give 15 g of rapidly absorbed carbohydrate (Box 51-3), wait 15 minutes, recheck the blood sugar, and administer another 15 g of glucose if the blood sugar is not above 70 mg/dL.

The nurse initiates or reinforces information the client must know to manage his or her condition independently. He or she refers the client to a diabetic educator if one is available; consultation with a dietitian may be appropriate. The extent of the teaching program depends on whether the client has been diabetic for some time or is newly diagnosed; even those who have had the disorder for years may have inaccurate ideas about their disorder and treatment regimen.

Before teaching begins, the nurse confers with the physician regarding:

* Type of diet for the client to follow
* Medication regimen (insulin, oral antidiabetic agents, adjuvant medications, or some combination)
* Materials for insulin administration, such as needle and syringe, insulin pen, insulin jet, or insulin pump
* Technique for monitoring blood glucose levels, self-testing devices (glucometer), and the suggested brand to use
* Materials for and frequency of urine testing

* Additional information, such as skin care, signs of diabetic ketoacidosis (DKA), HHNKS, and hypoglycemia (discussed later)

Whenever possible, the nurse includes the family in a diabetic teaching program because one or more family members may assume some or all responsibility for the treatment regimen. To allow the client and family member time to understand information, the nurse presents material in small increments. He or she may choose to begin teaching by explaining diabetes, why treatments are necessary, and the various methods of treatment. The nurse uses audiovisual materials to enhance learning. Because the treatment of diabetes is highly individualized, he or she emphasizes that the treatment of one person cannot be compared with that of another.

If the client requires insulin, the nurse identifies that the preferred site for injections is the abdomen and uses a chart to explain how to rotate injection sites. The American Diabetes Association, in its 2002 Position Statement, advocates rotating insulin injections in only one anatomic region to ensure consistent rates of absorption. Abdominal injections are absorbed most quickly and have the least rate variability. If the physician has recommended the use of a glucometer to monitor blood glucose levels, the nurse allows time for the client to use the glucometer and monitor his or her own blood glucose levels. Additional teaching topics include the following:

* Signs and symptoms of hyperglycemia and hypoglycemia
* The importance of weight reduction, if necessary
* Methods of terminating hypoglycemia with a rapidly absorbed carbohydrate, such as food or beverage sources, Prolycen (a commercial product containing glucose), glucose tablets, or glucose gel
* Problems that require contacting the physician, such as skin infection, pain in the extremities, visual problems, change in color or temperature of the skin of the extremities, frequent episodes of hypoglycemia, prolonged nausea and vomiting, and illness
* The importance of following an exercise regimen suggested by the physician. The nurse stresses that during exercise the client needs to have some food or other physician-approved form of glucose if symptoms of hypoglycemia occur. This is especially important for clients taking insulin or those subject to episodes of hypoglycemia while taking an oral antidiabetic agent.
* How to integrate the dietary exchange list throughout the day
* The information that is printed on food labels to promote compliance with the prescribed diet
* The definitions of products labeled as "low calorie" and "dietetic" and that these terms are not synonymous with "no sugar." They may contain sugar.
* The importance of drinking adequate water, especially in warm weather, when exercising and when perspiring
* Foot care
* The necessity for regular appointments with an ophthalmologist for comprehensive eye examinations
* The need to consult the physician regarding dosage adjustments for insulin or oral antidiabetic agent if the client becomes ill or cannot eat

NURSING CARE PLAN 51-1 | The Client With Diabetes Mellitus

Assessment

Determine the following:

- Evidence of polyuria, polydipsia, polyphagia
- Current weight; recent weight changes
- Vital signs, especially blood pressure in lying, sitting, and standing positions
- Blood glucose level before each meal and at bedtime
- Any ketones or albumin in the urine

- Serum electrolyte, cholesterol, lipid, triglyceride, blood urea nitrogen, and creatinine levels
- Condition of the skin and feet
- Any abnormal sensations such as pain, tingling, burning, numbness
- Visual acuity and last date of ophthalmic examination
- Knowledge of therapeutic management

Nursing Diagnosis: Imbalanced Nutrition: More than Body Requirements related to altered satiety, decreased activity, and habituation of preillness eating habits

Expected Outcome: Client will adhere to a prescribed calorie-controlled diet.

Interventions	Rationales
Provide three meals and snacks within prescribed caloric limits.	Restriction of calories promotes weight loss and balances glucose with naturally produced or parenterally administered insulin.
Suggest free foods such as up to 1 cup of raw vegetables like salad greens and sugar-free gelatin; unlimited sugar-free drinks; or low-sodium bouillon, if the client becomes hungry between meals or snacks.	Free foods contain fewer than 20 calories per serving; their consumption provides negligible calories.
Encourage client to drink 8 ounces of water before eating a meal.	Water is calorie free, distends the stomach, and provides a feeling of fullness.
Advise client to eat slowly and wait 15 seconds between chewing thoroughly, swallowing, and taking the next bite.	Slowed eating prolongs the pleasure of eating and allows time for the brain to sense satiation.

Evaluation of Expected Outcome

Client follows eats the prescribed diet and verbalizes understanding of restrictions and allowances.

PC: Hypoglycemia

Expected Outcome: The nurse will monitor for, manage, and minimize hypoglycemia.

Interventions	Rationales
Test capillary blood glucose level with a glucometer 30 minutes before each meal and at bedtime.	Hypoglycemia is more likely before the client consumes food.
Monitor for signs of hypoglycemia such as shakiness, diaphoresis, hunger, and disturbed cognition.	Low blood glucose level causes physiologic stimulation and diminishes the ability to think clearly.
Follow agency policy for administering a quick-acting source of simple carbohydrate to lower limit of blood glucose level.	Simple carbohydrates are absorbed quickly and tend to raise the blood glucose level within 15 minutes to eliminate the symptoms of hypoglycemia.
Recheck the capillary blood glucose level 15 minutes after treating a hypoglycemic episode.	Rechecking the level helps determine the client's response to the nursing intervention.
Repeat the administration of simple carbohydrate if the client continues to be symptomatic; reassess capillary blood glucose level.	The client may need additional simple carbohydrate to successfully raise blood glucose.
Notify the physician if the client's symptoms continue after two attempts to raise the blood sugar with oral substances.	Parenteral interventions to raise the blood glucose level are medically prescribed.
Offer client complex carbohydrates when hypoglycemia is controlled.	Complex carbohydrates are digested and absorbed more slowly than simple carbohydrates, which reduces the potential for another hypoglycemic episode.
Withhold insulin when the client must fast before laboratory or diagnostic procedures.	Eating and administration of insulin are timed according to insulin's onset, peak, and duration of action.
Ask a second nurse to double-check the vial of insulin and the number of units in the syringe before administering the injection.	Double-checking helps avoid errors in insulin administration. Giving more than the prescribed amount or mistaking rapid-acting or short-acting insulin for intermediate- or long-acting insulin can cause hypoglycemia.

NURSING CARE PLAN 51-1   The Client With Diabetes Mellitus (Continued)

Evaluation of Expected Outcome

Client's blood sugar is at least 70 mg/dl

PC: Hyperglycemia

Expected Outcome: The nurse will monitor for, manage, and minimize hyperglycemia.

Interventions	Rationales
Monitor capillary blood glucose levels before each meal and at bedtime; check urine for ketones if glucose levels are elevated.	Elevated blood glucose level before a client eats suggests that he or she is not compliant with the diet and may require a higher dose of an oral antidiabetic agent or coverage with rapid-acting or short-acting insulin. Ketonuria increases the potential for DKA.
Assess for clinical signs and symptoms of hyperglycemia such as thirst, increased urination, and sleepiness.	Hyperglycemia has a gradual onset with symptoms similar to the undiagnosed state; hyperglycemia can progress to DKA or HHNKS.
Administer insulin or oral antidiabetic agents as prescribed.	Insufficient insulin results in elevated blood glucose level.
Implement medical orders for insulin administration according to a sliding scale established by the physician.	Insulin lowers blood glucose level.
Notify the physician if the client with hyperglycemia is noninsulin dependent.	Modifications in the diet or changes in antidiabetic medications are medically prescribed.
Reinforce the importance of compliance with the prescribed diet, exercise, and medication regimen.	These measures manage hyperglycemia.

Evaluation of Expected Outcome

Blood glucose levels are within 80 to 120 mg/dL in a nonfasting state.

Nursing Diagnosis: Risk for Imbalanced Fluid Volume related to hyperglycemia and polyuria

Expected Outcome: Client will maintain proper fluid balance.

Interventions	Rationales
Monitor intake and output.	A deficit in fluid intake or excess urine output suggests a deficit in fluid volume.
Provide at least 1500 to 3000 mL of fluid per day.	The average fluid requirement per 24 hours is 1500 to 3000 mL.

Evaluation of Expected Outcome

Client is well-hydrated as evidenced by a fluid intake of between 1500 and 3000 mL with a similar urine output.

Nursing Diagnosis: Risk for Injury related to orthostatic hypotension and impaired vision secondary to neuropathy and retinopathy

Expected Outcome: Client will be free from injury.

Interventions	Rationales
Assist client when rising from a sitting or lying position.	Autonomic neuropathy causes orthostatic hypotension and the potential for fainting and falling.
Have client dangle on the side of the bed before ambulating.	Dangling allows a period during which blood flow is restored to the brain.
Keep the floor dry and the environment free of clutter.	Retinopathy may interfere with the client's ability to see potential safety hazards.

Evaluation of Expected Outcome

There is no evidence of trauma.

Nursing Diagnosis: Risk for Impaired Skin Integrity related to loss of sensation in feet and impaired blood circulation

Expected Outcome: Skin will remain intact.

(care plan continues on page 798)

NURSING CARE PLAN 51-1 The Client With Diabetes Mellitus (Continued)

Interventions	Rationales
Examine skin and feet daily.	Client may be insensitive to injuries and slow to heal because of peripheral neuropathy and vascular disturbances.
Assess skin for signs of breakdown, poor healing, change in color or temperature, or infection.	Impaired blood supply compromises the integrity of the integument.
Dry client's skin well after bathing, especially in areas of the body that are dark and moist.	Fungal infections are common in creases and folds of skin.
Rotate insulin injection sites; give each injection 1/2 to 1 inch away from the previous injection.	Rotating injection sites prevents lipoatrophy and lipohypertrophy.
Inspect inside the client's shoes for foreign objects or disrepair.	Friction or pressure can impair the integrity of the feet.
Provide foot care with daily hygiene.	Care of the feet prevents injury and skin breakdown.

Evaluation of Expected Outcome

Skin is warm, dry, and intact, with no evidence of tissue breakdown in the feet.

Nursing Diagnosis: Risk for Ineffective Management of Therapeutic Regimen related to insufficient knowledge regarding diabetes self-management

Expected Outcome: Client will verbalize and demonstrate knowledge of diabetes and self-management techniques.

Interventions	Rationales
Assess client's ability and willingness to learn about diabetes and self-management.	Teaching is more effective when the learner is capable and motivated to acquire information.
Teach client about insulin and how to self-administer using proper technique.	Clients learn in various ways: verbal explanations, reading information, seeing a demonstration, or using a hands-on application.
Allow client opportunities to practice administering insulin.	Practice promotes self-confidence and develops expertise.
Show client how to monitor blood glucose using a glucometer.	Using the same method as the client will use after discharge increases knowledgeable self-management.
Arrange for the dietitian to teach client about his or her nutrition therapy.	Dietitians are experts in nutrition therapy.
Review the importance of exercise and methods for daily activity.	Exercise reduces blood glucose level, helps with weight loss, and improves circulation.

Evaluation of Expected Outcome

Client demonstrates knowledge and skills to independently manage his or her disease.

ACUTE COMPLICATIONS OF DIABETES MELLITUS

Some clients, despite careful control of their disease, develop one or more serious complications over time. Some complications can be controlled when detected in the early stages.

BOX 51-3	Examples of 15 g of Rapidly Absorbed Carbohydrate

3–4 glucose tablets
1 small tube of glucose gel
1/2 cup fruit juice or regular soft drink
1 Tbsp honey or syrup
1 Tbsp of sugar or 5 small sugar cubes
6–8 LifeSavers™ candies
8 ounces of skim milk

DIABETIC KETOACIDOSIS

Diabetic ketoacidosis (DKA), a type of metabolic acidosis, occurs when there is an acute insulin deficiency or an inability to use whatever insulin the pancreas secretes.

Pathophysiology and Etiology

DKA can develop despite the client's compliance with the prescribed treatment regimen. Clients who develop DKA often have a severe, hard-to-control form of the disease (brittle or unstable diabetes). Occasionally, a client admitted to the hospital in DKA has undiagnosed diabetes. Other causes of this serious event are infection and noncompliance with the treatment regimen. (See the discussion of ketoacidosis under Pathophysiology and Etiology of Diabetes Mellitus.)

When the amount of glucose transported across cell membranes decreases, the liver increases its production of glucose. The blood glucose level becomes extremely elevated. The kidneys attempt to excrete the glucose, which is well beyond the renal threshold. In the process, excessive amounts of water, sodium, and potassium are excreted as well. The client becomes dehydrated; the skin is warm, dry, and flushed. Stored fat is broken down, causing ketones to accumulate in the blood and urine. As ketones mount, the pH of the blood becomes acidotic. The client begins breathing rapidly and deeply in an attempt to eliminate carbon dioxide and prevent it from forming carbonic acid, which would contribute even more to the acidotic state. If the condition is severe and prolonged, the client becomes comatose. Death results with untreated or ineffective treatment of DKA.

Assessment Findings

Early symptoms are vague and become more definite and serious as increasing ketones accumulate in the bloodstream. Weakness, thirst, anorexia, vomiting, drowsiness, and abdominal pain develop. The cheeks are flushed, and the skin and mouth are dry. The breath has an odor of acetone. Kussmaul respirations often are evident. The pulse is rapid and weak. The BP is low. The client may become unresponsive but restless. Blood glucose levels are elevated to 300 to 1000 mg/dL or more. Urine contains glucose and ketones. The blood pH ranges from 6.8 to 7.3. The serum bicarbonate level is decreased to levels from 0 to 15 mEq/L. The compensatory breathing pattern can lower the partial pressure of carbon dioxide in arterial blood ($PaCO_2$) to levels of 10 to 30 mm Hg. Serum sodium and potassium levels reflect the degree of dehydration (i.e., they may be elevated because they are concentrated in a low volume of body fluid); however, intracellular levels are low, but they are unmeasurable.

Medical Management

Treatment depends on the severity of DKA. The main goals of treatment are to (1) reduce the elevated blood glucose, (2) correct fluid and electrolyte imbalances, and (3) clear the urine and blood of ketones. To accomplish these goals, insulin is given intravenously. Insulin reduces the production of ketones by making glucose available for oxidation by the tissues and by restoring the liver's supply of glycogen. Regular insulin is added to an IV solution and infused continuously. The amount of insulin and the rate of infusion depend on the blood glucose levels, but the rate may be in the range of 5 Units per hour. Isotonic fluid is instilled at a high volume, for example, 250 to 500 mL per hour for several hours. The rate is adjusted once the client becomes rehydrated and diuresis is less acute. As insulin begins to lower the blood glucose level, the IV solution is changed to include one with glucose. This helps to avoid the potential for hypoglycemia. Potassium replacements are given despite elevated serum levels to raise intracellular stores. Periodic monitoring of serum electrolytes and blood glucose levels is necessary. The urine is tested for glucose and ketones.

Nursing Management

The nurse monitors IV infusions closely and takes vital signs frequently. Older adults and those with cardiopulmonary or renal disorders are prone to fluid overload. The nurse inserts an indwelling urinary catheter and monitors urine output to ensure that replaced potassium has a means for excretion. Besides checking serum electrolyte findings, the nurse attaches cardiac leads and observes the client's heart conduction pattern to detect evidence of hyperkalemia such as peaked T waves. Blood glucose level is measured frequently; the urine is similarly checked for the presence of ketones. He or she keeps the physician informed of the client's response, or lack of response, to therapy. See Nursing Care Plan 51-1 for additional nursing care.

HYPEROSMOLAR HYPERGLYCEMIC NONKETOTIC SYNDROME

Hyperosmolar hyperglycemic nonketotic syndrome (HHNKS), an acute complication of diabetes, is characterized by hyperglycemia without ketosis. It is not unusual to find the blood glucose level well over 500 mg/dL, but the pH of the blood remains within the normal range of 7.35 to 7.45. Fluid and electrolyte imbalances accompany HHNKS.

Pathophysiology and Etiology

HHNKS often results from a serious illness during which metabolic needs exceed the limits of available insulin. Because of persistent hyperglycemia, fluid moves from the intracellular compartment to the extracellular compartment. Diuresis occurs with a subsequent loss of sodium and potassium. Because the client still is secreting some insulin, which can transport glucose in the cells, fat metabolism is minimal or unaffected; hence, ketosis does not develop. HHNK syndrome is more common in undiagnosed or older clients with type 2 diabetes. It also occurs among clients who do not have diabetes who receive drugs that elevate blood glucose, or who require kidney dialysis or total parenteral nutrition.

Assessment Findings

Hypotension, mental changes, extreme thirst, dehydration, tachycardia, and fever develop. Neurologic signs include paralysis, lethargy, coma, and seizures. Symptoms of hypokalemia and hyponatremia usually are present. Physical examination reveals dry mucous membranes and poor skin turgor. Blood glucose levels are exceedingly high and serum potassium and sodium levels are low. The serum osmolarity is increased.

Medical Management

Treatment includes the administration of insulin and correction of fluid and electrolyte imbalances. A central catheter may be used to monitor the client's hemodynamic response to fluid replacement.

Nursing Management

The nurse measures the client's blood glucose level and assesses for electrolyte imbalances and dehydration. He or she implements medical orders for insulin, fluids, and electrolyte replacement and closely monitors the client's response to treatment. The nurse's priority areas for evaluation include hydration status, intake and output, skin turgor, vital signs, and electrolyte studies. The nurse observes the client's neurologic and cognitive symptoms; cognition may be significantly impaired in the early stages of care. The nurse protects the client's safety if cognition is impaired and judgment is poor. Additional management depends on symptoms (see Nursing Care Plan 51-1).

HYPOGLYCEMIA

Hypoglycemia, a low blood glucose level, is always a potential adverse reaction when administering medications for diabetes.

Pathophysiology and Etiology

When too much insulin (hyperinsulinism) is in the bloodstream relative to the amount of available glucose, hypoglycemia occurs. The blood glucose level falls below 70 mg/dL. Because glucose is the primary source of cellular energy, especially for the brain, hypoglycemia tends to manifest in neurologic changes such as confusion, difficulty processing information, anxious feelings, emotional irritability, and headache. The client feels hungry, a homeostatic mechanism to stimulate eating. If the condition is untreated, seizures, permanent brain damage, or death can occur.

Hypoglycemia occurs when a client with diabetes is (1) not eating at all and continues to take insulin or oral antidiabetic medications, (2) not eating sufficient calories to compensate for glucose-lowering medications, or (3) is exercising more than usual, which lowers available blood glucose. Alcohol consumption also interferes with the liver's ability to synthesize glucose from noncarbohydrates, placing clients with diabetes who drink at higher risk for hypoglycemia.

Assessment Findings

Signs and Symptoms

The pattern of symptoms varies somewhat depending on the degree of hypoglycemia, the individual reaction, and the type of insulin taken. Initial symptoms include weakness, headache, nausea, drowsiness, nervousness, hunger, tremors, malaise, and excessive perspiration. Some clients have characteristic personality or behavioral changes. Confusion and dizziness can occur. If hypoglycemia is not corrected, symptoms can progress to difficulty with coordination. The client may complain of double vision. If left untreated, unconsciousness and seizures can develop.

Although symptoms vary, each client tends to have a uniquely repetitive pattern when hypoglycemia develops. The manifestation of hypoglycemic symptoms usually is quite rapid, with unconsciousness or seizures occurring shortly after onset.

When a client with diabetes is found unconscious, DKA or hypoglycemia needs to be ruled out. These conditions are direct opposites: in ketoacidosis, the blood glucose level is high; in hypoglycemia, it is low. The nurse and client must be familiar with the symptoms of hypoglycemia and hyperglycemia to recognize and differentiate the complication as it is developing and treat it appropriately (Table 51-3).

Diagnostic Findings

Diagnosis is based on symptoms, client history, and blood glucose levels. The history is important in differentiating between DKA and hypoglycemia. If the client had insulin and has not eaten, it is most likely that hypoglycemia is present. If the client has eaten and has not taken or received insulin, DKA is more likely. Recognition of hypoglycemia must be immediate; therefore, a bedside glucometer test and sharp assessment skills are important.

Medical Management

The medical treatment for a hypoglycemic reaction is administration of 15 g of simple carbohydrate as soon as possible. If the client is unconscious, glucose gel can be applied in the buccal cavity of the mouth. If the client does not respond after two administrations of rapidly absorbed carbohydrate, the physician may order glucagon, a hormone that stimulates the liver to release glycogen, or 20 to 50 mL of 50% glucose is prescribed for IV administration. Once the hypoglycemic symptoms are relieved, the client with diabetes is given complex carbohydrates such as graham crackers and milk to sustain and prolong an adequate level of blood glucose.

Nursing Management

If the client is conscious and can swallow, the nurse gives an oral form of rapidly absorbed carbohydrate. He or she implements medical orders for parenteral medications such as IV glucose or parenteral glucagon. Whenever a client with diabetes mellitus is in a hospital unit, quick-acting carbohydrates are stocked and available. In a severe reaction, the nurse may provide more than an initial offering of

TABLE 51-3 Characteristics of Hyperglycemia and Hypoglycemia

CHARACTERISTIC	HYPERGLYCEMIA	HYPOGLYCEMIA
Predisposing factors	Insufficient or omitted insulin	Excessive insulin
	Concurrent infection	Unusual exercise
	Dietary indiscretion	Too little food
Onset	Slow; hours to days	Sudden; minutes
Mental status	Drowsy	Disoriented; eventually becomes comatose
Skin	Flushed, dry, hot	Pale, moist, cool
Blood pressure	Low	Normal
Pulse	Rapid, weak	Normal or slow, bounding
Respiration	Air hunger	Normal to rapid, shallow
Hunger	Absent	Often present
Thirst	Present	Absent
Vomiting	Present	May be absent
Urine glucose	Present in large amounts	Absent in second voided specimen
Response to treatment	Slow	Rapid

Adapted from Lilly Research Laboratories, Diabetes mellitus.

carbohydrate after monitoring the client's blood glucose level to evaluate the effect. If the symptoms do not abate and the blood glucose level remains low, the nurse collaborates with the physician concerning additional medical measures.

Above all, the nurse stays with the hypoglycemic client until the pronounced symptoms are corrected. When an episode of hypoglycemia occurs, the regulation of glucose metabolism may be tenuous for about 24 hours. The nurse observes the client at frequent intervals for further episodes of hypoglycemia.

The nurse can prevent hypoglycemia by:

- Ensuring that the meal is served within 15 minutes of administering rapid-acting insulin and within 30 minutes of giving short-acting insulin
- Ensuring that the client eats the prescribed diet and between-meal snacks
- Informing the physician immediately if nausea, vomiting, or diarrhea occur, or if the client refuses to eat
- Administering the correct type and dose of insulin at the prescribed times
- Asking a colleague to check the label on the insulin vial and the number of units in the insulin syringe against that which is ordered before administering insulin, to avoid a medication error

Additional nursing management of hypoglycemia depends on the symptoms presented (see Nursing Care Plan 51-1).

CHRONIC COMPLICATIONS OF DIABETES MELLITUS

Although clients with diabetes can develop many complications, extremely common ones include peripheral neuropathy, nephropathy, retinopathy, and vascular changes.

PERIPHERAL NEUROPATHY

Neuropathy is a general term that refers to pathologic changes in nerves. Neuropathies in clients with diabetes can affect motor, sensory, and autonomic nerves. Neuropathies develop 10 or more years after the onset of diabetes, but the incidence increases with the duration. Because their onset is gradual, the client usually is oblivious to the development in early stages.

Pathophysiology and Etiology

Neuropathy results from poor glucose control and decreased blood circulation to nerve tissue. Manifestations of peripheral neuropathies are more common among clients with diabetes who smoke and whose blood glucose level is poorly controlled. Because nitric acid dilates blood vessels, some believe that consistently elevated blood glucose levels lower nitric acid levels, impair circulation, and subsequently damage peripheral nerves. This may explain the development of erectile dysfunction in men with diabetes (see Chapter 55).

Motor Neuropathy

When motor nerves are affected, the muscles weaken and atrophy. Joint support is diminished. The feet widen. Eventually bone structure is affected, resulting in skeletal deformities, usually in the feet and ankles, with subsequent changes in gait. Areas of skin and soft tissue that are subjected to friction and pressure are prone to ulcerate (Fig. 51-9). If there is infection or impaired healing, portions of the affected extremity may require amputation (see Chap. 61).

Sensory Neuropathy

Neuropathy involving sensory nerves leads to *paresthesias,* abnormal sensations such as prickling, tingling, burning, or needle-like pain in the feet, legs, and sometimes hands. In severe cases, feeling is totally lost. This lack of sensitivity increases the potential for soft tissue injury without the client's awareness.

Autonomic Neuropathy

Neuropathy of autonomic nerves that affect organ functioning has several consequences. *Gastroparesis,* atony of the stomach, retards the movement of food from the stomach. If nerves that innervate the bladder are affected, the client does not sense the urge to void, and retained urine supports bacterial growth, causing frequent urinary tract infections. Incontinence also may occur when the bladder is overfilled. According to the American Diabetes Association, up to 50% of men with diabetes develop erectile dysfunction when nerves that promote erection become impaired. When autonomic nerves that affect cardiovascular function fail to function effectively, episodes of orthostatic hypotension occur. Clients with diabetes often do not sense the chest pain of angina as acutely as those without diabetes, which delays or interferes with prompt assessment and treatment of coronary artery disease and myocardial infarction.

Assessment Findings

Signs and Symptoms

Pain is one of the leading symptoms that accompany motor and sensory nerve changes. Skeletal muscles in the extremities become smaller. The feet swell and become insensitive

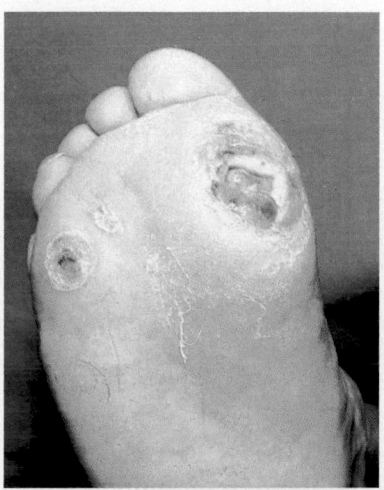

FIGURE 51-9. Neuropathic ulcers occur on pressure points in areas with diminished sensation in diabetic polyneuropathy. Pain is absent (and therefore the ulcer may go unnoticed). (From Smeltzer, S. C., et al. [2008]. *Brunner & Suddarth's textbook of medical–surgical nursing* [11th ed.]. Philadelphia: Lippincott Williams & Wilkins.)

to temperature or other tactile stimuli. Disturbing sensations develop that often are intensified by maintaining a position for an extended period, such as occupational tasks that require standing in place, holding the steering wheel while driving, or performing a repetitive motion such as knitting. The client may report digestive, urinary, and sexual dysfunction, and dizziness when rising.

Diagnostic Findings

A neurologic examination validates that when a tuning fork is in contact with the skin of the extremities, the client has diminished vibratory sense. Loss of protective sensation, the ability to sense and differentiate hot and cold, sharp and dull, and soft and rough stimuli, occurs. This is demonstrated with a screening test in which areas of the feet are touched with a nylon monofilament that delivers 10 g of force without the client's perception (Fig. 51-10). Electromyography studies demonstrate a slowed conduction of electrical stimulation along nerves (see Chap. 36).

Gerontologic Considerations

- Good foot care is especially important in older adults because other diseases common in this population, such as peripheral vascular disease and osteoarthritis, increase the risk of complications related to the feet. The client should consult a podiatrist at regular intervals.

Medical Management

Diet, exercise, and medication control blood glucose levels. Several medications can reduce pain, such as non-narcotic analgesics or a tricyclic antidepressant such as imipramine (Tofranil). Anticonvulsants such as gabapentin (Neurontin), carbamazepine (Tegretol), or phenytoin (Dilantin) also provide pain relief. Nonpharmacologic pain relief can be facilitated with transcutaneous electrical nerve stimulation. Elastic compression stockings, increasing dietary sodium, or

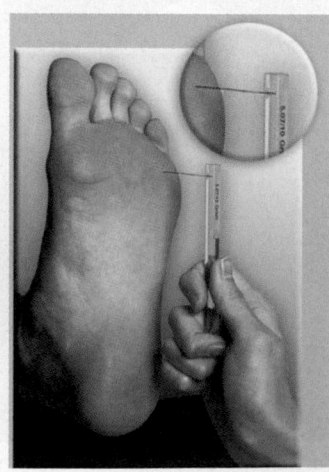

FIGURE 51-10. A strand of monofilament line is used to assess sensation in clients with diabetes. (Adapted from Cameron, B.L. [2002]. Making diabetes management routine. *American Journal of Nursing 102* [2]: 26–32.)

using fludrocortisone (Florinef), which increases fluid volume, or an antihypotensive agent such as midodrine (ProAmatine), help reduce orthostatic hypotension. Small, frequent meals or administration of metoclopramide (Reglan) are recommended for the relief of symptoms associated with gastroparesis. Antibiotic therapy, increased oral fluid intake, and urinating every 3 hours helps eliminate urinary tract infections. Various options are available for men who are concerned about erectile dysfunction (see Chap. 55).

Several pharmaceutical companies are developing drugs that might reverse diabetic neuropathies. Clinical trials include aldose reductase inhibitors (ARIs), which reduce the conversion of high blood glucose to sorbitol, known to damage nerve and renal cells, and insulin-like growth factor-1, a protein that promotes neural conduction and regrowth of nerve axons. Ranirestat, an ARI, has been shown to improve diabetic sensory neuropathy, and it is considered a promising agent for the treatment of complications of diabetes, especially neuropathy (Bril & Buchanan, 2006; Matsumoto et al., 2008).

Nursing Management

The nurse implements a teaching plan for the management of diabetes and its potential complications. If possible, the primary care nurse refers the client for classes with a diabetes educator. The nurse stresses foot care (Client and Family Teaching 51-1) and advises the client with peripheral autonomic neuropathy to rise slowly from a lying or sitting position, to drink generous fluids, and to wear knee-high or thigh-high elastic stockings during waking hours. The nurse emphasizes compliance with prescribed medications and warns the client to avoid taking more than the recommended doses of analgesics. For digestive problems, he or she explains that consuming a large volume of food at any one

Client and Family Teaching 51-1
Foot Care in Diabetes

The nurse instructs the client and family as follows:

- Inspect the feet daily for blisters, corns, calluses, long or ingrown nails, or any reddened areas; use a mirror if necessary to visualize all aspects of the foot.
- Wash the feet daily in warm (not hot) water.
- Dry the feet thoroughly, being careful to dry between the toes.
- Keep toenails short and cut straight across.
- Apply a moisturizer to feet daily.
- Do not use razor, abrasive, or commercial products to remove corns or calluses.
- Use lamb's wool between toes that overlap.
- Wear well-fitting shoes that fit comfortably when first worn; do not wear rubber, plastic, or vinyl shoes that cause the feet to perspire. Consult physician about wearing sneakers or canvas shoes.
- Never go barefoot.
- Visit a podiatrist regularly for foot care.
- Wash, dry, and cover any injuries with sterile gauze and call healthcare provider immediately for evaluation.
- Notify the physician about a blister, abrasion, or foot injury.

sitting and eating fatty foods delays stomach emptying. The nurse refers clients with erectile dysfunction to a urologist.

DIABETIC NEPHROPATHY

Diabetic nephropathy refers to the progressive decrease in renal function that occurs with diabetes mellitus. Clients with type 1 diabetes are more likely to develop diabetic nephropathy, but clients with type 2 diabetes also are affected.

Pathophysiology and Etiology

Nephropathy is a consequence of glomerular deterioration resulting in impaired filtration of blood during urine formation (see Chap. 57). There are five stages of nephropathy, each characterized by a successive progression of renal dysfunction (Table 51-4). Essentially, the glomeruli excrete serum proteins, especially albumin, and lose their ability to excrete nitrogen waste products.

Poor glucose control contributes to the onset of nephropathy. Although hypertension is an eventual consequence of diabetic nephropathy, when it occurs in the prediabetic or prenephropathic state, it accelerates the onset and progression of renal damage. Nephropathy is associated with retinopathy and systemic vascular changes (discussed later).

Assessment Findings

In the early stages, the client does not manifest any obvious signs and symptoms. Eventually, he or she notices swelling of the feet and hands, most likely from the loss of albumin, a colloid that pulls water into the vascular system. The BP increases gradually. The client feels tired and weak.

A routine urinalysis or dip with a chemical strip detects albumin in the urine. The blood urea nitrogen and serum creatinine become elevated. The renal creatinine clearance is decreased.

Medical Management

Controlling both blood glucose levels and hypertension can prevent or delay the development of diabetic nephropathy. The National Heart, Lung, and Blood Institute recommends that clients with diabetes maintain their BP at or below 130/85 mm Hg. The target BP of clients with diabetes who already have developed proteinuria is at or lower than 125/75 mm Hg. Angiotensin-converting enzyme (ACE) inhibitors such as captopril (Capoten) and angiotensin II receptor antagonists such as losartan (Cozaar) slow the progressive nature of nephropathy. A moderate reduction in dietary protein is beneficial. Smoking cessation is strongly recommended.

A new drug, aminoguanidine (Pimagedine), an advanced glycosylation end-product inhibitor, is under study. Results indicate that the yet-unapproved drug prevents or reduces damage to the glomeruli from excess glucose and decreases the urinary excretion of albumin. Research also has shown that aminoguanidine lowers blood lipid levels and slows retinal changes, raising the hope that, if the drug is approved, it can prevent or treat multiple complications of diabetes (Friedman, 2007).

Nursing Management

The nurse monitors the client's blood glucose and hemoglobin A1c results. He or she checks the urine with a test strip to detect evidence of albuminuria. The nurse provides additional teaching if the client's blood glucose level is not controlled. He or she refers the client to programs that assist with smoking cessation or discusses the possibility of nicotine patches or gum to control further habituation. The nurse explains the therapeutic regimen associated with prescribed antihypertensive drugs and dietary measures for lowering BP and complications from vascular disease (see Chap. 27). Because nephropathy is progressive, the nurse encourages the client to keep appointments for regular medical follow-up.

DIABETIC RETINOPATHY

Diabetic retinopathy refers to pathologic changes in the retina that are experienced by persons with diabetes. On average, it develops 10 or more years after the onset of diabetes. The earlier retinopathy develops, the more likely it is that vision will rapidly deteriorate.

Pathophysiology and Etiology

Diabetic retinopathy is a consequence of inadequately controlled blood glucose levels, which cause vascular changes in the retina (Fig. 51-11).

TABLE 51-4 Stages of Diabetic Nephropathy

STAGE	CHARACTERISTICS	EFFECTS	AVERAGE ONSET AFTER DIAGNOSIS OF DIABETES
Stage I	Hyperfiltration Glomerular hypertrophy	Blood flow through kidneys is increased. Kidneys are enlarged.	10 yr
Stage II	Microalbuminuria	Albumin, a blood protein, is excreted in small amounts.	
Stage III	Gross albuminuria	Large amount of albumin is excreted; urine consistently tests positive for its presence. Blood pressure becomes elevated. Excretion of nitrogen wastes is impaired.	15 yr
Stage IV	Advanced dysfunction	Severe impairment of glomerular filtration is evidenced by excessive proteinuria, hypertension, and rise in blood urea nitrogen and creatinine levels.	15–20 yr
Stage V	End-stage renal failure	Kidney functions are severely impaired; dialysis or renal transplantation is necessary.	20–25 yr

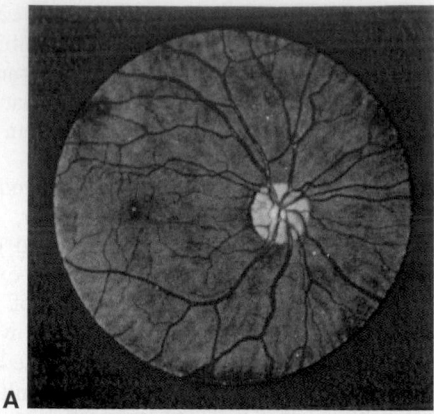

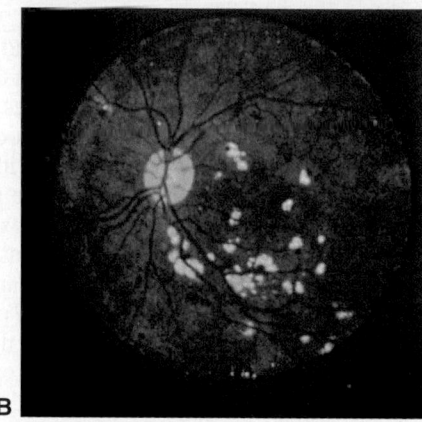

FIGURE 51-11. (**A**) In the normal eye, the light circular area over which several blood vessels converge is the optic disc, where the optic nerve meets the back of the eye. (**B**) In diabetic retinopathy, the fundus photograph shows characteristic waxy-looking lesions, microaneurysms, and hemorrhages.

There are two types: (1) nonproliferative retinopathy is the milder manifestation, and (2) proliferative retinopathy, the more severe form, can lead to blindness. In nonproliferative retinopathy, *microaneurysms,* outpouchings in retinal capillaries, develop from high vascular pressure and compromised circulation. The stasis of blood flow interferes with transferring substances between the retina and blood vessels. The deprived retinal cells swell.

In the more advanced, proliferative form, damaged blood vessels are replaced with new ones that grow along the surface of the retina. The newer blood vessels, however, are more fragile. They tend to rupture and leak blood into the vitreous, the gel-like fluid that fills the posterior portion of the eye. Inelastic scar tissue forms, which alters the shape of the retina, causes distorted vision, and pulls at the retina, increasing the potential for retinal detachment.

Assessment Findings

Clients with nonproliferative and proliferative retinopathy may not experience any visual changes for some time. When symptoms do occur, the client reports blurred vision, no vision in spotty areas, or seeing debris floating about the visual field.

Visual acuity is diminished. Ophthalmic examination reveals swelling near the macula of the eye, an area lateral to the optic nerve that provides acute central vision. Fluorescein angiography documents changes in retinal blood vessels photographically (see Chap. 42).

Medical Management

The client with diabetes is referred for an ophthalmic evaluation within 3 to 5 years after diagnosis. Some physicians may suggest yearly ophthalmic examinations. If there is evidence of retinal vessel changes, an ACE inhibitor such as lisinopril (Prinivil) is prescribed to dilate the retinal blood vessels and improve blood flow. If vitreous hemorrhage already has occurred, some physicians prefer to let the condition resolve on its own, which may take up to 18 months. A more expeditious technique is to seal leaking or newly forming blood vessels with laser photocoagulation. A vitrectomy, removal of bloodied vitreous, also improves the clarity of vision. In 2004, the FDA approved ovine hyaluronidase (Vitrase), a genetically engineered form of angiopoietin, a vascular growth factor that stimulates the repair of leaky retinal blood vessels. Vitrase has been shown to clear the bloodied vitreous after intraocular injection in approximately 1 month.

Nursing Management

The nurse encourages clients with diabetes to follow their therapeutic regimen to facilitate tight glucose control. He or she teaches clients about complications associated with diabetes and encourages regular ophthalmic examinations. When medications are prescribed, the nurse explains their purpose, techniques for self-administration, side effects, and symptoms that are important to report to the prescribing physician.

VASCULAR DISTURBANCES

Vascular disturbances affect many tissues and organs, as described in previous discussions of peripheral neuropathy, diabetic nephropathy, and retinopathy. In clients with diabetes, however, all the arteries and arterioles are more susceptible to accelerated atherosclerotic and arteriosclerotic changes than in clients without diabetes.

Pathophysiology and Etiology

A consistent finding in clients with diabetes is thickening of the arterial walls. The incidence of coronary artery disease also is increased. One possible explanation for obesity in clients with diabetes is that the brain may be insensitive to leptin, a chemical that signals satiation. A lack of response to leptin promotes overeating, which contributes to hyperlipidemia.

Assessment Findings

Peripheral vascular changes are one of the most common complications associated with diabetes (see Chap. 25). Because of a decreased blood supply, the extremities are pale and cool. Leg cramps can occur. Gangrene develops if blood supply to the extremities is markedly diminished. Uncontrolled infection leads to skin ulcers. Clients with diabetes are likely to develop chest discomfort when the coronary arteries are affected. Myocardial infarctions occur at a much earlier age than among the nondiabetic population.

Hyperlipidemia and elevated triglyceride levels correlate with the predisposition to atherosclerosis. Angiography and Doppler ultrasonic flow studies indicate peripheral vascular disease.

Medical and Surgical Management

Atherosclerosis is managed with lipid-lowering measures such as a low-fat diet, exercise, and medications. Vasodilators are prescribed to combat the effects of arteriosclerosis. Drugs that reduce platelet aggregation (e.g., aspirin) are prescribed prophylactically. Smoking cessation is advised. Impaired skin is managed with aggressive measures to promote healing (see Chap. 25). Uncontrolled gangrene of the extremities can result in amputation. The lower extremities are involved most often. Any type of surgery or hospitalization is an enormous stressor. The glucose levels of the client with diabetes increase, with a concomitant increased demand for insulin. The healthcare team closely monitors the client's blood glucose levels. Either higher doses of insulin or antidiabetic drugs are prescribed or elevated blood glucose levels are covered by administering rapid-acting or short-acting insulin before meals and at bedtime.

Nursing Management

Nursing management is geared toward the type of vascular disturbance and the signs and symptoms the client experiences.

CRITICAL THINKING EXERCISES

1. A client with diabetes mellitus has not followed the diet prescribed by the physician. What information would you include in a teaching plan for this client? What approach would you take to reinforce the importance of diet in the management of diabetes?
2. Explain the differences between the signs and symptoms of hyperglycemia and hypoglycemia.
3. A client's fasting blood sugar is 128 mg/dL and the glycosylated hemoglobin (hemoglobin A1c) is 8.8%. How would you explain the results of the laboratory tests to the client?
4. A client with diabetes says, "Nurse, I have diabetes, so why are you examining my feet?" What is an appropriate response from the nurse?

NCLEX-STYLE REVIEW QUESTIONS

1. When a client with type 1 diabetes comes to the clinic for a routine visit, which statement best indicates that the nurse is <u>assessing</u> for a complication related to the disease?
   1. "What does your blood pressure usually run"?
   2. "Have you had any heart palpitations"?
   3. "What is the color of your urine"?
   4. "Have you had your eyes checked recently"?
2. The prescribed treatment for a client with type 1 diabetes involves the self-administration of a combination of two insulins, short-acting insulin (Humulin R) and intermediate-acting insulin (Humulin N). Which action indicates that the client needs more practice?
   1. The client instills air into the short-acting and intermediate-acting insulin vials.
   2. The client withdraws the intermediate-acting insulin first and then the short-acting insulin. *(clear to cloudy)*
   3. The client rolls the vial of intermediate-acting insulin to mix it with its additive.
   4. The client inverts each vial prior to withdrawing the specified amount of insulin.
3. Which of the following are signs of hypoglycemia? Select all that apply.
   1. Flushed, warm skin
   2. Confusion
   3. Drowsiness
   4. Hunger
   5. Thirst
   6. Tremors
4. In addition to insulin, the physician has prescribed pramlintide (Symlin) 120 mcg subcutaneously before each meal. Pramlintide is supplied in 5 mL vials with a supply dosage of 600 mcg/mL. Fill in the blank with the volume the nurse should administer to the client? Round decimal points to one decimal place.
5. Which injection site is preferred for administering insulin?
   1. Upper arm
   2. Upper thigh
   3. Abdomen *absorbs more rapidly*
   4. Buttocks

$$\frac{120 \text{ mcg}}{600 \text{ mcg}} \times 1 \text{ mL} = 0.2 \text{ mL}$$

52

Introduction to the Reproductive System

Words To Know

breast self-examination
clinical breast examination
conization
digital rectal examination
dilatation and curettage
ejaculation
emission
erection
fertilization
genitalia
gynecologic examination
implantation
lactation
mammography
menarche
menopause
menstruation
oocytes
ovulation
ovum
Papanicolaou test
procreate
prostate-specific antigen
puberty
spermatocytes
spermatogenesis
spermatozoon
transillumination
tumor markers
vulva
zygote

Learning Objectives

On completion of this chapter, you will be able to:

1. Name the major external structures of the female reproductive system.
2. Name and give the function of four internal female reproductive structures.
3. Discuss the process of ovulation.
4. Explain the physiologic changes that lead to menstruation.
5. List at least five types of reproductive data that are obtained when taking a female's health history.
6. Discuss the purpose for the cytologic test known as a Papanicolaou test.
7. Review the instructions the nurse provides for a client who is scheduling a gynecologic examination and Papanicolaou test.
8. Name diagnostic tests used for diagnosing disorders of the female reproductive system.
9. Describe the anatomy and physiology of the breast.
10. Explain the differences between a clinical breast examination and breast self-examination.
11. Discuss the advantage of a mammographic examination.
12. Name three techniques for performing a breast biopsy.
13. Identify the major external structures of the male reproductive system.
14. Name and give the function of the chief internal male reproductive structures.
15. List three accessory structures of the male reproductive system.
16. Explain the terms: erection, emission, and ejaculation.
17. List at least five types of reproductive data that are obtained when taking a male's health history.
18. Name techniques for physically assessing male reproductive structures.
19. List methods that are used to diagnose prostate cancer.
20. Name two tests for determining infertility problems in males.

The reproductive systems of females and males form during embryonic development, and the external structures are evident at birth. However, the reproductive system does not become active and functional until **puberty** (the onset of sexual maturation). As the reproductive structures mature during adolescence, they facilitate the development of gender-specific physical characteristics and the ability to **procreate** (reproduce).

In both males and females, the reproductive system consists of external and internal **genitalia** (organs of reproduction). The breasts are included as part of the female's reproductive system because they are important for nourishing infants. This chapter reviews the anatomy and physiology unique to each gender and the assessment techniques used to determine normal and abnormal function. Subsequent chapters in this unit address common disorders of the reproductive system that occur among females and males, and the nurse's role in managing the care of clients who develop these disorders.

THE FEMALE REPRODUCTIVE SYSTEM

ANATOMY AND PHYSIOLOGY

External Structures

The major external structures of the female reproductive system include the *mons pubis*, vaginal orifice (opening), *labia majora, labia minora*, and *clitoris* (Fig. 52-1). These structures are also referred to as the **vulva** (collective term for external genitalia).

The *mons pubis* is a pad of fat located centrally in the lower pelvis. Once reproductive hormones are produced at puberty, the *mons pubis* develops a covering of hair. The *labia majora* and *minora* are the large and small hairless skin folds that, when separated, reveal the urethral and vaginal openings.

At the superior junction of the labia, there is a fleshy protrusion of tissue known as the *clitoris*. The clitoris is erectile tissue that enlarges and becomes extremely sensitive when stimulated by the penis or touching that accompanies sexual

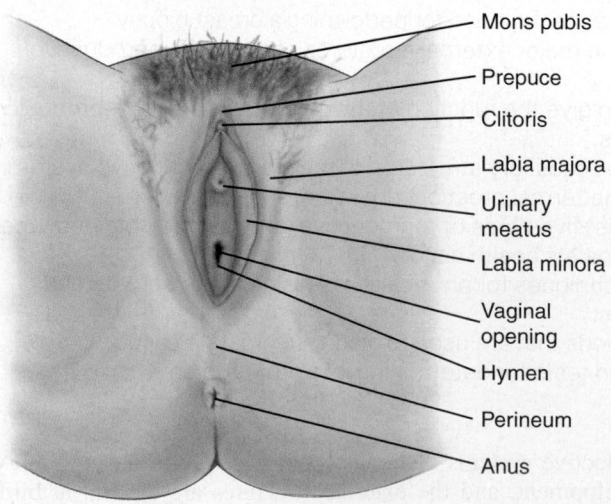

FIGURE 52-1. Female external genitalia.

- Mons pubis
- Prepuce
- Clitoris
- Labia majora
- Urinary meatus
- Labia minora
- Vaginal opening
- Hymen
- Perineum
- Anus

foreplay. On either side of the vaginal opening are mucus-secreting glands, called *Bartholin glands* or bulbourethral glands, that lubricate the vaginal opening during sexual arousal and facilitate penile penetration of the vagina during intercourse. The *fourchette* is the area beneath the vaginal opening at the base of the labia majora. Significant trauma to this tissue is often used as forensic evidence in rape trials.

The *hymen* (a mucosal membrane) is located at the vaginal opening. The hymen's absence does not necessarily confirm the loss of virginity. The hymen may rupture at the time of the first sexual intercourse, but it can be perforated by physical activity, insertion of a tampon, or pelvic examination.

Internal Structures

The internal female structures (Fig. 52-2) consist of the *vagina*, the *uterus*, two *fallopian tubes*, and two *ovaries*. The *vagina*, an expandable, tube-shaped structure, extends from the opening between the labia to the uterus. The vagina (1) provides a pathway for menstrual blood, (2) receives the penis and sperm during intercourse, and (3) serves as the structure through which an infant descends during the birth process. *Döderlein bacilli*, nonpathogenic bacteria residing in the vagina, use vaginal glycogen, a type of carbohydrate, to produce lactic acid. Routine douching of the vagina is discouraged because douching reduces the acidic medium, predisposing to the growth of infectious bacteria.

The *uterus*, the largest of the internal female reproductive structures, is approximately the size of a pear in the nonpregnant state. Various ligaments and muscles within the pelvis support and suspend the uterus, which is subdivided into the *corpus* (body), or major central portion; the *fundus*, or upper area; and a narrow neck, called the *cervix*. The cervix is lined with cells that secrete mucus, which is very thick except at the time of ovulation (discussed later). Thick mucus repels bacteria; thinner cervical mucus facilitates the movement of sperm (male sex cells) toward the **ovum** (pl., *ova*; matured female reproductive cell, or egg).

The uterine wall is composed of three layers: the *perimetrium*, the outer serous membrane; the *myometrium*, a smooth muscle layer that contracts to expel an infant during labor; and the mucosal *endometrium*, the innermost layer shed monthly during the menstrual cycle.

One or the other *fallopian tube* receives an extruded ovum every month and serves as the place where the ovum is most commonly fertilized. The sweeping motion of the *fimbriae*, which resemble fringes at the distal end of the fallopian tube, directs the released ovum into the fallopian tube.

The two ovaries (female gonads) lie behind and slightly below the ends of the fallopian tubes. Various ligaments hold the ovaries in place. In follicles of the cortex (outer layer) of each ovary, approximately one-half million **oocytes** (developing egg cells) are present in a female at birth. The ovaries also secrete two hormones: estrogen, which is responsible for secondary sexual characteristics such as breast development and the preparation of the uterus for conception, and progesterone (discussed later).

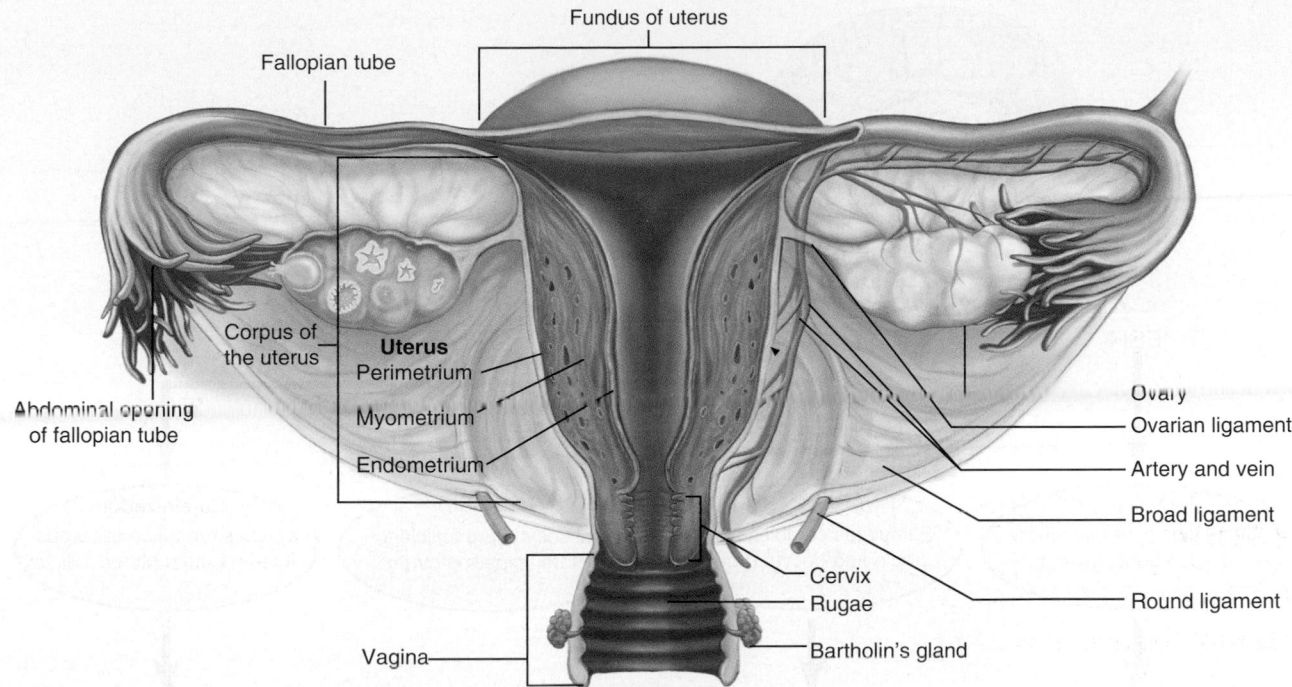

Fundus of uterus

Fallopian tube

Corpus of
the uterus

Uterus
Perimetrium

Myometrium

Endometrium

Abdominal opening
of fallopian tube

Ovary

Ovarian ligament

Artery and vein

Broad ligament

Cervix
Rugae

Round ligament

Vagina

Bartholin's gland

FIGURE 52-2. Internal female reproductive structures. The uterus, vagina, and a portion of the fallopian tube are shown in cross-section.

 Gerontologic Considerations

- The female genitalia change during the aging process.
Changes include thinning of pubic hair; decrease in the
size of the labia majora and minora, shortening and
narrowing of the vagina; and atrophy of Bartholin's glands,
which results in less lubrication. The cervix, uterus, fallopian
tubes, and vulva atrophy, causing a loss of vascularity and
elasticity, and resulting in irritation or excoriation of the
tissue.

▶ **Stop, Think, and Respond Exercise 52-1**

*What health teaching is appropriate when a client says
she self-administers a douche every week for the purpose of routine feminine hygiene?*

After puberty and until **menopause** (the termination of
female fertility; see Chapter 53), three processes occur: ovulation, pregnancy, and menstruation.

Ovulation

The roles of the internal structures are to release and transport the ovum and to support the development of a fertilized
ovum. **Ovulation** is the expulsion of an ovum from an
ovary. The cyclical release of the ovum is influenced by pituitary hormones. The anterior pituitary hormone known as
follicle-stimulating hormone (FSH) initiates ovulation
monthly. FSH triggers the maturation of a follicle in one of
the ovaries and an increased production of ovarian estrogen.
A second pituitary hormone, luteinizing hormone (LH),
causes the mature follicle to rupture, thereby releasing an
ovum from the ovary (Fig. 52-3).

After the ovum is released, movement of the fimbriae at
the end of the fallopian tube and the muscular contractions
of the tube itself draw the ovum into the tube and toward the
uterus. The cells surrounding the ruptured follicle transform
into the *corpus luteum* (yellow body), which secretes progesterone and estrogen. The endometrium, the inner lining of
the uterus, becomes thick and vascular in response to the
hormonal secretions.

Pregnancy

Pregnancy occurs as a result of fertilization and implantation.
Fertilization, the union of an ovum and a **spermatozoon** (pl.,
spermatozoa, the male reproductive cell), normally occurs in
the fallopian tube (Fig. 52-4). At the moment a sperm penetrates the ovum, the number of chromosomes is complete,
making it possible for an embryo to develop. The fertilized
ovum, or **zygote**, then proceeds down the uterus and attaches
itself in the endometrium (**implantation**). Once fertilization
and implantation occur, the pituitary production of FSH is
inhibited so that ovulation temporarily stops.

Menstruation

If the ovum is not fertilized, the production of progesterone
by the corpus luteum begins to decrease until it changes from
a yellow to a white spot on the ovary (corpus albicans).
Without the high level of progesterone, the endometrium
degenerates and sheds, a process referred to as **menstruation**, which begins about 2 weeks after ovulation (Fig. 52-5).
Menstrual flow usually lasts 4 to 5 days, with a normal loss
of 30 to 60 mL of blood. Women who have a heavy menses,
or menstrual flow, lose more blood. After menstruation, the
endometrium becomes thicker and more vascular again in
preparation for a possible pregnancy.

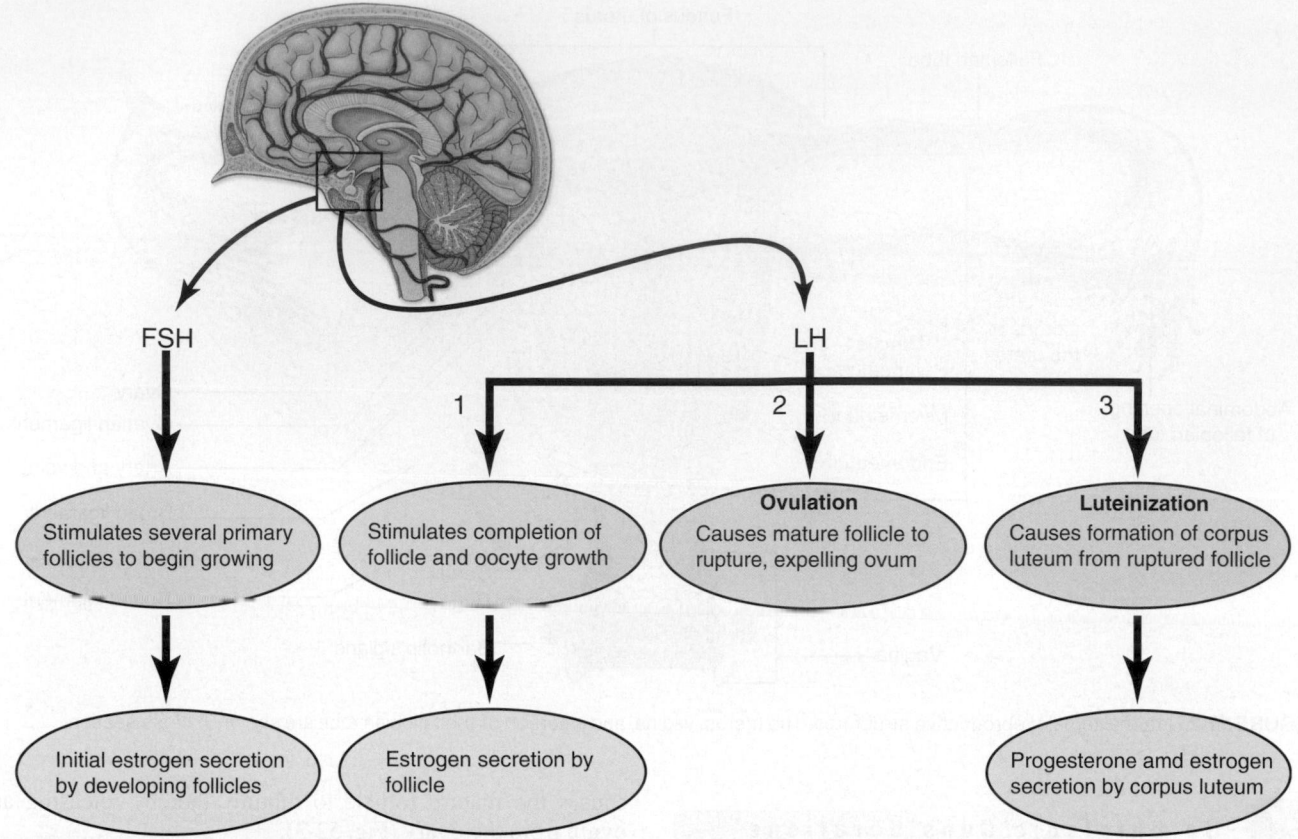

FIGURE 52-3. The effects of gonadotropins on the ovaries.

Because of these hormone-dependent changes, the microscopic characteristics of the uterus are in a cyclical state of transition. Thus, it is important that each gynecologic specimen sent to the laboratory be marked with the date of the beginning of the client's last menstrual period (LMP).

to regulate menstrual cycles, to interfere with tubal transport of sperm or a fertilized ovum, to suppress embryonic implantation, or to relieve symptoms caused by menstrual disorders.

 Pharmacologic Considerations

- Drugs containing estrogen and/or progestin are prescribed for females to suppress ovulation in an effort to prevent pregnancy,

 Gerontologic Considerations

- As women age, reproductive hormones produced by the pituitary gland and ovaries begin to decrease years before

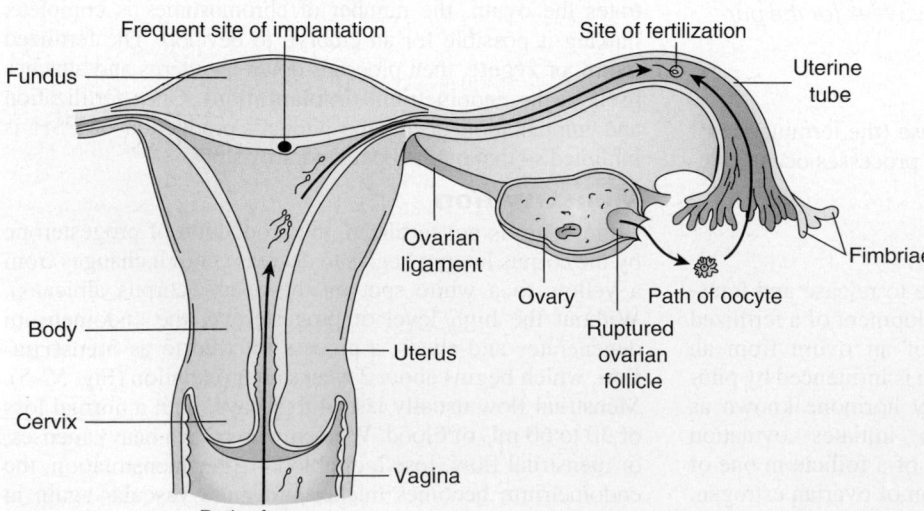

FIGURE 52-4. Schematic drawing of female reproductive organs, showing path of ovum from ovary into fallopian tube, path of spermatozoa, and the usual sites of fertilization and implantation.

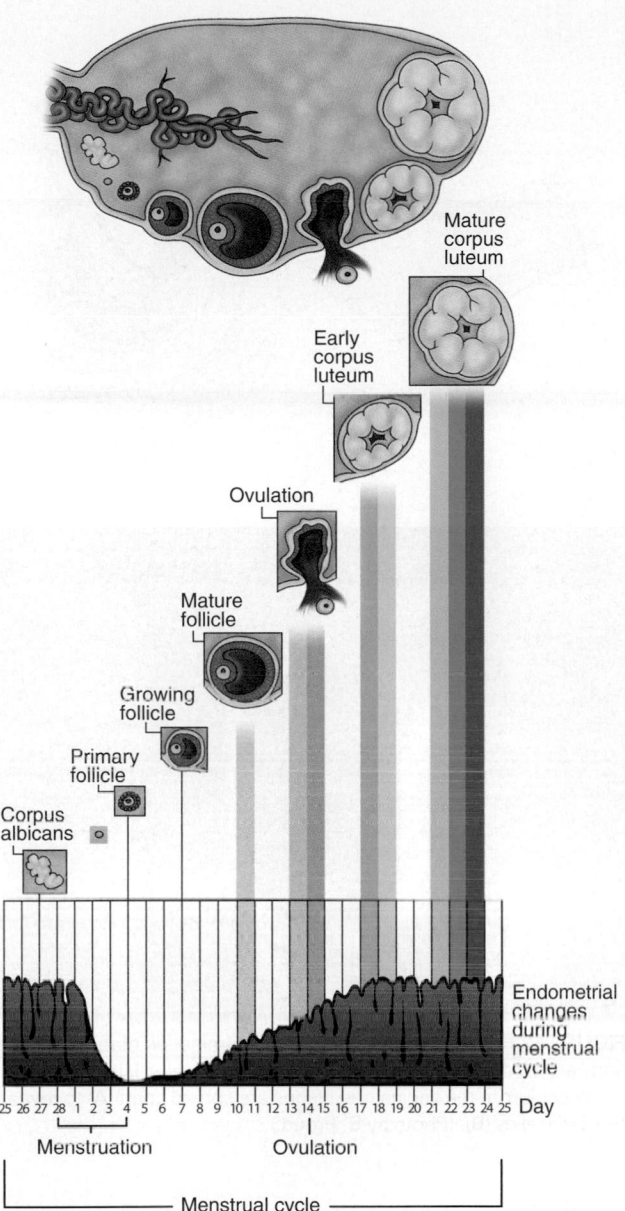

FIGURE 52-5. One menstrual cycle and the corresponding endometrial changes.

menses cease. Menopause on average occurs around age 50 in most females (see Chapter 53).

ASSESSMENT

Health History

To ensure a thorough baseline history, the nurse obtains the following information:

- General health and family history
- Age of **menarche**, the first menstruation
- Date of client's last menstrual period (LMP), description of the menstrual pattern and flow, other symptoms associated with menstruation
- Risks for sexually transmitted infections (see Chap. 56)

Nutrition Notes 52-1
Nutrition and Reproductive Health

- A severe reduction in body fat caused by extreme caloric restriction or excessive exercise can cause female reproductive abnormalities such as delayed or cessation of menstruation, small breasts, and impaired potential for implantation of a fertilized ovum. (Anderson, A., http://www.vanderbilt.edu/AnS/psychology/health_psychology/infert.htm). In males, the same factors can cause the genitals to appear or remain juvenile.
- Obese females may experience problems with subfertility or infertility. A cause of infertility in women is polycystic ovarian syndrome, a multiendocrine disordered linked to insulin resistance.

- Pregnancy history: number of pregnancies, live births, stillborn births; type of fetal abnormalities
- Abortion history
- Contraceptive practices
- Age of menopause, associated symptoms, and use of hormone replacement therapy (HRT)
- Date of last gynecologic and breast examination, including mammograms and Papanicolaou tests
- Prior treatments or surgery for a gynecologic disorder
- Drug, allergy, substance abuse, and smoking history
- Symptoms of present disorder, such as painful intercourse or characteristics of vaginal discharge, and duration

See Nutrition Notes 52-1 for nutrition factors that may influence reproductive health.

Gynecologic Examination (Pelvic Examination)

A physician, clinical nurse specialist, physician's assistant, or nurse practitioner performs the **gynecologic examination**, an inspection and palpation of pelvic reproductive structures. In preparation for the test, the nurse obtains examination gloves, lubricant, several sizes of bivalve speculums, a light source, and materials for obtaining a Papanicolaou test (discussed next). The nurse is sensitive to the fact that many women dislike having gynecologic examinations because they anticipate discomfort, are embarrassed, and have anxiety over possible diagnoses. Nursing Guidelines 52-1 provides suggestions on assisting the client undergoing a gynecologic examination.

Inspection of the external genitalia and adjacent structures occurs first, followed by the inspection of the vaginal wall and cervix, using a bivalve speculum (Fig. 52-6). Next, one or two fingers of a lubricated, gloved hand are placed into the vagina. By vaginal-abdominal palpation, the structures beyond the vaginal orifice are examined, and the position, size, and contour of the uterus, ovaries, and other pelvic structures are assessed (Fig. 52-7). At the end of the examination, a gloved finger is inserted into the rectum to palpate the posterior surface of the uterus.

NURSING GUIDELINES 52-1

Assisting the Client Undergoing a Pelvic Examination

- Have the client void before the examination.
- Ask client open-ended questions to promote verbalizing anxiety.
- Provide information on what to expect during the examination and when results from tissue samples will be available.
- Answer questions and use the opportunity to educate the client on health maintenance and health promotion activities.
- Have a blanket available.
- Assist client to assume a lithotomy position immediately before the examination.
- Put pleasing posters on the walls or ceiling to help distract the client.
- Guide the client to breathe deeply during the examination.

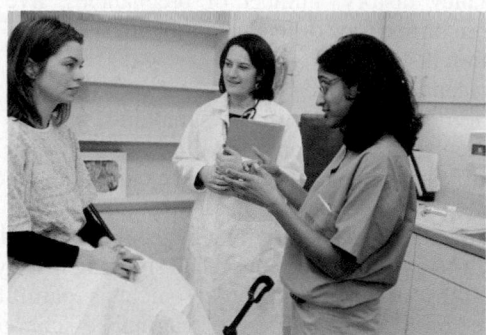

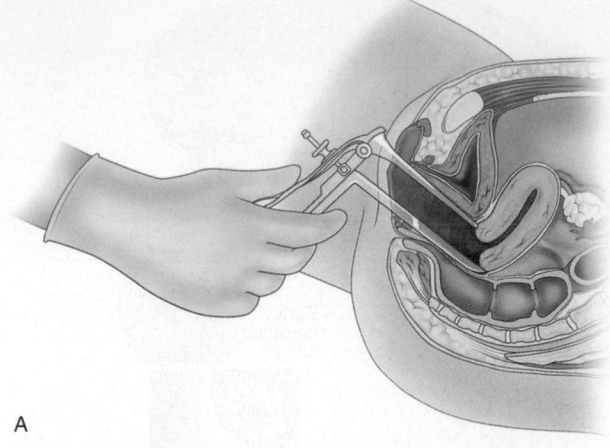

A

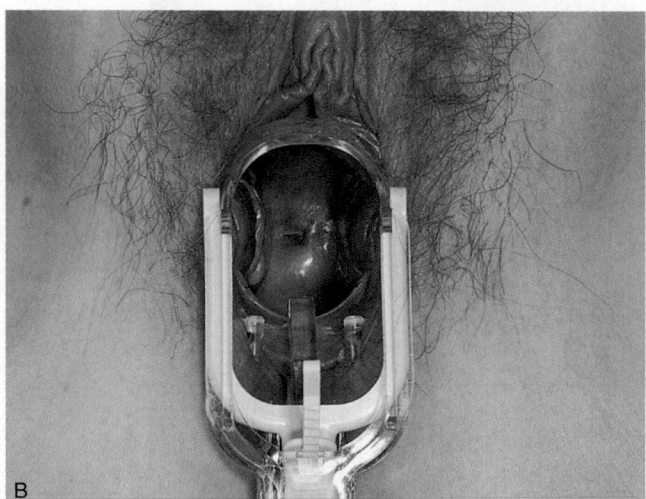

B

FIGURE 52-6. Technique for speculum examination of the vagina and cervix. After the examiner spreads the woman's labia and inserts the speculum in the vagina, the blades are spread apart (**A**) to reveal the cervical os (**B**). (Photo by B. Proud.)

Diagnostic Tests

Cytologic Test for Cervical Cancer (Papanicolaou Test)

A **Papanicolaou test** (Pap test), an important cervical cancer screening tool, involves obtaining a sample of exfoliated cells (dead cells that are shed). The specimens, which are best obtained 2 weeks after the first day of the LMP, are removed by scraping and brushing tissue during the pelvic examination (Fig. 52-8). The test is used mainly to detect early cancer of the cervix and secondarily to determine estrogen activity as it relates to menopause or endocrine abnormalities. Box 52-1 presents the classification system used to describe Pap test results.

The American Cancer Society (ACS) (2004) recommends that all women have an initial Pap test no later than 21 years of age or approximately 3 years after the onset of sexual intercourse. After an initial screening, a woman should undergo a Pap test with conventional cervical cytology smears annually with conventional cervical cytology or biennially with liquid-based cytology. At or after age 30, those women who have had three consecutive normal screening tests may be screened every 2 to 3 years unless they have high risk factors for developing cervical cancer.

Because a persistent infection with the human papilloma virus (HPV) is a major cause of cervical cancer, the ACS also recommends human papilloma virus (HPV) DNA testing. HPV testing should be done (1) for women who are 30 years of age or older every 3 years as an alternative to a cytologic examination, and (2) for women of any age who have an ambiguous Pap test (National Cancer Institute, 2008).

The nurse advises the client to schedule an appointment at a time other than during menstruation and before the appointment to (1) avoid intercourse for 2 days, (2) refrain from douching for 1 day, and (3) cease the use of vaginal medications for at least 48 hours. When assisting with the examination, the nurse obtains the required materials, prepares the client, and labels and preserves the specimens.

Cervical Biopsy

A cervical biopsy is performed when results from a Pap test are positive or questionable. Tissue is obtained by punching out multiple small samples or by performing **conization**, the process of removing a larger, cone-shaped section of cervical

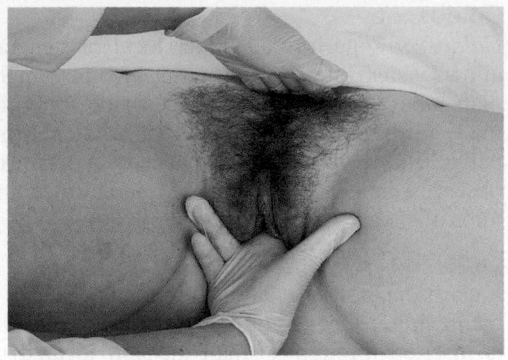
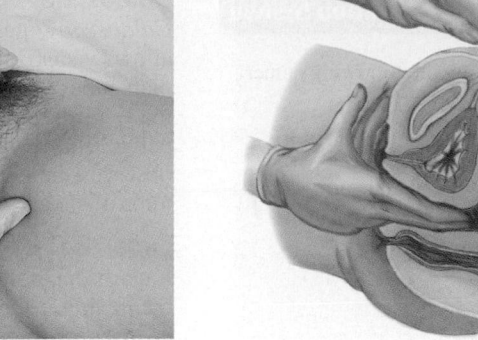

FIGURE 52-7. Bimanual examination of the pelvis.

tissue. Conization is an invasive surgical procedure performed on an outpatient basis; it also is used to treat early-stage cervical cancer.

If the client is premenopausal, the nurse schedules the biopsy for 1 week after the end of a menstrual period, when the cervix is least vascular. He or she tells the client that cramps and slight spotting may occur afterward. The nurse recommends a mild analgesic for discomfort and advises the client to report severe pain or heavy bleeding.

Endometrial Smears and Biopsy

Diagnosing cancer of the endometrium, the inner lining of the uterus, is accomplished by aspirating endometrial tissue specimens or performing an endometrial biopsy. Of the two, the endometrial biopsy is the more accurate method. A smear is obtained by inserting a flexible cannula through the cervix and into the uterine cavity. The cannula is attached to a syringe used to aspirate secretions. This procedure usually is performed without anesthesia.

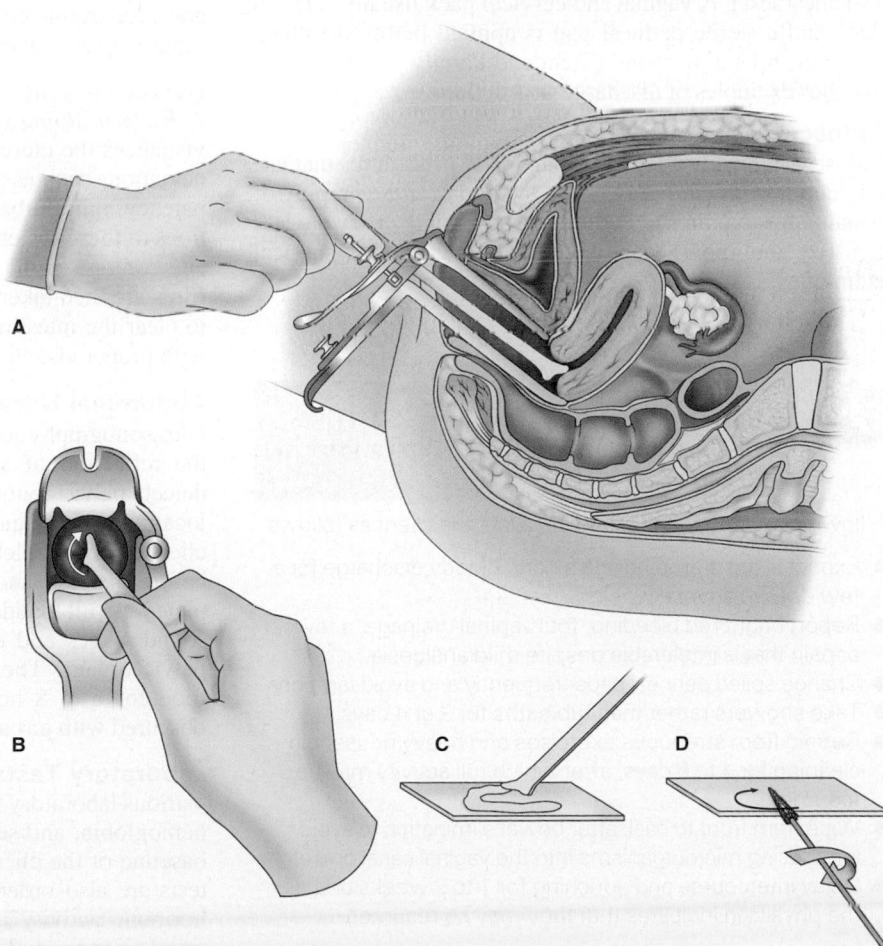

FIGURE 52-8. Specimen collection for Pap test. (**A**) With the speculum in place, the examiner uses a spatula to obtain cervical secretions. (**B**) He or she places the spatula tip in the cervical os and rotates the spatula 360°. (**C**) Examiner smears material that clings to the spatula smoothly on a glass slide and promptly places in a solution. (**D**) He or she rotates the cytobrush in the cervical os and rolls it onto a glass slide.

To obtain a biopsy specimen, a dilating instrument called a *uterine sound* is inserted through the cervical opening. A tissue sample is then obtained using a scraping instrument called a *curette* or by aspiration. This procedure can be performed without anesthesia in the physician's office.

Dilatation and Curettage

Dilatation and curettage (D and C) is a surgical procedure in which the cervix is stretched (dilatation) and the endometrium is scraped (curettage). Dilatation and curettage are performed to diagnose or treat various gynecologic problems (e.g., abnormal uterine bleeding) and to remove fetal and placental tissue. Samples of endometrial scrapings are obtained when the client is under general or light intravenous (IV) anesthesia. A vaginal and cervical pack usually is left in place and a sterile perineal pad is applied before the client leaves the operating room. Client and Family Teaching 52-1 provides examples of discharge instructions.

Endoscopic Examinations

Endoscopic examinations are diagnostic procedures that use a lighted instrument inserted into the body for the purpose of visualizing structures not otherwise accessible. They are less invasive and more economical than the use of surgical techniques.

Client and Family Teaching 52-1
Self-Care Instructions after Dilatation and Curettage

Following a D and C, the nurse instructs the client as follows:

- Expect slight cramping and a dark, bloody discharge for a few days to several weeks.
- Report bright red bleeding, foul vaginal drainage, a fever, or pain that is intolerable despite mild analgesia.
- Change soiled perineal pads frequently and avoid tampons.
- Take showers rather than tub baths for 3 or 4 days.
- Refrain from strenuous exercises and heavy household cleaning for 4 to 5 days, after which full activity may be resumed.
- Wipe from front to back after bowel elimination to avoid introducing microorganisms into the vaginal canal or urethra.
- Delay intercourse and douching for 1 to 2 weeks or until the physician indicates that they may be resumed.

Culdoscopy

Culdoscopy, performed under local or general anesthesia, allows visualization of the uterus, broad ligaments, and fallopian tubes by inserting an endoscope through an incision made in the posterior vaginal wall. Ectopic pregnancy and pelvic masses can be visualized. Afterward, the nurse observes the client for signs of internal bleeding and symptoms of shock.

Laparoscopy

Laparoscopy is an examination of the interior of the abdomen using a special endoscope called a *laparoscope*, which is inserted through a small incision located one-half inch below the umbilicus (Fig. 52-9). Two or 3 liters of carbon dioxide or nitrous oxide gas are introduced into the peritoneal cavity creating a pneumoperitoneum to separate the intestines from the pelvic organs and to facilitate visualization. Laparoscopy is used to detect an ectopic pregnancy, to perform a tubal ligation, to obtain ovarian tissue for biopsy, and to detect pelvic abnormalities.

The nurse can tell the client undergoing laparoscopy that she will experience discomfort in the shoulder as a result of the instillation of gas. Afterward, the nurse checks incisional sites for bleeding and relieves discomfort by administering a prescribed analgesic.

Colposcopy

A colposcopy is a procedure used to visualize the cervix and vagina. A speculum is inserted into the vagina, and the surface areas are examined with a light and magnifying lens (colposcope). A cervical biopsy and Pap test can be taken at this time.

Hysterosalpingogram

A *hysterosalpingogram* is a radiographic examination that visualizes the uterus and fallopian tubes. It is used to detect deviations such as adhesions and to determine fallopian tube patency, other tubal abnormalities, or congenital malformations of these structures. A cannula is inserted into the cervix and contrast media is injected. Fluoroscopic or radiographic films are then taken. Bowel preparation usually is necessary to clear the intestine of gas and fecal material that interfere with proper visualization of the uterus and fallopian tubes.

Abdominal Ultrasonography (Sonogram)

Ultrasonography aids in visualizing soft tissue by recording the reflection of sound waves. An abdominal ultrasound detects pelvic abnormalities such as tumors and the size and location of fetal and placental tissue. The nurse instructs the client to drink at least 1 quart of water 45 minutes to 1 hour before the test, and not to void until after the test is completed. A full bladder facilitates the transmission of the ultrasound waves and elevates the bowel away from the other pelvic organs. The client should restrict herself from solid food for 6 to 8 hours to avoid having images of her test obscured with gas and intestinal contents.

Laboratory Tests

Various laboratory tests, such as a complete blood cell count, hemoglobin, and serum electrolytes, are ordered to obtain a baseline of the client's health status. Culture and sensitivity tests are also ordered if an infection is suspected. Ovarian hormone activity is evaluated by total urine estrogen and urine pregnanediol tests.

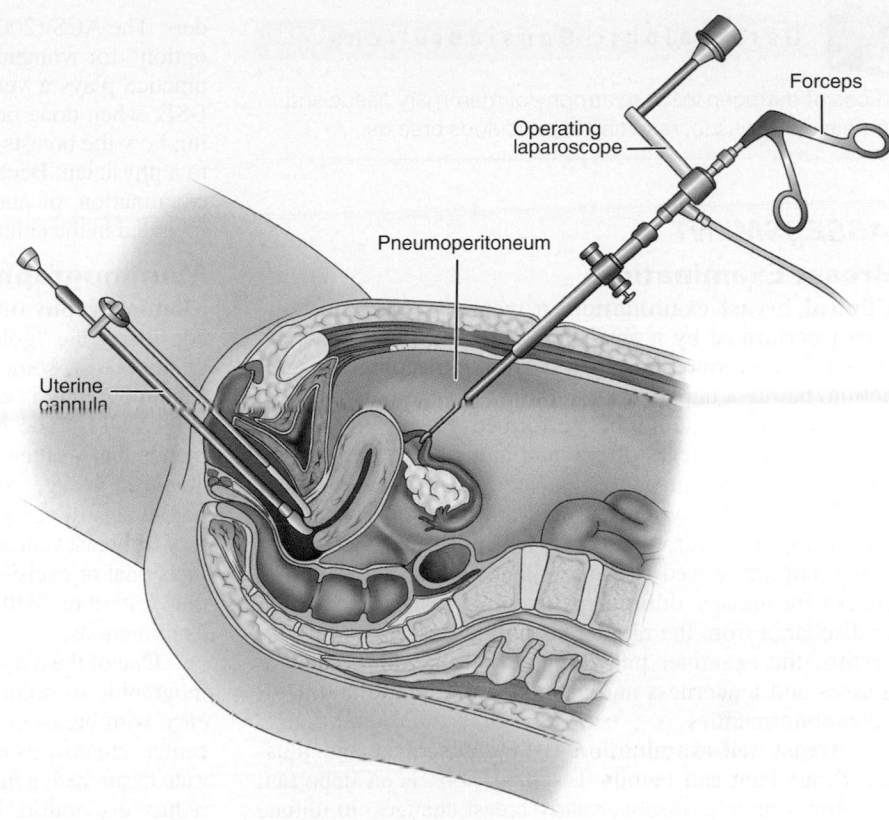

Forceps

Operating laparoscope

Pneumoperitoneum

Uterine cannula

FIGURE 52-9. Laparoscopy is used to visualize the interior of the abdomen.

THE BREASTS

ANATOMY AND PHYSIOLOGY

The breasts are modified sweat glands known as mammary glands that contain 15 to 20 lobes surrounded by fatty tissue. Each breast has a central nipple that is bordered by darker pigmented skin called the *areola*. Smooth muscle in the nipples contracts, causing the nipples to become erect when cold, touched, or sexually stimulated. The nipples are connected to an internal system of ducts where several lobules (subdivisions of a lobe) converge (Fig. 52-10). Although males and females have breasts, a primary function of the female breast is to produce milk, a process called **lactation**.

Estrogen secreted by the ovaries at the onset of puberty causes the growth and development of the female mammary system. The amount of fatty tissue determines the size of the breast. Further growth and development that occurs during pregnancy is hormone dependent. Prolactin promotes the production of milk from elements in the blood. Progesterone, secreted by the placenta, stimulates the development of alveoli, which secrete the milk. Estrogen, also secreted by the placenta, stimulates increased production of tubules and ducts to transport milk to the lactiferous duct, which drains at the nipple.

The breasts have an abundant supply of blood vessels and lymphatics. The axillary lymph nodes and the internal mammary lymph nodes drain venous blood from the breasts. It is through these blood vessels and lymphatics that cancer in the ducts of the breast spreads to distant areas of the body.

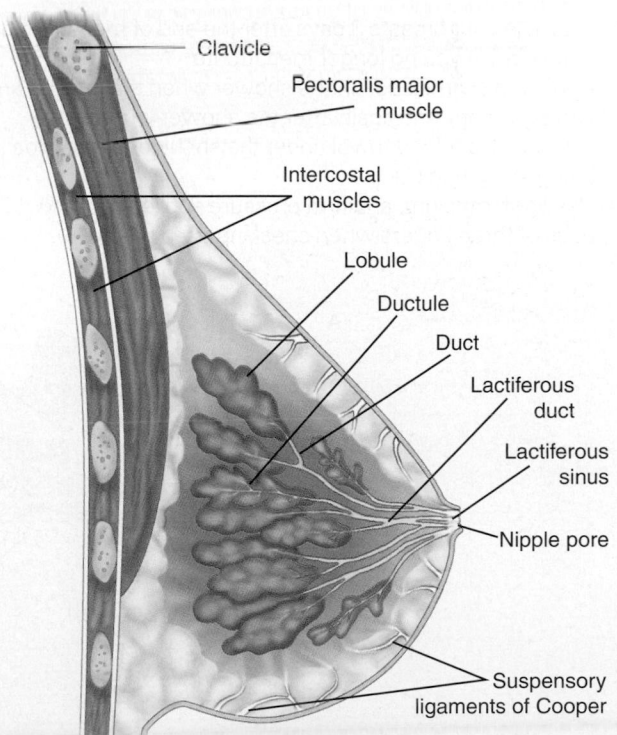

Clavicle

Pectoralis major muscle

Intercostal muscles

Lobule

Ductule

Duct

Lactiferous duct

Lactiferous sinus

Nipple pore

Suspensory ligaments of Cooper

FIGURE 52-10. Anatomy of the female breast (lateral view).

Gerontologic Considerations

- Loss of estrogen leads to atrophy of mammary tissue and increased fat tissue, resulting in pendulous breasts.

ASSESSMENT

Breast Examination

Clinical breast examination, a manual palpation of the breast performed by a physician, nurse, or physician's assistant, is performed during a client's gynecologic examination, before a mammogram, or during an annual physical examination. It should be performed every 3 years for women 20 to 39 years of age and annually for women 40 and older (American Cancer Society, 2003). The examiner notes breast size, symmetry, and any unusual changes in the skin of the breasts and nipples. With the client lying down and arm raised over the client's head, the examiner checks for masses, dimpling, flattening, rashes, ulceration, or discharge from the nipple. Using the flat part of the fingertips, the examiner palpates the breasts and axillae for masses and tenderness and examines the lymph nodes for other abnormalities.

Breast self-examination (BSE), described and illustrated in Client and Family Teaching 52-2, is an important way for women to discover early breast changes, to initiate early treatment, and to improve outcomes of breast disor-

ders. The ACS (2003) now states that a monthly BSE is "an option" for women who are 20 years and older because the practice plays a very small role in detecting breast cancer. BSE, when done occasionally, is still appropriate for learning how the breasts feel and look and reporting any changes to a physician. Because breast cancer can also occur in men, examination of the male breasts and axillae should be included in the annual physical examination.

Mammography

Mammography (mammogram) is a radiographic technique considered the "gold standard" for detecting cysts or tumors of the breast, some of which may be too small to palpate. Mammography is used as a screening test for breast cancer (Fig. 52-11). The National Cancer Institute (2002) recommends that women begin receiving annual mammograms at 40 years of age (Box 52-2). The need for mammograms before age 40 years depends on factors such as a family history of breast cancer, a past history of benign breast disease, incisional or excisional breast biopsies, and other conditions that interfere with accurate BSEs and clinical breast examinations.

One of the reasons why women avoid or postpone mammographic examination is the discomfort that they experience with breast compression. Some mammography testing centers are now using a radiolucent (allowing x-rays to penetrate tissue with a minimum of absorption) cushioning pad to reduce discomfort. Use of the pad does not compromise the quality of the mammographic image.

Client and Family Teaching 52-2
Breast Self-Examination

The nurse instructs the client as follows:

- Examine your breasts 3 days after the end of menstruation or anytime if you no longer menstruate.
- Begin the examination in the shower when the breasts are wet and soapy and again after the shower when lying down with a folded towel under the shoulder on the side being examined (A).
- Use light, medium, and firm pressure applied with the pads of three fingers when checking each breast (B).

- Move your fingers in circles, spokes of a wheel, or rows, but follow the same technique with each BSE.
- Feel every part of each breast, including the nipple area and the armpit to the collar bone.
- Raise your arms over your head and look at the breasts in a mirror.
- Look for changes in breast shape, size, and contour; puckering (dimpling) of the skin; or areas that appear red.
- Squeeze each nipple and look for liquid drainage.

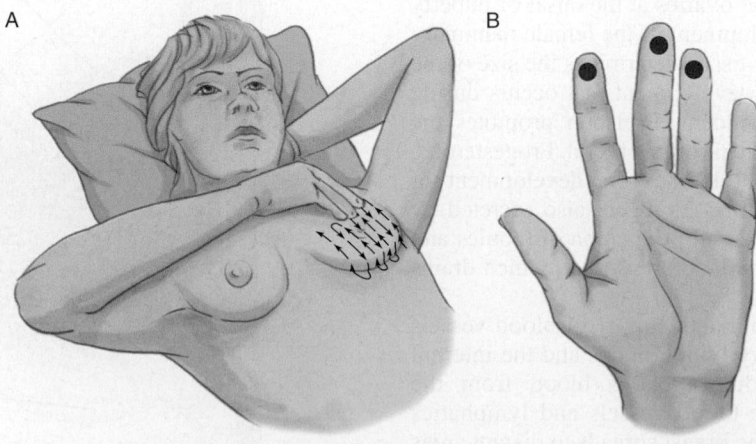

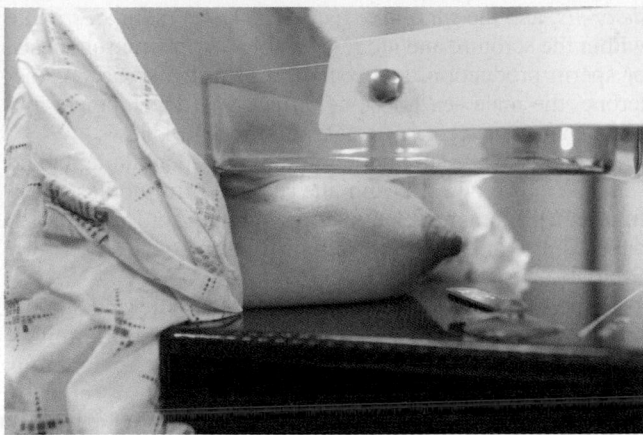

FIGURE 52-11. A client undergoing mammography.

When a mammogram is scheduled, the nurse explains the radiographic procedure and instructs the client to omit using a deodorant with aluminum hydroxide or body talc on the day of the test to avoid artifacts on the x-ray film. If the client forgets or fails to receive this information, the nurse provides a premoistened wipe to cleanse the axillae just before the test. The nurse determines how often the client performs BSEs and has her demonstrate or describe the technique. For women unfamiliar with BSE, the nurse instructs and demonstrates how to perform BSE. He or she ensures privacy throughout the examination, advises clients to have their mammograms at the same health agency, or arranges for records to be transferred so that previous mammogram results can be compared.

Ultrasonography

Ultrasonography (ultrasound) often is used with a mammogram to differentiate fluid-filled cysts from other types of breast lesions. The process involves the use of high-frequency sound waves to produce a visual picture. Ultrasonography has been useful for women with very dense breasts, especially younger women and those on HRT.

▶ **Stop, Think, and Respond Exercise 52-2**

A 52-year-old woman tells you she has never had a mammogram and has heard they are painful. How would you respond to her?

BOX 52-2 Guidelines for Mammography

The National Cancer Institute recommends that all women have a mammogram:

- Initially at age 40
- Every 1 to 2 years thereafter
- Women at higher than average risk of breast cancer should seek expert medical advice about screening before age 40 and the frequency of screening.

Source: National Cancer Institute. (2002). NCI Statement on Mammography Screening. (Online.) Available: http://www.cancer.gov/newscenter/mammstatement31jan02.

Breast Biopsy

A breast biopsy is performed to determine if a breast lesion is malignant. A specimen of tissue from the breast may be obtained through incisional biopsy, excisional biopsy, or aspiration biopsy.

Incisional Biopsy

Incisional biopsy is performed in the operating room, where one or more sections of tissue are removed. The specimen is frozen quickly and then examined microscopically by a pathologist while the client remains anesthetized. If the tissue is negative (i.e., benign), the remainder of the benign tissue is removed (if it has not been completely removed for biopsy), the incision is closed, and the client is sent to the recovery room. If the removed specimen is malignant, the surgeon may then perform the surgical procedure that offers the best chance of cure. The decision to operate immediately when there is a malignancy is thoroughly discussed with the client before surgery.

Excisional Biopsy

Some surgeons prefer an excisional biopsy, which is removal of the entire lesion. A pathologist examines the excised specimen later and more comprehensively. Clients may be discharged from the hospital before the results of the biopsy are obtained, or they may remain hospitalized. If the lesion is malignant, the biopsy results and the proposed treatment are discussed with the client.

Aspirational Biopsy

Aspirational biopsy, a procedure usually performed on an outpatient basis, uses a needle and syringe to obtain a sample of the suspect tissue. A local anesthetic is first injected around the area, and a sample of tissue is removed. A pathologist examines the tissue sample. Sometimes this procedure is done in the hospital under mammographic guidance to ensure an accurate sample of suspect tissue.

Nursing Management

The nurse allows the client time to ask questions and listens to concerns before the breast biopsy is performed. The client may have concerns about not only the procedure but also the results of the biopsy and possible diagnosis of cancer.

An aspiration biopsy usually causes minimal discomfort after the procedure, but there may be redness and soreness in the area. The nurse instructs the client to notify the physician if either drainage or bleeding from the biopsy site is more than slight or if increased redness, pain, or fever occurs. Incisional and excisional biopsies require sutures, but pain usually is minimal and relieved with a mild analgesic.

The nurse provides instructions regarding caring for the wound, using a mild analgesic, wearing a supportive brassiere, and timing of a follow-up appointment. He or she reviews the signs and symptoms that suggest wound infection.

THE MALE REPRODUCTIVE SYSTEM

ANATOMY AND PHYSIOLOGY

The anatomical structures and physiologic functions of the male reproductive system include the development of gender specific sexual characteristics and the manufacture and transportation of sperm and seminal fluid. The lower urinary tract and reproductive system structures are shared and closely associated with each other.

External Structures

The external male genitalia consist of the penis and scrotum. The *penis*, a cylindrical structure, contains the urethra through which both urine and sperm are eliminated. The penis contains nerves very sensitive to sexual stimulation. The tip of the penis is the *glans*. In an uncircumcised male, the *prepuce*, sometimes referred to as the foreskin, covers the glans. Three columns of erectile tissue run throughout the internal body, or shaft, of the penis. The pair on the dorsum is the *corpora cavernosa* (sing., corpus cavernosum), and the *corpus spongiosum* is on the ventral surface of the penis (Fig. 52-12).

The *scrotum* is the divided sac of skin that contains the right and left *testes* (male gonads), also called testicles. Since the testes cannot produce viable sperm when temperatures are at or above body temperature, their location within the scrotal sac ensures optimum conditions for sperm production. To maintain the temperature of the testes 3 degrees cooler than body temperature, smooth and skeletal muscles in the scrotum pull the tissue toward the body when external temperatures are cold. On the other hand, the smooth muscles relax, causing the scrotum to become loose and hang away from the body when environmental temperatures are hot (Marieb & Hoehn, 2007).

Gerontologic Considerations

- Loss of muscular tone with age causes the scrotum to become more pendulous. As the scrotum drops, there is an increased risk of trauma and injury to this area.

Internal Structures

The chief internal structures of the male reproductive system include the *testes, seminiferous tubules, epididymis, ductus deferens*, and the *spermatic cord*. The testes (sing., *testis*) lie within the scrotum and are responsible for **spermatogenesis**, or sperm production, and secretion of testosterone. Testosterone, the male sex hormone, affects the development and maintenance of secondary male sex characteristics.

The testes are subdivided into lobules containing coiled seminiferous tubules. Within the seminiferous tubules, **spermatocytes** (immature spermatozoa) form. Adult males produce approximately 400 million spermatocytes per day (Marieb & Hoehn, 2007).

Spermatogenesis is a result of both testosterone and the secretion of FSH, which is released by the anterior pituitary gland. Leydig cells in the spaces between the seminiferous tubules secrete testosterone. The secretion of testosterone is controlled by LH released by the anterior pituitary gland.

The epididymis collects the spermatocytes from the seminiferous tubules. The spermatocytes are nourished in the epididymis until they become motile. Mature spermatozoa (i.e., sperm) contain a head with a nucleus and 23 chromosomes, a midpiece that stores adenosine triphosphate (ATP) to supply energy during propulsion, and a tail that enables them to move toward the ovum.

The *vas deferens*, also called the *ductus deferens*, is connected to the epididymis. The vas deferens is joined with a network of blood vessels and nerves collectively referred to as the *spermatic cord*. The spermatic cord loops through the inguinal canal and into the pelvic cavity before it descends to the prostate gland. The wall of the vas deferens contains smooth muscle that moves sperm along the ductal pathway.

Accessory Structures

There are various accessory structures that support the transport and survival of sperm. They include the *seminal vesicles*, which join with the vas deferens to become the ejaculatory duct; the *prostate gland;* and the *bulbourethral glands*.

The *seminal vesicles* are a pair of glands that produce fluid with various substances that function to (1) nourish sperm, (2) enhance sperm motility by enzymatically

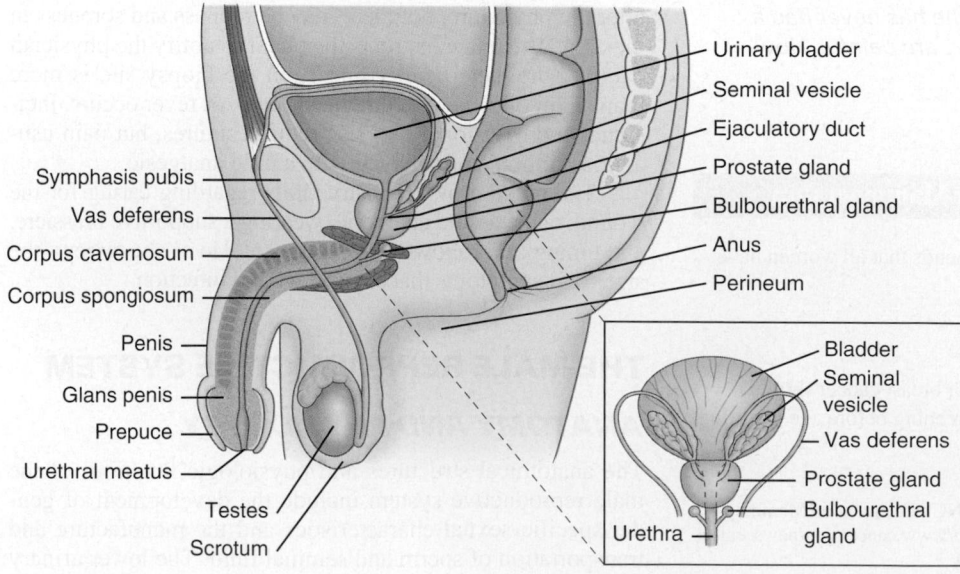

Symphasis pubis

Vas deferens

Corpus cavernosum

Corpus spongiosum

Penis

Glans penis

Prepuce

Urethral meatus

Testes

Scrotum

Urinary bladder

Seminal vesicle

Ejaculatory duct

Prostate gland

Bulbourethral gland

Anus

Perineum

Bladder

Seminal vesicle

Vas deferens

Prostate gland

Bulbourethral gland

Urethra

FIGURE 52-12. Anatomy of male reproductive system.

liquefying ejaculated semen (3) stimulate contraction of the uterus to help the sperm reach the ovum, and (4) resist sperm destruction by female antibodies (Marieb & Hoehn, 2007). Because seminal fluid fluoresces under ultraviolet light, criminologists are able to support charges of sexual assault when examining clothing or other fibers on which seminal fluid is present (Marieb & Hoehn, 2007).

The ejaculatory duct extends into the *prostate gland*, which encircles and empties into the urethra. The prostate gland contains secretory cells that produce alkaline fluid. The prostatic fluid mixes with sperm and fluid from the seminal vesicles during ejaculation. The alkalinity of the prostatic fluid neutralizes the acidic metabolic wastes released by sperm and counteracts the acid pH within the vagina to ensure mass survival of sperm.

Lastly, *bulbourethral glands*, also known as *Cowper's glands*, lie within the external urethral sphincter. Their function is similar to the Bartholin glands of the female; they secrete a mucous fluid that serves to facilitate penetration of the vagina by lubricating the head of the penis.

Gerontologic Considerations

- Older males experience individual differences in the decrease in testosterone and sperm (termed *andropause*). Although production of viable sperm decreases, the older man may continue to be able to reproduce.

- The prostate gland enlarges with age as fibrotic tissue replaces the glandular tissue. Prostate enlargement can compromise urination because it compresses the urethra.

Erection, Emission, and Ejaculation

Erection refers to a state in which the penis becomes elongated and rigid, facilitating its insertion into the female vagina. Erection takes place as a result of parasympathetic nerve activity. The parasympathetic nerves that innervate the penis cause the release of nitric oxide, a chemical with vasodilating properties. Dilation of the penile arteries compresses the veins within the penis, causing engorgement of blood within the tissue.

The movement of sperm and their mixture with fluid from the seminal vesicles and prostate gland into the urethra is called **emission**, a process mediated via the sympathetic nervous system.

Ejaculation is the discharge of semen, or fluid that contains sperm, from the penis. The process of ejaculation results from rhythmic contraction of the muscles of the vas deferens and the penis during orgasm and sexual climax. The normal volume of ejaculate is 2 to 6 mL, which contains an average of 60 to 100 million spermatozoa per mL. A count of fewer than 20 million spermatozoa per milliliter results in infertility (Smeltzer et al., 2008).

Following ejaculation, the sympathetic nervous system causes the arteries to constrict, allowing the accumulated blood to drain into the venous system. The penis then resumes its pre-erection state. Because the male sexual response is regulated via nervous system intervention, an absolute refractory period follows. This means that there is an interim period of time, ranging from a few minutes to several hours, which must elapse before a male can achieve a subsequent erection and ejaculation.

ASSESSMENT

History

The nurse obtains a general health and family history (see Chap. 4) and a detailed sexual history. A sexual history includes questions that elicit information about:

- Risks for sexually transmitted infections (STIs)
- Contraceptive practices
- Ability to achieve or sustain an erection
- Pain during sexual intercourse
- Premature ejaculation or other concerns of a sexual nature
- Inability of a sex partner to conceive
- Prior treatment (including drug therapy, diagnostic tests, or surgery) relative to the genitourinary system.

Pharmacologic Considerations

- Some types of medications, such as certain antihypertensives, can reduce a male's ability to achieve or sustain an erection.

Physical Examination

The nurse inspects the external genitalia, looking for abnormalities such as skin lesions and urethral discharge. He or she palpates the testes for tumors and examines the scrotum. **Transillumination**, shining a light through the scrotum, provides clues about the density of scrotal tissue. A **digital rectal examination** (DRE) is performed to assess the prostate for size as well as evidence of tumor (Fig. 52-13). Yearly DREs are recommended for men older than 40 to 50 years of age.

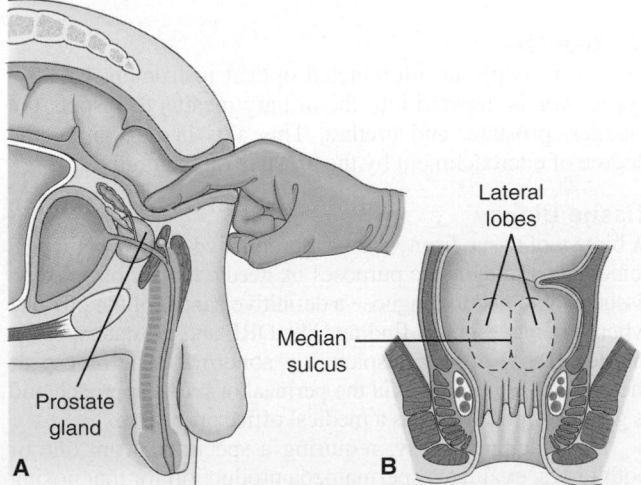

FIGURE 52-13. (**A**) Palpation of the prostate gland during digital rectal examination (DRE). (**B**) The prostate is round, with a palpable median sulcus or groove that separates the two lobes.

TABLE 52-1 Nursing Management of the Client Undergoing Genitourinary Diagnostic Testing

TEST	PREPROCEDURE CARE	POSTPROCEDURE CARE
All tests	Explain procedure, answer questions in a calm and reassuring manner. Use techniques of therapeutic communication to provide an opportunity for client to express concerns. Talk with client and inform him of each step as test proceeds.	Assist client to resume a comfortable position and clean up gels or lubricants. Answer questions about when test results will be available and when normal activity can resume. Provide written post-test instructions, if applicable.
Transrectal ultrasonography (ultrasound of prostate)	Assure client that test is not painful; administer or have client self-administer an enema; encourage client to focus on breathing slowly to reduce anxiety.	Assist client in removing excess lubricant. Explain that client may resume normal activities.
Cystoscopy	Inform client that he will experience bladder fullness and a strong desire to void. Inform client that an anesthetic lubricant will be instilled into the urethra to minimize discomfort and facilitate passage of cystoscope.	Instruct client to monitor voiding pattern and to report any bleeding or difficulty urinating. Inform client that prophylactic antibiotics will be given and stress that medication be taken as ordered.
Prostatic biopsy	Inform client that a local anesthetic may be used to minimize discomfort; administer or have client self-administer an enema if a rectal approach is used.	Provide information about site care. Instruct client that sitz baths and a mild analgesic will reduce discomfort. Tell client that a prophylactic antibiotic will be given and stress that medication be taken as ordered.
Testicular biopsy	Inform client that a local anesthetic will be administered.	In the case of an incisional rather than a needle biopsy, instruct the client to refrain from tub baths until the sutures are removed.

Diagnostic Tests

Several diagnostic tests commonly are performed to evaluate the male genitourinary tract. Table 52-1 describes appropriate nursing care for clients undergoing specific tests.

Transrectal Ultrasonography

Transrectal ultrasonography (TRUS) is a test in which a lubricated probe is inserted into the rectum to obtain a view of the prostate gland from various angles. The test is indicated in cases in which the prostate gland is enlarged or the blood level of prostate-specific antigen (see later discussion) is elevated.

Cystoscopy

In a cystoscopy, an illuminated optical instrument called a *cystoscope* is inserted into the urinary meatus to inspect the bladder, prostate, and urethra. This aids in evaluating the degree of encroachment by the prostate on the urethra.

Tissue Biopsy

A biopsy of tissue from various reproductive structures may be removed for diagnostic purposes. A needle biopsy of prostatic tissue is obtained to diagnose a definitive cancer of the prostate when other assessment findings like DRE and prostate-specific antigen (PSA) appear suspiciously abnormal. The biopsy of the prostate is obtained via the perineal or rectal approach and is generally performed as a medical office procedure.

A testicular biopsy, requiring a specimen from one or both testes, evaluates spermatozoa production for diagnosing infertility problems or testicular malignancy. Although this procedure can be done in the physician's office, it may also be performed in a hospital's ambulatory surgery department.

Cultures

Cultures are obtained from urethral secretions, skin lesions, or urine. Prostatic fluid can be expressed during a DRE and also sent for culture.

Fertility Tests

Fertility studies include a semen analysis to determine sperm count, sperm motility, and abnormal sperm. Other laboratory tests may include measuring the level of plasma LH, which is necessary for the release of testosterone from the testes. A decrease in the blood level of LH may be responsible for decreased testosterone production and infertility.

Tumor Markers

Tumor markers are substances synthesized by tumors that are released into the circulation in excessive amounts. The **prostate-specific antigen** (PSA) assay is a blood test that detects prostate cancer. Although an elevated PSA does not always indicate a malignancy, it now is possible to differentiate free PSA in total PSA. High percentages of free PSA are associated more often with benign disease, whereas, low percentages of free PSA indicate malignancy.

PSA screening can detect early-stage prostate cancer, but there is mixed and incomplete evidence that early detection improves healthy outcomes. Screening (using PSA levels) is associated with false positive results, unnecessary anxiety, biopsies, and potential complications of treatment of some cancers that may never have affected a client's health (American Cancer Society, 2008). There is insufficient evidence that the variations in PSA tests improve the accuracy of screening for prostate cancer. For males who are at least 50 years old or those younger who are at high risk, health care providers are advised to discuss the advantages and disadvantages of PSA screening and to offer the opportunity to decide for or against testing.

Other blood test findings that suggest cancer are elevated levels of alpha-fetoprotein, beta-human chorionic gonadotropin (bHCG), and total urine estrogens. Alkaline and acid phosphatase blood tests determine if prostatic cancer has spread to the bone.

▶ *Stop, Think, and Respond Exercise 52-3*

What health teaching is important to provide men to ensure early diagnosis and treatment of disorders that affect the male reproductive system?

 Pharmacologic Considerations

- Male and female athletes may self-administer anabolic steroids similar to testosterone to increase muscle mass and to facilitate physical endurance. However, such regimens have consequences for the reproductive system and general health. Males experience reduced and abnormal sperm production, atrophy of the testes, erectile dysfunction, breast enlargement, increased aggressiveness, depression, and suicidal tendencies. Females using steroids experience development of facial hair, breast reduction, cessation of menstruation, and hypertrophy of the clitoris. Both genders experience acne, risk of liver damage, and hypercholesterolemia.

CRITICAL THINKING EXERCISES

1. When a client says she has "female problems," what information is important to ask?
2. What nursing activities are appropriate when a woman has a pelvic examination during which a sample will be obtained for a Papanicolaou test?
3. A 50-year-old male is offered a PSA test, but refuses, following his physician's explanation concerning its advantages and disadvantages. Explain the rationale for the male's decision.

4. The sperm of the male partner of a couple experiencing infertility is examined. The male's volume of the semen specimen is 4 mL and contains a total of 300 million sperm. Explain the results of the test as it relates to the couple's fertility.

NCLEX-STYLE REVIEW QUESTIONS

1. What is the best answer when a client with a family history of breast cancer asks what method is best for detecting a tumor mass within the breasts?
   1. Clinical breast examination
   2. Breast self-examinations
   3. Mammography
   4. Ultrasonography
2. What instructions are essential when preparing a client for a mammogram? Select all that apply.
   1. Wear a supportive bra.
   2. Omit applying deodorant.
   3. Schedule the test within a week after menstruation.
   4. Perform a breast self-examination prior to the test
   5. Avoid body powder containing talc.
3. Discharge instructions from the nurse following a dilatation and curettage (D and C) should include notifying the physician if which of the following develops?
   1. Slight cramping
   2. Dark bloody discharge
   3. Elevated temperature
   4. Mild pain
4. During physical examination of the male reproductive system, which method would best provide the nurse information about the density of the client's scrotal tissue?
   1. Performing digital rectal examination
   2. Using transillumination
   3. Inspecting the size of the scrotum
   4. Using a scrotal radiography
5. Following a prostatic biopsy, what suggestion can the nurse provide to help relieve the client's discomfort?
   1. Take a sitz bath
   2. Void frequently
   3. Apply a scrotal support
   4. Sit on several pillows

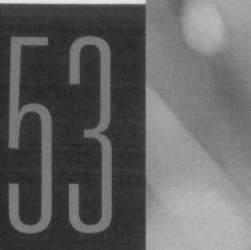

53

Caring for Clients with Disorders of the Female Reproductive System

Words To Know

amenorrhea
carcinoma in situ
cervicitis
cystocele
dysmenorrhea
dyspareunia
endometrial ablation
endometriosis
fibroid tumors
fistula
hormone replacement therapy
hysterectomy
Kegel exercises
libido
menorrhagia
menstrual diary
metrorrhagia
oligomenorrhea
oophorectomy
panhysterectomy
pelvic inflammatory disease
pessary
polycystic ovarian syndrome
premature ovarian failure
premenstrual syndrome
rectocele
salpingo-oophorectomy
sterility
toxic shock syndrome
vaginitis

Learning Objectives

On completion of this chapter, you will be able to:

1. Describe at least four conditions that deviate from normal menstrual patterns.
2. Describe the purpose of and how to keep a menstrual diary.
3. Give two examples of disorders characterized by amenorrhea and oligomenorrhea.
4. Discuss therapeutic techniques and nursing management for menstrual disorders.
5. List several physiologic consequences of menopause.
6. Give reasons for and against hormone replacement therapy.
7. Name four infectious and inflammatory conditions common in women and one cause for each.
8. Describe the signs and symptoms that differentiate three types of vaginal infections.
9. Discuss methods that may help prevent vaginal infections or their recurrence.
10. Describe the technique for inserting vaginal medications.
11. Name at least four aspects of nursing care for clients with pelvic inflammatory disease.
12. Give at least two suggestions that can help women avoid toxic shock syndrome.
13. List four structural abnormalities of the female reproductive system and their effects on fertility or sexuality.
14. Discuss methods the nurse can use to help a client select an appropriate treatment for endometriosis.
15. List three problems experienced by women who develop vaginal fistulas, and related nursing management.
16. Give examples of appropriate information when teaching a client to use a pessary.
17. Explain the term *carcinoma in situ* and how it applies to the prognosis of women with gynecologic malignancies.
18. Identify the most common reproductive cancers and methods for early diagnosis.
19. Discuss nursing diagnoses and potential complications among clients who undergo a hysterectomy and nursing interventions important to include in their care.
20. Give two reasons that explain the high lethality associated with ovarian cancer.
21. Name three possible causes of vaginal cancer.
22. Discuss the nursing management of and appropriate discharge instructions for a client who has a radical vulvectomy for vulvar cancer.

Diseases or disorders of pelvic reproductive structures can profoundly affect a woman's health and sexuality. This chapter discuss some common problems for which adult women seek healthcare, including disturbances in menstruation, infectious and inflammatory disorders, structural abnormalities, disorders affecting fertility, and benign and malignant tumors of the reproductive system. Menopause, although it is a normal physiologic process and not a disorder, is also discussed in this chapter because it often requires symptomatic management.

DISORDERS OF MENSTRUATION

PREMENSTRUAL SYNDROME

Premenstrual syndrome (PMS), and its more severe form known as *premenstrual dysphoric disorder* (PMDD), is a group of physical and emotional symptoms that occur in some women 7 to 10 days before menstruation. Its cause is unknown; however, it has been proposed that PMS results from excess estrogen, deficient progesterone, or both; hypothalamic-pituitary dysregulation; or the effect of reproductive hormones on brain chemicals such as endorphins, melatonin, and serotonin.

Women experience several symptoms, including weight gain, headache, nervousness, irritability, personality changes, depression, abdominal bloating, pain or tenderness of the breasts, breast enlargement, craving for sweets, swelling of the ankles, feet, and hands, anxiety, or increased physical activity. Diagnosis is based on data from a **menstrual diary** (Fig. 53-1) in which the client keeps daily recordings of her symptoms for at least 2 months. The classic finding is that the client is symptom-free during the period between the onset of menstruation and ovulation.

Treatment of PMS depends on the severity and type of symptoms experienced. Hormonal drug therapy aims at manipulating the cyclic fluctuation in estrogen and progesterone. This is accomplished with oral contraceptives, progesterone, synthetic androgens, or gonadotropin-releasing hormone (GnRH) analogs such as histrelin (Supprelin) and nafarelin (Synarel) for 6 months. In some instances, short-term therapy with tranquilizers or antidepressants such as fluoxetine (Prozac), which has been particularly beneficial, is indicated. Non-narcotic analgesics, such as mefenamic acid (Ponstel), ibuprofen (Motrin), and naproxen (Anaprox), are given for discomfort. Some vitamins and mineral supplements may also relieve PMS symptoms (Nutrition Note 53-1).

Diagnostic Diary A: Evaluation of PMS Symptoms

NAME _____

YEAR _____

Grading of Symptoms:
0—*No Symptoms*   2—*Moderate Symptoms*
1—*Mild Symptoms*   3—*Severe Symptoms (i.e., Disabling)*

DAY OF CYCLE	1	2	3	4	5	6	7	8	9	10	11	12	13	14	15	16	17	18	19	20	21	22	23	24	25	26	27	28	29	30	31
DATE																															
MENSES																															

PSYCHOLOGICAL SYMPTOMS

- Depression
- Anxiety
- Irritability
- Lethargy
- Insomnia
- Forgetfulness
- Confusion

PHYSICAL SYMPTOMS

- Swelling
- Breast tenderness
- Abdominal bloating
- Palpitations
- Weight gain
- Constipation
- Headache
- Rhinitis

PAIN SYMPTOMS (Usually NOT associated with PMS)

- Menstrual cramps
- Painful intercourse
- Pelvic pain
- Backache

Morning weight (lb)

FIGURE 53-1. Example of a diary kept by the client to track premenstrual symptoms. (From Chihal, H. J. [1990]. *Premenstrual syndrome: A clinic manual* [2nd ed., pp. 80–81]. Dallas, TX: Essential Medical Information Systems.)

Nutrition Notes 53-1
The Client With Premenstrual Syndrome

● Several vitamins and minerals taken on a daily basis may relieve symptoms associated with PMS, such as 100 mg vitamin B$_6$ to reduce irritability, fatigue, and depression; 400 IU of vitamin E to reduce breast tenderness; 1200 mg calcium in divided doses three times a day to relieve bloating and body aches; and 400 mg magnesium to relieve pain, water retention, and dysphoria (Gallagher, 2006).

● Some studies suggest that megadoses of vitamin B$_6$ relieve PMS symptoms, but large doses (i.e., 500 mg) can cause sensory neuropathy, which disappears after supplement use stops. Until the relationship between nutrients and PMS is more clearly defined, discourage self-medicating with megadoses of vitamins and minerals.

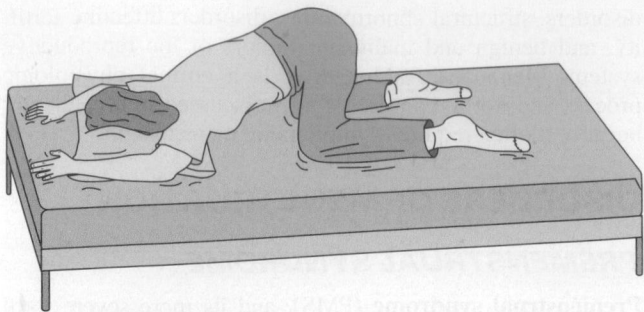

FIGURE 53-2. Knee-chest position.

To supplement medical treatment, the nurse encourages the client to make healthful lifestyle changes, such as:

• Keeping a regular schedule for meals rather than going for long periods without eating
• Eating 6 small meals per day that contain complex carbohydrates, fiber, and proteins, while reducing sugar and dietary fat
• Avoiding table salt and salty foods for several days before a menstrual period to alleviate bloating and fluid retention
• Reducing or eliminating caffeine to relieve irritability and ease breast tenderness
• Eliminating alcohol prior to menstruation to avoid depression or mood swings
• Exercising aerobically 3 to 5 times a week for 25 to 30 minutes
• Getting plenty of sleep each night
• Managing stress more effectively (American Academy of Family Physicians [2008])

The nurse explains how to maintain an accurate menstrual diary. The nurse also explains drug therapy using oral contraceptives. Because estrogen levels are pharmacologically suppressed, the client who takes a GnRH analog may experience vaginal dryness that can make intercourse uncomfortable and a loss of bone density similar to osteoporosis (refer to the Nursing Management section that accompanies the discussion of menopause for additional interventions). If the client takes nonsteroidal anti-inflammatory drugs (NSAIDs) to relieve pain, the nurse stresses the importance of taking the NSAIDs with food or after meals to avoid gastric distress.

DYSMENORRHEA

Dysmenorrhea is painful menstruation; it may be primary or secondary. Primary dysmenorrhea usually is idiopathic, and no abnormality is found. Secondary dysmenorrhea is a result of other disorders such as endometriosis, displacement of the uterus, or fibroid uterine tumors. Symptoms are lower abdominal pain and cramping, which may become more severe with fatigue, cold, and tension. Dysmenorrhea is treated with mild non-narcotic analgesics and by treating the underlying cause if one is identified.

For symptomatic relief of pain and discomfort, suggest local applications of heat, such as a warm shower, heating pad, or water bottle. Demonstrate how to assume a knee-chest position (Fig. 53-2) to relieve discomfort caused by retroversion (backward tilt) of the uterus. Encourage the client to obtain adequate rest, nutrition, and relief from stress to facilitate coping with periodic discomfort.

AMENORRHEA AND OLIGOMENORRHEA

Amenorrhea is the absence of menstrual flow. *Primary amenorrhea* is the term used when a woman of reproductive age has never menstruated. If menstruation stops after menstrual cycles have occurred, it is called *secondary amenorrhea*. Secondary amenorrhea occurs normally during pregnancy, after menopause, sometimes throughout lactation, and when the ovaries or uterus are surgically removed. **Oligomenorrhea** is infrequent menses. It is perfectly normal for adolescent females to experience oligomenorrhea for 1 year or more before they establish regular menses.

Oligomenorrhea and amenorrhea usually are caused by endocrine imbalances resulting from pituitary disorders or hypothyroidism, the stress response, or severely lean body mass. Female athletes, women with anorexia nervosa, or women with debilitating diseases can have such low levels of estrogen that menstruation ceases. Treatment focuses on correction of the underlying cause. Two reproductive system disorders that can cause oligomenorrhea and amenorrhea are premature ovarian failure and polycystic ovarian syndrome.

Premature Ovarian Failure

Premature ovarian failure (POF) is a disorder in which the ovaries cease to function in women younger than 40 years of age, some even early in their teens. It is characterized by irregular menses and symptoms that resemble natural menopause.

Although most women are born with approximately 2 million ovarian follicles with the potential to respond to stimulation by follicle-stimulating hormone (FSH), those with POF may not because their ovarian follicles are depleted or their follicles are unresponsive to FSH. In some women, the condition may result from an autoimmune attack that destroys the ovarian follicles. For most others, the follicle that is programmed to mature with stimulation of FSH lacks the support of other less mature follicles to help its development. The dominant follicle becomes luteinized, but it does not release an ovum (National Institute of Child Health and Human Development, 2007).

POF is diagnosed by determining the level of FSH in a sample of blood. A higher-than-normal level of FSH combined with the history of irregular menses or premature cessation of menstruation suggests POF.

Polycystic Ovarian Syndrome

Polycystic ovarian syndrome, a condition characterized by a cluster of signs and symptoms that include amenorrhea and oligomenorrhea, affects women between 20 and 40 years of age. Affected women generally consult a physician because of infrequent and irregular menses and a failure to become pregnant.

During a gynecologic examination, the physician palpates the ovaries that are enlarged from multiple fluid-filled cysts that form in the ovarian follicles. Vaginal ultrasonography and blood tests to measure hormone levels confirm the findings of the physical examination. The affected follicles neither secrete progesterone that suppresses menstruation nor release an ovum.

Polycystic ovarian syndrome is associated with multiple endocrine abnormalities such as overproduction and inefficient use of insulin and high testosterone levels. Women with this disorder tend to have problems including interference with menstruation and ovulation, weight gain, excessive growth of body hair, acne, thinning hair or baldness, abnormal lipid levels, and hypertension.

Treatment includes prescribing an oral contraceptive to offset the excess of testosterone and to regulate the menstrual cycle. For those women who want to conceive, the physician may prescribe an oral hypoglycemic agent such as metformin (Glucophage) and progestin-containing medications. Physicians prescribe lipid-lowering agents and antihypertensives to women who also manifest hyperlipidemia and high blood pressure.

MENORRHAGIA

Menorrhagia is excessive bleeding at the time of normal menstruation. It may be quantified as menstrual flow that lasts more than 7 days, that requires the use of an additional two pads per day, or that extends 3 or more days longer than usual. Menorrhagia can be caused by endocrine, coagulation, or systemic disorders.

Symptomatic relief is accomplished with NSAIDs, progestins, and oral contraceptives with combinations of estrogen and progestin. NSAIDs reduce prostaglandins, biologic chemicals that exist in endometrial tissue, where they exert a stimulating effect on the uterus. Progestins, natural and synthetic forms of progesterone, transform the proliferative endometrium into a secretory endometrium that simulates a pregnant state. When combination oral contraceptives are administered, they produce a "pill period," which is characterized by light menstrual bleeding.

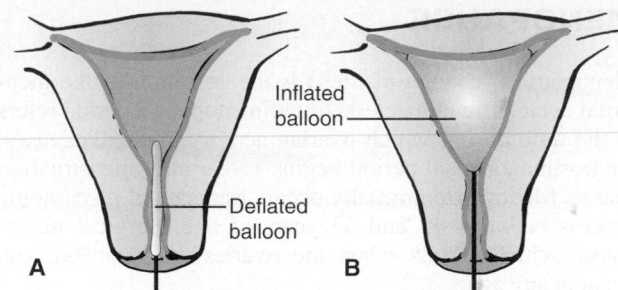

FIGURE 53-3. Uterine balloon therapy for menorrhagia. (**A**) Insertion of the catheter. (**B**) Infusion and heating of fluid within the balloon.

Dilation and curettage (D and C) is performed for symptomatic relief; however, effectiveness sometimes lasts only 1 to 2 months. **Endometrial ablation** (detachment of the lining of the uterus) by photodynamic therapy or uterine balloon therapy is a potential nonsurgical alternative. When photodynamic therapy is used, a photosensitive substance is applied to endometrial tissue, after which a laser probe is inserted through the cervix. The absorption of laser light by the tissue causes the endometrium to slough, in contrast to being removed with a surgical curette. Uterine balloon therapy produces the same effect by introducing a heated balloon into the uterus for 8 minutes (Fig. 53-3). Both of these procedures are gaining popularity because they are cost-effective. The post-treatment course is similar to that after a D and C (see Client and Family Teaching 52-1 in Chap. 52 for education guidelines).

METRORRHAGIA

Metrorrhagia is vaginal bleeding at a time other than a menstrual period. The amount of blood is not important; the fact that it occurs unexpectedly is significant. Irregular bleeding often results from an erratic stimulation of or response to pituitary or ovarian hormones, especially in adolescent girls and perimenopausal women. Some women "spot" for a day or two midway between menstrual periods. This functional bleeding is attributed to ovulation and is not considered abnormal. However, other causes for atypical bleeding include uterine malignancies, cervical irritation, or breakthrough bleeding that occurs with hormone replacement therapy or low-dose oral contraceptives. Intermenstrual or postcoital (after intercourse) bleeding needs to be evaluated promptly. Treatment depends on the underlying cause.

The nurse advises the client with unexplained bleeding to see a physician. For metrorrhagia or any menstrual disorder, the role of the nurse is the same: gather appropriate information; assist with gynecologic examinations; offer suggestions for relieving discomfort; instruct clients about their drug therapy; prepare clients for surgical interventions; care for them during recovery; and provide specific health-teaching instructions.

▶ *Stop, Think, and Respond Exercise 53-1*

What are the similarities and differences among primary and secondary amenorrhea, premature ovarian failure, and polycystic ovarian syndrome?

MENOPAUSE

Menopause ("change of life") is the cessation of the menstrual cycle. The climacteric or perimenopausal period refers to the time during which ovarian activity gradually ceases; the postmenopausal period begins 1 year after menstruation ceases. Menopause normally occurs as a natural physiologic process between 45 and 55 years of age. Surgical menopause, which results when the ovaries are removed, can occur at any age.

The changes in hormone levels that accompany menopause cause a variety of reproductive and systemic effects. Some women have symptoms so mild and transitory that they go unnoticed; other women experience severe symptoms. Some women seek healthcare to reduce the risk of osteoporosis and cardiovascular disease that occur when estrogen production decreases.

Physiology

Menopause occurs when ovarian function diminishes. Levels of estrogen and progesterone are reduced, ovulation gradually ceases, menstruation becomes irregular until it stops, and natural reproductive capacity ends. As the levels of estrogen and progesterone drop, the hypothalamus attempts to raise them by releasing GnRH, which stimulates the anterior pituitary gland to release FSH and luteinizing hormone (LH). The surge of hypothalamic-pituitary stimulation is thought to be responsible for alterations in temperature regulation, sleep disturbances, and disequilibrium in mood. Estrogen deficiency causes thinning of the vaginal walls, breast and uterine atrophy, and loss of bone density. The risks of heart disease and stroke increase with estrogen reduction. Depression, should it occur, is thought to be related more to an individual's perception of the social or psychological implications of menopause rather than to biologic factors.

Assessment Findings

Changing menstrual patterns, including irregular periods and scanty or sometimes unusually copious menstrual flow, signal the onset of menopause. During the perimenopausal period (the transitional period surrounding menopause), women may experience vasomotor disturbances such as hot flashes and sweats, sleep disturbance, irritability or depression, vaginal dryness, diminished **libido** (interest or desire for sex), or **dyspareunia** (discomfort during intercourse). These common symptoms often are the ones for which women seek treatment. A cytologic examination of vaginal and cervical smears (Pap test) shows a decrease in estrogen production.

Medical Management

The decision to administer **hormone replacement therapy** (HRT), or estrogen combined with progestin, is made for each client on an individual basis (Table 53-1). Findings from the Women's Health Initiative, a 15-year research study conducted by the National Heart, Lung, and Blood Institute, indicated that HRT with a combination of estrogen and progestin increased the risk of breast cancer, heart disease, blood clots, and stroke (http://www.nhlbi.nih.gov/whi/).

If HRT is indicated, it is prescribed in the lowest appropriate dose for a relatively short time. It is believed that estrogen in small doses can help prevent osteoporosis and relieve menopausal symptoms such as hot flashes, night sweats, and vaginal dryness. The risks of endometrial or breast cancer and the seriousness of future myocardial infarction and stroke may outweigh the potential benefit of preventing hip fractures and kyphosis that are secondary to osteoporosis.

It may be necessary to treat some of the symptoms associated with menopause. Vaginal itching and drying is prevented or reduced by drugs such as an estrogen or cortisone cream or ointment. Low-dose androgens are added to the hormone replacement regimen to restore an interest in sexual activity. Antidepressants or minor tranquilizers are prescribed for women experiencing emotional problems. Drugs such as bisphosphonates or selective estrogen receptor modulators (SERMs) (see Chap. 61), are available to reduce the potential of osteoporosis rather than prescribing HRT. Although there is little scientific evidence to support this, diets rich in phytoestrogens, such as isoflavones in soy products and lignans in flaxseed, may reduce menopausal symptoms, especially hot flashes. (Interestingly, women from Japan and China, where soy intake is high, report a low incidence of menopausal symptoms.)

TABLE 53-1 Risk and Benefits of Menopausal Hormone Replacement Therapy (HRT)

THERAPY	RISKS	BENEFITS
Estrogen alone*	Increased risk of fatal and nonfatal strokes Increased risk of endometrial cancer in women with a uterus	See below
Estrogen with or without progestin*	Increased risk of strokes and blood clots Increased risk of dementia in women 65 years or older Increased risk for gallbladder disease	Decreased potential for osteoporosis Relief from hot flashes, night sweats, and vaginal dryness
Estrogen with progestin*	Increased risk for breast cancer and heart attacks (but not with estrogen alone)	Decreased risk for colorectal cancer

*Estrogen and progestin are prescribed for women with a uterus; estrogen alone is prescribed for women with no uterus.

Source: National Institutes of Health. (2008). Women's Health Initiative (WHI) follow-up study confirms the health risks of long-term combination therapy outweigh benefits for postmenopausal women. Retrieved September 2008 from http://public.nhlbi.nih.gov/newsroom/home/GetPressRelease.aspx?id=2554.

Pharmacologic Considerations

- Estrogen therapy can cause nausea and vomiting, pigmentation of the nipple and areola, and uterine bleeding. Stress incontinence may occur. Sodium may be retained, leading to excessive storage of interstitial fluid and edema. Diuretics and a low-sodium diet help relieve this situation. Large doses of estrogen sometimes cause the mobilization of calcium into the bloodstream, damaging the kidney when it excretes the excess calcium.

- Chest pain and shortness of breath may be symptoms of a pulmonary embolus. Because synthetic estrogen hormones cause thromboemboli, instruct the client to contact the physician if tenderness, pain, swelling, or redness occurs in the legs. If vaginal bleeding occurs during hormonal therapy, the dose may need to be adjusted.

- When androgen therapy is prescribed, clients may have increased bone pain after the first few injections. As therapy continues, pain frequently lessens, some recalcification of bone occurs, and the client has an increased appetite and gains weight. Androgen therapy may cause fluid retention, increased libido, and distressing symptoms of virilization, such as deeper voice and increased facial and body hair.

  To prevent loss of bone mass in postmenopausal women, daily, weekly, or monthly oral medications such as alendronate (Fosamax), risedronate (Actonel), or ibandronate (Boniva) may be prescribed. These drugs act to prevent bone resorption. Do not give the oral drugs with milk or milk products because calcium inhibits absorption of the drug. The drugs are best absorbed when given with 8 ounces of water on arising in the morning. The client should avoid lying down and remain upright for at least 30 minutes after taking the drug to prevent dyspepsia and esophageal irritation.

- Raloxifene (Evista), given orally, and zoledronic acid (Reclast), given intravenously once a year, are SERMs that have some of the beneficial effects of natural estrogens, such as maintaining bone density and lowering lipid levels, yet have antiestrogen effects such as reducing the risk of uterine and breast cancer.

Nursing Management

The nurse collects a database that includes a menstrual, reproductive, and sexual history and prepares and supports the client during physical and diagnostic examinations. Health teaching addresses topics such as normal developmental changes during middle adulthood, coping strategies, health-promotion techniques, methods to achieve symptomatic relief, and treatment-related information.

Because normal and abnormal structural changes are easily confused, the nurse recommends regular gynecologic and breast examinations during and after menopause. The nurse also gives the following suggestions:

- Use bland skin creams or lotions to reduce skin dryness.
- Plan an exercise program to prevent weight gain and loss of calcium from the bones.

- Increase calcium intake by eating calcium-rich foods or by taking a supplement.
- Discuss with the prescriber the benefits, risks, and alternatives for HRT therapy.
- Discuss a schedule for routine gynecologic and breast examinations.
- Contact the physician if breakthrough vaginal bleeding or other symptoms occur while taking HRT. Changing the dosage, using a different combination of hormones, or substituting alternative medications may eliminate undesirable effects.
- Cultivate new interests and hobbies or resume those that have been abandoned because of other responsibilities.

INFECTIOUS AND INFLAMMATORY DISORDERS

VAGINITIS

Vaginitis is a condition in which the vagina is inflamed.

Pathophysiology and Etiology

Vaginal inflammation is caused by chemical or mechanical irritants such as feminine hygiene products, allergic reactions, age-related tissue changes (atrophic vaginitis with menopause), and the most common etiology, infections. The pathogenic microorganisms frequently associated with vaginitis are the bacterium *Gardnerella vaginalis*, the protozoan *Trichomonas vaginalis*, and the yeastlike fungus *Candida albicans* (see Chap. 56).

Although the vagina is self-protected by mucus-secreting cells and an acidic environment (pH of 3.5 to 4.5), the tissue still may become disrupted. Some situations predispose to vaginitis because they alter protective mechanisms. For example, antibiotics or frequent douching eliminate the bacilli that promote an acidic vaginal environment. Decreased estrogen at menopause reduces the thick, moist consistency of vaginal tissue. Pregnant women, those with unregulated diabetes, and those who take oral contraceptives containing estrogen have an excess of glycogen in vaginal mucus, which supports the growth of microorganisms.

Pharmacologic Considerations

- When antibiotics are taken for a long time or if repeated courses of antibiotic therapy are necessary, an overgrowth of *C. albicans* that usually exists in small numbers in the vagina can occur, resulting in vaginitis.

Gerontologic Considerations

- Vaginal flora change with age, causing the environment to become more alkaline and predisposing older women to vaginitis.

- Older women may develop perineal pruritus. To discover the cause, ask questions about diet, type of clothing worn, vaginal discharge, or other contributing factors. The client may be tested for glucose in the blood and urine, and a pelvic examination may be performed to rule out other abnormalities, such as cervicitis, cystocele, rectocele, or cancer of the vulva, cervix, or uterus which are discussed later.

Assessment Findings

An abnormal vaginal discharge is the primary symptom of vaginal infection, and the characteristics of the discharge often are indicative of the infecting organism (Table 53-2). The discharge often is accompanied by itching, burning, redness, and swelling of surrounding tissues. Diagnosis is confirmed by visual and microscopic examination of secretions.

Medical Management

Infectious vaginitis is remedied by using drugs to which the microorganism is particularly sensitive. They include antifungal, antiprotozoal, and antibiotic agents (Drug Therapy Table 53-1). In some cases, the sexual partner also is infected and the vaginitis recurs if both are not treated simultaneously.

Atrophic vaginitis is relieved with estrogen replacement administered as a topical cream. If the client has diabetes mellitus, regulating blood glucose is an important aspect of treatment.

Nursing Management

The nurse informs the client not to douche before the physical examination because washing away the secretions removes the characteristics of the vaginal discharge and interferes with obtaining an adequate diagnostic smear. After diagnosis, the nurse may insert the first dose of vaginal medication while teaching the client how to repeat the technique. Nonprescription drugs for the treatment of yeast infections are available. The nurse informs clients that although these drugs usually are effective, the initial diagnosis of vaginitis is best made by a physician. The nurse emphasizes the importance of completing the course of therapy.

The nurse also informs the client to avoid routine douching when asymptomatic, but to combat vaginitis, the client may douche daily for 10 to 14 days with a solution of 1 to 2 tablespoons of white vinegar in 1 pint of water (University of Maryland Medical Center, 2006). Taking *Lactobacillus acidophilus* in capsule form or eating yogurt containing active cultures of lactobacilli can replenish normal vaginal microorganisms. Sitz baths are recommended to relieve itching, burning, and swelling of the vulva and perineum. Skin protectants containing zinc oxide promote healing.

The nurse offers additional suggestions for preventing a recurrence of vaginal infections, as presented in Client and Family Teaching 53-1.

CERVICITIS

Cervicitis is an inflammation of the cervix.

Pathophysiology and Etiology

Cervical inflammation results from infectious microorganisms, decreased estrogen levels during menopause, or trauma during gynecologic procedures, or occurs as a consequence of inserting tampons or vaginal medication applicators. Streptococcal, staphylococcal, gonorrheal, and chlamydial (see Chap. 56) infections are the most common etiologies. The potential is greater during pregnancy and after childbirth, when the microorganisms can enter cervical tissue through small lacerations. The infection can travel upward through uterine and tubal structures, leading to pelvic inflammatory disease (see later discussion). Inflammation and subsequent formation of scar tissue increase the potential for ectopic pregnancy or difficulty conceiving. Chronic cervicitis decreases the amount and quality of cervical mucus and alters the pH, both of which are underlying causes of infertility.

Assessment Findings

Early cervicitis may fail to produce any symptoms. The client eventually spots or bleeds intermenstrually or develops a vaginal discharge. Dyspareunia (painful intercourse) or slight bleeding after sexual intercourse may occur. Severe cervicitis sometimes causes a sensation of weight in the pelvis.

Diagnosis is made by visual examination of the cervix. Microscopic examination of cervical smears identifies the causative microorganism.

Medical Management

Douches and local or systemic antibiotics are the treatment of choice for acute cervicitis. Chronic cervicitis is treated with electrocautery. Frank bleeding requires cervical or vaginal packing or electric coagulation of the bleeding vessel. Healing often takes 6 to 8 weeks. Severe chronic cervicitis is treated by conization (removal of the diseased portion of the cervical mucosa). This outpatient procedure uses an instrument that simultaneously cuts tissue and coagulates the

TABLE 53-2 Characteristics of Vaginal Infections

MICROORGANISM	COLOR OF DISCHARGE	CONSISTENCY	ODOR	OTHER SYMPTOMS
Candida albicans	Curdy white	Thick	Strong	Burning with urination
Trichomonas vaginalis	Yellow-white	Foamy	Foul	Severe itching
Gardnerella vaginalis	Gray-white	Watery	Fishy	More discharge after intercourse

DRUG THERAPY TABLE 53-1 Agents To Treat Vaginitis

Drug Category and Examples	Mechanism of Action	Side Effects	Nursing Considerations
Antiprotozoal metronidazole (*Flagyl*)	Antiprotozoal–trichomonacidal Mechanism of action unknown Used to treat trichomoniasis and Gardnerella vaginalis	Headache, dizziness, ataxia, unpleasant metallic taste, anorexia, nausea, vomiting, diarrhea, darkening of urine	This drug is contraindicated in first trimester of pregnancy. Sexual partner may need to be treated. Instruct client to complete therapy. Administer with food if gastrointestinal upset occurs. Advise client to avoid alcoholic beverages and alcohol-containing products—a severe reaction may occur. Alert client that darkening of the urine may occur.
Antifungal clotrimazole (*Gyne-Lotrimin*), miconazole (*Monistat*), terconazole (*Terazol*), tioconazole (*Vagistat*)	Disrupts fungal cell membrane, causing cell death Used in the treatment of candidiasis	Cramping, nausea, vomiting, slight urinary frequency, erythema, stinging	Obtain culture before initiating therapy. Administer cream or vaginal tablets high into vaginal canal; instruct client to remain recumbent for 10–15 min or administer at bedtime. Treatment continues through menses if necessary. Instruct partner to use a condom to prevent reinfection. Partner may need treatment. Client should use a sanitary pad to prevent staining underwear.
Antibiotic sulfisoxazole (*Gantrisin*)	Prevents cell replication by competing with the enzyme involved in the synthesis of intracellular proteins Used to treat vaginitis, *Chlamydia trachomatis*	Headache, nausea, vomiting, abdominal pain, agranulocytosis, photosensitivity, hematuria	Discontinue immediately if hypersensitivity reaction occurs. Administer medication on an empty stomach with a full glass of water Complete drug therapy as ordered. Inform client of potential side effects. Tell client to report blood in urine, rash, fever, difficulty breathing, drowsiness, nausea, vomiting, or diarrhea.

Client and Family Teaching 53-1
Preventing Vaginal Infections

The nurse teaches the client to do the following:

- Bathe daily with particular attention to perineal hygiene.
- Wipe from front to back after bowel movements.
- Avoid feminine hygiene products and douching more than once per week.
- Wear cotton undergarments and change them daily.
- Refrain from wearing layers of clothing, such as underwear plus pantyhose plus slacks, that increase warmth and interfere with air circulation about the genital area.
- Change from a wet swimsuit as soon as possible.
- Wash hands and devices that are inserted into the vagina, such as medication applicators, douche tips, and diaphragms, and store them in clean containers.
- Change sanitary pads before they become saturated; substitute a sanitary pad for a tampon at night.
- Use a condom or avoid intercourse if either client or her sex partner(s) has genitourinary symptoms.

bleeding area. Dilatation is done if there is cervical stenosis. Successful treatment eliminates the inflammation, relieves the symptoms, and aids fertility.

Nursing Management

The nurse schedules treatment procedures 5 to 8 days after the end of the menstrual period to reduce the potential for bleeding. The nurse positions the client as for a gynecologic examination and explains that a momentary cramping sensation may be felt during the electrocautery procedure. After electrocautery, the nurse instructs the client to:

- Rest more than usual for 1 to 2 days.
- Avoid straining or heavy lifting.
- Rest in bed and report if slight bleeding does occur; frank bleeding requires a return visit to the physician.
- Expect a grayish-green, malodorous discharge about 3 weeks after cautery.
- Anticipate slight bleeding about the 11th day.
- Return for a follow-up visit to the physician in 2 to 4 weeks.
- Abstain from sexual relations until tissues are healed.
- Expect that healing may take 6 to 8 weeks.

PELVIC INFLAMMATORY DISEASE

Pelvic inflammatory disease (PID) is an infection of the pelvic organs other than the uterus. These include the ovaries (oophoritis), fallopian tubes (salpingitis), pelvic vascular system, and pelvic supporting structures.

Pathophysiology and Etiology

Microorganisms enter pelvic structures through the cervix from the vagina (Fig. 53-4). The cause usually is bacterial, with gonococci and *C. trachomatis* being the most common pathogens. The infection travels up the uterus to the fallopian tubes (salpingitis) and ovaries (oophoritis) and can result in a pelvic abscess or peritonitis as pus from the infected tubes leaks into the abdomen.

Assessment Findings

Signs and symptoms include an infectious malodorous discharge, backache, severe or aching abdominal and pelvic pain, a bearing-down feeling, fever, dyspareunia, nausea and vomiting, menorrhagia, and dysmenorrhea. Some women experience milder symptoms such as pain during a pelvic examination. Severe infection may cause urinary symptoms.

Diagnosis is based on symptoms as well as a gynecologic examination. A culture and sensitivity test of the vaginal discharge is obtained to identify the causative microorganism. Ultrasonography, magnetic resonance imaging (MRI), or computed tomography (CT) may disclose a pelvic abscess.

Medical Management

Hospitalization with complete bed rest often is necessary. Parenteral or oral antibiotics are administered as soon as culture and sensitivity tests are obtained. Intravenous (IV) fluids are ordered if the client is dehydrated, and antipyretics are used if the temperature is elevated. A ruptured pelvic abscess requires emergency surgery.

Nursing Process for the Client With Pelvic Inflammatory Disease

Assessment

Obtain a complete medical, drug, and allergy history, and ask the client to describe all symptoms. A vaginal smear may be necessary.

If the client is an outpatient, instruct the client to refrain from douching for 48 hours before being examined. If the client is admitted to the hospital and a vaginal smear is ordered, inquire whether the client has douched within the last 48 hours.

Diagnosis, Planning, and Interventions

The nurse's role in caring for a client hospitalized with PID includes but is not limited to the following:

▸ **PC:** Sepsis related to systemic spread of pathogenic microorganisms

▸ **Expected Outcome:** The nurse will monitor to detect, manage, and minimize sepsis if it occurs.

- Monitor vital signs and results of white blood cell counts. *Increased temperature, pulse rate, and leukocytosis indicate an infectious process.*
- Maintain IV site and administer parenteral fluids and antibiotic therapy as scheduled. *The nurse implements prescribed medical therapy for treating an infectious process.*
- Keep the client in a semisitting position. *Keeping the upper body elevated facilitates pelvic drainage and minimizes upward extension of infection.*

▸ **Risk for Infection Transmission** related to direct or indirect contact with infectious microorganisms

▸ **Expected Outcome:** No nosocomial infections will occur among other clients or staff that can be traced to the client with the primary infection.

- Provide the client with a private room with a toilet and sink. *Separating the client from others confines the source of transmission to one location.*
- Follow contact isolation precautions. *Contact isolation is a category of transmission-based precautions for controlling the spread of infectious microorganisms found in wound drainage and other body fluids.*
- Wrap and dispose of soiled perineal pads in a lined biohazard container. *Confining objects that are heavily contaminated with infectious microorganisms reduces the potential for transmitting them to other susceptible people.*
- Bag soiled linen according to infection-control policies of the institution. *Linen that has been in contact with a person with*

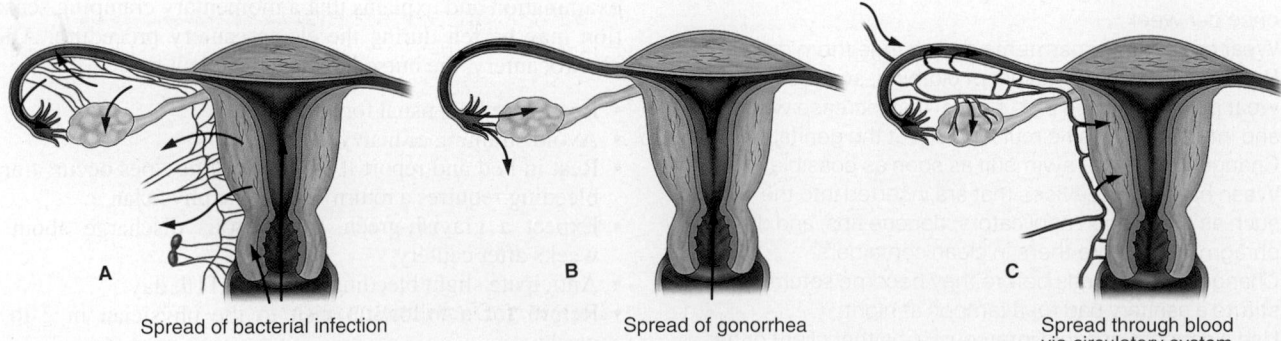

FIGURE 53-4. (A) Bacteria spread from the vagina and uterus through the lymphatics. **(B)** Gonorrhea spreads from the vagina and uterus through the tubes and ovaries. **(C)** Bacteria can also reach the reproductive organs through the bloodstream.

Spread of bacterial infection   Spread of gonorrhea   Spread through blood via circulatory system *infectious body fluids is contained in specially marked bags to avoid transmitting pathogens to personnel who handle laundry.*

- Leave a disposable stethoscope and thermometers in the room for assessments. *Instruments used for frequent assessments are restricted to the infectious client and then destroyed.*
- Perform hand hygiene after removing gloves. *Hand hygiene reduces the number of pathogens on the skin, which tend to grow and multiply in the warmth of latex or vinyl gloves.*
- Clean the cover on the blood pressure cuff with a disinfectant when the client is discharged. *A disinfectant destroys microorganisms on the surface of objects in the environment.*
- Instruct housekeeping personnel to damp mop the client's room after cleaning other clients' rooms and change the mop head when finished. *A principle of medical asepsis is to always clean the most heavily soiled area last. Changing the mop head prevents spreading microorganisms to other areas.*

▶ **Acute Pain** related to inflamed tissue and pelvic congestion

▶ **Expected Outcome:** Client's comfort will be maintained within a level of tolerance.

- Administer prescribed analgesic. *Analgesics relieve pain by various biochemical mechanisms.*
- Provide diversional activities to distract client from pain. *Distraction reduces pain perception by providing alternative stimuli to the brain.*
- Position for comfort and limit unnecessary activity. *An uncomfortable position and movement tend to increase pain intensity.*

▶ **Risk for Impaired Skin Integrity** related to excoriating potential of vaginal drainage

▶ **Expected Outcome:** Vulvar and perineal tissue will be intact.

- Wash the perineum well with soap and water every 4 hours. *Removing drainage from contact with the skin promotes skin integrity.*
- Pat or blot the skin dry. *Touching the skin gently rather than vigorously reduces trauma to the skin. Keeping the skin dry reduces the potential for maceration.*
- Change perineal pads frequently. *Changing perineal pads frequently increases the potential for absorbing and wicking drainage from the skin surface.*

Evaluation of Expected Outcomes

Expected outcomes are that vital signs and white blood cell count are normal. Infection control measures are effective. The client's pain or discomfort is relieved or eliminated. The genital tissue is free of redness and excoriation.

After discharge from the hospital, tell the client to temporarily abstain from sexual intercourse to prevent extending the infection and infecting the partner. In addition, explain that preventing subsequent episodes of PID can be accomplished by seeking medical attention when symptoms of infection, such as a feeling of pressure in the pelvic area, burning on urination, or vaginal drainage, first appear. Early treatment prevents the infection from moving up the reproductive tract, resulting in complications such as peritonitis, abscess formation, and obstruction of the fallopian tubes. When early treatment of acute PID is delayed or inadequate, the infection may become chronic.

TOXIC SHOCK SYNDROME

Toxic shock syndrome (TSS), a type of septic shock (see Chap. 17), is a life-threatening systemic reaction to the toxin produced by several kinds of bacteria. Some causative microorganisms include *Staphylococcus aureus, Streptococcus pyogenes*, and *Clostridium sordellii*. TSS also occurs in men and in nonmenstruating women with soft tissue and postoperative infections.

Pathophysiology and Etiology

TSS is associated with the use of superabsorbent tampons that are not changed frequently and internal contraceptive devices that remain in place longer than necessary. The syndrome occurs when virulent bacteria reproduce suddenly and abundantly in the body and remain unchecked by normal physiologic defense mechanisms. The bacteria produce chemicals that cause blood vessels to dilate, which keeps the major portion of the blood volume in the periphery, reduces cardiac output, and causes severe hypotension (shock). The toxin also seems to inhibit the ability of affected cells to use oxygen (Porth, 2008).

Assessment Findings

Signs and Symptoms

A sudden onset of high fever, chills, tenderness or pain in the muscles, nausea, vomiting, diarrhea, hypotension, hyperemia (increased redness and congestion) of vaginal mucous membranes, disorientation, and headache occurs. The skin is warm despite the fact that the client is in shock. A rash that first appears on the palms of the hands or the body a few hours after the infection later results in a shedding of the superficial layer of the skin (desquamation). The pulse is rapid and thready.

Diagnostic Findings

The infecting microorganism is found in cultures of specimens from the vagina, blood, urine, or other sites. The blood urea nitrogen, serum creatinine, and serum bilirubin levels are increased. The serum enzymes aspartate aminotransferase (AST) and alanine aminotransferase (ALT) are elevated. The platelet count may be decreased.

Medical Management

Circulation is supported with IV fluids while combating the infection with IV antibiotic therapy. Some drugs that are used include oxacillin (Prostaphlin), nafcillin (Nafcil), and methicillin (Staphcillin). Potent adrenergic drugs such as dopamine (Intropin) or dobutamine (Dobutrex) are given to counteract peripheral vasodilation and maintain renal perfusion. Oxygen is given to promote aerobic metabolism at the cellular level.

Nursing Management

The nurse frequently assesses vital signs. He or she administers the first dose of antibiotics immediately and as ordered thereafter. The nurse applies pressure to venipuncture or injection sites to control bleeding and oozing if the platelet count is low. He or she carefully measures intake and output and reports any sudden decrease in the urinary output or a urinary output of less than 500 mL/day to the physician.

Before discharge, the nurse teaches preventive measures such as using perineal pads rather than tampons or changing tampons frequently. He or she tells clients who use a diaphragm, vaginal sponge, or cervical cap for birth control to remove the device within 24 hours after use. The nurse emphasizes handwashing and keeping vaginal devices clean.

STRUCTURAL ABNORMALITIES

ENDOMETRIOSIS

Endometriosis is a condition in which tissue with a cellular structure and function resembling that of the endometrium is found outside the uterus. The atypical locations for endometrial tissue include the ovaries, the pelvic cavity, and occasionally the abdominal cavity.

Pathophysiology and Etiology

The cause of endometriosis is not clearly understood. It may result from remnants of embryonic tissue that remain in the abdominal cavity. Another possible cause is retrograde menstruation, in which the fallopian tubes expel fragments of endometrial tissue that eventually become implanted outside the uterus.

The ectopic tissue responds to stimulation by estrogen and, perhaps, to progesterone. The tissue bleeds when the endometrium of the uterus is shed, but unfortunately there is no outlet for the extrauterine bleeding. The trapped blood causes pain and ultimately adhesions in the peritoneal cavity. If the fallopian tubes are affected, they may become occluded and result in **sterility**, an inability to conceive. If endometrial tissue is enclosed in an ovary, a chocolate cyst (named because of its collection of dark blood) develops. Occasionally this cyst ruptures, spilling old blood and endometrial cells into the pelvic or abdominal cavity. The condition is relieved naturally when endometrial tissue atrophies after menopause or regresses during pregnancy.

Assessment Findings

Severe dysmenorrhea and copious menstrual bleeding are typical symptoms. The client may experience dyspareunia and pain on defecation. Rupture of a chocolate cyst results in severe abdominal pain that can mimic other abdominal pathologies such as appendicitis or bowel obstruction.

A pelvic examination reveals fixed, tender areas in the lower pelvis. Restricted mobility of the uterus from adhesions may be noted. A laparoscopy confirms the diagnosis.

Medical and Surgical Management

Endometriosis is cured by natural or surgical menopause. To preserve the potential for having children, many women are managed medically as long as possible. Estrogen-progestin contraceptives are administered to keep the client in a nonbleeding phase of her menstrual cycle for about 9 months. The goal is to control the ectopic tissue so that the client is symptom free for several years. The progestin norethindrone

(Norlutin) and the synthetic androgen danazol (Danocrine) are effective in causing atrophy of endometrial tissue.

Without destroying the possibility for childbearing, surgery is performed to remove the cysts, as much of the ectopic tissue as possible, and lyse adhesions caused by bleeding. Laparoscopy is used to remove small areas of endometrial tissue as well as relieve adhesions. Endometriosis that is widespread throughout the pelvic organs, however, may necessitate a **panhysterectomy**, removal of the uterus, both fallopian tubes, and ovaries.

Nursing Management

The nurse obtains a complete reproductive history, asking the client to describe all symptoms, including their duration, type and location of pain, number of days of menses, amount of menstrual flow, and regularity or irregularity of the menstrual cycle. He or she offers information on methods for relieving menstrual pain (see discussion of dysmenorrhea) and assists the client through the decision-making process as it applies to family planning and medical or surgical treatment of endometriosis before natural menopause. Some techniques for resolving decisional conflict include the following:

- Reinforce or clarify explanations of treatment options and the consequences of each option.
- Emphasize that the condition does not require an immediate decision and avoid giving advice or influencing the client's opinions.
- Suggest that the client include her significant other in discussion of options.
- Offer the option of seeking a second medical opinion.
- Suggest listing the pros and cons of each option to help determine which choice is most compatible with her values and goals.

The nurse emphasizes the importance of adhering to the prescribed medication schedule, if that is the client's choice, and the importance of regular gynecologic evaluations. He or she instructs the client to seek care if pain increases, the menstrual flow is extremely heavy, or pregnancy occurs. Refer to the information on nursing management of clients undergoing a hysterectomy (later in this chapter) for those who choose that treatment option.

VAGINAL FISTULAS

A **fistula** is an unnatural opening between two structures. The opening may be between a ureter and the vagina (ureterovaginal fistula), between the bladder and the vagina (vesicovaginal fistula), or between the rectum and the vagina (rectovaginal fistula; Fig. 53-5).

Pathophysiology and Etiology

Vaginal fistulas are caused by cancer, radiation treatment, surgical or obstetric injury, congenital anomaly, or a complication of ulcerative colitis. They result in the continuous drainage of urine or feces from the vagina. The vaginal wall and the external genitalia become excoriated and often infected. The client may not void through the urethra because urine does not accumulate in the bladder.

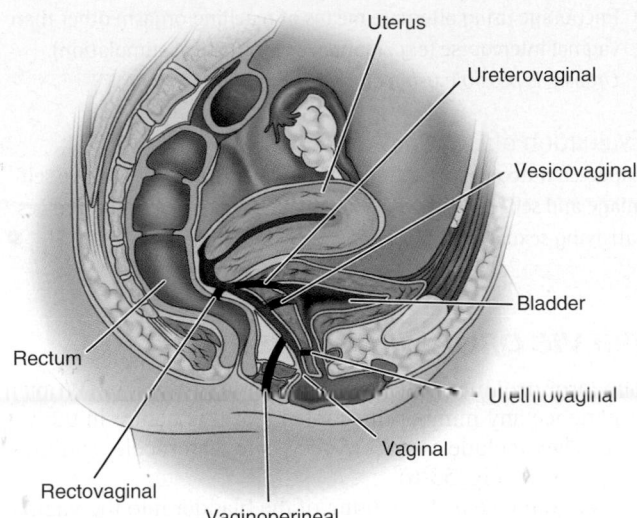

FIGURE 53-5. Types of vaginal fistulae.

Labels: Uterus, Ureterovaginal, Vesicovaginal, Bladder, Urethrovaginal, Vaginal, Rectum, Rectovaginal, Vaginoperineal

Assessment Findings

The client reports that urine or stool leaks from the vagina. Diagnosis is made by physical examination of the vaginal wall. A sterile probe is inserted if the fistula is easily seen or a dye (usually methylene blue) is used to detect the exact location of the fistula. When a vesicovaginal fistula is suspected, the colored dye is instilled into the bladder through a urethral catheter. A ureterovaginal fistula requires IV administration of the dye. An IV pyelogram (IVP) detects the flow of radiopaque dye through the lower genitourinary tract. A rectovaginal fistula is located by looking for fecal drainage on the posterior vaginal wall.

Medical and Surgical Management

Surgery is performed after inflammation and edema have disappeared. This may require months of treatment. Sometimes the tissues are in such poor condition that surgical repair is not possible. In the meantime, or if the fistula cannot be repaired, symptomatic treatment to reduce the risk for infection and manage skin excoriation is provided.

Nursing Process for the Client With a Vaginal Fistula

Assessment

Obtain the client's history and perform a physical assessment. Ask the client to describe the characteristics of the vaginal drainage. While wearing gloves, inspect the vaginal meatus and vault as well as the condition of the perianal skin. Help the client discuss the lifestyle changes that have accompanied the vaginal fistula.

Diagnosis, Planning, and Interventions

When managing the care of a client with a vaginal fistula, focus on implementing and teaching measures for maintaining skin integrity, helping the client maintain self-esteem, and offering suggestions for promoting sexuality if the client experiences sexual repercussions as a consequence of the condition. Before repair of a rectovaginal fistula, administer neomycin (Mycifradin), kanamycin

(Kantrex), or another prescribed antibiotic to clean the bowel of microorganisms. Provide a light, low-residue diet to keep stool soft, give an enema and a cleansing vaginal irrigation the morning of surgery, and insert an indwelling catheter to keep the bladder empty.

After surgery, serosanguineous vaginal drainage on the perineal pad is normal. No urine or feces from the vagina indicates healing of the repaired fistula. Prevent pelvic pressure and stress on the suture line by monitoring catheter drainage closely. The pressure of a full bladder from an obstructed catheter may break down the surgical repair and cause the fistula to reappear. Prevent and relieve pressure on perineal structures. Warm perineal irrigations and heat-lamp treatments are effective in promoting healing and lessening discomfort. Douches used during the postoperative period remove drainage, keep the suture area clean, and lessen chances of infection. About the 3rd or 4th postoperative day, a rectal suppository or a stool softener may be ordered to prevent straining during a bowel movement.

Specific diagnoses, expected outcomes, and interventions include but are not limited to the following:

▶ **Risk for Situational Low Self-Esteem** related to leaking of urine and stool and body and environmental odors

▶ **Expected Outcome:** Client's self-esteem will be maintained or restored as evidenced by a positive self-image and self-confidence.

- Recommend wearing disposable, absorbent incontinence briefs or perineal pads with protective panties, and changing and laundering clothing or bed linens as soon as possible. *Measures that absorb the drainage and keep clothing and the environment clean help to control odors that may be socially unacceptable.*
- Let the client know that commercial deodorizers are available for use in the home. *Pleasant fragrances disguise odors that may linger.*
- Recognize positive attributes when they are demonstrated. *Acknowledging the client's strengths elevates self-esteem.*
- Affirm that the client is capable of managing odor and elimination problems. *Instilling a sense of control increases self-esteem.*
- Provide genuine feedback on self-care and hygiene measures. *Compliments, when they are deserved, improve self-esteem.*

▶ **Risk for Impaired Skin Integrity** related to continuous skin contact with urine or stool

▶ **Expected Outcome:** Skin will remain intact or skin integrity will be restored.

- Advise daily bathing and frequent perineal hygiene with premoistened disposable wipes. *Removing drainage from contact with the skin promotes skin integrity.*
- Apply a skin protectant, such as collodion, over intact skin, or a skin barrier, such as zinc oxide or karaya paste, to excoriated skin. *Commercial skin products reduce contact with irritating drainage.*
- Teach the client how to take sitz baths and administer cleansing douches. *Water that is in motion helps to loosen debris and reduce contact with the skin.*
- Explain that mixing a perfumed scent with a fecal or urine odor may intensify the odor as well as irritate the area. *Colognes and*

perfumes contain alcohol, which promotes evaporation of drainage that contains unpleasant odors. Alcohol irritates excoriated skin.

- Inform the client that powders may cake and cause irritation or a superficial skin infection. The client may use a thin dusting of plain cornstarch but must wash it off thoroughly when the area becomes soiled with feces or urine. *Talc tends to attract moisture and take on the consistency of paste. Applying a light layer of cornstarch reduces friction when two skin surfaces move over one another.*

▸ Sexual Dysfunction related to embarrassment over vaginal drainage

▸ Expected Outcome: Client will engage in satisfying sexual activity.

- Recommend scheduling sexual intercourse to allow for hygienic preparation (e.g., bathing, perineal care). *Being clean promotes mutual sexual response between client and partner.*
- Point out that attractive lingerie, soft music, and scented candles may overcome emotional barriers to sex. *Modifications in clothing and the environment promote eroticism.*
- Suggest reclining on an absorbent, disposable pad. *Planning measures that prevent soiling of bed linen decreases self-consciousness.*
- Propose substituting the shower, private swimming pool, or a hot tub as a place for intercourse. *Having intercourse while water is flowing helps reduce attention on the drainage.*

- Encourage using alternate means of reaching orgasm other than vaginal intercourse (e.g., manual or mechanical stimulation). *Orgasm is possible using alternative methods.*

Evaluation of Expected Outcomes
Expected outcomes are that the client demonstrates a positive self-image and self-confidence. Skin remains intact. The client pursues satisfying sexual activities. ●

PELVIC ORGAN PROLAPSE

The term *prolapse* indicates a structural protrusion. Women experience any number of problems of this nature in the vagina. They include cystocele, rectocele, enterocele, and uterine prolapse (Fig. 53-6).

A **cystocele** is the bulging of the bladder into the vagina. A **rectocele** is a herniation of the rectum into the vagina. An *enterocele* is a protrusion of the intestinal wall into the vagina. A *uterovaginal prolapse* is the downward displacement of the cervix anywhere from low in the vagina to outside the vagina.

Pathophysiology and Etiology
Pelvic organ prolapse is a consequence of congenital or acquired weaknesses in the muscles and fascia that are needed to support pelvic structures. Common causes include unrepaired postpartum tears; stretching during pregnancy

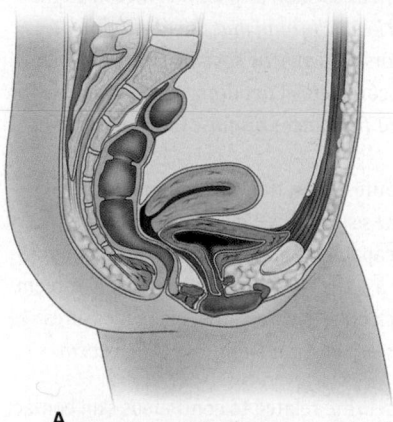
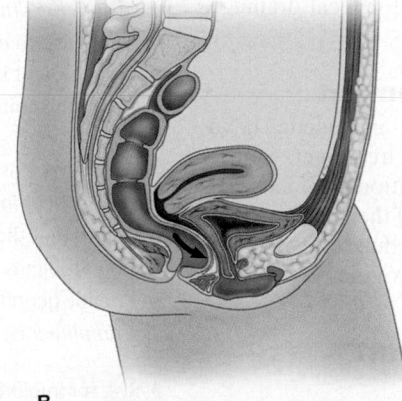
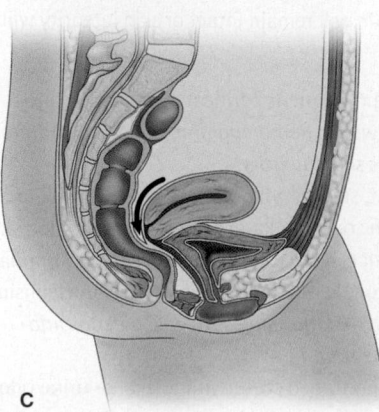
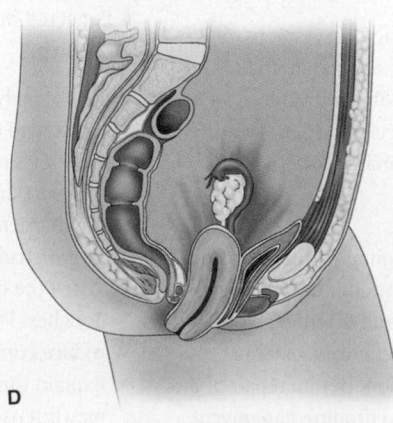

A

B

C

D

FIGURE 53-6. Types of pelvic organ prolapse. (**A**) Cystocele. (**B**) Rectocele. (**C**) Enterocele. (**D**) Uterine prolapse.

and childbirth or with tumorous masses, ascites, and obesity; and postmenopausal atrophy. As the pelvic floor relaxes, the uterus, rectum, intestine, and bladder, alone or in combination, herniate downward. Structural displacement of the bladder and bowel leads to alterations in urinary and bowel elimination. Uterine tissue that protrudes below the vaginal orifice is subject to irritation from clothing or rubbing against the thighs while walking; ulceration and infection frequently follow. Clients with severe uterovaginal prolapse are at greater risk for cervical cancer.

The functional consequences of pelvic organ prolapse can be disruptive. The client often experiences difficulty standing for long periods, walking with ease, lifting, and other activities that are hard to avoid.

Assessment Findings

Signs and Symptoms

Clients with a cystocele may experience stress incontinence—a little urine seeps every time the woman coughs, sneezes, laughs, bears down, or strains. Cystitis (inflammation of the bladder; see Chap. 59) results from the stagnation of urine in the bladder. With a rectocele, constipation often is a problem. In some instances, the client has to put her finger into the vagina and apply pressure to the posterior vaginal wall to reduce the herniation before being able to evacuate stool. Symptoms of a uterovaginal prolapse include backache, pelvic pain, fatigue, and a feeling that "something is dropping out," especially when lifting a heavy object, coughing, or standing for prolonged periods.

Diagnostic Findings

Diagnosis is confirmed during a pelvic examination and visual inspection of the vagina. Urinary tests are performed to reproduce stress incontinence or to determine the volume at which a client senses an urgent need to void. A Pap test determines the client's estrogen status.

Medical and Surgical Management

A **pessary**, which is a firm, doughnut-shaped or ring device, may be inserted in the upper vagina to reposition and give support to the uterus when surgery cannot be done or the client declines surgery. **Kegel exercises**, also known as *pelvic floor strengthening exercises* (see Chap. 59), are recommended when there is stress incontinence.

Surgical repairs are done transvaginally. The surgical repair of a cystocele is called *anterior colporrhaphy*. Repair of a rectocele is called *posterior colporrhaphy*. Repair of the tears (usually old obstetric tears) of the perineal floor is called *perineorrhaphy*. A vaginal hysterectomy (see later discussion) is done to remove a completely prolapsed uterus.

 Gerontologic Considerations

- Older women who experience uterine prolapse must carefully consider risks and benefits of surgery, especially if the surgery may impact other chronic conditions. A pessary is a nonsurgical option for treatment.

Nursing Management

The nurse obtains a comprehensive medical history, including the chief complaint and symptoms; inserts a catheter for diagnostic testing; assists with the pelvic examination and collection of specimens; and provides appropriate health teaching based on the physician's plan for treatment. He or she shows the client how to remove, clean, and reinsert a pessary, including the following information:

- Remove the pessary and thoroughly wash it with warm, soapy water, followed by rinsing and drying.
- Inspect the pessary to be sure that all secretions have been removed.
- Apply a sterile lubricant to the pessary before it is reinserted. Discomfort may indicate that it has been inserted incorrectly, the pessary has moved, or that it is causing irritation. Contact the physician if these problems occur.
- See the physician immediately if a white or yellow discharge from the vagina develops. It may indicate an infection.
- Assume the knee-chest position for a few minutes once or twice a day to keep the pelvic organs and the pessary in good position.
- Avoid heavy lifting and straining when having a bowel movement.

The nurse tells clients not wishing to manage their own pessary to see their physician at least every 2 months or sooner if vaginal discharge or changes in voiding develop.

After an anterior colporrhaphy, some women have temporary difficulty voiding or emptying the bladder completely. For this reason, clients are discharged with a retention catheter in place or are taught to perform clean intermittent catheterization (see Chap. 59) for 7 to 10 days until they can void sufficiently to empty the bladder. The client learns Kegel exercises after surgical repairs.

UTERINE DISPLACEMENT

In some women, the uterus, which normally is flexed about 45° anteriorly with the cervix positioned posteriorly, is displaced. *Retroversion*, the most common displacement, describes a uterus that tilts posteriorly with a cervix that tilts anteriorly. *Retroflexion* refers to a uterus that bends backward. *Anteversion* describes a uterus that bends forward as a whole unit (the opposite of retroversion). *Anteflexion* describes a uterus that is bent forward on itself (the opposite of retroflexion; Fig 53-7)

Pathophysiology and Etiology

Displacement usually is congenital; sometimes backward displacement is from childbearing or scar tissue that forms in clients who have endometriosis or PID. Positional displacement may not cause any noticeable problems, or it may be the underlying reason for discomfort during menstruation and intercourse. Some cases of infertility are caused by retrodisplacement of the uterus.

Assessment Findings

Clients with a malpositioned uterus describe having backache, dysmenorrhea, or dyspareunia. Sometimes the client

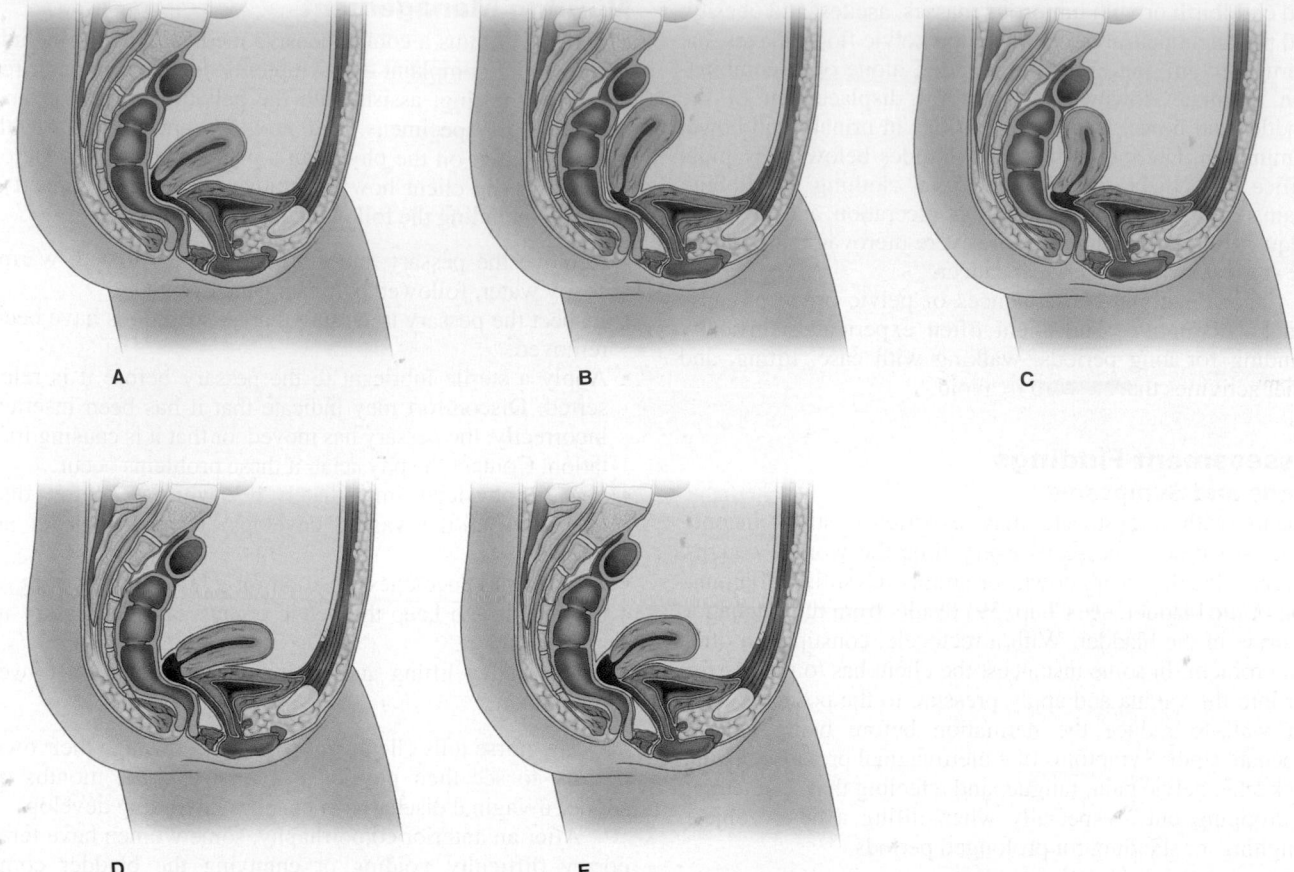

FIGURE 53-7. Variations in uterine position. (**A**) Normal. (**B**) Retroversion. (**C**) Retroflexion. (**D**) Anteversion. (**E**) Anteflexion.

seeks a medical examination to investigate the reason pregnancy has not occurred. A bimanual pelvic examination locates the abnormal position of the uterus.

Medical and Surgical Management

If the displacement causes severe discomfort, or if the sterility can be corrected, abdominal surgery is performed to relocate and suture the uterus to a more natural position. Age or complicating diseases sometimes make surgery too great a risk. Under such circumstances, the displacement is reduced by inserting a pessary, which repositions the uterus, and having the client assume the knee-chest position several times a day.

Nursing Management

The nurse performs an initial interview, collects pertinent data, and assists with the gynecologic examination. If surgery is performed, the nurse assesses the client for complications, manages wound drains, maintains patency of the indwelling catheter, inspects vaginal packing, and notes the condition of dressings. He or she includes deep breathing, pain management, and early ambulation in the postoperative management.

If a pessary is used to correct the prolapse, the nurse shows the client how to remove, clean, and reinsert it. He or she explains how to assume a knee-chest position and describes activity level and hygiene measures. The nurse schedules medical follow-up or instructs the client to do so.

> **Stop, Think, and Respond Exercise 53-2**
>
> Give examples of conditions that are associated with dysmenorrhea.

TUMORS OF THE FEMALE REPRODUCTIVE SYSTEM

UTERINE LEIOMYOMA

A *leiomyoma*, sometimes shortened to *myoma*, is a benign uterine growth principally consisting of smooth muscle and fibrous connective tissue. Myomas, which are the most common tumor in the female pelvis, often are referred to as **fibroid tumors**.

Pathophysiology and Etiology

Estrogen is believed to stimulate the development of fibroids. Tumors may be small or large, single or multiple. Growth usually is slow except during pregnancy. They shrink during and after menopause. Fibroids can occur in various locations in the uterus: subserous (below the serous membrane), intramural (within the wall), and submucosal (below the mucous membrane; Fig. 53-8). The latter are associated most frequently with excessive menstrual bleeding.

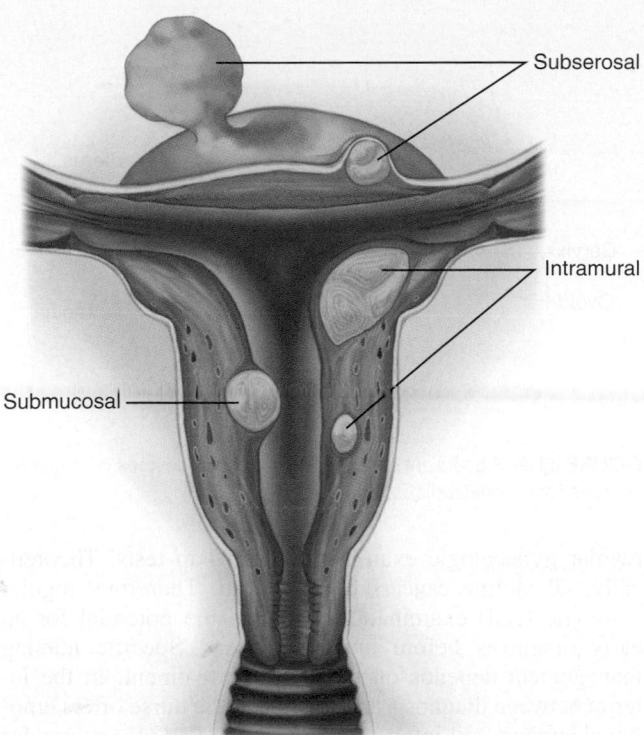

Subserosal

Intramural

Submucosal

FIGURE 53-8. Submucosal, intramural, and subserosal leiomyomas (fibroids). (From Ricci, S. S. [2009]. *Essentials of maternity, newborn, and women's health nursing* [2nd ed.]. Philadelphia: Lippincott Williams & Wilkins.)

Assessment Findings

When symptoms exist, menorrhagia is most common. There can be a feeling of pressure in the pelvic region, dysmenorrhea, anemia (from loss of blood), and malaise.

Benign uterine tumors may be detected during a pelvic examination. A Pap test is done to rule out a malignancy. A sonogram reveals uterine and fibroid size. Microscopic examination of the excised tumor confirms the diagnosis.

Medical and Surgical Management

Several factors govern the treatment of benign uterine tumors. A symptomatic tumor in a woman who wishes to have children is watched closely. The client receives a gynecologic examination every 3 to 6 months. A Pap test is repeated every 6 to 12 months.

When the client has abnormal bleeding, a D and C is performed to determine the cause of or to control the bleeding. Although a D and C does not remove the tumor, it may make more extensive surgery unnecessary. A myomectomy (surgical removal of the tumor only) through an abdominal incision or with a laparoscope inserted through the cervical canal preserves the uterus if a woman of childbearing years wishes to become pregnant in the future. A hysterectomy is performed when symptoms are severe and incapacitating, if the client is past childbearing years, or future pregnancy is not desired.

Nursing Management

The nurse assists with the gynecologic examination, reinforces medical explanations, and provides preoperative instructions. During the postoperative period, the nurse assists in the safe recovery of the client who undergoes surgery similar to that discussed for cervical and endometrial cancer.

CERVICAL AND ENDOMETRIAL CANCER

Cervical cancer, which affects the lowest portion of the uterus, is the second most frequent malignancy of the female reproductive system (breast cancer is first). Cancer of the endometrium affects the lining of the uterus, usually in the area of the fundus or corpus, and is more common in postmenopausal women.

Pathophysiology and Etiology

Cancer of the cervix has its peak incidence among women between 35 and 50 years of age and is associated with the following risk factors:

- Being born to mothers treated with diethylstilbestrol (DES) while pregnant
- Becoming sexually active at an early age
- Having multiple sexual partners or having intercourse with a high-risk man (one who has had multiple partners or penile condyloma [warts])
- Acquiring genital infections caused by the human papillomavirus (HPV)
- Having chronic cervicitis secondary to uterine prolapse
- Having a history of cigarette smoking
- Having had pelvic radiation

The risk of endometrial cancer increases after 50 years of age, especially in those women taking estrogens without the addition of progesterone for 5 or more years during and after menopause. Other risk factors include early menarche, late menopause, never having been pregnant (nulliparity), and obesity.

Cervical and endometrial cancers probably begin as premalignant lesions that later undergo malignant changes. The localized malignancy is referred to as **carcinoma in situ**. Untreated, it subsequently invades other areas of the uterus and adjacent tissue.

Assessment Findings

Signs and Symptoms

Bleeding is the earliest and most common symptom of both endometrial and cervical cancer. In early cervical cancer, spotting occurs first, especially after slight trauma such as douching or intercourse. The bleeding from endometrial cancer can be mistaken for menorrhagia in premenopausal women. Late symptoms for both include pain, symptoms of pressure on the bladder or bowel, and the generalized wasting associated with advanced cancer.

Diagnostic Findings

All vaginal bleeding is investigated, first by a gynecologic examination, then by diagnostic tests. Cervical cancer is detected with Pap tests and biopsies of suspect tissue. Cells obtained by endocervical aspiration or endometrial biopsy during a hysteroscopy identify abnormal cells higher in the uterus. Radiography, MRI, or CT scanning is used to determine if there is metastasis; a barium study or IVP is ordered

TABLE 53-3 Stages of Uterine Cancers

TYPE	STAGE	DESCRIPTION
Cervical	0	Carcinoma in situ
	I	Limited to the cervix
	II	Extends beyond the cervix to the upper two thirds of the vagina
	III	Involves the lower third of the vagina and is fixed to the pelvic wall
	IV	Involves the rectum, bladder, or extends beyond the true pelvis
Endometrial	0	Cancer in situ
	I	Confined to the corpus
	II	Involves the corpus and cervix
	III	Extends outside the uterus, but not the true pelvis
	IV	Involves the rectum, bladder, or extends outside the true pelvis

Adapted from the International Federation of Gynecology and Obstetrics.

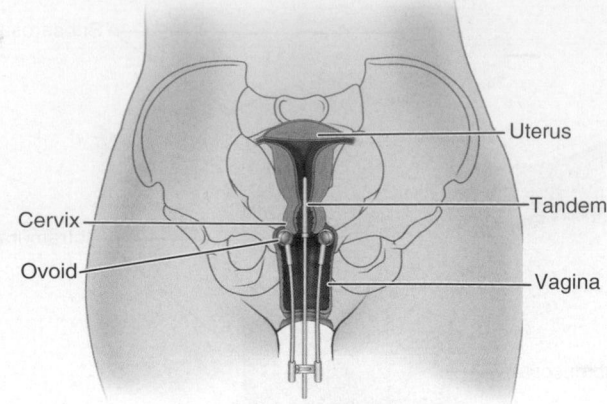

FIGURE 53-9. Placement of tandem and ovoids, devices containing sources for internal radiation therapy.

to determine bowel or bladder metastasis. Both types of cancer are classified according to stage (Table 53-3).

Medical and Surgical Management

Treatment of cervical and endometrial cancer depends on the stage of the tumor. Prognosis depends on how early the cancer is diagnosed. Methods for treating cervical and endometrial cancer include one of various types of **hysterectomy** (removal of uterus) (Box 53-1), external or internal radiation therapy (Fig. 53-9), and chemotherapy (see Chap. 18).

The uterus is removed using an abdominal or vaginal approach—the choice usually depends on the pathology and the client's condition. An abdominal approach always is used for a radical hysterectomy. The vaginal approach has fewer complications, reduced recovery time, and lower cost. Laparoscopically assisted vaginal hysterectomy, a combination of surgical and endoscopic techniques, is being used to perform vaginal hysterectomies that otherwise would have been performed abdominally.

Nursing Management

A major role of the nurse is to make women aware that a cervical cancer vaccine is available for females who are not yet sexually active (Box 53-2). All women should also have

regular gynecologic examinations and Pap tests. Theoretically, all uterine cancers begin in situ. Therefore, regular cytologic (cell) examinations increase the potential for an early diagnosis before invasion occurs. Specific nursing management depends on the selected treatment. In the interim between diagnosis and treatment, the nurse offers emotional support and information about the various options for treatment. See Chapter 18 for discussion of radiation therapy and chemotherapy and nursing management techniques.

Preoperative and Postoperative Care

Preoperative preparations vary depending on the surgeon's preference and the planned surgical approach (abdominal or vaginal). A douche is given before a vaginal hysterectomy, and an enema is given before either surgery. The nurse inserts an indwelling catheter before surgery and administers an antibiotic, usually one of the cephalosporins, during or after surgery to prevent infection. For general postoperative care, refer to perioperative standards of care discussed in Chapter 14; for postoperative care specific to an abdominal hysterectomy, refer to Nursing Care Plan 53-1.

BOX 53-1 **Types of Hysterectomies**

Total hysterectomy: Removal of the entire uterus and cervix

Subtotal hysterectomy: Removal of the uterus only, with a stump of the cervix left intact

Panhysterectomy: Removal of the uterus, fallopian tubes, and ovaries

Radical hysterectomy: Removal of the uterus, cervix, ovaries, and fallopian tubes; part of the upper vagina and some pelvic lymph nodes also may be removed at this time

Pelvic exenteration: Removal of all reproductive organs, rectum, colon, bladder, distal ureters, iliac blood vessels, and pelvic lymph nodes and peritoneum

---

BOX 53-2 **Cervical Cancer Vaccine**

- Gardasil is a vaccine that protects against four types of human papilloma virus (HPV), which cause 70% of cervical cancers and 90% of cervical warts (see Chap 56).
- The recommended age for administering the vaccine is 9 to 26 years of age (i.e., prior to becoming sexually active and possibly infected with HPV).
- The vaccine does not protect against types of HPV to which the person has already been infected.
- The vaccine consists of three injections over the course of 6 months.
- Side effects include injection site reactions, fever, nausea and vomiting, dizziness, and fainting.
- Routine cervical cancer screening is recommended regardless of vaccine use, because cervical cancer can develop from other causes, other strains of HPV not included in the vaccine, and from a prevaccination infection with one or more of the HPV vaccine strains.

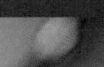

NURSING CARE PLAN 53-1 **The Client With a Total Abdominal Hysterectomy**

Assessment
- Assess vital signs and level of consciousness.
- Evaluate pain intensity.
- Monitor condition of the dressing, location of drains (nasogastric, wound), and patency of urinary catheter.

- Regularly check the type, volume, and rate of IV fluid, and the location and appearance of the IV site.
- Note the presence of antiembolic stockings.

Nursing Diagnosis: Acute Pain related to tissue trauma

Expected Outcome: Pain will be reduced to a tolerable level within 30 minutes of a nursing intervention.

Interventions	Rationales
Assess type of pain, intensity, and location each time you assess vital signs and as needed.	Pain assessment is the fifth vital sign.
Administer analgesics as ordered.	They reduce pain perception.
Implement nonpharmacologic interventions, such as distraction, imagery, and repositioning, to augment analgesia.	Substituting alternative stimuli to the brain decreases pain perception.

Evaluation of Expected Outcome
Client reports decreased discomfort; pain is adequately controlled.

PC: Thrombophlebitis

Expected Outcome: The nurse will monitor to detect, manage, and minimize thrombophlebitis.

Interventions	Rationales
Remove and reapply antiembolic stockings every 8 hours.	Antiembolic stockings support valves in veins and reduce venous stasis.
Encourage active leg exercises every 2 to 4 hours.	Skeletal muscle contraction propels venous blood toward the heart.
Assess for calf swelling and tenderness bilaterally every shift.	Calf tenderness and swelling are suggestive of a thrombus in the lower extremities.
Do not place pillows beneath the knees or raise the knees with the electric bed.	Bending the knees interferes with venous circulation and promotes venous stasis and clot formation.
Ambulate as much as possible.	Walking requires skeletal muscle contraction, which promotes venous circulation

Evaluation of Expected Outcome
No evidence thrombus formation.

PC: Urinary Retention

Expected Outcome: The nurse will monitor to detect, manage, and minimize urinary retention.

Interventions	Rationales
Measure intake and output every shift.	Intake and output facilitates assessment of fluid status.
Palpate the lower abdomen for distention.	The bladder is palpable when distended with urine.
Measure the volume of each voiding.	Voiding small amounts can indicate urinary retention with overflow.
Encourage a liberal fluid intake.	Urinary elimination is related to fluid intake.
Report bladder distention in the absence of voiding to the physician.	Medically prescribed interventions such as inserting a straight or indwelling catheter require an order from the physician.

Evaluation of Expected Outcome
Client voids in sufficient quantity.

PC: Abdominal Distention, Paralytic Ileus

Expected Outcome: The nurse will monitor to detect, manage, and minimize abdominal distention.

(care plan continues on page 040)

NURSING CARE PLAN 53-1 The Client With a Total Abdominal Hysterectomy (Continued)

Interventions	Rationales
Palpate the abdomen every 4 hours for signs of rigidity. Encourage ambulation.	The abdomen loses its soft quality as it distends with gas. Movement promotes intestinal peristalsis, which moves gas toward the rectum.
Report abdominal discomfort, nausea, abdominal distention, or diminished or faint bowel sounds to the physician.	Elimination of intestinal gas may be facilitated by using a rectal tube, which must be medically ordered.

Evaluation of Expected Outcome

Abdomen is soft; bowel sounds are normal; client passes flatus rectally.

PC: Vaginal Hemorrhage

Expected Outcome: The nurse will monitor to detect, manage, and minimize hemorrhage.

Interventions	Rationales
Record the number of perineal pads used.	Counting perineal pads facilitates the assessment of blood loss.
Assess blood pressure and pulse every 15 minutes if bleeding seems severe.	Blood pressure falls and pulse rate increases in relation to loss of circulating blood volume.
Record the color of bloody drainage.	Bright red bleeding correlates with arterial bleeding; dark red blood is more likely venous.
Report excessive bleeding or passage of blood clots to the physician.	A blood transfusion or an increased rate of IV fluid may be necessary to maintain blood volume to prevent shock.

Evaluation of Expected Outcome

Client has normal postoperative vaginal drainage; vital signs are within normal range.

Nursing Diagnosis: Risk for Disturbed Body Image related to misconceptions about physical and sexual consequences of hysterectomy

Expected Outcome: Client will maintain an accurate body image after surgery.

Interventions	Rationales
Give client an opportunity to verbalize perceptions and fears.	Clients are less apt to discuss personal problems or fears if they sense that the nurse does not have time to engage in a discussion.
Clarify that a hysterectomy does not physically compromise libido or ability to achieve orgasm or cause premature aging, depression, or masculinization.	Many women accept common myths and misperceptions as fact.

Evaluation of Expected Outcome

Client has a realistic understanding of the physical outcomes of surgery.

Nursing Diagnosis: Deficient Knowledge related to onset of menopause secondary to removal of ovaries in premenopausal women

Expected Outcome: Client will understand the consequences that accompany removal of the ovaries and methods for stabilizing reproductive hormone levels.

Interventions	Rationales
Discuss the physiologic effects of surgical menopause.	Besides the cessation of menstruation, hot flashes, emotional irritability, predisposition to osteoporosis, and increased cardiac risks also accompany some types of hysterectomy.
Explain the action, frequency of administration, side effects, and benefits of HRT.	Providing exogenous hormones reduces the deficit of endogenous hormone production.

Evaluation of Expected Outcome

Client accurately paraphrases health teaching related to surgical menopause.

Client and Family Teaching

Depending on the client's treatment, the teaching plan includes some or all of the following:

- Take any prescribed medications as ordered. Seek care if adverse drug effects occur.
- Avoid heavy lifting, sexual intercourse, vigorous physical exercise, and douching until permitted by the physician.
- Ambulate at intervals and avoid sitting in one position for a prolonged period.
- Clean the incision as directed.
- Seek medical care if any of the following signs and symptoms occurs: fever; redness, swelling, pain, or drainage of the incision; vaginal discharge that has a foul odor; vaginal bleeding; pain in the chest, abdomen, or legs.
- Avoid constipation and straining to have a bowel movement. Drink plenty of fluids. If constipation occurs, contact the physician.

OVARIAN CYSTS AND BENIGN OVARIAN TUMORS

A cyst is a membranous sac filled with fluid, cells, or both. Ovarian cysts, which are benign, are filled with fluid. Benign ovarian tumors are noncancerous growths of solid tissue.

Pathophysiology and Etiology

The exact etiologic mechanism for the variety of ovarian cysts and tumors is essentially unknown, but endocrine dysfunction has been implicated in some types. Follicular cysts are thought to develop when a ripening ovum fails to be released. Another type forms when the corpus luteum fails to regress after ovulation and continues to produce progesterone. Chocolate cysts are secondary to endometriosis. Ovarian cysts and benign tumors tend to affect menstruation and fertility, depending on the specific type. Some benign tumors have a potential to become malignant (Porth, 2008).

Assessment Findings

The client may experience pressure in the lower abdomen, backache, menstrual irregularities, and pain, which can be mistaken for appendicitis, ureteral stone, or other abdominal disorders. Clients with tumors associated with or influenced by hypothalamic, pituitary, or adrenal hormones can develop hirsutism (growth of facial hair), atrophy of the breasts, and sterility.

Tumors and cysts may be detected during a pelvic examination. Ultrasonography and laparoscopy are used to determine tumor size. Surgery is the only means for confirming a diagnosis of a benign tumor or cyst.

Medical and Surgical Management

Some ovarian cysts and benign tumors require no treatment or are treated with oral contraceptives to provide symptomatic relief. If the cyst ruptures, surgery, which can entail complete **oophorectomy** (removal of the ovary), oophorocystectomy (removal of the cystic tissue) only, or a **salpingo-oophorectomy** (removal of the ovary and fallopian tube), is required.

Nursing Management

The nurse explains measures for relieving menstrual discomfort and provides referrals to support groups that are devoted to infertile women. The preoperative preparation and postoperative management are the same as for any client having abdominal surgery and a general anesthetic (see Chap. 14). After surgery, some women develop abdominal distention, which is relieved by ambulating, inserting a rectal tube, or applying an abdominal binder. The nurse informs the client who has had surgery but not a hysterectomy to continue having regular gynecologic examinations and Pap tests because she is still at risk for uterine cancer.

CANCER OF THE OVARY

Although other types of female reproductive system cancers occur with greater incidence, ovarian tumors are the leading cause of death from gynecologic malignancies (American Cancer Society, 2008). Until recently, tumors of the ovary have been lethal largely because they present with nonspecific symptoms and therefore frequently are far advanced and inoperable by the time they are diagnosed.

Pathophysiology and Etiology

It is believed that some ovarian tumors have a hereditary link and that others arise from ovarian cysts. Recent research has shown that the more times a woman ovulates during her lifetime, the greater the risk of ovarian cancer. Women who are nulliparous, those with a family history of ovarian cancer, and those who have been diagnosed with other types of cancer such as endometrial, colon, or breast cancer tend to develop ovarian cancer more often than others.

Malignant tumors of the ovary are classified according to the type of cell from which they originate. Most are epithelial, followed by germ cell (an ovum) tumors. Other types are very rare.

Assessment Findings

In the beginning, clients experience vague lower abdominal discomfort. As the tumor grows larger, urinary frequency and urgency may develop because of pressure on the bladder. Later, ascites, weight loss, severe pain, and gastrointestinal symptoms occur. A mass may be felt during a pelvic examination. Many physicians believe that ovarian enlargement found on pelvic examination requires surgical exploration.

Laboratory studies measuring tumor marker antigens, such as alpha-fetoprotein, carcinoembryonic antigen, and CA 125, are ordered. Transvaginal and transabdominal ultrasound and Doppler imaging of ovarian vessels are used in an effort to detect early-stage ovarian cancer. A breakthrough in detecting early-stage ovarian cancer occurred in 2002 with the development of proteomic technology, the ability to study proteins inside cells. Proteomic technology uses artificial intelligence computer software to identify patterns of proteins. These methods are being used to detect patterns indicating ovarian cancer in serum blood samples. In the initial research, proteomic technology correctly detected early stage I ovarian cancer in all affected women in the sample study (National Cancer Institute, 2007). An abdominal CT scan, proctoscopy, barium study, chest radiograph, and IVP are performed to detect metastasis to other areas. A positive diagnosis is made by microscopic examination.

Medical and Surgical Management

Preventive measures recommended to at-risk populations include having at least two full-term pregnancies followed by breast-feeding and using oral contraceptives for more than 5 years. In addition, prophylactic bilateral oophorectomy is recommended for women at risk for hereditary ovarian cancer syndrome after they reach 35 years of age or after childbearing is completed. After diagnosis of a malignant tumor, the diseased ovary is removed. A total hysterectomy may or may not be performed. If both ovaries are removed, HRT may be prescribed.

Surgical treatment, which reduces the tumor load, is followed by chemotherapy. The current antineoplastic drug regimen of choice is a combination of cisplatin (Platinol) and paclitaxel (Taxol), although combinations of other drugs such as cyclophosphamide (Cytoxan) and carboplatin (Paraplatin) may be used as alternatives (National Institutes of Health, 2008; Garcia, 2007). The use of radiation therapy rather than chemotherapy is controversial at this time.

Nursing Management

Only a small percentage of clients with malignant tumors of the ovary survive 5 or more years despite intensive treatment. The emotional effects of the diagnosis require support and understanding on the part of the nurse and other members of the health team. Many of these clients are young, the treatment is difficult, and the prognosis is poor for those diagnosed with late-stage ovarian cancer. Women who are diagnosed in the early stage of the disease, when the cancer is still confined to the ovary, have a much better prognosis; more than 90% live 5 years or more after diagnosis. Unfortunately, only 19% of ovarian cancers are identified early (The New York Times Health Guide, 2008).

Preoperative and postoperative nursing care is similar to that of other clients who undergo abdominal surgery (see preoperative and postoperative care in the nursing management discussion of the client with cervical and endometrial cancer). See Nursing Care Plan 53-1 for nursing diagnoses and interventions for the client undergoing a total abdominal hysterectomy.

CANCER OF THE VAGINA

Cancer of the vagina is rare and usually seen in women older than 40 years of age.

Pathophysiology and Etiology

The incidence of vaginal cancer is higher among women infected with HPV, a sexually transmitted microorganism (see Chap. 56), and among those who use a pessary but neglect to remove and clean it. Studies have shown a relationship between the development of vaginal carcinoma in (young) adult female offspring whose mothers were administered DES early in their pregnancy. DES no longer is used to treat problems associated with pregnancy.

The upper posterior third of the vagina is the most common site of vaginal cancer. Metastatic lesions may occur in the cervix or adjacent areas such as the vulva, uterus, or rectum.

Assessment Findings

Abnormal vaginal bleeding usually is the predominant symptom. Dyspareunia also may occur. Visual examination of the vaginal canal discloses the lesion. A biopsy then confirms the diagnosis.

Medical and Surgical Management

Cancer of the vagina is treated according to the extent of the tumor. Most clients undergo laser photovaporization treatments, although a partial or total vaginectomy is a possibility. Radiation therapy also is used. Complications, such as fistulas and bleeding, arise from the tumor itself and from radiation therapy. These complications are difficult to correct and control.

Nursing Management

The poor prognosis and complications associated with vaginal cancer and its treatment present a nursing challenge. The nurse keeps the client as comfortable as possible and changes bedding and clothing frequently. Urine or fecal drainage from fistulas make odors difficult to control, but a room deodorizer and frequent gown and linen changes help.

The nurse encourages all women who took DES during a pregnancy to tell their daughters and advise them to have complete gynecologic examinations regularly. After treatment, clients may profit from techniques to reduce the discomfort during sexual intercourse that is caused by narrowing of the vagina. Some suggestions include using K-Y gel or prolonged foreplay to lubricate the vagina, having one's sex partner dilate the vagina with fingers before penetration with the penis, and taking a slower pace during sexual activities.

CANCER OF THE VULVA

Cancer of the vulva, the external female genitalia, is relatively rare. It usually occurs in women older than 60 years of age, but cases among younger women have arisen recently. Vulvar cancer is highly curable when diagnosed in an early stage.

Pathophysiology and Etiology

Infections with carcinogenic agents such as HPV and herpes simplex virus type 2 increase the risk of vulvar cancer (see Chap. 56). These infections are treatable but not curable, which explains the lifelong threat of genital cancer.

Atypical cells, which appear as white or pigmented raised patches, most commonly involve the labia majora. The cancer also occurs in the labia minora, clitoris, and Bartholin glands. Because of the widespread presence of the viruses in the vulvar epithelium and their potential for carcinogenesis, multiple cancerous sites may coexist or occur again after treatment. Although the cancer is slow growing, it can and does spread to the vagina, urethra, and anus through regional lymph nodes.

Assessment Findings

Pruritus and genital burning are the most frequent early symptoms. Later, a bloody discharge, enlarged lymph nodes, ulceration and swelling of the vulva, and a visible mass develop. Eventually, the client experiences severe pain. As the cancer ulcerates, a bloody and sometimes purulent discharge from the vulva occurs.

The lesions are first noted during inspection of the genitalia. Application of acetic acid tends to accentuate the abnormal tissue. Biopsy confirms the diagnosis.

Medical and Surgical Management

Vulvectomy (removal of the vulva) with or without the removal of lymph nodes (radical vulvectomy) is the standard for treatment. Laser photovaporization is being used as an alternative, however, to preserve the cosmetic appearance of the genitalia, especially if the lesions do not exceed a depth of 3 mm. The efficacy of preoperative chemotherapy plus radiation before surgery for advanced disease is being investigated.

When cancer of the vulva is inoperable, wet dressings and perineal irrigations with a deodorizing solution help control the odor and the infection that usually occur in the ulcerating neoplasm. Narcotic analgesics usually are necessary in the terminal stage of the disease.

▶ **Stop, Think, and Respond Exercise 53-3**

Which type of pelvic reproductive cancer has the highest incidence? Which reproductive cancer has the highest mortality rate?

Nursing Process for the Client With Cancer of the Vulva Undergoing Surgery

Assessment

Determine the location and level of discomfort or pain. Check for signs of infection and thrombophlebitis as well as the status of peripheral circulation and integrity of the skin. Discuss the client's perception of body image and explore concerns she may have about sexual function.

Diagnosis, Planning, and Interventions

Offer emotional support while the client awaits the results of the biopsy. If surgery is the selected method of treatment, provide appropriate preoperative and postoperative care.

Before surgery, instruct the client to begin initial skin preparation by washing the lower abdomen, genitalia, perineum, and upper thighs with antibacterial soap for several days before surgery. On the day of surgery, insert a Foley catheter and provide standard teaching for deep breathing and leg exercises. Antibiotic therapy may begin before the operative procedure.

Plan measures to prevent postoperative complications, manage pain, relieve edema in the lower extremities, prevent wound infection, and preserve and restore skin integrity. In addition, intervene therapeutically to assist the client in maintaining an acceptable body image, preparing for the resumption of sexual function,

and performing self-care activities after discharge. Refer to perioperative standards of care in Chapter 14.

Other nursing measures include, but are not limited to the following diagnoses, expected outcomes, and interventions:

▶ Acute Pain related to tissue trauma and swelling

▶ **Expected Outcome:** Pain will be relieved to a tolerable level within 30 minutes of a nursing intervention.

- Administer prescribed analgesics liberally. *Pain is best relieved by administering analgesia before pain becomes severe.*
- Place an air or egg crate mattress on the bed. *These mattresses promote comfort by distributing pressure more evenly.*
- Place client in a semirecumbent position. *It relieves pressure on the sutures.*
- Modify the client's position at least every 2 hours. *Any position becomes uncomfortable if maintained for a prolonged period.*
- Use as many pillows as necessary to promote comfort. *Pillows support, elevate, and relieve pressure.*
- When in a lateral position, bend and support the upper leg on pillows. *Bending and supporting the upper leg in a lateral position prevents tension on the operative area.*

▶ PC: Thrombophlebitis

▶ **Expected Outcome:** The nurse will monitor to detect, manage, and minimize risk for the development of thrombophlebitis.

- Assess for and report calf pain, swelling, or tenderness. *Calf pain, swelling, or tenderness indicates the possible development of a blood clot.*
- Remove and reapply antithrombotic stockings or pneumatic leg-compression device at regular intervals each day. *Compression of valves in the veins prevents venous stasis.*
- Ensure that the client performs leg exercises while in bed and ambulates as tolerated. *Skeletal muscle contraction promotes venous circulation.*
- Administer prescribed anticoagulants; monitor laboratory tests for therapeutic levels. *Anticoagulants interfere with blood clotting; dosages of anticoagulants are based on assessments of the partial thromboplastin time, prothrombin time, or international normalized ratio.*

▶ Ineffective Tissue Perfusion related to compromised lymphatic and venous circulation secondary to excision of lymph nodes and ligation of blood vessels

▶ **Expected Outcome:** Dependent edema will be absent by discharge.

- Elevate the lower extremities whenever possible. *Gravity promotes venous and lymphatic circulation.*
- Dangle the client's legs the evening of surgery and assist to ambulate daily. *Skeletal muscle movement that is required for ambulation promotes venous circulation.*

▶ Risk for infection related to compromised skin integrity in close proximity to the rectum

▶ **Expected Outcome:** Client will remain free of infection.

- Perform conscientious hand hygiene before caring for the wound. *Hand hygiene is the best method for preventing the transmission of microorganisms.*
- Inspect and change perineal dressing following principles of asepsis. *Using aseptic principles reduces the potential for transmitting pathogens.*
- Cleanse the anus with moistened antiseptic wipes after bowel elimination. *Stool contains pathogens that can be introduced into the wound.*
- Empty surgical drains and catheter drainage bag aseptically. *A tube or catheter provides a portal through which microorganisms can enter the body.*
- Observe and record the appearance and amount of drainage. *Evidence of purulent drainage suggests infection.*

▶ **Impaired Skin Integrity** related to unresolved tissue healing

▶ **Expected Outcome:** The wound will become approximated.

- Irrigate the wound with sterile saline, hydrogen peroxide, or a medically prescribed antiseptic solution at least three times daily. *Removing wound debris facilitates healing.*
- Dry the wound with a heat lamp or hair dryer. *Pressure or friction increases pain and can disrupt healing.*
- Give warm sitz baths after sutures have been removed. *Sitz baths increase circulation to the area and promote healing.*
- Cover intact skin with a transparent or air and water occlusive dressing. *Intact skin is protected from contact with moist drainage.*
- Support surgical drain during periods of ambulation. *An unsupported drain may be displaced from internal areas of the wound.*
- Explore the need to refer the client for home health nursing. *Home health nursing services are necessary if family or a significant member is unavailable for postdischarge wound care.*

▶ **Risk for Disturbed Body Image** related to emotional distress secondary to amputated genitalia

▶ **Expected Outcome:** Client will maintain a positive self-image.

- Ensure privacy when assessing the wound or carrying out treatment measures. *Privacy demonstrates respect for the client's dignity.*
- Keep the client clean, odor free, and well groomed. *Attention to personal appearance promotes feeling attractive.*
- Listen when the client expresses emotions regarding her changed appearance. *Verbalizing feelings relieves stress.*
- Encourage significant others to be genuinely attentive and to express acceptance through hand holding, sitting close, or other actions. *Touching is a nonverbal method for expressing continued regard for one another.*

▶ **Risk for Sexual Dysfunction** related to anatomic changes in external genitalia

▶ **Expected Outcome:** Client will find satisfactory techniques for experiencing sexual intimacy.

- Act as a liaison for information between the client and her surgeon as to the physical consequences of surgery. *Clients sometimes are reluctant to discuss sexual issues.*
- Role play or encourage discussions regarding sexual issues between the client and significant other. *Role playing can help client communicate about sensitive topics.*
- Explore the idea of using a vaginal dilator, liberal lubrication, and a side-lying position for intercourse once healing is complete. *Alternative sexual practices promote comfort and pleasure during sexual activities.*
- Suggest that the client seek a referral from her physician to a sexual counselor if sexual issues are unresolved. *Sexual counselors have expertise in helping clients resolve problems with sexuality.*

Evaluation of Expected Outcomes

Expected outcomes are that pain is reduced or eliminated. The calves are of normal size and not tender. There is no dependent edema. Temperature is normal, with no wound tenderness or purulent drainage; white blood cell count is normal. The wound heals and the skin becomes intact. The client interacts with others and resumes previous lifestyle activities. The client can experience sexual intimacy.

Before discharge, instruct the client on the following measures for self-care:

- Expect that wound healing may take as long as 6 months.
- Elevate the legs and wear antiembolic stockings to reduce dependent edema in the lower extremities.
- Eat a high-protein diet with sources of vitamin C to promote healing.
- Try to stand and straddle the toilet when attempting to void after the catheter is removed in 7 to 10 days so that urine is directed into the toilet rather than down the leg or perineum.
- After urination, cleanse the periurethral area with water or normal saline in a plastic container with a spout.
- Continue to take the prescribed stool softener after discharge.
- Take a sitz bath using a portable basin after each bowel movement.
- Report any unusual odor, fever, fresh bleeding, separation of the wound margin, inability to void or constipation, and perineal pain.

CRITICAL THINKING EXERCISES

1. What suggestions are helpful to help a young adult female maintain reproductive health?

2. A client reports that she becomes very moody every month and wonders if she has premenstrual syndrome (PMS). What additional information should the nurse obtain?

3. The parent of a young female asks why the cervical cancer vaccine is recommended for females from 9 through 26 years of age. What information can the nurse provide?

4. A woman who experiences severe dysmenorrhea has been diagnosed with endometriosis. What questions would you anticipate that this client may ask?

NCLEX-STYLE REVIEW QUESTIONS

1. A client has repeated vaginal infections. The symptoms suggest that the client has candidiasis caused by the yeastlike fungus, *Candida albicans*, and tests confirm that the infectious organism is indeed *C. albicans*. Which medical regimen is recommended?
   1. A nonprescription antifungal medication
   2. A prescription oral penicillin
   3. A prescription broad-spectrum antibiotic
   4. A vaginal douche of a mild soap solution

2. Three days after going to the clinic, a client who has become anemic due to menorrhagia, phones the health office and explains that she is having difficulty swallowing the large iron capsule. The physician orders a liquid iron preparation. The nurse instructs the client about administration of the liquid iron preparation. Which instruction is most appropriate?
   1. Mix it with milk.
   2. Use a straw.
   3. Pour it in a paper cup.
   4. Take it over ice.

3. A client with a vaginal fistula is at risk for low self-esteem because of leaking urine and stool and accompanying odors. Which of the following instructions from the nurse would be most helpful to address these problems?
   1. Wear disposable, absorbent incontinence briefs.
   2. Avoid the use of commercial deodorizers at home.
   3. Abstain from sexual intercourse.
   4. Avoid frequent douches.

4. Internal radiation therapy is used to treat a client with cancer of the cervix. An applicator containing radioactive material is inserted into the client's vagina. Because the client is receiving this type of radiation therapy, the nurse is most correct in adding which nursing order to the client's plan of care?
   1. Elevate the head of the bed to 90 degrees.
   2. Maintain strict bed rest.
   3. Offer nourishment every 2 hours.
   4. Weigh daily before breakfast.

5. A client with ovarian cancer is receiving antineoplastic chemotherapy following a total hysterectomy. Because many antineoplastic drugs affect bone marrow function, which laboratory test is most important to monitor for client safety?
   1. Complete blood count
   2. Differential cell count
   3. Total leukocyte count
   4. Mean cell volume

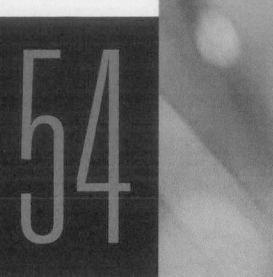

54

Caring for Clients with Breast Disorders

Words To Know

breast abscess
breast cancer
breast reconstruction
fibroadenoma
fibrocystic breast disease
lumpectomy
mammoplasty
mastalgia
mastectomy
mastitis
mastopexy
metastasis
modified radical mastectomy
partial (or segmental) mastectomy
reduction mammoplasty
sentinel lymph node mapping
simple (or total) mastectomy
subcutaneous mastectomy

Learning Objectives

On completion of this chapter, you will be able to:

1. List four signs and symptoms common in breast disorders.
2. Name two infectious and inflammatory breast disorders and explain how they are acquired.
3. Discuss health teaching that may help prevent or eliminate infectious and inflammatory breast disorders.
4. Compare and contrast two benign breast disorders.
5. Name groups at high risk for developing breast cancer.
6. List common signs and symptoms of breast cancer.
7. Describe four methods for treating cancer, including six surgical techniques used to remove a malignant breast tumor.
8. Give two criteria that are used when selecting a mastectomy procedure.
9. Name a serious complication of breast cancer treatment.
10. Discuss the nursing management of clients who undergo surgical treatment for breast cancer.
11. List four sites to which breast cancer commonly metastasizes.
12. Describe three elective cosmetic breast procedures for clients with a mastectomy.
13. Describe three cosmetic breast procedures that women with nondiseased breasts may elect.

The breasts are part of the female reproductive system, and they respond to the hormonal cycle associated with ovulation, menstruation, and pregnancy. Their primary function is the production of milk, a process referred to as *lactation*. This chapter discusses common disorders that affect breast tissue, which generally manifest with one or more of the following symptoms: breast tenderness or pain, breast mass, nipple discharge, and change in breast appearance. Also discussed are diagnostic and treatment methods and nursing management.

INFECTIOUS AND INFLAMMATORY BREAST DISORDERS

MASTITIS

Mastitis, an inflammation of breast tissue, can occur in one or both breasts. It is most common in women who are breast-feeding. Although mastitis can occur at any time, it is most common during the 2nd or 3rd week postpartum.

Pathophysiology and Etiology

Breast inflammation is caused or contributed to by one or more plugged lactiferous ducts or an infectious agent that enters through cracked or fissured nipples. Ducts become plugged as a consequence of infrequent nursing, failure to alternate breasts at each feeding, or an infant nursing weakly.

Lactating breasts have an elaborate blood supply and ductal system that easily supports microbial growth. If an infection develops, the most common causative microorganism is *Staphylococcus aureus*, which often is resistant to antibiotic therapy. The infectious process results from inadequate maternal hand washing, an infant infected by microorganisms on the hands of nursery personnel, or by organisms on the mother's skin.

Assessment Findings

Fever and malaise accompany breast tenderness, pain, and redness. The breast later becomes swollen, firm, and hard. A crack in the nipple or areola develops, and the axillary lymph nodes enlarge. Rarely a breast abscess will develop. A culture and sensitivity test on expressed breast milk identifies the infectious agent.

Medical Management

Drug therapy generally involves 10 days of an antibiotic from the penicillin group based on culture and sensitivity tests. For those clients allergic to penicillin, the physician may substitute erythromycin (E-mycin, Ilosone, Erythrocin). For organisms that are penicillin resistant, oxacillin (Prostaphlin), cephalosporins such as cefazolin (Kefzol), which are safe for women to take while breast-feeding, or vancomycin (Vancocin) are given. Analgesics are prescribed for pain. Heat also can be applied locally. To prevent engorgement and to maintain lactation, the breasts are emptied using a breast pump.

Nursing Management

The nurse assists with taking the health history (which includes identifying allergies to antibiotics), prepares the client for a physical examination, and collects the specimen of breast milk using Standard Precautions and aseptic principles. Client teaching includes information for self-administering antibiotic medications, principles of medical asepsis, and techniques to promote comfort and temporary alternatives to breast-feeding. Specific instructions to the client include the following:

- Take antibiotics as prescribed for the entire treatment period.
- Report side effects from the medication such as rash, gastrointestinal upset, and opportunistic infections in the mouth or vagina.
- Perform scrupulous hand hygiene before touching the breast.
- Bathe or shower regularly and apply lotion to dry or cracked nipples.
- Wear a supportive brassiere.
- Avoid wearing breast shields, which trap breast milk and moisture around the nipple.
- Apply warm soaks to the breast or let warm water from a shower flow over the breast.
- Express milk with a breast pump until the infection is resolved sufficiently to resume breast-feeding.

BREAST ABSCESS

A **breast abscess** is a localized collection of pus in breast tissue.

Pathophysiology and Etiology

An abscess occurring in the breast is most frequently a complication of postpartum mastitis. Purulent exudate accumulates in a confined, local area of breast tissue. *S. aureus* again is the most common cause.

Assessment Findings

The client experiences the signs and symptoms of mastitis; in the case of an abscess, however, pus may drain from the nipple. A physical examination of the breast determines diagnosis. A culture and sensitivity of nipple drainage identifies the infecting microorganism and indicates to which antibiotics it is sensitive.

Medical and Surgical Management

The client usually is hospitalized and placed on contact isolation precautions because the soiled dressings are highly infectious. The client is started on intravenous (IV) antibiotic therapy. The abscess may be incised, drained, and packed.

Nursing Management

The nurse removes and reapplies dressings following aseptic principles. To avoid irritating the skin from frequent removal of tape, the nurse uses a binder to hold the dressing in place. He or she applies zinc oxide to the surrounding skin to avoid maceration from irritating drainage or wound compresses. To reduce swelling, the nurse supports the arm and shoulder with pillows. He or she instructs the client not to shave axillary hair on the side with the abscess until healing is complete.

The mother who is temporarily separated from her newborn needs emotional support. The nurse helps the client to pump the client's breasts to remove milk and prevent engorgement. If the mother decides to terminate breast-feeding, the nurse applies a tight-fitting brassiere.

BENIGN BREAST LESIONS

FIBROCYSTIC BREAST DISEASE

Fibrocystic breast disease, also called *mammary dysplasia* (abnormal development of breast tissue) or *chronic cystic mastitis*, is a benign breast condition that affects women primarily between the ages of 30 and 50 years.

Pathophysiology and Etiology

Fibrocystic disease results from hormonal changes during the menstrual cycle. The use of caffeine and nicotine also may aggravate the condition.

When fibrocystic disease develops, single or multiple breast cysts appear in one or both breasts (Fig. 54-1). The cysts grow in size and become increasingly tender in proportion to the secretion of estrogen. Cyst formation tends to continue throughout the reproductive years. Some cysts disappear, although others can remain permanently. The condition resolves with menopause.

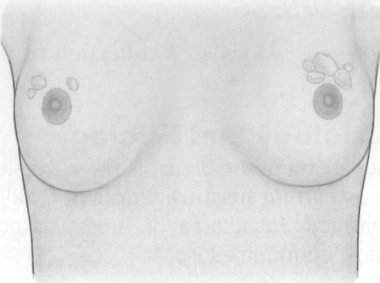

Breast cysts

FIGURE 54-1 Depiction of single and multiple breast cysts.

Although a correlation between fibrocystic disease and breast cancer was reported years ago, current studies have indicated no cause-and-effect relationship between these two conditions. Women with fibrocystic disease, however, may mistake a cancerous mass for a fibrocystic mass and delay medical diagnosis, perform breast self-examination (BSE) less vigorously because of breast tenderness, or fail to palpate a malignant mass disguised by scar tissue from a previous incisional biopsy.

Assessment Findings

Signs and Symptoms

Fibrocystic disease of the breast may produce no symptoms. However, many women report having tender or painful breasts and feeling one or more often multiple lumps within breast tissue. The symptoms are most noticeable just before menstruation and usually abate during menstruation. The size of the cyst often changes with the menstrual cycle, becoming larger before menstruation. Activities, such as weight training, can increase **mastalgia** (breast pain).

Diagnostic Findings

A preliminary diagnosis is made by examination of the breasts. The characteristic breast mass of fibrocystic disease is soft to firm, movable, and unlikely to cause nipple retraction. Fluid from the cysts is aspirated for cytologic examination, or an incisional biopsy is performed. If the results are questionable, mammography and ultrasonography are performed to distinguish a cystic lesion from a solid malignant tumor.

Medical and Surgical Management

Mild discomfort is relieved with an analgesic such as aspirin or ibuprofen (Advil). For severe symptoms, oral contraceptives or danazol (Danocrine), a synthetic androgen, and bromocriptine (Parlodel), a semisynthetic ergot derivative that mimics prolactin inhibitory factor, is prescribed (Drug Therapy Table 54-1).

Pharmacologic Considerations

- When a client is taking danazol (Danocrine), amenorrhea may occur, especially with higher doses. Treatment with danazol for fibrocystic disease usually continues for 4 to 6 months and may continue up to 9 months, if necessary, to eliminate cystic lesions. Inform the client to notify the healthcare provider if regular menses do not resume within 90 days after discontinuing the drug.

Occasionally, one or more cysts are removed surgically. Widespread disease that causes severe discomfort is treated with **partial or segmental mastectomy** (surgical procedure to remove part of the breast, axillary lymph nodes, pectoralis major and minor muscles, and in some instances, sternal lymph nodes). Care is taken to preserve the areola to provide a cosmetic appearance to the breast after surgery.

Nursing Management

The nurse obtains a health history and asks focused questions about the characteristics and timing of symptoms in relation to the menstrual cycle. During diagnostic examinations, the nurse prepares and supports the client, labels tissue or fluid specimens, and arranges for laboratory analysis.

The nurse teaches the client with fibrocystic disease to:

- Perform BSE using the same technique each time while becoming familiar with the feel and location of cystic masses.
- Schedule a breast examination with a physician every 6 months or whenever a new or unusual lump develops.
- Follow the guidelines of the National Cancer Institute (NCI) concerning mammography (see Chap. 52). The NCI is the lead agency for cancer research in the United States.
- Wear a well-fitting, supportive brassiere day and night.
- Take mild analgesics or prescription medications according to label directions.
- Apply cold compresses to the breasts when symptomatic.
- Avoid smoking, coffee, chocolate, and caffeinated soft drinks.
- Restrict activities that may cause trauma to the breasts such as playing soccer or other sports in which the breasts are unprotected.
- Consult with the physician about taking vitamin E supplement or oil of evening primrose (an herbal preparation), which some clients have found helpful.

FIBROADENOMA

A **fibroadenoma** is a solid, benign breast mass composed of connective and glandular tissue. This type of breast lesion usually occurs in women during late adolescence and early adulthood, but occasionally is found in older women.

Pathophysiology and Etiology

The cause of fibroadenomas is unknown. There may be a hormonal influence, however, because the mass grows during pregnancy and shrinks after menopause.

Classically, the benign tumor is a single nodule that grows slowly in nonpregnant women until it reaches a fixed, stable size. It usually does not enlarge and regress with each menstrual cycle, like those in fibrocystic disease, and it too is not considered precancerous.

Assessment Findings

A fibroadenoma presents as a painless, nontender lump in the breast. The lesion usually is encapsulated, mobile, and

DRUG THERAPY TABLE 54-1 Agents For Severe Fibrocystic Disease

Drug Category and Examples	Mechanism of Action	Side Effects	Nursing Considerations
Synthetic Androgen danazol (Danocrine)	Decreases estrogen and progesterone levels by suppressing follicle-stimulating hormone and luteinizing hormone	Acne, deepened voice, weight gain, flushing, vaginitis, enlarged clitoris, nervousness, emotional lability, fluid retention, headache, fatigue, liver dysfunction	Arrange for periodic history and physical exam; long-term use increases chances of side effects and medical supervision is required. Cancer should be ruled out before treatment is initiated. Client should begin taking the hormone during her menstrual period to ensure she is not pregnant. Instruct client to use a nonhormonal form of birth control. Inform client of possible side effects, that masculinizing can occur, and to report any unusual developments.
Progestins medroxyprogesterone (Provera, Amen)	Hinders estrogen's effect on breast tissue	Breakthrough bleeding, spotting, amenorrhea, rash, acne, weight gain, edema, depression, thrombophlebitis, migraine, loss of vision, photosensitivity	Arrange for periodic history and physical exam as noted above. Have client mark drug administration days on the calendar. Inform client of possible side effects, including signs and symptoms of thrombophlebitis and embolism. Instruct client to use a reliable method of birth control and sunscreen and to report any visual disturbances.
Estrogen and Progesterone Combinations estradiol and norethindrone (Ortho-Novum 10/11)	Oral contraceptives suppress ovarian secretion of estrogen and oppose estrogen's effect on breast tissue	Headache, dizziness, thromboembolism, nausea, breakthrough bleeding, depression, anxiety	Continued medical supervision is required; arrange for physical examination, Papanicolaou tests, and breast examinations at least yearly. Discuss side effects with client; instruct on signs and symptoms of thrombophlebitis and embolism. Instruct client not to smoke and to report any side effects.
Ergot Derivative bromocriptine (Parlodel)	Binds with prolactin- secreting cells of the anterior pituitary; inhibits the release of prolactin	Nausea, vomiting, diarrhea, constipation, headache, drowsiness, nasal congestion, hypotension	Administer initial dose at bedtime and with meals thereafter. Advise client to change positions slowly and to use a reliable contraceptive. Report any side effects.

firm when palpated. If the size of the mass is large, the breasts may appear asymmetric.

Ultrasound can reveal physical characteristics unique to a fibroadenoma versus malignant mass with a higher degree of accuracy than mammography. In the case of very young women—an atypical age for breast cancer—an excisional biopsy is performed only if the mass changes or becomes larger. If the mass is detected in a woman with a higher risk for developing breast cancer, such as one with a family history or of an older age, a biopsy is performed to confirm that the tissue is indeed benign.

Medical and Surgical Management

Based on the diagnostic findings, the client and her physician decide either to continue to observe the mass or excise it. Surgery involves removal of the benign tumor but not a **mastectomy** (excision of the breast). The client is discharged a few hours after recovery from anesthesia.

Nursing Management

The nurse provides emotional support while the diagnosis is tentative because finding a mass in the breast conjures up fears that it may be malignant. The nurse teaches the client as follows:

- Continue BSE and follow recommendations for mammography.
- Consult a physician if the characteristics of the mass change or if a pregnancy occurs.
- If surgery is performed, the nurse should include the following instructions to the client:
  - Keep the wound clean and covered until the incision heals.
  - Wear a firm, supportive brassiere to reduce incisional discomfort.
  - Follow label directions for taking a mild non-narcotic analgesic to relieve minor pain that may last 1 to 3 days.
  - Contact the surgeon to schedule a postoperative evaluation or call immediately if there is exceptional incisional pain or if swelling, wound drainage, or a fever develops.

MALIGNANT BREAST DISORDERS

CANCER OF THE BREAST

One woman in eight develops **breast cancer**, a mass of abnormal cells (American Cancer Society, 2008a; National Cancer Institute, 2008). The risk for breast cancer in women increases with age. Although breast cancer does occur in men, the male-female ratio is approximately 1:150. In terms of cancer-related deaths in women in the United States, breast cancer is second only to lung cancer. When the disease is discovered and treated early, the 5-year survival rate for small lesions is at least 80%.

Pathology and Pathophysiology

Certain factors appear to increase the risk of breast cancer. Being female, being older than 50 years of age, and having a family history of breast cancer are the most common risk factors. Relatives of women with breast cancer who carry a defective gene (BRCA1 or BRCA2) are very likely to develop breast cancer. Additional factors include exposure to ionizing radiation in childhood or adolescence, previous breast cancer, a history of colon or endometrial cancer, chronic alcohol consumption, early menarche, late menopause, obesity, and having no children or having children after 30 years of age. White women are at higher risk for breast cancer than African American women, but African American women are more likely to die of it. Most of the women diagnosed with breast cancer have none of the identified risk factors except being female or being older than 50 years of age (Mayo Clinic, 2007, National Cancer Institute, 2006).

Each normal breast contains 15 to 20 lobes connected by ducts to smaller lobules (refer to Fig. 52-10). The most common malignancy is ductal carcinoma (80%), followed by infiltrating lobular carcinoma (10%), medullary carcinoma, mucinous carcinoma, tubular ductal carcinoma, and inflammatory breast cancer, the rarest but most aggressive form of breast cancer (American Cancer Society, 2008b). Some malignant breast tumors are hormone dependent, meaning that estrogen or progesterone enhances tumor growth. Regardless of the type or its etiology, untreated cancer spreads elsewhere through the axillary lymph nodes to distant areas such as the lungs and brain.

Assessment Findings
Signs and Symptoms

The primary sign of breast cancer is a painless mass in the breast, most often in the upper outer quadrant (Fig. 54-2). The tumor may have been developing in situ, without invading the surrounding tissue, for as long as 2 years before becoming palpable. Other signs of breast cancer include a bloody discharge from the nipple, a dimpling of the skin over the lesion, retraction of the nipple, peau d'orange (orange peel) appearance of the skin, and a difference in size between the breasts (Fig. 54-3). The lesion may be fixed or movable, and axillary lymph nodes may be enlarged. Many of these signs depend on several factors, such as the type, location, and duration of the tumor.

> ### Gerontologic Considerations
>
> - With age, the breast tissue atrophies, causing pendulous breasts. Breast tissue becomes more fibrotic, which may be palpable or may cause some retraction of the nipple in older women but may not be a sign of cancer. Occasionally, preexisting breast tumors become more evident with age.

Diagnostic Findings

Mammography detects breast lesions earlier than they can be palpated. The radiologist often can differentiate a benign

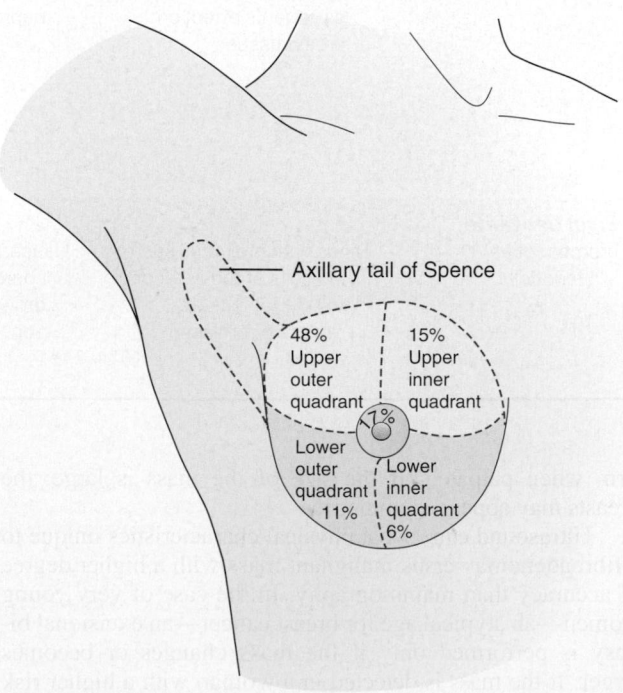

FIGURE 54-2 Locations of primary malignant breast tumors.

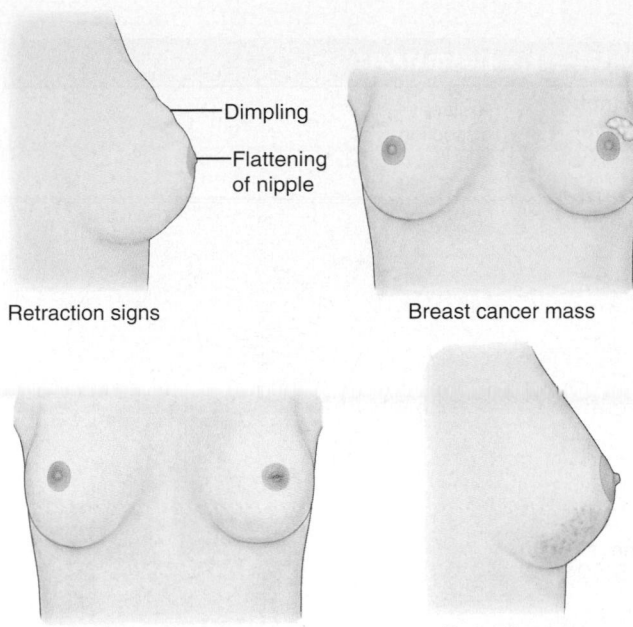

Dimpling

Flattening
of nipple

Retraction signs

Breast cancer mass

Nipple inversion

Peau d'orange

FIGURE 54-3 Signs and symptoms of breast cancer.

tumor from a malignant one on a radiograph. Even in women who are 65 years of age or older, regular mammograms ensure an early diagnosis and a decreased mortality rate from breast cancer. In addition to mammography, the American Cancer Society (ACS) recommends annual breast cancer screening with magnetic resonance imaging (breast MRI) for women at high risk for breast cancer (American Cancer Society, 2007). Biopsy and microscopic cell examination confirm the diagnosis.

Medical and Surgical Management

Treatment depends on the stage (Fig. 54-4) and type of breast tumor. It includes surgery, which may be combined with chemotherapy (including hormone therapy) and radiation therapy. Clinical trials using immunotherapy and vaccines are in progress.

Surgery

Surgery is performed immediately after obtaining the results of the biopsy or shortly thereafter. The type of surgery recommended depends on the stage of the tumor and the client's informed decision about treatment options (Table 54-1). The current trend is to perform the least disfiguring procedure necessary to obtain a favorable prognosis. Compared with more extensive types of mastectomy procedures, breast-conserving surgeries such as lumpectomy, partial mastectomy, and segmental mastectomy followed by radiation have demonstrated equivalent outcomes in terms of survival rate for treatment of early-stage breast cancer (Viani et al., 2007; McCloskey et al., 2006).

A new technique, sentinel lymph node mapping, determines whether complete removal of axillary lymph nodes is necessary. **Sentinel lymph node mapping** involves identifying the first (sentinel) lymph nodes through which the breast cancer cells would spread to regional lymph nodes in the axilla (Fig. 54-5). The sentinel lymph nodes are located by injecting a nuclear isotope around the breast tumor followed by the instillation of blue dye. After the breast tumor

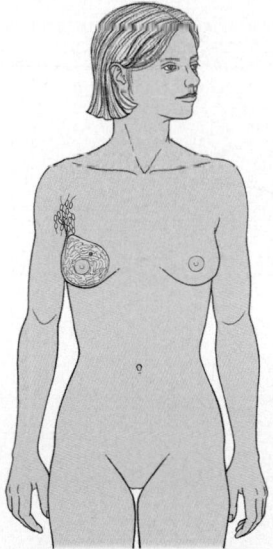

Stage 0: Tumor is confined to the milk duct or lobule.

Stage I: Tumor is less than 2 cm in diameter and confined to the breast.

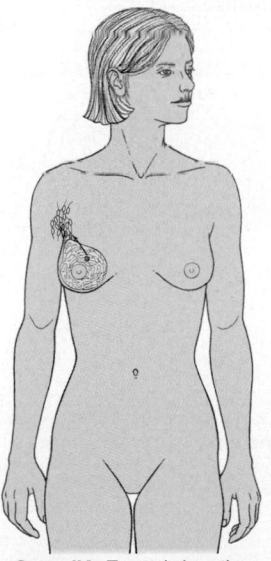

Stage IIA: Tumor is less than 5 cm, or tumor is smaller with 1, 2, or 3 axillary lymph node involvement.

Stage IIB: Tumor is greater than 5 cm. Up to 3 axillary lymph nodes may be involved.

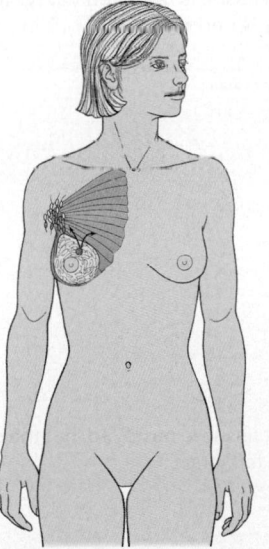

Stage IIIA: Tumor is greater than 5 cm and is confined to 4 to 10 lymph nodes.

Stage IIIB: Tumor, regardless of size, has spread to the chest wall or skin.

Stage IIIC: Tumor of any size with involvement of 10 or more lymph nodes, but no distant metastases.

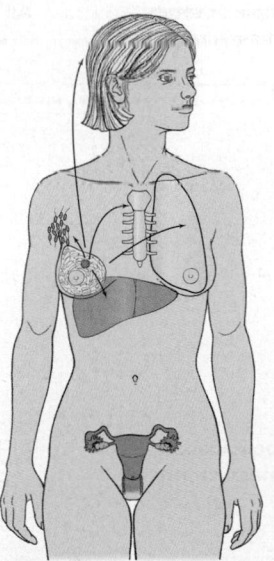

Stage IV: Tumor involves lymph nodes and there are distant metastases.

FIGURE 54-4 Breast cancer stages.

TABLE 54-1 Surgical Procedures for Breast Cancer

PROCEDURE	DESCRIPTION	ILLUSTRATION
Lumpectomy	Only the tumor is removed; some axillary lymph nodes may be excised at the same time for microscopic examination.	Axillary dissection
Partial or segmental mastectomy	The tumor and some breast tissue and some lymph nodes are removed.	
Simple or total mastectomy	All breast tissue is removed. No lymph node dissection is performed.	
Subcutaneous mastectomy	All breast tissue is removed, but the skin and nipple are left intact.	

TABLE 54-1 Surgical Procedures for Breast Cancer (Continued)

PROCEDURE	DESCRIPTION	ILLUSTRATION
Modified radical mastectomy	The breast, some lymph nodes, the lining over the chest muscles, and the pectoralis minor muscle are removed	Pectoralis minor muscle
Radical mastectomy	The breast, axillary lymph nodes, and pectoralis major and minor muscles are removed. In some instances, sternal lymph nodes also are removed.	Pectoralis minor muscle / Pectoralis major muscle

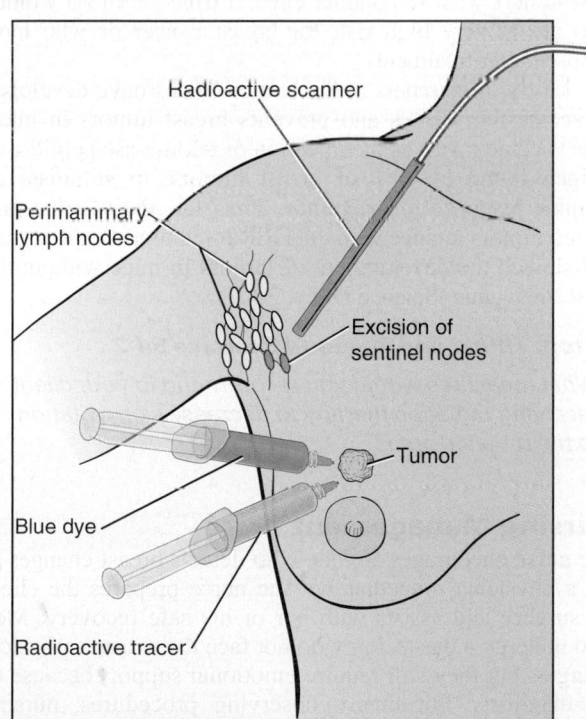

FIGURE 54-5 Sentinel lymph node mapping and excision to detect the spread of breast cancer to regional lymph nodes. The absence of cancer cells in sentinel lymph nodes suggests that the cancer is confined to breast tissue only.

is excised, a Geiger counter is passed over the perimammary tissue to find the area of most intense radioactivity. A small incision is made, and the blue dye is tracked to the sentinel lymph nodes. The sentinel lymph nodes are removed with a minimum of surrounding tissue and examined for cancer cells. An absence of cancer cells in the sentinel lymph nodes suggests that all lymph nodes are free of cancer cells. Validating the lack of lymph node metastasis allows the surgeon to preserve more breast, axillary tissue, and chest muscle. Leaving many normal lymph nodes intact reduces the potential for complications, such as lymphedema (discussed below), delayed wound healing, and altered skin sensation caused by the extensive disruption of lymphatic circulation.

Lymphedema, soft-tissue swelling from accumulated lymphatic fluid (see Chap. 32), occurs in some women after they have undergone breast cancer surgery. The condition, a consequence of removing or irradiating the axillary lymph nodes, is evidenced by temporary or permanent enlargement of the arm and hand on the side of the amputated breast. Impaired lymphatic circulation predisposes to disfigurement, reduced range of motion, heaviness of the limb, skin changes, infection, and, in severe cases, tissue necrosis that may require amputation of the limb.

Depending on circumstances, chemotherapy and chemotherapy plus radiation therapy are common surgical adjuncts. The choice depends on factors such as the type of cancer (e.g., sensitivity to estrogen; stage of the tumor; presence of metastasis; client's age). Bone marrow transplantation may be used if the breast cancer resists other forms of treatment.

> ### ▶ Stop, Think, and Respond Exercise 54-1
>
> *A client has had a modified radical mastectomy (a surgical procedure to remove the breast, some lymph nodes, the lining over the chest muscles, and the pectoralis minor muscle). While trying to teach her how to care for the incision, she avoids looking at the wound. How can you help her cope with the change in body image?*

Chemotherapy

The goal of chemotherapy is to destroy any cancer cells that may have escaped surgical removal. Recent drug research has affected chemotherapy recommendations and proposals for candidates who may benefit from them. Most women with stage I breast cancer who choose surgery only have an excellent prognosis. However, clinical trials suggest that clients with estrogen-sensitive tumors may benefit from the drug tamoxifen (Nolvadex), which blocks the tumor's ability to use estrogen, or a new category of drugs called aromatase inhibitors (AIs). AIs, such as anastrazole (Arimidex), exemestane (Aromasin), and letrozole (Femara), which lower the level of estrogen in the body, have delayed progression of breast cancer longer than tamoxifen. These agents have extended survival and prevented disease recurrence when used as primary adjuvant therapy (National Cancer Institute, 2007, 2006).

One or more of the following drugs are commonly given:

- An antiestrogen drug, such as tamoxifen (Nolvadex), for postmenopausal women whose tumors are hormone dependent. Although tamoxifen has been the mainstay of drug therapy for breast cancer since its approval in 1977, many women develop resistance to the drug; some physicians may prefer to give an AI initially or after a full course of tamoxifen, which generally is prescribed for 5 years (National Cancer Institute, 2008, 2007).
- An antiprogestin drug, mifepristone (RU486), which blocks progesterone-dependent breast cancers as determined by progesterone receptor assay on excised tissue.
- Androgen therapy for advanced breast cancer in postmenopausal women using testolactone (Teslac).
- Single or combined antineoplastic agents, such as cyclophosphamide (Cytoxan), doxorubicin (Adriamycin), 5-fluorouracil (5-FU), methotrexate (Folex), and prednisone (Deltasone). Antineoplastic drugs also are combined with drugs mentioned earlier that influence hormonal physiology.

Radiation Therapy

Radiation therapy can be given before or after surgery. If the surgeon finds that the axillary nodes contain cancer cells, that there is chest wall involvement, or that the tumor is larger than 5 cm, a series of radiation treatments usually is ordered prophylactically, even after a modified radical mastectomy. Side effects of radiation therapy include fatigue, skin redness similar to a bad sunburn, rash, minor discomfort, or pain (see Chap. 11). Some clients develop pneumonitis, rib fractures, and breast fibrosis.

Immunotherapy and Cancer Vaccines

A particular endogenous protein, known as HER2/neu, attaches to receptors in breasts to promote normal cell growth. However, an abundance of HER2/neu results in the growth of aggressive breast tumors. Researchers have developed trastuzumab (Herceptin), a monoclonal antibody that attaches to HER2/neu receptors, slows the growth of the cancerous cells, and reduces their metastases. In some cases, trastuzumab may work only briefly, and drug resistance follows.

Breast cancer vaccines are also being developed. One vaccine, the HER2 peptide E75 (NeuVax), is approaching phase III clinical trials. Thus far, the vaccine has reduced mortality by 50% (Gardner, 2008). A second vaccine, which is believed to be an improvement over NeuVax, is still being tested in mice. It also targets overexpressive HER2/neu cells, with an immune system stimulant. In mice, the vaccine prevented breast cancers from growing without evidence of toxicity. As the clinical trial proceeds, researchers will be monitoring the following: how effectively the vaccine treats HER2/neu–positive breast cancer, whether it restores drug sensitivity in those who have become drug resistant, whether it can prevent aggressive forms of breast cancer, and what specific side effects it has (Karmanos Cancer Institute, 2008).

Other experimental work on additional breast cancer vaccines is ongoing. Researchers in Italy have developed a breast cancer vaccine that stimulates the immune system to attack a protein called mammoglobin-A, which is found in 80% of breast cancer tumors (Narayanan et al., 2004; Quaglino, 2004). In preliminary experiments in mice bred to develop the HER2/neu breast cancer gene, the vaccine prevented 48% of the mice from developing the disease. Researchers want to conduct clinical trials on those women who are at very high risk for breast cancer or who have relapsed after treatment.

Lastly, researchers in the United States have developed a vaccine that delays and prevents breast tumors in mice. This vaccine involves the injection of telomerase peptide, an antigen found in 90% of breast tumors, to stimulate an immune response to the tumor. Thus far, the vaccine prevented tumors in mice with the HER2/neu breast cancer gene and slowed the development of tumors in mice without the HER2/neu gene (Science Daily, 2007).

> ### ▶ Stop, Think, and Respond Exercise 54-2
>
> *What measures would you recommend to your client receiving radiation therapy to decrease skin irritation to the radiated area?*

Nursing Management

The nurse encourages anyone who detects breast changes to see a physician immediately. The nurse prepares the client for surgery and assists with her or his safe recovery. Men who undergo a mastectomy do not face the extreme physical changes, but they still require emotional support because of the diagnosis. For breast-conserving procedures, nursing care focuses on wound management and discharge instructions. Nursing Care Plan 54-1 provides more specific information in managing the care of the client undergoing a modified radical mastectomy.

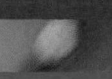

NURSING CARE PLAN 54-1 | The Client Undergoing a Modified Radical Mastectomy

Assessment

- Discuss the client's medical, drug, allergy, and family history.
- Take vital signs and weight.
- Determine the location of the breast lesion.

- Establish what diagnostic tests were performed before admission (if any).
- Discuss information the physician has given the client about the type and extent of surgery.

Nursing Diagnoses: Anxiety and **Fear** related to undergoing an unfamiliar experience and the potential consequences of the disease and its treatment

Expected Outcome: Client will indicate increased emotional comfort.

Interventions	Rationales
Provide an opportunity for the client to express feelings and discuss concerns.	Verbalizing helps the client deal openly with feelings.
Answer all questions; consult with other team members about matters that involve their expertise.	Presenting facts provides the client with reality-based information and reduces exaggerated perceptions.
Collaborate with physician on arranging for a visit from a Reach to Recovery or I Can Cope volunteer sponsored by the American Cancer Society.	People who have recovered from a similar diagnosis and surgery can serve as role models and answer questions from their own personal experiences.
Do not stifle crying; stay with client when emotions are overwhelming.	Crying relieves tension when a person can find no other coping strategy.
Encourage client's significant other or whomever the client turns to for support to remain with client as much and as long as possible.	The presence of others who provide emotional support reduces anxiety.
Keep client informed of the routine that will be followed in preparation for surgery and postoperative care.	Dealing with unexpected events heightens anxiety; knowledge facilitates a sense of control.

Evaluation of Expected Outcome

Anxiety is reduced.

Nursing Diagnosis: Deficient Knowledge related to surgical routines

Expected Outcome: Client will be able to paraphrase the preoperative and postoperative routine.

Intervention	Rationale
Explain that the arm on the surgical side may be elevated and movement away from the body (abduction) may be temporarily restricted.	Elevation reduces edema. Abduction is temporarily restricted until healing progresses.

Evaluation of Expected Outcome

- Client demonstrates an understanding of the type of surgery and potential postsurgical treatment modalities; preoperative preparations; and postoperative management, including coughing, deep breathing, and leg exercises.
- Client openly discusses and asks questions about surgery.

PC: Hemorrhage and **Shock**

Expected Outcome: The nurse will monitor to detect, manage, and minimize hemorrhage and shock.

Interventions	Rationales
Obtain vital signs according to agency routines. Do not take blood pressure on the arm on the side of the mastectomy.	The circulation of blood and lymph can be further compromised if the arm on the side of the mastectomy is used to measure blood pressure, to take blood specimens, or for intravenous (IV) infusions or injections.
Check color and amount of blood loss from the wound and drain, if one is present.	An increase in the volume or change to bright red color suggests excessive or arterial blood loss.
Feel underneath client's side or back for obscured bleeding.	Gravity can cause blood to drain posteriorly.
Administer IV fluids or blood transfusions at the rate prescribed.	Fluid replacement offsets fluid losses.

(care plan continues on page 856)

NURSING CARE PLAN 54-1   The Client Undergoing a Modified Radical Mastectomy (Continued)

Evaluation of Expected Outcome

Bleeding is controlled; shock does not occur.

Nursing Diagnosis: Risk for Ineffective Breathing Pattern and **Ineffective Airway Clearance** related to pain, weak cough, and bulky dressing

Expected Outcome: Client will breathe effortlessly and be well oxygenated.

Interventions	Rationales
Instruct client to deep breathe and cough every 2 hours during waking hours or use an incentive spirometer.	Deep breathing distends alveoli and promotes increased gas diffusion.
Splint incision to reduce discomfort.	Pain or fear of pain interferes with deep breathing.
Administer oxygen as prescribed.	Supplemental oxygen provides a higher concentration than found in room air.
Instruct client to self-administer analgesia before deep breathing and coughing if a patient-controlled analgesia (PCA) pump is available.	Pain is more adequately controlled when an analgesic is given before severe pain develops.

Evaluation of Expected Outcome

Gas exchange is adequate as evidenced by an SpO_2 of 90% or greater and clear lung sounds.

Nursing Diagnosis: Acute Pain related to tissue trauma

Expected Outcome: Discomfort will be controlled within a tolerable level.

Interventions	Rationales
Administer pain medication liberally according to prescribed dose and frequency.	Clients have the right to pain relief.
Avoid giving injections in the arm on the same side as the surgery.	Circulation of blood and lymph is impaired, which can affect the absorption of parenteral medication and increases the potential for infection.
Monitor response to analgesia 30 minutes after administration or more frequently if PCA is in use.	The nurse is obligated to use additional measures to reduce the client's pain until it is at her or his tolerable level.
Pin the tubing of the drain or the drain collection chamber to the client's gown.	Stabilizing the drain helps prevent it from pulling at the insertion site and increasing discomfort.
Implement nursing techniques such as changing positions, relaxation, distraction, and guided imagery (see Chap. 11).	Nonpharmacologic measures supplement or complement analgesia.
Collaborate with the physician if pain control is inadequate.	The nurse consults with the physician to determine possible changes in the type of analgesic, its dose, or frequency.

Evaluation of Expected Outcome

Pain is reduced.

Nursing Diagnoses: Impaired Skin Integrity and **Risk for Infection** secondary to surgical wound

Expected Outcome: The incision will heal; no infection will develop.

Interventions	Rationales
Limit movement, especially abduction, of the arm on the side of surgery until the wound edges are intact.	Activity can disrupt the approximation of the incision.
Inspect the wound for swelling, unusual drainage, odor, redness, or separation of the suture line.	Wound infections are accompanied by signs of inflammation and a delay in healing.
Empty and re-establish negative pressure in closed wound drains at least once per shift.	Negative pressure (suction) pulls fluid from the incisional area, which facilitates healing.
Administer antibiotic therapy as prescribed.	Antibiotics destroy or inhibit the growth of microorganisms.
Monitor the trend in temperature and white blood cell counts.	A fever and leukocytosis suggest that an infection is developing.
Allow the client to shower after the sutures and drains are removed.	Hygiene reduces the number of microorganisms on the skin.

NURSING CARE PLAN 54-1 **The Client Undergoing a Modified Radical Mastectomy** (Continued)

Evaluation of Expected Outcome

Incision heals without complications.

Nursing Diagnosis: Risk for Ineffective Tissue Perfusion (lymphedema) related to compromised flow of lymphatic fluid

Expected Outcome: Soft tissue in the arm on the side of surgery will be comparable with the opposite arm in color, size, and temperature.

Interventions	Rationales
Do not take blood pressures, give injections, administer IV infusions, or have blood drawn from the arm on the side of the mastectomy.	Procedures that affect the circulation in the affected arm can contribute to ineffective tissue perfusion.
Support and elevate the arm on the side of the mastectomy with pillows so it is kept higher than the heart.	Elevation promotes gravity drainage of fluid trapped in the soft tissue.
Place the arm in a sling when the client ambulates initially; eventually the arm can be positioned at the client's side.	A sling prevents stasis of fluid in distal areas of the arm.
Show the client how to squeeze and release a soft rubber ball or a rolled pair of cotton socks several times a day.	Venous blood and lymph circulate with contraction of skeletal muscles.
Remove and reapply an elastic roller bandage from the fingers to the axilla twice a day, or insert the affected arm into a pneumatic sleeve, an air-filled device that mechanically pumps the arm, for a half hour or the prescribed amount of time twice a day.	An elastic roller bandage or pneumatic sleeve compresses the valves in veins to promote circulation.
Assess the hand for swelling, dusky color, delayed nail blanching, coldness, and tingling and report abnormal findings.	The nurse is responsible for reporting abnormal findings to reduce the potential for complications.

Evaluation of Expected Outcome

The circulation is maintained in the operative arm; both arms are of comparable size.

Nursing Diagnosis: Impaired Physical Mobility related to alteration in pectoral chest muscles

Expected Outcome: Client will achieve full range of arm motion.

Interventions	Rationales
Start active exercises of the affected arm on the first or second postoperative day, or later if the physician indicates a need to postpone them (skin grafts may need additional time to heal).	Active exercise reduces the potential for contractures.
Begin with flexing and extending the fingers, wrist, and elbow. Later, encourage the client to use the affected arm to perform oral hygiene, hair combing, and face washing.	Exercise gradually restores the ability to flex, extend, and abduct the arm.
Show the client how to face and "finger-walk" up a wall in the room (see Client and Family Teaching 54-1). Mark the client's progress with masking tape so that the height can be exceeded with subsequent efforts.	Finger-walking increases the ability to raise the arm. Marking progress provides an incentive to meet or exceed heights during previous exercises.
Loop a rope or cord around a shower rod and raise and lower each arm in pulley fashion.	Modification in the technique for performing arm exercises facilitates rehabilitation.
Tie a string or rope to a doorknob and have the client turn the rope in a circular fashion.	Turning a rope promotes circumduction.

Evaluation of Expected Outcome

Client improves the use of the arm and hand of operative side. The client performs postmastectomy exercises.

Nursing Diagnosis: Risk for Injury related to change in center of gravity secondary to extensive removal of chest tissue

Expected Outcome: The client will not fall.

Interventions	Rationales
Assist the client during periods of ambulation.	The nurse supports the client when or if client loses balance.

(care plan continues on page 858)

NURSING CARE PLAN 54-1 The Client Undergoing a Modified Radical Mastectomy (Continued)

Interventions	Rationales
Walk on the client's unaffected side.	The client is more likely to drift toward the side of the body that is heavier.
Instruct the client to keep the shoulders level and the muscles relaxed when walking.	Clients tend to accommodate for the change in the center of gravity by leaning to the side.

Evaluation of Expected Outcome

The client remains injury free.

Nursing Diagnosis: Risk for Dysfunctional Grieving related to loss of breast

Expected Outcome: Client will express grief and deal with losses in an appropriate amount of time.

Interventions	Rationales
Avoid trying to diminish the significance of the loss.	Grief work involves dealing with the reality of a significant loss.
Acknowledge client's grief and reinforce that feeling angry or sad is normal and expected.	Validating client's feelings gives permission for him or her to experience true emotions.
Stay with client and ensure privacy during emotional periods.	The nurse's presence provides support.
Avoid administering prescribed sedatives or tranquilizers as a substitute for spending time with the client.	Ensuring privacy demonstrates respect for the client's dignity. Numbing the mind interferes with grieving.
Encourage sharing with those who can be empathic, such as another breast cancer survivor.	Sharing the significance of a loss with a person who has survived a similar experience provides a bond for healing.

Nursing Diagnoses: Risk for Disturbed Body Image, Ineffective Coping, and **Sexual Dysfunction** related to perceived loss of physical attractiveness and sexual desirability

Expected Outcome: Client will accept body changes, use positive coping strategies, and experience satisfactory sexual activity.

Interventions	Rationales
Suggest that client pad a bra with one or two cotton socks until a prosthesis is fitted in 6 to 8 weeks.	Padding a bra gives the outward appearance that the client has both breasts. Purchasing a prosthetic bra is delayed until the tissue heals.
Inform client that cosmetic breast reconstruction is an option to discuss with the surgeon.	Cosmetic breast reconstruction provides an alternative for simulating natural breast tissue.
Advocate that client and sexual partner openly express to each other how the surgery has affected them emotionally.	Open communication facilitates mutual understanding and acceptance of body change.
Discuss methods for dealing with the removed breast during sexual activities such as using no or low lighting during intercourse or wearing the upper portion of lingerie.	Modifying sexual activities reduces self-consciousness.

Evaluation of Expected Outcomes

Client adjusts to the loss of the breast.

The nurse prepares the client for common side effects of chemotherapy such as nausea, vomiting, changes in taste, alopecia (hair loss), mucositis, dermatitis, fatigue, weight gain, and bone marrow suppression. Some clients also experience mild short-term memory loss and difficulty with thought processes, known as "chemo-brain." It is not known whether this results from chemotherapy or the depression that frequently accompanies a cancer diagnosis. Administering antiemetics and anxiolytic medications before a chemotherapy treatment helps lessen the potential for vomiting. The nurse provides instructions regarding when and how the client should take medications at home to alleviate nausea and mouth sores and to boost the white blood cell or red blood cell

production. If alopecia is likely, the nurse offers the client a list of wig suppliers (usually provided through the ACS). Catalogs from which the client can purchase scarves, turbans, or hats to camouflage hair loss are available through the ACS.

Most clients are not hospitalized long after mastectomy. Therefore, providing early discharge instructions and making arrangements for home care are important interventions. Information that nurses commonly must address with the client includes the following:

- Explain wound and drain care or arrange for home health nursing.
- Assess the availability of family assistance at home.

- Look for and report any signs of infection or impaired wound healing such as drainage or significant pale or dusky appearance to the skin around the incision.
- Provide instructions for performing arm exercises and stress their continuation (Client and Family Teaching 54-1)
- Arrange for follow-up examinations by the surgeon.

- Instruct on the self-administration of prescribed drug therapy.
- Inform that some residual numbness or tingling on the chest wall and the inner side of the arm from the axilla to the elbow may occur and take as long as 1 year to resolve.

Client and Family Teaching 54-1
Performing Arm Exercises Following Surgery for Breast Cancer

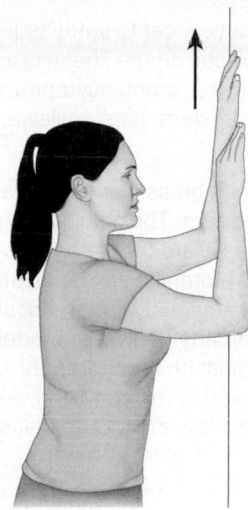

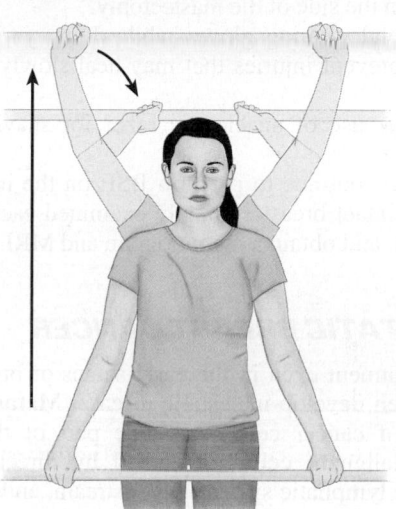

1. *Wall handclimbing.* Stand facing the wall with feet apart and toes as close to the wall as possible. With elbows slightly bent, place the palms of the hand on the wall at shoulder level. By flexing the fingers, work the hands up the wall until arms are fully extended. Then reverse the process, working the hands down to the starting point.

3. *Rod or broomstick lifting.* Grasp a rod with both hands, held about 2 feet apart. Keeping the arms straight, raise the rod over the head. Bend elbows to lower the rod behind the head. Reverse maneuver, raising the rod above the head, then return to the starting position.

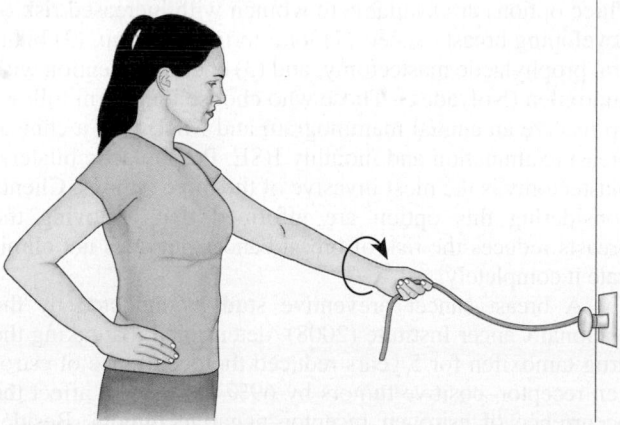

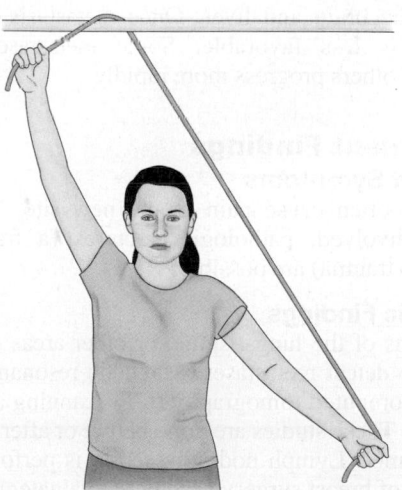

2. *Rope turning.* Tie a light rope to a doorknob. Stand facing the door. Take the free end of the rope in the hand on the side of the surgery. Place the other hand on the hip. With the rope-holding arm extended and held away from the body (nearly parallel with the floor), turn the rope, making as wide swings as possible. Begin slowly at first; speed up later.

4. *Pulley tugging.* Toss a light rope over a shower curtain rod or doorway curtain rod. Stand as nearly under the rope as possible. Grasp an end in each hand. Extend the arms straight and away from the body. Pull the left arm up by tugging down with the right arm, then the right arm up and the left down in a see-sawing motion.

- Suggest the application of cream or lotion to the arm if the skin tends to be dry.
- Explain that in the selection of a prosthesis, one filled with fluid assumes natural contours like the other breast, feels like normal breast tissue, and even radiates body warmth.
- Advise against lifting or carrying objects that weigh more than 15 lb. and making vigorous repetitive movements with the affected arm.
- Discourage sleeping on the affected arm or wearing constrictive clothing that impairs circulation.
- Reinforce that blood pressure measurements, injections, blood donations, and IV infusions are contraindicated in the arm on the side of the mastectomy.
- Recommend wearing gloves while doing yard or housework to prevent injuries that may heal slowly or become infected.
- Advise the use of an electric razor for shaving axillary hair.
- Instruct to continue to perform BSE on the intact breast, have the intact breast clinically examined each year by a physician, and obtain a mammogram and MRI.

METASTATIC BREAST CANCER

Despite treatment even in the early stages of breast cancer, some women develop metastatic disease. **Metastasis** is the migration of cancer cells from one part of the body to another. Malignant cells are spread by direct extension, through the lymphatic system, bloodstream, and cerebrospinal fluid.

Pathophysiology

Lymph nodes most commonly are involved in metastasis, and the skeletal and pulmonary systems may also be involved (in that order). In addition, metastases may be found in the brain and liver. Once metastasis occurs, the prognosis is less favorable. Some metastases progress slowly, but others progress more rapidly.

Assessment Findings

Signs and Symptoms

Metastases often cause pain in the new site. When bone becomes involved, pathologic fractures (a fracture after slight or no trauma) are possible.

Diagnostic Findings

Radiographs of the lungs, spine, or other areas of the body are used to detect metastases. Magnetic resonance imaging (MRI) or computed tomography (CT) scanning also may be performed. These studies are done before or after treating the primary tumor. Lymph node dissection is performed either at the time of breast surgery or later to evaluate metastasis to the lymph nodes draining the breasts.

Medical Management

Treatment aims at providing the greatest period of palliation (relieving symptoms without curing the disease) for the client. It varies with the physician and specific type of metastasis. Large doses of estrogen or testosterone sometimes alleviate the pain, weight loss, and malaise of meta-

static cancer. Intramuscular androgen (testosterone) therapy is used especially when metastases are to bone. All forms of treatment carry the possibility of unpleasant effects and complications. For palliative purposes, radiation therapy may be used to treat regional or distant metastases (especially to bone) or local tumor recurrence of the chest wall. Sometimes surgery, chemotherapy, and radiation are used to slow the growth of the new malignant site.

Pharmacologic Considerations

- Metastases of breast cancer to soft tissue and bone may respond to antineoplastic drugs. These drugs may cause bone marrow depression, granulocytopenia, anemia, nausea, vomiting, hypotension, dermatitis, malaise, diarrhea, and stomatitis.

- In treating clients with breast cancer metastases, pain management is important. The opioid analgesics morphine and fontanyl (Duragesic) are the drugs most often used for relief of cancer pain. Morphine can be given orally, rectally, subcutaneously, intravenously, intramuscularly, or by epidural catheter. Fentanyl is given transdermally. Clients taking these drugs must be monitored for adverse reactions, including excessive sedation, confusion, weakness, hypotension, constipation, dry mouth, nausea, vomiting, and anorexia.

Nursing Management

For nursing care of the client undergoing chemotherapy or radiation and caring for the terminally ill client with cancer, see Chapters 10 and 18.

BREAST CANCER PREVENTION

Three options are available to women with increased risk of developing breast cancer: (1) long-term follow-up, (2) bilateral prophylactic mastectomy, and (3) chemoprevention with tamoxifen (Nolvadex). Those who choose long-term follow-up receive an annual mammogram and MRI, with a clinical breast examination and monthly BSE. Prophylactic bilateral mastectomy is the most invasive of the three options. Clients considering this option are informed that removing the breasts reduces the risk of breast cancer but does not eliminate it completely.

A breast cancer preventive study, conducted by the National Cancer Institute (2008), determined that taking the drug tamoxifen for 5 years reduced the occurrence of estrogen receptor–positive tumors by 69% but did not affect the occurrence of estrogen receptor–negative tumors. Besides reducing the risk of breast cancer, tamoxifen preserves bone mineral density, thus preventing osteoporosis. It also lowers the low-density lipoprotein (LDL) cholesterol levels, although it is still unknown if it decreases the incidence of myocardial infarction in women. On the other hand, tamoxifen can have detrimental effects. It increases the incidences of endometrial cancer, deep vein thrombosis, pulmonary embolism, and cataracts. Other side effects include increased

Nutrition Notes 54-1
The Client at Risk for Breast Cancer

- There is limited but suggestive evidence that a high-fat diet increases the risk of postmenopausal breast cancer; there are no conclusions regarding the effect of fat intake on premenopausal breast cancer. However, there is convincing evidence that body fatness increases the risk of postmenopausal breast cancer, and abdominal fatness and adult weight gain are identified as probable risks (WCRF/AICR, 2007).
- Studies on the cancer-protective role of fruits and vegetables, soy, and fiber are inconclusive. The strongest link between diet and breast cancer is with alcohol; drinking more than one alcoholic drink per day may increase the risk of breast cancer by 40%.
- It is possible that the greatest effect of nutrition on breast cancer occurs during puberty or adolescence, when breasts are still forming.

hot flashes, cold sweats, vaginal discharge, genital itching, and pain with intercourse.

In 2006, the Multiple Outcomes of Raloxifene [MORE] trial showed that raloxifene (Evista), a drug used to prevent osteoporosis, reduced the risk of estrogen receptor–positive breast cancer by 55%. As with tamoxifen, no reduction in estrogen receptor–negative breast cancers was evident (Bevers, 2007). However, the risk of thromboembolic disease increased, because raloxifene is a selective estrogen receptor modifier (SERM).

The risk of breast cancer also decreases with regular use of nonsteroidal anti-inflammatory drugs (NSAIDS) when they are taken daily for at least 2 months (Barclay & Murata, 2007). Data from the Women's Health Initiative have determined that "the regular use of aspirin, ibuprofen, or other NSAIDs may have a significant chemoprotective effect against the development of breast cancer" (Harris et al., 2003). Women who took

two or more NSAID tablets per week for 5 to 10 years had a reduction in the incidence of breast cancer of 21% to 28% (American Cancer Society News Center, 2003).

Studies related to the role of diet in the development or prevention of breast cancer have been inconclusive (Nutrition Notes 54-1).

COSMETIC BREAST PROCEDURES

Some women undergo various cosmetic breast procedures, collectively referred to as **mammoplasty**, for several reasons, but primarily to improve their appearance.

BREAST RECONSTRUCTION

Breast reconstruction is a surgical procedure in which the area of a mastectomy is refashioned to simulate the contour of a breast and optionally to create a nipple and areola. The procedure is accomplished by using either an artificial implant filled with saline or autogenous (self) tissue. Reconstruction can begin at the time of mastectomy if sufficient skin is spared, or it can be performed later.

Artificial Implants

Before an implant can produce an optimum cosmetic appearance, the skin and tissue on the chest wall are expanded to provide a large enough space to fill and approximate the size of the remaining breast. Tissue expansion is achieved by stretching the chest wall over several months with an inflatable or saline-filled pocket (Fig. 54-6).

Some experts have alleged that silicone gel implants may be associated with connective tissue and autoimmune diseases. However, after years of data collection, the Food and Drug Administration (FDA, 2006) has determined that these implants are safe and effective despite high complication rates. For clients considering these devices, the FDA states that (1) breast implants are not expected to last a lifetime and one or more additional surgeries may be necessary; (2) changes in the breast are irreversible; (3) rupture of a

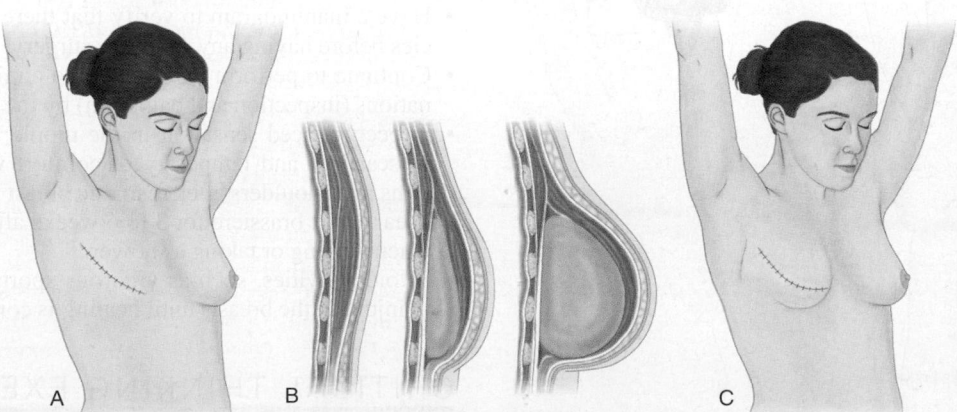

FIGURE 54-6 Breast reconstruction with tissue expander and artificial breast implant. (**A**) Mastectomy incision line before tissue expansion. (**B**) The expander is placed under the pectoralis muscle and is gradually filled with saline solution to stretch the skin. (**C**) The breast mound is restored. (The nipple and areola may be reconstructed later.) (Adapted from American Society of Plastic and Reconstructive Surgeons, Breast Reconstruction.)

silicone implant is most often "silent," and an initial MRI screening is recommended 3 years after implantation, followed by regular screenings every 2 years thereafter; (4) a ruptured implant requires surgical removal; and (5) the cost of regular lifetime MRI screenings may not be an insurance-covered benefit, which can result in costs that exceed those of the initial surgery. The FDA requires that manufacturers of silicone gel implants conduct studies on clients who received the implants for a 10-year period; this allows the FDA to track device failures and to have procedures in place to notify recipients of potential hazards.

Autogenous Tissue

Reconstructing the breast with autogenous tissue provides a more natural look and feel to the breast. The surgeon harvests tissue in a manner similar to a "tummy tuck" (abdominoplasty) from the rectus abdominis muscle along with its adjoining skin and fat (Fig. 54-7). Other donor sites, such as a portion of the latissimus dorsi or gluteal muscles, may be used. Removing donor tissue tends to leave a physical deformity, with some defects being more obvious than others.

If a woman desires a nipple, it is reconstructed from tissue from the opposite nipple, the ear, or toe. Tissue for the areola is selected from a site with a similar color, like the inner thigh or vaginal labia. It also may be created by pigmented tattoo.

REDUCTION MAMMOPLASTY

A **reduction mammoplasty** is an overnight surgical procedure in which glandular breast tissue, fat, and skin are removed bilaterally to decrease the size of large, pendulous breasts. Most candidates for a reduction mammoplasty wear a size D cup or larger brassiere and experience discomfort in the shoulders or back, skin irritation beneath the breasts, difficulty in finding suitable clothing, self-consciousness, or low self-esteem.

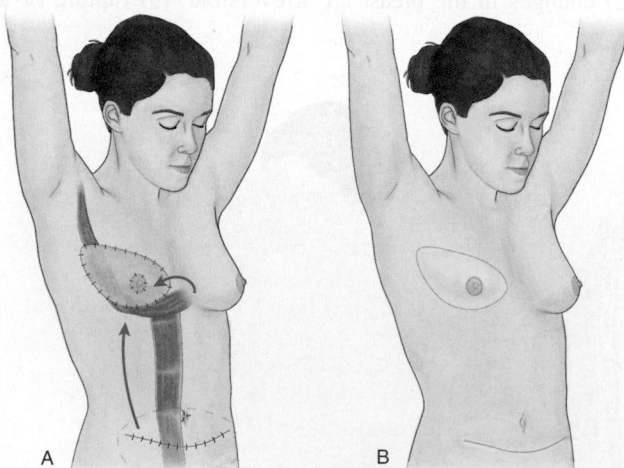

FIGURE 54-7 Autogenous breast reconstruction using the rectus abdominal muscle. (**A**) A breast mound is created by tunneling abdominal skin, fat, and muscle to the mastectomy site. (**B**) Final location of scars. (Adapted from American Society of Plastic and Reconstructive Surgeons, Breast Reconstruction.)

To reduce the size of the breasts, an incision is made around the nipple through which tissue is removed. The loose skin is tightened to reposition the areola and nipple. The client is discharged with a bulky chest dressing and sometimes a small wound drain.

OPPOSITE BREAST REDUCTION

The size of a reconstructed breast is limited by the amount of tissue that remains; thus, there may be potential asymmetry. Opposite breast reduction is a surgical procedure that is performed to reduce the volume of a healthy breast so it more closely resembles the size of a reconstructed breast. The procedure, although done for different reasons, is the same as a reduction mammoplasty.

BREAST LIFT

Ptosis, or drooping, of the breast(s) is corrected with a breast lift or, more technically, **mastopexy**. The sagging skin and low nipple placement that accompany weight loss or aging are corrected in a procedure similar to reduction mammoplasty, although the incision and scar line are smaller and the recovery time is shorter. In some cases, the size or contour of the breast is enhanced with breast augmentation techniques.

BREAST AUGMENTATION

Women who wish to enlarge their breasts may choose breast augmentation, which is similar to breast reconstruction using an artificial saline implant. When caring for women who undergo this procedure, the nurse maintains the client in a semi-Fowler's position after cosmetic breast surgery to promote drainage from the operative site. He or she gives analgesics for pain and inspects the operative site for changes in color and temperature. To minimize stretching of the tissues and suture line, the nurse maintains dressings and assists the client to use a support brassiere. He or she provides clients undergoing cosmetic breast surgery with information that applies to the type of surgery being performed. General guidelines include:

- Have a mammogram to verify that there are no malignancies before having any cosmetic surgery.
- Continue to perform BSE and have clinical breast examinations (inspection and palpation) by the physician.
- Expect reduced sensation in the nipple, a certain amount of scarring, and temporary discomfort when moving the arms and shoulders after cosmetic breast surgery.
- Wear a soft brassiere for 3 to 6 weeks after surgery except when bathing or taking a shower.
- Avoid activities, such as vigorous sports, that may result in injury to the breasts until healing is complete.

CRITICAL THINKING EXERCISES

1. How might the signs and symptoms differ among women with fibrocystic breast disease, a fibroadenoma, and malignant breast tumor?

2. What advice is appropriate for preventing breast cancer?

3. How does sentinel lymph node mapping contribute to breast conservation?

4. What information is appropriate for a client considering breast augmentation with silicone gel implants?

NCLEX-STYLE REVIEW QUESTIONS

1. A client makes an appointment with her physician because she has felt several lumps in her right breast. She is scheduled for a mammogram. The radiologist interprets the findings on the mammogram as benign fibrocystic disease. What nursing information is a correct explanation about when fibrocystic lesions usually become larger and more tender?
1. Nearer to beginning menopause.
2. Just before menstruation.
3. After the menstrual cycle.
4. Following sexual intercourse.

2. Which of the following groups of clients are at high risk for developing breast cancer? Select all that apply.
1. Women with a family history of breast cancer
2. Women who are obese
3. Women with multiple sex partners
4. Women who consume a high-fat diet
5. Women having had no pregnancies

3. Which of the following are current options for women at high risk for breast cancer? Select all that apply.

1. Long-term follow-up
2. Bilateral prophylactic mastectomy
3. Breast cancer vaccine
4. Chemoprotection with tamoxifen
5. Screenings with MRI of the breast

4. A client tells the nurse that she has been able to feel a lump in her left breast for 6 months. The physician recommends an excisional biopsy followed by an immediate modified radical mastectomy if the biopsy shows malignant cells. The woman tells the nurse that she would prefer to postpone the mastectomy until the biopsy has been more thoroughly examined. Which is the most appropriate initial nursing action?
1. Discourage her from opposing the physician.
2. Recommend that she seek a second opinion.
3. Explain that most biopsies are accurate.
4. Help advocate for her choice of treatment.

5. A client with a malignant breast tumor undergoes a left modified radical mastectomy. Which nursing order is most appropriate to add to the client's immediate postoperative plan for care?
1. Maintain the client in a dorsal recumbent position.
2. Limit oral fluid intake to no more than 2000 mL/day.
3. Use the right arm when assessing blood pressures.
4. Inspect the incision at least once each shift.

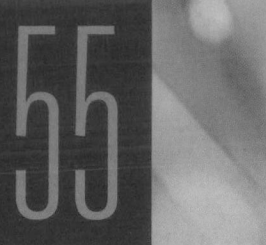

55

Caring for Clients with Disorders of the Male Reproductive System

Words To Know

benign prostatic hyperplasia
brachytherapy
cryptorchidism
epididymitis
erectile dysfunction
impotence
orchiectomy
orchiopexy
orchitis
prostatectomy
retrograde ejaculation
testicular self-examination
therapeutic vaccine
vasectomy

Learning Objectives

On completion of this chapter, you will be able to:

1. Give four examples of structural disorders that affect the male reproductive system.
2. Explain the technique and purpose for performing testicular self-examination.
3. List three infectious or inflammatory conditions and how they are acquired.
4. Discuss two erectile disorders and explain their effects on fertility and sexuality.
5. Identify two methods for treating erectile dysfunction.
6. Describe nursing care for a client being treated for erectile dysfunction.
7. Explain how prostatic hyperplasia compromises urinary elimination, and the symptoms it produces.
8. Discuss the nursing management of a client undergoing a prostatectomy.
9. Compare and contrast three male reproductive cancers in terms of age of onset, incidence, and treatment outcomes.
10. List home care instructions after a vasectomy.

A variety of conditions are threats to male reproductive health. This chapter provides information about genitourinary conditions that are specific to male clients such as congenital or acquired structural abnormalities, infectious and inflammatory conditions, erectile disorders, benign prostatic enlargement, and cancer.

STRUCTURAL ABNORMALITIES

Structural abnormalities of the male genitalia may be congenital or acquired. These various abnormalities, including cryptorchidism, torsion of the spermatic cord, disorders of the foreskin, and benign scrotal swelling, often require surgical repair. Nursing management after these surgeries is similar.

CRYPTORCHIDISM

Cryptorchidism is a condition in which one or both testes fail to descend into the scrotum. The undescended testis or testes may lie in the inguinal canal, in the abdominal cavity, or, rarely, in the perineum or femoral canal. The scrotum essentially is empty, but otherwise the client is asymptomatic. During childhood or at puberty, undescended testes occasionally find their way into the scrotum without treatment. At least one testis must be in the scrotum to ensure production of sperm.

The cause of undescended testes is unknown. The longer the testis remains undescended during childhood, however, the greater is the potential that fertility will be compromised. If the condition is not corrected by 2 years of age, the seminiferous tubules atrophy and fibrose. Some clients are treated with injections of human chorionic gonadotropin (hCG) twice weekly for 4 weeks after the infant is 6 months of age (Mayo Clinic, 2006). The hCG stimulates the testes to release testosterone, promoting their descent into the scrotum. If there is no response, which occurs in 80% of cases, surgery to secure the testis in the scrotum, called **orchiopexy** is performed, preferably between 1 and 2 years of age. If the problem remains uncorrected, the risk of testicular cancer is greater than 20% to 40% (see later discussion).

Nurses teach men, especially those who have had cryptorchidism, to perform **testicular self-examination** to detect any abnormal mass in the scrotum (Client and Family Teaching 55-1). Clients should examine the testicles monthly, preferably when warm, such as in the shower. The American Cancer Society does not currently recommend regular self-testicular examinations, except for those with specific testicular risk factors (American Cancer Society [2007]). The rationale for this guideline is that the incidence of testicular cancer is rare and is highly curable even if it develops, and

that imprecise examination leads to inaccurate high-positive results that can lead to unwarranted surgeries (Nichols, 2008). Men are advised to consult a physician if they detect a consistent, changing mass in a testis.

TORSION OF THE SPERMATIC CORD

Torsion means to twist. In this case, it is the spermatic cord that twists, kinking the artery and compromising blood flow to the testicle (Fig. 55-1). The condition occurs in prepubescent boys and in men whose spermatic cords are congenitally unsupported in the tunica vaginalis, the membrane surrounding the testes. Clients report a sudden, sharp testicular pain, with visible local swelling. The pain may be so severe that nausea, vomiting, chills, and fever occur. Torsion may follow severe exercise, but it also may occur during sleep or after a simple maneuver such as crossing the legs. Physical examination reveals an extremely tender testis. Elevation of the scrotum intensifies the pain by increasing the degree of twist.

Immediate surgery is necessary to prevent atrophy of the spermatic cord and preserve fertility. The torsion is reduced, excess tunica vaginalis is excised, and the testis is

---

 Client and Family Teaching 55-1
Performing Testicular Self-Examination

The nurse provides the following instructions:

1. Use both hands to palpate the testis. The normal testicle is smooth and uniform in consistency.
2. With the index and middle fingers under the testis and the thumb on top, roll the testis gently in a horizontal plane between the thumb and fingers (**A**).
3. Feel for any evidence of a small lump or abnormality.
4. Follow the same procedure and palpate upward along the testis (**B**).

5. Locate and palpate the epididymis (**C**), a cord-like structure on the top and back of the testicle that stores and transports sperm. Also locate and palpate the spermatic cord.
6. Repeat the examination for the other testis, epididymis, and spermatic cord. It is normal to find that one testis is larger than the other.
7. If you find any evidence of a small, pea-like lump or if the testis is swollen (possibly from an infection or tumor), consult your physician.

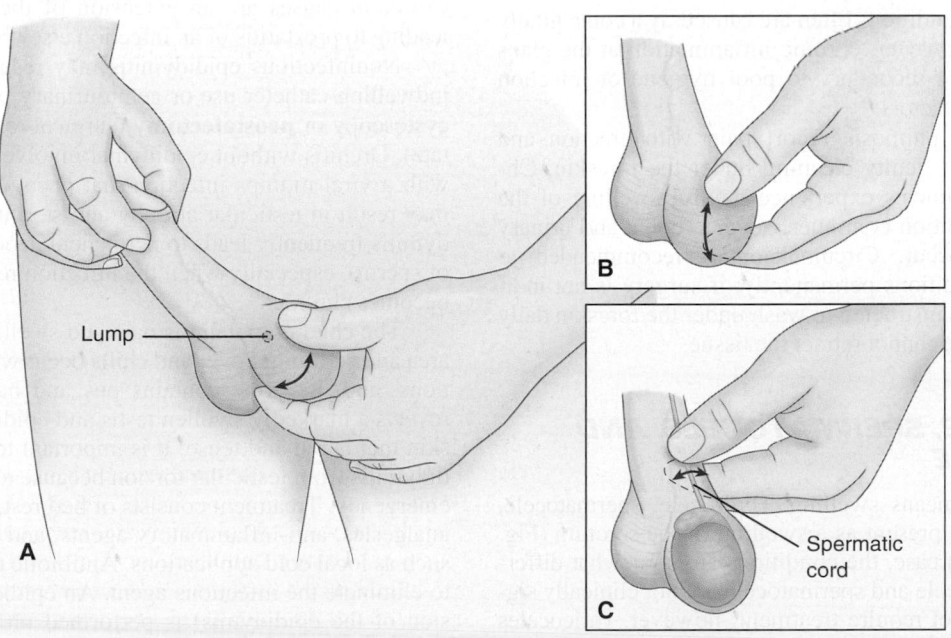

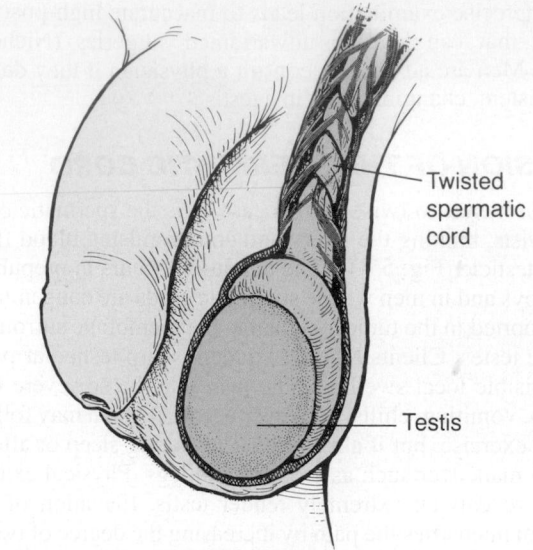

FIGURE 55-1 Torsion of the spermatic cord.

anchored with sutures in the scrotum. A prophylactic procedure may be performed on the opposite side.

Preoperatively, the nurse administers prescribed analgesia to relieve pain. After surgery, he or she applies a scrotal support, especially when the client is out of bed. The nurse inspects the dressing for signs of drainage and gives antibiotics if medically ordered. He or she reports any sudden onset of pain to the physician.

PHIMOSIS AND PARAPHIMOSIS

Phimosis and paraphimosis are conditions that occur among uncircumcised male clients when the opening of the foreskin is constricted. Phimosis refers to an inability to retract the foreskin (prepuce); paraphimosis is a strangulation of the glans penis from an inability to replace the retracted foreskin. These phimotic conditions often are caused by a congenitally small foreskin; however, chronic inflammation at the glans penis and prepuce secondary to poor hygiene or infection also are etiologic factors.

Clients with phimosis report pain with erection and intercourse and difficulty cleaning under the foreskin. Clients with paraphimosis experience painful swelling of the glans. If the condition continues, severe edema and urinary retention may occur. Circumcision is recommended to relieve these conditions permanently; if surgery is not indicated, the client is instructed to wash under the foreskin daily and seek care if he cannot retract the tissue.

HYDROCELE, SPERMATOCELE, AND VARICOCELE

The suffix *cele* means swelling. Hydrocele, spermatocele, and varicocele all present as a swelling of the scrotum (Fig. 55-2), but in each case, the conditions are somewhat different. Often, hydrocele and spermatocele are not clinically significant and do not require treatment; however, varicoceles are thought to be an underlying cause of male infertility and may be surgically repaired (Table 55-1).

- Pressure from a urologic tumor may precipitate congestion of blood in the scrotum in older men with new onset varicoceles.

INFECTIOUS AND INFLAMMATORY CONDITIONS

PROSTATITIS

Prostatitis is an inflammation of the prostate gland and is most often caused by microorganisms that reach the prostate by way of the urethra. *Escherichia coli* and microbes that cause sexually transmitted infections often are responsible (see Chap. 56), but in some instances no evidence of bacterial infection is found. Occasionally, a psychosexual problem may be the suspected cause of the client's symptoms. In any case, inflammation causes glandular swelling and tenderness. Because the prostate surrounds the urethra, a combination of genitourinary problems develops. Clients experience perineal pain or discomfort, an unusual sensation preceding or following ejaculation, low back pain, fever, chills, dysuria, and urethral discharge. Treatment consists of up to 30 days of antibiotic therapy, mild analgesics, and sitz baths.

The nurse stresses that sexual partners also need to be treated. He or she tells the client to avoid caffeine, prolonged sitting, and constipation, and regularly to drain the prostate gland through masturbation or intercourse. The nurse instructs the client to comply with antibiotic therapy and use a mild analgesic for pain.

EPIDIDYMITIS AND ORCHITIS

An inflammation of the epididymis (**epididymitis**) and testis (**orchitis**) occurs alone or concurrently (epididymo-orchitis). Common causes are an extension of the infectious agent, leading to prostatitis or an infection elsewhere in the body.

Noninfectious epididymitis may result from long-term indwelling catheter use or genitourinary procedures such as cystoscopy or **prostatectomy** (surgical removal of the prostate). Orchitis without epididymal involvement is associated with a viral mumps infection that occurs after puberty and may result in testicular atrophy and sterility. Bilateral epididymitis frequently leads to permanent azoospermia (absence of sperm), especially when the infection recurs frequently or becomes chronic.

The chief complaint is pain and swelling in the inguinal area and scrotum. Fever and chills occur with bacterial infections, and the urine contains pus and bacteria. Inspection reveals a markedly swollen testis and epididymis and scrotal skin that is red and tense. It is important to differentiate epididymitis from testicular torsion because torsion is a surgical emergency. Treatment consists of bed rest, scrotal elevation, analgesics, anti-inflammatory agents, and comfort measures such as local cold applications. Antibiotic therapy is initiated to eliminate the infectious agent. An epididymectomy (excision of the epididymis) is performed on clients who have recurrent, chronic, or intractable infections, but this results in sterility if it is performed bilaterally.

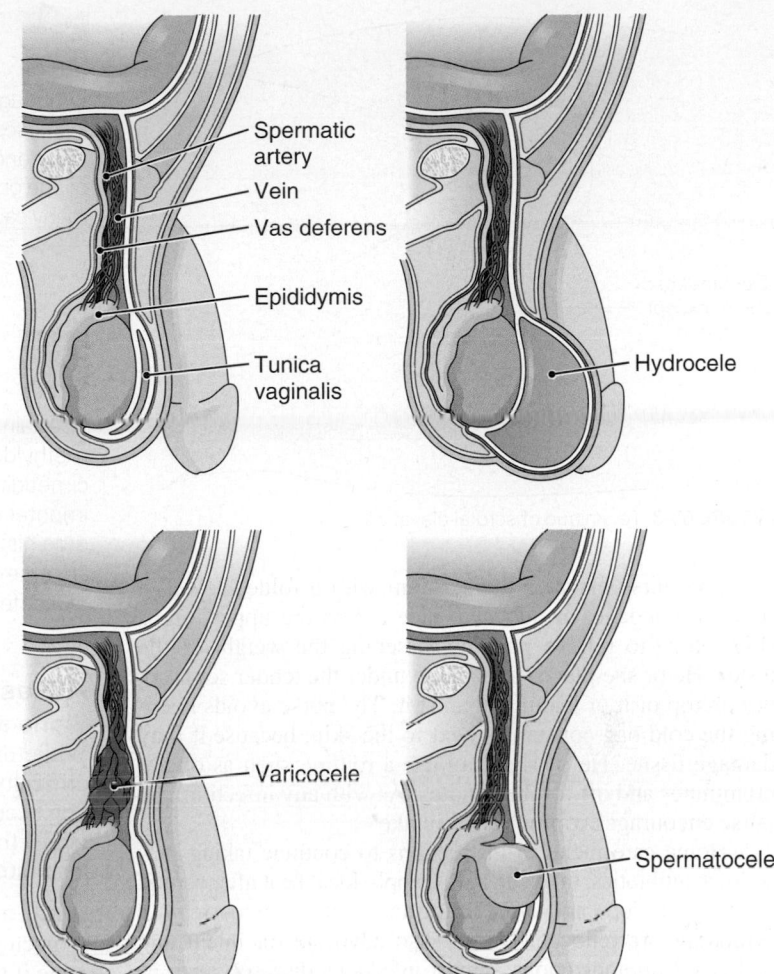

Spermatic
artery
Vein
Vas deferens
Epididymis
Tunica
vaginalis
Hydrocele
Varicocele
Spermatocele

FIGURE 55-2 Causes of scrotal swelling. Hydrocele is an accumulation of fluid around the testicle. Varicocele is characterized by dilation of the veins of the spermatic cord. Spermatocele is a self-contained cystic mass on the epididymis. (Image from Cohen, B. J. [2003]. *Medical terminology* [4th ed.]. Philadelphia: Lippincott Williams & Wilkins.)

TABLE 55-1 Comparison of Hydrocele, Spermatocele, and Varicocele

CONDITION AND ETIOLOGY	DESCRIPTION	SIGNS AND SYMPTOMS	DIAGNOSTIC AIDS	MEDICAL AND SURGICAL MANAGEMENT
Hydrocele Congenital defect, injury, infection, lymph obstruction, tumor, side effect of radiation, or unknown cause	Accumulation of as much as 100 mL of lymphatic fluid between the testis and tunica vaginalis	Swollen testicle, heaviness in scrotum or lower back; may be asymptomatic, pain if testicular blood flow is impaired	Palpation, transillumination	No treatment if asymptomatic; aspiration of fluid as a temporary measure; surgical excision of fluid-filled sac; treatment of primary condition (i.e., infection)
Spermatocele Unknown cause	Epididymal, sperm-containing cyst	Small, freely movable mass; usually asymptomatic, may be painful if large	Palpation, transillumination	No treatment unless cyst is large and causes pain
Varicocele Incompetent valves in the spermatic veins	Venous dilation with damage to elastic fibers and hypertrophy of vein walls	Feeling of heaviness in scrotum; may be asymptomatic or have pain and swelling	Palpation, auscultation of venous rush, ultrasound, blood flow studies	No treatment, surgical ligation, or sclerosing

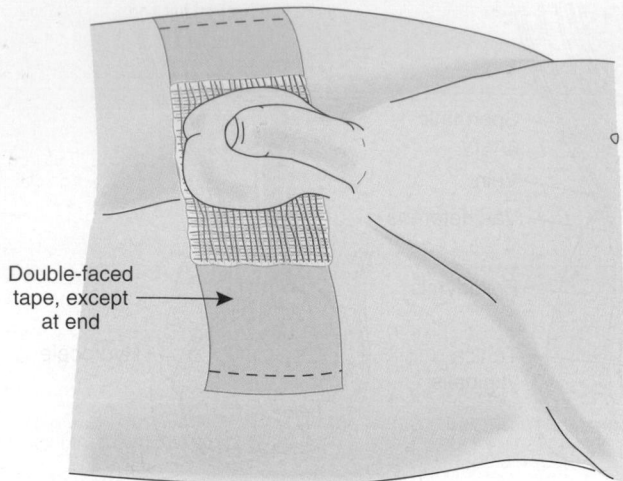

FIGURE 55-3 Technique of scrotal elevation.

The nurse elevates the scrotum with a folded towel, a four-tail bandage, or adhesive tape across the upper thighs (Fig. 55-3) to relieve pain by lessening the weight of the testes. He or she places an ice bag under the tender scrotum, not on top of it or leaning against it. The nurse avoids keeping the cold bag constantly next to the skin, because it may damage tissue. He or she may use a routine such as on for 60 minutes and off for 30 minutes. As with any infection, the nurse encourages copious fluid intake.

Home care includes instructions to continue taking prescribed antibiotics, take sitz baths, apply local heat after scrotal swelling subsides, and avoid lifting and sexual intercourse until symptoms are relieved. Nurses also advocate for infant and childhood immunizations against infectious diseases, such as mumps, to reduce potential adult complications such as orchitis.

ERECTION DISORDERS

ERECTILE DYSFUNCTION

Erectile dysfunction (ED), also known as **impotence**, is (1) the inability to achieve an erection, (2) the inability to achieve or maintain an erection that is sufficiently rigid for sexual activity, or (3) the inability to sustain erection for a satisfactory period of time. There must be multiple or persistent incidences of failed erection for the disorder to be considered pathologic.

Pathophysiology and Etiology

ED may have physical and psychological origins. Erection depends on three basic processes (see Chap. 52): appropriate neurologic stimulation; adequate arterial blood flow into blood vessels such as the cavernous artery, which expands penile tissue; and temporary trapping of venous blood so as to sustain an erection. When any one or more of these processes are ineffective or insufficient, ED occurs.

Common causes of ED include neurologic disorder such as spinal cord injury, perineal trauma, testosterone insufficiency, side effects of drug therapy, atherosclerosis, hypertension, and complications of diabetes mellitus. ED also may be related to anxiety or depression.

Gerontologic Considerations

- Although impotence is not a normal part of aging, incidence increases as men age; 15% to 25% of all men experience impotence by 65 years of age. More than half of all men 75 years of age or older are chronically impotent. Impotence may have many causes; contributing factors should be identified.

Pharmacologic Considerations

- Certain medications such as antihypertensive drugs (e.g., methyldopa, spironolactone), antidepressants, narcotics, and cimetidine can cause sexual dysfunction in men. If impotence or sexual dysfunction occurs, obtain a thorough drug history to determine if the sexual dysfunction is an adverse reaction to a drug and could be corrected by the use of a different medication.

Assessment Findings

Signs and Symptoms

While discussing a sexual health history, the client reports difficulty in achieving or maintaining an erection. If an erection occurs, the client may reveal that there is insufficient rigidity for penetrating the vagina or that intercourse is less than satisfactory because penetration cannot be sustained.

Diagnostic Findings

A nocturnal penile tumescence and rigidity test can determine if the client is experiencing spontaneous erections during sleep. The test involves applying sensors at the base and tip of the penis at bedtime for 1, 2, or 3 nights. The sensors detect the tumescence (enlargement) and firmness of the penis (Fig. 55-4). No spontaneous erections during sleep

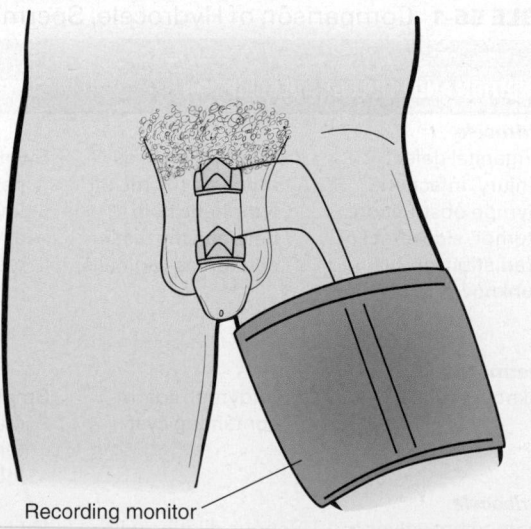

FIGURE 55-4 Nocturnal penile tumescence test. Sensing rings are located at the tip and base of the penis at night. The rings are attached to a monitor on the leg that records the force and duration of erections that occur during sleep.

suggests a physiologic etiology for ED. Evidence of spontaneous erections during sleep, but erectile dysfunction in a waking state, suggests a psychologic etiology. Test results may prove invalid, however, if the tester does not apply the sensors well or if the client sleeps restlessly.

Vascular ultrasound studies using a Doppler applied to the penis may quantify the perfusion of the penis with arterial blood during an erection.

Medical and Surgical Management

Several approaches exist to help restore sexual function. Substituting other drugs for those that cause impotence or treating the contributing cause may restore potency (erectile ability). The Consensus Panel on Health Care Clinician Management of Erectile Dysfunction has updated its recommendations (Montague et al., 2006). It recommends oral phosphodiesterase type 5 (PDE5) inhibitors as first-line therapy. If PDE5 therapy is unsuccessful, clients receive information about other available options for managing ED (Table 55-2).

The PDE5 inhibitors, such as sildenafil (Viagra), facilitate penile erection by producing smooth muscle relaxation in the corpora cavernosa, facilitating an inflow of blood. These drugs are taken 1/2 hour to 1 hour before sexual activity. They have no erectile effect without sexual stimulation. Apomorphine (Uprima), a dopamine agonist, an older drug used in the treatment of Parkinson's disease (see Chap.

37), is a possible alternative to phosphodiesterase inhibitors for the treatment of ED. This drug, which is administered as a nasal spray, has some advantages over sildenafil: (1) it acts within 15 to 25 minutes of administration, and (2) it is safer for men with coronary artery disease.

Some clients elect to facilitate penile engorgement by self-administering a urethral suppository of alprostadil or self-injecting drugs such as papaverine (Pavatine) with phentolamine (Regitine), or alprostadil (Caverject) into the corpora cavernosa to achieve an erection (Fig. 55-5). As an alternative, they may prefer to attach a vacuum device to the penis (Fig. 55-6).

Although vascular surgery is an option for some clients, many choose a surgically implanted penile prosthesis (Fig. 55-7). One type contains a saline reservoir that is pumped to fill the implant when sexual activity is desired; the other type maintains the penis in a semierect state at all times. The nurse informs the client before surgery that when a pump-type implant is inserted, the erect penis tends to be shorter than experienced in preillness erections because the cylinders do not fill the glans portion of the penis.

Nursing Management

If the client prefers to self-inject a vasodilator, the nurse provides instruction on technique, suggested frequency of injections, and side effects. If the client undergoes a penile implant, the nurse assesses for pain, swelling, bleeding, and

TABLE 55-2 Treatment Options For Erectile Dysfunction

TREATMENT	EFFECT	ADVANTAGES	DISADVANTAGES
Oral agents, such as phosphodiesterase (PDE5) inhibitors (sildenafil [Viagra], vardenafil [Levitra], tadalafil [Cialis])	Inhibition of PDE5 dilates arterial vessels in the corpus cavernosum producing an erection.	Easy to use Relatively short half-life for most	Expensive Must be taken 30–60 minutes prior to need, unless daily dose is used Contraindicated if taking nitrates May cause hypotension, headache, flushing, dyspepsia, nasal congestion, sensitivity to light, altered color perception, and blurred vision
Urethral suppository of alprostadil	Relaxes penile muscles, promoting vascular filling	Produces an erection within 15 minutes	Less effective than penile injection route May cause urethral burning and irritation Hypotension and dizziness may develop during initial therapy.
Self-injection with prostaglandin E1, alprostadil (Caverject), or papaverine HCl (Pavatine) phentolamine (Regitine)	Relaxes arterial blood vessels, resulting in increased blood flow into penis	Produces an erection in 5–20 minutes Erection is sustained up to 1 1/2 hours	Discomfort at injection site No more than 10 injections per month at equal intervals Painful, sustained erections lasting ≥4 hours are more likely to occur with papaverine and phentolamine
Vacuum constriction devices (VCDs)	Draws blood into the penis, producing an erection that is sustained with a tension band	Least expensive of treatment options Sustains erection for as long as 30 minutes Can be used daily	Some find the device cumbersome May cause pain and decreased sensation Obstructs ejaculation
Surgical implantation of semirigid or inflatable penile prosthesis	Provides penile rigidity sufficient for vaginal penetration	Permanent outcome; failure rate is 2.5%	Produces less penile enlargement compared with normal erections Requires 6 weeks to recover from surgery before sexual activity Besides the expense of surgery, there may be surgical complications such as infection, urethral or corporal perforation, prolonged pain, damage or malfunction, which may require additional surgery

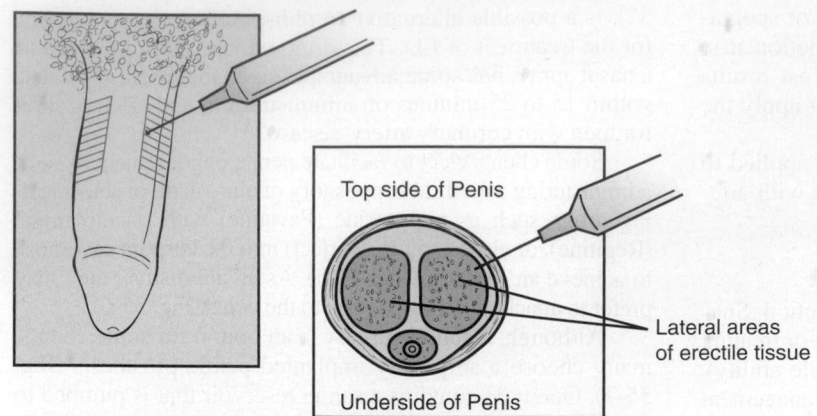

FIGURE 55-5 Penile injection technique. An injection site is selected on either of the lateral sides of the penis. The prescribed drug is injected into the erectile tissue at a 90-degree angle.

Top side of Penis

Lateral areas of erectile tissue

Underside of Penis

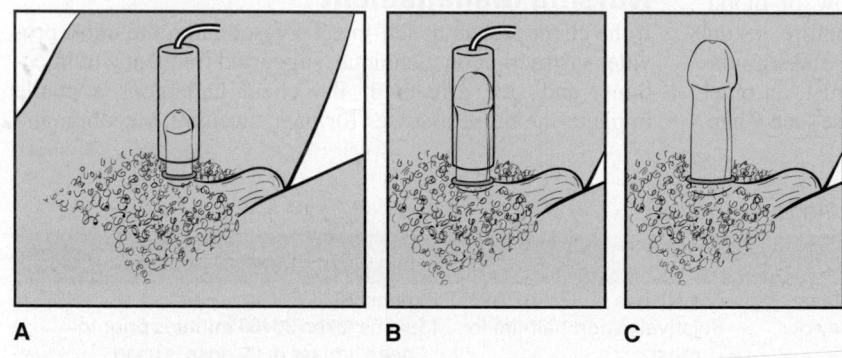

A   B   C

FIGURE 55-6 An erection is produced by (**A**) placing a vacuum device around the penis with a constricting attachment to the base of the penis. (**B**) The vacuum engorges the penis with blood. (**C**) When the vacuum device is removed, the constricting attachment prohibits the outflow of blood to sustain the erection.

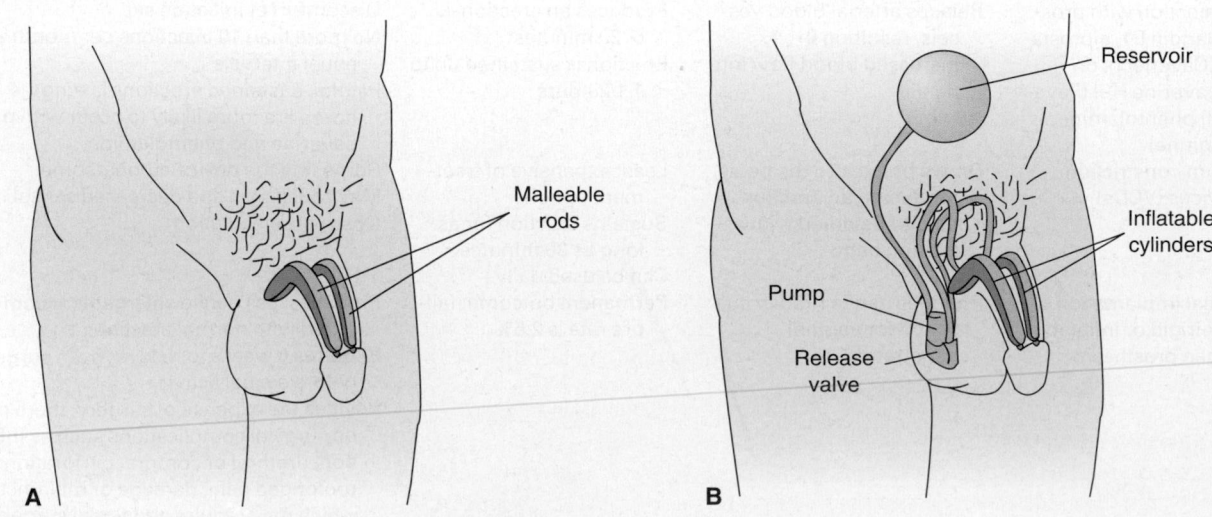

Malleable rods

Reservoir

Inflatable cylinders

Pump

Release valve

A   B

FIGURE 55-7 Examples of penile implants. (**A**) Semirigid. (**B**) Inflatable.

surgical complications such as infection. The nurse reinforces the information the physician identifies as possible complications after discharge, such as:

- Erosion of penile or urethral tissue from a mis-sized implant, pressure, and friction of the implanted cylinders, which is evidenced by seeing the implant through the skin
- Erosion of scrotal, bowel, or bladder tissue if an implant with a fluid reservoir is used, which is detected by changes in scrotal skin texture and elimination
- Migration of the cylinders, pump, or reservoir from their intended location, which is accompanied by pain, tenderness, and dysfunction of components that are part of the device
- Malfunction of the device characterized by underinflation, bulging of the cylinders during inflation, and loss of fluid from the implant, which can occur with migration, accidental trauma such as a fall, or aggressive or improper use of the device
- The nurse implements measures to ensure a safe recovery and provides instructions to promote self-care (Nursing Care Plan 55-1).

PRIAPISM

Priapism is a condition in which the penis becomes engorged and remains persistently erect without any sexual stimulation. The underlying etiology usually is a vascular problem, a medical condition that causes blood to thicken, or a side effect of medications, including those prescribed to treat impotence. The engorged penis produces significant discomfort and interferes with arterial blood flow and, in some cases, urinary elimination. If the erection lasts longer than 6 hours, the tissue may be sufficiently damaged to result in impotence.

Treatment options include administering vasoconstrictive medications such as terbutaline (Brethine) or phenylephrine (Neo-Synephrine) or draining the trapped blood with a needle placed in the side of the penis. If these interventions fail, emergency surgery is performed to shunt blood temporarily out of the corpora cavernosa. Healthcare providers must extend respect for the client's feelings and understandable embarrassment throughout interactions.

BENIGN PROSTATIC HYPERPLASIA

When the number of cells in a structure increases, the condition is referred to as *hyperplasia*. If the cells are nonmalignant, it is called *benign hyperplasia*. Thus, **benign prostatic hyperplasia** (BPH) indicates that the prostate gland contains more than the usual number of normal cells. When the gland enlarges, the condition is known as *benign prostatic hypertrophy*.

Pathophysiology and Etiology

BPH occurs as men age. The outward expansion of the gland is of no clinical importance. Inward encroachment, however, diminishes the diameter of the prostatic section of the urethra and interferes with emptying the bladder (Fig. 55-8).

Assessment Findings
Signs and Symptoms
The symptoms of BPH appear gradually. At first, the client notices that it takes more effort to void. Eventually, the urinary stream narrows and has decreased force. The bladder empties incompletely. As residual urine accumulates, the client has an urge to void more often and nocturia occurs. Because residual urine is a good culture medium for bacteria, symptoms of cystitis (inflammation of the bladder) may develop (see Chap. 59).

Diagnostic Findings
A digital rectal examination (DRE) reveals an enlarged and elastic gland. Cystoscopy exposes the extent of the infringement on the urethra and the effects on the bladder. Intravenous and retrograde pyelograms and blood chemistry tests give information about possible damage to the upper urinary tract from urinary retention. Measurement of a significant quantity of residual urine adds to the data that confirm the diagnosis. The prostate-specific antigen (PSA) test results may be slightly elevated. Transrectal ultrasonography indicates prostatic size and helps rule out the possibility that a malignancy is causing the enlargement.

Medical and Surgical Management
In the early stages of BPH, the progression of prostatic enlargement is monitored with periodic DREs. Drug therapy is the second line of treatment (Drug Therapy Table 55-1). Terazosin (Hytrin) or other alpha-adrenergic blockers help relax the muscles in the prostate and relieve urinary symptoms. Finasteride (Proscar, Propecia) and similar drugs that are androgen hormone inhibitors (also classified as 5-alpha reductase inhibitors) can be used to decrease symptoms and also appear to arrest the progression of prostate enlargement in some clients.

Some men have found that taking *saw palmetto*, an herbal substance from the fruit of the palm tree, or *Pygeum africanum*, an herb extracted from the bark of an African evergreen, relieves the symptoms of BPH. Saw palmetto interferes with the enzyme that converts testosterone to dihydrotestosterone. When dihydrotestosterone is inhibited, the stimulus for growth of the prostate gland is reduced. This herb also may inhibit cyclooxygenase, an enzyme that plays a role in inflammation, which may explain the manner in which the symptoms of prostatitis are relieved (Saper, Fletcher, & Rind, 2008). *P. africanum* probably reduces inflammation and removes cholesterol deposits within the prostate gland (Center for Holistic Urology, Columbia University Medical Center, 2006). Before self-administering any substance that is considered alternative therapy, clients should discuss the matter with their physicians.

Other forms of treatment are used when glandular enlargement results in pronounced symptoms. The aim of all surgical procedures for BPH is to enlarge the bladder outlet (Table 55-3). Surgeries preformed through the urethra include transcystoscopic urethroplasty, transurethral resection of the prostate (TURP), transurethral incision of the prostate (TUIP), and transurethral laser incision of the prostate (TULIP), and transurethral needle ablation (TUNA). Operations performed through an external incision include suprapubic, retroperitoneal, or perineal prostatectomy (Fig. 55-9). In almost all cases, a continuous bladder irrigation is ordered after TURP to remove blood clots and residual tissue.

After a TURP, between 66 and 75% of clients experience **retrograde ejaculation**, a condition in which the semen is deposited in the bladder rather than discharging through the urethra at the time of orgasm, rendering the client sterile.

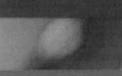

NURSING CARE PLAN 55-1 | **Postoperative Management of the Client With a Penile Implant**

Assessment

- Determine level of consciousness and vital signs.
- Check the condition of dressing and incision.
- Assess the client's level of pain.
- Evaluate the amount of penile and scrotal swelling.

- Check the status of the IV infusion (type of solution, drip rate, location of IV site).
- Note the urinary catheter and volume of urine elimination.
- Assess the client's knowledge of postoperative care and discharge instructions.

Nursing Diagnosis: Acute Pain related to tissue injury and swelling

Expected Outcome: Pain will be eliminated or reduced to the client's level of tolerance.

Interventions	Rationales
Assess level of discomfort as needed and whenever you assess vital signs.	An assessment of pain level is the fifth vital sign.
Administer analgesia as prescribed.	Clients have the right to pain relief.
Elevate genitalia with a rolled towel.	Elevation reduces swelling.
Apply an ice pack to the incision and replace as needed.	Facilitating vasoconstriction with an ice pack reduces swelling and pain.
Suspend linen over lower pelvis with a bed cradle.	A cradle prevents pressure on painful tissue from the weight of bed linen.

Evaluation of Expected Outcome

Pain is relieved and comfort is maintained.

PC: Risk for Bleeding related to inadequate hemostasis

Expected Outcome: The nurse will monitor for, manage, and minimize incisional bleeding.

Interventions	Rationales
Assess for frank bleeding or an enlarging hematoma around the incision, usually at the base of the penis where it joins the scrotum.	A large amount of obvious blood or its collection in the skin and underlying tissue indicates significant blood loss.
Ensure that the implant is semirigid.	Implant rigidity provides localized pressure that reduces bleeding.

Evaluation of Expected Outcome

Blood loss is minimal and swelling of the genitalia remains within acceptable limits.

Nursing Diagnosis: Risk for Urinary Retention related to urethral compression

Expected Outcome: Client will void without difficulty and empty his bladder with each voiding.

Interventions	Rationales
Monitor frequency and amount of each voiding.	Urinary retention is evidenced by the absence of voiding or voiding small, frequent amounts.
Palpate the lower abdomen.	The bladder is palpable when it is distended with urine.
Report an inability to void or lack of sufficient quantity per voiding.	Catheterization may be required to empty the bladder, or the physician may choose to order a medication to induce voiding.

Evaluation of Expected Outcome

Client voids in sufficient quantities; the bladder remains nonpalpable.

Nursing Diagnosis: Risk for Impaired Skin Integrity related to dermal deterioration secondary to a tight prosthesis

Expected Outcome: Skin in the operative area will remain supple and intact.

Interventions	Rationales
Look for pale, thin skin near the glans penis.	The prosthesis occupies space, stretches the skin, and reduces the diameter of blood vessels.
Report signs of inadequate capillary perfusion and skin erosion.	Prolonged interruption of blood flow causes tissue necrosis.

NURSING CARE PLAN 55-1   **Postoperative Management of the Client With a Penile Implant** (Continued)

Evaluation of Expected Outcome

Skin in the operative area will remain supple and intact.

Nursing Diagnosis: Risk for Situational Low Self-Esteem related to possible spectator curiosity concerning the outcome of the surgical procedure.

Expected Outcome: Client retains positive self-esteem.

Interventions	Rationales
Explain the purpose for genital inspection.	Genital inspection is performed for the purpose of assessing local tissue response rather than satisfying curiosity.
Provide privacy and draping during genital assessments.	The client has the right to privacy and to be treated with dignity.
Avoid unprofessional comments about the client's reasons for or outcome of surgery.	The client's decision for elective surgery is private and personal.
Provide opportunities for the client to privately share his feelings about his changed appearance.	Clients are more likely to openly discuss their feelings when they feel secure that others will not overhear the conversation.
Describe techniques for concealing the semierect appearance of the penis, such as wearing untucked shirts and pleated trousers or pants with an elastic waist.	Disguising the state of semierection decreases self-consciousness in social situations.

Evaluation of Expected Outcome

Client's self-esteem is undisturbed.

Nursing Diagnosis: Risk for Ineffective Therapeutic Regimen Management related to lack of knowledge concerning postoperative course after discharge

Expected Outcome: Client will acquire knowledge to ensure recovery without complications.

Interventions	Rationales
Explain that the penis should be taped against the skin in a straight position for 1 week or longer, but can be untaped for voiding.	Taping acts as a splint to keep the penis from moving about while healing takes place.
Identify the period for sexual abstinence (usually 3 to 6 weeks).	Sexual intercourse is safe once healing is complete.
Instruct on how to inflate and deflate an inflatable prosthesis.	An erect penis facilitates vaginal penetration; the client empties the penile implant after intercourse.
Inform client to avoid tight-fitting underwear.	Pressure and friction can cause tissue erosion and curvature of the penis.
Advise client to avoid contact sports.	The force of physical contact may alter the position or integrity of the penile implant.
Explain that the client must avoid heavy lifting for at least 3 weeks.	Straining can disrupt internal sutures and reconstructed tissue.
Emphasize the need to report persistent pain and swelling.	Pain and swelling are common signs of infection, erosion, and migration.

Evaluation of Expected Outcome

Client can verbalize discharge instructions and receives written information to which he can refer for self-care at home.

After a TURP and open prostatectomies, men may have temporary or permanent urinary incontinence, depending on the procedure used and the surgeon's technical skill. Perineal surgical approaches often result in permanent ED, although some nerve-sparing techniques are being developed.

Nursing Management

For the client who is not yet a candidate for surgery, the nurse teaches how to maintain optimal bladder emptying (Client and Family Teaching 55-2).

The surgical client requires support and information to allay anxiety and promote a postoperative period that is free of complications. The nurse teaches deep breathing and leg exercises and explains that the client will have continuous bladder irrigation for at least 24 hours after surgery.

Urethral catheterization before surgery is necessary for clients with sudden or acute retention. If difficulty is encountered while inserting a urethral catheter, a coude catheter, which has a curved tip, and instillable anesthetic lubricant are used to facilitate the procedure. If the catheter cannot be

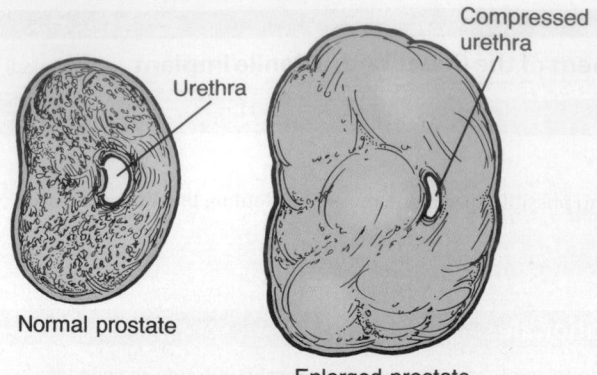

FIGURE 55-8 Comparison of normal prostate and enlarged prostate.

passed urethrally, a temporary suprapubic catheter, also called a cystostomy tube, is required to relieve bladder distention. For care after a prostatectomy, see Nursing Care Plan 55-2.

MALIGNANCIES OF THE MALE REPRODUCTIVE SYSTEM

CANCER OF THE PROSTATE

Prostatic cancer is second to skin cancer in frequency among American men. It ranks second as the cause of deaths from cancer. The incidence is higher in African Americans and men with a father or brother diagnosed with the disease at a young age. About 1 American male in 6 will be diagnosed with prostatic cancer, and 1 in 35 will die of the disease (American Cancer Society, 2008). The cancer grows slowly, however, and has a high survival rate. The survival rate 5 years after diagnosis is 100%; after 10 years, it is 92%; and after 15 years, it is 70% (American Cancer Society, 2008).

Pathophysiology and Etiology

The cause of prostatic cancer is unknown, but there seems to be a relationship with increased testosterone levels and a diet that is high in fat. A man with blood relatives who have prostatic cancer has an increased risk of developing the disease. Most prostatic carcinomas occur in the periphery of the gland. As it enlarges, it causes genitourinary symptoms similar to a variety of other conditions (e.g., BPH and cystitis). If untreated, tumor cells spread by way of the bloodstream and lymphatics to the pelvic lymph nodes and bone, particularly the lumbar vertebrae, pelvis, and hips.

Assessment Findings

Signs and Symptoms

At first, no symptoms occur, and none may develop for years. When the tumor grows large enough, it compromises urinary flow and causes frequency, nocturia, and dysuria (difficult or painful urination), hematuria (blood in the urine), hemospermia (blood in semen), and ED. The first symptoms of metastases may be back pain or pain down the leg from nerve sheath involvement. When pain develops, the disease often is in an advanced stage.

Diagnostic Findings

DRE detects a prostatic nodule. A PSA greater than 4 ng/mL is the basis for performing more definitive diagnostic procedures, and a PSA greater than 10 ng/mL indicates a prostatic malignancy. A PSA greater than 80 ng/mL indicates advanced metastatic disease. However, some men with normal PSA levels have prostatic cancer, whereas others with elevated PSA levels are cancer free.

When to use PSA screening is controversial. The U.S. Preventive Services Task Force (USPSTF) (2008) now believes that there is insufficient evidence for routine PSA screening in men older than 75 years of age. The rationale

DRUG THERAPY TABLE 55-1 Agents For Benign Prostatic Hyperplasia

Drug Category and Examples	Mechanism of Action	Side Effects	Nursing Considerations
Hormonal Agents finasteride (Proscar) dutasteride (Avodart)	Inhibit the conversion of testosterone into a potent androgen (dihydrotestosterone) on which the prostate depends; cause the gland to shrink	Loss of libido, impotence, decreased ejaculate, adverse effects on fetal development	Monitor urinary output. Avoid handling the drug if pregnant. Instruct to use a condom to prevent fetal exposure. Explain that sexual changes are reversible after drug is discontinued. Inform client that it may take 6 months or longer to achieve full benefit.
Alpha-Adrenergic Blockers terazosin (Hytrin) doxazosin (Cardura) tamsulosin (Flomax) alfuzosin (Uroxatral)	Reduce the tone of smooth muscle in the bladder neck and prostatic urethra	Hypotension, dizziness, nausea, urinary frequency, incontinence, edema, fatigue, headaches	Monitor urinary elimination patterns and postural blood pressure changes. Administer drug at bedtime to reduce orthostatic hypotension. Warn to change position slowly. Weigh regularly for evidence of fluid imbalance.

TABLE 55-3 Invasive Procedures for Prostatic Enlargement

PROCEDURE	DESCRIPTION
Transurethral Approaches	
Transcystoscopic urethroplasty	The balloon tip of a catheter is inflated for 10 to 20 minutes to stretch the prostatic urethra.
Urethral stent or coils	A flexible tube is permanently placed in the urethra to dilate the lumen.
Thermotherapy	A heated instrument inserted in a urethral catheter destroys prostatic tissue but preserves the urethra.
Transurethral resection of the prostate (TURP)	Part of the prostate is removed with a cutting instrument inserted through an endoscope.
Transurethral incision of the prostate (TUIP)	No tissue is removed; the bladder outlet is enlarged by making an incision in the prostate, which relieves pressure on the urethra.
Transurethral laser incision of the prostate (TULIP)	A laser is used to incise and destroy prostate tissue.
Transurethral needle ablation (TUNA)	Needles within the prostate deliver low-level radiofrequency energy to remove excess tissue.
Open Surgical Approaches	
Suprapubic prostatectomy	The prostate gland is removed by making a midline abdominal incision into the bladder. A suprapubic catheter, and a Foley catheter are inserted.
Retropubic prostatectomy	The prostate gland is removed through an abdominal incision, but the bladder is not entered.
Perineal prostatectomy	The prostate gland is removed through an incision made between the scrotum and anus.
Radical prostatectomy	The prostate gland and its capsule, seminal vesicles, and lymph nodes are removed through a retropubic or perineal incision; this procedure is reserved for clients with prostatic cancer.

for the recommendation is that some prostatic cancers grow so slowly, and the benefits of treatment may be minimal at an advanced age if they exist at all. In fact, there are potential quality-of-life consequences for treating prostatic cancer in men who would never have developed cancer-related symptoms during their lives. According to the USPSTF, there is inadequate evidence that PSA screening in men younger than 75 years of age actually improves health outcomes; treatment results after clinical detection with DRE are comparable (see Chap. 52). On the other hand, the American Cancer Society (2008) recommends that screening for prostatic cancer using

PSA and DRE should be offered to men beginning at 50 years of age who have at least a 10-year life expectancy; annual screenings should begin at age 45 for African Americans and men who have first-degree relatives with a history of prostatic cancer before 65 years of age.

Transrectal ultrasound confirms the presence of a mass. Definitive diagnosis is made by biopsy and microscopic examination of tissue. Sometimes the malignancy is detected after microscopic examination of tissue removed during a TURP or open prostatectomy for BPH.

Pelvic or spinal radiographs, bone scan, and magnetic resonance imaging (MRI) or computed tomography (CT) scanning detect metastases to bones. An elevated serum acid phosphatase is associated with bone metastasis. An intravenous pyelogram (IVP) and other renal function studies detect kidney damage caused by long-standing urethral obstruction and urinary retention (if present).

Medical and Surgical Management

The tumor size, microscopic characteristics (sometimes referred to as the *Gleason score*) and any metastases are used to establish the stage, which in turn determines treatment (Table 55-4). The client's age and general health status also are considered when planning treatment. Common treatment regimens include observation, which is sometimes called "watchful waiting," surgery, external radiation or brachytherapy (sealed source radiation), hormone therapy, or a combination of these.

Surgery

If the nodule is localized, an open suprapubic prostatectomy is the treatment of choice. A radical prostatectomy, performed through a perineal or retropubic approach, is the surgical preference if the tumor is large enough to be palpated or if it has spread to adjacent tissue.

Client and Family Teaching 55-2
Maintaining Optimal Bladder Function

The nurse instructs the client as follows:

- Void often and assist bladder emptying by leaning forward on toilet and "bearing down" (Valsalva maneuver), or pressing down on the bladder while seated on the toilet (Credé's maneuver).
- Drink frequent small volumes of oral fluids so that the bladder does not become extremely full at any one time.
- Limit alcohol and caffeine, which increase the urgency to urinate.
- Limit the use of cough, cold, or allergy medications containing decongestants, which can interfere with urination.
- Note any signs and symptoms of acute urinary obstruction and urinary infection such as distended bladder, lower abdominal discomfort, inability to urinate, small and frequent urination, fever and chills, and flank pain that indicate a need for medical attention.

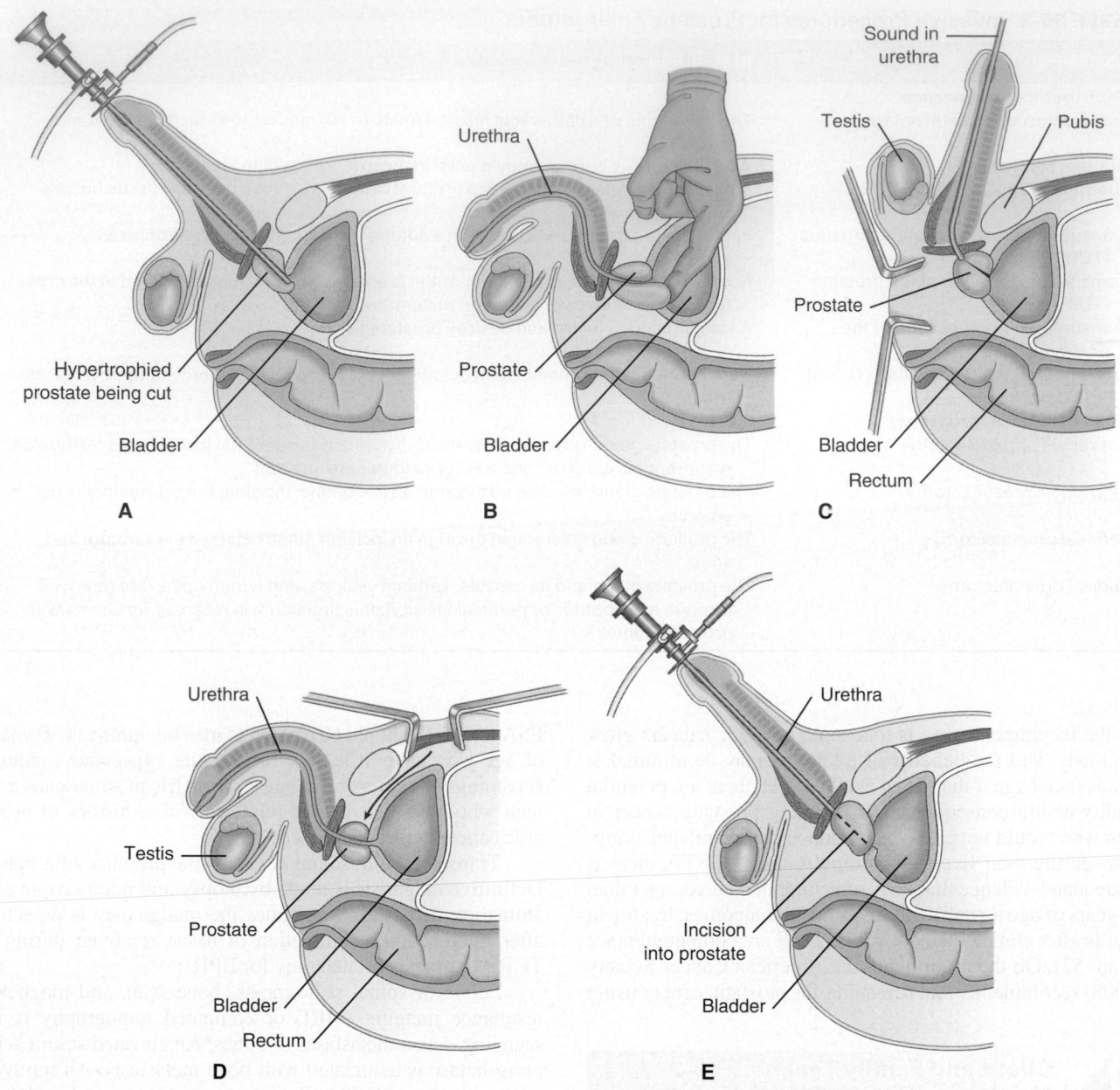

FIGURE 55-9 Examples of prostate surgery techniques. (**A**) Transurethral resection of the prostate (TURP). (**B**) Suprapubic prostatectomy. (**C**) Perineal prostatectomy. (**D**) Retropubic prostatectomy. (**E**) Transurethral incision of prostate (TUIP).

When a radical prostatectomy is performed, the entire prostate, its capsule, and the seminal vesicles are removed. The bladder neck is sutured to the membranous urethra over an indwelling urethral catheter, which is left in place for 10 to 14 days. Potential complications of this surgery include a 25% to 50% chance of impotence, difficulty with urinary control, and genital and lower extremity edema. A TURP may be performed if the client has urethral obstruction and his physical status is not amenable to treatment. Occasionally, permanent suprapubic urinary drainage may need to be established.

Removal of a cancerous prostate also can be performed laparoscopically. Although this procedure is technically more difficult, it has the same advantages as other similar, minimally invasive procedures: less pain, less blood loss, shorter recovery period, and quicker resumption of previous lifestyle. However, the American Cancer Society (2006) believes that more research is needed before this technique is considered comparable to other surgical methods for removing the prostate gland.

A bilateral **orchiectomy** (surgical removal of the testes) may be performed to eliminate the production of testosterone in men with advanced prostatic carcinoma (stage IV). Permanent side effects are impotence, loss of libido, hot flashes, and possible psychological disturbances. Many men do not accept surgical castration, and lower levels of testosterone are achieved with hormone therapy.

Radiation Therapy

Radiation therapy (see Chap. 18) may be used alone or in conjunction with other treatment modalities, especially when

NURSING CARE PLAN 55-2 | The Client Undergoing a Prostatectomy

Assessment
Determine the following before surgery:

- Medical, drug, and allergy history
- Symptoms such as urgency, frequency, hesitancy, nocturia, decreased urinary stream
- Previous episodes of urinary tract infections
- Discomfort that is associated with an acute, sudden episode of urinary retention because this problem may require immediate preoperative attention

- Vital signs
- Weight

Determine the following after surgery:

- Level of consciousness
- Vital signs
- Level of discomfort
- Location of urinary catheter(s)
- Volume and color of urine

PC: Risk for Hemorrhage related to inadequate hemostasis

Expected Outcome: The nurse will monitor to detect, manage, and minimize excessive bleeding.

Interventions	Rationales
Monitor vital signs every 15 minutes until stable and then every 4 hours.	Hypotension and tachycardia suggest a loss of blood volume.
Assess color of urine and status of dressing, if there is one, at least every 4 hours.	A change from burgundy to bright red, like catsup, suggests fresh bleeding.
Maintain traction on the urinary catheter for at least 6 hours after surgery.	Traction provides pressure on blood vessels, which facilitates hemostasis.
Discourage straining to have a bowel movement, attempts to void with the catheter in place, and lifting heavy objects.	Bearing down increases blood pressure, which can trigger fresh bleeding.
Report signs of hypovolemic shock to the physician.	The physician determines the medical measures such as administering blood transfusions and medications for stabilizing the client's condition.

Evaluation of Expected Outcome
Client's urine is light pink, clear, or amber.

PC: Anemia related to postoperative bleeding

Expected Outcome: The nurse will monitor to detect, manage, and minimize anemia.

Interventions	Rationales
Monitor laboratory test results when a complete blood count (CBC) is performed.	Low erythrocyte, hemoglobin, and hematocrit results indicate that the client may require the replacement of blood.
Assist with administering whole blood or packed cells as prescribed by the physician.	Transfusions of whole blood or packed cells replace depleted cells and intravascular fluid volume faster than the bone marrow can reproduce erythrocytes.

Evaluation of Expected Outcome
Client's hemoglobin is at least 10 g/dL.

Nursing Diagnosis: Risk for Urinary Retention related to obstruction of urinary catheter with tissue debris and blood clots or urethral stricture

Expected Outcome: Catheter will remain patent.

Interventions	Rationales
Instill bladder irrigation solution at a rate to maintain light pink or clear urine (Fig. 55-10).	Irrigating solution dilutes blood cells and tissue debris and facilitates removal from the bladder by gravity drainage.
Encourage client to drink about one glass of water every hour while awake.	A generous fluid intake keeps the urine dilute and the catheter patent.
Palpate bladder and assess true urine volume every 4 hours, whenever client complains of pain, or if urine leaks around catheter.	The bladder is not palpable unless distended. True urine volume is assessed by subtracting the volume of irrigating solution from the total urinary output. Pain and leaking fluid suggest accumulated urine with no appropriate outlet.

(care plan continues on page 878)

NURSING CARE PLAN 55-2 **The Client Undergoing a Prostatectomy** (Continued)

Interventions	Rationales
Avoid dependent loops and kinks in urinary catheter, never clamp urinary catheter, and do not allow client to lie on the drainage tubing.	Interference with gravity drainage results in urine accumulation in the bladder.
Keep drainage bag below the level of the bladder.	Fluid (urine in this case) flows by gravity from higher to lower locations. If the urinary drainage bag is above the bladder, urine flows backward into the bladder.

Evaluation of Expected Outcome

Urine drains freely from the catheter or with spontaneous voiding.

PC: Hyponatremia related to absorption of bladder irrigation solution

Expected Outcome: The nurse will monitor to detect, manage, and minimize hyponatremia.

Interventions	Rationales
Analyze if there is a realistic relationship between the amount of instilled irrigation solution and the drainage volume.	A deficit in irrigation volume suggests systemic absorption of a portion of the full amount.
Monitor and report if client develops weakness, muscle cramps, nausea, vomiting, confusion, seizures, or elevated blood pressure.	Hyponatremia is manifested in physical signs and symptoms.
Slow or interrupt the bladder irrigation if you suspect hyponatremia or fluid excess; report assessment data to the physician.	The nurse collaborates with the physician when management of the client's problems involves medical interventions.

Evaluation of Expected Outcome

Client's serum sodium level is 135–145 mEq/L.

Nursing Diagnosis: Acute Pain related to tissue injury or bladder spasms

Expected Outcome: Pain will be controlled within the client's level of tolerance.

Interventions	Rationales
Check that catheter is patent and draining before administering medication.	Obstruction in the flow of urine contributes to pain.
Administer a prescribed antispasmodic, such as a belladonna and opium suppository, or prescribed medications such as oxybutynin (Ditropan) or propantheline (Pro-Banthine), or an analgesic for incisional pain.	Anticholinergics relieve bladder spasms. Analgesics interfere with the perception of pain.
Explain that the large balloon holding the catheter in place, traction on the catheter, and the volume of instilling irrigant tend to produce the urge to void, but an effort to do so contributes to discomfort.	Offering the client an explanation helps alleviate the anxiety concerning the cause of discomfort.
Use nursing measures such as placing a rolled towel beneath the scrotum, assisting with the application of an athletic support, suggesting the use of a recliner rather than sitting on a hard surface, changing position, and diversional activities.	Alternative measures enhance the response to drug therapy.

Evaluation of Expected Outcome

Pain and discomfort are tolerable.

Nursing Diagnosis: Risk for Infection related to impaired tissue and potential contamination of catheters and incisional drains

Expected Outcome: Client will be free of infection as evidenced by progressive wound healing, no fever, no purulent drainage, expected white blood cell count, and urine free of bacteria.

Interventions	Rationales
Practice conscientious hand hygiene before providing nursing care.	Hand hygiene is the single most important method to reduce the potential for spreading microorganisms.

NURSING CARE PLAN 55-2 **The Client Undergoing a Prostatectomy** (Continued)

Interventions	Rationales
Keep ports used for emptying drainage clean.	A contaminated port provides a portal for microorganisms that can ascend to other structures in the urinary tract.
Reinforce or change moist dressings using surgical asepsis.	Moisture on a dressing wicks microorganisms into the wound.
Keep perineum clean after a bowel movement for clients with a perineal prostatectomy.	Stool contains many bacteria that can easily enter a perineal wound because of its close proximity to the anus.
Report tenderness, unusual drainage, foul odor, and fever.	An infection produces a cluster of common signs and symptoms.

Evaluation of Expected Outcome

There is no evidence of infection; vital signs are normal.

Nursing Diagnosis: Risk for Impaired Skin Integrity related to leaking urine from suprapubic catheter

Expected Outcome: Skin will remain free of redness and excoriation around the catheter site.

Interventions	Rationales
Clean skin around suprapubic catheter with mild soap and water; dry skin thoroughly (Nursing Guidelines 55-1).	Wet skin causes maceration of tissue. Strong soaps can irritate the skin.
Apply and change drain gauze around suprapubic catheter as it becomes moist.	A drain gauze absorbs moisture.
Enclose the suprapubic catheter in an ostomy appliance.	Ostomy equipment can be used as a means to collect urine and prevent contact between the skin and urine.
Consult an enterostomal therapist on substances such as karaya that can be applied to the skin.	Karaya provides a moisture-resistant barrier and protects the skin.

Evaluation of Expected Outcome

Skin remains intact or the wound heals normally.

Nursing Diagnosis: Urge or Total Urinary Incontinence related to altered urinary sphincter or nerve damage secondary to surgical procedure if nerves have been spared

Expected Outcome: Client will disguise incontinence or regain continence.

Interventions	Rationales
Provide absorbent pads or underwear.	Absorbing urine reduces embarrassment associated with incontinence.
Teach pelvic floor–strengthening exercises (Client and Family Teaching 55-3).	Pelvic floor exercises strengthen the muscles that promote urinary continence.
Suggest using a penile clamp, which is molded to comfortably fit around the shaft of the penis.	A penile clamp compresses the urethra externally, preventing incontinence.

Evaluation of Expected Outcome

Continence problems are controlled.

Nursing Diagnosis: Sexual Dysfunction related to structural changes secondary to surgical procedure

Expected Outcome: Sexual activity will be satisfactory.

Interventions	Rationales
Provide information on support groups.	Others who have experienced sexual dysfunction after prostatectomy may be both supportive and influential in solving sexual problems.
Clarify information concerning potential sexual consequences of the specific surgical procedure.	Sexual problems may be temporary or permanent depending on the type of prostatectomy that is performed.

Evaluation of Expected Outcome

Client resumes sexual activity, when appropriate, or adapts to sexual changes.

Nursing Diagnosis: Risk for Ineffective Therapeutic Regimen Management related to lack of knowledge about care after discharge

(care plan continues on page 880)

NURSING CARE PLAN 55-2 **The Client Undergoing a Prostatectomy** (Continued)

Expected Outcome: Client will refer to written instructions that correlate with drug teaching, wound and catheter care, and medical follow-up.

Interventions	Rationales
Emphasize ongoing medical care.	Medical follow-up ensures progressive recovery and monitoring for developing complications.
Advise client to avoid self-administering aspirin.	Aspirin interferes with platelet aggregation, which promotes bleeding.
Explain drug action, frequency of drug administration, and side effects of medications that will be taken after discharge.	Knowledge about discharge medications promotes compliance and safe use of prescribed drugs.
Demonstrate and have client return demonstration for catheter and wound care.	Appropriate catheter and wound care reduces the potential for infection.
Identify when client can resume activity, including sexual intercourse.	Physical exertion increases the potential for bleeding.
Suggest consuming 10–12 glasses of oral fluid each day, increasing dietary fiber, or using a mild laxative or stool softener.	Preventing constipation decreases the potential for bleeding if effort is required to eliminate stool.
Instruct client to immediately report pain in the pelvis or perineum, cloudy or bloody urine that persists despite drinking fluids, or fever or chills.	Unusual signs and symptoms indicate the possibility of a developing complication.

Evaluation of Expected Outcome

Client demonstrates an understanding of perineal exercises, medication schedule, activities to avoid, when to contact physician, and wound care.

---

there is local metastasis. Possible side effects include impotence, diarrhea, and urinary frequency and urgency.

Hormone Therapy

Men with stages III or IV carcinoma of the prostate are candidates for hormone therapy (Drug Therapy Table 55-2). With the use of antiandrogenic (male) hormones or estrogenic hormones, the progression of the malignancy may be retarded and there may be a prolonged period of palliation (comfort). Estramustine (Emcyt) is a combination of estrogen and an antineoplastic drug that also is used for palliative treatment.

Feminizing side effects occur with hormone therapy. The client's voice may become higher, hair and fat distribution may change, and breasts may become tender and enlarged. Libido and potency also are diminished. When estrogens are used in lower doses, the client may not experience these problems.

Immunotherapy

As this book goes to press, clinical trials are underway for an experimental therapeutic vaccine for advanced prostate cancer. A **therapeutic vaccine** is one that treats an existing disease as opposed to a prophylactic vaccine that prevents disease. The therapeutic vaccine for advanced prostate cancer that is closest to FDA approval is sipuleucel-T (Provenge). It stimulates the immune system to recognize and attack a protein known as prostatic acid phosphatase (PAP), a tumor associated antigen, which is found in about 95% of all prostate cancer cells. Researchers are examining whether the vaccine improves treatment outcomes better than standard therapies. There is hope that the vaccine may be able to improve quality and quantity of life for clients with advanced prostate cancer and avoid the more severe side effects of traditional antineoplastic drug therapy.

Trials to date have focused on men whose cancer has spread beyond the prostate gland and who are not benefitting from therapies that deprive the tumor of testosterone. Vaccine side effects seem to be minor and short-lived and include chills, fever, headache, fatigue, shortness of breath, vomiting, and mild tremor.

Client and Family Teaching 55-3
Performing Pelvic Floor–Strengthening Exercises

The nurse emphasizes the following points when teaching the client:

- Squeeze the pelvic floor muscles (those used to stop urination and hold back a bowel movement) for up to 10 seconds—longer is not better.
- Relax completely for 10 seconds—less is not better.
- Repeat sequence as many times as possible in 5 minutes or a cycle of 15 contractions followed by relaxation.
- Interrupt exercises when muscles can no longer be contracted tightly.
- Perform exercises in the morning and evening.
- Perform shorter pelvic floor exercises four or five times during the day:
  - Squeeze pelvic floor muscles and hold for 1 second.
  - Relax for 1 second.
  - Repeat five times in succession within 2 minutes.
- Continue long and short exercises for 3 to 4 months or until continent.

TABLE 55-4 Staging and Treatment of Prostatic Cancer

STAGE	DESCRIPTION	TREATMENT
Stage I	Cancer is small, grows slowly, and may never cause symptoms or other health problems	Observation or external radiation, or brachytherapy for asymptomatic males or older males with other serious health problems; for younger and healthier males, options include observation, radical prostatectomy, external radiation, or brachytherapy.
Stage II	Tumor is larger than stage I, yet confined to the prostate gland; if left untreated, the cancer is more likely to spread beyond the prostate and cause symptoms	For asymptomatic males or those who have other serious health problems, same treatment as for stage I, or radical prostatectomy, and radiation. For younger and otherwise healthy males, radical prostatectomy with removal of pelvic lymph nodes followed by external radiation if the cancer has spread at the time of surgery or the PSA level is still detectable several weeks after surgery. If there is a greater chance for reoccurrence based on pathology examination of the tissue and PSA scores, external or internal radiation (or both), several months of hormone therapy, and participating in a clinical treatment trial
Stage III	Tumor has spread beyond the prostate, but has not reached the bladder, rectum, lymph nodes or other organs; likely to recur after treatment	Observation for asymptomatic older males or those with other more serious illness; for others, hormone therapy alone or combined with external radiation, radical prostatectomy followed by radiation, participation in a clinical treatment trial
Stage IV	Tumor has spread to the bladder, rectum, lymph nodes, or distant organs such as the bones; not considered curable	Same as stage III; in addition: TURP to relieve symptoms, chemotherapy to manage a tumor that continues to grow and spread, and adjuvant treatment to relieve bone pain or other symptoms, immunotherapy once FDA approved.

Nursing Process for the Client With Prostatic Cancer

Assessment

Obtain a health history from the client and focus on identifying information such as changes in patterns of urinary elimination (frequency, urgency, and nocturia), hematuria, low back pain, and a family history of prostatic cancer. After extensive surgical treatment for prostatic cancer, assess the client for signs of infection, urinary incontinence, and sexual dysfunction and reinforce health teaching that aids in the detection of metastasis.

Diagnosis, Planning, and Interventions

Refer to Chapter 14 for general preoperative and postoperative standards of care. Radical prostatectomy is similar to other prostatectomy procedures and the same immediate postoperative nursing diagnoses and interventions apply. Diagnoses, expected outcomes, and interventions for clients with prostatic cancer include, but are not limited to, the following:

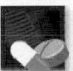

DRUG THERAPY TABLE 55-2 Hormonal Agents for Prostatic Cancer

Drug Category and Examples	Mechanism of Action	Side Effects	Nursing Considerations
Hormonal Oncologics diethylstilbestrol (DES)	Synthetic estrogen that reduces testosterone levels	Breast enlargement, nausea, vomiting, photosensitivity, elevated blood sugar	Offer small, frequent meals to offset nausea. Monitor blood sugar, especially in clients with diabetes mellitus. Recommend using a sunscreen or wearing protective clothing.
flutamide (Eulexin) bicalutamide (Casodex)	Blocks androgens	Breast enlargement, impotence, diarrhea, anemia, leukopenia, thrombocytopenia, jaundice	Instruct clients that periodic blood tests are required. Observe if urine is dark yellow.
goserelinxs (Zoladex) leuprolide (Lupron)	Inhibits pituitary gonadotropin secretion, which reduces testosterone to castration levels	Hot flashes, impotence, loss of libido	Administer as a monthly injection or subcutaneous implant. Use a local anesthetic before administering injection. Repeat injection every 28 days. Drug resistance occurs after 2 to 3 years of therapy.

▶ **Risk for Infection** related to home care of Foley catheter

▶ **Expected Outcome:** Client will be free of a urinary tract infection as evidenced by clear urine without bacteria or white blood cells.

- Tell the client to use soap and water to clean around the urethral meatus and several inches of the catheter at least twice a day. *Medical asepsis decreases the growth of microorganisms that can ascend upward into the urinary tract.*
- Demonstrate and have the client return the demonstration for keeping the connection between the catheter and leg bag clean when changing and replacing leg bags for routine cleaning. *Keeping connections and equipment clean reduces the portals for microbial entry into the urinary tract.*
- Tell the client or caregiver to clean the leg bag by using soap and water and then rinsing it with a 1:7 solution of vinegar and water. *Vinegar is a weak acid (acetic acid) that chemically interferes with the growth of microorganisms.*

▶ **Total Urinary Incontinence** related to surgical compromises to internal and external urinary sphincter muscles

▶ **Expected Outcome:** Urinary control will be re-established within 3 months after surgery or client will use equipment to collect urine.

- Teach pelvic floor retraining exercises (see Client and Family Teaching 55-3) if incontinence is not permanent. *Pelvic floor retraining exercises improve sphincter tone and bladder control.*
- For permanent incontinence, show the client how to apply a penile clamp or an external catheter connected to a leg bag. *Devising a method for mechanically controlling urinary incontinence or collecting urine unobtrusively decreases social embarrassment.*

▶ **Sexual Dysfunction** related to temporary impotence when pudendal nerve (responsible for erection and orgasm) is spared

▶ **Expected Outcome:** Client will use alternatives other than intercourse for sexual pleasure until potency resumes.

- Explain to the client and sexual partner that it may take from 3 to 12 months for sexual potency to return. *Providing a timeline helps the client and his sexual partner cope with temporary sexual dysfunction.*
- See interventions for impotence for additional suggestions. *Various alternatives to sexual intercourse may be useful for managing sexual dysfunction.*

▶ **PC: Impotence** related to pudendal nerve damage secondary to non-nerve-sparing radical perineal prostatectomy

▶ **Expected Outcome:** The nurse will assist the client and sexual partner to manage erectile dysfunction.

- Recommend demonstrating sexual feelings in ways other than intercourse. *Intimacy is communicated in many different ways. Becoming asexual is counterproductive.*
- Discuss the use of manual stimulation or a mechanical vibrator if it does not compromise the sex partner's moral values. *Stimulating the clitoris of the female manually or with a vibrator is an alternative method to sexual penetration for promoting female orgasm.*

▶ **PC: Metastasis**

▶ **Expected Outcome:** The nurse will assist the client to manage and minimize the possibility of a recurrence of the primary cancer or metastasis.

- Explain that the PSA level will decrease after prostatectomy; a subsequent rise indicates the cancer has reoccurred. *Having regular PSA levels after treatment aids in the early detection of cancer recurrence or metastasis. A phenomenon called a PSA "bounce," a rise in the PSA levels within 2 years of radiation therapy, is not pathologic; it may be caused by the release of PSA from dead and damaged cancer cells.*
- Clarify that repeat lymph node biopsies may be part of the surgical follow-up. *One method by which cancer cells are spread is the lymphatic system.*
- Inform the client that blood tests for measuring serum acid phosphatase are used to monitor evidence of bone metastasis. *A rise in acid phosphatase is a tumor marker for a client who has been treated for cancer of the prostate.*

Evaluation of Expected Outcomes

Expected outcomes for the client who is treated for cancer of the prostate are no evidence of infection and urinary continence. The client finds acceptable techniques for sexual expression when impotence is permanent. He identifies techniques that assist in monitoring for a recurrence of the primary cancer or its metastatic spread.

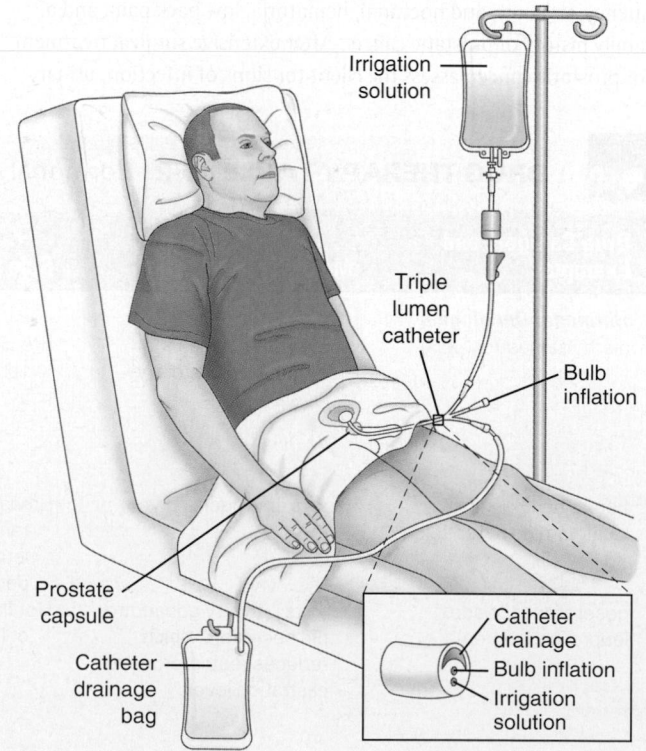

FIGURE 55-10 A three-way system for bladder irrigation.

Irrigation solution

Triple lumen catheter

Bulb inflation

Prostate capsule

Catheter drainage bag

Catheter drainage
Bulb inflation
Irrigation solution

As the client recovers, promote increased self-care and provide instructions for home management. The discharge plan of care includes, but is not limited to, the following:

- Maintain medical follow-up.
- Take medications as prescribed.
- Decrease dietary fat and increase fiber.
- Exercise regularly to increase lean body mass and decrease insulin levels, which is a catabolic hormone that promotes weight gain.
- Join a support group to learn more about the disease process and clinical research trials.
- Consult with the family physician or oncologist before self-treating with herbal supplements such as saw palmetto, which some believe is beneficial in relieving disorders of the prostate gland.

CANCER OF THE TESTES

Cancer of the testes is a malignancy seen in men between 18 and 40 years of age. Although this cancer is relatively rare, accounting for approximately 1% of cancers in men, it is the most common type in men between 15 and 34 years of age and is the leading cause of cancer deaths in men between 25 and 34 years of age. Significant advancement in treatment in recent years, however, has resulted in a 90% cure rate, even in clients with metastatic disease.

Pathophysiology and Etiology

The incidence of testicular cancer is higher in Caucasians and men with a history of cryptorchidism regardless of whether an orchiopexy was performed. Other clients who are at increased risk for testicular cancer include those with a family history of the disease, those who are human immunodeficiency virus (HIV)–positive or have developed acquired immunodeficiency syndrome (AIDS), and those who already have had cancer in one testicle. In most cases, only one testicle is affected, but the other may become cancerous if the tumor is not diagnosed early.

The exact etiology is unknown, but one possible explanation is that the cells in the undescended testis or testes degenerate earlier than occurs with natural aging. The degenerative process then leads to abnormal cellular changes.

Nearly all testicular tumors involve the sperm-forming germ cells. Those that consist of immature germ cells are called *seminomas; nonseminomas* develop among more mature, specialized germ cells. Nonseminomas grow more rapidly and tend to metastasize at a faster rate; therefore,

treatment is more aggressive. Testicular cancers tend to spread to the lungs, bone, and brain via the retroperitoneal lymph nodes or circulatory system (Nichols, 2008).

Assessment Findings

Gradual or sudden swelling of the scrotum or a lump felt on palpation always deserves prompt medical attention. The tumor usually presents as a hard, nontender nodule of the testis with additional coexisting symptoms (Box 55-1). Ultrasound of the testis may follow. Unless discovered early through testicular self-examination, the first symptoms such as unrelenting back pain or shortness of breath may be those of tumor metastasis.

Tumor markers include repeated elevations of alpha-fetoprotein and hCG. An IVP may show lymph node enlargement that displaces the ureters. Lymphangiography also is used to detect lymph node involvement. For detection of metastases, CT is preferred over MRI. Because biopsy risks spreading the highly malignant tumor cells, surgery is recommended immediately.

Medical and Surgical Management

Treatment of testicular tumors depends on the stage of the disease (Table 55-5) and includes surgery, chemotherapy, and radiation. Before medical or surgical treatment, however, the topic of sperm banking should be discussed to ensure future paternity. Locating a sperm bank and then collecting and banking sperm, which may take as long as 12 to 24 days, is omitted if the delay would jeopardize the outcome of treatment.

Surgery

A radical inguinal orchiectomy and removal of the spermatic cord are performed through an inguinal incision. The scrotal sac on the operative side looks and feels empty. It is possible to implant a testicular prosthesis filled with silicone gel at a later date.

Clients with nonseminomas usually undergo a radical, nerve-sparing, procedure known as retroperitoneal lymph

TABLE 55-5 Staging and Treatment of Germ Cell Tumors of the Testis

STAGE	DESCRIPTION	TREATMENT
Stage I	Tumor confined to the testis	Orchiectomy, retroperitoneal lymph node dissection
Stage II	Involvement of testis plus retroperitoneal nodes	Orchiectomy, retroperitoneal lymph node dissection, possible chemotherapy
Stage III	Distant metastasis	Orchiectomy, retroperitoneal lymph node dissection, four cycles of chemotherapy, surgery to resect residual masses

node dissection (RPLND) within 6 weeks of an orchiectomy as well. RPLND decreases potential metastasis from the testis and the need for chemotherapy. If only one testis is removed, sexual activity, libido, and fertility usually are unaffected. After a radical lymph node dissection, libido and erections are preserved, but unless the nerve-sparing procedure is performed, the surgery results in retrograde ejaculation.

Chemotherapy

A multiple antineoplastic drug regimen with combinations of bleomycin (Blenoxane), etoposide (Vespid), and cisplatin (Platinol), or others may be given depending on the type of tumor, stage of cancer, and surgery that was performed. Chemotherapy, which usually is aggressive initially, is modified as the tumor markers show a response. An autologous (self-donated) bone marrow transplantation may be recommended for recurrent disease or for clients who are resistant to drug therapy.

Sperm tend to be destroyed or mutated when exposed to toxic cancer drugs, but spermatogenesis eventually resumes months or years after chemotherapy. Men with low sperm counts prior to chemotherapy are less likely to recover sperm counts that are adequate for impregnation (Nichols, 2008).

Pharmacologic Considerations

- Bleomycin can cause pulmonary toxicity in those taking high doses of the drug or in those older than 70 years of age. Some clients taking bleomycin for testicular cancer have developed Raynaud's disease (see Chap. 25).

- Cisplatin is extremely nephrotoxic, and the client must be kept well hydrated. Administration of at least 3000 mL of fluid per 24 hours is necessary if the client's condition permits. Report any evidence of fluid retention such as edema, weight gain, difficulty breathing, or bubbly lung sounds. Irreversible ototoxicity can occur. Audiometric testing is recommended before the first dose and before each subsequent dose. Ototoxicity can occur after a single dose.

- Administration of antiemetic drugs before chemotherapy can reduce or eliminate the incidence of nausea and vomiting. Some chemotherapeutic agents, such as cisplatin, however, can cause severe nausea and vomiting that does not respond well to antiemetics, and that can persist for up to 7 days after treatment.

- All chemotherapeutic agents are capable of causing an anaphylactoid reaction. Report any of the following symptoms to the primary healthcare provider: any skin rash, hives, difficulty breathing, wheezing, tachycardia, or hypotension.

- Chemotherapy for cancer increases the risk of infection, anorexia, vomiting, and hair loss.

- Drugs such as epoetin (Epogen, Procrit) and filgrastim (Neupogen) or pegfilgrastim (Neulasta) can stimulate the development of red and white blood cells whose production has been suppressed with antineoplastic drugs.

NURSING GUIDELINES 55-1

Managing the Care of a Client With a Suprapubic Catheter*

Purpose: To drain urine from the bladder through a catheter that is inserted through the anterior abdominal wall and anchored with external skin sutures. The client may or may not have a urethral (Foley) catheter as well.

- Stabilize the catheter by taping it to the skin of the abdomen.
- Keep the catheter connected to a sterile drainage system.
- Keep the drainage system below the level of the insertion site.
- Empty the urine from the bag periodically to reduce tension on the catheter and skin.
- Record the urine output from the suprapubic catheter separate from voided urine output or output from another catheter.
- Keep the skin clean and dry at the insertion site to avoid skin irritation and compromised skin integrity.
- For "trial voiding":
  - Clamp the catheter for 4 hours.
  - Have the client void naturally.
  - Unclamp the suprapubic catheter.
  - Measure the residual urine.
- Collaborate with the physician on removing the suprapubic catheter when the residual urine is repeatedly <100 mL.
- To remove the catheter:
  - Offer an analgesic 30 minutes before proceeding.
  - Wash hands and don gloves.
  - Empty the urinary drainage and record amount.
  - Position the client on his back.
  - Free the tape from the skin.
  - Remove gloves, rewash hands.
  - Open a suture removal kit.
  - Don sterile gloves.
  - Remove the skin sutures.
  - Pull gently on the catheter until it is free.
  - Place a sterile dressing over the insertion site.
  - Remove gloves and wash hands.
  - Change the dressing when it becomes moist until the site heals in approximately 2 days.

*A suprapubic catheter also may be called a *cystostomy tube*.

Radiation

Seminomas are sensitive to radiation, and most clients receive radiation to the retroperitoneal lymph nodes. Shielding of the remaining testis minimizes impairment of sperm production. For clients with nonseminomas, radiation is considered an adjunct to lymphadenectomy and chemotherapy.

Nursing Management
Preoperative Period

One of nursing's chief concerns is responding to the client's emotional distress over having a life-threatening diagnosis, being unfamiliar with the surgical experience, and confronting alterations in body image and sexuality. All clients are understandably concerned over the potential change in their sexual image and fertility; however, it may be of even greater concern to men in the age group most often affected. The nurse provides private opportunities for the client to ask questions and uses therapeutic communication techniques to encourage the client to verbalize his feelings.

Postoperative Period

Refer to Chapter 14 for postoperative standards of care. After an orchiectomy the nurse applies a scrotal support. If drains have been inserted, they are connected to closed (Jackson-Pratt) or open (machine) suction. The nurse gives prophylactic antibiotics to prevent infection. He or she manages pain, which may be severe after a radical lymph node dissection, with narcotic analgesics. If pain is not relieved and nursing measures to augment the effect of analgesics are inadequate, the nurse collaborates with the physician to modify drug therapy.

As the client's comfort improves, the nurse may discuss the effects of the diagnosis and treatment and again provide opportunities for the safe expression of anxiety, fear, and grief. The nurse provides the client with names of local support groups and encourages him to contact them for emotional support after discharge.

A teaching plan includes the following instructions for home care:

- Drink plenty of fluids and eat a well-balanced diet to avoid constipation.
- Obtain adequate rest; avoid fatigue and heavy lifting.
- Wash the incision with warm soap and water. Report any redness, drainage, pain, or swelling of the incision or scrotum.
- Take any prescribed medication exactly as directed.
- Perform self-examination of the remaining testicle every month and immediately report any changes.
- Seek care if any of the following occur: fever, chills, adverse drug effects, weight loss, or anorexia.

For clients who are concerned about future reproduction, the nurse discusses issues as appropriate for the client's particular situation. If a client has banked sperm, the nurse informs him that normal pregnancies have occurred with sperm stored up to 10 years. For clients for whom treatment has proceeded without collecting and storing sperm, the nurse identifies other options, such as donor insemination or adoption. He or she may suggest contacting the department of social services to become a foster parent, volunteering as a Big Brother, or leading a scout troop or youth group to compensate for the inability to raise biologic children.

CANCER OF THE PENIS

Penile cancer is rare and occurs more often in men who are uncircumcised. The cause is unknown but it is thought that chronic irritation leads to a precancerous skin lesion that eventually undergoes malignant changes. Medical attention is sought when the lesion, which typically has been present for years, becomes infected. Biopsy confirms the existence of malignant cells and lymphangiography identifies if the lymph nodes are involved. The tumor is staged using MRI and CT scanning.

Treatment includes tumor excision, chemotherapy, external or interstitial radiation therapy, or all three. In some cases, the penis is partially or completely amputated and the scrotum and testes excised. Full amputation of the penis requires the insertion of a permanent drainage tube in the perineal tissue to empty the bladder. The 5-year survival rate for cancer of the penis is 65%.

ELECTIVE STERILIZATION

A **vasectomy** is a minor surgical procedure done in a physician's office or clinic. It involves the ligation of the vas deferens and results in permanent sterilization by interrupting the pathway that transports sperm (Fig. 55-11). On occasion, the client may complain of impotence, although the procedure has no effect on erection or ejaculation. It may take several weeks or more after surgery before the ejaculatory fluid is free of sperm, and the client is informed to use a reliable method of contraception until sperm no longer are present. The client may wish to consider banking sperm before undergoing the procedure. Some men feel ambivalent about having this procedure, and the nurse provides the client with an opportunity to express these feelings.

The nurse reinforces the following important information for home care after a vasectomy:

- Expect some bruising and incisional soreness after the local anesthetic wears off.
- Apply ice packs to the scrotum to reduce swelling; remove the cold application after 20 minutes and replace again after the tissue rewarms.
- Take a mild analgesic, such as aspirin or acetaminophen, for discomfort.
- Wear an athletic support for several days for comfort.
- Resume usual activities in 2 to 3 days, but avoid strenuous exercise for up to 5 days.
- Resume sexual activity when comfort allows, usually in 1 week.
- Use a reliable method of contraception until the physician indicates that sperm no longer are present, which may be determined after 10 or more ejaculations.
- Report severe pain, fever, or swelling at the top of the testes.

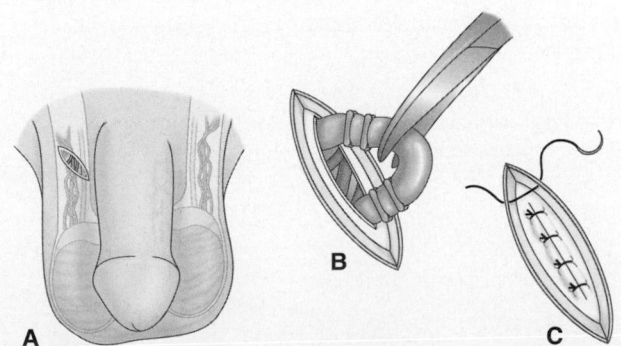

FIGURE 55-11 Vasectomy procedure. (**A**) An incision is made to expose the vas deferens. (**B**) The vas deferens is isolated and severed. (**C**) The severed ends are occluded with sutures or sealed with electrocautery, and the incision is closed.

A vasovasostomy is a surgical attempt to reverse a vasectomy by restoring patency and continuity to the vas deferens; a vasoepididymostomy connects the stump of the vas deferens directly to the epididymis. It may take from 3 to 6 months after reversal procedures before sperm counts and motility are normal. Lack of success usually is the result of either scar formation or sperm leakage from the surgical connection.

CRITICAL THINKING EXERCISES

1. Assume you are attending a team conference to plan the care of a client who is having a suprapubic prostatectomy. What nursing interventions are appropriate?
2. Describe the typical client who acquires benign prostatic hypertrophy versus one who develops testicular cancer.
3. What information can the nurse provide to a male who is experiencing erectile dysfunction?
4. A male is considering a vasectomy but is worried that the procedure will affect his sexuality. How would the nurse respond?

NCLEX-STYLE REVIEW QUESTIONS

1. An client describes experiencing nocturia. To gather more information about symptoms associated with benign prostatic hypertrophy, which question is most important to ask next?
   1. "Have you noticed any changes in sexual function?"
   2. "Have you felt any lumps in your scrotum recently?"
   3. "Do you have difficulty starting to void?"
   4. "Do you have problems controlling urination?"
2. A nurse is assigned to care for a client following a suprapubic prostatectomy. The client has a catheter in the urethra and another in an abdominal incision. When documenting the urinary output in the medical record, what is the most correct nursing documentation?
   1. Record only the output from the urethral catheter.
   2. Record only the output from the wound catheter.
   3. Record the output from each catheter separately.
   4. Record the combined output from both catheters.
3. Which nursing intervention is most important to add to the plan for care following the removal of a suprapubic catheter?
   1. Reposition the client every 2 hours.
   2. Change abdominal dressing when wet.
   3. Ambulate the client with assistance.
   4. Encourage deep breathing hourly.
4. Why would the nurse advise a client who has been prescribed sildenafil (Viagra) for erectile dysfunction to avoid taking a nitrate such as sublingual nitroglycerin (Nitrostat)?
   1. The combination interferes with an erection.
   2. Sildenafil counteracts vasodilation by nitroglycerin
   3. The client is likely to experience hypotension
   4. Priapism is likely to occur when used together
5. What factor is most likely responsible for a client's development of orchitis?
   1. The client was never immunized for mumps.
   2. The client is an active homosexual.
   3. The client has multiple sexual partners.
   4. The client is a military veteran.

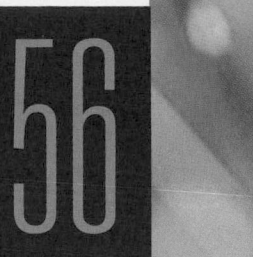

56

Caring for Clients with Sexually Transmitted Infections

Words To Know

autoinoculation
chancre
chancroid
Charcot's joints
chlamydia
condylomata
genital herpes
genital warts
gonorrhea
granuloma inguinale
herpes simplex virus type 2
human papillomavirus
lymphogranuloma venereum
neuropathic joint disease
syphilis
tabes dorsalis
venereal diseases

Learning Objectives

On completion of this chapter, you will be able to:

1. Name five common sexually transmitted infections (STIs) and identify those that are curable.
2. List five STIs that by law must be reported.
3. Give two reasons why statistics on reportable STIs are not totally accurate.
4. Discuss several factors contributing to the transmission of STIs.
5. Give two reasons why women acquire STIs more often than men.
6. Name the most common and fastest-spreading STI.
7. Explain two ways STIs are spread.
8. Discuss methods that are helpful in preventing STIs.
9. Discuss information that is important to teach clients about using condoms.
10. Name the type of infectious microorganism that causes each of the common STIs.
11. Identify complications that are common among clients who acquire each of the most common STIs.
12. Name drugs used to treat common STIs.

Sexually transmitted infections (STIs), also known as *sexually transmitted diseases (STDs)* or **venereal diseases**, are a diverse group of infections spread through sexual activity with an infected person. The term *STI* is increasingly used to emphasize that a person can be infected without experiencing symptoms of disease. STIs are a significant public health problem. Some, such as acquired immunodeficiency syndrome (AIDS; see Chap. 35), hepatitis (see Chap. 47), and skin infestations with lice and mites (see Chap. 65), are spread by additional routes as well. The pathogens that cause STIs include bacteria, fungi, parasites, protozoans, and viruses. Besides AIDS, the five most common STIs are chlamydia, gonorrhea, syphilis, genital herpes, and genital warts. Of these, chlamydia, gonorrhea, and syphilis are easily cured with early and adequate treatment. Social, sexual, and biologic factors contribute to the high incidence of STIs and include the following:

- Ignorance of how STIs are transmitted or prevented
- Asymptomatic sexual partner(s)
- Casual sex with partner(s) about whom little is known
- Sex with high-risk partner(s), such as those who use intravenous (IV) drugs, are bisexual, or have sex with prostitutes
- Multiple concurrent or sequential sexual partner(s)
- Failure to use contraceptive techniques that also reduce the risk of acquiring STIs
- Sexual contact during the period between infection and the manifestation of symptoms

- Failure to seek early treatment
- Noncompliance with treatment or failure to refrain from sexual contact until treatment is complete
- Mutation and resistance of microorganisms to antimicrobial drug therapy

EPIDEMIOLOGY

Epidemiology is the study of the occurrence, distribution, and causes of human diseases. The Centers for Disease Control and Prevention (CDC) has the challenging task of gathering disease statistics such as the incidence of STIs. Determining the exact incidence of these diseases is difficult because only a few are reportable by law. Of the reportable diseases, some are undiagnosed and untreated, some are treated and unreported, and some are misdiagnosed.

Reporting of new STI cases is the responsibility of either the healthcare provider or the testing laboratory. This reporting is kept confidential, and it is protected from subpoena. The reported incidence of STIs is disproportionately higher in racial and ethnic minorities. This disparity may be the result of (1) limited access to healthcare, (2) poverty, (3) actual higher rate of disease occurrence, or (4) more reporting by public health clinics where many in these respective populations seek treatment (CDC, 2007).

Table 56-1 lists data on the reportable STIs in the United States in 2006 according to statistics compiled by the CDC. Other STIs such as genital herpes, hepatitis B, venereal warts (condylomata acuminata), granuloma inguinale, and lymphoma venereum are not reportable by law. Therefore, it is difficult to document the statistics pertaining to these diseases. STIs occur more often in women than in men, probably because the moist, warm vaginal environment is conducive to microbial growth and because the vagina, as a receptive orifice, is more readily traumatized during sexual activity.

Obtaining a sexual history (Box 56-1) is a crucial component of assessment of clients presenting with signs or symptoms of an STI. Asking questions nonjudgmentally is essential.

TABLE 56-1 Incidence of Reportable STIs in the United States in 2006

DISEASE	NUMBER OF NEW CASES IN U.S. (2006)	RATE OF INCREASE FROM 2005
Chlamydia	1,030,911	5.6%
Gonorrhea	358,366	5.5%
Syphilis	9,756	13.8%
Chancroid	33	48.4%
HIV/AIDS	56,300	Generally stable since 1990s

From: Centers for Disease Control and Prevention. (2007). Trends in Reportable Sexually Transmitted Disease in the United States, 2006. http://www.cdc.gov/STD/STATS06/trends2006.htm;? Centers for Disease Control and Prevention. (2007). STD Surveillance 2006. http://www.cdc.gov/std/STATS06/toc2006.htm; Centers for Disease Control and Prevention. (2008). Estimates of New HIV Infections in the United States. http://www.cdc.gov/hiv/topics/surveillance/resources/factsheets/incidence.htm.

BOX 56-1 Questions to Ask When Obtaining a Sexual History from the Client With an STI

- Have you had new or multiple sexual partners in recent weeks?
- Do you use a condom during sexual activity?
- Do you have a history of an STI?
- Have you engaged in vaginal, anal, or oral sex?
- Were you the receptive partner in anal or oral sex?
- Do you have a history of infection with human immunodeficiency virus (HIV)?
- Do you have a history of employment as a sex worker?
- DO you use drugs or alcohol when engaging in sex?
- Is there a possibility of pregnancy?

Gerontologic Considerations

- The stereotype that older adults are not sexually active is inaccurate. A health history for older adults should include questions about sexuality and behaviors that put clients at risk for STIs.

- Some older adults with STIs may have limited knowledge of STIs or may be embarrassed to discuss symptoms. Not recognizing symptoms may cause them to delay seeking healthcare. Therefore, a thorough history and physical and psychosocial assessment are important, and education should include explanations of treatments and avoidance of sexual behaviors until treatment is completed in order to prevent infection of the partner.

- Older adults in nonmonogamous relationships who are no longer concerned about an unplanned pregnancy are at risk for STIs if they fail to use barrier or chemical contraceptive methods at the time of sexual intimacy.

In addition to curing the infection when possible (some STIs are not curable), treatment consists of education and counseling to reduce the client's risk of contracting an STI in the future (Client and Family Teaching 56-1). Screening counseling, and, if indicated, treating his or her sexual partner(s) is essential.

COMMON SEXUALLY TRANSMITTED INFECTIONS

CHLAMYDIA

Chlamydia is the most common and fastest-spreading bacterial STI in the United States. The number of new cases totals 2.8 million per year (Centers for Disease Control and Prevention (CDC), 2007).

Pathophysiology and Etiology

The causative microorganism is a bacterium, *Chlamydia trachomatis*, that lives inside the cells it infects. The disease is spread by sexual intercourse or genital contact without penetration.

Client and Family Teaching 56-1
Methods for Reducing the Risk of STIs

The nurse emphasizes the following methods to reduce risk:

● Abstain from sexual activities.
● Have monogamous sex with an uninfected partner.
● Use latex condoms with nonoxynol-9 (a spermicide) when having oral, vaginal, or anal intercourse.
● Combine the use of male condoms with a spermicide when having vaginal intercourse, or use a female condom.
● Urinate and wash the genital and perineal areas before and immediately after having sexual intercourse.
● Wash your hands and any areas where there has been direct contact with semen or vaginal mucus.
● Refuse or terminate sexual activity that causes trauma to the genitals, internal reproductive structures, anus, and elsewhere.
● If infected, report the information to all sexual partners and encourage them to seek medical diagnosis and treatment.
● Avoid unprotected sex until you and sexual partners have completed treatment.

The microorganism invades the reproductive structures (see discussion of pelvic inflammatory disease [PID] in Chap. 53), the urethra in women, and the urethra and epididymis in men (see discussion of urethritis in this chapter). The tissue irritation, which may be permanent despite successful eradication of the bacteria, puts those with chlamydial infections at greater risk for acquiring other STIs, such as AIDS.

Untreated chlamydia can cause sterility in infected women; infected pregnant women can transmit the microorganism to their infants during birth.

Chlamydial infections also can be spread to the eyes by **autoinoculation** (self-transmission to another area of the body), usually by unwashed hands. Ophthalmic infections, which are more common in underdeveloped countries where flies are the vector for transmitting the microorganism, can cause granulation of the cornea and blindness.

Assessment Findings

As many as 75% of all infected women and 25% of all infected men are asymptomatic. Symptoms, if they occur, may appear 1 to 3 weeks after infection. They include a sparse, clear urethral discharge, redness and irritation of the infected tissue, burning on urination, lower abdominal pain in women, and testicular pain in men.

Diagnosis is made by microscopic examination and culture of secretions. A test kit is available that identifies the microorganism in approximately 15 minutes. The CDC (2007) recommends annual screening for chlamydia in all sexually active women younger than 26 years of age and in women with new or multiple sexual partners to reduce the incidence of PID. It is a common practice to test clients for chlamydia, gonorrhea, as well as syphilis, because it is not unusual for clients to have concurrent infections with more than one STI.

Medical Management

Antimicrobial drugs, such as a single oral dose of azithromycin (Zithromax) or a 7-day regimen of doxycycline (Vibramycin), erythromycin (E-Mycin), ofloxacin (Floxin), or levofloxacin (Levaquin) are used for treatment.

Pharmacologic Considerations

- It is important to obtain an allergy history before administration of any antimicrobial agent. Inform the physician of a client's allergy to any antimicrobial agent, so that he or she can order an alternative drug.

- Both doxycycline and azithromycin are contraindicated during pregnancy.

Nursing Management

The nurse sensitively obtains a sexual history, follows precautions for preventing infection transmission, assists in collecting a specimen for microscopic analysis, explains the course of treatment, and discusses methods for preventing transmission and reinfection (Nursing Care Plan 56-1 and Client and Family Teaching 56-2).

GONORRHEA

Gonorrhea is the second most frequently reported communicable disease in the United States (CDC, 2007). Its highest incidence occurs in the 15- to 24-year-old age group. Many women are asymptomatic, a factor that contributes to the spread of the disease.

Pathophysiology and Etiology

The infection is caused by a bacterium, *Neisseria gonorrhoeae*, which can be transmitted heterosexually or homosexually. The microorganism invades the urethra, vagina, rectum, or pharynx, depending on the nature of sexual contact; it can spread throughout the body.

In untreated men, the localized infection may spread to the prostate, seminal vesicles, and epididymis. Urethral strictures may develop, requiring periodic dilation of the urethra or, possibly, reconstructive urethral surgery. In women, the infection may progress upward to the cervix, endometrium, and fallopian tubes, and symptoms of PID (see Chap. 53) may develop. Data suggests that gonorrhea facilitates human immunodeficiency virus (HIV) transmission (CDC, 2007). Gonorrhea also can be transmitted to an infant's eyes at the time of birth.

Assessment Findings
Signs and Symptoms

In men, symptoms usually appear 2 to 6 days after infection. Urethritis with a purulent discharge and pain on urination are the most common signs and symptoms. A small proportion of men are asymptomatic. More than half of infected women experience no symptoms. When symptoms do occur, women have a white or yellow vaginal discharge, intermenstrual

NURSING CARE PLAN 56-1 | The Client With an STI

Assessment

Determine the following:

- Vital signs
- Health history with a focus on the onset and course of current symptoms
- Similar symptoms in sexual partner(s)
- Presence of oral, vaginal, rectal, or genitourinary lesions

- Characteristics of discharge (vaginal, urethral, rectal), if any is evident
- Evidence of skin rash or abnormal appearance of integument
- Accompanying symptoms such as joint or abdominal pain or pain during intercourse
- Failure to become pregnant if pregnancy is desired
- Drug and allergy history

Nursing Diagnosis: Situational Low Self-Esteem related to shame or guilt about acquiring an STI

Expected Outcome: Client's self-esteem will be positive.

Interventions	Rationales
Avoid being judgmental.	Negative responses from others lower self-esteem.
Affirm client's good judgment in seeking treatment.	Acknowledging a positive action helps increase client's self-esteem.
Assure client that medical information is confidential and, although some STIs are reported, access to such information is carefully guarded.	Keeping personal information confidential helps the client avoid any public ridicule.
Refer client to a support group for people who have acquired a similar STI.	Members of support groups have similar problems and help others cope with medical, emotional, and social issues.

Evaluation of Expected Outcome

Client's self-esteem improves or remains at the same level as before he or she required medical treatment for STI.

Nursing Diagnosis: Acute Pain related to inflammation and changes in the skin and mucous membranes

Expected Outcome: Pain will be relieved to client's level of tolerance.

Interventions	Rationales
Provide a prescribed analgesic.	Analgesics relieve pain by various physiologic mechanisms.
Administer prescribed antimicrobials specific to the infectious microorganism.	Discomfort usually is relieved when the infection resolves.
Advise regular bathing.	Bathing removes irritating drainage.
Recommend wearing loosely woven cotton underwear and full-cut, nonconstricting outer clothing.	Cotton is a natural fiber that wicks drainage away from the body. Nonconstricting clothing allows air to circulate between the skin and outerwear and avoids friction.

Evaluation of Expected Outcome

Client is comfortable; symptoms are reduced or relieved.

Nursing Diagnoses: Impaired Skin Integrity and **Impaired Mucous Membranes** related to inflammation of local tissues and scratching secondary to infectious process

Expected Outcomes: (1) Skin lesions will heal. (2) Integrity of mucous membranes will be restored.

Interventions	Rationales
Provide information on appropriate topical skin applications.	Various over-the-counter and prescription medications can be applied to the skin to relieve inflammation, reduce itching, lubricate the skin, and dry lesions.
Advise client to pat rather than rub skin dry.	Patting reduces friction and the itch-scratch-itch cycle.
Reinforce compliance with medical treatment.	Taking prescribed medications according to directions ensures eradication or control of the infecting microorganism.

NURSING CARE PLAN 56-1 The Client With an STI (Continued)

Evaluation of Expected Outcomes

Skin and mucous membranes are intact; no lesions are evident.

Nursing Diagnosis: Risk for Infection Transmission related to infectious drainage and viral shedding

Expected Outcome: The infection will remain confined and not be transmitted to any other susceptible host.

Interventions	Rationales
Follow Standard Precautions before diagnosis and Contact Precautions after diagnosis is confirmed.	Standard Precautions reduce the risk of transmission of a blood-borne infection before a diagnosis is made. Transmission-based precautions interfere with the routes by which specific pathogens are spread.
Advise client to have all sexual partners tested and treated.	STIs often are transmitted between both sexual partners; to eradicate the infection, sexual partners must be treated as well.
Identify methods for preventing STIs such as abstinence, barrier and chemical types of contraceptives, and voiding and washing after sexual intercourse.	STIs are spread by direct contact; methods that prevent direct contact reduce the potential for disease transmission.
Recommend early prenatal care to pregnant women.	Some STIs can be transmitted during childbirth.
Explain how to manage articles used for personal hygiene and items to avoid sharing with noninfected people.	Keeping personal hygiene items separate from others and preventing indirect contact with contaminated items can reduce the potential for disease transmission.
Direct client to take medications as prescribed and return for medical follow-up.	Compliance and medical follow-up help ensure that the infection responds to treatment.

Evaluation of Expected Outcome

No other person acquires the STI from the infected person.

Nursing Diagnosis: Anxiety related to possible consequences of STI

Expected Outcome: Client will feel comfortable when he or she acquires realistic information.

Interventions	Rationales
Explain the cause of the STI and how to avoid potential consequences or complications.	Accurate knowledge dispels inaccurate beliefs and misconceptions.
Instruct client infected with carcinogenic (cancer-causing) viruses to have regular cancer screening examinations.	These examinations in risk-prone clients facilitate early diagnosis and optimistic prognosis.

Evaluation of Expected Outcome

Client feels self-assured and confident about managing the STI.

Nursing Diagnosis: Ineffective Sexuality Patterns related to shame about revealing the risk for an STI to sexual partner(s)

Expected Outcome: Client will resume sexual relationships with modifications that help to avoid STI transmission.

Interventions	Rationales
Role-play situations in which client communicates his or her STI status to a significant other.	Role-playing with an uninvolved person helps a person rehearse and prepare for a situation that evokes anxiety.
Suggest that the client and sexual partner(s) discuss and select methods that will facilitate sexual activity without transmitting the STI.	Open communication facilitates a mutual plan for reducing the potential for disease transmission.

Evaluation of Expected Outcome

Client discusses and implements modifications for sexual expression.

Nursing Diagnoses: Risk for Ineffective Therapeutic Regimen Management and **Risk for Noncompliance** related to lack of knowledge or abandoning recommendations

Expected Outcomes: (1) Client will understand the regimen for curing or controlling the STI. (2) Client will comply with the plan of care.

(care plan continues on page 892)

NURSING CARE PLAN 56-1   The Client With an STI (Continued)

Interventions	Rationales
Provide specific client teaching that is appropriate for the particular STI.	STIs result from various pathogens; treatment varies.
Emphasize completing the full course of drug therapy.	Drug therapy may cure or slow the progression of the STI and relieve symptoms.
Provide client with a telephone number for obtaining objective and authoritative information.	Clients may be more inclined to ask questions about an STI and its treatment if their identity can remain anonymous.
Schedule an appointment for follow-up care.	Medical follow-up promotes compliance with therapeutic regimen.

Evaluation of Expected Outcomes

Client paraphrases the plan for treatment and carries out prescribed interventions.

bleeding due to cervicitis, and painful urination. An anal infection is accompanied by painful bowel elimination and a purulent rectal discharge; the throat is sore when the pharynx is infected. If the microorganism disseminates (scatters) throughout the body, the client may manifest a skin rash, fever, and painful joints.

Diagnostic Findings

Specimens of drainage from infected tissue are examined microscopically immediately after they are collected or are inoculated on a culture medium and incubated to reveal the causative organism.

Medical Management

The microorganism *N. gonorrhoeae* has become increasingly resistant to penicillin, tetracyclines, and fluoroquinolones. Therefore, the current CDC (2006) recommendation for treating gonorrhea is a single intramuscular dose of a broad-spectrum cephalosporin such as ceftriaxone (Rocephin) or oral dosing with cefixime (Suprax). Coinfection with chlamydia is common; therefore, clients also are given a single dose of oral azithromycin (Zithromax) or oral doxycycline (Vibramycin) for 7 to 10 days. Clients with complicated gonococcal infections, as in PID or disseminated infection, are hospitalized and treated with IV multiple-drug therapy. Repeat therapy with different antibiotics may be required.

Nursing Management

The nursing management and client teaching are similar for those clients with chlamydia. However, when a culture is collected from a woman, the vaginal speculum is moistened with water rather than lubricated, because lubricant may destroy the gonococci and cause inaccurate test results. See Nursing Care Plan 56-1 for additional nursing management.

 Pharmacologic Considerations

- Explain the prescribed drug regimen to the client. Information includes the number of capsules or tablets per dose, the time of day to take the drug, food restrictions (if any), and possible adverse effects. Emphasize the importance of completing a course of therapy.

SYPHILIS

Syphilis is a curable STI that also can be transmitted from the blood of an infected person, directly from the lesion, or across the placenta to an unborn infant. The incidence of syphilis in the United States has been increasing for the past 6 years, especially among women, newborns of infected mothers, African Americans, and men having sex with men (CDC, 2007).

Pathophysiology and Etiology

The spirochete *Treponema pallidum* is the causative microorganism of syphilis. The time between infection and the first occurrence of symptoms is about 21 days. If untreated, syphilis progresses through three distinct stages: primary, secondary, and tertiary. Syphilis is infectious only during the primary and secondary stages. In the third stage, the client becomes demented and dies from complications involving other organ systems.

 Client and Family Teaching 56-2
The Client With an STI

The nurse emphasizes the following points when teaching the client:

● Take prescribed medication according to label directions for the full length of time that it is prescribed.
● Stop having sex until retesting indicates that the infection is gone.
● Urge any and all sexual partners to be examined and follow through with concurrent treatment.
● Use a condom, a contraceptive barrier device, consistently and correctly (Client and Family Teaching 56-3) before any and all sexual contact after completing medical treatment.
● Do not assume that successful treatment means there is any permanent immunity; reinfection can and does occur if preventive sexual practices are not implemented.
● Seek treatment as soon as possible if the symptoms continue or if they recur after successful treatment.

Client and Family Teaching 56-3
Proper Use of Condoms

The nurse emphasizes the following points when teaching the client:

- Purchase condoms that are made in the United States because they are of higher quality and have been tested for reliability.
- Select condoms that are lubricated with a spermicide or silicone.
- Do not use natural-membrane condoms, which act as a barrier to sperm but allow viruses to pass through
- Keep condoms in a cool, dry place.
- Discard condoms beyond their expiration date or if they are more than 5 years old.
- Never unroll or examine a condom before its use or use one that appears to have deteriorated.
- Pinch the space at the condom tip (Fig. A) while unrolling the condom over the erect penis (Fig. B). Unroll the condom all the way to the base of the penis.
- Use additional water-based lubricant to reduce friction and prevent tearing the condom; avoid oil-based lubricants, which can weaken latex.
- Remove the condom from the vagina before the penis becomes limp.

- Dispose of the condom in a lined container.
- Apply a new condom before each sex act.
- Use a silicone-based lubricant to prevent the condom from breaking; silicone does not deteriorate latex.
- Understand that breakage and slipping rates may be higher during anal sex.

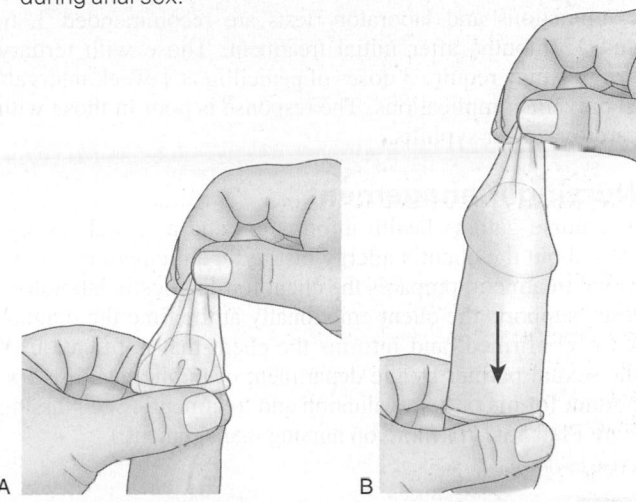

A   B

(Adapted from American Social Health Association. [1999–2008]. How to use a condom—Do's and don'ts. Available: http://www.ashastd.org/condom/condom_overview.cfm)

Assessment Findings

Signs and Symptoms

In the primary (early) stage, a **chancre** (painless ulcer) appears on the genitals, anus, cervix, or other parts of the body (Fig. 56-1). At first, the lesion resembles a small papule, which later ulcerates. The chancre heals in several weeks and, if treatment has not been initiated, the client progresses to the secondary stage of syphilis.

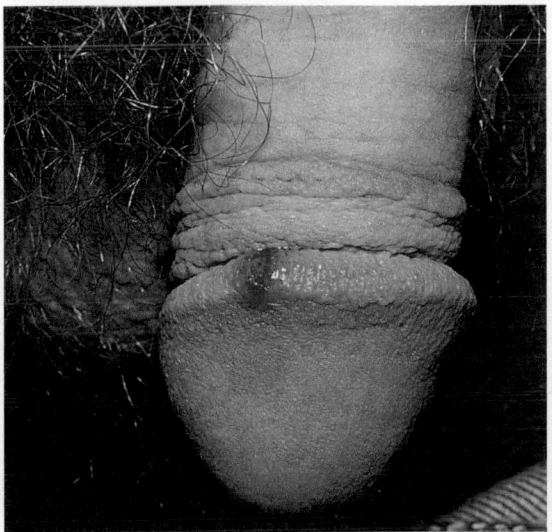

FIGURE 56-1 Syphilitic chancre on the penis. (From Rubin, R., & Strayer, D. S. [2008]. *Rubin's pathology: Clinicopathologic foundations of medicine.* [5th ed.]. Philadelphia; Lippincott Williams & Wilkins.)

Symptoms of secondary syphilis include fever, malaise, rash, headache, sore throat, and lymph node enlargement. Late, or tertiary, syphilis is noninfectious because the microorganism has invaded the central nervous system (CNS) as well as other organs of the body. Symptoms of tertiary syphilis include **tabes dorsalis** (a degenerative condition of the CNS that results in loss of peripheral reflexes and of vibratory and position senses), ataxia, and **neuropathic joint disease**, also called **Charcot's joints**. Cardiovascular complications include aortic aneurysm and aortic valve insufficiency.

Gerontologic Considerations

- Syphilis causes approximately 10% of cases of heart disease in clients older than 50 years of age. The most frequently seen valvular disorder that results from syphilis is aortic insufficiency. Damaged valves may need to be replaced with a ball-valve prosthesis. Dementia may be a complication of tertiary syphilis.

Diagnostic Findings

Diagnosis is made by detecting the spirochete in microscopic examination of scrapings from the chancre, by a positive Venereal Disease Research Laboratory (VDRL) test or rapid plasma reagin (RPR) on blood serum, and a positive fluorescent treponemal antibody absorption test (FTA-ABS). Occasionally, the FTA-ABS test is falsely positive in clients with systemic lupus erythematosus, a connective tissue disease; and rheumatoid arthritis. When a person develops CNS symptoms, the cerebrospinal fluid is examined.

Medical Management

A single dose of parenterally administered penicillin G (Pfizerpen, Wycillin) is used to treat primary and secondary syphilis. Clients who are allergic to penicillin are given a 14-day regimen of tetracycline or doxycycline. Follow-up examinations and laboratory tests are recommended 3, 6, and 12 months after initial treatment. Those with tertiary syphilis may require 3 doses of penicillin at 1-week intervals to prevent complications. The response is poor in those with cardiovascular syphilis.

Nursing Management

The nurse gathers health information and a sexual history, asks about the client's allergy history in anticipation of antibiotic treatment, prepares the client for diagnostic laboratory tests, supports the client emotionally at the time the diagnosis is confirmed, and informs the client that notification of the sexual partner by the department of public health is important for his or her evaluation and treatment. (See Nursing Care Plan 56-1 for more on nursing management.)

Pharmacologic Considerations

- Monitor clients receiving penicillin for at least 30 minutes after a parenteral injection to watch for a possible allergic reaction. Symptoms of an allergic reaction include pruritus, difficulty breathing, hypotension, sweating, and tachycardia.

HERPES INFECTION

Herpes infection is a highly contagious STI that is controllable but not curable. Presently, herpes affects at least 50 million people in the United States (CDC, 2006). It increases the risk of cervical cancer and infection with HIV.

Pathophysiology and Etiology

Although **herpes simplex virus type 2** (HSV-2), also known as **genital herpes**, is primarily responsible for genital and perineal lesions, herpes simplex virus type 1 (HSV-1), associated with cold sores around the nose and lips, also can cause anogenital lesions. One in five people older than 12 years of age is infected with the virus that causes genital herpes; at the current rate of infection, approximately 40% to 50% of Americans may be infected by the year 2025 (American Social Health Association, 2006). Transmission of the herpes viruses is by either direct contact with oral or genital secretions from a person during an active stage of the disease, sexual contact during periods of asymptomatic viral shedding, or autoinoculation. Transmission also can occur from mother to infant during a vaginal birth and carries a neonatal mortality rate of 50%. HSV-1 and HSV-2 may be introduced into the eye, the mouth, the genital area, or a skin site.

Herpes recurs because after the initial infection, the virus remains dormant in the ganglia of the nerves that supply the area. Symptoms usually are more severe with the initial outbreak. Subsequent episodes usually are shorter and less intense. When the virus is active, shedding viral particles are infectious.

Most clients with genital herpes have at least one outbreak per year, and many clients report 5 to 10 outbreaks per year. Some clients note that stress, emotional situations, exposure to sunlight, menstruation, and fever reactivate the disease.

Assessment Findings

After a short incubation period, HSV-2 causes single or multiple vesicles on the penis, prepuce, buttocks, thighs, introitus, or cervix (Fig. 56-2). The HSV-2 lesions burn and itch before becoming fluid-filled blisters. The vesicles rupture in 1 to 3 days and are followed by painful, reddened ulcers that scab over and eventually disappear. The outbreak may be accompanied by swelling of the inguinal lymph nodes, flu-like symptoms, and headache. The initial attack lasts 3 to 4 weeks; subsequent attacks usually last 10 days.

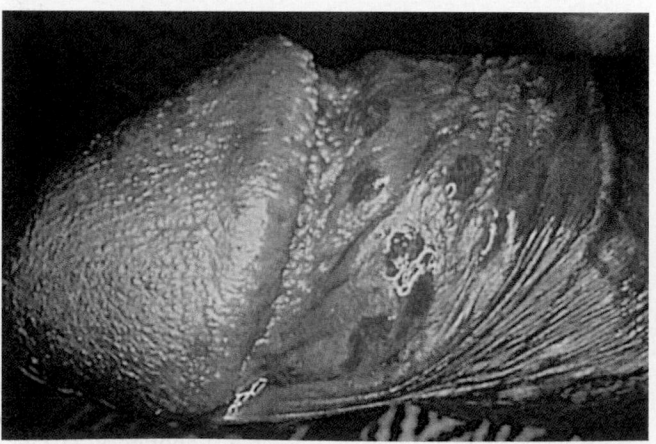
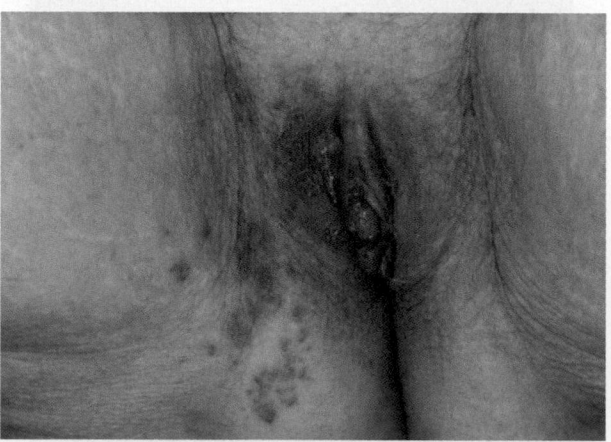

A   **B**

FIGURE 56-2 Genital herpes lesions (**A**) on the penis and (**B**) on the vulva. (Photo *A* from Goodheart, H. P. [2009]. *Goodheart's photoguide to common skin disorders: Diagnosis and management.* [3rd ed.]. Philadelphia: Lippincott Williams & Wilkins. Photo *B* © Dr. P. Marrazi/Photo Researchers, Inc.)

Diagnosis of HSV-1 and HSV-2 infection is tentatively made by inspecting the lesions. Smears and scrapings from the lesions are examined microscopically using special stains to confirm the clinical impression.

Medical Management

Because an outbreak of HSV-1 infection often is self-limiting, treatment may be unnecessary. If treated, either type of herpes responds to the antiviral drugs acyclovir (Zovirax), valacyclovir (Valtrex), and famciclovir (Famvir) (Drug Therapy Table 56-1). The client may take oral antiviral medications episodically for 3 to 5 days to shorten the duration of lesions or continuously as suppressive therapy to reduce the frequency of outbreaks by as much as 70% to 80%. Episodic therapy begins within 1 day of lesion onset or during the period immediately preceding an outbreak, when the client is aware of early symptoms. IV acyclovir is used if there is a severe episode of HSV-2 or if the client is immunocompromised. Cesarean delivery is performed on pregnant women with active lesions to prevent transmission to the newborn. Antiviral drug therapy does not necessarily prevent viral shedding. Infected clients compliant with drug therapy may still transmit the virus. Topical applications of antiviral drugs offer minimal clinical benefit for HSV-2 infections, and are not recommended (CDC, Sexually Transmitted Diseases Treatment Guidelines, 2006).

The frequency of recurrent outbreaks in many clients diminishes over time. Consequently, the physician may suggest discontinuing suppressive therapy to evaluate the client's need for continuous medication.

Nursing Management

The nurse collects appropriate health and sexual data, uses Standard Precautions when inspecting lesions, obtains specimens, and provides related health teaching. More on nursing management appears in Nursing Care Plan 56-1.

The nurse instructs clients with HSV-2 infections to:

- Inform all potential sexual partners of the HSV infection, even if it is in an inactive state.
- Use a condom during sexual activity even if the disease is dormant.
- Avoid sexual contact if there is any question that the infection is active; condoms do not protect skin and mucous membrane that is left exposed.
- Keep lesions dry using alcohol, peroxide, witch hazel, and warm air from a hair dryer.
- Check with the physician about taking warm baths with Epsom salts or baking soda to relieve discomfort.
- Wear loose clothing that promotes air circulation about the genitals.
- Perform thorough handwashing after direct contact with lesions, and keep any personal hygiene articles, like a towel, separate to avoid inadvertent use by others.
- Use a separate towel to pat lesions dry and another when drying other body parts to avoid autoinoculation.
- Have annual Papanicolaou tests to detect cervical cancer.
- Investigate stress management strategies because reducing stress tends to decrease the frequency of outbreaks.

GENITAL WARTS

Genital warts, also called **condylomata**, are an STI that tends to recur even after treatment. Anyone can become infected with genital warts, but people with AIDS as well as others with an immunodeficiency are particularly susceptible. One fourth of the people in the United States carry the virus and are infectious but do not manifest symptoms. Untreated genital warts may resolve on their own, remain unchanged, or increase in size or number.

Pathophysiology and Etiology

The **human papillomavirus** (HPV)—strains 6, 11, 16, 18, 31, 33, and 35—causes genital warts. However, many of the 20 million people infected with these strains do not develop genital warts. HPV is transmitted by genital-genital, genital-anal, or genital-oral contact with an infected person. Sexual penetration is not necessary to transmit HPV, and the warts also can be spread to other body areas by autoinoculation. The virus is contagious as long as the warts are present. Warts can grow in the mouth and throat of infants infected at birth. HPV infection is associated with uterine cervical abnormalities, which may lead to cervical and other pelvic reproductive types of cancer (see Chap 53). The strains of HPV that cause genital warts are different than those that cause cervical cancer, however.

Assessment Findings

Genital warts usually are painless and appear as a single lesion or cluster of soft, fleshy growths on the genitalia (Fig. 56-3) or cervix, in the vagina, or on the perineum, anus, throat, or mouth. Sometimes the warts are so small that they are inconspicuous; however, they can become large and raised—resembling a cauliflower. Large genital warts may narrow or obstruct the urethra, vagina, anus, or throat.

Genital warts turn white when vinegar is applied to the lesion. The highlighted tissue is then examined with a magnifying glass.

Medical and Surgical Management

If the warts are not extensive, and the client can reach them, the physician may prescribe podofilox (Condylox) solution or gel, or imiquimod (Aldara) cream for self-application. Treatment may involve twice-daily applications of podofilox for 3 days, followed by nontreatment for 4 days. The client repeats the cycle up to four times, if necessary. Imiquimod cream requires application at bedtime, three times a week. The client removes the ointment with soap and water in the morning. The treatment period with imiquimod cream can extend to 16 weeks.

If the genital warts are of substantial size or are in an anatomic location that is difficult to reach, the client may defer treatment to a nurse or physician. Physician-administered treatment involves removing the warts in one or more of the following methods: surgical excision with scalpel or scissors, laser therapy, electrocautery (heat), cryotherapy (freezing) with liquid nitrogen, local applications of chemicals, or parenteral administration of natural or recombinant interferon.

The major chemicals used to eradicate the warts include: local applications of trichloroacetic acid, bichloroacetic acid, podophyllum resin in tincture of benzoin (Pod-Ben-25), or

DRUG THERAPY TABLE 56-1 Agents Used To Treat STIs

Drug Category and Examples	Use	Side Effects	Nursing Considerations*
Antibiotics			
All antibiotics		Allergy, anaphylaxis (applies to all antibiotics listed below)	Inquire about allergies and past reactions to medications. Be aware that clients allergic to cephalosporins also may be allergic to penicillin antibiotics. Inform client to seek treatment if rash, hives, fever, or difficulty breathing occur.
penicillin G	Syphilis, gonorrhea	Allergy, stomatitis, nausea, vomiting, diarrhea, rash, fever, wheezing, pain at injection site	Give intramuscularly into gluteus maximus only. Massage site. Have client wait for 30 min after injection in case allergic reaction occurs.
erythromycin	Syphilis, gonorrhea, chlamydia, chancroid, lymphogranuloma venereum, prophylactically to prevent eye infection in newborns	Allergy, abdominal cramps, diarrhea, vomiting, rash, emotional lability, altered thinking, ototoxicity, hepatitis	Reassure client that emotional and cognitive side effects, should they occur, are temporary. Report tinnitus and jaundice.
doxycycline	Syphilis, gonorrhea, granuloma inguinale, lymphogranuloma venereum	Allergy, anorexia, nausea, vomiting, diarrhea, sensitivity to light, liver failure, discoloration of developing teeth, liver damage	Suggest taking with meals if gastrointestinal upset occurs. Inform client to report dark-colored urine or light-colored stools. Use a sunscreen. Strongly encourage client to return for all follow-up visits to ensure that organism has been eradicated.
ceftriaxone	Gonorrhea	Allergy, anorexia, nausea, vomiting, diarrhea, rash, fever, decreased hematocrit, disulfiram-like reaction with alcohol	Avoid alcohol during and for 3 days after drug therapy. Inform client of possible side effects and to report unusual fatigue.
tetracycline	Syphilis, gonorrhea, chlamydia	Allergy, nausea, vomiting, diarrhea, discoloration of developing teeth, phototoxicity, superinfections	Take on an empty stomach. Avoid antacids, dairy products, and iron supplements. Do not use outdated drugs because they are nephrotoxic. Use a sunscreen. Report appearance of oral or vaginal yeast infections.
ciprofloxacin	Gonorrhea	Headache, dizziness, nausea, diarrhea, vomiting	Take on an empty stomach and avoid antacids within 2 hr of antibiotic dose. Drink plenty of water. Report any side effects.
Antivirals			
acyclovir	Herpes (decreases severity and frequency of outbreaks)	Headache, nausea, vomiting, diarrhea, acute renal failure with other nephrotoxic drugs or renal disease	Inform client that drug does not cure the disease. Clients should avoid sexual activity during outbreaks and wear a condom at other times.

DRUG THERAPY TABLE 56-1 Agents Used To Treat STIs (Continued)

Drug Category and Examples	Use	Side Effects	Nursing Considerations*
Caustics podophyllum resin	Genital warts	Peripheral neuropathy, thrombocytopenia and leukopenia when absorbed systemically, irritation of normal tissue	Highly toxic and should be applied only by the physician. Surrounding skin may be protected with petroleum jelly. Use minimal amount possible. Warn client that local irritation may occur in 12–48 hr.

*Strongly encourage all clients to return for all follow-up visits to ensure that the organism has been eradicated.

5-fluorouracil (5-FU) cream. The warts will most likely be eradicated after three to six cycles of treatment (CDC, Sexually Transmitted Diseases Treatment Guidelines, 2006). Eradication does not mean the condition is cured; the person is temporarily noncontagious once the warts are destroyed.

Pharmacologic Considerations

- Podofilox or podophyllin resin should not be used by pregnant women, because it may cause birth defects

Nursing Management

Nurses provide information about transmission of STIs to sexually active people and prepare people with possible STIs for medical examination, diagnosis, and treatment. Nursing management is discussed further in Nursing Care Plan 56-1.

The nurse tells clients with HPV to:

- Avoid intimate contact until the warts are removed.
- Advise all sexual contacts to be examined and treated.

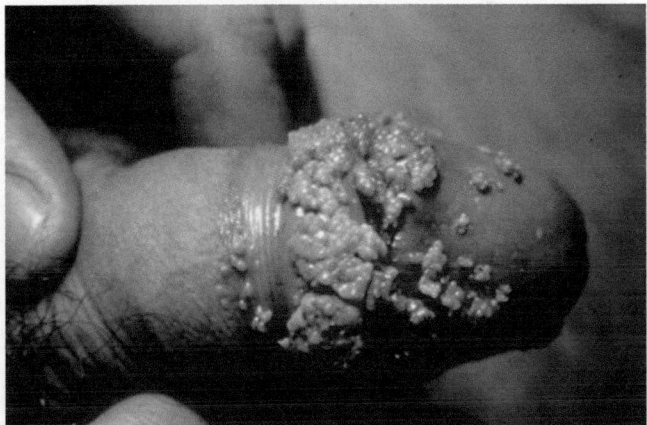

FIGURE 56-3 Genital warts on the penis. The warts may resemble small cauliflowers. (From Goodheart, H. P. [2009]. *Goodheart's photoguide to common skin disorders: Diagnosis and management* [3rd ed.]. Philadelphia: Lippincott Williams & Wilkins.)

- Seek treatment at an STD/STI clinic or with a private physician when, and if, the warts return.
- Use a condom even when the lesions are absent (see Client and Family Teaching 56-2), and suggest that the sexual partner wash his or her genitals or other skin areas immediately after intimate contact.
- Provide information about the diagnosis and treatment in future health histories, especially if a pregnancy occurs.
- Avoid stress and genital trauma, which appear to be factors in reactivating the virus (Porth, 2006).
- Obtain yearly examinations for the possibility of reproductive cancers.

> **Stop, Think, and Respond Exercise 56-1**
>
> *Which STI is associated with the following signs?*
>
> 1. *Painless ulceration on the genitals or other areas of sexual contact*
> 2. *Discharge from the vagina, urethra, or both; burning on urination; and abdominal pain in women*
> 3. *Cluster of soft, fleshy growths about the genitals or other places of sexual contact*
> 4. *Burning and itching about the genitals before an outbreak of multiple vesicles that become painful after rupture*

OTHER SEXUALLY TRANSMITTED INFECTIONS

GRANULOMA INGUINALE

Granuloma inguinale, or donovanosis, is caused by *Calymmatobacterium granulomatis* and is relatively uncommon in the United States. The infection is characterized by lesions in the genital, inguinal, and anal areas; it is treated with antimicrobials, usually tetracycline or sulfisoxazole (Gantrisin).

CHANCROID

Chancroid is caused by the *Haemophilus ducreyi* bacillus. The infection, which was reported in 33 people in the United States in 2006, is characterized by the appearance of a macule, followed by vesicle-pustule formation, and, finally, a painful genital ulcer and enlarged, tender lymph nodes in the inguinal area. It is treated and cured with azithromycin, ceftriaxone, ciprofloxacin, or erythromycin.

LYMPHOGRANULOMA VENEREUM

Lymphogranuloma venereum, caused by a strain of *C. trachomatis*, is characterized by a small erosion or papule and enlargement of adjacent lymph nodes. The affected lymph nodes can become necrotic. The usual site of infection is the genital area. The infection is treated with doxycycline or erythromycin.

CRITICAL THINKING EXERCISES

1. Discuss STI information that is appropriate to provide for a person who confides that he or she is having unprotected sexual intercourse with more than one person.
2. Explain information that a client who has never used a male condom should know.
3. A female tests positive for chlamydia. The physician could treat the client with a single dose of azithromycin (Zithromax) or a 7-day regimen of doxycycline (Vibramycin) taken twice a day. Which drug treatment is more advantageous than the other? Support your answer.
4. What might the nurse tell a client with chlamydia who says, "Well, this isn't as serious as having gonorrhea or syphilis"?

NCLEX-STYLE REVIEW QUESTIONS

1. A male client reports symptoms that are suggestive of a gonorrhea infection. If a culture is ordered to detect the causative organism, which body substance does the nurse collect?
   1. Venous blood
   2. Sterile urine
   3. Ejaculated semen
   4. Urethral drainage

2. When a nurse counsels a female client with HPV-2 infection, which information is accurate?
   1. Being infected means that any children you have in the future will be immune to the disease.
   2. If you take your medicine as prescribed, you will not infect anyone else.
   3. Have a Pap test at least every 6 months.
   4. Avoid vaginal intercourse for at least 6 months.

3. A nurse is assessing a male client with tertiary syphilis. Which finding is most associated with this stage of the disease?
   1. Sharp leg pains
   2. Red skin rash
   3. Penile ulcers
   4. Patchy hair loss

4. When the nurse teaches a client who has been diagnosed with a chlamydia infection, which statement is accurate?
   1. Males manifest symptoms, but infected women do not.
   2. This is a rare type of STI.
   3. Your sexual partner(s) need simultaneous treatment.
   4. There is no known cure for this kind of infection.

5. A nurse refers a client with genital warts to a gynecologist, who confirms that they are caused by the human papillomavirus. What is the most correct response when the client asks if there is any danger associated with this condition?
   1. Genital warts can be treated with an antibiotic, such as penicillin or tetracycline.
   2. Genital warts increase the risk of cancer of the vulva, vagina, and cervix.
   3. Genital warts can be prevented if the individual takes birth control pills.
   4. Genital warts are of no danger to the client and need not be treated at this time.

UNIT 14
Caring for Clients with Urinary and Renal Disorders

57

Introduction to the Urinary System

Words To Know

blood urea nitrogen
costovertebral angle
creatinine
creatinine clearance test
cystogram
cystometrogram
cystoscope
cystoscopy
excretory urogram
intravenous pyelogram
postvoid residual
renal arteriogram
retrograde pyelogram
ultrasonography
urinalysis
urine osmolality
urine protein test
urine specific gravity
urodynamic studies
uroflowmetry
urography
voiding cystourethrogram

Learning Objectives

On completion of this chapter, you will be able to:

1. Name the parts of the urinary system.
2. Define the primary functions of the kidney and other structures in the urinary system.
3. List tests performed for the diagnosis of urologic and renal system diseases.
4. Identify laboratory tests performed to diagnose urologic and renal system diseases.
5. Discuss nursing management for a client undergoing diagnostic evaluation of the urinary tract.

The urinary system consists of the kidneys, renal pelves (sing., *pelvis*), ureters, urinary bladder, and urethra. The kidneys have many functions (Box 57-1), including excreting excess water and nitrogenous waste products of protein metabolism; assisting in maintenance of acid-base and electrolyte balance; producing the enzyme *renin,* which helps regulate blood pressure; and producing the hormone *erythropoietin,* which stimulates red blood cell production. The remainder of the urinary system is involved in the transport (ureters and pelves), storage (bladder), and excretion (urethra) of urine.

Urologic nursing assessment focuses on changes in urine production, transport, storage, and elimination. Other responsibilities of urologic nurses involve caring for clients with conditions that affect the reproductive systems, discussed in Chapters 53 and 55.

ANATOMY AND PHYSIOLOGY

The upper urinary tract is composed of the kidneys, renal pelves, and ureters. The lower urinary tract consists of the bladder, urethra, and pelvic floor muscles (Fig. 57-1).

Kidneys, Renal Pelvis, and Ureters

The two kidneys are paired, bean-shaped organs located in the upper abdomen on either side of the vertebral column. They span from the level of the 12th thoracic vertebra to the 3rd lumbar vertebra. A thin, fibrous capsule encloses each kidney; the peritoneum separates the kidney from

BOX 57-1 Functions of the Kidney

- Urine formation
- Excretion of waste products
- Regulation of electrolytes
- Regulation of acid-base balance
- Control of water balance
- Control of blood pressure
- Renal clearance
- Regulation of red blood cell production
- Synthesis of vitamin D to active form
- Secretion of prostaglandins
- Regulates calcium and phosphorus balance
- Activates growth hormone

(From Smeltzer, S. C., et al. [2008]. *Brunner & Suddarth's textbook of medical–surgical nursing* [11th ed.]. Philadelphia: Lippincott Williams & Wilkins.)

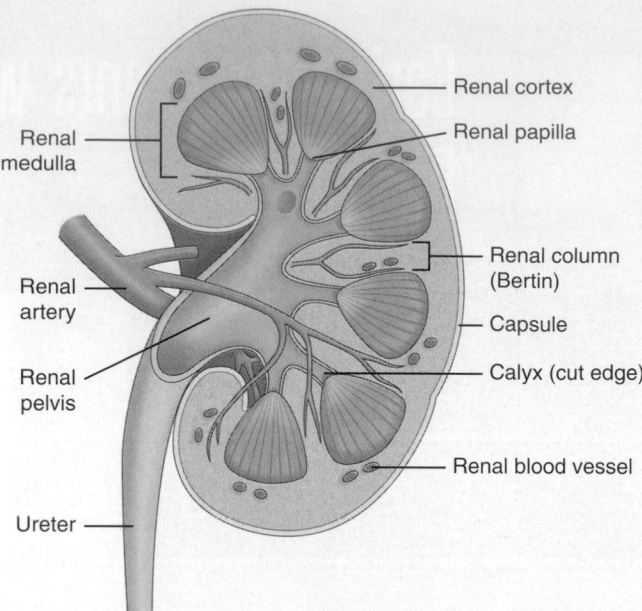

FIGURE 57-2 Internal structure of the kidney.

the abdominal cavity anteriorly. The blood supply to each kidney consists of a renal artery and renal vein. The renal artery arises from the aorta and the renal vein empties into the vena cava. The kidneys receive 25% of the total cardiac output.

A cross-section of the kidney (Fig. 57-2) helps to illustrate the inner structures. The two main areas are the renal pelvis and the parenchyma. The *parenchyma* is made up of a cortex (outer layer) and a medulla (inner core). Within each cortex are microscopic nephrons that carry out the functions of the kidneys. Each kidney contains about 1 million *nephrons,* which are the smallest functioning units of the kidney. Each nephron consists of the *glomerulus, afferent arteriole, efferent arteriole, Bowman's capsule, distal* and *proximal*

convoluted tubules, the *loop of Henle,* and the *collecting tubule* (Fig. 57-3). The medulla contains calyces (pyramids), cone-shaped structures that open to the renal pelvis, a large funnel-like structure in the center of the kidney. The renal pelvis then empties into the ureter, which carries urine to the bladder for storage.

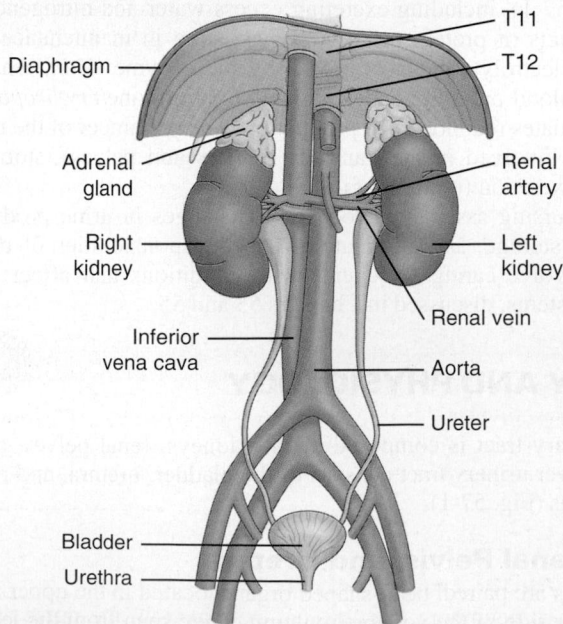

FIGURE 57-1 Kidneys, ureters, and bladder. The right kidney is usually lower than the left.

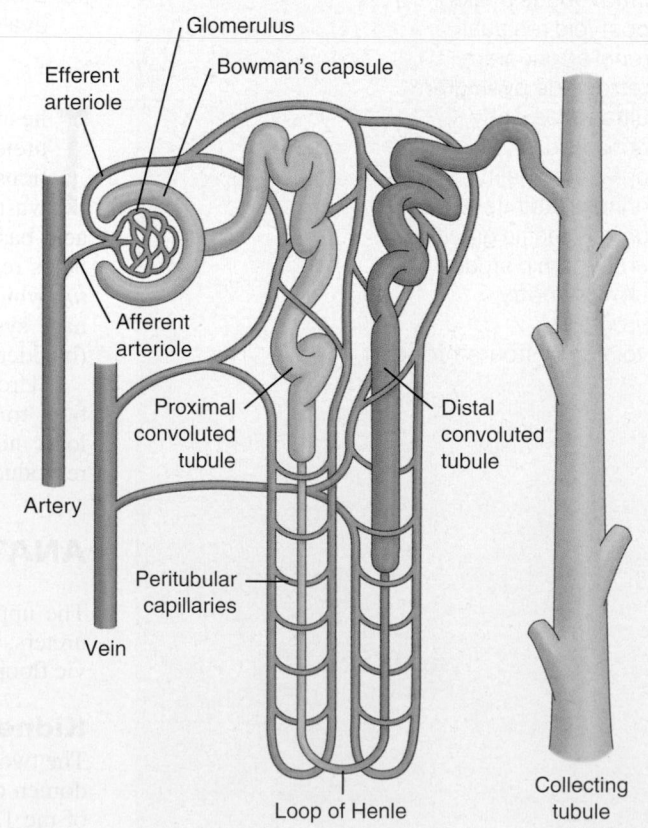

FIGURE 57-3 Representation of a nephron.

Bladder, Urethra, and Pelvic Floor Muscles

The bladder, urethra, and pelvic floor muscles form the urethrovesical unit. The urinary bladder, located just behind the pubis, is a hollow, muscular organ. Its shape and size vary with the amount of urine it contains as well as the person's age. In general, adult bladders hold 300 to 500 mL of urine.

The urethra is a hollow tube that begins at the bladder neck and ends at the external meatus. It serves as a conduit during urination and has a sphincter mechanism to prevent urine leakage. The male urethra extends approximately 24 cm (10 inches) from the bladder neck through the prostate and the penile shaft to the glans penis. The female urethra extends about 4 cm (1.5–2 inches) from the bladder neck to the external meatus, anterior to the vagina.

The pelvic floor muscles constitute the final part of the urethrovesical unit. These muscles form a sling that supports the bladder and urethra, rectum, and some reproductive organs.

Urine Formation

There are three steps in the complex process of urine formation:

1. *Glomerular filtration*—involves the filtration of plasma by the glomerulus (see Fig. 57-3). Filtered substances include water, sodium, chloride, bicarbonate, potassium, glucose, urea, creatinine, and uric acid.
2. *Tubular reabsorption*—the filtrate enters Bowman's capsule and then moves through the tubular system of the nephron and is either reabsorbed (placed back into the systemic circulation) or excreted as urine.
3. *Tubular secretion*—the formed urine drains from the collecting tubules, into the renal pelvis, and down each ureter to the bladder.

The filtrate that is secreted as urine usually contains water, sodium, chloride, bicarbonate, potassium, urea, creatinine, and uric acid. Amino acids and glucose typically are reabsorbed and not excreted in the urine. Protein molecules, except for periodic small amounts of globulins and albumin, also are reabsorbed. Transient proteinuria in small amounts (<150 mg/dL) is not considered a problem. Persistent and elevated proteinuria may indicate glomerular damage. Glycosuria (glucose in the urine) occurs when the glucose concentration in the blood and glomerular filtrate exceeds the ability of the tubules to reabsorb the glucose (Porth, 2007; Smeltzer et al., 2008).

Gerontologic Considerations

- Age-related changes in kidney function, such as decreased renal blood flow and glomerular filtration rate and thickening of the renal tubules, can alter the excretion of drugs in older adults, increasing the risk of drug toxicity.

- Decreased ability to concentrate urine may lead to increased susceptibility to dehydration, further complicated by a deficit in thirst.

Urine Elimination

Urine flows from the renal pelvis through the ureter into the bladder. Peristaltic waves help to move the urine to the bladder. Normally, urine flows in one direction because of this peristaltic action and because the ureters enter the bladder at an oblique angle. Reflux of urine (urine that flows backward) can occur secondary to an overdistended bladder or other problems, and may cause infections (see Chapter 59).

The desire to urinate comes from the feeling of bladder fullness. A nerve reflex is triggered when approximately 150 mL of urine accumulates. During urination, the bladder muscle contracts and the sphincter muscles relax, forcing urine out of the bladder and urethra through the urethral meatus. If there is any interference or abnormality of these muscles, the bladder may not empty completely or empty uncontrollably (incontinence).

Gerontologic Considerations

- Urine formation increases during the night, when leg elevation promotes blood return to the heart and kidneys, and may interrupt sleep patterns. Older persons may need to drink more fluids throughout the day to allow for limiting their intake after the evening meal.

> **Stop, Think, and Respond Exercise 57-1**
> *What factors influence the amount of urine produced?*

ASSESSMENT

History

The nurse obtains information about general health, childhood and family illnesses, past medical history, allergies, sexual and reproductive health, exposure to toxic chemicals or gas, and history of present complaint (Box 57-2). Table 57-1 describes risk factors for renal or urologic disorders. In addition to the client's chief complaint and medical history, a medication history is important. Older clients in particular may be taking multiple medications, which may affect renal function. The nurse also obtains information about voiding patterns, which may indicate renal or urologic problems (Table 57-2).

Pharmacologic Considerations

- Nephrotoxicity may occur with the administration of certain drugs and is potentially serious because it decreases urinary excretion of the drug and increases the risk of drug toxicity.

Physical Examination

Before beginning the physical examination, the nurse asks the client to void. Inspection includes observing the abdomen for scars, symmetry, abdominal movements, and

BOX 57-2 **Assessing the Chief Complaint Related to the Urinary System**

The nurse collects information about the following:

- Voiding changes or disturbances
- Urine volume changes
- Irritative voiding symptoms (frequency, urgency, nocturia, dysuria)
- Obstructive voiding symptoms (hesitancy, straining, residual urine, retention, urinary stream force and size)
- Urinary incontinence (total overflow, stress, urge, functional)
- Urine characteristics changes (color, hematuria, clarity, odor, pH)
- Systemic manifestations (fever, weight loss)
- Gastrointestinal signs and symptoms (nausea, vomiting, diarrhea, abdominal cramping, distention)
- Pain (type, location, severity, local, referred, colic, spasms)
- Masses of the flank, abdomen, or genital areas (polycystic kidneys, hydronephrosis, renal cell carcinoma)
- Abnormal abdominal or genital appearance
- Sexual or reproductive dysfunction

pulsations. Examining the back and noting any bulging, bruising, or scars are important steps.

The experienced examiner auscultates the abdomen for bruits (abnormal vascular sounds heard over a blood vessel). In addition, he or she percusses the area over the bladder beginning 2 inches above the symphysis pubis and moving toward the base of the bladder. Percussion usually produces a tympanic sound; it produces a dull sound if the bladder is filled. The nurse can palpate the suprapubic area but can palpate the bladder only if it is moderately distended (Fig. 57-4). Assessing the kidneys for tenderness or pain is done by lightly striking the fist at the **costovertebral angle** (CVA), which is the area where the lower ribs meet the vertebrae (Fig. 57-5). Normally, the client experiences a dull

thud. Pain or tenderness may indicate a renal disorder. The nurse also assesses for signs of electrolyte and water imbalances (see Chap. 16).

In addition to evaluating the client's general health, the nurse evaluates the client for signs or symptoms of:

- Periorbital edema (swelling around the eyes)
- Edema of the extremities
- Cardiac failure
- Mental changes

All of these signs or symptoms may indicate urinary tract disorders. The nurse also obtains vital signs and weight.

Diagnostic Tests

In the male client, diseases and disorders of the reproductive system also affect the urinary system. In addition to the diagnostic tests discussed in the following sections, tests that may be performed on the male client are discussed in Chapters 55 and 56.

Radiography

An x-ray study of the abdomen includes x-rays of the kidneys, ureters, and bladder (KUB). It is performed to show the size and position of the kidneys, ureters, and bony pelvis as well as any radiopaque urinary calculi (stones), abnormal gas patterns (indicative of renal mass), and anatomic defects of the bony spinal column (indicative of neuropathic bladder dysfunction). An x-ray of the pelvis, chest, or other area may reveal metastatic bone lesions that could be a result of renal or bladder tumors.

Ultrasonography

Renal **ultrasonography** identifies the kidney's shape, size, location, collecting systems, and adjacent tissues. Other uses include identification of renal cysts or obstruction sites, assistance in needle placement for renal biopsy or nephrostomy tube placement, and drainage of a renal abscess. There are no contraindications to this procedure. It is not invasive, does not require the injection of a radiopaque dye, and does

TABLE 57-1 Risk Factors for Various Renal or Urologic Disorders

RISK FACTOR	POSSIBLE RENAL OR UROLOGIC DISORDER
Childhood diseases: strep throat, impetigo, nephrotic syndrome	Chronic renal failure
Advanced age	Incomplete emptying of bladder, leading to urinary tract infection
Instrumentation of urinary tract, cystoscopy, catheterization	Urinary tract infection, incontinence
Immobilization	Kidney stone formation
Occupational, recreational, or environmental exposure to chemicals (plastics, pitch, tar, rubber)	Acute renal failure
Diabetes mellitus	Chronic renal failure, neurogenic bladder
Hypertension	Renal insufficiency, chronic renal failure
Systemic lupus erythematosus	Nephritis, chronic renal failure
Gout, hyperparathyroidism, Crohn's disease	Kidney stone formation
Sickle cell anemia, multiple myeloma	Chronic renal failure
Benign prostatic hypertrophy	Obstruction to urine flow, leading to frequency, oliguria, anuria
Radiation therapy to pelvis	Cystitis, fibrosis of ureter, or fistula in urinary tract
Recent pelvic surgery	Inadvertent trauma to ureters or bladder
Obstetric injury, tumors	Incontinence
Spinal cord injury	Neurogenic bladder, urinary tract infection, incontinence

TABLE 57-2 Problems Associated With Changes In Voiding

PROBLEM	DEFINITION	POSSIBLE ETIOLOGY
Frequency	Frequent voiding—more than every 3 hours	Infection, obstruction of lower urinary tract leading to residual urine and overflow, anxiety, diuretics, benign prostatic hyperplasia, urethral stricture, diabetic neuropathy
Urgency	Strong desire to void	Infection, chronic prostatitis, urethritis, obstruction of lower urinary tract leading to residual urine and overflow, anxiety, diuretics, benign prostatic hyperplasia, urethral stricture, diabetic neuropathy
Dysuria	Painful or difficult voiding	Lower urinary tract infection, inflammation of bladder or urethra, acute prostatitis, stones, foreign bodies, tumors in bladder
Hesitancy	Delay, difficulty in initiating voiding	Benign prostatic hyperplasia, compression of urethra, outlet obstruction, neurogenic bladder
Nocturia	Excessive urination at night	Decreased renal concentrating ability, heart failure, diabetes mellitus, incomplete bladder emptying, excessive fluid intake at bedtime, nephrotic syndrome, cirrhosis with ascites
Incontinence	Involuntary loss of urine	External urinary sphincter injury, obstetric injury, lesions of bladder neck, detrusor muscle dysfunction, infection, neurogenic bladder, medications, neurologic abnormalities
Enuresis	Involuntary voiding during sleep	Delay in functional maturation of central nervous system (bladder control usually achieved by 5 years of age), obstructive disease of lower urinary tract, genetic factors, failure to concentrate urine, urinary tract infection, psychological stress
Polyuria	Increased volume of urine voided	Diabetes mellitus, diabetes insipidus, diuretics, excess fluid intake, lithium toxicity, certain types of kidney disease (hypercalcemic and hypokalemic nephropathy)
Oliguria	Urine output less than 400 mL/day	Acute or chronic renal failure (see Chap. 58), inadequate fluid intake
Anuria	Urine output less than 50 mL/day	Acute or chronic renal failure (see Chap. 58), complete obstruction
Hematuria	Red blood cells in the urine	Cancer of genitourinary tract, acute glomerulonephritis, renal stones, renal tuberculosis, blood dyscrasia, trauma, extreme exercise, rheumatic fever, hemophilia, leukemia, sickle cell trait or disease
Proteinuria	Abnormal amounts of protein in the urine	Acute and chronic renal disease, nephrotic syndrome, vigorous exercise, heat stroke, severe heart failure, diabetic nephropathy, multiple myeloma

not require fasting or bowel preparation for a renal or bladder sonogram.

Computed Tomography Scan and Magnetic Resonance Imaging

A computed tomography (CT) scan or magnetic resonance imaging (MRI) of the abdomen and pelvis may be obtained to diagnose renal pathology, determine kidney size, and evaluate tissue densities with or without contrast material. An iodine-based contrast medium may be injected intravenously (IV) after the initial scan to enhance the images, especially when vascular tumors are suspected. The CT scan also is useful in identifying calculi, congenital abnormalities, obstruction, infections, and polycystic disease. An MRI produces sharp images of the kidneys and can delineate the renal cortex from the medulla. It also is useful in identifying bladder tumors, staging renal cell carcinoma, and imaging the vascular system.

Angiography

A renal angiogram (**renal arteriogram**) provides details of the arterial supply to the kidneys, specifically the location and number of renal arteries (multiple vessels to the kidney are not unusual) and the patency of each renal artery. A catheter is passed up the femoral artery into the aorta to the level of the renal vessels. Contrast medium is then injected into the catheter and serial x-rays are taken. The radiopaque dye first outlines the aorta in the area of the renal artery, then enters the renal artery and the kidney. A series of x-rays is taken. The catheter tip also may be passed into each renal artery for additional images. The procedure lasts 30 to 90 minutes. This procedure is contraindicated if a client is allergic to iodine contrast material.

The nurse must ask the client about allergy to iodine or seafood and any previous dye reactions. He or she reviews pertinent laboratory tests (blood urea nitrogen [BUN], creatinine) to assess renal function, records vital signs, and

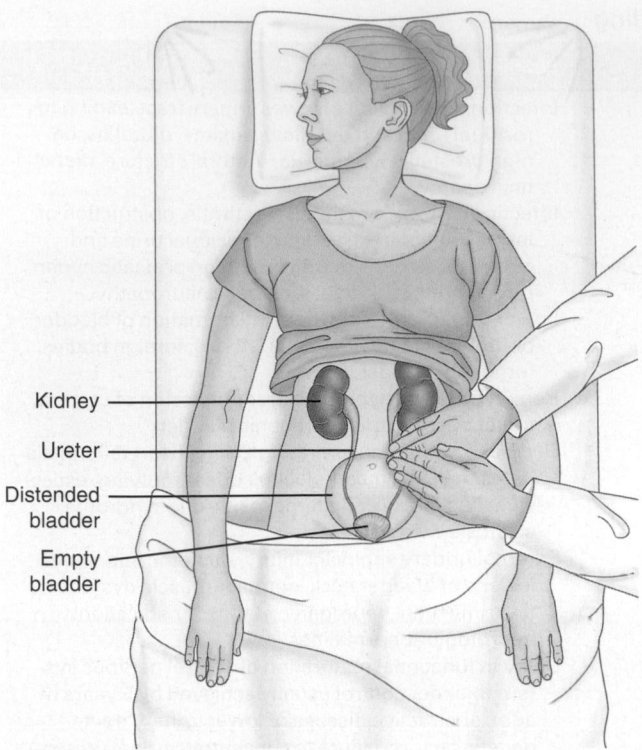

FIGURE 57-4 Palpation of the bladder.

Client and Family Teaching 57-1
Undergoing a Renal Angiography

The nurse reviews the following points with the client undergoing this test:

● Drink extra fluids on the day before the test; do not eat any food or fluids (per protocol) before testing; IV fluids will be given before, during, and after the test; medication will be given to promote relaxation; local anesthesia is administered.
● Expect a burning sensation or feeling of heat, pain, or nausea while contrast material is injected. These reactions are normal and transient.
● Remain on strict bed rest for 4 to 8 hours or more as per protocol. A urinal or bedpan must be used in the meantime.
● Drink extra fluids (2000 to 3000 mL over the 24-hour postprocedure period).

assesses peripheral pulses. The nurse instructs the client to void before the procedure. If ordered, he or she administers a sedative to promote relaxation before the procedure. After the procedure, the physician applies a pressure dressing to the femoral area, which remains in place for several hours. The nurse palpates the pulses in the legs and feet at least every 1 to 2 hours for signs of arterial occlusion. Monitoring the pressure dressing is important to note frank bleeding or hematoma formation. If either condition occurs, the nurse immediately notifies the physician. Another important

assessment is for hypersensitivity responses to contrast material. Clients remain on bed rest for 4 to 8 hours. The nurse also monitors and documents intake and output. Client and Family Teaching 57-1 outlines education points.

Cystoscopy

Cystoscopy is the visual examination of the inside of the bladder using an instrument called a *cystoscope*. When the urethra is examined, the procedure is called *cystourethroscopy*. The **cystoscope** consists of a lighted tube with a telescopic lens (Fig. 57-6). Cystoscopy is used to identify the cause of painless hematuria, urinary incontinence, or urinary retention. It is useful in the evaluation of structural and functional changes of the bladder. The cystoscope is inserted through the urethra into the bladder. Local anesthesia is usual; however, spinal or general anesthesia also may be used. The procedure lasts 30 to 45 minutes. The size of the cystoscope is graded in the French (F) scale; usually, one

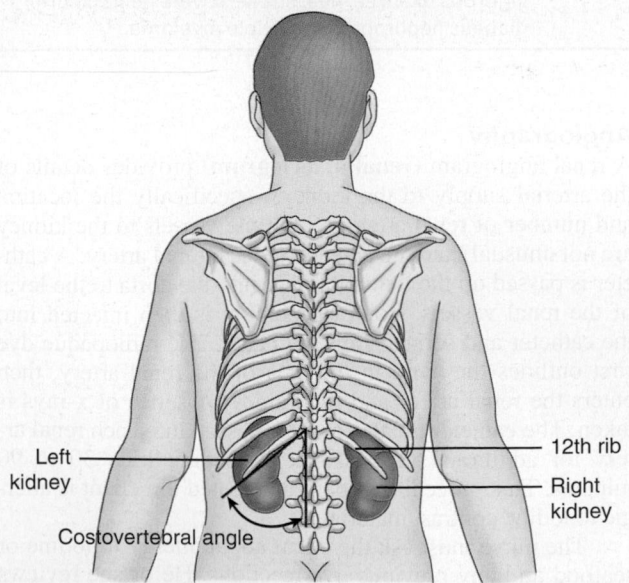

FIGURE 57-5 Location of the costovertebral angle (CVA). The CVA is the area used to assess the kidneys for tenderness or pain.

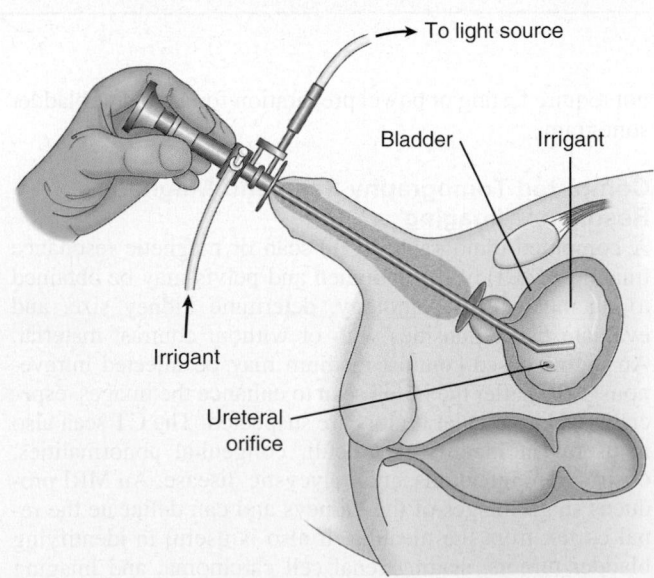

FIGURE 57-6 Cystoscopic examination.

that is 20 to 24 F is used in adults. Biopsy samples (tissue examination), cell washings (cytologic analysis), and urine samples may be obtained.

Preoperative sedatives or antispasmodics may be ordered. Cystoscopy can aggravate any abnormality of the urinary tract. A urine culture should be obtained before testing. If a urinary infection was present before the cystoscopy, chills, fever, and possibly septicemia may occur. The nurse observes the client for these and other symptoms and reports findings to the physician. Clients receive antibiotics after a cystoscopy. The nurse records vital signs before and after the procedure. If general anesthesia is used, he or she should monitor vital signs every 15 to 30 minutes until the client is stable. Significant prostatic obstruction may result in pain and complete urinary retention after a cystoscopy. The nurse administers medications for pain or bladder spasms postprocedure as ordered.

▶ Stop, Think, and Respond Exercise 57-2

A client having a cystoscopy has the potential for complications. What are these?

Intravenous Pyelogram and Retrograde Pyelogram

An **intravenous pyelogram** (IVP), also known as **excretory urogram** or IV **urography**, is a radiologic study used to evaluate the structure and function of the kidneys, ureters, and bladder. It locates the site of any urinary tract obstructions and is helpful in the investigation of the causes of flank pain, hematuria, or renal colic. It is based on the ability of the kidneys to excrete a radiopaque dye (also called a *contrast medium*) in the urine. The IV radiopaque dye outlines the kidney pelves, ureters, and bladder as the blood containing the dye passes through the urinary tract. After the IV injection of contrast material, radiographs of the urinary tract are taken after 1 minute (kidney visualization), at 3 to 5 minutes (renal collecting system visualization), at 10 minutes (ureters visualization), and at 20 to 30 minutes (bladder filling visualization). A postvoiding radiograph shows the emptying of the bladder.

Because radiopaque dye usually contains iodine, the physician may inject a minute amount of the radiopaque dye IV and observe the client for 5 to 10 minutes to determine any allergy to iodine. Radiopaque dyes that do not contain iodine, called *nonionic contrast agents,* are available and produce fewer allergic reactions.

A **retrograde pyelogram** may be performed if better visualization of the complete ureter and renal pelvis is needed. A flexible radiopaque ureteral catheter is inserted in each ureteral orifice (opening at the terminal end of the ureter), which lie on the lower posterior wall of the bladder. This is done during a cystoscopy. Visualization of the ureters and renal pelves is possible after sterile contrast medium is instilled into the renal collecting system. This procedure also is used to evaluate ureteral stent or catheter placement. Retrograde pyelography carries the risks of sepsis and severe urinary tract infection.

An IVP is scheduled before any barium test or gallbladder series that uses contrast material (iodine). If the client already is scheduled for barium studies of the upper or lower gastrointestinal tract, these diagnostic tests probably will be delayed until urologic studies are completed. It may take several days for barium to be removed from the gastrointestinal tract, and its presence can distort IVP findings. Nursing Guidelines 57-1 provide information on the care of the client undergoing a pyelogram.

After the IVP or retrograde pyelogram, the nurse instructs the client to consume an adequate fluid intake. In addition, the client continues to receive IV fluid replacement.

NURSING GUIDELINES 57-1

Caring for the Client Undergoing Intravenous or Retrograde Pyelogram

- Check the client's allergy history, especially to intravenous contrast dye (iodine) or seafood. Inquire about previous reactions to x-ray studies that used contrast media. Report allergies to the physician or radiology department personnel.
- Instruct the client to fast from food for 8 to 12 hours before the pyelogram. Fluids are permitted.
- Cleanse the bowel per physician order so that there is no interference with visualization of the kidneys on the radiographic film. It is important that the bowel preparation be effective because poor cleansing of the intestinal tract may require that the test be repeated. Clients with a peptic ulcer or ulcerative colitis usually require modification of the bowel-cleansing preparation.
- Document baseline vital signs.
- Explain the procedure and its purpose. Tell clients that a series of x-rays will be taken after injection or instillation of IV contrast material and that the entire test requires 1 to 1½ hours to complete.

- Caution clients that they may experience burning, hot flushing sensations, unpleasant (metallic) taste in the mouth, or nausea or vomiting as the contrast is given. Half the clients experience nausea or vomiting. Reassure clients that these reactions are transient.
- Encourage adequate fluid intake postprocedure and voiding within 8 hours postprocedure. A burning sensation on voiding and small amounts of blood-tinged urine are normal and should disappear after the third voiding.
- Advise the use of warm tub baths to decrease urethral discomfort or spasms after a retrograde pyelogram. These reactions should disappear within 24 hours.
- Instruct the client to abstain from alcohol 48 hours postprocedure to avoid irritating the bladder.
- Discuss taking antibiotics for 1 to 3 days postprocedure. Teach the client to report flank pain, chills, fever, dysuria, or bleeding. Advise client to notify physician should symptoms present.

The nurse monitors and documents the intake and output, making sure that urine output is at least 30 mL/hour. Clients who are dehydrated are at high risk for renal failure from the toxic effect of the contrast medium on the kidney tissues. The nurse also monitors vital signs. If additional radiographs are to be taken in the next 24 hours (if the excretory function of the kidney is abnormal), the physician or radiology department provides instructions regarding the food and fluid intake.

The client undergoing a retrograde pyelogram may experience a dull ache caused by distention of the renal pelves with the radiopaque dye. The nurse observes the client for signs and symptoms of pyelonephritis (see Chap. 58) 24 to 48 hours postprocedure because of the instrumentation and injection of material. If there are any symptoms, the nurse reports them to the physician and obtains a urine specimen for culture and analysis. Antibiotic agents are administered as directed.

Biopsy

Biopsies of urinary tract tissue are taken to diagnose cancer, assess prostatic enlargement, diagnose and monitor progression of renal disease, and assess and evaluate treatment of renal transplant rejection. Bladder biopsies are obtained during cystoscopy. Information about prostate biopsy can be found in Chapter 55. Table 57-3 describes renal biopsy techniques. Renal biopsy carries the risk of postprocedure bleeding because the kidneys receive up to 25% of the cardiac output each minute.

The nurse reassures the client undergoing a renal biopsy and explains the procedure and its purpose. In addition, he or she records vital signs and reviews pretest coagulation studies, urinalysis, IVP, and renal scan. After the procedure, the client remains on bed rest. The nurse observes the urine for signs of hematuria. It is important to assess the dressing frequently for signs of bleeding, monitor vital signs, and evaluate the type and severity of pain. Severe pain in the back, shoulder, or abdomen can indicate bleeding. The nurse notifies the physician of these signs and symptoms immediately. He or she also assesses the client for difficulty voiding. The nurse needs to encourage the client to have adequate fluid intake after the biopsy. If the client is to be discharged the following day, the nurse instructs him or her to:

- Maintain limited activity for several days to avoid bleeding.
- Complete prophylactic antibiotic therapy as indicated.
- Notify the physician immediately if experiencing signs and symptoms of systemic infection (fever, malaise), urinary tract infection (dysuria, frequency, discolored urine, malodorous urine), or bleeding (hematuria, lightheadedness, flank pain, or rapid pulse).

Cystogram and Voiding Cystourethrogram

A **cystogram** evaluates abnormalities in bladder structure and filling through the instillation of contrast dye and radiography. A **voiding cystourethrogram** (VCUG) is similar to a cystogram except the client is instructed to void (the urine contains the radiopaque dye), and a rapid series of x-rays are taken. Urinary tract infection is a contraindication to a cystogram or VCUG.

Urodynamic Studies

Urodynamic studies evaluate bladder and urethral function and are performed to assess causes of reduced urine flow, urinary retention, and urinary incontinence. Two of the main tests are uroflowmetry and cystometrogram.

Uroflowmetry (determination of the urinary flow rate) is performed to evaluate bladder and sphincter function. This noninvasive procedure measures the time and rate of voiding, the volume of urine voided, and the pattern of urination. Results are compared with normal flow rates and urinary patterns. Results vary by age and sex. Table 57-4 lists normal uroflowmetry values. The client usually is catheterized afterward for the postvoid residual. A **postvoid residual** is the amount of urine left in the bladder after voiding and provides information about bladder function. Normal postvoid residual is 0 to 30 mL; however, retention of up to 100 mL may be acceptable in the older adult.

A **cystometrogram** (CMG) evaluates the bladder tone and capacity. A retention catheter is inserted into the bladder after the client voids. The bladder is slowly filled with sterile saline and the client indicates at what point the first urge to void is felt and when the bladder feels full. These measurements indicate whether the client's bladder capacity is normal. Most clients feel a mild urge to void at approximately 120 mL and a strong urge to void at about 250 mL. By comparison, clients with a neurogenic bladder (see Chap. 59) may not feel an urge to void until 500 mL or more has been instilled. In many instances the client with a neurogenic bladder never feels an urge to void, and instillation is terminated at this point. The client is assessed for bladder contractions that he or she cannot control, leakage around the catheter, or leakage of urine when asked to cough. Pressures within the bladder are also assessed. The client may be given antibiotics for a day or two after a CMG.

TABLE 57-3 Techniques for Renal Biopsy

TYPE OF BIOPSY	DESCRIPTION
Needle biopsy	• Minimally invasive • Renal tissue is removed through a needle • Useful when CT or MRI findings are inconclusive
Fine-needle aspiration biopsy	• Minimally invasive • Performed under local anesthesia in the operating room • Needle placement guided by fluoroscopy
Open biopsy	• Small incision made into flank • Usually performed if needle biopsy tissue samples are not satisfactory

TABLE 57-4 Normal Urine Flow Rates

GENDER	YOUNG ADULT	MIDDLE-AGED ADULT	OLDER ADULT
Male	21 mL/second	12 mL/second	9 mL/second
Female	18 mL/second	15 mL/second	10 mL/second

Laboratory Tests

Urinalysis

Much information about systemic diseases and the condition of the kidneys and lower urinary tract can be learned by **urinalysis,** a study of the components and characteristics of the urine. Urinalysis also is useful in monitoring the effects of treatment of known urinary or renal conditions. The characteristics of normal urine and possible causes contributing to abnormal results are listed in Table 57-5. A clean-catch midstream specimen from the first voiding of the morning is

TABLE 57-5 Urinalysis Characteristics

CHARACTERISTIC AND NORMAL VALUE	ABNORMAL FINDINGS	POSSIBLE CAUSES
Color: yellow	Colorless	Overhydration, diabetes insipidus, chronic renal disease, diuretic therapy, diabetes mellitus
	Red, pink	Hematuria, foods (beets, rhubarb, blackberries), drugs (phenothiazines, rifampin)
	Dark yellow or orange	Bilirubin, dehydration, drugs (multiple vitamins, pyridium, azogantrisin)
	Green	*Pseudomonas* infection, bilirubin, drugs (methylene blue, amitriptyline, vitamin B complex)
	Brown	Dehydration, urobilinogen, drugs (Cascara, Flagyl)
	Dark brown to black	Melanin, drugs (Macrodantin, Quinine, Methyldopa)
Clarity: clear	Cloudy	Phosphaturia
	Turbid	Pyuria, bacteriuria, parasitic disease
	Hazy	Mucus
	Smoky, milky	Prostatic fluid, sperm, lipids
	Pinkish precipitates	Hyperuricemia
Specific gravity: 1.003–1.029	Dilute (1.00–1.010) or concentrated (1.029–1.030)	Low: diabetes insipidus, kidney disorders
		High: false reading due to pus, albumin, protein, glucose, or dextran in urine
Urine osmolality: 50–1200 mOsm/kg considered normal; 500–800 mOsm/kg average	Elevated	Fluid volume deficit
	Decreased	Fluid volume excess
		Renal disease
pH: 4.5–7.5	>7.5	Urinary tract infection, metabolic acidosis, Cushing's syndrome, low-protein diet with large vegetable intake, diet high in dairy and citrus fruit, drugs (sodium bicarbonate, thiazides)
Ketones: none	Ketonuria	Starvation, fasting, abnormal carbohydrate metabolism, diabetes mellitus, pregnancy, pernicious anemia, vomiting, high-protein diet (Nutrition Notes 57-1)
Protein: none	Proteinuria	Cancer, severe heart failure, renal disease, glomerulonephritis, nephrotic syndrome, trauma, fever, heavy exercise
Glucose: none	Glycosuria	Diabetes mellitus, gestational diabetes
Red blood cells: 0–3 RBCs/ high-power field	>3 RBCs/high-power field	Renal disorders (glomerulonephritis, calculus, cancer, trauma, cysts), systemic disease (lupus, sickle cell, hypertension)
White blood cells: 0–4/ high-power field	>4/high-power field	Urinary tract infection (acute pyelonephritis, cystitis, urethritis), renal disease, urinary stones
Bilirubin: none	Bilirubinuria	Hepatitis, biliary obstruction
Urobilinogen: <1 mg/dL	>1 mg/dL	Hepatitis, cirrhosis, congestive heart failure, hemolytic anemia
Casts: 0–2 hyaline casts/low-power field	>2/low-power field	Granular casts (glomerulonephritis, renal disease); fatty casts (nephrotic syndrome); cellular casts (glomeruli or tubule infection); hyaline casts (fever, strenuous exercise, congestive heart failure)
Crystals: none to few	Many	Urolithiasis, chronic renal failure, gout, urinary tract infection
Bacteria: negative per high-power field	Positive	Urinary tract infection, pyelonephritis, cystitis

preferred. The nurse teaches the client how to collect a clean-catch specimen (Client and Family Teaching 57-2).

Pharmacologic Considerations

- Some drugs may have an effect on the outcome of urinary tract tests as well as the appearance of the urine. For example, nitrofurantoin may color the urine brown and methylene blue may color the urine a pale blue-green. Contamination of urine with povidone-iodine can cause a false-positive hematuria result (dipstick method). Other drugs can affect urine pH, such as ammonium chloride and mandelic acid, both of which can cause acidic urine, whereas sodium bicarbonate, thiazide diuretics, acetazolamide, and potassium citrate promote alkaline urine.

Urine Culture and Sensitivity

When infection is suspected, a urine specimen may be taken for culture by collecting a clean-catch midstream specimen or by urinary catheterization. It is important that the urine specimen not be contaminated by skin bacteria. The container is labeled with the client's name and the time and date of the voiding. To prevent the growth of bacteria in the urine and decomposition, the nurse ensures delivery of the urine specimen immediately to the laboratory or refrigerates it promptly until it can be taken to the laboratory.

24-Hour Urine Collection

Sometimes the entire 24-hour volume of urine is collected, such as a 24-hour urine for 17-ketosteroids. The client is

Client and Family Teaching 57-2
Obtaining a Clean-Catch Midstream Urine Specimen

The nurse teaches the client as follows:

● Wash your hands and remove the lid from the specimen container without touching the inside of the lid.
● Open antiseptic towelette package and cleanse the urethral area.
  ● *Females:* Hold labia apart with one hand. Wipe down one side of the urethra with the first towelette and discard, wipe down the other side with the second towelette and discard, and wipe down the center with the third towelette and discard. Wipe one time only with each towelette, from front to back.
  ● *Males:* Retract foreskin if uncircumcised. Clean the urethral meatus in a circular motion using each towelette one time.
● Begin voiding into the toilet, urinal, or bedpan; females, continue to hold labia apart while voiding.
● Void 30 to 50 mL of the midstream urine into the collection container and then finish urinating into the toilet, bedpan, or urinal. Be careful not to contaminate the container.
● Carefully replace the lid, dry the container if necessary, and wash your hands.

initially instructed to void and discard the urine. The collection bottle is marked with the time the client voided. Thereafter, all the urine is collected for the entire 24 hours. The last urine is voided at the same time the test originally began. The entire specimen is refrigerated to prevent bacterial growth. To prevent any part of the specimen from being lost or contaminated, the nurse tells the client to use separate receptacles for voiding and defecation. If any urine is discarded by mistake or lost while defecating, the nurse stops the test, because the loss of even a small amount of urine can invalidate the test.

Urine Specific Gravity

Urine specific gravity is a measurement of the kidney's ability to concentrate and excrete urine. The specific gravity measures urine concentration by measuring the density of urine and comparing it with the density of distilled water. The density of distilled water is 1 (1 mL of distilled water weighs 1 g). The number, weight, and size of urine solutes (particles) determine its specific gravity (density). Normally, the specific gravity is inversely proportional to urine volume. On a hot day, a person who is perspiring profusely and taking little fluid has low urine output with a high specific gravity. Conversely, a person who has a high fluid intake and who is not losing excessive water from perspiration, diarrhea, or vomiting has copious urine output with a low specific gravity. When the kidneys are diseased, the ability to concentrate urine may be impaired and the specific gravity remains relatively constant, no matter what the water needs of the body are or how much the client drinks.

Urine Osmolality

Urine osmolality reflects the ability of the kidney to concentrate and dilute urine, through measurement of the number of particles in a kilogram of solution. Osmolality of the urine and kidney is done at the same time in order to determine the client's fluid status. Urine osmolality normally ranges from 50 to 1200 mOsm/kg, averaging 500 to 800 mOsm/kg. Serum osmolality is 275 to 300 mOsm/kg. A client with kidney disease does not concentrate urine effectively, if at all, resulting in a decreased urine osmolality.

Urine Protein

The **urine protein test** is used to identify renal disease. Normally, protein is minimally present in the urine. An increase in urine protein levels also may be seen with salt depletion, strenuous exercise, fever, or dehydration. Proteinuria in an individual urine specimen may be detected by dipping a test reagent stick (dipstick method) in the urine and comparing color changes with the provided color chart.

Creatinine Clearance Test

A **creatinine clearance test** is used to determine kidney function and creatinine excretion. **Creatinine** is a substance that results from the breakdown of phosphocreatine (an amino acid waste product), which is present in muscle tissue. It is filtered by the glomeruli and is excreted at a fairly constant rate by the kidney. The total amount of excreted creatinine is called *creatinine clearance.* The renal tubules increase creatinine secretion with any decrease in glomerular filtration (renal failure). Muscle necrosis and atrophy greatly increase urinary creatinine due to accompanying protein catabolism. For this test, a 4-, 12-, or 24-hour urine specimen and a sample of blood (serum creatinine) are collected. The blood sample is obtained either at the midpoint or at the beginning and end of urine collection (varies per protocol). Both urine and blood samples are sent to the laboratory.

Blood Chemistries

When the nephrons fail to remove waste products efficiently from the body, the blood chemistry is altered. Deterioration in renal function is manifested by rises in the **blood urea nitrogen** (BUN) and creatinine values, both of which are protein breakdown products. Table 57-6 shows normal values of common blood studies performed on clients with signs and symptoms of a urinary system disorder, as well as renal implications regarding abnormal results. A moderate decrease in renal function occurs, however, before these values rise.

Pharmacologic Considerations

- Aminoglycosides such as gentamicin can result in increased levels of BUN and serum creatinine, indicating nephrotoxicity. Signs of nephrotoxicity may not occur until the client has received 5 or more days of therapy. Nephrotoxicity from the use of the aminoglycosides is reversible if the drug is discontinued as soon as the symptoms appear.

- Diuretic therapy can result in increased sodium, chloride, and magnesium levels with 24-hour urine electrolyte testing.

Nursing Process for the Client Undergoing Diagnostic Testing for a Renal or Urologic Disorder

Assessment

Interview the client to determine past experience with the test or other urologic procedures. Ask the client to discuss the nature of

Nutrition Notes 57-1
Nutrition and Urinary Health

- Dietary intake can affect urine characteristics as well as urinary tract disorders and their management.
- A high-protein, low-carbohydrate diet can cause ketonuria.
- Megadoses of vitamin C can interfere with certain laboratory tests, such as for glycosuria and fecal occult blood.
- Asparagus has a weak diuretic action and produces a pungent urine odor.

past experiences and expectations for the current tests. If the client had preparations before the test, check to see that preparations are complete. Also review the client's history and determine if there is any allergy history to contrast agents, if applicable.

Take the client's vital signs and weigh the client if required. Depending on the test, ask the client to void. If informed consent is required (necessary for invasive procedures), check for the signed consent form. Client and family members need teaching and reassurance about the purpose of the test and what the procedure involves. They also need to know the care required after the procedure.

Diagnosis, Planning, and Interventions

Clients undergoing diagnostic testing often are anxious and worried. Clients having urologic testing may feel embarrassed and afraid that the testing will be painful. Provide privacy, reassurance, and information and maintain a professional and empathic attitude.

▸ **Anxiety and Fear** related to uncertainty of outcomes of diagnostic testing and the undertaking of an unfamiliar experience

▸ **Expected Outcome:** Client will verbalize reduced apprehension about diagnostic testing.

• Assess client's level of anxiety. *A high level of fear interferes with learning and cooperation.*

TABLE 57-6 Normal Serum Values and Renal Disease

PARAMETER	NORMAL VALUE	CHANGE SEEN IN RENAL DISEASE
Calcium	8.8–10 mg/dL	Decreased in renal failure
Carbon dioxide combining power	23–30 mmol/L	Decreased in acute renal failure
Magnesium	1.3–2.1 mEq/L	Decreased in chronic renal disease
Phosphate, inorganic phosphorus	2.7–4.5 mg/dL	Increased in renal failure
Potassium	3.5–5.0 mEq/L	Increased in renal failure
Total protein	6.0–8.0 g/dL	Increased in poor renal function; decreased in nephrotic syndrome
Sodium	135–148 mmol/L	Decreased in severe nephritis; increased in renal disease
Blood urea nitrogen	7–18 mg/dL	Increased in renal disease and urinary obstruction
Creatinine	Male: 0.7–1.3 mg/dL Female: 0.6–1.1 mg/dL	Increased in renal disease or insufficiency
Albumin	>60 yr: 3.4–4.8 g/dL <60 yr: 3.5–5 g/dL	Decreased in renal failure
Chloride	98–107 mEq/L	Decreased in renal failure (onset)
Uric acid	Male: 4.5–8 ng/dL Female: 2.5–6.2 ng/dL	Increased in renal failure

- Explain or re-explain the test, diagnostic procedure, equipment, tubes, or drains to be used. *Thorough understanding of what is expected promotes compliance and cooperation and decreases fear.*
- Use simple language with client or significant others, especially with outpatient procedures or tests. *Using words and language that the client can understand promotes understanding and cooperation.*
- Answer questions about testing or consult with other health team members in matters that involve their expertise. *Additional information provides clarification, promotes understanding, and reduces anxiety.*
- Acknowledge appropriateness of client's feelings; correct any misinterpretations. Avoid false reassurances. Encourage client to verbalize thoughts and feelings. *Acknowledgment of a client's fears conveys acceptance of the client and allows him or her to focus on instructions and what is expected.*
- Provide a calm, nonthreatening environment. Respond to client's needs as quickly as possible. Encourage significant other(s) to stay with the client. *These measures convey calm and promote client's ability to cope.*
- Administer sedative medications as ordered. *Medication reduces anxiety and assists the client to proceed with the test.*

▶ Deficient Knowledge related to diagnostic procedures, tests, and preprocedure and postprocedure care

▶ Expected Outcome: Client will be able to demonstrate or verbalize an understanding of diagnostic procedure, test, and precare and postcare.

- Provide for physical comfort and quiet atmosphere for the client (or significant other) without disruptions. *Doing so allows for concentration on topic and limits distractions.*
- Assess client's knowledge base; explain the purpose of and discuss the procedure or test. *These steps incorporate prior knowledge and promote learning.*
- Move from general to specific details (i.e., radiologic site, required medications, equipment, IV lines, anesthesia, precare and postcare, catheters or drains used). *Doing so provides a foundation of knowledge and proceeds to more specific information.*
- Discuss home care (i.e., fluid intake, medication use, signs and symptoms of genitourinary infection) and postprocedure conditions requiring physician follow-up (i.e., frank bleeding, inability to urinate, increased pain, or fever). *The nurse provides essential information for home care and builds on the foundation of information about the procedure.*
- Discuss concerns about radiographic exposure or refer concerns to the physician or radiologist. *Expressing concerns reduces their effects and provides a means to access other resources.*
- Encourage questions, repetition of information, and return demonstration (as appropriate) from the client or significant other. *Repetition of information and return demonstrations internalize information and behaviors.*

Evaluation of Expected Outcomes

The client reports a decrease in his or her fear and demonstrates a better understanding of the tests, procedures, or both. The client complies with instructions.

CRITICAL THINKING EXERCISES

1. A client is admitted with dehydration. What urinalysis results would support this diagnosis?
2. A client who is scheduled for an intravenous pyelogram later in the day mentions that he is allergic to shrimp. What action should the nurse take?
3. A client who was hospitalized for abdominal surgery had a Foley catheter for several days. It was removed. The nurse noticed that the client's first voided urine was concentrated and cloudy and had a strong odor. What actions does the nurse need to initiate?
4. What explanation would you provide for a client who has to have a postvoid residual?

NCLEX-STYLE REVIEW QUESTIONS

1. Which of the following interventions would best help the nurse detect signs of arterial occlusion in a client following renal angiography?
   1. Assess the client's pain level every 4 hours.
   2. Monitor the client's intake and output every 4 hours.
   3. Assess the client's pressure dressing once a shift.
   4. Palpate the pulses in the legs and feet every hour.
2. The physician orders a 24-hour urine collection for a client who develops signs and symptoms that resemble Cushing's syndrome. The nurse is most accurate in instructing the client that the urine collection will begin at what time?
   1. At noontime
   2. With the client's next voiding
   3. After the client's next voiding
   4. At midnight
3. The nurse assesses the client with diarrhea for signs of fluid volume deficit. Which assessment finding best indicates that the client is becoming dehydrated?
   1. The client's blood pressure is elevated.
   2. The client's heart rate is irregular.
   3. The client's mucous membranes are pink.
   4. The client's urine is dark yellow.
4. A client with type 1 diabetes mellitus consults a physician because the client has been experiencing urinary problems. When the nurse instructs the client about the technique for collecting a clean-catch midstream urine specimen for routine urinalysis, which statement is most accurate?
   1. Cleanse the urethral area using several circular motions.
   2. Void into the plastic liner that is under the toilet seat.
   3. After voiding a small amount, collect a sample of urine.
   4. Mix the antiseptic solution with the collected urine specimen.

5. The client who is being treated for pyelonephritis is scheduled for an intravenous pyelogram (IVP). When the nurse prepares the client for the IVP, which of the following is the best explanation for administering a laxative?

1. Emptying the bowel improves the ability to visualize the urinary structures.

2. Emptying the bowel also aids in examining the lower gastrointestinal tract.

3. Emptying the bowel prevents accidental stool incontinence during the x-ray.

4. Emptying the bowel reduces the potential for constipation or impaction.

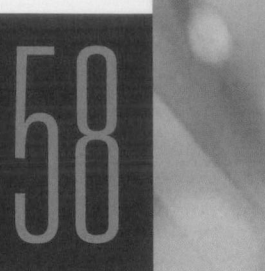

58 Caring for Clients with Disorders of the Kidneys and Ureters

Learning Objectives

On completion of this chapter, you will be able to:

1. Differentiate pyelonephritis and glomerulonephritis.
2. Name problems the nurse manages when caring for clients with glomerulonephritis.
3. Explain the pathophysiology and associated renal complications of polycystic disease.
4. Give examples of conditions that predispose to renal calculi.
5. Identify methods for eliminating small renal calculi and larger stones.
6. Discuss the nursing management of a client with a nephrostomy tube.
7. Describe conditions that cause a ureteral stricture.
8. Explain the classic triad of symptoms associated with renal cancer.
9. Discuss problems the nurse manages when caring for a client with a nephrectomy.
10. Differentiate acute and chronic renal failure.
11. Explain pathophysiologic problems associated with chronic renal failure.
12. Describe sources of organs for kidney transplantation.
13. Identify nursing methods for managing pruritus.
14. Explain the purposes and methods of dialysis.
15. Discuss nursing assessments performed when caring for clients undergoing dialysis.

The most common urologic disorders are infectious and inflammatory conditions. Those that affect the kidneys are extremely dangerous because damage to the nephrons can result in permanent renal dysfunction. The same is true of other upper urinary tract disorders such as kidney and ureteral stones and tumors. The consequences can lead to acute or chronic renal failure.

INFECTIOUS AND INFLAMMATORY DISORDERS OF THE KIDNEY

Infectious and inflammatory disorders of the kidney affect structures such as the renal pelvis, the nephrons, or both.

PYELONEPHRITIS

Pyelonephritis is an acute or chronic bacterial infection of the kidney and the lining of the collecting system (kidney pelvis). *Acute pyelonephritis* presents with moderate to severe symptoms that usually last 1 to 2 weeks. If the treatment of acute pyelonephritis is unsuccessful and the infection recurs, it is termed *chronic pyelonephritis*.

Pathophysiology and Etiology

Bacteria ascend to the kidney and kidney pelves by way of the bladder and urethra. Normal fecal flora such as *Escherichia coli, Klebsiella pneumoniae, Proteus mirabilis, Streptococcus fecalis, Pseudomonas aeruginosa,* and *Staphylococcus aureus* are the most common bacteria that cause acute pyelonephritis. *E. coli* accounts for about 85% of infections. Additional risk factors for chronic pyelonephritis, such as urinary obstruction and reflux (Fig. 58-1), are listed in Box 58-1.

 Gerontologic Considerations

- Urinary obstruction is the most common cause of pyelonephritis in the older adult. When present, the older adult may not experience the fever and difficulty voiding common in younger adults.

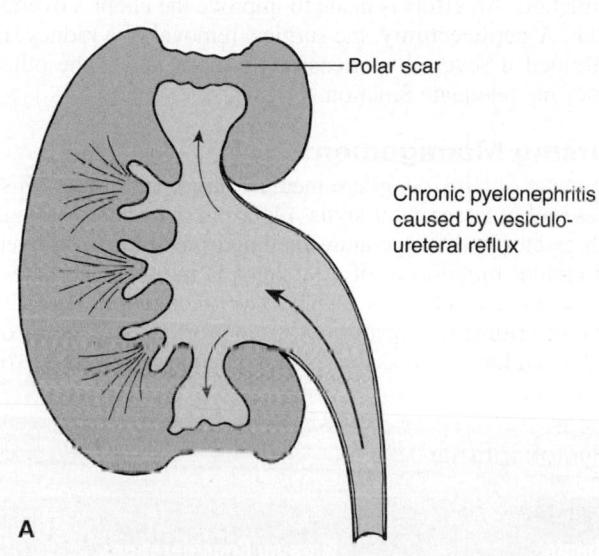

Polar scar

Chronic pyelonephritis caused by vesiculo-ureteral reflux

A

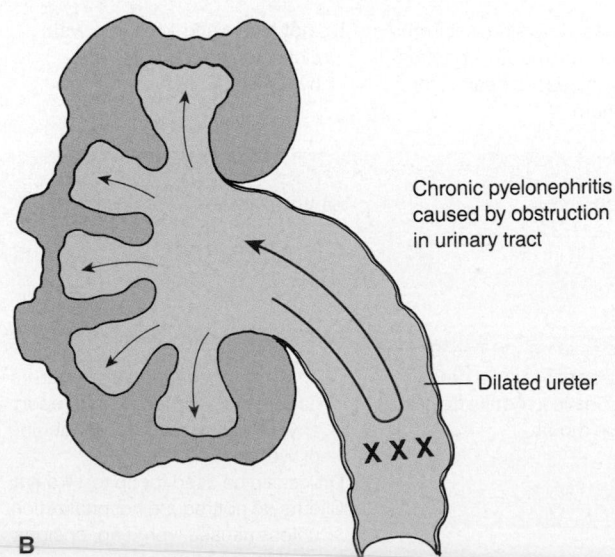

Chronic pyelonephritis caused by obstruction in urinary tract

Dilated ureter

B

FIGURE 58-1. Causes of chronic pyelonephritis include (**A**) vesicoureteral reflux and (**B**) urinary tract obstruction.

BOX 58-1	Risk Factors for Pyelonephritis

Acute Pyelonephritis
- Instrumentation of the urethra and bladder (catheterization, cystoscopy, urologic surgery)
- Inability to empty the bladder
- Pregnancy
- Urinary stasis
- Urinary obstruction (tumors, strictures, calculi, prostatic hypertrophy)
- Diabetes mellitus
- Other renal disease (polycystic kidney disease)
- Neurogenic bladder (stroke, multiple sclerosis, spinal cord injury)
- Women with increased sexual activity, diaphragm, spermicide use, failure to void after intercourse, history of recent urinary infection
- Men who perform anal intercourse, infection with HIV

Chronic Pyelonephritis
- Recurrent episodes of acute pyelonephritis
- Chronic obstruction (e.g., strictures and stones)
- Reflux disorders that allow urine to flow backward up the ureters

In acute pyelonephritis, the inflammation causes the kidneys to grossly enlarge. The cortex and medulla develop multiple abscesses. The renal calyces and pelves also can become involved. Resolution of the inflammation results in fibrosis and scarring. Chronic pyelonephritis develops after recurrent episodes of acute pyelonephritis. The kidneys manifest irreversible degenerative changes and become small and atrophic. If destruction of nephrons is extensive, renal failure develops. Renal dysfunction may not occur for 20 or more years after the onset of the disease. About 10% to 15% of clients with chronic pyelonephritis require dialysis.

▶ Stop, Think, and Respond Exercise 58-1

Explain why a client with an indwelling catheter is at risk for acute pyelonephritis.

Assessment Findings

Signs and Symptoms

Flank pain or tenderness, chills, fever, and malaise occur in clients with acute pyelonephritis. Frequency and burning on urination are present if there is accompanying cystitis (bladder infection). Some clients with chronic pyelonephritis are asymptomatic; others have a low-grade fever and vague gastrointestinal complaints. Polyuria and nocturia develop when the tubules of the nephrons fail to reabsorb water efficiently.

Diagnostic Findings

A urinalysis demonstrates multiple abnormalities. The chief abnormality is **pyuria**, or pus (a combination of bacteria and leukocytes) in the urine (Box 58-2). A urine culture identifies the causative microorganism. The physician initially may perform an ultrasound or computed tomography (CT) scan to determine if there is obstruction in the urinary tract. A cystoscopy, or intravenous pyelogram (IVP) or retrograde

BOX 58-2 **Urinalysis Results with Pyelonephritis**

Acute Pyelonephritis
- Bacteria and bacterial casts
- Leukocytes (large)
- Casts (leukocytes, granular, renal tubular)
- Red blood cells (few)
- Low specific gravity
- Slightly alkaline pH
- Proteinuria (minimal to mild)
- Urine culture: organism colony count of >100,000 organisms/mm^3 urine

Chronic Pyelonephritis
- Leukocytes (increased)
- Proteinuria (absent, minimal, or intermittent)
- Bacteria
- Casts (present in early stages and absent in late stages)
- Low specific gravity

pyelogram, demonstrates obstruction or damage to structures of the urinary tract. An IVP is not usually done if acute pyelonephritis is suspected because the IVP is generally unremarkable in 75% of clients (Smeltzer et al., 2008). An x-ray of the kidneys, ureters, and bladder may reveal calculi, cysts, or tumors in the kidney or other urinary structures. The diagnosis of chronic pyelonephritis is based on a history of repeated acute pyelonephritis. Serum creatinine and blood urea nitrogen (BUN) levels, if elevated, indicate impaired renal function.

Medical and Surgical Management

Treatment of acute pyelonephritis includes relieving fever and pain and prescribing antimicrobial drugs such as trimethoprim-sulfamethoxazole (TMP-SMZ, Septra), gentamycin with or without ampicillin, cephalosporin, or ciprofloxacin (Cipro) for 14 days. Two weeks after the client completes initial treatment, a follow-up urine culture is done. Antispasmodics and anticholinergics such as oxybutynin (Ditropan) and propantheline (Pro-Banthine) are additional pharmacologic interventions that relax the smooth muscles of the ureters and bladder, promote comfort, and increase bladder capacity (Drug Therapy Table 58-1). Symptoms usually disappear within a few days of antibiotic therapy. Four to 6 weeks of drug therapy are prescribed for clients with a history of frequent relapsing infections with the same microorganism.

The goal of treatment for chronic pyelonephritis is to prevent progressive kidney damage. When possible, any urinary tract obstruction is relieved to save the kidney from destruction. An effort is made to improve the client's overall health. A **nephrectomy**, the surgical removal of a kidney, is performed if severe hypertension develops and if the other kidney has adequate function.

Nursing Management

The nurse obtains complete medical, drug, and allergy histories and assesses vital signs, reporting abnormal findings such as elevated temperature or blood pressure. Continued and regular monitoring of vital signs is important to detect any evidence of changes. A physical examination helps the nurse determine the location of discomfort and any signs of fluid retention such as peripheral edema or shortness of

DRUG THERAPY TABLE 58-1 Agents to Treat Pyelonephritis

Drug Category and Examples	Mechanism of Action	Side Effects	Nursing Considerations
Antispasmodics oxybutynin chloride (Ditropan) flavoxate (Urispas), belladonna and opium suppositories	Inhibit the action of acetylcholine and relaxes smooth muscle of the ureters and bladder	Dizziness, drowsiness, blurred vision, dry mouth, constipation, increased heart rate, delirium	Do not administer to clients with closed-angle glaucoma or hypotension.
Antispasmodics with Anticholinergic Properties propantheline (Pro-Banthine), hyoscyamine (Levsinex), tincture of belladonna	Reduce spasms and smooth muscle contractions by inhibiting the effects of acetylcholine, thereby increasing bladder capacity	Same as above	Same as above
Oral Antibiotics trimethoprim-sulfamethoxazole (Bactrim, Septra), ciprofloxacin (Cipro)	Inhibit bacterial growth and destroys microorganisms	Same as above; sulfa drugs may leave a metal aftertaste in the mouth	Clients should complete the entire course of drug therapy and report any further symptoms, continuing or worsening. Drugs can be used for up to 14 days. Clients do not require hospitalization unless nausea, vomiting, or signs of septicemia develop.

breath. The nurse observes and documents the characteristics of the client's urine. A clean-catch urine specimen is collected for urinalysis and urine culture. The nurse measures intake and output and recommends, if not contraindicated, a liberal daily fluid intake of approximately 3000 to 4000 mL, to flush infectious microorganisms from the urinary tract. The nurse also administers prescribed medications. He or she evaluates laboratory test results such as BUN, creatinine, serum electrolytes, and urine culture to determine the client's response to therapy. If chronic pyelonephritis develops, the treatment often is lengthy. Poor health and prolonged medical therapy are discouraging. The nurse urges the client to follow the recommendations of the physician and adhere to the prescribed medication regimen. Client and Family Teaching 58-1 outlines important teaching points.

 Pharmacologic Considerations

- Use caution when giving drugs excreted by the kidney to those with renal disease. If the drug is deemed necessary, it may be given in lower than normal doses; observe the client closely for any changes in renal status if normal doses are necessary. Pay special attention to the client's urinary output, because this method is a way to determine a change in renal status.

ACUTE GLOMERULONEPHRITIS

The term *nephritis* describes a group of inflammatory but noninfectious diseases characterized by widespread kidney damage. **Glomerulonephritis** is a type of nephritis that occurs most frequently in children and young adults; however, it can affect people of any age. The exact incidence of the disease is unknown, but it occurs twice as often in men as in women. Most clients recover spontaneously or with minimal therapy without sequelae. Some develop chronic glomerulonephritis, and there is a risk of kidney failure for some clients.

Pathophysiology and Etiology

Glomerulonephritis can occur as a result of infections from group A beta-hemolytic streptococcal infections, bacterial endocarditis, or viral infections such as hepatitis B or C or human immunodeficiency virus (HIV). The relationship between the infection and acute glomerulonephritis is not clear. Microorganisms are not present in the kidney when symptoms appear, but the glomeruli are acutely inflamed. Most believe that the inflammatory response is from antigen–antibody stimulation in the glomerular capillary membrane. The disruption of membrane permeability causes red blood cells (RBCs) and protein molecules to filter from the glomeruli into Bowman's capsule and eventually become lost in the urine. Figure 58-2 outlines the sequence of events in acute glomerulonephritis.

 Client and Family Teaching 58-1
Acute Pyelonephritis

The teaching plan for the client with acute pyelonephritis includes the following recommendations:

- Review information about the disease, its cause, related risk factors, treatment, and preventive measures.
- Read about the purpose, dosage, side effects, and toxic effects of all prescribed medications.
- Complete the entire regimen of antimicrobial therapy as indicated, even if symptoms abate.
- Drink a large volume of oral fluids daily.
- Consume acid-forming foods such as meat, fish, poultry, eggs, grains, corn, lentils, and cranberries, prunes, plums, and their juices to prevent calcium and magnesium phosphate stone formation.
- Avoid alcohol and caffeine products if bladder spasms are present or until a clinical response to therapy is verified.
- Demonstrate how to collect a clean-catch midstream urine specimen for subsequent medical follow-up at 2 weeks and 3 months after treatment.
- Have your blood pressure monitored intermittently.
- Consult the primary care provider if you experience signs of recurring or worsening pyelonephritis or lower urinary tract infection (frequency, urgency, burning, cloudy urine, and fever).
- Practice methods to prevent reinfection—women should wipe from front to back after defecation and wear cotton undergarments. Void every 2 to 3 hours when awake and before and after intercourse.

Assessment Findings
Signs and Symptoms

About 50% of clients with glomerulonephritis have no symptoms. Early symptoms may be so slight that the client does not seek medical attention. Occasionally the onset is sudden, with pronounced symptoms such as fever, nausea, malaise, headache, generalized edema, or **periorbital edema**, puffiness around the eyes. Some clients experience pain or tenderness over the kidney area and mild to moderate hypertension. In some instances, a routine physical examination reveals the disorder. More often, the client or family notices that the person's face is pale and puffy and that slight ankle edema occurs in the evening. The appetite is poor, and **nocturia** (urination during the night) may be present. Irritability and shortness of breath also develop. As the condition progresses, the client develops **hematuria** (blood in the urine), anemia (from the hematuria), convulsions associated with hypertension, congestive heart failure, **oliguria** (low urine output of 100 to 500 mL/day), and perhaps **anuria** (<100 mL of urine over 24 hours). Fluid retention and hypertension contribute to visual disturbances, often as a result of papilledema or hemorrhage in the eye, and epistaxis (nosebleeds).

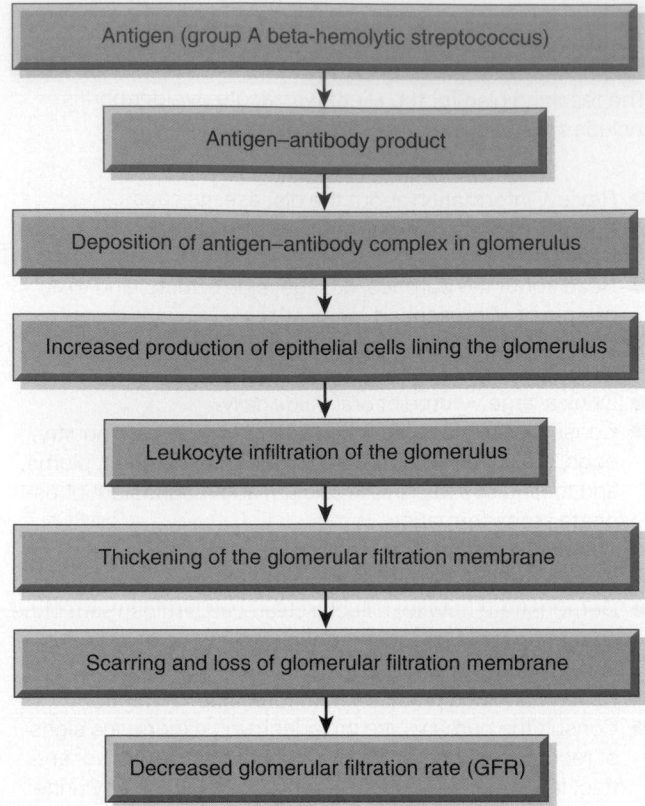

FIGURE 58-2. Sequence of events in acute glomerulonephritis.

Gerontologic Considerations

- Acute glomerulonephritis in the older adult usually occurs in those with preexisting chronic glomerulonephritis, often caused by streptococcus or gram-negative bacteria. Glomerulonephritis may occur as immunity declines; as an immunologic reaction to another system disease, such as lupus (lupus erythematosus); or as the result of unknown causes. Symptoms in the older adult are subtle and nonspecific (e.g., nausea, malaise, arthralgia, exacerbation of preexisting illness), and therefore may go undetected. Heart or renal failure symptoms may accompany the presentation.

Diagnostic Findings

Gross or microscopic hematuria gives the urine a dark, smoky, or frank bloody appearance. Laboratory findings include proteinuria (primarily as albumin in the urine) and an elevated anti-streptolysin O titer from the recent streptococcal infection. There are decreased hemoglobin, slightly elevated BUN and serum creatinine levels, and an elevated erythrocyte sedimentation rate. If renal insufficiency develops, serum electrolyte levels indicate hyperkalemia, hypermagnesemia, hypocalcemia, and dilutional hyponatremia. Percutaneous renal biopsy reveals cellular changes characteristic of an antigen-antibody response and the extent of damage that already has occurred.

Medical Management

No specific treatment exists for acute glomerulonephritis. Treatment is guided by the symptoms and the underlying abnormality. Treatment may consist of bed rest, a sodium-restricted diet (if edema or hypertension is present), and antimicrobial drugs to prevent a superimposed infection in the already inflamed kidney. Penicillin may be used to abolish any remaining streptococci from the recent infection. Diuretics to reduce edema and antihypertensive agents for severe hypertension may be necessary. Vitamins are added to the diet to improve general resistance, and oral iron supplements may be needed to counteract anemia. Corticosteroids and immunosuppressive agents may be given to treat a rapidly progressive inflammatory process. Any increase in hematuria, proteinuria, or blood pressure indicates a need for aggressive treatment. The client is not considered cured until the urine is free of protein and RBCs for 6 months. Return to full activity usually is not permitted until the urine is free of protein for 1 month.

Nursing Management

The client must maintain bed rest when the blood pressure is elevated and edema is present. The nurse collects daily urine specimens to assist with evaluating the client's response to treatment. He or she assesses blood pressure every 4 hours or as ordered. Encouraging adequate fluid intake and measuring intake and output are important nursing interventions. Although the diet may be restricted in sodium and protein, it is necessary for the client to have adequate carbohydrate intake to prevent the catabolism of body protein stores.

Client teaching aims to accomplish the following:

- Identify the specific amount of sodium that is allowed and sources of sodium to avoid.
- Explain the purpose of diuretic therapy or other prescribed medications, the dosing regimen, and side effects.
- Recommend regular blood pressure monitoring.
- Caution client to avoid contact with persons who have infections.
- Emphasize compliance with medical appointments and the necessity for repeated urinalyses.
- Advise client to contact the physician if urinary volumes diminish, there is unexplained weight gain, or headaches or nosebleeds occur.

CHRONIC GLOMERULONEPHRITIS

Chronic glomerulonephritis is a slowly progressive disease characterized by inflammation of the glomeruli, causing irreversible damage to the nephrons. The course of the disease is highly variable. Some clients live for years with no or occasional symptomatic episodes. In other clients, the disease is rapidly fatal unless they receive dialysis to take care of the renal failure.

Pathophysiology and Etiology

A small number of those with chronic glomerulonephritis are known to have had repeated acute glomerulonephritis, but many do not have that history. Complications of autoimmune connective tissue disorders, such as lupus erythematosus (see Chap. 63) and Goodpasture's syndrome (a rare disease that includes progressive glomerulonephritis, hemoptysis, and marked RBC destruction), also may cause chronic glomerulonephritis.

The chronic inflammation leads to ever-increasing bands of scar tissue that replace nephrons, the vital functioning units of the kidney. Decreased glomerular filtration eventually can lead to renal failure. Chronic glomerulonephritis accounts for approximately 40% of people on dialysis.

Assessment Findings
Signs and Symptoms
Some clients do not experience symptoms until renal damage is severe. Generalized edema known as **anasarca** is a common finding. Anasarca is caused by the shift of fluid from the intravascular space to interstitial and intracellular locations. The fluid shift results from depletion of serum proteins, particularly albumin, which are lost in the urine. Clients remain markedly edematous for months or years. They may feel relatively well, but the kidney continues to excrete albumin. The fluid burden and subsequent renal failure contribute to fatigue, headache, hypertension, dyspnea, and visual disturbances.

Diagnostic Findings
Low RBC volume is detected through complete blood counts. Its underlying cause is the excretion of erythrocytes in the urine and reduced production of erythropoietin. **Azotemia**, accumulation of nitrogen waste products in the blood, is evidenced by elevated BUN, serum creatinine, and uric acid levels. The urine contains protein (albumin), sediment, **casts** (deposits of minerals that break loose from the walls of the tubules), and red and white blood cells. The urinary creatinine clearance is reduced. Serum electrolyte changes indicate nephron dysfunction.

Chest radiography and echocardiography evaluate cardiac size because cardiac enlargement is common. A percutaneous kidney biopsy may be performed in the early stage to confirm the diagnosis and to determine the severity of the disorder. In late stages, the kidneys are too small to safely perform a biopsy.

Medical Management
Treatment is nonspecific and symptomatic. Management goals include the following:

- Controlling hypertension with medications and sodium restriction
- Correcting fluid and electrolyte imbalance
- Reducing edema with diuretic therapy
- Preventing congestive heart failure
- Eliminating urinary tract infections (UTIs) with antimicrobials

Renal failure eventually may necessitate dialysis or kidney transplantation, discussed later in this chapter.

Nursing Process for the Client with Chronic Glomerulonephritis

Assessment
Monitor fluid and electrolyte balance by checking blood values, intake and output, and skin turgor, and look for any edema. Also assess the client's neurologic, cardiac, and mental status.

Diagnosis, Planning, and Interventions
Caring for the client with chronic glomerulonephritis involves close observation for changes in fluid and electrolyte status and kidney function. Clients may experience anxiety or depression and require emotional support. Diagnoses, expected outcomes, and interventions include, but are not limited to, the following:

▶ **Excess Fluid Volume** related to decreased glomerular filtration

▶ **Expected Outcomes:** Client will maintain a fluid volume within normal limits as evidenced by urine output greater than 500 mL/day, systolic blood pressure less than 140 mm Hg, reduced proteinuria, and no crackles, gurgles, or S_3 heart sounds.

- Weigh client daily at the same time on the same scale with client wearing similar clothing each time. *Changes in body weight reflect changes in body fluid volume. Consistent conditions provide a baseline and database for observing changes and determining treatment.*
- Measure intake and output. *Accurate measurements provide a database for evaluating fluid balance.*
- Plan with client to proportionately distribute restricted fluid volumes over 24 hours. *The nurse must carefully plan fluid restriction to maintain intravascular volume and cardiac workload. Involving the client in planning promotes his or her compliance with restrictions.*
- Monitor blood pressure, heart rate, and lung and heart sounds each shift. Notify the physician of significant changes. *Changes in these parameters indicate changes in fluid volume.*
- Assess for edema, tight rings or shoes, or clothes that do not fit comfortably. *Renal failure causes dependent edema, as evidenced by pitting edema and tight rings or shoes.*
- Request that the dietitian instruct the client on sodium restriction and adequate caloric intake. *Restricted sodium promotes excretion of excess fluid. Clients require adequate caloric intake to maintain energy levels and proper nutrition.*
- Suggest herbs or spices that increase the palatability of food. *Decreased sodium reduces the flavor of food. Adding herbs and spices helps enhance food flavor.*
- Administer prescribed diuretics. *They promote diuresis, decrease edema, and increase renal blood flow.*

▶ **Activity Intolerance** related to fatigue, anemia, retention of waste products, and generalized edema

▶ **Expected Outcome:** Client will demonstrate the need to balance rest and activity.

- Avoid clustering nursing tasks and physical activities. *Spacing activities conserves energy.*
- Provide periods of rest and promote uninterrupted sleep at night. *Adequate rest conserves energy levels and decreases fatigue.*
- Facilitate an adequate nutritional intake that includes some complete protein and iron-rich foods. *Complete proteins provide a positive nitrogen balance needed for growth and healing. Although some protein is necessary for complete nutrition,*

clients with decreased kidney function have difficulty excreting waste products from protein metabolism, so there is need to restrict protein intake. Iron-rich foods enhance hemoglobin formation, increasing the blood's oxygen-carrying capacity and enhancing energy levels and activity tolerance.

- Eliminate any unnecessary activities of daily living (ADLs). Assist client with ADLs when he or she shows evidence of tachycardia or dyspnea. *Reducing activities and providing assistance decrease oxygen consumption and conserve energy.*

Evaluation of Expected Outcomes

Urine output is 650 mL/day. Systolic blood pressure is 132 mm Hg. Bilateral breath sounds are clear and heart sounds are normal. The client plans rest periods in the day and reduces commitments. He or she also demonstrates understanding of appropriate diet, as evidenced by food choices.

The nurse evaluates the client's ability to manage home care and the availability of a support system before developing discharge plans. If the client lacks a support system from the family or extended family members, the nurse consults with the physician for a referral to a social agency or home health care agency. Client and Family Teaching 58-2 provides important discharge instructions.

CONGENITAL KIDNEY DISORDERS: POLYCYSTIC DISEASE

Individuals may be born with various malformations of renal structures. Most of these are unpredictable because they are

---

| **Client and Family Teaching 58-2** |
| **Chronic Glomerulonephritis** |

The nurse teaches the client and family as follows:

- Follow the diet and fluid regimen recommended by the physician and as outlined by the dietitian.
- Take medications exactly as directed on the container label. Do not omit or discontinue any medication unless ordered to do so by the physician. Do not take nonprescription drugs unless a physician approves their use.
- Monitor and record temperature and weight daily. (In some instances, clients may be asked to monitor their blood pressure.)
- Follow the physician's recommendations as to physical activity and exercise. Take frequent rest periods if fatigue occurs.
- Contact the physician if there are questions about medications; if symptoms become worse; or if fever, chills, blood in the urine, weight gain, swelling of the arms or legs or periorbital edema, difficulty in breathing, difficulty in thinking, severe fatigue, excessive sleepiness, constipation, loss of appetite, or an upper respiratory infection occurs.
- Emphasize that frequent follow-up visits and laboratory tests are necessary to monitor response to treatment.

---

the result of errors in fetal development. Polycystic disease, however, is the result of a hereditary trait.

The two manifestations of polycystic disease are the infantile and adult forms. The infantile form is rare. It may cause fetal death (before delivery), early neonatal death, or renal failure during childhood. The adult form has its onset between 30 and 50 years of age and insidiously progresses to renal insufficiency. Once renal failure develops, polycystic disease usually is fatal within 4 years, unless the client receives dialysis treatment or an organ transplant. Women and men are affected equally. Death usually results from renal failure or the complications of hypertensive cardiovascular disease.

Pathophysiology and Etiology

Adult polycystic kidney disease is inherited as an autosomal dominant trait, which means that an affected parent passes the gene for the disease to his or her children. Each child has a 50:50 chance of acquiring the defective gene (Fig. 58-3). This is opposed to autosomal recessive inheritance, in which a child has a 25% chance of being affected.

As the name implies, this disorder is characterized by the formation of multiple bilateral kidney cysts (Fig. 58-4). The cysts interfere with kidney function and eventually lead to renal failure. The fluid-filled cysts cause great enlargement of the kidneys, from their normal size of a fist to that of a football. As the cysts enlarge, they compress the renal blood vessels and cause chronic hypertension. Bleeding into cysts causes flank pain. People with polycystic disease are much more susceptible to kidney infections and kidney stones. Beside renal failure, other complications include cysts on the pancreas and liver, an enlarged heart, mitral valve prolapse, and brain aneurysm.

Assessment Findings

Hypertension is present in approximately 75% of affected clients at the time of diagnosis. Other symptoms, such as pain from retroperitoneal bleeding, lumbar discomfort, and

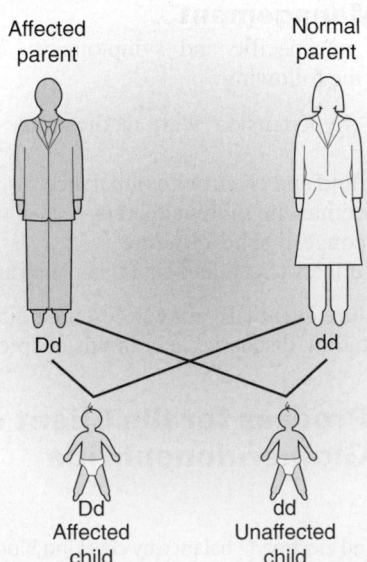

FIGURE 58-3. Inheritance of an autosomal dominant disorder.

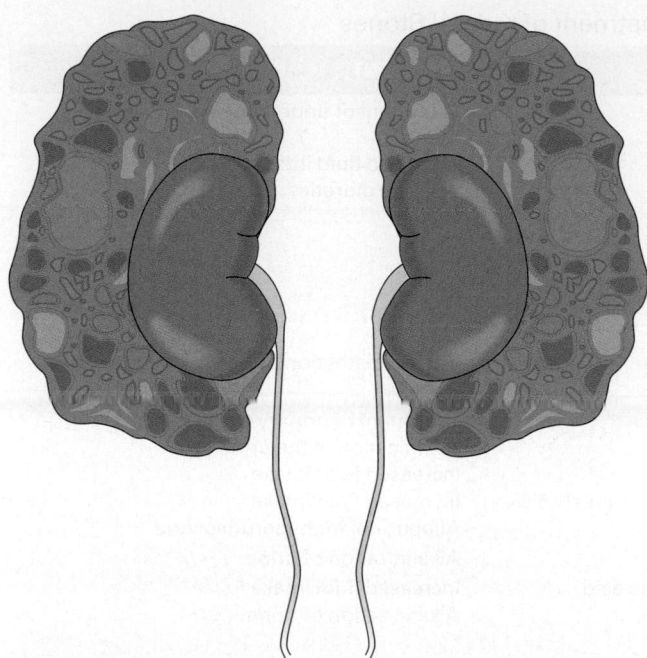

FIGURE 58-4. Normal kidneys in comparison with polycystic kidneys.

abdominal tenderness are caused by the size and effects of the cysts. The client may experience **colic** (acute spasmodic pain) when there is ureteral passage of clots or calculi. Many clients with this disorder also have hematuria because of UTIs and ruptured cysts. Renal stones are also common.

A family history of affected members is a presumptive diagnostic indicator. Urinalysis shows mild proteinuria, hematuria, and pyuria. A complete blood count may show decreased or increased RBCs and hematocrit; an increase is seen because erythropoietin production sometimes is accelerated. Abdominal ultrasound, CT scan, magnetic resonance imaging (MRI), and IVP reveal enlarged kidneys with indentations caused by cysts. Laboratory tests such as BUN and serum creatinine indicate the degree of current kidney dysfunction.

Medical and Surgical Management

Polycystic disease has no cure, but some interventions reduce the rate of progression. Hypertension is treated with antihypertensive drugs, diuretic medications, and sodium restriction. Despite these interventions, the hypertension is difficult to control. When and if urinary infections develop, they are treated promptly with antibiotics. Low RBC counts are treated with iron supplements, injections of erythropoietin (Epogen), or blood transfusions. Nephrotoxic medications, such as nonsteroidal anti-inflammatory drugs (NSAIDs) and cephalosporin antibiotics, are avoided at all costs.

 Pharmacologic Considerations

- Nephrotoxic drugs are not administered to a client with renal disease unless the client's life is in danger and no other therapeutic agent is of value.

Dialysis substitutes for kidney function when renal failure occurs and while the client awaits an organ transplant. Surgical removal of one or both kidneys may be required. Animal research is being conducted using the antineoplastic drug, paclitaxel (Taxol), steroids such as methylprednisolone (Depo-Medrol), and an antihyperlipidemic agent, lovastatin (Mevacor) to evaluate if these drugs slow the rate of disease progression.

Nursing Management

Many clients with polycystic disease are treated as outpatients by primary care physicians or nephrologists, physicians who specialize in the diagnosis and treatment of renal diseases. When hospitalization is necessary, the nurse assesses vital signs, especially blood pressure, and reports any significant elevations. He or she monitors laboratory test results for indicators of renal function. The nurse inspects the urine for signs of bleeding or infection. He or she measures and documents intake and output at least every 8 hours. The nurse reports any decrease in or absence of urine output. For further information about complications or advanced stages, refer to Nursing Process for the Client With Renal Calculi and the Nursing Management sections in the discussions of the client with renal failure and dialysis.

OBSTRUCTIVE DISORDERS

Urinary obstruction at any point in the urinary tract can occur in clients of all ages for various reasons. Obstructing conditions include urinary tract stones, strictures, and tumors. Table 58-1 lists causes of urinary tract obstruction.

KIDNEY AND URETERAL STONES

Urolithiasis refers to a condition of stones (**calculus;** pl. *calculi*) in the urinary tract. A calculus is a precipitate of mineral salts that ordinarily remain dissolved in urine. About 70% to

TABLE 58-1 Causes of Urinary Tract Obstruction

LEVEL OF OBSTRUCTION	CAUSE
Renal pelvis	Renal calculi
	Papillary necrosis
Ureter	Renal calculi
	Pregnancy
	Tumors that compress the ureter
	Ureteral stricture
	Congenital disorders of the uretero-vesical junction, and ureteropelvic junction strictures
Bladder and urethra	Bladder cancer
	Neurogenic bladder
	Bladder stones
	Prostatic hyperplasia or cancer
	Urethral strictures
	Congenital urethral defects

(From Porth, C. M. [2007]. *Essentials of Pathophysiology: Concepts of altered health states* [2nd ed.]. Philadelphia: Lippincott Williams & Wilkins.)

TABLE 58-2 Composition, Contributing Factors, and Treatment of Kidney Stones

TYPE OF STONE	CONTRIBUTING FACTORS	TREATMENT
Calcium (oxalate and phosphate)	Hypercalcemia and hypercalciuria	Treatment of underlying conditions
	Immobilization	Increased fluid intake
		Thiazide diuretics
	Hyperparathyroidism	
	Vitamin D intoxication	
	Diffuse bone disease	
	Milk-alkali syndrome	
	Renal tubular acidosis	
	Hyperoxaluria	Dietary restriction of foods high in oxalate
	Intestinal bypass surgery	
Magnesium ammonium phosphate (struvite)	Urea-splitting urinary tract infections	Treatment of urinary tract infection
		Acidification of the urine
		Increased fluid intake
Uric acid (urate)	Formed in acid urine with pH of approximately 5.5	Increased fluid intake
	Gout	Allopurinol for hyperuricosuria
	High-purine diet	Alkalinization of urine
Cystine	Cystinuria (inherited disorder of amino acid metabolism)	Increased fluid intake
		Alkalinization of urine

80% of renal calculi in the United States are composed of calcium oxalate, calcium phosphate, or both (Porth, 2007). Others are composed of calcium phosphate, uric acid, cystine, and magnesium ammonium phosphate, or struvite (Table 58-2). Stones may be smooth, jagged, or staghorn shaped (Fig. 58-5).

Calculi can occur anywhere in the urinary tract from the kidney pelvis and beyond. When a stone forms, the condition is called *urolithiasis*. **Nephrolithiasis** refers to a kidney stone, the size of which may range from microscopic to several centimeters. **Ureterolithiasis** is a stone in the ureter. Ureteral stones usually are small; some may be no larger than a grain of sand.

Pathophysiology and Etiology

The reason urinary calculi form is not fully understood. Predisposing factors include the following:

*   **Calciuria**, excessive calcium in the urine, as may accompany hyperparathyroid disease, administration of calcium-based antacids, and excessive intake of vitamin D
*   Dehydration
*   UTI with urea-splitting organisms such as *P. mirabilis,* which makes urine alkaline, a condition that promotes precipitation of calcium
*   Obstructive disorders, such as an enlarged prostate gland, which foster urinary stasis
*   Metabolic disorders, such as gout, in which uric acid crystallizes
*   Osteoporosis, in which bone is demineralized
*   Prolonged immobility from paralysis secondary to spinal injuries or other incapacitating conditions that result in sluggish emptying of urine from the urinary tract

Calculi traumatize the walls of the urinary tract and irritate the cellular lining, causing pain as violent contractions of the ureter develop to pass the stone along. But the ureteral

spasms may just as easily hold a stone in place. If a stone totally or partially obstructs the passage of urine beyond its location, pressure increases in the area above the stone. The pressure contributes to pain, and urinary stasis promotes secondary infection. The retained urine distends the renal pelvis, a condition called **hydronephrosis**. Eventually, there

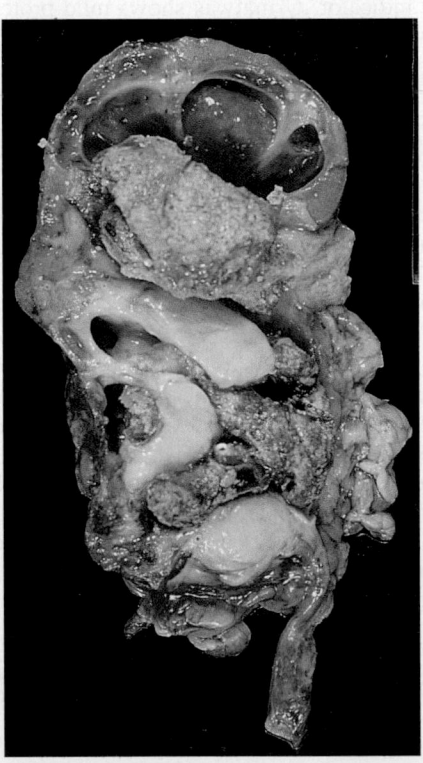

FIGURE 58-5. Staghorn calculi. The kidney shows hydronephrosis and stones that are casts of the dilated calyces. (From Rubin, R., & Strayer, D. S., eds. [2008]. *Pathology: Clinicopathologic foundations of medicine* [5th ed.]. Philadelphia: Lippincott Williams & Wilkins.)

may be compression of the glomeruli and tiny arterioles that supply blood to the kidney, which can result in permanent kidney damage.

Assessment Findings
Signs and Symptoms
Symptoms of a kidney or ureteral stone vary with size, location, and cause. Small stones may pass unnoticed; however, sudden, sharp, severe flank pain that travels to the suprapubic region and external genitalia is the classic symptom of urinary calculi. The pain is accompanied by renal or ureteral colic, painful spasms that attempt to move the stone. The pain comes in waves that radiate to the inguinal ring, the inner aspect of the thigh, and to the testicle or tip of the penis in men, or the urinary meatus or labia in women. The severity of the pain usually is inversely proportional to the size of the stone. Smaller stones travel more rapidly down the ureter, causing more forceful ureteral spasm and, therefore, greater pain. The severity of the pain can cause nausea, vomiting, and shock.

If an infection develops, the client may experience chills, fever, and serious hypotension. Urinary retention or dysuria may accompany obstruction. The kidney pelvis and ureter may become markedly enlarged as a consequence of urinary obstruction, and a mass may be palpated. The client also may experience renal tenderness.

Diagnostic Findings
Urinalysis shows evidence of gross or microscopic hematuria from trauma as the calculus tears at tissue as it moves downward. In addition, the urinalysis may show a pH conducive to stone formation, increased specific gravity, mineral crystals, and casts. Leukocytes in the urine and an elevated white blood cell count indicate an infectious process. A urine culture identifies specific infectious microorganisms.

Radiography identifies most translucent kidney stones. If visualization is inconclusive, an IVP shows dye-filling defects caused by a stone. The dye stops at a certain point in the ureter and demonstrates enlargement above the obstruction. Kidney ultrasonography also detects obstructive changes. Depending on how long the stone has been present, some blood chemistry values, such as serum creatinine, BUN, and serum uric acid, may be elevated. Analysis of the stone content is useful in preventing recurrence.

Medical Management
Small calculi are passed naturally with no specific interventions. If the stone is 5 mm or less in diameter and moving, the pain is tolerable, and if there is no obstruction, the client is managed medically with vigorous hydration, analgesics (including opioids and NSAIDs), antimicrobial therapy, and drugs that dissolve calculi or eventually alter conditions that promote their formation.

For larger stones, **extracorporeal shock wave lithotripsy** (ESWL), a procedure that uses 800 to 2400 shock waves aimed from outside the body toward soft tissue to dense stones (Fig. 58-6A), may be used. The stones are shattered into smaller particles that are passed from the urinary tract. ESWL is administered with the client in a water bath or surrounded by a soft cushion while under light anesthesia or sedation. Stones also can be pulverized with laser lithotripsy.

To do so, a fine wire, through which the laser beam passes, is inserted into the ureter by means of a cystoscope. Repeated bursts of the laser reduce the stone to a fine powder, which is then passed in the urine.

Other stone removal procedures are performed with ureteroscopic approaches in which the endoscope is inserted from the urethra into the upper urinary tract under anesthesia to grasp, crush, and remove stones from the kidney pelvis or ureter (see Fig. 58-6B). Afterward, a catheter or **ureteral stent**, a slender supportive device, is left in place for 3 days to splint the ureter or divert the urine past any possible tear in the ureteral wall (Fig. 58-7). If the stone cannot be removed, a ureteral catheter is left in place for 24 hours to dilate the ureter in the hope that the stone will pass through it or that it will be pulled into the bladder when the catheter is removed.

Pharmacologic Considerations

- Sodium bicarbonate (baking soda), usually in tablet form, may be used to alkalize the urine of clients with kidney stones to prevent stone recurrence.

Stop, Think, and Respond Exercise 58-2
For healthcare personnel to perform ESWL, the client must be in a clean water bath or surrounded by soft cushions. What concerns might the client have? What are your best responses?

Surgical Management
Calculi that are large or complicated by obstruction, ongoing UTI, kidney damage, or constant bleeding require surgical removal. Surgical options include a percutaneous nephrolithotomy, ureterolithotomy, pyelolithotomy, and nephrolithotomy.

A *percutaneous nephrolithotomy* is an endoscopic procedure. A nephroscope is tunneled into the kidney through a tiny skin incision while the client is under general anesthesia (see Fig. 58-6C). Ultrasound is used to crush the stone. The fragments are removed through the endoscope.

For *ureterolithotomy*, *pyelolithotomy*, or *nephrolithotomy*, a suprapubic abdominal or flank incision is made and the stone is removed under direct visualization while the client is anesthetized. A **pyeloplasty**, surgical repair of the ureteropelvic junction or other anatomic anomalies, may be performed at the same time. The additional surgery is done to correct conditions that contribute to the development of stones and prevent their recurrence.

A nephrectomy is indicated if a stone has permanently and severely damaged a kidney beyond adequate function. The other kidney must be fully functional.

After any of these surgical procedures, drainage of urine from the affected kidney is accomplished with a nephrostomy tube during the healing process. A **nephrostomy tube**, also called a *pyelostomy tube*, is a catheter inserted through the skin into the renal pelvis. A nephrostomy tube is used to

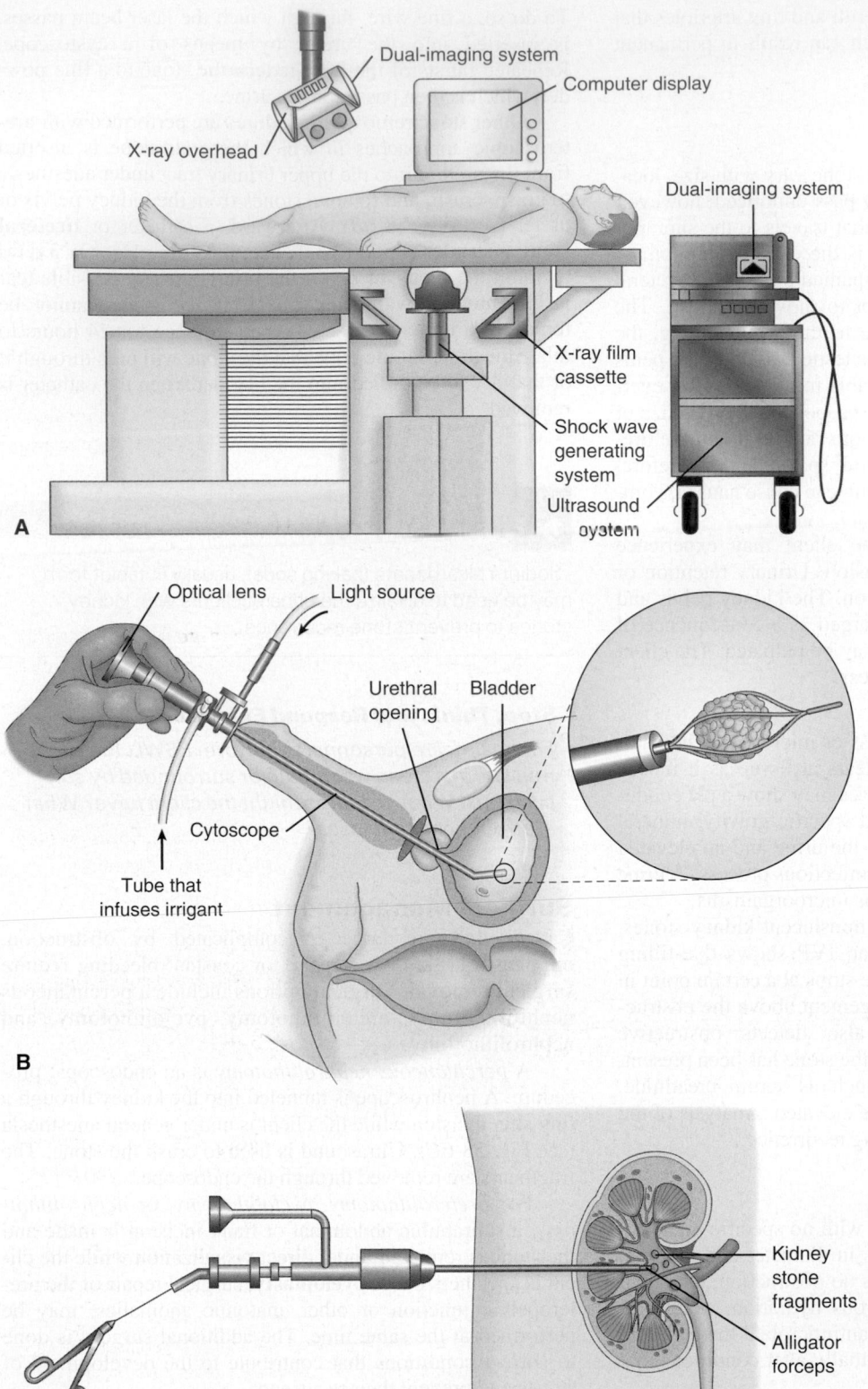

FIGURE 58-6. Methods of treating renal stones. (**A**) Extracorporeal shock wave lithotripsy (ESWL). (**B**) Cystoscopy. (**C**) Percutaneous nephrolithotomy.

manage any obstruction to urine flow above the bladder. The tube is kept in place with a suture through the skin. Unlike the bladder, the kidney pelvis can hold only 5 to 8 mL of urine. If a blood clot or kinking or compression of the tubing impairs urinary drainage for even a short time, hydronephrosis and damage to surgically repaired tissue can result. The client complains of pain if the renal pelvis becomes distended with urine.

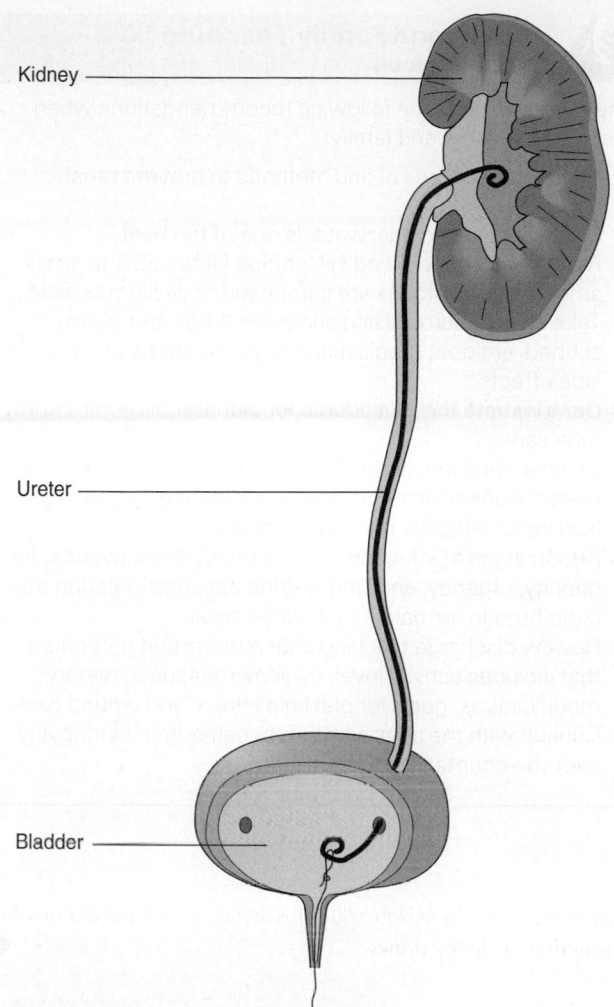

Kidney

Ureter

Bladder

FIGURE 58-7. Example of a ureteral stent; in this case, a double J stent.

Nursing Process for the Client with Renal Calculi

Assessment

Obtain a complete history, including a drug and allergy history, family history, history of immobility, episodes of dehydration, UTIs, and diet. Assess pain intensity and location and associated symptoms such as nausea and vomiting. In addition, monitor vital signs and assess all urine for stones by straining it through a gauze or wire mesh and closely inspecting it. Save solid material for laboratory analysis. Urine may show evidence of hematuria. In some instances, the client may experience anuria related to bilateral obstruction and have abdominal distention.

Diagnosis, Planning, and Interventions

Three goals when caring for a client with urinary calculi include improving urinary output, relieving pain, and preventing or treating infection. Clients often are frightened because of the excruciating pain, and thus require emotional support as well as pain management. Typical diagnoses, expected outcomes, and interventions include, but are not limited to, the following.

▶ **Acute Pain** related to increased pressure in the renal pelvis or renal colic

▶ **Expected Outcome:** Pain will decrease within 30 minutes of a nursing measure.

- Administer prescribed narcotic analgesic. *It assists in decreasing pain related to ureteral colic during an acute episode and promotes muscle relaxation.*
- Provide supplemental nonpharmacologic interventions such as a comfortable position, guided imagery, and distraction. *These measures promote relaxation, redirect attention, and enhance coping ability.*
- Encourage ambulation and liberal fluid intake when the client is comfortable. *The supine position can increase colic; ambulation relieves it. Increased fluid intake promotes the passage of a stone and prevents urinary stasis or the formation of new stones.*

▶ **PC: Hydronephrosis** related to ureteral obstruction

▶ **Expected Outcome:** The nurse will manage and minimize hydronephrosis.

- Monitor intake and output. *This record provides information about kidney function and indicates any complications such as hydronephrosis.*
- Administer antibiotics as ordered. *Antimicrobials treat the cause of UTI associated with urolithiasis and urinary stasis.*
- Manage a nephrostomy tube by following Nursing Guidelines 58-1. *Proper management ensures that the nephrostomy tube remains in place, urine drains properly, and infection is prevented.*

▶ **Risk for Infection** related to urinary stasis

▶ **Expected Outcome:** Urinary tract infection will not develop, as evidenced by urine free of pus and microorganisms and normal temperature and white blood cell count.

- Administer antimicrobial therapy as prescribed. *UTIs potentiate stone formation. Antibiotics treat the infection.*
- Encourage fluid intake to 3000 mL/day unless contraindicated. *Increased hydration flushes bacteria, blood, and other debris, and may expedite stone passage.*
- Maintain patency of all catheters or encourage client to void every 2 to 3 hours. *Adequate urinary flow or frequent voiding prevents urinary stasis and eliminates bacteria, blood, and other particles.*
- Follow aseptic principles when changing dressings or urinary drainage equipment. *Strict asepsis prevents introduction of microbes into the urinary tract.*

▶ **Risk for Ineffective (Renal) Tissue Perfusion** related to increased fluid pressure in ureter and kidney pelvis

▶ **Expected Outcome:** Kidney will remain adequately perfused with blood, as evidenced by normal serum creatinine, BUN, and distribution of radiopaque dye after IVP.

NURSING GUIDELINES 58-1

Managing a Nephrostomy Tube

- Connect the nephrostomy tube to a closed drainage system.
- Have a second nephrostomy tube available at the bedside for the physician's use in case the present one is displaced.
- Secure the tube to the client's flank with tape to ensure that it does not become dislodged.
- Keep the urine collection bag below the level of insertion.
- Never clamp the nephrostomy tubing.
- Check that the nephrostomy and drainage tubing are not kinked or that the client is not compressing the tubing.
- Use no more than 5 to 8 mL of sterile normal saline to maintain patency if an irrigation is medically ordered.
- Record the urine output from the nephrostomy tube separately from other urinary volumes.
- Assess the tube insertion site for bleeding and drainage.
- Change the dressing around the nephrostomy tube if and when it becomes damp. Apply a skin barrier ointment around the incision to prevent excoriation.
- Notify the physician immediately if the nephrostomy tube becomes dislodged or if there is an absence of urinary drainage.

- Monitor laboratory and diagnostic test results. *Elevated BUN, creatinine, and electrolyte levels indicate kidney dysfunction and assist in evaluating hydration status and effectiveness of other interventions.*
- Prepare client safely but quickly for treatment measures that promote urinary drainage if it becomes apparent that kidney function is compromised. *Prompt intervention may prevent serious complications.*

Evaluation of Expected Outcomes

Pain is reduced. Urine output is balanced with intake. Urine is clear. The client is afebrile. Findings from urine and blood tests indicate adequate renal function. For clients undergoing surgical procedures, the nurse explains the procedure and follows standards for perioperative care in Chapter 14. After lithotripsy, endoscopy, or surgery, the nurse assesses vital signs, measures fluid intake and output, and inspects the color of urine, which may be grossly bloody for a time. After ESWL, the nurse should inspect the flank for ecchymosis, which is expected. The nurse documents the location of discoloration. Clients require analgesics for postprocedural discomfort.

If a ureteroscopy is performed and a urethral catheter is in place, the nurse attaches the catheter to a closed drainage system. Pink-tinged urine may be seen, but if frank blood appears in the urine or the client complains of severe abdominal pain, the nurse must notify the physician immediately. If a ureteral stent is present, the nurse checks for the suture, which extends from the urinary meatus and is used for stent removal. It is important that the client maintain a total daily fluid volume of approximately 3000 mL. For more information, see Client and Family Teaching 58-3. In addi-

Client and Family Teaching 58-3
Renal Calculi

The nurse includes the following recommendations when teaching the client and family:

- Review the causes of and methods to prevent renal calculi.
- Drink plenty of liquids; water is one of the best.
- Restrict foods identified in Nutrition Notes 58-1 to small amounts if the stones are composed of calcium oxalate.
- Take all antimicrobial and analgesic drugs and, if prescribed, antigout medications as prescribed and report any side effects.
- Demonstrate the procedures for catheter or nephrostomy tube care.
- Strain urine if the stone or its fragments have not passed.
- Report signs of acute obstruction immediately, such as inability or difficulty in voiding, or pain.
- Report signs of infection such as fever, chills, dysuria, frequency, urgency, and cloudy urine because infection may contribute to formation of urinary calculi.
- Review discharge teaching after a treatment procedure that includes activity level, hygiene measures, dietary modifications, goals for oral fluid intake, and wound care.
- Consult with the physician before self-administering any over-the-counter medications.

tion, refer to Nutrition Notes 58-1 for dietary recommendations for prevention of kidney stones.

Nutrition Notes 58-1
The Client at Risk for Kidney Stones

The following dietary recommendations are appropriate for prevention of kidney stones:

- Consume a normal protein diet; a high-protein diet promotes urinary excretion of calcium, oxalate, and uric acid.
- Restrict sodium to 2 to 3 g/day because sodium competes with calcium for reabsorption in the kidneys.
- Consume a normal calcium intake balanced throughout the day. A low-calcium diet may increase the risk of stone formation by increasing urinary oxalate excretion: with less calcium available in the GI tract to bind with oxalate, more oxalate is absorbed and urinary oxalate increases.
- Restrict oxalate-containing foods such as dark leafy green vegetables, berries, rhubarb, tea, nuts, chocolate, beans (green, wax, and dried), tofu, sweet potatoes, wheat bran, and draft beer.
- Avoid vitamin C supplements because vitamin C degrades to oxalate.

(Adapted from Smeltzer, S. C., et al. [2008]. *Brunner & Suddarth's textbook of medical-surgical nursing* [11th ed.]. Philadelphia: Lippincott Williams & Wilkins, p. 1591.)

URETERAL STRICTURE

A stricture is a narrowing of a lumen. A ureteral stricture is the narrowing of a ureter.

Pathophysiology and Etiology

A ureteral stricture is relatively rare, but the incidence is higher among those with chronic ureteral stone formation. Recurrent inflammation and infection cause scar tissue to accumulate in the ureter. Other conditions that can interfere with urine passing through the ureter are congenital anomalies or conditions that mechanically compress the ureter, such as pregnancy or tumors in the abdomen or upper urinary tract.

In many instances, the ureter is only partially narrowed. Symptoms develop over time as the area of the ureter above the stricture dilates with urine (*hydroureter*) and the kidney pelvis slowly enlarges. Stasis of urine promotes an upper UTI.

Assessment Findings

Flank pain or discomfort and tenderness at the costovertebral angle from enlargement of the renal pelvis often develop. The client experiences back or abdominal discomfort, which tends to increase during periods of elevated fluid intake. A voiding cystourethrogram and ultrasonography help to identify structural changes consistent with impaired passage of urine.

Medical and Surgical Management

Various measures are used to treat strictures. Management depends on the location, the density, and the length of the stricture. The ureter can be stretched by inserting a dilator called a *filiform* or *urethral sound,* a curved metal rod, followed by others that are sequentially larger.

If the obstruction persists, the physician performs a **ureteroplasty**, removal of the narrowed section of ureter and reconnection of the patent portions. This is the preferred procedure for a mid-ureteral stricture. A ureteral stent is placed in the ureter to provide support to the walls of the ureter, relieve the obstruction, and maintain the flow of urine through the ureter and into the bladder. Lower ureteral strictures are treated by removing the narrowed portion of the ureter and reimplanting the remaining section into the bladder wall.

Besides correcting strictures, ureteral surgery is performed to remove tumors, repair accidental ligation of the ureter during abdominal surgery (the highest incidence is seen in hysterectomies), and to extricate a ureteral stone that cannot be removed by other means.

Nursing Management

The nurse follows the standards of care for the perioperative client if the client undergoes surgery (see Chap. 14). If a ureteral catheter is inserted before surgery, the nurse measures the urine output from the catheter hourly. He or she must immediately report lack of urine output from the ureteral catheter.

On return from surgery, all urinary drainage tubes and catheters are connected to a closed drainage system or to the type of drainage system ordered by the physician. The main complication associated with ureteral surgery is failure of the ureter to transport urine from the kidney to the bladder. The nurse must contact the physician if:

- Signs of shock appear.
- Urinary output from the ureteral catheter is decreased or absent.
- The client complains of significant abdominal pain, which may indicate leakage of urine into the peritoneal cavity.
- Signs of a UTI develop, such as fever and chills, or the urine is cloudy or has a foul odor.

Depending on the surgical procedure, the client may need instruction in the care of the ureteral or urethral catheter(s), the management of the drainage collection system, incision care, and a review of the prescribed diet and medication schedule.

TUMORS OF THE KIDNEY

Tumors of the kidney are almost always cancerous. Renal cell carcinoma is the most common type of kidney cancer in adults. A second type of kidney cancer is transitional cell cancer. In both types men are affected more than women.

Pathophysiology and Etiology

The cause of kidney tumors is unknown. The incidence is higher in older adults, which suggests chronic exposure to a carcinogen whose metabolites involve renal excretion. Bladder cancer (see Chap. 59) is associated with the carcinogenic effects of long-term cigarette smoking. It is possible that renal tumors are similarly initiated through this mechanism or exposure to some other environmental toxin (e.g., asbestos) or volatile solvent (e.g., gasoline). Box 58-3 lists risk factors for renal cancer.

Because the kidneys are deeply protected in the body, tumors can become quite large before causing symptoms. As the tumor enlarges, it occupies space, extending into adjacent renal structures and interfering with urine outflow. Tumor cells tend to metastasize by way of the renal vein and vena cava to the lungs, bone, lymph nodes, liver, and brain. Lung metastases predominate. Sometimes, the first symptom occurs when the tumor has metastasized to other organs.

BOX 58-3 Risk Factors for Renal Cancer

- Age: risk increases with age; most renal cancers occur after age 60
- Gender: Affects men more than women
- Tobacco use
- Occupational exposure to industrial chemicals, such as petroleum products, heavy metals, and asbestos
- Obesity
- Unopposed estrogen therapy
- Polycystic kidney disease
- Treatment for kidney failure, including clients on dialysis and those receiving a kidney transplant

Assessment Findings

In early stages, renal cancers rarely cause symptoms. In later stages, clients generally present with painless hematuria, which can be intermittent and microscopic or continuous and visible (Smeltzer et al., 2008). In addition, clients may experience persistent back pain that does not go away, weight loss, malaise, and unexplained fever. In some clients a mass is palpable. Colic-like discomfort during the passage of blood clots may also occur.

An abdominal mass found on a routine physical examination or on radiographic examination for other purposes suggests a kidney tumor. An IVP, cystoscopy with retrograde pyelograms, ultrasonography, MRI, renal angiography, and CT scan are used to locate the tumor. Sequential urine samples contain RBCs as well as malignant cells.

Medical and Surgical Management

Radical nephrectomy, including removal of the tumor, adrenal gland, surrounding perinephric fat, and fascia, is the treatment for a malignant renal tumor. For clients who have early stage renal cancer or have only one kidney, the tumor may be removed from the kidney, leaving the kidney and surrounding tissue intact. A laparoscopic nephrectomy may be done on clients with early stage carcinoma. When a tumor arises in the collecting system or the ureter, a complete nephroureterectomy (removal of the kidney and ureter) is done. A cuff of bladder tissue is removed as well because the recurrence rate in any stump of ureter left behind is high. Surgery may be followed by radiation therapy, chemotherapy, hormonal therapy, and/or immunotherapy while the client is still in the hospital or on a postdischarge basis.

For some clients, surgery may be too risky. In these cases, treatment may involve embolization or cryoablation. Embolization involves occlusion of the renal artery to kill the tumor cells. Cryoablation uses special needles called cryoprobes to freeze and then thaw cancer cells, eventually destroying the cancerous cells. CT scans are used to monitor the process.

If extensive metastases are found, only palliative treatment is given. In these cases, the physician explains to the client and family that the treatment measures are not curative.

Nursing Management

In addition to the standard preoperative preparations, the nurse implements other prescribed procedures that facilitate the postoperative assessment and recovery of the client, such as inserting a urethral catheter and nasogastric tube.

Nursing Process for the Client Recovering From a Nephrectomy

Assessment

On the client's return from surgery, assess vital signs frequently. Inspecting and identifying the type and location of drains or catheters are important measures. The indwelling (Foley) catheter drainage system is placed below the level of the bed. Drains in or around the incision may drain by closed negative pressure (i.e., Jackson-Pratt) or low mechanical suction.

Diagnosis, Planning, and Interventions

▶ **PC: Internal Hemorrhage** related to bleeding from the ligated renal artery or vein

▶ **Expected Outcome:** The nurse will manage and minimize hemorrhage.

• Monitor blood pressure and pulse rate every 1 to 4 hours for the first 24 to 48 hours after surgery. *Decreased intravascular volume results in hypotension and tachycardia. Frequent monitoring assists in detecting changes in intravascular volume.*

• Report decreased blood pressure, increased pulse, restlessness, or sudden onset of flank pain. *Death can occur quickly unless the client is immediately returned to surgery to control the bleeding.*

• Administer IV fluids and blood transfusions as ordered. *Isotonic fluids and blood replacement help to restore and maintain intravascular volume.*

• Note and record the color of drainage from each tube and catheter. *Assessment findings direct interventions and provide a means for further comparison and evaluation.*

• Follow the physician's orders concerning postoperative positioning. *Keeping the client from lying on the operative side avoids interference with wound drainage.*

• Contact the surgeon about any frank bleeding or a sudden decrease in urine output. *Although pink-tinged drainage is normal for several days after surgery, frank bleeding, sudden decreased urine, or both indicate complications.*

▶ **Acute Pain** related to tissue trauma and pressure from urinary obstruction

▶ **Expected Outcome:** Pain will be relieved to a tolerable level within 30 minutes of an intervention.

• Keep drainage catheters unclamped, unkinked, and below the level of insertion. *Unobstructed urine flow promotes urine elimination and prevents pain related to obstruction.*

• Secure all tubings to reduce movement at the site of insertion or displacement. *This measure reduces pain at the insertion site and promotes comfort.*

• Encourage oral fluids as soon as allowed and tolerated without causing nausea or vomiting. *Fluids dilute the urine and prevent catheter obstruction from sediment or small blood clots, thus reducing potential for pain and discomfort.*

• Irrigate tubings as ordered. *Irrigation promotes urinary flow and reduces potential for pain.*

• Administer prescribed analgesia and supplement drug therapy with nursing measures that promote comfort. *Analgesics and nonpharmacologic methods assist in reducing pain and promote the client's sense of control and participation in self-care.*

• Splint the incision when repositioning the client or during efforts to cough and deep breathe. *Splinting reduces tension on the surgical site and prevents or reduces pain-related movement.*

- Risk for Ineffective Breathing Pattern related to incisional pain and restricted positioning; Risk for Ineffective Airway Clearance related to weak cough secondary to incisional pain

- **Expected Outcomes:** Breathing rate and depth will be sufficient to maintain blood oxygen saturation (SpO$_2$) at 90% or above. Secretions will be raised. Lung sounds will be clear in all lobes.

- Encourage client to breathe deeply and cough every 2 hours. Use an incentive spirometer to evaluate effectiveness. *These efforts increase alveolar ventilation and assist in clearing secretions.*

- Use two hands to apply firm support of the incision when the client coughs or performs deep breathing exercises. *This technique splints the incision, reducing pain and promoting the client's ability to breathe deeply and cough.*

- Auscultate the lungs daily; notify the physician of any abnormal or absent breath sounds. *Breath sounds should be clear. Fine, scattered crackles at bases indicate that the client should be more vigorous in deep breathing and coughing. Coarser crackles indicate fluid in the airway; wheezes indicate a partial obstruction. Absent breath sounds require prompt intervention.*

- Risk for Infection related to impaired skin integrity and stasis of urine

- **Expected Outcome:** Client will be free of infection as evidenced by normal findings in temperature, urine culture, and white blood cell count.

- Monitor temperature every 4 hours. *Fever usually is the first and only sign of infection.*

- Contact the physician if the client's temperature is above 101°F (38.3°C) or he or she experiences chills, or if purulent drainage or redness, swelling, and warmth at the incision are noted. *Elevated temperatures and incisional signs indicate an infection that requires intervention.*

- Use aseptic technique when changing the surgical dressing or managing the catheter and drainage systems. *Asepsis prevents introduction of microorganisms to the urinary tract or to areas where skin integrity has been lost.*

- Administer antibiotic therapy as prescribed. *Antibiotics treat infections, reducing the risk of further infection.*

Evaluation of Expected Outcomes

The client shows no evidence of hemorrhage. Interventions reduce or eliminate pain. Breathing rate and depth maintain the SpO$_2$ at 90% or above. The client raises secretions, and lung sounds are clear in all lobes. No infections develop.

Clients who have had a nephrectomy usually have the drains (if any) removed before discharge. A dressing over the incision may or may not be required. If the physician orders a dressing applied and changed at home, the nurse shows the client and family how to change the dressing and provides a list of the necessary materials for dressing changes (Client and Family Teaching 58-4).

Client and Family Teaching 58-4
Home Care After Nephrectomy

The teaching plan should include the following instructions:

- Change the dressing as ordered by the physician.
- Wash hands thoroughly before and after each dressing change.
- Drink plenty of fluids and follow the diet recommended by the physician.
- Avoid exposure to others who have possible infections.
- Take prescribed medication as directed on the container. Do not omit a dose.
- Contact the physician immediately if pain, fever, or chills occurs or if the urine becomes bloody, cloudy, or foul smelling.

RENAL FAILURE

Renal failure is the inability of the nephrons in the kidneys to maintain fluid, electrolyte, and acid-base balances; excrete nitrogen waste products; and perform regulatory functions such as maintaining calcification of bones and producing erythropoietin. There are two types of renal failure: acute and chronic. **Acute renal failure** (ARF) is characterized by a sudden and rapid decrease in renal function. ARF potentially is reversible with early, aggressive treatment of its contributing etiology. **Chronic renal failure** (CRF) is characterized by progressive and irreversible damage to the nephrons. It may take months to years for CRF to develop.

Pathophysiology and Etiology

Acute Renal Failure

Renal failure can develop as a consequence of prerenal, intrarenal, and postrenal disorders (Table 58-3). Prerenal disorders are nonneurologic conditions that disrupt renal blood flow to the nephrons, affecting their filtering ability. This is the most common type of ARF. Intrarenal conditions are conditions in the kidney itself that destroy nephrons. Postrenal disorders usually are obstructive problems in structures below the kidney(s) that have damaging repercussions for the nephrons above.

ARF progresses through four phases:

1. Initiation phase
2. Oliguric phase
3. Diuretic phase
4. Recovery phase

Initiation Phase

The initiation phase begins with the onset of the contributing event. It is accompanied by reduced blood flow to the nephrons to the point of acute tubular necrosis. **Acute tubular necrosis** refers to the death of cells in the collecting tubules of the nephrons, where reabsorption of water, electrolytes, and excretion of protein wastes and excess metabolic substances occurs.

TABLE 58-3 Causes of Acute Renal Failure

PRERENAL	INTRARENAL	POSTRENAL
Hypovolemic shock	Ischemia	Ureteral calculi
Cardiogenic shock secondary to congestive heart failure	Nephrotoxicity secondary to drugs such as aminoglycosides	Prostatic hypertrophy
Septic shock	Acute and chronic glomerulonephritis	Ureteral stricture
Anaphylaxis	Polycystic disease	Ureteral or bladder tumor
Dehydration	Untreated prerenal and postrenal disorders	
Renal artery thrombosis or stenosis	Myoglobinuria secondary to burns	
Cardiac arrest	Hemoglobinuria secondary to transfusion reaction	
Lethal dysrhythmias		

Oliguric Phase

The oliguric phase is associated with the excretion of less-than-adequate urinary volumes. This phase begins within 48 hours after the initial cellular insult and may last for 10 to 14 days or longer (Porth, 2007). Fluid volume excess develops, which leads to edema, hypertension, and cardiopulmonary complications. Azotemia, the marked accumulation of urea and other nitrogenous wastes such as creatinine and uric acid in the blood, creates a potential for neurologic changes such as seizures, coma, and death.

Currently there is better treatment of many prerenal causes of ARF. For that reason, some clients excrete urinary volumes greater than 500 mL/day. The urine has a very low specific gravity, however, because it lacks normal amounts of excreted substances such as excess potassium and hydrogen ions, to maintain homeostasis. Consequently, hyperkalemia, metabolic acidosis, and **uremia**, a toxic state caused by the accumulation of nitrogen wastes, develop regardless of the excreted water volume.

Diuretic Phase

Diuresis begins as the nephrons recover. Despite an increased water content of urine, the excretion of wastes and electrolytes continues to be impaired. The BUN, creatinine, potassium, and phosphate levels remain elevated in the blood.

Recovery Phase

It may take 1 or more years of recovery while normal glomerular filtration and tubular function are restored. Some clients recover completely, whereas others develop varying degrees of permanent renal dysfunction.

Gerontologic Considerations

- The older adult is at high risk for acute renal failure because of a decline in the glomerular filtration rate, loss of nephrons, and reduced glomeruli. Prognosis is favorable, and treatment for older adults is the same as for younger adults.

Chronic Renal Failure

CRF is associated more often with intrarenal conditions or is a complication of systemic diseases such as diabetes mellitus and disseminated lupus erythematosus. In CRF, the kidneys are so extensively damaged that they do not adequately remove protein by-products and electrolytes from the blood and do not maintain acid-base balance. The National Kidney Foundation (2008) identifies several stages of CRF (Box 58-4), beginning with an increased risk stage, which refers to clients with risk factors for CRF. Clients progress from Stage 1 to Stage 5, or from reduced renal reserve (40% to 75% loss of nephron function), to renal insufficiency (75% to 90% loss of nephron function) to **end-stage renal disease** (less than 10% of nephron function). In end-stage renal disease, a regular course of dialysis or kidney transplantation is necessary to maintain life.

Because damage to the nephrons is slow, declining renal function is less apparent until the end stage. The BUN and serum creatinine levels gradually rise. Hyponatremia is a reflection of diluted sodium ions in an excess volume of water in the blood. Actual electrolyte imbalances include hyperkalemia, hyperphosphatemia, hypermagnesemia, and hypocalcemia. The skin becomes the excretory organ for the substances the kidney usually clears from the body. A precipitate, referred to as **uremic frost**, may form on the skin.

Metabolic acidosis develops because the tubules cannot convert carbonic acid in the blood to water and bicarbonate ions. Erythropoietin production is inadequate, causing anemia. Susceptibility to infection increases as a result of a

BOX 58-4 Stages of Chronic Renal Disease

Stage 1: Slight kidney damage with normal or increased filtration: a glomerular filtration rate (GFR) of more than 90 [*]

Stage 2: Mild decrease in kidney function with a GFR of 60–89

Stage 3: Moderate decrease in kidney function with GFR of 30–59

Stage 4: Severe decrease in kidney function with GFR of 15–29

Stage 5: Kidney failure (ESRD) requiring dialysis or transplantation with GFR less than 15

* GFR measured as mL/min/1.73m^2.
(Adapted from National Kidney Foundation [2008]. Stages of Chronic Kidney Disease. Available at http://www.kidney.org/professionals/kls/pdf/icd9codes.pdf. Accessed on September 26, 2008.)

deficient immune system, particularly cellular immunity (see Chap. 33), as well as a decrease in the white blood cell count. Edema and hypertension are consequences of impaired urinary elimination. **Osteodystrophy**, a condition in which the bones become demineralized, occurs from hypocalcemia and hyperphosphatemia. The parathyroid glands secrete more parathormone to raise blood calcium levels.

Assessment Findings

Signs and Symptoms

In both ARF and CRF, the client has elevated blood pressure and weight gain. Urine output usually is decreased. Those with CRF develop other symptoms as the disease worsens. Facial features appear puffy from fluid retention. The skin is pale. Ulceration and bleeding of the gastrointestinal tract may occur. The oral mucous membranes bleed, and blood may be found in the feces. The client reports vague symptoms such as lethargy, headache, anorexia, and dry mouth. Later, other problems develop such as pruritus and dry, scaly skin. The breath and body may have an odor characteristic of urine. Muscle cramps, bone pain or tenderness, and spontaneous fractures can develop. Mental processes progressively slow as electrolyte imbalances become marked and nitrogenous wastes accumulate. The client may experience seizures. Table 58-4 lists the systemic manifestations of CRF.

Diagnostic Findings

Laboratory blood tests reveal elevations in BUN, creatinine, potassium, magnesium, and phosphorus. Calcium levels are low. The RBC count, hematocrit, and hemoglobin are decreased. The pH of the blood is on the acidotic side. Urinalysis reveals a decreased specific gravity. An IVP provides evidence of renal dysfunction. In clients with severe renal failure, dye excretion usually is delayed. A percutaneous renal biopsy shows destruction of nephrons. Radiography and ultrasonography demonstrate structural defects in the kidneys, ureters, and bladder. Renal angiography identifies obstructions in blood vessels.

Medical Management

Prevention of ARF is an important function of physicians. Clients at risk for dehydration are adequately hydrated. Risks for dehydration include surgery, diagnostic studies that require fluid restriction and contrast agents, and treatment for cancer or metabolic disorders. Shock and hypotension are treated as quickly as possible with replacement fluids and blood. Treating infections promptly and thoroughly also is important, and greatly assists in preventing sepsis. Continuous monitoring of renal function is very important for clients at risk for ARF. Nurses are crucial in monitoring renal function, as well as preventing toxic drug effects (Smeltzer et al., 2008).

In ARF, measures are taken to quickly remedy the primary cause of renal failure. Renal damage can be limited by aggressively administering parenteral fluids to increase plasma volume, giving vasodilating and diuretic drugs, and infusing dopamine (Intropin) to improve cardiac output and perfuse the renal arteries.

To reduce complications and keep the client alive during the 2 or 3 weeks while the tubules are regenerating, hemodialysis (discussed later), a technique in which the blood is filtered externally with a machine, is performed. When hemodialysis is a temporary measure, the blood is removed and returned through a double-lumen catheter or twin central venous catheters (Fig. 58-8). Continuous renal replacement therapy (CRRT) is the filtration of blood

TABLE 58-4 Systemic Complications of Chronic Renal Failure

BODY SYSTEM	COMPLICATION
Cardiovascular	Congestive heart failure, hypertension, cardiac dysrhythmias, edema
Metabolic	Electrolyte imbalance, metabolic acidosis
Respiratory	Shortness of breath, pulmonary edema
Gastrointestinal	Malnutrition, vitamin deficiencies, anorexia, nausea, bleeding
Integumentary	Dry skin, pruritus
Neurologic	Lethargy, confusion, depression, seizures, coma
Sensory	Peripheral neuropathies
Musculoskeletal	Bone demineralization, muscle cramps, joint pain
Immunologic	Impaired immune function, decreased antibody production, increased incidence of hepatitis B and other infections

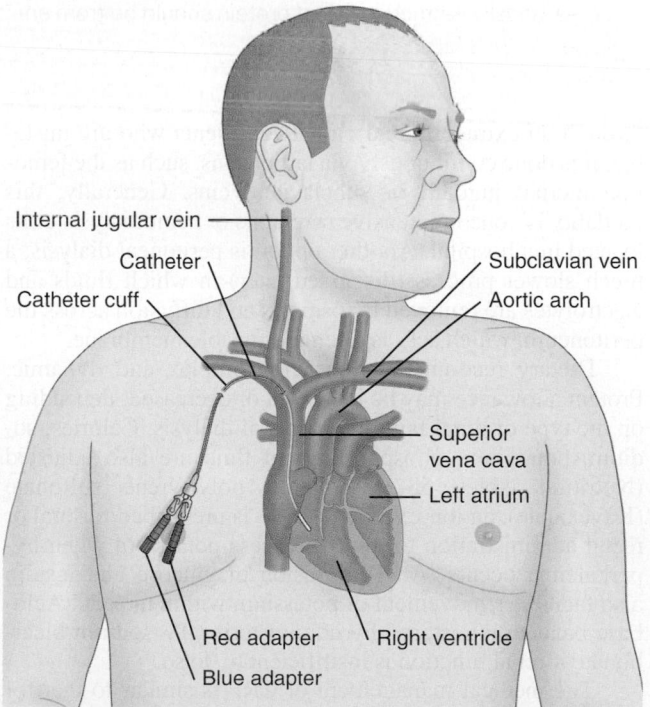

FIGURE 58-8. Double-lumen, cuffed catheter used for emergency hemodialysis. Red adapter attaches to blood line through which blood is pumped from the client to the dialyzer. After the blood passes through the dialyzer, it returns to the client through the blue adapter.

Nutrition Notes 58-2
The Client with Renal Failure

Acute Renal Failure

- The goal of nutrition therapy for acute renal failure is to prevent or minimize malnutrition. Nutrition therapy is likely to be beneficial, but has not been proven to speed recovery of renal function or improve survival.
- Protein recommendations range from 0.8 to 1.2 g/kg for clients who are not catabolic and are not receiving dialysis to 1.2 to 1.5 g/kg for clients who are catabolic and/or receiving dialysis. The normal RDA for protein is 0.8 g/kg.
- For both sodium and potassium, allowances range from 2 to 3 g/day. During the diuretic phase, potassium intake is liberalized to replenish losses.
- Calories, phosphorus, and calcium allowances are individualized.
- Fluid allowance equals the volume of urine produced plus 500 mL to compensate for insensible losses.

Chronic Renal Failure

- The objectives of nutrition therapy for chronic kidney disease are to reduce serum nitrogen levels, reduce hypertension and edema, prevent body catabolism, improve renal function, and prevent or delay the onset of complications. Dietary interventions frequently are adjusted according to the client's laboratory values and clinical symptoms.
- Protein restriction, the cornerstone of nutrition therapy, ranges from 0.6 to 0.75 g/kg. Because most Americans consume almost twice as much protein as needed, however, many clients who must follow the diet view it as unrealistically restrictive. Most protein should be from ani-

mal sources, which in general have a higher biologic value than plant proteins. Pure sugars and heart healthy fats are used liberally for calories to spare body and dietary protein.
- Multiple and complicated restrictions in protein, sodium, potassium, and fluid, compounded by anorexia and taste alterations, make dietary compliance difficult to achieve and maintain. Strong social support, frequent self-monitoring of protein intake, the use of specially formulated low-protein foods, and adequate guidelines for increasing calorie intake may improve dietary compliance.
- Renal diet food lists, called "choices" to distinguish them from diabetic "exchanges," are used to simplify meal planning. Foods are grouped into lists according to their protein, sodium, and potassium content; phosphorus and fluid also may be considered. Portion sizes are specified so that all servings in a list have approximately the same amount of protein, sodium, and potassium. An individualized meal plan specifies the number of choices allowed from each list for each meal and snack; any item may be chosen in a list, but items from one list cannot be substituted for another. The complexity and composition of choice lists vary greatly among institutions.
- Once dialysis begins, protein restrictions are liberalized to 1.2 to 1.3 g/kg to account for nutritional losses through the dialysate. Clients receiving peritoneal dialysis need to adjust their calorie intake downward to compensate for the calories absorbed from the glucose in the dialysate. Potassium, sodium, and fluid allowances are determined on an individual basis.

---

through an extracorporeal circuit for clients who are unstable. It is done continuously via large veins, such as the femoral, internal jugular, or subclavian veins. Generally, this modality is done in intensive care units or hemodialysis units located in a hospital. Another option is peritoneal dialysis, a much slower process (discussed later) in which fluids and electrolytes are removed by osmosis and diffusion across the peritoneum, which acts as a semipermeable membrane.

Dietary recommendations are complex and dynamic. Protein allowance may be increased or decreased, depending on the type of renal failure and use of dialysis. Calories, sodium, potassium, phosphorus, and fluid are also adjusted (Nutrition Notes 58-2). Sodium polystyrene sulfonate (Kayexalate), an ion-exchange resin, is prescribed for oral or rectal administration to remove excess potassium when hyperkalemia occurs. An IV infusion of glucose and insulin also facilitates movement of potassium within the cell. Acid-base balance is restored by administering IV sodium bicarbonate if renal function is insufficient to do so.

The medical management of CRF is similar to that for ARF, except the period of treatment is lifelong (unless a kidney transplantation is performed). Rather than administer blood transfusions to correct chronic anemia, erythropoetin (Epogen) is administered to stimulate bone marrow production of RBCs.

Surgical Management

Some clients in the end stage of CRF are candidates for kidney transplantation. One healthy kidney can perform the work of two. Donors for a transplant are selected from compatible living donors who may or may not be relatives or from organ donors who are brain dead and whose next of kin give permission for harvesting organs. Any potential donor with a history of hypertension, malignant disease, or diabetes is excluded from donation. To facilitate matching a recipient with a donor, a client is placed on a national computerized transplant waiting list. Whenever an organ becomes available, the computer searches for the recipient who is the best match.

When a transplantation is performed, the donor kidney is inserted through an abdominal incision and the nonfunctioning kidneys are left in place unless the client is extremely hypertensive. The blood vessels from the donor kidney are sutured to the iliac artery and vein and the ureter is implanted in the bladder (Fig. 58-9).

Even a perfect match does not guarantee that a transplanted organ will not be rejected. Ironically, even some less-than-perfectly matched transplanted organs are successful primarily because of immunosuppressive drugs such as:

- Azathioprine (Imuran)
- Corticosteroids (prednisone)

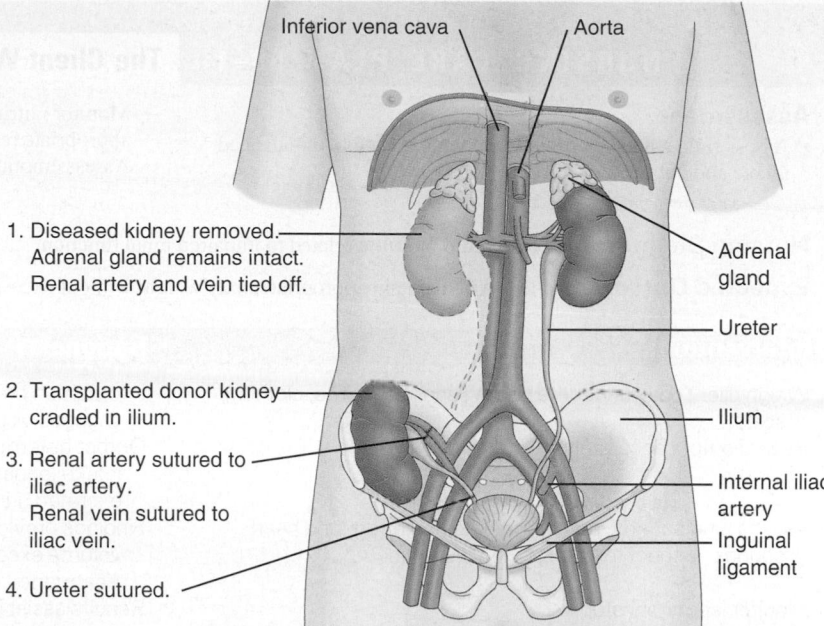

1. Diseased kidney removed.
   Adrenal gland remains intact.
   Renal artery and vein tied off.

2. Transplanted donor kidney
   cradled in ilium.

3. Renal artery sutured to
   iliac artery.
   Renal vein sutured to
   iliac vein.

4. Ureter sutured.

Inferior vena cava

Aorta

Adrenal gland

Ureter

Ilium

Internal iliac artery

Inguinal ligament

FIGURE 58-9. Transplanted kidney and ureter.

- Cyclosporine—available as a microemulsion (Neoral), which provides a more sustained concentration
- Tacrolimus (Prograf)—similar to cyclosporine but more potent
- Other combinations, including:
  - Mycophenolate mofetil (CellCept)—specifically for preventing kidney transplant rejection
  - Sirolimus (Rapamune)
  - Antithymocyte mofetil (Thymoglobulin) (Smeltzer et al., 2008)
- Muromonab-CD3 (Orthoclone OKT3)—a monoclonal antibody

If rejection occurs, the client resumes hemodialysis and waits for another transplant.

Nursing Management

Before conducting an initial interview and physical assessment, the nurse attempts to learn the cause (if known), type (acute versus chronic), and prognosis of the renal disorder. Clients may be unable to give an accurate history because of the effect of renal failure on the thought processes or because they are acutely ill. It may be necessary to obtain information from the family. The nursing care for the client undergoing renal transplantation is complex and specialized. Standard postoperative nursing interventions are applicable (see Chap. 14), with the added consideration of assessing for signs of rejection and prevention of infection. Box 58-5 describes signs and symptoms of transplant rejection.

Nursing care for clients with renal failure is extensive. See Nursing Care Plan 58-1 and Client and Family Teaching 58-5 for more information.

▶ **Stop, Think, and Respond Exercise 58-3**

Clients who have a kidney transplant are at risk for infection. What nursing measures help to prevent infection?

DIALYSIS

Dialysis is a procedure for cleaning and filtering the blood. It substitutes for kidney function when the kidneys cannot remove the nitrogenous waste products and maintain adequate fluid, electrolyte, and acid-base balances.

During dialysis, the client's blood is filtered by diffusion and osmosis (see Chap. 16). Substances such as water, urea, creatinine, and dangerously high levels of potassium move from the blood through the semipermeable membrane to the **dialysate**, the solution used during dialysis that has a composition similar to normal human plasma. Dialysis is performed by hemodialysis and peritoneal dialysis. Either technique can be performed at home or in a dialysis center. Each type has advantages and disadvantages (Table 58-5).

HEMODIALYSIS

Hemodialysis requires transporting blood from the client through a **dialyzer**, a semipermeable membrane filter in a machine (Fig. 58-10). The dialyzer contains many tiny

---

BOX 58-5 **Signs and Symptoms of Kidney Transplant Rejection**

Hypertension
Edema
Oliguria
Fever
Abdominal pain
Swelling or tenderness over the transplanted kidney
Shortness of breath
Weight gain
Increase in serum creatinine levels

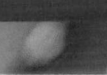

NURSING CARE PLAN 58–1 The Client With Chronic Renal Failure

Assessment

- Assess fluid status, including problems related to unbalanced intake and output.
- Monitor nutritional status, making sure the client follows the appropriate restrictions.
- Assess emotional status to provide relevant support.

Nursing Diagnosis: Excess Fluid Volume related to impaired renal function.

Expected Outcome: Client will maintain appropriate body weight without excess fluid.

Interventions	Rationales
Weigh client daily under the same conditions: time, clothing, scale.	Information provides a baseline and database for monitoring changes. A gain of 1 kg (2.2 lb) equals 1 L of fluid.
Record output accurately.	Output determines intake. Usually, client is allowed 500 mL intake (equals insensible fluid losses) plus the volume of excreted urine per day.
Assess lung sounds, respiratory rate and effort, and heart sounds. Inspect for jugular vein distention.	Findings provide a baseline and database to determine fluid volume excess, needed interventions, and effects of treatments. Fluid overload may cause pulmonary edema.
Monitor laboratory studies.	Results assist in identifying fluid excess and promote earlier interventions.
Administer prescribed diuretics and antihypertensives.	These drugs reduce fluid excess and decrease cardiac workload.
Prepare client for dialysis.	Dialysis reduces uremic toxins, corrects electrolyte imbalances, and decreases fluid overload.

Evaluation of Expected Outcome

Client demonstrates appropriate urine output/fluid balance as evidenced by stable weight, vital signs within normal range for the client, no edema, and only slightly elevated electrolyte levels.

Nursing Diagnosis: Imbalanced Nutrition: Risk for Less than Body Requirements related to anorexia, increased metabolic needs, and dietary restrictions

Expected Outcome: Client will maintain adequate nutritional intake.

Interventions	Rationales
Monitor and record client's dietary intake.	Findings provide a database for nutritional changes and effects of interventions.
Provide frequent small feedings.	They minimize nausea and anorexia and promote the intake of high-calorie, nutritious foods.
Encourage client to be involved with food choices and times for meals.	Involving the client promotes interest and control and considers dietary habits and preferences.
Explain restrictions and provide a list of nutritional needs and acceptable food choices.	Doing so promotes client's understanding of the relationship between food intake and kidney disease and provides a positive approach to dietary restrictions.

Evaluation of Expected Outcome

Client maintains weight, unrelated to fluid volume, following dietary needs and restrictions.

Nursing Diagnosis: Risk for Impaired Tissue Integrity related to restricted oral intake and increased nitrogenous wastes in body fluids such as saliva

Expected Outcome: The oral mucosa and lips will remain moist and intact.

Interventions	Rationales
Assess mouth for inflammation, ulceration, or bleeding.	Findings provide a database for intervention and evaluation of treatment effectiveness.
Instruct or assist client to provide mouth care after each meal and at bedtime or every 4 hours while awake. Encourage client to swish but not swallow water frequently as desired.	Frequent mouth care removes debris, rinses away nitrogenous wastes in saliva, prevents accumulation of bacteria, and keeps mucous membranes moist.
Provide lanolin-based lip balm for use as needed.	It keeps lips moist and promotes integrity, preventing bleeding and introduction of microorganisms.

(Continued)

NURSING CARE PLAN 58-1   The Client With Chronic Renal Failure (Continued)

Evaluation of Expected Outcome

Client performs frequent mouth care. Mucous membranes and lips remain moist and intact.

Nursing Diagnosis: Activity Intolerance related to fatigue, anemia, weakness, retention of nitrogenous waste products, and dialysis procedure

Expected Outcome: Client will participate in activities as tolerated.

Interventions	Rationales
Determine cause of activity intolerance.	Knowing the cause assists in planning appropriate interventions.
If able, encourage client to increase activity slowly. Perform range-of-motion exercises as tolerated.	Activity and exercises help maintain or improve muscle tone, strength, and endurance.
Provide periods of rest between activities.	Rest decreases oxygen consumption and improves energy levels.

Evaluation of Expected Outcome

Client participates in activities and can do ADLs with minimal assistance.

PCs: Hypertension, Azotemia, Electrolyte Imbalances, Anemia

Expected Outcome: Nurse will minimize and manage potential complications.

Interventions	Rationales
Administer prescribed antihypertensive and diuretic medications as ordered.	They lower blood pressure and increase urine output from partially functional kidneys.
Restrict protein intake to foods that are complete proteins (contain all essential amino acids) within prescribed limits.	Complete proteins provide positive nitrogen balance needed for healing and growth.
Provide sufficient calories from carbohydrates and fats.	Doing so prevents catabolism of muscle and body stores of protein.
Monitor cardiac rhythm.	Hyperkalemia and other electrolyte imbalances can cause dangerous dysrhythmias.
Restrict sources of potassium usually found in fresh fruits and vegetables.	Hyperkalemia can cause life-threatening changes.
Be prepared to administer glucose and regular insulin.	They promote transfer of potassium from extracellular to intracellular locations.
Restrict sodium intake as ordered.	Doing so prevents excess sodium and fluid accumulation.
Administer calcium supplements, vitamin D supplements, and phosphate binders (Amphogel); at same time, limit phosphorus-containing foods such as dairy products, dried beans, and soft drinks.	CRF causes numerous physiologic changes that affect calcium, phosphorus, and vitamin D metabolism, requiring supplementation and dietary restrictions.
Administer prescribed iron and folic acid supplements or Epogen.	Iron and folic acid supplements are needed for RBC production. Epogen stimulates bone marrow to produce RBCs.

Evaluation of Expected Outcome

Blood pressure is 140/90 mm Hg. BUN and creatinine levels are slightly elevated. Serum electrolyte levels are minimally elevated. RBC and hemoglobin levels are within normal levels.

Nursing Diagnosis: Risk for Impaired Skin Integrity related to scratching secondary to pruritus

Expected Outcome: Skin will remain intact and free of crystals.

Interventions	Rationales
Instruct client to limit bathing to less than 1/2 hour, using lukewarm water and glycerin-based soap. Add emollient to skin two to three times a day.	These measures reduce skin drying while rinsing away nitrogenous waste products. Emollients restore moisture. All measures help to maintain skin integrity.
Keep the environment humidified.	Humidification provides moisture to the skin and prevents drying.
Institute measures that prevent client from scratching, such as keeping fingernails short and encouraging client to use soft clothing and bedding.	These measures prevent trauma to the skin and maintain skin integrity.

NURSING CARE PLAN 58-1   The Client With Chronic Renal Failure (Continued)

Evaluation of Expected Outcome

Client maintains intact skin without evidence of crystals.

Nursing Diagnosis: Risk for Infection related to compromised immune defenses

Expected Outcome: Client will remain free of infection.

Interventions	Rationales
Monitor temperature at least every shift. Monitor for signs and symptoms of infection.	Clients with kidney failure are very prone to infection. Chills, malaise, sore throat, redness, drainage, and elevated temperature are all signs of infection.
Restrict contact with family, friends, or staff who may have an infectious disorder.	Doing so prevents spread of microorganisms to immunocompromised client.
Ensure that all who come in contact with client practice appropriate aseptic technique.	Handwashing, clean environment, and asepsis prevent the spread of microorganisms.

Evaluation of Expected Outcome

Client is afebrile and demonstrates no signs or symptoms of infection.

Nursing Diagnosis: Situational Low Self-Esteem related to change in body image, dependency, and role change.

Expected Outcome: Client will seek help as needed and demonstrate improved self-concept.

Interventions	Rationales
Demonstrate acceptance and respect for client.	They promote client's self-acceptance.
Assess client's relationships with significant others.	Doing so identifies client's strengths and support systems.
Encourage client and significant others to discuss changes produced by the disease and its treatments.	Identifying concerns and questions helps arrive at solutions.
Provide information about support groups.	They give an opportunity for clients and families to receive support and understanding. They also assist with coping.

Evaluation of Expected Outcome

Client demonstrates improved self-concept as evidenced by positive coping skills, ability to express concerns, and ability to seek support.

hollow fibers. Blood moves through the hollow fibers. Water and wastes from the blood move into the dialysate fluid that flows around the fibers, but protein and RBCs do not. The filtered blood is returned to the client. The entire cycle takes 4 to 6 hours and is performed three times a week.

Client and Family Teaching 58-5
The Client With Chronic Renal Failure

Develop a teaching plan based on the following:

- Follow the diet and fluid intake recommended by the physician. Do not use salt substitutes (which often contain potassium) unless allowed by the physician.
- Take medications exactly as prescribed by the physician.
- Do not use any nonprescription drug unless use is approved by the physician.
- Measure and record fluid intake and urine output. Limit fluids as recommended.
- Avoid exposure to those with any type of infection (e.g., colds, sore throats, flu).
- Monitor blood pressure as recommended by the physician.
- Keep skin clean and dry. Take brief showers with tepid water, pat skin to dry, use moisturizing lotions or creams like Eucerin, Nivea, Alpha Keri, or Lubriderm. Avoid scratching.
- When doing laundry, use a mild laundry detergent. Use an extra rinse cycle to remove all detergent or add 1 tsp of vinegar per quart of water to the rinse cycle to remove detergent residue.
- Keep a record of daily weight, and report any rapid weight gain to the physician.
- Take frequent rest periods; avoid heavy exercise.
- If any of the following occurs, contact the physician immediately: inability to urinate, slow decrease in daily urine output, weight gain (more than 5 lb or amount recommended by physician), chills, fever, sore throat, cough, blood in the urine or stool, easy bleeding or bruising, lethargy, extreme fatigue, persistent headache, nausea, vomiting, or diarrhea.

TABLE 58-5 Comparison of Hemodialysis and Peritoneal Dialysis

TYPE OF DIALYSIS	ADVANTAGES	DISADVANTAGES
Hemodialysis	Rapid removal of solutes and water Takes less time No risk for peritonitis Personnel perform procedure in a dialysis center	Bulge from fistula or graft is obvious Risk for vascular complications, infection, distal ischemia, carpal tunnel syndrome, hypotension, and disequilibrium Strict fluid and dietary restrictions Life-style revolves around dialysis appointments Home hemodialysis requires space for the machine and training to use it
Peritoneal	Simple to perform Facilitates independence Easier access No anticoagulation Fewer problems with hypotension or disequilibrium Less rigid dietary and fluid restrictions More flexibility in life-style and activities	More time-consuming Weight gain from glucose in the dialysate Peritonitis is a potential complication Requires training and motivation

Vascular Access

There are several methods for facilitating the removal and return of the client's dialyzed blood. One technique using tunneled central venous catheter access has already been described. Two others more commonly used for clients with CRF are (1) arteriovenous (AV) fistula and (2) AV graft.

Arteriovenous Fistula

An **arteriovenous fistula** is a surgical anastomosis (connection) of an artery and vein lying in close proximity (Fig. 58-11). The vessels usually joined are the cephalic vein and the radial artery or the cephalic vein and brachial artery. Fistulas are preferred over grafts because they have a better record of remaining patent and have fewer complications, such as thrombosis and infection, compared with other access options. They require from 1 to 4 months to mature, however, before being used. Consequently, some fistulas are created prematurely so they are ready when a client eventually requires dialysis.

At the time of dialysis, two venipunctures are performed at either end of the fistula. The distal venipuncture is used to remove blood that is transported to the machine. The proximal needle puncture is used to return the dialyzed blood. When dialysis is completed, the needles are removed and pressure dressings are applied for several hours.

Blood samples are taken before and after dialysis. The client's predialysis and postdialysis weights are compared. Sometimes as much as 10 lbs of fluid is removed. Examples of postdialysis laboratory studies include BUN, creatinine, sodium, potassium, chlorides, and hematocrit. These are used as indicators of the efficiency of dialysis.

Arteriovenous Graft

An **arteriovenous graft** is a type of vascular access method that uses a tube of synthetic material (e.g., Gore-Tex or polytetrafluoroethylene) to connect a vein and artery in the upper or lower arm (see Fig. 58-11). The graft pulsates with blood flow. AV grafts can be used 14 days after their insertion. Although the graft reseals after each needle puncture, the expected life of the graft is 3 to 5 years with repeated use.

Other Forms of Hemodialysis

There are several types of hemodialysis generally used for ARF or short-term use. These include:

- *Continuous renal replacement therapy (CRRT)* – This is generally used in critical care units for clients who have ARF or are too unstable to manage aggressive hemodialysis. Portable equipment pumps blood from the client through a hemofilter and back of the client in a slow continuous mode.
- *Continuous venovenous hemofiltration (CVVH)* – Used for ARF, blood from a double-lumen venous catheter is pumped through a hemofilter; does not require arterial access.
- *Continuous venovenous hemodialysis (CVVHD)* – With this technique, blood is pumped from a double-lumen venous catheter through a hemofilter and a concentration gradient that removes even more uremic toxins and fluids; also does not require arterial access (Smeltzer et al., 2008).

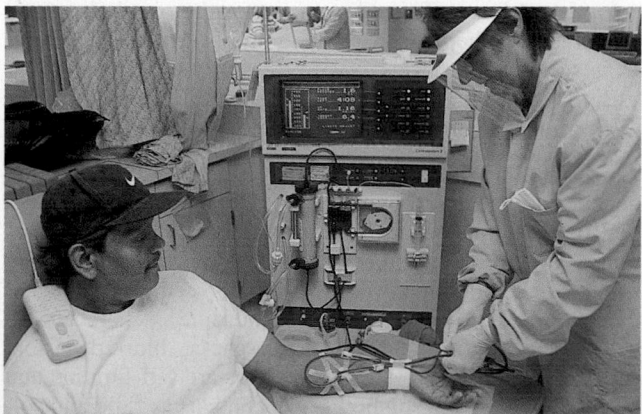

FIGURE 58-10. During hemodialysis the client's blood flows to the hemodialysis machine, through a dialyzer (where filtering takes place), and back to the client's body.

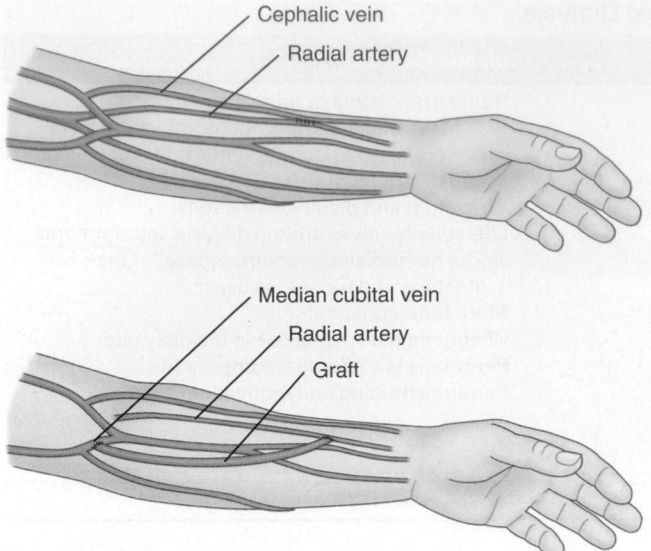

FIGURE 58-11. An internal arteriovenous fistula (*top*) is created by a side-to-side anastomosis of the artery and vein. A graft (*bottom*) can also be established between the artery and vein.

Nursing Management

The nurse assesses and records vital signs before and after hemodialysis as well as weighing the client and obtaining blood for laboratory testing. To prepare for vascular access the nurse:

- Inspects the skin over the fistula or graft for signs of infection.
- Palpates for a **thrill** (vibration) over the vascular access or listens for a **bruit**, a loud sound caused by turbulent blood flow. If absent, the nurse postpones further use and reports findings.
- Notes the color of skin and nailbeds and mobility of fingers.
- Washes the skin over the fistula or graft with soap and water or antiseptic.
- Avoids puncturing the same site that was used previously.
- After dialysis is completed, does not administer injections for 2 to 4 hours. This allows time for the metabolism and excretion of heparin, which is administered during dialysis, to reach safe levels.
- Before discharging the client, observes for disequilibrium syndrome, a potential complication.

Disequilibrium syndrome is a neurologic condition believed to be caused by cerebral edema. The shift in cerebral fluid volume occurs when the concentrations of solutes in the blood are lowered rapidly during dialysis. Decreasing solute concentration lowers the plasma osmolality. Water then floods the brain tissue. The syndrome is characterized by headache, disorientation, restlessness, blurred vision, confusion, and seizures. The symptoms are self-limiting and disappear within several hours after dialysis as fluid and solute concentrations equalize. The syndrome can be prevented by slowing the dialysis process to allow time for gradual equilibration of water.

The nurse teaches the client undergoing hemodialysis the following:

- Avoid carrying heavy items in the arm with the fistula or graft.
- Wear clothing with loose sleeves or made of fabrics that will not obstruct blood flow.
- Do not sleep on the vascular access arm.
- Do not permit venipunctures, injections, or blood pressures in the arm with the vascular access.
- Wash the skin over the vascular access daily.
- Assess for a thrill or bruit daily.
- Report signs of an infection or signs of impaired blood flow to dialysis personnel or physician immediately.

PERITONEAL DIALYSIS

Peritoneal dialysis uses the peritoneum, the semipermeable membrane lining the abdomen, to filter fluid, wastes, and chemicals (Fig. 58-12). The dialysate is similar in composition to normal plasma but made hypertonic by dextrose. Higher concentrations of dextrose increase the osmotic effect, thus increasing the amount of water removed from the client's bloodstream. The dialysate is instilled and drained from the abdominal cavity by means of a catheter. Substances or solutes pass from the tiny blood vessels in the peritoneal membrane into the dialysate by means of diffusion, because the dialysate becomes an area of low concentration drawing from an area of high concentration. The catheter, which has many perforations, is sutured in place and a dressing is applied.

There are three types of peritoneal dialysis: (1) continuous ambulatory peritoneal dialysis (CAPD), (2) continuous cyclic peritoneal dialysis (CCPD), and (3) intermittent peritoneal dialysis (IPD), often referred to as nocturnal intermittent peritoneal dialysis (NIPD).

Continuous Ambulatory Peritoneal Dialysis

When CAPD is performed, approximately 2000 mL of dialysate is instilled by gravity through the catheter in 30 to 40 minutes. The catheter is clamped and the solution may dwell for 4 to 10 hours. The instillation bag is lowered below the

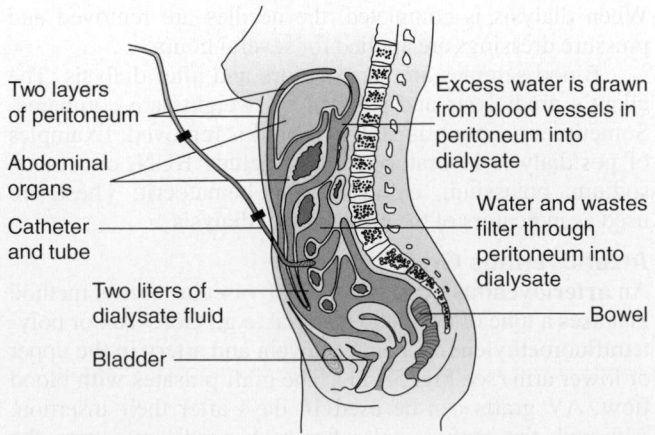

FIGURE 58-12. Peritoneal dialysis.

level of the catheter and unclamped for 30 to 40 minutes to allow time for gravity drainage. The process is repeated three to four times a day on a continuous basis.

Gerontologic Considerations

- CAPD may be an appropriate treatment option for older clients who do not meet the qualifications for kidney transplant. Planning with the older adult and family or caregivers should include monitoring.

Continuous Cyclic Peritoneal Dialysis

In CCPD, a machine is connected to the dialysis catheter. It automatically fills and drains dialysate from the abdomen when the person sleeps. CCPD is performed during a 10- to 12-hour period. The peritoneum is filled with solution during the daytime, but it allows the client to go about activities during the day without performing exchanges of dialysate solutions.

Intermittent Peritoneal Dialysis

Treatments for IPD are performed with the same type of machine as that used for CCPD; however, the process occurs periodically, with perhaps several days between dialysis treatments. When IPD is done, sessions may last 24 hours. The total time spent on IPD is between 36 and 42 hours per week.

Nursing Management

The nurse obtains and reviews laboratory test findings before dialysis and records vital signs and weight. If the client is acutely ill, it may be necessary to use a bed scale. It also may be necessary to weigh the client as often as every 8 hours while the procedure is in progress. Peritonitis is a major complication of peritoneal dialysis. The nurse monitors and reports fever, nausea, vomiting, and severe abdominal pain, rigidity, or tenderness before, during, or after dialysis.

▶ *Stop, Think, and Respond Exercise 58-4*

Consider why a client may not be a good candidate for CAPD.

Instillation

Dialysate solution is warmed approximately to body temperature. The nurse adds prescribed drugs such as an antibiotic to the dialysate. He or she attaches the bag of dialysate and administration tubing to the abdominal catheter. The nurse instills the solution and clamps the tubing. If the infusion is slow, the nurse asks the client to move from side to side. If this maneuver is unsuccessful, the physician may need to reposition the catheter. Pain in the left shoulder, if it occurs, may be the result of diaphragmatic irritation caused by the high concentration of glucose.

The nurse records the instillation time, the volume and type of dialysate, plus any medications added. He or she monitors blood pressure and pulse frequently. A drop in blood pressure and increased pulse rate are associated with rapid shifts in fluid that may happen because the dialysate has a high concentration of glucose. As long as the client is stable, he or she can change positions, eat, and drink.

Drainage

At the end of the dwell time, the nurse lowers the empty bag used to instill the solution and opens the clamp. He or she observes the appearance of the siphoned fluid—it should be relatively clear. The nurse must report drainage that is cloudy or tinged with blood. The next instillation may relieve abdominal pain at the end of the drainage period. The nurse notifies the physician if marked abdominal distention accompanies pain. In such a case, the nurse must delay the next dialysis cycle until a physician examines the client.

The nurse measures the difference between the volume instilled and the volume removed. If there is a drainage deficit, he or she notifies the physician before instilling more fluid. The nurse weighs the client after the last cycle of drainage.

Nursing Guidelines 58-2 provides information related to performing peritoneal dialysis. Client and Family Teaching 58-6 lists important instructions for the client performing a peritoneal dialysis at home.

NURSING GUIDELINES 58-2

Performing Peritoneal Dialysis

- Use strict aseptic technique, including wearing a mask. The client will need to wear a mask whenever there is a procedure involving the peritoneal dialysis catheter.
- Check dialysate for correct concentration and amount.
- Warm prescribed dialysate to body temperature, using a commercial warmer.
- Follow prescribed times for infusing the dialysate—the infusion clamp is opened during infusion and clamped after infusion.
- Let dialysate dwell for prescribed time.
- When dwell time is done, open drain clamp and let fluid drain by gravity into drainage bag.
- Document the characteristics and amount of outflow of effluent.
- Monitor client's vital signs, especially when draining effluent.
- Document total fluid intake and output; record positive and negative balances after each exchange.
- Monitor serum electrolyte, glucose, and lipid levels as ordered.
- Do not:
  - use expired or cloudy dialysate.
  - warm dialysate in microwave.
  - proceed with infusion if client has signs/symptoms of peritonitis or infection at insertion site.
  - break sterile technique.

Client and Family Teaching 58-6
Performing a Peritoneal Dialysis at Home

The nurse instructs the client as follows:

- Keep dialysis supplies in a clean area away from children and pets.
- Avoid using any dialysate solutions that are expired and look cloudy, discolored, or contain sediment.
- Wash hands before handling the catheter.
- Prevent infection by using sterile gloves during cleaning and exchanges of dialysate.
- Wear a mask when performing exchanges if you have an upper respiratory infection.
- Clean the catheter insertion site daily with an antiseptic such as povidone-iodine (Betadine).
- Inspect the catheter insertion site for signs of infection.
- Keep the catheter stabilized to the abdomen above the belt line to avoid constant rubbing.
- Avoid using scissors during dressing changes to prevent puncturing or cutting the catheter.
- Call the physician if:
  - a fever develops.
  - there is redness, pain, or pus draining around the catheter.
  - the external length of the catheter increases.
  - nausea, vomiting, or abdominal pain develop.

CRITICAL THINKING EXERCISES

1. A client with a ureteral stone is experiencing severe pain. Another nurse believes the client has a low pain tolerance. What action is appropriate at this time? Why?

2. A client who had a left nephrectomy is having discomfort when coughing, deep breathing, and changing positions. What nursing measures could relieve her discomfort?

3. If you had CRF and must decide to have either hemodialysis or peritoneal dialysis when end-stage renal disease develops, explain which choice you would make and the reasons for that choice.

4. A client is diagnosed with ARF. If you were caring for this client, describe the signs and symptoms that you would expect to see when the client is in the recovery phase.

NCLEX-STYLE REVIEW QUESTIONS

1. A client has undergone a nephrectomy and insertion of a urethral catheter. As part of the nursing care plan, the nurse records the color of drainage from each tube and catheter. Which of the following is the best rationale for this nursing intervention?
   1. Restore and maintain intravascular volume.
   2. Provide a means for further comparison and evaluation.
   3. Avoid interference with wound drainage.
   4. Prevent pain related to obstruction.

2. A client who has chronic glomerulonephritis has deteriorated to the early stages of renal failure. In assessing the client for the progression of renal failure, the nurse is most correct to assess for which of the following?
   1. Anemia
   2. Anorexia
   3. Diabetes
   4. Hyperthyroidism

3. A client who has chronic glomerulonephritis has deteriorated to the early stages of renal failure. If this client is similar to others in the oliguric phase of renal failure, the nurse is most likely to find the urine output is within what range?
   1. Between 50 and 100 mL per hour
   2. Between 100 and 150 mL per hour
   3. Between 500 and 1000 mL per day
   4. Between 100 and 500 mL per day

4. Because of impaired urine elimination, the nurse is concerned about which potential skin problems that will require additional team planning for the client in renal failure?
   1. Extreme oiliness
   2. Loss of skin turgor
   3. Pronounced itching
   4. Reduced perspiration

5. The client with urolithiasis is scheduled for extracorporeal shock wave lithotripsy (ESWL) to pulverize the stone. Which statement is the best evidence that the client who will undergo ESWL understands the scheduled procedure?
   1. "A laser beam will be aimed at my kidneys."
   2. "I will be submerged in a tank of water."
   3. "I will experience a tingling sensation."
   4. "Radiation will be focused on my bladder."

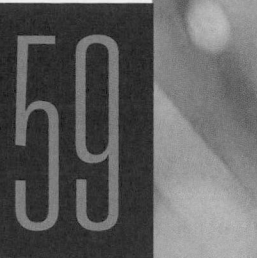

59

Caring for Clients with Disorders of the Bladder and Urethra

Learning Objectives

On completion of this chapter, you will be able to:

1. Explain urinary retention and appropriate nursing management.
2. Discuss urinary incontinence and appropriate nursing management.
3. Describe the pathophysiologic changes seen in cystitis, interstitial cystitis, and urethritis.
4. Explain the symptoms associated with bladder stones.
5. Discuss the cause and treatment of urethral strictures.
6. Identify the most common early symptom of a malignant tumor of the bladder, and outline treatment and nursing care.
7. Describe various types of urinary diversion procedures.
8. Identify components of a teaching plan for a client having a urinary diversion procedure.

Disorders of the bladder and urethra are common and can be the source of severe problems that become chronic, altering a client's lifestyle. Many disorders affecting the bladder and urethra are treated on an outpatient basis; the more serious disorders require hospitalization.

VOIDING DYSFUNCTION

Urinary retention and urinary incontinence are voiding dysfunctions. Urinary **retention** is the inability to urinate or effectively empty the bladder. Urinary **incontinence** is the inability to control the voiding of urine. Clients experiencing either retention or incontinence face temporary or permanent alterations in their ability to urinate normally. These conditions require individualized approaches to solving the problem and sensitivity to the client's needs, both physiologic and psychosocial.

URINARY RETENTION

Pathophysiology and Etiology

Urinary retention may be either acute or chronic. Acute urinary retention is seen in complete urethral obstruction, after general anesthesia, or with the administration of certain drugs such as atropine or a phenothiazine. Chronic urinary retention often is seen in clients with disorders such as prostatic enlargement or neurologic disorders that result in a **neurogenic bladder** (a bladder that does not receive adequate nerve stimulation).

The client with acute urinary retention usually cannot void at all. The client with chronic urinary retention may be able to void but does not completely empty the bladder (retention with overflow) and has a large residual volume. The **residual urine** is urine retained in the bladder after the client voids. The amount may vary from 30 mL to several hundred milliliters.

Assessment Findings

Symptoms of acute urinary retention are sudden inability to void, distended bladder, and severe lower abdominal pain and discomfort. Chronic urinary retention may not produce symptoms because the bladder has stretched over time and accommodates large volumes without producing discomfort. The overstretched bladder does not contract effectively, and the client is unaware that the bladder is not emptying completely. If the amount of residual urine is large, the client may void frequently in small amounts. Signs of a bladder infection (e.g., fever, chills, pain on urination) and dribbling of urine also may be present.

Urinalysis may show an increased number of white blood cells, indicating an acute or chronic bladder infection. Catheterization or ultrasound can determine postvoid residual volume. Urodynamic testing uses video radiography; radiopaque contrast dye is instilled in the bladder via a small catheter, and bladder pressures are measured during filling and voiding. Electromyography (EMG) determines the activity of the external sphincter during voiding. X-rays show the bladder's anatomy, and if there are any problems.

Medical and Surgical Management

Acute urinary retention requires immediate catheterization. If a catheter cannot be inserted through the urethra, special urologic instruments that dilate the urethra may be used.

Chronic retention is managed by permanent drainage with a urethral catheter, suprapubic **cystostomy** tube (a catheter inserted through the abdominal wall directly into the bladder), or clean intermittent catheterization (CIC). Permanent catheterization of the bladder carries the risk of bladder stones, renal disease, bladder infection, and **urosepsis,** a serious systemic infection from microorganisms in the urinary tract invading the bloodstream. Because the incidence of complications is lower, CIC is the preferred treatment. Other methods, particularly for clients who have lost nervous system control secondary to disease or injury, are to use Credé's Maneuver or manual voiding, or abdominal strain (Valsalva Maneuver voiding; Box 59-1) Clients may combine these methods with timed voiding, which means that clients void according to a schedule, not waiting to feel the urge.

<table>
<tr><td colspan="2">**B O X 5 9 - 1** **Credé or Valsalva Voiding**</td></tr>
<tr><td colspan="2">

Credé's Maneuver (Manual)

Apply gentle downward pressure to the bladder during voiding. This maneuver may be done by the client or family member. The client also may do this by sitting on the toilet and rocking back and forth gently.

Valsalva Maneuver

Instruct the client to bear down as with defecation. Do not teach this method to a client with cardiac problems or who may be adversely affected by a vagal response (heart rate slows).
</td></tr>
</table>

CIC may not be possible for clients who lack the mobility or cognitive functioning to perform the procedure. Some male clients who cannot perform CIC can avoid the complications of permanent indwelling catheters by undergoing surgery to release the urethral sphincters. Urine then drains freely out the urethra and the client wears a condom catheter. Nursing Guidelines 59-1 provides instructions about the application of a condom catheter. If it is possible to remove the cause, such as excising excess prostatic tissue, surgery is performed. However, surgery does not always result in restoration of normal voiding.

External collection systems for women are available but proper fit is a problem. Women who cannot accomplish CIC usually are treated with a permanent indwelling catheter.

Nursing Management

The conscious client is able to verbalize the pain and discomfort associated with urinary retention. Clients with Alzheimer's disease or psychiatric disorders, or the comatose, anesthetized, or spinal cord–injured client may be unable to communicate or feel the pain and discomfort associated with acute urinary retention. An important nursing responsibility is measuring intake and output, palpating the abdomen for a distended bladder, promoting complete urination, and monitoring the voiding pattern of clients.

NURSING GUIDELINES 59-1

Applying a Condom Catheter

- Assess the penis for swelling or skin breakdown.
- Verify client's willingness to use a condom catheter.
- Wash and dry the penis well.
- Wrap the adhesive strip in an upward spiral about the penis, taking care not to wrap it tightly.
- Roll the wider end of the sheath toward the narrow catheter tip (most condom catheters are packaged this way—rolling the condom is not necessary).
- Hold approximately 1–2 inches (2.5–5 cm) of the lower sheath below the tip of the penis and unroll the sheath upward.
- Secure the upper end of the unrolled sheath to the skin with a second strip of adhesive or a Velcro strap, but not so tightly as to interfere with circulation.

- Connect the catheter drainage tip to a drainage bag.
- Keep the penis positioned in a downward position.
- Assess the penis at least every 2 hours; also check the catheter to make sure it has not become twisted.
- Empty leg bag (if one is used) when it becomes partially filled, so that the weight of the collected urine does not dislodge the condom.
- Remove or change the condom catheter daily, or more often as needed, to check skin integrity.
- Substitute a waterproof garment during periods of nonuse of a condom catheter.
- Wash the catheter and collection bag with mild soap and water and rinse with a 1:7 vinegar-and-water solution.

▶ *Stop, Think, and Respond Exercise 59-1*

If the priority nursing diagnosis for a client with urinary retention is Urinary Retention related to high urethral pressure secondary to prostate enlargement, which of the following is a priority nursing intervention?

1. *Obtain a history from the client about the duration of this problem.*
2. *Ask the client if he has any problems with bowel elimination.*
3. *Initiate a bladder log, which includes information about urine output and fluid intake.*
4. *Catheterize the client to relieve a full bladder and to measure urine output.*

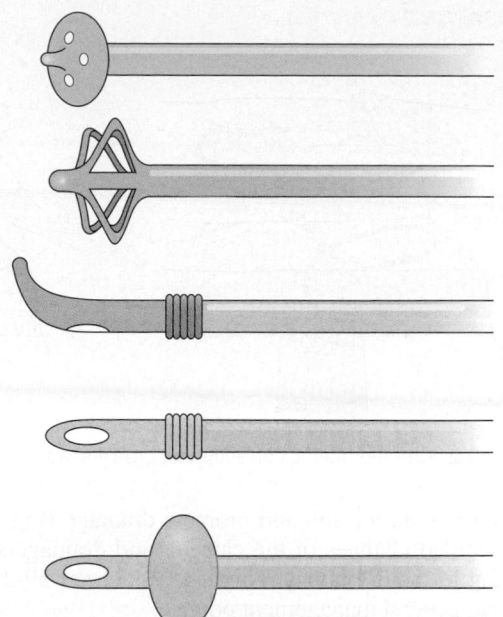

FIGURE 59-1. Catheter tips (*top to bottom*): de Pezzer catheter, Malecot catheter, coudé catheter, Foley catheter, Foley catheter with balloon inflated. The de Pezzer and the Malecot catheters are inserted by the physician with a stylet that temporarily straightens the tip. The Foley and coudé catheters are retained by inflating the balloon.

Acute Urinary Retention

Acute retention that is likely to resolve quickly (e.g., after anesthesia) probably will be treated by intermittent catheterization. Clients with acute retention unlikely to resolve without surgical intervention (e.g., retention caused by an enlarged prostate) probably will have an indwelling catheter.

The nurse collaborates with the physician to determine (1) if the catheter is to be left in place or removed after the bladder is emptied, and (2) the size and type of catheter to be used. Catheters are sized according to the French system (e.g., 14 F to 24 F); the higher the number, the larger the diameter of the catheter. Examples of the various types of catheter tips are shown in Figure 59-1.

Clients with an obstruction may be more easily catheterized with a coudé catheter. The curved tip slides over obstructing tissue more readily than the straight-tipped catheter. The nurse selects the appropriate catheter and inserts it under sterile conditions, noting the characteristics and volume of urine returned. If the volume of urine is large (>700 mL), it may be necessary to clamp the catheter before the bladder has emptied completely to prevent bladder spasms or loss of bladder tone. This practice varies, so it is important to check agency policy.

If the client is going to be managed by CIC, the client and the nurse establish the schedule. Clients are catheterized every 4 to 6 hours, depending on the amount of urine obtained and the fluid intake. The bladder should not be allowed to get distended beyond 350 mL because bladder overdistention results in loss of bladder tone, decreased blood flow to the bladder, and reduction in the layer of mucin that protects the bladder mucosa. CIC continues until the postvoid residual volume is less than 30 mL. To obtain accurate residual volumes, it is important that clients have the opportunity to void first and that catheterization occur immediately after the attempt. The nurse records both the volume voided (even if it is zero) and the volume obtained by catheterization. Postoperative urinary retention usually resolves within 24 to 48 hours.

Chronic Urinary Retention

Chronic urinary retention may go unrecognized. The nurse should ask all clients during an initial health assessment about voiding frequency, the amount (e.g., small, moderate, large) of urine passed each time, the presence of pain or dis-

comfort in the lower abdomen, pain or discomfort on voiding, and difficulty in starting the urinary stream. The examiner gently palpates or percusses the lower abdomen to determine if the bladder is distended. In addition, the nurse obtains a complete medical, drug, and allergy history and reports suspected chronic urinary retention to the physician.

Intermittent Catheterization

Intermittent catheterization performed in the hospital setting is a sterile procedure. When performed by clients or family members in the home, clean rather than aseptic technique is used. A commercially prepared straight catheterization kit is available in hospitals. The kit includes a straight-tipped catheter, sterile gloves, lubricant, and a sterile collection container. At home, the client uses a red rubber catheter that can be washed and reused for 2 to 3 months before replacing. Gloves are not required, but clients must wash their hands thoroughly before and after the procedure. The client can drain the urine into a clean container or directly into the toilet bowl. The schedule is usually three to four times per day, although the frequency can be increased depending on residual volume. If more than 400 mL is returned, the client should be catheterized more often. Client education in technique, catheter care, and follow-up care is an important function of the nurse both in the acute and home care settings.

Indwelling Catheters

A urethral indwelling catheter is one route for permanent bladder catheterization. A cystostomy tube, also called a *suprapubic catheter,* is an alternative that is inserted through an abdominal incision into the bladder. Clients require catheter care, including careful cleansing of the urethral meatus or cystostomy site and proximal catheter, maintenance of the integrity of the closed drainage system, proper anchoring of

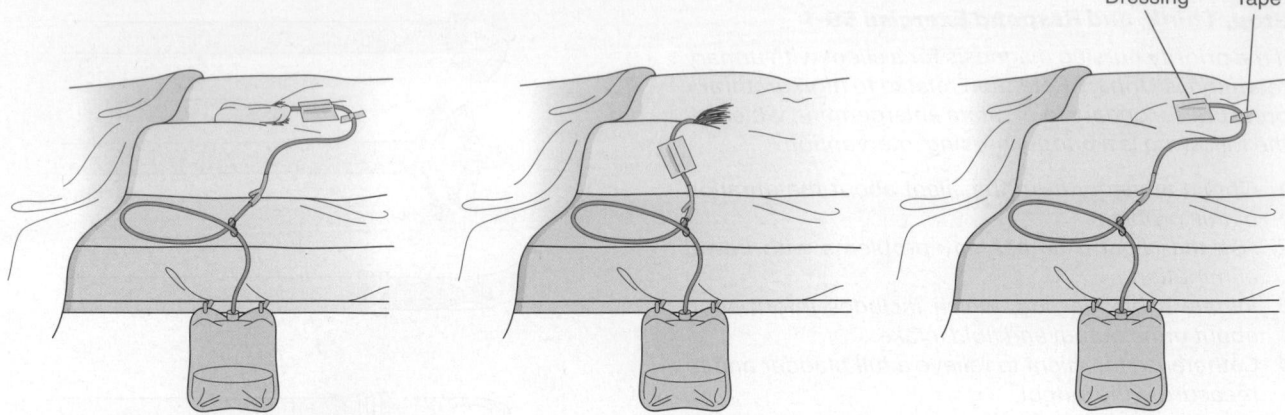

FIGURE 59-2. Catheter tubing correctly anchored and attached to closed drainage system. (**A**) Male. (**B**) Female. (**C**) Suprapubic.

the tube to avoid tension and promote drainage (Fig. 59-2), and scheduled changes of the catheter and drainage system according to facility policy. Nursing Guidelines 59-2 offers additional general management points.

▸ **Stop, Think, and Respond Exercise 59-2**

What methods should a nurse use to prevent the occurrence of a nosocomial infection in the catheterized client?

URINARY INCONTINENCE

Urinary incontinence affects many clients and is a major healthcare concern. It is estimated that at least one third of older adults living in the community and one half of older clients in institutions suffer from incontinence. Not only is incontinence a psychosocial problem, it is a physical problem in that skin breakdown and urinary tract infection may result from incontinence. Table 59-1 describes the different types of incontinence.

Pathophysiology and Etiology

Urinary incontinence may result from either bladder or urethral dysfunction (or both). Box 59-2 identifies risk factors for urinary incontinence. The bladder can contract without warning, fail to accommodate adequate volumes of urine, or fail to empty completely and become overstretched, resulting in overflow incontinence. These conditions result from neurologic disease, bladder outlet obstruction, or trauma in all clients; bladder prolapse or low estrogen levels in women; and prostatic enlargement in men.

Another cause of incontinence is failure of the urethral sphincters to hold urine in the bladder. This may result from trauma, prostate surgery, or relaxed pelvic muscles. Impingement of the spinal nerves, such as in tumors of the spinal cord, herniated disk, or spinal cord injuries, can

NURSING GUIDELINES 59-2

General Principles of Catheterization and Catheter Care

The following general principles apply to the insertion and maintenance of urethral or suprapubic catheters:

- Always use aseptic technique for insertion.
- Thoroughly cleanse the urethral meatus before insertion of a catheter.
- An adult urethra usually takes a size 14-F to 18-F indwelling catheter. A smaller size may be used for intermittent (straight, single) catheterization.
- When inserting an indwelling catheter, test the balloon before insertion.
- Lubricate the catheter with a sterile, water-soluble lubricant and insert.
- Never force a catheter if resistance is felt.
- Never reinsert an indwelling catheter that accidentally becomes dislodged; replace it with a new sterile catheter.
- Catheters are connected to a sterile closed drainage system.
- Keep the drainage bag lower than the catheter.

- Change indwelling urethral catheters according to the physician's orders or agency policy.
- Provide urethral catheter care twice a day and after bowel movements.
- Inspect the cystostomy tube site for leakage of urine around the catheter, bleeding, or signs and symptoms of infection.
- Change the cystostomy dressing once per shift or more often if necessary.
- If a permanent vesicocutaneous (bladder to skin) fistula forms, the size of the cystostomy tube may need to be increased to prevent leakage of urine.
- Unless contraindicated by heart failure or renal disease, encourage clients to drink plenty of fluids (2000–3000 mL), especially those that acidify the urine, such as cranberry juice.
- Monitor client for signs and symptoms of urinary tract infection: fever, chills, hypotension, and confusion.
- Monitor fluid balance and laboratory tests that measure kidney function.

TABLE 59-1 Types of Urinary Incontinence

TYPE OF INCONTINENCE	SYMPTOMS	CAUSES
Transient incontinence	Occurs suddenly; temporary; lasts less than 6 months	Temporary delirium or confusion; infection; increased urine production related to metabolic conditions; effects of some medications such as diuretics, anticholinergics, or antidepressant
Stress incontinence	Client has involuntary loss of urine from intact urethra, which results from sudden increase in intra-abdominal pressure, such as with sneezing or coughing.	Decreased pelvic muscle tone, primarily seen in women, and associated with multiple pregnancies, obstetric injuries, obesity, menopause, or pelvic disease
Urge incontinence	Client experiences urge to void but cannot control voiding in time to reach a toilet.	Bladder irritation related to urinary tract infections, bladder tumors, radiation therapy, enlarged prostate, or neurologic dysfunction
Overflow incontinence	Involuntary loss of urine related to overdistended bladder; clients void small amounts frequently; dribbling	Obstruction from fecal impaction or enlarged prostate; smooth muscle relaxants that relax the bladder and increase capacity; impaired ability of bladder to contract related to neurologic abnormalities, such as spinal cord lesions or tumors, or obstruction to urine output
Functional incontinence	Client has intact function of the lower urinary tract but cannot identify the need to void or ambulate to the toilet	Cognitive impairments, such as brain injury or Alzheimer's disease, or physical limitations, such as rheumatoid arthritis or musculoskeletal injuries
Reflex incontinence	Bladder has uninhibited contractions; involuntary reflexes produce spontaneous voiding, with partial or complete loss of sensation of bladder fullness or urge to void.	Impaired conduction of impulses above reflex arc level secondary to spinal cord injury, tumor, or infection
Mixed incontinence	Client has features of two or more types of incontinence	As an example, older adults often experience two different types such as stress and overflow incontinence
Total incontinence	Urine is continuously and unpredictably lost from the bladder.	Results from surgery, trauma, or anatomic malformation

interfere with the impulse conduction to the brain, resulting in a neurogenic bladder and incontinence. A neurogenic bladder may be spastic, causing incontinence, or it may be flaccid, causing retention.

Assessment Findings

Clients complain of urgency, frequency, leaking small amounts when coughing or sneezing, or complete inability to control urine, depending on the underlying cause. Tests such as a urine culture and sensitivity, cystoscopy, or urodynamics are used to determine the type of incontinence.

Gerontologic Considerations

- Asking older adults about involuntary urine loss may provide more information than asking about incontinence, due to possible embarrassment, the belief that incontinence is a part of aging, or fear of institutionalization. Any new onset of urinary incontinence should be a priority in nursing care plans.

- Carefully assess the cause of incontinence in the older adult. Older adults may be incontinent simply because environmental or physical conditions prevent them from maneuvering quickly enough to get to the bathroom before urination occurs. In these situations, a change in the

environment or an assistive device may alleviate the incontinence. Incontinence may also result from alcohol or drug use, impacted stool, peripheral venous insufficiency, arthritis, or cognitive changes.

BOX 59-2 Risk Factors for Urinary Incontinence

Pregnancy: vaginal delivery, episiotomy
Menopause
Genitourinary surgery
Pelvic muscle weakness
Incompetent urethra as a result of trauma or sphincter relaxation
Immobility
High-impact exercise
Diabetes mellitus
Stroke
Age-related changes in the urinary tract
Morbid obesity
Cognitive disturbances: dementia, Parkinson's disease
Medications: diuretics, sedatives, hypnotics, opioids
Caregiver or toilet unavailable

Medical and Surgical Management

Treatment is aimed at correcting the disorder causing incontinence (when possible), providing medication to control incontinence, correcting the situational problems that contribute to functional incontinence, or instituting a bladder-retraining program. Pharmacologic agents that can improve bladder retention, emptying, and control include anticholinergic drugs such as oxybutynin chloride (Ditropan), which reduces bladder spasticity and involuntary bladder contractions; tolterodine tartrate (Detrol), with similar action to oxybutynin chloride; and phenoxybenzamine hydrochloride (Dibenzaline), which may be useful in treating problems with sphincter control. Bethanechol (Urecholine) helps to increase contraction of the detrusor muscle, which assists with emptying of the bladder. Some tricyclic antidepressant medications (amitriptyline (Elavil), nortriptyline (Pamelos), and amoxapine (Asendin)) are useful in treating incontinence because they decrease bladder contractions and increase bladder neck resistance (Smeltzer et al., 2008). Pseudoephedrine (Sudafed) may help stress incontinence. Estrogen may be useful in restoring mucosal, vascular, and muscular integrity of the urethra for postmenopausal incontinence, but treatment may only be effective for about a year (Smeltzer et al., 2008). Sometimes medication to control incontinence results in retention and must be discontinued. Occasionally clients who can easily perform CIC may opt for medication-induced retention and CIC because it allows them to stay dry.

Surgeries to improve urinary control include:

- Bladder augmentation—a procedure that increases the storage capacity of the bladder
- Periurethral bulking—placement of small amounts of collagen in urethral walls to aid the closing pressure
- Implantation of an artificial sphincter that can be inflated to prevent urine loss and deflated to allow urination (Fig. 59-3)
- Surgeries to provide better support for urinary structures, such as:
  - Retropubic suspension—an open abdominal procedure that involves lifting and anchoring the bladder and urethra to the pelvic wall through the vagina and pubic ligaments; usually done in conjunction with another open abdominal surgery such as a hysterectomy.
  - Anterior repair—a procedure that increases support to the bladder by tightening the vaginal wall under the urethra.
  - Transvaginal needle suspension—a procedure in which the bladder and urethra are attached to the pubic bone or fibrous tissue of the rectum through two vaginal incisions and a midline suprapubic incision.
  - Sling procedures—a procedure in which a small vaginal incision is used to place a piece of synthetic or natural (harvested from the inner thigh or abdomen) material under the bladder neck; it is secured to the abdominal wall or pelvic bone to create a hammock-type lifting of the urethra (Bray, Van Sell & Miller-Anderson, 2007).
  - Sacral nerve stimulator implantation—implantation of a small device, similar to a pacemaker, that acts on nerves that control bladder and pelvic floor contractions. It is

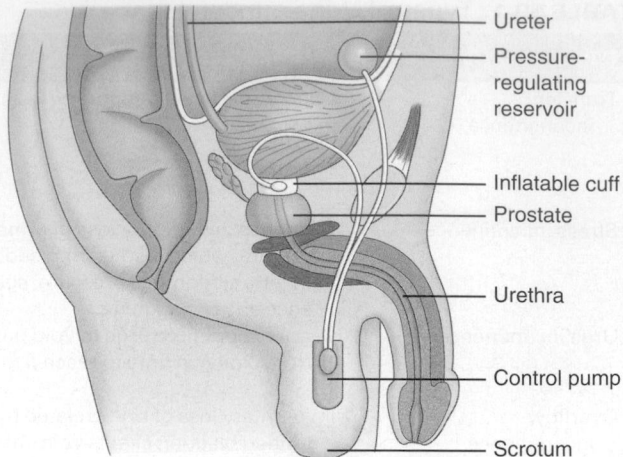

FIGURE 59-3. Artificial urinary sphincter. An inflatable cuff is inserted surgically around the urethra or bladder neck. To empty the bladder, the cuff is deflated by squeezing the control pump located in the scrotum.

implanted under the skin in the abdomen. A wire connected to a sacral nerve emits electrical pulses to stimulate the nerve and help control the bladder. The client does not experience pain and is relieved from heavy leaking in many cases.
- Surgical correction of anatomic problems
- Urethroplasty—surgery to repair structures damaged by trauma

Nursing Management

Goals when caring for a client with urinary incontinence include maintaining continence as much as possible, preventing skin breakdown, reducing anxiety, and initiating a bladder-training program. It must be determined if the client is truly incontinent or if situations prevent the client from getting to the bathroom. Such situations include impaired mobility, physical restraints, and use of sedatives. In addition to assessing for functional causes of incontinence, the nurse obtains details regarding the pattern of incontinence and use of medications that may play a role in the problem. It is important to assess for skin breakdown and determine methods the client has used to manage incontinence.

Instruction centers on exercises to increase muscle tone and voluntary control (Kegel exercises), techniques to assist bladder emptying, and bladder training. Client and Family Teaching 59-1 outlines instructions for Kegel exercises. Success of a bladder-retraining program depends not only on the cause of incontinence but on the motivation of the client and the amount of skillful help and encouragement received from the healthcare team. Some clients respond very well to scheduled voiding, usually at 2- to 4-hour intervals. Another method is referred to as prompted voiding (Specht, 2005), which combines scheduled voiding with prompting and praising. It is used for cognitively intact clients who require encouragement with self-initiated voiding and cognitively impaired clients who gradually become accustomed to being taken to the bathroom regularly.

Client and Family Teaching 59-1
Performing Kegel Exercises

Initial Instructions

1. Sit or stand with legs slightly apart.
2. Draw in perivaginal muscles and anal sphincter as when controlling voiding or defecating.
3. Hold this position of contraction for 5 seconds (instruct client to count or time with a watch).
4. Relax contraction for at least 10 seconds.
5. Repeat exercises 5 to 6 times, increasing slowly to 25 times.
6. Repeat the sequence of exercises three to four times a day.
7. Gradually do the exercises for a total of 200 repetitions.

Advanced Instructions

1. Sit on the toilet and begin to urinate.
2. Stop the flow of urine by doing a Kegel exercise.
3. Hold this position for 5 seconds.
4. Relax and begin voiding.
5. Repeat this sequence five times with each voiding.

Bladder Training

One method of bladder training for the client with an indwelling urethral catheter is to alternately clamp and unclamp the catheter. The clamping and unclamping of the catheter begins to re-establish normal bladder function and capacity. In the beginning, the catheter may be unclamped for 5 minutes every 1 or 2 hours. The length of time is gradually increased to every 3 or 4 hours, giving the bladder a chance to fill more completely. When possible, the nurse teaches the client to release the clamp at scheduled times. The catheter eventually is removed.

At this point, or when training clients who have not had an indwelling catheter, the nurse instructs the client to try to void every hour. Usually the client is not able to retain urine longer than an hour, and frequent voiding is necessary to prevent incontinence. Gradually the client lengthens the interval between voidings to 2, 3, or 4 hours. At first, many clients do not empty the bladder, and they must be catheterized after voiding to remove residual urine. When the client is catheterized for residual urine, the nurse records the amount removed.

When a client is unable to control the storage and passage of urine or when a bladder-training program fails, clients may exhibit varying degrees of anxiety and depression. The nurse needs to offer constant encouragement throughout the bladder-training program. Anxiety may be reduced once the client notes the effort, concern, and interest of the healthcare team. If an accident occurs, it is important to change the bed linen promptly and assure the client that accidents are to be expected during the retraining process. Reducing anxiety may, in some instances, contribute to the success of a bladder-training program.

Barrier Garments and External Collection Devices

If it is not possible to establish a voiding routine and incontinence persists, the healthcare team works with the client to devise a system of collecting the urine. Male clients can use a condom catheter over the penis and connect the tubing to a closed drainage system or disposable urinary drainage bag. External drainage systems are available for women, but it is difficult to get the devices to fit securely. Male and female clients may choose to wear protective pants with a plastic outside layer and absorbent material inside. These pants can be pinned or snapped in place. Liners also are available and are worn next to the skin. They are nonabsorbent, and thus the urine passes through them to the absorbent layer. For this reason, the liners dry quickly and leave the skin dry and free of urine, even though the absorbent material is soaked.

Clients who are incontinent may have problems with odor and maintaining skin integrity. Urea-splitting microorganisms, such as *Micrococcus ureae,* cause the urea in urine to react with water, creating ammonia and causing urine odor, skin breakdown, and ammonia dermatitis. One way to protect the skin is to avoid any contact with urine. When contact is unavoidable, the nurse instructs the client to use soap and water after each episode to clean the skin thoroughly. It also is important to dry the skin completely and apply a skin barrier or moisture sealant to protect the skin. When possible, the nurse encourages the client to expose the affected area to air.

Client and Family Teaching

The nurse encourages clients to actively participate in whatever methods are used to empty the bladder. In addition, the nurse demonstrates procedures as needed for the client and family to understand. Refer to Client and Family Teaching 59-2 for more strategies that assist clients to manage urinary incontinence.

Gerontologic Considerations

- Any client's physical and cognitive abilities must be considered when instituting a bladder rehabilitation program. However, older adults may have more involuntary relaxation of the bladder sphincter than younger clients, necessitating shorter time periods between voiding attempts (e.g., 1 to 1.5 hours rather than 2 hours). It is important for all healthcare providers, family members, or other caregivers to adhere to the client's individual schedule in order to prevent episodes of incontinence, which can impact the person's self-esteem.

INFECTIOUS AND INFLAMMATORY DISORDERS

Infections and inflammations of the bladder and urethra are common. Although usually able to be treated on an outpatient basis, urinary tract infections (UTIs) are a potential source of more complex problems requiring invasive treatment.

CYSTITIS

Pathophysiology and Etiology

Cystitis is an inflammation of the urinary bladder. The inflammation usually is caused by a bacterial infection.

Client and Family Teaching 59-2
Managing Urinary Incontinence

The nurse recommends the following strategies to clients coping with urinary incontinence, modifying instructions to address clients' individual needs:

- Be aware of the amount and timing of fluid intake.
- Avoid taking diuretics after 4 PM.
- Avoid bladder irritants, including caffeine, alcohol, and aspartame (NutraSweet).
- Avoid constipation—adequate fluids, fiber, exercise, and stool softeners if recommended.
- Void regularly—every 2–3 hours:
  - First thing in the AM
  - Before each meal
  - Before going to bed
  - During the night as needed
- Perform kesel exercises as recommended.
- Stop smoking—frequent coughing increases incontinence.
- Control odors by frequent cleansing of the perineum, changing clothes and incontinence briefs (e.g., Attends, Depends) when they become wet, and using an electric room deodorizer.
- Avoid using perfume or scented powders, lotions, or sprays. Mixing a perfumed scent with a urine odor may intensify the odor, irritate the skin, or cause a skin infection.
- Wash garments as soon as possible in warm, soapy water.
- Use plastic to cover objects, such as a mattress and chairs, to prevent staining and lingering odors. The plastic must be washed with mild soapy water daily or more often if needed.
- Place a sheet or blanket between the skin and the plastic.
- Follow the recommendations of the physician about clamping and unclamping the catheter (when this method is prescribed) or changing the catheter or cystostomy tube.
- Keep a record of fluid intake. Drink plenty of fluids during waking hours. Drink most of the required fluids in the morning and early afternoon hours and decrease the intake toward evening.
- Follow the recommended bladder-training program. Time is required to achieve success.
- Contact the physician if any of the following occurs: increased discomfort, rash around the perineal area, pain in the lower abdomen, fever, chills, or cloudy urine.

Bacteria can invade the bladder from an infection in the kidneys, lymphatics, and urethra (Fig. 59-4). Because the urethra is short in women, ascending infections or microorganisms from the vagina or rectum are more common. Causes of cystitis include urologic instrumentation (e.g., cystoscopy, catheterization), fecal contamination, prostatitis or benign prostatic hyperplasia, indwelling catheters, pregnancy, and sexual intercourse.

The lining of the bladder provides a natural resistance to most bacterial invasions by preventing an inflammatory reaction from occurring. If bacteria do survive in the bladder, however, they adhere to the mucosal lining of the bladder and multiply. The surface of the bladder becomes edematous and reddened, and ulcerations may develop. When urine contacts these irritated areas, the client experiences pain and urgency, which is magnified in the presence of even slight bladder distention.

Assessment Findings
Signs and Symptoms

The symptoms of cystitis include urgency (feeling a pressing need to void although the bladder is not full), frequency, low back pain, dysuria, perineal and suprapubic pain, and hematuria, especially at the termination of the stream (terminal hematuria). If bacteremia is present, the client also may have chills and fever. Chronic cystitis causes similar symptoms, but usually they are less severe.

Diagnostic Findings

Microscopic examination of the urine reveals an increase in the number of red and white blood cells. Culture and sensitivity studies are used to identify the causative microorganism and appropriate antimicrobial therapy. If repeated episodes occur, intravenous pyelogram (IVP) or cystoscopy with or without retrograde pyelograms may be

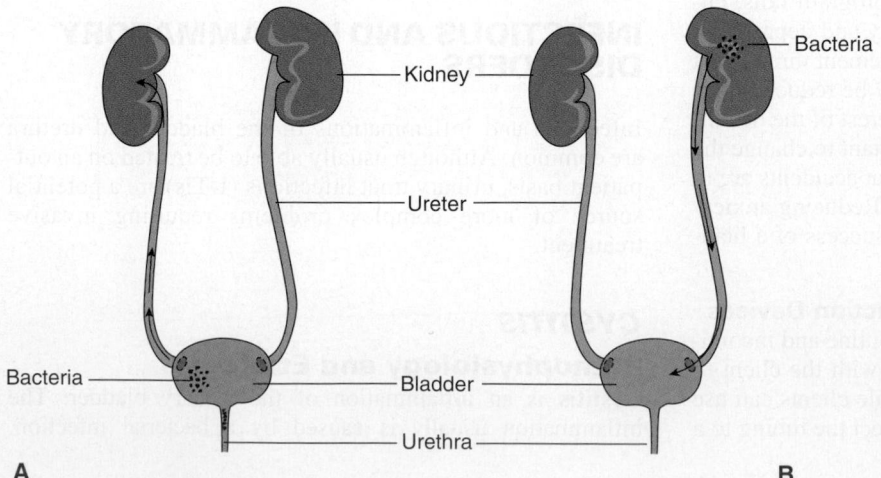

FIGURE 59-4. Urinary tract infection. **(A)** Microorganisms invade the bladder and ascend to the ureter and kidney. **(B)** Microorganisms in the kidney descend the ureter to the bladder.

needed to identify the possible cause, such as chronic prostatitis or a bladder **diverticulum** (weakening and out-pouching of the bladder wall), which encourages urinary stasis and infection.

Medical Management

Medical management includes antimicrobial therapy and correction of contributing factors. Examples of drugs that may be used include trimethoprim-sulfamethoxazole (TMP-SMZ, Septra, Bactrim) and nitrofurantoin macrocrystals (Macrodantin). Cranberry juice or vitamin C may be recommended to keep the bacteria from adhering to the wall of the bladder and thus promoting their excretion and enhancing the effectiveness of drug therapy. When there is a partial urethral obstruction, no treatment of cystitis is fully effective until adequate drainage of urine is restored by the removal of the obstruction (see discussion of urethral strictures). In some instances, treatment may be prolonged and may need to be repeated.

Pharmacologic Considerations

- Antibiotics and sulfonamides are drugs commonly used to treat urinary tract infections (UTIs). Other drugs used are furan derivatives, nitrofurantoin macrocrystals (Macrodantin) and nitrofurantoin (Furadantin), and the acids methenamine mandelate (Mandelamine) and nalidixic acid (NegGram). An azo dye, phenazopyridine (Pyridium), may be ordered for its soothing effect on bladder mucosa and often is used in conjunction with urinary antimicrobial drugs.

- Instruct clients who receive drugs for UTIs to finish the course of therapy even though they may feel improved and be symptom free after several days of therapy. A completed course of therapy is essential to be sure the infection is under control.

- Advise clients to follow their physicians' instructions about the medication, such as drinking extra fluids.

Nursing Management

The nurse advises the client to drink extra fluids. Cranberry juice provides a less favorable climate for bacterial growth. It is important to emphasize the importance of finishing the prescribed course of therapy. The nurse also instructs the client in the prevention of repeated cystitis (Client and Family Teaching 59-3).

▶ Stop, Think, and Respond Exercise 59-3

Your 30-year-old client tells you that she has had four urinary tract infections (UTIs) in the past 6 months. What information should you get before providing the client with instructions about preventing future UTIs?

INTERSTITIAL CYSTITIS

Pathophysiology and Etiology

Interstitial cystitis (IC) is a chronic inflammation of the bladder mucosa. It is more common in women than men.

Client and Family Teaching 59-3
Preventing Cystitis

The nurse instructs the client as follows:

● Increase fluid intake to 2 to 3 L a day.
● Avoid coffee, teas, colas, and alcohol.
● Shower rather than bathe in a tub.
● Cleanse perineum after each bowel movement with front-to-back motion.
● Avoid irritating substances such as bubble bath, bath salts, perineal lotions, vaginal sprays, nylon underwear, scented toilet paper.
● Wear cotton underwear.
● Void every 2 to 3 hours while awake.
● Empty bladder completely with each voiding.
● Void after sexual intercourse.
● Notify physician of the following: urgency, frequency, burning with urination, difficulty urinating, or blood in the urine.
● Take medication exactly as prescribed.

The bladder wall contains multiple pinpoint hemorrhagic areas that join and form larger hemorrhagic areas that may progress to fissuring and scarring of the bladder mucosa. Superficial erosion of the bladder mucosa (Hunner's ulcer) may develop. Eventually, the bladder shrinks from scarring. The cause of IC is unknown, but it has been suggested that there may be a hormonal link because flare-ups appear to occur before menstruation. Another theory is that IC may be an autoimmune disorder or part of a systemic condition because some persons have a history of migraine headaches, ulcerative colitis, endometriosis, or chronic fatigue syndrome.

Assessment Findings

Symptoms mimic other disorders such as cystitis, bladder cancer, or a sexually transmitted infection (STI). Frequent, painful urination and passing a small volume of urine are the most common symptoms. The pain may be described as searing or burning. The client reports an onset of pain and the need to void as soon as a small amount of urine is present in the bladder. Many clients report painful intercourse.

Cystoscopy reveals a markedly inflamed bladder mucosa with pinpoint hemorrhages and a bladder capacity that is smaller than normal. Filling the bladder during cystoscopy to improve visualization usually results in severe pain.

A voiding cystourethrogram also demonstrates a small bladder capacity. Results of urinalysis usually are normal, but if cystitis is present, an increase in the number of red and white blood cells may be seen; urine cultures are negative. A record of the number of voidings and the amount voided over a 2- or 3-day period, along with the symptoms, help to confirm the diagnosis. A biopsy of the bladder mucosa reveals an inflammatory process with scarring and hemorrhagic areas, and confirms the diagnosis.

Medical and Surgical Management

There is no single effective specific therapy for IC. Elmiron (pentosan polysulfate), a bladder protectant, is the most effective medication. It provides relief of the bladder pain associated with IC. Antidepressant drugs may also relieve pain as well as treat the depression that can accompany the disorder. Other therapies include bladder instillation of DMSO (dimethyl sulfoxide) or silver nitrate. A more recent treatment uses a laser, inserted into the abdominal cavity with a laparoscope, to sever the sensory (pain) fibers of the bladder. This procedure is used to relieve the severe pain associated with IC. Severe IC can be incapacitating, and a urinary diversion procedure (see later discussion) may offer the only relief of symptoms for a selected group of clients.

Nursing Management

The nurse advises the client to avoid spicy and acidic foods because they may contribute to pain and discomfort. Psychological support is necessary because many times IC has gone undiagnosed and the client has been told that there is nothing wrong. Clients with IC often have their lives severely disrupted by pain and frequent trips to the bathroom, sometimes several times an hour. Some clients are unable to hold jobs because of the severity of symptoms. Sexual activity is avoided because of fear of pain, straining their relationships and interfering with intimacy. Clients should be referred to a chronic pain center to cope with the pain and to an IC support group.

URETHRITIS

Pathophysiology and Etiology

Urethritis (inflammation of the urethra) is seen more commonly in men than in women. Urethritis caused by microorganisms other than gonococci is called *nongonococcal urethritis.* Gonorrhea, an STI, is a specific form of infection that can attack the mucous membrane of a normal urethra (see Chap. 56).

In women, urethritis may accompany cystitis but also may be secondary to vaginal infections. Soaps, bubble baths, sanitary napkins, or scented toilet paper also may cause urethritis.

In men, a common cause of urethritis is infection with *Chlamydia trachomatis* or *Ureaplasma urealyticum,* which causes an STI. The distal portion of the normal male urethra is not totally sterile. Bacteria that normally are present cause no difficulty unless these tissues are traumatized, usually after instrumentation such as catheterization or cystoscopic examination. Under such conditions, bacteria may gain a foothold to cause a nonspecific urethritis. Other causes of nonspecific urethritis in men include irritation during vigorous intercourse, rectal intercourse, or intercourse with a woman who has a vaginal infection.

Assessment Findings

Infection of the urethra results in discomfort on urination varying from a slight tickling sensation to burning or severe discomfort and urinary frequency. Fever is not common, but fever in the male client may be due to further extension of the infection to areas such as the prostate, testes, and epididymis.

The client's history and symptoms often provide a tentative diagnosis. In men, a urethral smear is obtained for culture and sensitivity to identify the causative microorganism. In women, a urinalysis (clean-catch midstream specimen) may identify the causative microorganism.

Medical Management

Treatment includes appropriate antibiotic therapy, liberal fluid intake, analgesics, warm sitz baths, and improvement of the client's resistance to infection by a good diet and plenty of rest. If urethritis is due to an STI, it is treated with appropriate antibiotic therapy (see Chap. 56). Failure to seek treatment for gonococcal urethritis may result in a urethral stricture in men.

Nursing Management

The nurse reinforces the need to complete antibiotic therapy, drink plenty of fluids, and take warm sitz baths and analgesics for pain. Urethritis may be seen in clients with indwelling urethral catheters. To prevent or decrease urethritis, the nurse needs to be vigilant with sterile technique, as well as to exercise gentleness when changing catheters. It also is essential to provide frequent perineal care, especially if the client is incontinent of feces. In addition to washing around the anus and buttocks, the nurse also cleans the meatus and labia of the female client. When cleaning the anal area, wiping away from the urethra ensures that there is no contamination. If cotton pledgets are used, the nurse wipes from the urethral meatus to the anus in a single stroke and discards the pledget. Client teaching information is included in the Nursing Process section that follows.

Nursing Process for the Client With an Infection of the Bladder or Urethra

Assessment

Ask the client about present symptoms, specifically seeking information related to the presence of pain and changes in urination, including frequency, urgency, and burning with urination. Assess the client's sexual practices, including methods of contraception and personal hygiene. Ask the client to void. When the client voids, measure the volume and check the urine for color, cloudiness, concentration, odor, and presence of blood.

Diagnosis, Planning, and Interventions

▶ **Acute Pain** related to infection and inflammation of the bladder and/ or urethra

▶ **Expected Outcome:** The client will express relief of pain and discomfort.

• Assure the client that pain and discomfort will decrease with treatment. *Antibacterial and antispasmodic medications are quickly effective in relieving the pain and discomfort associated with UTIs.*

• Administer analgesics and antispasmodics as indicated. *Prompt administration of prescribed medications ensures that effective blood levels are maintained for treatment of infection. Antispasmodics relieve bladder irritability.*

- Encourage the client to use warm sitz baths two or three times a day to relieve discomfort. *Promotes relief of pain and reduces spasm.*
- Encourage the client to increase daily fluid intake to at least 8 large glasses, excluding coffee, tea, alcohol, and colas. *Promotes renal blood flow and flushes bacteria from the urinary tract. Coffee, tea, alcohol, and colas are urinary tract irritants.*
- Instruct the client to void at regular intervals, even if uncomfortable. *Frequent voiding promotes emptying the bladder, which contributes to lower bacterial counts, reduction of urinary stasis, and prevention of reinfection.*

▶ Anxiety related to pain, discomfort, and frequent urination

▶ Expected Outcomes: (1) Client will verbalize anxiety related to symptoms. (2) Client will state self-care measures to relieve anxiety.

- Encourage client to talk about his or her symptoms and fears related to the disorder. *Providing an opportunity for the client to discuss concerns and fears assists in relieving anxiety.*
- Provide information that assists in alleviating fears. *Accurate information alleviates fear and corrects misconceptions.*

▶ Deficient Knowledge regarding inflammation and infection of the bladder and urethra related to disease process and treatment

▶ Expected Outcomes: (1) Client will verbalize understanding of condition, prognosis, and treatment. (2) Client will participate in the treatment regimen.

- Review the treatment plan. *Doing so provides a time for the client to ask questions.*
- Instruct client about medications, dosage, frequency, expected effects, and possible side effects. *Providing clients with accurate information promotes adherence to drug regimen.*
- Emphasize the need to complete the entire course of medications, even after symptoms have subsided. *Complete antibiotic therapy eradicates infection and prevents recurrence.*
- Teach client the importance of increased fluid intake. *Increased fluid intake flushes the urinary tract and removes bacteria.*
- If the client is on a special diet (e.g., a low-sodium or diabetic diet), check with the physician regarding drinking juices or beverages or eating foods that are liquid at room temperature. Teach client modified fluid guidelines as needed. *Some liquids either must be considered part of the daily dietary allowances or may not be allowed because they contain substances that must be eliminated from the diet. In some diets, a limited amount of certain liquids may be allowed.*
- Teach about possible benefits of including one or more glasses of 100% cranberry juice (not cranberry juice cocktail) in daily fluid intake. *Cranberry juice may prevent bacteria from adhering to the lining of the urinary tract. However, not all bacteria are sensitive to the juice, and protection lasts only as long as the juice is consumed regularly.*
- Review client's hygiene practices. *Poor hygiene practices, such as back-to-front perineal cleansing, especially after a bowel move-*

ment, or soaking in dirty bath water, can contribute to the introduction of bacterial contaminants to the urinary tract.

- Instruct the client to notify the physician if symptoms persist after the course of drug therapy is completed, if the symptoms become worse, or if fever or chills occur. *Persistent or worsening symptoms may indicate that the treatment is ineffective or inadequate and requires further medical attention.*
- Teach client methods to prevent future infections. *Appropriate personal hygiene, increased fluid intake (promotes voiding and dilution of urine), and frequent voiding prevent UTI.*

Evaluation of Expected Outcomes

The client reports relief of pain and discomfort and states that he or she is adhering to the medication regimen. The client states that he or she is not anxious and feels much better now that there are no symptoms. He or she demonstrates understanding of the treatment plan as evidenced by intake of at least 2 L of water, frequent voiding, and appropriate personal hygiene practices. ●

OBSTRUCTIVE DISORDERS

Obstruction of the lower urinary tract is a blockage in the bladder or in the urethra. Many obstructions are related to congenital anomalies, but in adults, obstructions occur from stones that block the passage of urine, or from a narrowing that occurs as a result of a trauma, inflammation, or infection. Box 59-3 lists general signs of an outflow obstruction.

BLADDER STONES

Pathophysiology and Etiology

Stones may form in the bladder or originate in the upper urinary tract and travel to and remain in the bladder. Large bladder stones develop in those with chronic urinary retention and urinary stasis. Clients who are immobile (e.g., the unconscious client or those with paraplegia or quadriplegia) also may have a tendency to form bladder stones.

Assessment Findings

Symptoms of bladder stone formation include hematuria, suprapubic pain, difficulty starting the urinary stream, symptoms of a bladder infection, and a feeling that the bladder is not completely empty. Some clients may have few or no symptoms.

Cystoscopy, a kidney-ureter-bladder (KUB) study, IVP, or ultrasound studies detect the presence of bladder stones.

BOX 59-3	Signs of Obstructed Urine Flow

- Straining to empty bladder
- Feeling that bladder does not empty completely
- Hesitancy
- Weak stream
- Frequency
- Overflow incontinence
- Bladder distention

Blood chemistries and 24-hour urine collection for serum calcium and uric acid may identify the possible cause of stone formation.

Medical and Surgical Management

Bladder stones may be removed through the transurethral route, using a stone-crushing instrument (lithotrite). This procedure, called a **litholapaxy,** is suitable for small and soft stones and is performed under general anesthesia. Larger, noncrushable stones must be removed through a surgical (suprapubic) incision into the bladder.

When it is possible to determine the chemical composition of stones that have passed or been removed, dietary treatment is based on the primary component of the stone. A low-purine diet is used for uric acid stones, although the benefits are unknown. Clients with a history of calcium oxalate stone formation need a diet that is adequate in calcium and low in oxalate (see Nutrition Notes 58-1). Only clients who have type II absorptive hypercalciuria—approximately half of the clients—need to limit calcium intake (Smeltzer et al, 2008). Usually, clients are told to increase their fluid intake significantly, consume a moderate protein intake, and limit sodium (Nutrition Notes 59-1). Despite dietary changes, some clients continue to form stones in the urinary tract.

Nursing Management

The nurse obtains a complete medical, drug, and allergy history, asking the client to describe the symptoms, including the type and location of the pain. Determining if the client is allergic to iodine or seafood is essential because iodine-containing radiopaque substances may be used during diagnostic tests to locate the obstruction. The nurse monitors vital signs every 4 hours or as ordered, and notifies the physician if the client's temperature is higher than 101°F (38.3°C) orally. Intake and output and the color of the urine are documented in the medical record.

Nutrition Notes 59-1
The Client With Bladder Stones

● Encourage clients with bladder stones to drink 8 ounces of fluid hourly during waking hours, or at least 2 L of fluid daily.

● A low-purine diet, used for uric acid stones, limits organ meats (brain, kidney, liver, sweetbreads), game meat, gravies, anchovies, herring, mackerel, sardines, and scallops. All meats, fish, and poultry contain significant amounts of purines, so compliance is difficult.

● Clients with calcium oxalate stones should consume adequate calcium (e.g., 3 cups of milk daily) because calcium binds with oxalate in the GI tract to lower urinary oxalate levels. Foods high in oxalates should be avoided: dark leafy green vegetables, berries, rhubarb, tea, nuts, chocolate, beans (green, wax, and dried), tofu, sweet potatoes, wheat bran, and draft beer. Avoiding excessive protein intake is associated with lower urinary oxalate and lower uric acid levels. Reducing sodium intake can lower urinary calcium levels.

If there is any evidence of gross hematuria, the nurse reports it immediately. Encouraging the client to drink fluids (unless contraindicated by heart failure or renal disease) is important because extra fluids help pass stones and reduce the chance of infection or inflammation. The nurse filters the urine for stones by straining all urine through gauze or wire mesh. If solid material is found, it is sent in a labeled container to the laboratory for analysis. If the client has moderate to severe pain, the nurse administers a narcotic analgesic as ordered. If the analgesic fails to relieve at least some of the pain or if the pain becomes worse despite administration of an analgesic, the nurse notifies the physician, and provides details regarding the effects of medical or surgical procedures.

If a litholapaxy successfully removes the stone, a urethral catheter may be left in place to keep the bladder continuously empty for 1 to 2 days after the procedure. The nurse administers antibiotics as ordered. Once oral fluids are tolerated, it is important to encourage the client to drink extra fluids to reduce inflammation of the bladder mucosa. In addition, the nurse monitors the urine output and voiding pattern.

If open removal is required, the bladder is incised and the stone removed. A urethral catheter may be left in place for a week or more to keep the bladder empty and prevent tension on the bladder sutures. In addition to standard postoperative care (see Chap. 14), nursing management involves providing the same care as for the client having a suprapubic prostatectomy (see Chap. 55). The nurse closely monitors the client's voiding once the catheter is removed to prevent urinary retention.

The nurse teaches the client to:

• Strain urine and send any stone found to the laboratory for examination.
• Follow the dietary recommendations.
• Take the prescribed medications as directed.
• Contact the physician if symptoms return.
• Drink plenty of fluids (at least 10 large glasses each day) and exercise regularly.
• Contact the physician if hematuria, burning, chills, fever, or pain occurs.

URETHRAL STRICTURES
Pathophysiology and Etiology

Strictures of the urethra are caused by infections such as untreated gonorrhea or chronic nongonococcal urethritis. Other causes include trauma to the lower urinary tract or pelvis, such as accidents, childbirth, intercourse, or surgical procedures. Urethral strictures may be congenital.

A **stricture** (narrowing) in the urethra obstructs the flow of urine and can cause complications in the bladder or upper urinary tract. The kidney pelves can become distended with the backflow of urine. The bladder distends when the urethra is obstructed and a diverticulum (outpouching) of the muscular bladder wall may form (Fig. 59-5). In some instances, more than one diverticulum may be seen. Urine becomes trapped in the diverticulum, stagnates, and becomes a culture medium for bacteria. For this reason, infection occurs often

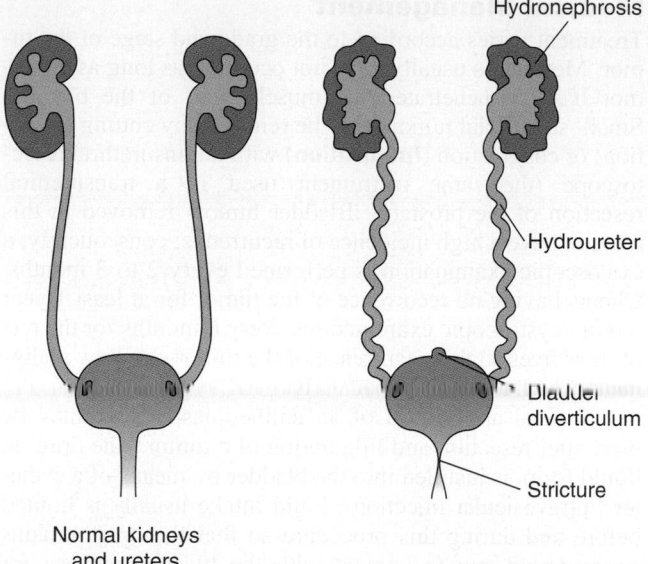

FIGURE 59-5. Urethral stricture can result in hydroureters, hydronephrosis (dilation of the ureters and kidney), and bladder diverticulum.

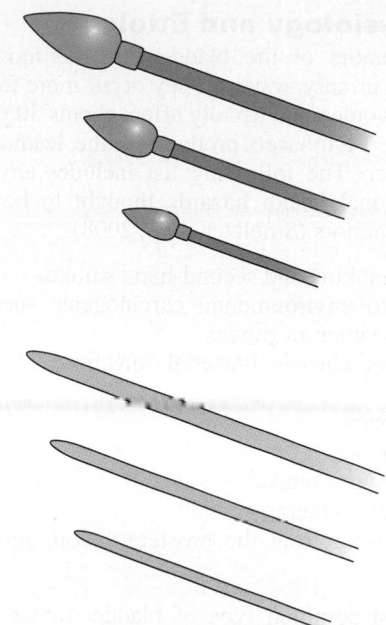

FIGURE 59-6. Bougies (**A**) and filiforms (**B**) are used to dilate the urethra.

and is difficult to control until the obstruction is corrected. Men experience urethral stricture more frequently than women, secondary to the anatomic differences and the length of the urethra. A urethral stricture may result in acute or chronic urinary retention.

Assessment Findings

Symptoms include.

- Slow or decreased force of stream of urine
- Hesitancy
- Burning
- Frequency
- Nocturia
- Retention of residual urine in the bladder—may lead to bladder distention and infection

The client may be able to pass more urine after voiding and waiting a few minutes. The final quantity of urine comes from the diverticulum and may be malodorous.

The stricture may be seen on cystoscopy, retrograde pyelogram, and IVP. A voiding cystourethrogram also may show the stricture as well as the presence of a bladder diverticulum.

Medical and Surgical Management

Urethral strictures are treated by dilatation, which is the use of specially designed instruments called *bougies, sounds, filiforms,* and *followers* (Fig. 59-6) that are passed gently into the urethra. Although done gently, the procedure usually is painful. Because forceful stretching of the urethra may cause bleeding and further stricture formation, dilatation begins with a 6-F or 8-F urethral dilator. During subsequent treatments, the physician increases the size of the dilator until 24 F or 26 F can be tolerated. Depending on the cause of the stricture and the response to the therapy, the condition may subside after one or two treatments. However, periodic

dilatations usually are required indefinitely or until the condition is corrected surgically.

If dilatation is unsuccessful, a **urethroplasty** (surgical repair of the urethra) may be attempted. The urine is diverted from the urethra by a cystostomy tube until the urethra has been repaired. In one method of reconstructing the urethra, the constricted area is resected, and a mucosal graft (which may be taken from the bladder) is inserted to restore the continuity of the urethra. After surgery, the client has a splinting catheter in the urethra that remains until healing has occurred. This operation may be performed in two stages: urinary diversion at the first operation and plastic repair at the second.

Nursing Management

The nurse advises the client that the urine may be blood tinged after urethral dilatation and that it may burn when voiding. Sitz baths and non-narcotic analgesics may relieve discomfort. The nurse encourages the client to drink extra fluids for several days after the procedure. It is important for the client to keep appointments for follow-up dilatations and not to wait until there is a marked reduction in the urinary stream or other symptoms of obstruction to return. The nurse instructs the client to take all of the antibiotics and to contact the physician if difficulty voiding or frank bleeding occurs.

If a urethroplasty is performed, it is most important that the urethral catheter remain in place and securely anchored. After surgery, turning and repositioning requires special attention to prevent excessive tension on the urethral catheter.

MALIGNANT TUMORS OF THE BLADDER

Malignant tumors of the bladder are frightening for clients. Bloody urine often is the first sign of a problem and the reason clients seek medical attention.

Pathophysiology and Etiology

Malignant tumors of the bladder are the most common tumors in the urinary system. They occur more frequently in men than in women and usually affect clients 50 years of age or older. Use of tobacco products is the leading cause of bladder cancer. The following list includes environmental and occupational health hazards thought to be associated with bladder tumors (Smeltzer et al., 2008):

- Cigarette smoking and second-hand smoke
- Exposure to environmental carcinogens, such as dyes, paint, ink, leather, or rubber
- Recurrent or chronic bacterial infections of the urinary tract
- Bladder stones
- High urinary pH
- High cholesterol intake
- Pelvic radiation therapy
- Cancers arising from the prostate, colon, and rectum in men

The most common type of bladder tumor is a transitional cell carcinoma, which develops in the bladder's epithelial lining. The tumors are classified as papillary or nonpapillary. Papillary lesions are superficial and extend outward from the mucosal layer. Nonpapillary tumors are solid growths that grow inward, deep into the bladder wall. This type is more likely to metastasize, usually to the lymph nodes, liver, lungs, and bone. Other types include squamous cell carcinoma and adenocarcinoma.

Assessment Findings

Signs and Symptoms

The most common first symptom of a malignant tumor of the bladder is painless hematuria. Additional early symptoms include UTI with symptoms such as fever, dysuria, urgency, and frequency. Later symptoms are related to metastases and include pelvic pain, urinary retention (if the tumor blocks the bladder outlet), and urinary frequency from the tumor occupying bladder space. If bleeding has been present for some time, the client also may have symptoms of anemia (fatigue, shortness of breath) caused by blood loss.

▶ **Stop, Think, and Respond Exercise 65-4**

A 55-year-old man is admitted with blood in the urine. The medical diagnosis is "Rule out bladder cancer." When the nurse admits this client, what is an important question to ask?

Diagnostic Findings

The tumor usually is seen by cystoscopic examination and confirmed by microscopic biopsy. A retrograde pyelogram may be obtained to detect any kidney damage if the tumor is obstructing one of the ureteral orifices. A computed tomography scan and radiographs of the pelvis may show a tumor shadow or bony metastases. Ultrasonography also may show tumor size and location. Routine laboratory tests may be performed to evaluate kidney function and determine the degree of anemia due to persistent hematuria. Urine cytology is done to determine if there are cancer cells in the urine.

Medical Management

Treatment varies according to the grade and stage of the tumor. Metastases usually have not occurred as long as the tumor has not penetrated the muscle wall of the bladder. Small, superficial tumors may be removed by cutting (resection) or coagulation (**fulguration**) with a transurethral resectoscope (the same instrument used in a transurethral resection of the prostate). Bladder tumors removed in this manner have a high incidence of recurrence; consequently, a cystoscopic examination is performed every 2 to 3 months. Clients having no recurrence of the tumor for at least 1 year require cystoscopic examinations every 6 months for the rest of their lives so that recurrence of the tumor or a new malignant growth can be detected early.

Topical application of an antineoplastic drug may be used after resection and fulguration of a tumor. The drug, in liquid form, is instilled into the bladder by means of a catheter (intravesicular injection). Fluid intake usually is limited before and during this procedure so that the drug remains concentrated and in contact with the bladder mucosa for about 2 hours. The client then voids and is given extra oral fluids to flush the drug from the bladder.

Intravesicular injection of BCG (bacillus Calmette-Guérin) Live, a weakened strain of *Mycobacterium bovis,* also may be used. It appears that BCG causes an inflammatory reaction in the bladder wall that in turn destroys malignant cells. Another form of therapy includes the administration of interferon alfa-2a (Roferon-A) injected intravenously (IV) or directly into the bladder. Interferon appears to stimulate the production of lymphocytes and macrophages that may destroy malignant cells.

Photodynamic therapy also may be used in the treatment of bladder cancer. This experimental treatment involves the IV injection of a photosensitizing agent that is absorbed in concentration by malignant cells. A laser, inserted through a cystoscope, is used to destroy those cells that have a high concentration of the photosensitizing agent.

Radiation therapy may be done if surgery is planned for the client. This reduces the size and extent of the tumor and decreases the risk of metastasis.

Surgical Management

A **cystectomy** (surgical removal of the bladder) and a urinary diversion procedure often are necessary when the tumor has penetrated the muscle wall. When a cystectomy is performed, the bladder and lower third of both ureters are removed. If the tumor has extended through the bladder wall, the surgeon may perform a radical cystectomy.

In women, a radical cystectomy usually includes removal of the bladder, lower third of both ureters, uterus, fallopian tubes, ovaries, anterior vaginal wall, and urethra. In men, a radical cystectomy usually includes removal of the bladder, lower third of both ureters, prostate, and seminal vesicles.

Once a cystectomy is performed, urine must be diverted to another collecting system. This is called a **urinary diversion.** Although urinary diversion procedures are used for the treatment of bladder tumors, they also are used for extensive pelvic malignancies and severe traumatic injury to the bladder. Some urinary diversions require external ostomy bags to

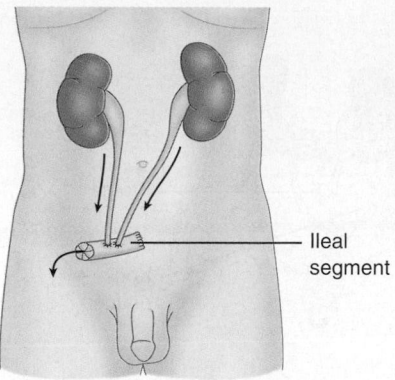

A: Conventional ileal conduit.
The surgeon transplants the ureters to an isolated section of the terminal ileum (ileal conduit), bringing one end to the abdominal wall. The ureter may also be transplanted into the transverse sigmoid colon (colon conduit) or proximal jejunum (jejunal conduit).

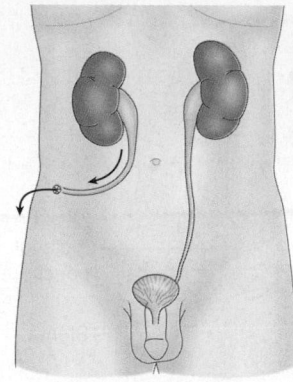

B: Cutaneous uroterostomy.
The surgeon brings the detached ureter through the abdominal wall and attaches it to an opening in the skin.

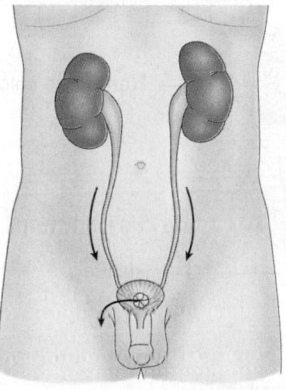

C: Vesicotomy.
The surgeon sutures the bladder to the abdominal wall and creates an opening (stoma) through the abdominal and bladder walls for urinary drainage.

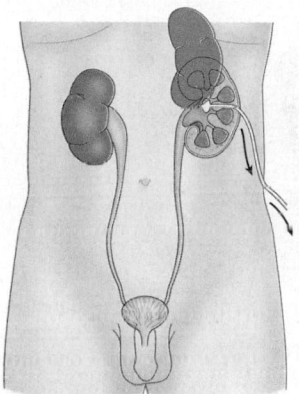

D: Nephrostomy.
The surgeon inserts a catheter into the renal pelvis via an incision into the flank or, by percutaneous catheter placement, into the kidney.

FIGURE 59-7. Types of cutaneous diversions include (**A**) the conventional ileal conduit, (**B**) cutaneous ureterostomy, (**C**) vesicostomy, and (**D**) nephrostomy.

collect the urine—referred to as *cutaneous urinary diversions* (Fig. 59-7). Other types create a reservoir within the body and the reservoir is catheterized to drain the urine—these are called *continent urinary diversions* (Fig. 59-8). In some instances the urine is diverted to the colon and the client voids rectally—this also is referred to as a continent urinary diversion. Each of the procedures has advantages and disadvantages. The type of procedure used depends on many factors, such as the age and physical condition of the client, the procedure that can produce the best results for the client, and the extent of metastases.

Nursing Management

Preoperative Period

The nurse obtains a complete medical, drug, and allergy history on admission and asks the client or family member to describe all symptoms. The assessment also includes an evaluation of general physical and emotional status, vital signs, and weight.

Caring for a client during the preoperative period includes reducing anxiety and increasing understanding of the preparations for surgery and postoperative care. The client may display various emotional responses before surgery. Some may appear depressed; others show a mixture of anxiety and depression. The client faces drastic changes in the manner of excreting urine from the body, the diagnosis of cancer, and the changes in body image. The nurse encourages the client to talk about the surgery and the changes that will occur. He or she may suggest a visit from a member of a local ostomy group to provide emotional support as well as information. The enterostomal therapist should meet with the client to discuss placement of the stoma and collection devices. Photographs or drawings are useful in showing the placement of the stoma and urostomy pouch.

The nurse determines the client's ability to manage stoma care or self-catheterization by assessing manual dexterity, level of understanding, and vision. Assessing the client's social support and resources, including whether insurance will cover ostomy supplies, is important. The

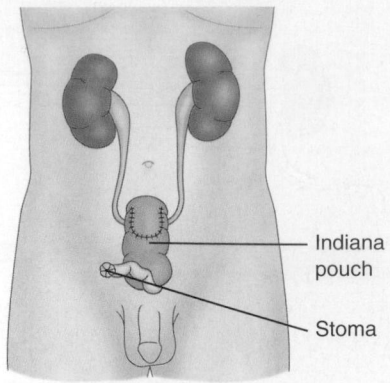

A: Indiana pouch.
The surgeon introduces the ureters into a segment of ileum and cecum. Urine is drained periodically by inserting a catheter into the stoma.

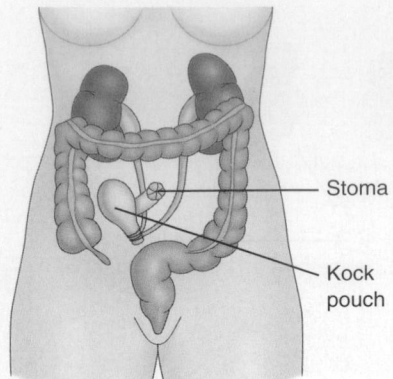

B: Continent ileal urinary diversions (Kock pouch). The surgeon transplants the ureters to an isolated segment of small bowel, ascending colon, or ileocolonic segment and develops an effective continence mechanism or valve. Urine is drained by inserting a catheter into the stoma.

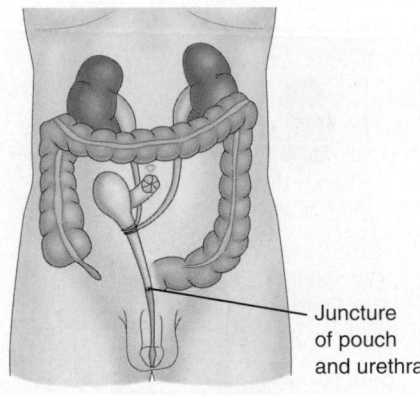

C:
In male patients, the Kock pouch can be modified by attaching one end of the pouch to the urethra, allowing more normal voiding. The female urethra is too short for this modification.

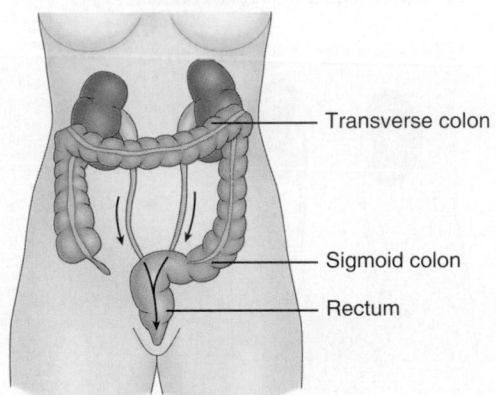

D: Ureterosigmoidostomy.
The surgeon introduces the ureters into the sigmoid colon, thereby allowing urine to flow through the colon and out of the rectum.

FIGURE 59-8. Types of continent urinary diversions include (**A**) the Indiana pouch, (**B** and **C**) the Kock pouch, also called a continent ileal diversion, and (**D**) a ureterosigmoidostomy.

nurse explains all preoperative preparations to the client and family and gives them time to ask additional questions about the surgery, preparations for surgery, and management after surgery.

Depending on the extent and type of surgery, preoperative preparations may include insertion of a nasogastric tube, placement of IV and central venous pressure lines, administration of cleansing enemas, and adherence to a low-residue diet several days before surgery. Laxatives and enemas and a drug such as kanamycin (Kantrex) or neomycin (Mycifradin) may be given if a ureterosigmoidostomy (see Fig. 59-8D) is to be performed. These agents decrease the number of microorganisms in the bowel and lessen the possibility of infection as a complication of connecting the ureters to the bowel. Clients scheduled for an ileal conduit (see Fig. 59-7A) or continent urinary diversion procedure (see Fig. 59-7) also may have the bowel prepared in this manner.

Postoperative Period
Clients undergoing urinary diversion are subject to the same conditions and complications as any surgical client. Refer to Chapter 14 for nursing diagnoses and interventions for managing standard postoperative care. Management issues related specifically to urinary diversion procedures include observing for leakage of urine or stool from the anastomosis, maintaining renal function, assessing for signs and symptoms of peritonitis, maintaining integrity of the urinary diversion and urine collection devices, maintaining skin and stomal integrity, promoting a positive body image, and teaching the client how to manage the diversion.

The nurse checks the client's chart for information regarding the type and extent of surgery and orders for connection of catheters or drains, IV fluids, and analgesics. Clients will have multiple drainage tubes, ureteral stents, and a nasogastric tube. All urinary drainage tubes must be labeled, and the urine output from each catheter or stoma must be measured and recorded hourly.

Maintaining accurate intake and output measurements during the postoperative period is important because it indicates both renal function and the integrity of the urinary diversion structures. Obstruction of urine flow can severely damage the kidneys. If urinary drainage stops or decreases to less than 30 mL/hour, or if the client complains of back pain, the nurse needs to notify the physician immediately. Inspection of the urine includes checking for color, clarity, and presence of blood. It is essential immediately to report concentrated, cloudy, or bloody urine to the physician. Ureteral stents remain in place for several days after surgery.

The nasogastric tube is connected to low intermittent suction. This prevents distention and pressure on the suture line due to the collection of gas in the bowel. The nasogastric tube is removed once peristalsis has returned and the diet can be advanced. All laboratory reports are reviewed as soon as they are received and abnormalities reported to the physician promptly. The following sections address management issues specific to the most common procedures.

Ileal Conduit

A transparent ostomy bag is applied over the stoma to make stomal assessment easier. The nurse contacts the physician immediately if there is excessive bleeding, changes in the color of the stoma (e.g., from a normal to a cyanotic color), or separation of the stoma edges from the surrounding skin. The nurse uses gauze pads to clean mucus away from the stoma. Because the intestinal anastomosis can leak fecal material or the ileal conduit may leak urine into the peritoneal cavity, he or she observes for and promptly reports symptoms of peritonitis (e.g., abdominal tenderness or distention, fever, severe pain). Management of the urinary stoma is similar to management of a fecal stoma (see Chap. 48). The skin needs protection, the surgical dressings must be changed promptly when they become wet, and the appliances need care and cleansing. Each time he or she changes a temporary drainage bag, the nurse inspects the skin around the stoma for signs of infection and skin breakdown.

Continent Urinary Diversion (Kock Pouch, Indiana Pouch)

The nurse inspects the stoma for bleeding or cyanosis. He or she may irrigate the pouch, if ordered, to prevent mucous plugs or blood clots. The nurse teaches the client how to perform intermittent self-catheterization. Initially this is done every 1 to 2 hours but eventually will be performed every 4 to 6 hours.

Ureterosigmoidostomy

A catheter is inserted in the rectum to drain urine continuously. The nurse checks the amount and color of drainage from the rectal catheter every 1 or 2 hours and inspects the anal and gluteal areas for signs of early skin breakdown. The catheter is removed when peristalsis returns. Because the sigmoid colon reabsorbs urinary constituents, clients are prone to fluid and electrolyte imbalances throughout the postoperative period (as well as for the rest of their lives). Observation for signs of electrolyte losses is essential. The nurse teaches the client exercises to improve sphincter control. Once good control is achieved, the nurse instructs the client to void (rectally) every 2 hours to prevent reabsorption of fluid and electrolytes. Clients must never have enemas, suppositories, or laxatives.

Nursing Process for the Psychosocial Care of the Client Undergoing Urinary Diversion

Assessment

Assess the client's knowledge about the effects of surgery on sexual function. Up to 85% of men experience erectile dysfunction after urinary diversion. Women may have painful intercourse and lack lubrication. Ask the client about his or her current level of social activity and what changes he or she thinks will occur after surgery. Assess the client's understanding of long-term postoperative care.

Diagnosis, Planning, and Interventions

▶ **Risk for Ineffective Sexuality Patterns** related to erectile dysfunction (male) or dyspareunia (female)

▶ **Expected Outcome:** Client will regain erectile function or ease painful intercourse.

- Tactfully ask the client if he or she has any questions. *Asking provides an opportunity to discuss sexuality issues.*
- Encourage client and partner to share their feelings about alteration in sexual function. *Acknowledging the importance of sexual function and expression may assist the client and partner to seek sexual counseling and to explore alternative methods of expressing sexuality.*
- Discuss alternatives to sexual intercourse such as closeness and giving pleasure to a partner. Provide information about penile prosthesis for men and water-soluble lubricants for women. Inform women that Kegel exercises may ease painful intercourse. Discuss masturbation, either individual or mutual, as an option. *Alternatives to sexual intercourse enable and enhance sexual satisfaction that physical limitations may otherwise impede.*

▶ **Disturbed Body Image** related to change in appearance and function

▶ **Expected Outcome:** Client will accept altered appearance and perform self-care.

- Assess client's willingness to look at the stoma. Accept client's response and reinforce that anxiety is normal. Reassure client that nursing staff will provide care until he or she is ready. *Gradual exposure is part of rehabilitation. The nurse supports the client's process.*
- Discuss change in function and let client know what to expect when recovery from surgery is complete. Suggest a visit from an ostomate who can provide valuable personal information, support, and resources. *Providing information and group support assists the client to know that he or she is not alone and will be prepared to care for himself or herself.*
- Help client gain independence by reinforcing that self-care is quite manageable and providing time for practice. *Encouragement and support promote confidence and move the client from a dependent to an independent role.*

▶ Risk for Social Isolation related to fear of accidents or urine odor

▶ **Expected Outcome:** Client will maintain social relationships.

- Explain that odor-proof pouches or pouches with carbon filters or other odor barriers are available. A few drops of liquid deodorizer or diluted white vinegar also may assist in controlling odors. Suggest avoiding odor-producing foods, such as asparagus, eggs, or cheese. *A client may become socially isolated from the odors produced by the urinary diversion. Information about how to control odors will assist the client to implement measures and then to feel that friends, coworkers, and acquaintances will accept him or her.*
- Oral ascorbic acid may help to control odors. *Ascorbic acid helps to acidify urine and suppress urine odors.*
- Teach client to care for the pouch and to change it every 3 days if it is a one-piece pouch or every 4 to 7 days if it is a two-piece pouch. *Appropriate care assists in reducing odors and contributes to the client's level of confidence.*
- Tell client to empty the bag before it gets half full to prevent tension on the adhesive wafer and to eliminate source of odors. Inform the client to carry a spare pouch in case adhesive loosens while away from home. *These measures prevent accidents or embarrassment and provide the client with a sense of control and positive well-being.*
- Suggest drinking cranberry juice or using an appliance deodorant. *These measures reduce odors and assist the client to feel in control.*
- Suggest that the client contact the urostomy association for suggestions and additional support in alleviating anxiety. Instruct client with a ureterosigmoidostomy to avoid gas-forming foods. *Receiving support and accurate information contributes positively to a client's sense of well-being.*

▶ Risk for Ineffective Management of Therapeutic Regimen related to inadequate knowledge about stomal care

▶ **Expected Outcome:** Client will demonstrate ability to change ostomy pouch.

- Explain procedure for removing the old pouch and fitting and applying a new one. Tell client to change the pouch in the morning before consuming liquids and to insert a tampon or rolled gauze into the stoma to absorb urine during appliance change. Make sure the appliance fits well and the skin is completely dry when applying adhesive wafer. *Knowledge of specific procedures and treatment regimen increases a client's understanding and promotes responsibility for self-care.*
- Picture-frame the wafer with paper tape to seal edges. Show the client how to empty the pouch and attach it to an overnight drainage system. *These measures provide more control over the outcome and improve the client's ability to care for himself or herself.*
- Teach client to inspect the peristomal skin each time he or she changes the pouch. Advise using a liquid skin barrier to protect the skin. If abdominal skin must be shaved, use an electric razor. *These strategies prevent skin breakdown and promote early*

intervention. They also provide the client with the skill and knowledge to adequately care for himself or herself.

▶ Risk for Ineffective Management of Therapeutic Regimen related to inadequate knowledge about intermittent catheterization of continent urinary diversions (Kock pouch, Indiana pouch)

▶ **Expected Outcome:** Client will demonstrate ability to catheterize the pouch.

- Identify need for continuous drainage and frequent catheterizations in early postoperative period. Explain need for irrigations (to flush mucus and prevent plugging of catheter). *Understanding the rationales for the procedures promotes learning and ability for self-care.*
- Teach client to self-catheterize by lubricating catheter, inserting it into pouch, and allowing urine to drain into the toilet bowl. *Demonstration of procedures assists the client to develop competence and confidence in the self-care activities.*

Evaluation of Expected Outcomes

The client discusses methods for resuming sexual activity and alternatives to sexual intercourse. He or she states methods to avoid accidents and control urine odor. The client verbalizes a willingness to maintain social activity. He or she correctly changes the ostomy appliance and successfully self-catheterizes continent pouch. Client and Family Teaching 59-4 outlines information to include in a teaching plan. ●

TRAUMA

Trauma to the bladder or urethra is potentially harmful and frequently requires surgical intervention.

Pathophysiology and Etiology

Various types of injury can affect the urinary tract. Gunshot and stab wounds, crushing injuries, and forceful blows can result in tears, hemorrhage, or penetration of one or more parts. Some penetrating bladder injuries are small, whereas others are large, with a rapid collection of urine in the peritoneal cavity. Injuries to the kidney area may result in bruising or tearing of the kidney and its capsule. Depending on the severity of the injury, blood and urine may leak into the peritoneal cavity.

Assessment Findings

Signs and Symptoms

Symptoms vary according to the area affected and the type of injury. Anuria, hematuria, pain in the abdomen (which may indicate bleeding or leakage of urine into the abdominal cavity), pain in the bladder or kidney areas, and symptoms of shock may be indicators of urinary tract injury. During treatment of a client with extensive injury, an indwelling catheter may be inserted, and hematuria or lack of urine output may be the first sign of a traumatic injury to the urinary tract. Certain other types of injuries, such as stab or gunshot

Client and Family Teaching 59-4
Management of a Urinary Diversion

Material included in a client teaching plan is specific to the type of surgery, the surgeon's specific discharge orders, or both. Consider the following:

- Watch for signs and symptoms of fluid and electrolyte imbalances as instructed.
- Keep closed collection containers below the level of the stoma. Keep tubing that connects the catheter or collection appliance to the closed drainage system straight to prevent urine from collecting in a curve of the tube. Avoid kinks that prevent the drainage of urine.
- Drink adequate fluids. Note color of the urine. If urine appears darker than usual, more fluids may be needed. Call physician if urine is dark in spite of an adequate fluid intake.
- Take medications as prescribed by the physician. Do not omit or stop taking the drugs. Do not take or use any non-prescription drug without first checking with the physician. Clients with an ureterosigmoidostomy must not use laxatives or enemas.
- Control odors with cranberry juice, yogurt, or buttermilk. Avoid foods that may impart an odor to the urine, such as asparagus, cheese, or eggs.
- Consult with an enterostomal therapist regarding skin care techniques. Keep skin clean. When changing the adhesive

wafer (to which the urostomy collection bag is attached), remove all remaining adhesive before applying a new wafer.
- Drain the continent urostomy four times a day or as directed by the physician.
- Wash the urinary collection pouch thoroughly after changing. Rinse the pouch with or soak in a solution of vinegar and water if crystals form in the pouch.
- Contact physician if any of the following occur:
  - Fever
  - Chills
  - Blood in the urine
  - Failure of a stoma or catheter to drain urine
  - Skin problems around the stoma
  - Weight loss (>5 lbs)
  - Loss of appetite (more than a few days)
  - Inability to insert the catheter in the continent urostomy
  - Pain in the flank (kidney area or lower abdomen)
  - Signs of fluid or electrolyte imbalance
  - Any unusual symptom or problem

---

wounds, may be immediately identified because of outward signs of injury (e.g., entry wounds on skin surface).

Diagnostic Findings
Injury to the urinary tract initially may be overlooked when the client has incurred widespread, massive injuries. Abdominal x-rays, cystoscopy, IVP, and exploratory surgery may be used to identify the type and location of the injury.

Surgical Management
Treatment depends on the type, location, and extent of injury as well as on the condition of the client. For example, a stab wound in the kidney area may require emergency exploratory surgery. Once the kidney is exposed, the physician needs to determine if the trauma to the kidney can be repaired or if the kidney must be removed immediately. Examples of surgeries that may be performed for urinary tract trauma include cystostomy (temporary or permanent), nephrectomy, insertion of a nephrostomy tube, repair (reanastomosis) of the ureter, and cystectomy.

Nursing Management
The most important nursing task is recognition of abnormal findings. Lack of urinary output, diffuse and severe abdominal pain, and hematuria are examples of signs and symptoms that may indicate an injury to the urinary tract. In some instances, the injury may be such that symptoms do not appear for several hours or days after the initial trauma.

Other nursing management depends on the surgical interventions performed and the symptoms the client experiences. In addition, the nurse needs to focus on the client's physical and emotional needs related to the trauma.

CRITICAL THINKING EXERCISES

1. A client has recurrent cystitis. Her physician wants to perform a cystoscopy and retrograde pyelograms. She asks you why she needs these tests because the medication she took in the past cured her problem. What explanation would you give?
2. Discuss the possible psychosocial effects of interstitial cystitis.
3. A client has an ureterosigmoidostomy. What teaching will you do regarding long-term follow-up and care?
4. A client had a radical cystectomy with an ileal conduit. When the LPN observes the ileal conduit through the transparent urostomy pouch, she notes that the stomal opening is red and draining urine with mucus. What action should the LPN take?

NCLEX-STYLE REVIEW QUESTIONS

1. A client has just undergone a surgical procedure for removal of a malignant tumor. As a result, the client's urine is diverted to a stomal pouch. Which of the following

diet-related suggestions would the nurse be most likely to suggest so that the client remains odor free?
1. Eat spicy foods.
2. Eat eggs, asparagus, or cheese.
3. Drink cranberry juice.
4. Drink tea, coffee, and colas.

2. A client who undergoes litholapaxy for removing bladder stones is anxious to know how long the urethral catheter should be kept in place. The nurse most correctly responds that catheters generally remain in place for how long?
1. 6 to 7 days
2. 1 to 2 days
3. 2 to 3 days
4. 3 to 4 days

3. If a client says she does the following, which one indicates the best measure for preventing a urinary tract infection?
1. Drying the perineum thoroughly after bowel elimination
2. Performing appropriate handwashing after bowel elimination
3. Using a feminine hygiene spray after bowel elimination
4. Wiping away from the urinary meatus after bowel elimination

4. The physician prescribes a urinary anti-infective combination of trimethoprim (Proloprim) and sulfamethoxazole (Bactrim) twice a day for a client with acute pyelonephritis. Which nursing instruction is most appropriate for preventing crystal formation in the urine?
1. Avoid carbonated soft drinks.
2. Drink 3 quarts of water daily.
3. Eat more acidic citrus fruits.
4. Take the medication with food.

5. A client whose bladder cancer has been unresponsive to treatment will have his bladder surgically removed and an ileal conduit will be created to facilitate urinary elimination. When the client asks the nurse to clarify the surgeon's explanation of the procedure, which statement is most correct?
1. "Urine will be eliminated with stool from the rectum."
2. "Urine will drain from an abdominal opening."
3. "Your urine will be deposited in your small intestine."
4. "Your urine will empty from a special catheter."

60

Introduction to the Musculoskeletal System

Learning Objectives

On completion of this chapter, you will be able to:

1. Describe major structures and functions of the musculoskeletal system.
2. Discuss elements of the nursing assessment of the musculoskeletal system.
3. Identify common diagnostic and laboratory tests used in the evaluation of musculoskeletal disorders.
4. Discuss the nursing management of clients undergoing tests for musculoskeletal disorders.

The musculoskeletal system consists of bones, muscles, joints, tendons, ligaments, cartilage, and bursae. It supports the body and facilitates movement. Other functions include storage of calcium, phosphorus, magnesium, and fluoride; production of blood cells in the bone marrow; and protection and support to body organs, such as the lungs, heart, and brain. Injury to or disease in any part of the musculoskeletal system can cause pain, immobility, or disability and potentially affect quality of life.

ANATOMY AND PHYSIOLOGY

Bones

The human body has 206 bones. The bones of the skeleton are classified as:

- *Short bones,* such as those in the fingers and toes
- *Long bones,* such as the femur and ulna
- *Flat bones,* such as the sternum
- *Irregular bones,* such as the vertebrae

There are two types of bony tissue. The first is **cancellous bone**, or spongy bone, which is light and contains many spaces. The second is **cortical bone,** or compact bone, which is dense and hard. Both types are found in varying amounts in all bones. Cancellous bone is found at the rounded, irregular ends, or **epiphyses,** of long bones. Cortical bony tissue covers bones and is found chiefly in the long shafts, or **diaphyses,** of bones in the arms and legs. The combination of the two types of bony tissue provides strength and support, yet keeps the skeleton light to promote endurance during activity.

Bone is composed of cells, protein matrix, and mineral deposits. The three types of bone cells are osteo*blasts,* osteo*cytes,* and osteo*clasts.* Cells that build bones are called **osteoblasts**. These cells secrete bone matrix (mostly collagen), in which inorganic minerals, such as calcium salts, are deposited. This process of *ossification* and *calcification* transforms the osteoblasts into mature bone cells, called **osteocytes,** which are involved in maintaining bone tissue. During times of rapid bone growth or bone injury, osteocytes function as osteoblasts to form new bone. **Osteoclasts** are the cells involved in the destruction, resorption, and remodeling of bone.

During growth, bones primarily lengthen. The diameter also increases when osteoclasts break down previously formed bone, however, making the central canal wider. When skeletal growth is complete, the osteoclasts, which are part of the mononuclear phagocyte system (blood cells involved in ingesting particulate matter—or recycling old cells), continue with the remodeling of bones by balancing bone *resorption* with new bone cell replacement. Bone formation and resorption continue throughout life. The greatest activity occurs from birth through puberty. Box 60-1 reviews factors that affect bone formation.

A layer of tissue called **periosteum** covers the bones (but not the joints). The inner layer of periosteum contains the osteoblasts necessary for bone formation. The periosteum is rich in blood and lymph vessels and supplies the bone with nourishment.

Inside the bones are two types of bone marrow: red and yellow. **Red bone marrow,** found primarily in the sternum, ileum, vertebrae, and ribs, manufactures blood cells and hemoglobin. Long bones have **yellow bone marrow,** which consists primarily of fat cells and connective tissue. If the blood cell supply becomes compromised, the yellow marrow may take on the characteristics of red marrow and begin producing blood cells.

Muscles

There are three kinds of muscles: skeletal, smooth, and cardiac. **Skeletal muscles** are voluntary muscles; impulses that travel from efferent nerves of the brain and spinal cord control their function. The skeletal muscles promote movement

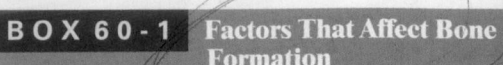

BOX 60-1 Factors That Affect Bone Formation

Bone Formation Facilitators
Calcium
Phosphorus
Estrogen
Testosterone
Calcitonin
Vitamins A, C, D
Growth hormone
Exercise
Insulin

Bone Formation Retardants
Estrogen/androgen deficiency
Vitamin deficiency
Starvation
Diabetes
Steroids
Inactivity/immobility
Heparin
Excess parathyroid hormone

of the bones of the skeleton. Examples of skeletal muscles are the biceps in the arms and the gastrocnemius in the calves.

Skeletal muscle is composed of muscle cells or fibers that contain several myofibrils. Sliding filaments called *sarcomeres* make up myofibrils. They are the contractile units of skeletal muscle. Impulses from the central nervous system cause the release of acetylcholine at the motor end plate of the motor neuron that innervates the muscle. As a result, calcium ions are released, and the release stimulates actin and myosin in the sarcomeres to slide closer together, resulting in contraction of the muscle. When calcium is depleted, the actin and myosin fibers move apart, causing relaxation of the sarcomeres, and thus the muscle.

Smooth and cardiac muscles are involuntary muscles; their activity is controlled by mechanisms in their tissue of origin and by neurotransmitters released from the autonomic nervous system. Smooth muscles are found mainly in the walls of certain organs or cavities of the body, such as the stomach, intestine, blood vessels, and ureters. Cardiac muscle is found only in the heart.

TABLE 60-1 Types and Characteristics of Joints

TYPE	CHARACTERISTIC	EXAMPLE
Synarthrodial joints	Immovable	At the suture line of skull between the temporal and occipital bones
Amphiarthrodial joints	Slightly movable	Between the vertebrae
Diarthrodial joints (also called *synovial joints*)	Freely movable	Gliding joint: fingers
		Hinge joint: elbow
		Pivot joint: ends of radius and ulna
		Condyloid joint: between the wrist and forearm
		Saddle joint: between the wrist and metacarpal bone of the thumb
		Ball-and-socket joint: hip

Joints

A **joint** is the junction between two or more bones. Table 60-1 outlines types and characteristics of joints. Free moving joints, or diarthrodial joints, make up most skeletal joints. They allow certain movements. Terms related to diarthrodial joint movement are presented in Box 60-2. The surfaces of diarthrodial joints are covered with hyaline cartilage, which reduces friction during joint movement. The space between is the joint cavity, which is enclosed by a fibrous capsule lined with synovial membrane. This membrane produces synovial fluid, which acts as a lubricant.

Tendons

Tendons are cordlike structures that attach muscles to the periosteum of the bone. A muscle has two or more attachments. One is called the *origin* and is more fixed. The other is called the *insertion* and is more movable. When a muscle contracts, both attachments are pulled, and the insertion is drawn closer to the origin. An example can be found in the biceps of the arm, which has two origin tendons, attached to the scapula, and one insertion tendon, attached to the radius. When the biceps contracts, the lower arm (with the insertion tendon) moves toward the upper arm (with the origin tendons).

Ligaments

Ligaments consisting of fibrous tissue connect two adjacent, freely movable bones. They help protect the joints by stabilizing their surfaces and keeping them in proper alignment. In some instances, ligaments completely enclose a joint.

Cartilage

Cartilage is a firm, dense type of connective tissue that consists of cells embedded in a substance called the *matrix*. The matrix is firm and compact, thus enabling it to withstand pressure and torsion. The primary functions of cartilage are to reduce friction between articular surfaces, absorb shocks, and reduce stress on joint surfaces.

Hyaline or articular cartilage covers the surface of movable joints, such as the elbow, and protects the surface of these joints. Other types of cartilage include costal cartilage, which connects the ribs and sternum; semilunar cartilage, which is one of the cartilages of the knee joint; fibrous cartilage, found between the vertebrae (intervertebral discs); and elastic cartilage, found in the larynx, epiglottis, and outer ear.

Bursae

A **bursa** is a small sac filled with synovial fluid. Bursae reduce friction between areas, such as tendon and bone and tendon and ligament. Inflammation of these sacs is called *bursitis*.

ASSESSMENT

History

The focus of the initial history depends on whether the client has a chronic disorder or a recent injury. If the disorder is long-standing, the nurse obtains a thorough medical, drug, and allergy history. If the client is injured, the nurse finds out when and how the trauma occurred. He or she

---

BOX 60-2 **Glossary of Diarthrodial Movement**

Adduction: Movement toward the midline of the body
Abduction: movement away from the midline of the body

Dorsiflexion: Movement that flexes hand back toward body or foot toward leg

Flexion: Bending of a joint
Extension: Return movement from flexion
Hyperextension: Extension beyond straight or neutral position

Supination: Rotation of the forearm so that palm of hand is up
Pronation: Rotation of forearm so that palm of hand is down

Rotation: Turning or movement of a part around its axis
External (outward) rotation: Movement away from the center
Internal (inward) rotation: Movement toward the center

compiles a list of symptoms that includes information about the onset, duration, and location of discomfort or pain. Determining whether activity makes the symptoms better or worse is important. The nurse also identifies associated symptoms, such as muscle cramping or skin lesions, and asks the client if the problem interferes with activities of daily living. If the client has an open wound, the nurse ascertains when the client last received a tetanus immunization.

The nurse must obtain a history of past disorders and medical or surgical treatments as soon as possible. Attention to chronic or concurrent disorders, such as diabetes mellitus, is essential. In addition, the nurse obtains a family history, especially when relatives have had similar symptoms, and an occupational history. Nutrition Notes 60-1 outlines the role of nutrition in the client's musculoskeletal health.

▶ **Stop, Think, and Respond Exercise 60-1**

A neighbor calls you and states that he tripped and fell, spraining his ankle. When you arrive to help him, what questions should you ask? What should you observe?

Nutrition Notes 60-1
Nutrition and Musculoskeletal Health

● Although bone formation and resorption continue throughout life, net bone loss exceeds net bone gain in all people after peak bone mass is attained, sometime between ages 30 and 35 years. An adequate calcium intake before that time helps maximize peak bone mass; the denser the bones, the less susceptible they are to fracture.

● Calcium intake recommendations are set at 1000 mg/day for adults younger than 50 years of age and 1200 mg/day for those over age 50. This translates to about four servings from the dairy group each day. Clients who cannot or are unwilling to consume ample dairy products are not likely to meet their calcium requirement through diet alone.

● Nondairy sources of calcium include dark green leafy vegetables, sardines, canned salmon with bones, broccoli, and calcium-fortified orange juice. With the exception of calcium-fortified orange juice, the body does not absorb calcium from nondairy sources well.

● Vitamin D protects against bone loss and decreases the risk of fracture by facilitating the absorption of calcium from food and supplements. Without adequate vitamin D, calcium is excreted, not absorbed, even if calcium intake is adequate. Many people do not consume enough vitamin D because dietary sources are limited. Many people do not make adequate vitamin D because synthesis is impaired by northern latitude, sunscreen, dark skin, and aging.

● Vitamin K, magnesium, and potassium—nutrients found in fruits and vegetables—help maintain bone density.

Physical Examination

For a general musculoskeletal assessment, the nurse observes the client's ability to ambulate, sit, stand, and perform activities requiring fine motor skills, such as grasping objects. General inspection includes examining the client for symmetry, size, and contour of extremities and random movements. A spinal inspection includes identifying spinal curvatures (Fig. 60-1):

- *Kyphosis*—exaggerated convex curvature of the thoracic spine (humpback)
- *Lordosis*—excessive concave curvature of the lumbar spine (swayback)
- *Scoliosis*—lateral curvature of the spine

The nurse palpates the muscles and joints to identify swelling, degree of firmness, local warm areas, and any involuntary movements. To test the client's muscle strength, the nurse applies force to the client's extremity as the client pushes against that force. The nurse also must perform a neurovascular assessment (Table 60-2), which includes assessing range of motion for the joints, taking care not to force movement. The nurse notes any abnormal muscle movements such as spasms or tremors. In addition, the nurse:

- Looks for abnormal size or alignment and symmetry, comparing one side with the other.

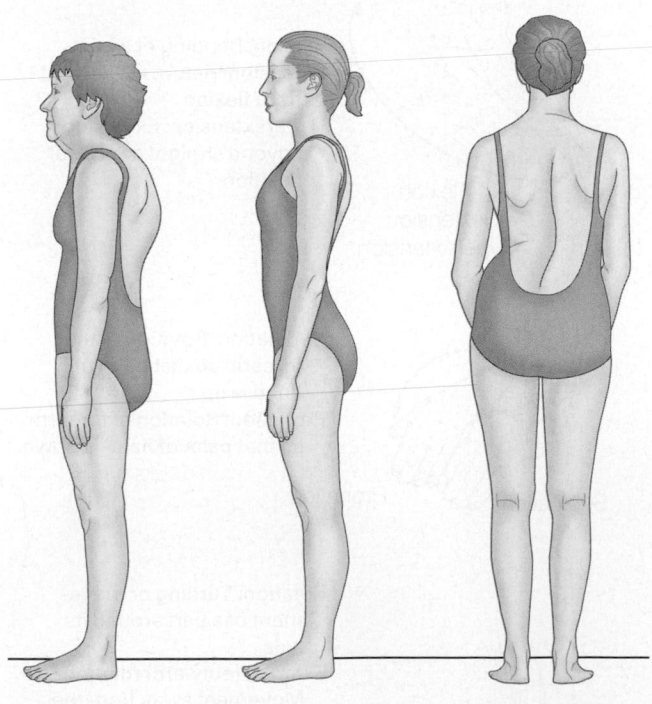

A: Kyphosis   **B:** Lordosis   **C:** Scoliosis

FIGURE 60-1 Common spinal curvatures include kyphosis, lordosis, and scoliosis.

TABLE 60-2 Neurovascular Assessment Findings in Musculoskeletal Assessment

ASSESSMENTS	NORMAL FINDINGS	ABNORMAL FINDINGS
Circulation		
Distal pulses	Present and strong	Absent or weak
Capillary refill	Color returns to compressed nailbed within 3 seconds	Nailbed stays blanched after 3 seconds
Skin color	Similar to color in other body areas	Pale or dusky
Skin temperature	Warm	Cold
Local edema	Absent	+1 to +4 swelling
Sensation		
Arm injury	Can identify pressure applied to the tip of the index finger (median nerve) and the fifth finger (ulnar nerve), web between the thumb (radial nerve)	Numb to touch or feels abnormal sensation, like tingling or burning
Leg injury	Can identify pressure applied to great toe (peroneal nerve) and sole of the foot at the base of the toes (posterior tibial nerve) without observing the stimulus	Same as above
Mobility		
Arm injury	Can spread fingers on affected hand (ulnar nerve)	Weak or cannot move fingers
	Can press thumb to last digit on affected hand (median nerve)	Cannot approximate thumb to finger
		Cannot extend thumb
	Demonstrates the "hitchhiker's sign" with affected hand, can flex and extend wrist (radial nerve)	Wrist-drop is apparent.
Leg injury	Can flex and extend ankle (peroneal and posterior tibial nerves)	Foot-drop is apparent.
Pain	Proportional to injury but relieved with analgesia or nursing interventions	Constant or increased despite implementation of pain-relieving techniques

- Inspects and palpates for pain, tenderness, swelling, and redness.
- Observes the degree of movement and range of motion, but never persists beyond the point of pain.
- Tests for muscle strength.
- Inspects for muscle wasting.

Depending on the symptoms and findings, additional assessments may include looking for changes in gait and body posture, favoring one side over the other, and ability to bend and twist the trunk, head, and extremities. As clients age, they experience many changes in the musculoskeletal system. After 35 years, people generally experience loss of bone mass and height and changes in the structure of the spine and joints. Table 60-3 describes musculoskeletal changes related to aging. It is essential to assess clients for musculoskeletal changes because of their potential impact on activities of daily living.

 Gerontologic Considerations

- Changes in structure, function, chemical composition, and heridiraty genetic patterns affect the musculoskeletal system in older adults. With age, the fibrocartilage of intervertebral disks becomes thinner and drier, causing compression of the disks of the spinal column, and the water content of joint cartilage decreases, leading to a height loss of as much as 1 to 2 cm every 2 decades, and possible formation of dorsal kyphosis.

- In both men and women, the amount of bone formed during remodeling decreases with age. Bone resorption occurring more rapidly than bone formation increases the risk for skeletal fractures.

- Age-related declines of estrogen and testosterone production cause bone loss. Prolonged immobilization, hypercalciuria, malabsorption, cigarette smoking, or alcoholism may accelerate loss of bone mass.

- Maintaining an active lifestyle and obtaining adequate calcium and vitamin D can delay the decline in muscle strength and bone mass among older adults.

If the client has a traumatic injury, physical assessment begins with taking vital signs. Further assessment depends on the type and area of injury. As the nurse conducts the assessment, he or she maintains standard precautions. The nurse needs to cut the clothing from around an injured area if there is no other way to examine the client. Comparing structures and assessment findings on one side of the body with those on the opposite side assists the nurse in determining the degree of injury. Although the nurse must be thorough, it

TABLE 60-3 Age-Related Musculoskeletal Changes

STRUCTURE	STRUCTURAL CHANGE	FUNCTIONAL CHANGE	SIGNS AND SYMPTOMS
Bones	Gradual, progressive loss of bone mass after age 35 Vertebral collapse	Increased bone fragility; fracture-prone—most commonly vertebrae, hip, and wrist	Loss of height Posture changes Kyphosis Flexion of hips and knees Back pain Osteoporosis Fracture
Muscles	Increased collagen—results in fibrosis Decreased muscle mass (atrophy); wasting Decreased tendon elasticity	Loss of strength and flexibility Weakness and fatigue Stumbling Falls	Loss of strength Diminished agility Decreased endurance Prolonged response time or decreased reaction time Decreased muscle tone Increased frequency of falls Broad base of support
Joints	Cartilage progressively deteriorates Intervertebral discs thin	Stiffness and reduced flexibility Pain Difficulty performing ADLs	Decreased range of motion Decreased flexibility Stiffness Loss of height
Ligaments	Relaxed ligaments (decreased strength; weakness)	Postural joint abnormality Weakness	Joint pain with movement—improves with rest Crepitus Joint swelling/enlargement Degenerative joint disease (osteoarthritis)

also is important to be gentle, recognizing that assessment techniques may increase the client's pain. The examination includes the following:

- Observing for swelling, external bleeding, or bruising
- Palpating the peripheral pulses
- Evaluating peripheral circulation; assessing peripheral pulse (rate and character), skin coloration (pink, gray, pale, ashen), temperature, and capillary refill time
- Checking the sensation of the injured part
- Looking for broken skin, open wounds, superficial or embedded debris in or around the wound, protrusion of bone or other tissue from the wound
- Examining for injury beyond the original area; for example, auscultating the chest and abdomen if an abdominal or thoracic injury occurred or checking the pupils and mental status if a head injury occurred
- Looking for malalignment of the injured limb
- Assessing for pain, noting the type and location

The physician needs to examine the client before the nurse touches, cleans, or disturbs open wounds and before moving the injured extremity.

Diagnostic Tests
Imaging Procedures
Radiographic films, computed tomography (CT), and magnetic resonance imaging (MRI) help identify traumatic disorders,

such as fractures and dislocations, and other bone disorders, such as malignant bone lesions, joint deformities, calcification, degenerative changes, osteoporosis, and joint disease.

An **arthrogram** is a radiographic examination of a joint, usually the knee or shoulder. The physician first injects a local anesthetic and then inserts a needle into the joint space. Fluoroscopy may be used to verify correct placement of the needle. The synovial fluid in the joint is aspirated and sent to the laboratory for analysis. A contrast medium is then injected, and x-ray films are taken. After undergoing arthrography, the client is informed that he or she may hear crackling or clicking noises in the joint for up to 2 days. Noises beyond this time are abnormal; the client should report them.

▶ *Stop, Think, and Respond Exercise 60-2*
Review your knowledge of MRIs. What precautions need to be adhered to before a client undergoes MRI?

Arthroscopy
Arthroscopy is the internal inspection of a joint using an instrument called an *arthroscope*. The most common use of arthroscopy is visualization of the knee joint, a common site of injury. After administering a local or general anesthetic, the physician inserts a large-bore needle into the joint and injects sterile normal saline solution to distend the joint.

After inserting the arthroscope, the examiner inspects the joint for signs of injury or deterioration. Joint fluid may be removed and sent to the laboratory for examination. Depending on the findings, the physician sometimes can use the arthroscope to perform therapeutic procedures, such as removing bits of torn or floating cartilage.

Afterward, the client's entire leg is elevated without flexing the knee. A cold pack is placed over the bulky dressing covering the site where the arthroscope was inserted. A prescribed analgesic is administered as necessary. Nursing Guidelines 60-1 outlines the nurse's role in assisting the client undergoing arthroscopy.

Arthrocentesis

Arthrocentesis is the aspiration of synovial fluid. The client receives local anesthesia just before this procedure. The physician inserts a large needle into the joint and removes the fluid. Synovial fluid may be aspirated to relieve discomfort caused by an excessive accumulation in the joint space or to inject a drug, such as a corticosteroid preparation. The removed synovial fluid may be sent to the laboratory for microscopic examination or for culture and sensitivity studies. Arthrocentesis also may be performed during an arthrogram or arthroscopy.

Synovial Fluid Analysis

Synovial fluid is aspirated and examined to diagnose disorders such as traumatic arthritis, septic arthritis (caused by a microorganism), gout, rheumatic fever, and systemic lupus erythematosus. Normally, synovial fluid is clear and nearly colorless. Laboratory examination of synovial fluid may include microscopic examination for blood cells, crystals, and formed debris that may be present in the joint space after an injury. If an infection is suspected, culture and sensitivity

studies are ordered. A chemical analysis for substances such as protein and glucose also may be performed.

Bone Densitometry

Bone densitometry estimates bone density. Radiography of the wrist, hip, or spine helps to determine bone mineral density (BMD). Bone density scanning or dual-energy x-ray absorptiometry (DXA or DEXA) uses advanced radiographic technology to measure BMD. DEXA is most often done on the lower spine and hips. Portable DEXA devices use x-rays or ultrasound to measure the quantity and quality of wrist, finger, or heel bone and to provide an estimate of bone density.

Bone Scan

A **bone scan** uses the intravenous injection of a radionuclide to detect the uptake of the radioactive substance by the bone. A bone scan may be ordered to detect metastatic bone lesions, fractures, and certain types of inflammatory disorders. The radionuclide is taken up in areas of increased metabolism, which occur in bone cancer, metastatic bone disease, and osteomyelitis (bone infection).

Electromyography

Electromyography tests the electrical potential of the muscles and nerves leading to the muscles. It is done to evaluate muscle weakness or deterioration, pain, and disability and to differentiate muscle and nerve problems. The physician inserts needle electrodes into selected muscles and uses electrical current to stimulate the muscles. An oscilloscope records responses to the electrical stimuli. If the client experiences discomfort after the study, warm compresses to the area help relieve the discomfort.

Biopsy

A biopsy is done to identify the composition of bone, muscle, or synovium. The specimen may be removed with a needle or excised surgically while the client is under general anesthesia. Afterward, the nurse observes the site for signs of bleeding or swelling, assesses for pain, applies ice to the site, and administers analgesics as indicated.

Blood Tests

A complete blood count (which includes a red blood cell count, hemoglobin level, white blood cell count, and differential) may be ordered to detect infection, inflammation, or anemia. Examples of other diagnostic blood tests and findings of various musculoskeletal disorders include:

- Elevated alkaline phosphatase level, which may indicate bone tumors and healing fractures
- Elevated acid phosphatase level, which may indicate Paget's disease (a disorder characterized by excessive bone destruction and disorganized repair) and metastatic cancer
- Decreased serum calcium level, which may indicate osteomalacia, osteoporosis, and bone tumors

 NURSING GUIDELINES 60-1

Assisting the Client Through Arthroscopy

Before the Procedure

- Explain the procedure.
- Ensure that the client has signed the informed consent form.
- Verify that the client has been NPO for at least 6 hours.
- Administer preoperative medications, if ordered.

After the Procedure

- Instruct client to report unusual pain, bleeding, drainage, or swelling at the arthroscopic site.
- Advise client to resume usual diet as tolerated.
- Review discharge instructions with the client and explain medication regimen.
- Inspect dressing before discharge.

- Increased serum phosphorus level, which may indicate bone tumors and healing fractures
- Elevated serum uric acid level, which may indicate gout (treated or untreated)
- Elevated antinuclear antibody level, which may indicate systemic lupus erythematosus, a connective tissue disorder

Urine Tests

When ordered, the nurse collects 24-hour urine samples for analysis to determine levels of uric acid and calcium excretion. In gout, the 24-hour excretion of uric acid is elevated. Elevated calcium levels are found in metastatic bone lesions and in clients with prolonged immobility.

NURSING MANAGEMENT

Some diagnostic tests are performed while the client is assessed in the emergency department, on an outpatient basis, or after admission for treatment of the disorder. The nurse implements protocols necessary to prepare the client for the diagnostic examination, identifies and sends collected specimens to the laboratory, and manages the client's safe recovery after invasive procedures.

If the client has a chronic disorder, the nurse obtains a general medical history and a description of the current symptoms. He or she compiles drug and allergy histories. An allergy to iodine and seafood may be a contraindication to performing an arthrogram or other test in which a contrast medium is instilled.

No special care is required after most laboratory tests, general radiography, or a bone scan. If the client has had an invasive joint examination, the nurse inspects the area for swelling and bleeding or serous drainage. He or she changes or reinforces dressings as needed. If the client has severe pain in the area, the nurse must notify the physician, who may order the application of ice and an analgesic for pain or discomfort.

In the case of a traumatic injury, the nurse obtains information regarding the injury from the client, the person accompanying the client, or paramedics and ambulance personnel. He or she takes vital signs during the initial examination and at frequent intervals until the client's condition stabilizes. The nurse also checks the neurovascular status of the affected limb, including circulation, motion, and sensation. Keeping the client calm and promoting comfort are essential measures. For example, if the client has an injury of the arm, the nurse prepares a sling to ease pain until treatment can be initiated.

Nursing Process for the Client With a Musculoskeletal Injury

Assessment

Assess the client's injury in terms of its location, nature, and effects on mobility. Also determine the circulatory status to the injured area by checking circulation, sensation, and mobility, if it is not

Client and Family Teaching 60-1
Musculoskeletal Care

The nurse includes the following information:

- Report signs and symptoms, such as excessive pain or throbbing, prolonged or fresh bleeding, swelling, skin color changes, decrease in sensation, or purulent drainage
- Maintain any special body position that the nurse instructs you to take.
- Resume bathing and activity as directed by physician.
- Resume work and other activities per physician's orders.
- Review purpose of prescribed drugs, how to take them, and possible side effects
- Arrange date for a follow-up appointment with the physician, if one is required
- Demonstrate how to remove and reapply dressings, and how to apply an immobilizer or sling, if one is used
- Demonstrate safe crutch-walking gait, if crutches are temporarily needed

contraindicated. Assessing the client's level of pain is essential. Monitor the client's vital signs and closely observe for signs of shock.

Diagnosis, Planning, and Interventions

Provide a brief, broad overview of diagnostic tests or treatments, because the client will find it difficult to comprehend details while anxious. Provide the client and family with information about how long the test or examination will take, where it will be done, and what preparations (if any) are necessary. Allow the client an opportunity to ask questions or make comments as he or she processes the information. Before carrying out any preliminary activities before a diagnostic test, describe what is about to be done.

Invasive procedures, such as arthroscopy, and treatment procedures require the client to sign a consent form. The physician is responsible for explaining the purpose of the procedure, its risks and benefits, and available alternatives. Repeat or clarify the physician's explanations. After an outpatient procedure, the physician often gives the client special instructions for self-care. Because recalling information from memory can lead to confusion or injury, however, also provide written discharge instructions. Client and Family Teaching 60-1 discusses further education points. Additional diagnoses, expected outcomes, and interventions include the following:

▶ Acute Pain related to tissue injury

▶ Expected Outcome: Client will have relief from pain.

- Minimize or avoid moving the painful body part. *Doing so prevents increased pain and helps the client to relax.*
- If the client must be moved from a stretcher, wheelchair, or an examination table, request sufficient help and support the

joints above and below the area of discomfort during transfer. *Sufficient support prevents pain and avoids increasing discomfort.*

- Support an acutely or chronically inflamed joint in a comfortable position. *Maintaining a neutral position reduces pain.*
- Elevate a swollen extremity as long as doing so does not potentiate the trauma from an injury. Alternatively, cradle a painful arm in a sling when the client is up and about. *These measures reduce swelling and, subsequently, pain.*
- Observe for signs of respiratory depression if administering a prescribed narcotic analgesic for pain relief. *Opioids may cause respiratory depression and lead to sedation in a client susceptible to shock after a traumatic injury.*
- Notify physician if pain increases or is unrelieved. *Persistent pain may indicate further injury or sequelae to trauma.*

▶ **Risk for Impaired Tissue Perfusion** related to swelling, inflammation, or inactivity imposed by injury

▶ **Expected Outcome:** Client will maintain tissue perfusion in the injured area as evidenced by normal neurovascular assessment findings.

- Keep a swollen body part above the level of the heart. *This position promotes venous circulation and relieves edema.*
- Consult with the physician about applying a cold pack if an injury is recent. *Cold reduces circulation to the affected area and may impair neurovascular health.*
- In cases of head injury, elevate the client's head slightly while keeping the neck neutral. *Such positioning reduces the risk of further injury.*
- Report the absence of a peripheral pulse and severe pain immediately. *These findings may indicate ischemia.*

▶ **Anxiety** related to pain and injury, its treatment, and the potential for altered mobility

▶ **Expected Outcome:** Client's anxiety will be reduced as evidenced by vital signs within normal range and no signs of being overly alert or easily startled.

- Relieve discomfort as much as possible. *Doing so eliminates at least one aspect of the client's concerns.*
- Call the client by name; be empathic and attentive. *Attention to the client's needs promotes relaxation and comfort.*
- Instill confidence by demonstrating technical skill and competence in explanations or preparations for tests or treatments. *A confident nurse can help reduce a client's anxiety.*
- Speak quietly in simple sentences that the client can understand. *Understanding reduces anxiety.*
- Allow a supportive family member to stay with the client if possible. *This measure can comfort the client.*

Evaluation of Expected Outcomes

The client states that medication and positioning have relieved pain. Neurovascular status remains intact, as evidenced by good perfusion, strong pulses, ability to tense muscles, and appropriate sensation. The client has a calm demeanor and states that he or she feels less anxious. ●

CRITICAL THINKING EXERCISES

1. A client for whom you are caring in a nursing home falls. What assessments would you make?
2. What signs and symptoms would indicate that the tissue in an injured extremity is not being adequately perfused?
3. The nurse is conducting an assessment of the client's physical mobility and wants to determine the client's ability to abduct the fingers in each hand. What instructions should the nurse give the client?
4. Consider your acquired knowledge related to mobility and immobility. A client has injured his ankle. What initial steps should you take to prevent swelling and further injury?

NCLEX-STYLE REVIEW QUESTIONS

1. A client is admitted to a medical unit. The admitting nurse recognizes that which of the following situations place this client at risk for fractures? Select all that apply.
   1. The client drinks three glasses of milk daily.
   2. The client has a decreased intake related to cancer treatments.
   3. The client has a history of diabetes mellitus.
   4. The client periodically takes steroids for a long history of asthma.
   5. The client claims to walk 1 mile every day.
2. A nurse is assessing a client's range of motion. To determine the client's ability to pronate the forearm, what question should the nurse ask the client?
   1. "Can you extend the elbow in a straight position?"
   2. "Can you flex your wrist toward the forearm?"
   3. "Can you move the elbow away from your body?"
   4. "Can you turn the hand so that the palm is down?"
3. The nurse is assessing the client's circulation in the right leg following an injury. Which findings need further action?
   1. Capillary refill is longer than 3 seconds.
   2. Peripheral pulses in right leg are strong.
   3. Skin temperature is warm to touch.
   4. There is no edema present.
4. A client is a resident in an assisted living facility. The home health nurse, in planning care for this client, is correct in stating this client is at risk for falls related to which of the following age-related factors? Select all that apply.
   1. Slowed daily activities
   2. Decreased appetite
   3. Decreased range of motion
   4. Increased bone fragility
   5. Loss of muscle strength

5. A nurse is providing discharge instructions following an arthroscopy. The nurse recognizes that the client does not understand the instructions when the client makes which of the following statements?
1. "I understand that I can resume a normal diet."
2. "I need to wait to call the doctor because a high level of pain is normal."
3. "I must call the doctor if there is blood on the dressing."
4. "I will resume my medications per your instructions."

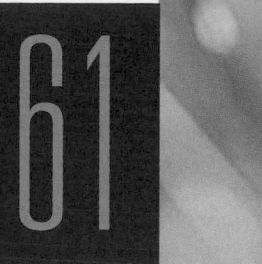

61

Caring for Clients Requiring Orthopedic Treatment

Words To Know

arthroplasty
avascular necrosis
brace
cast
closed reduction
external fixation
internal fixation
open reduction
prosthesis
splint
subluxation
traction

Learning Objectives

On completion of this chapter, you will be able to:

1. Differentiate types of casts.
2. Discuss the nursing management for a client with a cast.
3. State the reasons for using splints or braces.
4. Identify the principles for maintaining traction and describe nursing care for the client in traction.
5. Differentiate between closed reduction and open reduction and between internal fixation and external fixation.
6. Describe nursing care for the client with a fracture reduction.
7. Identify the reasons for performing orthopedic surgery.
8. Discuss the nursing management for a client undergoing orthopedic surgery.
9. Describe the positioning precautions after a conventional total hip replacement.
10. Explain the nursing needs of the client undergoing total knee replacement.
11. Discuss amputation, including reasons it may be performed and appropriate nursing management of the client.

Musculoskeletal disorders are common in any client population and contribute to temporary or permanent disability. Clients with orthopedic disorders often cannot meet all of their activities of daily living (ADLs). Management of musculoskeletal disorders involves the use of casts, splints and braces, traction, and various types of orthopedic surgery. Amputation may also be done following a traumatic injury or because of disease or disability.

CASTS

A **cast** is a rigid mold that immobilizes an injured structure while it heals. There are basically three types of casts. A *cylinder cast* encircles an arm or leg, leaving the fingers or toes exposed. A *body cast* is a larger form of a cylinder cast that encircles the trunk from about the nipple line to the iliac crests. A *hip spica cast* surrounds one or both legs and the trunk. It may be strengthened by a bar that spans a casted area between the legs (Fig. 61-1). This type of cast is trimmed open in the anal and genital areas to facilitate elimination. Other types of casts are described in Box 61-1.

To keep aligned bone fragments from becoming displaced, the cast is applied from the joint above the break to the one below it. The joint is slightly flexed to decrease stiffness. Some fractures (e.g., a stress fracture) do not require surgical reduction or manual manipulation to realign the bone because the fractured bone still remains perfectly aligned. If a closed or open reduction is required, the client receives an analgesic or a general or local anesthetic to relieve pain.

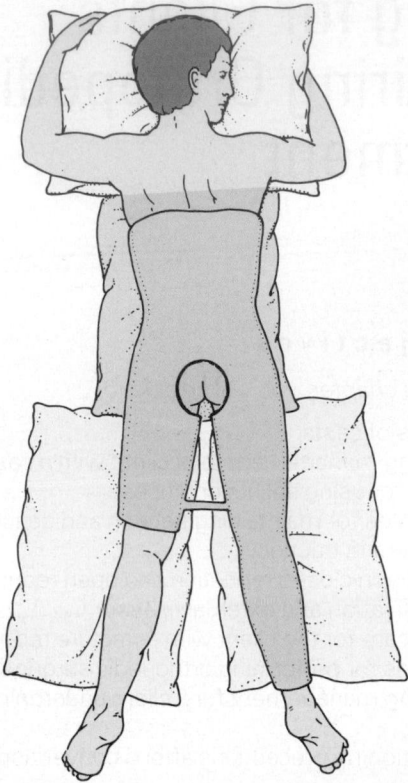

FIGURE 61-1. Spica cast. This client with a spica cast is resting on pillows until the cast dries. His feet are positioned so that they support the desired body alignment. Note the bar, ensuring adequate space between the casted legs.

Cast Composition

Nonplaster or synthetic casts are usually made of polyurethane material, generally known as fiberglass. Water activates the hardeners that impregnate the open weave fabric

to form a rigid cast within minutes. Depending on the degree of swelling at the site of the fracture, this type of cast may be used initially or a plaster of Paris cast may be used until the swelling subsides and then a fiberglass cast may be applied. Plaster casts require a longer time for drying, but mold better to the client, and are initially used until the swelling subsides. Fiberglass casts dry more quickly, are lighter in weight, longer-lasting, and breathable. Clients with synthetic casts have fewer skin problems and may bear weight soon after the cast is applied, depending upon the type of fracture.

When applying the cast, the physician positions the client to ensure proper alignment of the part to be immobilized. The client's buttocks may be supported on a casting frame when a body cast or spica cast is applied so the casting material can be wrapped around the client's trunk. A nurse or an assistant holds the arm or leg in place during application of a cylinder cast (Box 61-2). If the client is awake, healthcare providers explain that the cast material will feel warm during application as a result of being mixed with water.

A wet cast must be kept uncovered so that water can evaporate. Most physicians prefer natural evaporation but may order a cast dryer to speed evaporation. Intense heat is never used. There is a danger not only of burning the client but also of cracking the outside of the cast while leaving the inside damp and hospitable to mold. The drying cast should be supported on pillows. If necessary, healthcare personnel can reposition the casted arm or leg with the palms of the hands. Using the fingertips or compressing the cast on a hard surface can lead to a pressure sore later.

Cast Windows

After the cast dries, a cast window, or opening, may be cut. This usually is done when the client reports discomfort under the cast or has a wound that requires a dressing change. The window permits direct inspection of the skin, a means to check the pulse in a casted arm or leg, or a way to change a dressing. Once a window is cut, the solid piece of cast is replaced in its original site and secured with adhesive tape or a roller bandage. Leaving the window open may allow the skin and soft tissue to bulge through the opening.

BOX 61-1 **Examples of Types of Casts**

Short arm cast: Extends from below the elbow to the palmar crease and is secured around the base of the thumb. If the thumb is also casted, it is referred to as a *thumb spica* or *gauntlet* cast.

Long arm cast: Extends from the upper level of the axillary fold to the proximal palmar crease. The elbow is usually immobilized at a right angle.

Short leg cast: Extends from below the knee to the base of the toes. The foot is flexed at a right angle in a neutral position.

Long leg cast: Extends from the junction of the upper and middle third of the thigh to the base of the toes. The knee may be slightly flexed.

Walking cast: A short or long leg cast reinforced for strength

Body cast: Encircles the trunk

Shoulder spica cast: A body cast that encloses the trunk and the shoulder and elbow

Hip spica cast: Encloses the trunk and a lower extremity. A double hip spica cast includes both legs.

(Adapted from Smeltzer, S.C., et al. [2008]. *Brunner & Suddarth's textbook of medical-surgical nursing* [11th ed.]. Philadelphia: Lippincott Williams & Wilkins, p. 2355.)

BOX 61-2 **Applying a Cast**

In general, the physician or nurse practitioner applies a cast as follows:
- Clean and dry the skin surface of the part to be casted.
- Cover the skin with stockinette, a tubular knitted material.
- Wrap padding around the limb, especially over bony prominences.
- Apply rolls or strips of plaster or nonplaster cast material evenly over the stockinette and padding.
- Smooth the layers and edges of the cast.
- Fasten the stockinette in cufflike fashion to the outside of the cast.
- Arrange for an x-ray study after casting to check bone alignment.

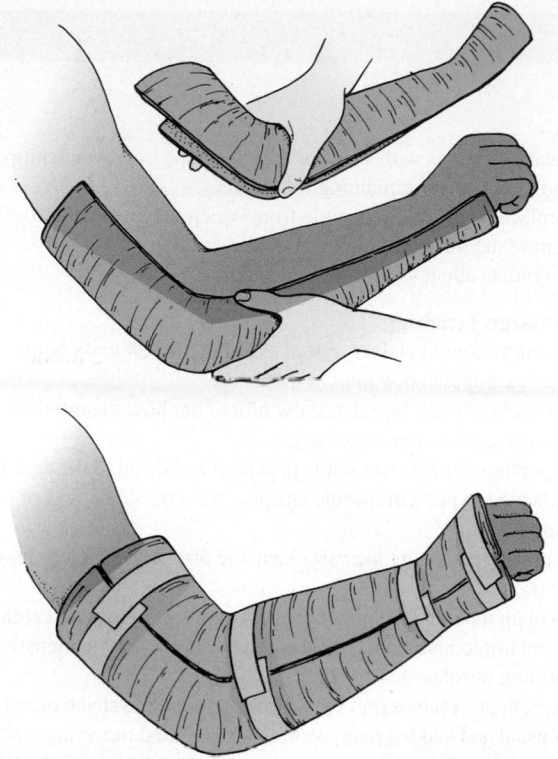

FIGURE 61-2. (**A**) A bivalved cast. (**B**) The two halves are rejoined.

Bivalve Casts

Once a cast has been applied, it may be bivalved, or cut in two (Fig. 61-2). This may be necessary if the arm or leg swells, causing the rigid cast to compress the tissue and interfere with its blood supply. A bivalved cast also may be used for a client who is being weaned from a cast, when a sharp radiograph is needed, or as a splint for immobilizing painful joints when a client has arthritis.

Cast Removal

Casts are removed with a mechanical cast cutter. Cast cutters are noisy and frightening, and the client needs reassurance that the machine will not cut into the skin. Once the cast is off, the skin appears mottled and may be covered with a yellowish crust composed of accumulated body oil and dead skin. The client usually sheds this residue in a few days. Lotions and warm baths or soaks may help to soften the skin and remove debris.

The now uncasted limb feels surprisingly light, and the client may report weakness and stiffness. For some time, the limb will need support. An elastic bandage may be wrapped on a leg, the client may use a cane, and an arm may be kept in a sling until progressive active exercise and physical therapy help the client regain normal strength and motion.

Nursing Guidelines 61-1 provides information about caring for a client with a cast. Nursing care includes teaching clients with casts to the lower extremities how to ambulate with crutches.

SPLINTS AND BRACES

A **splint** immobilizes and supports an injured body part in a functional position. The client would use a splint when a musculoskeletal condition:

- Does not require rigid immobilization.
- Causes a large degree of swelling.
- Requires special skin treatment.

Splints can be made of plaster or a more pliable thermoplastic material. They should be padded so that they do not cause pressure or skin abrasions and breakdown. The healthcare professional fits the client with a splint and then overwraps it with an elastic bandage applied in a spiral mode. This helps to promote circulation and maintain the position of the splint. Other types of splints include canvas splints, soft or hard ready-made splints, soft variety splints that support an injured upper extremity, and commercial soft splints padded and contoured to fit a client's extremity. Velcro straps on the splint attach the splint to the injured extremity.

Braces provide support, control movement, and prevent additional injury for more long-term use (Smeltzer et al., 2008). Made of plastic materials, canvas, leather, or metal, braces are custom fit to each client. The nurse must provide instruction to the client and family on how to apply the brace and to administer scrupulous skin care to prevent irritation and injury.

▶ *Stop, Think, and Respond Exercise 61-1*

A client with a brace on his lower-right extremity tells you that the brace is cutting into his ankle bone. What is your best action?

REDUCING FRACTURES

Clients experiencing a disruption in the functional continuity of a bone have sustained some form of a fracture (refer to Chapter 62 for more discussion of fractures). Reducing a fracture involves restoring proper alignment to the injured bone. Treatment of fractures includes one or more methods: traction, closed or open reduction, internal or external fixation, or cast application (see previous discussion). The treatment method depends on several factors, including the first aid given, the location and severity of the break, and the age and overall physical condition of the client.

Traction

Traction is a method of pulling structures of the musculoskeletal system. For traction to achieve its purpose, it requires *counter traction*, a force opposite to the mechanical pull. Counter traction usually is supplied by the client's own weight. Traction is used to relieve muscle spasm, align bones, and maintain immobilization. The two most common types are skin traction and skeletal traction.

Skin traction is achieved by applying devices to the skin that indirectly affect the muscles or bones. An example is Buck's traction (Fig. 61-3A); another example is Russell traction (see Fig. 61-3B). Skeletal traction is applied directly to a bone by using a wire (Kirschner), pin (Steinmann), or cranial tongs (Crutchfield). General or local anesthesia may

NURSING GUIDELINES 61–1

Caring for the Client With a Cast

Before Cast Application

- Inspect the condition of the skin that will be covered with a cast.
- Assess circulation, sensation, and mobility to establish a baseline.
- Evaluate the client's pain level.
- Remove clothing that will be difficult to remove after the cast is applied.
- Explain the procedure to the client. Remember to tell the client that the cast will feel warm—even hot—as it is applied, but that it will not burn the skin.

After Cast Application

- Leave the cast uncovered.
- Assess circulation, sensation, and mobility in exposed fingers and toes every 1 to 2 hours.
- Monitor for signs of complications related to cast application. Report abnormal findings immediately.
- Handle wet cast with the palms of the hands, not the fingers.
- Elevate casted extremity so that it is higher than the heart.
- Reposition the client frequently while cast is drying so that the cast dries as evenly as possible.
- Apply ice packs to the cast where surgery was performed.
- Circle areas where blood seeped through and write the time on the circle.

- Petal cast edges with strips of adhesive tape to prevent chipping and to cover any remaining rough areas.
- Replace windows in the hole from which they were cut to prevent tissue from bulging through the opening.
- Ambulate client as soon as indicated.

Discharge Teaching

- Instruct client to elevate casted extremity for 24 to 48 hours after cast application, and as indicated.
- If the client has a leg cast, show him or her how to ambulate safely (see illustration below).
- Teach how to exercise joints proximal and distal to the cast as indicated to prevent muscle atrophy, weakness, and loss of joint mobility.
- Emphasize keeping the cast clean and dry. A damp cloth may be used.
- Explain that the skin under the cast may feel itchy, and caution client not to insert objects like straws, combs, eating utensils, knitting needles, and the like.
- The client should report the following to the physician or nurse: unusual and sudden pain, painful or decreased movement, or persistent pain; fever, foul odors, or increased warmth of extremity; drainage from under the cast; changes in circulation, mobility, or sensation (burning, numbness, tingling, or cold).

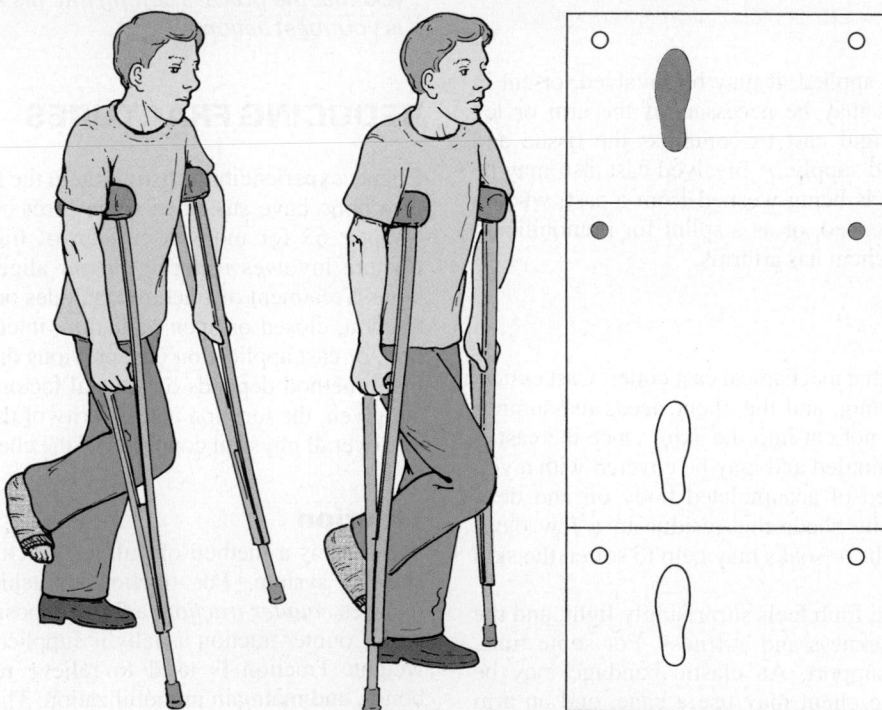

Crutch-walking using the three-point, non-weight-bearing gait pattern (three blocks at right). At left, the client positions himself at the bottom of a triangle composed of each crutch and the unaffected leg. In the center, the client advances his unaffected leg forward by supporting himself on the hand grips of the crutches and swinging his hips and the unaffected leg through the crutch opening.

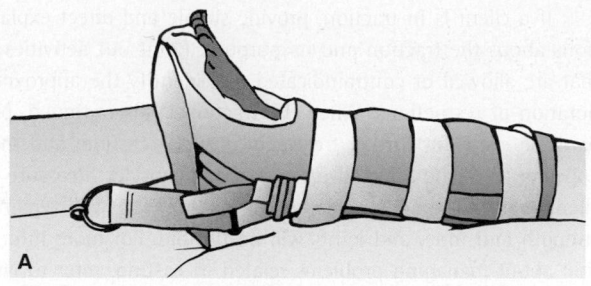

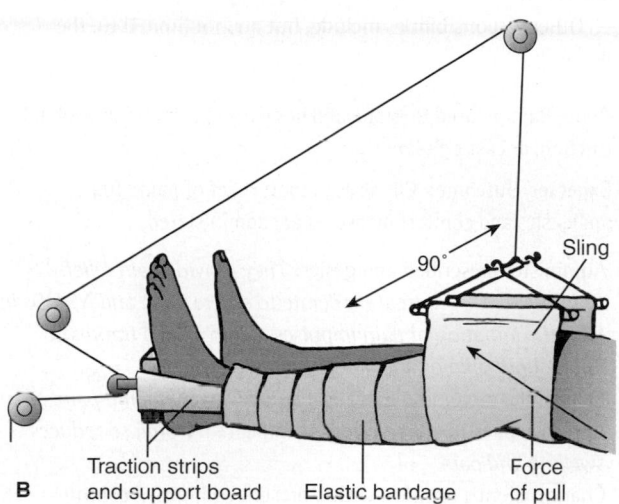

FIGURE 61-3. Two examples of skin traction: (**A**) Buck's traction and (**B**) Russell traction.

be used when inserting these devices. The pull is achieved by connecting the attachment from the client to a system of ropes, pulleys, and weights on an orthopedic bed frame. A Thomas splint with a Pearson attachment often is used to suspend a leg in traction. This is referred to as *balanced suspension traction.* Figure 61-4 presents an example of skeletal traction (Thomas splint) with balanced suspension. The principles for maintaining effective traction are discussed in

Box 61-3. Nursing care measures for a client in traction are presented in Nursing Guidelines 61-2.

Closed Reduction

In a **closed reduction**, the bone is restored to its normal position by external manipulation. A bandage, cast, or traction then immobilizes the area. X-ray films are taken to ensure correct alignment of the bone. Depending on the site and type of fracture, the client receives a local (nerve block) or general anesthetic for this procedure.

Open Reduction

In an **open reduction**, which is performed in the operating room, the bone is surgically exposed and realigned. Usually the client receives a general or spinal anesthetic. Radiographic studies, taken while the client is still anesthetized, show whether re-alignments are needed.

Internal Fixation

If **internal fixation** is needed to stabilize the reduced fracture, the surgeon secures the bone with metal screws, plates, rods, nails, or pins. A cast or other method of immobilization is then applied. Figure 61-5 depicts examples of internal fixation techniques. Open reduction is required when:

- Soft tissue, such as nerves or blood vessels, is caught between the ends of the broken pieces of bone.
- The bone has a wide separation.
- Comminuted fractures are present.
- Patella and other joints are fractured.
- Open fractures are evident.
- Wound debridement is necessary.
- Internal fixation is needed.

External Fixation

In **external fixation**, the surgeon inserts metal pins into the bone or bones from outside the skin surface and then attaches a compression device to the pins (Fig. 61-6). Some complex or comminuted fractures may require an external

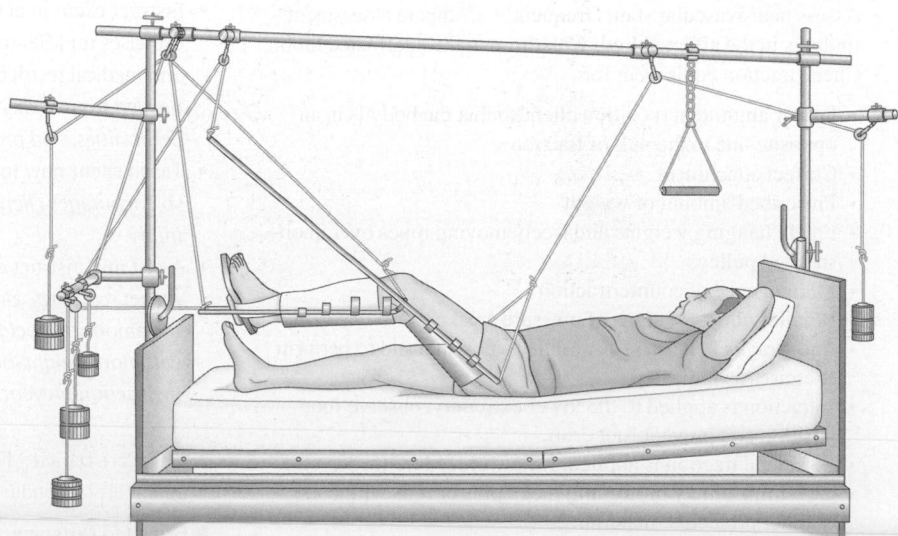

FIGURE 61-4. Skeletal traction with balanced suspension and Thomas leg splint.

BOX 61-3 Principles of Effective Traction

- Ensure continuous traction.
- Maintain countertraction.
- See that the pull of traction and countertraction are in opposite directions but in straight alignment.
- Suspend splints and slings without interference.
- Be sure that ropes move freely through each pulley.
- Apply the exact amount of weight prescribed.
- Make sure that the weights hang freely.

---

fixation device to stabilize and position the bone. Because the pin sites are an entry for infection, monitoring for redness, drainage, and tenderness is necessary. Nursing Guidelines 61-3 describe pin care for an external fixation device.

Nursing Process for the Client With a Fracture Reduction

Assessment

When caring for the client with a fracture, assess the client for neurovascular and systemic complications.

Diagnosis, Planning, and Interventions

General nursing measures include administering analgesics, providing comfort measures, assisting with ADLs, preventing constipation, promoting physical mobility, preventing infection, maintaining skin integrity, and preparing the client for self-care. Because the client may be discharged shortly after application of an immobilization device or a cast, review needed care with the client and family. In addition, reinforce instructions regarding exercise and ambulatory activities.

NURSING GUIDELINES 61–2

Managing the Care of the Client in Traction

- Assess neurovascular status frequently. Compare assessment findings in the affected limb with those in the unaffected limb.
- Check traction equipment for:
  - Proper alignment (position client so that the body is in an opposite line to the pull of traction)
  - Correct attachment
  - Prescribed amount of weight
  - Freely hanging weights and freely moving ropes over unobstructed pulleys
  - Maintenance of countertraction
- Monitor client for signs of pressure areas.
- Encourage client to be as mobile as possible and to perform exercises as indicated.
- If traction is applied to the lower extremity, observe foot position and prevent foot drop.
- If skeletal traction is applied, follow procedure for pin care.
- Cover tips of any protruding metal pins or rods with corks or other protective material.

If a client is in traction, provide simple and direct explanations about the traction and its purpose. Point out activities that are allowed or contraindicated and identify the approximate duration of restrictions. When the traction is discontinued, prepare the client for further treatment, such as casting, and the appearance of the affected area—skin and muscles. Reassure the client that with gradual exercise and use, muscles will regain strength and tone, and joints will be flexible. For more information about managing problems related to casting, refer to Nursing Guidelines 61-1. For information about clients with specific fractures, such as those affecting the clavicle or knee, refer to Table 61-1.

Other responsibilities include, but are not limited to, the following:

▶ **Acute Pain** related to tissue and bone trauma, swelling, skeletal traction, or cast pressure

▶ **Expected Outcome:** Client will report relief of pain after analgesics and comfort measures are administered.

- Administer prescribed analgesics. *They provide pain relief. Opioids are used to treat moderate to severe pain, and NSAIDs inhibit the initiation of pain impulses. Often after a traumatic injury, both opioids and NSAIDs are prescribed.*
- Elevate the extremity. *Elevation reduces swelling and pain.*
- Apply ice pack to site of injury as indicated. *Doing so reduces swelling and pain.*
- Change client's position within prescribed limits. *Position changes relieve pressure on bony prominences and promote comfort.*

▶ **Impaired Physical Mobility** related to pain, swelling, surgical procedure, or immobilization from traction, cast, or splint

▶ **Expected Outcomes:** (1) Client will regain or maintain maximum mobility and optimal functional position. (2) Client will have increased strength and function in the affected limb.

- Assess level of mobility. *These data provide a baseline for comparison.*
- Instruct client in active and passive range-of-motion (ROM) exercises for affected and unaffected extremities, within physical and medical restrictions. *ROM exercises strengthen muscles needed for mobility and function, prevent contractures and deformities, and promote circulation.*
- Teach client how to turn safely, adhering to restrictions. *Doing so encourages client's active participation and prevents further injury.*
- Assist and instruct client in the use of mobility aids (wheelchair, walker, crutches, canes) as needed. *The client must be aware of the amount of weight bearing allowed. Ambulatory aids assist with non-weight-bearing or partial weight-bearing restrictions. Instruction prevents injury from unsafe use.*

▶ **Self-Care Deficit: Feeding, Hygiene, Dressing, Toileting** related to immobility secondary to traction or casts

▶ **Expected Outcome:** Client will maintain maximum self-care.

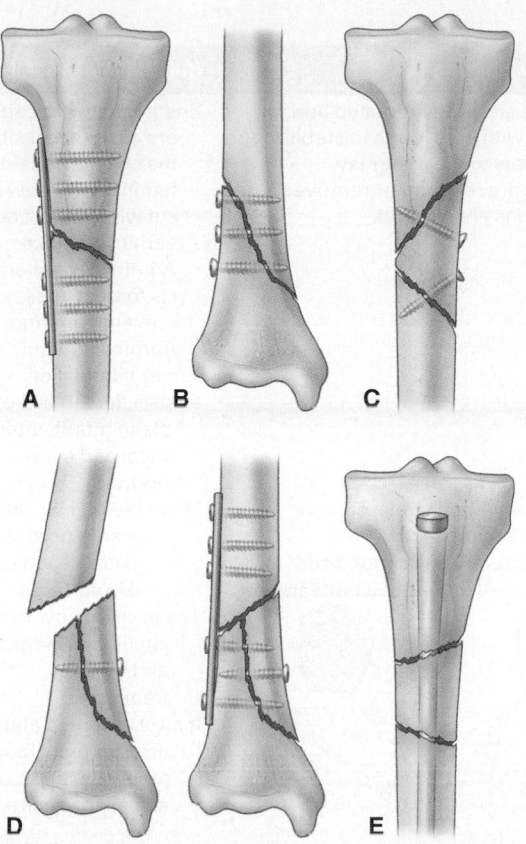

FIGURE 61-5. Techniques of internal fixation. (**A**) Plate and six screws for a transverse or short oblique fracture. (**B**) Screws for a long oblique or spiral fracture. (**C**) Screws for a long butterfly tragment. (**D**) Plate and six screws for a short buttertly tragment. (**E**) Medullary nail for a segmental fracture.

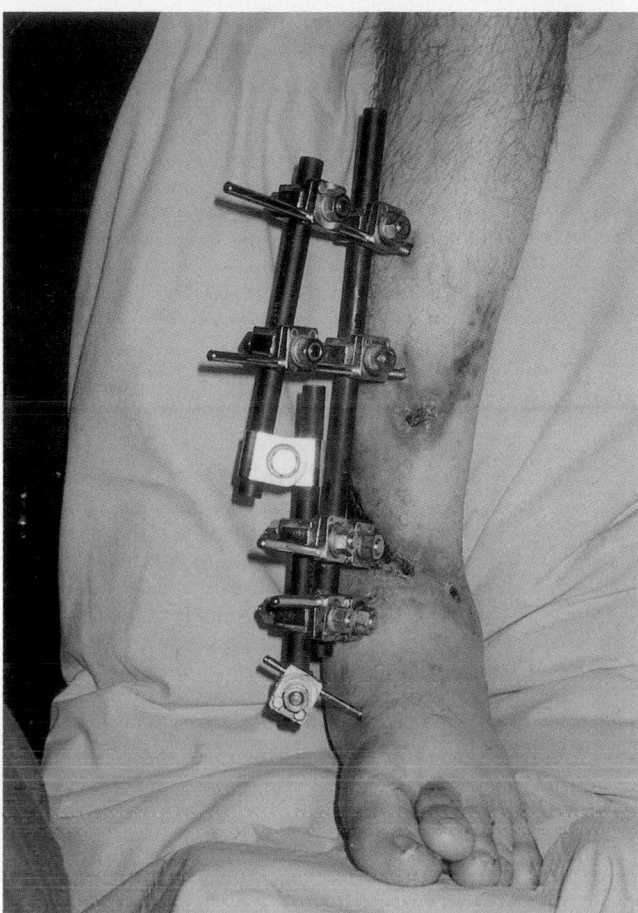

FIGURE 61-6. External fixation device.

- Assist client to meet self-care needs as indicated. *Limited mobility and ROM prevent client from safely providing self-care; assistance promotes safety.*
- Instruct client to perform self-care activities as much as possible. *Doing so promotes independence.*
- Provide assistive devices as indicated. *They help the client to be as independent as possible.*
- Allow client to plan self-care that best meets ongoing needs. *Doing so involves client in care and helps him or her to have control.*

▶ **Impaired Tissue Integrity** related to puncture wound; compound fracture; pins, wires, screws, or other surgical intervention; or physical immobility

▶ **Expected Outcomes:** (1) Client will demonstrate adequate wound healing without infection. (2) Skin will remain intact.

- Provide pin care. *It assists in monitoring client for infection and maintains a clean environment.*
- Report any signs of infection in the pin care sites, wounds, or surgical incisions. *Doing so promotes early intervention and prevents further infection.*
- Administer antibiotics as indicated. *Antibiotics treat infection and prevent complications, such as osteomyelitis.*

NURSING GUIDELINES 61-3

Providing Pin Care

Scrupulous pin care assists in preventing localized infection at the pin sites and systemic infection and osteomyelitis:

- Assess pin sites for redness, swelling, increased tenderness, and drainage.
- Examine pins for signs of breakage, bending, or shifting.
- Wearing gloves, use cotton-tipped applicators and saline or other prescribed solution, such as chlorhexidine solution, to cleanse pin sites.
- Use at least one applicator per pin—do not use applicator more than once.
- Clean pin site from pin outward.
- Unless there are obvious signs of infection, leave crusts around pin sites intact, as they provide a normal protective barrier.
- Avoid applying ointment to pin sites unless specifically ordered.
- Obtain culture if purulent drainage is present.
- Teach client not to touch pin sites.
- Instruct family member in pin care if client is discharged.

TABLE 61-1 Nursing Care for Specific Fractures

SITE OF FRACTURE	SIGNS AND SYMPTOMS	TREATMENT	NURSING MANAGEMENT
Mandible	Inability to close mouth after trauma to jaw Chin displaced from midline Teeth absent, loose, or broken Lacerations to mouth and tongue Oral pain, swelling, bruising, and bleeding	Fractures are surgically reduced and immobilized with wire loops to stabilize the lower jaw to the upper jaw. Broken teeth are repaired or removed. Oral lacerations are sutured.	Ensure that wire cutters are easily accessible at the client's bedside. Be familiar with how to cut wire loops if client vomits or chokes. Administer antiemetics to treat nausea and prevent vomiting. Administer liquid or semiliquid diet. Assist client to thoroughly clean mouth after each meal and every 2 hours.
Clavicle	After fracture or dislocation, arm on the affected side held close to the chest to reduce pain Affected shoulder appears to slope downward and droop inward Motion restricted Muscle spasm common	Motion can be limited with a sling or clavicular strap. Displaced fractures are immobilized with a figure-8 or Velpeau bandage. Velpeau bandage	Use a layer of stockinette or soft, porous material between skin surfaces. Teach client how to assess circulation, sensation, and mobility frequently. Instruct client to abduct arms or rest elbows on table or chair to relieve axillary pressure.
Rib	Additional injuries—to the lungs, subclavian arteries or veins, liver, or spleen Severe chest pain on inspiration and shallow respirations. The client has other symptoms if other injuries are present.	Clients are treated for the pain that accompanies fractured ribs, especially when breathing. A rib belt or elastic bandage is used to support the injured rib cage, although this restricts chest movement and may cause further lung problems.	Assess for signs and symptoms of pneumonia and atelectasis (collapsed lung) secondary to shallow respirations. Encourage deep breathing. Administer pain medications as indicated.
Upper extremity (fractures ranging from uncomplicated to complex and involving the bone ends, joints, tendons, and ligaments)	Pain Compartment syndrome, common complication of forearm fractures, possibly leading to Volkmann's contracture, a clawlike deformity of the hand	Extent of injury determines treatment: • Cast with or without closed reduction • Open reduction with internal fixation • Hanging heavy cast that pulls a fractured humerus into alignment Hanging arm cast	Assess neurovascular status frequently. Report abnormal findings immediately. Implement measures to relieve pain and swelling. Pad skin around neck if the client has a hanging cast.

TABLE 61-1 Nursing Care for Specific Fractures (continued)

SITE OF FRACTURE	SIGNS AND SYMPTOMS	TREATMENT	NURSING MANAGEMENT

Wrist, hand, or finger	Typically results from a fall
	May involve only the lower radius (e.g., a Colles' fracture in which the distal end of the radius breaks off and becomes displaced)
	Pain and swelling in the affected area
	Deformed-looking hand, wrist or finger
		Closed reduction with a cast
		  Open reduction with internal fixation
		  Splints applied to fractured fingers
			Show client how to use a sling.
			Teach client how to do active ROM exercises in fingers of affected hand.

Spine	May follow severe injury; if compression fracture, may result from osteoporosis Pain radiating to the leg Tenderness at injury site Muscle spasms Deformity of spinal column Neurologic deficits	Bed rest for an uncomplicated fracture Spinal brace Laminectomy with fusion Cast Head traction: halo brace with rigid vest that allows client to move but immobilizes vertebraes	Teach client to log roll if on bed rest, and as indicated. Assess client's sensation, mobility, and strength in the extremities. Administer pin care if client has a halo brace.
Pelvis (fractures range from minor to severe or crushing injuries)	Tenderness, swelling, and ecchymoses, or more severe symptoms if internal injuries accompany fracture Severed nerves Loss of lower limb function Internal bleeding	Minor fractures: bed rest and comfort measures Severe injuries: multiple-system approach related to the nature of the injuries Pelvic slings, spica casts, or open reduction with internal or external fixation	Assess circulation, sensation, and mobility in the lower extremities. Monitor elimination patterns. Insert an indwelling catheter as necessary. Provide a fracture bedpan. Administer suppositories or small volume enemas as indicated. Assess skin frequently for signs of breakdown. Provide frequent skin care. Administer pain medications as prescribed.
Knee (involving kneecap or the ends of the femur or tibia; injuries to the ligaments or tendons)	May follow falls or blows or athletic competition (particularly tears of the cruciate ligaments) Pain, swelling, ecchymoses Inability or limited ability to move or bend the joint	Immobilization with a leg splint Leg immobilizer Arthroscopic surgery to remove bone fragments or to repair ligament tears Open reduction and insertion of wire sutures Removal of patella if fragmented extensively Skeletal traction	Assist client to use ambulatory aids, such as crutches or walker. Teach client to perform active ROM exercises within limitations.

(table continues on page 978)

TABLE 61-1 Nursing Care for Specific Fractures (continued)

SITE OF FRACTURE	SIGNS AND SYMPTOMS	TREATMENT	NURSING MANAGEMENT
Lower leg (fibula fracture usually occurs with tibial fracture)	Usually results from fall or trauma Pain and swelling Inability to bear weight Ecchymoses and possible deformity Bleeding and protrusion of bone fragments (in compound fractures)	Closed reduction with cast Open reduction with internal fixation	Assess signs and symptoms of compartment syndrome. Urge client to perform active and passive ROM exercises frequently. Assist client to use ambulatory aids.
Ankle	Severe pain Difficulty bearing weight Swelling Protruding bone fragments (severe fractures)	Cast or splint Open or closed reduction and internal fixation followed by casting	Administer pain medications as prescribed. Implement methods to reduce swelling. Assist client to use ambulatory aids. Assess for signs and symptoms of compartment syndrome.
Feet and toes (can occur alone or with other lower extremity fractures)	Pain, swelling, ecchymosis, and difficulty bearing weight Inability to wear shoe Protrusion of small bones (in crushing injuries)	Casting Open reduction with internal fixation Fusion (bones with multiple fractures) Supportive measures: analgesics, cold applications, elevation of foot, and loose-fitting shoes	Assess neurovascular status frequently. Provide cast care as needed. Assist client to use ambulatory aids. Instruct client in safety measures to prevent additional injuries (using nightlights, avoiding narrowed pathways, removing throw rugs, clearing stairways).

- Protect bony prominences from pressure by using pressure-relieving techniques under elbows, heels, and coccyx. Massage bony prominences and skin surfaces subjected to pressure unless they remain red when pressure is relieved. *These measures prevent further injury and potential infection and promote circulation to the area.*
- Assess traction frequently to ensure proper alignment and to prevent pressure areas. *Doing so prevents mechanical injury to the skin and tissues.*
- Petal cast edges with waterproof tape. *This measure protects skin from abrasion* (see Nursing Guidelines 61-1).

Evaluation of Expected Outcomes

Pain is reduced or relieved. The client regains mobility and function and achieves the maximum level of self-care. Wounds heal without infection, and the skin is intact. Nutrition Notes 61-1 highlights nutrition considerations for the client receiving orthopedic treatment.

ORTHOPEDIC SURGERY

Orthopedic surgery is performed for various reasons: to correct a deformity, remove a primary bone tumor, align

fractured bones (open reduction), repair or replace a joint, insert a bone graft to promote bone healing, or stabilize a bone internally (using rods, pins, screws, nails, or wires).

Open Reduction Internal Fixation

If surgery for a fracture cannot be performed right away, Buck's traction or other skin traction may be applied to relieve muscle spasm and pain until surgery is performed. Open reduction-internal fixation (ORIF), accomplished with wire, nails, plate, and/or an intramedullary rod (a rod inserted into the center of the bone with wires around the bone for stabilization), is done to hold bone fragments in place until bone healing is complete.

Nutrition Notes 61-1
The Client Receiving Orthopedic Treatment

- Protein requirements increase during prolonged immobility to correct negative nitrogen balance, promote healing, and help prevent skin breakdown and infections. A protein intake of 1.2 g/kg body weight is recommended; the client needs adequate calories to spare protein.
- A high fiber intake helps prevent constipation.

Surgical Procedures to Correct Joint Dysfunction

Several surgical techniques, described in Box 61-4, may be done to minimize or correct joint dysfunction. Clients with arthritis, trauma, hip fracture, or a congenital deformity may have an **arthroplasty**, or reconstruction of the joint. This procedure uses an artificial joint that restores previously lost function and relieves pain. Reconstructive joint surgery is performed when mobility and quality of life are compromised. The two joints most frequently replaced are the knee and hip. Other joints that may be replaced are the shoulder, ankle, wrist, and finger joints.

The materials used in an artificial joint (**prosthesis**) are metal and high-density polyethylene (Fig. 61-7), although Silastic is used for finger prostheses. Special bone cement or a specialized coating on the prosthesis pieces, which promotes bone growth on the implant, holds the prosthesis parts in place. There are problems with the prosthesis loosening due to failure of the cement, so in many instances porous-coated cementless joint components are used. These allow the bone to grow into the prosthesis and thus securely fix the joint replacement in place. Clients having this type of prosthesis must have adequate blood supply in healthy bone (Smeltzer et al., 2008).

Postoperative complications include hemorrhage; **subluxation**, or dislocation of the artificial joint; infection; thromboembolism; and **avascular necrosis**, or death of bone tissue due to diminished or absent blood supply. A cemented prosthesis may loosen many years later.

Depending on the type of joint replacement, clients may be asked to donate their own blood preoperatively for use postoperatively if a transfusion is required. Anticoagulant therapy and early ambulation are very important for clients who have knee or hip replacement. These clients often use a continuous passive motion (CPM) machine after surgery. This machine promotes healing and flexibility in the knee and hip joint and increases circulation to the operative area. The physician orders the amount of extension and flexion produced by the machine as well as the frequency of use. Clients with knee replacements have the amount of flexion

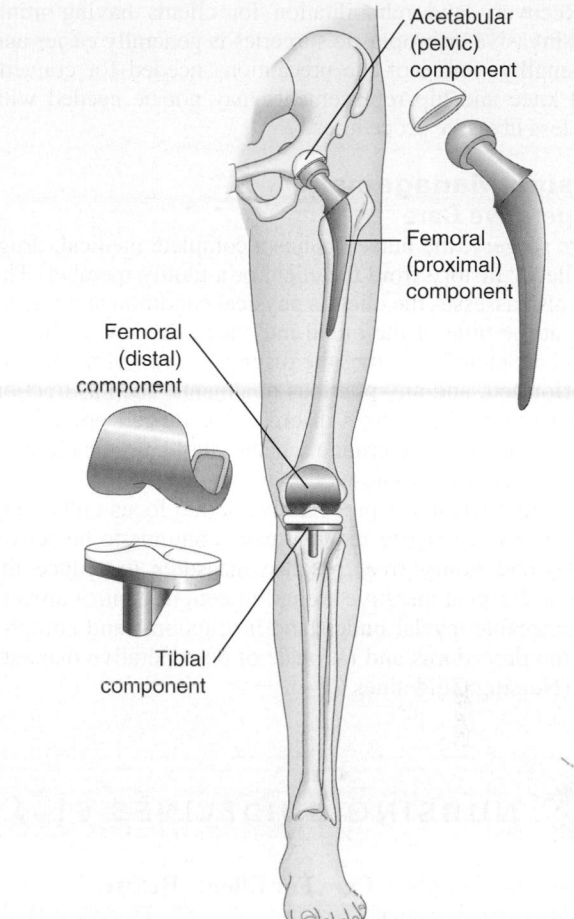

FIGURE 61-7. Hip and knee replacement.

and the frequency of use increased daily while hospitalized. The goal is for the client to have the ability to bend the knee 90° by discharge. The amount of flexion for clients with hip replacements should never exceed 30° in a CPM machine.

Minimally invasive joint replacement surgeries are beginning to replace conventional joint replacement surgeries. The differences involve the following:

- Much smaller incision(s), often one quarter to one half the size of conventional arthroplasties
- Smaller prostheses in some instances
- No cement, only porous-surfaced prostheses
- No surgical cutting of muscle or tendon; surgeons work around these structures by splitting and dividing muscles whenever possible
- Resurfacing, a technique in which only the worn surfaces of the joint are replaced or covered; this technique is used more in younger, active clients who do not have any deformities
- Computer-assisted surgery for some joint replacements, which involves computer-guided imagery that assists orthopedic surgeons to better align the prosthesis and promotes better long-term effectiveness
- Procedures take longer, requiring longer periods of time that a client is having anesthesia, thus increasing anesthesia-related risks

---

B O X 6 1 - 4 | **Surgical Procedures to Correct Joint Deformity**

Arthrodesis: Fusion of a joint (most often the wrist or knee) for stabilization and pain relief

Arthroplasty: Total reconstruction or replacement of a joint (most often the knee or hip) with an artificial joint to restore function and relieve pain

Hemiarthroplasty: The replacement of one of the articular surfaces in a joint, such as the femoral head but not the acetabulum

Total arthroplasty: The replacement of both articular surfaces within one joint

Osteotomy: Cutting and removal of a wedge of bone (most often the tibia or femur) to change the bone's alignment, thereby improving function and relieving pain

Recovery and rehabilitation for clients having minimally invasive arthroplastic surgeries is generally easier and less lengthy. Some of the precautions needed for conventional knee and hip replacements may not be needed with these less invasive procedures.

Nursing Management

Preoperative Care

Before surgery, the nurse obtains a complete medical, drug, and allergy history from the client or a family member. The nurse also assesses the client's physical condition and mental status at the time of the initial interview. Review of the client's chart includes noting the diagnosis, type of surgery to be performed, and any previous treatments, such as traction or drug use. If the client's disorder was treated previously, the nurse needs to determine whether any complications or problems occurred because of or during treatment.

Client goals in the preoperative period focus on helping the client to experience reduced pain; continue to be active, mobile, and injury free; practice measures to reduce the potential for postoperative wound infection; control anxiety at manageable levels; understand instructions; and comprehend the procedures and rationale of postoperative management (Nursing Guidelines 61-4).

NURSING GUIDELINES 61–4

Ensuring Complete Care For Clients Before Orthopedic Surgery

- Review the operation and the reason for it.
- Administer prescribed analgesics.
- Relieve the client's discomfort through positioning and joint immobilization.
- Support painful joints and be gentle when moving the client.
- Allow ample time for physical activities, because the client with a musculoskeletal disorder needs more time to carry out preoperative routines. Allow the client to use any ambulatory aid that was brought from home.
- Demonstrate use of the overbed trapeze and encourage its use.
- Demonstrate and have the client perform necessary postoperative activities, such as coughing and deep-breathing exercises.
- Provide preoperative skin care as indicated by agency policy and procedure. If the client has initiated skin preparation at home, check to be sure the procedures were performed.
- Obtain adequate help when transferring a sedated client who is not in traction from the bed to the surgical stretcher. However, keep a client who is in traction in the hospital bed. Then, without lifting or removing the traction weights, transport the bed to the operating room.
- Administer the IV prophylactic antibiotic if ordered before surgery. (Although laminar airflow in the operating suite has reduced the incidence of postoperative infection, a great risk for infection remains for every client having orthopedic surgery. The number of personnel in the operating room may need to be limited to reduce a potential reservoir of infecting microorganisms.)

Postoperative Care

Ideally, postoperative nursing management begins before surgery with demonstrations of deep-breathing and coughing exercises and descriptions and demonstrations of the incentive spirometer (if that is likely to be used after surgery). Even if the client will have postoperative physical therapy, the nurse explains and helps the client practice active and isometric leg exercises. He or she also describes other devices that may be used after surgery, such as intravenous infusions of fluid and blood, oxygen, a wound drain, elastic stockings, or roller bandages. It also is necessary to include a discussion of the possible use of traction or the CPM machine.

If a client is scheduled for joint replacement or other surgery, the nurse withholds aspirin before surgery to reduce the risk for excessive bleeding. It is essential to monitor the complete blood count, prothrombin time, and bleeding and clotting times to ensure that the client's ability to control bleeding is not compromised. If the client will use a CPM machine after surgery, it is useful for the client to be fitted for this before surgery.

When the client returns from surgery, the nurse reviews the physician orders concerning movement, turning, or positioning of the extremities. Usually, the head of the bed remains at 45° or less. The client with a total hip replacement needs to have legs abducted and extended because the opposite positions of adduction and flexion beyond 90° can dislocate the prosthetic femoral head from the acetabulum. Clients with a total hip replacement need to sit in an elevated chair or on a seat raised by pillows, so that the flexion remains less than 90°. Ice packs help reduce pain and inflammation to the incisional site (particularly after knee surgery). Box 61-5 provides information about avoiding hip dislocation after total hip replacement.

If CPM devices are prescribed to promote gentle flexion and extension of the knee after knee replacement, the nurse or physical therapist increases the flexion as indicated up to the goal of 90°. If CPM devices are used after hip surgery, the flexion should not exceed 30°.

| BOX 61-5 | Avoiding Hip Dislocation After Conventional Replacement Surgery |

Until the hip prosthesis stabilizes after hip replacement surgery, the client needs to learn about proper positioning so that the prosthesis remains in place. Dislocation of the hip is a serious complication of surgery that causes pain and necessitates reoperation to correct the dislocation. Desirable positions include abduction, neutral rotation, and flexion of less than 90°. When the client is seated, the knees should be lower than the hip. Guidelines for avoiding displacement are as follows:
- Keep the knees apart at all times.
- Put a pillow between the legs when sleeping.
- Never cross the legs when seated.
- Avoid bending forward when seated in a chair.
- Avoid bending forward to pick up an object on the floor.
- Use a raised toilet seat.
- Do not flex the hip to put on clothing such as pants, stockings, socks, or shoes.

Preventing postoperative complications after joint replacement is an important role of the nurse. Table 61-2 presents strategies to prevent postoperative complications after joint replacement surgery. Nursing Care Plan 61-1 provides more information related to nursing management of a client who requires surgery.

Client and Family Teaching

The nurse talks with the client, family, and other significant caregivers about the support system that will be available after discharge. It is important to explore the kinds of assistance the client needs for moving and walking, preparing meals, getting to the physician's office or physical therapy department, and performing other household tasks. The nurse tries to identify modifications that will be necessary in the home environment, such as relocating the bed to a ground floor level. In addition, he or she provides information about renting home care equipment, arranging for home delivery of meals through a community agency or church service group, or scheduling transportation with an agency that has a medical van or hydraulic lift available. The nurse may refer the client to a home healthcare agency or extended-care facility. He or she provides printed discharge instructions for future reference and covers the following general points:

- Follow the directions of the physician. Do not resume any activity that has been restricted until told to do so.
- Perform exercises exactly as prescribed by the physician and physical therapist.

- Use the recommended device (walker, cane, crutches) for walking.
- Wear supportive shoes when using crutches, walker, or cane.
- Eliminate safety hazards in the home, such as scatter rugs.
- Eat a nutritious diet and drink plenty of fluids.
- Take prescribed medications as directed; do not use or take any nonprescription drugs unless the physician has approved them.
- Notify the physician if the incision has unusual drainage or if fever, chills, sudden onset of pain, redness, or swelling occurs.

AMPUTATION

Amputation is the removal of a limb. It may occur as a result of trauma (traumatic amputation) or in an effort to control disease or disability (therapeutic amputation).

Etiology

The following are conditions for which an amputation may be performed:

- Malignant tumors
- Long-standing infections of bone and tissue that prohibit restoration of function
- Extensive trauma to an extremity

TABLE 61-2 Preventing Postoperative Complications After Joint Replacement Surgery

POTENTIAL COMPLICATION	POTENTIAL RISK FACTORS	PREVENTION STRATEGIES
Dislocation of prosthesis	Positioning beyond recommended flexion or extension Malfunction of prosthesis	Position client as prescribed. Instruct client to maintain appropriate position. Use pillows, splints, immobilizers, or slings to maintain prescribed position. Report increased pain, swelling, or change in mobility.
Infection	Older, debilitated clients Malnourishment Other infections such as urinary tract infections or dental abscesses Incision, wound drains, catheters, or IVs Hematoma	Monitor vital signs. Assess wound appearance and drainage. Practice aseptic technique when changing dressings and emptying drainage devices. Administer prophylactic antibiotics as prescribed. Teach client that for at least 3 months after surgery there is a potential for infection; he or she may require prophylactic antibiotics for dental cleaning or other invasive procedures. Report increased pain, elevated temperature, redness, swelling, or change in drainage from the incision.
Neurovascular compromise	Trauma Edema Immobilization devices	Assess neurovascular status frequently, including color, temperature, capillary refill, pulses, edema, pain, mobility, and sensation. Report client complaints of deep, unrelenting pain; feelings of tightness; numbness; and decreased mobility. Elevate extremity. Release constricting dressings, wraps, casts, or immobilizers.
Deep vein thrombosis	Surgical procedure Immobility	Apply elastic stockings/wraps as prescribed. Assess peripheral pulses. Change position frequently as allowed. Increase activity as indicated. Encourage client to perform passive ROM exercises. Prevent pressure on popliteal vessels.

NURSING CARE PLAN 61-1 | The Client Undergoing Orthopedic Surgery

Assessment

- When the client returns from surgery, review orders in the chart regarding immobilization, movement or turning, and positioning of the arm or leg. Inspect the dressing over the incision. If a wound drain is present, assess the patency of the drain and the type and amount of drainage in the collection receptacle. Assess the neurovascular status of the affected extremity. Monitor vital signs frequently until they stabilize, and routinely thereafter. Maintain the infusing IV fluids as ordered. Assess respiratory status. Encourage the client to identify pain levels and the effectiveness of analgesics.
- Within the first 24 to 72 hours after orthopedic surgery, a complication such as a fat embolus may occur (see Table 62-1) The symptoms are similar to those of a pulmonary embolus. In addition, petechial hemorrhages may appear on the skin of the chest. Report severe chest pain or unrelieved incisional pain to the physician immediately.

Nursing Diagnosis: Risk for Ineffective Breathing Pattern related to mucus and inability to mobilize secretions from the airway

Expected Outcome: Client will demonstrate effective respiratory rate and depth with clear breath sounds.

Interventions	Rationales
Instruct client to deep breathe and cough every 2 hours until he or she can ambulate.	These measures expand the lungs and mobilize mucus, preventing pooling of secretions.
Encourage client to use an incentive spirometer to increase deep breathing. Evaluate client's efforts.	Increasing respiratory effort improves client's respiratory status.
Turn client at least every 2 hours and encourage activity within prescribed limits.	Movement facilitates lung expansion and prevents pooling of secretions.
Auscultate lung sounds every 4 hours.	Immobility can cause hypoventilation, predisposing a client to atelectasis, pooling of respiratory secretions, and pneumonia.

Evaluation of Expected Outcome

Client effectively deep breathes and coughs. Lung sounds are clear.

Nursing Diagnosis: Acute Pain related to surgery

Expected Outcome: Client will report relief of pain.

Interventions	Rationales
Gently move client or adjust position.	Gentle handling minimizes discomfort.
Administer analgesics as prescribed. Instruct client in the use of patient-controlled analgesia if prescribed.	Regular administration of analgesics controls and prevents escalation of pain.
Elevate affected extremity and use cold applications.	These measures reduce swelling.
Report client's complaints of severe or sudden and unrelenting pain.	These findings may indicate a complication of surgery (see Table 62-1)

Evaluation of Expected Outcome

Client reports pain relief with analgesics and positioning.

Nursing Diagnosis: Risk for Disuse Syndrome related to immobility imposed by casting, traction, and non-weight-bearing status

Expected Outcome: Client will maintain full ROM of unaffected joints, intact skin, good peripheral blood flow, and normal bowel and bladder function.

Interventions	Rationales.
Encourage client to do ROM exercises as indicated.	ROM exercises help to maintain muscle strength and tone and prevent contractions.
Position client so that joints are in anatomic alignment.	Proper positioning prevents joint deformities and damage to peripheral nerves and blood vessels.
Get client up as soon as indicated, either in chair, ambulating, or on tilt table.	Early mobilization prevents complications related to prolonged bed rest.
When getting client up after bed rest, do so slowly. monitoring for signs of postural hypotension, tachycardia, nausea, diaphoresis, or syncope.	When sitting or standing after even 3 to 4 days of bed rest, a client can experience postural hypotension.
Turn client every 2 hours; inspect skin for signs of pressure.	Frequent turning relieves pressure and identifies problems, allowing for early intervention.
Apply antiembolism stockings as indicated.	They help prevent deep vein thrombosis (DVT).

NURSING CARE PLAN 61-1 The Client Undergoing Orthopedic Surgery (Continued)

Interventions	Rationales.
Monitor peripheral circulation, particularly noting skin color, pulses, or any swelling.	Prolonged bed rest, orthopedic surgery, and venous stasis can cause DVT and pulmonary embolism. Capillary refill should be brisk (within 3 seconds), skin should be warm and normally colored, and the client should be able to move the extremity. Diminished or absent pulses, pale or mottled skin, cool or cold skin, or increased pain (especially with movement) can indicate arterial obstruction. Changes in sensation such as numbness, tingling, or prickling may indicate nerve compression and damage, compartment syndrome, or both.
Monitor bowel function daily. Provide increased fluids and fiber.	Immobilization causes constipation secondary to inactivity and inappropriate food intake. Decreased fluid intake contributes to constipation.
Encourage client to increase fluid intake to 2000 mL/day unless contraindicated.	Increased intake promotes normal bladder function and prevents constipation, kidney stones, and other related complications of prolonged bed rest.

Evaluation of Expected Outcomes

- Client can maintain full ROM of unaffected joints.
- Skin remains intact without signs of pressure or breakdown.
- Peripheral circulation is adequate to sustain tissue perfusion.
- Client has adequate urine output and regular bowel movements.

Nursing Diagnosis: **Risk for Infection** related to compromised skin integrity

Expected Outcome: Client will remain free of infection.

Interventions	Rationales
Inspect pins or wire sites used in traction or external fixation devices and the surgical incision, or beneath a cast window for signs of infection.	Regular inspection promotes early detection of and prompt intervention for infection.
Practice Standard Precautions and conscientious handwashing.	These measures prevent infection.
Use aseptic principles when changing dressings and performing pin care.	Asepsis prevents the introduction of microorganisms into wounds and incisions.
Keep wound drainage system below the level of the incision.	Doing so prevents backflow of drainage into the incision.
Administer prescribed antibiotics.	They reduce microorganisms and control infection.
Report purulent wound drainage, elevated temperature, chills, and increased white blood count.	These are signs of infection that require intervention.

Evaluation of Expected Outcome

Client is free of infection, as evidenced by normal temperature, clean incisions and pin sites, and no purulent drainage.

Nursing Diagnosis: **Self-Care Deficit: Bathing and Hygiene, Feeding, Dressing, and Toileting** related to musculoskeletal impairment

Expected Outcome: Client will gradually perform ADLs as independently as possible.

Interventions	Rationales
Collaborate with client to determine tasks that he or she may perform independently.	Doing so promotes independence and provides client with a sense of control.
Plan activities and rest.	Doing so conserves energy and prevents fatigue.
Consult with physical therapist (PT) and occupational therapist (OT) about client's needs related to ADLs.	PT and OT will determine adaptive equipment needed, as well as client's strengths and abilities to master self-care tasks.
Provide pain medication 45 minutes before activity.	Pain relief promotes participation in self-care.

Evaluation of Expected Outcome

Client can partially bathe and feed himself or herself, dress upper body, and use the bedside commode.

- Death of tissues from peripheral vascular insufficiency or peripheral vasospastic diseases such as Buerger's and Raynaud's diseases
- Thermal injuries
- Deformity of a limb, rendering it a useless hindrance
- Life-threatening disorders, such as arterial thrombosis and gas bacillus infections

Medical and Surgical Management

Unless emergency surgery is performed, the client is treated for any disorder that may influence healing (e.g., uncontrolled diabetes mellitus, dehydration, infection, electrolyte imbalances, poor nutrition, chronic respiratory disorders). When it is decided that amputation must be performed as a lifesaving measure, the following factors help the surgical team decide at which level to amputate the arm or leg (e.g., above or below the knee, above or below the elbow):

- Amount of tissue that must be removed to eliminate the disorder
- Level at which the blood supply is adequate to preserve circulation to tissue that will remain
- Number of joints that can be preserved
- Length of residual limb that will promote fitting a prosthesis, an artificial limb, for rehabilitation

The levels of some commonly planned amputations include below the knee (BK), above the knee (AK), below the elbow (BE), and above the elbow (AE). The surgical objective is to create a gently tapering stump with muscular padding over the end. Occasionally, knee disarticulations (amputation through a joint), disarticulation at the ankle joint, and partial foot amputations are performed.

Amputation Methods

An amputation may be performed using an open or closed method. In an open amputation (guillotine amputation), the end of the residual limb (or stump) is temporarily open with no skin covering it. Open amputations usually are performed in cases of infection. Skin traction is applied, and the infected area is allowed to drain. The traction must be continuous. The surgeon may arrange the traction so that the client can turn over in bed.

In the more common closed amputation (flap amputation), skin flaps cover the severed bone end. Clients with a closed amputation return from surgery with either a soft compression dressing or rigid plaster shell covering the residual limb. The compression dressing consists of gauze over which elastic roller bandages are wrapped to create pressure to control bleeding. There may be a walking pylon, a type of temporary prosthesis composed of a metal post and molded foot, attached to the rigid plaster shell (Fig. 61-8). It may be weeks before the postoperative client is referred to a prosthetist, a professional who creates and fits artificial limbs.

A *staged amputation* is planned when a client has severe infection and gangrene. The guillotine method is first used, and then a few days later, after the infection is treated and the client is stable, a more definitive, closed amputation is done.

Arm Amputation

The arms have highly specialized functions. Consequently, the amputation of an arm, particularly the arm with the

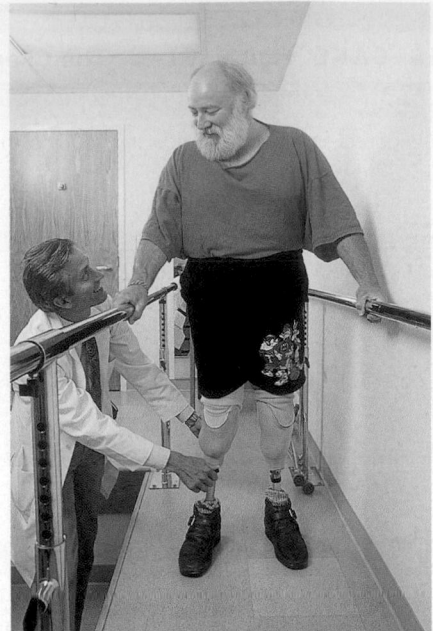

FIGURE 61-8. Many amputees receive prostheses soon after surgery and begin learning how to use them with the help and support of the rehabilitation team, which includes nurses, physicians, physical therapists, and others.

dominant hand, requires great physical and emotional adjustment during the preoperative as well as postoperative periods. Fortunately, most clients with arm amputations can be measured for a prosthesis shortly after the surgical scar heals.

Three types of prostheses are available for arm amputees: a shoulder harness with cables that attach to a mechanical terminal device, referred to as a *hook;* a semifunctioning cosmetic hand that can be substituted for the hook; and a myoelectric arm.

The hook performs the functions of the hand and fingers when the amputee moves the scapula and expands the chest, activating the cables attached from a shoulder harness to the mechanical device. The mechanical terminal device is strong, sturdy, and functional. The cosmetic hand, which can be attached to the same cables as the hook, has the appearance of a natural hand, but it lacks the capacity for performing fine motor skills. The myoelectric arm has a realistic-looking hand that is activated by electrical impulses from muscles in the upper arm. The electrical activity is relayed from electrodes in the shell of the prosthesis to microcircuits in the prosthetic fingers. The myoelectric arm has three advantages: it eliminates the need to wear a harness, the terminal device looks natural, and it has somewhat better function than the cosmetic hand. Despite its advantages, the myoelectric arm is not rugged enough to do the work of the mechanical terminal device.

Leg Amputation

Amputation of a leg is a more common operation than amputation of an arm. The AK amputation is more disabling than a BK amputation; therefore, unless evidence suggests that the knee cannot be saved, every attempt is made to amputate below the knee.

The trend is to have a temporary prosthesis attached to the plaster shell covering the residual lower limb immediately after surgery. It reduces psychological trauma for the client because it promotes a more intact sense of body image after surgery. Also, the walking pylon facilitates early ambulation. Almost immediately, the client is allowed to stand and place a limited amount of weight on the residual limb. As the stump heals and edema disappears, a second cast may be re-applied or a temporary socket made of lightweight polypropylene may be constructed. Ultimately, a conventional prosthesis is custom-made to conform to the stump as well as to the client's needs. Leg prostheses may be held in place by means of a pelvic belt or suction.

Complications

Hematoma, hemorrhage, and infection are potential complications in the immediate postoperative period. Potential complications late in the postoperative course include chronic osteomyelitis (after persistent infection) and, rarely, a burning pain (causalgia), the cause of which is unknown. Pain may result from a stump neuroma, which is formed when the cut ends of nerves become entangled in the healing scar. A neuroma is treated with injections of procaine, a local anesthetic, or re-amputation.

Phantom Limb and Phantom Pain

The surgeon informs the client of the potential phenomenon of phantom limb sensation, which is a feeling that the amputated portion of the limb still remains. It is a normal, frequently occurring physiologic response after amputation. Phantom sensations can persist for months or decades, or can come and go. Although clients are aware of phantom sensations, they usually learn to ignore them.

Phantom pain is pain or other discomfort, such as burning, tingling, throbbing, or itching, in the missing limb. Pain felt from the phantom limb can be an extremely serious problem in relation to the client's emotional status and ability to use a prosthesis. Severe, prolonged phantom limb pain may require surgical removal of nerve endings at the end of the stump.

Rehabilitation

The success of the amputee's rehabilitation depends on variables such as age, type of amputation, condition of the stump, physical status, condition of the remaining limb, concurrent debilitating illness, visual motor coordination, motivation, acceptance, and cooperation. Clients vary greatly in their learning capacity and ability to master the use of a prosthesis. The period allotted for training also varies with each client. It is vital that the physician, the nurse, the physical and occupational therapists, the family, and the client maintain realistic expectations throughout the rehabilitation period.

Presurgical Nursing Management

Nursing management of an amputee can be segmented into two key functions: those before surgery and those after surgery. In general, presurgical nursing management involves considerations for any surgery, specifically taking a complete medical, drug, and allergy history and evaluating the client for mental and emotional acceptance of the surgical procedure.

Assessing motor strength and flexibility of other joints is important to determine potential problems involving rehabilitation. If the client is acutely ill, such as with a gangre-nous limb and related fever, disorientation, and electrolyte imbalances, the nurse monitors circulation in the limb for changes, such as severe pain, color changes, and lack of peripheral pulses. It is crucial that the nurse inform the physician of problems as they occur because surgery may become an emergency.

Nursing interventions aim to reduce pain and anxiety and support the client as he or she begins to grieve the loss of the limb and adapt to potential changes. The nurse administers narcotic analgesics before surgery to clients with severe pain. Other comfort measures include handling the painful limb gently, elevating a swollen limb, encouraging family presence and support, being available, especially at times when the client is alone, helping the client to express concerns, and clarifying misperceptions.

Before surgery, the nurse explains all the routine preoperative preparations and reinforces what the physician has discussed with the client and family regarding the extent of physical disability; the psychological, aesthetic, social, and vocational implications; and the realistic possibilities for prosthetic restoration. The nurse must exercise care in answering questions about prosthetic devices and their use because it always is possible that the amputation may need to involve more of the limb than originally anticipated. In addition, the nurse reviews the postoperative management, such as deep breathing, coughing, positioning, and routine exercises and encourages the client to practice the exercises if time and the client's condition permit.

Clients vary in their reactions to the impending loss of a limb. The amount of grief is thought to be proportional to the symbolic significance of the part and the resultant degree of disability and deformity. Anger and depression are common emotions. The nurse acknowledges the client's feelings and remains objective and nonjudgmental as the client expresses negative emotional responses. Reassuring the client that his or her reaction is normal may provide comfort. The nurse should not shame, criticize, or trivialize the client's behavior.

How well the client can cope usually depends on prior experience and how he or she has dealt with previous losses. The nurse protects the client from additional sources of stress. While the client is preoccupied with the potential loss, the nurse should not make unnecessary demands or expect full participation in the plan of care. The nurse provides assistance with activities that at any other time the client could carry out independently. The nurse also promotes adequate sleep and discusses coping techniques that have been used successfully in the past and encourages their repetition. Fostering communication with family members or friends promotes support.

Nursing Process for the Client After a Limb Amputation

Assessment

Monitor vital signs to determine any changes, particularly elevations in temperature (indicating possible infection), pulse, and blood pressure. Reviewing the client's medical record provides information about the reason for and type and level of the amputation. Inspect the dressing or plaster shell and, when changing the dressing, assess the wound for signs of infection, excessive drainage, or separation of wound edges. In addition, evaluate the client's general condition as well as level of pain and discomfort, and implement measures to relieve it.

Diagnosis, Planning, and Interventions

Nursing management involves all concerns addressed after any orthopedic surgery (see Nursing Care Plan 61-1). Implement measures to prevent infection, promote healing, and avoid skin breakdown. See Nursing Guidelines 61-5 for stump care and bandaging. Care also includes, but is not limited to, the following:

▶ **Risk for Self-Care Deficit (specify bathing/hygiene, dressing/ grooming, feeding, toileting)** related to impediments imposed by amputation

▶ **Expected Outcome:** Client will participate in self-care and recuperative measures to the fullest extent possible.

- Encourage clients with leg amputations to assume some of their own care 1 or 2 days after surgery. *Incorporating the client's abilities increases self-care independence.*
- Assist clients with an arm amputation, especially on the dominant side, until they can use the opposite extremity. *It takes time for clients to adjust to having only one upper extremity.*
- Exercise and position the client in proper alignment. *Correct positioning prevents contractures after amputation, maintains skeletal alignment, and promotes active movement of the uninvolved limbs.*
- Work with the physical therapist to implement a program of active and isometric exercises. *These exercises increase the client's abilities and strengths.*

▶ **Risk for Disuse Syndrome** related to altered mobility after amputation

▶ **Expected Outcomes:** (1) Client will become progressively mobile and independent. (2) Client will maintain intact skin, adequate tissue perfusion, and normal pulmonary function. (3) Client will not develop complications related to immobility.

- Place client with a leg amputation in the prone position several times a day. *This position promotes stump extension and prevents contractures.*
- Position client so that he or she is in normal anatomic alignment at all times. *Improper positioning may injure peripheral nerves and blood vessels and cause joint deformities.*
- Use a trochanter roll to prevent external rotation of the hip and knee. Avoid placing pillows between the legs. *These measures prevent abduction deformity.*
- Advise the client who is lying on the stomach to adduct the stump so it presses against the other leg. *Adduction stretches flexor muscles and prevents abduction deformity.*
- On the 1st or 2nd postoperative day, assist client to stand to regain a sense of balance. Stepping on the floor with the temporary prosthesis and weight bearing of about 10% of body weight usually is permitted at this time. *These measures promote strength and balance while preventing injury.*

- Expect the client with a temporary prosthesis to progress to walking with crutches or a walker or in parallel bars 2 to 4 days after the amputation with a high degree of safety (full weight bearing on the unaffected leg). *This measure promotes independence.*
- Provide client with assistive devices. *They help client to be more independent and maintain more mobility.*
- Use antiembolism stockings. *They prevent deep vein thrombosis.*
- Monitor pulmonary status and implement deep-breathing and coughing exercises. *Decreased mobility can result in hypoventilation and may lead to atelectasis and pooling of secretions. Pulmonary exercises improve lung expansion and mobilize secretions.*
- Increase fluid intake to 2000 mL (if permitted). *This intake promotes urine output and prevents constipation.*

▶ **Grieving** related to loss of body part

▶ **Expected Outcome:** Client will state that he or she is beginning to resolve loss and develop strategies for coping without an arm or leg.

- Listen actively and empathetically. *Doing so facilitates communication.*
- Allow clients time to talk about their loss and express feelings of grief, anger, depression, and anxiety. *Grief is hard work and needs time.*
- Discuss each new challenge as it arises. *Providing information and listening to client's feelings assists the client to face new issues.*
- Allow client time to process information. *Providing time allows the client to adjust to new situations.*
- Implement changes gradually. *Doing so gives client time to adjust and adapt.*
- Reinforce progress that has been made. *Doing so provides encouragement and support.*
- Remain available to the client for physical and emotional support. *The nurse can serve as a consistent support system.*
- Foster family involvement because their encouragement often helps motivate a client to face each new problem, accept failure, and develop a determination to overcome obstacles. *Support from significant others can have a positive effect.*
- Ambulate the client with a leg amputation as soon as possible. *Doing so dispels the doubt that permanent disability will prevail.*
- Explore the possibility of a meeting with a rehabilitated amputee. *Someone who has endured a similar experience can serve as a support network.*

▶ **Disturbed Body Image** related to loss of body part and function

▶ **Expected Outcome:** Client will progressively adjust to the change in body image.

- Keep in mind that the attitude of staff and family members bears greatly on how clients perceive themselves. *A positive approach promotes a client's positive self-image.*
- Do not treat the client as less than competent. *Focusing on client's strengths and abilities promotes his or her self-image.*

NURSING GUIDELINES 61–5

Stump Care and Bandaging

Stump Care

- Assess the covering over the stump frequently to determine the type and amount of drainage from the incision. Expect some oozing of blood, but if a gauze dressing is used, it may need to be reinforced.
- Keep a tourniquet in plain view at bedside and if hemorrhage occurs, apply it and notify the physician.
- Generally, elevate the stump for the first 24 to 48 hours to prevent edema. In some cases, such as an AK amputation, a slight Trendelenburg position is preferred to elevating the stump on pillows because bending the hip promotes a flexion contracture. A bed board or a firm mattress provides skeletal support.
- If the client has a rigid plaster cast with walking pylon, loosen the harness, which suspends the cast from the waist, when the client is in bed. Slightly tighten the harness when the client is ambulatory.

Bandaging

Before a permanent prosthesis can be made, the stump must shrink and be shaped. This is done with elastic bandages that are wrapped about the stump. Unlike leg stumps, arm stumps do not need as massive a shrinkage over as long a period. Various bandaging techniques are appropriate, but several principles are observed:

- Remove and rewrap the bandage at least twice during the day and before the client retires for the night.
- Bandage joints in a way that promotes a neutral or extended position.
- Avoid circular turns, which act like a tourniquet and interfere with blood flow.

Client and Family Teaching 61-1
Home Care After Limb Amputation

If the client has to bandage the stump at home, the nurse teaches both the client and the family how to apply the bandage and how to care for the stump and provides other general instructions:

- Wash the bandages, rinse them well, and lay them flat to dry because hanging tends to decrease the elasticity.
- When the bandages are dry, they must be rolled without stretching.
- Follow the physician's recommendations regarding caring for the stump, applying a stump dressing, washing the stump, and elevating the stump when sitting.
- Do not apply nonprescription drugs (ointments, creams, topical pain relievers) to the stump unless the physician has approved the use of a specific product.
- Adhere to the plan of scheduled exercises and complete each group of exercises as outlined by the physical therapist.
- Do not exceed the physician's recommendations regarding weight bearing and joint flexion.
- Eat well-balanced and nutritious meals or follow the diet recommended by the physician. Avoid gaining excess weight during the recovery period because weight gain may interfere with use of a leg prosthesis.
- Expect that phantom limb sensation, if present, may persist for some time, which is normal.
- Avoid injury to the stump, even though it appears to be healed. Report any skin impairment immediately.
- Continue deep-breathing exercises until fully mobile.
- Contact the physician if fever, chills, productive cough, bleeding or oozing from the stump, purulent drainage from the incision, new or different pain in the stump, or any change in the appearance of the stump occurs.

- Avoid nonverbal implications that the client, the stump, or the prosthesis is repulsive. *Being aware of nonverbal behavior indicates how the client feels about himself or herself.*
- Make a point to visit the client frequently, especially when no particular nursing activity must be performed. *Such visits encourage client to feel more positively about himself or herself.*
- Make eye contact during verbal interactions. *The nurse must treat all clients with the same respect.*
- Sit close to the client's bedside and lean forward when talking. *Doing so communicates a personal interest in the client.*
- Offer praise when the client successfully accomplishes a task. *Praise builds self-esteem and self-confidence.*
- If appropriate, explore the client's reasons for refusing to use a prosthesis. *If the problem is amenable to change, the nurse can enlist the help of the surgeon, physical therapist, or prosthetist.*

Evaluation of Expected Outcomes

By discharge, the client reports reduced and manageable pain, no infection, and intact skin; he or she demonstrates optimal participation in self-care. The client experiences increasing mobility along with increasing resolution of grief, greater self-acceptance, and acceptance of current situation. He or she experiences no postoperative complications. The client does not withdraw from social situations, has a positive attitude about the future, and can demonstrate adequate independent self-care.

Discharge teaching depends on many factors, including the length of hospitalization, the type and location of the amputation, the age and physical condition of the client, and the type of dressing or prosthesis the client wears. Factors related to the home environment influence the plan for rehabilitation after discharge. Some clients need to modify their living arrangements, use a wheelchair, or make other accommodations or changes. See Client and Family Teaching 61-1 for discharge instructions. ●

CRITICAL THINKING EXERCISES

1. A male client had a total hip replacement 3 days ago and wants to use the toilet for a bowel movement. Explain how to assist this client.

2. A female client has just returned from the recovery unit after an AK amputation. Fresh blood has saturated the

stump dressing. What actions should you take at this time?

3. A young man, admitted with a fractured radius, complains of increasing pain in his hand after a cast was applied, despite having received a narcotic analgesic 30 minutes ago. What assessments are important to make at this time?

4. A client asks the nurse why the cast on his fractured left tibia extends on to his foot and over his knee. What would you tell him?

NCLEX-STYLE REVIEW QUESTIONS

1. While backpacking with a youth group, a client sustains an injury to the lower leg. A nurse who is accompanying the group suspects a fracture of the tibia. To immobilize the suspected fracture, where is the best location to apply the splint?
   1. above the ankle to below the knee.
   2. above the knee to below the hip.
   3. below the ankle to above the knee.
   4. below the knee to above the hip.

2. Postoperatively, before turning the client with the hip prosthesis onto the nonoperative side, what would the nurse do first?
   1. Elevate the head of client's bed.
   2. Flex client's knee on the affected side.
   3. Have client point toes downward.
   4. Place pillows between the client's legs.

3. A plaster arm cast will be applied to an adult client with a compound fracture of the radius. When preparing the client for the cast application, what does the nurse explain to the client?
   1. The client may experience itching while the cast is wet.
   2. The client's arm will feel warm as the wet plaster sets.
   3. The cast will feel tight as it is applied.
   4. There will be a foul odor until the cast is dry.

4. A plaster arm cast is applied to an adult client with a compound fracture of the radius. While the physician wraps the arm with rolls of wet plaster, where should the nurse support the wet cast?
   1. On a firm surface
   2. On a soft mattress
   3. With the palms of the hands
   4. With the tips of the fingers

5. A plaster cast has been applied to an adult client with a compound fracture of the radius. Which method is best for assessing the circulation of the casted extremity?
   1. Ask the client if he or she can wiggle the fingers.
   2. Depress the nail bed and document the time it takes for the color to return.
   3. Feel the cast to determine if it is unusually hot or cold.
   4. See if there is enough room to insert a finger between the cast and the extremity.

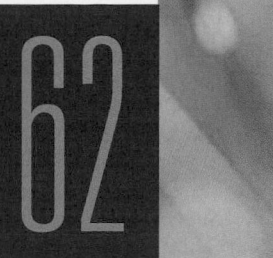

62

Caring for Clients with Traumatic Musculoskeletal Injuries

Words To Know

avascular necrosis
avulsion fracture
callus
carpal tunnel syndrome
compartment syndrome
contusion
dislocation
ecchymosis
epicondylitis
fasciotomy
fracture
ganglioncyst
menisectomy
palsy
rotator cuff
sprain
strain
subluxation
tendonitis
Volkmann's contracture

Learning Objectives

On completion of this chapter, you reader will be able to:

1. Differentiate strains, contusions, and sprains.
2. Define joint dislocations.
3. Discuss the nursing management of various types of sports or work-related injuries.
4. Identify the stages of bone healing after a fracture.
5. Describe the signs and symptoms of a fracture.
6. Explain the nursing management for clients with various types of fractures.
7. Discuss methods used to prevent complications associated with fractures.
8. Discuss potential complications associated with a fractured hip.

Injuries to the musculoskeletal system affect more than just a muscle or bone. A fractured bone or other injury can potentially cause dysfunction to the surrounding muscle and injury to the blood vessels and nerves. Treatment of musculoskeletal trauma involves immobilization of the injured area until it has healed. It also requires prevention of further injury and complications.

STRAINS, CONTUSIONS, AND SPRAINS

A **strain** is an injury to a muscle when it is stretched or pulled beyond its capacity. A **contusion** is a soft tissue injury resulting from a blow or blunt trauma. **Sprains** are injuries to the ligaments surrounding a joint.

Pathophysiology and Etiology

A strain results from excessive stress, overuse, or overstretching. Small blood vessels in the muscle rupture, and the muscle fibers sustain tiny tears. The client experiences inflammation, local tenderness, and muscle spasms.

In contusions, injury is confined to the soft tissues and does not affect the musculoskeletal structure. Many small blood vessels rupture, causing bruises (**ecchymosis**) or a hematoma (collection of blood). Applying cold packs helps to alleviate local pain, swelling, and bruising. A contusion usually resolves within 2 weeks.

Areas most subject to sprains are the wrist, elbow, knee, and ankle. A sprain of the cervical spine is commonly called a *whiplash injury*. Sprains result from sudden, unusual movement or stretching about a joint, which is common with falls or other accidental injuries. The force twists the joint in a direction it was not designed for or displaces it beyond its normal range of motion (ROM) by partially tearing or rupturing the attachment of ligaments. The damage usually is confined to the ligaments and adjacent soft tissue. In severe traumatic sprains, however, a chip of bone to which the ligament is attached may become detached.

At this point, the injury becomes an **avulsion fracture.** A hematoma that may develop subsequently contributes to the pain because the mass exerts additional pressure on nerve endings in the area.

Assessment Findings

The injured area becomes painful immediately, and swelling usually follows. The person typically avoids full weight bearing or using the injured joint or limb. Later, ecchymoses may appear. In cases of extensive ligamental tearing, the joint may be unstable until it heals.

In most cases, diagnosis is made by examination of the affected part and symptoms. Radiographic films may show a larger-than-usual joint space and rule out or confirm an accompanying fracture. Arthrography demonstrates asymmetry in the joint as a result of the damaged ligaments, or arthroscopy may disclose trauma in the joint capsule.

Medical and Surgical Management

Treatment consists of applying ice or a chemical cold pack to the area to reduce swelling and relieve pain for the first 24 to 48 hours. Elevation of the part and compression with an elastic bandage also may be recommended. The acronym RICES refers to *r*est, *i*ce, *c*ompression, *e*levation, and *s*tabilization—a method for remembering the treatment for strains, contusions, and sprains (Lasowski-Jones, 2006). After two days, when swelling no longer is likely to increase, applying heat reduces pain and relieves local edema by improving circulation. Full use of the injured joint is discouraged temporarily. Nonsteroidal anti-inflammatory drugs (NSAIDs) ease discomfort.

Continued trauma during healing may result in a permanently unstable joint or the formation of fibrous adhesions that may limit full ROM. Occasionally, a removable splint or light cast is applied for several weeks. A soft cervical collar limits motion if the client has a neck sprain. When sufficient healing has occurred, progressively active exercises are prescribed.

▶ **Stop, Think, and Respond Exercise 62-1**

You are at a playground when you notice a man, who has been playing basketball with his son, fall and grab his ankle. He says his ankle hurts very badly, and he does not think that he can walk. What action should you take?

DISLOCATIONS

Dislocations occur when the articular surfaces of a joint are no longer in contact. The shoulder, hip, and knee commonly are affected. A partial dislocation is referred to as a **subluxation.**

Pathophysiology and Etiology

In adults, trauma usually causes dislocations. Occasionally, diseases of the joint result in dislocations when the ligaments supporting a joint are torn, stretched, or relaxed. Separation of adjacent bones from their articulating joint interferes with normal use and produces a distorted appearance. The injury may disrupt local blood supply to structures such as the joint cartilage, causing degeneration, chronic pain, and restricted movement. **Compartment syndrome** (a condition in which a structure such as a tendon or nerve is constricted in a confined space) also may develop. The syndrome affects nerve innervation, leading to subsequent **palsy** (decreased sensation and movement). If compartment syndrome occurs in an upper extremity, it may lead to **Volkmann's contracture,** a clawlike deformity of the hand resulting from obstructed arterial blood flow to the forearm and hand. The client is unable to extend his or her fingers and complains of unrelenting pain, particularly if attempting to stretch the hand. There also are signs of compromised circulation to the hand.

Another possible complication of dislocations during the healing process involves an insufficient deposit of collagen during the repair stage. The end result is that the ligaments may have reduced tensile strength and future instability, leading to recurrent dislocations of the same joint.

Assessment Findings

The client often reports hearing a "popping" sound when the dislocation occurs. Another common complaint is that the joint suddenly "gave out," implying that it became unstable or nonsupportive. If the dislocation results from trauma, the client usually experiences considerable pain from the injury or the resultant muscle spasm.

On inspection, the structural shape is altered. A depression may be noted about the joint's circumference, indicating that the bones above and below are no longer aligned. If the dislocation affects an extremity, the arm or leg may be shorter than its unaffected counterpart as a result of the displacement of one of the articulating bones. ROM is limited. Evidence of soft-tissue injury includes swelling, coolness, numbness, tingling, and pale or dusky color of the distal tissue.

Radiographic films show intact yet malpositioned bones. Arthrography or arthroscopy may reveal damage to other structures in the joint capsule.

Medical and Surgical Management

The physician manipulates the joint or reduces the displaced parts until they return to normal position, then immobilizes the joint with an elastic bandage, cast, or splint for several weeks. Doing so allows the joint capsule and surrounding ligaments to heal. The client may receive a local or general anesthetic before the manipulation is performed. Some dislocations may require surgery, either to correct the dislocation or to repair damage caused by the injury.

Nursing Management

The nurse relieves the client's discomfort by administering prescribed analgesics, elevating and immobilizing the affected limb, and applying cold packs to the injury. He or she performs neurovascular assessments every 30 minutes for several hours, and then at least every 2 to 4 hours for the next 1 or 2 days to detect complications such as compartment syndrome. See Chapter 60 (Table 60-3) for more information about neurovascular assessments. Client and Family Teaching 62-1 describes preventive strategies for sports and/or work-related activities.

> ### Client and Family Teaching 62-1
> ### Preventing Sports and/or Work-Related Injuries
>
> The nurse teaches the client the following preventive measures:
>
> ● Use proper equipment at work and during participation in athletic activities.
> ● At work, look at ways to modify the environment to prevent injury. (Some work settings consult with ergonomic experts to modify the environment.)
> ● Exercise regularly to maintain joint and muscle strength.
> ● Maintain a healthy weight.
> ● Prepare for athletic activities by doing gradual warm-up exercises and stretching following the warm-up.
> ● At work, take a few minutes every 2 hours to relax, stretch muscles, and change position.
> ● Following exercise, allow for "cool-off" time and stretching so that the body has time to adapt to the change in activity level.
> ● If body symptoms such as pain or discomfort with movement occur, rest that body part until symptoms subside and then gradually re-introduce the activity.
> ● If symptoms persist, seek medical advice.

SPECIFIC INJURIES TO UPPER AND LOWER EXTREMITIES

Frequent sites of injury and pain in the extremities include the shoulder, elbow, wrist, knee, and ankle. Some of the injuries include acute injuries, such as those described above, and fractures (see later discussion). Other disorders occur more gradually as a result of repeated or overuse of a particular joint related to sports and exercise and work-related injuries. These include tendonitis, stress fractures, and other related injuries.

TENDONITIS

Tendonitis is the inflammation of a tendon caused by overuse. There are several types of tendonitis that commonly occur as a result of repeated sports and/or work activities. Epicondylitis, ganglions, and carpal tunnel syndrome are recurrent injuries that are frequently seen. **Epicondylitis** (tennis elbow) is a painful inflammation of the elbow. A **ganglioncyst** is a cystic mass that develops near tendon sheaths and joints of the wrist. **Carpal tunnel syndrome** is a term for a group of symptoms located in the carpal tunnel of the wrist, a narrow, inelastic canal through which the carpal tendons and median nerve pass.

Pathophysiology and Etiology

The primary causes of these injuries are trauma and repeated stress. Injury also is responsible for epicondylitis, which occurs when the tendons of the medial or lateral radial and ulnar epicondyles sustain damage. The injury typically follows excessive pronation and supination of the forearm, such

as that which occurs when playing tennis, pitching ball, or rowing. Ganglion cysts form through defects in the tendon sheath or joint capsule and occur most commonly in women younger than 50 years of age.

Carpal tunnel syndrome results from repetitive wrist motion that traumatizes the tendon sheath or ligaments in the carpal canal. The trauma produces swelling that compresses the median nerve against the transverse carpal ligament. Those affected tend to be in occupations that perform repetitive hand movements, such as cashiers, typists, musicians, assemblers, and all who spend many hours using a computer keyboard and mouse.

Assessment Findings
Signs and Symptoms

These injuries are marked by pain and inflammation, which can spread to surrounding tissues. In epicondylitis, clients report pain radiating down the dorsal surface of the forearm and a weak grasp. Clients with ganglion cysts experience pain and tenderness in the affected area. Clients with carpal tunnel syndrome describe pain or burning in one or both hands, which may radiate to the forearm and shoulder in severe cases. The pain tends to be more prominent at night and early in the morning. Shaking the hands may reduce the pain by promoting movement of edematous fluid from the carpal canal. Sensation may be lost or reduced in the thumb, index, middle, and a portion of the ring finger. The client may be unable to flex the index and middle fingers to make a fist. Flexion of the wrist usually causes immediate pain and numbness.

Diagnostic Findings

In general, x ray studies are used to identify abnormalities and rule out fracture and other problems. In carpal tunnel syndrome, results of electromyography, which relies on a mild electrical current to stimulate the nerve, show a delay in motor response in muscles innervated by the median nerve. Other tests are Tinel's sign, which is a test that elicits tingling, numbness, and pain for clients with carpal tunnel syndrome, and Phalen's sign, which involves having the client flex the wrist for 30 seconds to determine if pain or numbness occurs (a positive sign for carpal tunnel syndrome). The examiner percusses the median nerve, located on the inner aspect of the wrist, to elicit this response.

Medical and Surgical Management

Treatment of these disorders includes applications of cold (ice) and heat, exercise, steroidal anti-inflammatory medications, local injection of corticosteroids, analgesics, NSAIDs, and rest. Surgical intervention may be necessary to repair tears and ruptures. In many cases, clients with injuries of the shoulder or other portions of the upper extremity are referred for physical therapy. Treatment for epicondylitis may include splinting to rest and support the joint structures. Corticosteroids may be injected locally. Treatment of the ganglion cyst includes aspiration of the ganglion, corticosteroid injection, and surgical excision.

Carpal tunnel treatment involves resting the hands when possible and splinting the hand and wrist. NSAIDs and periodic injections of a corticosteroid preparation may relieve the inflammation and discomfort. If conservative treatment fails, surgery to release the pressure of the ligament on the median nerve may be performed.

Nursing Management

The nurse provides information about medications. If the client is taking NSAIDs, the nurse stresses to take these medications with food. If corticosteroid injections are ordered, he or she explains what the client can expect and mentions that the injection itself may cause some discomfort.

 Pharmacologic Considerations

- The most common adverse effects of NSAIDs are related to the gastrointestinal (GI) tract: nausea, vomiting, diarrhea, and constipation. GI bleeding, which in some cases is severe, has been reported with the use of these drugs.

The nurse shows clients how to use and care for prescribed splints and perform related ROM exercises. Some clients find that hand exercises are less painful if performed with the hand under warm water. Additional management activities involve exploring ways to perform activities of daily living (ADLs) or alter job responsibilities to relieve stress and reduce injury to joints.

Key teaching points include the following:

• Rest the joint in a position that reduces stress.
• Support the affected arm joint on pillows while sleeping.
• Apply cold for the first 24 to 48 hours to reduce swelling and pain.
• Gradually increase joint movement.
• Avoid working or lifting above shoulder level. Do not push objects with the arm joint, particularly the shoulder.
• Perform ROM and strengthening exercises as prescribed by the physician or physical therapist.

ROTATOR CUFF TEAR

The **rotator cuff** is made up of a complexity of muscles and tendons that connect the proximal humerus, clavicle, and scapula, which in turn connect with the sternum and ribs

(Porth, 2007). Rotator cuff injuries can occur as a result of a traumatic injury or from chronic overuse or irritation of the shoulder joint. Clients experience pain with movement and limited mobility of the shoulder and arm. They especially have difficulty with activities that involve stretching their arm above their head. Many clients find that the pain is worse at night and that they are unable to sleep on the affected side. The diagnosis is based on physical examination—generally, there is tenderness on the acromioclavicular joint. Radiography, arthrography, and magnetic resonance imaging (MRI) can evaluate the extent of the rotator cuff tear and any soft tissue injury.

Initial treatment begins with the use of NSAIDs. The physician will advise clients to modify their activities and to rest the joint. Physicians may also recommend corticosteroid injections into the shoulder joint, with progressive passive and active exercises and stretching. Surgical procedures include (Smeltzer et al., 2008):

• Arthroscopic debridement of devitalized tissue
• Arthroscopic tendon repair
• Open acromioplasty with tendon repair

Clients have to immobilize the shoulder for several days to weeks and then undergo physical therapy for several weeks to months. Generally, clients will have full recovery postoperatively within 6 to 12 months.

LIGAMENT AND MENISCAL INJURIES

Ligament and meniscal injuries to the knee occur as a result of a traumatic injury. Figure 62-1 depicts the knee ligaments and menisci (cartilages in the knee). Injuries can occur to the lateral or medial collateral knee ligaments (these ligaments provide stability to the sides of the knee) or to the anterior or posterior cruciate ligaments (ACL or PCL) (these ligaments provide stability to forward and backward movements). In addition, menisci can become injured, disrupting the stability of the leg when flexed or extended.

Pathophysiology and Etiology

Injury to the ligaments of the knee occurs at a time when the client is standing firmly and receives a blow or twists in a different direction while hyperextending the knee. The client

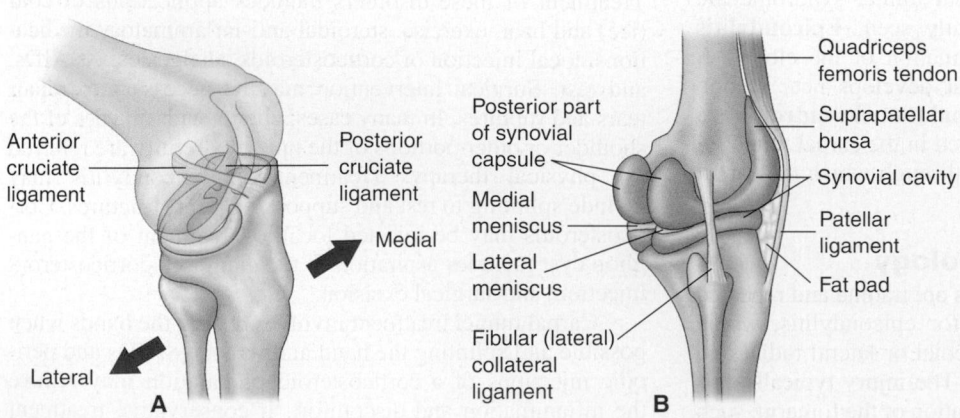

FIGURE 62-1. Knee ligaments and menisci. (**A**) Anterolateral view. (**B**) Posterolateral view.

Anterior cruciate ligament

Posterior cruciate ligament

Medial

Lateral

Posterior part of synovial capsule

Medial meniscus

Lateral meniscus

Fibular (lateral) collateral ligament

Quadriceps femoris tendon

Suprapatellar bursa

Synovial cavity

Patellar ligament

Fat pad

experiences pain, instability of the joint, and ambulatory difficulty. When the ACL or PCL tears, the client may report a popping sound or tearing sensation. Meniscal injuries occur with twisting of the knee or repeated squatting. Clients report that their knee "gave way" and may experience a click in their knee as they ambulate. In some instances, the knee locks because the cartilage moves as it tears and prevents full flexion and extension (Smeltzer et al., 2008).

Medical and Surgical Management

Treatment depends on the extent of the injury. Initial treatment involves immobilizing the joint and limiting weight bearing. The physician may recommend NSAIDs, as well as the use of ice during the first 48 hours. Gradual introduction of activity assists the client to progress without causing further injury. Surgical procedures include repair of the ligaments and tendons involved. For torn menisci, the surgeon removes the damaged cartilage (**meniscectomy**). Following surgery the physician will immobilize, prescribe NSAIDs, and recommend the application of cold therapy. Physical rehabilitation includes exercises, gradual weight bearing, and the use of any ambulatory devices. Recovery is generally complete within 3 to 12 months, depending on the nature of the injury and the type of surgery.

RUPTURED ACHILLES TENDON

Rupture of the Achilles tendon occurs secondary to trauma. As the client engages in an activity, the calf muscle contracts suddenly while the foot is grounded firmly in place. There is often a loud pop, and the client experiences severe pain and inability to plantar flex the affected foot. The client usually requires surgical repair for complete healing to occur. Following surgery, the client wears a cast or brace for 6 to 8 weeks. Physical therapy is necessary for the client to regain mobility, strength, and full ROM.

The nurse teaches the client about activity restrictions, the use of ambulatory aids, and pain management. Clients who have surgery need to have preoperative and postoperative instructions. Refer to Nursing Care Plan 61-1 in Chapter 61 for more information relevant to orthopedic surgery.

FRACTURES

A **fracture** is a break in the continuity of a bone. Fractures may affect tissues or organs near the bones as well. Fractures are classified according to type and extent (Box 62-1).

Pathophysiology and Etiology

When force applied to a bone exceeds maximum resistance, the bone breaks. Sudden direct force from a blow or fall causes most fractures; however, some result from indirect force—for example, from a strong muscle contraction, such as during a seizure. A few fractures result from underlying weakness created by bone infections, bone tumors, or more bone resorption than production (as occurs in clients who are inactive or aging).

For 10 to 40 minutes after a bone breaks, the muscles surrounding the bone are flaccid. Then they go into spasm, often increasing deformity and interfering with the vascular

---

BOX 62-1	Types of Fractures

Avulsion: a pulling away of a fragment of bone by a ligament or tendon and its attachment

Comminuted: a fracture in which bone has splintered into several fragments

Compound: a fracture in which damage also involves the skin or mucous membranes

Compression: a fracture in which bone has been compressed (seen in vertebral fractures)

Depressed: a fracture in which fragments are driven inward (seen frequently in fractures of skull and facial bones)

Epiphyseal: a fracture through the epiphysis

Greenstick: a fracture in which one side of a bone is broken and the other side is bent

Impacted: a fracture in which a bone fragment is driven into another bone fragment

Oblique: a fracture occurring at an angle across the bone (less stable than transverse)

Pathologic: a fracture that occurs through an area of diseased bone (bone cyst, Paget's disease, bony metastasis, tumor); can occur without trauma or a fall

Simple: a fracture that remains contained; does not break the skin

Spiral: a fracture twisting around the shaft of the bone

Transverse: a fracture that is straight across the bone

---

and lymphatic circulations. The tissue surrounding the fracture swells from hemorrhage and edema. Healing begins (Fig. 62-2) when blood in the area clots and a fibrin network forms between the broken bone ends. The fibrin network changes into granulation tissue. Osteoblasts, which proliferate in the clot, increase the secretion of an enzyme that restores the alkaline pH. As a result, calcium is deposited and true bone forms. The healing mass is called a **callus**. It holds the ends of the bone together but cannot endure strain. Bone repair is a local process. About 1 year of healing must pass before bone regains its former structural strength, becomes well consolidated and remodeled (re-formed), and possesses fat and marrow cells.

Although fractures are common, they are associated with various complications, particularly when they are very complex. Table 62-1 briefly describes the types of possible complications, which include compartment syndrome, thromboembolism, fat embolism, delayed healing, nonunion, malunion, infection, and **avascular necrosis** (death of bone from an insufficient blood supply). In addition, any client who is inactive during convalescence is prone to pneumonia, thrombophlebitis, pressure sores, urinary tract infection, renal calculi, constipation, muscle atrophy, weight gain, and depression.

Gerontologic Considerations

- Older adults are more prone to skeletal fractures because bone resorption takes place more rapidly than bone formation (see Chap. 60).

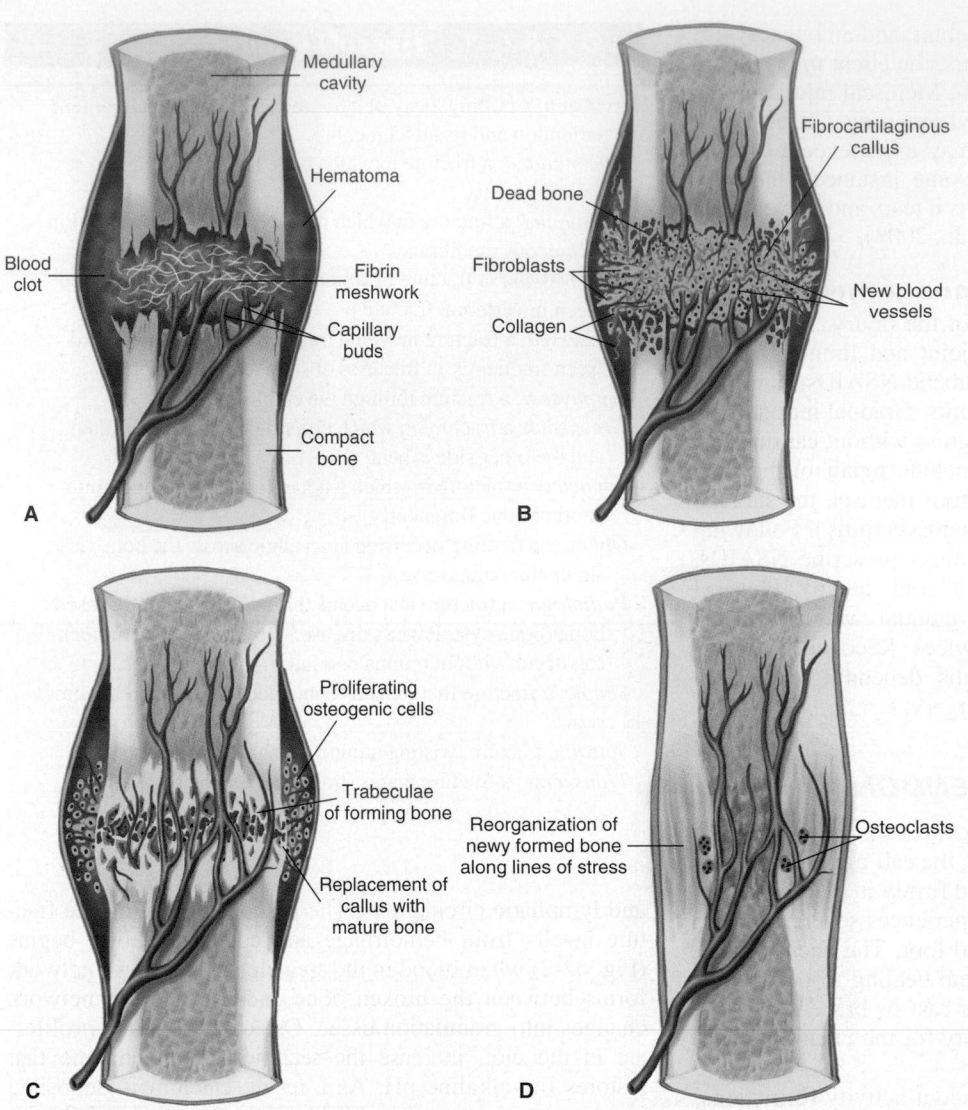

FIGURE 62-2. Process of bone healing. (**A**) Immediately after a bone fractures, blood seeps into the area, and a hematoma (blood clot) forms. (**B**) After 1 week, osteoblasts form as the clot retracts. After about 3 weeks, a procallus forms and stabilizes the fracture. (**C**) A callus with bone cells forms in 6 to 12 weeks. In 3 to 4 months, osteoblasts begin to remodel the fracture site. (**D**) If the fractured bone has been accurately aligned during healing, remodeling will be complete in about 12 months. (From Porth, C. M. [2007]. *Essentials of pathophysiology: Concepts of altered health states.* [2nd ed.]. Philadelphia: Lippincott Williams & Wilkins.)

Assessment Findings

Signs and Symptoms

The signs and symptoms of a fracture vary, depending on the type and location. They include the following:

- Pain—One of the most consistent symptoms of a fracture is pain, which may be severe. Attempts to move the part and pressure over the fracture increase pain.
- Loss of function—Skeletal muscular function depends on intact bone.
- Deformity—A break may cause an extremity to bend backward or to assume another unusual position.
- False motion—Unnatural motion occurs at the site of the fracture.
- Crepitus—The grating sound of bone ends moving over one another may be audible (this term also refers to a popping sound caused by air trapped in soft tissue).
- Edema—Swelling usually is greatest directly over the fracture.
- Spasm—Muscles near fractures involuntarily contract. Spasm, which accounts for some of the pain, may cause a limb to shorten when the fracture involves a long bone.

If sharp bone fragments tear through sufficient surrounding soft tissue, there is bleeding and black and blue discoloration of the area. If a nerve is damaged, paralysis may result.

▶ ***Stop, Think, and Respond Exercise 62-2***

You are cross-country skiing with a friend and notice that a person ahead of you has fallen. When you get closer, this person tells you that she has hurt her arm. What signs would indicate that this woman probably has a fractured humerus?

Diagnostic Findings

One or more radiographic views of the area almost always demonstrate altered bone structure. Stress fractures may not be apparent radiographically for a few weeks. A bone scan usually can identify a nondisplaced or stress fracture before radiographic changes are evident. In some instances, a computed tomography (CT) scan or MRI may be necessary.

TABLE 62-1 Complications of Fractures

COMPLICATION	DESCRIPTION	NURSING IMPLICATIONS
Shock	Hypovolemic shock related to blood loss and loss of extracellular fluid from damaged tissue. If untreated, the client's condition will deteriorate.	Administer blood and fluid volume replacements as prescribed to prevent further losses.
Fat embolism	Fat globules released after fractures of pelvis or long bones, or after multiple injuries or crushing injuries. Globules combine with platelets to form emboli. Onset is rapid, with client experiencing respiratory distress and cerebral disturbances.	Monitor client for symptoms, which usually occur within 48–72 hours. To prevent fatty emboli, provide early respiratory support, ensure rapid immobilization of fracture, and observe client closely for signs of respiratory and nervous system problems.
Pulmonary embolism	Thromboembolism may occur after fracture or surgery to repair fractures. These lead to pulmonary emboli in some clients and can be fatal.	Promote circulation and prevent venous stasis to avoid pulmonary embolism. Administer low-dose heparin subcutaneously as prescribed to prevent clot formation.
Compartment syndrome	Tissue perfusion in the muscle compartment (muscle covered by inelastic fascia) is compromised secondary to tissue swelling, hemorrhage, or a cast that is too tight. If circulation is not restored, ischemia and tissue anoxia lead to permanent nerve damage, muscle atrophy, and contracture.	Monitor client for signs and symptoms of compartment syndrome such as unrelenting pain, unrelieved by analgesics. Elevate the extremity, apply ice, and perform neurovascular checks to help prevent this complication. As indicated, relieve pressure by loosening cast or preparing the client for a **fasciotomy** (surgical incision of fascia and separation of muscles).
Delayed bone healing	Bone fails to heal at the expected rate. Delayed healing may result from nonunion, characterized by the ends of the fractured bone failing to unite and heal, or it may result from malunion, characterized by the ends of the fractured bone healing in a deformed position.	Delayed union may require surgical intervention to promote bone growth, and correct the incorrect union. If necessary, prepare the client for use of electrical stimulation measures that promote bone growth, or for a bone graft.
Infection	The potential for infection increases with compound fractures, application of skeletal traction, or surgical procedures.	Perform careful assessments and maintain aseptic technique to prevent infections. Monitor for early signs of infection because early detection promotes early correction of the problem.
Avascular necrosis	This condition occurs from interruption of the blood supply to the fracture fragments after which the bone tissue dies; most common in the femoral head.	Be alert for client reports of pain and decreased function of the affected limb. If necessary, prepare the client for surgery, such as bone graft, bone prosthesis, joint replacement, joint fusion, or amputation.

Medical and Surgical Management

The goal is to re-establish functional continuity of the bone. Treatment includes one or more methods: traction, closed or open reduction, internal or external fixation, or cast application. The treatment method depends on many factors, including the first aid given, the location and severity of the break, and the age and overall physical condition of the client. Chapter 61 describes medical and surgical modalities used for clients with orthopedic injuries, including fractures.

Nursing Management

When caring for the client with a fracture, the nurse assesses for neurovascular and systemic complications. General nursing measures include administering analgesics, providing comfort measures, assisting with ADLs, preventing constipation, promoting physical mobility, preventing infection, maintaining skin integrity, and preparing client for self-care.

Because the client may be discharged shortly after application of an immobilization device or a cast, the nurse reviews care with the client or family. In addition, he or she reinforces instructions regarding exercise and ambulatory activities.

If a client is in traction, he or she requires simple and direct explanations about the traction and its purpose. The nurse points out activities that are allowed or contraindicated and identifies the approximate duration of the restrictions. When traction is discontinued, the nurse prepares the client for further treatment, such as casting, and for the appearance of the affected area—skin and muscles. He or she reassures the client that, with gradual exercise and use, muscles will regain strength and tone, and joints will be flexible. For more information about managing problems related to casting, refer to Nursing Guidelines 61-1 in Chapter 61. For information about clients with specific fractures, such as those affecting the clavicle or knee, refer to Table 61-1 in Chapter 61.

FRACTURED FEMUR

A fracture of the femur commonly occurs in automobile accidents but may also occur in falls from ladders or other high places, or in gunshot wounds. Multiple injuries often accompany fractures of the femur, because they usually occur with severe trauma.

Assessment Findings

Severe pain, swelling, and ecchymosis may be seen. The client usually cannot move the hip or knee. If a compound fracture has occurred, an open wound or a protrusion of bone is seen. Radiographic films show the type and location of the fracture.

Medical and Surgical Management

Fractures of the femur usually are treated initially with some form of traction to prevent deformities and soft-tissue injury. Skeletal traction or an external fixator is used to align the fracture in preparation for future reduction if the fracture occurred in the lower two thirds of the femur. Once the femur is aligned, a spica cast may be used to maintain the corrected position.

Nursing Management

Because the client is confined to bed, the nurse implements measures to prevent complications of immobility and inactivity. He or she positions the client in line with the pull exerted by the traction. The nurse cleans pin sites with a prescribed agent to prevent infection (see Nursing Guidelines 61-3).

FRACTURED HIP

Usually a hip fracture affects the proximal end of the femur. This type of fracture commonly results from a fall and occurs more frequently in older adults with osteoporosis. Usually the falls are not very traumatic, but the client's condition contributes to the resulting fracture. Fractures may occur in the femoral neck (intracapsular or inside the hip joint capsule), between the trochanters (intertrochanteric-extracapsular or outside the hip joint capsule), or below the trochanters (subtrochanteric-extracapsular). Figure 62-3 illustrates regions of the proximal femur.

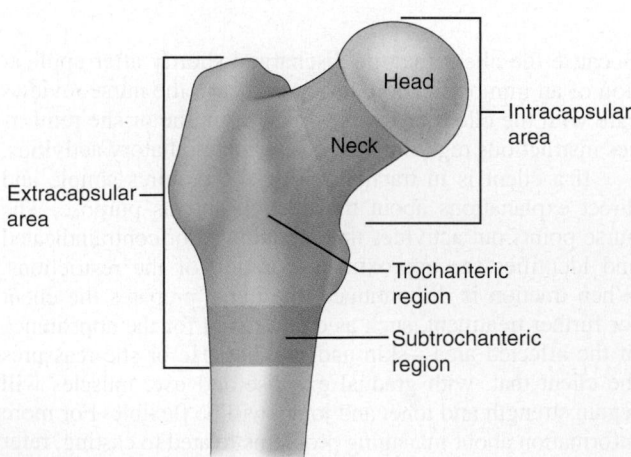

FIGURE 62-3. Regions of the proximal femur where hip fractures may occur.

Assessment Findings

The client reports severe pain that increases with leg movement. The pain frequently radiates to the knee, and the client may have a sensation of pressure in the outer aspect of the hip. Discontinuity of the bone and muscle spasm cause shortening and external rotation of the leg. A large blood loss may accompany subtrochanteric and intertrochanteric fractures, leading to hypovolemic shock. There also may be extensive bruising and swelling in the hip, groin, and thigh. Femoral neck fractures are intracapsular, so bleeding is more likely to be contained within the joint capsule. Radiographic studies reveal the exact location of the fracture, which may be within or outside the joint capsule.

Medical and Surgical Management

Chapter 61 describes general medical and surgical management for clients with fractures. Intracapsular hip fractures are prone to nonunion and avascular necrosis from the disrupted blood supply. Therefore, the fractured head and neck may be removed and replaced with a metal device such as an Austin-Moore or Thompson prosthesis. This procedure is referred to as *hemiarthroplasty*. The bone heals around the metallic device, which in the meantime holds the bone together. Thus, the bone is united immediately, and clients are mobilized much earlier than they are with traction. Plates, bands, screws, and pins may be removed after the bone has healed. More often, they are left in place permanently. The precautions with hemiarthroplasty are greater because the surgeon must dislocate the hip to replace the femoral head. Clients may have a total hip arthroplasty (see Chapter 61).

Nursing Management

Most clients with a fractured hip are older adults and are prone to complications. After surgery, the nurse implements measures to prevent skin breakdown, wound infection, pneumonia, constipation, urinary retention, muscle atrophy, and contractures. The client usually has a wound drain in place for 1 to 2 days after surgery. The nurse monitors the drainage and administers antibiotics as prescribed.

The nurse must show the client how to use the overhead trapeze safely for independent movement and activity. When the client is recumbent, the nurse places a trochanter roll beside the hip to maintain a neutral position so that the repaired hip stays in place. He or she places abductor pillows between the client's legs when turning the client from side to side. Refer to Chapter 61 for more information about nursing management of a client following insertion of a hip prosthesis. Nursing Care Plan 61-1 provides additional nursing management strategies for postoperative orthopedic clients.

If a hip prosthesis has been inserted, the nurse instructs the client to avoid adduction of the affected leg until it has healed. The client must use abductor pillows at all times. Soon after surgery, the nurse or physical therapist assists the client to transfer from the bed to a chair. The chair must have an elevated seat, either with its structure or with pillows, so that the client does not flex the hips beyond 90°. The client usually requires much encouragement and assistance. Eventually the client progresses to ambulating with a walker. Before discharge, the nurse needs to explore ways to ensure safety in the client's home to avoid future injuries and falls.

CRITICAL THINKING EXERCISES

1. A client is admitted to a surgical floor with an open fracture of the right arm. What are important priorities when caring for this client?

2. The nurse tells the client who sprained her left ankle 2 hours ago that she needs to apply an ice pack to the injured area. What explanation should the nurse give for this action?

3. Describe factors that can interfere with bone healing.

4. What factors can contribute to rotator cuff injuries?

NCLEX-STYLE REVIEW QUESTIONS

1. A graphic designer, who spends hours working on the computer, complains of slight pain in the right hand. The pain tends to be more prominent at night and early in the morning. The client is diagnosed with a mild form of carpal tunnel syndrome; the condition is not yet serious. Which of the following would the nurse recommend to help reduce the pain? Select all that apply.
1. Flexing the affected wrist
2. Shaking the affected hand
3. Resting the hands when possible
4. Physical therapy
5. Surgical intervention

2. A client presents in the emergency room with a shoulder injury after falling from a stepladder. When the nurse assesses the client's injuries, which finding best indicates that the client has dislocated the shoulder?
1. The affected arm is longer than the other.
2. The client is experiencing intense pain.
3. The client is hesitant to move the affected arm.
4. There is obvious swelling about the joint.

3. An x-ray of an injured client's leg reveals a comminuted fracture of the distal tibia. The nurse correctly informs the client that a comminuted fracture means that:
1. A portion of the bone is split away.
2. One bone end is driven into the other.
3. The bone is splintered into pieces.
4. There is no open break in the skin.

4. A client with a fractured tibia undergoes surgery to realign the bones. After surgery, the client experiences signs and symptoms of a fat embolism. What is one of the signs that the nurse recognizes?
1. Abdominal distention.
2. Difficulty swallowing.
3. Respiratory distress.
4. Swelling at the incision site.

5. A client is hospitalized with a fractured right hip. What is the most typical sign of an intertrochanteric fracture of the hip seen during the nurse's admission assessment?
1. Bruising of the affected leg.
2. External rotation of the leg.
3. Lengthening of the affected leg.
4. Paralysis of the affected leg.

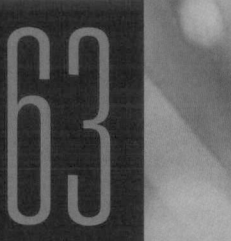

63

Caring For Clients with Orthopedic and Connective Tissue Disorders

Words To Know

ankylosing spondylitis
ankylosis
arthritis
arthroplasty
Bouchard's nodes
bursitis
degenerative joint disease
fibromyalgia
gout
hallux valgus
hammer toe
Heberden's nodes
hyperuricemia
involucrum
Lyme disease
mallet toe
osteomalacia
osteomyelitis
osteoporosis
Paget's disease
pannus
rheumatoid arthritis
rheumatic disorders
sequestrum
synovectomy
synovitis
systemic lupus erythematosus
tophi

Learning Objectives

On completion of this chapter, you will be able to:

1. Explain the difference between rheumatoid arthritis and degenerative joint disease (osteoarthritis) and describe nursing management.
2. Describe the clinical manifestations of temporomandibular disorder (TMD).
3. State the pathophysiology of gout, fibromyalgia, bursitis, and ankylosing spondylitis.
4. Delineate the nursing care required for clients with gout, fibromyalgia, bursitis, and ankylosing spondylitis.
5. Discuss the multisystem involvement associated with systemic lupus erythematosus.
6. Identify the causes of osteomyelitis.
7. Explain the inflammatory process associated with Lyme disease.
8. Identify risk factors for development of osteoporosis.
9. Distinguish the pathophysiology of osteomalacia and Paget's disease.
10. Differentiate between bunions and hammer toe.
11. Discuss characteristics of benign and malignant bone tumors.

The musculoskeletal system consists of structures the body uses for support and movement. It also protects body organs. Disorders affecting the musculoskeletal system affect the person's ability to perform activities of daily living (ADLs) and to remain active, mobile, and physically fit. Many clients with musculoskeletal disorders are treated as outpatients. A few may require hospitalization in the acute phase of the disorder, for surgery on a degenerative joint, or for other medical or surgical therapies.

INFLAMMATORY DISORDERS

Arthritis is a general condition characterized by inflammation and degeneration of a joint. **Rheumatic disorders** include more than 100 different types of recognized inflammatory disorders, making this collective group the most common orthopedic problem. These disorders involve inflammation and degeneration of connective tissue structures, especially joints. They have the potential to interfere with mobility and ADLs. Clients with inflammatory disorders may need assistance with tasks that most people take for granted. These disorders affect a client's physical, psychological, and social functions.

The discussion in this chapter is limited to rheumatoid arthritis, osteoarthritis, temporomandibular disorder, gout, fibromyalgia, ankylosing spondylitis, and lupus erythematosus.

RHEUMATOID ARTHRITIS

Rheumatoid arthritis (RA) is a systemic inflammatory disorder of connective tissue/joints characterized by chronicity, remissions, and exacerbations. The potential for disability with RA is great and related to the effects on joints, as well as the systemic problems.

Pathophysiology and Etiology

The nature of RA, a crippling disease, is not fully understood. Its cause is unknown, although it is believed to be an autoimmune disease. Genetic predisposition and other factors may be involved. RA strikes in the most productive years of adulthood, usually between 20 and 40 years of age. The disorder also can be found in young children and older adults. Young adult women appear to be affected more than men, but the incidence equalizes as adults age. Typically, RA affects small joints early and involves large joints later (Bullock & Henze, 2000).

The autoimmune reaction from RA occurs primarily in the synovial tissue. Approximately 70% to 80% of people with RA have a substance called *rheumatoid factor* (RF), an antibody that reacts with a fragment of immunoglobulin G (IgG). This self-produced (autologous) antibody forms immune complexes (IgG/RF). It is uncertain why. Theories include genetic predisposition or viral infections that alter the IgG so that it is seen as foreign. In many individuals there

is also a strong genetic association of human leukocyte antigen (HLA) with RA (Porth, 2007).

The autoimmune reaction is described in Figure 63-1. Basically, it seems that lymphocytes in the inflammatory infiltrate of the synovial tissue produce RF. Polymorphonuclear leukocytes, monocytes, and lymphocytes are attracted to the area and cause phagocytosis of the immune complexes. During this process, lysosomal enzymes are released, which cause destructive changes in the joint cartilage (Fig. 63-2). The changes produce more inflammation, which perpetuates the entire process of RA:

1. The inflammatory process (**synovitis**) advances as the congestion and edema develop in the synovial membrane and joint capsule.
2. Synovial tissue experiences reactive hyperplasia.
3. Vasodilation and increased blood flow cause warmth and redness.
4. Increased capillary permeability causes swelling.
5. Rheumatoid synovitis advances, leading to **pannus** formation (destructive vascular granulation tissue, characteristic of RA).
6. Pannus destroys adjacent cartilage, joint capsule, and bone.
7. Pannus eventually forms between joint margins, reducing joint mobility and leading to potential **ankylosis** (joint immobility).

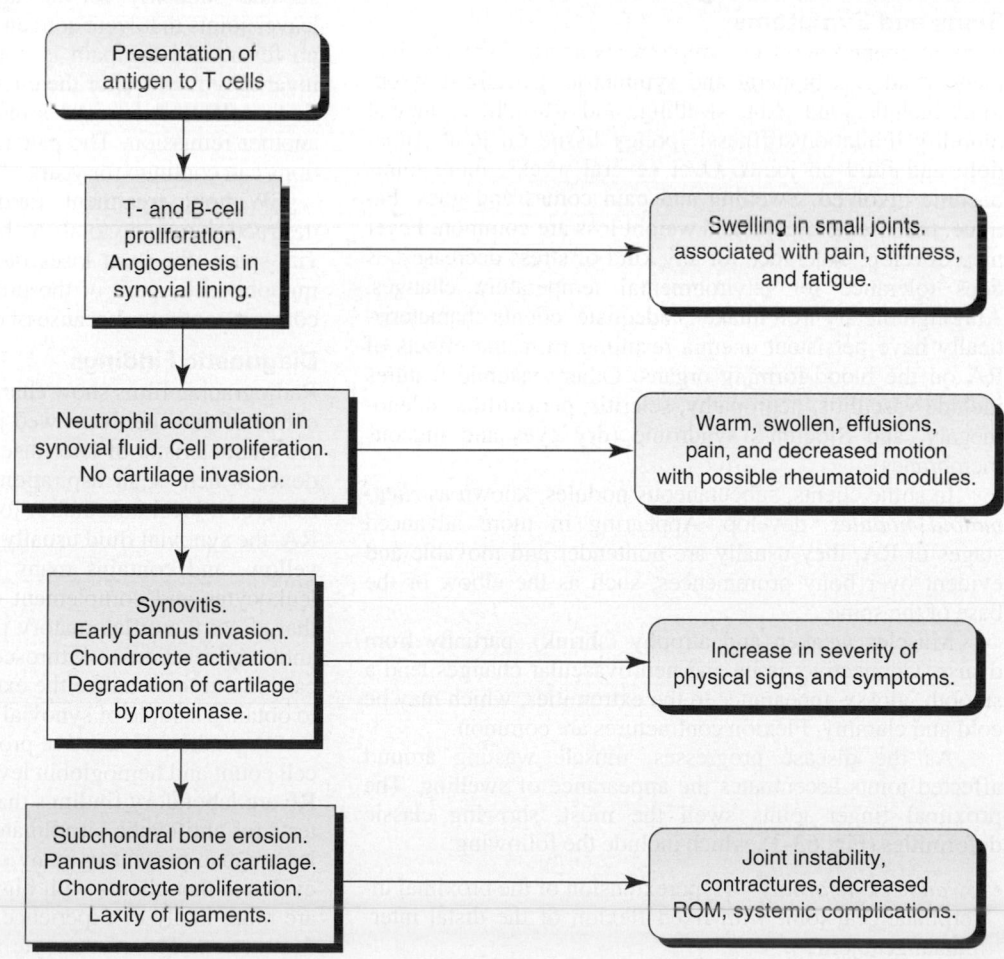

FIGURE 63-1. Pathophysiology and associated physical signs of rheumatoid arthritis.

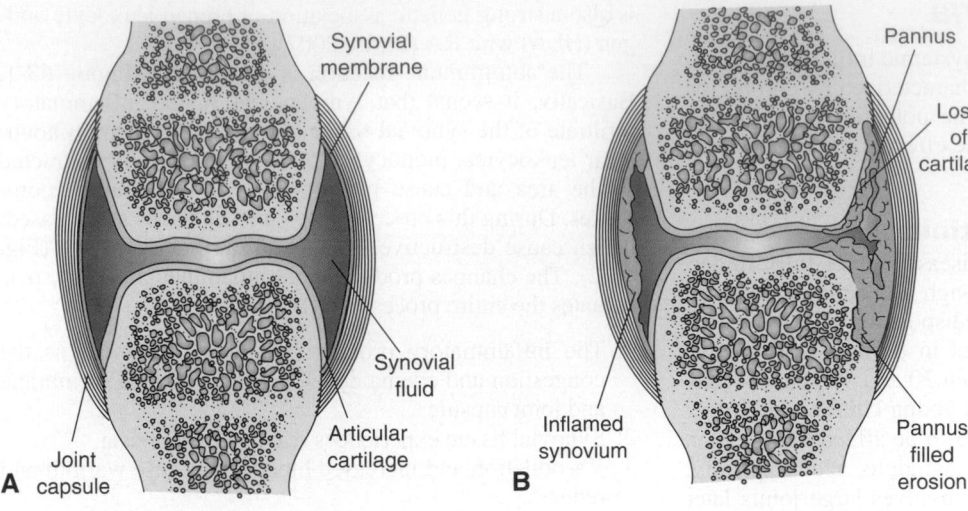

FIGURE 63-2. **(A)** Normal joint structures. **(B)** Joint changes in rheumatoid arthritis. The left side of the drawing denotes early changes occurring within the synovium. The right side shows progressive disease that leads to erosion and formation of pannus.

8. Disease progression causes further inflammation and structural changes (Bullock & Henze, 2000; Porth, 2007).

Most clients with RA experience exacerbations and remissions. For some clients, the progression is steady, relentless, and not necessarily responsive to therapy. Box 63-1 lists articular and extra-articular manifestations of RA.

Assessment Findings

Signs and Symptoms

In most clients, onset of symptoms is acute. Joint involvement usually is bilateral and symmetric. Localized symptoms include joint pain, swelling, and warmth; erythema; mobility limitation/stiffness; spongy tissue on joint palpation; and fluid on joints. Over several weeks, more joints become involved. Swelling and pain comes and goes. Fatigue, malaise, anorexia, and weight loss are common. Fever may develop. Tolerance for any kind of stress decreases, as does tolerance for environmental temperature changes. Although dietary iron intake is adequate, clients characteristically have persistent anemia resulting from the effects of RA on the blood-forming organs. Other systemic features include vasculitis, neuropathy, scleritis, pericarditis, splenomegaly, and Sjögren's syndrome (dry eyes and mucous membranes).

In some clients, subcutaneous nodules, known as *rheumatoid nodules*, develop. Appearing in more advanced stages of RA, they usually are nontender and movable and evident over bony prominences, such as the elbow or the base of the spine.

Muscles weaken and atrophy (shrink), partially from disuse. Connective tissue and neurovascular changes lend a smooth, glossy appearance to the extremities, which may be cold and clammy. Flexion contractures are common.

As the disease progresses, muscle wasting around affected joints accentuates the appearance of swelling. The proximal finger joints swell the most, showing classic deformities (Fig. 63-3), which include the following:

- *Swan neck deformity*—Hyperextension of the proximal interphalangeal joint with fixed flexion of the distal interphalangeal joint

- *Boutonnière deformity*—Persistent flexion of the proximal interphalangeal joint with hyperextension of the distal interphalangeal joint
- *Ulnar deviation*—Fingers deviating laterally toward the ulna

Whether resting or moving, clients in this stage of the disease have considerable chronic pain, which typically is worse in the morning after a night's rest. The symptoms may subside suddenly for no apparent reason. Inflammation leaves joints that were sore and red; the client is not stiff, has no fever, and the pain is gone. Yet the symptoms almost invariably return after the client has had a symptom-free period. Inflammation causes more joint damage, followed by another remission. The pattern of remissions and exacerbations can continue for years.

Without treatment (and sometimes with it), joint destruction may be total. As bony growth replaces the synovial space, the joint loses motion. Once the joint becomes immobile, the pain of the inflammation decreases, but discomfort continues because of contractures and immobility.

Diagnostic Findings

Radiographic films show characteristic joint changes and the extent of damage. Narrowed joint spaces and bony erosions are characteristic of later disease. An arthrocentesis may be done, which is an aspiration of synovial fluid (the client receives a local anesthetic) for microscopic examination. In RA, the synovial fluid usually appears cloudy, milky, or dark yellow, and contains many inflammatory cells, including leukocytes and complement (a group of proteins in blood that affect the inflammatory process and influence antigen–antibody reactions). Arthroscopic examination also may be carried out to visualize the extent of joint damage as well as to obtain a sample of synovial fluid.

A positive C-reactive protein (CRP) test, low red blood cell count and hemoglobin levels in later stages, and positive RF are laboratory findings that support the diagnosis. Blood tests for anti-cyclic citrullinated peptide (anti-CCP) antibodies are also present in many clients with RA. There is some evidence that clients with higher levels of RF and anti-CCP are more likely to experience increased problems with joint destruction. The erythrocyte sedimentation rate (ESR) may

BOX 63-1 **Articular and Extra-articular Manifestations of Rheumatoid Arthritis**

- *Subcutaneous nodules:* Firm, freely movable, rubbery or granular nodules caused by deposition of extra-articular granulation tissue. Usually found at joint points such as knuckles and elbows.
- *Synovial cysts:* Called *Baker's cysts* in popliteal fossa; filled with synovial fluid that may be found in periarticular areas in elbow, shoulder, or small joints.
- *Arthritis:* Bilateral involvement of the small joints and later the large joints; hands joints usually are swollen and may be red. Inflammation leads to disability from destruction of cartilage, bone, and tendons. Flexion contractures are common. Osteoporosis, vertebral compression fractures, and avascular necrosis of the femoral head are common and may relate to treatment with corticosteroids. Usually at least three joint areas are involved.
- *Systemic rheumatoid vasculitis:* Immune complex–mediated inflammation in small and medium-sized arteries. It may be life-threatening if in a critical area. Causes pericardial, cardiac, pulmonary, and other types of lesions. Digital necrosis is common.
- *Compression neuropathy:* Mainly causes peripheral nerve entrapment with carpal tunnel syndrome. Paresthesias, pain, burning, muscle wasting, and weakness are common symptoms.
- *Cardiac disease:* Pericardial lesions and effusions are common and may or may not be symptomatic. Conduction system abnormalities from blockages due to rheumatic nodules around the atrioventricular node may cause heart block.
- *Pleuropulmonary disease:* Pleural effusions or pleuritic chest pain are relatively common. Pulmonary fibrosis or progressive interstitial lung disease may be seen with or without rheumatoid nodules in the lung parenchyma.
- *Episcleritis and scleritis:* Episcleritis is an inflammatory condition of the connective tissue between the sclera and conjunctiva. Scleritis is an inflammatory condition of the sclera and can cause scleral perforation.
- *Sicca syndrome:* A condition of dry eyes and dry mouth that can result from infiltration of the lacrimal and salivary glands with lymphocytes.

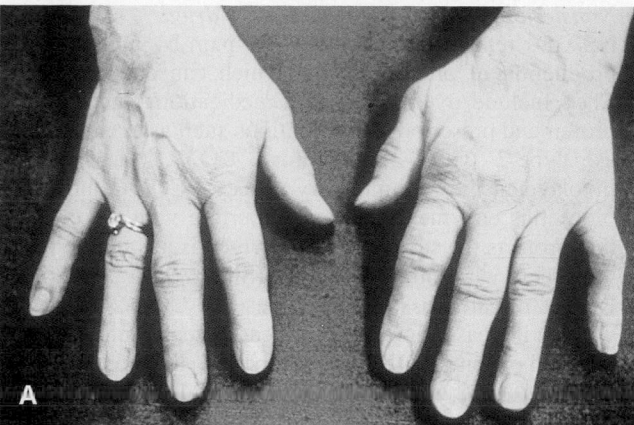

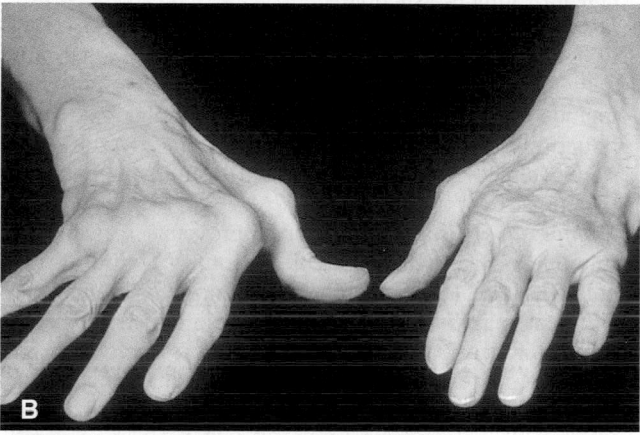

FIGURE 63-3. Rheumatoid arthritis. (**A**) Early. (**B**) Advanced.

one of the few truly therapeutic steps medicine has to offer. Rest, systemic and local, is balanced carefully with exercise. Unless the client has other medical complications, such as diabetes or hypertension, the diet need not be modified (Nutrition Notes 63-1).

Drug Therapy

Drug therapy is not curative but helps relieve pain and, in some instances, suppresses the inflammatory process. In general, the following classes of drug therapy may be ordered:

Nutrition Notes 63-1
The Client with Rheumatoid Arthritis

- No conclusive evidence has shown that nutrition therapy can prevent or cure RA.
- Omega-3 fatty acids found in fatty fish (e.g., mackerel, herring, salmon) and, to a lesser extent, in flaxseed, olive, and canola oils relieve joint tenderness and fatigue in some people, possibly by inhibiting the inflammatory response of certain prostaglandins. The use of fish oil supplements is not recommended, but eating more dietary sources of omega-3 fatty acids may be beneficial.
- Malnutrition is common among clients with RA; monitor weight changes.
- Discourage quack "cures" and self-prescribed supplements.

be elevated, particularly as the disease progresses. C4 complement component is decreased. Antinuclear antibody (ANA) test results also may be positive. Serum protein electrophoresis may disclose increased levels of gamma and alpha globulin but decreased albumin.

Medical and Surgical Management

Although RA cannot be cured, much can be done to minimize damage. Treatment goals include decreasing joint inflammation before bony ankylosis occurs, relieving discomfort, preventing or correcting deformities, and maintaining or restoring function of affected structures. Early treatment leads to the best results.

Optimal health conditions must be maintained because supporting the resistance of the body to the inflammation is

Celebrex

- *Nonsteroidal anti-inflammatory drugs (NSAIDs)*—NSAIDs relieve inflammation and pain by inhibiting the production of prostaglandins, which can damage joints. They include over-the-counter medications such as ibuprofen and prescription medications such as cyclooxygenase type-2 (COX-2) inhibitors. COX is an enzyme involved in the inflammatory process; COX-2 inhibitors block this enzyme, but do not interfere with the enzyme that protects the stomach lining, which is a common problem seen with other NSAIDs (Smeltzer et al., 2008). Recent research associated the use of COX-2 inhibitors with an increased incidence of heart disease and led to the removal of some COX-2 inhibitors from the market.
- *Steroids*—Drugs such as prednisone and methylprednisolone (Medrol) are used to reduce pain and inflammation and slow joint destruction.
- *Disease-modifying antirheumatic drugs (DMARDs)*—DMARDs reduce the amount of joint damage and slow damage to other tissues as well. Common DMARDs include hydroxychloroquine (Plaquenil), the gold compound auranofin (Ridaura), sulfasalazine (Azulfidine), minocycline (Dynacin, Minocin) and methotrexate (Rheumatrex).
- *Immunosuppressants*—Immunosuppressants calm the immune system, which is typically out of control for clients with RA. Drugs such as cyclosporine or azathioprine (Imuran) may be added to enhance the effects of methotrexate or may be used in clients with severe classic RA that does not respond to more conventional therapies.
- *TNF-alpha inhibitors*—TNF-alpha is a cytokine that is an inflammatory for clients with RA; TNF-alpha inhibitors block the cytokine, thus reducing pain and inflammation. They often are given in conjunction with methotrexate. TNF inhibitors approved for treatment of rheumatoid arthritis are etanercept (Enbrel), infliximab (Remicade) and adalimumab (Humira).
- Drugs used for RA from other drug classes include:
  - Anakinra (Kineret)—similar to interleukin-1-receptor antagonist, a naturally occurring chemical in the body that stops the inflammation associated with RA
  - Abatacept (Orencia)—inactivates T cells and reduces pain, inflammation, and joint damage
  - Rituximab (Rituxan)—reduces the number of B cells in the body, which are involved with the inflammatory process

Drug Therapy Table 63-1 provides for more information about drugs used for RA. For many clients, combination therapy is initiated. Recommendations from the American College of Rheumatology (2008) include hydroxychloroquine, azathioprine, and methotrexate or gold plus methotrexate, in addition to an NSAID. As symptoms abate and remission occurs, drug doses are tapered. Local applications of heat and cold are used concurrently with drug therapy to relieve swelling and pain.

Pharmacologic Considerations

- Instruct clients taking aspirin for arthritis not to substitute buffered aspirin or enteric-coated aspirin for regular aspirin unless the physician approves the change. Aspirin cannot be used in clients with ulcers, a history of ulcers, or bleeding disorders.

- The most common adverse effects of NSAIDs are related to the GI tract: nausea, vomiting, diarrhea, and constipation. GI bleeding, which in some cases is severe, has been reported with the use of these drugs.

- Caution clients with diseases of the bones and joints against discontinuing their drugs if and when they begin to feel improved.

Nondrug Therapy

A nondrug therapy approved for clients with advanced RA is Prosorba column therapy. This method uses a protein A immunoadsorption column called Prosorba. Blood is taken from one arm and run through an apheresis machine to separate plasma from red blood cells and other blood components. The plasma then passes through the Prosorba column, where some of the antibodies associated with RA are removed. The plasma, red blood cells, and other components are rejoined and returned to the client in the other arm. The procedure is done in 12 weekly sessions for 2 to 2 1/2 hours each session. About 30% of the clients who receive these treatments experience limited relief (Arthritis Foundation, 2008; Smeltzer et al., 2008).

Another newer treatment is the injection of viscosupplements (Hyalgan, Synvisc, and Supartz). Viscosupplements act as a lubricant, substituting for hyaluronic acid, the substance that provides joint fluid viscosity. Pain relief appears to last 6 to 13 months. Side effects include swelling, redness, or heat at the injection site. Clients allergic to eggs should not receive these injections (Arthritis Foundation, 2008).

Surgery

Several surgical techniques may be performed to minimize or correct the joint deformities of RA (refer to Box 61-4). Many individuals with various types of arthritis undergo an **arthroplasty**, or reconstruction of the joint, using an artificial joint that restores previously lost function and relieves pain. Refer to Chapter 61 for a more in-depth discussion of reconstructive joint surgery. In addition, clients with RA may have a **synovectomy**, which is a procedure to remove the lining of the joint. This procedure is performed when the lining is inflamed and adding to the pain the client is experiencing.

Nursing Management

Nursing management involves teaching clients about the disease and providing information about maintaining general health, relieving pain, reducing stress, decreasing the inflammatory process, and preserving joint mobility. The nurse also instructs clients about the medication regimen, particularly therapeutic and adverse effects. Other nursing activities center on how to apply heat and cold packs locally or how to use a transcutaneous electrical nerve stimulation (TENS) unit to relieve pain in a particular joint. A TENS unit has electrodes that are applied to the skin from a portable stimulation unit that the client learns to operate.

DRUG THERAPY TABLE 63-1 Agents for Rheumatoid Arthritis

Drug Category and Examples	Mechanism of Action	Nursing Considerations
Nonsteroidal Anti-inflammatory Drugs (NSAIDs)		
diclofenac sodium (Voltaren), fenoprofen (Nalfon), ibuprofen (Motrin), indomethacin (Indocin), naproxen (Naprosyn), piroxicam (Feldene), sulindac (Clinoril)	Blocks undesirable effects of prostaglandins, which contribute to the inflammatory response Reduces pain and inflammation	Give with food or milk. Monitor client for decreased RBC and blood in urine. Assess client for abdominal pain, unusual bleeding or bruising, and tinnitus. Advise client not to take other NSAIDs or salicylates.
Salicylates aspirin	Relieves mild to moderate pain Interferes with the inflammatory response	Give with food or milk. Monitor for tinnitus, GI distress, unusual bleeding or bruising, dark-colored stools.
Cyclooxygenase-2 (COX-2) Inhibitors celecoxib (Celebrex)	Blocks the enzyme involved in inflammation, thus relieving pain and inflammation	Do not administer with other NSAIDs. These drugs are less likely to cause gastric symptoms or unusual bleeding or bruising. There is an increased risk of CV events in clients receiving long-term celecoxib therapy according to a new FDA warning.
Disease-Modifying Antirheumatic Drugs (DMARDs)		
Gold Salts auranofin (Ridaura)	Anti-inflammatory, antiarthritic, and immunomodulating	Take with milk or food. May cause abdominal cramps, nausea, vomiting, loose stools, or sun sensitivity. Never give IV; if given IM, give deep IM.
Immunosuppressant Agents azathioprine (Imuran), cyclosporine	Suppresses lymphocyte proliferation, interfering with the inflammatory response	These drugs decrease ability to fight off infection; report fever, chills, or cough.
Antineoplastic Agents methotrexate (Rheumatrex)	Interferes with purine metabolism, which then releases adenosine, which is an anti-inflammatory	These drugs may cause nausea and vomiting, loss of appetite, diarrhea, hair loss, unusual bleeding and bruising.
Antirheumatic penicillamine (Cuprimine, Depen)	Suppresses immune response by lowering immunoglobulin M associated with rheumatoid factor	Give on empty stomach; withhold food and drugs for 1 hr after administering. Assess for fever after 2–3 wk of therapy. These drugs diminish taste. Use with caution in clients who are allergic to penicillin. Monitor for rash or other skin changes.
Anti-tumor necrosis factor-alpha (Anti-TNF-alpha) adalimumab (Humira), etanercept (Enbrel), infliximab (Remicade)	Work against the TNF found in the joint spaces of clients with RA. Suppress the immune response associated with TNF.	May be used alone or in combination with other drugs. Monitor for secondary infections and teach clients about increased risk related to compromised immune systems. These drugs are used in severe cases of RA; cover all precautions and potentials with the client.
Antimalarials hydroxychloroquine (Plaquenil)	Reduces inflammation	Give with food or milk. Monitor blood counts. Do not give with other anti-inflammatories or gold compounds. Consult with physician before giving to clients with ophthalmic, neurologic, hepatic, or GI disorders. Inform client that urine will appear brown. Monitor for muscle weakness, visual changes, skin lesions, hypotension, and electrocardiographic changes.

(drug table Continues on page 1004)

DRUG THERAPY TABLE 63-1 Agents for Rheumatoid Arthritis (Continued)

Drug Category and Examples	Mechanism of Action	Nursing Considerations
Glucocorticoids prednisone (Meticorten), hydrocortisone (Cortef)	Anti-inflammatory and immunosuppressant	Give with food or milk. Decrease dose and frequency gradually. With long-term therapy monitor for GI distress, hyperglycemia, edema, poor wound healing, personality changes, or pathologic fractures.
Biologic-Response Modifiers etanercept (Enbrel), infliximab (Remicade)	Reduces inflammatory responses	Do not give live vaccines if client is receiving these medications. Discontinue if client gets a serious infection. Give with caution to clients with multiple sclerosis or other demyelinating disorders.

Nurses collaborate with occupational therapists to provide equipment, utensils, and instruction regarding energy conservation and maintenance of joint alignment. Physical therapists (PTs) plan an appropriate exercise regimen. Home care planning involves providing nursing assistance for ADLs and ensuring that the home environment is safe. Out of consideration for the typical pain and morning stiffness, the nurse teaches the nursing assistant to allow extra time for completing hygiene or other procedures.

When joints are severely inflamed, the use of a splint may reduce but not totally eliminate active motion. Even during an acute episode, the nurse encourages the client to move affected parts gently to help lessen the possibility of ankylosis, muscle wasting, osteoporosis, and the debilitating effects of prolonged rest. Clients must avoid positions of flexion.

The nurse continues to urge the client to eat nutritious, well-balanced meals despite anorexia. As joints become deformed and destroyed, the techniques and equipment used to perform ADLs may require modification. Clients need assistance to deal with chronic pain, changes in function, changes in appearance, and related depression and feelings of helplessness. Education about the disease is essential because many people spend large sums of money on unscientific treatments in hopes of a cure.

▶ **Stop, Think, and Respond Exercise 63-1**

A 35-year-old woman recently diagnosed with RA asks you if her disease happened because she experimented with marijuana and drank a lot of alcohol in her adolescence. How would you respond?

DEGENERATIVE JOINT DISEASE

Degenerative joint disease (DJD), also referred to as osteoarthritis (OA), is the most common form of arthritis. It also is known as the "wear and tear" disease and typically affects the weight-bearing joints. It is characterized by a slow and steady progression of destructive changes in weight-bearing joints and those that are repeatedly used for work. Unlike RA, DJD has no remissions and no systemic symptoms, such as malaise and fever. Table 63-1 compares OA and RA.

Pathophysiology and Etiology

A lifetime of repeated trauma leads to degenerative joint changes. Hips, knees, the spine, and the distal interphalangeal joints in the hands commonly are affected. Risk factors include increasing age, previous joint injury, obesity, congenital and developmental disorders (such as Legg-Calvé-Perthes disease), hereditary factors, and decreased bone density. OA may be classified as *primary*, which is disease without a known etiology, or *secondary*, when OA has an underlying cause such as injury or a congenital disorder (Bullock & Henze, 2000).

The degenerative process begins when the cartilage that covers the bone ends becomes thin, rough, and ragged. Malacia or soft spots develop. The cartilage no longer springs back into shape after normal use. As the cartilage wears away, the joint space decreases, so that the bone surfaces are closer and rub together. In an attempt to repair the damaged surface, new bone develops in the form of bone spurs, bone cysts, or osteophytes, which are extended margins of the joints. The joint becomes deformed, and the client experiences pain and limited joint movement. Ankylosis does not occur, but the resulting deformity may partially dislocate the joint. Structures around the affected joint, such as the joint, capsule, synovial membrane, and ligaments, demonstrate degenerative changes. (Bullock & Henze, 2000, p. 832). Figure 63-4 depicts the joint changes seen in osteoarthritis.

Assessment Findings

Early symptoms are brief joint stiffness and pain after a period of inactivity. The pain usually increases with heavy use

TABLE 63-1 Comparison of Rheumatoid Arthritis and Osteoarthritis

	RHEUMATOID ARTHRITIS	OSTEOARTHRITIS
Age	Usually between ages 20 and 50	Usually after age 40
Sex	More common in women than men	Before age 45, more common in men; after age 45, more common in women, especially in the hands
Onset	May develop suddenly (weeks or months)	Develops slowly over many years
Symptoms		
Pain	General achiness; nocturnal pain; pain at rest	Deep, aching pain with motion early in the disease; later, pain at rest
Stiffness	Morning stiffness that lasts at least 1 hr	Stiffness localized to involved joints, which rarely exceeds 20 min; often related to weather
Joint motion	Decreased	Limited
Other	Depression, fatigue, low-grade fever, anorexia, malaise, weakness, weight loss	Instability of weight-bearing joints; crepitus; crackling
Physical signs	If multiple joints involved, usually symmetric	One or many joints involved; asymmetric
	Joints typically involved are hands (small joints), feet (small joints), wrists, elbows, knees, ankles, shoulders.	Joints typically involved are hands (first carpometacarpal joint), feet (first metatarso-phalangeal joint), hips, knees, cervical and lumbar spine
	Hand deformities include ulnar deviation and subluxation of metacarpophalangeal joints	Joints—bony proliferation or occasional synovitis; local tenderness; crepitus; muscle atrophy; effusions
	Joints may be tender, swollen, and red.	
	Synovial fluid is thin and cloudy with elevated protein and polymorphonuclear cell levels.	Synovial fluid—high viscosity with mild leukocytosis (<2000 WBC:mm3)
Laboratory values	Rheumatoid factor (RF) elevated in 80% of clients with RA	No specific test
	Elevated ESR	ESR and hematologic survey results are normal
	Decreased RBC and C4 complement	No systemic manifestations

and is relieved by rest. Later, even rest may not adequately relieve the pain. Eventually the joint undergoes enlargement and increased limitation of movement. When DJD afflicts the hands, the fingers frequently develop painless bony nodules on the dorsolateral surface of the interphalangeal joints: **Heberden's nodes** (bony enlargement of the distal interphalangeal joints; Fig. 63-5) and **Bouchard's nodes** (bony enlargement of the proximal interphalangeal joints). Crepitus may be heard and felt when the joint is moved. The ROM of the affected joint becomes progressively limited, and stiffness and pain increase.

Radiographic films demonstrate disruption of the joint cartilage and bony changes. Some clients may have a slightly elevated ESR.

Medical and Surgical Management

Nonpharmacologic treatment includes local rest of the affected joints, which is emphasized more than total body rest. Heat applied to the painful part may afford some relief. Weight loss is recommended for obese clients. Splints, braces, canes, or crutches may reduce discomfort, relieve pain, and prevent further destruction of the affected joints. An

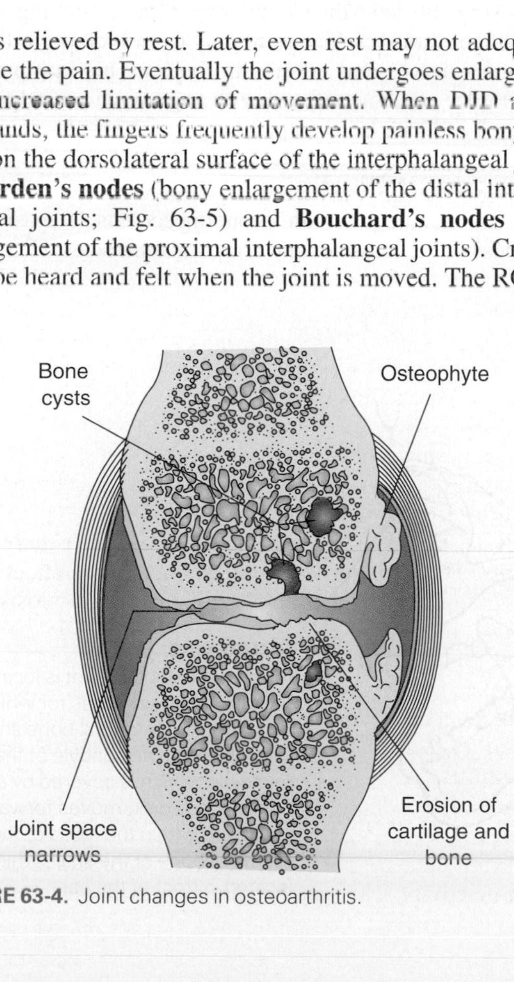

FIGURE 63-4. Joint changes in osteoarthritis.

Bone cysts

Osteophyte

Joint space narrows

Erosion of cartilage and bone

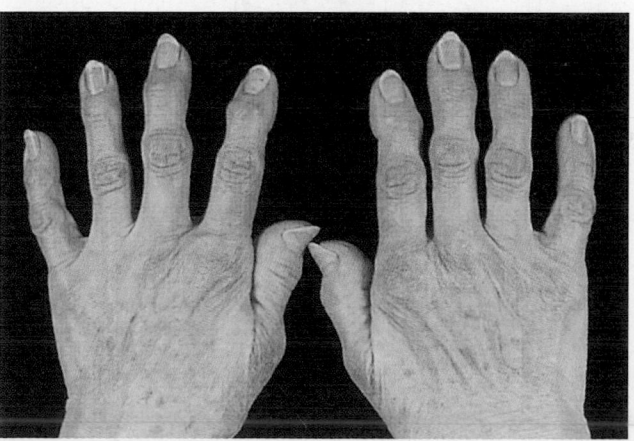

FIGURE 63-5. Heberden's nodes.

exercise program helps to preserve joint ROM and strength. Clients should not engage in activity that places excessive stress on affected joints. A TENS unit may help reduce joint pain.

Large doses of acetaminophen may be used initially along with nonpharmacologic treatments. If acetaminophen is ineffective, however, systemic anti-inflammatory drugs, such as aspirin and NSAIDs, are prescribed. Although these drugs do not prevent or cure DJD, they may decrease its severity. Corticosteroids may be injected into acutely inflamed joints with limited success. When possible, long-term use of these agents is avoided. Use of narcotics is deferred because of the disorder's chronic nature. Newer pharmacologic approaches include glucosamine and chondroitin. These medications theoretically increase tissue function and interfere with the breakdown of cartilage. The intra-articulation injection of hyaluronic acid, referred to as viscosupplementation, theoretically improves cartilage function and interferes with its breakdown (Arthritis Foundation, 2008).

Many clients eventually have reconstructive joint surgery, particularly at a time when mobility and quality of life are compromised. The most frequently replaced joints include the knee and the hip; other joints also replaced are the shoulder and finger joints. Refer to Chapter 61 for more information about reconstructive surgery.

Nursing Management

The nurse teaches about the purpose of drug therapy, administration times, and therapeutic and side effects. Because aspirin and NSAIDs can cause gastric bleeding, the nurse advises clients to take the medication with food. It is important that the client maintain moderate activity, with instructions about how to regulate the type, vigor, and frequency according to the symptoms experienced. If the client is overweight, he or she needs explanations about dietary changes that promote weight loss. The nurse may need to remind the client to assume good posture to avoid unusual stress on a joint. If the client needs ambulatory aids such as crutches, a cane, or a walker, he or she will need a referral to a PT for fitting and practice.

Pharmacologic Considerations

- Warn clients with arthritis about drugs, health foods, and certain food substances available in drug form that are promoted as cures for arthritis, although no evidence supports these claims.

TEMPOROMANDIBULAR DISORDER

Temporomandibular disorder (TMD) is a cluster of symptoms localized near the jaw.

Pathophysiology and Etiology

Causes of TMD include degenerative arthritis of the mandibular joint, malocclusion of the teeth, bruxism (grinding of the teeth), and dislocation of the jaw during endotracheal intubation.

TMD occurs when the meniscus, or cartilaginous disk, between the condyle (end of the mandible) and the temporal bone becomes displaced from the fossa (socket) of the temporal bone (Fig. 63-6). Because facial muscles such as the masseter and temporalis muscles move this gliding joint, the client develops jaw pain from muscle spasms. If the cartilage wears away, there is a grating sensation when opening and closing the jaw; the client may hear a clicking sound when the joint moves. The joint may even lock periodically. Sometimes nerves and arteries in the area are compressed. The disorder can be confused with trigeminal neuralgia and migraine headache (see Chap. 37).

Assessment Findings

Symptoms include jaw pain, pronounced muscle spasm, and tenderness of the masseter and temporalis muscles. Headache,

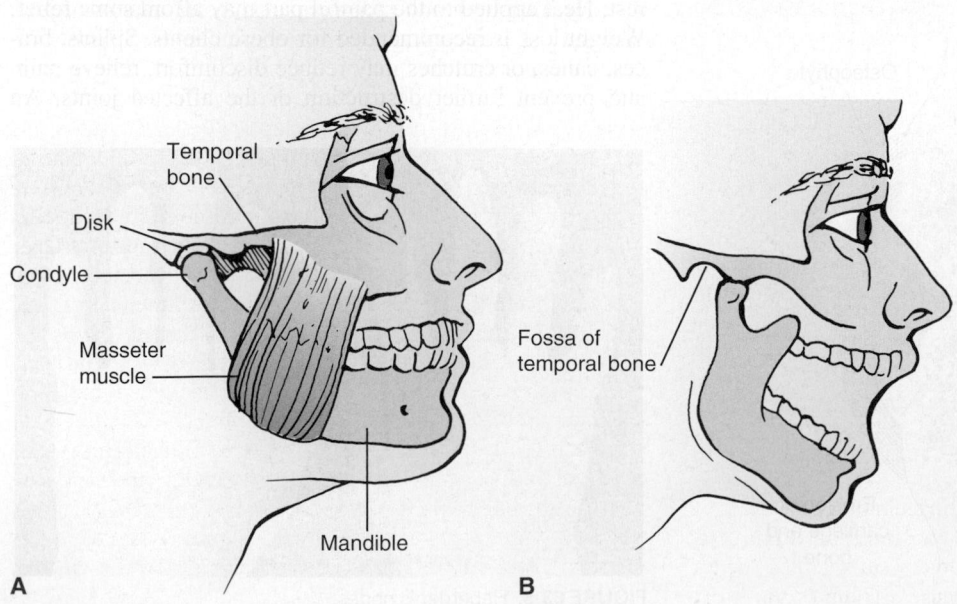

FIGURE 63-6. (A) The temporomandibular joint is located between the two bones for which it is named: the temporal bone and mandible. **(B)** The condyle of the mandible, which is covered by a cartilaginous disk, moves forward and backward within the fossa of the temporal bone of the skull, which is located in front of the ear.

Temporal bone
Disk
Condyle
Masseter muscle
Mandible
Fossa of temporal bone

A

B

tinnitus (ringing in the ears), and ear pain accompany the localized discomfort. The client experiences clicking of the jaw when moving the joint, or the jaw can lock, which interferes with opening the mouth. Special dental radiographs often reveal evidence of joint displacement.

Medical and Surgical Management

Treatment is referral to a dentist who has experience managing clients with TMD. Analgesics are prescribed or recommended; the client wears a custom-fitted mouth guard during sleep. Transcutaneous electrical nerve stimulation, injection of a local anesthetic to relieve muscle spasm, and oral irrigations with ice water also are used to reduce and relieve discomfort. Reconstructive surgery of the temporomandibular joint is available if conservative treatment is ineffective.

Nursing Management

The nurse monitors the client's weight and ability to consume food. If indicated, the nurse obtains a nutritional consultation with the dietitian. With the help of the dietitian, the nurse modifies the diet to include soft rather than coarse food, which is easier to chew. He or she provides nutritional liquid supplements and assists the client to acquire skills that control pain, such as using a bite guard during sleep.

GOUT

Gout, a painful metabolic disorder involving an inflammatory reaction in the joints, usually affects the feet (especially the great toe), hands, elbows, ankles, and knees.

Pathophysiology and Etiology

The disorder tends to be inherited and affects more men than women. Gout may occur secondary to other diseases marked by decreased renal excretion of uric acid. It also has been identified among clients who have received organ transplants and the antirejection drug cyclosporine.

Gout is characterized by **hyperuricemia** (accumulation of uric acid in the blood), caused by alterations in uric acid production, excretion, or both. Hyperuricemia occurs from one or a combination of the following pathologies:

- Primary hyperuricemia
  - Severe dieting or starvation
  - Excessive ingestion of purines (organ meats, shellfish, sardines)
  - Heredity
- Secondary hyperuricemia
  - Abnormal purine metabolism
  - Increased rate of protein synthesis with overproduction or underexcretion of uric acid
  - Increased cellular turnover, as in leukemia, multiple myeloma, and other cancers; some anemias; and psoriasis
  - Altered renal tubular function related to use of diuretics and salicylates and excessive alcohol intake, leading to underexcretion of uric acid (Smeltzer et al., 2008)

Urate (a salt of uric acid) crystallizes in body tissues and is deposited in soft and bony tissues, causing local inflammation and irritation. Collections of urate crystals, called **tophi**, are found in the cartilage of the outer ear (pinna), the great toe, hands, and other joints, ligaments, bursae, and tendons. As these deposits accumulate, they destroy the joint, producing a chronically swollen, deformed appearance. The uric acid also may precipitate in urine, causing renal stones.

Assessment Findings
Signs and Symptoms

A gout attack is characterized by a sudden onset of acute pain and tenderness in one joint. The skin turns red and the joint swells so that it is warm and hypersensitive to touch. Fever may be present. Tophi may be palpated around the fingers, great toes, or earlobes, particularly if the client has chronic and severe hyperuricemia. The attack may last for 1 or 2 weeks, but moderate swelling and tenderness may persist. A symptom-free period usually is followed by another attack, which may occur any time. Repeated episodes in the same joint may deform the joint.

Diagnostic Findings

Diagnosis usually is based on the obvious clinical signs and hyperuricemia. Synovial fluid aspirated from the joint during arthrocentesis contains urate crystals. The urate deposits also may be identifiable with a radiographic examination. Elevated uric acid levels in serum and urine (24-hour urine collection) correlate with gout, but these findings are common to other disorders as well.

Medical and Surgical Management

Although gout cannot be cured in the sense of removing the basic metabolic difficulty of constant or recurrent hyperuricemia, the attacks usually can be controlled. The aim of treatment is to decrease sodium urate in the extracellular fluid so that deposits do not form.

Two main treatment approaches involve (1) using uricosuric drugs that promote renal excretion of urates by inhibiting the reabsorption of uric acid in the renal tubules, and (2) decreasing ingestion of purine. The regimen is individualized and may be changed in response to the changes in the course of the disease.

Pain during a severe acute attack may require NSAIDs, such as ibuprofen and indomethacin. Acute attacks of gout also may be treated with colchicine or phenylbutazone. Colchicine is administered every 1 or 2 hours until the pain subsides or nausea, vomiting, intestinal cramping, and diarrhea develop. When one or more of these symptoms occurs, the drug should be stopped temporarily. Drugs used for long-term gout management include colchicine, allopurinol (Zyloprim), probenecid (Benemid), indomethacin (Indocin), and sulfinpyrazone (Anturane). To prevent future attacks, drug therapy continues after the acute attack subsides (Drug Therapy Table 63-2). Salicylates inactivate uricosurics, and clients with a history of gout should not use them.

It is now known that the body can synthesize purines; thus, emphasis on strict diet restriction has decreased, with more focus on the use of uricosuric drugs. The prescribed diet includes adequate protein, with limitation of purine-rich foods to avoid contributing to the underlying problem. The diet prescription also is relatively high in complex carbohydrates and low in fats because carbohydrates increase urate excretion and fats retard it. Overweight clients are encouraged to lose weight. A high fluid intake helps increase

DRUG THERAPY TABLE 63-2 Selected Antigout Medications

Drug	Mechanism of Action	Nursing Considerations
colchicine	Lowers the deposition of uric acid and interferes with leukocytes and kinin formation, thus reducing inflammation Does not alter serum or urine levels of uric acid Used in acute and chronic management	Acute management: Administer when attack first begins. Dosage is increased until pain is relieved or diarrhea develops. Chronic management: Prolonged use may decrease vitamin B12 absorption. Drug causes GI upset in most clients.
probenecid (Benemid)	Uricosuric agent; inhibits renal reabsorption of urates and increases the urinary excretion of uric acid Prevents tophi formation	Be alert for nausea, rash, and constipation.
pllopurinol (Zyloprim)	Xanthine oxidase inhibitor; interrupts the breakdown of purines before uric acid forms Inhibits xanthine oxidase because it blocks uric acid formation	Be alert for side effects, including bone marrow depression, vomiting, and abdominal pain.

excretion of uric acid. Nutrition Notes 63-2 outlines additional considerations.

Surgery may be performed to remove the large tophi of advanced gout. Surgery also may be used to correct crippling deformities that may result from treatment delays or to fuse unstable joints and increase their function.

Nursing Management

The nurse places a bed cradle over the affected joint to protect it from the pressure of the bed linen. If colchicine is prescribed, he or she explains about the hourly administration until side effects occur or acute pain subsides. The nurse instructs the client to report gastrointestinal (GI) symptoms. He or she measures intake and output, especially when diarrhea accompanies colchicine therapy for acute gout. The nurse provides clear explanations of long-term drug and diet therapy before discharge.

Nutrition Notes 63-2
The Client with Gout

- During an acute attack, high purine foods are avoided, including organ meats, gravies, meat extracts, anchovies, herring, mackerel, sardines, and scallops.
- Gradual weight loss helps reduce serum uric acid levels in clients with gout. Clients should avoid fasting, low-carbohydrate diets, and rapid weight loss because these measures increase the likelihood of ketone formation, which inhibits uric acid excretion.
- A high-carbohydrate diet promotes urate excretion, as does a low-fat diet. These modifications are recommended even if weight loss is not attempted.
- To reduce the risk of renal calculi, a complication of prolonged immobility and gout, advise clients to drink at least 2 quarts of fluid daily. Drinking fluid before bed and during the night helps keep the urine dilute.
- Alcohol is eliminated because it can contribute to an attack.

Pharmacologic Considerations

- Clients with gout need detailed instructions about their medical regimens in relation to the drugs to take and the importance of increasing their fluid intake to reduce the possibility of calculi formation in the urinary tract.

FIBROMYALGIA

Fibromyalgia is a chronic syndrome of pain, fatigue, and sleep disturbances. The pain is widespread, affecting muscles, ligaments, and tendons.

Pathophysiology and Etiology

There is not any definitive pathophysiology identified with fibromyalgia. One theory of central pain syndromes states that the central nervous system becomes sensitized to a stimulus, increasing the client's sensitivity to pain signals (FitzGibbons, 2007). It is believed that repeated nerve stimulation results in abnormal levels of neurotransmitters that signal pain. The pain receptors in the brain develop a memory of the pain and are more sensitive to the signals. This process of central nervous system sensitization theoretically lowers a client's pain threshold. There are areas of pain on touch called tender points that can be identified on people with fibromyalgia that other people without this condition do not have. There is currently no explanation as to why this occurs.

Approximately 10 million people in the United States are diagnosed with fibromyalgia (National Fibromyalgia Association, 2009). Women, in particular middle-aged women, are most vulnerable to fibromyalgia, but the syndrome does affect men, women, and children. Although it seems more prevalent and common today, fibromyalgia has been in existence for hundreds of years, but was never accurately diagnosed. In 1990, the American College of

Rheumatology (2008) identified criteria for the diagnosis of fibromyalgia.

Assessment Findings

Signs and Symptoms

Widespread and chronic pain is the most common finding. The American College of Rheumatology identifies 18 tender points on palpation that are particularly sensitive. If a client has 11 out of 18 tender points, that is considered diagnostic for fibromyalgia. However, many clients with fibromyalgia have lower pain thresholds everywhere, not just at the identified tender points (FitzGibbons, 2007).

Other signs and symptoms include:

- Fatigue and sleep disturbances
- Irritable bowel syndrome
- Chronic headaches and temporomandibular joint (TMJ) dysfunction
- Heightened sensitivity to lights, noise, and touch
- Depression and/or anxiety
- Cognitive or memory impairment, referred to as "fibro-fog" (Dellwo, 2008)

Diagnostic Findings

Diagnosis is often difficult and involves ruling out other diseases and conditions. The presence of widespread and chronic pain in all four quadrants of the body, but most especially the axial chest, neck, and back is particularly a hallmark for diagnosing fibromyalgia (FitzGibbons, 2007). Initial tests are done for blood counts, chemistry profile, thyroid levels, Lyme disease titer, and C-reactive protein, mostly to rule out other conditions. Identifying 11 of the 18 tender points identified by the American College of Rheumatology is useful, but not considered definitive by many physicians. Generally, clients are diagnosed based on all of their symptoms and not so much through specific tests.

Medical Management

Analgesics, including acetaminophen and NSAIDs, are prescribed to alleviate some of the painful symptoms of fibromyalgia. Tramadol (Ultram), a prescription pain reliever, may be taken with or without acetaminophen. Muscle relaxants such as cyclobenzaprine (Flexeril) may be prescribed short-term at bedtime to help with muscle aches. Pregabalin (Lyrica), an antiseizure medication also used to treat some types of pain, is the first drug approved by the Food and Drug Administration to treat fibromyalgia. It is used to reduce pain and fatigue and improve sleep quality for people with fibromyalgia. Tricyclic antidepressants (TCAs), especially amitriptyline, are used with some success for chronic pain. Dual serotonin norepinephrine reuptake inhibitors, such as venlafaxine (Effexor XR) and duloxetine (Cymbalta), are ordered to treat pain, sleep disorders, cognitive impairment, and mood changes (FitzGibbons, 2007). Other medications are prescribed for treatment of specific symptoms a client may experience with fibromyalgia, such as antiepileptics for burning pain, and corticosteroids as anti-inflammatory agents.

Some clients benefit from acupuncture treatments, massage therapy, cognitive behavior therapy, biofeedback, aquatherapy, and hypnotherapy. FitzGibbons (2007) states that clinical trials for vagus nerve stimulation are being conducted on clients with fibromyalgia. The vagus nerve is involved in central pain processing.

Nursing Management

Nursing care focuses on providing support to clients. Often clients have endured disturbing symptoms for a long period of time and feel that they were not believed. Encouraging clients to live a healthy lifestyle is important. This includes a healthy diet, avoidance of caffeine and alcohol, regular exercise, decreased stress, and adequate sleep. A support group may prove helpful, so that clients can share their experiences. It is important to refer clients to reliable sources for fibromyalgia, such as the National Fibromyalgia Association, and to remind them not to engage in treatments that have not been verified.

BURSITIS

Bursitis is an inflammation of the bursa, a fluid-filled sac that cushions bone ends to enhance a gliding movement. The elbow, shoulder, and knee are common sites of bursitis.

Pathophysiology and Etiology

Trauma is the most common cause of acute bursitis. Other causes include overuse, stress, infection, and secondary effects of gout and RA. Typical of any inflammation, pain and swelling occur with compromised function.

Assessment Findings

Painful movement of a joint, such as the elbow or shoulder, is the most common symptom. A distinct lump may be felt. If the bursa ruptures, tissue in the area may become edematous, warm, and tender.

An x-ray study may reveal a calcified bursa, and aspiration of fluid may demonstrate the following:

- A few leukocytes in transparent fluid if the etiology is trauma
- A large collection of leukocytes if the cause is sepsis
- Colonies of staphylococcal or streptococcal microorganisms
- Urate crystals in bursitis secondary to gout
- Cholesterol crystals, common in clients with bursitis and RA, which may cause the fluid from the bursa to appear cloudy

Medical and Surgical Management

Joint rest usually is recommended. Salicylates or NSAIDs may be prescribed. If the problem persists, a corticosteroid preparation may be injected into the joint to reduce inflammation. After pain and inflammation are reduced, ongoing therapy involves mild ROM exercises. If infection is the cause, antibiotics will be ordered.

 Pharmacologic Considerations

- Tell clients taking large doses of salicylates the signs of GI bleeding and salicylism, and the possibility of easy bruising and other bleeding tendencies. Signs of salicylism include headache, nausea, vomiting, tinnitus, increased pulse and respiratory rates, fever, mental confusion, and drowsiness.

- Large doses of salicylates can interfere with the blood's clotting mechanism. Instruct clients taking these drugs to inform their physicians and dentists of their prolonged and high-dose ingestion of salicylates.

Nursing Management

The nurse reviews the prescribed medication and exercise regimens with the client and allows time for questions and answers. He or she advises the client not to traumatize or overuse the recovering joint but to use it normally. Failure to use the joint after pain and inflammation are controlled may result in partial limitation of joint motion.

ANKYLOSING SPONDYLITIS

Ankylosing spondylitis, or Marie-Strümpell disease, is a chronic connective tissue disorder of the spine and surrounding cartilaginous joints, such as the sacroiliac joints and soft tissues around the vertebrae. Characteristics include spondylosis and fusion of the vertebrae.

Pathophysiology and Etiology

Ankylosing spondylitis usually begins in early adulthood and is more common in men than in women. Its etiology is unknown, although some theorize that an altered immune response occurs when T-cell lymphocytes mistake human cells for similar-appearing bacterial antigens. There also is a strong familial tendency for some affected individuals. Once the inflammation begins, it continues, causing progressive immobility and fixation (ankylosis) of the joints in the hips, and ascends the vertebrae. Respiratory function may be compromised if kyphosis (a hunchback-like spinal curve) develops. In a few cases, there may be extra-articular (nonjoint) manifestations, such as aortitis (inflammation of the aorta), iridocyclitis (inflammation of the iris and ciliary body of the eye), and pulmonary fibrosis.

Assessment Findings
Signs and Symptoms
The most common symptoms are low back pain and stiffness. As the disease progresses, the spine and hips become more immobile, thus restricting movement. The lumbar curve of the spine may flatten. The neck can be permanently flexed and the client appears to be in a perpetual stooped position. Aortic regurgitation or atrioventricular node conduction disturbances may occur. Lung sounds may be reduced, especially in the apical areas. The client may experience fatigue, anorexia, and weight loss.

Diagnostic Findings
Evidence of inflammation is demonstrated by an elevated ESR. A culture of synovial fluid, however, is negative for causative microorganisms. Elevations of alkaline phosphatase and creatinine phosphokinase levels are common. An HLA test, used for determining inherited tissue markers for immune functions, demonstrates the presence of HLA-B2 in 90% of clients with this disorder. X-ray films or computed tomography (CT) scans show erosion, ossification, and fusion of the joints in the spine and hips.

Medical and Surgical Management

Treatment is supportive, the major goal being to maintain functional posture. NSAIDs such as naproxen or indomethacin are usually prescribed for relieving inflammation and pain. Drugs used to treat RA may also be prescribed, such as DMARDs and tumor necrosis factor (TNF) blockers. Sleeping on a firm mattress (preferably without a pillow) and following a prescribed exercise program may help delay or prevent spinal deformity, especially if begun in the early stages of the disease. A back brace also may be prescribed for some clients. Severe hip involvement may be treated with a total hip replacement.

Nursing Management

The nurse administers prescribed drugs and clarifies information about the disease. He or she encourages the client to perform ADLs as much as possible. The nurse teaches the client to perform mild exercises that reduce stiffness and pain. He or she provides emotional support, recognizing that the client must deal with pain, skeletal changes, and impaired mobility.

SYSTEMIC LUPUS ERYTHEMATOSUS

Systemic lupus erythematosus (SLE) is a diffuse connective tissue disease. As the name implies, it affects multiple body systems such as the skin, joints, kidney, serous membranes of the heart and lungs, lymph nodes, and GI tract.

Pathophysiology and Etiology

SLE is more common in women than in men. Most clients have this disorder in the 3rd or 4th decade of life, but it may be seen in young children and in middle-aged and older adults. It is believed to be autoimmune, but the triggering mechanism is still unknown. There is a strong familial tendency, suggesting that certain inherited cellular antigenic markers confuse the ability of T cells to distinguish self from nonself. By mistake, helper T cells alert B cells to produce antibodies against normal cells, or suppressor T cells may be ineffective in controlling a B-cell response once it has been initiated. The disease may have periods during which it is in a subacute form or even in remission. Exposure to ultraviolet light is a factor in reactivating the disease.

Antibodies destroy connective tissues of the body. Affected structures undergo inflammation, fibrosis, scarring, and dysfunction. Polymorphonuclear leukocytes (neutrophils) engulf the nuclei of attacked cells. Laboratory studies confirm this finding, which is considered diagnostic.

Assessment Findings
Signs and Symptoms
According to Porth (2007), SLE is known as the *great imitator* because the clinical signs resemble many other conditions (Box 63-2). SLE is also marked by remissions and

BOX 63-2 Clinical Manifestations of Systemic Lupus Erythematosus

SLE is known as the *great imitator*, with manifestations that resemble many other diseases.

- *Constitutional:* fevers, fatigue, anorexia, weight loss
- *Musculoskeletal:* arthritis, muscle weakness and atrophy, avascular necrosis
- *Dermatologic:* alopecia, photosensitivity, rash, skin lesions that appear or worsen in sunlight; mouth sores
- *Cardiovascular:* chest pain, pericarditis, systolic murmurs, valvular complications, Raynaud's phenomenon, easy bruising
- *Pulmonary:* shortness of breath, pleuritis, pneumonitis, pulmonary hypertension
- *Renal:* nephritis, glomerulonephritis
- *Neuropsychiatric:* cognitive dysfunction, depression, anxiety, psychosis
- Dry eyes

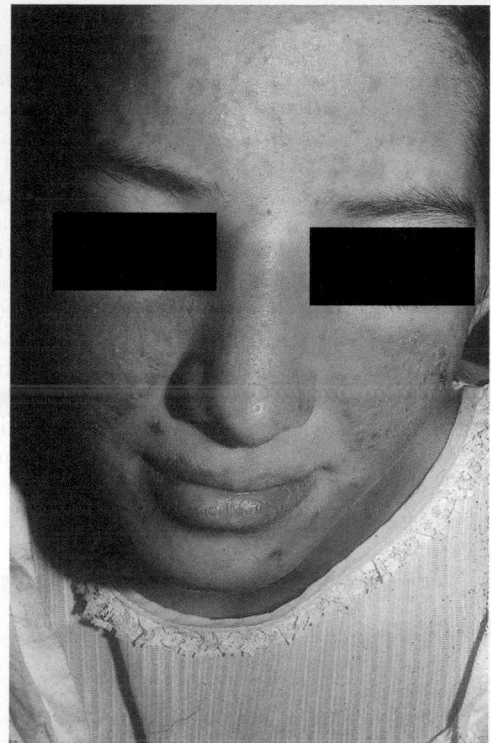

FIGURE 63-7. Characteristic malar or butterfly rash seen in systemic lupus erythematosus. (From Goodheart, H. P. [2009]. *Goodheart's photoguide to common skin disorders: Diagnosis and management.* [3rd ed.]. Philadelphia: Lippincott Williams & Wilkins.)

exacerbations (referred to as flares). Early signs and symptoms of SLE may include fever, weight loss, pain in the joints (arthralgia), malaise, muscle pain, and extreme fatigue. These symptoms are vague and may persist for several months to 2 years before more prominent symptoms develop and the client seeks medical advice.

A prominent sign for about half of the clients with SLE is a red, butterfly-shaped rash known as malar rash, on the face over the bridge of the nose and the cheeks (Fig. 63-7). The word *lupus* means "wolf." The term may have been used as a description for the facial rash that, to some, resembled the mask of reddish-brown fur on a wolf.

Two other types of skin manifestations may occur with SLE. The first is discoid lupus erythematosus (DLE), which involves a chronic rash with erythematous papules or plaques and scaling. Eventually DLE can lead to scarring and pigmentation changes. The symptoms of DLE are related only to the skin, the most prominent symptom being the appearance of the facial rash. Skin manifestations of the disorder also may be found on the forehead, earlobes, and scalp. Scalp involvement usually results in patchy loss of hair (alopecia). These symptoms also may be seen in people with SLE. The second type is subacute cutaneous lupus erythematosus, which presents with papulosquamous lesions.

Clients also may exhibit behavioral disturbances (confusion, hallucinations, irritability), chest pain (as a result of involvement of the pleura or pericarditis), fluid retention, proteinuria, and hematuria (as a result of renal involvement), progressive weight loss, nausea and vomiting, and, in women, irregular or heavy menses. Other signs of the disease include the following:

- Nonspecific electrocardiographic changes
- A pericardial friction rub
- Pulmonary changes seen on radiographic studies
- Enlargement of the spleen and lymph nodes
- Raynaud's phenomenon (vasospasm of the smaller vessels of the hands and feet resulting in blanching of the skin and, at times, pain and cyanosis of the extremities)

- Musculoskeletal problems, such as arthralgias and arthritis, including joint swelling, tenderness, pain on movement, and morning stiffness

Diagnostic Findings

Diagnosis of SLE is based on presenting symptoms and blood tests. Blood studies show anemia, thrombocytopenia, leukocytosis or leukopenia, and positive serum antinuclear antibody (ANA). Anti-double-stranded DNA (anti-dsDNA) antibody test is a test that shows high titers of antibodies against native DNA. This is very specific for SLE because this test is not positive for other autoimmune disorders. Approximately 60% to 70% of people with SLE have positive anti-dsDNA. Anti-Smith (anti-Sm) antibodies are specific for SLE, but are found in only 20% to 30% of clients with SLE (Rooney, 2005). Other laboratory studies may indicate multisystem involvement, such as an elevated creatinine level with kidney involvement. Additional tests, such as a renal biopsy and urinalysis, may be performed to determine the effect of the disorder on other body systems.

The American College of Rheumatology (2008) has identified 11 criteria for SLE. Clients presenting with four of these criteria at one time or individually over time are diagnosed with probable SLE. These criteria are: malar rash, discoid rash, photosensitivity, oral ulcers, arthritis, pleuritis or pericarditis, renal disorder, neurological disorders such as seizures, hematologic disorder such as thrombocytopenia, immunologic disorder as indicated by tests such as positive anti-dsDNA, and positive ANA test.

Medical Management

There is no specific treatment for this disorder. Medical management aims at producing a remission and preventing or treating acute exacerbations of the disorder. High doses of corticosteroids are used initially. Those with severe disease or for whom steroid-related side effects are problematic may be treated with cytotoxic drugs such as azathioprine (Imuran) and cyclophosphamide (Cytoxan). Simple analgesics such as aspirin or an NSAID may be prescribed for fever and joint discomfort. Topical corticosteroids may be used for skin manifestations. Hydroxychloroquine (Plaquenil) and chloroquine (Aralen), which are antimalarials, have been found to be effective medications for clients with SLE. These drugs are used when clients present with symptoms, but they are also useful in preventing flares. Renal impairment may be treated with dialysis or kidney transplantation. Cardiac, GI, and central nervous system complications are treated symptomatically.

Nursing Process for the Client With Systemic Lupus Erythematosus

Assessment

Review the medical record and diagnostic findings to evaluate the stage of disease and appropriate interventions. Assess the client's understanding of the nature of the disorder, its treatment, and the limitations imposed by the disease process. Inspect the skin for rashes, purpuric lesions, and other skin changes and ask about the client's degree of sensitivity to sunlight. Inspect for ulcerations in the mouth and throat (signs of GI involvement). In addition, listen to the heart for pericardial friction rub and to the lungs for abnormal sounds, which might suggest pleural involvement.

Diagnosis, Planning, and Interventions

Nursing management focuses on measures to minimize exacerbations and to alleviate symptoms. Administer prescribed medications and monitor for side effects. Before discharge, client education efforts involve reminding the client of the need for close medical follow-up and thorough medication instruction (i.e., never abruptly discontinue taking a prescribed corticosteroid without consulting the physician, and follow the dosage regimen exactly, particularly if the drug dose is being decreased gradually).

Because the disease and drugs alter body image, assist the client to verbalize feelings and implement effective coping mechanisms. If the client desires, arrange a referral to the Lupus Foundation of America, which is dedicated to providing information about the disease, or to a local support or self-help group.

Since SLE is a chronic disease and treated mainly on an outpatient basis, much nursing management revolves around teaching. Clients and their families need accurate and complete information about the disease, its treatment and prognosis, and self-care measures to increase comfort and promote health. Specific measures are discussed in Client and Family Teaching 63-1.

Other nursing care involves, but is not limited to, the following diagnoses, expected outcomes, and interventions.

▶ **Chronic Pain** related to inflammation and disease progression

Client and Family Teaching 63-1
Systemic Lupus Erythematosus

The nurse typically addresses the following with the client:

- Lifestyle modifications are necessary as related to musculoskeletal restrictions and systemic involvement. For example, because sunlight tends to exacerbate the disease, avoid sunlight and ultraviolet radiation. When outdoors, apply effective sunscreens with a sun protection factor (SPF) of 15 or higher and wear clothing that covers the arms and legs and a wide-brimmed hat to shade the face. Sunlamps and tanning booths are taboo.
- Pace activities. Because fatigue is a major issue, allow for adequate rest along with regular activity to promote mobility and prevent joint stiffness. Avoid activities that cause severe pain or discomfort.
- Maintain a well-balanced diet and increase fluid intake to raise energy levels and promote tissue healing.
- Avoid crowds when possible and people with known infections, such as colds.
- Periodically review the medication program with your healthcare providers, particularly the effects and adverse effects of medications and related signs and symptoms that require attention and should be reported to the physician (increased severity of symptoms, involvement in other joints or areas of the body, weight loss, prolonged anorexia, nausea, vomiting, fever, cough, shortness of breath, difficult urination, infection, or any other unusual occurrence).
- Take medications exactly as directed and do not stop the medication if symptoms are relieved unless advised to do so by the physician.
- If symptoms become worse, do not increase the dosage unless advised to do so by the physician. Do not use over-the-counter drugs unless a physician approves their use.
- Use nonpharmacologic comfort measures. For instance, a moist form of heat may relieve joint stiffness. Use warm, not hot, soaks, wraps, or towels hot from the clothes dryer and take care not to burn the skin.
- Inform physicians and dentists of current therapy before any treatment, surgery, or drugs are prescribed.

▶ **Expected Outcomes:** (1) Client will experience relief from pain and discomfort. (2) Client will adhere to the prescribed pharmacologic regimen. (3) Client will demonstrate use of alternative methods to reduce pain.

- Administer prescribed analgesic and anti-inflammatory medications. *Pain and discomfort respond to combination drug regimens, which promote comfort and reduce the disease's inflammatory effects.*
- Review the rationale for adhering to the prescribed regimen. *Teaching promotes the client's compliance and may prevent the client from trying unsafe and ineffective therapies.*
- Elevate swollen and painful joints and apply heat or cold as indicated. *Nonpharmacologic methods decrease swelling and promote comfort.*

- Monitor the client if he or she uses braces or splints. *They promote rest to inflamed joints but may cause skin irritation. Frequent monitoring prevents skin breakdown.*
- Balance activity with rest. *Alternating rest and activity conserves energy and promotes productivity and control.*
- Move painful joints gently and slowly while supporting the extremity above and below the joint. *Doing so promotes optimal mobility and reduces pain.*
- Avoid heavy blankets or clothing. *They increase pressure and pain.*

▶ Impaired Physical Mobility related to inflammation, joint problems, pain, or decreased muscle strength

▶ Expected Outcomes: (1) Client will maintain maximal physical function within limitations. (2) Client will increase muscle strength in affected areas or in areas that compensate for physical limitations. (3) Client will retain function with limitation of contractures.

- Assist client to maintain appropriate body alignment and neutral positioning during periods of inactivity. *Doing so prevents contractures and increases mobility.*
- Encourage moderate and progressive exercise as indicated. *Exercise promotes mobility and reduces fatigue.*
- Advise client to use moist heat before performing ROM exercises. *Moist heat relaxes muscles and reduces resistance to ROM exercises.*
- Urge client to wear supportive shoes and to use assistive devices for ambulation as needed. *These measures improve mobility.*
- Recommend sitting in elevated chairs that have arm rests that can help client to stand up. *These chairs improve the client's ability to be more independent.*
- Encourage client to maintain erect posture when sitting, standing, and walking. *Appropriate posture promotes optimal mobility and enhances muscle strengthening.*

▶ Self-Care Deficit (specify bathing/hygiene, dressing/ grooming, feeding, toileting) related to exacerbation of disease, inflammation, and decreased mobility

▶ Expected Outcomes: (1) Client will perform self-care activities at highest possible level. (2) Client will identify methods that assist her or him to meet self-care needs.

- Modify clothing so that the client can easily put it on and take it off (e.g., use Velcro fasteners instead of buttons, front fasteners rather than back zippers, elastic shoe laces, cardigan sweaters instead of pullovers). *Ease in changing clothes promotes independence in self-care.*
- Pad handles for easy grasping. *Doing so enhances self-care abilities.*
- Suggest an electric toothbrush, which is easier to handle than a manual toothbrush. *This helps encourage the client to care for self.*
- Provide cooking and eating utensils designed to promote a good grip (particularly useful for clients with hand deformities). *This measure enhances self-care abilities.*

- Identify equipment resources and dealers for wheelchairs, elevated commode seats, and other assistive devices. *Doing so assists the client to plan for changes in lifestyle.*

▶ Disturbed Body Image related to change in appearance and inability to perform tasks and activities

▶ Expected Outcomes: (1) Client will verbalize increased confidence when dealing with changes in appearance and functional abilities. (2) Client will establish realistic future goals.

- Accept client without reservation. *Nonverbal behavior expresses feelings. Facial expressions, tone of voice, or other behaviors promote acceptance or nonacceptance.*
- Avoid nonverbal messages that convey impatience with the client's disabilities. *Clients with disability require more time to finish tasks. Patience promotes independence.*
- Assist client only as needed or requested. *Doing so encourages client to perform self-care as much as possible.*
- Do not overprotect client or increase dependency. *A client involved with his or her own care can make decisions and is better able to identify when he or she needs help.*
- Focus on what the client can do rather than not do. *Emphasizing strengths is essential.*
- Assist client to identify strengths. *Doing so promotes a positive self-image.*
- Encourage client to express fears, misgivings, or other concerns. *Acknowledging feelings assists client to identify resources and use coping mechanisms.*
- Acknowledge feelings of grief and hostility. *Doing so provides an atmosphere of acceptance.*
- Refer client for counseling if he or she withdraws, shows signs of denial, or otherwise exhibits maladaptive behavior. *Doing so provides other resources to increase coping skills.*

Evaluation of Expected Outcomes

The client reports relief of pain and discomfort, adheres to prescribed drug therapy, and uses alternative methods to reduce pain. He or she demonstrates maximal physical function within limitations, showing evidence of increased muscle strength function. The client can perform self-care at the highest possible level and has a plan for meeting future self-care needs as independently as possible. He or she reports self-confidence and acceptance in the face of altered physical appearance and function and states realistic future goals. The client copes realistically and well with the chronicity of the disease. ●

MUSCULOSKELETAL INFECTIOUS DISORDERS

The musculoskeletal system is subject to infections that can profoundly impact a person's mobility, ability to perform ADLs, and quality of life. This section focuses on osteomyelitis, a condition that affects bone, and Lyme disease, an illness that affects multiple systems including the musculoskeletal system.

OSTEOMYELITIS

Osteomyelitis is an infection of the bone. Limited blood supply, inflammation of and pressure on the tissue, and formation of new bone around devitalized bone tissue make osteomyelitis a difficult and challenging condition to treat. In adults, osteomyelitis may become chronic, greatly affecting quality of life.

Pathophysiology and Etiology

Staphylococcus aureus causes 70% to 80% of bone infections. Other organisms include *Proteus vulgaris* and *Pseudomonas aeruginosa*, as well as *Escherichia coli*. According to Smeltzer et al. (2008) "The incidence of penicillin-resistant, nosocomial, gram-negative, and anaerobic infections is increasing" (p. 2413). Osteomyelitis results from bacteria reaching the bone through the bloodstream. Acute localized osteomyelitis occurs when bone is contaminated directly by trauma, such as penetrating wounds or compound fractures. Occasionally, surgical contamination or direct extension of bacteria from an infected area adjacent to the bone, such as the pin sites of skeletal traction, can cause osteomyelitis.

Microorganisms appear to migrate to the area just below the epiphysis of a long bone where the blood supply is more generous, but circulation through the area is limited. As the microorganisms multiply, they spread down to the bone shaft. The pressure from the collecting exudate elevates the periosteum. New bone cells (**involucrum**) are deposited on the periosteum while the underlying bone becomes necrotic. The pocket of necrotic bone (**sequestrum**) may remain sequestered for years or eventually drain by forming a sinus tract through to the skin. The infection tends to linger in a chronic state because it is difficult to penetrate the infected tissue by administering systemic antibiotic drugs.

In its weakened condition, the infected bone is prone to pathologic fracture. The diseased bone may lengthen as bone growth is stimulated, or it may shorten because of the destruction of the epiphyseal plate. Other complications of osteomyelitis include septicemia, thrombophlebitis, muscle contractures, pathologic fractures, and nonunion of fractures.

Assessment Findings

Evidence of an acute infection appears suddenly: high fever, chills, rapid pulse, tenderness or pain over the affected area, redness, and swelling. Chronic infection may be characterized by a persistent draining sinus.

With acute osteomyelitis, laboratory tests usually show an elevated leukocyte count, an elevated ESR, and possibly a blood culture positive for infective organisms. Identification of the causative organism may require an aspiration of subperiosteal pus for culture and sensitivity. Radiographic findings may be inconclusive in the early stages of infection, but later studies demonstrate irregular bone decalcification, bone necrosis, elevation of the periosteum, and new bone formation. Bone scans and MRI are useful in definitive diagnoses.

Radiographic studies for chronic osteomyelitis show large cavities, sequestra or dense bone formations, and raised periosteum. Areas of infection are delineated by bone scan. Blood studies reveal a normal leukocyte count and ESR and possible anemia.

Medical and Surgical Management

Management of osteomyelitis includes the following:

- Immobilization with a cast or immobilizer to decrease pain and prevent fracture. The cast may be windowed to provide access for wound care.
- Application of warm saline soaks to the affected area for 20 minutes several times a day to increase circulation to the affected area
- Identification of the causative organism to initiate appropriate and ongoing antibiotic therapy for infection control. Intravenous (IV) antibiotic therapy is administered for 3 to 6 weeks. Oral antibiotics then follow for as long as 3 months.
- Surgical debridement of the necrotic tissue and sequestrum to remove the infected areas
- Closed irrigation with saline or an antibiotic solution and low suction to the affected area to flush away necrotic tissue
- Antibiotic-impregnated beads may be directly applied in the wound for 2 to 4 weeks
- Bone grafts for the debrided cavity to stimulate bone growth
- Muscle flaps grafted to the affected area to enhance blood supply

Nursing Management

Clients with osteomyelitis experience pain, inflammation, swelling, and impaired mobility because of pain and the inability to bear weight. Caretakers must handle the arm or leg or related area gently to prevent additional pain or fracture. They must protect the infected area from injury. The nurse instructs the client to elevate the area and to bear weight only as indicated. Nursing management includes protecting the skin from breakdown, administering the prescribed antibiotics and pain medications, and informing the client about the expected therapeutic effects and possible side effects. Clients with chronic osteomyelitis require extensive emotional support, related to the long-term nature of this illness.

> **Stop, Think, and Respond Exercise 63-2**
>
> *Which of the following clients is at greatest risk for osteomyelitis?*
>
> 1. *A 65-year-old client recently diagnosed with osteoarthritis*
> 2. *A 70-year-old client who recently sustained an open compound fracture of the tibia after a motor vehicle accident*
> 3. *A 40-year-old client diagnosed with Lyme disease*

LYME DISEASE

Lyme disease (Lyme borreliosis) gained wide recognition in the 1970s, when residents of Lyme, Connecticut, experienced an epidemic of progressive symptoms, beginning with a characteristic rash and eventually involving the cardiac, neurologic, and musculoskeletal systems.

Pathophysiology and Etiology

Typically, Lyme disease is prevalent during warmer months, when ticks are abundant, but it may occur at any time. It is most common in the northeast and mid-Atlantic states, and in other northern areas of the United States, where deer ticks (*Ixodes dammini*) are more prevalent. The ticks feed on white-tailed deer or white-footed mice, and then become carriers of the spirochetal bacterium *Borrelia burgdorferi*. When ticks bite humans, they transmit the bacteria, which results in a chronic inflammatory process and multisystem disease.

Assessment Findings

Signs and Symptoms

If untreated, the disease moves through three stages. Early stage 1 symptoms for about one third of clients include a red macule or papule at the site of the tick bite, a characteristic bull's-eye rash (called erythema migrans) with round rings surrounding the center, headache, neck stiffness, and pain. Secondary pruritic lesions may accompany fever, chills, and malaise. The initial papule may not develop until 20 to 30 days after the bite. Some clients experience nausea, vomiting, and sore throat.

Midstage symptoms occur as the organism proliferates throughout the body and cardiac and neurologic involvement becomes evident. Cardiac problems include dysrhythmias and heart block. Neurologic symptoms such as facial palsy, meningitis, and encephalitis are possible. Some clients have problems with weakness, pain, and paresthesia (abnormal sensations).

Later symptoms (at least 4 weeks after the bite) include arthritis and other musculoskeletal problems. Joints, particularly knees, become warm, swollen, and painful. Joint erosion may result from the inflammatory process.

Diagnostic Findings

Diagnosis is based on the presenting signs and symptoms. The enzyme-linked immunosorbent assay (ELISA) test detects antibodies to *Borrelia burgdorferi*. This test can have false positive results, so other tests may be used. The Western blot test is done if the ELISA is positive. It detects antibodies to several proteins of *Borrelia burgdorferi*. The polymerase chain reaction (PCR) test detects bacterial DNA in fluid aspirated from an infected joint. This test is done on clients with chronic Lyme arthritis. It can also be done on cerebrospinal fluid for clients with nervous system symptoms.

Medical and Surgical Management

Treatment includes administering antibiotics and supportive measures. If the disease is treated early, the prognosis is favorable. Permanent multisystem problems may occur if treatment is delayed.

Nursing Management

Nursing management involves teaching the client and family about the disease and its treatment. It is extremely important to educate clients about avoiding Lyme disease (Client and Family Teaching 63-2).

Client and Family Teaching 63-2
Tips for Avoiding Lyme Disease

The nurse teaches the client and family measures to avoid Lyme disease:

Personal Protection

- Wear light-colored clothing to increase tick visibility.
- Wear long-sleeved shirts and long pants (tuck pants into socks or boots).
- Treat clothing with tick repellant.
- Wear a hat; pull long hair back so that it does not brush against shrubs or other vegetation.
- Walk in the center of a path surrounded by grass, brush, or woods.
- Do a tick check after being outside—ticks are particularly attracted to hairy areas such as the scalp, groin, and armpits, as well as the back of knees and neck.

Environmental Protection

- Remove leaf, grass, and brush litter.
- Clear brush and tall grass from around house and other structures, as well as gardens and flower beds.
- Keep grass mowed.
- Place a 3-foot wood chip barrier along lawn edges that border woods.
- Erect fences to keep deer away from houses and gardens.
- Prune low-lying shrubs to let in more sunlight.
- Keep woodpiles neat, dry, and off the ground.
- Keep ground bare under bird feeders, place them away from house, and suspend feeding when ticks are most active.

(Adapted from Wade, C. F. [2000]. Keeping Lyme disease at bay. *American Journal of Nursing*, 100[7], 26–31.)

STRUCTURAL DISORDERS

Structural disorders of the musculoskeletal system involve metabolic conditions that alter bone structure. These alterations result in pain, bone deformity, and fracture.

OSTEOPOROSIS

Osteoporosis, a loss of bone density, occurs principally in older adults and affects more women than men.

Pathophysiology and Etiology

Normally, the processes of bone formation and bone reabsorption occur evenly. In osteoporosis, however, loss of bone substance exceeds bone formation. The total bone mass and density is reduced, resulting in bones that become progressively porous, brittle, and fragile. Compression fractures of the vertebrae are common. Aging contributes to osteoporosis (the loss of bone mass) in the following ways:

- Levels of calcitonin, which inhibits bone reabsorption and promotes bone formation, decrease with aging.

- Levels of estrogen, which inhibits bone breakdown, decrease in postmenopausal women.
- Levels of parathyroid hormone, which increases bone reabsorption, increase with aging.

Gerontologic Considerations

- Estrogen deficiency, which occurs at menopause, is considered the leading factor in osteoporosis among aging women.

Small-framed, thin white women are at greatest risk for osteoporosis. African American women have a greater bone density and thus are less susceptible to osteoporosis. Men have an increased bone mass and do not have hormonal changes, and thus do not acquire osteoporosis as frequently and get it at a later age (Smeltzer et al., 2008).

Other causes of osteoporosis, which may occur in any age group and both sexes, include a family history of osteoporosis, chronic low calcium intake, excessive intake of caffeine, tobacco use, Cushing's syndrome, prolonged use of high doses of corticosteroids, prolonged periods of immobility, hyperthyroidism, hyperparathyroidism, eating disorders, malabsorption syndromes, breast cancer (especially if treated with chemotherapy that suppresses estrogen, excluding Tamoxifen, which may reduce the risk of fractures), renal or liver failure, alcoholism, lactose intolerance, and dietary deficiency of vitamin D and calcium. Some medications interfere with the body's ability to use and metabolize calcium, including thyroid supplements, anticonvulsants, isoniazid, aluminum-containing antacids, tetracycline, selective serotonin reuptake inhibitors (SSRIs), and heparin.

Assessment Findings

Clients with osteoporosis frequently complain of lumbosacral pain, thoracic back pain, or both. The bone pain or tenderness results from tiny compression fractures in the vertebrae. Accompanying loss of height is known as *progressive kyphosis* (Fig. 63-8).

Radiographic examination of the bones shows bone loss once it is 25% or more. Bone deformities (especially in the spine), such as kyphosis and lordosis, and pathologic fractures in long bones also may be seen. Dual energy x-ray absorptiometry (DEXA) is a test that measures bone mineral density (BMD) at the spine and hip. Quantitative ultrasonic studies (QUS) (bone sonometer) measure heel density and provide baseline information for diagnosing osteoporosis and predicting risk of fracture. Results of laboratory studies usually are normal, but such studies may be performed to rule out other disorders such as multiple myeloma, hyperparathyroidism, or metastatic bone lesions.

Medical Management

A diet rich in calcium and vitamin D throughout life can prevent osteoporosis. Osteoporosis cannot be treated directly, but medical management can slow the rate of bone reabsorption. Bone pain or tenderness may respond to mild analgesics such as aspirin. Oral calcium preparations (calcium gluconate, calcium lactate, calcium carbonate, or dibasic

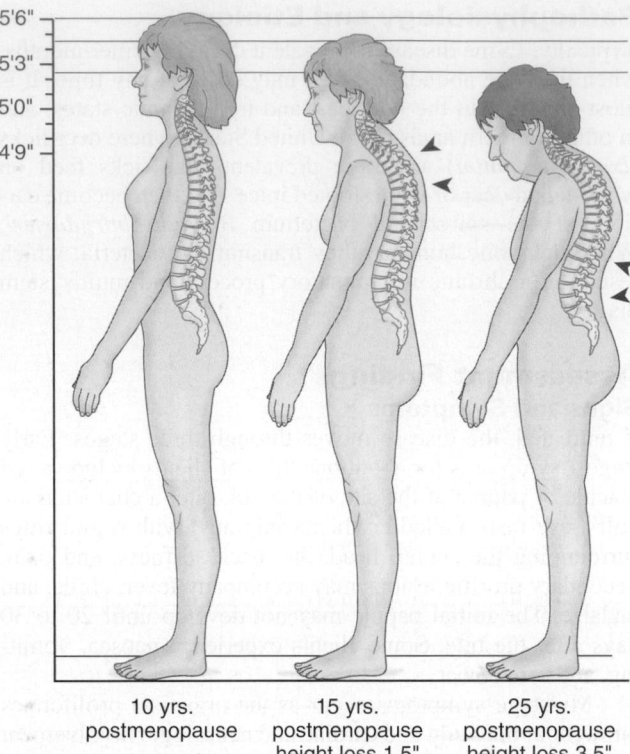

10 yrs.
postmenopause

15 yrs.
postmenopause
height loss 1.5"

25 yrs.
postmenopause
height loss 3.5"

FIGURE 63-8. Typical loss of height associated with osteoporosis and aging.

calcium phosphate) may be recommended to supplement dietary calcium. Some of these preparations also contain vitamin D, which is needed for absorption of calcium in the intestine.

Pharmacologic Considerations

- Oral calcium preparations with vitamin D are better absorbed than those without. Clients should not take oral calcium preparations with other oral drugs because calcium may alter or block their absorption. For example, calcium decreases absorption of tetracycline and phenytoin. Clients should take other drugs 1 to 2 hours after calcium carbonate.

- Clients may take oral calcium with meals to enhance absorption and minimize gastric distress.

Medications used in the treatment of osteoporosis include the following:

- Bisphosphonates, including alendronate sodium (Fosamax) and risedronate (Actonel), inhibit bone resorption. These drugs may be taken once a week or monthly, which reduces the gastroesophageal side effects. Zoledronic acid (Reclast) is another bisphosphonate that is given intravenously once a year.
- Calcitonin inhibits bone reabsorption and slows bone loss. This medication is usually administered as a nasal spray, but may be administered subcutaneously.

- Selective estrogen receptor modifiers (SERMs), such as raloxifene (Evista), preserve BMD and thus reduce the risk for osteoporosis. SERMs do not have the risks associated with estrogen, such as increased risk of uterine cancer.
- Hormone replacement therapy (HRT) was the treatment of choice at one time. However, the potential risks of uterine cancer and heart disease and the availability of other treatments have changed the use of HRT. Instead of oral forms of HRT, women may choose patches, creams, or the vaginal ring.
- Teriparatide (Forteo) is a powerful drug, similar to parathyroid hormone, that stimulates new bone growth. It is used to treat osteoporosis in people who are at high risk of fractures. Teriparatide is given once a day by injection under the skin on the thigh or abdomen.
- Tamoxifen (Nolvadex) is used primarily by women with breast cancer or with a high risk of developing breast cancer; it has an estrogen-like effect on bone cells and apparently reduces the risk of fractures.

Other treatment focuses on relieving pain and preventing injury. Exercise programs are initiated to improve muscle strength and increase weight-bearing activity. Outdoor activity is encouraged so that the client enhances his or her ability to produce vitamin D. A physical therapy program is showing promise in reducing back pain, improving posture, and reducing fall risk in clients with osteoporosis and kyphosis. It uses a combination of a spinal weighted kypho-orthosis (WKO), which is a weighted harness, with specific back extension exercises (Tencer, 2005).

Nursing Management

In providing care for clients with osteoporosis, the nurse emphasizes the need for a nutritious, well-balanced diet that is high in calcium, vitamin D, and protein—all recommended to delay or prevent osteoporosis (Nutrition Notes

Nutrition Notes 63-3
The Client with Osteoporosis

- It is possible to fulfill vitamin D requirements by taking a daily 15-minute walk in the sun. However, significant rates of low vitamin D status are documented in studies of healthy adults and children in the United States and other countries. Winter, living in northern latitudes, black race, and older age are associated with low vitamin D synthesis. A dietary source is considered essential because few people meet optimal conditions.
- Vitamin D occurs naturally in a few food sources, namely, fatty fish, fish liver oils, and egg yolks. Foods fortified with vitamin D include milk and breakfast cereals and a few brands of orange juice, yogurt, margarine, and hot cereals.
- Diets rich in fruits and vegetables provide vitamin K, magnesium, and potassium, nutrients known to help maintain bone density.
- Diets high in salt, caffeine, and sugar are associated with bone loss and should be avoided.

63-3). The nurse especially advises women to drink three glasses of milk daily or eat other dairy products to acquire approximately 1000 to 1500 mg of calcium; those who smoke cigarettes may require more. Orange juice fortified with calcium is a nutritious alternative. If the client takes antacids, the nurse suggests those containing calcium. He or she recommends activity that promotes bone formation, such as regular, weight-bearing aerobic exercise (e.g., walking).

▶ Stop, Think, and Respond Exercise 63-3

A 45-year-old female client tells you that she has never liked milk and usually avoids dairy products because she thinks they are too fattening. What do you need to assess to ascertain if she is at risk for osteoporosis? What teaching does she need?

OSTEOMALACIA

Osteomalacia, a metabolic bone disease, is a softening of bones generally caused by Vitamin D deficiency.

Pathophysiology and Etiology

The defect in osteomalacia results from insufficient calcium absorption caused by insufficient calcium intake or resistance to the action of vitamin D. Alternatively, it may occur from phosphate deficiency related to increased renal losses or decreased intestinal absorption. Large amounts of new bone fail to calcify. The bone mass is structurally weaker and bone deformities occur. Additional risk factors are identified in Box 63-3.

Assessment Findings

Clients with osteomalacia experience bone pain and weakness. They also complain of tenderness if the bones are palpated. Bone deformities, such as kyphosis and bowing of the legs, occur as the disease advances. Clients exhibit a waddling type of gait, putting them at risk for falls and fractures.

Radiographic studies demonstrate demineralization of the bone. A bone scan detects increased and decreased areas of bone metabolism. Serum levels of calcium and phosphorus are low. Alkaline phosphatase levels typically are elevated.

B O X 6 3 - 3	Risk Factors for Osteomalacia

Dietary deficiencies
Malnutrition, particularly low calcium intake
Malabsorption
Gastrectomy
Chronic renal failure
Anticonvulsant therapy (phenytoin, phenobarbital)
Insufficient vitamin D (no supplements in food and lack of sunlight)
Poverty
Food fads
Lack of nutritional knowledge

Medical and Surgical Treatment

Treatment aims at correcting the underlying cause. This includes supplements of calcium, phosphorus, and vitamin D; adequate nutrition; exposure to sunlight; and progressive exercise and ambulation. Bone deformities may require braces or surgery for correction.

Nursing Management

The nurse is in a primary role of educating the client about the disease and its treatment and therefore includes teaching in the care plan. He or she teaches the client about methods and medications used to relieve pain and discomfort. The nurse allows the client to verbalize self-concept issues related to deformities and activity restrictions.

PAGET'S DISEASE

Paget's disease (osteitis deformans) is a chronic bone disorder characterized by abnormal bone remodeling. It affects adults older than 60 years of age. The most common areas of involvement are the long bones, spine, pelvis, and skull.

Pathophysiology and Etiology

In Paget's disease, some skeletal bones are unaffected; other bones are marked by a disturbance in the ratio between bone formation and reabsorption. The excessive osteoclastic activity causes the bones to become soft and bowed initially. Later, the bones thicken when compensatory osteoblastic activity resumes. The process of bone turnover continues, resulting in a classic mosaic pattern of bone matrix development. The new bone has high mineral content but is not well formed. This causes the bones to be weak and prone to fracture.

Although the cause of Paget's disease is unknown, the process by which clients with this disorder deposit collagen, a protein in connective tissue, is thought to be defective. This is based on the fact that the affected bones are high in mineral content but poorly constructed. A family history of the disorder is not uncommon. Additional findings indicate a possible link between the disease and a previous viral infection.

Complications include pathologic fractures, paralysis from spinal cord compression, cranial nerve damage, such as deafness from compression of the skull, and kidney stones. Occasionally, the lesions undergo malignant changes.

Assessment Findings

Some clients are asymptomatic, with only some mild skeletal deformity. Other clients have marked skeletal deformities, which may include enlargement of the skull, bowing of the long bones, and kyphosis. Bone pain and tenderness on pressure may be elicited. Paget's disease may go undiscovered until an x-ray for another problem reveals the disorder.

Radiographic examination discloses bones in various stages of resorption and remodeling with a mosaic appearance to the bone structure. Pathologic fractures appear and the bones are curved and enlarged. Bone scans usually are done. An elevated serum alkaline phosphatase level and increased urinary hydroxyproline (an amino acid found in collagen) excretion are common. Calcium levels usually are normal.

Medical and Surgical Management

Clients without symptoms usually do not need treatment. Those with symptoms may benefit from drug therapy. Analgesics such as aspirin or NSAIDs usually can control pain. Those with moderate to severe pain may benefit from treatment with calcitonin (Calcimar), a hormone that appears to block the resorption of bone by reducing the number of osteoclasts and decreasing the rate of bone turnover. Treatment with calcitonin usually results in a drop in the serum alkaline phosphatase level and urinary excretion of hydroxyproline, followed by regression of the lesions. Although not an analgesic, calcitonin reduces pain because it seems to promote the regression of lesions. The client still may require analgesics, however, until bone pain is relieved.

Pharmacologic Considerations

- Calcitonin is administered subcutaneously or as a nasal spray. Some adverse effects associated with this drug include nausea (with or without vomiting), inflammation at the injection site, increased urinary frequency, anorexia, diarrhea, and abdominal pain.

Bisphosphonates, such as etidronate disodium (Didronel), given orally or IV, or alendronate sodium (Fosamax) may be given to reduce the activity of Paget's disease and hopefully induce long-term remission of the disease. These drugs reduce normal and abnormal bone resorption and secondarily reduce bone formation that is coupled to bone resorption.

Surgery may be performed to repair pathologic fractures, replace damaged joints, realign deformed bones, or relieve neurologic complications.

Nursing Management

The nurse implements prescribed drug therapy and monitors for side effects. If self-care is limited, the nurse assists the client with ADLs. Client safety is a priority because strength and balance may be compromised. As appropriate, the nurse also teaches the client how to use ambulatory aids (e.g., a walker or cane), self-administer prescribed drugs, and implement measures to reduce falls within the home. For nursing management of a client who requires surgery, refer to Nursing Care Plan 62-1 in Chapter 62.

DISORDERS OF THE FEET

Many foot disorders are treated on an outpatient basis or encountered by nurses when caring for clients with other disorders. Foot disorders that commonly affect clients and for which surgery may be performed are bunions and hammer toes.

Hallux valgus, also called a *bunion*, is a deformity of the great (large) toe at its metatarsophalangeal joint (Fig. 63-9A).

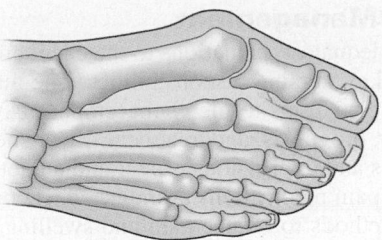

A Hallux valgus (bunion)

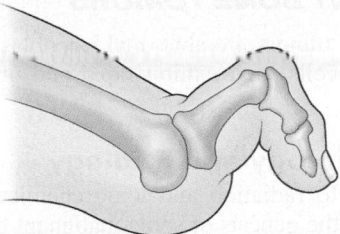

B Hammer toe

FIGURE 63-9. Common foot problems: (**A**) Hallux valgus or bunion; (**B**) hammer toe.

Hammer toe is a flexion deformity of the proximal interphalangeal (PIP) joint and may involve several toes (see Fig. 63-9B). **Mallet toe** is a flexion deformity of the distal interphalangeal joint (DIP) and also can affect several toes. Although the affected joints for hammer toe and mallet toe differ, the symptoms and treatment are basically the same.

Pathophysiology and Etiology

Bunions are associated with heredity, arthritis, or improperly fitting shoes. Women tend to be affected more than men. The first metatarsal bone enlarges on the medial side. The metatarsal bone protrudes at an acute angle toward the midline of the body while the great toe points laterally. There is an overgrowth of soft tissue (bursa), which actually is the bunion. The foot widens and the arch flattens. The malalignment results in pain from the stress on the joint, improper support and distribution of body weight, and inflammation of the bursa.

Like bunions, hammer toe and mallet toe also result from wearing poorly fitting shoes. Toes are pulled upward by the shoe, as the ball of the foot is pulled down. Corns (small, round, elevated overgrowths of epidermis) usually develop on top of the toes. Calluses (wide, thickened layer of skin) form under the metatarsal area.

Assessment Findings

The malalignment typical of bunions results in pain from the stress on the joint, improper support and distribution of body weight, and inflammation of the bursa. The client complains of pain on walking or flexing the foot, tenderness, and redness of the joint. The typical appearance of the foot deformity is obvious. In hammer toe and mallet toe, the foot deformity is also evident. Corns and calluses are easily seen. The client complains of discomfort with ambulation.

Radiographic films of the foot reveal the degree of joint deformity.

Medical and Surgical Management

No treatment is necessary for bunions if pain is not severe and the client has little or no difficulty. Low-heeled, properly fitted shoes are recommended. A bunionectomy, the surgical procedure to remove the bunion and correct the deformity, may be performed when the individual has pain and difficulty walking. Treatment of hammer toe and mallet toe includes exercises, wearing properly fitting or open-toed shoes, use of pads to protect the joints, and surgery to correct the malalignment. Surgeries for repair of foot disorders are performed on an outpatient or short-term admission basis, with the client discharged in the late afternoon or the following morning. Rest, elevation of the foot, and analgesics are prescribed.

Nursing Management

Nursing management of foot disorders includes relieving pain and discomfort, improving mobility, and instructing clients about the necessity for proper foot attire. Many clients are treated in an outpatient setting. Nurses in these settings usually are charged with teaching the client about the foot condition, treatment, medications, and postoperative care if the client had surgery (Client and Family Teaching 63-3).

Client and Family Teaching 63-3
Home Care After Foot Surgery

The nurse provides the following instructions for the outpatient client:

Pain Management—Methods to Reduce Pain

- Elevate foot
- Apply ice as instructed
- Take pain medications as prescribed
- Call physician for pain not relieved

Signs of Impaired Circulation to Report to Physician

- Change in sensation
- Inability to move toes
- Toes or foot cool to touch
- Toes or foot are pale or blue

Mobility

- Use assistive devices appropriately
- Adhere to weight-bearing restrictions
- Wear protective shoe over wound dressing

Wound Care

- Keep dressing or cast clean and dry
- Report signs of wound infection—pain, drainage, fever
- Take antibiotics as prescribed
- Change dressing as prescribed

(Adapted from Smeltzer, S. C., et al. [2008]. *Brunner and Suddarth's textbook of medical-surgical nursing* [11th ed.]. Philadelphia: Lippincott Williams & Wilkins.)

BONE TUMORS

Bone tumors may be benign or malignant. Benign tumors of the bone are more common than malignant bone tumors. Malignant tumors are primary, originating in the bone, or secondary, originating from elsewhere in the body (e.g., breast, lung, prostate, or kidney) and traveling to the bone (metastasis). Secondary or metastatic bone tumors are more common than primary bone tumors.

BENIGN BONE TUMORS

Benign bone tumors have the potential to cause fractures of bones. However, they are not life-threatening and usually cause few symptoms.

Pathophysiology and Etiology

Benign tumors usually are the result of misplaced or overgrown clusters of normal bone or cartilage cells that cause the structure to enlarge and impair local function. They grow slowly and do not metastasize. Their growth can weaken the bone structure by compressing or displacing the normal tissue. Types of bone tumors include (Smeltzer et al., 2008):

- *Osteochondroma*—occurs as a large projection of bone at the ends of long bones, developing during growth periods and then becoming a static bone mass
- *Enchondroma*—a hyaline cartilage tumor that develops in the hand, ribs, femur, tibia, humerus, or pelvis
- *Bone cysts*:
  - Aneurysmal bone cysts—painful, palpable mass found in long or flat bones and vertebrae
  - Unicameral bone cysts—may cause pathologic fractures in the humerus or femur
- *Osteoid osteoma*—painful tumor surrounded by reactive bone tissue
- *Osteoclastoma*—giant cell tumors that may invade local tissue; usually soft and hemorrhagic; may become malignant

Assessment Findings

Clients with benign bone tumors may experience pain or discomfort that worsens when bearing weight. The bone appears deformed and swelling may appear over the involved area. If the tumor is in a bone of the extremities, movement may be decreased and pathologic fractures may occur easily.

Radiography, bone scans, and biopsy of the tumor determine the diagnosis.

Medical and Surgical Management

Medical management includes treating pain and preventing fractures. Surgery is performed if the tumor does not stop growing, bone deformity is present or the pain is interfering with ADLs and mobility.

Curettage (scraping) or local excision is the usual procedure. Bone grafts may need to be done to promote bone growth and healing. Splints or casts are applied until the bone heals. Clients require close monitoring after surgery because benign bone tumors can recur.

Nursing Management

Providing adequate explanations to the client and alleviating anxiety are key nursing responsibilities. The nurse provides adequate explanations to the client, emphasizing the nature of the tumor, prognosis, and treatment. He or she allows time for questions and expressions of fear and anxiety. The nurse administers pain medications as indicated. He or she teaches the client methods to reduce pain and swelling and encourages the client to elevate the affected extremity.

MALIGNANT BONE TUMORS

Malignant bone tumors are abnormal osteoblasts or myeloblasts (marrow cells) that exhibit rapid and uncontrollable growth.

Pathophysiology and Etiology

Prior exposure to radiation and toxic chemicals has been associated with the genesis of some malignant bone tumors. A hereditary link in which a tumor suppressor gene may be absent or impaired also is suspected, because the same type of tumor may appear among siblings in the same family. Primary tumors include osteosarcoma, Ewing's sarcoma, chondrosarcoma, and fibrosarcoma.

Malignant bone tumors usually are located around the knee in the distal femur or proximal fibula; a few are found in the proximal humerus. As the tumor expands, it lifts the periosteum in much the same way as osteomyelitis. Metastasis occurs through the circulatory or lymphatic system. Metastasis to the lungs is common.

Assessment Findings

A pathologic fracture may be the event that leads the client to seek treatment. Clients with malignant tumors of the bone complain of persistent pain, swelling, and difficulty in moving the involved extremity. A limp or abnormal gait may be noted when the client walks. By the time the client experiences symptoms, however, the tumor usually has spread beyond its primary site.

The bone appears abnormal on radiographic examination, MRI, or bone scan. Biopsy identifies abnormal cells. A malignancy of the skeletal system is associated with an elevated serum alkaline phosphatase level.

Medical and Surgical Management

Treatment of primary malignant bone tumors may involve surgical removal of the tumor by amputating the extremity or by wide local resection. However, limb-sparing surgery is much more common today, because chemotherapy before surgery and advanced surgical techniques make this possible. Chemotherapy and radiation therapy after surgery aims to destroy tumor cells that escape from the original tumor site. Clients with osteosarcoma will most likely have a prosthesis or transplant of bone from another part of the body.

Nursing Management

Clients with malignant bone tumors require extensive emotional support and information about the disease, treatment, and prognosis. The nurse implements preoperative and postoperative measures for clients who are having surgery. For clients who must have an amputation, refer to the section on amputation in Chapter 61 for specific nursing care. As in other orthopedic surgeries, general nursing responsibilities include keeping the affected extremity elevated to reduce swelling, assessing neurovascular status frequently (see Chap. 60), and monitoring closely for complications if the affected limb is immobilized after surgery.

CRITICAL THINKING EXERCISES

1. A 50-year-old woman tells you that her mother has had two hip replacements secondary to degenerative joint disease. She is worried that her current hip pain will lead to the same problem. What suggestions would you make?
2. What differentiates osteomalacia from Paget's disease?
3. When teaching a client with SLE, what should a primary goal be?
4. A client is being evaluated for possible fibromyalgia. What factors make it difficult to establish a diagnosis?

NCLEX-STYLE REVIEW QUESTIONS

1. When planning care for the client with rheumatoid arthritis, when will the nurse expect that the client will need more time and assistance with activities of daily living?
   1. at noontime
   2. before bedtime
   3. in late afternoon
   4. in the early morning
2. The nurse instructs the client with osteoarthritis in his left hip that stress on painful joints can be minimized by which of the following measures?
   1. Applying a topical analgesic cream.
   2. Becoming more physically active.
   3. Maintaining a normal weight.
   4. Soaking in a tub of hot bath water.
3. A client diagnosed with osteomalacia has been told that his condition may improve with the addition of vitamin D. In addition to recommending the consumption of foods that are fortified with vitamin D, what is the most appropriate recommendation for the nurse to give the client?
   1. Consume bright orange vegetables.
   2. Eat meat from growth-stimulated cattle.
   3. Get more direct exposure to sunlight.
   4. Purchase organically grown produce.
4. Which statement made by the client with rheumatoid arthritis indicates that further instruction regarding corticosteroid therapy is necessary?
   1. "I am susceptible to getting infections."
   2. "I may become very depressed and perhaps suicidal."
   3. "I may develop low blood sugar and need glucose"
   4. "I should never stop taking my medication abruptly."
5. The client with osteoarthritis in his left hip uses a cane when ambulating. When the nurse observes him walk, which assessment finding indicates that he needs more instruction regarding the use of his cane?
   1. The client holds his head up and looks straight ahead.
   2. The client uses the cane on his painful side.
   3. The client wears athletic shoes with nonskid soles.
   4. The tip of the cane is covered with a rubber cap.

UNIT 16
Caring for Clients with Integumentary Disorders

64

Introduction to the Integumentary System

Words To Know

apocrine glands
debridement
dermis
eccrine glands
epidermis
hyphae
integument
keratin
melanin
pheromones
pressure sores
sebaceous glands
sebum
shearing
skin tear
stratum corneum
subcutaneous tissue
sweat glands
Wood's light

Learning Objectives

On completion of this chapter, you will be able to:

1. Name the structures that form the integument.
2. List four functions of the integumentary system.
3. Identify the purpose of sebum and melanin.
4. Differentiate between eccrine and apocrine glands.
5. Name at least three facts about the integument that are pertinent to document when obtaining a health history.
6. Give the characteristics of normal skin.
7. Describe the criteria for staging pressure sores.
8. List characteristics of hair assessed during a physical examination.
9. Describe the characteristics of normal nails.
10. Name four diagnostic tests performed to determine the etiology of skin disorders.
11. Describe seven medical and surgical techniques for treating skin disorders.

The **integument** includes structures that cover the body's exterior surface. The primary structure is the skin, which contains sebaceous and sweat glands and sensory nerve endings (Fig. 64-1). The integument also includes accessory structures such as the hair and nails. The structures that make up the integument protect the body from environmental injuries, help regulate body temperature, serve as sensory organs, and facilitate the synthesis of vitamin D.

ANATOMY AND PHYSIOLOGY

Skin

The skin is composed of two layers: the **epidermis**, the outermost layer, and the **dermis**, which lies below the epidermis. The epidermis contains an outer layer of dead skin cells, the **stratum corneum**, that forms a tough protective protein called **keratin**. The epidermis is constantly shed and replaced with epithelial cells from the dermis every day. The epidermis is totally replaced approximately every 35 to 45 days; the average person sheds 40 pounds of dead skin cells in his or her lifetime (Marieb, Mallatt, & Wilhelm, 2007).

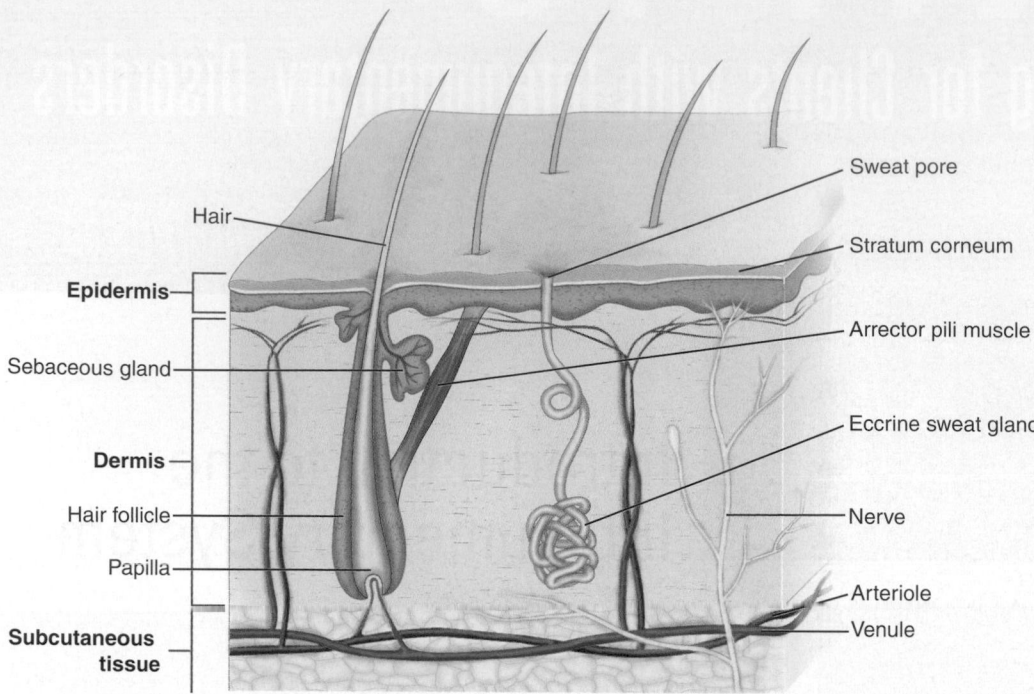

FIGURE 64-1. A cross-section of the skin.

The dermis, or true skin, consists of connective tissue and contains elastic fibers, blood vessels, sensory and motor nerves, sweat and sebaceous (oil) glands, and hair follicles (roots). The superficial dermal layer on the ventral surface of the hands and feet contains ridges and indentations that create a unique pattern of fingerprints, palm prints, and footprints. In addition to providing a means of identification, the dermal ridges facilitate the ability to grip and hold objects.

The **subcutaneous tissue,** the layer of skin attached to muscle and bone, is composed primarily of connective tissue and fat cells. Skin has a tremendous capacity to stretch with little subsequent damage, as is evident during pregnancy and after soft-tissue injury.

The color of the skin is determined by a pigment called **melanin,** which is manufactured by melanocytes located in the epidermis. The production of melanin is under the control of the middle lobe (pars intermedia) of the pituitary gland, which secretes melanocyte-stimulating hormone. The more melanin found in the epidermis, the darker the skin color. Exposure to ultraviolet light temporarily stimulates the production of melanin to absorb harmful radiation.

The skin has four major functions: protection, temperature regulation, sensory processing, and chemical synthesis.

Protection

The skin forms a protective barrier between the outside world and underlying organs and structures of the body. This barrier prevents microorganisms and other foreign substances from reaching the structures below the epidermis. It also prevents structures below the surface of the skin from losing water.

Areas of the skin subjected to friction, such as where a pencil is held repeatedly, have accelerated rates of epidermal cell production. A *callus,* which is a thick layer of epidermal cells, forms in response to recurring friction on an area of skin. Intense friction causes a blister to develop.

Temperature Regulation

To maintain a relatively consistent body temperature, the skin heats or cools the structures below. The body continuously produces internal heat during cellular metabolism. Erector muscles around shafts of hair contract to generate heat and prevent heat loss at the body's surface. Elevation of skin hairs interferes with local air circulation and maintains the warmth of the skin.

Heat dissipates through the skin and through respiration. Heat is lost by four methods (Fig. 64-2):

- *Radiation* is the transfer of surface heat in the environment. An example of radiant heat loss is the escape of heat from the surface of warm skin into cooler air.
- *Conduction* is the transfer of heat through contact. An example of conductive heat loss is placing a cool cloth on warm skin.
- *Evaporation* is the loss of moisture or water. Water on the surface of the body is warmed. As the moisture vaporizes, the body is cooled. Evaporation occurs unnoticed (insensible loss) and when there is obvious perspiration.
- *Convection* is the transfer of heat by means of currents of liquids or gases in which warm air molecules move away from the body. An example of convection is a cool breeze that blows across the body surface.

When the temperature and humidity outside the body rise, radiation, evaporation, and convection are ineffective. The alternative method by which heat is transferred under these conditions is by conduction. This is why exposure to warm temperatures and densely saturated moist air can raise the body temperature and result in heat stroke.

Sensory Processing

The skin combined with body hair serves as a means of monitoring the outside environment, as well as warning of

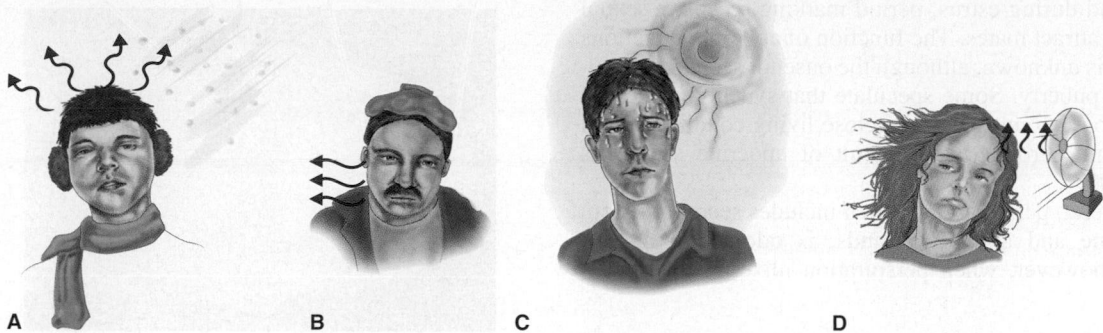

FIGURE 64-2. Methods of heat loss. (**A**) radiation, (**B**) conduction, (**C**) evaporation, and (**D**) convection.

danger. Specialized nerve endings in the skin respond to pressure, pain, heat, and cold.

Chemical Synthesis

The skin forms a chemical substance called 7-dehydrocholesterol, which facilitates the synthesis of vitamin D when the skin is exposed to ultraviolet light (sunlight). Vitamin D is necessary for the formation of healthy bones and teeth. Dark-skinned people do not synthesize vitamin D as readily as light-skinned people. Cloudy environments and air pollutants that block sunlight also interfere with vitamin D synthesis. Therefore, vitamin D is added to some food sources, such as milk.

Gerontologic Considerations

- Multiple changes of aging contribute to loss of skin elasticity, resulting in wrinkle formation on various body areas. Other changes include an increase in skin dryness and a decline in the function of skin as a barrier and first line of defense. Wound healing is slowed due to decreased immunologic responsiveness, and loss of subcutaneous fat impacts thermoregulation. The aging process may also impact vitamin D production and alter the absorption of some topical drugs. Age-related changes result in reduced sensation of light touch, with an increase in cutaneous pain threshold.

▶ **Stop, Think, and Respond Exercise 64-1**

Discuss the importance of keeping the skin intact.

Hair

Hair originates in the hair follicles in the dermis. It covers all parts of the body except the palms, soles, dorsum of the fingers, lips, penis, labia, and nipples. There are two types of hair: (1) *vellus* hair, which has a wooly or wispy texture, and (2) *terminal* hair, a coarser variety that develops at puberty under the influence of androgen hormones, in the axillae, pubic region, face of men, arms, chest, and legs. Men of some ethnic groups (e.g., Native Americans and Asians) have less facial and body hair than their Anglo-American counterparts.

Hundreds of strands of keratin link together with amino acids to form hair. Scalp hair grows more rapidly than hair in other locations. At midlife, hair growth slows, and hair texture is lost. After menopause, some women develop sparse terminal hairs about their face as the ratio of estrogen to androgen hormones decreases.

Melanin, produced by melanocytes in the hair root, influences hair color. The three types of melanin are brown, black, and yellow. Types of melanin are genetically inherited, as are hair texture, shape, and rate of growth. Melanin production decreases with age, causing the hair to become gray or white. Illness, hormone levels, nutrition, aging, and other factors can affect hair growth, texture, and loss (see Chapter 65 for a discussion of baldness).

Sebaceous and Sweat Glands

Sebaceous glands are connected to each hair follicle and secrete an oily substance called **sebum**, which is a lubricant that prevents drying and cracking of the skin and hair. As sebum fills the glandular duct, it enters the hair follicle, from which it eventually is released. During puberty, sebaceous glands in the forehead, nose, chest, and back become more active. Excess sebum may plug the gland. The plugged gland at first appears white, but it later blackens as the sebum oxidizes. Bacterial growth that breaks down the sebum into irritating fatty acids converts the "blackhead" to a pustule and localized area of inflammation that is characteristic of acne (see Chap. 65).

The two types of **sweat glands** are eccrine and apocrine. **Eccrine glands** release water and electrolytes, such as sodium and chloride, in the form of perspiration. The rate of perspiration is related to body temperature. Adults can produce as much as 3 L under extremely hot conditions. The pH of perspiration is slightly acidic, which helps provide a hostile environment for microbial colonization. Frequent washing with alkaline soaps removes sebum and reduces the acid mantle of protection.

Apocrine glands are found around the nipples, in the anogenital region, in the eyelids (Moll's glands), in the mammary glands of the breast, and in the external ear canals—where the secretion is referred to as *cerumen*. In some animal species, the apocrine glands release **pheromones**, hormone-like chemicals that communicate reproductive and social information among the species. For example, dogs release pheromones during urination to mark their territory and during estrus, period marking receptive sexual activity, to attract mates. The function of apocrine secretions in humans is unknown, although the onset of secretions coincides with puberty. Some speculate that synchronization of menstruation among women in close living conditions such as a dormitory room is the result of apocrine secretions (Bhutta, 2007).

In general, perspiration, which includes secretions from both eccrine and apocrine glands, is odorless. An odor develops, however, when perspiration mixes with bacteria on the skin.

Gerontologic Consideration

- In older adults, reduced sebum production leads to skin dryness and roughness.

- A decline in the number of eccrine glands, along with decreased cutaneous vascularity, causes a decrease in spontaneous sweating with age; this makes older persons more vulnerable to heat.

Nails

Fingernails and toenails are layers of hard keratin that have a protective function. In primates and humans, the nails may be a biologic diversification of claws. Animal species that have claws use them to catch and tear prey, whereas primates and humans developed nails on their fingers and toes because they had a greater biologic need for grasping and manipulating primitive tools or utensils.

The nail root lies buried beneath the nail's exposed surface in a fold of skin (Fig. 64-3). The nails have an abundant capillary blood supply, resulting in their pink semitransparent appearance that facilitates circulatory assessment. The exception to the pink appearance is the actively growing base, where the nail is so thick that the pink color is obscured by the white moon-shaped area known as the *lunula*.

ASSESSMENT

History

Initial assessment of the client begins with a thorough history. The history is based on symptoms. The nurse includes the following questions:

- When did the disorder first begin and where did it first appear?
- Where are the lesions located?
- Have there been any changes in the disorder since it first appeared (an increase or decrease in symptoms; in appearance or color; in location)?
- Has the problem spread?
- What are the physical sensations pertaining to the disorder (pain, itching, burning, and intensity)?
- Do other physical or emotional problems appear to be associated with the disorder?
- Was a specific event associated with the onset of the disorder?

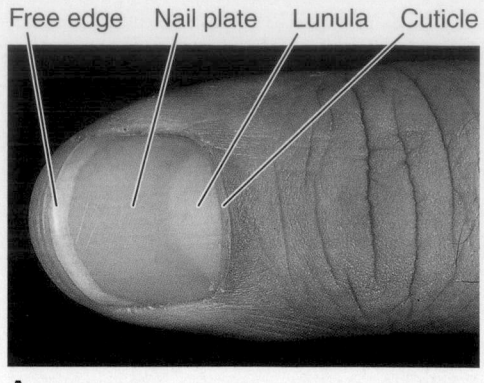

A

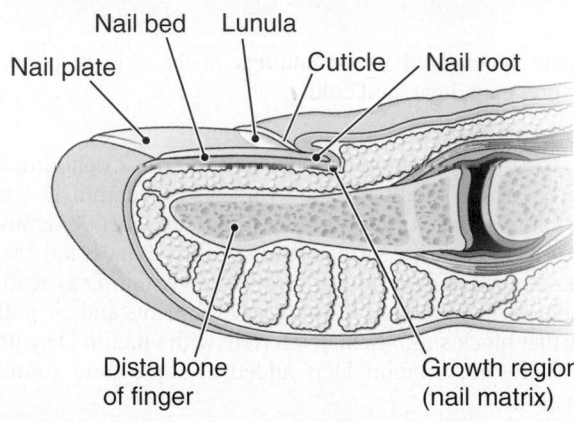

B

FIGURE 64-3. External (**A**) and cross-sectional (**B**) views of a nail.

- What factors appear to make the condition better or worse?
- Do you or anyone in your family have known or suspected allergies?
- What prescription and nonprescription medications have you taken recently?
- Have you made changes in personal products, such as soaps, deodorants, and cosmetics?
- Have there been recent changes in your work or living environment, such as pets, plants, sprays, dust, and pollutants, that might have precipitated this problem?

Physical Examination

During a physical examination, the nurse inspects and palpates the structures of the integument.

Skin Assessment

The nurse examines the skin on all areas of the body. He or she can do so during the head-to-toe assessment or as a focused assessment. Good lighting is essential. The skin should be smooth, unbroken, of uniform color according to the person's ethnic or racial origin, warm, and resilient. It should feel neither wet nor unusually dry.

Color deviations have several possible causes (Table 64-1). While examining the skin, the nurse may detect changes in its structure or integrity such as those listed in Table 64-2. The nurse documents the sites of any abnormalities.

TABLE 64-1 Common Skin Color Variations

COLOR	TERM	POSSIBLE CAUSES
Pale, regardless of race	Pallor	Anemia, blood loss
Red	Erythema	Superficial burns, local inflammation, carbon monoxide poisoning
Pink	Flushed	Fever, hypertension
Purple	Ecchymosis	Trauma to soft tissue
Blue	Cyanosis	Low tissue oxygenation
Yellow	Jaundice	Liver or kidney disease, destruction of red blood cells
Brown	Tan	Racial variation, sun exposure, pregnancy, Addison's disease

Pharmacologic Considerations

- Suspect a drug allergy whenever the client has a skin rash.

Gerontologic Considerations

- Older persons who have had increased sun exposure may develop skin lesions and should be taught careful self-examination. Small, brown, pigmented, benign lesions, known as *liver spots* or *senile lentigines,* form on the hands and forearms of older people. Small, yellow or brown raised lesions, called *senile keratoses,* may appear on the face and trunk. Senile keratoses are precancerous and require close observation for any change in size, color, or form. These lesions may be removed by freezing, chemical peel, cauterization, or topical creams.

The nurse assesses temperature by placing the dorsum of the hand on the surface of the skin. He or she can detect moisture with the palmar surface. The nurse determines the quality of skin turgor by grasping the skin, such as that over the sternum, between the thumb and forefinger. Normally, the skin returns to its original position immediately after being released. Tight, shiny skin suggests fluid retention; loose, dry skin may indicate dehydration. Poor nutrition can lead to changes in skin integrity and turgor.

Pressure Sore Staging

Pressure sores, also known as *decubitus ulcers,* occur when capillary blood flow to an area is reduced. This may happen when the skin over a bony prominence is compressed between the weight of the body and a supporting surface for a prolonged period. Common locations include the skin over the coccyx and sacrum in the lower spine, the hips, heels, elbows, shoulder blades, ears, and back of head (Fig. 64-4).

Prevention of pressure sores first involves identifying persons who are at greatest risk (Box 64-1). Once the nurse has identified at-risk clients, he or she implements measures that reduce conditions under which pressure sores are likely to form. Some examples are as follows:

- Turning and repositioning the client frequently
- Keeping client's skin clean and dry
- Massaging bony prominences if the client's skin blanches with pressure relief
- Using a moisturizing skin cleanser rather than soap
- Applying pressure-relieving devices to the bed and chairs
- Padding body areas that are subject to pressure and friction
- Avoiding **shearing**, a physical force that separates layers of tissue in opposite directions, such as when a seated client slides downward

Pressure sores are categorized into one of four stages (Fig. 64-5) depending on the extent of tissue injury.

Stage I
Stage I pressure sores are characterized by redness of the skin. The reddened skin of a beginning pressure sore fails to resume its normal color, or blanch, when pressure is relieved.

Stage II
A stage II pressure sore is red and is accompanied by blistering or a shallow break in the skin, sometimes described as a **skin tear**. Impairment of the skin leads to microbial colonization and infection of the wound.

Stage III
Pressure sores classified as stage III are those in which the superficial skin impairment progresses to a shallow crater that extends to the subcutaneous tissue. Stage III pressure sores may be accompanied by serous drainage from leaking plasma or purulent drainage (white or yellow-tinged fluid) caused by a wound infection. Although a stage III pressure sore is a significant wound, the area is relatively painless.

Stage IV
Stage IV pressure sores are the most traumatic and life-threatening. The tissue is deeply ulcerated, exposing muscle and bone. The dead tissue produces a rank odor. Local infection, which is the rule rather than the exception, easily spreads throughout the body, causing a potentially fatal condition referred to as *sepsis.*

Nutrition Notes 64-1 outlines nutritional considerations for pressure sore healing.

Scalp and Hair Assessment
The nurse assesses the scalp by separating the hair at random areas and inspecting the skin. The scalp normally is smooth, intact, and free of lesions.

Hair assessment applies not only to the head, but to other locations such as the eyebrows, eyelashes, chest, arms,

TABLE 64-2 Terms for Various Skin Lesions

TYPE OF LESION	DESCRIPTION	EXAMPLES	DEPICTION
Macule	Flat, round, colored	Freckles, rash	 Macule
Papule	Elevated, obvious raised border, solid	Wart	 Papule
Vesicle	Elevated, round, filled with serum	Blister	 Vesicle
Wheal	Elevated, irregular border, no free fluid	Hives	 Wheal
Pustule	Elevated, raised border, filled with pus	Boil	 Pustule
Nodule	Elevated solid mass, extends into deeper tissue	Enlarged lymph node	 Nodule
Cyst	Encapsulated, round, fluid-filled or solid mass beneath the skin	Tissue growth	 Cyst

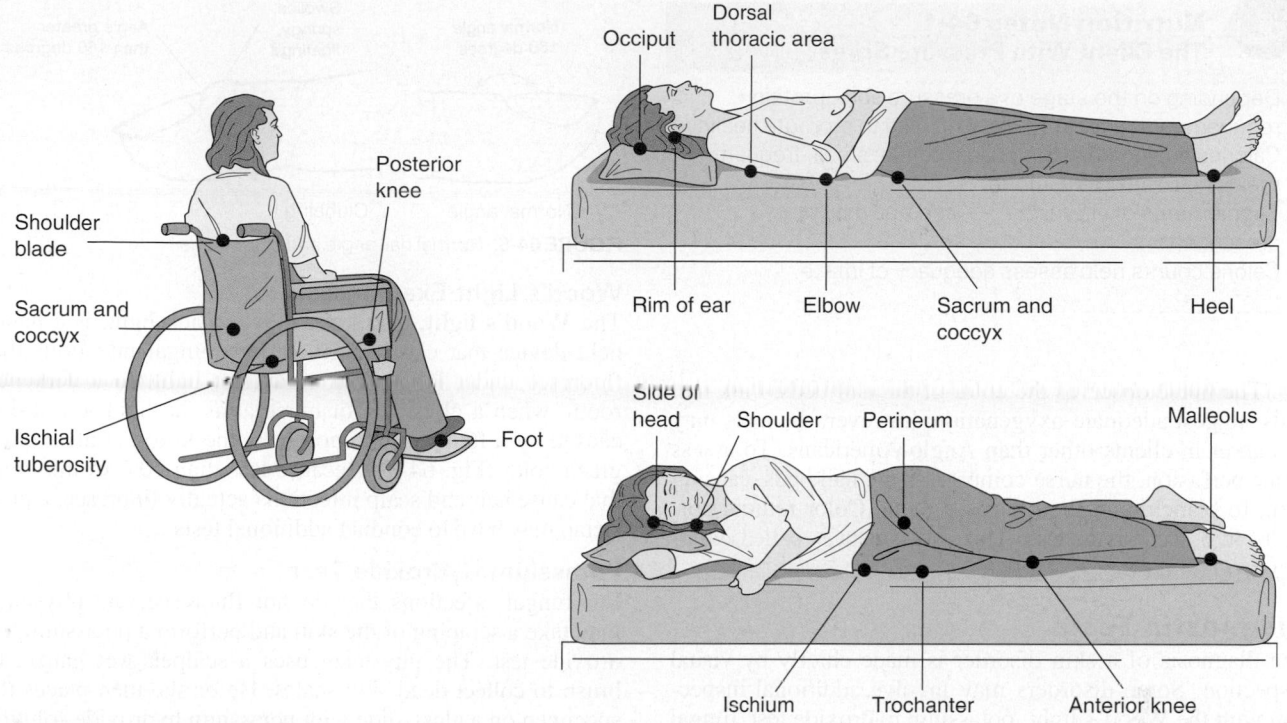

FIGURE 64-4. Common locations for pressure sores in supine, lateral, and sitting positions.

▶ *Stop, Think, and Respond Exercise 64-2*

What type of skin lesion does a client have if it is described as follows:

1. Elevated, round, and filled with serum?
2. Flat, round, and red?
3. Elevated, solid, with a raised border?
4. Elevated, round, raised border, filled with pus?

pubis, and legs. The nurse notes the color, texture, and distribution, keeping sex- and age-related variations in mind. Hair may become brittle and thin as a result of poor nutrition. The presence of nits and eggs from a louse infestation (see Chap. 65), as well as scales and flaking skin, are also abnormal findings.

Nail Assessment

Normal nails appear slightly convex with a 160° angle between the nail base and the skin. Concave-shaped nails,

referred to as *spooning* because of their characteristic appearance, are a sign of iron-deficiency anemia. Clubbing of the nails, evidenced by an angle greater than 160 degrees, suggests long-standing cardiopulmonary disease (Fig. 64-6). Although the thickness of the nail varies from 0.3 to 0.65 mm (van de Kerkhof et al., 2005), nails thicken when there is a fungal infection and poor circulation. There may be evidence of other nail abnormalities (Fig. 64-7).

| BOX 64-1 | Risk Factors for Developing Pressure Sores |

- Dehydration
- Diaphoresis
- Emaciation
- Immobility
- Inactivity
- Incontinence
- Localized edema
- Malnutrition
- Sedation
- Vascular disease

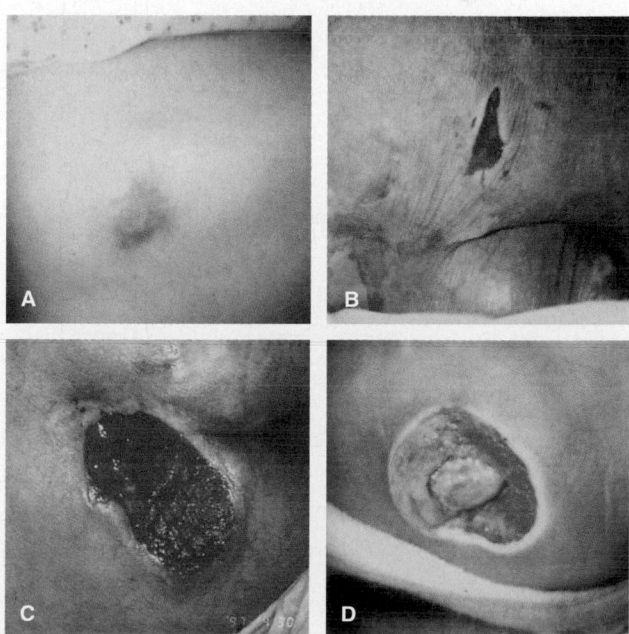

FIGURE 64-5. Pressure sore stages: (**A**) stage I, (**B**) stage II, (**C**) stage III, and (**D**) stage IV.

Nutrition Notes 64-1
The Client With Pressure Sores

● Depending on the stage of a pressure sore, protein requirements range from 1 to 1.6 g/kg to promote healing.
● Calories are increased to spare protein; small, frequent meals help maximize intake.
● Supplements of vitamins A, C, and zinc may be prescribed.
● Calorie counts help assess adequacy of intake.

FIGURE 64-6. Normal nail angle and clubbed nail.

The nurse observes the color of the nail beds. Pink nail beds suggest adequate oxygenation; however, the nails may be darker in clients other than Anglo-Americans. To assess tissue perfusion, the nurse compresses the nail beds, causing them to blanch, and then releases them. Color returns normally in 3 seconds or less. This assessment is called *capillary refill time.*

Diagnostic Tests

The diagnosis of a skin disorder is made chiefly by visual inspection. Some disorders may involve additional inspection with the Wood's light, potassium hydroxide test, fungal culture, and skin biopsy. Culture and sensitivity tests are performed on lesions that are suspected or known to contain bacteria. Allergy tests by intradermal injection, the scratch test, and the patch test are used to confirm an allergy to one or more substances (see Chapter 34).

Wood's Light Examination

The **Wood's light**, also known as a black light, is a handheld device that can identify certain fungal infections that fluoresce under long-wave ultraviolet light. In a darkened room, when a physician or nurse aims the light at a lesion caused by a fungus that fluoresces, the lesion emits a blue-green color (Fig. 64-8). Because less than 10% of the fungi that cause hair and scalp infections actually fluoresce, a physician may have to conduct additional tests.

Potassium Hydroxide Test

For fungal infections that do not fluoresce, the physician may take a scraping of the skin and perform a potassium hydroxide test. The physician uses a scalpel, wet gauze, or brush to collect dead skin scales. He or she then places the specimen on a glass slide with potassium hydroxide solution and applies heat. The heated solution dissolves the skin and hair cells but does not affect any fungal cells. The physician microscopically examines the slide to check for any **hyphae** (threadlike filaments within the cells of most fungi). This test confirms that a fungal infection has caused the lesion, but

Onychorrhexis
• Brittle, fragile, uneven nail edge
• Associated with malnutrition, overhydration, thyrotoxicosis, chemical damage, radiation, aging

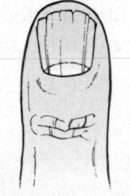
Onychorrhexis

Splinter Hemorrhages
• Blood streaks
• Associated with heart disease, hypertension, rheumatoid arthritis, neoplasms, trauma

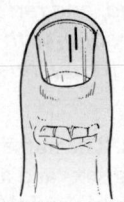
Splinter hemorrhage

Onychauxis
• Nail hypertrophy
• Associated with trauma, aging, fungal infections

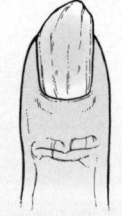
Onychauxis

Subungual Hematoma
• Blood clot
• Associated with trauma

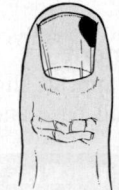
Subungual hematoma

Beau's Lines
• Tranverse furrows in nail plate
• Associated with malnutrition, severe illness

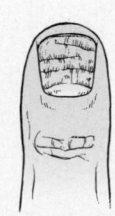
Beau's lines

FIGURE 64-7. Nail abnormalities.

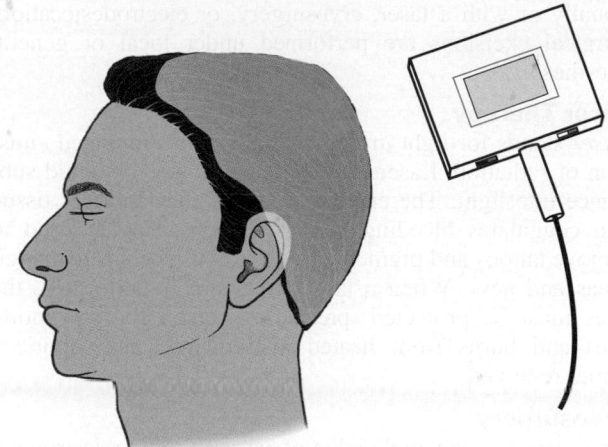

FIGURE 64-8. Fungal organisms glow under Wood's light illumination.

the physician may need a culture to identify the specific species of fungus.

Fungal Culture

The procedure for obtaining a specimen for fungal culture is similar to that for a potassium hydroxide test. The physician places the scraped cells into a sterile container and sends it to the laboratory, where an analyst spreads the cells on the surface of a nutritive medium such as agar. The specimen requires incubation at room temperature for 2 to 3 weeks. Once a sufficient colony exists, the analyst examines it microscopically to identify the type of fungus causing the infection.

Skin Biopsy

A physician obtains a biopsy of skin tissue to identify malignant, premalignant, and nonmalignant skin lesions as well as chronic skin disorders such as Hansen's disease (leprosy). After injecting a local anesthetic, the physician obtains skin cells for the biopsy in one of three ways: (1) scraping the lesion parallel with the skin with a scalpel or razor blade, (2) excising the lesion partially or entirely with scissors or a scalpel, or (3) using the punching instrument to remove a cylindrical core of tissue (Fig. 64-9). The physician preserves the specimen in formaldehyde, and the pathologist examines it microscopically to identify any abnormal cells. Depending on the type of biopsy, the client may require some sutures to close the skin and control bleeding.

MEDICAL AND SURGICAL TREATMENT OF SKIN DISORDERS

Various types of therapies are used in the treatment or management of skin disorders. They include drug therapy, wet dressings, therapeutic baths, surgical excision, radiation therapy, photochemotherapy, hyperbaric oxygenation, and lifestyle changes.

Drug Therapy

Topical and systemic medications are used to treat skin disorders. Some examples are as follows:

- Corticosteroids are applied topically or administered systemically (orally, intramuscularly, intravenously) to relieve inflammatory and allergic symptoms. When used systemically, corticosteroids can have serious side effects; therefore, they are used primarily to relieve acute problems. Continued long-term use brings greater risk and is justified only when the disease itself is serious and other treatments cannot relieve it. Used as directed, topical application of a corticosteroid does not result in the pronounced adverse effects seen with systemic administration, and can be used for longer periods.
- Antihistamines frequently are prescribed when allergy is a factor in causing the skin disorder. They relieve itching and shorten the duration of the allergic reaction.
- Antibiotic, antifungal, and antiviral agents are used to treat infectious disorders. They are applied topically or administered systemically.
- Scabicides and pediculicides are used in the treatment of infestations with the scabies mite and lice (see Chap. 65).
- Local (topical) anesthetics are applied to relieve minor skin pain and itching.
- Emollients, ointments, powders, and lotions, which may be combined with other agents, soothe, protect, and soften the skin.
- Antiseborrheic agents are applied directly to the scalp or incorporated into shampooing products. They are used to control dandruff (see Chap. 65).
- Antiseptics are used to reduce bacteria on the skin.
- Keratolytics dissolve thickened, cornified skin such as warts, corns, and calluses. Their action causes the treated area to soften and swell, facilitating removal.

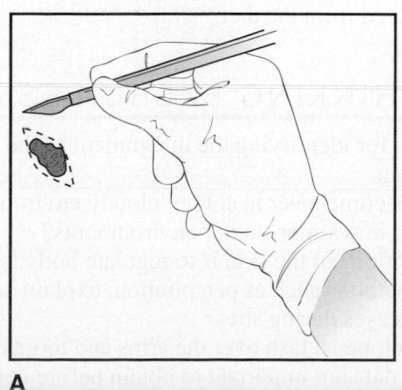

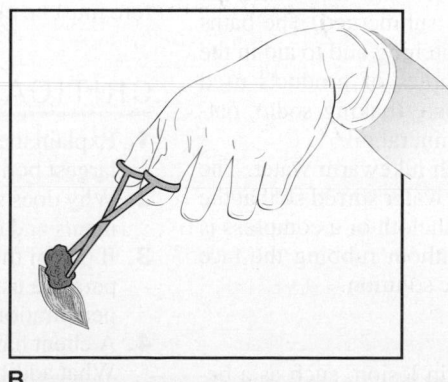

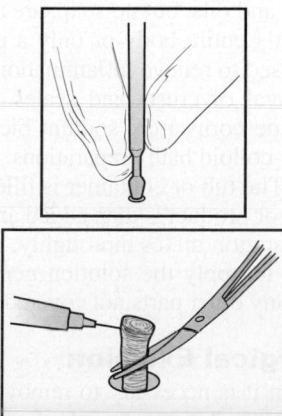

A   B   C

FIGURE 64-9. Three techniques for obtaining a skin biopsy: (**A**) scrape, (**B**) surgical excision, and (**C**) punch.

Nurses use Standard Precautions when applying any topical medication to impaired skin or changing dressings that cover an open lesion. Infected, draining, or weeping lesions may require contact precautions as well (see Chap. 12). It is important to apply topical medication as prescribed, such as a thin layer evenly spread over the area, or a thick layer dabbed on the area. The nurse takes care in applying medication so that lesions are not broken or skin surfaces abraded.

 Pharmacologic Considerations

- Instruct clients taking antibiotic, antiviral, or antifungal agents to complete the entire prescription, even if the condition resolves before he or she finishes all the medication.

- As with any medication, drug interactions may occur. If the client is taking medication for another disorder, list all medications the client takes to rule out potential drug interactions.

Wet Dressings

Wet dressings are used to apply a solution to a skin lesion. They have a cooling and soothing effect. The nature of the skin lesion (open or intact) determines whether sterile technique is required. A dry dressing consisting of gauze or other porous material is first applied to the area. Cotton is not used because of its tendency to stick to wound surfaces. The dressing is then saturated with the prescribed liquid. Dressings can be temporarily anchored with nonallergenic tape or roller gauze.

Some wet dressings are left in place until dry as a method of **debridement**, a technique for removing damaged tissue from a wound. When the dried gauze is removed, it usually contains bits of trapped debris in the gauze mesh. Removing dead and dying tissue provides an environment that fosters and promotes regeneration of healthy tissue and closure of the wound.

Therapeutic Baths

A therapeutic bath is one in which various solutions, powders, and oils, but no soap, are added to water into which the client's entire body or only a part is submerged. The baths are used to relieve inflammation and itching and to aid in the removal of crusts and scales. Examples of products used include cornstarch, sodium bicarbonate (baking soda), oatmeal-colloid bath preparations, and mineral oil.

The tub or container is filled with lukewarm water. The drug or product is then added and the water stirred so that the preparation mixes thoroughly. A washcloth or a compress is used to apply the solution gently without rubbing the face and any other parts not covered by the solution.

Surgical Excision

When it is necessary to remove a skin lesion, such as a benign or malignant growth, the tissue may be excised conven-tionally or with a laser, cryosurgery, or electrodesiccation. Surgical excisions are performed under local or general anesthesia.

Laser Therapy

Laser stands for *l*ight *a*mplification by the *s*timulated *e*mission of *r*adiation. Lasers convert a solid, gas, or liquid substance into light. The energy of laser light vaporizes tissue and coagulates bleeding vessels. Lasers also are used to remove tattoos and pigmented skin lesions such as hemangiomas and nevi. When a laser procedure is performed, the eyes must be protected, precautions taken for preventing fires and burns from heated instruments, and vaporized fumes removed.

Cryosurgery

Cryosurgery is the application of extreme cold to destroy tissue. Liquid nitrogen circulates through a probe that is touched to the skin or inserted to the center of the lesion. After application of extreme cold, the area thaws and becomes gelatin-like in appearance. A scab forms at the site. Healing takes approximately 4 to 6 weeks.

Electrodesiccation

Electrodesiccation (or electrosurgery) is the use of electrical energy converted to heat, which destroys the tissue. Plantar warts and skin tumors are examples of disorders treated by this method.

Radiation Therapy

Radiation therapy is used to treat malignant skin lesions. For more information on radiation therapy, see Chapter 18.

Photochemotherapy

Photochemotherapy involves a combination of psoralen methoxsalen and type A ultraviolet light. It is one method used to treat psoriasis, a chronic skin condition (see Chapter 65). The psoralen methoxsalen is taken 1 to 2 hours before exposure to ultraviolet A.

Lifestyle Changes

Some skin disorders such as psoriasis (see Chapter 65) and herpes simplex infections (see Chapter 56) grow worse when the person is tired or under emotional stress. Therefore, rest and sleep are an important part of treatment. Diet also is an important part of treatment because certain foods contribute to or aggravate skin disorders in some individuals and therefore must be eliminated from the diet.

CRITICAL THINKING EXERCISES

1. Explain the basis for identifying the integument as the largest body organ.
2. Why does skin become paler in colder, cloudy environments and darker in warmer, sunny environments?
3. If one of the functions of the skin is to regulate body temperature using methods such as perspiration, explain why perspiration increases during stress.
4. A client has developed a rash over the arms and thorax. What additional data are important to obtain before contacting the physician?

NCLEX-STYLE REVIEW QUESTIONS

1. The nurse examines a client who slipped and fell while climbing stairs and now has swelling of one ankle and pain on movement. If the nurse documents that the client's ankle shows signs of ecchymosis, this indicates that the skin is which of the following?
   1. freckled
   2. mottled
   3. bruised
   4. blanched

2. Which of the following are factors that cause wrinkles among older adults? Select all that apply.
   1. Loss of skin elasticity
   2. Decrease in melanin
   3. Loss of subcutaneous tissue
   4. Deficiency of vitamin D
   5. Altered production of sebum

3. During a routine assessment, the nurse notes that a client's fingernails have a clubbed appearance. What does this finding indicate?
   1. The client's fingernails are normal.
   2. The client may have chronic cardiopulmonary disease.
   3. The client may have a fungal infection in the nail beds.
   4. The client may have iron-deficiency anemia.

4. Which of the following assessment techniques helps the nurse determine the quality of the client's skin turgor?
   1. Feeling the skin with the palmar surface of the hand.
   2. Grasping a fold of skin over the sternum.
   3. Placing the dorsum of the hand on the skin.
   4. Depressing the skin over a bony prominence.

5. During a physical assessment, the nurse notes that the skin over bony prominences of the coccyx and shoulders is becoming red. Which measure for preventing impaired skin integrity is appropriate to add to the plan of care at this time?
   1. Using a bed board for support
   2. Changing position every 2 hours
   3. Rubbing reddened areas every 2 hours
   4. Adding alcohol to the bath water

6. An elderly bedridden client frequently slides to the bottom of the bed with the feet touching the footboard. The nurses reposition the client on a regular basis. Which of the following is the most likely outcome of the client's downward movement in bed?
   1. The client is at risk for a traumatic fracture if a fall occurs.
   2. The client is at risk for hypothermia because of skin exposure.
   3. The client is at risk for bruising because of contact with the footboard.
   4. The client is at risk for skin impairment because of shearing forces.

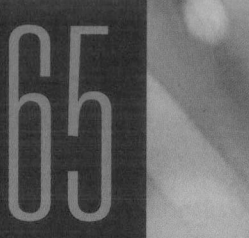

65 Caring for Clients with Skin, Hair, and Nail Disorders

Words To Know

acne vulgaris
alopecia
body piercing
carbuncle
comedone
dermabrasion
dermatitis
dermatome
dermatophytes
dermatophytoses
erythema
furuncle
furunculosis
granuloma
herpes zoster
nits
onychocryptosis
onychomycosis
pediculosis
photochemotherapy
podiatrist
pruritus
psoriasis
rhinophyma
rosacea
scabies
shingles
tattoo

Learning Objectives

On completion of this chapter, you will be able to:

1. Identify risks associated with tattooing and body piercing.
2. Describe general care following tattooing and body piercing.
3. Define and name two types of dermatitis.
4. Explain factors that lead to acne vulgaris.
5. Describe characteristics of rosacea.
6. Differentiate between a furuncle, furunculosis, and carbuncle.
7. Describe the appearance and cause of psoriasis.
8. Describe the process for eradicating a skin mite infection using a scabicidal medication.
9. Identify locations on the body where parasitic fungi known as dermatophytes are most likely to infect.
10. Describe the characteristics of an outbreak of shingles.
11. Discuss factors that promote skin cancer as well as measures that help prevent it.
12. Name two conditions characterized by hair loss, and the etiology for each.
13. Describe the appearance of head lice and nits and explain how to remove them.
14. Discuss factors that promote fungal infections of the nails.
15. Name techniques for preventing onychocryptosis (ingrown toenails).

Disorders of the skin, hair, and nails are common. Because self-image is inextricably related to how a person looks, complications from body ornamentation and disorders of the integumentary system not only affect appearance, but also have personal and social implications. In addition to requiring medical or surgical treatment, clients with disorders of the skin, which is the focus of this chapter, need empathic support while they cope with complications associated with tattooing or body piercing or chronic or acute conditions affecting the integument.

BODY ORNAMENTATION

Historically, people have altered normal skin for ornamental, cosmetic, and utilitarian reasons. Physicians have used a form of tattooing known as micropigmentation as an adjunct to medical procedures such as breast reconstruction surgery (see Chap. 54) and to recreate the appearance of eyebrows on people who have lost facial hair. Some people have tattoos applied as a form of permanent makeup to save time or to compensate for a physical disability that interferes with the hand dexterity required for daily application. Recently, however, there is a trend among adolescents and younger adults to alter the skin with ornamental tattooing, body piercing, and graphic designs using permanently colored pigments.

TATTOOS

A **tattoo** is pigmentation of the dermal layer of skin with needles containing dye. Tattoo artists inject the skin with an electrical vibrating instrument that injects pigment 50 to 3000 times per minute into the dermis of the skin at a depth of 1/64 to 1/16 of an inch (Freyenberger, 1998; peer reviewed by Eland, 2004).

Reputable tattoo studios require a signed parental consent for minors; however, not all tattooists ask for the signed consent form, despite the fact that some states require it. Some people ask a friend to perform the tattooing or they tattoo themselves with substances such as India ink, using nonsterile objects such as pins or the tips of ink pens.

If a person makes known his or her intention to receive a tattoo, the nurse can recommend that the selected tattooist at least be certified by the Alliance for Professional Tattooists. Members of this organization follow infection-control guidelines developed in conjunction with the U. S. Food and Drug Administration (FDA) (2008). Currently, however, people who perform invasive body art procedures are not required to adhere to any federal safety standards designed to prevent transmission of bloodborne pathogens (Smith, 2007). Tattooists are regulated by local jurisdictions only (FDA, 2008).

Risks Associated With Tattooing

Pigment inks are cosmetics that require approval according to the Federal Food, Drug, and Cosmetic Act. Although these inks are approved for cosmetic use, none is approved by the FDA for injection into the skin. The number of adverse reactions and potential health risks is increasing; therefore, the FDA is investigating tattoo inks and additional color additives that adulterate tattoo pigment products. The current consensus is that the pigments used in ornamental tattooing inks for nonmedical use are associated with various health risks.

Once applied, the pigments are difficult or impossible to remove. Allergies to tattoo pigments also can occur. Tattoos also interfere with the quality of magnetic resonance imaging (MRI) because of the interaction of metallic compounds within the pigment. Some people have experienced swelling or burning in the area of the tattoo when undergoing an MRI (FDA, 2008). Infection is also a potential complication from a tattoo. Unless the tattooist sterilizes the equipment, including components that hold the needles, potential for transmitting bloodborne infectious diseases, such as hepatitis B and C (see Chap. 47) and human immunodeficiency virus (HIV) (see Chap. 35), exists. The tattooist should discard even the ink after each use, but, in reality, he or she may return the ink to the supplier's bottle for the next customer. For these reasons, the American Association of Blood Banks rejects potential blood donors who have received a tattoo within 1 year.

Other consequences of tattooing are physiologic responses to traumatized integument. A **granuloma**, an inflammatory nodular lesion, may form as a result of a cellular attack waged against the particles in the tattoo pigment, which the body senses as foreign (see Chap. 33). Some people, especially those with darkly pigmented skin, tend to form keloids, an overgrowth of scar tissue (see Chap. 4).

Another common problem is that the person regrets having gotten a tattoo or feels dissatisfied with its appearance.

Skin Care Following a Tattoo

The trauma created by a tattoo is similar to that of a minor burn. The priority of care is preventing infection, supporting regeneration of tissue, and protecting the skin from concurrent and future damage. The nurse advises the client to do the following (Mayo Clinic, 2008; Freyenberger, 1998; peer reviewed by Eland, 2004):

- Temporarily avoid swimming, soaking in a hot tub, and touching the newly tattooed skin.
- Cover the new tattoo with antibiotic ointment and a sterile gauze dressing for 12 hours.
- Perform handwashing before caring for the tattooed skin.
- Remove the dressing after 12 hours, while showering or after wetting the gauze, to soften the drainage that may adhere to the dressing.
- Wash the tattooed area with antibacterial soap at least 3 times a day, taking care to pat the skin dry until the skin heals.
- Repeat the applications of antibacterial ointment after each skin cleansing for 5 days.
- Apply a moisturizing skin lotion that is free of perfume and color additives for 2 weeks after discontinuing the antibiotic ointment.
- Avoid direct sunlight on the skin for at least 4 weeks and always use a waterproof sunscreen with a sun protection factor (SPF) of 30 or higher thereafter; cover the tattoo if using a tanning bed.

Tattoo Removal

Although tattoos can be removed, the skin rarely returns to its pre-tattooed appearance. Some techniques for changing the skin's appearance include the following:

- Laser treatments, which tend to lighten tattoos
- Dermabrasion, which mechanically abrades the skin layers with a sanding disc or wire brush, sometimes leaving scar tissue in its place
- Salabrasion, which uses a salt solution to abrade the skin
- Scarification of the skin with an acid solution
- Plastic surgery, in which the surgeon inserts fluid-filled balloons under the skin to stretch it so that he or she can remove the tattooed skin, approximate the wound edges, and retattoo the skin to camouflage the existing tattoo

BODY PIERCING

Body piercing is the insertion of a metal ring or barbell, which is a straight or curved rod, into a body part (Fig. 65-1). Common locations for body piercing include lips, ear cartilage, cheeks, nose, tongue, eyebrows, navel, nipples, or genital area. Although there is great potential for infection and other medical complications, no federal regulations or certification programs exist for body piercers (Armstrong, 2004). Consequently, people who perform body piercings vary widely in their knowledge of asepsis and the anatomy of the tissue that they pierce. Some belong to the Association of Professional Piercers, an organization that advocates for educating and encouraging regulations for body piercing.

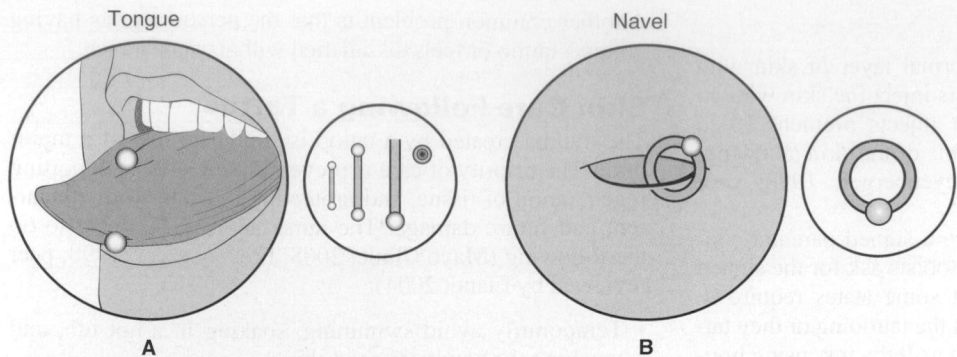

Tongue   Navel

A   B

FIGURE 65-1. Examples of body piercing. (**A**) The straight barbell comes in various gauges and lengths. (**B**) The ends of the ring are inserted into a captive bead.

Risks Associated With Body Piercing

One in three college students has a pierced body part, and approximately 17% to 45% of people with body piercing experience complications; in certain body sites, the incidence of complications is even higher (Smith, 2007). No reliable estimates are available, because statistics do not account for unreported and self-treated complications.

Tissue trauma, swelling, and bleeding, especially of the tongue, are initial risks associated with body piercing. The soft-tissue injury is increased if a piercing gun is used, because the spring-loaded device drives the body jewelry through the tissue with intense compressive force. The piercing jewelry must be long enough to allow for initial swelling. In some tongue piercings, the airway may become obstructed from swelling.

Later, piercing jewelry in and about the mouth and nose may interfere with resuscitation efforts that require oral or nasal intubation. There are dental implications with oral jewelry as well. Metallic devices can chip or crack teeth and may cause artifacts on dental x-rays or conceal pathology. Oral devices can interfere with speaking and swallowing and cause respiratory complications if metallic parts become inhaled (American Dental Association, 2005). Piercings around the genitals may complicate urinary catheterization and vaginal delivery. Piercings can affect breast feeding if a nipple has piercing jewelry. Also, allergic reactions to brass and nickel jewelry have occurred. Noncorrosive metal, such as surgical stainless steel, niobium, titanium, or solid 14K gold, are safest for piercings.

Perhaps one of the major risks with body piercing is infection. The potential for infection exists until the pierced body part heals, which may take from 2 weeks to 9 months, depending on the tissue (Table 65-1). The risk is greater with a piercing gun, which is difficult to sterilize. The risk is compounded with poor asepsis on the part of the piercer.

Like tattooing, body piercing carries a risk for transmitting hepatitis and HIV. Reports of tetanus and tuberculosis have been attributed to ear piercing (Ferringer, Pride, & Tyler, 2008). Because the mouth is teeming with microorganisms, oral piercings provide a potential for causing or exacerbating endocarditis, an inflammatory disorder of the heart and heart valves (see Chap. 23).

Site Care Following a Body Piercing

Site care for oral piercings of the tongue or lip is unique. The recipient of the piercing must keep the mouth as clean as possible and should use a soft-bristled toothbrush to avoid additional oral injury. In addition, he or she should rinse the mouth for 30 to 60 seconds with an antibacterial, alcohol-free mouthwash after eating food until the piercing heals. The recipient can substitute an antifungal mouthwash or salt water if a superinfection of candidiasis develops from the antibacterial mouthwash.

After a body piercing in other areas, the nurse instructs the person to care for the site as follows (Mayo Clinic, 2008; Armstrong, 2004; Freyenberger, 2002):

- After handwashing, clean the site with antibacterial soap and water twice a day or more often to remove perspiration and body fluids.
- During washing, move the piercing jewelry back and forth to help clean the pierced tract.
- After cleaning, rinse the site with plain water.
- Avoid alcohol and hydrogen peroxide, which dry the skin; povidone iodine Betadine, which discolors gold jewelry; and ointments, which prevent oxygen from reaching the impaired tissue.
- Restrict use of public pools and hot tubs while the pierced area heals.
- Eliminate the application of cosmetics and makeup around facial piercings until the piercings have healed.
- Wear clean, loose clothing to facilitate air circulation; change bed linens at least weekly.
- Check that the piercing jewelry is secured and intact, especially before eating and sleeping.

TABLE 65-1 Healing Time According to Site of Body Piercing

SITE	HEALING TIME
Clitoris	2–6 weeks
Coronal ridge (penis)	6–8 weeks
Ear lobe and auricle	6–8 weeks
Eyebrow	6–8 weeks
Glans penis	3–9 months
Labia majora	2–4 months
Labia minora	2–6 weeks
Lip	6–8 weeks
Navel	Up to 9 months
Nipple	2–4 months
Scrotum	2–3 months
Tongue	3–6 weeks
Urethral meatus	2–4 weeks

Source: Meltzer, D.I. (2005). Complications of body piercing. Available at http://www.aafp.org/afp/20051115/2029.html. Accessed October 2008.

Removal of Body-Piercing Jewelry

The site where the person inserts body-piercing jewelry will close if he or she removes the jewelry before healing is complete. The person must remove the jewelry, however, if a localized or serious infection does not respond to antibiotic therapy. The person can keep the piercing tract patent by inserting a temporary retainer or suture material through the pierced tissue. Special jeweler's tools are generally needed for removal. The person can remove a barbell by stabilizing the rod and twisting the spherical ends in opposite directions. For circular jewelry connected with a captive bead, the ends can be pried apart, taking care not to lose the bead (Armstrong, 2004).

SKIN DISORDERS

DERMATITIS

Dermatitis is a general term that refers to an inflammation of the skin. It is a common sign of many skin disorders accompanied by a red rash. An associated symptom is **pruritus**, or itching. Dermatitis and pruritus may be localized or generalized. Because both are nonspecific symptoms, it is essential that the cause be diagnosed and definitively treated. Two common types are allergic and irritant dermatitis.

Pathophysiology and Etiology

Allergic contact dermatitis develops in people who are sensitive to one or more substances, such as drugs, fibers in clothing, cosmetics, plants (e.g., poison ivy), and dyes. Primary irritant dermatitis is a localized reaction that occurs when the skin comes into contact with a strong chemical such as a solvent or detergent.

In clients with allergies, sensitized mast cells in the skin release histamine, causing a red rash, itching, and localized swelling (see Chap. 34). An allergy, however, does not cause irritant dermatitis. Rather, the caustic quality of the substance damages the protein structure of the skin or eliminates secretions that protect it.

 Gerontologic Considerations

- A decrease in epidermal replacement rates contributes to excessive drying of older person's skin, leading to pruritus and infection. Daily bathing is not necessary, and lotion or cream may be helpful in soothing dry areas. Early assessment and treatment of any type of skin lesion helps prevent infection and complications.

Assessment Findings

The skin response is characterized by dilation of the blood vessels, causing redness and swelling, and sometimes by *vesiculation* (blister formation) and oozing (Fig. 65-2). Itching is a prominent symptom. Primary irritant dermatitis may cause soreness or discomfort from irritation, itching, redness, swelling, and vesiculation.

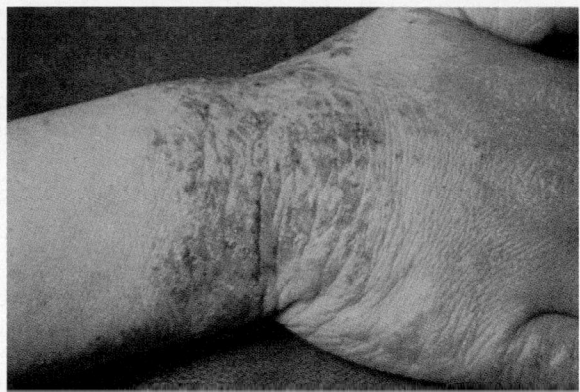

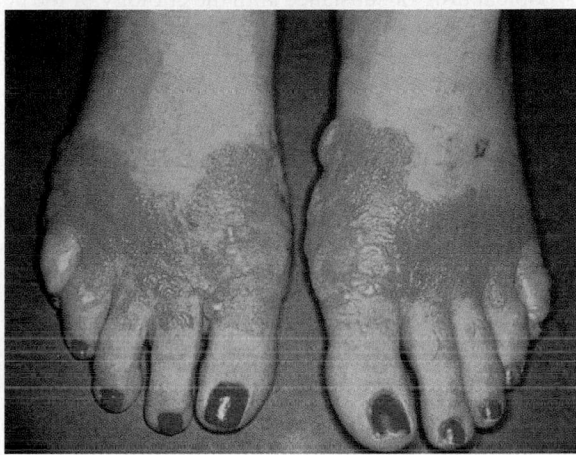

FIGURE 65-2. Contact dermatitis of the (**A**) wrist and (**B**) feet from shoe material. (B courtesy of Glaxo-Wellcome Co.)

Diagnosis is made by visual examination of the area. A detailed and thorough history helps identify the offending substances as well as the type of dermatitis. In difficult cases, a skin patch test may identify an allergic substance.

Medical Management

Treatment of both types of dermatitis is to remove the substances causing the reaction. This is done by flushing the skin with cool water. Topical lotions, such as calamine, or systemic drugs, such as diphenhydramine (Benadryl) or cyproheptadine (Periactin), are prescribed to relieve itching. Moisturizing creams with lanolin restore lubrication. In more severe cases, wet dressings with astringent solutions, such as Burow's solution (aluminum acetate), are prescribed. Corticosteroids taken orally or applied topically also provide relief.

 Pharmacologic Considerations

- Ointments, creams, and lotions prescribed for dermatologic disorders must be applied exactly as the physician directs (e.g., sparingly or a thick or thin coat covering the lesion). Remind the client that, unless he or she applies the drug exactly as ordered, it may not be of therapeutic value. If the client uses an excessive amount, he or she is wasting the drug.

- Drugs prescribed for dermatologic conditions may relieve symptoms but do not necessarily cure the disease. Skin disorders may require long-term therapy, often with a periodic change in prescriptions. This can be discouraging to the client. Encourage persistence in following the physician's instructions.

Nursing Management

The nurse advises clients to wear rubber gloves when coming in contact with any substance such as soap or solvents, put all clothes through a second rinse cycle when laundering to remove soap residue, and avoid the use of cosmetics or any topical drug or substance until the etiology of the dermatitis is identified. Measures that reduce itching or preserve the integrity of the skin are presented in Client and Family Teaching 65-1.

ACNE VULGARIS

Acne vulgaris, which tends to coincide with puberty, is an inflammatory disorder that affects the sebaceous glands and hair follicles. The severity of the condition varies from minimal to severe.

Pathophysiology and Etiology

Acne is believed to be related to the rise in androgen hormone levels that occur when secondary sex characteristics are developing. Androgens increase the size and activity of sebaceous glands within the skin. The overproduction of sebum provides an ideal environment for bacterial growth. Any correlation with specific food items (e.g., chocolate) is more myth than fact.

Sebum, keratin, and bacteria accumulate and dilate the follicle. The collective secretions form a **comedone**, or what most refer to as a *blackhead* (Fig. 65-3). The dark appearance is the result of oxidation of the core material. The follicle becomes further distended and irritated, causing a raised papule in the skin. If the follicular wall ruptures, the

Client and Family Teaching 65–1
Reducing Itching with Dermatitis

The nurse emphasizes the following points when teaching the client:

● Keep nails short and clean.
● Use light cotton bedding and clothing that allow normal evaporation of moisture from the skin (avoid wool, synthetics, and other dense fibers).
● Wear white cotton gloves if prone to scratching during sleep.
● Avoid regular soap for bathing; hypoallergenic or glycerin soaps can be used without causing skin irritation or itching.
● Use tepid bath water; pat rather than rub the skin dry.
● Inform the physician if the drug therapy fails to restore skin integrity or relieve itching.

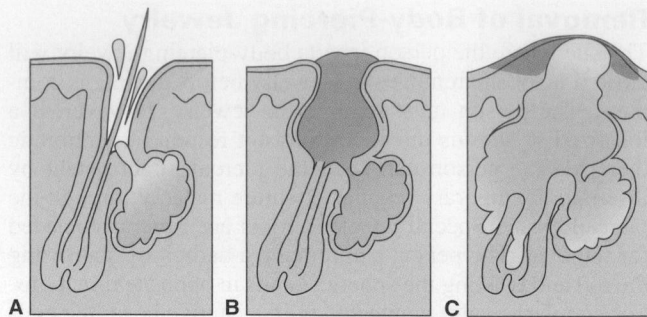

FIGURE 65-3. Acne vulgaris. (**A**) Normal sebaceous gland and hair follicle. (**B**) Comedone formation. (**C**) Pustule formation.

inflammatory response extends into the marginal areas of dermis. In serious cases, inflamed nodules and cysts develop. The skin lesions are aggravated by cosmetics as well as picking and squeezing blemishes. Severe acne, if neglected, leads to deep, pitted scars that leave the skin permanently pockmarked. Acne vulgaris improves after adolescence.

Assessment Findings

Comedones and pustules appear on the face, chest, and back, where the skin is excessively oily (Fig. 65-4). Oiliness of the scalp often accompanies acne. Diagnosis is made by visual examination of the affected areas.

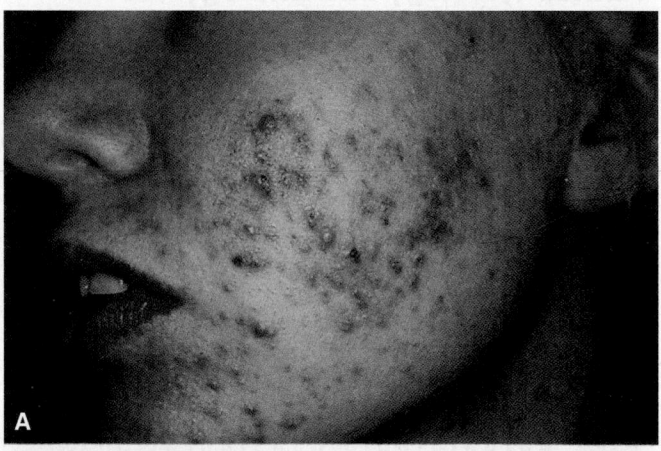

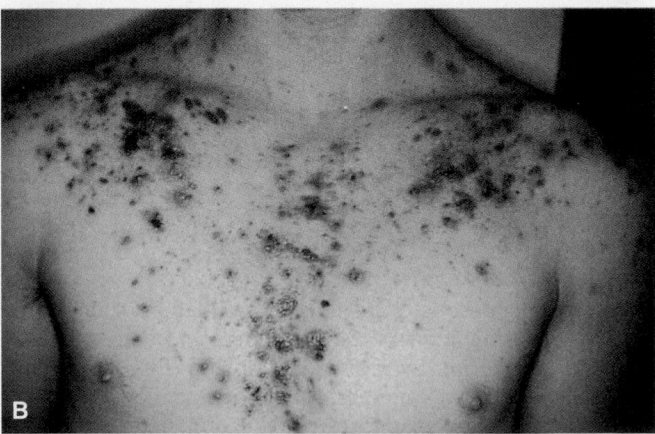

FIGURE 65-4. Acne of (**A**) the face and (**B**) the chest.

Medical Management

Mild cases of acne improve with gentle facial cleansing and nonprescription drying agents containing benzoyl peroxide. Drug therapy includes the topical application of tretinoin (Retin-A) or tazarotene (Tazorac), or oral administration of isotretinoin (Accutane). Topical and systemic antibiotics such as tetracycline and erythromycin, in low doses, also are used for severe acne and have produced good results. The comedones can be removed and the pustules drained with special instruments.

 Pharmacologic Considerations

- Warn clients using acne preparations containing benzoyl peroxide that this ingredient is an oxidizing agent and may remove the color from clothing, rugs, and furniture. Thorough handwashing after drug use may not remove all the drug, and permanent fabric discoloration may still occur. Users of products containing benzoyl peroxide should wear disposable plastic gloves when applying the drug.

- The dosage of isotretinoin (Accutane) in the treatment of severe acne is determined by weight. Warn clients not to increase the dosage of the drug if the acne becomes worse or does not respond to treatment.

Surgical Management

Dermabrasion is a method of removing surface layers of scarred skin. It is useful in lessening scars such as the pitting from severe acne. The outermost layers of the skin are removed by sandpaper, a rotating wire brush, chemicals (chemical face peeling), or a diamond wheel. A local anesthetic, such as an ethyl chloride and Freon mixture, is used during the procedure. Afterward, the skin looks and feels raw and sore, and some crusting from serous exudate occurs. Clients frequently say that the discomfort is much like that from a burn. The client is instructed to avoid washing the area until it has healed sufficiently. The client also must refrain from picking and touching the area because contact with the fingers might cause infection or scarring from secondary trauma.

Nursing Management

The nurse advises the client to keep the face and hair clean and avoid cosmetics that contribute to oily skin. He or she explains that, above all else, manipulating the lesions worsens the condition. For female clients, the nurse warns about the risk of birth defects associated with systemic oral isotretinoin. He or she explains that women for whom this drug is prescribed must (1) have a negative pregnancy test 2 weeks before beginning therapy, (2) comply with contraceptive measures while taking the drug and for 1 month after discontinuing therapy, and (3) check with a physician about risks to an infant while breastfeeding.

The nurse should also instruct the client to keep the hair short and away from the face and forehead. Washing the hair frequently is beneficial; daily shampooing does not damage hair. The nurse also tells the client to avoid using makeup, lotions, hair sprays, and skin-care products unless approved by a physician.

ROSACEA

Rosacea, a chronic skin disorder that manifests in a variety of ways, is generally characterized by a rosy appearance. This condition is the fifth most prevalent skin disorder; it affects approximately 14 million generally fair-skinned Americans who are 30 to 60 years of age (National Institute of Arthritis and Musculoskeletal and Skin Diseases, 2005). Healthcare professionals sometimes refer to it as adult acne or acne rosacea because the skin manifestations are somewhat similar. Rosacea is totally unrelated to acne vulgaris, however, and may worsen if treated similarly. It is incurable, but manageable, and may progress in severity.

Pathophysiology and Etiology

The cause of rosacea is unknown, but several hypotheses have been proposed, including genetics, immunological factors, exposure to ultraviolet (UV) light, bacterial skin infection with *Helicobacter pylori,* and mite infestation of the facial hair follicles (Dermatology Information System, 2008). The mite *Demodex folliculorum* is a normal inhabitant of the skin; however, it is more abundant among people with rosacea. It is still unclear whether the skin mite provokes an inflammatory or allergic reaction or blocks skin follicles, which facilitates survival of the mite.

Most believe that the disorder results from a genetically inherited vascular anomaly that initially causes episodic blushing about the face. The blushing is attributed to changes in connective tissue that fail to provide support for superficial blood vessels (Mascai et al., 1996).

The loss of support causes a prolonged state of vasodilation lasting hours or days. Eventually, the facial capillaries and arterioles become chronically dilated, appearing as visible linear streaks on the skin, a condition known as *telangiectases.* The chronic vasodilation causes the dermal tissue and sebaceous glands to hypertrophy and develop elevated papules and pustules. The skin across the nose and cheeks becomes unevenly thickened and distorted. If vascular structures of the eyes and eyelids become affected, there may be a bloodshot appearance accompanied by decreased tearing.

Assessment Findings

The earliest sign of rosacea is frequent, intermittent blushing across the nose, forehead, cheeks, and chin. Factors that contribute to vasodilation or irritation of the skin may trigger blushing; examples include consuming hot beverages, spicy food, or alcohol; exposure to sun, wind, or cold; bathing with hot water; stress, or use of skin care products (National Rosacea Society, 2008). As the condition progresses, the skin remains red, appearing like a persistent sunburn. The inflamed tissue may sting and feel chronically irritated; solid papules or pustules form. The face appears swollen and baggy, and large facial pores produce a texture resembling an orange peel. The nose becomes permanently enlarged, red, nodular, and bulbous, a condition known as

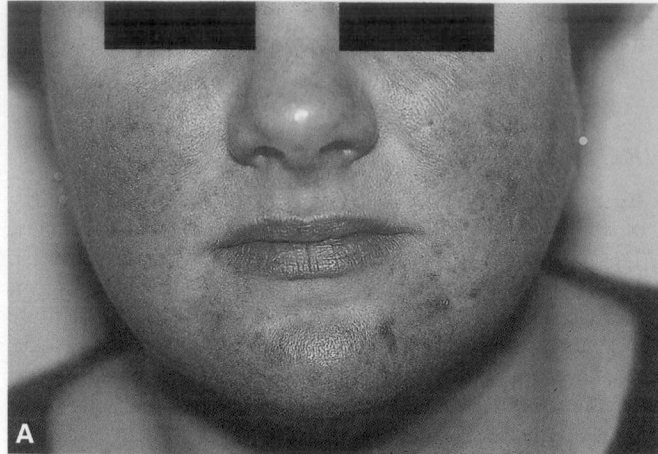

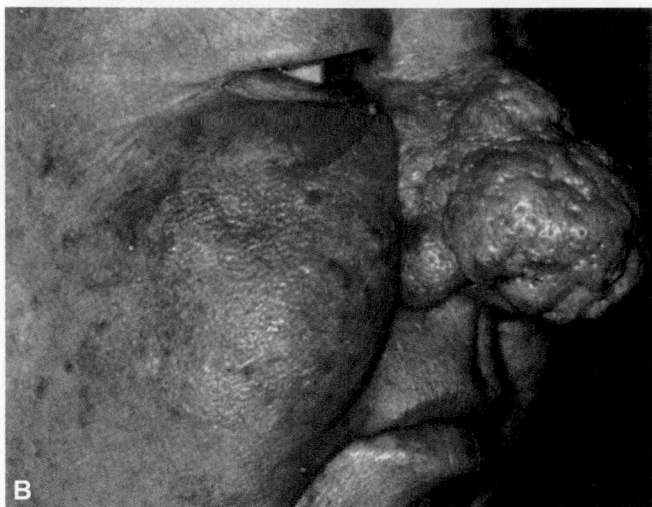

FIGURE 65-5. (**A**) Rosacea causes areas of erythema, papules, and pustules on the face. (**B**) Chronic rosacea with rhinophyma. (A from Goodheart, H. P. [2009]. *Goodheart's photoguide to common skin disorders* [3rd ed.]. Philadelphia: Lippincott Williams & Wilkins. B courtesy of Hoechst-Roussel Pharmaceuticals, Inc.)

rhinophyma (Fig. 65-5). The eyes, if affected, appear inflamed. The client may report that he or she cannot wear contact lenses or that the eyes feel as though a foreign body is present.

Medical and Surgical Management

Treatment goals include minimizing the symptoms and promoting a more acceptable appearance. Physicians treat rosacea initially with oral antibiotics such as minocycline (Minocin), a tetracycline, or erythromycin (Ilosone), a macrolide, to subdue the associated inflammation. Once inflammation is controlled, the physician may prescribe topical medications such as metronidazole (MetroGel, Noritate) or sulfacetamide (Sodium Sulamyd) with or without sulfur to sustain the anti-inflammatory effect. The treatment regimen might include topical retinoids, derivatives of vitamin A, such as isotretinoin (Accutane), provided that the client is not pregnant and takes measures to avoid pregnancy. Healthcare professionals believe that retinoids can shrink sebaceous glands and reduce dermatologic inflammation. Topical drug therapy may be long-term to promote a remission of symptoms.

Other approaches can improve the client's appearance. A series of two to four laser treatments reduces excessive tissue, especially about the nose, and permanently obliterates telangiectases by sealing blood vessels. Pulsed light (Photo-Derm™) is light energy used to eliminate vascular lesions. In the case of rosacea, the energy penetrates the dermis without disrupting the epidermis to stimulate growth of collagen and to rejuvenate the skin's appearance.

Nursing Management

The nurse encourages the client to maintain a diary documenting lifestyle practices and events that trigger symptoms. Establishing a cause-and-effect relationship between specific foods and beverages, for example, helps the client avoid exacerbations. In addition, the nurse advises the client to minimize sun exposure and always to use sunscreen of SPF 15 or higher. The nurse suggests protecting the skin in cold or windy weather with a scarf or ski mask and applying a skin moisturizer. The nurse teaches the client to pace physical activity to avoid overheating, which is accompanied by vasodilation. The nurse reviews a basic skin-care regimen that includes washing the face with lukewarm water and a gentle cleanser; avoiding the use of a face cloth, which may be too abrasive; blotting the skin dry; and waiting 5 to 30 minutes after cleansing before applying medication to reduce potential discomfort. He or she cautions the client to avoid self-treatment with acne medications, especially those containing benzoyl peroxide, which tend to irritate affected skin further. The nurse explores alternative stress-management techniques with the client and encourages implementing new coping strategies (see Chap. 67) to complement the therapeutic medical regimen.

FURUNCLES, FURUNCULOSIS, AND CARBUNCLES

A **furuncle** is a boil. **Furunculosis** refers to having multiple furuncles. A **carbuncle** is a furuncle from which pus drains.

Pathophysiology and Etiology

The cause of furuncles and carbuncles is skin infections with organisms that usually exist harmlessly on the skin surface. When an injury such as that caused by squeezing a lesion impairs the integrity of the skin, microorganisms can enter and colonize in the skin. Furunculosis also is associated with diabetes mellitus because an elevated blood glucose level promotes microbial growth. Other factors that predispose to these conditions include poor diet and general health and any disorder that lowers resistance.

Assessment Findings

The lesion, which may appear anywhere on the body, but especially around the neck, axillary, and groin regions, appears as a raised, painful pustule surrounded by erythema. The area feels hard to the touch. After a few days, the lesion exudes pus and later a core. The client also may experience a fever, anorexia, weakness, and malaise. A culture of the exudate identifies the infectious organism.

Medical and Surgical Management

Hot wet soaks are used to localize the infection and provide symptomatic relief. It may be the only treatment necessary. Antibiotics are used in some instances, especially when a fever is present or if the lesion is a carbuncle. Surgical incision and drainage may be necessary.

Nursing Management

The nurse follows strict aseptic technique when applying or changing a dressing to prevent the spread of the infection to other parts of the body or to others. He or she teaches the client also to do so. The nurse informs the client to never pick or squeeze a furuncle—drainage is infectious, and this practice favors spread of the infection to surrounding tissues or even to the bloodstream. In addition, the client should wash hands thoroughly before and after applying topical medications, keep hands away from infected areas, and use face cloths and towels separate from those used by others. It is important to wash clothing, towels, and face cloths in hot water and bleach separately from family laundry.

PSORIASIS

Psoriasis is a chronic, noninfectious inflammatory disorder of the skin that affects both men and women. Its onset is in young and middle adulthood. Although there are many types of psoriasis, the most common is plaque psoriasis (Fig. 65-6). Periods of emotional stress, hormonal cycles, infection, and seasonal changes appear to aggravate the condition.

Pathophysiology and Etiology

The cause of psoriasis is unknown, but a genetic predisposition is likely because many report a family history of the disorder. Although the predisposition exists, the disorder seems to require a triggering mechanism such as systemic infection, injury to the skin, vaccination, or injection. This also suggests a link with the immune system. The fact that the disorder has periods of exacerbation and remission strengthens this hypothesis.

In psoriasis, skin cells called *keratinocytes* behave as if there is a need to repair a wound. The cells of the epidermis proliferate faster than normal—so fast, in fact, that the upper layer of cells cannot be shed fast enough to make room for the newly produced cells. The excessive cells accumulate and form elevated, scaly lesions called *plaque*. The area around the lesion becomes red from the increased blood supply needed to nourish the rapidly developing skin cells.

Assessment Findings

Psoriasis is characterized by patches of **erythema** (redness) covered with silvery scales, usually on the extensor surfaces of the elbows, knees, trunk, and scalp. Itching usually is absent or slight, but occasionally it is severe. The lesions are obvious and unsightly, and the scales tend to shed.

Diagnosis is made by visual examination of the lesions. A skin biopsy reveals increased proliferation of epidermal cells.

Medical Management

Psoriasis has no cure. Symptomatic treatment to control the scaling and itching includes the use of topical agents such as coal tar extract, corticosteroids, or anthralin. Anthralin, a distillate of crude coal tar, is applied to thick plaques; it tends to irritate unaffected skin areas. Topical corticosteroids, topical retinoids, and analogs of vitamin D have proved beneficial. Methotrexate, an antimetabolite used in the treatment of cancer, is prescribed for clients with severe disease that does not respond to other forms of therapy. This drug inhibits the production of cells that divide rapidly (cancer cells, cells composing the skin and mucous membranes) and is capable of reducing plaque formation. Dosage is carefully individualized because the drug causes serious adverse effects.

Etretinate (Tegison) is related to retinoic acid and retinol (vitamin A) and is used to treat psoriasis that does not respond to other therapies. Its use is recommended only for those clients who can reliably understand and carry out the treatment regimen, are capable of complying with mandatory contraceptive measures, and do not intend to become pregnant. Another method of treatment is the injection of triamcinolone acetonide (Kenacort), a corticosteroid, into isolated psoriatic plaques. This method of treatment is successful in some cases.

Recently, healthcare professionals have used biologic therapy techniques that alter immune system responses, administering humanized monoclonal antibodies such as efalizumab (Raptiva) and infliximab (Remicade), which have been approved for the treatment of rheumatoid arthritis and other autoimmune disorders. These drugs modify the activities of T-cells (see Chap. 39) and reduce inflammation and hyperplasia of the epidermis in clients with psoriasis, resulting in rapid and significant improvement. Unfortunately, these drugs also are associated with anaphylaxis and serious infections. Consequently, they are reserved for severe cases (Pariser, 2003).

Photochemotherapy, a combination of UV light therapy and a photosensitizing psoralen drug such as methoxsalen (Oxsoralen-Ultra), also has been used for severe,

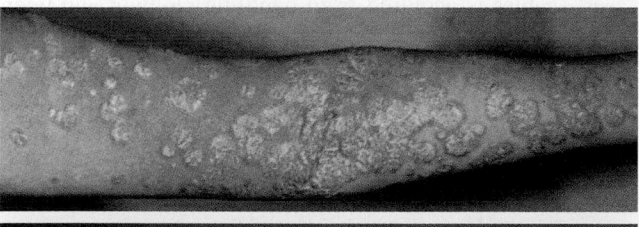
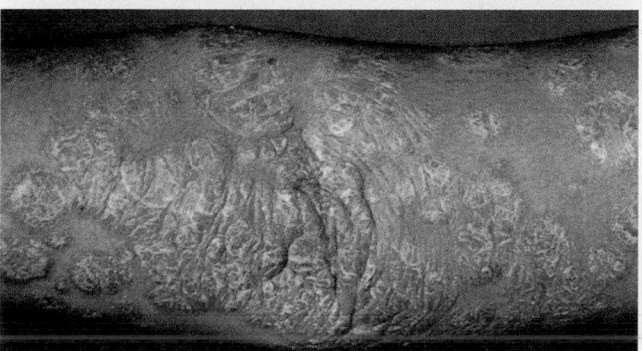

FIGURE 65-6. Psoriasis on the elbows (Roche Laboratories).

disabling psoriasis that does not respond to other methods of treatment. The extent of exposure is based on the client's skin tolerance. Treatments are given once every other day or less because phototoxic reactions may appear 48 hours or more after light exposure. Once the psoriasis clears, the client is placed on a maintenance treatment program.

Some clients respond well to treatment; others receive only minor relief. The condition tends to recur.

Pharmacologic Considerations

- Clients receiving photochemotherapy for severe psoriasis must follow the physician's directions regarding the timing of taking the drug methoxsalen because a therapeutic effect from photochemotherapy depends on an effective tissue concentration in the skin during irradiation.

Nursing Process for the Client With Psoriasis

Assessment
Inspect and evaluate the integrity of the skin in a well-lit environment. Compare the pathologic appearance of the affected skin with the characteristics of normal skin. Ask the client whether there is a family history of psoriasis and determine the onset, duration, and possible triggering factors.

Diagnosis, Planning, and Interventions
Show acceptance of clients with skin lesions, who need a great deal of understanding and emotional support. Explain that treatment usually is for a lifetime and that it is necessary to follow the plan of therapy. Reassure clients for whom more than one form of treatment has failed that other, untried modalities may offer improved control of symptoms. Instruct the client receiving photochemotherapy to avoid exposure to sunlight for 8 hours after treatment because it takes that long for the body to excrete methoxsalen.

Diagnoses, outcomes, and interventions for clients with psoriasis include, but are not limited to, the following.

▶ Impaired Skin Integrity related to decreased protective function of epidermal tissue

▶ Expected Outcome: Client will achieve smoother skin with control of lesions and increased protective skin function.

- Instruct the client that repeated trauma to the skin (cuts, abrasions, sunburn) may exacerbate psoriasis. *Giving facts provides a means by which the client can help manage the disorder.*
- Advise the client not to pick or scratch lesions. *Disruption of the lesions causes secondary skin trauma.*
- Inspect the skin regularly for signs of infection. *Impaired skin integrity provides a portal through which pathogens can enter.*
- Wash the affected area with warm water and pat dry. Apply moisturizing or medicated topical ointments as ordered. *Clean, moisturized skin that is not irritated by friction during drying helps maintain skin integrity.*

▶ Disturbed Body Image related to embarrassment of skin appearance and self-perception of uncleanliness

▶ Expected Outcome: Client will acquire self-acceptance regarding skin changes.

- Inform the client that psoriasis has no permanent cure but that the condition usually can be controlled or cleared. *The reality of the prognosis facilitates the development of mechanisms for coping with the skin disorder.*
- Assist the client to carry out cosmetic efforts to decrease visibility of lesions. *Camouflaging the skin lesions reduces self-consciousness.*
- Encourage the client to join a psoriasis support group. *A support group helps the client understand that many others have the same disorder and similar problems. Group work facilitates coping better than working alone.*

Evaluation of Expected Outcomes
Expected outcomes are improved integrity and appearance of the skin. Itching is reduced or eliminated. The client understands clearly what the diagnosis of psoriasis means in terms of duration and length of treatment. He or she copes effectively with the altered appearance.

SCABIES
Scabies is a fairly common infectious skin disease.

Pathophysiology and Etiology
Scabies is caused by infestation with the itch mite (*Sarcoptes scabiei*). Anyone can acquire scabies; it is erroneous to assume that infected people have poor personal hygiene. Outbreaks are common where large groups of people are confined, such as nursing homes, military barracks, prisons, boarding schools, and childcare centers.

The mites are spread by skin-to-skin contact. In rare cases, scabies is acquired from handling clothing and linen in recent contact with an infected person. Scabies mites do not survive off the body more than 2 days.

Assessment Findings
Signs and Symptoms
Itching is intense, especially at night. Commonly affected areas include the webs and sides of fingers and around the wrists, elbows, armpits, waist, thighs, genitalia, nipples, breasts, and lower buttocks. Excoriation from scratching accompanies the itching. Skin burrows are caused by the female itch mite, which invades the skin to lay her eggs.

Diagnostic Findings
Diagnosis is made by examining the affected areas. Providers, however, often confuse scabies with other skin conditions. Therefore, the American Academy of Dermatology recommends an examination using mineral oil or ink. After dropping sterile mineral oil on the lesion, the skin is scraped onto a slide and examined microscopically to detect the mites, their eggs, or feces. The ink test is performed by

applying a blue or black felt-tipped pen to the lesion, which highlights the burrows when the skin surface is wiped.

Medical Management

Scabicides, chemicals that destroy mites, such as lindane (cream or lotion), permethrin cream, and crotamiton cream or lotion, are prescribed. The medication is applied to the skin from the neck down in a thin layer, left on for 8 to 12 hours, and then removed by washing. Thorough bathing, clean clothing, and the avoidance of contact with others who have scabies are essential in preventing recurrence.

Nursing Management

Before any treatment begins, the nurse advises the client to bathe thoroughly. The nurse then reviews the directions for applying the scabicide medication included with the product. He or she emphasizes the importance of following the directions for complete eradication of the scabies mite. The nurse instructs the client, after bathing and applying the medication, to don clean clothing and launder preworn clothing, towels, and bed linen in hot water as soon as possible. He or she tells the client to vacuum furniture and other unwashable items. Last, the nurse explains that itching may continue for 2 to 3 weeks after treatment.

 Gerontologic Considerations

- Although all clients should be carefully assessed for scabies and head lice discussed later, it is especially important for older adults who are frail or have cognitive limitations. These clients may be unable to inform the nurse of symptoms or may manifest atypical symptoms, including increased confusion or agitation.

DERMATOPHYTOSES

Dermatophytoses (tinea) are superficial fungal infections; they have been given many unscientific names. For example, a common term for one dermatophytosis is *ringworm,* which is a misnomer because a worm does not cause the infection. Other examples are *athlete's foot* for a foot infection and *jock itch* for an infection in the groin.

Pathophysiology and Etiology

Dermatophytes (also called *tinea*) are parasitic fungi that invade the skin, scalp, and nails (discussed later). The terms *tinea pedis, tinea capitis, tinea corporis,* and *tinea cruris* identify the skin areas of infection, namely, feet, head, body, and groin, respectively.

Assessment Findings

Tinea corporis appears as rings of papules or vesicles with a clear center in nonhairy areas of the skin (Fig. 65-7). Several clusters of rings may be found in the same general location. The affected skin often itches and becomes red, scaly, cracked, and sore. In tinea pedis, the infection begins in the skin between the toes and spreads to the soles of the feet. Tinea capitis, which is more common in children, invades the hair shaft below the scalp, followed by breaking of the hair, usually close to the scalp.

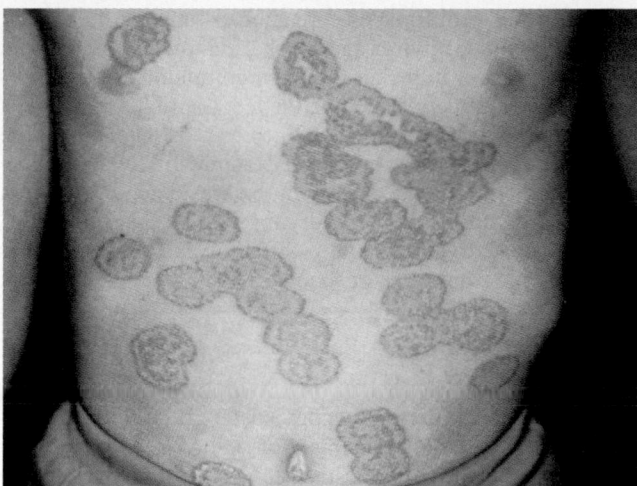

FIGURE 65-7. Tinea corporis, which is commonly referred to as ringworm because of its circular appearance. (From Hall, J. C. [1999]. *Sauer's manual of skin diseases* [8th ed.]. Philadelphia: Lippincott Williams & Wilkins.)

Diagnosis is made by visual examination of the affected areas. The lesions are scraped and examined microscopically. When a Wood's light is used, the affected areas fluoresce a green-yellow color.

Medical Management

Treatment of tinea pedis includes the topical use of antifungal agents, such as benzoic and salicylic acid ointment (Whitfield's ointment), Burow's solution, undecylenic acid, and tolnaftate (Tinactin). Oral griseofulvin (Grisactin), a systemic antifungal agent, also is useful in treatment. The drug may be required for many weeks to eradicate the infection. Tinea capitis may be treated with oral griseofulvin, which is taken with meals. A topical antifungal agent also may be prescribed to destroy fungi present on the hair shafts above the surface of the scalp. Treatment of tinea corporis includes the use of topical antifungal agents for less severe infections. Oral griseofulvin is prescribed for more severe infections. Tinea cruris often responds to topical application of tolnaftate or miconazole (Micatin). Tinea onychomycosis (discussed later) may respond to oral griseofulvin, but long-term therapy usually is necessary.

Nursing Management

If an oral or topical antifungal agent is prescribed, the nurse reviews the directions for use. He or she explains that the infected person must use separate towels, washcloths, grooming articles, and clothing because the disorder is contagious. The nurse stresses that keeping the affected areas dry reduces the spread of the infection. The nurse recommends thoroughly drying all areas of the body after a bath or shower, including the skin folds. To prevent infection and reinfection of tinea cruris, the nurse suggests avoiding excessive heat and humidity, not wearing tight-fitting clothing or nylon next to the skin (in hot, humid weather), and keeping the skin as dry as possible.

To avoid acquiring or spreading a fungal infection of the feet, the nurse advises against sharing towels and slippers or going barefoot in locker rooms or community bathrooms. He or she recommends keeping the feet (particularly the area between the toes) dry, which increases resistance to the infection. For clients whose feet perspire freely, the nurse advises applying powder between the toes, keeping the area dry, washing and thoroughly drying the feet daily, and putting on clean, dry socks and a different pair of shoes after coming home from work or school.

SHINGLES

Shingles, also known as **herpes zoster**, is a skin disorder that develops years after an infection with varicella (chickenpox). It is more frequent in middle-aged to older adults, as well as in people who are immunocompromised.

Pathophysiology and Etiology

Herpes zoster is an acute reactivation of the varicella-zoster virus, which lies dormant in nerve roots. When aging, cancer, drugs, or acquired immunodeficiency syndrome suppresses a client's immune system, the virus migrates along one or more cranial or spinal nerve routes. Viral reactivation produces inflammatory symptoms in the **dermatome**, a skin area supplied by the nerve (Fig. 65-8). Raised, fluid-filled, and painful skin eruptions accompany the inflammation.

If herpes zoster affects the ophthalmic branch of the trigeminal nerve (third cranial nerve), corneal (eye) ulcerations may occur. Involvement of the vestibulocochlear nerve (eighth cranial nerve) can lead to vertigo and permanent hearing loss. Cerebral vasculitis (inflammation of cerebral vessels) is the most serious complication, because involvement of the internal carotid arteries can result in a stroke. Rarely, the virus spreads to the brain, resulting in encephalitis.

Susceptible people who are exposed to someone in the early stages of herpes zoster infection can acquire varicella. The virus is contagious until the crusts from ruptured lesions have dried and fallen off the skin. Herpes zoster infection also can recur.

Assessment Findings

Initial symptoms include a low-grade fever, headache, and malaise. An area of skin along a dermatome develops a red, blotchy appearance that begins to itch or feel numb. In about 24 to 48 hours, vesicles appear on the skin along the nerve's pathway. Usually the eruptions are unilateral (one side) on the trunk, neck, or head. They become severely painful. Severe itching soon follows. Like chickenpox lesions, the vesicles rupture in a few days and crusts form. Scarring or permanent skin discoloration is possible. Pain (postherpetic neuralgia) and itching may persist for months or as long as 2 years or more. Secondary skin infections may occur from scratching the area.

Diagnosis is made primarily by examination of the lesions and symptoms.

Medical Management

Oral acyclovir (Zovirax), when taken within 48 hours of the appearance of symptoms, reduces their severity and prevents

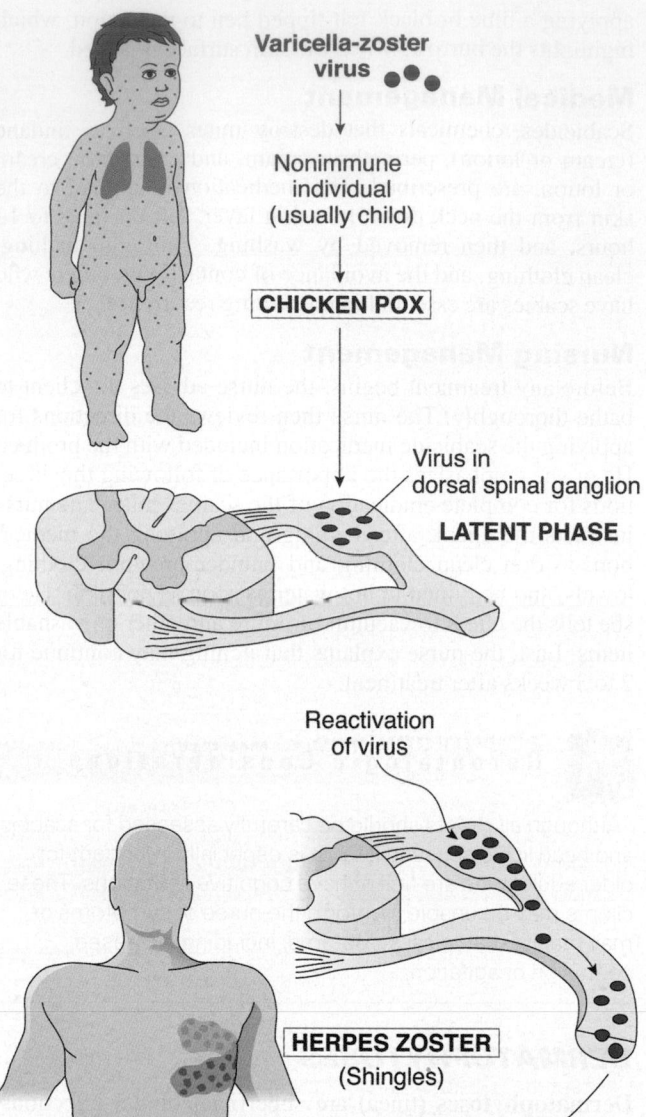

FIGURE 65-8. Varicella-zoster virus (chickenpox) and herpes zoster (shingles). After a person has had chickenpox (usually as a child), the varicella-zoster virus resides in a dorsal spinal ganglion, where it remains dormant for many years. When reactivated, it spreads to peripheral nerves of sensory dermatomes, causing shingles. (From Rubin, R., & Strayer, D.S., eds. [2008]. *Rubin's pathology: Clinicopathologic foundations of medicine* [5th ed.]. Philadelphia: Lippincott Williams & Wilkins.)

the development of additional lesions. Topical acyclovir also may be applied to the lesions. A brief course of corticosteroid therapy reduces pain. Lesions of the ophthalmic division of the trigeminal nerve require immediate examination and treatment by an ophthalmologist.

Additional treatment is symptomatic. Analgesics and liquid preparations with a drying or antipruritic effect are applied to the affected area once the crusts have fallen off. The skin may be so sensitive that any clothing or application of topical drugs intensifies pain or itching. A narcotic analgesic such as codeine often is necessary during the first few days to weeks.

Nursing Management

A supervisory nurse reassigns nursing personnel who have not had chickenpox to avoid contact with a client with herpes zoster. The nurse instructs clients with crusted lesions to avoid contact with immunocompromised people and those who have not had chickenpox. He or she advises the client that application of cool or warm compresses or warm showers may relieve pain and itching; it may be necessary to experiment with both to determine which provides the most relief. The nurse advises the client to wear loose clothing and avoid scratching the area. If oral acyclovir is prescribed, the nurse reviews the dose regimen, as printed on the prescription label.

SKIN CANCER

Skin cancer is the most common type of cancer in the United States; in 2008, more than one million new cases were diagnosed (National Cancer Institute, 2008). This disease can involve any one of three types of cells in the epidermis: squamous cells that are flat and scaly; basal cells that are round; and melanocytes, cells that contain color pigment.

Pathophysiology and Etiology

Increased exposure to UV radiation, especially UVB and UVC, harmful components in the spectrum of sunlight, predisposes to malignant skin changes and other health risks, including cataracts and premature aging of the skin. Fair-skinned people are more susceptible to skin cancer than dark-skinned people.

Several factors predispose to malignant changes in the skin.

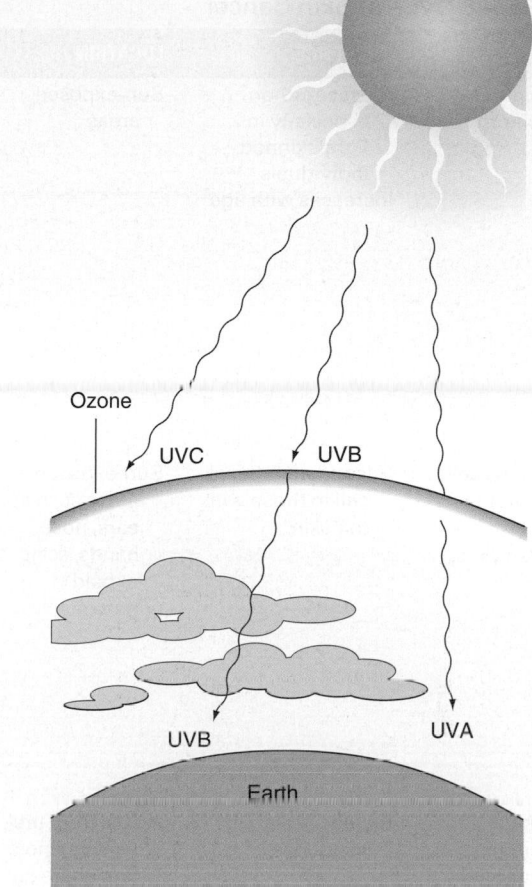

FIGURE 65-9. A layer of ozone shields or reduces the harmful spectrum of ultraviolet wavelengths known as UVC and UVB.

- Thinning ozone layer. Ozone, a naturally occurring atmospheric gas, absorbs UVB and UVC radiation (Fig. 65-9). Ozone depletion occurs primarily as a result of the release of chlorofluorocarbons (CFCs) in refrigerants, aerosol propellants, and other industrial pollutants.
- Residence in high-altitude areas where the atmosphere is thinner than at sea level or in areas with a regular cloud cover because people are less likely to use sun protective precautions.
- Decreased melanin in skin, especially in people who sunburn easily and tan minimally; black- or brown-skinned people rarely are affected (Porth, 2006).
- Prolonged, repeated exposure to UV rays in those who do farming, fishing, road construction, and so on, or those who frequent tanning salons and use sunlamps
- Prior radiation therapy for an unrelated form of cancer
- Ulcerations of long duration and scar tissue (both prone to malignant changes)

Malignant growths of the skin (Table 65-2) usually are primary lesions; that is, they originate in the skin. Prompt removal of the malignant tissue prevents its spread to other parts of the body or tissues.

Assessment Findings

Symptoms vary, but usually the new appearance of a growth or a change in color of the skin is the first symptom the client notices. The lesion can be smooth or rough, flat or elevated, and itchy or tender. It may bleed. Diagnosis is made by visual inspection and confirmed by biopsy.

Medical and Surgical Management

Depending on the size and the location of the lesion, treatment of squamous cell and basal cell carcinomas may involve electrodesiccation, surgical excision, cryosurgery, or radiation therapy. The client is followed regularly for at least 3 to 5 years to be sure regrowth has not occurred.

The treatment of melanoma involves radical excision of the tumor and adjacent tissues, followed by chemotherapy. The administration of melphalan (Alkeran) and prednisone is an example of an initial antineoplastic therapy regimen. Interferon alfa-n3 (Alferon N) has controlled metastases in some persons. Clinical trials of other types of therapies are being conducted. In some instances, skin grafting may be necessary to replace large areas of defect when a wide excision of the tumor is necessary.

Nursing Management

The nurse examines and measures abnormal-appearing skin lesions, especially those in sun-exposed areas such as the face, nose, lips, and hands. The nurse determines facts about the lesion, including when the lesion first was noticed, whether the lesion has undergone any recent changes, and, if

TABLE 65-2 Type of Skin Cancer

TYPE	INCIDENCE	LOCATION	APPEARANCE	CHARACTERISTICS
Basal cell carcinoma	Most common, especially in light-skinned individuals Increases with age	Sun-exposed areas	Small, shiny, gray or yellowish plaque that undergoes central ulceration	Slow growing, rarely metastasizes; commonly recurs
Squamous cell carcinoma	Second after basal cell in those with fair skin	Sun-exposed areas such as ears, nose, hands, scalp of bald persons	Scaly, elevated lesion with an irregular border; shallow, large ulcerations form in untreated advanced lesions	Can metastasize through blood and lymph
Malignant Malignan Malignan melanoma	Increasing in incidence	Arises from pre-existing mole anywhere on the body	Raised brown or black lesion In some cases, satellite lesions occur adjacent to the primary cancer	Poor prognosis because of distant metastases

so, what kind. He or she also teaches the client how to perform a skin self-examination (Client and Family Teaching 65-2).

Surgery for a malignant melanoma may involve structures of the head and neck, trunk, or extremities. The specific nursing management of those having radical surgery for this malignancy depends on the original site of the tumor and the extent of surgery. The nurse gives emotional support to those having disfiguring surgery.

The nurse encourages all people with any type of skin change to seek medical attention. He or she advises those in high-risk groups for malignant skin lesions to examine all areas of their body and scalp for new lesions or changes in moles, other growths, or pigmented lesions. If a client notes any change, he or she should make an appointment for a medical examination as soon as possible.

The nurse educates clients about measures to prevent skin cancer, some of which include the following:

• Always use a sunscreen with an SPF of at least 15; higher SPFs are beneficial for clients who sunburn easily.

• Reapply sunscreen at least every 2 hours or more often if swimming or perspiring.
• Use a lip balm with sunscreen.
• Wear a hat with a wide brim and cover the back of the neck.
• Stay in the shade when outdoors.
• Wear tightly woven, but loose-fitting clothing.
• Avoid prolonged sun exposure between 10:00 am and 4:00 pm.
• Avoid artificial tanning.

The nurse also recommends that at-risk clients consult the UV Forecast, a daily report that rates the UV conditions from 0 to 10+ in 30 metropolitan areas. The U.S. Environmental Protection Agency releases the forecast, which radio and television stations broadcast during weather reports as a public service. Depending on the numerical rating, called the UV Index, sun-sensitive people are advised to take protective measures (Fig. 65-10). A sensometer, a credit card–sized device, also is available so that a person can determine the UV level in his or her immediate locale.

Client and Family Teaching 65–2
Performing a Skin Self-Examination

The nurse emphasizes the following points when teaching the client and family:

- Allow time after a shower or bath for the examination.
- Ensure that there is adequate light to facilitate inspection.
- Use a full-length mirror and hand-held mirror.
- Examine the skin from head to toe, including the back, scalp, genital area, and between the buttocks.
- Commit the location, appearance, and feel of birthmarks, moles, and other skin lesions to memory or photograph them for future comparisons.
- Look for any changes in previous skin characteristics or the development of something new.
- Inspect the scalp by moving the hair with a comb or blow dryer; when examining the posterior scalp, another person may be helpful.
- Look at the front and back of the body as well as the left and right sides. It is also important to check the fingernails, toenails, soles of the feet, and between the toes.
- Report information about the skin examination to a physician.

Adapted from: National Cancer Institute. (2005). How to do a skin self-exam. http://www.cancer.gov/cancertopics/wyntk/skin/page13. Accessed October 2008.

SCALP AND HAIR DISORDERS

Some conditions are unique to the scalp and hair. They include inflammatory and noninflammatory scalp conditions and disorders that cause hair loss.

SEBORRHEA, SEBORRHEIC DERMATITIS, AND DANDRUFF

Seborrhea and dandruff are noninflammatory conditions that usually precede or accompany seborrheic dermatitis. Seborrheic dermatitis has an inflammatory component.

Pathophysiology and Etiology

Seborrhea is a dermatologic condition associated with excessive production of secretions from the sebaceous glands. Although seborrhea is not always confined to the scalp, it is one of the primary sites. *Seborrheic dermatitis* presents as red areas covered by yellowish, greasy-appearing scales. *Dandruff*, on the other hand, is loose, scaly material of dead, keratinized epithelium shed from the scalp in clients who may or may not have seborrheic dermatitis. Dermatologists believe that a tiny fungus known as *Pityrosporum ovale* causes dandruff. Most people harbor this fungus, yet only some people develop dandruff. Some possible factors for this phenomenon include excessive perspiration, inadequate diet, stress, and hormone activity.

Scalp conditions cause more of a cosmetic rather than a health problem. They usually necessitate retreatment. They do not progress or transform into other serious skin disorders.

Assessment Findings

Clients note that the hair is unusually oily. There may be red or scaly patches on the scalp. White flakes fall from the hair and become more obvious when they collect on the shoulders of dark clothing. The inflamed areas may itch.

No diagnostic testing is necessary unless the condition does not respond to treatment. In that case, a skin biopsy or laboratory blood work is performed to eliminate the possibility that the condition was misdiagnosed.

Medical Management

Frequent shampooing with or without a medicated product helps reduce oil in the scalp and hair. Effective medicated shampoos contain tar, zinc pyrithione, selenium sulfide, sulfur, or salicylic acid. Some clients require topical applications of corticosteroids.

Nursing Management

The nurse explains the underlying cause. He or she reviews the directions and frequency for using medications. The nurse informs clients that the disorder may recur and that persistent treatment is necessary to control the condition.

ALOPECIA

Alopecia means "baldness." The condition affects the hair follicles and results in partial or total hair loss. It is normal to shed 50 to 100 hairs a day, which are replaced by new ones from the same hair follicles. In some cases, however, hair loss is excessive, which may be temporary or permanent.

Alopecia is not life-threatening; however, whenever men or women lose their hair, most experience self-consciousness and lose self-confidence. Many spend great sums of money on unscientific methods for restoring hair growth. Although not everyone can be helped, several options are available to clients with hair loss.

Pathophysiology and Etiology

Hair loss can develop for several reasons. In cases of temporary hair loss, possible causes include medications such as antineoplastic drugs, inadequate diet, thyroid disease, tinea infection, improper application of hair care products, and hair styles that pull the hair tightly.

Alopecia areata and androgenetic alopecia are two chronic conditions that are difficult to reverse. Alopecia areata is believed to be an autoimmune disorder characterized by patchy areas of hair loss about the size of a coin. It can progress to total hair loss and even loss of hair from the entire body. Antibodies attack and destroy the hair follicle.

Androgenetic alopecia is a genetically acquired condition; many refer to it as *male pattern baldness*. The term is somewhat inaccurate because it also affects women, although to a milder degree. A person inherits androgenetic alopecia from his or her mother or father. When testosterone, an androgenic hormone, combines with an enzyme, 5-alpha-reductase, in the hair follicle, hair production stops. This condition begins in adolescence or early adulthood and progresses with age.

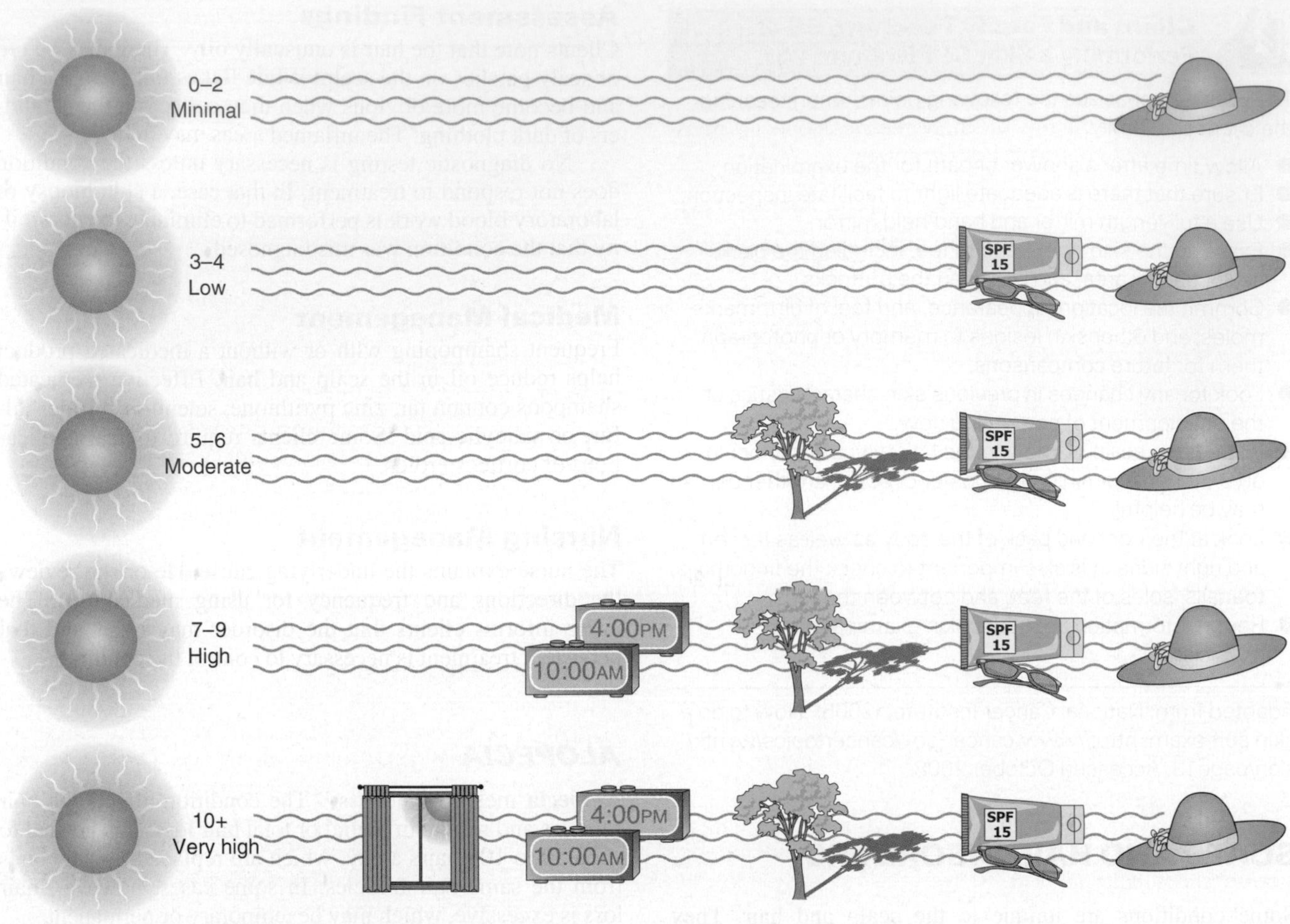

FIGURE 65-10. Sun protection measures based on the UV index.

Assessment Findings

Clients note that their hair is thinning or falling out in patches in several areas of the scalp. Those with a family history of baldness tend to lose hair in the lateral frontal areas or over the vertex of the head (Fig. 65-11). Women report thinning in the frontal, parietal, and crown regions. Primary hair loss is not associated with any other physical health problems.

Diagnostic tests are performed to determine any physical disorder that is contributing to the hair loss. When results are negative, the family history and pattern of hair loss suggest hereditary baldness or an autoimmune disorder.

Medical Management

If a medical disorder causes hair loss, relieving the cause usually restores hair growth. Some drugs can retard hair loss

and promote hair growth. Examples of drugs for alopecia include minoxidil (Rogaine) and finasteride (Propecia); however, the hair growth that is stimulated has a downy texture. If a client discontinues minoxidil or finasteride, hair growth stops and baldness recurs. Finasteride is contraindicated for use by women because it is an androgenic inhibitor. Young clients who begin drug therapy when hair loss is minimal obtain the best results. A hair addition is a technique for giving the appearance of more hair by attaching extra hair to the client's natural hair.

Surgical Management

Some clients who are balding prefer a more permanent solution with hair replacement surgery or other surgical techniques. Hair grafting is a technique for transplanting

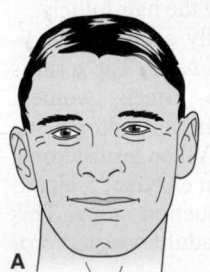 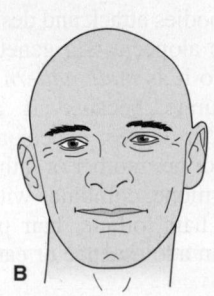 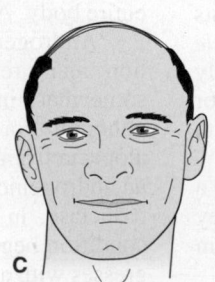 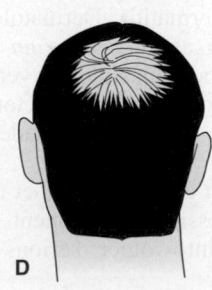

FIGURE 65-11. Patterns of hair loss. (**A** and **B**) Alopecia areata; (**C** and **D**) androgenetic alopecia.

hair-bearing scalp from the back and sides of the head into bald areas. Each graft contains from one to eight hairs. A bald area that is approximately 3 inches square requires approximately 500 to 600 hair grafts. Unfortunately, because of the progressive nature of androgenetic alopecia, transplanted hairs may not survive permanently.

A procedure that disguises hair loss is a scalp reduction that surgically removes a bald area. A scalp reduction usually is performed along with hair grafts. Another surgical technique is to transfer a skin flap. The flap transfers the greatest amount of hair in a short amount of time. However, the scalp may have to be expanded before surgery to stretch the flap area because the flap remains attached in its original location at one end.

Nursing Management

The nurse supports clients who may not have the financial means for medical or surgical treatment. He or she reassures them that they can cope with hair loss. The nurse suggests consulting a cosmetologist who can provide a haircut and style that minimizes the appearance of hair loss. He or she tells women to opt for loose styling rather than ponytails or braids. The nurse recommends using a conditioner or detangler after shampooing to avoid pulling hair from the head and a wide-toothed comb or brush with smooth tips.

HEAD LICE

An infestation with lice is called **pediculosis**. Although lice can infest any hairy parts of the body such as the pubic area, they are more likely to be found on and in the hair on the head.

Pathophysiology and Etiology

Lice are crawling brown insects about the size of sesame seeds; they do not fly or jump (Fig. 65-12). Nymphs look like moving dandruff, but they may appear red after feeding. Adult lice and nymphs creep over the skin and feed on human blood. The bites result in itching. Eggs, or **nits**, laid by adult females, are tightly cemented to the side of hair shafts. They look like small, yellowish-white ovals. Nits

hatch in 7 to 10 days. Lice have a life span of approximately 30 days, during which time one female can lay 100 to 400 nits. Researchers believe that lice are developing strains that resist chemical extermination.

Lice are transmitted through direct contact. They cannot survive longer than about 24 hours without blood. Sharing clothing, combs, and brushes promotes transmission. Anyone can acquire lice, but infestations among school children tend to be difficult to arrest. Many schools have a "zero tolerance" policy for lice infestation; that is, they bar an infected child from attending school until the hair and scalp are free of lice and nits.

Assessment Findings

Itching of the scalp is the most common complaint. Intense scratching can lead to a secondary infection. The adult forms of lice are difficult to see because they quickly move away from light. The nits cling to hairs close to 1/20 to 1/4 inch from the scalp.

Diagnosis is made by scalp and hair inspection. Live lice are retrieved with tweezers or the adhesive side of tape.

Medical Management

Nonprescription shampoos, gels, and liquids containing pediculicides are effective. One example is permethrin liquid (Nix), which kills adult forms of lice. Other over-the-counter products such as RID, Pronto, and A-200 contain pyrethrin, a natural insecticide from the chrysanthemum, and piperonyl butoxide. The National Pediculosis Association opposes the use of strong chemicals such as lindane (Kwell), which is neurotoxic, and those that contain benzene, which is carcinogenic, especially in children. Pediculicides are contraindicated for some individuals (see Client and Family Teaching 65-3). Nits and live lice are removed mechanically with a fine-toothed combing tool such as the LiceMeister.

Nursing Management

The nurse teaches school volunteers and parents how to detect and recognize lice and nits. Those who have not learned this measure may mistake other hair and scalp conditions for lice and unnecessarily stigmatize children who are dismissed from school. The nurse removes nits and lice and teaches the family to do likewise using the information in Client and Family Teaching 65-3.

The nurse instructs the client or family not to shampoo or rinse with a conditioner before applying the pediculicide. Conditioner coats the hair and protects the nits. The nurse instructs clients to follow the label directions on the pediculicide; leaving the chemical(s) on for longer than 10 minutes or covering the head with a shower cap does not increase effectiveness and, in fact, may increase the potential for toxicity.

Nurses, especially those employed in school systems, can provide clients with important information on detection, elimination, and prevention of reinfestation. Some facts to include are as follows:

- Anyone can become infected; infestation is no reflection on hygiene or living conditions.

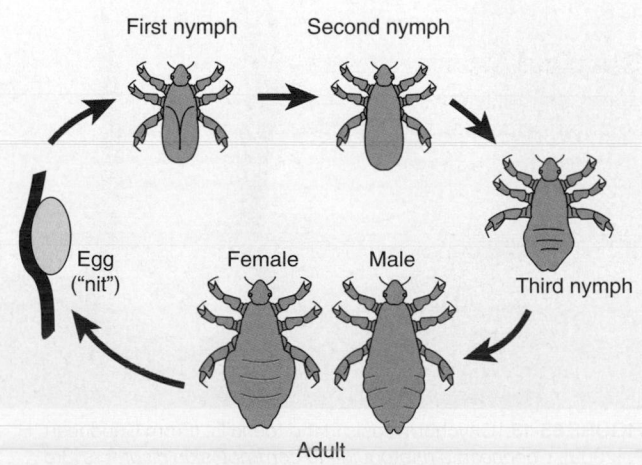

FIGURE 65-12. The life cycle of head lice.

Client and Family Teaching 65-3
Removing Nits and Lice

The nurse provides the following instructions:

- Cut long hair to make it more manageable.
- Apply the pediculocide to the hair.
- Seat the infested client where there is good light.
- Comb the hair free of tangles while the hair is damp.
- Divide the hair into sections.
- Lift a 1-inch strand of hair from a hair section.
- Use a special lice comb that has narrow stainless steel teeth (available from the National Pediculosis Association).
- Start at the crown and comb firmly, deeply, and evenly away from the scalp to the end of the hair.
- Pin back or secure the combed strand and hair section before going to another area.
- Redampen the uncombed hair if it begins to dry.
- Dip the comb in water or wipe it with a paper towel periodically to remove dead lice and their eggs, or pull dental floss through the teeth of the comb.
- Deposit debris in a sealable plastic bag.
- Unfasten the sectioned hair and rinse the head thoroughly.
- Assume that some lice will be missed.
- Repeat combings daily until there no longer is any evidence of lice or nits.

- Perform hair inspection whenever there is an outbreak (even if asymptomatic). However, there is no value in using a pediculicide prophylactically.
- Know how to treat a lice infestation. If everyone who is infested with lice follows the prescribed treatment, the outbreak can be controlled and eliminated. Manual removal is one of the best and safest options for eliminating lice and nits.
- Do not use pediculicides in women who are pregnant or nursing. These agents are also contraindicated in children younger than 2 years of age and in clients who have health conditions such as open wounds, epilepsy, or asthma.
- Never use a pediculicide on the eyebrows or eyelashes.
- Do not use pediculicides on pets—they do not harbor lice.
- Wash clothing and vacuum furniture, bedding, and carpets.

> **Stop, Think, and Respond Exercise 65-1**
>
> What information is helpful for parents whose children acquire head lice?

NAIL DISORDERS

The nails, especially toenails, are subject to disorders. Two common conditions include fungal infections, known as *onychomycosis,* and ingrown toenails, technically called *onychocryptosis.*

ONYCHOMYCOSIS

Onychomycosis is a fungal dermatophyte infection of the fingernails or toenails. A fungus is a tiny, plantlike parasite that thrives in warm, dark, moist environments. Fungi can spread unchecked from one nail to another. They more commonly affect the toenails because conditions inside shoes are perfect for breeding fungi.

Pathophysiology and Etiology

Onychomycosis and tinea pedis (athlete's foot) often occur together. Older adults and immunocompromised clients are at greater risk for fungal infections. The incidence of fungal fingernail infections has increased among women who have artificial nails. Unsanitary cleansing of nail-application utensils between customers in salons seems to be the mode of transmission.

The fungi relocate themselves from the surrounding skin to beneath the nail plate. The fleshy portion underneath the nail becomes inflamed. The nail becomes elevated, thickens, loosens, and changes color. Eventually the nail plate is destroyed. The longer the infection is present, the more difficult it is to cure.

Assessment Findings

One or more nails appear grossly different from normal. They are much thicker, causing them to be elevated and distorted. They are yellowed and friable (Fig. 65-13). Because they are difficult to trim, the infected nail(s) may be long and jagged. The pressure and friction from thickened toenails can lead to pain because shoes do not fit comfortably and socks may wear through.

Diagnosis usually is made on the basis of appearance. Microscopic examination of nail scrapings, however, can confirm the diagnosis.

Medical and Surgical Management

Treatment involves prolonged systemic drug therapy with either of two antifungal agents: itraconazole (Sporanox) and terbinafine (Lamisil). Both drugs inhibit fungal enzymes that regulate cell membrane permeability and result in fungal death. Clients take the medications daily for 2 weeks for

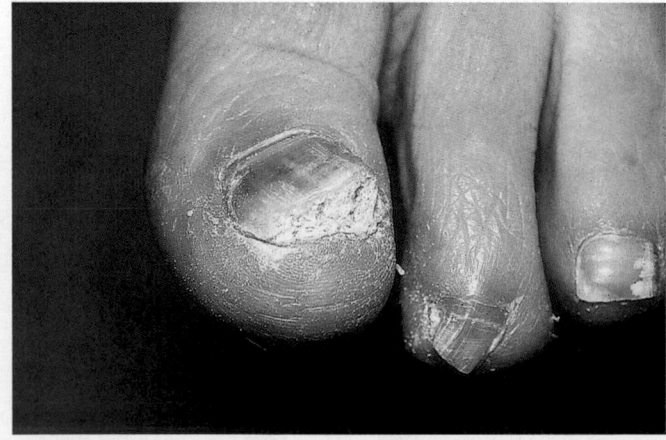

FIGURE 65-13. Onychomycosis in the toenails. (From Goodheart, H. P. [2009]. *Goodheart's photoguide to common skin disorders* [3rd ed.]. Philadelphia: Lippincott Williams & Wilkins.)

fingernail infections and 3 weeks for toenail infections. Terbinafine also can be administered in a pulse-dosing regimen consisting of 1 week of medication followed by a 3-week rest period. Repeated pulse dosing is necessary to eradicate the infection. Drug therapy is more than 50% effective. Because nails grow slowly, it may take as long as 12 months before the nail appears normal.

A more radical solution involves removal of the infected nail. This usually is a last resort because it causes permanent cosmetic changes. Surgery is considered when the condition results in chronic pain or causes difficulty in wearing shoes.

Nursing Management

The nurse reinforces that the condition is chronic and to remain compliant with drug therapy for the duration of treatment. He or she explains the dosing regimen, side effects that may develop, and drug interactions. To prevent reinfection, the nurse reminds clients to:

- Alternate pairs of shoes daily.
- Purchase leather shoes that promote evaporation of foot moisture.
- Never go barefoot.
- Wear footwear at communal pools or when showering in gyms or fitness centers.
- Avoid any damage to the skin around the nail, which makes it easier for fungi to colonize.

ONYCHOCRYPTOSIS

Onychocryptosis is the medical term for an ingrown toenail. This common condition can affect all people, although some are more predisposed than others. It usually affects the inside edge of the great toe. Recurrence tends to be a significant problem.

Pathophysiology and Etiology

Some people have an inherited trait that causes a curvature in the growing nail plate. These clients have a higher incidence of ingrown toenails despite the fit of their shoes or methods for keeping the nails trimmed. The latter two factors, along with fungal nail infections, explain why most others acquire ingrown toenails. Athletes or those who are physically active seem to have repeated episodes as a result of recurring trauma.

When the nail curves during growth, a corner of the nail becomes trapped under the skin. As the nail grows, it cuts into the flesh at the lateral border of the nail. The trauma causes local inflammation. The impaired skin provides an opportunity for bacteria secondarily to invade the traumatized tissue.

Assessment Findings

The client feels local pressure from the abnormal nail growth. Redness, swelling, and pain occur where the nail pierces the adjacent tissue (Fig. 65-14). The corner of the upper nail is embedded in tissue. Purulent drainage and an odor are evident if the tissue is infected. Some people develop compensatory gait and postural changes in an effort to relieve the pain. Physical examination is sufficient for diagnosis.

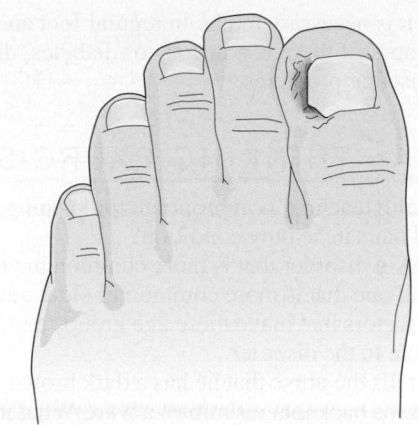

FIGURE 65-14. Infected ingrown toenail.

Medical and Surgical Management

Treating the infection, if present, is as important as correcting the nail disorder. Local or systemic antibiotic therapy sometimes is prescribed. Applications of hydrogen peroxide are used to loosen and remove exudate. To promote healing, the foot is soaked in warm water and Epsom salts, followed by thorough drying. A wedge of cotton may be inserted to lift the corner of the nail. Clients with diabetes or peripheral vascular disease are referred to a **podiatrist**, a person trained to care for feet. Older clients and those with chronic diseases are especially susceptible to traumatic complications that can impair circulation and necessitate amputation.

For persistent or recurrent ingrown toenails, surgery is indicated. Various techniques are used to remove the nail border, not the entire nail, and its root. Surgical procedures are done in the physician's office using local anesthesia or a laser to vaporize the abnormal tissue. Chemical cauterization controls bleeding, and no sutures are required. The client temporarily may need to wear a slipper or shoe from which the toe has been cut out until the swelling and discomfort subsides, but he or she can resume most activities immediately.

Nursing Management

The nurse explains how to perform foot-soaking regimens and techniques to relieve the pressure around the ingrown nail. If surgery is performed, the nurse instructs the client how to change the dressing, the frequency of dressing changes, and signs of infection or compromised circulation to report immediately to the surgeon.

The nurse provides the following information to affected clients:

- Wear wide shoes and loose socks with sufficient room for the toes.
- Use nail clippers rather than scissors to trim toenails. Toenails should be trimmed so that they are slightly longer than the end of the toes, without rounding off of the corners.
- Keep the feet clean and dry.
- Avoid physical activities that involve sudden stops, such as playing basketball, which jams the toes into the front of the shoe.

In addition, it is necessary to obtain regular foot and nail care from a podiatrist if there is a history of diabetes, diminished vision, or vascular problems.

CRITICAL THINKING EXERCISES

1. What health teaching is appropriate for keeping the skin, hair, and nails in healthy condition?
2. Name a skin disorder that is more common in younger adults and one that is more common in older adults. Discuss the factors that make these age groups particularly susceptible to the disorder.
3. A client tells the nurse that he has a dark brown raised lesion on his back that resembles a wart. What information can the nurse provide?
4. A child is sent home from school with a note about being infested with head lice. What can the nurse tell the mother?

NCLEX-STYLE REVIEW QUESTIONS

1. Which area of health teaching is essential when a female client is prescribed isotretinoin (Accutane) for treating acne vulgaris?
   1. Prevention of sexual transmitted infec-tions
   2. Methods for predicting ovulation
   3. Breast self-examination techniques
   4. Techniques for avoiding pregnancy

2. When a client with shingles (herpes zoster) asks what causes the disease, what is the most correct reply?
   1. It is caused by a vector-borne insect, such as a tick.
   2. It is caused by a toxin from a bacterial infection.
   3. It is caused by the reactivation of a dormant virus.
   4. It is caused by an antigen-antibody response.

3. A nurse assesses a client with psoriasis at a dermatology clinic. When examining the skin of this client, what is the nurse is most likely to observe?
   1. A red rash containing raised pustules.
   2. Weeping skin lesions on the trunk of the body.
   3. Red skin patches covered with silvery scales.
   4. Fluid-filled blisters surrounded by crusts.

4. What is the best nursing advice for people who have frequent outbreaks of tinea pedis (athlete's foot)?
   1. Never go barefoot when outdoors.
   2. Cut the nails straight across.
   3. Wear different shoes each day.
   4. Avoid wearing white cotton socks.

5. A biopsy of a scalp lesion of an Anglo-American client reveals the presence of a basal cell carcinoma. Which of the following characteristics most likely contributes to developing skin cancer?
   1. Chronic cigarette smoking
   2. Male pattern baldness.
   3. Eating very few vegetables
   4. Bathing with a deodorant soap

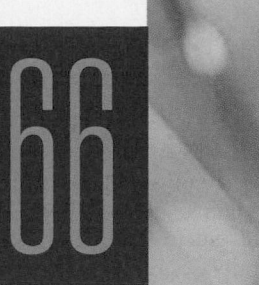

66

Caring for Clients with Burns

Learning Objectives

On completion of this chapter, you will be able to:

1. Explain how the depth and percentage of burns are determined.
2. Name three life-threatening complications of serious burns.
3. Differentiate between open and closed methods of wound care for burns.
4. Name three sources of skin grafts.
5. Describe nursing management for the client with a burn injury.

Approximately 1 million people in the United States seek treatment for burn injuries, most of which are minor (Naradzay & Alson, 2006). The incidence of burns is decreasing (American Burn Association, 2000), but approximately 40,000 people sustain a major burn and require hospitalization (American Burn Association, 2007). The American Burn Association (2007) estimates that 4000 people die from burns each year. The risk for acquiring a burn injury is highest among children and adults older than 60 years of age. The most common causes of thermal burns in older adults are scalding and home fires; these fires are secondary to smoking, alcohol ingestion, or flammable substances that ignite materials (National Fire Protection Association, 2008, Van Houten, 2007).

This chapter reviews types of burns, their physiological consequences, essential assessments of caring for clients with burns, and the principles and techniques of burn management.

BURN INJURIES

A burn is a traumatic injury to the skin and underlying tissues. Heat, chemicals, or electricity cause burn injuries. Burns caused by electricity are characteristically the most severe because they are deep. Furthermore, electricity moving through the body follows an undetermined course from entrance to exit, causing major damage in its path.

Pathophysiology and Etiology

The immediate initial cause of cell damage is heat. The severity of the burn is related to the temperature of the heat source, its duration of contact, and the thickness of the tissue exposed to the heat source. The location of the burn also is significant. Burns in the perineal area are at increased risk for infection from organisms in the stool. Burns of the face, neck, or chest have the potential to impair ventilation. Burns involving the hands or major joints can affect dexterity and mobility.

Thermal injuries cause the protein in cells to coagulate. Chemicals such as strong acids, bases, and organic compounds yield heat during a reaction with substances in cells and tissue. They subsequently liquefy tissue and loosen the attachment to nutritive sublayers in the skin. Electrical burns and lightning also produce heat, which is greatest at the points of entry to and exit from the body. Because deep tissues cool more slowly than those at the surface, it is difficult initially to determine the extent of internal damage. Cardiac dysrhythmias and central nervous system complications are common among victims of electrical burns.

The initial burn injury is further extended by inflammatory processes that affect layers of tissue below the initial surface injury. For example, protease enzymes and chemical oxidants are proteolytic, causing additional injury to healing tissue and deactivation of tissue growth factors. Neutrophils, whose mission is to phagocytize debris, consume available oxygen at the wound site, contributing to tissue hypoxia. Injured capillaries thrombose, causing localized ischemia and tissue necrosis. Bacterial colonization, mechanical trauma, and even topically applied antimicrobial agents further damage viable tissue.

Serious burns cause various neuroendocrine changes within the first 24 hours. Adrenocorticotropic hormone (ACTH) and antidiuretic hormone (ADH) are released in response to stress and hypovolemia. When the adrenal cortex is stimulated, it releases glucocorticoids, which cause hyperglycemia, and aldosterone, a mineralocorticoid, which causes sodium retention. Sodium retention leads to peripheral edema as a result of fluid shifts and oliguria. The client eventually enters a hypermetabolic state that requires increased oxygen and nutrition to compensate for the accelerated tissue catabolism.

After a burn, fluid from the body moves toward the burned area, which accounts for edema at the burn site. Some of the fluid is then trapped in this area and rendered unavailable for use by the body, leading to intravascular fluid deficit. Fluid also is lost from the burned area, often in extremely large amounts, in the forms of water vapor and seepage. Decreased blood pressure follows. If physiologic changes are not immediately recognized and corrected, irreversible shock is likely. These changes usually happen rapidly and the cli-

ent's status may change from hour to hour, requiring that clients with burns receive intensive care by skilled personnel.

Fluid shifts, electrolyte deficits, and loss of extracellular proteins such as albumin from the burn wound affect fluid and electrolyte status. Anemia develops because the heat literally destroys erythrocytes. The client with a burn experiences hemoconcentration when the plasma component of blood is lost or trapped. The sluggish flow of blood cells through blood vessels results in inadequate nutrition to healthy body cells and organs.

Myoglobin and hemoglobin are transported to the kidneys, where they may cause tubular necrosis and acute renal failure.

The release of histamine as a consequence of the stress response increases gastric acidity. The client with a burn is prone to developing gastric ulcers.

Inhalation of hot air, smoke, or toxic chemicals, accompanying injuries such as fractures, concurrent medical problems, and the client's age increase the mortality rate from burn injuries.

 Gerontologic Considerations

- Burns can result in serious complications in older adults because aging is associated with diminished renal, cardiac, and respiratory function. Client teaching should include information about reducing flame and scald burns that occur in home settings.

Depth of Burn Injury
One method for determining the extent of injury is to assess the depth of the burn. Burn depth is classified as follows (Fig. 66-1):

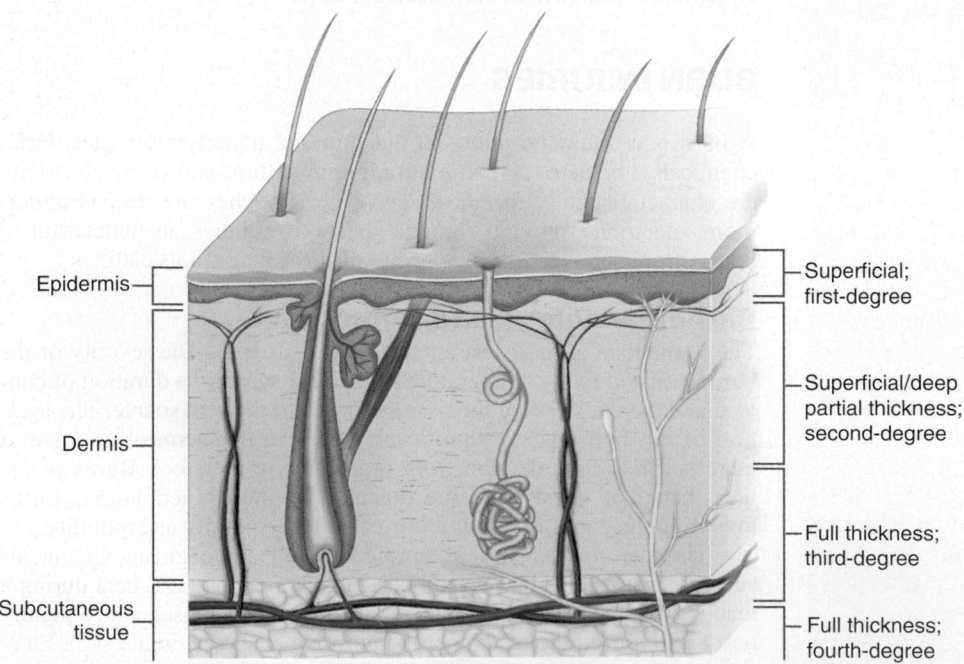

Epidermis

Dermis

Subcutaneous tissue

Superficial; first-degree

Superficial/deep partial thickness; second-degree

Full thickness; third-degree

Full thickness; fourth-degree

FIGURE 66-1. Depths of burn injury.

TABLE 66-1 Depth of Burn Injuries

TYPE	DEPTH	CHARACTERISTICS
Superficial (first degree)	Epidermis and part of dermis	Painful with pink or red edema, but subsides quickly; no scarring
Superficial partial thickness (second degree)	Epidermis and dermis, hair follicles intact	Mottled pink to red, painful, blistered or exuding fluid, blanches with pressure
Deep partial thickness (second degree)	Deeper layer of the dermis with damage to sweat and sebaceous glands	Variable color from patchy red to white, wet or waxy dry, does not blanch with pressure, sensitive to pressure only
Full thickness (third degree)	Epidermis, dermis, subcutaneous tissue	Red, white, tan, brown, or black; leathery covering (eschar); painless
Full thickness (fourth degree)	Epidermis, dermis, subcutaneous tissue; may include fat, fascia, muscle, and bone	Black; depressed; painless; scarring

1. Superficial (first degree)
2. Superficial partial thickness and deep partial thickness (second degree)
3. Full thickness (third and fourth degree)

Burn depth is determined by assessing the color, characteristics of the skin, and sensation in the area of the burn injury (Table 66-1).

A *superficial burn* is similar to a sunburn. The epidermis is injured, but the dermis is unaffected. Although the burn is red and painful, it heals in less than 5 days, usually spontaneously with symptomatic treatment. Infection, increased metabolism, and scarring do not occur.

A *partial-thickness burn* is classified as either superficial or deep partial thickness, depending on how much dermis is damaged. A *superficial partial-thickness burn* heals within 14 days, with possibly some pigmentary changes but no scarring; it requires no surgical intervention (Fig. 66-2 *A*). A *deep partial-thickness burn* takes more than 3 weeks to heal, may need debridement, is subject to hypertrophic scarring, and may require skin grafts (see Fig. 66-2 *B*).

A *full-thickness burn* destroys all layers of the skin and consequently is painless (Fig. 66-3). The tissue appears charred or lifeless. If not debrided, this type of burn injury leads to sepsis, extensive scarring, and contractures. Skin grafts are necessary for a full-thickness burn because the skin cells no longer are alive to regenerate. The most serious burn can involve muscle and bone.

Zones of Burn Injury

Determining the depth of a burn is difficult initially because there are combinations of injury zones in the same location (Fig. 66-4). The *zone of coagulation,* which is at the center of the injury, is the area where the injury is most severe and usually deepest. The area of intermediate burn injury is referred to as the *zone of stasis.* It is here that blood vessels are damaged, but the tissue has the potential to survive. If circulation is secondarily impaired, however, injured tissue in the zone of stasis can convert to a zone of coagulation. The *zone of hyperemia* is the area of least injury, where the epidermis and dermis are only minimally damaged. Because the early appearance of the burn injury can change, the estimate of burn depth may be revised in the first 24 to 72 hours.

Extent of Burn Injury

Besides determining the burn depth and zones, the severity of a burn also is determined by assessing the percentage of

burn injury. The "Rule of Nines" (Fig. 66-5) is a quick initial method of estimating how much of the client's skin surface is involved. Another quick assessment technique is to compare the client's palm with the size of the burn wound. The palm is approximately 1% of a person's total body surface area (TBSA).

Special charts and graphs, such as the one shown in Figure 66-6, provide more precise estimates for determining the percentage of the TBSA that is burned. A computerized assessment tool is available that calculates percent TBSA,

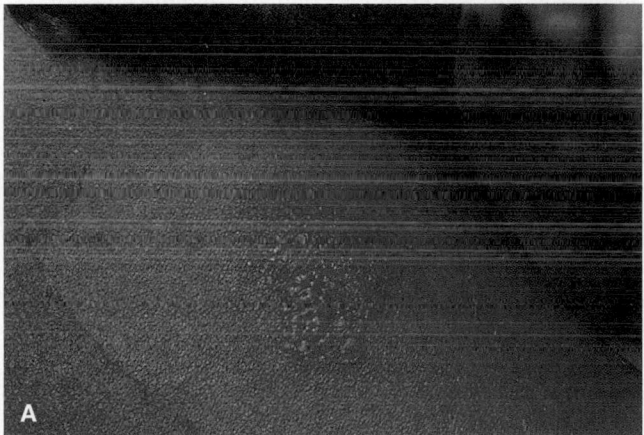

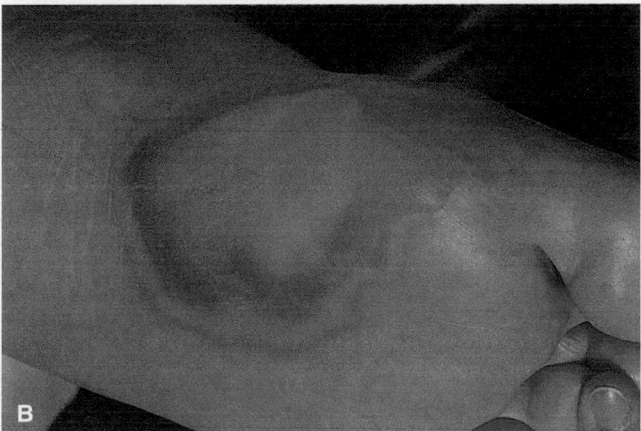

FIGURE 66-2. (A) Superficial partial thickness burn. **(B)** Deep partial-thickness burn.

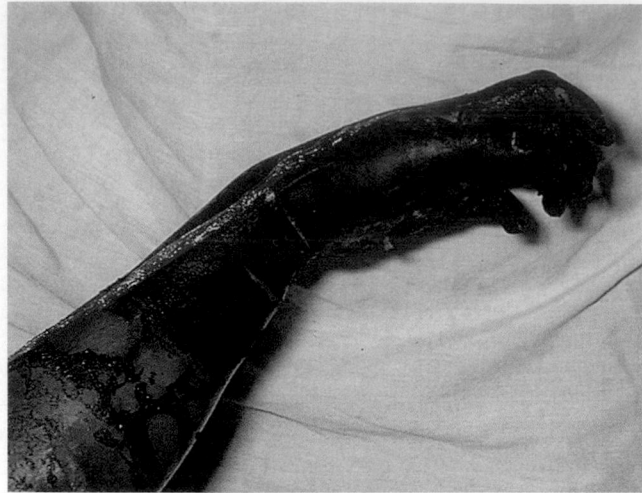

FIGURE 66-3. Full-thickness burn.

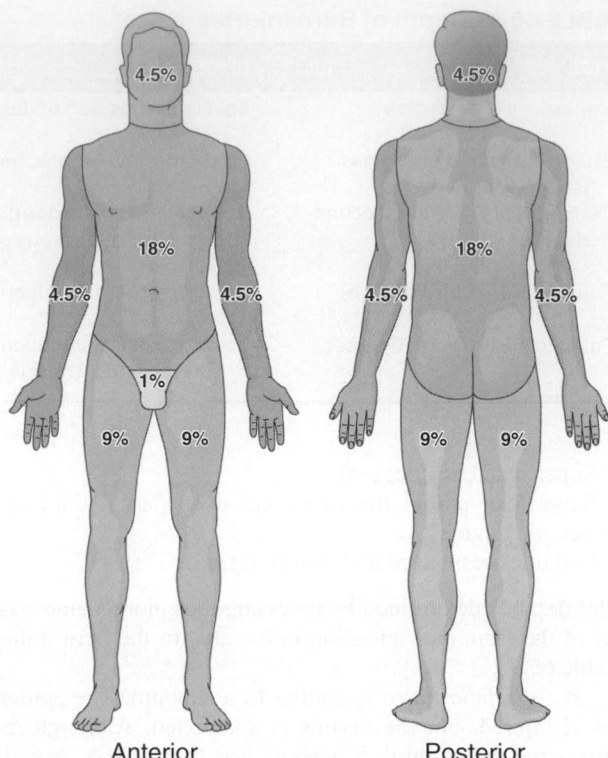

FIGURE 66-5. Rule of Nines. This method is used to estimate the percentage of total body surface area (TBSA) affected by a burn injury.

fluid resuscitation requirements for burns exceeding 20% using the Parkland formula (discussed later), and wound coverage for skin grafting (http://www.sagediagram.com).

▶ *Stop, Think, and Respond Exercise 66-1*

Using the Rule of Nines, calculate the TBSA that is burned if the burn includes one arm and the anterior chest.

Assessment Findings

Skin color ranges from light pink to black, depending on the depth of the burn. There may be edema or blistering. The client experiences pain in all areas except those affected by full-thickness burns. Clients with extensive burns may exhibit symptoms of hypovolemic shock, such as hypotension,

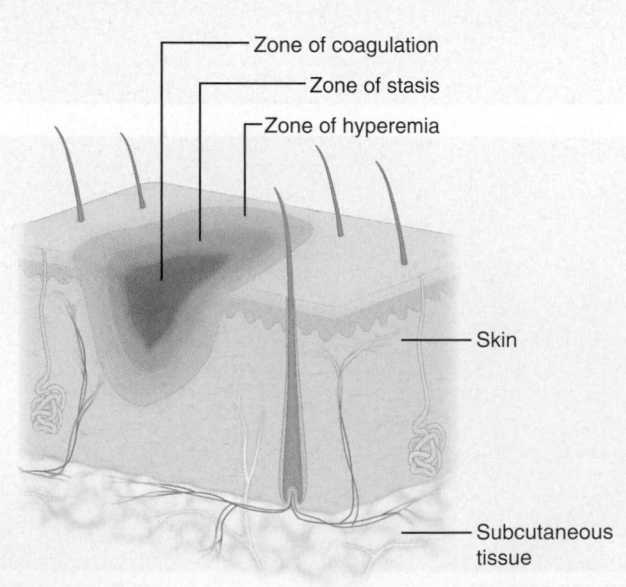

FIGURE 66-4. Zones of burn injury.

tachycardia, oliguria, or anuria. Breathing may be compromised (Box 66-1). In electrical burns, there usually are entrance and exit wounds.

Diagnosis is made by physical inspection. Radiographs identify secondary injuries such as fractures or compromised lung function in inhalation injuries.

Medical Management

The outcome of a burn injury depends on the initial first aid provided and the subsequent treatment in the hospital or burn center. Any one of three complications—inhalation injury, hypovolemic shock, and infection—can be life-threatening. Clients with major burns are transported to a regional burn center (Box 66-2).

Initial First Aid

At the scene of a fire, the first priority is to prevent further injury to the affected person. If the clothing is on fire, the client is placed in a horizontal position and rolled in a blanket to smother the fire. Laying the client flat prevents the fire, hot air, and smoke from rising toward the head and entering the respiratory passages. The client is taken to a hospital immediately thereafter for examination. During transport, other people who have been burned around the face or neck or who may have inhaled smoke, chemicals, steam, or flames are observed closely for respiratory difficulties. Inhalation of such substances can damage or severely irritate the mucous membrane lining the respiratory passages, resulting in edema of the respiratory tract. In addition, secretion of mucus may be excessive, which also makes

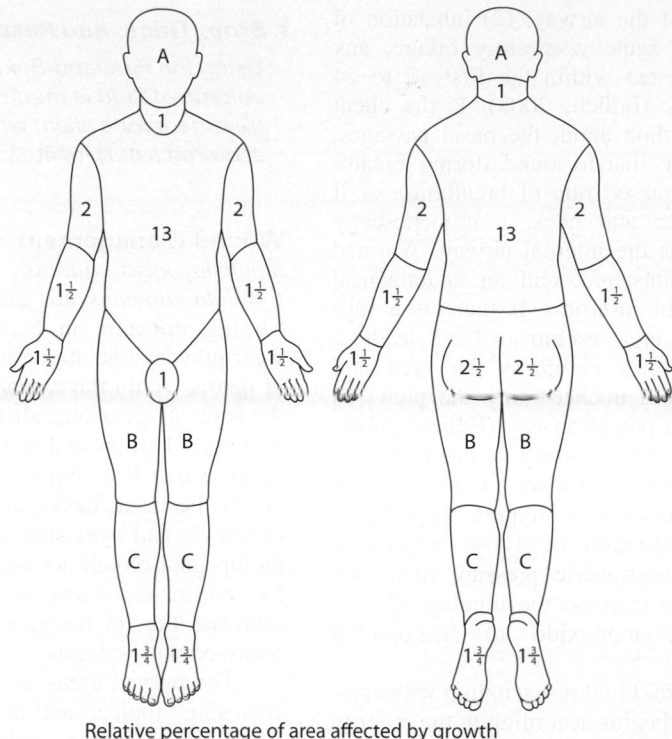

Relative percentage of area affected by growth

Age in years	0	1	5	10	15	Adult
A-1/2 of head	9 1/2	8 1/2	6 1/2	5 1/2	4 1/2	3 1/2
B-1/2 of one thigh	2 3/4	3 1/4	4	4 1/4	4 1/2	4 3/4
C-1/2 of one leg	2 1/2	2 1/2	2 3/4	3	3 1/4	3 1/2

	Superficial	Deep
	%	%
Region		
Ant. head (face)		
Post. head		
Neck		
Ant. trunk		
Post. trunk		
Right arm		
Left arm		
Right hand		
Left hand		
Buttock		
Genitalia		
Right leg		
Left leg		
Right foot		
Left foot		
Subtotals		
Totals		

FIGURE 66-6. The Lund and Browder burns assessment chart is the most accurate method for estimating percentage of body surface area burned according to age and growth size.

breathing difficult. Oxygen is administered, and intravenous (IV) fluid therapy is begun en route.

Acute Care

When the client with a burn arrives, the medical team works quickly to assess the extent of burn injury and additional trauma such as fractures, head injury, and lacerations. Team members implement several aspects of burn treatment, including maintaining adequate ventilation and initiating fluid resuscitation. Impaired ventilation is associated with a burn involving the upper airway and

---

BOX 66-1 **Signs of Heat or Smoke Inhalation Injury**

- Sore throat
- Singed nasal hairs, eyebrows, eyelashes
- Hoarseness
- Carbon in sputum
- Soot around mouth or nose
- Shortness of breath
- Stridor

BOX 66-2 **American Burn Association Referral Criteria**

- Partial- or full-thickness burn greater than 10% TBSA for those younger than 10 or older than 50 years of age
- Partial- or full-thickness burn greater than 20% TBSA in other age groups
- Partial- or full-thickness burn involving the face, hands, feet, genitalia, perineum, and major joints
- Full-thickness burn greater than 5% TBSA in any age group
- Electrical burn, including one caused by lightning
- Chemical burn
- Inhalation injury
- Burn injury with a preexisting medical disorder (e.g., diabetes, heart disease)
- Burn complicated by trauma
- Burn victim taken first to a hospital without qualified personnel or equipment for the care of burned children
- Burn injury in children who will require social/emotional and/or long-term rehabilitation, including cases involving suspected child abuse or substance abuse

results from (1) swelling of the airway, (2) inhalation of carbon monoxide, and (3) acute respiratory failure, any or all of which are manifested within the first 12 to 24 hours after the burn injury (Edlich, 2008). If the client has soot or evidence of carbon about the nasal passages, difficulty breathing, **stridor** (harsh sound during breathing), or **tachypnea** (an increased rate of breathing), or if there is edema of the face and neck, a bronchoscopy may be performed to assess the internal airway. Warmed humidified oxygen is administered, and an endotracheal tube should be available for insertion. If there is a full-thickness burn in the neck area, **eschar** (a hard, leathery crust of dehydrated skin) may compress the neck and pull it into flexion, making a tracheostomy the preferred technique for maintaining a patent airway (Edlich, 2008). Mechanical ventilation may be necessary to maintain normal blood gases and prevent respiratory failure. Victims of carbon monoxide poisoning may require **hyperbaric oxygen treatment** (administration of 100% oxygen at three times greater than atmospheric pressure in a specially designed chamber) to increase the binding of oxygen rather than carbon monoxide to hemoglobin molecules.

Blood samples are drawn. Fluid resuscitation with crystalloid and colloid solutions begins according to the severity of the burn injury (Table 66-2). The fluid-replacement regimen is calculated from the time the burn injury occurred; any fluid infused by emergency medical personnel is factored into the replacement volume. The goals of fluid resuscitation include (1) restoration of intravascular volume, (2) prevention of tissue and cellular ischemia, and (3) maintenance of vital organ functions. Successful fluid resuscitation is gauged by a urinary output of 0.3 to 0.5 mL/kg/ hour via an indwelling catheter. A low-dose infusion of dopamine (Intropin) may be necessary to ensure renal perfusion (Edlich, 2008).

IV analgesics are administered for pain, which often is severe. Morphine sulfate is generally the drug of choice. Doses as high as 50 mg/hr may be necessary in adults who are severely burned (Eldich, 2008). If respiratory depression develops, the physician will administer naloxone (Narcan), an opiate antagonist. A tetanus immunization is also administered.

> ▶ **Stop, Think, and Respond Exercise 66-2**
>
> Using the Parkland-Baxter formula, determine what volume of fluid is required during the first 24 hours of treatment for a client who weighs 168 lbs and has acquired a burn of 40% TBSA.

Wound Management

Staphylococcus aureus, Pseudomonas aeruginosa, and *Candida albicans* are the most common microorganisms causing infection in burned tissue. Healthcare providers wear powder-free sterile gloves to reduce the accumulation of debris within the wound, which may complicate healing. As soon as possible, all the client's clothing is removed. The body hair around the perimeter of the burns is shaved, because hair is a source of bacterial wound contamination. When the head, neck, and upper chest are burned, singed eyebrows and eyelashes are clipped, scalp hair is shaved, the lips and mouth are cleansed, and the lips are lubricated. Eye ointments or irrigations are used to remove dirt and to lubricate the lid margins. Blisters that have ruptured are removed with scissors.

The burned areas are cleansed to remove debris. After cleansing, topical antimicrobial medications are applied. Wound management includes the **open method**, in which the wound is left uncovered, or the **closed method**, in which the wound is covered. The closed method involves the use of one or more types of dressing materials (Table 66-3). The final step is closing the wound with a skin graft or skin substitute or applying cultured skin.

Open Method

The open method (exposure method), which exposes the burned areas to air, has been virtually abandoned since the advent of effective topical antimicrobials. It still is used on a small scale, however, for burned areas such as the face and perineum, where it is difficult to apply dressing materials.

If the open method is used, the client is placed in isolation in a bed with sterile linen. Health team members and visitors wear sterile gowns and masks. The skin of the client

TABLE 66-2 Fluid Resuscitation Formulas

FORMULA	FLUIDS	AMOUNT*	EXAMPLE FOR 220-LB VICTIM WITH 50% BURN
Brooke (modified)	Lactated Ringer's	2 mL/kg/% burn	10,000 mL†
	Second 24 hours	0.3–0.5 mL/kg/% burn	1500–2500 mL
	Colloid (plasma, albumin, dextran)	Approximate evaporative losses	2000 mL (avg.)
	5% Glucose/water		
Parkland-Baxter	Lactated Ringer's	4 mL/kg/% burn	20,000 mL†
Evans	Saline	1 mL/kg/% burn	5000 mL
	Colloid	1 mL/kg/% burn	5000 mL
	5% Glucose/water	Approximate evaporative losses	2000 mL (avg.)

*Goal: Establish urine output of 50 mL/hour.

†Half of fluid volume given in first 8 hours; remaining half in next 16 hours; time is calculated from time of burn injury, not time fluid resuscitation begins.

TABLE 66-3 Open and Closed Methods of Burn Care

TYPE	ADVANTAGES	DISADVANTAGES
Open method	Reduces labor-intensive care Causes less pain during wound care Facilitates inspection Decreases expense	Contributes to wound desiccation (dryness) Promotes loss of water and body heat Exposes wound to pathogens Contributes to pain during repositioning Compromises modesty
Closed method	Maintains moist wound Promotes maintenance of body temperature Decreases cross-contamination of wound Provides wound debridement during dressing removal Keeps skin folds separated Reduces pain during position changes	Requires more time Adds to expense Enhances growth of pathogens beneath dressings Interferes with wound assessment Causes more blood loss with removal Can interfere with circulation if tightly applied

with a burn is sensitive to drafts and temperature changes; therefore, a bed cradle or sheets are placed over the client. The room is kept warm and humidified.

A hard crust forms over a partial-thickness burn in 2 or 3 days, and **epithelialization** (regrowth of skin) is completed in about 2 or 3 weeks. At this time, the crust falls off, is debrided, or is loosened by whirlpool baths. Eschar forms in areas of full-thickness burns. If the eschar constricts the area and impairs circulation, an **escharotomy** (an incision into the eschar) is done to relieve pressure on the affected area (see Fig. 66-3). A dressing may be used to cover the exposed areas as the eschar is removed. New skin cannot grow beneath eschar.

Closed Method

The closed method is the current preferred method of wound management. First, the burn area is covered with nonadherent and absorbent dressings, which consist of gauze impregnated with petroleum jelly or ointment-based antimicrobials and fluffed gauze pads. The final covering is an occlusive or semiocclusive dressing made of polyvinyl, polyethylene, polyurethane, and hydrocolloid materials. Occlusive dressings prevent bacteria from contact with the wound but are minimally permeable to water and oxygen. Various topical antimicrobials are applied to the burn wound to discourage the growth of pathogens or control or eliminate any infection that develops. The trend is to change the wound dressing once a day to minimize pain. More frequent dressing changes occur when the wound is infected or when there is significant saturation with wound exudates.

▶ **Stop, Think, and Respond Exercise 66-3**

If a person is seriously burned, which method of wound management would you expect the burn unit to use? Give at least three reasons for your answer.

Antimicrobial Therapy

Three major antimicrobials are used to treat burns: silver sulfadiazine (Silvadene) 1% ointment is the most commonly used antimicrobial, followed by mafenide (Sulfamylon), and silver nitrate ($AgNO_3$) 0.5% solution (Drug Therapy Table 66-1). Acticoat is a dressing that contains a thin, soluble film coat of silver and can remain on the burn for up to 5 days,

which greatly reduces the pain associated with dressing changes. Aquacel Ag is a topical dressing to which silver has been added for the management of partial-thickness burns. It is rated as better than silver sulfadiazine, the most commonly used topical antimicrobial. It releases the silver within the dressing for up to 2 weeks, thus requiring fewer dressing changes; this translates into a reduction in nursing care time and client discomfort. The dressing generates a faster rate of epithelialization, produces less burning or stinging, and reduces scar height (Mishra et al., 2007).

Other commonly used drugs are povidone-iodine (Betadine), gentamicin (Garamycin) 0.1% cream, nitrofurazone (Furacin), mupirocin (Bactroban), clotrimazole (Lotrimin), and ciclopirox (Loprox). Povidone-iodine is contraindicated with some skin substitutes (discussed later) because it can damage new tissue growth in the wound bed.

Topical antimicrobials have various advantages and disadvantages (See Drug Therapy Table 66-1). All drugs are applied using sterile technique. Because infection is the rule rather than the exception, the client may require systemic antibiotics and antifungals. Some examples include amphotericin B (Fungizone) and penicillin G (Pfizerpen).

Surgical Management

Additional treatment modalities to promote healing include debridement, skin grafting, application of a skin substitute, and application of cultured skin.

Debridement

Wound **debridement** is the removal of necrotic tissue. Debridement is accomplished in one of four ways:

- Naturally as the nonliving tissue sloughs away from uninjured tissue
- Mechanically when dead tissue adheres to dressings or is detached during cleansing
- Enzymatically through the application of topical enzymes to the burn wound
- Surgically with the use of forceps and scissors during dressing changes or wound cleansing

A disadvantage of surgical debridement is bleeding. Burn victims already have secondary problems with healing

DRUG THERAPY TABLE 66-1 Topical Antimicrobial Agents for Burn Injuries

Drug	Considerations for Use	Advantages	Disadvantages
silver sulfadiazine (Silvadene)	Topical cream containing antimicrobials, silver, and a sulfonamide, to prevent or manage infections in burn wounds	Cream with broad-spectrum properties Relatively painless when applied Easy to apply using sterile gloved hands	Minimal penetration of eschar May cause a rash or allergic reaction in those sensitive to sulfonamides Transient leukopenia Forms a gelatinous cover over the burn wound that can be removed Bacterial resistance can develop
mafenide acetate (Sulfamylon)	Topical antimicrobial cream to control or prevent bacterial gram-positive or gram-negative infections within the burn wound and on skin grafts requiring moist dressings	Most effective antimicrobial because it penetrates eschar Can be used as an open method of burn management or with closed method Preferred for electrical burns	Causes severe burning for 20 minutes post-application, which requires premedication Contraindicated in clients who are hypersensitive to mafenide acetate Use may result in metabolic acidosis when applied to extensive partial- or full-thickness burns
silver nitrate	Broad-spectrum agent for bacteriostatic use in partial- and full-thickness burns Currently being replaced by dressings impregnated with silver such as Acticoat and Aquacel Ag	Solution for application Low cost Not associated with bacterial resistance	Does not penetrate eschar Requires frequent dressing changes or repeated saturation of dressings Hypotonic solution may decrease electrolyte level Stains the skin and burn wound black as well as anything it contacts; staining interferes with wound assessment

because of preexisting low red blood cell counts that the accompanying blood loss potentiates.

After dead tissue is removed, it is imperative that the healthy tissue be covered with a skin graft, a temporary skin substitute, or cultured skin.

Skin Grafting

Superficial burns heal when keratinocytes from the periphery and beneath the dermis proliferate to regenerate the epidermis. Skin grafting is necessary for deep partial-thickness and full-thickness burns because the skin layers responsible for regeneration have been destroyed. Unassisted healing, that is, healing without the use of skin grafts or skin substitutes, results in the proliferation of granulation tissue. Granulation tissue contains fibroblasts, which create hypertrophic scars that contract and pull the edges of the wound together, causing contractures. Large burns may not be able to granulate fully, resulting in chronic open wounds.

The purposes of a skin graft are to:

- Lessen the potential for infection
- Minimize fluid loss by evaporation
- Hasten recovery
- Reduce scarring
- Prevent loss of function

Sources of Skin Grafts

Several sources are available for skin grafting. An **autograft** uses the client's own skin, which is transplanted from one part of the body to another. Only autograft or skin transplanted from one identical twin to another can become a permanent part of the client's own skin.

An **allograft** or homograft is human skin obtained from a cadaver. Allografts temporarily cover large areas of tissue. Although allografts slough away after approximately 1 week, they last for the critical period until the client's own skin can be used for skin grafting. Cadaver skin usually is in short supply; although the tissue is screened for human immunodeficiency virus and hepatitis, concerns remain that it could be a source of other pathogens.

A **heterograft** or xenograft is obtained from animals, principally pigs. Like allografts, heterografts temporarily cover large sites. Allografts and heterografts are rejected in days to weeks and must be removed and replaced at that time.

Types of Autografts

Human skin from the client with a burn is harvested under general anesthesia. Either a split-thickness or full-thickness graft is removed. In a **split-thickness graft**, the epidermis and a thin layer of dermis are harvested from the client's skin. Split-thickness autografts vary in thickness (0.008–0.024 inch), size, and shape and usually are obtained from the buttocks or thighs. A dermatome, a scalpel, or another special instrument is used to remove the skin from the donor site. Split-thickness autografts have more successful outcomes than other types; however, their cosmetic appearance is less than desirable, they are less elastic, and hair does not grow from their surface.

A **full-thickness graft**, which may be 0.035-inch thick, includes epidermis, dermis, and some subcutaneous tissue. This type of graft is used when the burned area is fairly small or involves the hands, face, or neck. Full-thickness grafts are more comparable in appearance to normal skin and can tolerate more stress once they become permanently attached to the burn wound.

A **slit graft** (also called a *lace* or an *expansile graft*) is used when the area available as a donor site is limited, as in clients with extensive burns. The skin is removed from the donor site and passed through an instrument that slits it; thus, a smaller piece of skin is stretched to cover a larger area (Fig. 66-7).

Harvesting the client's own tissue has several disadvantages: (1) it compounds the client's pain because it creates a new wound, (2) the donor site has the potential for scarring and atypical pigment changes, (3) there is a potential for donor site infection, (4) there is a delay in wound closure while waiting for the donor site to heal and be reharvested, and (5) delays caused by waiting for harvest sites to heal increase costs and challenge the client's ability to cope with a prolonged hospitalization. It may be virtually impossible to harvest sufficient skin to close totally a full-thickness burn wound that is greater than 60% TBSA (Schulz et al., 2000). Regardless of the source of the skin grafts, it is imperative to limit movement for some time to prevent disrupting the graft.

Once the skin graft heals, pressure garments made of elasticized cloth or plastic are applied over the grafted area (Fig. 66-8). These garments smooth the grafted skin, reducing scarring and the potential for wound contractures. The client may need to wear a pressure garment for up to 2 years (Client and Family Teaching 66-1).

The client is also advised to use sunscreen with a high sun protection factor (SPF) when outdoors to prevent permanent pigment changes in the healing skin. Scarring can be further reduced by applying Mederma, a topical gel, to the skin 3 to 4 times a day for up to 6 months, or Cica-Care, a silicone gel sheet. One gel sheet can be used for up to 28 days. Manufacturers of these products claim that they minimize the visibility of scars by reducing their dark pigmentation and flattening the raised scar tissue (Burn Survivor Resource Center, 2002).

Skin Substitutes

Scientists are creating alternative materials referred to as *skin substitutes* that cover the wound and promote healing. These

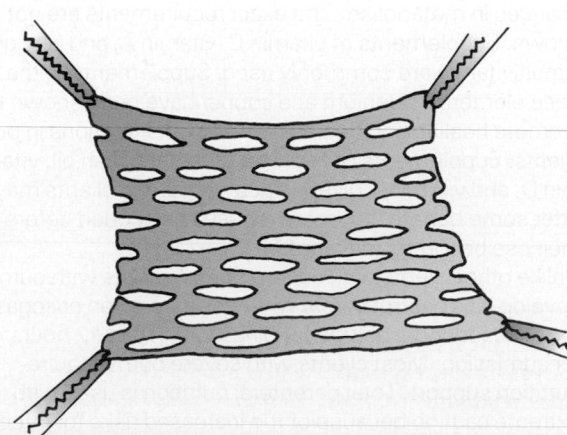

FIGURE 66-7. A slit graft. The slits allow for stretching to cover a larger area of tissue.

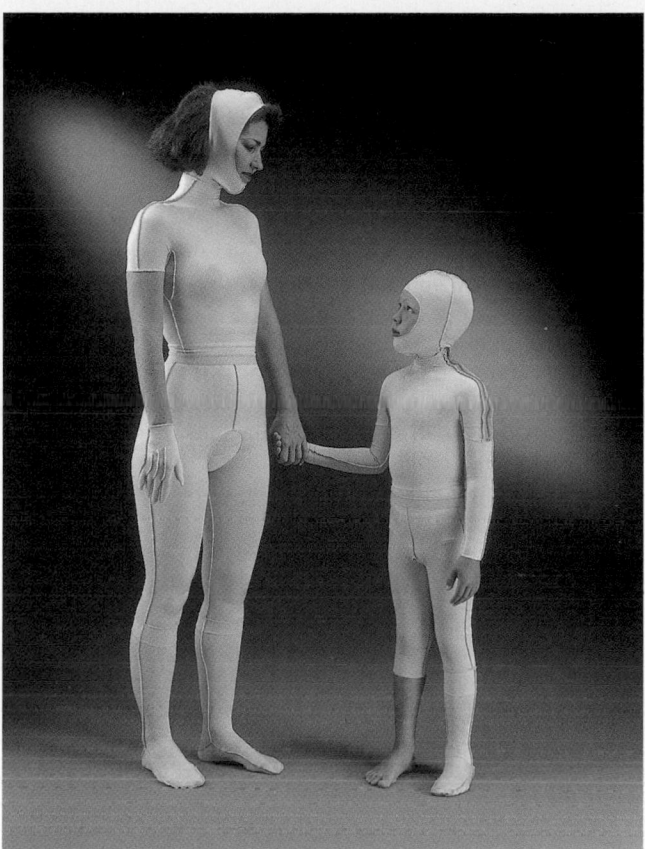

FIGURE 66-8. Elastic pressure garments. (Used with permission of Jobst Institute, Inc., Toledo, OH.)

 Client and Family Teaching 66-1
Use of a Pressure Garment

The nurse teaches the client and family to:

- Wear the pressure garment at least 23 hours each day.
- Follow the manufacturer's instructions for donning and removing the pressure garment.
- Contact the physician or physical therapist if the garment causes discomfort or does not seem to fit properly.
- Ensure that holes or nonfunctioning zippers are repaired immediately or as soon as possible.
- Hand-wash the pressure garment daily with a mild laundry detergent.
- Rinse the garment thoroughly to remove detergent residue, salt water, or chlorinated water from a swimming pool.
- Squeeze and roll the garment in a towel to remove as much moisture as possible; do not wring the garment.
- Hang the garment to dry at room temperature away from direct heat; do not dry the garment in the sun or in a clothes dryer.
- Massage any moisturizers, lotions, creams, petroleum-based ointments completely into the skin, because these can cause deterioration of the garment.

Adapted from Burn Survivor Resource Center, Medical care guide: Pressure garments. Available at http://www.burnsurvivor.com/presure_garments.html. Accessed October 2008.

bioengineered coverings promote wound healing by interacting directly with body tissues. Skin substitutes can be applied all over the burn wound as soon as the skin is cleaned and debrided instead of having to wait until enough skin is available for grafting purposes.

Several skin substitutes are available. Biobrane is a nylon-silicone membrane coated with a protein derived from pig tissue (Fig. 66-9). TransCyte is created by culturing human fibroblasts from the dermis with a biosynthetic semipermeable membrane attached to nylon mesh. Integra consists of a two-layer membrane: one is a synthetic epidermal layer, and the other contains cross-linked collagen fibers that mimic the dermal layer of skin. The pseudodermal layer becomes a permanent cover; the outer layer, which provides a barrier against pathogens, is removed in 2 to 3 weeks and replaced with a thin autograft. The thin autograft heals in only a few days and provides a better cosmetic appearance.

Cultured Skin

Another alternative for covering the wound, especially if it is massive, is to culture the client's skin in a laboratory. Cultured skin is a wound-closure product that is developed by growing the client's own skin cells in a laboratory culture medium. From a piece of postage stamp–sized skin, it is possible to grow sufficient skin to cover nearly the entire body in 3 weeks. A skin substitute is used to cover the burn wound while the skin culture is growing.

Once sufficient cultured cells are available, they are combined with a fabric material made from collagen that dissolves after it is applied to the wound. The burn wound heals in 2 to 3 weeks without traditional skin grafting. The only current disadvantage to this method of using cultured skin is that the pigmentation does not perfectly match the original skin color; however, scientists are working on eliminating this problem. At the Cincinnati Shriners Hospital for Children, researchers are attempting to modify cultured skin genetically (1) to reduce infection during healing, (2) to allow for the formation of sweat glands and hair follicles, and (3) to allow for the production of pigment

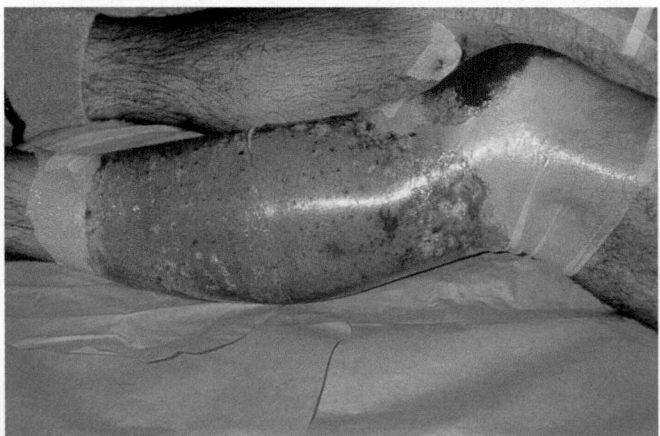

FIGURE 66-9. Biobrane dressing applied to lower extremity partial-thickness burn. (Used with permission of Dow Hickam Pharmaceuticals.)

(Singer, 2007). In the United Kingdom, physicians are taking a postage suspension of cultured skin cells then spraying it on the burned area. The advantages of the latter include increased rate of healing as well as improved overall function and cosmetic appearance (Petherick & Harder, 2005).

Nursing Management

Nursing management focuses on assessing the wound and determining how the burn injury has affected the client's status. The nurse calculates fluid-replacement requirements and infuses the prescribed volume according to the agency's protocol. He or she quickly recognizes and efficiently treats signs of shock (see Chap. 17). The nurse administers prescribed analgesics to relieve or reduce pain. He or she cleans the wound, applies an antimicrobial agent, and covers the wound with the prescribed dressing. The nurse monitors the wound to determine any infection. He or she helps the client and family cope with the change in body image and encourages the client to perform exercises that minimize contractures. The nurse encourages adequate nutrition and provides supplements as ordered (Nutrition Notes 66-1). Before discharge, the nurse teaches the client about the use of a pressure garment and methods for skin care. Refer to Nursing Care Plan 66-1 for additional nursing management.

Nutrition Notes 66-1
The Client With a Burn Injury

- Extensive burns are one of the most severe forms of stress that a person can experience. Calorie needs may increase to 4000 to 5000 calories/day. Protein needs are typically 2.0 to 2.5 g/kg, especially if burns are >10% of TBSA. Calorie and protein needs increase if complications develop, and they lessen as wound healing progresses.

- Although it is generally agreed that vitamin needs increase in burn clients because of losses from wounds and changes in metabolism, the exact requirements are not known. Supplements of vitamin C, vitamin A, and zinc plus a multivitamin are commonly used. Supplements of the trace elements selenium and copper have been shown to promote healing and decrease the risk of infections in burn clients. Supplements of arginine, glutamine, fish oil, vitamin D, and vitamin K given to acutely burned clients may offer some benefit, but more research is needed before their use becomes mainstream.

- Unlike other clients with severe stress, clients with burns develop less gastroparesis when they are given nasogastric or nasoduodenal tube feedings within 8 to 12 hours after admission. Most clients with severe burns require nutrition support. Total parenteral nutrition is used with extreme caution because of the increased risks for infection and sepsis.

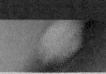

NURSING CARE PLAN 66-1 | The Client With Burns

Assessment

- Determine the type of burn (thermal, chemical, electrical) and when it occurred.
- Assess vital signs.
- Look for evidence of inhalation injury.
- Determine the oxygen saturation and respiratory effort.
- Evaluate pain intensity.
- Determine the volume and characteristics of urine.
- Note the percentage and depth of burn.
- Auscultate bowel sounds.
- Assess for concurrent medical problems, and review the results of laboratory tests.

Depending on the extent and degree of burns, some or all of the following nursing diagnoses may apply. Diagnoses change as the client progresses through treatment and the stages of healing.

Nursing Diagnoses: Risk for Ineffective Airway Clearance related to increased airway secretions; **Risk for Impaired Gas** Exchange related to edema of airway and inhalation of carbon

Expected Outcomes: (1) The airway will be patent. (2) Gas exchange will be adequate as evidenced by clear lung sounds, blood oxygen saturation (SpO_2) greater than 90%, and arterial oxygen pressure (PaO_2) greater than 80 mm Hg.

Interventions	Rationales
Monitor characteristics of respirations and lung sounds frequently.	Frequent focused assessments of respiratory function facilitate early detection of compromised ventilation.
Check respiratory rate before and after administering an opioid analgesic.	Narcotic analgesics depress the respiratory center in the brain.
Measure SpO_2 with a pulse oximeter or analyze arterial blood gas (ABG) results.	The PaO_2 can be determined deductively from the SpO_2; an SpO_2 of 90% or greater suggests that the PaO_2 is at least 80 mm Hg. ABGs provide objective measurements of serum O_2, CO_2, and bicarbonate levels.
Administer oxygen as prescribed.	Supplemental oxygen increases the percentage of inhaled oxygen above that in room air.
Suction the airway cautiously if edema is present.	Suctioning removes accumulated secretions, but the trauma of catheter insertion can worsen edema.
Facilitate ventilation with artificial airways, such as with an endotracheal tube and ventilator.	An artificial airway and ventilator facilitate the maintenance of adequate gas exchange.
Be prepared to assist with an escharotomy if there is a circumferential burn of the chest.	An escharotomy releases constriction and allows greater chest expansion.

Evaluation of Expected Outcomes

Client breathes effortlessly and is well oxygenated.

PC: Hypovolemic Shock

Expected Outcome: Nurse will monitor to detect, manage, and minimize hypovolemia.

Interventions	Rationales
Monitor vital signs every 15 minutes.	Hypotension and tachycardia suggest impending shock.
Measure intake and output hourly.	Hourly measurements facilitate early detection of mismatches between fluid intake and output.
Weigh the client daily at the same time with similar dressings.	A loss of 2 lb in 24 hours suggests a 1-L deficit in fluid.
Administer fluids according to the fluid resuscitation formula.	A large volume of fluid is necessary to prevent hypovolemic shock.
Report urine output of <50 mL/hour.	Urine output < 50 mL/hour suggests inadequate renal perfusion due to hypovolemia or other causes.

Evaluation of Expected Outcome

Client does not experience hypovolemic shock.

Nursing Diagnosis: Acute Pain related to tissue injury

Expected Outcome: Pain will be within client's level of tolerance.

(Continued)

NURSING CARE PLAN 66-1 **The Client With Burns** (Continued)

Interventions	Rationales
Assess pain intensity as needed and whenever you measure vital signs.	Assessing pain is the fifth vital sign.
Administer prescribed IV analgesia.	The IV route facilitates drug distribution when absorption is impaired at other parenteral routes.
Give analgesics prophylactically 30 minutes before dressing changes or débridements.	Preventing severe pain is easier than relieving it.

Interventions	Rationales
Implement nonpharmacologic methods of pain relief: imagery, self-hypnosis, and distraction.	Alternative methods for relieving pain supplement pharmacologic methods.
Place client on a CircOlectric bed or other type of turning frame to facilitate turning and repositioning.	Pain is reduced when the bed turns the client mechanically and passively.
Exercise caution and gentleness when removing and reapplying dressings.	Pain is intensified when movement stimulates intact sensory nerves.

Evaluation of Expected Outcome

Client responds to pain-relieving techniques.

Nursing Diagnosis: Hypothermia related to impaired ability to regulate body temperature

Expected Outcome. Temperature will be in normal range.

Interventions	Rationales
Reduce evaporation from burn wound by humidifying the environment, preventing drafts, and covering the burn wound with ointment, creams, and dressings.	Impaired skin cannot regulate body temperature; reducing the potential for heat loss helps maintain body temperature.

Evaluation of Expected Outcome

Temperature is normal.

PC: Infection related to impaired skin integrity

Expected Outcome: Nurse will monitor to detect, manage, and minimize infection.

Interventions	Rationales
Assess temperature every 4 hours; monitor results of blood counts and cultures.	Fever, leukocytosis, and bacterial growth from a wound culture indicate infection.
Use sterile or clean linen.	Surgical and medical asepsis reduce the potential for infection.
Wear sterile or clean caps, gowns, and masks.	Using outer garments reduces the transmission of pathogens from contaminated clothing to the client.
Restrict infectious people from visiting or caring for client.	Limiting contact with sources of infection protects a susceptible host.
Apply and administer prescribed antimicrobial and antibiotic therapy.	Antimicrobials and antibiotics suppress the growth of pathogens.
Inspect burn areas for healing, drainage, formation of eschar, infection, and stability of the skin graft or wound covering.	Direct observation of the wound and comparing normal and abnormal findings help determine the client's response to treatment.
Accurately record all findings.	

Evaluation of Expected Outcome

Wound infections are eliminated, and the wound heals.

PC: Skin Graft Disruption

Expected Outcome: Nurse will monitor to detect, manage, and minimize skin graft disruption.

Interventions	Rationales
Avoid excessive pressure on grafted area; minimize movement.	Relief of pressure and restricting movement promote vascularization.
Assist physician with dressing changes.	Graft disruption is minimized when the nurse assists the physician and client.
Monitor color and odor in the area of grafted tissue.	A pale color suggests ischemia. A dark appearance suggests poor venous outflow. A foul odor suggests colonization with bacteria.

NURSING CARE PLAN 66-1   The Client With Burns (Continued)

Evaluation of Expected Outcome

The burn wound is covered; skin grafts are viable.

PC: Gastric and Intestinal Paresis (Hypomotility) and Peptic Ulcer

Expected Outcome: Nurse will monitor to detect, manage, and minimize gastrointestinal hypomotility and peptic ulcer.

Interventions	Rationales
Assess for abdominal distention and status of bowel sounds.	Abdominal distention and diminished or absent bowel sounds suggest impaired peristalsis.
Insert a prescribed nasogastric tube; connect it to low intermittent suction.	Negative pressure removes gas and secretions from the upper gastrointestinal tract.
Administer IV histamine antagonists and drugs such as metoclopramide (Reglan).	Histamine antagonists raise the pH of gastric secretions and reduce the potential for gastric mucosal irritation. Metoclopramide promotes stomach emptying.
Instill antacid through nasogastric tube; clamp for 30 minutes before reconnecting to suction.	Antacids neutralize stomach acid.
Assess pH of gastric secretions every shift; report if pH is less than 3.	Drug therapy should raise gastric pH above 3; if not, the physician may choose to include a proton pump inhibitor such as omeprazole (Prilosec) or a cytoprotective agent such as misoprostol (Cytotec).

Evaluation of Expected Outcome

Bowel sounds are active in all abdominal quadrants; client experiences no epigastric distress.

Nursing Diagnosis: Risk for Constipation related to fluid loss, decreased oral nutrition, inactivity, and narcotic analgesia

Expected Outcome: Client will pass stool regularly and with ease.

Interventions	Rationales
Monitor bowel elimination.	Infrequent and difficult bowel elimination with passage of dry hard stool indicates constipation.
Provide a generous volume of oral liquids, fresh fruit and vegetables, and whole grains when the client is allowed oral intake.	Cellulose is undigested fiber and pulls water into the intestine creating a bulkier, moist stool that is easy to eliminate.
Administer prescribed stool softener or laxatives.	Laxatives promote bowel elimination by increasing intestinal bulk and stimulating motility. Stool softeners draw water into the fecal mass, easing elimination.
Remove any fecal impactions.	Impacted stool is difficult to pass and may require digital removal.

Evaluation of Expected Outcome

Bowel movements are regular; stool is moist and easily passed.

PC: Anemia related to destruction of red blood cells (RBCs) and blood loss from stress ulcer

Expected Outcome. Nurse will monitor to detect, manage, and minimize anemia.

Interventions	Rationales
Monitor hemoglobin and hematocrit laboratory results.	Decreased hemoglobin and hematocrit values suggest blood loss.
Check gastric secretions and stool for occult or frank blood.	Identifying the source of blood loss helps the physician prescribe additional medical interventions to alleviate the problem.
Administer whole blood or packed RBCs as prescribed.	Administration of blood helps replace depleted RBCs.
Provide iron-rich food or supplements when it is safe to use the oral route.	The heme component of hemoglobin contains iron.

Evaluation of Expected Outcome

Erythrocyte, hemoglobin, and hematocrit values are within normal ranges.

Nursing Diagnosis: Risk for Imbalanced Nutrition: Less than Body Requirements related to increased caloric requirements and inability to ingest food orally

Expected Outcome: Nutritional intake will compensate for a hypercatabolic state.

(Continued)

NURSING CARE PLAN 66-1 **The Client With Burns** (Continued)

Interventions	Rationales
Administer total parenteral nutrition (TPN) until tube or oral feedings are initiated.	TPN provides calories and essential nutrients that meet metabolic needs.
Monitor weight loss or gain.	Weighing the client helps determine if dietary management is adequate.
Provide high-protein, iron-rich foods in small, frequent feedings when oral nourishment is allowed.	Protein facilitates cellular growth and repair. Iron prevents nutritional anemia. Small, frequent meals are likely to provide sufficient calories.

Evaluation of Expected Outcome

Client maintains weight, with no evidence of malnutrition, vitamin deficiencies, electrolyte imbalance, or muscle wasting.

Nursing Diagnosis: Impaired Physical Mobility related to pain, bulky dressings, and contracted skin secondary to scar formation

Expected Outcome: Range of motion and muscle strength will be preserved or restored.

Interventions	Rationales
Keep joints in burned areas neutral: extended rather than flexed.	A neutral position facilitates functional use.
Exercise uninvolved joints actively; exercise involved joints during hydrotherapy.	Exercise promotes muscle tone and strength. Exercising in water reduces resistance to work.
Encourage performance of activities of daily living (ADLs), such as brushing teeth and eating.	Performing ADLs is a form of active exercise that maintains the flexibility of joints and muscle tone.

Evaluation of Expected Outcome

Client regains functional use of joints in burn areas.

Nursing Diagnosis: Risk for Disturbed Thought Processes related to reduced mental stimulation, sleep deprivation, social isolation, fluid and electrolyte imbalance, narcotic administration, and sepsis

Expected Outcome: Client will remain oriented and have realistic perceptions.

Interventions	Rationales
Assess mental status every shift.	Focused assessments facilitate the early detection of problems.
Reorient the confused client.	Providing facts helps the client reorder thinking.
Have a calendar and clock within client's view.	Environmental cues help prevent disorientation.
Discuss current events; encourage visits from family.	Interacting with others and staying aware of current events help stimulate the mind.
Cluster nursing activities to facilitate continuous sleep.	Sleep deprivation contributes to confusion and disorientation.

Evaluation of Expected Outcome

Client logically processes verbal and environmental cues.

Nursing Diagnoses: Risk for Ineffective Coping and **Risk for Ineffective Family Coping: Disabled or Compromise** related to inadequate emotional resources for managing multiple stressors

Expected Outcome: Client and family will adapt and use strategies for effective coping.

Interventions	Rationales
Explain methods and reasons for treatment.	Information helps clarify the plan and assists the client to strive to meet goals.
Acknowledge signs of progress.	Objective evidence of progress sustains motivation.
Involve client and family in long-range planning, physical therapy, and vocational rehabilitation.	A client and family who feel they are part of a team willingly participate in achieving goals.
Refer family to counseling for assistance in managing conflicts.	Health professionals with specialized expertise can help clients and family members solve problems.

Evaluation of Expected Outcome

Client and family cope effectively and use resources wisely to manage client's care.

CRITICAL THINKING EXERCISES

1. Discuss methods used to reduce the potential for infection in a burn wound.
2. While caring for a burn client, the nurse determines the following problems: pain, coughing carbonaceous sputum, and no urinary output since admission 2 hours ago. What should be the nurse's highest priority?
3. Which type of skin graft is best for healing a burn wound?
4. A client who is recovering from a major burn reports that the elastic pressure garment is "too warm" and therefore resists wearing it. How might the nurse respond to this comment by the client?

NCLEX-STYLE REVIEW QUESTIONS

1. A nurse stops to give first aid to a burn victim running from a home that is on fire. The nurse rolls the victim on the ground to smother the flames. The chest and neck of the victim are burned. What is the next priority for the nurse?
   1. Determine the extent of the burn.
   2. Identify the victim's next of kin.
   3. Obtain the victim's pulse and blood pressure.
   4. Monitor the victim for respiratory distress.
2. In the emergency department, it is determined that a burn victim has deep partial- and full-thickness burns over 35% of the upper body. During the nursing assessment of the burn injury, the initial appearance of the full-thickness burn could be described as which of the following?
   1. Mottled and wet
   2. White and leathery
   3. Pink and blistered
   4. Red and painful
3. The blood pressure of a burn victim has stabilized. What is the best means of assessing the client's response to the initial burn treatment?
   1. Range of motion
   2. Urinary output
   3. Level of pain
   4. Body temperature
4. The treatment plan for a burn victim includes using the open method of burn wound management. What is most appropriate for the nurse to monitor when caring for a client being treated by the open method?
   1. Infection
   2. Hyperthermia
   3. Depression
   4. Malnutrition
5. A burn wound periodically is debrided using hydrotherapy. What nursing action is essential shortly before each debridement?
   1. Keep the client in a fasting state.
   2. Witness a signed consent form.
   3. Administer a prescribed analgesic.
   4. Weigh the client on a bed scale.

UNIT 17
Caring for Clients with Psychobiologic Disorders

67

Interaction of Body and Mind

Words To Know

brain mapping
coping mechanisms
distress
eustress
general adaptation syndrome
hardiness
immunopeptides
mental status examination
neuropeptides
neurotransmitters
placebo
placebo effect
psyche
psychobiologic disorders
psychobiology
psychoneuroendocrinology
psychoneuroimmunology
psychosomatic disorders
receptors
soma
stress
stress management
stress-related disorders

Learning Objectives

On completion of this chapter, you will be able to:

1. Discuss new areas of neuroscience being studied to learn more about mind-body connections and their effect on health.
2. Name chemical substances transmitted between neurons, giving examples of each.
3. Explain why mental illnesses are now considered psychobiologic disorders.
4. Name biologic and psychologic components that contribute to disorders affecting the body and mind.
5. List examples of techniques used to assess clients with psychobiologic disorders.
6. Describe treatment and nursing care for psychobiologic disorders.
7. Distinguish between stress, eustress, and distress.
8. Describe the general adaptation syndrome, naming its three stages.
9. Explain the purpose of coping mechanisms and the outcomes that may result from their use.
10. List the defining features of hardiness.
11. Discuss techniques that the nurse can suggest for helping clients cope with stressors.
12. Discuss the rationale for a mind–immune system connection.
13. Discuss four explanations for the development of psychosomatic disorders.
14. Describe treatment and nursing care for psychosomatic disorders.
15. Explain the placebo effect.

The mind and the body were once thought of as completely separate structures. Now more than ever, they are viewed as a single communicating entity. Recent research has uncovered anatomic and chemical links between the body and the mind, and new fields of science have emerged (Box 67-1). This chapter examines the links between the body and mind and their effects on health. The rest of the chapters in this unit discuss disorders that were, and still are by many, considered purely psychological or psychosocial—that is, separate from physiology. Yet evidence supports that these disorders are **psychobiologic disorders,** conditions in which evidence supports a connection between abnormalities in the brain and altered cognition, perception, emotion, behavior, and socialization.

THE BRAIN AND PSYCHOBIOLOGIC FUNCTION

The brain is a complex organ made up of the cerebrum, brain stem, and cerebellum (Fig. 67-1). The *cerebrum* is the brain's largest component. It is the basis for sensory perception, voluntary movement, personality, intelligence, language, thoughts, judgment, emotions, memory, creativity, and motivation. The outer layer of the cerebrum receives, processes, integrates, and relays information to appropriate functional areas of the brain. The *cerebral cortex* is the major pathway of physiologic intercommunication.

The *limbic system* is a network in the brain that contains structures involved in emotions and related physiologic functions. It includes the *thalamus*, which connects many brain centers and modulates movement, sensation, behavior, and emotions. The limbic system also includes the *hypothalamus*, which controls the autonomic nervous system and

coordinates the endocrine and immune systems through pituitary–adrenocortical connections (Porth, 2006). Because of its neuroendocrine and neuroimmunologic roles, the limbic system affects and determines many psychobiologic activities (see Chap. 68).

> **Stop, Think, and Respond Exercise 67-1**
>
> *Which two structures in the brain play the greatest role in connecting the mind with physiologic functions?*

Receptors

Receptors are structures found on the surface of cells throughout the body and brain. Each cell has millions of different receptors. These receptors sense and pick up chemical messengers that arrive in the extracellular fluid. A chemical messenger may be thought of as a specific key that fits into and binds with a specific receptor. Only those messengers that have molecules in exactly the right shape can bind with specific receptors. For example, opiate receptors can bind only with chemicals in the opiate group, such as heroin, morphine, or endorphins. Once binding occurs, the message is received and the cell begins to respond. Chemical messengers may be natural or synthetic, and the message may cause the cell to perform any number of activities. Neurotransmitters are the messengers that play a significant role in regulating all physical, emotional, and mental processes.

Neurotransmitters

Neurotransmitters (Table 67-1) are natural endogenous chemical messengers. They communicate information that affects thinking, behavior, and bodily functions across the synaptic cleft between neurons (Fig. 67-2). The chemicals, which are synthesized in the neurons and then stored in vesicles in the axons, are released and attach themselves (bind) momentarily to the receptors on postsynaptic neurons. After the chemicals have transmitted their information, they are either:

- Broken down into inactive substances by enzymes such as monoamine oxidase, acetylcholinesterase, and so on
- Recaptured by the releasing neuron for later use, a process called *reuptake*
- Weakened by becoming diluted in intercellular fluid.

Neurons are classified by the type of neurotransmitter they release; for example, cholinergic neurons release acetylcholine, and dopaminergic neurons release dopamine.

Neuropeptides are a separate type of neurotransmitter. They include endogenous chemicals such as:

- Substance P, which transmits the sensation of pain (see Chap. 11).
- Endorphins and enkephalins, morphine-like neuropeptides that interrupt the transmission of substance P and promote a feeling of well-being.
- Neurohormones released by interactions between the hypothalamus, pituitary, and the endocrine glands they stimulate.

Different areas of the brain contain different types of neurons with specific neurotransmitters. Each neurotransmitter

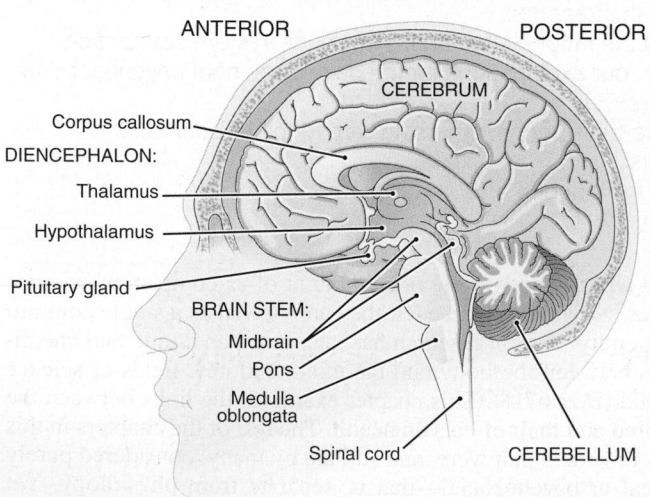

FIGURE 67-1. Brain structures.

TABLE 67-1 Selected Neurotransmitters

NEUROTRANSMITTER	ABBREVIATION	EXAMPLES OF FUNCTIONS
Serotonin (5-hydroxytryptamine)	5-HT	Stabilizes mood Induces sleep Regulates temperature Controls appetite
Dopamine	DA	Integrates thoughts Promotes movement in concert with ACH Stimulates hypothalamic endocrine activity Enhances judgment
Norepinephrine	NE	Affects attention and concentration Raises energy level Heightens arousal
Acetylcholine	ACH	Assists memory storage Promotes movement in concert with DA Prepares for action
Gamma-aminobutyric acid	GABA	Reduces arousal and aggression Inhibits excitatory neurotransmitters like NE and DA Decreases seizure potential
Glutamate	GT	Promotes neuronal excitation Acts as a neurotoxic mediator in various neurologic disorders

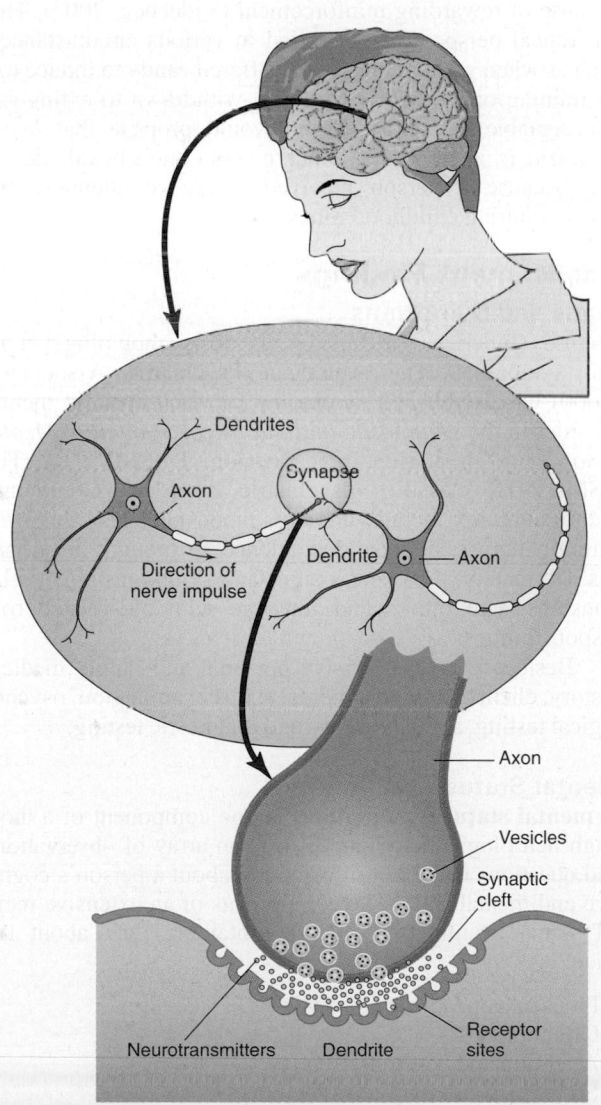

FIGURE 67-2. Neurotransmitter anatomy.

has either a stimulating or inhibiting effect on neurons. All brain function, including thoughts, emotions, or messages to organs and muscles, depends on these neurotransmitters.

Receptors for neurotransmitters and neuropeptides are located not only throughout the CNS, but also in the endocrine and immune systems. This finding suggests that these systems communicate with each other through chemical messages. This concept has tremendous implications for how the mind and emotions can affect physical well-being and how physical status can affect the mind.

PSYCHOBIOLOGIC ILLNESS

Historically, many believed that mental illness resulted from character defects, demonic possession, or punishment by God. These myths persist, which explains why individuals with mental illness sometimes are feared and stigmatized. The study of brain structure, chemistry, and genetics has begun to replace ignorance and misinformation about mental illness with facts. Brain pathology is now seen as the major factor contributing to mental illnesses, now called *psychobiologic disorders*. Some examples of psychobiologic disorders are stress-related/anxiety disorders (see Chap. 68), mood disorders (see Chap. 69), eating disorders (see Chap. 70), chemical dependence (see Chap. 71), and thought disorders (see Chap. 72).

Pathophysiology and Etiology

Biologic Factors

The neurotransmitters dopamine, norepinephrine, epinephrine, serotonin, and acetylcholine often are implicated in the psychobiology of mental illness. Because the neurotransmitters are concentrated in different areas of the brain, disruption of a neurotransmitter system results in the specific symptoms associated with that area of the brain. For example, dopamine influences movement, memory, thoughts, and judgment. The disorganized thought patterns and bizarre behavior of schizophrenia have been correlated with excess levels of dopamine; the impaired balance and uncontrolled tremors of Parkinson's disease have been linked with low levels of dopamine. Serotonin is found in areas that regulate sleep, appetite, sexual behavior, and mood. Imbalances in serotonin are thought to be responsible for depression, eating disorders, sleep disturbances, and obsessive-compulsive disorder. Excessive levels of the neuroexcitatory neurotransmitter glutamate have been implicated in neurodegenerative diseases such as amyotrophic lateral sclerosis, Huntington's disease, and the sequelae of strokes (Sheldon, 2007; Schmidt & Reith, Eds., 2005).

Other insights into brain physiology came from observing the effects of medications on behavior and symptoms (psychopharmacology). The theory that depression results from decreased levels of norepinephrine and serotonin was first suggested when the monoamine oxidase inhibitors, which block the inactivation of norepinephrine and serotonin (see Chap. 69), were found to alleviate depression. Similarly, antianxiety medications such as the benzodiazepines (see Chap. 68) activate gamma-aminobutyric acid (GABA) receptors that inhibit arousal, excitement, and aggression. Riluzole (Rilutek), an antiglutamate drug, has shown therapeutic benefits for the treatment of amyotrophic lateral sclerosis, also known as Lou Gehrig's disease (Sanofi Aventis, 2009).

▶ **Stop, Think, and Respond Exercise 67-2**

If norepinephrine binds to its receptor site on cells, what effects would occur?

Psychological Factors

Psychological factors (forces that shape behavior) also influence psychological equilibrium and may be tied to brain chemistry as well. Some researchers propose that the neurotransmitter network links emotion, memory, and learned behavior (Pert, 1997). Psychological factors have long been components of psychiatric theory and include intrapersonal development, interpersonal interactions, and learning.

Intrapersonal Development

Sigmund Freud proposed that disordered behavior is the result of intrapersonal (within oneself) conflicts that arise during particular stages of development that occur between infancy and adolescence. For example, Freud correlated compulsive neatness and stinginess with rigid toilet training. Freud greatly emphasized sexual aspects of behaviors between an infant and mother, conflicts surrounding toilet training, awareness of gender differences and genital pleasure, rivalry with the same-sex parent, investment of energy in intellectual pursuits, and efforts to establish relationships with members of the opposite sex. Although many of Freud's theories have been questioned, negated, rejected, revised, and expanded, he provided the foundation for the current fields of psychiatry and psychology, and thus many of his tenets have withstood the test of time.

▶ **Stop, Think, and Respond Exercise 67-3**

What do you think may be the physiologic and psychological consequences if an infant is not held very much, is not talked to affectionately, or is ignored when hungry?

Interpersonal Interaction

Other theorists, such as Erik Erikson and Harry Stack Sullivan, proposed that mental health or illness is a consequence of social relationships and interpersonal interactions (Videbeck, 2007). Some theorists go further, suggesting that a person's mental stability is affected not only by relationships with significant others, but also is influenced by social systems, such as neighborhood, city, and country where a person resides. The more positive the social system, the better the chances are that a person will be mentally healthy and well adjusted.

Learning

The psychologist B. F. Skinner proposed the theory that adaptive and maladaptive behaviors are learned and repeated because of rewarding reinforcement (Videbeck, 2007). This theoretical perspective is applied in various circumstances, such as when young children are offered candy to induce toilet training or when privileges are withdrawn to extinguish unacceptable behaviors. Some would propose that *hypochondriasis,* an abnormal concern about one's health, develops because a person received excessive attention and concern during childhood illnesses.

Assessment Findings

Signs and Symptoms

Brain dysfunction can cause a mix of psychobiologic signs and symptoms. The American Psychiatric Association (2000) has established symptoms for each specific mental disorder in the *Diagnostic and Statistical Manual of Mental Disorders* (4th edition, text revision; DSM-IV-TR). The DSM-IV-TR classifies psychiatric disorders. Commonly seen symptoms include anxiety, mood changes, abnormal eating patterns, chemical dependence, or thought disturbances. Ultimately, the client's signs and symptoms affect relationships with others and interfere with age-related role responsibilities.

Besides a comprehensive personal and family medical history, clients undergo a mental status examination, psychological testing, and laboratory and diagnostic testing.

Mental Status Examination

A **mental status examination** is one component of a thorough neurologic examination. It is an array of observations and questions that elicit information about a person's cognitive and mental state. The components of an extensive mental status examination include obtaining data about the client's:

- Physical appearance
- Orientation
- Attention and concentration
- Short-term and long-term memory
- Movement and coordination

- Speech patterns
- Mood
- Intellectual performance
- Perception
- Insight
- Judgment
- Thought content

Nurses regularly conduct Mini-Mental Status Examinations (Box 67-2). Changes in the total score are used to evaluate changes in the client's condition.

Gerontologic Considerations

- Older adults vary in the ability to accurately complete a Mini-Mental Status Examination, depending on cognitive abilities and educational levels.

Psychological Tests
Psychological tests are administered to detect personality characteristics, interpersonal conflicts, and self-concept. Table 67-2 gives examples of various psychological tests.

Diagnostic Findings
Measuring levels of neurotransmitters and neuropeptides is difficult, expensive, and sometimes impossible. Unfortunately, a definitive diagnosis for many psychobiologic disorders usually is achieved by ruling out other diseases that manifest similar symptoms. Chapter 36 provides a description of tests such as electroencephalography (EEG), computed tomography (CT) scan, magnetic resonance imaging (MRI), and positron emission tomography (PET) scan.

One of the newest diagnostic tools, brain mapping, suggests that the future diagnosis of psychobiologic disorders will be more efficient. **Brain mapping** is a technique that compares a client's brain activity patterns (from an EEG or other electronic image) with a computerized database of electrophysiologic abnormalities (Crossroads Institute, 2008). A growing database of distinctive patterns for seizure disorders, schizophrenia, depression, dementia, anxiety disorders, atten-

tion deficit/hyperactivity disorder, and others now exists for comparison.

Medical and Nursing Management
Treatment of psychobiologic disorders depends on the specific diagnosis. Modalities include drug therapy, psychotherapy, cognitive therapy, and behavior modification (see Chaps. 68 through 72). Drug therapy aims at correcting the underlying biochemical abnormality and is particularly useful with mood disorders (see Chap. 69), anxiety disorders (see Chap. 68), and schizophrenia (see Chap. 72). The goals of psychotherapy, cognitive therapy, and behavior modification are to uncover repressed thoughts and emotions and identify healthier coping mechanisms. Nurses play an active role in all aspects of treatment, including administering and monitoring response to drug therapy, implementing behavior modification plans, and providing individual and group counseling.

THE BRAIN AND PSYCHOSOMATIC FUNCTION

In addition to the study of the biologic basis of mental illness, brain chemistry and its effects on physical health are being widely researched as well. Emotions, which originate in brain structures and chemicals, can powerfully influence an individual's health and sense of well-being.

According to Selye's theory (1956), **stress** is a physiologic response to biologic stressors such as surgical trauma or infection, psychological stressors such as worry and fear, or sociologic stressors, including a new job or increased family responsibilities. Stress has been implicated in the development or exacerbation of autoimmune diseases, anorexia nervosa, obsessive-compulsive disorder, panic attacks, thyroid conditions, heart disease, functional and inflammatory disorders of the gastrointestinal tract, chronic pain conditions, and diabetes.

Stress is not an entirely negative concept. Just the right amount of stress, called **eustress**, is what maintains a healthy balance in life. Eustress helps individuals to pursue goals, learn to solve problems, or manage life's predictable and unpredictable crises. Excessive, ill-timed, or unrelieved stress is called **distress**. It triggers the **general adaptation syndrome**, a nonspecific physiologic response to a stressor (Fig. 67-3). This response, which can cycle many times through the alarm and resistance stages before reaching the exhaustion stage, occurs through the neuroendocrine and autonomic nervous systems.

Physiologic Stress Response
The autonomic nervous system consists of the sympathetic and the parasympathetic divisions (see Chap. 36). The most common pathway for the stress response is through the sympathetic division, which uses norepinephrine to stimulate body systems, arousal, and anxiety in response to stress. This response overrides the control of the parasympathetic nervous system, which slows many metabolic processes. A few individuals respond to stressors through the parasympathetic

---

BOX 67-2 · Sample Mini-Mental Status Examination Questions

- What is the year?
- What is today's date?
- In what city (town) are we?
- Spell "globe" backward.
- Repeat the following statement: "A rolling stone gathers no moss."
- Write a sentence of your own choice. (Nurse evaluates whether sentence has a subject, predicate [verb], and object.)

From Folstein, M. E., Folstein, S. E., & McHugh, P. R. (1975). Mini-Mental State: A practical method for grading the cognitive state of patients for the clinician. *Journal of Psychiatric Research, 12*(189). Used with permission.

TABLE 67-2 Psychological Tests

TEST	DESCRIPTION
Minnesota Multiphasic Personality Inventory (MMPI)	This true-or-false test of 550 questions is used to analyze which of nine clinical personality traits are manifested by the client's responses.
Beck Depression Inventory	Client rates self according to statements that concern mood.
Draw-a-Person (tree, house, family) Test	Client's drawing is analyzed for symbolism about his or her self-perception or other emotional data.
Word Association Test	Client is asked to quickly provide a response to words, such as "mother . . . work . . .", etc. Responses are analyzed for psychological significance.
Thematic Apperception Test (TAT)	Client is asked to look at pictures and then tell a story about them. Recurring themes in the stories suggest the underlying basis of emotional problems.
Rorschach Test	The client is asked to indicate what he or she sees in each of 10 separate inkblots.

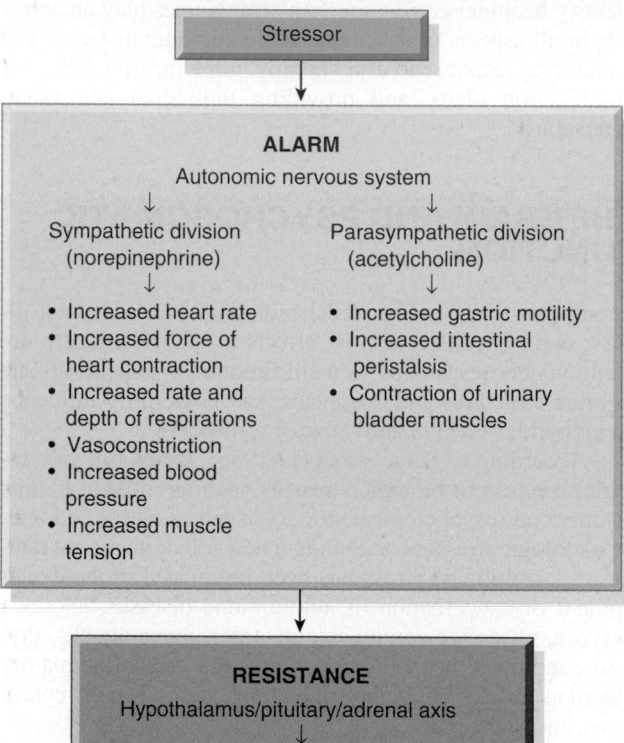

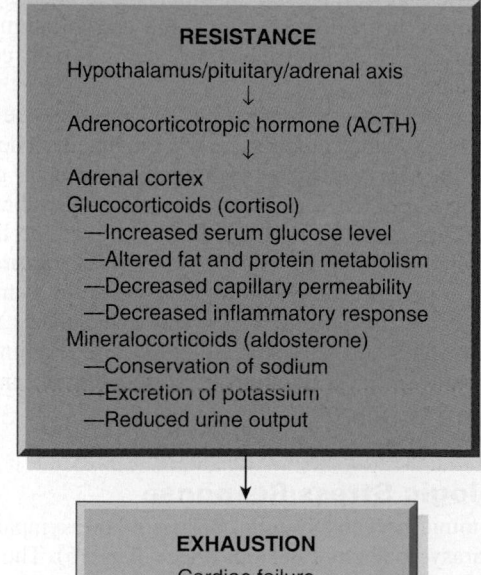

FIGURE 67-3. General adaptation syndrome, a nonspecific neuroendocrine response to an actual or a perceived stressor.

pathway. Instead of being stimulated to fight or flee, parasympathetic responders become frozen by fear. Becoming motionless is beneficial among various animals. For example, possums "play dead" when a predator is nearby, which causes the predator to lose interest in its potential prey. Some theorists argue that taking a similarly less aggressive stance could help humans to avoid confrontation.

Psychological Stress Response

Just as the body responds to stressors, the **psyche**, or mind, also reacts to stress. **Coping mechanisms** are unconscious tactics humans use to protect themselves from feeling inadequate or threatened. These mechanisms function like psychological first aid by helping temporarily to avoid the emotional effects of a stressful situation. When used appropriately and in moderation, coping mechanisms allow maintenance of psychological equilibrium and lead to psychological growth. If a person overuses coping mechanisms, however, he or she becomes dysfunctional. In addition, some individuals develop maladaptive coping mechanisms, such as abusing alcohol or other substances.

Some people have developed a particularly effective coping style called **hardiness** (Kobasa, 1979). Characteristics of hardiness are as follows:

- A commitment to something meaningful versus a sense of alienation
- A sense of having control over sources of stress versus a feeling of helplessness
- The perception of life events as a challenge rather than a threat

Nursing Guidelines 67-1 outlines interventions that can foster effective coping skills and a sense of hardiness.

 Gerontologic Considerations

- Older clients who have learned positive coping skills continue to cope well as they age. However, age-related changes, progression of chronic conditions, and transitions in living arrangements may overwhelm the coping resources of some older adults. Nursing care and discharge planning that allows the older adult to demonstrate characteristics of hardiness (commitment, control, and challenge) can minimize feelings of helplessness and hopelessness.

NURSING GUIDELINES 67-1

Fostering Effective Coping Skills

- Explore the coping strategies the client has found helpful in the past and encourage their continued use.
- Encourage clients to reestablish priorities and to strike a healthy balance between work and play.
- Suggest cultivating relationships with family and friends who are supportive.
- Teach the client assertiveness skills by role-playing how to (1) clearly state feelings, and (2) say "no" to unreasonable requests.
- Discuss time-management techniques like (1) getting up earlier, (2) avoiding procrastination, (3) performing stressful tasks when the client has maximum energy, and (4) eliminating or delegating unwanted tasks.
- Recommend a daily exercise program to reduce stimulating neurotransmitters and release endorphins and enkephalins such as (1) beginning with a 5- to 10-minute workout, (2) increasing the duration by 5 minutes each day, and (3) building up to a 30- to 45-minute period of exercise.
- Tell the client to avoid using alcohol or other nonprescribed sedative drugs as forms of self-treatment.
- Suggest writing about feelings in a diary if verbalizing traumatic or angry thoughts is difficult.
- Suggest stress management education and joining a support group.

PSYCHOSOMATIC ILLNESSES

Psyche refers to the mind, and **soma** refers to the body. The term *psychosomatic* means "pertaining to the mind-body relationship," and psychosomatic illness refers to illnesses influenced by the mind. In the past, *psychosomatic* had a negative connotation, suggesting that a client's illness was not medically legitimate. Psychoneuroimmunologic research since the early 1980s, however, has given the term a much more holistic meaning, reflecting the concept that the mind and the body are not separate. **Psychosomatic disorders**, also known as **stress-related disorders** (Box 67-3) are bona fide medical conditions associated with or aggravated by stress. Many healthcare providers now believe that all illnesses, if not psychosomatic in origin, have psychosomatic components.

Pathophysiology and Etiology

Biologic Factors

In addition to the known effects of stress on the autonomic nervous system, studies show that stressful events, such as preparing for examinations or undergoing job strain, also affect the immune system. The purpose of the immune system is to defend the body against cancer and invading microorganisms. Stress can lower the numbers of white blood cells, the immune system's disease fighters. Research also shows that chronic stress or very intense stress, such as the death of a spouse, has a greater effect on health than

BOX 67-3 Stress-Related Diseases and Disorders

Allergic and hypersensitivity disorders
Anovulation
Bronchial asthma
Bruxism
Cancer
Cardiac dysrhythmias
Connective tissue disorders
Eczema
Hair loss
Herpes simplex infection
Hypertension
Infertility
Irritable bowel syndrome
Low back pain
Multiple sclerosis
Psoriasis
Rheumatoid arthritis
Temporomandibular joint disorder
Tension headaches
Tic disorders

temporary stressors. This finding seems to be particularly true when a person lacks supportive relationships. A connection seems to exist between poorer immune function and loneliness; when individuals share emotions with others, immune functions improve.

 Gerontologic Considerations

- Social isolation, multiple losses, and grieving may increase an older adult's vulnerability and reaction to stressors.

Support for a biologic connection between the mind and the immune system is found in research that demonstrates that the immune system and the brain communicate with each other through the chemical messenger system using neurotransmitters and immunopeptides. **Immunopeptides** (or immunotransmitters) are called *cytokines* (see Chap. 33) and function in the same way as neurotransmitters; they relay messages throughout the immune system and the brain (Pert, 1997). Immune cells also can secrete small quantities of neurochemicals. In addition, nerve cells connecting the organs of the immune system (thymus, spleen, and lymph nodes) to the brain have been identified. This ability to communicate through chemicals implies that the immune system can make the brain aware of processes at distant sites in the body and that the brain can send messages directing the immune system's actions. The powerful actions of neurotransmitters, especially in states of excess or depletion, suggest that the psychological state can significantly affect immune function.

Many stress-related diseases involve allergic, inflammatory, or altered immune responses (see Chap. 34). They are characterized by physical symptoms that cycle through periods of *remission,* or absence, and *exacerbation,* or recurrence, with the symptomatic episodes often occurring when the client is under stress. The brain–immune system connection suggests that changes in body chemistry during periods of stress trigger an autoimmune (self-attacking) response or result in immunosuppression. Invasion of the body by cancer cells or disease-causing microorganisms, however, is not sufficient cause for disease; disease occurs when defenses are compromised or cannot recognize unnatural cells or pathogens. For this reason, psychological variables that influence immunity have the potential to influence the onset and progression of immune system–mediated diseases.

Psychological Factors

The association of certain psychological characteristics with an increased incidence of illness has been observed for centuries. Research suggests that there may be a generic, disease-prone personality with character traits that include anger and hostility, depression, anxiety, and other features (Pelletier, 1977, 1995). The type of disease that develops is related to an individual's health habits, environmental exposure, family history, and other socioeconomic factors.

Anger

Although anger is a normal emotion, some people fail to express it, perhaps feeling threatened by possible retaliation. They expend vast amounts of energy maintaining a facade of being happy and well adjusted. The effect of chronically suppressing anger and the neurochemical changes that accompany it, however, may be the triggering mechanism for a dysfunctional immune response.

Conversely, evidence suggests that the excess expression of hostility and anger is correlated with an increased incidence of heart attacks and may result from low levels of serotonin. The frequent activation of the sympathetic nervous system in persons prone to anger and hostility is another factor implicated in the development of heart disease.

Dependence

Some propose that unmet dependency needs and fears of rejection or abandonment provoke feelings of insecurity among some individuals with psychosomatic disorders (Townsend, 2009). Helplessness is related to dependence, and numerous studies have shown that people who feel powerless in their lives have more illnesses than those who have a sense of control.

Ambivalence

Ambivalence means feeling or acting in two opposing ways at the same time. For example, an individual may feel hostility toward the persons from whom they most want love and approval, or he or she may act independently and yet desire dependence. These unresolved conflicts may affect neurotransmitter and immune functioning and may be another key to the development of physical disorders.

Assessment Findings

Signs and Symptoms

Many stress-prone individuals seek medical attention when they experience symptoms in one or more organs affected by the autonomic nervous system. Clients may present with heart palpitations, pounding headaches, breathlessness,

tightness in the chest, chest pain, chronic pain, irritability, epigastric pain, abdominal discomfort and bloating, or constipation alternating with diarrhea. Many other illnesses, including cancer and cardiovascular disease, are not so obviously related to stress but are thought to have a psychosomatic component. The biopsychosocial effects of stress and mental state should be considered in the evaluation and treatment of all illnesses.

Gerontologic Considerations

- The cumulative effects of years of chronic psychosomatic disorders may lead to debilitating conditions in late adulthood.

Diagnostic Findings

Diagnostic tests are done to determine the extent of the disease and all physical causes for the client's symptoms. Because other conditions such as excessive intake of caffeine, cocaine use, mitral valve prolapse, hyperthyroidism, hypoglycemia, and lactose intolerance, to name a few, can mimic the signs and symptoms of some stress-related diseases, it is important to conduct tests before assuming that the disorder is stress induced.

Medical and Nursing Management

Treatment involves standard medical care pertinent to the diagnosis, control of the physical symptoms, and implementation of methods effective in managing stress and supporting the immune system. Nurses have an important role in participating in the treatment and education of clients regarding these methods. Stress management and other techniques have gained acceptance based on studies that suggest psychological factors can reduce the effects of stressors on the immune system and facilitate healing. **Stress management** programs offer instruction in relaxation techniques and effective coping strategies, including assertiveness training and developing a network of social support. Nutrition Notes 67-1 outlines nutritional considerations for clients with psychosomatic disorders.

Nutrition Notes 67-1
The Client with a Stress-Related Disorder

- Some people overeat in response to stressors, whereas others deny normal hunger. Assess for changes in appetite, eating patterns, and weight. Encourage clients to eat at regular intervals to avoid both overeating and undereating.
- Dietary interventions for some stress-related disorders may be necessary only during periods of exacerbation, such as avoiding lactose during acute episodes of diarrhea. For other stress-related disorders, such as irritable bowel syndrome, dietary interventions are recommended regardless of symptoms.

Pharmacologic Considerations

- Obtain a complete current medication history for each client, including nonprescription drugs. Some people who experience stress take illegally obtained stimulants and tranquilizers that they may not mention unless asked.

- Anti-inflammatory drugs and corticosteroids often are given to treat the symptoms of various psychosomatic diseases. Drug treatment is considered symptomatic rather than curative.

PSYCHOBIOLOGIC INTERVENTION: THE PLACEBO EFFECT

Psychobiologic intervention refers to those techniques that use the mind and body to alter disease. Some examples of the mind-body connection are discussed in Chapter 9 as they relate to alternative and complementary therapies. The placebo effect often is used as an example of how the mind and body are connected. A **placebo** is an inert or inactive substance that by its very nature cannot alter physiology, yet does so in a significant number of people. The **placebo effect** refers to the healing or improvement that takes place simply because the individual believes a treatment method will be effective.

The placebo effect was first observed during drug research. In most clinical drug trials, half the research volunteers receive the drug being studied, whereas the other half receive a placebo. None of the volunteers or the researchers knows which subjects are receiving the actual drug, a process referred to as a double-blind study. When the results of the studies are analyzed, researchers typically find that 30% or more of the individuals who receive a placebo experience improvement. This is thought to show how a person's belief system can positively influence health and that a purely psychological basis for recovery exists. In other words, when clients believe in the treatment regimen or have faith in the prescriber, it potentiates a positive outcome. Harnessing the psychological forces that create a placebo effect by communicating caring, optimism about treatment, and the belief that the client has the ability to recover can significantly affect wellness.

CRITICAL THINKING EXERCISES

1. What would you say to someone who characterizes mental illness as the manifestation of a poor or weak character?

2. What suggestions would you offer to someone who has a stress-related (psychosomatic) disorder?

3. How might failing one test in school be considered *eustress* but failing several tests be considered *distress*?

4. Based on the premises of the placebo effect, what response would you expect if you gave 100 people a red-colored candy resembling a pill that you said would increase their desire for sex?

NCLEX-STYLE REVIEW QUESTIONS

1. When faced with a stressor, which of the following are sympathetic nervous system responses? Select all that apply.
1. Increased heart rate
2. Elevated blood pressure
3. Increased peristalsis
4. Decreased gastric motility
5. Increased muscle tension

2. Which one of the following brain structures plays a major role in experiencing emotions and responding emotionally?
1. Hypothalamus
2. Brain stem
3. Limbic system
4. Cerebellum

3. Which one of the following is an assessment tool that nurses can perform to provide a wide overview of a client's psychoneurologic functioning?
1. Mental status examination
2. Word association test
3. Hamilton anxiety scale
4. Rorschach test

4. Which one of the following is the best outcome of effective coping?
1. Eustress
2. Hardiness
3. Resistance
4. Control

5. What is the most common effect on a client who overuses coping mechanisms?
1. The client becomes mentally ill.
2. The client becomes distressed.
3. The client becomes dysfunctional.
4. The client becomes hyperactive.

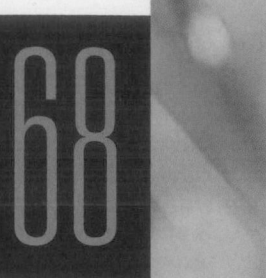

68

Caring for Clients with Anxiety Disorders

Words To Know
agoraphobia
anxiety
anxiety disorders
anxiolytics
behavioral therapy
cognitive therapy
compulsion
desensitization
fear
flashbacks
generalized anxiety disorder
limbic system
obsession
obsessive–compulsive disorder
panic disorder
phobic disorders
post-traumatic stress disorder
psychic numbing
psychotherapy
social phobia

Learning Objectives

On completion of this chapter, you will be able to:

1. Differentiate anxiety from fear.
2. Name four levels of anxiety, explaining the differences among the various levels.
3. Give six areas of nursing management that apply to the care of anxious clients.
4. Name examples of anxiety disorders.
5. List categories of drugs used to treat anxiety disorders.
6. Name and discuss two types of psychotherapy used to treat anxiety disorders.
7. List six nursing interventions that are helpful for reducing anxiety.
8. Discuss areas of teaching for clients with anxiety disorders.

Although anxiety and fear are normal human responses, anxiety disorders are not. Questions remain whether anxiety disorders are strictly biologic, learned, the result of unconscious emotional conflicts, or a combination of all three. Probably both physical and psychological factors play a role. A person is first genetically predisposed to an anxiety disorder and then manifests a disorder when exposed to situational triggers.

This chapter explores anxiety and fear and discusses how to intervene when a client is anxious. It also explores anxiety disorders and nursing care of those who have them.

ANXIETY AND FEAR

Anxiety differs from fear, but these terms often are used interchangeably. **Anxiety** is a vague uneasy feeling, the cause of which is not readily identifiable. It is evoked when a person anticipates nonspecific danger. **Fear** is a feeling of terror in response to someone or something specific that a person perceives as dangerous or threatening. Because it is common for clients to be anxious in an unfamiliar environment, or to be fearful of pain, suffering, or death, both reactions are common in hospitals and other healthcare facilities.

Because many medical and surgical clients temporarily feel vulnerable, they are prime candidates for experiencing anxiety. Recognizing the signs of escalating anxiety, understanding its consequences, and intervening appropriately are important interventions.

Levels of Anxiety
Anxiety may occur at several levels (Table 68-1). It may be mild, which is constructive and prepares a person to take action in appropriate situations. For example, mild anxiety before a test causes most people to study.

TABLE 68-1 Levels of Anxiety

LEVEL	BEHAVIORAL MANIFESTATIONS	PHYSICAL MANIFESTATIONS
Mild	Attention is heightened. Sensory perception is expanded. Focus is on stimuli. Reality is intact. Information processing is accurate. Person feels in control.	Muscle tone increases. Heart rate, blood pressure, and breathing slightly increase. Perspiration is noticeable.
Moderate	Person is more easily distracted. Concentration is slightly impaired. Person can redirect attention. Learning takes more effort. Perception narrows. Problem-solving becomes difficult. Person is irritable and feels inadequate.	Muscles are tense. Slight leg or hand tremors may occur. Rate, pitch, and volume of speech change. Respiratory depth and vital signs increase. Sleep is disturbed.
Severe	Attention span decreases. Person cannot concentrate or remain focused. Perception is reduced. Ability to learn is impaired. Information processing is inaccurate or incomplete. Person is aware of extreme discomfort. Effort is needed to control emotions. Person feels incompetent.	Symptoms include hyperventilation, dizziness, tachycardia, heart palpitations, and hypertension. Fine motor movement is impaired. Communication is limited.
Panic	Person exaggerates details. Perception is distorted. Learning is disabled. Thoughts are fragmented. Person cannot control emotions and feels helpless.	Speech is incoherent. Movements are haphazard, usually in an effort to escape. Symptoms include dyspnea, fainting, tremors, and diaphoresis.

Anxiety may be moderate or severe as well. Panic may even develop. Moderate, severe, and panic levels of anxiety are counterproductive; they provoke responses that interfere with well-being. As a person's level of anxiety escalates:

- Physiologic changes occur, such as elevation of blood pressure and racing heart.
- Perception of information and events narrows.
- Thinking becomes increasingly disorganized and distorted.
- Physical and emotional fatigue develops from the investment of energy in worrying.

▶ **Stop, Think, and Respond Exercise 68-1**

Give examples of situations that provoke mild anxiety and the appropriate outcomes that usually result. Discuss situations that may trigger more extreme levels of anxiety and their potential consequences.

Nursing Management

The nurse can assist the anxious client by implementing interventions that maintain or restore a sense of calm and control.

Building Trust

Building trust is especially critical to developing a therapeutic relationship with an anxious client. Being available and attentive to the client's needs contributes to this trust. The nurse should not leave an anxious client alone, especially during a new or potentially frightening experience.

Restoring Comfort

The nurse's interventions are guided by what will bring relief to a particular person. The nurse should ask the client to suggest methods that may be personally comforting. For example, some clients find it helpful for the nurse to give support in nonverbal ways, such as remaining with them without talking, holding a hand, or stroking the skin. Others prefer to talk about how they feel but are more relaxed if the nurse remains physically distant (Fig. 68-1).

Modifying Communication

The nurse should avoid interrupting anxious clients when they talk. Although verbalizing does not always relieve

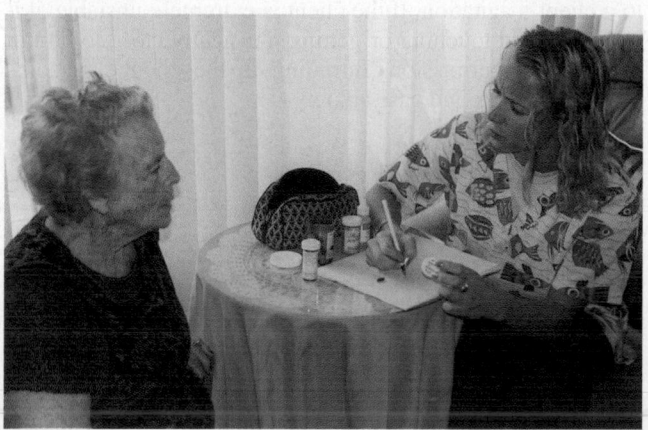

FIGURE 68-1. A nurse listens to an anxious client.

anxiety, it can be beneficial. Talking helps in processing information and exploring methods for dealing with problems. Some clients prefer not to discuss their anxiety and fears with the nurse. In such cases, the nurse respects the client's right to privacy. Offering a referral to a health professional such as a psychiatrist or medical social worker with counseling expertise, however, is appropriate.

Adjusting Teaching

Because an anxious client's attention and concentration are limited, directions or explanations must be simple, brief, and repeated frequently. To determine a client's level of comprehension, asking the person to paraphrase what he or she has been taught is helpful. The client also benefits from reductions in sensory stimulation such as dimming the lights and eliminating as much noise and interruptions as possible. The nurse must avoid expecting the client to show a great deal of self-reliance or independence until the client feels more relaxed and secure.

Helping Problem-Solve

Anxiety impairs problem-solving ability, and clients may look to the nurse for advice in decision-making. Nurses avoid influencing their clients' choices. Instead, they help clients follow a step-by-step problem-solving process to formulate decisions:

1. Identifying problems
2. Determining their causes
3. Exploring possible solutions
4. Examining the pros and cons of each option
5. Selecting the choice that is most compatible with personal values

Once the client arrives at a decision, the nurse advocates on the client's behalf for its implementation—even if it is not one the nurse would personally choose. The nurse also respects the client's right to change his or her mind at any time.

Ensuring Safety

People who are experiencing panic-level anxiety can act impulsively and endanger their safety (e.g., jumping out of a window, running into the street). The nurse remains calm to help such people reduce anxiety to a more manageable level. Having only one nurse interact with the client usually is best, because responding to multiple sources of stimulation adds to a client's agitation. If the client is extremely unstable, it is wise to avoid touching or getting physically close to him or her without permission. Intruding in the client's personal space is likely to increase anxiety.

ANXIETY DISORDERS

Anxiety disorders are a group of psychobiologic illnesses that result from activation of the autonomic nervous system, chiefly the sympathetic division. They tend to be chronic and sometimes appear without any logical explanation.

Types

Some examples of anxiety disorders include generalized anxiety disorder, panic disorder, phobic disorders, post-traumatic

---

BOX 68-1 Examples of Conditions That Resemble Generalized Anxiety Disorder

- Mitral valve prolapse
- Hypoglycemia
- Hyperthyroidism
- Premenstrual syndrome
- Menopause
- Dementia
- Abuse of psychostimulants (cocaine, caffeine, weight loss drugs)
- Sedative (alcohol, opioids, barbiturates) withdrawal

---

stress disorder, and obsessive-compulsive disorder. Anxiety disorders sometimes lead to other psychobiologic conditions such as depression, substance abuse, and binge-eating disorder and compulsive overeating, which are discussed in subsequent chapters.

Generalized Anxiety Disorder

Generalized anxiety disorder is characterized by chronic worrying on a daily basis for 6 or more months. There usually is more than one focus of worry. For example, a person may be worried about finances, job performance, and personal health. Often, the worrying is out of proportion with reality. In addition to worrying, other signs and symptoms of anxiety accompany the client's distress. When the client seeks medical attention, test results fail to reveal physical disorders that produce signs and symptoms similar to anxiety (Box 68-1).

 Gerontologic Considerations

- Older adults on fixed incomes often experience anxiety due to financial problems related to housing and medical expenses. Feelings of vulnerability, limitations associated with age, and fear of the unknown future may also contribute to anxiety in older adults.

Panic Disorder

Panic disorder is the most extreme manifestation of anxiety. People who are affected experience an abrupt onset of physical symptoms and terror that include intense apprehension; tachycardia, palpitations, chest pain, smothering or choking sensations; hyperventilation; lightheadedness; feeling of impending doom; and fear of fainting, dying, losing control, or going insane.

Episodes of panic may last minutes to less than 1 hour and then spontaneously subside. The episodes are often referred to as *attacks* because they interrupt a period during which the client is asymptomatic. The first instinct during a panic attack is to escape to a safer place. The unexplained flight from work, school, or the like that ensues often strains relationships with others who observe the client's behavior as strange.

The person who experiences a panic attack often is at a loss to identify its cause but associates the location or concurrent activity as the precipitating event. Most affected people cope with their disorder by avoiding situations or places where attacks have occurred. As the attacks recur in a variety of circumstances, however, people with panic disorder often develop agoraphobia. **Agoraphobia** is a fear of experiencing a panic attack in a place where the person may be publicly humiliated by his or her behavior or help may be unavailable. Consequently, many of those with panic disorder permanently confine themselves to their homes, where they feel safe.

Phobic Disorders

Phobic disorders are those conditions in which a person manifests an exaggerated fear. Many people are irrationally afraid of insects, animals, or various life experiences, such as riding on a roller coaster or flying in an airplane, some of which are potentially dangerous. When a person with a phobic disorder is exposed to the phobic stimulus, however, he or she experiences symptoms of anxiety that may reach severe or panic levels. He or she usually goes to extremes to avoid the object of the phobia or painfully endures the phobic stimulus despite the fact that it causes severe distress. Most people with phobic disorders are aware of how illogical the phobia is and how unrealistic their disabling response has become.

One common phobic disorder is social phobia. People with **social phobia**, also known as *social anxiety,* fear those situations in which they must perform in front of or may capture the attention of others. Examples of situations that may induce social phobia include speaking publicly, entertaining theatrically or musically, eating in a restaurant or at a banquet, attending a party, or being asked to explain a concept in an academic setting. The greatest worry for people with social phobia, which is for the most part imagined, is that they will be embarrassed or criticized for failing to meet acceptable standards.

Post-traumatic Stress Disorder

Post-traumatic stress disorder (PTSD) is a condition that involves a delayed anxiety response 3 or more months after an emotionally traumatic experience (Box 68-2). Although traumatic experiences are somewhat relative, they must be extraordinarily severe to cause PTSD. The circumstances of the traumatic event involve actual or threatened death or injury to self or others and produce fear, helplessness, or horror. Some people feel guilty for having survived such an event when others just as deserving of life died.

Initially, the affected person avoids dealing with the tragedy and detaches himself or herself from others using a technique that is referred to as **psychic numbing**. Eventually, however, the person no longer can stifle his or her memories. Months or years later, the memories may resurface in recurrent nightmares or **flashbacks**, in which the person feels as if he or she is reliving the precipitating event. This feeling may also occur when the person is exposed to a situation that resembles the original trauma, such as associating the explosive sound of fireworks with military gunfire.

To relieve symptoms of guilt, grief, anger, or sadness, some clients with PTSD abuse substances such as alcohol or other mind- and mood-altering drugs. When such coping strategies prove ineffective, they may act out aggressively. They may respond violently if startled from sleep. Those who suspect that they may have PTSD should consult a mental health professional for a definitive diagnosis.

> ▶ ***Stop, Think, and Respond Exercise 68-2***
> *Discuss how nurses who care for seriously burned clients may develop PTSD.*

Obsessive–Compulsive Disorder

Obsessive-compulsive disorder (OCD) is manifested by the performance of an anxiety-relieving ritual (**compulsion**) to terminate a disturbing, persistent thought (**obsession**). Obsessions may involve concerns about potential danger or being contaminated with germs. They are intrusive, and people with OCD cannot dismiss them from their consciousness. To relieve their anxiety, clients with OCD repetitively perform a tension-relieving compulsion that usually falls into one or more of the following categories:

- Cleaning, such as repetitiously scrubbing the surface of a dining table
- Washing, such as repeated bathing or handwashing
- Checking, such as verifying that doors have been locked or an iron has been unplugged even though the person has already checked
- Counting, such as a bank teller repeatedly making sure that the money in a cash drawer is accurate
- Touching, such as feeling to make sure that a lucky charm is on one's person or having to touch the door frame before entering a room

Clients with OCD may feel compelled to perform the same act repeatedly for a specific number of times or in a prescribed sequence. The more the person resists performing the compulsive act, the more the anxiety escalates. The same is true if another person interrupts, alters, or forbids the ritual. Because the rituals are often excessive and time-consuming, they may lead to problems in social relationships, failure in school, or loss of employment. Most clients with OCD recognize that their thoughts and behaviors border on the ridiculous, but they are helpless to stop independently.

BOX 68-2	**Traumatic Events Associated With Post-traumatic Stress Disorder**

- Witnessing a murder or violent crime
- Watching the torture of a person or animal
- Escaping a fiery crash (car, plane, train) or industrial explosion
- Seeing military friends or public servants killed in the line of duty
- Being raped or abused
- Surviving a natural disaster such as a flood, earthquake, or tornado
- Being trapped in an automobile, elevator, subway, or underground cave
- Being taken hostage by criminals or terrorists

Pathophysiology and Etiology

Genetic studies suggest that many anxiety disorders have familial patterns. This finding can imply an inherited faulty physiology, maladaptive learning, or acquisition of personality traits modeled after those displayed by significant others.

Symptoms are manifested because the neurotransmitter norepinephrine floods the limbic system; a minority of people respond to stress through the parasympathetic route, in which case the neurotransmitter acetylcholine causes symptoms. The **limbic system**, a ring of neural structures is buried within the cerebrum (see Chap. 67). It is made up of portions of the thalamus, hypothalamus, amygdala, and interconnections with other structures such as the cingulate gyrus, fornix, and parahippocampal gyrus (Fig. 68-2). The limbic system is a physiologic network for emotions, survival and behavioral responses, motivation, and learning. The biochemical changes brought on by the autonomic nervous system trigger physical arousal in the cortex and the neuroendocrine pathways involving the hypothalamus, pituitary, and adrenal glands.

Other biochemical mechanisms also may contribute to the development of anxiety disorders. A dysregulation of gamma-aminobutyric acid (GABA), a neurotransmitter that should buffer or extinguish the activity of norepinephrine, is one possibility. The second possibility is depletion of serotonin, which would explain why some clients with anxiety disorders develop depression or improve when receiving treatment with antidepressant drugs (see Chap. 69).

Assessment Findings

Signs and Symptoms

Although anxiety causes behavioral, cognitive, and emotional effects, most clients seek treatment for physical signs and symptoms (cardiovascular, respiratory, neuromuscular, gastrointestinal, integumentary problems; Table 68-2). For example, clients may be concerned about palpitations, breathlessness, chronic fatigue, tension headaches, and sleep disturbances. In many clients, blood pressure is elevated and heart rate is increased. Some clients acknowledge having unrealistic worries or fears or exaggerated startle reactions, experiencing flashbacks of previously traumatic events,

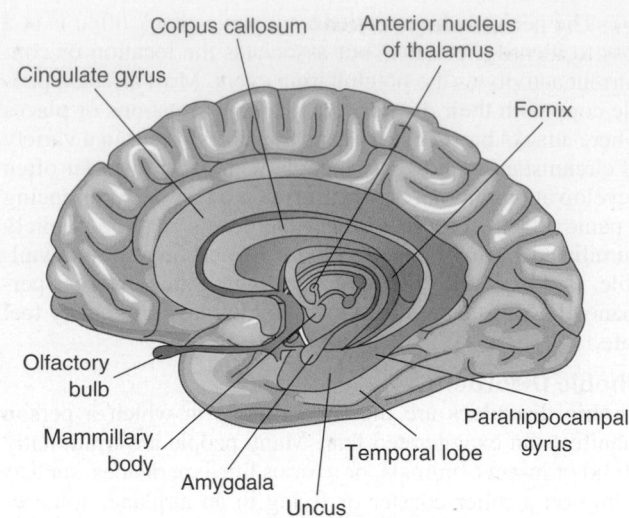

FIGURE 68-2. The limbic system is the center for emotions.

avoiding situations that provoke symptoms, or performing ritualistic behaviors.

Gerontologic Considerations

- Anxiety may be manifested in the older adult as confusion, behavior changes, or withdrawal. Assessment should include questions about the older adult's loss of significant others, relocation, and fears about future self-care abilities.

Diagnostic Findings

Findings from laboratory blood tests and diagnostic tests such as electrocardiography are essentially normal. Positron emission tomography (PET) and computed tomography (CT) scans have shown abnormal brain use of glucose in clients with anxiety disorders. Magnetic resonance imaging (MRI) has demonstrated atrophy in some brain areas in selected anxiety disorders. Diagnosis of most clients with anxiety disorders, however, is based on symptomatology and history.

TABLE 68-2 Common Signs and Symptoms of Anxiety

RESPONSES	SIGNS AND SYMPTOMS
Physical	
Cardiovascular	Hypertension, tachycardia, palpitations, fainting*
Respiratory	Dyspnea, rapid breathing, hyperventilation, choking sensation, tightness in the chest
Neuromuscular	Tremors, restlessness, insomnia, muscle tension, excessive sleep,* generalized weakness, dizziness
Gastrointestinal	Anorexia, nausea, diarrhea,* constipation, feeling of fullness
Urinary	Frequency and urgency of urination*
Integumentary	Diaphoresis, sweaty palms, pallor, blushing,* dry mouth
Behavioral	Crying, rapid speech or mutism, hypervigilance, being easily startled or accident-prone, social isolation, physical escape, avoidance, loss of interest in sexual activity, pacing, fidgeting, nail-biting, picking at skin, seeking comfort in food or alcohol, absenteeism, failure to complete or poor performance of tasks
Cognitive	Forgetfulness, poor judgment, lack of motivation, confusion, nightmares, intrusive thoughts, preoccupation, decreased attention and concentration, inability to recall information
Emotional	Unrealistic fears, mood swings, easily angered, impatient, intolerant, nervous

*Indicates a parasympathetic rather than a sympathetic nervous system response.

Medical Management

The medical management of anxiety disorders includes drug therapy combined with cognitive and behavioral psychotherapy. Drug therapy relieves the symptoms associated with anxiety, but it does not eliminate causative factors. Once drug therapy is implemented, however, clients are more capable of dealing with issues affecting their daily lives.

Drug Therapy

Drugs that (1) reduce or block levels of norepinephrine or (2) normalize levels of serotonin are most commonly prescribed for anxiety disorders. They include anxiolytics, beta-adrenergic blockers, central-acting sympatholytics, and occasionally antidepressants (Drug Therapy Table 68-1).

DRUG THERAPY TABLE 68-1 Drugs Used To Treat Anxiety

Drug Category and Examples	Mechanism of Action	Side Effects	Nursing Considerations
Benzodiazepines alprazolam (Xanax), lorazepam (Ativan), diazepam (Valium)	Exact mechanism of action not understood, but is thought to increase the inhibitory effects of GABA, making the cells less responsive to norepinephrine	Transient mild drowsiness, sedation, fatigue, lightheadedness, constipation, diarrhea, nausea, dry mouth, drug dependence	Instruct client to avoid alcohol and other CNS depressants. Warn client that cimetidine, disulfiram, omeprazole, valproic acid, and oral contraceptives increase the effects of these drugs. Tell client to avoid operating machinery, report all side effects, and avoid stopping the drug abruptly.
Nonbenzodiazepine anxiolytics buspirone (BuSpar), paroxetine (Paxil), fluvoxamine (Luvox)	Exact mechanism unknown but does bind with serotonin and dopamine receptors	Dizziness, nervousness, insomnia, headache, lightheadedness, dry mouth, abdominal distress, vomiting, palpitations, chest pain, hyperventilation	Instruct client to avoid alcohol and other CNS depressants and operating machinery, and to report side effects. Inform client that frequent small meals and sucking on ice chips will alleviate GI disturbances and dry mouth.
Beta-adrenergic blockers propranolol hydrochloride (Inderal), atenolol (Tenormin), metoprolol (Lopressor)	Decrease the effects of the sympathetic nervous system by reducing CNS sympathetic outflow and blocking beta-adrenergic receptors	Fatigue, nausea, vomiting, diarrhea, flatulence, constipation, bradycardia, hypotension, congestive heart failure, dysrhythmias, erectile dysfunction, decreased libido, decreased activity tolerance	Monitor heart rate, blood pressure, and postural changes. Instruct client to avoid alcohol, to report all side effects, and not to discontinue the drug abruptly. Review all medications because propranolol can interact with many other drugs. Administer with food. Warn clients with diabetes that propranolol may obscure signs and symptoms of hypoglycemia and thus to manage serum glucose carefully.
Central-acting sympatholytics clonidine hydrochloride (Catapres), methyldopa (Aldomet), guanabenz (Wytensin)	Decrease the sympathetic outflow from the CNS and inhibit sympathetic nervous system effects	Drowsiness, sedation, dizziness, constipation, dry mouth, anorexia, erectile dysfunction, weight gain, weakness, nightmares	Monitor blood pressure and postural changes. Instruct client to avoid alcohol. Inform client to take drug as prescribed and not to miss doses or abruptly discontinue use. Tell client to report any side effects and that side effects will disappear once the drug is discontinued.

CNS = central nervous system; GABA = gamma-aminobutyric acid.

Anxiolytics

Anxiolytics are drugs that relieve the symptoms of anxiety. Sometimes they are referred to as *minor tranquilizers* to differentiate them from major tranquilizers or antipsychotic drugs used to treat thought disorders such as schizophrenia. Anxiolytics include benzodiazepines such as alprazolam (Xanax), lorazepam (Ativan), and diazepam (Valium) and nonbenzodiazepine drugs such as buspirone (BuSpar).

Pharmacologic Considerations

- Benzodiazepines such as alprazolam (Xanax) and diazepam (Valium) are used in the short-term treatment of anxiety. Long-term treatment is not recommended because prolonged use can result in drug dependence.

- Buspirone, a nonbenzodiazepine, also is recommended for short-term treatment of anxiety. It does not produce muscle relaxation or cause sedation. It can take up to 3 to 4 weeks to produce the full effect. Nonbenzodiazepines are sometimes preferred when a client has a history of alcoholism or abuse of other sedative drugs.

- Antianxiety drugs may cause drowsiness or blurred vision. Advise the client to use caution while driving or performing tasks requiring mental alertness.

Gerontologic Considerations

- Antianxiety drugs may cause short periods of memory impairment that can aggravate an already existing cognitive disorder. These drugs may also cause dizziness or lightheadedness, increasing the risk of falling in older adults. In addition, before administering a benzodiazepine to an older adult, assess for sleep problems, especially snoring. These drugs have the potential to exacerbate sleep apnea.

- The kidneys excrete most antianxiety agents; therefore, older adults with impaired kidney function are at increased risk for drug toxicity when taking these medications.

- Short-acting benzodiazepines, such as alprazolam, are preferred in older adults because they are less likely than longer-acting benzodiazepines to cause toxicity, leading to excessive sedation and depression.

- Buspirone is commonly used to treat anxiety in older adults. The drug does not produce dependence or interact with benzodiazepines or alcohol. A decrease in anxiety may occur in approximately 1 week; however, the drug may take up to 4 weeks before a full therapeutic response occurs.

▶ ***Stop, Think, and Respond Exercise 68-3***

What health teaching is appropriate when a client begins taking an anxiolytic drug?

Beta-Adrenergic Blockers

Receptors for norepinephrine are referred to as *alpha-adrenergic* and *beta-adrenergic receptors.* Beta-adrenergic receptors are located primarily in the heart and lungs. When norepinephrine stimulates beta-adrenergic receptors, heart rate, forcefulness of heart contraction, and dilation of bronchi all increase. The ultimate outcome is that the body is prepared for "fight or flight," a function of the sympathetic nervous system. In anxiety disorders, norepinephrine prepares the body for a similar response. Blocking the beta-adrenergic receptors with drugs such as propranolol (Inderal), atenolol (Tenormin), or metoprolol (Lopressor) reduces the sympathetic nervous system stimulation that causes some symptoms associated with anxiety.

Beta-adrenergic blockers frequently are prescribed for people with social phobia. This category of drugs does not cause sedation, tolerance, or addiction. These drugs do, however, lower blood pressure and subsequently can cause episodes of dizziness or fainting when the client rises quickly from a lying or sitting position. Other major side effects include bradycardia and elevated blood glucose level. Those taking a nonselective beta-adrenergic blocker—one that interferes with bronchodilation—may experience fatigue, dyspnea, and wheezing.

▶ ***Stop, Think, and Respond Exercise 68-4***

Beta-adrenergic blockers should be cautiously prescribed or avoided for clients with which kinds of concurrent medical conditions?

Central-Acting Sympatholytics

Central-acting sympatholytics block alpha-2 receptors for norepinephrine in the brain stem. Consequently, they reduce heart rate and blood pressure. Examples of drugs in this category include clonidine (Catapres), methyldopa (Aldomet), and guanabenz (Wytensin). Although these drugs are prescribed more often to control primary hypertension, they potentially have beneficial effects in anxious people with elevated blood pressure. Clonidine also is used to control hypertension in people who experience withdrawal symptoms when abruptly abstaining from alcohol or anxiolytic therapy.

Side effects associated with central-acting sympatholytics include sedation, dizziness, dry mouth, constipation, urinary retention, elevated blood glucose, fatigue, erectile dysfunction, and diminished libido. Some people may have a rash or experience depression. Blood pressure should be monitored on a regular basis. The client must learn to rise slowly from a sitting or lying position to avoid postural (orthostatic) hypotension. Clients with diabetes may need to adjust their medication regimen to maintain normal ranges in blood glucose level.

Antidepressants

Obsessive-compulsive disorder seems to respond to the administration of selective serotonin reuptake inhibitors (SSRIs)—antidepressants such as fluvoxamine (Luvox), sertraline (Zoloft), paroxetine (Paxil), and fluoxetine (Prozac); or tricyclic antidepressants (TCAs) such as clomipramine (Anafranil). Sertraline also has been approved for the treatment of social phobia. The symptoms of PTSD are somewhat relieved by some SSRIs such as citalopram (Celexa) and TCAs such as amitriptyline (Elavil) and imipramine (Tofranil). These antidepressants sustain levels of serotonin, which perhaps is the mechanism by which these medications treat selected anxiety disorders. Antidepressants are discussed in more detail in Chapter 69.

Psychotherapy
Psychotherapy involves talking with a psychiatrist, psychologist, or mental health counselor. Some clients respond better when therapy sessions are conducted one on one; others, such as those with PTSD, respond better to group interactions.

Cognitive Therapy
One type of psychotherapy useful in treating clients with anxiety disorders is cognitive therapy. **Cognitive therapy** is a type of psychotherapy in which the therapist helps clients alter their irrational thinking, correct their faulty belief systems, and replace negative self-statements with positive ones. This therapy is based on the theory that it is not events per se that provoke anxiety but rather the person's interpretation of events. By reshaping a person's viewpoint, the disorder can be minimized or eliminated.

Behavioral Therapy
Behavioral therapy attempts to extinguish undesirable responses by learning other adaptive techniques. One example that is sometimes used with clients who have phobic disorders or OCD is desensitization. **Desensitization** involves providing emotional support while gradually exposing a person to whatever it is that provokes anxiety. If anxiety escalates, the therapist coaches the client to engage in some form of distraction or perform relaxation or breathing exercises to overcome symptoms. Eventually, the client can tolerate the anxiety provoking experience independently by learning methods for eliminating physical and emotional discomfort.

Nursing Process for the Client With an Anxiety Disorder

Assessment
Observe for evidence of various levels of anxiety: pacing, talking excessively, complaining, crying, being withdrawn, or trying to run away. Ask the client to express anxiety with open-ended questions such as "How are you feeling now?" It is helpful to have the client rate his or her anxiety level using a scale from 0 to 10. Determine the level at which the client feels that anxiety is tolerable. Inquire if the client has an effective method for controlling anxiety and document the response. Observe the client's mood for signs of concurrent depression and explore the client's use of and knowledge about medications to treat the disorder. Obtain a complete current medication history for each client, including nonprescription drugs. Many people who experience anxiety take over-the-counter drugs, herbal remedies, stimulants, and tranquilizers that they may not mention unless asked. Nutrition Notes 68-1 lists assessment considerations related to the client's diet.

> ### Nutrition Notes 68-1
> ### The Client With an Anxiety Disorder
>
> - Clients with anxiety should avoid caffeine because it contributes to and potentiates the physiologic stimulation experienced with anxiety.
> - Although some clients with anxiety lose their appetite, others may react to stress by overeating. Therefore, it is important to regularly assess the client's current weight and monitor weight fluctuations over time.

Diagnosis, Planning, and Interventions

▶ **Anxiety** related to perception of danger

▶ **Expected Outcome:** The client's anxiety will return to a tolerable level.

- Reduce as many external stimuli, such as noise, bright lights, and activity, as possible. *Numerous stimuli escalate anxiety because they interfere with attention and concentration. Dealing simultaneously with multiple stimuli can tax the client's energy.*
- Maintain a calm manner when interacting with the client. *Anxiety is communicated; an anxious nurse can increase anxiety in a client. Modeling a controlled state promotes a similar response in the client.*
- Take a position at least an arm's length away from the client. *Invading an anxious client's personal space may increase his or her discomfort.*
- Avoid touching the client without first asking permission. *An anxious client may misinterpret unexpected touching as a threatening gesture.*
- Establish trust by being available to the client and keeping promises. *Insecurity can be relieved if the client knows he or she can depend on assistance from the nurse.*
- Advise the client to seek out the nurse or another supportive person when feeling the effects of anxiety. *The earlier that anxiety is de-escalated, the sooner the client will experience relief of symptoms.*
- Stay with the client during periods of severe anxiety. *The nurse's presence can help the client stay in control or restore control to a more comfortable level.*
- Follow a consistent schedule for routine activities. *Unpredictability heightens anxiety; consistency helps a client manage time and cope with personal demands.*
- Encourage the client to identify what he or she perceives to be a threat to emotional equilibrium. *Processing situations verbally may give the client perspective on perceived threats so that they are more realistic and less exaggerated.*
- Use a soft voice, short sentences, and clear messages when exchanging information. *Anxious clients have a short attention span and reduced ability to concentrate; they may be unable to follow lengthy or complicated information.*
- Provide specific, succinct directions for tasks the client should complete or assist the client who becomes agitated. *Anxious clients have difficulty following instructions and performing tasks in correct sequence. Assistance relieves unnecessary distress.*

- Instruct and help the client with moderate or severe anxiety to perform one or more of the following until anxiety is within a tolerable level:
  - Count slowly backward from 100. *Distraction redirects the client's attention from distressing physiologic symptoms to the task at hand.*
  - Breathe slowly and deeply in through the nose and out through the mouth. *Slowing respirations aborts hyperventilation and subsequent potential for fainting, peripheral tingling, and numbness from respiratory alkalosis.*
  - Offer a warm bath or back rub. *Warm running water promotes relaxation; massage relaxes muscles and possibly releases endorphins, natural chemicals that promote a sense of well-being.*
  - Progressively relax groups of muscles from the toes to the head. *Consciously relaxing muscles relieves tension and fatigue.*
  - Repeat positive statements such as "I am in control," "I am safe," "I am relaxed." *Positive self-talk can be transformed into reality.*
  - Visualize a pleasant, relaxing place. *Imagery can transform a person's aroused state to one that is more relaxed.*
  - Listen to a relaxation tape or soothing music. *Distraction helps to refocus attention to less anxiety-provoking stimuli.*
  - Engage in a large-muscle activity such as riding an exercise bicycle or going for a brisk walk. *Activity uses norepinephrine and can reduce it to a more manageable amount.*
- Administer antianxiety medication that has been prescribed on an as-needed (prn) basis if nonpharmacologic approaches are ineffective. *Medication may be necessary to ensure the client's or others' safety if there is a potential for loss of control or violent acting out.*

▶ **Risk for Ineffective Therapeutic Regimen Management** related to knowledge deficit of drug and dietary modifications

▶ **Expected Outcome:** The client will safely manage his or her own self-care.

- Explain the routine for self-administering prescribed medications and side effects associated with prescribed drugs. *Identifying the frequency and approximate time during the day when medications should be taken ensures safe self-care. Knowing what to expect as side effects reduces the potential for noncompliance or harm.*
- Emphasize that the client must avoid alcohol and other sedating drugs when taking anxiolytic drugs. *Combining two drugs that cause sedation may have dangerous consequences.*
- Encourage compliance with drug therapy, although it may take several weeks for the client to feel a beneficial effect. *Making the client aware that symptoms will not disappear immediately may create motivation for remaining compliant.*
- Advise the client to first discuss discontinuing drug therapy for whatever reason with the prescribing physician. *Abrupt discontinuation of benzodiazepines can cause withdrawal symptoms that mimic anxiety.*
- Tell the client to avoid caffeine, nicotine, or stimulating drugs such as nonprescription diet pills and cold and allergy

medications. *These drugs contain chemicals that stimulate the sympathetic nervous system, which interferes with the desired effect of anxiolytic drug therapy.*

- Inform the client of the process for arranging follow-up appointments with his or her physician. *The client needs periodic contact with the treating physician for further assessment, evaluation of treatment outcomes, or adjustment of the therapeutic regimen.*
- Provide information on self-help groups for anxiety. *Interacting with others who share similar problems can help clients cope.*

Evaluation of Expected Outcomes

After successful nursing interventions, the client deals with anxiety-provoking stimuli realistically and implements measures to decrease anxiety. He or she has extended periods during which anxiety is at a tolerable level and participates in normal activities without becoming incapacitated by anxiety.

The client accurately repeats information on the dose, frequency, potential side effects, and duration of drug therapy. He or she verbalizes possible consequences if an anxiolytic drug is discontinued abruptly and lists drugs, foods, and beverages that are contraindicated when taking anxiolytic medication. Finally, the client has written instructions for follow-up care and is aware of community-based groups that may help in the management of his or her disorder. ●

CRITICAL THINKING EXERCISES

1. Discuss nursing interventions that would be appropriate when a client tells you that he or she feels anxious about upcoming surgery.
2. What interventions should a nurse implement if a client suddenly experiences a panic attack?
3. What suggestions from a nurse could help reduce anxiety in older adults?
4. What health teaching should the nurse provide to a client who has been prescribed a benzodiazepine for managing symptoms of anxiety?

NCLEX-STYLE REVIEW QUESTIONS

1. A client who has been experiencing chest pain is scheduled to undergo a cardiac catheterization and coronary arteriogram. Which of the following nursing actions is best for reducing the client's anxiety?
   1. Teach the client how coronary artery disease is usually treated.
   2. Listen to the client express his or her feelings about cardiac disease.
   3. Explain to the client how well other people have handled these tests.
   4. Avoid discussing the cardiac catheterization procedure until the client is relaxed.
2. For which of the following drugs used to manage anxiety is it most important for the nurse to monitor the client for hypotension? Select all that apply.
   1. Alprazolam (Xanax)
   2. Propranolol (Inderal)

3. Lorazepam (Ativan)
4. Buspirone (BuSpar)
5. Clonidine (Catapres)

Anti-Hypertensives

3. A client receives a prescription for antianxiety medication. Why should the nurse tell the client to avoid drugs such as caffeine, nicotine, nonprescription diet pills, and cold and allergy medications?

1. They potentiate the action of antianxiety medications.
2. They cause withdrawal symptoms that mimic anxiety.
3. They release endorphins that decrease a sense of well-being.
4. They stimulate the sympathetic nervous system.

4. When caring for a client with panic level of anxiety, which is the most important nursing action?

1. Remain with the client indefinitely.
2. Relocate the client to a visitors' room.
3. Offer the client a cup of coffee or tea.
4. Notify the physician of the client's symptoms.

5. A client receives a prescription for a benzodiazepine. Why should the nurse advise this client to use caution when driving or performing tasks requiring mental alertness?

1. Benzodiazepines may cause confusion.
2. Benzodiazepines may cause behavior changes.
3. Benzodiazepines may cause sleep disorders.
4. Benzodiazepines may cause drowsiness.

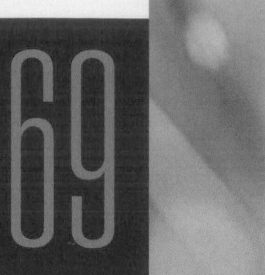

69

Caring for Clients with Mood Disorders

Words To Know
affect
bipolar disorder
deep brain stimulation
delusions
dexamethasone (cortisol) suppression test
dopamine
electroconvulsive therapy
euthymic
gamma-aminobutyric acid
hallucinations
hypertensive crisis
major (unipolar) depression
mania
melatonin
monoamine hypothesis
mood
mood disorders
norepinephrine
photoperiods
phototherapy
psychomotor agitation
psychomotor retardation
psychotherapy
psychotic depression
reactive (secondary) depression
reuptake
seasonal affective disorder
serotonin
serotonin syndrome
transcranial magnetic stimulation
vagus nerve stimulation

Learning Objectives

On completion of this chapter, you will be able to:

1. Discuss common signs and symptoms of mood disorders.
2. Name three neurotransmitters that, when imbalanced, affect mood.
3. Identify the types of drugs that are used to treat depression and nursing considerations related to their administration.
4. Discuss the causes, manifestations, and management of serotonin syndrome.
5. Identify the reasons electroconvulsive therapy is used in the management of depression.
6. Name three interventions that are alternatives to electroconvulsive therapy for recurrent depression.
7. Give three criteria that indicate a high risk for suicide.
8. Discuss nursing measures that are useful in preventing suicide.
9. Discuss the nursing management of clients with depression.
10. Describe seasonal affective disorder, its treatment, and nursing management.
11. Explain bipolar disorder and describe its treatment and nursing management.

The term **mood** refers to a person's overall feeling state. Mood is displayed in a person's **affect**, the verbal and nonverbal behavior that communicates feelings (Table 69-1). This chapter discusses a variety of mood disorders, their management, and their nursing care.

THE MOOD CONTINUUM AND MOOD DISORDERS

Mood may be thought of as a continuum, with extremes of emotion existing at both ends or poles (Fig. 69-1). People with normal moods are referred to as **euthymic**; they are capable of experiencing a variety of feelings, all of which are situationally appropriate. *Dysthymia*, a feeling of unremitting sadness, is similar to but less severe than major depression which is discussed later. *Cyclothymia*, alternating sad and elated moods, resembles bipolar disorder, but the extremes of mood are less pronounced. **Mania** refers to the frenzied state of euphoria exhibited by persons during the manic phase of bipolar disorder which is defined and discussed later.

People who have what psychologists and psychiatrists call **mood disorders** experience an extreme persistent mood or severe mood swings that interfere with social relationships. The primary mood disturbances include major (unipolar) depression and bipolar disorder, formerly called *manic-depressive syndrome*. In **psychotic depression**, an extreme form of depressive disorder, some individuals experience **hallucinations**, sensory phenomena such as hearing voices or seeing

TABLE 69-1 Examples of Mood and Affect

MOOD	AFFECT
Happy	Smiling
	Briskly walking
	Paying attention to appearance
	Showing a positive attitude
	Being cooperative, creative, gregarious
Depressed	Looking gloomy
	Being inactive
	Neglecting appearance
	Feeling empty
	Showing no initiative
	Being insensitive to others' feelings, or isolated

images that do not objectively exist, and **delusions**, fixed false beliefs that often are persecutory or guilt-ridden in nature. **Seasonal affective disorder** (SAD) is a mood disorder characterized by depression that develops during darker winter months and then disappears in the spring.

MAJOR DEPRESSION

Everyone experiences depression at some point. In most cases, transient depression is a normal reaction to loss, such as the death of a loved one; disappointment, such as being fired from a job; or overwhelming events, such as being heavily in debt. A sad feeling that can be directly attributed to a situation or cause is referred to as **reactive (secondary) depression**. Usually, reactive depression is self-limiting; when circumstances change or supportive others provide help, depression is relieved. Nevertheless, many people experience **major (unipolar) depression**, a sad mood with no obvious relationship to situational events. Millions of Americans report feeling depressed; however, the actual incidence of major depression in adults is believed to be approximately 19 million (Holmberg, 2006). Depression is also a comorbid (coexisting) condition among people with anxiety disorders and substance abuse (see Chaps. 68 and 71).

Pathophysiology and Etiology

Brain function, and consequently mood, depends on the dynamic interplay of neurotransmitters (see Chap. 67). Moods are most likely generated by the limbic system, which is the center for emotions (see Chap. 68). Several possible explanations exist for the causes and mechanisms that trigger major depressive symptoms. The most solid evidence

at present suggests that mood disorders are related to genetics, dysregulation of neurotransmitters, and neuroendocrine imbalance. Psychological and social theories suggest that infantile rejection or neglect, learned feelings of helplessness, chronic exposure to discrimination, or distorted or false perceptions about oneself contribute to depression. Although these latter factors should not be dismissed, research in brain chemistry gives more support to biologic explanations.

Genetics

Mood disorders tend to be prevalent among close blood relatives, which suggests a genetic link. Even when raised separately, each identical twin has a higher incidence of depressive episodes when the other is affected (Kelsoe, 2004). Researchers are studying the DNA of fairly homogeneous groups (e.g., the Amish) for variations in chromosome patterns in relatives who have mood disorders and those who do not. Preliminary evidence shows that differences exist in at least two chromosomes, but research must continue before a definite conclusion can be reached (Videbeck, 2007).

▶ *Stop, Think, and Respond Exercise 69-1*

Besides genetics, What other reason might explain why people who are related manifest similar disturbances in mood?

Neurotransmitter Dysregulation

The most widely accepted psychobiologic theory for depression is the **monoamine hypothesis**, which proposes that depression results from imbalances in one or more of the monoamine neurotransmitters: serotonin, norepinephrine, and dopamine. The hypothesis is based on the fact that levels of a metabolite of **serotonin**, 5-HIAA, measured in cerebrospinal fluid, are lower in depressed people than in samples taken from euthymic people. Second, **norepinephrine** levels may be low or high among people affected by depression. Low levels of norepinephrine help explain why some depressed people develop **psychomotor retardation**, which is characterized by a lack of energy, increased sleep, and little interest in daily events or responsibilities. On the other hand, some depressed people may have excessive norepinephrine. They are more likely to experience **psychomotor agitation** with such stimulating manifestations as insomnia, pacing, and distractibility, rather than lethargy. Third, the symptoms of some clients who are depressed suggest an excess of **dopamine**, which is associated with distortion of thoughts. In moderate to severe depression, this may be evidenced as over-reactive guilt, self-blame, self-pity, and low self-worth. Refer to Nutrition Notes 69-1 for dietary considerations.

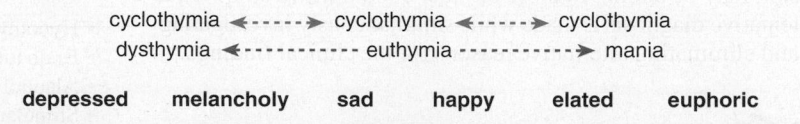

cyclothymia ◄----► cyclothymia ◄----► cyclothymia

dysthymia ◄----------- euthymia -----------► mania

depressed   melancholy   sad   happy   elated   euphoric

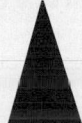

FIGURE 69-1. Mood continuum.

Nutrition Notes 69-1
The Client With Depression

● Carbohydrates from any source, such as cereals, pasta, fruit, and sugar, stimulate a temporary increase in serotonin production by increasing the amount of tryptophan in the brain; tryptophan is the amino acid precursor of serotonin.
● The results can range from a mild feeling of calmness after eating a carbohydrate snack to drowsiness after eating a large carbohydrate-rich meal.

Neuroendocrine Imbalance

Interactions of the pituitary, adrenal cortex, thyroid gland, and ovaries also may play a role in producing depression by altering levels of hormones. These endocrine glands are stimulated and suppressed through the hypothalamus, a structure in the limbic system. Abnormal levels of cortisol, a hormone produced by the adrenal cortex, and variations in thyroid hormones are accompanied by changes in mood and motor activity. The hypothalamus also influences the pituitary gland's stimulation of reproductive hormones. The latter hormonal relationships help to explain the altered mood states associated with premenstrual syndrome, late luteal phase dysphoric disorder (see Chap. 53), menopause, and postpartum depression.

Gerontologic Considerations

- Impaired regulation of neurotransmitters in older adults suggests biological predisposition to depression and thought disorders.

- Alterations in hormone production (i.e., adrenal, pituitary, thyroid) that occur with vascular changes of aging may impact the feedback loop (refer to Chap. 49) for other hormone production and may therefore impact emotional equilibrium.

Assessment Findings

Signs and Symptoms

The predominant feature of major depression is a persistent sad mood accompanied by multiple physiologic and cognitive (thought) changes, represented by the acronym SAD IMAGES (Box 69-1). Because the manifestations of depression may be similar to those of other conditions (Box 69-2), a tentative diagnosis is made while simultaneously investigating and eliminating alternative reasons for the clinical findings.

Gerontologic Considerations

- Cognitive impairment in the depressed older adult can be easily confused with dementia (i.e., pseudodementia). Careful assessment is necessary to distinguish between the

BOX 69-1 | Signs and Symptoms of Major Depression

Sad mood
Appetite change (increased or decreased)
Disturbed sleep (insomnia or hypersomnia)
Inability to concentrate
Marked decrease in pleasure
Apathy, including lack of interest in sex
Guilty feelings
Energy changes (restlessness or inactivity)
Suicidal thoughts

two because depression usually can be treated successfully in older adults.

- Older adults may be reluctant to admit depressive feelings if they view depression as a character weakness rather than a chemical imbalance. Older adults who seek treatment for subacute physical symptoms, such as loss of appetite, trouble sleeping, lack of energy, and weight loss, may actually be depressed. Attempts at self-medicating with alcohol or herbal preparations should also be assessed.

Diagnostic Findings

Studies that identify 5-HIAA in cerebrospinal fluid and the metabolite of norepinephrine in urine are financially prohibitive except for research purposes. Blood levels of serotonin can be measured more easily, but there is some question whether the level in blood correlates with the level necessary for normal mood in the brain. Furthermore, some managed care groups consider diagnostic laboratory tests of neurotransmitter levels unnecessary. Third-party payers often maintain that a diagnosis of depression can be confirmed or ruled out by the client's clinical presentation and by performing other standard tests for disorders that mimic depression. Findings that would indicate alternative diagnoses to depression include low thyroid function test results, suggesting hypothyroidism (see Chap. 50); abnormal blood glucose levels, suggesting diabetes mellitus (see Chap. 51); low hemoglobin levels, indicative of anemia (see Chap. 31); and detection of drug abuse in a urine drug screen (see Chap. 71).

Occasionally, physicians order a **dexamethasone suppression test** (DST), also called a **cortisol suppression test**.

BOX 69-2 | Conditions That Mimic Depression

• Hypothyroidism
• Brain tumor
• Alcohol or sedative abuse
• Stimulant withdrawal
• Chronic hypoxia
• Side effects of drug therapy such as corticosteroids, antihypertensives such as reserpine (Serpasil), methyldopa (Aldomet), propranolol (Inderal)

This blood test theoretically indicates major depression if cortisol levels remain elevated despite the administration of an oral dose of dexamethasone, a corticosteroid, the day before. Under normal conditions, increased blood levels of corticosteroid should suppress the pituitary gland's secretion of corticotropin through a negative feedback loop. Statistics show, however, that the level of cortisol remains elevated in clients who are depressed, suggesting that cortisol is a chemical marker for depression. Many physicians, however, do not believe that the DST is significant; therefore, it is not widely ordered.

Neurologic imaging tests such as computed tomography (CT) or magnetic resonance imaging (MRI) may be performed to eliminate diagnoses such as brain tumor or cerebrovascular accident as causes for a client's altered mood. A positron emission tomography (PET) scan may show a change in activity in the prefrontal cortex suggestive of a mood disorder (Fig. 69-2). The physician may omit imaging tests if he or she thinks the clinical evidence strongly supports the diagnosis of depression.

Medical Management

The most commonly used treatments for depression are drug therapy (Drug Therapy Table 69-1), psychotherapy, and, in severe cases, electroconvulsive therapy. Some new forms of treatment include vagus nerve stimulation, deep brain stimulation, and transcranial magnetic stimulation.

Drug Therapy

The three main categories of drugs that relieve the symptoms of depression are tricyclic antidepressants (TCAs); monoamine oxidase inhibitors (MAOIs); and multiple reuptake inhibitors such as selective serotonin reuptake inhibitors (SSRIs), serotonin norepinephrine reuptake inhibitors (SNRIs; sometimes called selective serotonin norepinephrine reuptake inhibitors [SSNRIs]), and atypical antidepressants that affect levels of norepinephrine and dopamine; see Drug Therapy Table 69-1.

Most antidepressants increase or potentiate levels of serotonin. **Serotonin syndrome** is a potentially life-threatening condition that results from elevated levels of serotonin in the blood secondary to drug therapy. Manifestations include fever, sweating, shivering, feelings of intoxication, confusion, restlessness, anxiety, disorientation, ataxia, tachycardia, hypertension, tremors, and muscular spasms and rigidity. The following factors place a client at risk for serotonin syndrome:

- Antidepressants from different classes such as MAOIs and SSRIs are coprescribed.
- The time between weaning from one antidepressant drug to initiating another is inadequate.
- Other serotonergic agonists, drugs that stimulate serotonin receptors, are combined with antidepressant therapy. Serotonergic agonists include dextromethorphan (Benylin, Pertussin, Delsym), meperidine (Demerol), and lithium (Eskalith, Lithane).

Temporarily withholding the antidepressant is recommended initially. In severe cases, symptoms can be managed with anxiolytic drugs such as diazepam (Valium), beta-adrenergic blockers such as propranolol (Inderal), or skeletal muscle relaxants such as dantrolene (Dantrium), while supporting breathing with mechanical ventilation.

Tricyclic Antidepressants

The TCAs such as amitriptyline (Elavil) and imipramine (Tofranil) were the first group of drugs used to treat depression; they occasionally are prescribed for clients with chronic pain (see Chap. 11). Tricyclics were so named because they have three chemical attachments in their organic molecular structure. Many variations of drugs in this category have been developed since the first tricyclics. The subsequent modifications are referred to as *bicyclics* and even *heterocyclics,* according to the changes in their molecules. Collectively, they may be called *cyclic* antidepressants.

Cyclic antidepressants block the **reuptake** of serotonin and norepinephrine (Fig. 69-3). In other words, they interfere

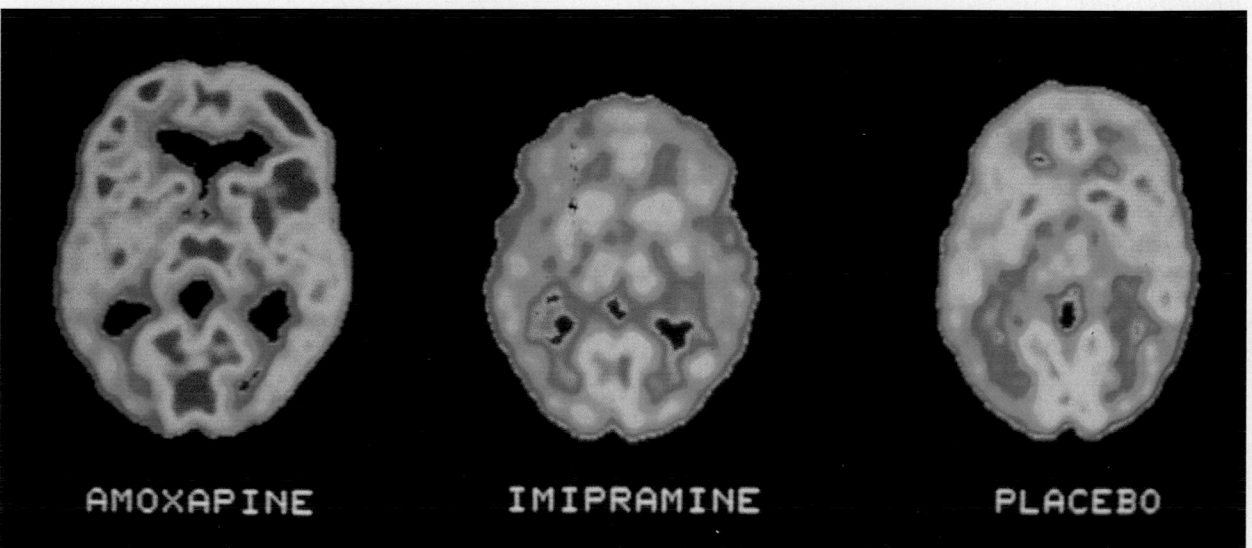

FIGURE 69-2. PET scanning is useful in revealing metabolic changes in the cortex on unmedicated and medicated clients. (Courtesy of Monte S. Buchsbaum, MD, The Mount Sinai Medical Center and School of Medicine, New York, NY. From Videbeck, S. [2007]. *Psychiatric mental health nursing,* 4th ed. Philadelphia: Lippincott Williams & Wilkins.)

DRUG THERAPY TABLE 69-1 Antidepressant Drug Therapy

Drug Category and Examples	Mechanism of Action	Side Effects	Nursing Considerations
Tricyclic antidepressants (TCAs) amitriptyline (Elavil), nortripty-line (Pamelor), imipramine (Tofranil)	Block the reuptake of sero-tonin and norepinephrine	Orthostatic hypotension, sedation, dry mouth, blurred vision, weight gain, constipa-tion, urinary retention, cardiac dysrhythmias	Inform client that maximum relief may not occur for 2–4 weeks or longer. Caution client to rise slowly from a lying or sitting position. Inform client that blurred vision and dry mouth will decrease over time. Discuss the increased potential for suicide as energy increases before depression resolves. Discontinue the drug gradually.
Monoamine oxidase inhibitors (MAOIs) phenelzine (Nardil), tranylcypro-mine (Parnate)	Block the enzyme that breaks down monoamines	Headache, insomnia, severe hypertension with certain foods and drugs, orthostatic hypotension, transient erectile dysfunction, constipation or diarrhea, dry mouth, blurred vision	Provide information on diet and drug restrictions to avoid hy-pertensive crisis. Advise client to wear a Medic Alert bracelet. Educate client about potentially lethal interaction with meperidine (Demerol) Explain that there may be a 2- to 6-week delay before symptoms improve. Advise client to take last dose earlier than bedtime to avoid sleep disturbances. Allow at least a 14-day interval between discontinuing a TCA and initiating an MAOI.
Selective serotonin reuptake inhibitors (SSRIs) fluoxetine (Prozac), sertraline (Zoloft), paroxetine (Paxil)	Block the reuptake of sero-tonin and lesser amounts of norepinephrine	Weight loss, insomnia, tremor, nervousness, headache, decreased libido, erectile dysfunction, interference with liver enzymes that potentiates the risk for altered metabolism of other drugs	Instruct client to avoid caffeine and other foods or drugs that are cardiac stimulants. Monitor blood pressure and heart rate. Allow at least 14 days before switching to an MAOI. Monitor for serotonin syndrome, which can result from a drug-drug interaction.
Serotonin norepinephrine reuptake inhibitors (SNRI) duloxetine (Cymbalta), desvenla-faxine (Pristiq)	Block reuptake of serotonin and norepinephrine and reduce sensitivity to glutamate	Weight gain or loss, (associated with the depressive symp-toms); insomnia, nervousness, headache, decreased libido, erectile dysfunction, chest pain/heart palpitations	Avoid use of caffeine and alcohol. Allow 14 days between changing from or to a MAOI. Monitor for mood changes and signs of serotonin syndrome. Educate in cases of severe depression to monitor for suicidal ideations.

DRUG THERAPY TABLE 69-1 Antidepressant Drug Therapy (*Continued*)

Drug Category and Examples	Mechanism of Action	Side Effects	Nursing Considerations
Atypical Antidepressant Drugs bupropion (Wellbutrin) maprotiline (Ludiomil)	Bupropion blocks reuptake of dopamine and norepinephrine and slight effect on serotonin; maprotiline blocks reuptake of norepinephrine	Weight loss or gain, nervousness, anxiety, decreased libido with maprotiline, potential interaction with other medications	Avoid use of caffeine and alcohol when taking medications. Allow 14 days between switching medications to or from an MAOI; monitor for mood changes.

with the reabsorption of these two neurotransmitters by the releasing presynaptic neuron, thereby creating a sustained effect.

One disadvantage of cyclic antidepressants is the lag time between the initiation of drug therapy and relief of the depressive symptoms. It may take from 10 to 28 days or longer, depending on the specific cyclic drug, before a client notes any change in mood. Another disadvantage is that cyclics are highly lethal if taken in an overdose. Because suicide is not uncommon in clients who are depressed, the physician must consider limiting the number of individual TCAs that are filled in any one prescription. Regardless of the prescribed class of antidepressant, clients with psychomotor retardation may attempt suicide once their level of energy increases. Nurses should not be lulled into thinking that a client who is depressed is necessarily nonsuicidal just because he or she is more active. In fact, close observation is even more important at this time.

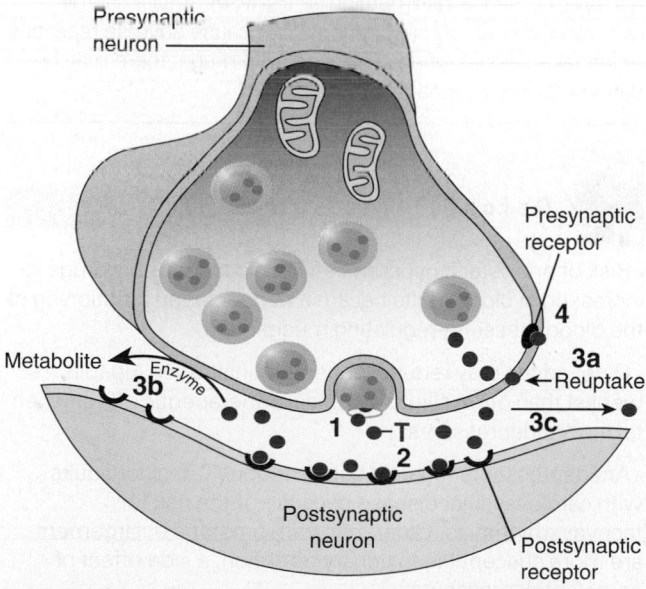

FIGURE 69-3. Schematic illustration of (**1**) neurotransmitter (T) release, (**2**) binding of transmitter to postsynaptic receptor; termination of transmitter action by (**3a**) reuptake of transmitter into the presynaptic terminal, (**3b**) enzymatic degradation, or (**3c**) diffusion away from the synapse; and (**4**) binding of transmitter to presynaptic receptors for feedback regulation of transmitter release. (From Rhoades, R. A. & Tanner, G. A. [1996]. *Medical physiology.* Boston: Little, Brown, p. 46.)

Side effects of cyclic antidepressants, such as postural hypotension, tachycardia, cardiac dysrhythmias, blurred vision, dry mouth, urinary retention, and constipation, make them particularly undesirable for older adults. Some cyclic antidepressants are more sedating than others. Signs of liver toxicity and bone marrow depression require frequent monitoring. The seizure threshold may also be lowered, causing a convulsion in clients who never experienced one before. There must be sufficient time (2–4 weeks) between tapering the dosage of a cyclic antidepressant and initiating drug therapy with an MAOI or SSRI.

Monoamine Oxidase Inhibitors

Monoamine oxidase is an enzyme that breaks down monoamine neurotransmitters. Inhibiting this enzyme allows the neurotransmitters to continue stimulating receptor sites for norepinephrine, serotonin, and, to some extent, dopamine. MAOIs such as tranylcypromine (Parnate) and phenelzine (Nardil), however, are the least prescribed category of antidepressants because they have a high potential for food drug and drug-drug interactions (Box 69-3). When an MAOI is combined with foods containing tyramine, another monoamine, clients are likely to develop a potentially fatal **hypertensive crisis**, with symptoms such as elevated blood pressure, headache (often an occipital headache), nausea, vomiting, sweating, palpitations, visual changes, neck stiffness, sensitivity to light, and tachycardia. The nurse, therefore, has a grave responsibility for teaching clients about dietary and drug restrictions, which the client must follow for at least 2 weeks after discontinuing the MAOI.

The physician usually prescribes a low dose at the beginning of MAOI drug therapy and increases the dose according to the client's tolerance of side effects, which include dry mouth, blurred vision, constipation, urinary retention, postural hypotension, insomnia, weight gain, and sexual dysfunction. The lag time before the client experiences a therapeutic effect is approximately 3 to 6 weeks after beginning MAOI therapy (Fortinash & Holoday-Worret, 2007). Dosages must be tapered when the client no longer needs the drug. At least 2 weeks should elapse after the last dose of a cyclic antidepressant and the initiation of an MAOI.

▶ ***Stop, Think, and Respond Exercise 69-2***

What information would you offer to a person who has just started MAOI therapy and plans to go out for pizza and beer?

BOX 69-3	Food, Beverage, and Drug Restrictions During Monoamine Oxidase Inhibitor Drug Therapy

Food and Beverages to Avoid
Aged, hard cheese
Chocolate
Pickled herring
Overripe bananas
Chicken liver
Dried fish
Fermented meat (salami)
Yogurt
Pepperoni, sausage
Sour cream
Broad beans (fava beans)
Monosodium glutamate
Beer
Soy sauce
Red wine
Meat tenderizer

Drugs to Avoid
Cold and allergy medications
Appetite suppressants
Antiasthmatics
Antihypertensives
Meperidine (Demerol)
Antidepressants in other categories
Local anesthetics with epinephrine

Multiple Reuptake Inhibitors

Three newer categories of drugs may be classified as multiple reuptake inhibitors: SSRIs, SNRIs, and atypical antidepressants.

Selective Serotonin Reuptake Inhibitors. The SSRIs, as their name implies, interfere primarily with the reabsorption of serotonin. They also inhibit reuptake of norepinephrine, but to a lesser degree. The accumulated serotonin prolongs the stimulation of neuroreceptor sites. SSRIs are the newest and currently most prescribed group of drugs used to treat depression. They are widely used for several reasons: (1) they have milder side effects; (2) they are unlikely to cause death in cases of overdose; (3) dosages do not need much adjustment after initiation of therapy; and (4) the lag time is short, perhaps 3 to 10 days.

Although SSRIs cause side effects such as nausea, weight loss, insomnia, nervousness, tremor, and headache, these problems tend to dissipate within weeks of starting drug therapy. If the side effects do not resolve, they can be managed with additional medications such as a mild hypnotic for sleep. Unfortunately, sexual dysfunction (e.g., reduced desire for sex, erectile and ejaculatory dysfunction, inability to reach orgasm) is a frequent and undesirable side effect. Alterations in sexual activity are a leading cause of noncompliance. Lowering the dose of SSRIs can reduce sexual side effects, but many clients, especially men, are reluctant to discuss changes in their sexuality with the prescribing physician.

Recently, concern regarding the use of SSRIs in the treatment of depression in children and adolescents has pro-

liferated. Clinical evidence has shown that clients in this age range experience increased risk of suicidal thoughts and behavior (National Institute of Mental Health, 2005). Although this class of medication clearly provides therapeutic benefits for children and adolescents who are depressed, the U.S. Food and Drug Administration (FDA) (2008) has issued a "black box" prescription drug-warning label. The warning advises the close monitoring of children and adolescents for worsening depression, thoughts or attempts of suicide, or significant changes in behavior, such as social withdrawal.

Serotonin Norepinephrine Reuptake Inhibitors. SNRIs such as duloxetine (Cymbalta) and desvenlafaxine (Pristiq) potentiate the action of both serotonin and norepinephrine by interfering with neuronal reuptake. To reduce the incidence of side effects, the physician may start the client on a low dose and increase it gradually. SNRIs provide rapid relief of symptoms with fewer sexual side effects compared with SSRIs.

Atypical Antidepressants. Several other drugs such as bupropion (Wellbutrin) relieve depression by stabilizing levels of dopamine and norepinephrine. Maprotiline (Ludiomil) and nefazodone (Serzone) inhibit the reuptake of neurotransmitters and also block nerve cell receptors, causing a greater availability of neurotransmitters to the brain. The atypical drugs are used as alternatives for clients who do not respond to trials with other classes of antidepressants.

Pharmacologic Considerations

- Anyone who takes an antidepressant, mood-stabilizing drug, or any other prescribed medication should consult a physician before self-medicating with St. John's wort, ginkgo biloba, kava, tyrosine, or S-adrenosylmethionine (SAM-e) SAM-e. Herbal remedies and dietary supplements can cause adverse reactions when taken alone; when combined with drugs, there may be dangerous interactions.

Gerontologic Considerations

- Risk of orthostatic hypotension from psychotropic drugs is increased in older adults because of decreased functioning of the blood pressure–regulating mechanism.

- Older adults may require longer administration (up to 8 weeks) than other clients to obtain a therapeutic effect when taking antidepressants.

- Antidepressants must be used cautiously in older adults with cardiovascular disease because of the risk for tachydysrhythmias. Older men with prostatic enlargement are more susceptible to urinary retention, a side effect of some antidepressants.

▶ **Stop, Think, and Respond Exercise 69-3**

How would you respond to a client who reports feeling just as depressed as when he or she began antidepressant drug therapy 4 days earlier?

Psychotherapy

Psychotherapy, talking with a psychiatrist, psychologist, or mental health counselor, promotes coping with emotional problems, gaining insight into behaviors, and learning techniques that can improve well-being. Various types of psychotherapy are available:

- *Psychodynamic psychotherapy* is patterned after a Freudian model. Clients discuss their early life experiences to raise repressed feelings to a conscious level. Clients often are in psychodynamic psychotherapy for months to years. This form of therapy can be tedious and expensive, but traumatic events buried deep in the unconscious may require extensive therapy.
- *Interpersonal psychotherapy* is facilitated by a bond that develops between the therapist and client. The empathy and trust help clients gain an understanding of their condition and the courage and support to overcome it.
- *Supportive psychotherapy* helps clients learn about their disorder and treatment techniques, improve or develop new social skills, obtain positive reinforcement for progress, and gain encouragement to persevere.
- *Cognitive therapy* helps clients replace negative, and often illogical, ways of thinking with more positive outlooks. For example, the therapist might encourage a person who believes a friend purposely avoided speaking to him or her in a store to consider other possibilities (e.g., the friend was preoccupied and did not actually notice the client, the friend did not recognize the client, the friend was in a hurry and could not spend time socializing).
- *Behavioral therapy* endeavors to change unhealthy ways of behaving. Clients are rewarded verbally or in some other way when they alter their behavior positively. For example, when a person who is often taken advantage of at work asserts himself or herself, the therapist praises the client's action. The praise and recognition encourage the client to continually repeat the healthy behavior. Gradually, the resulting changes increase self-esteem and promote further improvement.

Psychotherapy often is more productive after clients who are depressed respond to antidepressant drug therapy. Clients should be advised that if they feel uncomfortable or dissatisfied with a particular practitioner or style of therapy, they can be referred elsewhere.

Electroconvulsive Therapy

Electroconvulsive therapy (ECT) uses the application of an electric stimulus to one or both temporal regions of the head to produce a brief, generalized seizure. Although the exact mechanism of action is unknown, the belief is that ECT achieves its effect by either increasing circulating levels of monoamine neurotransmitters or by improving transmission to the receptor site. ECT usually is reserved for clients who are depressed and:

- Have not responded to drug therapy
- Are intolerant of the side effects of antidepressant medications
- Are so seriously suicidal that waiting for antidepressants to become effective jeopardizes their safety

Except for clients who are extremely suicidal, ECT can be administered on an ambulatory, outpatient basis. Many clients experience aftereffects, including headache; soreness of skeletal muscles; temporary confusion; short-term, patchy memory loss; and brief learning disability. ECT usually is contraindicated for clients with cardiac or neurovascular diseases.

Therapeutic Alternatives for Chronic or Treatment-Resistant Depression

Three surgical or device-based interventions can be used to relieve depression in clients who have exhausted drug therapy and have not responded to ECT.

Vagus Nerve Stimulation

Vagus nerve stimulation (VNS) was first used to treat epilepsy. Anecdotally, clients with epilepsy who were treated with VNS reported an improvement in their mood. As a result, in 2005, the FDA approved the use of VNS for intractable depression.

The VNS device consists of an electrode that is tunneled beneath the skin at the neck. One end of the electrode is attached to the vagus nerve, a cranial nerve that exits the brain stem, travels through the neck, and moves down to supply the chest and abdomen. The other end of the electrode is connected to a pulse generator implanted in the chest, similar to a cardiac pacemaker (Fig. 69-4). The pulse generator sends intermittent electrical impulses directed toward the brain via the vagus nerve. VNS can be turned off or reprogrammed by using a hand-held magnetic wand over the pulse generator.

After insertion, a client may experience hoarseness, cough, or some shortness of breath during the time of stimulation. Relief of depressive symptoms may take 9 to 12 months (Schlaepfer et al., 2008).

Deep Brain Stimulation

Deep brain stimulation (DBS), a more invasive procedure, has been used to help manage the tremors caused by Parkinson's disease (see Chap. 37) and other neurologic conditions. It is believed that sending continuous electrical signals via DBS can alter brain circuitry and relieve depression. DBS involves implanting an electrode in the brain through a small opening in the skull. The distal end of the electrode is passed under the skin of the head, neck, and shoulder, eventually connecting to a neurostimulator implanted under the skin near the clavicle, chest, or abdomen. A magnet can be used

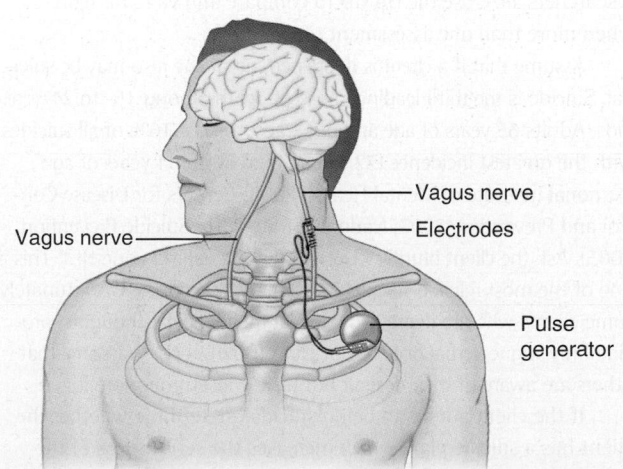

FIGURE 69-4. Vagus nerve stimulation (VNS) sends pulsed waves of energy from a pacemaker-like device under the skin to electrodes attached to a branch of the left vagus cranial nerve. These energy waves subsequently stimulate the areas of the brain that influence mood.

to adjust the neurostimulator. Battery replacement is necessary every 3 to 5 years (Neurosurgerytoday.org, 2007).

Among the effects that clients may experience are temporary tingling in the face or limbs, speech or vision problems, jolting or shocking sensations, dizziness, reduced coordination, and difficulty concentrating.

Transcranial Magnetic Stimulation

Transcranial magnetic stimulation (TMS) is a noninvasive method of stimulating the brain to treat depression. Stimulation is achieved by delivering short pulses of energy through an electromagnetic coil placed against the scalp near the forehead. The energy is aimed at brain cells within the limbic system. Therapy requires administering 3000 pulses a minute for 40 minutes five times a week for 2 to 6 weeks (Mayo Clinic, 2008). Although TMS is expensive (about $6,000 to $10,000 per person), the procedure has proven to be very safe.

Headaches have been the most frequently reported complaint of TMS. Muscle contraction within the scalp or jaw during the procedure may occur (CBS News, 2008).

Nursing Process for the Depressed or Suicidal Client

Assessment

Assess the client physically and monitor mood and affect. Use various standard assessment questionnaires as a database for quantifying a person's mood state and for tracking changes that occur during treatment. Examples are the Beck Depression Inventory, a self-assessment tool that contains 22 multiple-choice questions that the client reads and answers independently, and the Hamilton Rating Scale for Depression (HAMD), which is administered by a mental health worker. Usually the scores on the Beck Depression Inventory correlate closely with the HAMD. The HAMD is used more widely for determining the severity of depression. The National Institute of Mental Health has used the HAMD to evaluate responses to pharmacologic drug treatment; pharmaceutical companies use the HAMD when submitting research results for new antidepressant approval by the FDA; and practitioners and researchers alike use the HAMD to compare and validate scores when more than one assessment tool is used.

Assume that if a client is depressed, he or she also may be suicidal. Suicide is the third leading cause of death among 15- to 24-year-olds. Adults 65 years of age and older account for 16% of all suicides, with the greatest incidence (22.9%) in men 80 to 84 years of age (National Institute of Mental Health, 2008; Centers for Disease Control and Prevention, 2007; National Strategy for Suicide Prevention, 2005). Ask the client bluntly, "Do you feel like killing yourself?" This is one of the most reliable suicide assessment techniques. Unfortunately, some clients who are depressed conceal their suicidal thoughts, provide only vague verbal or behavior clues (Box 69-4), or assume that others are aware of their despair but have chosen to ignore it.

If the client admits to being suicidal, determine whether the client has a suicide plan, which increases the seriousness of the risk. Assess if the plan is feasible and determine whether it is of high or low lethality. High-lethality methods are those from which the possibility of rescue is remote. Some examples include shooting

BOX 69-4 Clues of Suicidal Intentions

Clear Verbal Clues
"I'm planning to kill myself."
"I wish I were dead."

Vague Verbal Clues
"I just can't stand it any longer."
"Nobody needs me anymore."
"Life has lost its meaning for me."
"You won't be seeing me anymore."
"I'm getting out."
"Everybody would be better off without me."

Behavioral Clues
Giving away a valued possession
Donating large sums of money to charity
Putting personal affairs in order
Writing poetry with morbid themes
Composing a suicide note
Making funeral arrangements
Buying a gun; stockpiling pills
Lifting of depressed mood (may indicate a plan and energy to carry it out)

or hanging oneself; jumping from a bridge or building; throwing oneself in front of a train or truck; and driving into a tree, into a wall, or off a cliff. Low-lethality methods are those that allow a window of time for the person who attempts suicide to be found and rescued. They include overdosing on medications, cutting the wrists, or inhaling carbon monoxide. In almost all cases, people who are suicidal are ambivalent—they would choose life rather than death if they held some hope for the future. Despite conscientious efforts to prevent suicide, some people cannot be stopped.

Determine the level at which the client who is depressed can carry out activities of daily living. People who are depressed may not eat, bathe, shave, or shampoo or style their hair. In some cases, they neglect self-care because they lack energy. They also may ignore cleanliness and grooming because of low self-esteem or little concern for social acceptance.

Gerontologic Considerations

- The rate of suicide is extremely high in older adults. Older adults who are depressed often use a high-lethality method to ensure successful suicide. Losses such as death of family/friends or relocation, physical and emotional changes of aging, and lack of control over chronic or terminal illness may trigger feelings of hopelessness, which increase the risk of suicide.

- Behaviors such as putting personal affairs in order, giving away possessions, and making funeral plans are a sign of good judgment in older adults and do not necessarily convey suicidal ideation. Other indicators, such as unsatisfactory relationships, poor or failing health, divorce, losing one's spouse or partner, or addiction may be stronger indicators of suicide in older adults.

Diagnosis, Planning, and Interventions

▶ **Risk for Suicide** related to feelings of hopelessness

▶ **Expected Outcomes:** (1) The client will not harm self. (2) The client will identify a reason for living.

- If hospitalized, move the client close to the nursing station. *Doing so facilitates close and frequent observation.*
- Encourage a client who is not hospitalized to contact a friend or relative rather than remain alone. *The presence of another supportive person can deter a suicide attempt.*
- Talk to a nonhospitalized client on the phone as long as possible while contacting a 911 operator. *Communication with a comforting person can delay a potential suicide attempt or provide time to obtain assistance from emergency personnel who can intervene.*
- Make a verbal or written contract with the client that he or she will not attempt suicide. *Clients often honor such commitments.*
- Confiscate any objects that the client may use for self-harm, such as belts, shoelaces, safety razors, sharp combs, keys, or knives. *Limiting access to items that the client can use for self-destruction reduces the resources he or she has for attempting suicide.*
- Inspect the client's mouth, looking under the tongue and within the buccal cavity, after administering medications. *Suicidal clients may conceal and hoard medications until they stockpile sufficient numbers for an overdose.*
- Observe the client's whereabouts at least every 15 minutes, and spend time interacting with him or her. *These measures reduce the client's potential time for attempting or completing suicide and increase the response time available to resuscitate a person who has attempted suicide.*
- Keep the client busy and involved in activities. *Activity shifts the client's attention away from his or her emotional pain and hopelessness.*

▶ **Ineffective Coping** related to feelings of helplessness and worthlessness

▶ **Expected Outcome:** The client will identify one or more alternatives to suicide.

- Acknowledge the client's feeling of despair. *Recognizing a client's mood demonstrates that the nurse has noticed the person and is perceptive.*
- Indicate that you want to help. *Offering assistance is characterized as a therapeutic use of self. Doing so reassures the client that you will not abandon him or her and that he or she is worthy of help.*
- Emphasize hope, previous positive experiences, and outcomes. *Such discussion reinforces that the client has the potential to overcome current difficulties based on past success.*
- Explore other courses of action rather than suicide. *Alternatives help the client consider options for dealing with the current situation.*
- Appeal to the client's ambivalence by indicating that current feelings are likely to change given additional time. *Most suicidal clients will delay or dismiss suicidal activities if they believe that they will feel better eventually.*
- Discuss previous coping strategies and encourage using some that were effective in the past. *Reusing previous methods for managing problems offers the possibility that similar actions can achieve a positive result.*
- Develop a plan for maintaining future safety such as talking with a trusted friend or calling a crisis hotline. *If a plan is developed, there is a possibility that the client will implement it.*

▶ **Disturbed Sleep Pattern** related to depression

▶ **Expected Outcome:** The client will sleep a maximum of 8 hours during the night with no napping during the day.

- Keep the client busy during the day, and discourage napping or going to bed early. *Left alone, depressed clients are likely to become more vegetative (i.e., they withdraw by sleeping).*
- Include active exercise during the day, but not before bedtime. *Exercise relieves anxiety, but it may cause stimulation when performed at night.*

Evaluation of Expected Outcomes

Expected outcomes are that the client's suicidal feelings pass. The client implements new or previously successful coping strategies to manage emotional problems. At night, the client falls asleep easily and does not awaken for 6 to 8 hours.

SEASONAL AFFECTIVE DISORDER

Seasonal affective disorder (SAD) is a mood disorder that has its onset during darker winter months and spontaneously disappears in the spring. SAD is more prevalent among people living in states north of 40 to 50° of latitude, such as Washington, Oregon, Minnesota, Michigan, New York, and the New England states. Native Alaskans do not manifest the disorder as much as those who move there.

Pathophysiology and Etiology

The best explanation for SAD is that it is a primitive biologic response triggered by **photoperiods**, daytime hours that are short because of fewer hours of sunlight. The condition actually resembles the characteristics of hibernating animals. Theorists believe that light rays follow a visual pathway to the hypothalamus, the center for regulating sleep, hunger, libido, and mood. The hypothalamus relays the light-sensing data to the pineal gland, which regulates the production of a hormone called melatonin. **Melatonin**, which also affects regulation of serotonin, induces sleep during dark hours and is suppressed by daylight (Fig. 69-5). When hours of daylight become fewer, the production of melatonin is extended. In northern latitudes, melatonin secretion is sustained until spring, when days become brighter and longer.

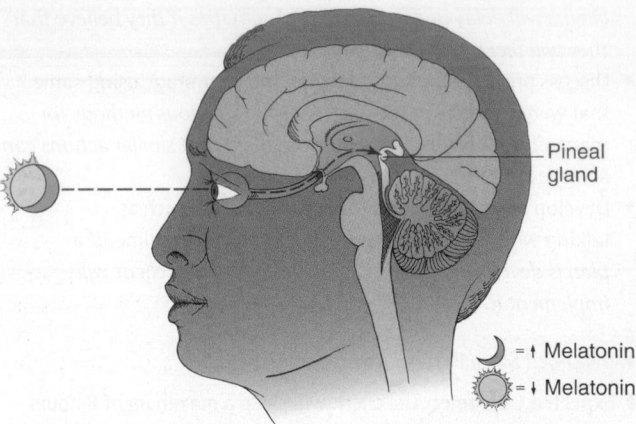

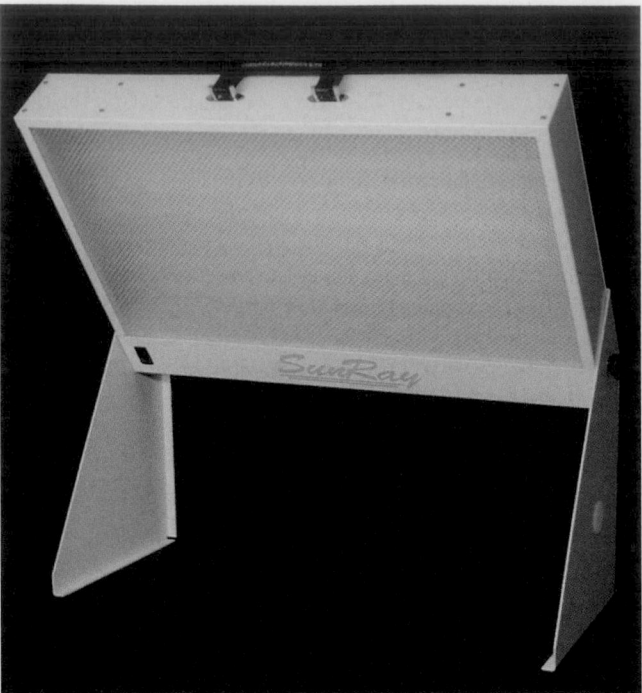

FIGURE 69-5. Melatonin (and subsequently serotonin) levels depend on exposure to sunlight. Melatonin induces sleep during dark hours and is suppressed by daylight. Dark months result in seasonal affective disorder for some people.

Assessment Findings

Clients with SAD use the terms *sleepy, fatigued,* and *lethargic* to describe themselves in the winter. The lack of energy crosses over into feeling irritable, unable to concentrate, worthless, guilty, depressed—even suicidal. Some also report cravings for carbohydrates, which leads to weight gain, much like an animal preparing to sleep through the winter. As clients with SAD become more depressed and irritable, they are less inclined to interact socially. Many tend to stay indoors and dread leaving home.

The depression is bimodal; it cycles with the seasons. After a prolonged period of winter depression, most report a lifting of spirits in the spring. Some also describe feeling energetic, more motivated, hyperactive, and even euphoric. The cheery mood or absence of depressive symptoms tends to be sustained until late fall, when the depressive pattern repeats itself.

At this time, no diagnostic tests can confirm SAD. Physicians rely on clients' reports of cycling moods that correlate with the ratio of sunlight.

Medical Management

For those who cannot move to a sunnier location, phototherapy is the best alternative for treating SAD. **Phototherapy** involves using artificial light that simulates the intensity of sunlight. The artificial light is produced by fluorescent bulbs at 2,500 to 10,000 lux, the international measurement of illumination. Ten thousand lux is approximately 10 to 20 times as bright as ordinary indoor light.

The frequency and duration for phototherapy can vary, but a common prescription is to sit by the light source from 30 minutes to 2 hours per day, preferably in the early morning hours (Fig. 69-6). The client need not stare at the fluorescent light; in fact, it is best not to look directly at it. Glancing periodically at the light is sufficient to relieve symptoms in 1 to 2 weeks. Other models are available as well. A head-mounted light that shines on the face during daytime activities facilitates mobility. Bedroom phototherapy lights can be set with an automatic timer to come on at a predawn schedule. Even though the sleeper's eyes are closed, it is

FIGURE 69-6. Phototherapy products such as a light box relieve the symptoms of seasonal affective disorder. (Courtesy of Light Therapy Products.)

believed that the light penetrates the eyelids, which triggers a decline in melatonin—much like daybreak naturally activates arousal from sleep.

Nursing Management

Because most clients with SAD are outpatients or may soon become so, the nurse provides information on how to implement phototherapy and how to supplement its beneficial effects. One of the most important principles to stress is that natural sunlight is brighter and better than any artificial substitute. The nurse also should teach measures found in Client and Family Teaching 69-1.

Client and Family Teaching 69-1
Seasonal Affective Disorder (SAD)

The nurse teaches the client who experiences SAD and his or her family the following:

● Avoid the use of eyeglasses or contact lenses that are coated to shield ultraviolet radiation, because the coating interferes with light transmission to the pineal gland.
● Add more lamps and bright fixtures at home and work.
● Install skylights.
● Trim shrubs and trees from around windows.
● Use translucent curtains or shades rather than heavy drapes.
● Sleep and work in an east-facing room.
● Take brief walks outside around noon without sunglasses.
● Jog after sunup and before sundown.
● Take up an outdoor winter sport.

BIPOLAR DISORDER

The several types of **bipolar disorder** all involve cycling among depressive, euthymic, and euphoric moods (Types of Bipolar Disorder, 2008). Typically, people with *bipolar I disorder* experience severely dysfunctional moods lasting several months; depressive phases tend to be longer than manic phases. Some clients with bipolar I disorder may also manifest psychotic symptoms such as delusions and hallucinations (see Chap. 72) from time to time. People with *bipolar II disorder* have severe depression alternating with hypomania, a milder degree of mania, between periods of euthymia. People with bipolar II disorder never have psychotic symptoms. In *cyclothymic disorder*, a subtype of bipolar II disorder, people have milder mood swings, which occur abruptly and are of short duration. However, clients with cyclothymic disorder are never free of symptoms for more than 2 months. Ironically, in *mixed bipolar disorder*, mania and depression occur simultaneously. People feel grandiose and have a great deal of energy, but they are irritable and are quick to anger. Clients with *rapid cycling bipolar disorder* experience at least four episodes of mania and depression per year, whereas those with *ultra-rapid cycling bipolar disorder* have alternating moods that may occur within a month or less.

 Gerontologic Considerations

- As people with bipolar disorder age, depressive episodes may increase in frequency and last longer. The functional decline may lead to relocation to a long-term care setting.

Pathophysiology and Etiology

Extremes in levels of monoamines—excessive in mania and inadequate during depression—seem to be responsible for the symptoms of bipolar disorder. In severe cases, excess dopamine may cause distorted thinking and hallucinations. Another possibility is that there is insufficient **gamma-aminobutyric acid** (GABA), an inhibitory neurotransmitter, to counteract the effects of the monoamines. Altered blood calcium levels also may contribute to the development of bipolar disorder because calcium is required for exciting neurons. Genetic predisposition also is implicated in the development of bipolar disorder.

Assessment Findings

Signs and Symptoms

Signs and symptoms of the depressive phase of bipolar disorder are the same as those for major depression. During the manic phase, clients are hyperactive and often display an exaggerated sense of their own importance. They can quickly become angry and aggressive with those who attempt to restrain their burst of energy and wild ideas. Because judgment is impaired—another characteristic of the disorder—reckless and impulsive behavior such as sexual promiscuity, criminal activity, spending sprees, gambling, and risky business transactions can occur. The surge of norepinephrine allows clients who are experiencing the manic phase to go without sleep for long periods. It also causes rapid thinking accompanied by racing speech. When extremely ill, some people experience psychotic features such as hallucinations. Combined with delusions, which are illogical false beliefs, clients with bipolar disorder can become homicidal or suicidal.

Diagnostic Findings

It eventually may be possible to predict which people will develop bipolar disorder with the use of gene mapping. At present, however, no objective tests are available, and the diagnosis is based on the client's history. The key indicator is the client's pattern of emotional "highs" and "lows." A family member with bipolar disorder is a risk factor, as is a history of substance abuse, because undiagnosed people naively attempt to self-medicate to relieve the depressive episodes.

Medical Management

Bipolar disorder is managed by the administration of one or more mood-stabilizing medications (Drug Therapy Table 69-2). Lithium (Eskalith, Lithane, Lithobid), a chemical element, usually is the initial drug of choice. It controls both depressive as well as manic symptoms in clients who respond to lithium monotherapy (single-drug treatment). The American Psychiatric Association's Practice Guideline for the Treatment of Bipolar Disorder (2002) also recommends the use of anticonvulsants such as valproic acid derivatives (Depakote, Depakene, Valproate), carbamazepine (Tegretol), or oxcarbazepine (Trileptal), alone or in combination with lithium, for controlling mood swings. Antipsychotics such as olanzapine (Zyprexa) or risperidone (Risperdal) (see Chap. 71) also may be prescribed for a brief period to induce sedation and control hallucinations and delusions. Benzodiazepines such as lorazepam (Ativan) may be used as an adjunctive drug during initial symptom management. Some have proposed using calcium channel blockers, but little research supports the application of their use for managing bipolar disorder.

Lithium

Lithium is a naturally occurring element found in stone and spring water that flows from underground sources. Pharmaceutical preparations are available for those who are lithium-deficient. When ingested, lithium moves easily through cell membranes, but it is less easily removed. Some believe that this feature may stabilize cell membranes, leading to the equalization of moods. Another possibility is that lithium regulates the activity between neurotransmitters such as serotonin, norepinephrine, dopamine, and their receptor sites. However, lithium:

- May be ineffective for some.
- Has a delay of 5 to 14 days in achieving therapeutic benefits.
- Has a narrow range of safety between a therapeutic serum level (0.8–1.2 mEq) and toxic levels (1.5 mEq).
- May be nontherapeutic or dangerously elevated when taken in combination with other drugs (Box 69-5).
- Causes side effects that challenge compliance.
- Requires periodic laboratory tests to monitor serum blood levels.

Lithium crosses the placental barrier; therefore, its use is contraindicated in pregnant women. Furthermore, lithium is

DRUG THERAPY TABLE 69-2 Mood-Stabilizing Medications

Drug Examples	Mechanism of Action	Side Effects	Nursing Considerations
lithium carbonate (Eskalith, Lithane, Lithobid)	Alters sodium transport in nerve and muscle cells; increases intraneural stores and inhibits release of norepinephrine and dopamine	Hand tremors, nausea, vomiting, diarrhea, thirst, polyuria, sedation, thyroid dysfunction, wrist and ankle edema at therapeutic level	Administer with meals. Withhold if serum level is ≥1.5 mEq. Female clients should use contraception and avoid breast-feeding.
valproic acid (Depakote)	May increase levels of GABA	Drowsiness, mild tremor, ataxia, nausea, vomiting, diarrhea, blood dyscrasias, liver toxicity	Administer with meals. Caution client to avoid activities that require alertness and coordination. Monitor blood for therapeutic level.
oxcarbazepine (Trileptal)	Decreases rate of neuronal impulse transmission	Dizziness, drowsiness, unsteady gait, nausea, vomiting, skin rash, liver toxicity, hyponatremia, ankle swelling, birth defects	Administer with meals. Caution client to avoid activities that require alertness and coordination. Monitor blood for therapeutic levels. Female clients should use contraceptives.
clonazepam (Klonopin)	May increase brain levels of GABA	Drowsiness, dizziness, unsteady gait, nausea, vomiting, constipation, blood dyscrasias, dry mouth, liver toxicity	Collaborate with the physician on baseline blood tests before initiating therapy. Administer drug with food or milk. Drowsiness may be potentiated if combined with alcohol or other sedative drugs. Monitor laboratory findings during therapy and withhold drug if there is bone marrow suppression or serious elevation in liver enzymes. Advise sucking on hard candy or more frequent oral hygiene to relieve dry mouth. Advise women that incidence of birth defects increases if drug is taken during pregnancy, and to use a reliable contraceptive while taking this drug. Never discontinue the drug abruptly.

GABA = gamma-aminobutyric acid.

water soluble and present in all body fluids, including breast milk. Lithium administered to infants through breast milk can cause toxicity; thus, breast-feeding mothers should also avoid use. Loss of body fluid from diarrhea, diuretics, and excessive perspiration can lead to concentrated blood levels and lithium toxicity. Because the body always attempts to balance cations with anions, lithium may be retained if sodium levels are low. Providers must stress the importance of maintaining an adequate ingestion of salt to all clients who rely on lithium to control their disorder.

Pharmacologic Considerations

- Monitor for signs and symptoms of lithium toxicity: diarrhea, vomiting, nausea, drowsiness, muscular weakness, twitching, and lack of coordination.

- Polyuria can occur with administration of lithium. Unless contraindicated because of a disease condition, the client

may require an increase in fluids up to 3000 mL/day to maintain fluid balance.

BOX 69-5	Drugs Affecting Serum Lithium Levels

Increase Serum Lithium Level
Tetracycline
Thiazide diuretics
Loop diuretics
Nonsteroidal anti-inflammatory drugs (NSAIDs)
Haloperidol

Decrease Serum Lithium Level
Theophylline
Aminophylline
Carbamazepine
Sodium bicarbonate
Osmotic diuretics

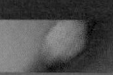

NURSING CARE PLAN 69-1 — The Client With Bipolar Disorder/Acute Manic Phase

Assessment

- It may be necessary to perform the initial assessment and physical examination in brief increments. Bipolar clients have short attention spans and poor concentration; they become easily frustrated if their activity is curtailed. As an alternative, use the family as a more objective resource for necessary information. Their information is valuable because the client's symptoms have usually created multiple crises.
- Determine what types of prescribed medications the client takes and if he or she has been compliant with the medication regimen. Sometimes antidepressants can trigger manic symptoms because they raise mono amine neurotransmitter levels.
- Ask about the client's use of alcohol or other controlled substances because many clients with bipolar disorder attempt to self-medicate to control their moods or they use drugs recreationally because of their poor judgment.

- Obtain information about the client's recent sleep patterns, hydration, and dietary intake.
- Observe the client's attention to hygiene and manner of dress. Check the female client's last date of menstruation and if she has consistently used contraception.
- Prepare the client for laboratory and diagnostic tests that are likely to include an electrocardiogram, thyroid function studies, and a profile of blood chemistry tests. Note if the client is voiding in sufficient quantities and inquire as to the client's bowel elimination patterns, including the date of the last bowel movement.
- Record baseline vital signs.
- Listen to the client's thought content during verbal interactions. The client is likely to speak loudly and rapidly. At the very least, bipolar clients express expansive and elaborate ideas or schemes. Some may have paranoid ideas or inflate their own importance. They may be experiencing hallucinations.

Nursing Diagnosis: Disturbed Thought Processes related to excessive levels of monoamines

Expected Outcome: Client will be oriented and accurately perceive circumstances surrounding admission.

Interventions	Rationales
Orient client to person, place, time, and events.	Racing thoughts often interfere with comprehension.
Provide information in small amounts, using brief sentences.	Brief discussions accommodate for short attention span.
Reduce distracting stimuli such as noise and stimulation.	External stimuli potentiate client's internal activity.
Present reality when client is delusional; do not press the issue if it causes agitation.	Failing to present reality reinforces that client's delusions are real. Persistence may create conflict or cause client to act out violently.
Monitor client's whereabouts to ensure that he or she does not wander from unit or healthcare agency.	Bipolar clients are impulsive and resist being confined. Healthcare personnel are responsible for safety at all times.

Evaluation of Expected Outcome

- Client becomes oriented.
- Client interacts appropriately for the situation.

Nursing Diagnosis: Risk for Other-Directed Violence and **Risk for Self-Directed Violence**

Expected Outcome: Client will not injure self or others.

Interventions	Rationales
Take client to a room or other secluded area when he or she shows signs of aggression.	Decreased stimulation may restore self-control.
Set firm limits for behavioral expectations using a modulated and controlled tone of voice.	Client remains informed of the kinds of behavior that will not be tolerated. A modulated, controlled voice is less likely to provoke a confrontation.
Offer client a large-muscle activity like playing basketball or riding an exercise bicycle.	Exercise releases energy and reduces the potential for an angry outburst.
Administer a prescribed short-acting sedative if aggressive behavior escalates and endangers others.	A sedate client is more responsive to directions from others and less likely to become physically violent.
Obtain an order to seclude or restrain if client becomes violent.	Legally, restraints must be avoided unless absolutely necessary to protect others because clients have the right to the least restrictive treatment.
Initiate suicide precautions if data suggest vulnerability for self-harm.	The client's safety is a priority of care.

Evaluation of Expected Outcome

- Client has no angry outbursts.
- Client demonstrates self-control.

(care plan continues on page 1102)

NURSING CARE PLAN 69-1 **The Client With Bipolar Disorder/Acute Manic Phase** (Continued)

Nursing Diagnosis: Imbalanced Nutrition: Less than Body Requirements related to increased activity and distraction from eating

Expected Outcome: Client will maintain admission weight.

Interventions	Rationales
Consult the dietitian about increasing calories at meal times.	Loading calories without loading quantities of food may help maintain weight and nutrition.
Offer liquid nutritional supplements at least three times a day.	Each container of liquid nourishment may provide 350 or more calories. Consuming liquids does not require sitting at a table and interrupting activity.
Provide finger foods that the client may consume throughout the day.	Frequent snacking increases caloric intake and nourishment.

Evaluation of Expected Outcome

Client consumes sufficient food to maintain weight.

Nursing Diagnosis: Risk for Imbalanced Fluid Volume related to polyuria secondary to lithium therapy and inattention to thirst

Expected Outcome: Client will be adequately hydrated insert period

Interventions	Rationales
Monitor intake and output if possible.	Urine output of 1500 to 3000 mL indicates an adequate fluid volume.
Offer at least 25000 to 3000 mL of fluid per day.	An adequate volume compensates for polyuria that can occur with lithium therapy. Urination ensures excretion of lithium.
Monitor electrolyte laboratory results.	Electrolytes become elevated when fluid intake is low.

Evaluation of Expected Outcome

- Client consumes sufficient fluids to maintain hydration.
- Client has moist mucous membranes, light-colored urine, and normal body temperature.

Nursing Diagnosis: Bathing/Hygiene Self-Care Deficit related to decreased attention and concentration

Expected Outcome: Client will be clean and groomed each day.

Interventions	Rationales
Prepare necessities for bathing, grooming, and hygiene for client. Supervise hygiene and provide assistance if needed.	Distractibility may interfere with client's ability to organize hygiene items. Client may be less thorough without nurse's supervision.
Spread uncompleted hygiene tasks throughout remainder of the day.	All hygiene needs may not be met at one time.
Help client to dress appropriately and remain dressed.	Bipolar clients may dress flamboyantly or seductively unless supervised. Poor judgment may result in episodes of nudity.

Evaluation of Expected Outcome

Client resumes independent responsibility for self-care and activities of daily living.

 Gerontologic Considerations

- Older adults taking lithium for bipolar disorder require careful monitoring of lithium levels. The kidneys eliminate lithium, and age-related changes may reduce renal clearance, predisposing older clients to lithium toxicity.

Anticonvulsants

Anticonvulsants may achieve their therapeutic effects by enhancing the action of GABA in much the same way that benzodiazepines reduce anxiety (see Chap. 68). One of the first anticonvulsants used to treat bipolar disorder was carbamazepine (Tegretol). It still is used to manage the symptoms of clients at the onset of acute mania. In addition, it is efficacious for decreasing the incidence and frequency of mood swings among rapid cyclers. However, because carbamazepine stimulates drug metabolism by the liver, maintaining consistent therapeutic drug levels is difficult. Clients who take carbamazepine also are at risk for infection because the drug impairs white blood cell formation. Consequently, serum drug levels and leukocyte counts must be monitored periodically.

Valproic acid derivatives such as Depakote are preferred to carbamazepine most of the time. These derivatives also enhance GABA activity. Clients who take valproic acid tend to experience gastrointestinal symptoms such as nausea, vomiting, and diarrhea. Some experience sedation and ataxia, putting them at risk for injury. Periodic assessment of liver function, serum ammonia, and blood cell counts is necessary. Although valproic acid is unsafe during pregnancy, it can be combined with lithium and used for the long-term management of bipolar disorder.

Nursing Management

Nursing Care Plan 69-1 provides a detailed discussion of care for the client with bipolar disorder. Before discharge, the nurse educates the client and his or her significant others on these aspects:

- The disease process
- How prescribed drugs help in symptom management
- Drug effects and side effects
- Signs of drug toxicity and actions to take
- Frequency of blood tests
- The advantages of wearing a MedicAlert bracelet

In addition to arranging outpatient therapy, the nurse informs the client and others of support groups that can continue the educational and therapeutic processes. Both the client and those who live in the same environment need to understand the signs of relapse, such as an inability to sleep for several days in a row, or increasingly impulsive behavior, such as making unnecessary purchases. The nurse also reviews the signs of cycling into a depressed mood so that indications for reinitiating medical care are clear.

CRITICAL THINKING EXERCISES

1. Two clients who are depressed are in a psychiatric hospital. One feels suicidal but has no plan for carrying out the suicide. The other indicates that he would kill himself with a gun but has none. Describe the similarities and differences in their nursing care.
2. What physical consequences might occur for the client in a manic episode?

3. What problems might family members experience as a result of living with a person with a mood disorder?
4. Based on what is known about seasonal affective disorder, explain why people with this condition feel energized in the spring and are unmotivated when winters have prolonged prolonged periods of cloudy, rainy weather.

NCLEX-STYLE REVIEW QUESTIONS

1. Immediately after administering an antidepressant to a client who is at risk for suicide, which of the following nursing interventions is most appropriate?
   1. Observing the client at least every 15 minutes
   2. Inspecting the client's mouth and oral cavity
   3. Spending time interacting with the client
   4. Exploring alternatives to suicide with the client

2. A cyclic antidepressant is prescribed for a client with major depression. What information should the nurse include in the health teaching for the client and family? Select all that apply.
   1. The client should rise slowly to avoid hypotension.
   2. It may take 2 to 3 days before noting any change in mood.
   3. Seasonal affective disorder may develop.
   4. This drug is highly lethal if an overdose is taken.
   5. Convulsions are a potential side effect.

3. Electroconvulsive therapy is usually reserved for which group of depressed clients? Select all that apply.
   1. Those who have no history of a seizure disorder
   2. Those who are intolerant of side effects of antidepressants
   3. Those who are severely suicidal
   4. Those who are prone to hypertensive crisis
   5. Those who have not responded to drug therapy

4. Which of the following instructions should a nurse provide to a client who depends on lithium to control bipolar disorder? Select all that apply.
   1. Ensure adequate exercise.
   2. Drink ample amounts of fluid.
   3. Ensure an adequate intake of salt.
   4. Have regular laboratory tests.
   5. Do not eat aged, hard cheese.

5. When reviewing the lithium level of a client with bipolar disorder, which laboratory finding indicates a therapeutic level?
   1. 0.3 mEq
   2. 0.5 mEq
   3. 1.2 mEq
   4. 1.8 mEq

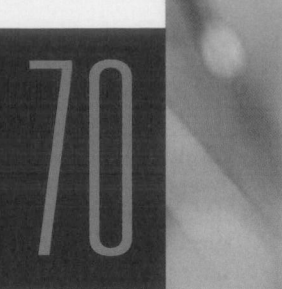

70

Caring for Clients with Eating Disorders

Words to Know

adipocytes
anorexia nervosa
binge eating disorder
body mass index
bulimarexia
bulimia nervosa
compulsive overeating
corticotropin-releasing factor
eating disorders
endocannabinoids
food binges
lanugo
leptin
melanin-concentrating hormone
normal eating
orexin A and B
purging
satiety
water loading

Learning Objectives

On completion of this chapter, you will be able to:

1. Differentiate normal eating from an eating disorder.
2. Name four types of eating disorders.
3. Describe two forms of anorexia nervosa.
4. Name the neurotransmitters, neurohormones, and other chemicals that affect the appetite and satiety center in the brain.
5. Discuss two reasons why most people with anorexia nervosa induce self-starvation.
6. Identify the tool used to evaluate a person's size in relation to norms within the adult population.
7. Give the healthy range for body mass index.
8. List four components of treatment for clients with anorexia nervosa.
9. Discuss the nurse's role in managing the care of a client with anorexia nervosa.
10. Give two examples of how people with bulimia nervosa compensate for binging.
11. Name two problems, besides nutrition, that are the nursing focus when caring for clients with bulimia nervosa.
12. Differentiate between binge eating disorder and compulsive overeating.
13. Discuss at least three psychosocial problems that may accompany overeating syndromes.
14. Describe nursing care for a client with binge eating disorder or compulsive overeating.

A rich variety of foods, sufficient for energy needs, growth and repair of cells, and maintenance of weight, is required to preserve health. Depending on such variables as gender, age, physical condition, activity level, and height, normal eating involves consuming approximately 1,500 to 2,500 calories per day, usually spread over three meals and two to three snacks. **Normal eating** occurs in response to hunger and ceases when **satiety** (a feeling of comfortable fullness) is attained. This chapter deals with conditions that involve eating disorders.

Collectively, **eating disorders** involve eating that

- Is outside the range of normal
- Is accompanied by anxiety and guilt
- Results in physiologic imbalances or medical complications

Eating disorders affect 7 million women and 1 million men of all ethnicities and socioeconomic levels (National Association of Anorexia Nervosa and Associated Disorders, 2008). These conditions are more prevalent in young women between 12 and 25 years of age.

Often, clients with eating disorders strive to keep their illness secret; family and friends may become aware of the problem only when emotional and behavioral symptoms become repeatedly noticeable

TABLE 70-1 Signs and Symptoms of Eating Disorders

EATING DISORDER	PHYSICAL	EMOTIONAL	BEHAVIORAL
Anorexia nervosa	Decrease of 25% in body weight; weight is 85% or less of normal; lanugo; alopecia; cold intolerance; amenorrhea; constipation; abdominal pain	Distorted body image; hatred of a particular body part; low self-esteem; depression; isolation; perfectionism	Restriction of food choices and intake; ritualistic handling of food (e.g., cutting into tiny pieces, arranging food in a certain way); weighing oneself frequently; denial of hunger
Bulimia nervosa	Inability to interpret accurately hunger and fullness signals; swelling of parotid glands ("chipmunk cheeks"); frequent weight fluctuations; irregular menses	Feeling unable to control eating; depressive mood and frequent mood swings; black-and-white thinking; exaggerated concern about weight	Excessive exercise, use of diuretics, and laxatives; secret eating of high-calorie, high-carbohydrate foods; alternately binging and fasting
Binge eating and compulsive overeating	Obesity; discomfort after eating	Preoccupation with weight, eating, and dieting; attributes professional and social success and failure to weight; feels disgust or guilt after eating; feels lack of control over eating	Frequent dieting; restricts activities because of embarrassment about weight; eating when not hungry; rapid eating; eating alone

(Table 70-1) or when serious health consequences develop. Box 70-1 is a self-test that can assist people in determining if an eating pattern is abnormal.

Gerontologic Considerations

- Eating disorders in the older population are often overlooked or inaccurately diagnosed and may result in death. Accurate diagnosis is complicated by age related changes such as loss of appetite due to diminished taste or smell or medication side effects; physical disabilities that interfere with obtaining, preparing, or eating foods; and effects of chronic comorbidities.

Anorexia nervosa, bulimia nervosa, binge eating, and compulsive overeating are eating disorders. Obesity is a consequence of overeating; therefore, some clients who are obese also have an eating disorder.

ANOREXIA NERVOSA

Anorexia nervosa is an eating disorder characterized by an obsession for thinness that is achieved through self-starvation. It occurs more often in women. One of 200 girls 12 to 18 years of age develops anorexia nervosa. Although men also have eating disorders, they are less likely to disclose this type of information to a health professional, and when they do, the information is often dismissed, untreated, and unreported.

People with anorexia nervosa consume an average of 600 to 900 calories per day, and often less. They feel hunger but control the urge to eat because of a morbid fear of becoming fat. Almost universally, people with anorexia consider themselves obese despite appearing emaciated.

There are two types of anorexia: (1) severe restriction of caloric intake, and (2) **bulimarexia**, of extended self-

starvation and a period of extended binging and purging which cycle at alternate times.

Pathophysiology and Etiology

The exact cause of anorexia nervosa is unknown. Many authorities believe that anorexia and other eating disorders result from a combination of cultural, social, psychological, and physiologic factors. More and more evidence is strengthening the connection between genetics and altered physiology.

Culturally and socially, young women and men are influenced by role models in the media—people who are extremely thin. It is suggested that thinness is linked to attractiveness and success. However, the image being portrayed as ideal is, for most people, unhealthy and unrealistic. Self-starvation or rigorous physical activity is sometimes the only way to achieve a similar appearance. Some athletes such as gymnasts, ice skaters, and even ballet dancers restrict food intake, assuming that low body weight will improve performance.

Physiological influences play a major role in the development of eating disorders. Research suggests that neurotransmitters and neurohormones, which may be genetically altered, influence normal and abnormal eating patterns by binding with receptors in the appetite center of the hypothalamus. People with anorexia may experience a dysregulation of serotonin and dopamine. Increased serotonin levels contribute to restricted eating; the brain is fooled into believing satiety has occurred (Kaye, 2008). Support for this phenomenon is evident by the fact that drugs that increase serotonin such as some selective serotonin reuptake inhibitors (SSRIs; see Chap. 69) produce weight loss as a side effect. High serotonergic activity also may relate to overcontrol of eating, obsessive thinking, and perfectionism. Normal levels of dopamine influence both realistic thinking and pleasure. An excess of dopamine may interfere with the ability to recognize and respond appropriately to the potential health hazards from self-starvation. Although thinking about food and

BOX 70-1 **Eating Behavior Self-Test**

_____ Even though people tell me I'm thin, I feel fat.

_____ I get anxious if I can't exercise.

_____ My menstrual periods are irregular or absent. (female)

_____ My sex drive is not as strong as it used to be. (male)

_____ I worry about what I will eat.

_____ If I gain weight, I get anxious or depressed.

_____ I would rather eat by myself that with family or friends.

_____ Other people talk about the way I eat.

_____ I get anxious when people urge me to eat.

_____ I don't talk much about my fear of being fat because no one understands how I feel.

_____ I enjoy cooking for others, but I don't usually eat what I've cooked.

_____ I have a secret stash of food.

_____ When I eat I'm afraid I won't be able to stop.

_____ I lie about what I eat.

_____ I don't like to be bothered or interrupted when I'm eating.

_____ If I were thinner, I would like myself better.

_____ I have missed work or school because of my weight or eating habits.

_____ I tend to be depressed and irritable.

_____ I feel guilty when I eat.

_____ I avoid some people because they bug me about the way I eat.

_____ My eating habits and fear of food interfere with friendships or romantic relationships.

_____ I cut my food into tiny pieces, eat it on special plates, make patterns on my plate with it, or spit it out before swallowing it.

_____ I am hardly ever satisfied with myself.

_____ I have taken laxatives to control my weight.

_____ I have vomited to control my weight.

_____ I want to be thinner than my friends.

_____ I have said or thought, "I would rather die than be fat."

_____ I have fasted to lose weight.

_____ In romantic moments I cannot let myself go because I am worried about my fat and flab.

If you answer yes to any of these questions, discuss your eating habits with your physician.

Adapted from Anorexia Nervosa and Related Eating Disorders, Inc. Are you at risk? Take a self-test. (2002). Available online at: http://www.eatingdisorderanswers.com/id25.html.

preparing it for others may contribute to feelings of pleasure, an excess of serotonin restricts consumption of food (Olson, 2006). People with bulimarexia may experience feelings of euphoria at the time of a binge (Murphy, 2007).

Recently, investigators have located receptors in the human brain for **melanin-concentrating hormone** (Souers, 2007). In animal studies, low levels of this hormone caused weight loss, and high levels promoted obesity. **Leptin**, a substance produced by fat cells known as **adipocytes**, has added another piece to the puzzle of eating disorders. Leptin acts on receptors in the hypothalamus, where high levels inhibit food intake. In addition, some speculate that there are

interrelated endocrine disturbances in pituitary, adrenal, thyroid, and reproductive hormones. For example, **corticotropin-releasing hormone** (CRH) acts as a major anorexic signal that limits the consumption of calories, increases energy expenditure, and promotes sustained weight loss (Inui, 2001). The question is whether the various hormonal disturbances are a cause or a result of starvation.

At the psychological end of the spectrum, it has been noted that people with anorexia nervosa are often perfectionists, have low self-esteem, and possess an intense desire to please others. Refusal to eat also is considered a form of self-control used to cope with stressful life experiences or dysfunctional family relationships (Murphy, 2007).

Complications

Failure to consume adequate nourishment eventually deprives all body systems of the nutritional elements required for homeostasis, growth, and cellular repair. Low levels of serum estrogen also lead to osteopenia (low bone mass) and premature osteoporosis (severe demineralization of bones), both of which result in stress fractures, particularly of the spine and hips. Starvation can lead to vitamin deficiencies, fluid and electrolyte imbalances, and finally, death from cardiac failure or arrhythmia.

Assessment Findings

Signs and Symptoms

Clients with anorexia nervosa may appear skeleton-like and may weigh 85% or less than others of similar build, age, and height. In addition, they develop a growth of fine body hair called **lanugo**; in the absence of subcutaneous fat, this helps maintain body temperature by preventing heat loss. In addition, clients with anorexia tend to be hypotensive and may have an irregular, low pulse rate. Severe malnutrition causes clients to be constipated, feel cold most of the time, have frequent infections, and cease menstruating. Many conceal their starvation by hiding or disposing of food and dressing in bulky clothing. When clients with anorexia are confronted with the fact that they are in danger of dying, they deny the seriousness of others' concerns.

 Pharmacologic Consideration

- Clients with anorexia nervosa who also have insulin-dependent (type 1) diabetes mellitus, often adolescent girls, sometimes reduce their dose of insulin to promote weight loss. This practice is medically unsafe.

 Gerontologic Considerations

- Older adults with significant weight loss should be assessed for major depression, which may manifest with severe weight loss.

- Older adults sometimes simply refuse to eat as a form of protest or in an effort to seek validation of self-worth, resulting in self-starvation. Self-starvation may also be a reaction to health problems such as cognitive decline, terminal disease, or inability to cope with other losses. Self-starvation is related to major depression or faulty coping skills and is *not* classified as an eating disorder.

Diagnostic Findings

Body mass index (BMI), a mathematical computation based on height and weight (Box 70-2), is used to evaluate a person's size in relation to norms within the adult population. In people with anorexia, the BMI is typically 16 or less. Anemia is usually present, and electrolyte levels, especially potassium and sometimes sodium, are often dangerously low. Deficiencies in serum proteins are reflected in low albumin, transferrin, and ferritin levels. Cardiac irregularities are identified by electrocardiography. Bone densitometry studies are used to determine whether osteopenia is present, and if so, how severe it has become.

▶ ***Stop, Think, and Respond Exercise 70-1***

Besides having weight that is less than normal for height, what other findings suggest that an underweight person has anorexia nervosa?

Medical Management

Treatment of anorexia nervosa involves nutritional therapy, drug therapy, psychotherapy, and family counseling. Nutritional therapy includes providing nourishing meals, supplemental vitamins and minerals, intravenous fluids and electrolytes, tube feedings, or total parenteral nutrition. Once the client's weight improves or stabilizes, outpatient treatment begins.

B O X 7 0 - 2	Body Mass Index Formula, Calculation, and Interpretation

Formula

$$BMI = \frac{weight \ (kg)}{height \ (m^2)}$$

Calculation

1. Divide weight in pounds by 2.2 to convert to weight in kilograms (kg).
2. Divide height in inches by 39.4 to convert to height in meters (m).
3. Square the answer in step 2 by multiplying the number times itself; this gives the height in m².
4. Divide the weight (kg) by the height (m²).

Interpretation

Anorectic	BMI = ≤ 16
Underweight	BMI = 16–18.5
Healthy	BMI = 18.5–24.9
Overweight	BMI = 25–29.9
Obese	BMI = 30–34.9
Severely obese	BMI = 35–39.9
Extremely obese	BMI = ≥40

The resumption of normal eating behaviors, not simply restoring body weight, is the focus of nutritional treatment. Initially, as few as 1500 calories may be prescribed, because large amounts of food, as well as high-fat foods and "gassy" vegetables, may cause gastrointestinal discomfort and constipation. No foods are restricted, but so-called diet foods (e.g., artificially sweetened beverages, fat-free foods) should be avoided. Ongoing nutritional counseling may be needed throughout the maintenance period.

To promote compliance with the weight gain regimen, behavioral therapy (see Chap. 68) is instituted. By eating, the client earns privileges for having visitors and participating in social and physical activities. The privileges are used to reinforce desired behavior.

Antidepressant medications such as selective serotonin reuptake inhibitors (SSRIs) are administered to manage depressive and obsessive symptoms. Atypical antipsychotics such as olanzapine (Zyprexa), aripiprazole (Abilify), and others block dopamine receptors, resulting in a reduction of altered perception of weight, fears about gaining weight, denial of the seriousness of low body weight, and actual promotion of weight gain (Crawford et al., 2008; Cassels, 2008). Supplemental vitamins and minerals such as those containing iron, potassium, and calcium may be included in the therapeutic regimen to compensate for natural sources that are not being consumed as a result of the client's self-imposed fast. Stool softeners or laxatives may be necessary to counteract the constipation due to absence of dietary fiber.

Individual, group, and cognitive psychotherapy (see Chap. 68) is used to help clients gain insight into their distorted perceptions of thinness and the motivations for persisting in weight-loss behaviors. Counseling and involvement in self-help groups for several years are often indicated.

Family counseling is aimed at relieving the power struggle between the client and those who try to convince the client to eat. It also focuses on learning skills for undoing enmeshment—a pattern in which two or more people lack limits that separate one person from another, resulting in a loss of personal identity and exclusion of others.

Nursing Process for the Client with Anorexia Nervosa

Assessment

Perform a physical assessment, being careful to note signs of malnutrition such as absence of body fat, dry skin, and scalp hair, the presence of fine hair covering the body, edema from hypoproteinemia, and cold hands and feet. Monitor vital signs on a regular basis to detect hypothermia, bradycardia, and hypotension. Use cardiac monitoring to detect dysrhythmias caused by hypokalemia. Weigh the client as accurately as possible with minimal clothing, and calculate the BMI (see Box 70-2). Obtain a nutritional history. Ask the client about whether he or she restricts food intake or combines it with purging. Keep in mind that excessive exercise is also a form of purging. Ask the female client for the date of her last menstrual period. Observe the client's mood and anxiety level. Ask the client about family dynamics and other stressors.

Diagnosis, Planning, and Interventions

The nurse counsels and educates the family of a person with anorexia nervosa (Client and Family Teaching 70-1). The nurse's role in caring for the client with anorexia includes, but is not limited to the following.

▶ **Imbalanced nutrition: Less than body requirements** related to fear of gaining weight

▶ **Expected Outcomes:** (1) The client will gain 2 to 5 lb by a mutually agreed target date; (2) the client will attain and maintain a BMI of at least 18.5.

• Consistently assign the same few nurses to the client's care. *Limiting staff relationships promotes a therapeutic alliance, consistency, and reduces the potential for manipulation.*

• Establish a contract with the client for expected weight restoration and target date; include the rewards for reaching goals and consequences for failure to reach goals. *Participating in setting goals promotes self-involvement and a sense of ownership in the plan. Identifying positive and negative consequences makes the client aware of how outcomes in the therapeutic plan will be managed.*

• Weigh the client regularly, but randomly. *Random weights are generally more accurate. They prevent the client from water loading, a technique in which clients with anorexia attempt to demonstrate weight gain by consuming a large volume of water and avoiding urination before being weighed.*

• Work with the dietitian to provide at least 6 to 8 meals each day with a total caloric value between 1500 to 2000 calories, then gradually increase the total calories to between 2500 to 4000 calories/day. *The client is much more likely to work toward weight gain if food is offered frequently and is not heavily calorie loaded. To gain 1 lb of weight, a person must consume 3500 calories that are not utilized for basic metabolism and activities.*

• Set a limit of 30 minutes to consume the meal. *People with anorexia practice various rituals such as cutting food into small pieces and rearranging the food on the plate without actually*

Client and Family Teaching 70-1
Anorexia Nervosa

The nurse counsels and educates family members by offering the following suggestions:

● Focus on the person with anorexia rather than on the eating disorder itself.
● Give unconditional love to the person with anorexia.
● Avoid making the person with anorexia feel guilty for the family distress that the disorder causes in daily living.
● Give the person with anorexia the power to make decisions and facilitate changes in matters other than eating.
● Avoid being manipulated by the person with anorexia.
● Demonstrate united support for one another and the plan for the client's treatment.
● Prepare for rehospitalization if the client becomes medically unstable or experiences a relapse.

eating the food. Informing clients of the time limit may provide an incentive to consume food.

• Observe or sit with the client during meals. *Being observed prevents the client from hiding food rather than eating it.*

• Remove the dietary tray after 30 minutes without commenting on food that has not been eaten. *Removal of the food at the designated time avoids a power struggle. Negative comments reinforce that the client was victorious in resisting the urge to eat. Withholding any comments avoids an adversarial image.*

• Record the type and amount of food consumed. *Documentation provides information on which to evaluate the progress of the client and helps the dietitian calculate the client's caloric intake.*

• Restrict the client's use of the bathroom for 2 hours after meals or accompany the client to the bathroom. *A two-hour restriction allows time for consumed food to enter the small intestine for absorption rather than being vomited.*

• Give the client a liquid nutritional supplement for the uneaten calories at meals. *Clients may consume calorie-loaded liquids in place of solid food.*

• Implement behavioral rewards or consequences consistently and fairly. *Deviation from guidelines or their inconsistent application reduces the effectiveness of the plan of care.*

• Administer prescribed drug, vitamin, and mineral therapy, and ensure that the client attends group and individual psychotherapy. *Resistance to the therapeutic regimen is common. Anorexia requires management with medical, nutritional, and psychological modalities.*

▶ **Disturbed body image** related to unrealistic body size.

▶ **Expected Outcome:** The client will develop a realistic perception of self and insight into the motivation for thinness.

• Encourage the client to talk about perceptions of body image, but avoid opposing the client's views. *Disagreeing tends to further entrench the client's beliefs.*

• Offer the observation that the fixation with weight control diverts attention and energy needed to deal with real issues surrounding psychosocial conflicts. *Awareness is raised by offering an alternative view.*

• Help the client clarify issues underlying the need to control weight gain and promote weight loss. *Self-examination helps develop insight.*

• Suggest that perfection is not possible and that no body image is worth dying for. *Calling attention to the seriousness of the health problem may promote a modification in the client's behavior.*

Evaluation of Expected Outcomes

The client consumes nutritious food, resulting in a gradual weight gain and a BMI that is greater than 18.5. The client no longer perceives himself or herself as fat. There is evidence of insight on the part of the client, based on his or her self-disclosure that withholding the consumption of food created a feeling of power and that it served as a means of controlling family stressors and achieving an unrealistic image of perfection.

BULIMIA NERVOSA

Bulimia nervosa is characterized by a minimum of two episodes of secret **food binges** — rapid consumption of a large number of calories — per week followed by behaviors intended to prevent weight gain. For the condition to be considered true bulimia, the abnormal eating pattern must have persisted for at least 6 months. There are two different manifestations of bulimia: (1) binging followed by **purging**, elimination of nutrients, using self-induced vomiting, laxatives, enemas, or diuretics, and (2) binging followed by fasting, using diet pills, or engaging in excessive exercise (see Binge Eating Disorder later in this chapter).

In contrast to clients with anorexia nervosa, clients with bulimia nervosa

1. are generally older at the onset of the disorder
2. are overweight or normal weight
3. admit that their eating behavior is abnormal
4. are ashamed of habitually binging and purging

Pathophysiology and Etiology

It is believed that the hypothalamus is the center for appetite regulation. When the lateral area of hypothalamus is stimulated, people feel like eating; when the ventromedial area of the hypothalamus is stimulated, they feel satiated (full) and eating behavior ceases (Rolls, 2005). These two areas of the hypothalamus are turned on and off by neurotransmitters. Research suggests that people with bulimia have a biochemically induced compulsion to eat as a result of increased sensitivity to norepinephrine within the hypothalamus and reduced levels of serotonin, which disguise the point of satiety. Because serotonin is synthesized from the essential amino acid tryptophan, it is believed that binge eating acts as a mechanism to supply tryptophan so as to increase serotonin levels, similar to how thirst stimulates drinking water or beverages to correct a deficit in fluid volume.

Two neurohormones, called **orexin A** and **orexin B** after the Greek word, *orexis*, meaning appetite, have been discovered. When laboratory animals were injected with orexin hormones, which attach to receptors in the lateral hypothalamus, the animals consumed 8 to 10 times the normal amount of food. This has led to the hypothesis that the levels of orexin A and B contribute to binge eating and obesity in humans. Leptin, a substance manufactured in human fat cells, is believed to suppress orexigenic (appetite-stimulating) chemicals. Therefore, binge eating may occur in the absence of leptin or reduced receptors for leptin (Baranowska et al., 2005).

Whatever the cause, once a binge begins, it is difficult to control. During a binge, people with bulimia consume 3,500 to 11,500 calories of food in 2 hours or less. Eating is terminated by one of the following:

- Abdominal pain
- Interruption (discovery by others)
- Sleeping

After the eating frenzy, bulimics feel so guilty that they purge, fast (abstain from food, but not days on end such as someone with bulimarexia), or exercise.

Complications

Repetitive regurgitation of gastric acids due to self-induced vomiting and use of emetics such as ipecac damage teeth by eroding the dental enamel. Abuse of laxatives and enemas contributes to constipation. The nonprescribed use of diuretics and diet pills predisposes to fluid, electrolyte, and cardiac problems. Some people with bulimia also compulsively abuse drugs or alcohol. The shame and guilt may trigger suicidal thoughts or attempts.

Assessment Findings

Signs and Symptoms

Clients with bulimia tend to be of normal weight or slightly overweight; however, their weight can fluctuate as much as 10 lb in a week. Self-induced vomiting results in hoarseness, inflammation of the esophagus and oral pharynx, calluses on the back of the hand and fingers from repeatedly stimulating the gag reflex, erosion of tooth enamel, and swollen parotid glands.

Diagnostic Findings

Diagnosis is based on the clinical findings and a history of persistent binging and purging. Serum electrolytes may be altered, depending on the time that has elapsed since the last purge. A radiograph of the upper gastrointestinal tract shows an overstretched or stenotic esophagus from frequent regurgitation and inflammation followed by scarring.

Medical Management

Treatment of bulimia nervosa includes drug therapy with antidepressants (see Chap. 69), individual and group psychotherapy, and behavior modification techniques (see Chap. 68). Most clients are managed on an outpatient basis.

Nursing Process for the Client with Bulimia Nervosa

Assessment

Obtain the client's history and current health information. Weigh the client, and calculate the BMI (see Box 70-2). Inspect the teeth to detect dental damage. Examine the conjunctiva for ruptured blood vessels caused by the rise in blood pressure during forced vomiting. Ask questions concerning (1) the frequency of binging and purging episodes, (2) the client's state of mind prior to a binge, (3) the types and amounts of food that are consumed during a binge, and (4) the nature of the purge. Take an inventory of medications, such as emetics, diuretics, and laxatives, that are used for purging. If exercise is the technique the client uses to purge, identify the type of activity and average duration of exercise.

Diagnosis, Planning, and Interventions

Like people with anorexia, clients with bulimia nervosa need to resume normal eating behaviors and avoid restrictive practices. They may also need to accept a body weight higher than they would like. Identify and correct clients' fears and misconceptions about food and weight; clients who are persuaded to occasionally eat small amounts of high-caloric foods are less likely to binge later. Advise clients not to skip meals or snacks, to use appropriate utensils, to not pick at food, and to not feel guilty about occasional planned indulgences.

Provide emotional support and health teaching. Some important areas to reinforce during teaching include:

- Follow a dietary plan that is compatible with MyPyramid, developed by the U.S. Department of Agriculture and the U.S. Department of Health and Human Services (Fig. 70-1)
- Eat at a slow pace
- Eat only in the presence of others

Other aspects of the nurse's role in caring for clients with bulimia nervosa includes, but is not limited to, the following.

- **Imbalanced nutrition:** **More than body requirements** related to compulsion to binge.
- **Expected Outcomes:** (1) The client will delay the urge to binge or purge. (2) The client will consume no more than 2000 to 3000 calories per day divided among three meals plus or minus snacks. (3) The client will maintain a stable weight.

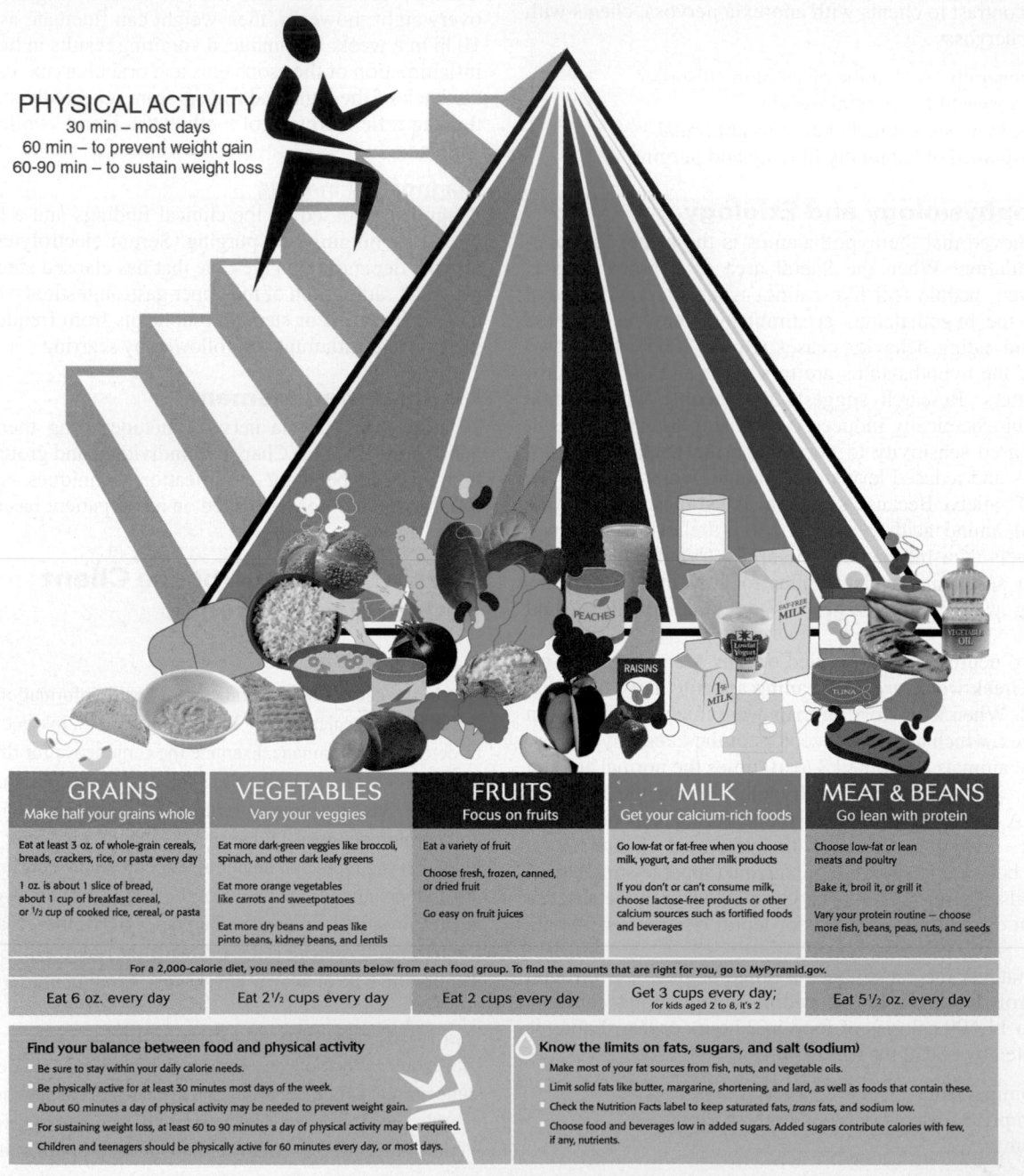

PHYSICAL ACTIVITY
30 min – most days
60 min – to prevent weight gain
60-90 min – to sustain weight loss

GRAINS	VEGETABLES	FRUITS	MILK	MEAT & BEANS
Make half your grains whole	Vary your veggies	Focus on fruits	Get your calcium-rich foods	Go lean with protein
Eat at least 3 oz. of whole-grain cereals, breads, crackers, rice, or pasta every day 1 oz. is about 1 slice of bread, about 1 cup of breakfast cereal, or ½ cup of cooked rice, cereal, or pasta	Eat more dark-green veggies like broccoli, spinach, and other dark leafy greens Eat more orange vegetables like carrots and sweetpotatoes Eat more dry beans and peas like pinto beans, kidney beans, and lentils	Eat a variety of fruit Choose fresh, frozen, canned, or dried fruit Go easy on fruit juices	Go low-fat or fat-free when you choose milk, yogurt, and other milk products If you don't or can't consume milk, choose lactose-free products or other calcium sources such as fortified foods and beverages	Choose low-fat or lean meats and poultry Bake it, broil it, or grill it Vary your protein routine – choose more fish, beans, peas, nuts, and seeds

For a 2,000-calorie diet, you need the amounts below from each food group. To find the amounts that are right for you, go to MyPyramid.gov.

Eat 6 oz. every day	Eat 2½ cups every day	Eat 2 cups every day	Get 3 cups every day; for kids aged 2 to 8, it's 2	Eat 5½ oz. every day

Find your balance between food and physical activity
- Be sure to stay within your daily calorie needs.
- Be physically active for at least 30 minutes most days of the week.
- About 60 minutes a day of physical activity may be needed to prevent weight gain.
- For sustaining weight loss, at least 60 to 90 minutes a day of physical activity may be required.
- Children and teenagers should be physically active for 60 minutes every day, or most days.

Know the limits on fats, sugars, and salt (sodium)
- Make most of your fat sources from fish, nuts, and vegetable oils.
- Limit solid fats like butter, margarine, shortening, and lard, as well as foods that contain these.
- Check the Nutrition Facts label to keep saturated fats, *trans* fats, and sodium low.
- Choose food and beverages low in added sugars. Added sugars contribute calories with few, if any, nutrients.

FIGURE 70-1. MyPyramid is a tool that Identifies foods in five major food groups that provides most, but not all, of the nutrients an adult needs. Foods in one group cannot replace those in another. No one major food group is more important than another. (Source: U.S. Department of Agriculture and U.S. Department of Health and Human Services, 2005.)

- Help the client identify feelings, situations, or foods that trigger binging episodes. *Raising an awareness of triggering events can break the cycle of binging and purging.*
- Explore alternative coping strategies with the client for dealing with triggering stimuli. *Developing techniques for controlling impulses can abort a binging episode.*
- Explain to the client that starving leads to binging. *Eating slowly and regularly, in controlled amounts, reduces hunger.*
- Tell the client to restrict eating to the kitchen or dining room only at specific times. *Restricting the location for eating and the time during which food is eaten interferes with the usual patterns of binge eating. Private binges often take place in locations other than the usual places for eating, such as in the living room while watching television.*
- Instruct the client to wait at least one hour after a meal before succumbing to a binge. *Delaying a binge helps the client separate normal eating from abnormal eating and from turning a normal meal into a binge.*
- Discuss alternatives for aborting or interrupting the eating binges, such as eating with a family member or friend, calling a friend for support if alone, leaving the binging location, and stocking low-calorie food. *Binging takes place when the client with bulimia is alone and when there is a low potential for being discovered. Consuming low-calorie foods may create less anxiety and reduce the potential for purging.*
- Suggest that the client adulterate a known binge food such as dropping it in dirt or soaking it in vinegar if all else fails. *Making the food unpalatable is a behavior modification technique, called negative reinforcement, that may abort a binge.*

▶ Ineffective Coping related to managing guilty feelings by purging

▶ Expected Outcome: The client will implement effective coping mechanisms for dealing with guilt and stressors.

- Acknowledge and compliment the client when binging or purging is controlled. *Positive reinforcement increases the potential that the behavior will be repeated.*
- Remain nonjudgmental when the client reports having binged or purged. *Increasing or adding to the client's shame reinforces the client's guilt.*
- Encourage the client to forgive herself or himself for binging and purging. *People with bulimia judge themselves severely after binging or purging.*
- Formulate a contract with the client to seek out the nurse or another support person when the client feels the urge to purge. *A contract is a useful tool for obtaining the client's compliance. Reducing the incidence of purging decreases the guilt a client feels.*
- Have the client discard all purging paraphernalia such as medications and enema equipment. *The inability to purge reduces potential guilt.*

▶ Situational Low Self-Esteem related to poor impulse control and ineffective methods to control weight.

▶ Expected Outcome: The client will report increased self-esteem.

- Discuss keeping a diary or journal where entries describe incidents when the urge to binge or purge was overcome. *A written record is an objective resource for self-evaluation of the client's progress.*
- Encourage the client to read previous diary or journal entries whenever negative thoughts intrude. *The client's own statements are self-affirming evidence that progress is being made.*
- Help dispel the faulty perception that losing control over binging and purging means the client is a total failure. *Clients tend to overlook their positive attributes and condemn themselves because of a single weakness.*
- Refer the client to a dietitian. *Loss of weight without purging increases self-esteem. A dietitian has the expertise to develop a personalized plan for meeting nutritional needs while facilitating gradual weight loss.*

Evaluation of Expected Outcomes

Binging and purging are reduced or eliminated, and the client's caloric intake is in accordance with her or his metabolic needs. The client successfully implements alternative strategies for managing compulsive behaviors and has a positive regard for herself or himself. ●

▶ *Stop, Think, and Respond Exercise 70-2*
Where is the appetite center and what substances stimulate or suppress the appetite center?

BINGE EATING DISORDER AND COMPULSIVE OVEREATING

Binge eating disorder is characterized as the inability to control overeating, accompanied by a guilty feeling. However, people do not engage in compensating behaviors to prevent weight gain. **Compulsive overeating** is characterized as eating in the absence of hunger or regardless of feeling full. Some people have both problems simultaneously. Either may result in obesity.

Pathophysiology and Etiology

The cause of overeating syndromes is still unknown. Because people with eating disorders suffer from anxiety, depression, and compulsive behavior, there is growing evidence that biochemical factors are involved in binge eating and compulsive overeating. Similarly to anorexia and bulimia nervosa, there is likely an imbalance of neurotransmitters such as norepinephrine and serotonin, or neurohormones such as orexin A and B or leptin, which affect the appetite center in the brain. There also may be additional neuroendocrine disequilibrium involving cortisol, a hormone released by the adrenal cortex in response to stress (see Chap. 67); reduced cholecystokinin, a hormone secreted by the mucosa of the upper small intestine that causes laboratory animals to stop eating when they feel full; and imbalances in neuropeptides Y and YY, psychoactive chemicals that stimulate eating behavior in research animals.

In 2001, scientists located brain receptors for **endocannabinoids**, natural chemicals with marijuana-like properties, that activate the appetite center (Kirkham, 2007; Di Marzo, 2005). The existence of endocannabinoids helps explain why marijuana users develop ravenous hunger, called "the munchies," and why dronabinol (Marinol), synthetic tetrahydrocannabinol (THC) — the active ingredient in marijuana — helps clients with cancer and acquired immunodeficiency syndrome (AIDS) gain weight. Increased amounts of endocannabinoids or an increased sensitivity to their presence may explain some syndromes characterized by overeating. Also, the fact that many overeaters state they use food as a way of coping with stress should not be overlooked.

Complications

Ultimately, overeating leads to many physical and emotional problems. As a consequence of obesity, many people develop hyperlipidemia (elevated blood fat levels), hypertension, type 2 diabetes, degenerative arthritis, and sleep apnea. There is a higher risk of gallbladder disease, heart disease, and some types of cancer. Many people feel unhappy, ashamed, and disgusted with themselves. They tend to become socially isolated to avoid being noticed and possibly rejected.

Assessment Findings

Signs and Symptoms

Overeaters are typically overweight and have a history of unsuccessful attempts at dieting. Clients tend to eat in the absence of hunger. They have preferences for high-sugar and high-fat foods that they may nibble over several hours or gorge on until they feel uncomfortably full. Some report that they overeat or binge when they are angry, sad, bored, or anxious. They often have a history of other compulsive behaviors such as alcohol or drug abuse. Some reveal that they have considered suicide or have performed self-mutilation, such as cutting and burning themselves, pulling their hair, and interfering with wound healing to cope with their intense feelings, to punish themselves, or to experience physical pain to counteract the consequences of feeling emotionally numb.

Diagnostic Findings

People with overeating syndromes generally have a BMI of 30 or above. Other laboratory and diagnostic tests reflect secondary complications from obesity such as elevated blood sugar, cholesterol, and serum lipid levels.

Medical Management

A comprehensive approach to treating overeating syndromes involves weight reduction, psychotherapy, and self-help support groups. The first step is a sensible weight loss regimen prescribed by a dietitian. Strict dieting is discouraged, because it tends to worsen binge eating. To help clients lose weight and remain compliant, short-term drug therapy may be used. Prescribed medications include antidepressants such as SSRIs (e.g., fluoxetine [Prozac]), which promote weight loss (see Chap. 69).

Because it produces favorable health benefits and is more likely to be maintained, attaining a weight loss goal of 10% to 20%, rather than an "ideal" weight, should be encouraged. It is estimated that 95% of people who lose weight regain it within 5 years, and some dieters gain back more than they originally lost. The newer approaches to weight management stress that all foods are acceptable and teach clients to recognize and differentiate between physiologic and psychological hunger.

Support groups, such as Overeaters Anonymous (see Nursing Resources in Appendix A), or group therapy in eating disorder clinics are helpful adjuncts to individual psychotherapy. In some cases, surgery is an option for severely obese clients with medical complications (see Chap. 45).

Nursing Process for the Client Who Compulsively Overeats

Assessment

Interview the client with sensitivity to the client's self-consciousness about weight and emotional problems. Perform a comprehensive physical assessment and calculate the client's BMI (see Box 70-2). Provide privacy when measuring weight and height.

Diagnosis, Planning, and Interventions

Client and Family Teaching 70-2 may be helpful in management of a client with an overeating disorder. The nurse's role in caring for

---

Client and Family Teaching 70-2
Overeating Syndromes

The nurse counsels clients with overeating syndromes to:

- Obtain treatment from professionals who are experienced in treating eating disorders, and continue with this therapy.
- Follow the label directions for taking prescribed medications; report any untoward effects.
- Avoid popular nonprescription diet pills. These generally contain phenylpropanolamine (PPA) and caffeine, which are central nervous system stimulants. They can increase heart rate and blood pressure and cause dizziness, irritability, insomnia, and dry mouth.
- Strict dieting or fasting is the leading cause of binging.
- Exercise on the advice of a physician to reduce the appetite and increase weight loss.
- Avoid nutritional and weight loss centers, because they generally do not offer the comprehensive services most clients need to keep from gaining weight once the target weight is reached.
- Read food labels, and understand that those that say "sugar free" or "contains no cholesterol" do not mean that the ingredients are calorie free or even low calorie.
- Talk to a close friend or support person about feelings about food.
- Attend Overeaters Anonymous meetings. This is a free self-help group that is modeled after the 12-step program of Alcoholics Anonymous.
- Remember that recovery is a day-by-day process; it is self-defeating to dwell on the lack of previous success or relapses that may occur.

clients with overeating syndromes includes, but is not limited to the following:

▸ **Imbalanced Nutrition: More than Body Requirements** related to insensitivity to satiety.

▸ **Expected Outcome:** The client will consume only the prescribed number of calories per day.

- Advise the client to follow the meal plan for three meals and three snacks each day that has been developed by a dietitian in conjunction with nutritional counseling. *Compliance with a nutritious food plan promotes gradual weight loss. Avoiding extremely restrictive low-calorie diets decreases preoccupation with food and weight and the risk of binge eating.*
- Teach the client to avoid "trigger" foods, those substances that contribute to cravings and overeating. *Eating can be self-regulated by reducing the unique food stimuli that lead to unrestrained eating.*
- Emphasize that the client should not deviate from the food plan. *Deviation leads to overeating.*
- Recommend that the client use a scale and measuring utensils to comply with portion sizes. *Estimating amounts increases the potential for consuming more calories than the food plan allows.*
- Remind the client to prepare a shopping list and purchase only the size and amount of food that is needed. *Impulse shopping or having leftovers increases the potential for eating more than the planned amount.*
- Suggest that the client plan activities throughout the day that involve others. *Isolation provides an opportunity for secretive binging.*

▸ **Risk for Loneliness** related to self-consciousness concerning appearance and eating behavior.

▸ **Expected Outcome:** The client will participate in social relationships and activities.

- Accept the client for herself or himself. *Rejection encourages isolation.*
- Seek the client out for verbal interactions. *Attention from others reinforces that the client is a worthwhile person.*
- Encourage the client to contact friends or support persons or join social or self-help groups. *Activities that involve other people reduce feelings of loneliness.*
- Suggest that the client cultivate leisure activities that can be shared with others. *Mutually shared activities provide opportunities for social relationships.*

Evaluation of Expected Outcomes:

The client complies with the food plan and loses weight gradually. The client takes part in group activities and develops a network of friends. ●

CRITICAL THINKING EXERCISES

1. Based on MyPyramid, what amounts from various food groups should be consumed on a daily basis for a 2000-calorie diet of a nonpregnant adult?
2. Calculate the body mass index of a person who weighs 175 lbs and is 63" tall. What conclusion is appropriate based on your calculation?
3. What weight loss strategies are appropriate to recommend and discourage for an obese client who is a compulsive overeater?
4. Name some consequences of self-starvation secondary to anorexia nervosa.

NCLEX-STYLE REVIEW QUESTIONS

1. Which of the following signs and symptoms are associated with anorexia nervosa? Select all that apply.
   1. Growth of fine body hair
   2. Club-shaped fingertips
   3. Hypoactive bowel sounds
   4. Conjunctival hemorrhages
   5. Low blood pressure
2. When reviewing the data obtained following the assessment of a client diagnosed with bulimia, which finding is most related to this eating disorder?
   1. Extremely low body weight
   2. Erosion of dental enamel
   3. Cessation of menstruation
   4. Patchy loss of hair
3. Which nursing goal is the highest priority when managing the care of a client with anorexia nervosa?
   1. To improve the client's distorted body image
   2. To help the client use healthier coping techniques
   3. To restore normal nutrition and health
   4. To help the client develop assertiveness
4. What is the best guidance the nurse can give a nursing assistant who reports that a client with anorexia rearranges the food on the dietary tray but does not eat any of it?
   1. Blend the food and administer it by tube feeding.
   2. Remind the client that the intake is being recorded.
   3. Review the treatment goals with the client again.
   4. Remove the food without making any comments.
5. Which nursing action is most appropriate when the nurse observes a client with anorexia nervosa drinking a full pitcher of water just before being weighed?
   1. Postpone weighing the client until later.
   2. Confront the client about what was observed.
   3. Say nothing and weigh the client as usual.
   4. Subtract 2 lb (0.9 kg) from the client's weight.

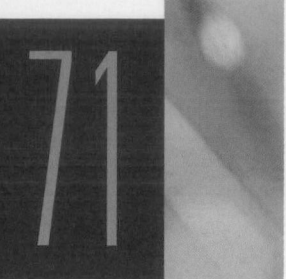

71

Caring for Clients with Chemical Dependence

Words To Know

alcoholism
aversion therapy
blackouts
central nervous system depressants
central nervous system stimulants
chemical dependence
cross-tolerance
detoxification
environmental tobacco smoke
methadone maintenance therapy
opiate dependence
polydrug abuse
rapid opiate detoxification
relapse
Rule of One Hundreds
substance abuse
tolerance
withdrawal

Learning Objectives

On completion of this chapter, you will be able to:

1. Discuss the health and social consequences of substance abuse.
2. Name four commonly abused addictive substances and at least three other categories of abused drugs.
3. Discuss the meaning of withdrawal.
4. Explain tolerance and give two mechanisms by which it occurs.
5. List four steps in the progression toward chemical dependence.
6. List two physiologic explanations and two psychosocial factors for the development of chemical dependence.
7. Explain two ways abused drugs produce their effects.
8. Define alcoholism and list three accompanying symptoms.
9. Describe treatment and nursing management for clients with alcoholism.
10. List five potential health consequences of tobacco use.
11. Discuss the components of a successful smoking cessation program.
12. Discuss elements of recovery programs.
13. Describe signs and symptoms of cocaine and methamphetamine abuse as they relate to the manner of use.
14. Describe treatment and nursing management for clients addicted to cocaine and methamphetamine
15. Discuss methods for managing opiate dependence.

Substance abuse and chemical dependence, which are discussed in this chapter, are serious public health and social problems. They contribute significantly to *morbidity* (incidence of disease) and *mortality* (deaths) from liver damage, cardiopulmonary disease, and infectious diseases such as hepatitis and acquired immunodeficiency syndrome (AIDS). Alcohol and drug abuse also are major contributors to domestic violence and child abuse, crime, traffic and boating fatalities, assaults, and murders.

SUBSTANCE ABUSE AND CHEMICAL DEPENDENCE

Substance abuse is the use of a drug for a purpose that is different from its intended use. Usually, it is the consequences of inappropriately taking drugs—primarily mind-altering and mood-altering substances—that are of major concern. Commonly abused drugs include alcohol, cocaine, heroin, hallucinogens, amphetamines, marijuana, barbiturates, volatile hydrocarbons such as those found in glue, and nicotine.

Gerontologic Considerations

- Older adults may abuse over-the-counter and prescription drugs or alcohol rather than illicit drugs.

Because of their widespread use and harmful effects, alcohol and nicotine contribute most to morbidity and mortality, and thus are considered the most harmful substances. Tobacco use is so widely accepted and its psychoactive properties are so subtle that its negative social and occupational effects seem minor. Yet tobacco is an addictive substance that contributes annually to the deaths of 438,000 people—as many as are caused by alcohol, cocaine, heroin, suicide, homicide, motor vehicle accidents, fire, and AIDS combined (Centers for Disease Control and Prevention, 2007).

Pharmacologic Considerations

- Obtain a careful drug history from chemically dependent clients because abuse of multiple substances is common.

Withdrawal refers to the physical symptoms and craving for a drug that occur when a person abruptly stops using an abused substance (Table 71-1). **Chemical dependence** means that a person must take a drug to avoid withdrawal symptoms. *Addiction* sometimes is used interchangeably with *dependence*, but addiction more accurately refers to the drug-seeking behaviors that interfere with work, relationships, and normal activities (Box 71-1). **Tolerance** refers to the reduction in a drug's effect that follows persistent use. Tolerance results because the body develops mechanisms for using the drug more effectively or inactivating the drug more efficiently. Consequently, a person must take increasing amounts of the substance to obtain the desired effect.

Pathophysiology and Etiology

The causes of chemical dependence are complex and involve many psychobiologic factors. Substance abuse often begins with curious experimentation and progresses to habituation, psychological and physical dependence, and finally addiction (Table 71-2). One factor that explains substance abuse is the self-reinforcing pleasurable effects that some substances produce in the limbic system of the brain, depending on the type of substance. **Central nervous system stimulants**

TABLE 71-1 Commonly Abused Substances

DRUG	EFFECTS	SIGNS AND SYMPTOMS OF TOXICITY	SIGNS AND SYMPTOMS OF WITHDRAWAL
Alcohol	Central nervous system depressant • Lethargy • Slurred speech • Slowed motor reaction • Impaired judgment • Decreased social inhibition	Nausea and vomiting, loss of coordination, belligerence, stupor, coma	Anxiety, agitation, elevated vital signs, hyperactive reflexes, tremors, diaphoresis, insomnia, hallucinations, seizures
Cocaine and methamphetamine	Central nervous system stimulants • Tachycardia • Hypertension • Increased energy • Feeling of well-being • Insensitivity to pain and fatigue • Weight loss	Restlessness, paranoia, irritability, auditory and tactile hallucinations, convulsions, respiratory or cardiac arrest	Depressed mood, lethargy, impaired concentration, craving for drug
Heroin and other opiates	Central nervous system depressant • Initial brief rush of euphoria • Sedation • Reduced motivation, attention, and concentration • Altered sensitivity to stressors • Pain relief • Lowered vital signs, especially respiratory rate • Slowed peristalsis • Constricted pupils • Decreased interest in sex	Respiratory depression, hypothermia, pinpoint pupils, coma	Yawning, runny nose, perspiration, goose bumps, anorexia, vomiting, diarrhea, dilated pupils, insomnia, elevated vital signs, drug craving
Nicotine	Central nervous system stimulant • Tachycardia • Increased BP • Alertness • Feeling of well-being	Inhaled toxins cause hypoxemia, carcinogenesis Signs of acute nicotine poisoning (most often in a child who ingests the drug) include nausea, vomiting, abdominal pain, diarrhea, salivation, seizures	Craving, reduced concentration, emotional irritability, nervousness, fatigue, disturbed sleep, increased appetite

| **BOX 71-1** | **Signs of Alcohol or Drug Addiction** |

BOX 71-1   Signs of Alcohol or Drug Addiction

- Regularly drinking or taking more than was originally planned
- Unsuccessfully attempting to reduce or regulate use
- Spending excessive time obtaining, consuming, or recovering from the effects of the drug
- Continuing use despite negative consequences
- Drinking or consuming drugs in solitary
- Failing to fulfill major role obligations at work, school, or home
- Exhibiting tolerance to alcohol and sedative drugs
- Displaying withdrawal symptoms when drug is not consumed

are chemical agents that temporarily accelerate physical and mental functions. Stimulants such as caffeine (the most widely used CNS stimulant), nicotine, cocaine, and amphetamines affect levels of norepinephrine, dopamine, and acetylcholine. **Central nervous system depressants** are chemical agents that slow brain and physiologic activity. Depressant drugs such as alcohol, heroin and other opiates and barbiturates cause effects similar to those of gamma-aminobutyric acid (GABA), endorphins, and enkephalins. These drugs either mimic the neurotransmitters by attaching to their receptor sites or block their reuptake (see Chap. 67).

Psychosocial dynamics also are a component in substance use and abuse. Observing family members, peers, and role models who use alcohol, tobacco, and other drugs influences impressionable teenagers and youngsters. The promotion of alcohol in U.S. culture also fosters its use and abuse. Many people abuse drugs in a dysfunctional effort to cope with psychosocial stressors.

Treatment

Initiating treatment is one of the most difficult hurdles in treating chemical dependence. Clients deny their addiction, rationalize substance use, or blame life situations for their drug and drinking habits. Often, dependent people must "hit bottom" before they seek help. Once they seek treatment and withdrawal is managed, recovering people must learn new methods of coping with stressors, repair relationships damaged by addiction, and develop new interests and activities to fill the time once devoted to using drugs or alcohol.

Although some people quit taking abused substances unassisted, most benefit from chemical detoxification and a treatment plan that involves abstinence, counseling, and

support of peers through a 12-step program. Twelve-step programs are free and provide specific guidelines (steps) for becoming and staying drug or alcohol free. Frequent (daily, if necessary) attendance at meetings is encouraged. During meetings, members share their experiences and discuss the 12 steps and other topics related to recovery.

ALCOHOL DEPENDENCE

Alcoholism is a chronic, progressive, multisystem disease characterized by an inability to control the consumption of alcohol. Unchecked, alcoholism is fatal. Serious medical consequences of alcoholism are dose related; that is, the more alcohol a person consumes, the sooner he or she experiences life-threatening health problems, such as portal hypertension, esophageal varices, and cirrhosis of the liver (see Chap. 47). On a drink-by-drink comparison, women are more likely to experience health problems earlier than men because in general they weigh less than men. Consequently, the same amount of alcohol is more concentrated and more toxic to women than to men.

Pathophysiology and Etiology

Genetic factors may play a role in alcoholism. Children of alcoholics are three to five times more likely to develop alcoholism than children of nonalcoholics, indicating a possible genetic link. In addition, there is evidence suggesting that a genetically determined component alters metabolism of alcohol in those with the disease. The abnormal metabolism produces a substance called tetrahydroisoquinoline (THIQ) (Box 71-2) (Alcohol and Drug Treatment, 2006; Olms, 1983). Studies have shown that THIQ creates an intense craving for alcohol in rats and remains in the animal brain even during abstinence. Some believe that the lifelong presence of THIQ explains why (1) there is no cure for alcoholism, (2) why people with alcoholism are prone to relapse, and (3) why people with alcoholism are quick to resume their previous addictive drinking patterns after periods of sobriety.

The presence of THIQ in humans with alcoholism continues to be debated, and research has turned to other genetic possibilities. For example, variant genes for dopamine and dopamine receptors have been identified, as well as geneticbased deficiencies in serotonin or serotonin receptors in people with the disease (Alcohol and Drug Treatment, 2006; Edenburg & Foroud, 2006). Dopamine is a neurotransmitter that locks onto receptors, triggering sensations of pleasure

TABLE 71-2 Patterns of Substance Abuse

EXPERIMENTATION	HABITUATION	DEPENDENCE	ADDICTION
Initial use	Repeated use	Frequent use	Unremitting use
Low dose	Uniform doses	Doses increase	High doses
Finds experience pleasurable	Seeks to re-experience pleasure	Craves ongoing pleasure from drug	Needs drug to feel "normal"
No discomfort from abstinence	No discomfort from abstinence	Experiences minor physical discomfort if drug is not used	Experiences severe withdrawal symptoms if drug is not used

BOX 71-2 Normal and Alcoholic Metabolism of Alcohol

Ethyl alcohol
↓
Acetaldehyde + dopamine → Tetrahydroisoquinoline
↓   (THIQ)
Acetic acid (vinegar)
↓
Carbon dioxide + water

Altered alcohol metabolism shown in purple

and reward, which may explain its relationship to addictive behaviors.

Assessment Findings

Signs and Symptoms

Although the client may emphatically deny problem drinking, he or she typically has a history of increasing alcohol consumption. The person may hide containers of alcohol and drink privately at any time during the day. Many clients manifest a great tolerance for alcohol and a **cross-tolerance** (reduced effect) for sedative-hypnotic drugs. **Blackouts**, periods of amnesia involving events and activities during drinking, occur even in the early stages. Family and friends note alcoholic behaviors, and social or legal repercussions occur. A history of marital, financial, and occupational problems reflects the person's inability to control drinking despite negative consequences. Many clients with alcoholism have been arrested for driving under the influence of alcohol.

Gerontologic Considerations

- Older adults may use alcohol as self-treatment or may begin taking over-the-counter medication with an alcohol base; progressive use or amounts compounded by a slowed metabolism may lead to alcoholism or alcohol toxicity.

- Alcoholism may be difficult to identify in older adults because symptoms such as tremors, unsteady gait, or memory loss mimic changes associated with aging.

- Older adults who drink alcohol exhibit greater impairment and neurologic deficits such as confusion, ataxia, and loss of cognitive ability than younger adults and recover more slowly.

- Dementia may be associated with heavy ingestion of alcohol for 10 or more years, or with ingestion of other toxic substances, including heavy metals.

People who are acutely intoxicated may enter the tertiary care hospital with altered mental status or acute gastric bleeding, or as victims of trauma or violence. When hospitalization occurs, management of alcohol withdrawal is as important as management of the related conditions. Withdrawal from alcohol results in nervous system stimulation manifested by tremors, sweating, hypertension, tachycardia, heart palpitations, craving for alcohol, seizures, and hallucinations.

▶ **Stop, Think, and Respond Exercise 71-1**

What assessment findings suggest that a person who consumes alcohol is an alcoholic rather than a social drinker?

Complications

A host of alcohol-related physical symptoms can accompany persistent drinking. Esophagitis, gastritis, enlarged liver, esophageal and rectal bleeding, and pancreatitis are common. Memory is impaired, and clients may experience erectile dysfunction or decreased libido. Studies also implicate alcohol in liver cancer, cerebrovascular accident, metabolic deficiencies, aspiration pneumonia, cardiomyopathy, blood dyscrasias, and neurologic disorders. Infants born to women who consumed alcohol during pregnancy sometimes have fetal alcohol syndrome, which causes physical and intellectual deficits.

Diagnostic Findings

A blood alcohol level measures the percentage of alcohol in the blood, indicating the extent of alcohol intoxication at the time of measurement (Table 71-3). However, tolerance for alcohol may decrease the physiologic effects of accumulating blood alcohol levels in people who are chronic drinkers. Elevated levels of gamma-glutamyl transpeptidase (GGTP), aspartate aminotransferase (AST), and alanine aminotransferase (ALT) reflect alcohol-induced liver disease. High levels of pancreatic enzymes (amylase and lipase) may indicate pancreatitis, which develops secondarily to alcoholism.

TABLE 71-3 Blood Alcohol Level and Associated Impairment

BLOOD ALCOHOL LEVEL	PERCENTAGE OF BLOOD ALCOHOL	PHYSICAL AND BEHAVIORAL EFFECTS
50 mg/dL	0.05%	Mood changes, loosening of inhibition, decreased judgment, slight euphoria
80–100 mg/dL	0.08–0.1%	Reduced muscle coordination, decreased reaction time, impaired vision
200 mg/dL	0.2%	Staggering, poor control of emotions, easily angered
300 mg/dL	0.3%	Mental confusion, stupor
400 mg/dL	0.4%	Coma
500 mg/dL	0.5%	Respiratory depression, death

Medical Management and Rehabilitation

To break the progression of alcoholism, clients undergo detoxification, nutritional therapy, psychotherapy, and drug therapy. They are encouraged to continue rehabilitation by joining a support group such as Alcoholics Anonymous (AA).

Detoxification

Alcohol withdrawal without detoxification is a potentially fatal process. **Detoxification** ("detox") involves stabilizing the client with a sedative drug while the alcohol is metabolized from his or her system. Withdrawal symptoms are controlled until they subside. Drugs used in detoxification are lorazepam (Ativan), diazepam (Valium), and chlordiazepoxide (Librium); Drug Therapy Table 71-1). Initially, these medications are administered frequently and in high doses to compensate for the client's cross-tolerance; they are then tapered and discontinued. A beta-adrenergic blocker such as propranolol (Inderal) is given to reduce the dangerously elevated heart rate and blood pressure that can occur during withdrawal. Alcoholism may result in thiamine deficiency, which can lead to dementia. Because thiamine is necessary for the metabolism of glucose, glucose solutions must be avoided until thiamine is administered. Once thiamine is administered, intravenous (IV) hydration with glucose and additional vitamins, such as folic acid, supports the client metabolically until the condition stabilizes.

Nutritional Therapy

People with alcoholism often are undernourished and have deficiencies of B vitamins. Injections of thiamine for 3 days followed by oral administration and folic acid supplements often are prescribed. Vitamin therapy prevents neurologic complications, known as Wernicke's encephalopathy and Korsakoff's psychosis, that affect memory and cognitive functions. Nutrition Notes 71-1 outlines additional nutrition considerations.

Psychotherapy

Individual or group psychotherapy helps the client to gain greater insight into the emotional problems that have led to or resulted from alcohol dependence. Family therapy with the spouse and children provides an opportunity to share how alcoholism has affected each person so that psychosocial healing may begin.

Nutrition Notes 71-1
The Client With Alcoholism

- For clients with moderate to severe pancreatitis, the preferred route of delivering nutrition has shifted away from parenteral nutrition toward enteral nutrition delivered into the jejunum. Jejunal feedings do not stimulate pancreatic secretions, are well tolerated, and are less likely than parenteral nutrition to cause complications.
- For clients with chronic pancreatitis, a low-fat diet may help minimize pain after eating.
- Sodium and fluid restrictions are indicated for ascites, a consequence of liver damage.
- A soft diet is used for esophageal varices.

Drug Therapy

Disulfiram (Antabuse) is a drug given to people recovering from alcoholism who cannot control the compulsion to drink. It is a form of **aversion therapy** because it deters drinking by causing unpleasant physical reactions when alcohol is consumed or absorbed through the skin. For clients who are prescribed disulfiram, health teaching includes a list of products that contain alcohol such as liquid cough suppressants (Box 71-3). The client must be informed that life-threatening cardiopulmonary complications and even death can occur when disulfiram and alcohol are combined.

Pharmacologic Considerations

- A reaction to disulfiram can occur up to 2 weeks after discontinuing the drug. Inform the client to avoid all forms of alcohol (e.g., cough syrups, elixirs, topical applications of personal care products such as after-shave lotion, food flavoring extracts) for at least 2 weeks after discontinuing disulfiram.

Gerontologic Considerations

- Caution is necessary when administering disulfiram to older adults. This drug interferes with the actions of several drugs (e.g., warfarin, nitroglycerin) that are often a part of the older adult's medication regimen.

Acamprosate calcium (Campral) is a newer drug that acts on the neurotransmitter glutamate to alleviate the physiological and psychological distress following withdrawal from alcohol (see Drug Therapy Table 71-1). Naltrexone (Trexan, ReVia), a narcotic antagonist, is also used as an adjunct in people who are recovering from alcoholism. It reduces the pleasure associated with drinking alcohol, should the person **relapse** (return to drinking).

Support Groups

Alcoholics Anonymous was the first 12-step self-help program. Founded in 1926 by an alcoholic physician, AA is composed of and run by recovering alcoholics to help people who are dependent on alcohol get and stay sober. AA emphasizes personal accountability, spirituality, and

BOX 71-3 Obscure Sources of Alcohol

- Liquid cough and cold medications
- Liquid sleep medications
- Flavoring extracts
- Mouthwash
- Rubbing alcohol
- Aftershave lotions
- Fruitcake with alcohol

powerlessness over alcohol. Family members of clients with alcoholism may benefit from attending meetings of Al Anon, Alateen, or Adult Children of Alcoholics to learn more about how alcoholism affects them.

> ### Stop, Think, and Respond Exercise 71-2
>
> Explain why the first of AA's 12 steps leading to recovery from alcoholism is "We admitted we were powerless over alcohol—and that our lives had become unmanageable."

Nursing Process for the Client With Alcohol Dependence

Assessment

Examine the client from head to toe; note any signs of fall-related injuries, abdominal enlargement, jaundiced skin or sclera, and blood in any body fluids or stool that may indicate complications from liver damage or portal hypertension (see Chap. 47). Question the client about the use of alcohol when establishing the client's database. The CAGE Screening Test is helpful in detecting alcoholic behaviors (Box 71-4). If the client admits to consuming alcohol, determine the type, how much, and when the last drink was consumed. The latter information is important because withdrawal symptoms occur within 3 to 72 hours after a client's last drink. When appropriate, administer a breath-alcohol concentration test or blood alcohol level as soon as possible to obtain an approximation of the client's current alcohol level. Determine if the client has a history of seizures or other severe symptoms in previous withdrawals merits close observation of the client for a similar reaction the client for a similar reaction.

Monitor the client for signs and symptoms of withdrawal. If a standardized symptom withdrawal flow sheet is unavailable, use the **Rule of One Hundreds** as an indicator of escalating withdrawal. The Rule of One Hundreds refers to a body temperature of at least 100°F, a pulse rate of at least 100 beats per minute, or a diastolic blood pressure of at least 100 mm Hg. The rise in any one of these three vital signs suggests the need for sedative medication, because the physiologic consequences of withdrawal may be extremely difficult to counteract once they have begun.

> **BOX 71-4** **CAGE Questionnaire for Alcoholism**
>
> 1. Have you ever felt that you ought to **C**ut down on your drinking?
> 2. Have people **A**nnoyed you by criticizing your drinking?
> 3. Have you ever felt **G**uilty about your drinking?
> 4. Have you ever had a drink first thing in the morning to steady your nerves or get rid of a hangover (**E**ye-opener)?
>
> From Ewing, J. A. [1984] Detecting alcoholism: The CAGE questionnaire. *Journal of the American Medical Association*, 252, 1905–1907.

Diagnosis, Planning, and Interventions

▶ **PC: Alcohol Withdrawal**

▶ **Expected Outcome:** The nurse will manage and minimize alcohol withdrawal.

- Assess the client's vital signs and other data, such as hand tremors, hyperactive tendon reflexes, diaphoresis, anxiety, insomnia, and disorientation, that suggest physiologic stimulation. *As the body metabolizes alcohol, it releases norepinephrine, causing autonomic nervous system stimulation.*
- Consult with the physician regarding the need for a detoxification drug. *The physician is responsible for prescribing a drug for detoxification and the dose, route, and frequency of administration according to assessment data the nurse obtains.*
- Administer prescribed detoxification medication. *Minor tranquilizers maintain a controlled level of intoxication so withdrawal is less rapid and dangerous.*
- Repeat assessments for withdrawal at least every 2 hours. *Administration of a detoxification drug should control physiologic stimulation; if not, administration of another dose is warranted.*
- Monitor for seizure activity, hallucinations, extreme tremors, and agitation. *If early and minor symptoms of alcohol withdrawal are not managed effectively, the client's withdrawal will progress in severity because of norepinephrine and dopamine stimulation.*
- Restrict caffeine during withdrawal.
- Caffeine is a central nervous system stimulant that heightens the symptoms of withdrawal.

▶ **Imbalanced Nutrition: Less Than Body Requirements** related to inadequate dietary intake

▶ **Expected Outcome:** The client will consume at least 75% of the food that is served.

- Obtain a baseline weight. *Documenting the client's current weight provides a means of evaluating if the client's subsequent nutritional intake maintains or increases the current weight.*
- Determine the client's food preferences. *A person is more likely to consume food that he or she likes.*
- Collaborate with the dietary department to provide six small meals each day and an ample variety of snacks. *The client is likely to consume more food if the quantity is distributed throughout the day.*
- Monitor dietary intake and record data in the medical record. *Documentation provides an objective means for evaluating the client's progress.*

▶ **Anticipatory Grieving** related to loss of alcohol use and related social activities and social contacts

▶ **Expected Outcomes:** (1) The client will verbalize that alcohol abuse is an illness that requires ongoing treatment and support. (2) The client will understand the connection between alcohol and its associated activities and develop non–alcohol-related interests and contacts.

- Let the client express feelings concerning potential losses. *Discussing the effects of abstinence is the first step in working through grief.*

- Explore alternatives that may substitute for potential losses. *Identifying activities and other people with whom to socialize may substitute for the void caused by abstaining from alcohol.*
- Encourage the family or significant others to support one another. *The physical and emotional burden associated with life-altering changes can be lightened if shared among many people who are meaningful to the client.*
- Promote sharing of experiences between the client and others who are further ahead in their recovery. *Role models who are dealing with similar issues can motivate and encourage the client.*

▶ **Health–Seeking Behavior: Abstinence From Alcohol** related to a desire to manage a chronically, fatal disease

▶ **Expected Outcome:** The client will formulate a plan for attaining and maintaining sobriety.

- Provide the locations of AA meetings. *Knowing the locations and times of meetings allows the client to make personal choices in pursuing his or her recovery.*
- Explain that a sponsor may be selected from among those who attend AA meetings. *A sponsor provides social and emotional support throughout recovery.*
- Recommend that the client begin reading the "Big Book" of AA. *This book, titled* Alcohol Anonymous, *describes the traditional 12 steps that lead to recovery.*
- Prepare the client for possible relapse by role-playing situations that may entice him or her to drink. *Role-playing helps the client prepare for possible barriers to recovery and provides an opportunity to simulate methods for dealing with them.*

Evaluation of Expected Outcomes

Vital signs are stable, and symptoms of withdrawal are controlled. The client eats a well-balanced diet and sleeps an adequate number of hours per night. The client demonstrates a willingness to cope with losses associated with overcoming dependence on alcohol. He or she also moves forward with measures to remain sober, such as participating in AA. ●

Gerontologic Considerations

- Nurses and caregivers must avoid age-related stereotypes and support older adults' efforts to overcome or prevent chemical dependence by promoting social networks and reducing isolation that may accompany growing older.

NICOTINE DEPENDENCE

Nicotine, the stimulant drug in tobacco, is the most heavily used addictive, mood-altering substance in the United States. The drug is absorbed by inhaling the tobacco in cigarettes, cigars, and pipes, or through the mucous membranes of the mouth from loose tobacco.

Pathophysiology and Etiology

A person's dependence on tobacco develops gradually and progresses through six stages (Rossie et al., 2004):

- Precontemplation: lacks ideas about personally using tobacco
- Contemplation: entertains the possibility of using a tobacco product
- Initiation: uses a tobacco product for the first time
- Experimentation: uses tobacco sporadically
- Regular smoking: establishes a pattern of consistent use
- Established habit: requires regular and increased use of tobacco

The addictive quality of tobacco occurs because of nicotine, an active ingredient in tobacco. Nicotine mimics the neurotransmitter acetylcholine, which intensifies the release of dopamine in the brain, promoting an experience of pleasure and reward. As the body adjusts to the dopamine stimulation from nicotine, tolerance develops, and the person needs to smoke more and more. Dependence develops as a result of experiencing a combination of pleasure, reward, and tolerance (Rossie et al., 2004).

Pleasurable psychological effects are offset by nicotine's pathological consequences. Smoking raises carbon monoxide levels in the blood and causes constriction of peripheral blood vessels, which contributes to cardiovascular disease. Tobacco smoke disrupts the structure of alveoli, causing them to become overstretched and inelastic, as in emphysema. It is implicated in the development and recurrence of gastric ulcers. The smoke in inhaled tobacco products contains more than 40 carcinogenic chemicals. Smokeless tobacco (chewing tobacco) exposes the oral cavity to carcinogens, inhaled tobacco targets the lungs and distant organs, and cigars or pipes repeatedly expose the oral cavity and esophagus to harmful substances.

Although smoking and tobacco use have decreased in recent decades, approximately 21% of adults use tobacco (Chong, 2007; CDC, 2005). Estimates of associated medical costs are $50 billion annually. Passive absorption of smoke also can cause disease in nonsmokers. Nicotine produces tolerance, resulting in increased use over time and withdrawal symptoms when use is discontinued. Users light up or chew to maintain blood and brain drug levels; nicotine is then distributed throughout the body, metabolized in the liver, and excreted by the kidneys. Frequency of tobacco use also is governed by conditioned, learned responses, meaning that past patterns of use reinforce the habit of smoking; for example, smoking may follow a meal or accompany talking on the telephone or consuming coffee. This factor is important, in that smoking-cessation strategies must target both the physical dependence and the conditioned related behaviors.

Consequences

Smoking is responsible for 90% of deaths from lung cancer and from chronic obstructive lung disease. It also causes a significant number of cancers that affect the mouth, larynx, esophagus, and bladder. The rate of coronary heart disease in smokers is 2 to 4 times that in nonsmokers. Smokers are 10 times more likely to develop peripheral vascular disease than nonsmokers. There also is a correlation between cigarette smoking and premature delivery and low-birth-weight infants (CDC, 2008; National Cancer Institute, 2008).

Gerontologic Considerations

- The bones of postmenopausal women who smoke are less dense, and these women are at higher risk for fractures, especially of the hip, as they age.

Breathing **environmental tobacco smoke** (also called *secondhand smoke* or *passive smoke*), the smoke given off by the burning end of a cigarette, pipe, or cigar and the exhaled smoke from the lungs of a smoker, is potentially injurious to others. *Epidemiologists,* scientists who study the incidence and causation of illnesses, have identified that breathing secondhand smoke causes headaches and eye, nose, and throat irritation. Nonsmokers exposed to environmental tobacco smoke have increased rates of heart disease, lung and other types of cancer, and lower respiratory tract infections. Risk of sudden infant death syndrome is increased in infants whose mothers smoked throughout pregnancy and after delivery. Children with asthma have an increased frequency of and more severe attacks when exposed to an environment with secondhand smoke.

Medical Management

All smokers and tobacco users are advised to quit and should be provided with materials that inform them of methods to do so. Various levels of intervention are available and include minimal approaches such as brief counseling and follow-up or more intense measures such as enrollment in behavior-modification programs. These programs help clients manage temptation and extinguish preconditioned cues to smoke. They also provide rewards for goal achievement. Pharmacologic therapy using drugs for smoking cessation includes non-nicotine medications such as bupropion (Zyban) and varenicline (Chantix), which are dopamine uptake inhibitors that help suppress nicotine's addicting reinforcement, and nicotine substitutes (gum, patch, inhaler), which allow dopamine to be released but at a lower rate than occurs with smoking (see Drug Therapy Table 71-1). The nicotine substitutes are gradually tapered and stopped; they help clients avoid withdrawal symptoms and are an adjunct to other interventions.

Pharmacologic Considerations

- Young children are particularly sensitive to the effects of even small doses of nicotine. Discarded nicotine patches contain enough nicotine to cause serious adverse reactions in children. Advise clients to store nicotine gum out of children's reach and to dispose of mixtures of saliva and smokeless tobacco products, which may cause acute nicotine poisoning if consumed. If a child chews or swallows nicotine gum, contact the physician or local poison control center.

Relapse is common, because withdrawal symptoms begin within several hours after the last cigarette is smoked and peak 2 to 3 days later. More than 75% of people who attempt to stop smoking resume smoking within 3 months. About 10% to 15% of smokers who quit remain tobacco free for 1 year. Attempts to quit, however, are a predictor of eventual success; 60% of those who try and fail ultimately do succeed sometimes after trying six to seven times (Rossie et al., 2004).

Nursing Management

Nurses help clients who smoke by counseling them to quit and providing them with information on various smoking cessation products and programs. Nurturing the client's belief that he or she can be successful is an important supportive measure. Because many clients fear gaining weight after smoking cessation, the nurse informs them that typical weight gain in the year after cessation is 5 to 10 lbs (Mirken, 2008). The nurse then helps the client plan strategies to offset the tendency for weight gain, such as beginning a walking program, substituting fruits for high-calorie desserts, and reducing dietary fat. Sucking on sugarless hard candy or chewing sugarless gum also may help by keeping the client's mouth busy without adding calories. If the client is unwilling to contemplate quitting, the nurse informs him or her of the dangers of secondhand smoke to others and encourages abstinence from smoking in the presence of nonsmokers, especially children. The nurse also actively promotes individual and community health by learning smoking-cessation techniques and providing seminars to the public.

Based on recommendations from the U.S. Environmental Protection Agency, the nurse can advise nonsmokers on techniques for reducing the inhalation of secondhand smoke:

- Do not permit others to smoke in one's home or workplace.
- If smoking takes place in the home, increase ventilation by opening windows or using exhaust fans.
- Avoid riding in a car with someone who smokes; the small area contributes to a high concentration of toxic smoke, which increases exposure.

COCAINE AND METHAMPHETAMINE DEPENDENCE

Cocaine and methamphetamine are CNS stimulants. Although the actions of methamphetamine are stronger and last longer than those of cocaine, the physiologic and psychologic effects of the two substances are comparable because of the rapid and excessive release of norepinephrine, dopamine, and serotonin. Each drug is associated with some unique health problems that develop from use and abuse.

Cocaine is a CNS stimulant obtained from the leaves of the coca plant. The powder form of cocaine is snorted (inhaled through the nose) or dissolved and injected intravenously. Crack, a purified form of cocaine with a crystalline or rocklike appearance, makes a crackling sound when it is heated; it is smoked either by placing it in a pipe or by sprinkling it onto or mixing it with tobacco or marijuana. Cocaine may be freebased, which reduces the drug to its purest form.

DRUG THERAPY TABLE 71-1 Drugs Used in the Recovery from Chemical Dependence

Drug Category and Examples	Mechanism of Action	Side Effects	Nursing Considerations
Benzodiazepine lorazepam (Ativan)	Occupies GABA receptors or increases GABA so as to depress the central nervous system	Sedation, confusion, restlessness, bradycardia, tachycardia, urinary retention or incontinence, drug dependence	If giving IV, monitor vital signs carefully. Intramuscular injection can be quite painful; dilute with equal volume for IV administration, assess injection sites, administer slowly. Observe client for excessive sedation, and use cautiously in clients with impaired kidney or liver function.
Antialcoholic Agent disulfiram (Antabuse)	Blocks oxidation of alcohol, resulting in the accumulation of acetaldehyde	*If alcohol is used:* flushing, throbbing headaches, dyspnea, vomiting, tachycardia, hypotension, blurred vision; severe reactions can result in convulsions, myocardial infarction, death *Disulfiram alone:* drowsiness, headache, dermatitis	Do not administer until at least 12 hours have elapsed since last exposure to alcohol. Inform client to avoid all sources of alcohol and to wear a medical identification bracelet. Arrange for follow-up liver and blood studies. Inform client of potential side effects and to report them to a healthcare provider.
acamprosate (Campral)	Modulates the neurotransmitter glutamate to restore neuronal balance; it alleviates the physiological and psychological distress during the postacute withdrawal period, making it easier not to drink.	Hypersensitivity to acamprosate, weakness, diarrhea, flatulence, nausea, pruritus, headache, change in sexual desire or decreased sexual ability, anxiety, dizziness, insomnia	Does not eliminate or diminish withdrawal symptoms; monitor for symptoms of depression or suicidal thinking. May impair judgment, thinking, and motor skills.
Smoking Deterrents nicotine transdermal (Nicotrol)	Binds to nicotinic receptors in central and peripheral nervous system	Headache, insomnia, diarrhea, constipation, pharyngitis, burning and itching at site, backache, chest pain, dysmenorrhea	Explain application, site rotation, and disposal of used patches so that pets or children do not come in contact with product. Inform client of side effects and to report any that occur.
varenicline (Chantix)	Nicotine agonist that binds to nicotine receptor sites, reducing the severity of withdrawal symptoms	Nausea, flatulence, constipation, sleep disturbance, vivid dreams, agitation, depressed mood, suicidal thoughts	Begin administering 1 week prior to smoking cessation. Administer on a full stomach with full glass of water to prevent nausea. Duration of therapy is no more than 12 weeks. Expect a lower dose for clients with renal disease. Not to be used with other smoking cessation products.
bupropion (Zyban)	Increases norepinephrine and dopamine by blocking their neuronal reuptake reducing the desire for nicotine and reducing nicotine withdrawal	Nausea, insomnia, dry mouth, constipation, tremor, anxiety, lowers seizure threshold.	Begin administering 1 week prior to smoking cessation. Monitor blood pressure if using concurrently with nicotine replacement therapy Advise to swallow tablet whole; never chew, crush, or break. Contraindicated in seizure, eating, and bipolar disorders, pregnancy, and breastfeeding.
Narcotic Antagonists naloxone (Narcan)	Blocks opioids at their receptor sites	Abrupt reversal of opioid depression may result in acute opiate withdrawal	Monitor for improved respiratory function within 2 minutes of drug administration. Continue monitoring after arousal as the duration of

DRUG THERAPY TABLE 71-1 Drugs Used in the Recovery from Chemical Dependence (*Continued*)

Drug Category and Examples	Mechanism of Action	Side Effects	Nursing Considerations
			naloxone is less than that of opioids; repeat doses may be required. May repeat administration at 2–3 minute intervals up to a cumulative dose of 10 mg.
naltrexone hydrochloride (Trexan, ReVia)	Blocks the effects of opioids and aids in the abstinence from alcohol	Insomnia, anxiety, nervousness, low energy, abdominal pain, nausea, vomiting, decreased sexual potency, delayed ejaculation, rash, joint and muscle pain, increased thirst	Induces sudden withdrawal so do not use until 7 to 14 days have elapsed since last exposure to opioids. Inform client that small doses of opioids will have no effect. Larger doses may overcome the inhibiting effect, but coma or death may occur. Tell the client to report any side effects.
Narcotic Agonist Analgesic			
methadone (Dolophine)	Binds with opioid receptors in the CNS and produces euphoria, analgesia, and sedation	Light-headedness, dizziness, sedation, nausea, vomiting, respiratory depression, circulatory depression, shock, cardiac arrest	A single liquid oral dose is used for maintenance. Constipation may be severe; ensure that client is taking a stool softener. Use with caution in clients receiving sedatives, hypnotics, tranquilizers, tricyclic antidepressants, and monoamine oxidase inhibitors—respiratory depression, hypotension, and coma can occur.

A person smokes freebased cocaine by sprinkling it onto a cigarette or inhaling it through a pipe. Freebased cocaine provides an intense physical experience as the drug is absorbed, more so than when it is taken by other routes. It also increases the risk of toxic effects and overdose reactions. Metabolism of cocaine, which is rapid, usually is followed by an intense craving to use the drug again. Cravings can recur months or years after abstinence.

Methamphetamine, also known as "meth," is an addicting stimulant that is made by combining over-the-counter medications containing ephedrine and pseudoephedrine with other chemicals such as ammonia, acetone, and lye. The finished substance is generally smoked or injected intravenously. When self-administered, the user experiences extreme pleasure, euphoria, and CNS stimulation similar to that associated with cocaine use.

Assessment Findings

Signs and Symptoms

Signs and symptoms of each drug's effect may be brief (see Table 71-1) because of the rapid metabolism and the powerful craving to use the drug again. Signs correlate with its route of administration and consequences of chronic use. For example, ulceration of the nasal mucosa and perforation of the nasal septum are found in people who snort cocaine. Needle marks are found along the pathways of veins in those who inject cocaine intravenously. Those who smoke or freebase cocaine

may have burns on their faces, fingertips, or eyebrows from using or leaning over a lighted pipe. Smoking cocaine can cause a chronic cough and pulmonary congestion.

Methamphetamine users may develop acne and be covered with multiple scratched lesions. Some users have tactile hallucinations and believe that insects are crawling under their skin, which causes them to scratch their face, hands, and arms. The constriction of blood vessels makes the resulting lesions slow to heal. Methamphetamine use also causes the salivary glands to dry out, leading to a wearing away of the tooth enamel from acids in the mouth. Oral tissues decay from impaired blood supply. This condition is sometimes referred to as "meth mouth" because of the characteristic appearance of broken, discolored, and rotting teeth. Extreme weight loss is also common.

Clients who are addicted to cocaine and methamphetamine often have a problem with **polydrug abuse**, abuse of more than one substance. It is common for them also to take sedative drugs such as alcohol, minor tranquilizers, barbiturates, and marijuana to offset their agitation and irritability.

Complications

Long-term abusers of cocaine and methamphetamine experience anorexia, weight loss, memory impairment, personality and behavioral changes, paranoia, psychosis, and hallucinations. Medically, stimulant abuse can cause rapid and severe hypertension, cardiac dysrhythmias, seizures, cerebral hemorrhage (stroke), myocardial infarction (heart attack), and respiratory arrest. Newborns also can experience withdrawal symptoms if their mothers recently used CNS stimulants.

Methamphetamine users are also at higher risk for contracting human immunodeficiency virus (HIV) and hepatitis B because the surge of neurotransmitters increases sexual drive and decreases judgment. Consequently, sexual activity, especially among gay men, may be more aggressive and prolonged, thus increasing the potential for anogenital bleeding and the transmission of blood-borne viruses.

Diagnostic Findings

Drug toxicology tests are done on blood and urine. Metabolites of cocaine can be found in a urine drug screen for up to 36 hours. Metabolites of methamphetamine can be found for up to 3 to 6 days. Other abused substances also are identified.

Medical Management and Rehabilitation

Cocaine toxicity (see Table 71-1) requires immediate treatment because the condition is life-threatening. Referral to Cocaine Anonymous, which is based on the same principles as AA, provides a source of ongoing support for those addicted to cocaine. Participation in individual and group psychotherapy and Cocaine Anonymous is encouraged to help the client eliminate all forms of drug abuse. The recreational use of other drugs can lead to relapse.

To help the person addicted to cocaine with recovery, medications such as bromocriptine (Parlodel) and amantadine (Symmetrel) are used temporarily. They increase or mimic the effects of dopamine, the neurotransmitter that is most likely responsible for the rewarding and reinforcing effects of addicting substances. Antidepressants are prescribed to relieve the dysphoria (depression) that occurs during withdrawal. Amino acid precursors such as phenylalanine and tyrosine, the substances from which the neurotransmitters norepinephrine and dopamine are made, are included in drug therapy to replace levels depleted by chronic use.

A research project presently in phase III clinical trials is an anticocaine vaccine developed by Xenova Pharmaceuticals in England. The vaccine, which is currently called TA-CD, promotes the development of antibodies that bind with cocaine and prevent the drug from reaching the brain (National Institute on Drug Abuse, 2008).

Unfortunately, recovery from methamphetamine abuse is more difficult. It may take years of antidepressant drug therapy and behavior modification techniques.

Nursing Management

The nurse assesses the client's history of drug use and his or her current physical condition. The nurse also looks for signs of toxicity and withdrawal. He or she implements medical treatment during a life-threatening emergency. Later, the nurse explains the effects of drug abuse and the risks for continuing drug-taking behaviors. Monitoring the client for suicidal ideation (see Chap. 69) and administering medications that provide support during withdrawal are essential nursing interventions.

OPIATE DEPENDENCE

Opiate dependence is an addiction to narcotics, CNS-depressant drugs that are either derived from or chemically similar to opium. *Opioid* is a term for synthetic opiate narcotics. Some examples of opiate drugs include heroin (diacetylmorphine), codeine, morphine, meperidine (Demerol), methadone, hydromorphone (Dilaudid), oxycodone (OxyContin), and opium, as in tincture of paregoric. Opiates produce sedation after initial euphoria. The rate of tolerance and chemical dependence is related to the drug, dose, and frequency of use.

Assessment Findings

Refer to heroin in Table 71-1 for the effects of opiates. The pupils usually are pinpoint in size. Constipation is associated with slowed peristalsis. Chronic use is evidenced by anorexia, weight loss, constipation, malnutrition, needle marks, and scarring (tracks) along the paths of veins.

Respiratory depression can lead to unconsciousness and death. Sharing needles during the IV administration of any abused substance can lead to AIDS, hepatitis, and septicemia. Abscesses may develop in punctured skin and veins. General debilitation increases susceptibility to tuberculosis and anemia. Neonates in withdrawal are observed to have a high-pitched cry, tremors, insomnia, increased respirations, vomiting, diarrhea, dehydration, and convulsions.

A urine drug screen reveals evidence of opiate use. Rapid recovery (within 2–5 minutes) from lethargy, hypotension, and respiratory depression after the IV administration of a narcotic antagonist such as naloxone (Narcan) supports the diagnosis of narcotic overdose.

Medical Management and Rehabilitation

Withdrawal symptoms are treated with the alpha-adrenergic blocker clonidine (Catapres) to inhibit the release of norepinephrine. Methadone (Dolophine), a synthetic narcotic, may be used to eliminate or control withdrawal symptoms.

One method for helping those addicted to heroin avoid IV or street-supplied narcotics is methadone maintenance therapy. **Methadone maintenance therapy** involves substituting one addicting drug for another. The advantage is that because methadone is a synthetic drug prepared by a pharmaceutical company, the drug is untainted and the dose is reliable. The rationale behind methadone maintenance therapy is that it forestalls withdrawal, avoids a toxic overdose, reduces the potential for blood-borne infections, and theoretically reduces crime because the drug is provided legally. Some addicts, however, have been known to combine methadone with their depressant drug of choice, which increases the potential of overdose and death. The practice of testing the urine before providing methadone is one way of screening and eliminating those who are abusing the system.

Naltrexone (Trexan, ReVia), an opiate antagonist, also is used for opiate addiction. Naltrexone blocks endorphin receptors; if clients return to opiate abuse while taking naltrexone, they do not experience the previous level of opiate effects. Naltrexone is administered IV for **rapid opiate detoxification**, a procedure for accelerating opiate drug withdrawal within 4 to 8 hours while the client is under anesthesia. Rapid detoxification eliminates the physical discomfort of opiate withdrawal; however, it increases the risks associated with prolonged anesthesia with mechanical ventilation and is more expensive than traditional detoxification protocols.

Psychotherapy is an important aspect of rehabilitation. It involves treating the complex web of social problems that accompanies the addiction. Clients also are referred to Narcotics Anonymous, a self-help organization modeled after AA.

Nursing Management

The nurse's role is similar to that discussed for other types of chemical dependence, with a few exceptions that apply to administering drug therapy. If naltrexone is prescribed as an opiate deterrent, the client must be opiate free for at least 7 days before administration begins. The nurse advises the client who takes methadone to tell healthcare providers or wear a MedicAlert tag in case the client needs a narcotic, tranquilizer, or barbiturate. Because methadone is a narcotic, lower doses of other sedative drugs are necessary because the combination can potentiate their depressant action.

OTHER ABUSED SUBSTANCES

Various other substances are abused and addictive. Some examples include hallucinogens, amphetamines, marijuana, barbiturates, tranquilizers, and volatile hydrocarbons. Signs and symptoms follow the same pattern as with previously discussed substances: experimental use progresses through stages of increased use until dependence and addiction occur; there is failure to meet social, familial, or occupational obligations, with increased defensive mechanisms to explain behavior; disturbances in mood and physical function occur as the result of drug abuse. Treatment and recovery include withdrawal, abstinence, and ongoing participation in a support group.

CRITICAL THINKING EXERCISES

1. What information would you offer to a smoker who claims that "smoke free environments" violate his or her right to smoke?
2. From which type of substance could a person be withdrawing if the following assessments are made? The client has a runny nose and tearing eyes, and he or she yawns frequently. The pilomotor muscles around the hair follicles cause "goose bumps" to appear. Nausea, vomiting, abdominal cramps, and diarrhea are present.
3. Explain why people recovering from alcoholism who have reached an extensive period of sobriety refer to themselves as "recovering" alcoholics rather than "recovered" alcoholics.
4. Why might an alcoholic with a blood alcohol level of 0.425% manifest physical and behavioral effects characteristic of a much lower blood alcohol level?

NCLEX-STYLE REVIEW QUESTIONS

1. Which one of the following abused substances is associated with the development of esophageal varices?
   1. Heroin
   2. Cocaine
   3. Alcohol
   4. Methamphetamine
2. What is the best description of a "blackout" experienced by a person with alcoholism?
   1. A period of lost consciousness.
   2. A period of temporary amnesia.
   3. A period of impaired vision.
   4. A period of dusky skin coloration.
3. Which of the following neurotransmitters is released when a person uses methamphetamine? Select all that apply.
   1. Gamma aminobutyric acid
   2. Norepinephrine
   3. Glutamate
   4. Serotonin
   5. Dopamine
4. Which vitamin is essential for the nurse to provide to help prevent neurologic complications associated with chronic alcoholism?
   1. Ascorbic acid (vitamin C)
   2. Calciferol (vitamin D)
   3. Thiamine (vitamin B_1)
   4. Pyridoxine (vitamin B_6)
5. Which drug can the nurse anticipate will be prescribed when a client has taken an overdose of an opiate?
   1. Lorazepam (Ativan)
   2. Acamprosate (Campral)
   3. Bupropion (Zyban)
   4. Naloxone (Narcan)

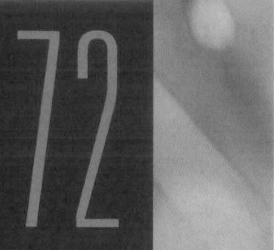

72

Caring for Clients with Dementia and Thought Disorders

Learning Objectives

On completion of this chapter, you will be able to:

1. Differentiate between delirium and dementia, and give an example of a condition that causes each.
2. List five etiologic factors linked to Alzheimer's disease.
3. Discuss the pathophysiologic changes associated with Alzheimer's disease.
4. Name the first symptom of Alzheimer's disease.
5. Identify two methods for diagnosing Alzheimer's disease.
6. Explain the mechanism of drug therapy in Alzheimer's disease.
7. Describe nursing management for clients with Alzheimer's disease.
8. Name three characteristics of schizophrenia.
9. Describe two psychobiologic explanations for schizophrenia.
10. Differentiate between positive and negative symptoms of schizophrenia, and give two examples of each.
11. Discuss the medical management of most people with schizophrenia.
12. Name three examples of antipsychotic drugs and their mechanisms of action.
13. Explain the term *extrapyramidal symptoms,* and list four examples.
14. Describe a technique to prevent noncompliance with drug therapy in clients with schizophrenia.
15. Describe the nursing management of clients with schizophrenia.

Changes in **mentation**, or mental activity, can occur anytime during the life cycle. **Cognitive functions**, such as short-term memory and learning ability, change gradually as people get older, but many acute, chronic, reversible, and irreversible conditions that impair thinking processes can occur at any age. Although older adults are at greatest risk for cognitive impairment, one should never assume that such impairment is necessarily a normal consequence of aging nor that it is untreatable. Depression and other medical disorders, such as hypothyroidism, can manifest as mental dysfunction. Consequently, mental changes require aggressive investigation to determine what, if anything, can reverse the symptoms that clients experience. This chapter discusses conditions that are characterized by dementia and thought disorders.

DELIRIUM AND DEMENTIA

Delirium is a sudden, transient state of confusion. The period of confusion depends on the cause of the delirium. Clients with delirium may have difficulty processing information. They may be disoriented as to the date, time of day, and location. Their judgment may be impaired, or they may be unable to perform intellectually at the same capacity as in the past. Some clients with delirium may be suspicious or frightened or behave inappropriately.

Delirium can result from high fever, head trauma, brain tumor, drug intoxication or withdrawal, metabolic disorders (e.g., liver or renal failure), or inflammatory disorders of the central nervous system (CNS), such as meningitis or encephalitis. Treating the underlying medical condition usually restores mental functions.

 Gerontologic Considerations

Delirium in older adults may occur as the presenting symptom for infections such as pneumonia or urinary tract infections or from fecal impaction. Delirium may present as hyperactivity (e.g., picking at bedcovers or clothing, nervous behaviors) or as hypoactivity (e.g., refusing to make eye contact or verbal exchanges, lethargy).

Dementia, which more commonly affects older adults, refers to conditions in which decline in memory, thinking, and reasoning is severe enough to affect the daily life of an alert person. Various disorders are characterized by dementia. Alzheimer's disease is the leading example, followed by cerebrovascular disorders (see Chap. 38) and Parkinson's disease (see Chap. 37). In contrast to delirium, dementia is manifested by a gradual, irreversible loss of intellectual abilities. Although clients with dementia display signs and symptoms similar to those of delirium, several differences exist (Table 72-1).

▶ *Stop, Think, and Respond Exercise 72-1*

In the descriptions that follow, which client is manifesting delirium, and which is manifesting dementia?

- *Client A is 60 years of age. He developed a headache and high fever 24 hours ago. When he is aroused, he thinks he is in the city in which he spent his boyhood. He calls for his mother who has been dead for more than 10 years.*
- *Client B is 60 years old. He got lost driving home from work last week. Lately he has had difficulty remembering where he put his keys and wallet. His wife believes that he is more argumentative than usual.*

ALZHEIMER'S DISEASE

Alzheimer's disease is a progressive, deteriorating brain disorder. Two types exist: early onset (before age 60 years) and late onset (after age 60 years), with late onset being more common. The incidence of Alzheimer's disease doubles every 5 years after the age of 65. Nearly 30% of all adults older than 85 years of age manifest Alzheimer's disease, and the prediction is that it will affect 13 million Americans by the year 2050 (Medical University of South Carolina, 2008). The National Center for Health Statistics (2008) lists this disease as the sixth leading cause of death in the United States.

Pathophysiology and Etiology

Having a first-degree relative with Alzheimer's disease nearly doubles the risk for acquiring a familial form of dementia. The strongest Alzheimer's markers are located on chromosome 14. Presenilin genes (PSEN1 and PSEN2) on chromosomes 1 and 14 correlate with early-onset Alzheimer's. These markers and other abnormalities on chromosomes 10, 19, and 21 are associated with the disease (Fisher Center for Alzheimer's Research Foundation, 2008).

The abnormal genes lead to Alzheimer's disease by initiating a process that is believed to progress in the following way:

- **Amyloid precursor protein** (APP), a normal neuronal protein consisting of three parts, resides partially inside and outside the neuron's membrane (Fig. 72-1A).
- Beta-secretase, a cellular enzyme, cuts the external portion of APP, forming a fragment called sAPPβ (soluble amyloid precursor protein beta).
- Gamma-secretase, a second enzyme, cuts the internal portion of sAPPβ, causing the middle portion to become a free-floating fragment of **beta amyloid,** a starchy protein (see Fig 72-1B).
- Beta amyloid injures neurons in the area of the brain responsible for producing **acetylcholine**, the neurotransmitter that is critical for memory and cognition.
- As more and more beta amyloid accumulates from increasing numbers of released APP fragments, the particles begin to stick together, forming **amyloid plaques.**
- Accumulating amyloid plaques produce toxic effects on neurons by stimulating an excessive amount of the neurotoxic neurotransmitter **glutamate,** a contributing factor in neuronal cell death.

TABLE 72-1 Comparison of Dementia and Delirium

	DEMENTIA	DELIRIUM
Onset	Gradual	Sudden
Presentation	Alert	Blunted
	Attentive	Inattentive
Course	Stable	Unstable
	Progressive deterioration	Fluctuations in function
	Extended	Brief
Duration	Permanent	Temporary
Treatment	Symptomatic or supportive	Specific
Outcome	Incurable	Curable

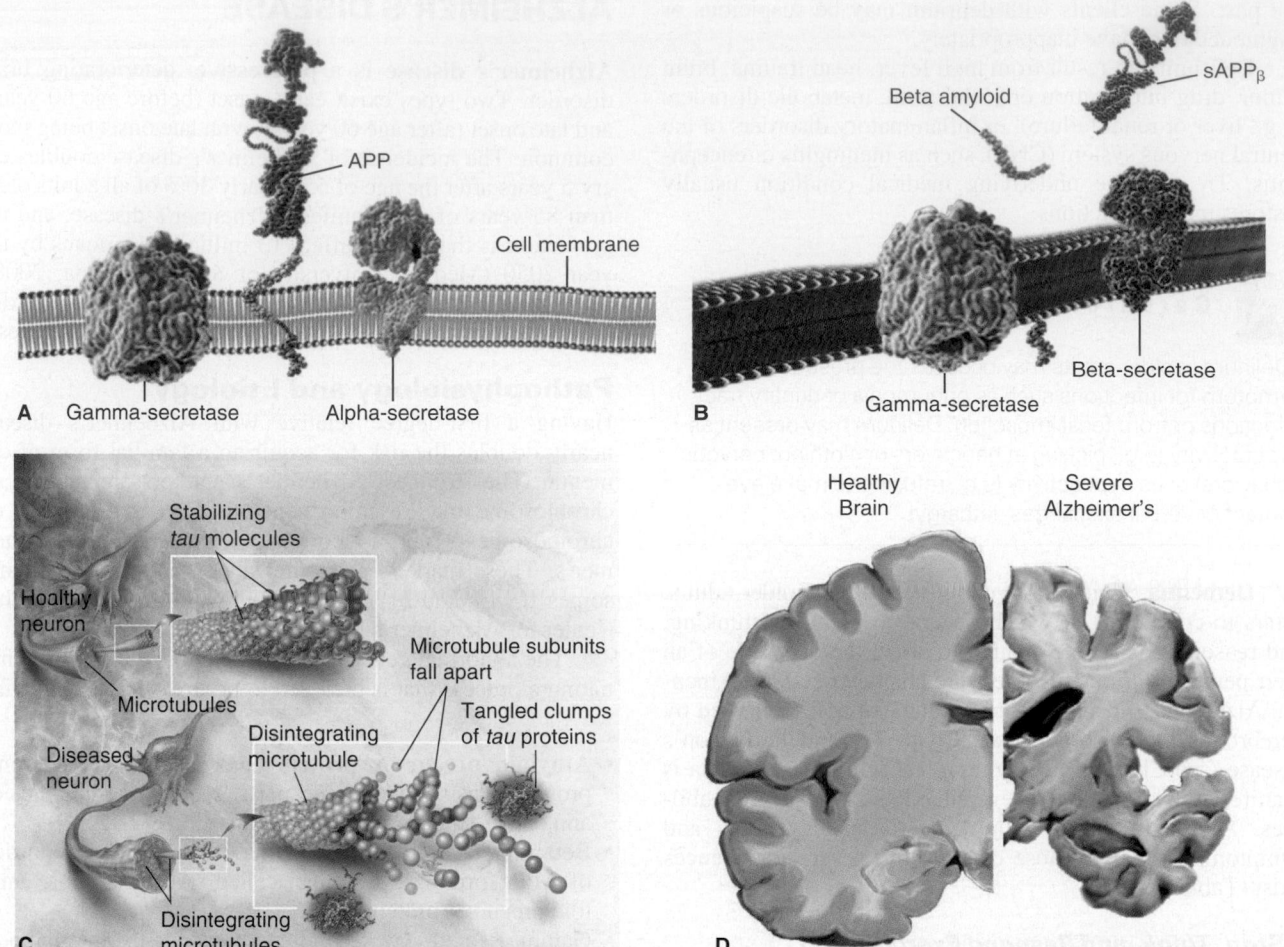

FIGURE 72-1. Selected pathophysiologic processes in Alzheimer's disease. **(A)** Amyloid precursor protein (APP) is embedded in the neuron's cell membrane. **(B)** Enzymes beta- and gamma-secretase sever sAPPβ, releasing a fragment that becomes beta amyloid. **(C)** Neurofibrillary tangles of tau proteins in microtubules form. **(D)** As microtubules disintegrate and more and more neurons die, the brain atrophies (note differences in the healthy and Alzheimer's affected brain). (Images courtesy of the Alzheimer's Disease Education and Referral Center, a service of the National Institute on Aging.)

- Meanwhile, inside the neuron, an abnormal protein called *tau* causes the neuron's microtubules to clump together, forming **neurofibrillary tangles** (see Fig. 72-1C). The microtubules are responsible for transporting nutrients from the cell body to the axon.
- Eventually the microtubules disintegrate, and the neuron dies because the transport system is destroyed.
- As more and more neurons die, the brain atrophies (National Institute on Aging, 2008) (see Fig. 72-1D).

Although inherited, mutated genes are implicated in the development of early-onset Alzheimer's, the etiology of late-onset Alzheimer's disease is not as clear. It may be a combination of genetic, environmental, and lifestyle factors. The decreased size of the cerebral cortex and hippocampus together with acetylcholine deficiency and glutamate toxicity explain the cognitive deficits and alterations in emotions that accompany the disease. The degree to which amyloid plaque and neurofibrillary tangles are present is directly related to the severity of disease manifestations.

Assessment Findings

Signs and Symptoms

Alzheimer's disease progresses through seven distinct stages that correspond with those identified in the Global Deterioration Scale (Table 72-2). Progression from one stage to another can occur at different rates in different people. The early stages may last 2 to 4 years or longer, or it may take as long as 5 to 10 years before a person needs constant care.

Onset usually is insidious, and symptoms may develop slowly over years. Memory loss, the classic symptom, is confined at first to recent information. Eventually, long-term memory and the ability to make appropriate judgments and problem-solve become impaired as well. Disturbances in behavior, personality changes, and depression also occur. As the disease advances, memory, cognition, awareness, and the ability to care for self deteriorate markedly. Clients may wander and become lost. Periodic incidences of violent behavior are possible. Problems with speaking (**aphasia**), reading (**alexia**), writing (**agraphia**), and calculating (**acalculia**)

TABLE 72-2 Global Deterioration Scale

STAGE	CHARACTERISTIC	MANIFESTATIONS
1	Normal mentation	None
2	Forgetfulness	Concern for self-identified memory changes such as forgetting location of items and familiar names
		No objective demonstration of memory deficit
		No social consequences for minor memory loss
3	Early confusion	One or more of the following: Getting lost in an unfamiliar location
		Decline in work performance noticed by others
		Deficit in word and name finding
		Little retention of what has been read
		Difficulty remembering names of new acquaintances
		Loss or misplacement of valuable objects
		Impaired ability to concentrate
		Objective demonstration of memory deficit
		Denial of memory and cognitive deficits
		Mild to moderate anxiety
4	Late confusion	Deficits in the following areas: Current and recent events
		Personal history
		Counting backward in series of numbers
		Traveling and handling finances
		Inability to perform complex tasks such as preparing dinner for guests
		Strong denial of impairment
		Blunted affect
		Retreat from challenges
5	Early dementia	Assistance of others needed
		Memory loss for important information like address and telephone number
		Some disorientation to time or place
		Difficulty counting backward by 4s or 2s
		May have difficulty choosing proper clothing
6	Middle dementia	May forget name of spouse or significant others
		Unaware of recent events and experiences
		Memory of past sketchy
		Unaware of date and surroundings
		Difficulty counting backward and sometimes forward in 10s
		Requires assistance with activities of daily living
		May be incontinent
		Needs assistance to travel
		Confuses day and night
		Personality and emotional changes such as:Delusional thinking
		Repetition of cleaning
		Anxiety, agitation, violence
		Cannot keep a thought long enough to carry it out
7	Late dementia	Loss of verbal ability
		Grunting may be evident
		Incontinent; requires help with toileting and feeding
		Loss of motor skills for walking, sitting, head control, and smiling

Adapted from Reisberg, B., et al. [1982]. The global deterioration scale (GDS): An instrument for the assessment of primary degenerative dementia. *American Journal of Psychiatry, 139,* 1136–1139.

develop. Inability to recognize objects and sounds (visual, tactile, and auditory **agnosia**), difficulty walking (**ataxia**), and tremors occur. In the final stage of the disease, an inability to accomplish activities of daily living (ADLs; **apraxia**), such as grooming, toileting, and eating, despite intact motor function, makes the client totally dependent on others.

Diagnostic Findings
Ruling out Alzheimer's disease in clients who are experiencing similar signs and symptoms can spare them emotional agony, as well as saving time and money spent on nonspecific tests. The diagnosis of Alzheimer's usually is made by excluding other causes for the client's symptoms. A computed tomography (CT) scan shows shrinking of the cerebral cortex, but this is not apparent in the early stages of the disease. Positron emission tomography (PET) and magnetic resonance imaging (MRI) provide structural and metabolic information about the brain. Electroencephalography detects slower-than-normal brain waves. None of these diagnostic tests is specific for Alzheimer's disease, which, until

recently, could be confirmed only during a postmortem examination of the brain.

A new diagnostic test called Nymox AD7C detects evidence of beta amyloid protein in cerebrospinal fluid. Genetic studies identify mutations on chromosomes 1, 14, and 21, which detect the early-onset form of Alzheimer's disease. Fluorescence imaging microscopy is being used to image the molecular biochemical activities in various cells of people with a family history of early-onset Alzheimer's disease (National Institute on Aging, 2008).

Medical Management

No cure exists for Alzheimer's disease; treatment is mainly supportive, using one of various drugs currently available, but newer therapeutic advances show promise. Although it is best to maintain the client's independence in the familiar environment of his or her home for as long as possible, the client's safety and burden on the primary caregiver, usually the spouse, may become an issue. Eventually, clients may be referred to an extended care facility, many of which have a unit dedicated to the care of clients with Alzheimer's disease or other forms of dementia.

Current drugs approved for the treatment of dementia of the Alzheimer's type include cholinesterase inhibitors such as tacrine (Cognex), donepezil (Aricept), rivastigmine (Exelon), and galantamine hydrobromide (Razadyne) (Drug Therapy Table 72-1). These drugs increase acetylcholine by inhibiting cholinesterase, the enzyme that degrades it. When administered in the early to middle stages of Alzheimer's disease, some clients improve, some stay the same, some progress more slowly, and some fail to respond. All clients eventually get worse over time.

The newest drug, memantine (Namenda), has a different mechanism of action than the cholinesterase inhibitors. Memantine is a neuroprotective drug classified as an N-methyl-d-aspartate (NMDA) antagonist. By blocking NMDA receptors, the drug protects neurons from excessive stimulation by glutamate, an excitatory neurotransmitter responsible for neuronal death. Clients in advanced stages of Alzheimer's disease experienced less deterioration when taking memantine than others who were given a placebo.

Antidepressants or tranquilizers may help agitated or depressed clients. Valproic acid (Depakene, Depakote, Valproate), which is generally prescribed for seizure disorders,

DRUG THERAPY TABLE 72-1 Agents for Treating Alzheimer's Disease

Drug Category and Examples	Mechanism of Action	Side Effects	Nursing Considerations
Cholinesterase Inhibitors			
donepezil (Aricept)	Inhibits the breakdown of acetylcholine	Nausea, vomiting, diarrhea, bradycardia, possible exacerbations of asthma and chronic obstructive pulmonary disease, muscle cramps, loss of appetite	Tell client that frequent small meals may minimize gastrointestinal upset. Monitor heart rate, and report bradycardia (heart rate <60 beats per minute).
tacrine (Cognex)	Provides for increased levels of acetylcholine in the cortex by inhibiting cholinesterase, the enzyme that breaks down acetylcholine	Headache, fatigue, confusion, seizures, dizziness, nausea, vomiting, diarrhea, gastrointestinal upset, abdominal pain, loss of appetite, skin rashes, hepatotoxicity	Administer on an empty stomach on an around-the-clock schedule. Do not abruptly discontinue. Arrange for regular blood tests to determine aminotransferase levels. Inform client and family of side effects and to report any that occur. Tell client to exercise caution if performing tasks that require alertness.
galantamine hydrobromide (Razadyne)	Increases concentration of acetylcholine by blocking action of acetylcholinesterase	Nausea, vomiting, anorexia, diarrhea, weight loss	Tell client to take drug at morning and evening meals.
N-Methyl-D-Aspartate (NMDA) Antagonist			
memantine (Namenda)	Blocks NMDA receptors	Allergic reactions, dizziness, headache, confusion, constipation	Avoid with renal disease and alkaline urine. Give with full glass of water. Can be taken with or without food. Caution client about driving or performing hazardous activities.

bipolar disorder, and schizophrenia, may be effective. It is being studied to determine whether it may delay agitation and memory problems in those who are in the early stages of Alzheimer's disease (Qing et al., 2008).

An orally administered inhibitor of gamma-secretase, currently identified as LY450139 dihydrate, is in clinical trials. If effective, the gamma-secretase inhibitor may prevent the release of APP fragments, thus preventing the development of amyloid plaques (Alzheimer Research Forum, 2008). Other potential Alzheimer drug therapies target the prevention of neurofibrillary tangles caused by abnormal *tau* protein. The two drugs under study include AL-108, which is incorporated in a nasal spray, and methylthioninium chloride (MTC), both of which have been shown to improve memory (Kennedy & Leon, 2008).

An immunotherapeutic approach, which some refer to as a vaccine, is currently also in clinical trials (Medical News Today, 2008). This method involves the administration of six intravenous infusions containing bapineuzumab, a monoclonal antibody (see Chap. 18). It is expected that the antibodies will target, bind, and remove beta amyloid from the brain of humans with mild to moderate Alzheimer's disease just as successfully as they did in animal studies.

Ketasyn, a product referred to as a "medical food," may soon become available with a physician's prescription. A medical food is defined by the U.S. Food and Drug Administration (FDA) as a substance formulated to be consumed by or administered enterally to people with an impaired capacity to digest, absorb, or metabolize ordinary foods or certain nutrients. The hypothesis for its use is that there is a metabolic dysfunction in the brains of those with Alzheimer's disease that (1) interferes with the neurons' ability to utilize glucose for energy, (2) impairs the utilization of fat, (3) reduces the production of acetylcholine, and (4) interferes with the clearance of amyloid producing protein. When taken orally, Ketasyn is metabolized into ketones, which the brain can use as an alternative to glucose thus improving cognitive function (Levine, 2008).

Nursing Management

The major focus of nursing management is to help the client and caregiver maintain the highest possible quality of life by supporting mental and physical functions and ensuring safety. Most clients initially receive care in their homes, and home health nurses can instruct the family about physical care, the disease process, and treatment. They also provide emotional support and intervene if family caregivers become overburdened. As the disease progresses, the client's nutritional needs must be considered (Nutrition Notes 72-1). When it becomes necessary to transfer the client from the home to an extended care facility, the nurse meets the client's physical needs on a full-time basis and helps the family cope during the client's deterioration. See Nursing Care Plan 72-1 and Client and Family Teaching 72-1 for additional information.

Gerontologic Considerations

- Cognitive changes alter older adults' roles and relationships, impacting clients' self-worth and evoking fear of the

Nutrition Notes 72-1
The Client with Alzheimer's Disease

- Alzheimer's disease can devastate nutritional status. Forgetfulness, alterations in smell and taste, and decreasing ability to self-feed impair intake. Weight loss is common. Choking may occur if the client forgets to chew food thoroughly or hoards food in his or her mouth.
- Increased agitation significantly increases calorie requirements. Nutritionally dense foods that are easy to consume, such as finger foods and liquid supplements, help maximize intake. Minimize distractions at meals and offer one food at a time to avoid overwhelming the client.
- Clients in the later stages of Alzheimer's disease may be unable to swallow or may not know what to do when food is placed in their mouths. When such a situation occurs, a decision regarding nutritional support (e.g., percutaneous endoscopic gastrostomy tube feedings) must be made (see Chap 45).

progression of the disease. Older adults with few or no family members or significant others are at high risk for loss of identity. Photographs from younger years may help provide a sense of identity.

- Older adults often experience painful co-morbidities such as neuropathy or arthritis. Assessment for pain in the presence of cognitive decline requires careful observation of facial expressions and body positioning and collaboration with caregivers and significant others. Altered cognition does not negate the person's need for comfort.

SCHIZOPHRENIA

Schizophrenia is a thought disorder characterized by deterioration in mental functioning, disturbances in sensory perception, and changes in affect (emotion). Clients with schizophrenia improve with drug therapy but, unfortunately, never fully recover. Because the condition is lifelong and appears in young adulthood, it causes considerable anguish for families who must deal with both the burden of healthcare costs and the responsibility for caring for a loved one with this illness.

Pathophysiology and Etiology

Schizophrenia, historically attributed to emotional dysfunction, is now categorized as a psychobiologic disease because of recent findings in brain and neurotransmitter chemistry. Many neurotransmitter imbalances are involved in schizophrenia. Dopamine excess is believed to be the major cause of the symptoms, with imbalances of norepinephrine, serotonin (5-HT), and gamma-aminobutyric acid (GABA; see Chap. 67) also playing a role. The disease is known to have a familial or genetic component. Other theories suggest that the anatomic and physiologic changes associated with schizophrenia result from a viral infection experienced by the affected individual's mother during pregnancy. The

NURSING CARE PLAN 72-1 | The Client With Alzheimer's Disease

Assessment

- Interview both client and family because the client may be unable to give a complete or objective history regarding memory, sleep patterns, moods, and self-care activities. Assess the caregiver's strengths, limitations, and ability to manage caregiving activities.

- Perform a complete head-to-toe physical examination. Be especially attentive to muscular strength, balance, and gait.
- Determine the client's mental status. Identify level of orientation, short-term and long-term memory, social behavior, emotional status, cognitive and motor skills, and ability to perform ADLs.

Nursing Diagnosis: Caregiver Role Strain related to being overwhelmed by responsibilities, fatigue, and depression

Expected Outcome: Caregiver will experience less anxiety as knowledge about implementing plans that will provide needed relief increases.

Interventions	Rationales
Assess caregiver's strengths, limitations, and ability to manage caregiving activities.	The spouse (who is the usual caregiver) may experience sleep deprivation, physical injury, and social isolation if no one else is available to assist with client care.
Suggest scheduling **respite care,** brief relief from caregiving responsibilities, with family and friends on a regular rotating basis.	Dividing caregiving responsibilities promotes physical endurance and emotional stability.
Provide a list of agencies that offer social services such as the county's commission on aging and Social Security and Medicare agencies.	Clients may be unaware of services available for assistance or how to contact them.
Develop a list of people to contact in an emergency, including a 24-hour hotline for the home health nursing agency.	Having a plan helps clients obtain assistance in a crisis.
Recommend that caregiver and client take care of legal matters such as wills, transferring titles, and preparing an advanced directive (see Chap. 10).	Attending to legal matters before severe cognitive changes occur is best.
Suggest establishing **durable power of attorney,** designating who may make decisions regarding finances or healthcare when the client becomes **incompetent,** the legal term for the inability to understand the risks or benefits of decisions.	Such measures ensure that the client's spouse or caregiver has access to unencumbered funds and follows the client's wishes regarding healthcare decisions.
Advise caregiver to obtain **guardianship** or **conservatorship,** court-appointed responsibility, for managing the client's care and assets if the client already is incompetent.	The client's financial assets may be frozen unless the court stipulates that another person can have access to private accounts.
Encourage the caregiver to temporarily place the client in a long-term nursing facility to take a well-deserved vacation.	Giving the caregiver a temporary option for a vacation may help to sustain his or her ability to continue caring for the client.

Evaluation of Expected Outcomes

- Caregiver seeks relief from responsibilities at least 1 or 2 days a week.
- Caregiver and client take care of legal issues.

Nursing Diagnosis: Risk for Interrupted Family Processes related to guilt over placing the client in a care facility

Expected Outcome: Family will remain united and supportive over the decision to transfer the client's care to others.

Interventions	Rationales
Acknowledge and empathize with the family's ambivalent feelings.	Family is more likely to accept transfer of the client's care if the nurse demonstrates empathy.
Emphasize skills and services that the facility provides.	Knowledge that the facility offers many services to promote and maintain the client's well-being enhances acceptance of the decision.
Let the family participate in developing and revising the plan of care.	Family participation promotes a team approach to managing the client's care.
Keep the family informed of the client's progress or lack thereof.	Communication often is the key to good interpersonal relationships.
Encourage the family to visit and participate in the client's care as much as they want.	Promoting continued interactions conveys a sense that family is included rather than excluded from the client's life.

NURSING CARE PLAN 72-1 **The Client With Alzheimer's Disease** (Continued)

Interventions	Rationales
Allow the family privacy during interactions with the client, and make an area available to them for special occasions like birthdays.	Making special accommodations for family activities individualizes care.
Keep a current list of family phone numbers, listing the relationships of members to the client and indications for which they prefer to be called.	Accurate information is important when communication is necessary.
Prepare the family for the client's likely deterioration.	Realistic preparation for the progression of the disease promotes anticipatory grieving and acceptance of the client's potentially terminal condition.

Evaluation of Expected Outcomes

- Family members reconcile themselves to the difficult decision to transfer the care of the client to a nursing care facility.
- They remain involved in the client's care and understand the changes that accompany the disease process.

Nursing Diagnosis: Impaired Memory related to global cognitive deficits

Expected Outcome: Client will be reoriented and participate in life experiences to his or her potential.

Interventions	Rationales
Orient client frequently to person, place, and time.	Frequent reminders accommodate for impairment in memory.
Place a large-faced clock and calendars at multiple places in the client's environment.	External clues help the client maintain orientation or become oriented with minimal effort.
Assign consistent caregivers, and maintain a structured daily routine.	Repetition and consistency reduce episodes of confusion.
Attach something the client can recognize to the door of his or her room.	The client is more likely to find his or her room by looking for a familiar clue like his or her name printed in large letters or a brightly colored bow.
Make sure the client wears an identification bracelet with an address and telephone number.	Clients with Alzheimer's disease are known to wander and not recall their current residence.
Maintain a current photograph in the medical record.	Having the means to identify the client aids in search-and-rescue efforts.

Evaluation of Expected Outcome

Client becomes reoriented with techniques such as verbal reminders and environmental clues like a large-faced clock and calendar and can participate in activities that occur at consistent times throughout the day.

Nursing Diagnosis: Risk for Trauma related to ataxia and propensity for wandering

Expected Outcome: Client will move about freely and safely in the healthcare facility but will not leave the facility unsupervised.

Interventions	Rationales
Help the client don supportive walking shoes when out of bed.	Supportive shoes promote a stable gait and posture.
Provide assistance with ambulation. Remove hazards, such as foot stools, small tables, or liquid spills, from the ambulatory area.	Assistance reduces the potential for falls. Removing obstacles and slippery surfaces promotes safer ambulation.
Keep the environment well lighted.	The ability to see helps the client avoid environmental hazards.
Maintain the bed in low position.	Should a fall occur, the bed's low position reduces the potential for serious injury.
Use **restraint alternatives,** protective or adaptive devices for fall protection and postural support.	Physical restraints increase the potential for injury; clients have the right to the least restrictive intervention.
Place a bed monitor under the client's mattress.	Bed monitors alert caregivers when a client gets out of bed without signaling for assistance.
Install alarms on exit doors, and respond immediately when one sounds.	An alarm alerts caregivers when someone leaves who is unauthorized to do so.

Evaluation of Expected Outcomes

- No injuries occur.
- The client's whereabouts are known at all times.

(Continued)

NURSING CARE PLAN 72-1 **The Client With Alzheimer's Disease** (Continued)

Nursing Diagnosis: Disturbed Sleep Pattern related to confusion between day and night

Expected Outcome: Client will sleep uninterrupted for at least 6 hours or return to sleep after awakening during the night.

Interventions	Rationales
Keep client active during daytime hours, but avoid excessive fatigue.	Remaining awake during daytime hours helps enhance normal circadian rhythm.
Restrict consumption of coffee, tea, and cola.	Caffeine, a CNS stimulant, interferes with sleep.
Make sure that the room is comfortably warm or cool and that the client has urinated and satisfied his or her thirst just before bedtime.	Meeting basic comfort needs promotes sleep once the client retires for the night.
Dim the lights and reduce unnecessary noise.	A darkened environment increases production of melatonin, which promotes sleep; a quiet environment reduces stimulation of the cerebral cortex.
Provide a lighted clock at the bedside.	A clock provides an environmental clue as to whether it is time to sleep or awaken.
Redirect the client gently, but firmly, to return to bed if night-time wandering occurs.	Caregivers help reinforce appropriate behavior.

Evaluation of Expected Outcome

Client returns to bed after awakening and wandering and sleeps until an appropriate time for the day's activities.

Nursing Diagnosis: Impaired Verbal Communication related to expressive or receptive aphasia

Expected Outcome: Client will communicate with healthcare professional at whatever level is possible.

Interventions	Rationales
Approach from the front, make eye contact, and look for a response to your voice.	Obtaining the client's attention promotes verbal interaction.
Get the client's attention by using the name to which he or she is most likely to respond.	Using a client's name increases cognitive awareness and potential for social interaction.
Keep explanations or directions short and simple.	Being succinct makes it easier for the client to process information and respond appropriately.
Give gentle reminders or model the desired response.	Reminding and modeling compensate for failing memory or loss of language skills.
Involve client in one idea or task at a time.	Keeping ideas and tasks to a minimum promotes attention and concentration.
Reduce environmental stimuli like noise and activity.	Excess stimulation interferes with attention and concentration and may agitate the client.
Promote interactions that tap into the client's long-term memory such as reminiscing; offer client verbal cues such as, "1 understand you were . . . (a school teacher)."	Long-term memory is retained more than short-term memory; recalling information promotes social interaction and elevates self-esteem.
Give client plenty of time to respond to questions. Try to understand what client wants to convey.	Impaired language skills make communication more difficult.
Repeat information that you believe the client is trying to communicate.	Rephrasing or paraphrasing helps ensure accurate interpretation of the client's thoughts.
Include client in small group activities, even if there is little or no socialization.	Despite the appearance of being uninvolved, participation may stimulate the client's awareness.
Change activities or distract the client if he or she becomes angry, hostile, or uncooperative.	The nurse is responsible for ensuring the safety of the client, other clients, and staff.

Evaluation of Expected Outcome

Client understands spoken works and responds verbally.

neurochemical imbalance produces a variety of manifestations characterized by **delusions** (disturbed thinking), with themes that may include suspiciousness; persecution; being controlled; grandiosity (belief in one's importance); religious fixation; or preoccupation with sex, a love interest, illness, or a body part. **Hallucinations** (sensory experiences only the client perceives) that are usually auditory or visual may be experienced.

Client and Family Teaching 72–1
Caring for a Family Member with Dementia

The nurse emphasizes the following points when teaching the family and caregivers.

● Support, interact with, and cognitively stimulate the client.
● Minimize situations that contribute to the client's confusion and frustration such as noise and distractions from a television—even mirrors may unduly disturb the client.
● Allow the client to remain as independent as possible.
● Follow a consistent routine throughout each day.
● Do not leave the person with an advanced cognitive disorder alone; investigate the services of a day care facility for occasional respite.
● Park the car in a location where the client cannot see or gain access to it.
● Keep a means of identification on the client's person at all times in case of wandering.
● Install an on-off safety switch on the stove and oven.
● Store household chemicals in cupboards with safety latches.
● Lock up lighters, matches, and knives.
● Disable locks on bathroom doors.
● Use the services of a social worker.
● Access crisis telephone numbers if problems arise and coping skills are tested.
● Become involved with the local community mental health association.
● Join and attend meetings of a support group for caretakers of those who are cognitively impaired.

BOX 72-1 Positive and Negative Symptoms of Schizophrenia

Positive

• *Delusions,* false beliefs that cannot be changed by logical reasoning
• *Hallucinations,* sensory experiences that others do not perceive; can be auditory, visual, tactile, olfactory, or gustatory (involving taste)
• *Loose associations,* a sequence of ideas that are slightly connected
• *Inappropriate affect,* a display of emotional feeling inconsistent with the situation
• Peculiarities in speech like *echolalia,* repeating what others say; *rhyming; word salad,* using unrelated words in a sentence; or *neologisms,* inventing new words
• Bizarre behavior such as *stereotopy* (repetitive movement) and *echopraxia* (mimicking the movements of others)

Negative

• *Concrete thinking,* an inability to explain abstract ideas
• *Thought blocking,* an inability to recall information for a time
• *Symbolism,* attaching significance to an insignificant object or idea
• *Blunted* or *flat affect,* little or no display of feeling
• *Anhedonia,* inability to experience pleasure
• *Catatonia,* immobility
• *Posturing,* assuming statuesque positions
• *Autism,* social withdrawal
• Self-neglect of hygiene, eating, work, finances, and the like
• *Poverty of thought,* lacking any opinions or ideas

Assessment Findings

Symptoms usually begin during late adolescence to early adulthood. Clients manifest a range of symptoms categorized as positive or negative. **Positive symptoms** include delusions, hallucinations, and fluent but disorganized speech. **Negative symptoms**, sometimes called *defect symptoms,* are marked by impoverished speech and an inability to enjoy relationships or express emotions (Box 72-1). Positive symptoms are more easily managed (with drugs) than negative symptoms. Classic symptoms are inexplicable sensory experiences such as hearing voices or seeing apparitions of people who are not there. These occur in combination with peculiar patterns of speaking and odd motor behaviors. The client also tends to abandon relationships and interactions with others and loses motivation for working, going to school, or engaging in other goal-driven behaviors. Hygiene and appearance tend to lose their previous importance.

The diagnosis is made primarily on the symptomatology and by ruling out other possible causes. CT and PET scans, MRIs, and brain mapping (see Chap. 67) may show decreased brain size and activity, especially in the frontal and temporal lobes.

Medical Management

Clients with schizophrenia are referred to the care of psychiatrists. Once the client is in the mental health system, every effort is made to avoid institutionalization. The exception is when the client is dangerous to self or others. In general, community mental health services are selected that meet the client's needs for psychotherapy, drug administration, and social needs, such as housing, job assistance, and money management.

Antipsychotic drugs are the mainstay of treatment. These drugs, also called *major tranquilizers* or *neuroleptics,* belong to several different chemical families, but all block receptors for dopamine. Newer antipsychotic drugs block dopamine receptors and also are antagonists of serotonin. Some examples of older antipsychotic drugs are haloperidol (Haldol) and fluphenazine (Prolixin) as well as the more recent antipsychotics risperidone (Risperdal), clozapine (Clozaril), and olanzapine (Zyprexa). See Drug Therapy Table 72-2.

Risperidone, clozapine, and olanzapine, newer drugs called *atypical antipsychotics,* produce their effects with reduced incidence of **extrapyramidal symptoms** (EPS), movement disorders associated with traditional antipsychotics (Box 72-2). Clozapine, however, has the potential adverse effect of dangerously depressing bone marrow function, and clients who take clozapine must have a blood count weekly or biweekly. If the white blood cell count drops too low, the drug is discontinued to reduce the potential for infection. Anticholinergic drugs such as trihexyphenidyl

DRUG THERAPY TABLE 72-2 Agents to Treat Schizophrenia

Drug Category and Examples	Mechanism of Action	Side Effects	Nursing Considerations
Antipsychotics haloperidol (Haldol)	Blocks postsynaptic dopamine receptors	Drowsiness, pseudoparkinsonism, dystonia, akathisia, neuroleptic malignant syndrome, dysrhythmias, suppression of cough reflex, anaphylactoid reactions, anemia, dry mouth, constipation, urinary retention	Monitor older clients for dehydration and aspiration potential. Withdraw drug gradually. Tell client to avoid driving. Instruct client to drink fluids and report any side effects.
fluphenazine (Prolixin)	Blocks postsynaptic dopamine receptors	Drowsiness, extrapyramidal syndromes, dysrhythmias, suppression of cough reflex, dry mouth, constipation, urinary retention	Tell client to avoid alcohol. Do not mix oral concentrate with caffeine-containing beverages, teas, or apple juice. Monitor older clients for signs of dehydration. Tell client to drink plenty of fluids and to report any side effects.
risperidone (Risperdal)	Blocks dopamine and serotonin receptors in the brain	Insomnia, agitation, headache, anxiety, drowsiness, nausea, vomiting, constipation, tardive dyskinesia, neuroleptic malignant syndrome, seizures	Monitor client for seizures when initiating therapy or increasing dose. Increase dose gradually until therapeutic effect is achieved. Tell client not to stop taking drug abruptly or to make up missed doses, but to contact the healthcare provider. Instruct client not to take this drug during pregnancy and to report any side effects.
olanzapine (Zyprexa)	Blocks dopamine and serotonin receptors	Dizziness, drowsiness, headache, weight gain, orthostatic hypotension, extrapyramidal symptoms	Instruct clients in measures to offset orthostatic hypotension, such as rising slowly and doing ankle pumps before standing. Monitor for extrapyramidal symptoms. Initiate anticholinergic drugs to control EPS. Decrease, discontinue, or switch medications as directed.

(Artane) and benztropine (Cogentin) are given to prevent or relieve EPS. Antipsychotics sometimes are combined with anticonvulsant drugs such as clonazepam (Klonopin) and carbamazepine (Tegretol).

Noncompliance with drug therapy is the leading cause of the return of disease symptoms and the need for short-term hospitalization. For this reason, some nonhospitalized clients are given **depot injections**, intramuscular injections of antipsychotic drugs in an oil suspension that are gradually absorbed. These injections are repeated every 2 to 4 weeks.

Pharmacologic Considerations

- Monitor the client taking an antipsychotic drug for symptoms of neuroleptic malignant syndrome. Notify the primary healthcare provider immediately if a high fever,

increased confusion, dyspnea, tachycardia, hypertension, severe muscle stiffness, or loss of bladder control occurs.

- Advise clients to take all antipsychotic drugs as directed, to avoid double dosing if they miss a dose, and not to stop antipsychotic drugs abruptly.

Gerontologic Considerations

- Older adult clients require lower dosages of antipsychotic drugs. They also may experience comorbidities of psychosis, dementia, and depression, requiring careful examination of treatment efficacy for each.

- Haloperidol (Haldol) should be used only with extreme caution in older adults due to risk for dehydration, falls, and

BOX 72-2 **Extrapyramidal Side Effects (EPS)**

EPS associated with traditional antipsychotic drugs include the following movement disorders:
- *Akinesia* (pseudoparkinsonism): The client appears to have symptoms of Parkinson's disease (see Chap. 37) such as hand tremors, stooped posture, stiff shuffling gait.
- *Akathisia:* The client cannot sit or stand still.
- *Dystonia:* Sudden severe muscle spasm occurs, usually in the neck, tongue, or eyes.
- *Tardive dyskinesia:* The client makes involuntary muscle movements, usually in the face, such as tongue thrusting, continuous chewing, grimacing, lip smacking, blinking; irreversible once manifested.

cognitive changes. Report confusion, falls, lethargy, decreased thirst, weakness, and dry mucous membranes.

- Older adults are particularly susceptible to tardive dyskinesia because of the long-term administration of typical antipsychotics. Report symptoms immediately because the drug must be discontinued to prevent further dyskinesia.

Nursing Process for the Client With Schizophrenia

Assessment

When caring for clients in acute care or community mental health settings, perform a Mini-Mental Status Examination (see Chap. 67) during the initial contact and periodically thereafter to monitor for changes. Assess the client for positive and negative symptoms of schizophrenia, including delusions, bizarre speech patterns, hallucinations, agitation, stupor, and social withdrawal. Also assess the client's physical status, including hygiene and nutritional condition.

Diagnosis, Planning, and Interventions

▶ **Disturbed Thought Processes** related to brain changes as manifested by illogical beliefs

▶ **Expected Outcome:** The client's thoughts will be reality-based as evidenced by a decrease in or absence of delusions.

- Administer antipsychotic drugs as prescribed. *Antipsychotics block dopamine and/or serotonin receptors and usually reduce or relieve positive symptoms such as delusions.*
- Do not argue about the validity of the client's delusions or try to convince him or her otherwise, but indicate that you do not share the client's delusional belief. *Clients may become more fixated on their delusions, defensive, or hostile if others challenge their delusions. Stating that you do not share the client's belief prevents the client from assuming that the delusion is plausible.*
- Shift the client's focus to what is real in the "here and now" when he or she dwells on the delusion. *Redirecting the client's thoughts to present reality interrupts delusional thinking.*

- Direct and stay with the client in a quiet place when he or she becomes agitated. *Reduced stimuli help restore calm and prevent loss of control.*

▶ **Disturbed Sensory Perception** (Specify: Auditory, Visual, Olfactory, Tactile, Gustatory) related to brain changes as manifested by hallucinations

▶ **Expected Outcome:** The client will acknowledge that hallucinations are not real or will minimize their importance.

- Intervene when it appears that the client is experiencing a hallucination such as assuming a listening pose or laughing or talking when others are absent or uninvolved in interaction. *Hallucinations may frighten the client. The presence of another person helps the client cope.*
- State that you do not hear or see anyone, but acknowledge that the experience must seem real and frightening to the client. *Stating that you do not share the content of the hallucination helps the client understand that it is not real.*
- Stay with the client throughout the hallucination. *The presence of another trusted person relieves anxiety, facilitates coping, and protects the client from acting dangerously.*
- Avoid touching the client without warning. *Unexpected touching may cause the client to respond violently to what he or she perceives as a threat.*
- Call auditory hallucinations "the voices" rather than using a personal pronoun such as "they" or "them." *Personifying the voices suggests the words are coming from real people.*
- Ask the client to share the content of the hallucination. *Obtaining specific information about the hallucination helps to determine if the safety of the client or others is in jeopardy.*
- Distract the client from attending to the hallucination. *Distraction interrupts the perception of the hallucination, thereby reducing the accompanying emotional distress.*
- Teach the client the technique of **voice dismissal**, which refers to saying "stop" or "be gone." *Voice dismissal is a method the client can use to halt the hallucination.*

▶ **Self-Care Deficit** (Specify type: Bathing/Hygiene, Dressing/Grooming, Feeding, Toileting) related to lack of motivation, illogical fears, emotional withdrawal

▶ **Expected Outcome:** The client will independently perform ADLs.

- Explain where hygiene is performed and how to obtain soap, shampoo, and toothpaste. *Informing the client of the location and resources for bathing and hygiene promotes self-care.*
- Direct the client to care for himself or herself at an appropriate time. *Gentle direction facilitates cooperation.*
- Assist if the client cannot initiate or complete self-care. *The nurse implements a therapeutic use of self when a client is incapable of total self-care.*
- Praise any worthy accomplishments. *Praise is a form of positive reinforcement, which increases the possibility that the client will repeat the activity.*
- Monitor food and fluid intake and toileting patterns. *Data collection facilitates problem identification.*

- Provide nutritious snacks if the client eats insufficiently. *Eating nutritious foods promotes a stable weight and well-being.*

▶ **Impaired Social Interaction** related to autism as evidenced by absence from group meetings and reluctance to participate in group activities

▶ **Expected Outcome:** The client will interact independently with one person initially and more than one person as his or her comfort level improves and symptoms are managed.

- Accompany the client to group meetings and activities. *Support from a trusted other may help the client participate in situations that he or she perceives as threatening or causing social discomfort.*
- Sit by the client, but do not manipulate the client into participating. *The nurse's physical presence reduces anxiety. Pressure to participate may increase the client's anxiety.*
- Share time with the client after the group interaction, and use open-ended questions to explore his or her perception of the experience. *Private discussions promote the client's ability to process the group event and his or her comfort level.*
- Verbally compliment the client when deserved for speaking voluntarily with others or acting appropriately in a social situation. *Approval from someone the client respects empowers the client to make further efforts to interact with others.*
- Suggest ways the client can improve interactions with others. *The nurse acts as a mentor to help the client modify social skills.*

Evaluation of Expected Outcomes

Expected outcomes are that the client thinks rationally and realistically and reports fewer delusions and hallucinations. Communication is coherent and understandable. The client manages self-care, takes responsibility for other ADLs, socializes, and interacts in group activities. ●

▶ ***Stop, Think, and Respond Exercise 72-2***

Discuss appropriate nursing interventions when a client with schizophrenia expresses a delusional belief or experiences a hallucination.

CRITICAL THINKING EXERCISES

1. Discuss the similarities and differences between Alzheimer's disease and schizophrenia.

2. In what ways are the interventions for altered mentation different for a client with Alzheimer's disease and schizophrenia?

3. Which neurotransmitters are generally imbalanced in Alzheimer's disease and schizophrenia?

4. Why is the incidence of Alzheimer's disease continuing to rise?

NCLEX-STYLE REVIEW QUESTIONS

1. A client with dementia is admitted to the Alzheimer's unit in an extended-care facility. What pathology occurs in Alzheimer's disease that distinguishes it from other dementias?
1. Destruction of brain cells from hypoxia
2. Destruction of brain cells from a stroke
3. Neurofibrillary tangles and plaques in the brain
4. Superficial infection in the meninges of the brain

2. When a client with Alzheimer's disease is observed to wander about a facility, which nursing intervention is most appropriate for the client's safety?
1. Make sure the client is dressed appropriately for the environment
2. Keep the client confined to a nearby room in the facility
3. Attach an identity tag to the client with a phone number
4. Lock all the outside doors within the facility

3. What approach is best when managing the care of a client with dementia who insists on always carrying a purse?
1. Find out why the client feels the need for a purse
2. Inform the client that the purse may be lost
3. Ask the client where the purse can be stored
4. Ensure the client has the purse at all times

4. What is the best nursing action for preventing frustration and agitation when an older client with dementia asks about his or her mother, who is deceased?
1. Explain that the client's mother has been dead several years.
2. Tell the client that his or her mother will visit a little later.
3. Say "You miss your mother. What was she like?"
4. Ask when the client last saw his or her mother.

5. For what side effect should the nurse closely monitor clients with schizophrenia who are receiving clozapine (Clozaril)?
1. Signs of infection
2. Elevated blood pressure
3. Extrapyramidal symptoms
4. Hypoglycemia

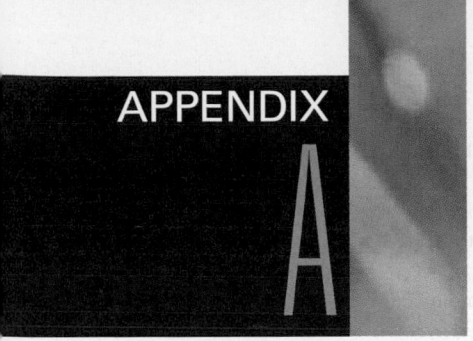

APPENDIX A

Nursing Resources

Unit 1: Nursing Roles and Responsibilities

Centers for Medicare and Medicaid Services
http://www.medicare.gov/publications
NANDA International
http://www.nanda.org/
National Council of State Boards of Nursing (NCSBN)
https://www.ncsbn.org

Unit 2: Client Care Concerns

CHAPTER 7: Nurse–Client Relationships

Alexander Graham Bell Association for the Deaf and Hard of Hearing
http://www.agbell.org
American Association of Managed Care Nurses, Inc.
http://aamcn.org
American Speech-Language-Hearing Association
http://www.asha.org/
Animated American Sign Language Dictionary
http://commtechlab.msu.edu/sites/aslweb/browser.htm
AT&T Language Line Services
http://www.languageline.com
Joint Commission
http://jointcommission.org
National Association of the Deaf
http://www.nad.org
National Council on Interpreting in Health Care
http://www.hospitals.unm.edu/ILS/Documents/NCIHC.pdf
National Institute on Deafness and Other Communication Disorders
http://www.nidcd.nih.gov
Nursing World
http://nursingworld.org/

CHAPTER 8: Cultural Care Considerations

Language Line Services
http://www.languageline.com/

CHAPTER 9: Complementary and Alternative Therapies

American Association of Acupuncture and Oriental Medicine
http://www.aaaomonline.org/
American Holistic Health Association
http://www.ahha.org
American Holistic Nurses Association
http://www.ahna.org
American Self-Help Clearinghouse
http://www.selfhelpgroups.org

Association for Applied Psychophysiology and Biofeedback
http://aapb.org
Association for Integrative Medicine
http://www.integrativemedicine.org
International Society for Holistic Health
http://www.internationalsocietyforholistic-health-care.htm
Johns Hopkins Center for Complementary and Alternative Medicine
http://www.hopkinsmedicine.org/cam/
Mayo Clinic, Alternative Medicine Center
http://www.mayoclinic.com/health/alternative-medicine/CM99999
National Cancer Institute, Complementary and Alternative Medicine
http://www.cancer.gov/cancertopics/factsheet/Therapy/CAM
National Center for Complementary and Alternative Medicine
http://nccam.nih.gov

CHAPTER 10: End-of-Life Care

American Hospice Foundation
http://www.americanhospice.org/

Unit 3: Foundations of Medical-Surgical Nursing

CHAPTER 11: Pain Management

American Academy of Pain Management
http://aapainmanage.org
American Chronic Pain Association
http://www.theacpa.org
American Pain Foundation
http://www.painfoundation.org
American Pain Society
http://ampainsoc.org
American Pharmacists Association, Pain Management Partnership
http://www.pharmacist.com/AM/Template.cfm?Section=Pain_Management_Partnership
American Society for Interventional Pain Physicians
http://asipp.org
American Society for Pain Management Nursing
http://www.aspmn.org
Holistic Nursing Institute
http://www.holisticnursinginstitute.org
Hospice and Palliative Nurses Association
http://www.hpna.org
International Association for the Study of Pain
http://www.iasp-pain.org
National Chronic Pain Outreach Association
http://neurosurgery.mgh.harvard.edu/ncpainoa.htm
Pain.com – A World of Information on Pain
http://www.pain.com

CHAPTER 12: Infection

Association for Professionals in Infection Control and Epidemiology
http://www.apic.org

Centers for Disease Control and Prevention
http://cdc.gov

Healthcare Infection Control Practices Advisory Committee
http://www.cdc.gov/ncidod/dhqp/hicpac.html

Hospital Infection Society
http://www.his.org.uk/

International Federation of Infection Control
http://www.theific.org

Joint Commission/Infection Control Initiatives
http://www.jointcommission.org/PatientSafety/Infection
Control

National Center for Environmental Health
http://www.cdc.gov.nceh/default.htm

National Committee for Quality Assurance
http://www.ncqa.org

National Patient Safety Foundation
http://www.npsf.org

Pan American Health Organization
http://www.paho.org

Society for Healthcare Epidemiology of America
http://www.shea-online.org

Surgical Infection Society
http://www.sisna.org

U.S. Food and Drug Administration
http://fda.gov

World Health Organization
http://who.int/

CHAPTER 13: Intravenous Therapy

Canadian Intravenous Nurses Society
http://www.cina.ca

Infusion Nurses Society
http://www.ins1.org

Infusion Therapy and Vascular Access Courses
http://www.hadawayassociates.com

International Sharps Injury Prevention Society
http://www.isips.org/cina.php

League of Intravenous Therapy Education
http://www.lite.org

LVN Intravenous Therapy Certification
http://www.avc.edu/academics/ccs/class%20descriptions/
LVN_Intravenous_Therapy_Certificate.htm

CHAPTER 14: Perioperative Care

American Academy of Ambulatory Care Nursing
http://www.aaacn.org

American Academy of Medical-Surgical Nurses
http://www.medsurgnurse.org

American Association of Nurse Anesthetists
http://www.aana.com

American College of Surgeons
http://www.facs.org/

American Operating Room Nurses
http://www.aorn.org

American Society of PeriAnesthesia Nurses
http://www.aspan.org

Association of Perioperative Registered Nurses, Inc.
http://www.aorn.org.

CHAPTER 15: Disaster Situations

Centers for Disease Control and Prevention. Abstract: Consensus statement: Smallpox as a biological weapon: Medical and public health management.
http://www.emergency.cdc.gov/agent/smallpox/
smallpoxconsensus.pdf

Centers for Disease Control and Prevention; Bioterrorism readiness plan: A template for healthcare facilities.
http://www.cdc.gov/ncidod/dhqp/pdf/bt/13apr99APIC-
CDCBioterrorism.PDF

Centers for Disease Control and Prevention, Emergency Preparedness & Response Site
http://www.bt.cdc.gov

Centers for Disease Control and Prevention. Emergency Preparedness & Response, Bioterrorism Agents/Diseases.
http://www.bt.cdc.gov/agent/agentlist.asp

Centers for Disease Control and Prevention. Facts about cyanide.
http://emergency.cdc.gov/agent/cyanide/basics/facts.asp

Centers for Disease Control and Prevention. Fact sheet, preparing for a terrorist bombing: A common sense approach.
http://www.bt.cdc.gov/masstrauma/pdf/preparingterrorist-
bombing.pdf

Centers for Disease Control and Prevention. Frequently asked questions about a nuclear blast.
http://www.bt.cdc.gov/radiation.nuclearfaq.asp

Centers for Disease Control and Prevention. Radiological Terrorism Emergency Management Pocket Guide for Clinicians
http://www.cal-pen.org/calpen/tool_kit_docs/
Print_Radiation_CDC_clinicianpocketguide.pdf

Terrorism and Other Public Health Emergencies
http://www.hhs.gov/disasters/press/newsroom/mediaguide/
HHSMediaReferenceGuideFinal.pdf

Unit 4: Caring for Clients with Multisystem Disorders

CHAPTER 16: Caring for Clients with Fluid, Electrolyte, and Acid–Base Imbalances

American Association for the Advancement of Science
http://www.aaas.org/

American Physiological Society
http://www.the-aps.org/

CHAPTER 17: Caring for Clients in Shock

American Academy of Emergency Medicine
http://www.aaem.org/

American Association of Critical Care Nurses
http://www.aacn.org/

American College of Emergency Physicians
http://www.acep.org/

American Trauma Society
http://www.amtrauma.org

Emergency Nurses Association
http://www.ena.org/

CHAPTER 18: Caring for Clients with Cancer

American Cancer Society
http://www.cancer.org

Unit 5: Caring for Clients With Respiratory Disorders

American Lung Association (ALA)
  http://www.lungusa.org.
American Sleep Apnea Association (ASAA)
  http://www.sleepapnea.org
Asthma and Allergy Foundation of America (AAFA)
  http://www.aafa.org.
CancerCare National Office
  http://www.lungcancer.org.
Cystic Fibrosis Foundation
  http://www.cff.org.
International Association of Laryngectomees (IAL)
  http://www.theial.com/ial/
Lung Cancer Alliance
  www.lungcanceralliance.org

Unit 6: Caring for Clients with Cardiovascular Disorders

Alliance of Cardiovascular Professionals
  http://www.acp-online.org/
American Association of Echocardiography
  http://asecho.org/
American College of Cardiovascular Nursing
  http://www.accn.net
American Heart Association
  http://www.americanheart.org/
Biorobotics Laboratory
  http://brl.ee.washington.edu/BRL/
Cardiac Arrest Survivor Network
  http://www.casn-network.com
Health Resources and Services Administration, Division of Transplantation
  http://www.hrsa.gov/OSP/dot/dotmain.htm
International Academy of Cardiology
  http://cardiologyonline.com/
International Society for Endovascular Specialists
  http://iscsonline.org/
National Heart, Lung, and Blood Institute
  http://www.nhlbi.nih.gov/index.htm
North American Society for Cardiac Imaging
  http://www.nasci.org/
Perivascular Nurse Consultants. Inc.
  http://www.pncnurse.com
Preventive Cardiovascular Nurses Association
  http://www.pcna.net/
Research Center for Stroke and Heart Disease
  http://www.stroke-heart.org/
Society for Cardiovascular Pathology
  http://scvp.net/
Society for Vascular Nursing
  http://www.svnnet.org/
Society for Geriatric Cardiology
  http://www.sgcard.org/
World Heart Federation
  http://www.worldheart.org/

Unit 7: Caring For Clients With Hematopoietic and Lymphatic Disorders

American Society of Hematology
  http://www.hematology.org/

Blood and Marrow Transplant Information Network
  http://www.bmtinfonet.org/
International Association of Sickle Cell Nurses and Physician Assistants
  http://www.emory.edu/PEDS/SICKLE/parnpage.htm
Joint Center for Sickle Cell and Thalassemic Disorders
  http://sickle.bwh.harvard.edu
Leukemia and Lymphoma Society, Inc.
  http://www.leukemia.org/
Leukemia Research Foundation
  http://leukemia-research.org/
Lymphoma Research Foundation
  http://www.lymphoma.org/
Management and Therapy for Sickle Cell Disease
  http://www.nhlbi.nih.gov/index.htm
National Hemophilia Foundation
  http://www.hemophilia.org/home.htm
National Lymphedema Network
  http://lymphnet.org/
National Marrow Donor Program
  http://www.marrow.org/
Sickle Cell Disease Association of America, Inc.
  http://www.sicklecelldisease.org/

Unit 8: Caring for Clients with Immune Disorders

AIDS Drug Assistance Programs (ADAP)
  http://www.critpath.org/docs/adap.htm
AIDS Treatment Data Network
  http://www.atdn.org/
AIDS Virus Education and Research Trust (AVERT)
  http://www.avert.org/
Allergic and Nonallergic Rhinitis
  http://www.njc.org/
American Academy of Allergy, Asthma, and Immunology
  http://www.aaaai.org/
American Association of Immunologists
  http://www.aai.org/
American Foundation for AIDS Research
  http://www.amFAR.org/
American Society for Histocompatibility and Immunogenetics
  http://www.ashi-hla.org/
Asthma and Allergy Foundation of America
  http://www.aafa.org/
The CFIDS (Chronic Fatigue Immune Dysfunction Syndrome) Association of America
  http://www.cfids.org/
Health and Human Services Minority HIV/AIDS Initiative
  http://www.omhrc.gov/OMH/AIDS/aidshome_new.htm
The National Chronic Fatigue Immune Dysfunction Foundation
  http://www.ncf-net.org/
National Institute of Allergy and Infectious Disease
  http://www.niaid.nih.gov
Project Inform (Information, Inspiration, and Advocacy for People Living with HIV/AIDS)
  http://www.projinf.org/

Unit 9: Caring For Clients With Neurologic Disorders

American Academy of Neurology and Orthopaedic Surgeons
  http://www.aan.com

American Academy of Neurology
http://www.aan.com
American Association of Neuroscience Nurses
http://aann.org/
American Association of Spinal Cord Injury Nurses
http://www.aascin.org
American Board of Electroencephalography and Neurophysiology
http://www.ecnsociety.com/ec_aben.htm
American Council for Headache Education
http://www.achenet.org/
American Spinal Injury Association
http://www.asia-spinalinjury.org/
American Stroke Association: A Division of the American Heart Association
http://www.strokeassociation.org/
Amyotrophic Lateral Sclerosis Association of America
http://www.alsa.org/
Association for Rehabilitation Nurses
http://www.rehabnurse.org/
Brain Aneurysm Foundation
http://neurosurgery.mgh.harvard.edu.baf
Brain Surgery Organization
http://brainsurgery.org/
Christopher Reeve Foundation
http://www.paralysis.org
Consortium for Spinal Cord Medicine
http://www.scicpg.org/
Epilepsy Foundation of America
http://www.efa.org/
Federation of Spine Associations
http://www.aaos.org/
Guillain-Barré Syndrome Foundation International
http://www.gbs.cidp.org/
Information Center for Individuals with Disabilities
http://www.disability.net
Intracranial Hypertension Research Foundation
http://www.IHRFoundation.org/
Multiple Sclerosis Foundation
http://www.msfacts.org/
Myasthenia Gravis Foundation of America
http://www.med.unc.edu/mgfa
National Aphasia Association
http://www.aphasia.org/
National Association of Rehabilitation Agencies
http://www.naranet.org/
National Headache Foundation
http://www.headaches.org/
National Institute of Neurological Disorders and Stroke
http://www.ninds.nih.gov/
National Multiple Sclerosis Society
http://www.nmss.org/
Organization for Understanding Cluster Headaches
http://www.clusterheadaches.org/
The National Parkinson Foundation, Inc.
http://www.parkinson.org/
National Rehabilitation Association
http://www.nationalrehab.org/
National Spinal Cord Association
http://www.spinalcord.org/
National Stroke Association
http://www.stroke.org/

Society for Neuroscience
http://www.sfn.org/

Unit 10: Caring for Clients With Sensory Disorders

Acoustic Neuroma Association
http://www.anausa.org.
American Academy of Ophthalmology
http://www.geteyesmart.org.
American Foundation for the Blind
http://www.afb.org.
American Speech-Language-Hearing Association (ASHA)
http://www.asha.org.
Association for Macular Diseases, Inc.
http://www.macular.org
Glaucoma Research Foundation
http://www.glaucoma.org
International Society of Refractive Surgery of the American Academy of Ophthalmology (ISRS/AAO)
http://www.aao.org/isrs
Macular Degeneration Foundation
http://www.eyesight.org
National Eye Institute
http://www.nei.nih.gov/health/
National Federation of the Blind (NFB)
http://www.nfb.org

Unit 11: Caring For Clients With Gastrointestinal Disorders

American Association of Enterostomal Therapists
http://www.wocncb.org/
American Gastroenterological Association
http://www.gastro.org/
American Liver Association
http://www.liverfoundation.org/
Colon Cancer Alliance
http://www. Ccalliance.org
Crohn's and Colitis Foundation of America
http://www.ccfa.org/
Hepatitis Foundation International
http://www.hepfi.org/
International Foundation for Functional Gastrointestinal Disorders
http://www.iffgd.org/
International Ostomy Association
http://www.ostomyinternational.org/
National Digestive Diseases Information Clearing House
http://www.niddk.nih.gov/health/digest/nddic.htm
United Ostomy Association
http://www.uoa.org/
Wound Ostomy and Continent Nurses Society
http://www.wocn.org/

Unit 12: Caring for Clients with Endocrine Disorders

American Association of Clinical Endocrinologists
http://www.aace.com/
American Association of Diabetes Educators
http://www.aadenet.org/

American Association of Endocrine Surgeons
http://www.endocrinesurgeons.org/
American Diabetes Association
http://www.diabetes.org/
American Foundation of Thyroid Patients
http://www.thyroidfoundation.org/
American Thyroid Association
http://www.thyroid.org/
Diabetes Action Research and Education Foundation
http://diabetesaction.org/
The Endocrine Society
http://www.endo-society.org/
The Insulin-Free World Federation
http://www.insulin-free.org/
Joslin Diabetes Center
http://www.joslin.harvard.edu
National Adrenal Diseases Foundation
http://medhelp.org/nadf/
National Diabetes Information Clearinghouse
http://www.niddk.nih.gov/health/digest/niddic.htm
National Institute of Diabetes and Digestive and Kidney Diseases
http://www.niddk.nih.gov/
Pituitary Network Association
http://www.pituitary.com/
Thyroid Foundation of America, Inc.
http://www.allthyroid.org/
The Thyroid Society
http://www.the-thyroid-society.org/
Women in Endocrinology
http://www.women-in-endo.org/

Unit 13: Caring for Clients with Breast and Reproductive Disorders

Adopt a Special Kid
http://www.adoptaspecialkid.org/
Adoption Service Information Agency, Inc.
http://www.asia-adopt.org/
Adopt World, Inc.
http://adoptionworld.org/
The Association for the Cure of Cancer of the Prostate
http://www.capcure.org/
Breast Implants Information
http://www.fda.gov/cdrh/breastimplants/index.html
The Education Center for Prostate Cancer Patients
http://www.ecpcp.org/
Endometriosis Association
http://endometriosisassn.org/
Hysterectomy Educational Resources & Services
http://www.ccon.com/hers/
National Council for Adoption
http://www.ncfa-usa.org/
Organization of Parenting Through Surrogacy
http://www.opts.com
RESOLVE: (National Infertility Support Group)
http://www.resolve.org/
Sex Information and Education Council of the United States (SIECUS)
http://www.siecus.org/
Us Too (Support group for prostate cancer)
http://www.ustoo.com/

Y-ME National Breast Cancer Organization
http://www.y-me.org/

Unit 14: Caring for Clients With Urinary and Renal Disorders

American Association of Kidney Patients
http://www.aakp.org
American Foundation for Urologic Disease
http://www.afud.org
American Urological Association
http://www.auanet.org
National Association for Continence
http://www.nafc.org
National Kidney Foundation
http://www.kidney.org

Unit 15: Caring for Clients With Musculoskeletal Disorders

American College of Rheumatology
http://www.rheumatology.org
Arthritis Foundation
http://www.arthritis.org.
Lupus Foundation of America, Inc.
http://www.lupus.org.
National Amputation Foundation
http://www.nationalamputation.org
National Association of Orthopaedic Nurses (NOAN)
http://www.orthonurse.org.
National Fibromyalgia Association
http://www.fmaware.org.
National Osteoporosis Foundation
http://www.nof.org
The American Fibromyalgia Syndrome Association (AFSA)
http://www.afsafund.org.
The Paget Foundation
http://www.pagct.org

Unit 16: Caring for Clients with Integumentary Disorders

American Academy of Cosmetic Surgery
http://www.cosmeticsurgery.org/
American Academy of Dermatology
http://www.aad.org/
American Association of Tissue Banks
http://www.aatb.org/
American Burn Association
http://www.ameriburn.org/
American Hair Loss Council
http://www.ahlc.org/
American Society for Dermatologic Surgery
http://www.asds-net.org/
American Society of Plastic Surgeons
http://www.plasticsurgery.org/
Burn Surgery Organization
http://burnsurgery.org/
Dermatology Nurses' Association
http://www.dnanurse.org

International Myeloma Foundation
  http://www.myeloma.org/
National Fire Protection Association
  http://www.nfpa.org/
National Institute of Arthritis and Musculoskeletal and Skin Diseases
  http://www. niams.nih.gov
National Pediculosis Association, Inc.
  http://www.headlice.org/
National Psoriasis Foundation
  http://www.psoriasis.org/

Unit 17: Caring for Clients with Psychobiologic Disorders

The Academy for Guided Imagery
  http://www.healthynet.agi/
Academy of Psychosomatic Medicine
  http://www.apm.org/
Action on Smoking and Health
  http://ash.org/
Administration on Aging
  http://www.aoa.dhhs.gov/
Al-Anon Family Group Headquarters, Inc.
  http://www.al-anon.alateen.org/
Alcoholics Anonymous
  http://www.alcoholics-anonymous.org/
Alliance for Aging Research
  http://www.agingresearch.org/
Alzheimer's Association
  http://www.alz.org/
Alzheimer's Disease Education and Referral Center
  http://www.alzheimers.org/
American Dietetic Association
  http://www.eatright.org/
American Psychiatric Association
  http://www.psych.org/
American Psychological Association
  http://www.apa.org/
American Psychosomatic Society
  http://www.psychosomatic.org/
Anxiety Disorders Association of America
  http://www.adaa.org/
Association for the Advancement of Behavior Therapy
  http://www.aabt.org/
Center for Food Safety and Applied Nutrition
  http://vm.cfsan.fda.gov/list.html
Center for the Study of Anorexia and Bulimia
  http://www.4woman.gov/nwhic/references/mdreferraks/csab.htm
Children of Aging Parents
  http://www.caps4caregivers.org/
Eldercare Locator
  http://www.eldercare.gov/

The Gerontological Society of America
  http://www.geron.org/
The Mind/Body Medical Institute
  http://www.mbmi.org/home/
Mothers Against Drunk Driving
  http://www.madd.org/
Narcotics Anonymous
  http://www.na.org/
National Aging Information Center
  http://aoa.dhhs.gov/naic/
National Alliance for the Mentally Ill
  http://www.nami.org/
National Anxiety Foundation
  http://lexington-on-line.com/naf.html
National Association for Anorexia and Associated Disorders
  http://www.anad.org/
National Association of Area Agencies on Aging
  http://www.n4a.org/
National Clearing House for Alcohol and Drug Information
  http://www.samhsa.gov/centers/clearinghouse/clearinghouses.html
National Council on Alcoholism and Drug Dependence
  http://www.ncadd.org/
National Depressive and Manic Depressive Association
  http://ndmda.org/
National Eating Disorders Association
  http://www.nationaleatingdisorders.org/
National Foundation for Depressive Illness
  http://www.depression.org/
National Institute of Mental Health
  http://www.nimh.nih.gov/
National Institute on Aging
  http://www.nia.nih.gov/
National Institute on Alcohol Abuse and Alcoholism
  http://www.niaaa.nih.gov/
National Institute on Drug Abuse
  http://www.nida.nih.gov/
National Mental Health Association
  http://ww.nmha.org/
National Mental Health Consumers' Self-Help Clearinghouse
  http://ww.mhselfhelp.org/
Organization for Human Brain Mapping
  http://www.humanbrainmapping.org/
Overeaters Anonymous
  http://www.overeatersanonymous.org/
Recovery, Inc.
  http://www.recovery-inc.com/
Schizophrenia.com
  http://www.schizophrenia.com
Society for Light Treatment and Biological Rhythms
  http://www.sltbr.org/

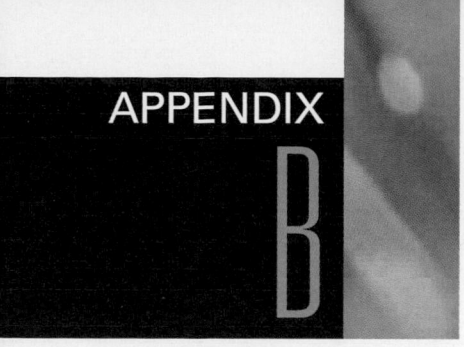

Commonly Used Abbreviations and Acronyms

3DCRT = Three-dimensional conformal radiation therapy
5-DHT = 5-alpha-reductase
5-HT = serotonin
AA = Alcoholics Anonymous
ABG = arterial blood gas
ACC = American College of Cardiology
ACE = angiotensin-converting enzyme
ACF = acute renal failure
ACLS = advanced cardiac life support
ACOA = Adult Children of Alcoholics
ACS = American Cancer Society
ACTH = adrenocorticotropic hormone
AD = Alzheimer's disease
ADH = antidiuretic hormone
ADC = AIDS dementia complex
ADLs = activities of daily living
AE = above the elbow
AED = automatic electrical defibrillator
AFP = alpha fetoprotein
AHA = American Heart Association
AI = adequate intake
AICD = automatic implanted cardiac defibrillator
AIDS = acquired immunodeficiency syndrome
AK = above the knee
ALL = acute lymphocytic leukemia
ALP = alkaline phosphatase
ALS = amyotrophic lateral sclerosis
ALT = alanine aminotransferase
AMA = American Medical Association
AMD = age-related macular degeneration
AML = acute myelogenous leukemia
ANA = American Nurses Association
ANA = antinuclear antibody
ANCAs = antineutrophil cytoplasmic antibodies
ANP = atrial natriuretic peptide
APACHE = Acute Physiology, Age, and Chronic Health
    Evaluation
APP = amyloid precursor protein
ARDS = acute respiratory distress syndrome
ARI = aldose reductase inhibitor
ARS = acute radiation syndrome
ASCAs = antisaccharomyces antibodies
ASHA = The American Speech-Language-Hearing Association
ASL = American sign language
ASO = antistreptolysin-O
AST = aspartate aminotransferase
ATN = acute tubular necrosis
ATP = adenosine triphosphate
AV = atrioventricular
BAL = blood alcohol level; British anti-lewisite

BCG = bacilli Calmette-Guérin
BE = below the elbow
BhCG = beta human chorionic gonadotropin
BK = below the knee
BMI = body mass index
BMR = basal metabolic rate
BP = blood pressure
BPH = benign prostatic hyperplasia
BRAT = bananas, rice, applesauce, toast
BRM = biologic response modifier
BSE = breast self-examination
BUN = blood urea nitrogen
CABG = coronary artery bypass graft
CAD = coronary artery disease
CAP = community-acquired pneumonia
CAPD = continuous ambulatory peritoneal dialysis
CAT = computed axial tomography
CBC = complete blood count
CCPD = continuous cyclic peritoneal dialysis
CDC = Centers for Disease Control and Prevention
CDCA = chenodeoxycholic acid
CEA = carcinoembryonic antigen
CF = cystic fibrosis
CFC = chlorofluorocarbon
CFS = chronic fatigue syndrome
CFTCR = cystic fibrosis transmembrane conductance regulator
CHF = congestive heart failure
CIC = clean intermittent catheterization
CIS = carcinoma in situ
CJD = Creutzfeldt-Jakob disease
CK = creatine kinase
CK-MB = creatine kinase isoenzyme MB
CLL = chronic lymphocytic leukemia
CMG = cystometrogram
CML = chronic myelogenous leukemia
CMV = cytomegalovirus
CNA = certified nurse's aide
CNS = central nervous system
CNV = choroidal neovascularization
CO = cardiac output
COPD = chronic obstructive pulmonary disease
CPAP = continuous positive airway pressure
CPM = continuous passive motion
CPR = cardiopulmonary resuscitation
CRF = chronic renal failure
CRH = corticotropin-releasing hormone
CRP = c-reactive protein
CRT = cardiac resynchronization therapy
CSF = cerebrospinal fluid; colony-stimulating factor
CST = cortisol suppression test

CT = computed tomography
CTZ = chemoreceptor trigger zone
CVA = cerebrovascular accident; costovertebral angle
CVP = central venous pressure
D and C = dilation and curettage
D_5W = 5% dextrose in water solution
DASH = Dietary Approaches to Stop Hypertension
DBS = deep brain stimulation
DCA = directional coronary atherectomy
DES = diethylstilbestrol
DEXA = dual-energy x-ray absorptiometry
DIC = disseminated intravascular coagulation
DJD = degenerative joint disease
DKA = diabetic ketoacidosis
DLE = discoid lupus erythematosus
DMARD = disease-modifying antirheumatic drugs
DMAST = Dyna Med Anti-Shock Trousers
DMSO = dimethyl sulfoxide
DNA = deoxyribonucleic acid
DNR = do not resuscitate
DPT = diphtheria, pertussis, tetanus
DRE = digital rectal examination
DRG = diagnosis-related group
DSM-IV-TR = *Diagnostic and Statistical Manual of Mental Disorders*, 4th edition, text revision
DSP = distal sensory polyneuropathy
DSRP = distal splenorenal shunt
DST = dexamethasone suppression test
DUIL = driving under the influence of liquor
DVT = deep vein thrombosis
DWI = driving while intoxicated
EBCT = electron beam computed tomography
ECF = eosinophil chemotactic factor
ECG = electrocardiogram
ECMO = extracorporeal membrane oxygenator
ECT = electroconvulsive therapy
ED = emergency department
EECP = enhanced external counterpulsation
EEG = electroencephalography
EGD = esophagogastroduodenoscopy
ELISA = enzyme-linked immunosorbent assay
EMG = electromyelogram
ENG = electronystagmography
EPA = eicosapentaenoic acid
EPS = extrapyramidal symptoms
ERCP = endoscopic retrograde cholangiopancreatography
ESR = erythrocyte sedimentation rate
ESRD = end-stage renal disease
ESWL = extracorporeal shock wave lithotripsy
EUG = excretory urogram
FAS = fetal alcohol syndrome
FDA = Food and Drug Administration
FEMA = Federal Emergency Management Agency
FES = functional electrical stimulation
FSH = follicle-stimulating hormone
FTA-ABS = fluorescent treponemal antibody absorption test
GABA = gamma aminobutyric acid
GAD = generalized anxiety disorder
GCS = Glasgow coma scale
GERD = gastroesophageal reflux disease
GH = growth hormone

GHB = gamma hydroxybutyrate
GI = gastrointestinal
GHRH = growth hormone-releasing hormone
GnRH = gonadotropin-releasing hormone
GVHD = graft-versus-host disease
GTT = glutamyltransferase
GVHD = graft-versus-host disease
HAAT = highly active antiretroviral therapy
HAMD = Hamilton Rating Scale for Depression
HAP = hospital-acquired pneumonia
HAV = hepatitis A virus
Hb = hemoglobin
HbA = hemoglobin A
HbF = fetal hemoglobin
HbS = hemoglobin S
HBV = hepatitis B virus
HCl = hydrochloric acid
Hct = hematocrit
HCV = hepatitis C virus
HDL = high-density lipoprotein
HDV = hepatitis D virus
HEV = hepatitis E virus
HHNKS = hyperosmolar hyperglycemic nonketotic syndrome
HiB = *Haemophilus influenzae* B
HIV = human immunodeficiency virus
HLA = human lymphocyte antigen
HMO = health maintenance organization
HPA = hypothalamus pituitary adrenal
HPI = history of present illness
HPV = human papilloma virus
HRT = hormone replacement therapy
HSV-1 = type-1 herpes simplex virus
HSV-2 = type-2 herpes simplex virus
IABP = intra-aortic balloon pump
IBD = inflammatory bowel disease
IBS = irritable bowel syndrome
IC = interstitial cystitis
ICD = integrated delivery system
ICF = intermediate care facility
ICP = intracranial pressure
ICSH = interstitial cell-stimulating hormone
IDDM = insulin-dependent diabetes mellitus
Ig = immunoglobulin
IGF-1 = insulin-like growth factor
IGFBP-3 = insulin-like growth factor binding protein-3
IL = interleukin
IICP = increased intracranial pressure
IL-2 = interleukin-2
IM = intramuscular
IMA = internal mammary artery
INR = international normalized ratio
IOL = intraocular lens
IOP = intraocular pressure
IORT = intraoperative radiation therapy
IPD = intermittent peritoneal dialysis
IPG = impedance plethysmography
IPV = inactivated poliomyelitis
IUG = intravenous urography
IV = intravenous
IVAC = implanted vascular access
IVP = intravenous pyelogram

IVU = intravenous urography

JCAHO = Joint Commission on Accreditation of Healthcare Organizations

KI = potassium iodide

KUB = kidney, ureter, bladder

LASIK = Laser-assisted in situ keratomileusis

LES = lower esophageal sphincter

LDH = lactate dehydrogenase

LDL = low-density lipoprotein

LEP = limited English proficiency

LH = luteinizing hormone

LMP = last menstrual period

LOC = level of consciousness

LPN = licensed practical nurse

LVEDP = left ventricular end diastolic pressure

LVN = licensed vocational nurse

MAB = monoclonal antibodies

MAOI = monoamine oxidase inhibitor

MAST = military anti-shock trousers

MCH = mean cell hemoglobin

MCHC = mean cell hemoglobin concentration

MCO = managed care organization

MCT = medium-chain triglycerides

MCV = mean cell volume

MDI = metered-dose inhaler

MH = malignant hyperthermia

MHC = major histocompatibility complex

MI = myocardial infarction

MIDCAB = minimally invasive direct coronary artery bypass

MMR = measles, mumps, rubella

MAb = monoclonal antibodies

MPHG = metabolite of norepinephrine

MRCP = magnetic resonance cholangiopancreatography

MRI = magnetic resonance imaging

MS = multiple sclerosis

MSG = monosodium glutamate

MTBE = methyl-*tert*-butyl ether

MUGA = multiple gated acquisition scan

NADH = nicotinamide adenine dinucleotide

NANDA = North American Nursing Diagnosis Association

NCCAM = National Center for Complementary and Alternative Medicine

NCI = National Cancer Institute

NCLEX-PN = National Licensing Examination for Practical Nurses

NCSBN = National Council of State Boards of Nursing

NFT = neurofibrillary tangle

NIDDM = non–insulin-dependent diabetes mellitus

NIH = National Institutes of Health

NK = natural killer (cell)

NMDA = *N*-methyl-D-aspartate

NMH = neurally mediated hypotension

NNRTI = non-nucleoside reverse transcriptase inhibitor

NPO = nothing by mouth

NRC = Nuclear Regulatory Commission

NRTI = nucleoside reverse transcriptase inhibitor

NS = normal saline

NSAID = nonsteroidal anti-inflammatory drug

OA = osteoarthritis

OAF = osteoclastic-activating factor

OCD = obsessive-compulsive disorder

OIA = optical immunoassay

OPCAB = off-pump coronary artery bypass

OR = operating room

ORIF = open reduction internal fixation

OSHA = Occupational Safety and Health Administration

OT = occupational therapist

PA = pulmonary artery

PAC = premature atrial contraction

PACAB = port access coronary artery bypass

$PaCO_2$ = partial pressure of carbon dioxide

PACU = postanesthesia care unit

PaO_2 = partial pressure of oxygen

PAP = pulmonary artery pressure

PASG = pneumatic anti-shock garment

PC = potential complication

PCA = patient-controlled analgesia

PCP = pneumocystis pneumonia

PCR = polymerase chain reaction

PCV = pneumococcal conjugate vaccine

PCWP = pulmonary capillary wedge pressure

PDP = prescription drug plan

PE = pulmonary embolus

PEEP = positive end-expiratory pressure

PEG = percutaneous endoscopic gastrostomy

PENS = percutaneous electrical nerve stimulation

PET = positron emission tomography

PIC = peripheral indwelling catheter

PICC = peripherally inserted central catheter

PID = pelvic inflammatory disease

PIP = proximal interphalangeal joint

PMI = point of maximum impulse

PMS = premenstrual syndrome

PNS = peripheral nervous system

PPD = purified protein derivative

PPO = preferred provider organization

PPS = prospective payment systems

PR = peripheral resistance

PRK = photorefractive keratectomy

PRN = prescribed on an as-needed basis

PSA = prostate-specific antigen

PT = physical therapist; prothrombin time

PTC = percutaneous transhepatic cholangiography

PTCA = percutaneous transluminal coronary angioplasty

PTCRA = percutaneous transluminal catheter rotational ablation

PTSD = post-traumatic stress disorder

PTT = partial thromboplastin time

PTU = propylthiouracil

PUD = peptic ulcer disease

PVC = premature ventricular contraction

QI = quality indicators

RA = rheumatoid arthritis

RAI = radioactive iodine

RAST = radioallergosorbent blood test

RBC = red blood cell

RDA = recommended dietary allowance

RF = rheumatoid factor

RK = radial keratotomy

RLQ = right lower quadrant

RN = registered nurse

RNA = ribonucleic acid

ROM = range of motion

RPR = rapid plasma reagent

RSV = respiratory syncytial virus
RT = reverse transcriptase
RUQ = right upper quadrant
SA = sinoatrial
SAD = seasonal affective disorder
SCLE = subacute cutaneous lupus erythematosus
SIADH = syndrome of inappropriate antidiuretic hormone
SIDS = sudden infant death syndrome
SIV = simian (monkey) immunodeficiency virus
SLE = systemic lupus erythematosus
SLIT = sublingual-swallow immunotherapy
SNF = skilled nursing facility
SNRI = selective norepinephrine reuptake inhibitor
SPECT = single-photon emission computed tomography
SPF = sun protection factor
SpO_2 = saturated oxygen
SIRS = systemic inflammatory response syndrome
SRS = stereotactic radiation therapy
SRS-A = slow-reactive substance of anaphylaxis
SSI = surgical site infection
SSNRI = selective serotonin norepinephrine reuptake inhibitor
SSRI = selective serotonin reuptake inhibitor
STD = sexually transmitted disease
STI = sexually transmitted infection
SVT = supraventricular tachycardia
T_3 = triiodothyronine
T_4 = tetraiodothyronine
TB = tuberculosis
TBSA = total body surface area
TCA = tricyclic antidepressant
TDD = telecommunication device for the deaf
TE = transluminal extraction
TEE = transesophageal echocardiography
TENS = transcutaneous electrical nerve stimulation
TEP = tracheoesophageal puncture

THBO = topical hyperbaric oxygen
THC = tetrahydrocannabinol
TIA = transient ischemic attack
TIPS = transjugular intrahepatic portosystemic shunt
TIQ = tetrahydroisoquinoline
TMD = temporomandibular disorder
TMJ = temporomandibular joint
TMR = transmyocardial revascularization
TMS = transcranial magnetic stimulation
TNF = tumor necrosis factor
TPA = tissue plasminogen activator
TPN = total parenteral nutrition
TRH = thyrotropin releasing hormone
TSE = transmissible spongiform encephalopathy
TSH = thyroid-stimulating hormone
TSS = toxic shock syndrome
TUIP = transurethral incision of the prostate
TULIP = transurethral laser incision of the prostate
TUR = transurethral resection
TURP = transurethral resection of the prostate
TZD = thiazolidinedione
UAP = unlicensed assistive personnel
UDCA = ursodeoxycholic acid
UES = upper esophageal sphincter
URI = upper respiratory infection
UTI = urinary tract infection
UNOS = The United Network for Organ Sharing
UV = ultraviolet
VAD = ventricular assist device
VCUG = voiding cystourethrogram
VDRL = Venereal Disease Research Laboratory
VNS = vagus nerve stimulation
WBC = white blood cell
WHO = World Health Organization
WOCN = wound, ostomy and continent nurses

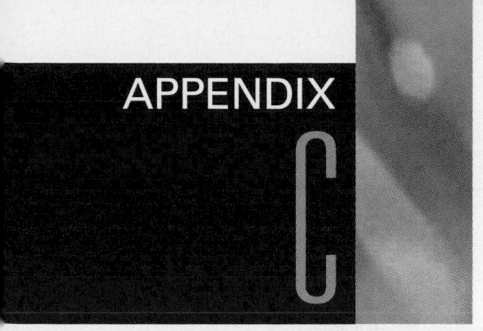

Laboratory Values

Laboratory values vary somewhat in different references. Laboratory technique also may alter values. The nurse is responsible for checking reported laboratory values against the normal ranges provided by the laboratory.

Abbreviations

cu	cubic
daL	decaliter (10 L)
dL	deciliter (100 mL)
g	gram
HPF	high powered field
L	liter
LPF	low-power field
mcg	microgram
mcL	microliter
mcm	micron (micrometer)
mcm^3	cubic micrometer
mEq	milliequivalent
mg	milligram
mL	milliliter
mm	millimeter
mm^3	cubic millimeter
mm Hg	millimeter of mercury
mmol	one-thousandth of a mole
mOsm	milliosmole
ng	nanogram (one billionth of a gram)
pg	picogram (one trillionth of a gram)
torr	measurement equivalent to 1 mm Hg

Symbols

> greater than
≥ greater than or equal to
< less than
≤ less than or equal to
/ per
± plus or minus

Coagulation Tests

	Values
Bleeding time (Ivy, Duke)	3–10 minutes
Partial thromboplastin time (PTT)	60–70 seconds
Activated partial thromboplastin time (APPT)	30–40 seconds
Prothrombin time (PT)	10–14 seconds or 70%–100% of control
International normalized ratio (INR)	Therapeutic range 2.0–3.0; high therapeutic range 3.0–4.5; over 4.5 critical

Hematology

	Values
Platelet count	150,000–350,000/mcL
Reticulocyte count	0.5%–2.5%
Sedimentation rate (ESR)	
Male	0–15 mm/hr

Hematology

	Values
Female	0–20 mm/hr
Complete blood count (CBC)	
Hematocrit	
Male	40%–54%
Female	37%–47%
Hemoglobin	
Male	13.5–17.5 g/dL
Female	12–16 g/dL
Red cell count	
Male	4.6–5.4 million/mcL
Female	3.6–5.0 million/mcL
White cell count	5,000–10,000/mcL
Neutrophils	60%–70% (3000–7000/mcL)
Eosinophils	1%–4% (50–400/mcL)
Basophils	0.5%–1% (23–100/mcL)
Lymphocytes	20%–40% (1000–4000/mcL)
Monocytes	2%–6% (100–600/mcL)
Erythrocyte indices	
Mean corpuscular volume (MCV)	$87–103 mcm^3$
Mean corpuscular hemoglobin (MCH)	26–34 pg/cell
Mean corpuscular hemoglobin concentration (MCHC)	31–37 g/dL

Blood Volume

Plasma volume	30–45 mL/kg
Red cell volume	20–35 mL/kg (higher in men than in women)
Total blood volume	55–80 mL/kg

Blood Chemistries

	Values
Alanine aminotransferase (ALT) (formerly SGPT)	10–35 units/L
Ammonia	14–45 mcg/dL
Amylase	50–150 units/L; 25–130 International Units/L by enzymatic method
Aspartate aminotransferase (AST) (formerly SGOT)	6–20 units/L
Bilirubin, total	0.2–1.0 mg/dL
Bilirubin, total direct (conjugated)	0.0–0.2 mg/dL
Bilirubin, indirect (unconjugated)	0.2–08. mg/dL
Anion gap (or R factor)	±12 mEq/L
Blood gases	
pH	7.35–7.45

Blood Chemistries	Values
$PaCO_2$	35–45 mm Hg
SaO_2	95% or higher arterial blood
PaO_2	80–100 mm Hg
HCO_3	22–26 mEq/L
Base excess (BE)	± 2 mEq/L
Blood urea nitrogen (BUN)	7–18 mg/dL
Calcium (total)	8.8–10 mg/dL
Calcium (ionized)	4.4–5.4 mg/dL
Carbon dioxide (CO_2 content)	23–30 mmol/L
Carcinoembryonic antigen (CEA)	up to 2.5 ng/mL
Cephalin flocculation	negative to 1+
Chloride	98–106 mmol/L
Cholesterol	desirable range ≤ 200 mg/dL
Coagulant factor assay	
Factor VIII	55%–145% of normal
Factor IX	60%–140% of normal
Creatine kinase (CK)	38–174 units/L
CK isoenzymes	
MM (muscle)	94%–100%
MB (heart)	0%–6%
BB (brain)	0%
Creatinine	0.6–1.2 mg/dL
Ferritin	15–300 ng/mL
Folic acid (Folate)	3–17 ng/mL
Glucose (fasting, serum)	70–110 mg/dL
Glucose (postprandial)	<120 mg/dL
High-density lipoprotein (HDL)	≥40 mg/dL
Insulin	6–24 micro-units/mL
Ketone bodies	negative
Lactic acid dehydrogenase (LD)	95–200 milliunits/mL (results vary)
LD isoenzymes	
LD-1	14%–26%
LD-2	29%–39%
LD-3	13%–26%
LD-4	8%–16%
LD-5	6%–16%
Lipase	10–180 units/L
Low-density lipoproteins (LDL)	desirable: <130 mg/dL
Magnesium	1.3–2.1 mEq/L
Phosphatase, acid	0–3.1 ng/mL
Phosphatase, alkaline	17–142 Units/L
Phosphate, inorganic phosphorus	2.7–4.5 mg/dL
Potassium	3.5–5.3 mEq/L
Proteins, total	6.0–8.0 g/dL
Albumin	3.8–5.0 g/dL
Globulin	2.3–3.5 g/dL
Prostate-specific antigen (PSA)	0–4.0 ng/mL
Sodium	135–145 mEq/L
T_3 (free triiodothyronine)	260–480 pg/dL
T_4 (free thyroxine)	0.8–2.4 ng/dL
Triglycerides	desirable: <150 mg/dL
Uric acid	3.5–7.2 mg/dL
Vitamin B_{12}	100–700 pg/mL
Vitamin B_{12} (unsaturated binding capacity)	743–1632 pg/mL

Urine	Values
Acetoacetic acid	negative
Acetone	negative
Albumin (quantitative)	negative
Aldosterone (24-hr specimen)	5–22 mcg/24 hr
Casts	rare/HPF
Color	pale yellow to dark amber

Urine	Values
Creatinine clearance	
Male	<0.8–1.8 g/24 hr
Female	<0.6–1.6 g/24 hr
Glucose	negative
Ketones	negative
Bilirubin	negative
17 hydroxycorticosteroid (as 17-ketogenic steroids or 17 KGS)	male: 3–10 mg/24 hr female: 2–6 mg/24 hr
17-ketosteroids	male: 5–24 mg/24 hr female: 5–15 mg/24 hr
Microscopic examination	RBC—0–1/HPF WBC—0–4/HPF casts—rare/HPF
pH	4.6–8.0
Protein	0–trace
Protein (24 hr)	25–150 mg/ 24 hr
Specific gravity	1.003–1.035
Turbidity	usually clear (cloudiness not always abnormal)
Volume	600–1600 mL/24 hr

Cerebrospinal Fluid	Values
Cell count	0–5 WBC/mL
Chloride	118–132 mEq/L
Color	clear, colorless
Glucose	40–70 mg/dL
Protein	15–45 mg/dL

Serology	Values
Antistreptolysin-O titer (ASLO)	<160 Todd units
Cold agglutinins	<1:16
C-reactive protein (CRP)	6.8–820 mcg/DL
Fluorescent treponemal antibodies (FTA)	negative
Hepatitis-associated antigen (HAA or HBAg)	negative
Heterophile antibody titers	<1.28
VDRL	nonreactive

Drugs	Values
Ethanol	0.08%–0.1% (50–100 mg/dL) under influence of alcohol
	0.1.%–0.15% (100–150 mg/dL) reaction time affected
	0.15%–0.25% (150–250 mg/dL) intoxication
	0.25%–0.3% (250–300 mg/dl) severe intoxication
	0.3%–0.4% (300–400 mg/dL) comatose
	0.4%–0.5% (400–500 mg/dL) fatal
Salicylates	5–30 mg/dL therapeutic range
	30–50 mg/dL mildly toxic range
	50–60 mg/dL severely toxic range
	>60 mg/dL lethal
Digitoxin	20–35 ng/mL therapeutic range
	>40 ng/mL toxic range
Digoxin	0.5–2.0 ng/mL therapeutic range
	>2.5 ng/mL toxic range
Lidocaine	1.5–6.0 mcg/mL therapeutic range
	>6 mg/mL toxic range

Tests for HIV/AIDS	Values
ELISA (enzyme-linked immunosorbent assay)	positive if antibodies to HIV present
Western blot (WB)	positive if antibodies to HIV present
P24 antigen	negative if noninfected with HIV or in early stage of infection
PCR (polymerase chain reaction)	negative if uninfected or performed earlier than 28 days following HIV infection; 95% accuracy after 28 days of infection

Tests for HIV/AIDS	Values
T-cell count	1500–4000 cells/mm^3 (normal)
T4 cells	450–1400 cells/mm^3 (normal)
T8 cells	190–725 cells/mm^3 (normal)
T4/T8 ratio	1.0–3.5 (normal)
HIV viral load (nucleic acid amplification test)	40–500 copies/mL (low viral load)
	5000–10,000 copies/mL (high viral load)

Glossary

A

Abdominoperineal resection surgical procedure involving wide excision of the rectum and the creation of a sigmoid colostomy.

ABO system method by which blood is identified as one of four blood types: A, B, AB, or O.

Acalculia neurologic impairment of a person's ability to perform calculations.

Accelerated hypertension markedly elevated blood pressure accompanied by hemorrhages and exudates in the eyes.

Acceptance fifth stage of Elisabeth Kübler-Ross' five stages of grief, in which a dying client accepts his or her fate and makes peace spiritually and with those with whom he or she is close.

Accommodation process in which the lens of the eye changes shape to view objects that are near or distant.

Accountability being answerable for the consequences of one's actions or inactions.

Acetylcholine neurotransmitter released at the nerve endings of parasympathetic nerve fibers, at some nerve endings in the sympathetic nervous system, and at nerve endings of skeletal muscles; also critical for memory and cognition.

Acetylcholinesterase enzyme that inactivates acetylcholine.

Acidosis excessive accumulation of acids or an excessive loss of bicarbonate in body fluids; can occur as a result of either metabolic or respiratory alterations.

Acids substances that release hydrogen.

Acne vulgaris inflammatory disorder that affects the sebaceous glands and hair follicles.

Acoustic neuroma benign Schwann cell tumor that progressively enlarges and adversely impacts cranial nerve VIII, which consists of the vestibular and cochlear nerves.

Acquired immunodeficiency syndrome (AIDS) infectious and eventually fatal syndrome that profoundly weakens the immune system and that is acquired from a pathogen known as the human immunodeficiency virus (HIV).

Acromegaly condition in which growth hormone is oversecreted after the epiphyses of the long bones have sealed.

Active transport use of energy to move chemicals from an area of low concentration to an area of higher concentration.

Actual diagnosis nursing diagnosis that identifies an existing problem. See also *possible diagnosis* and *risk diagnosis*.

Acuity the gravity and degree to which a person's medical condition changes.

Acupuncture technique of healing in which a needle is placed in one or more acupoints to restore the balance and free flow of energy within the body.

Acute bronchitis inflammation of the mucous membranes that line the major bronchi and their branches.

Acute chest syndrome type of pneumonia triggered by decreased hemoglobin and infiltrates within the lungs.

Acute coronary syndrome any group of clinical symptoms compatible with acute myocardial ischemia.

Acute heart failure sudden change in the heart's ability to contract.

Acute pain discomfort that has a short duration (from a few seconds to less than 6 months) and is associated with tissue trauma, including surgery, or some other recent identifiable etiology.

Acute radiation syndrome effect on those exposed to radiation, which may result in death in as little as 10 hours or may last up to 5 weeks.

Acute renal failure sudden and rapid decrease in the ability of nephrons within the kidneys to maintain fluid, electrolyte, and acid base balance, excrete nitrogen waste products, and perform regulatory functions such as maintaining calcification of bones and producing erythropoietin.

Acute retroviral syndrome syndrome that occurs in some cases of primary HIV infection that is often mistaken for "flu" or some other common illness.

Acute tubular necrosis death of cells within the collecting tubules of the nephrons, where reabsorption of water and electrolytes, and excretion of protein wastes and excess metabolic substances occur.

Addiction repetitive pattern of drug seeking and drug use to satisfy a craving for a drug's mind-altering or mood-altering effects.

Addisonian crisis life-threatening endocrine emergency when corticosteroid therapy is abruptly discontinued.

Adenohypophysis anterior lobe of the pituitary gland.

Adenoidectomy surgical removal of the adenoids.

Adenoiditis inflammation of the adenoids.

Adenoids lymphoid tissue located in the nasopharynx that protect the body from infection.

Adjuvant drugs medications that are co-administered when treating pain (e.g., improving analgesic effect without increasing dosage, controlling concurrent symptoms, moderating side effects).

Administrative law body of law that creates and enforces rules and regulations concerning the health, welfare, and safety of citizens.

Adrenal cortex outer portion of the adrenal glands; manufactures and secretes glucocorticoids, mineralocorticoids, and small amounts of sex hormones.

Adrenal glands glands located above the kidneys; the outer portion is the cortex, and the inner portion is the medulla.

Adrenal insufficiency decreased adrenal cortical function.

Adrenal medulla inner portion of the adrenal glands; secretes epinephrine and norepinephrine, two hormones released in response to stress or threat to life.

Adrenalectomy surgical removal of the adrenal gland(s), usually to remove a cancerous tumor.

Adrenocorticotropic hormone (ACTH) substance secreted by the pituitary that stimulates the adrenal glands to secrete corticosteroid hormones.

Advance directives documents in which a client states in advance his or her wishes regarding life-sustaining treatment and other medical care.

Advocacy (1) promoting the cause of another person or organization and (2) safeguarding of a client's rights and the supporting of his or her interests.

Affect verbal and nonverbal behavior that communicates feelings.

Affective learner person who processes information best when it appeals to his or her feelings, beliefs, and values.

Affective touch personal contact with a client that is used to communicate concern, caring, and support. See also *task-oriented touch*.

Afterload force that the ventricle must overcome to empty its diastolic volume.

Agnosia neurologic impairment of a person's ability to recognize objects and sounds.

Agoraphobia fear of experiencing a panic attack in a public place, which often leads to its victims permanently confining themselves to their homes.

Agranulocytes leukocytes that do not contain granules.

Agranulocytosis decreased production of granulocytes, including neutrophils, basophils, and eosinophils.

Agraphia neurologic impairment of a person's ability to write.

AIDS dementia complex neurologic condition that causes degeneration of the brain, especially in areas that affect mood, cognition, and motor functions.

AIDS drug assistance programs state based programs partially funded by Title II of the Ryan White CARE Act that help low- and middle-income clients obtain expensive AIDS medications.

Alcoholism chronic, progressive multisystem disease characterized by an inability to control the consumption of alcohol.

Aldosterone hormone that causes retention of sodium and water.

Alexia neurologic impairment of a person's ability to read.

Alkalosis excessive accumulation of base or a loss of acid in body fluids; can occur as a result of either metabolic or respiratory alterations.

Allergen antigen that can cause an allergic response.

Allergic disorder disorder characterized by a hyperimmune response to weak antigens that are usually harmless.

Allodynia exaggerated pain response due to increased sensitivity to stimuli such as air currents, pressure of clothing, vibration

Allograft skin graft that uses human skin obtained from a cadaver to temporarily cover large areas of tissue until the client's own skin can be used for skin grafting.

Alloimmunity immune response waged against transplanted organs and tissues that carry nonself antigens.

Alopecia condition that affects the hair follicles and results in partial or total hair loss.

Alpha fetoprotein serum protein normally produced during fetal development that is a marker indicating a primary malignant liver tumor.

Alternative medical systems healthcare techniques that evolved from non-Western cultures.

Alternative therapy treatment used instead of conventional medical treatment.

Alveolus (pl., alveoli) small, clustered sac that begins where the bronchioles end and is the location for the exchange of oxygen and CO_2.

Alzheimer's disease progressive, deteriorating brain disorder.

Ambulatory care also referred to as *outpatient care;* care delivered on an outpatient basis.

Ambulatory surgery surgery that requires fewer than 24 hours of hospitalization; sometimes referred to as same-day or outpatient surgery.

Amenorrhea absence of menstrual flow, usually caused by endocrine imbalances resulting from pituitary disorders or hypothyroidism, the stress response, or severely lean body mass.

Amyloid plaques clusters of amyloid protein fragments that stick together and damage neurons in the brain.

Amyloid precursor protein normal protein that resides partially inside and outside the cell membranes of neurons in the brain.

Anaerobic metabolism inefficient mechanism for meeting energy requirements used when the amount of oxygen reaching the cells decreases.

Analgesic substance that interferes with pain perception.

Anaphylactic shock severe allergic reaction that occurs after exposure to a substance to which a person is extremely sensitive.

Anaphylaxis rapid and profound allergic response characterized by shock, laryngeal edema, wheezing, stridor, tachycardia, and generalized itching.

Anasarca generalized edema caused by the shift of fluid from the intravascular space to interstitial and intracellular fluid locations.

Anastomosis surgical connection between two structures.

Androgogy principles of teaching adult learners.

Anecdotal record handwritten, personal account of an incident made at the time of occurrence and updated as needed; used to refresh a nurse's memory.

Anemia deficiency of either erythrocytes or hemoglobin.

Anergy inability to mount an immune response.

Anesthesia partial or complete loss of the sensation of pain with or without the loss of consciousness; may be general, regional, or local.

Anesthesiologist physician who has completed 2 years of residency in anesthesia and is responsible for administering anesthesia to a client and for monitoring a client during and after the surgical procedure.

Anesthetist person who administers anesthesia under the supervision of an anesthesiologist.

Aneurysm stretching and bulging of an arterial wall, usually caused by weakening of the vessel.

Anger second stage in Elisabeth Kübler-Ross' five stages of grief in which a client responds angrily to impending death and may displace this anger onto others, such as the physician, nurses, family, or God.

Angina pectoris chest pain of cardiac origin.

Angiocardiography diagnostic procedure in which a radiopaque dye is injected into a vein and its course through the heart is recorded by a series of radiographic pictures taken in rapid succession.

Angiogenesis regeneration of blood vessels.

Angioneurotic edema acute swelling of the face, neck, lips, larynx, hands, feet, genitals, and internal organs.

Anion gap difference between sodium and potassium cation (positive ion) concentrations and the sum of chloride and bicarbonate anions (negative ions) in the extracellular fluid.

Anions negative ions.

Ankylosing spondylitis chronic, connective tissue disorder of the spine and surrounding cartilaginous joints, such as the sacroiliac joints and soft tissues around the vertebrae.

Ankylosis joint immobility.

Annuloplasty surgical repair of the mitral valve leaflets and their fibrous ring.

Anorexia lack of appetite.

Anorexia nervosa eating disorder characterized by an obsession for thinness that is achieved through self-starvation.

Anthrax disease caused by a spore-forming bacterium known as *Bacillus anthracis.*

Antibodies chemical substances that destroy foreign agents such as microorganisms.

Anticipatory grieving grieving that occurs before death, often when the dying client and family begin to consider the impact of their potential loss.

Antidiuretic hormone (ADH) substance secreted by the pituitary in response to low blood volume that promotes reabsorption of water that the kidneys would ordinarily excrete.

Antigens protein markers on cells.

Antineoplastic type of drug used to treat cancer that works by interfering with cellular function and reproduction.

Antioxidants chemicals that block the chemical reactions that cause free radicals.

Anuria urine output of <100 mL of urine over 24 hours.

Anxiety vague uneasy feeling, the cause of which is not readily identifiable and which is evoked when a person anticipates non-specific danger.

Anxiety disorders group of psychobiologic illnesses that result from the activation of the autonomic nervous system, chiefly the sympathetic division.

Anxiolytics drugs that relieve the symptoms of anxiety; sometimes referred to as minor tranquilizers.

Aortic regurgitation backward flow of blood that occurs when the aortic valve does not close tightly.

Aortic stenosis narrowing of the aortic valve's opening when its cusps become stiff and rigid.

Aortic valve heart valve (opening) between the left ventricle and aorta that prevents blood from flowing back into the ventricle after the heart contracts.

Aortography diagnostic procedure that detects aortic abnormalities such as aneurysms and arterial occlusions by injecting contrast medium and taking radiographic films of the abdominal aorta and major arteries in the legs.

Aphasia neurologic impairment of a person's ability to speak.

Apheresis process of separating blood into its components.

Aphonia complete loss of voice.

Apitherapy medicinal use of bee venom.

Aplasia failure to develop.

Apocrine glands sweat glands found around the nipples, in the anogenital region, in the eyelids (Moll's glands), in the mammary glands of the breast, and in the external ear canals.

Apolipoproteins proteins on the surface of cholesterol molecules that bind to enzymes which direct cholesterol to sites for metabolism.

Appendectomy surgical removal of the appendix.

Appendicitis inflammation of a narrow, blind protrusion called the vermiform appendix located at the tip of the cecum in the right lower quadrant of the abdomen.

Appliance device worn over a stoma for the collection of feces or urine.

Apraxia inability to accomplish activities of daily living, such as grooming, toileting, and eating, despite intact motor function.

Arachnoid middle membrane lying directly below the dura that protects the brain.

Aromatherapy use of scents to alter emotions and biologic processes.

Arteries blood vessels that carry oxygenated blood.

Arteriography diagnostic procedure that involves instilling dye, referred to as contrast medium, into an artery.

Arterioles smallest oxygen carrying blood vessels.

Arteriosclerosis loss of elasticity or hardening of the arteries.

Arteriovenous fistula surgical anastomosis (connection) of an artery and vein lying in close proximity.

Arteriovenous graft type of vascular access method that uses a tube of synthetic material or polytetrafluoroethylene to connect a vein and artery in the upper or lower arm.

Arthritis general condition characterized by inflammation and degeneration of a joint.

Arthrocentesis aspiration of synovial fluid.

Arthrodesis fusion of a joint, most often the wrist or knee, for stabilization and pain relief.

Arthrogram radiographic examination of a joint, usually the knee or shoulder.

Arthroplasty surgical reconstruction of a joint, using an artificial joint that restores previously lost function and relieves pain.

Arthroscopy internal inspection of a joint by means of an instrument called an arthroscope.

Artificially acquired active immunity immunity that results from the administration of a killed or weakened microorganism or attenuated toxin.

Asbestosis fibrous inflammation or chronic induration of the lungs caused by the inhalation of asbestos.

Ascites collection of fluid in the peritoneal cavity.

Assessment step in the nursing process that involves the careful observation and evaluation of a client's health status.

Assisted living type of living arrangement that provides care to residents who require assistance with up to three activities of daily living but also maintains their privacy and dignity.

Asthma reversible obstructive disease of the lower airway characterized by inflammation of the airway and a hyper-responsiveness of the airway to internal or external stimuli.

Astigmatism visual distortion caused by an irregularly shaped cornea.

Asystole absence of heart contraction; cardiac arrest.

Ataxia neurologic impairment of a person's ability to walk.

Atelectasis disorder in which the alveoli collapse.

Atherectomy surgical removal of fatty plaque from arteries by inserting a cardiac catheter with a cutting tool at the tip or performing laser angioplasty.

Atheroma fatty mass within the arterial wall.

Atherosclerosis condition in which the lumen of the artery fills with fatty deposits, chiefly composed of cholesterol.

Atria upper chambers of the heart; *atrium* (singular).

Atrial fibrillation cardiac rhythm disorder in which several areas in the right atrium initiate disorganized, rapid impulses causing the atria to quiver rather than contract.

Atrial flutter cardiac rhythm disorder in which a single atrial impulse outside the sinoatrial node causes the atria to contract at an exceedingly rapid rate (200 to 400 times/min).

Atrioventricular valves openings between the atria and ventricles.

Audiometry precise measurement of hearing acuity.

Aura sensation, either of weakness, numbness or a hallucinatory odor or sound, that occurs immediately before a generalized tonic-clonic seizure.

Auscultation listening with a stethoscope for normal and abnormal sounds generated by organs and structures such as the heart, lungs, intestines, and major arteries.

Autoantibodies antibodies against self-antigens.

Autocratic leadership style of leadership characterized by strong control by the manager over a work group.

Autograft skin graft that uses a client's own skin, which is transplanted from one part of the body to another.

Autoimmune disorder disorder in which killer T cells and autoantibodies attack or destroy natural cells.

Autoinoculation self-transmission of an infection to another area of the body.

Autologous blood self-donated blood.

Automatic implanted cardiac defibrillator internal electrical device used to restore a life-sustaining cardiac rhythm.

Automaticity ability of heart tissue to initiate electrical stimulus independently.

Automatisms inappropriate, automatic, repetitive movements such as lip smacking and picking at clothing or objects.

Autonomic dysreflexia exaggerated sympathetic nervous system response resulting from a spinal cord injury above T6. Characteristics include severe hypertension, slow heart rate, pounding headache, nausea, blurred vision, flushed skin, sweating, goosebumps, nasal stuffiness, and anxiety.

Autoregulation ability of the brain to provide sufficient arterial blood flow despite rising intracranial pressure.

Avascular necrosis death of bone from an insufficient blood supply.

Aversion therapy technique that deters a behavior by causing unpleasant physical reactions when the behavior occurs.

Avulsion fracture severe traumatic sprain in which a chip of bone to which a ligament is attached becomes detached.

Axon nerve fiber that projects and conducts impulses away from the neuron's cell body.

Ayurvedic medicine system of medicine with roots in India whose object is to help individuals become unified with nature to develop a strong body, clear mind, and tranquil spirit.

Azotemia accumulation of nitrogen waste products in the blood, evidenced by elevated BUN, serum creatinine, and uric acid levels.

B

Bacteremia condition resulting from microorganisms escaping the lymph nodes and reaching the bloodstream, which may lead to sepsis.

Balloon tamponade tube that is inserted through the esophagus into the stomach, then inflated to compress esophageal varices and control hemorrhage.

Balloon valvuloplasty invasive, nonsurgical procedure to enlarge a narrowed heart valve using a deflated balloon that is threaded through a peripheral blood vessel into the stenotic valve, then inflated to stretch the opening.

Bargaining third stage in Elisabeth Kübler-Ross' five stages of grief in which a client attempts to negotiate a delay in dying with God or some higher power, usually until after a particularly significant event.

Barium enema radiographic study used to identify polyps, tumors, inflammation, strictures, and other abnormalities of the colon after instilling barium solution rectally.

Barium swallow fluoroscopic observation of a client swallowing a flavored barium solution and its progress down the esophagus to detect structural abnormalities of the esophagus as well as swallowing discoordination and oral aspiration.

Baroreceptors stretch receptors in the aortic arch and carotid sinus that signal the brain to release ADH when blood volume decreases, systolic blood pressure falls, or the right atrium is underfilled, and to suppress ADH when blood volume increases, systolic blood pressure rises, or the right atrium is overfilled.

Bases chemical substances that bind with hydrogen.

Basophils granulocytes that are active in allergic contact dermatitis and some delayed hypersensitivity reactions.

Battle's sign bruising of the mastoid process behind the ear.

Behavioral therapy type of psychotherapy that attempts to extinguish undesirable responses through the learning of other adaptive techniques.

Benign type of tumor that is not invasive or spreading.

Benign prostatic hyperplasia condition in which the prostate gland contains more than the usual number of normal cells.

Beta amyloid starchy component that accumulates in the brains of clients with Alzheimer's disease and injures neurons in the area of the brain responsible for producing acetylcholine, the neurotransmitter that is critical for memory and cognition.

Bicarbonate-carbonic acid buffer system regulates plasma pH by adding hydrogen ions to increase acidity and removing them to promote alkalinity.

Bicuspid valve opening between the left atrium and left ventricle; also known as the *mitral valve.*

Bigeminy cardiac rhythm pattern in which every other heart beat is a premature ventricular contraction.

Biliary colic upper abdominal pain that may radiate to the back and shoulders.

Binge eating disorder inability to control overeating.

Biocultural ecology examines biologic cultural differences.

Biofeedback technique in which an individual voluntarily controls one or more physiologic functions such as body temperature, heart rate, blood pressure, and brain waves.

Biologic disaster an event in which pathogens or their toxins cause harm to many humans and other living species.

Biologically based practices (therapies) use of natural products to treat illness. Examples include botanicals, animal-derived extracts, vitamins, minerals, fatty acids, amino acids, and proteins.

Bipolar disorder disorder characterized by cycling between depression, euthymia, and mania.

Blackouts periods of amnesia involving events and activities while consuming alcohol.

Blistering agents (or vesicants) chemicals that damage exposed skin and mucous membranes on contact.

Blood dyscrasias abnormalities in the numbers and types of blood cells.

Blood products components extracted from blood and administered to clients who need specific blood substances but not all the fluid and cellular components in whole blood.

Blood urea nitrogen protein breakdown product; deterioration in renal function is manifested by a rise in its values.

Board of nursing state organization governing the nursing profession responsible for protecting the public, reviewing and approving nursing education programs in the state, forming criteria for granting licensure, overseeing procedures for licensure examinations, issuing or transferring licenses, and implementing disciplinary procedures.

Boarding homes small homes with individual rooms where residents pay for room and board and minimal nursing services.

Body mass index mathematical computation based on height and weight to evaluate a person's size in relation to norms within the adult population.

Body piercing act of inserting a metal ring or barbell, which is a straight or curved rod, into the lips, ear cartilage, cheeks, nose, tongue, eyebrows, navel, nipples, or genital area.

Bone scan study that uses the intravenous injection of a radionuclide to detect the uptake of the radioactive substance by the bone.

Botulism disease that develops from the neurotoxin produced by *Clostridium botulinum,* an anaerobic bacillus.

Bouchard's nodes bony enlargement of the proximal interphalangeal joints.

Braces supports made of plastic materials, canvas, leather, or metal that are custom fit to each client, provide controlled movement, and prevent additional injury.

Brachytherapy direct internal application of a high dose of radiation within a sealed source on or within a tumor.

Bradydysrhythmia slow abnormal cardiac rhythm.

Bradykinesia slowness in performing spontaneous movements.

Brain mapping technique that compares a client's brain activity patterns (from an EEG or other electronic image) with a computerized database of electrophysiologic abnormalities.

Brain stem part of the central nervous system consisting of the midbrain, pons, and medulla oblongata.

Breakthrough pain acute pain that occasionally develops in those who have chronic pain.

Breast abscess localized collection of pus within breast tissue.

Breast cancer mass of abnormal cells in the breast.

Breast reconstruction surgical procedure in which the area of a mastectomy is refashioned to simulate the contour of a breast and optionally to create a nipple and areola.

Breast self-examination technique for examining one's own breasts for lumps and suspicious changes.

Bronchiectasis chronic obstructive pulmonary disease characterized by chronic infection and irreversible dilation of the bronchi and bronchioles.

Bronchioles smaller subdivisions of bronchi.

Bronchus (pl., bronchi) one of the two main branches of the trachea.

Brudzinski's sign assessment finding in which flexion of the neck produces flexion of the knees and hips.

Bruit purring or blowing sound caused by blood flowing over the rough surface of one or both carotid arteries.

B-type natriuretic peptide (BNP) cardioprotective neurohormone that functions to decrease blood pressure by increasing excretion of sodium and water, promoting arterial dilation, and counteracting renin, angiotensin, and aldosterone.

Bulimia nervosa eating disorder characterized by food binges of a large number of calories followed by measures to prevent weight gain.

Bulimarexia eating disorder characterized by periods of food restriction and periods of binging followed by purging.

Bursa small sac filled with synovial fluid that reduces friction between tendon and bone and between tendon and ligament.

Bursitis inflammation of the bursa, a fluid-filled sac that cushions bone ends to enhance a gliding movement.

C

Calcification process in which inorganic minerals, such as calcium salts, are deposited in body tissues.

Calcitonin hormone that inhibits the release of calcium from bone into the extracellular fluid.

Calciuria excessive calcium in the urine.

Calculus precipitate of mineral salts that ordinarily remain dissolved in urine.

Callus healing mass that forms after a bone is fractured, which holds the ends of the bone together but cannot endure strain.

Caloric stimulation test test that assesses the vestibular reflexes of the inner ear that control balance.

Cancellous bone bony tissue that is light and contains many spaces.

Cancer disease characterized by abnormal, disorganized cell proliferation.

Candidiasis yeast infection caused by the *Candida albicans* microorganism that may develop in the oral, pharyngeal, esophageal, or vaginal cavities or within folds of the skin.

Capillaries blood vessels that connect arterioles to venules.

Capitation type of financial management of an insurance plan that pays a preset fee per member per month to a healthcare provider, usually a hospital or hospital system, that covers all medical costs incurred and is paid regardless of whether the member requires healthcare services.

Capsid double layer of lipid material that surrounds the genetically incomplete HIV.

Caput medusae dilation of the veins over the abdomen.

Carbuncle deep skin and subcutaneous abscess from which pus drains.

Carcinogenesis process of malignant transformation and altering of the genetic structure of DNA within the cells.

Carcinogens factors or agents that contribute to the development of cancer.

Carcinoma in situ localized malignancy that, if untreated, will subsequently invade other areas.

Cardiac catheterization diagnostic test performed in an operative setting during which a catheter is inserted from a peripheral blood vessel in the groin, arm, or neck into one of the great vessels and then into the heart.

Cardiac cycle contraction (systole) and relaxation (diastole) of both atria and both ventricles.

Cardiac index calculation that reflects the cardiac output in relation to a particular client's body size.

Cardiac output volume of blood ejected from the left ventricle per minute.

Cardiac rehabilitation program following a cardiac event that combines exercise and educational activities to speed recovery and reduce or prevent recurring episodes.

Cardiac resynchronization therapy technique that restores synchrony in the contractions of the right and left ventricles using a biventricular pacemaker.

Cardiac tamponade acute compression of the heart.

Cardiogenic shock shock that occurs when contraction of the heart is ineffective and cardiac output is reduced.

Cardiomyopathy chronic condition characterized by structural changes in the heart muscle.

Cardiomyoplasty surgical procedure in which a client's own chest muscle is grafted to the aorta and wrapped around the heart to augment ineffective myocardial muscle contraction.

Cardioplegia intentional stopping of the heart for a surgical procedure.

Cardiopulmonary bypass technique in which blood is mechanically circulated and oxygenated outside the body.

Caregiver person who performs health-related activities that a sick person cannot perform independently.

Carina lower part of the trachea.

Carpal tunnel syndrome term for a group of symptoms located in the wrist where the median nerve passes through a narrow, inelastic canal formed by the carpal bones.

Carpopedal spasm involuntary contraction of hand muscles.

Carrier human or animal that harbors an infectious microorganism but does not show active evidence of the disease.

Cartilage firm, dense connective tissue whose primary functions are to reduce friction between articular surfaces, absorb shocks, and reduce stress on joint surfaces.

Case management system of healthcare delivery in which a case manager plans and coordinates a client's progress through the various phases of care to avoid delays, unnecessary diagnostic testing, and overuse of expensive resources.

Case method historically early system of nursing care in which one nurse provided all the services that a particular client required, accompanying the client to the hospital, providing care in the home, and performing many household duties as well.

Cast rigid mold that immobilizes an injured structure while it heals.

Casts deposits of minerals that break loose from the walls of renal tubules.

Cataract disorder in which the lens of the eye becomes opaque.

Catecholamines neurotransmitters that stimulate responses by the sympathetic nervous system.

Cation positive charged electrolyte.

Cauda equina small sections of spinal nerves that begin after the end of the spinal cord between the first and second lumbar vertebrae.

Cell-mediated response process that occurs when T cells survey proteins in the body, actively analyze the surface features, and respond to those that differ from the host by directly attacking the invading antigen.

Central nervous system part of the nervous system consisting of the brain and spinal cord.

Central nervous system depressants chemical agents that slow brain and physiologic activity.

Central nervous system stimulants chemical agents that accelerate physical and mental functions.

Central venous infusions infusions that deliver solutions into a large central vein, such as the vena cava.

Central venous pressure pressure produced by venous blood in the right atrium.

Central vision ability to discriminate letters, words, and the details of any image.

Cephalalgia aching in the head.

Cerebellum part of the brain located behind and below the cerebrum that controls and coordinates muscle movement.

Cerebral hematoma bleeding within the skull that forms an expanding lesion.

Cerebral infarction death of brain tissue.

Cerebrovascular accident prolonged interruption in the flow of blood through one of the arteries supplying the brain.

Cerebrum part of the brain consisting of two hemispheres connected by the corpus callosum.

Certified interpreter person who is certified by a professional organization through rigorous testing based on appropriate and consistent criteria

Cervicitis inflammation of the cervix.

Chancre painless ulcer that accompanies first-stage syphilis.

Chancroid sexually transmitted infection caused by the *Haemophilus ducreyi* bacillus and characterized by the appearance of a macule, followed by vesicle-pustule formation and, finally, a painful ulcer.

Charcot's joints neuropathic joint disease, a common finding in tertiary syphilis.

Chemical cardioversion use of drugs to eliminate a dysrhythmia.

Chemical dependence condition of needing to take a drug to avoid withdrawal symptoms.

Chemical disaster result of a release of toxic man-made substances with a potential for causing mass casualties.

Chemonucleolysis procedure in which the enzyme chymopapain is injected into the nucleus pulposus to shrink or dissolve a ruptured intervertebral disk and relieve pressure on spinal nerve roots.

Chemoreceptors structures that are sensitive to the pH, CO_2, and oxygen in the blood and regulate sympathetic nervous system stimulation or inhibition.

Chemotaxis process of attracting migratory cells to a particular area within the body.

Chemotherapy technique that uses antineoplastic (anti-cancer) agents to treat cancer cells locally and systemically.

Cheyne-Stokes respirations pattern of respiration in which shallow, rapid breathing is followed by a period of apnea.

Chief complaint that which the client perceives to be the health problem that needs treatment.

Chinese medicine medical system developed in China and other Asian countries that views health as the balancing of opposite forces and views illness as a consequence of imbalance.

Chiropractic technique of performing spinal manipulation as a generic method for curing neuromuscular disorders and a host of other diseases.

Chlamydia sexually transmitted infection caused by a bacterium, *Chlamydia trachomatis,* which lives inside the cells it infects; the disease is spread by sexual intercourse or genital contact without penetration and is the most common and fastest spreading bacterial STI in the United States.

Chlorine liquid respiratory toxin that becomes a gas when released into the atmosphere.

Cholangiography test used to determine the patency of the ducts from the liver and gallbladder using a dye that is usually instilled intravenously.

Cholecystitis inflammation or infection of the gallbladder.

Cholecystography test used to identify the presence of stones in the gallbladder or common bile duct and tumors or other obstructions, by observing the ability of the gallbladder to concentrate and store an iodine-based, radiopaque contrast medium.

Choledocholithiasis disorder in which gallstones are located within the common bile duct.

Cholelithiasis disorder in which stones are formed in the gallbladder.

Cholestasis ineffective bile drainage.

Cholesterol fatty (lipid) substance.

Choreiform movements uncontrollable writhing and twisting of the body.

Chronic bronchitis prolonged (or extended) inflammation of the bronchi, accompanied by a chronic cough and excessive production of mucus for at least 3 months each year for two consecutive years.

Chronic fatigue syndrome complex of symptoms primarily characterized by profound lack of energy with no identifiable cause that worsens with physical activity and does not improve with rest.

Chronic heart failure disorder in which the heart's ability to pump effectively is compromised for an extended period of time.

Chronic obstructive pulmonary disease broad, nonspecific term that describes a group of pulmonary disorders with symptoms of chronic cough and expectoration, dyspnea, and impaired expiratory airflow.

Chronic pain discomfort that lasts longer than 6 months.

Chronic renal failure progressive and irreversible decrease in the ability of nephrons within the kidneys to maintain fluid, electrolyte, and acid-base balance, excrete nitrogen waste products, and perform regulatory functions such as maintaining calcification of bones and producing erythropoietin.

Chvostek's sign assessment finding in which a client's mouth twitches and jaw tightens following the tapping of the facial nerve.

Cilia hair-like processes whose action moves substances like mucus to prevent irritation to and contamination of the lower airway.

Circulatory overload fluid volume that exceeds what is normal for the intravascular space and has the potential to compromise cardiopulmonary function if it remains unresolved.

Cirrhosis degenerative liver disorder caused by generalized cellular damage.

Civil law body of law that is concerned with disputes between individual citizens and that protects each individual's personal freedoms and property rights.

Client term used for the recipient of healthcare services that emphasizes the recipient's personal responsibility for health and active partnership in healthcare.

Client database collection of information from the client's medical and nursing history, physical examination, and diagnostic studies.

Clinical breast examination inspection of the breast in which an examiner notes breast size and symmetry and any unusual changes in the skin of the breasts and nipples and palpates the breasts and axillae for masses, lymph nodes, tenderness, and other abnormalities.

Clinical pathways guidelines that standardize important aspects of care such as diagnostic work-ups, nursing care, education, physical therapy, and discharge planning for specific diagnoses or procedures.

Closed head injury injury to the head in which an intact layer of scalp covers the fractured skull.

Closed method burn wound management technique in which the wound is covered. The closed method involves the use of one or more types of dressing materials.

Closed questions questions asked during a client interview that require only "yes" or "no" answers. See also *open-ended questions*.

Closed reduction procedure in which a fractured bone is restored to its normal position by external manipulation, then immobilized with a bandage, cast, or traction.

Coagulopathies bleeding disorders that involve platelets or clotting factors.

Cochlear implant device that is surgically placed in the inner ear and connected to a receiver in the bone behind the ear to improve hearing.

Codons points on HIV genes where mutations occur.

Cognitive functions abilities of a person involving knowledge, understanding, and perception.

Cognitive learner person who processes information best by listening to or reading facts and descriptions.

Cognitive therapy type of psychotherapy in which a therapist helps a client by altering his or her interpretation of events.

Colectomy partial or complete surgical removal of the colon.

Colic acute spasmotic pain.

Collaboration use of a team effort to achieve client care outcomes.

Collaborative problems complications with a physiologic origin that nurses manage using physician-prescribed and nursing-prescribed interventions.

Collaborator person who works with others to achieve a common goal.

Collateral circulation circulation formed by smaller blood vessels branching off from or near larger occluded vessels.

Colloid solutions solutions containing water and molecules of suspended substances such as blood cells and blood products (e.g., albumin).

Colonoscopy procedure in which an endoscope is used to visually examine the inner surface of the colon.

Colony stimulating factors cytokines that regulate the production, maturation, and function of blood cells.

Colostomy surgically created opening between the colon and the skin.

Comedone skin condition commonly called a blackhead; formed when sebum, keratin, and bacteria accumulate and dilate a hair follicle.

Comfort zone that area of a client's personal space which, when intruded, does not create anxiety.

Commissures area where the cusps of a cardiac valve contact each other.

Commissurotomy surgical procedure in which adhesions are opened in the cardiac valve cusps.

Common law system of laws that uses earlier court decisions, judgments, and decrees as precedents for interpretation of laws; also known as judicial law.

Community-acquired infections diseases that are transmitted from one infected person or reservoir to another, such as TB and meningitis.

Compartment syndrome symptoms such as severe pain that develop when a tendon or nerve is compressed within a confined space.

Compensation acceleration of regulatory processes in the lungs and kidneys when an imbalance in acids or bases occurs.

Compensation stage first stage of shock, during which several physiologic mechanisms attempt to stabilize the spiraling consequences of shock.

Complement system immune process in which many different proteins are activated in a chain reaction when an antibody binds with an antigen.

Complementary therapy treatment used in addition to conventional medical treatment.

Complex decongestive physiotherapy activity that includes (1) distal to proximal massage of edematous areas to facilitate lymphatic drainage into collateral vessels; (2) application of compression dressings to relieve edema by reducing the excess volume of fluid in the interstitial space; (3) active exercise to promote lymphatic circulation and maintain functional use of the limb; and (4) care and maintenance of skin and nails vulnerable to secondary complications.

Compulsion anxiety-relieving ritual.

Compulsive overeating disorder characterized by eating when not hungry or regardless of feeling full.

Concept mapping method that links important ideas about the care a client requires and provides a means for students and nurses to consider all the client's problems and develop a plan to treat them.

Concussion injury resulting from a blow to the head that jars the brain and results in diffuse and microscopic injury to it.

Conduction system neural tissue that sustains the electrical activity of the heart.

Conductive hearing loss hearing loss that is due to interference in the transmission of sound waves to the inner ear.

Conductivity ability of cardiac tissue to transmit an electrical stimulus from cell to cell within the heart.

Condylomas sexually transmitted genital warts which are usually painless and appear as a single lesion or cluster of soft, fleshy growths on the genitalia or cervix, within the vagina, or on the perineum, anus, throat, or mouth.

Congestive heart failure accumulation of blood and fluid within organs and tissues as a result of ineffective heart contraction.

Congregate housing residential center made up of free-standing apartments, private rooms, or both, that provides independent to minimal assistance for seniors or disabled adults.

Conization surgical removal of a large cone-shaped section of cervical uterine tissue.

Conjunctivitis inflammation of the conjunctiva.

Conservatorship responsibility for managing a client's care and assets appointed by a court when the client is incompetent.

Constitutional law fundamental freedoms and rights granted by the Constitution to all citizens of the United States.

Continent ileostomy (Kock pouch) creation of an internal reservoir for the storage of GI effluent.

Contractility ability of cardiac tissue to stretch as a single unit and recoil.

Contrecoup injury result of trauma to the head from force that is strong enough to send the brain ricocheting to the opposite side of the skull, resulting in dual bruising.

Contusion (1) soft tissue injury resulting from a blow or blunt trauma; (2) injury to the head that leads to gross structural injury to the brain and results in bruising and, sometimes, hemorrhage of superficial cerebral tissue.

Conventional (allopathic) medicine practices that embody traditional Western treatment of diseases

Convulsion seizure characterized by spasmodic contractions of muscles.

Coping mechanisms unconscious tactics people use to protect themselves from feeling inadequate or threatened.

Cor pulmonale disorder in which pulmonary disease causes the right ventricle to enlarge or fail.

Corneal transplantation replacement of abnormal corneal tissue with healthy donated corneal tissue.

Corneal trephine surgical procedure in which a small hole is produced at the junction of the cornea and sclera to provide an outlet for aqueous fluid.

Coronary arteries blood vessels that supply oxygenated blood to cardiac muscle.

Coronary artery bypass graft surgical procedure that improves myocardial oxygenation by bypassing or detouring around the occluded portion of one or more coronary arteries with a relocated blood vessel from a healthy leg vein or chest artery.

Coronary artery disease arteriosclerotic and atherosclerotic changes in the coronary arteries supplying the myocardium.

Coronary occlusion obstruction of a coronary artery that reduces or totally interrupts blood supply to the distal muscle area.

Coronary ostia openings to the coronary arteries; *ostium* (singular).

Coronary stent small, metal coil with mesh-like openings placed within the coronary artery during PTCA that prevents the coronary artery from collapsing.

Coronary thrombosis blood clot within a coronary artery.

Corpus callosum band of white fibers that acts as a bridge for transmitting impulses between the left and right hemispheres of the brain.

Cortical bone bony tissue that is dense and hard.

Corticosteroid hormones chemicals secreted by the adrenal cortex.

Corticosteroids collective term for the glucocorticoids, mineralocorticoids, and small amounts of sex hormones manufactured and secreted by the adrenal cortex.

Coryza rhinitis or the common cold.

Costovertebral angle area where the lower ribs meet the vertebrae.

Coup injury trauma to the brain caused when the head is struck directly

Couplets two premature ventricular contractions in a row.

Craniectomy surgical procedure in which a portion of a cranial bone is removed.

Cranioplasty surgical procedure in which a defect in a cranial bone is repaired using a metal or plastic plate or wire mesh.

Craniotomy surgical procedure in which the skull is opened to gain access to structures beneath the cranial bones.

Creatinine substance that results from the breakdown of phosphocreatine (amino acid waste product), which is present in muscle tissue, is filtered by the glomeruli, and is excreted at a fairly constant rate by the kidney.

Creatinine clearance test study used to determine kidney function and creatinine excretion.

Credé's maneuver technique in which the client bends at the waist or presses inward and downward over the bladder to increase abdominal pressure and facilitate emptying the bladder.

Criminal law body of law concerned with offenses that violate the public's welfare.

Critical thinking intentional, contemplative, outcome-directed thinking.

Crohn's disease chronic inflammatory bowel condition that can occur in any portion of the GI tract but predominantly affects the terminal portion of the ileum.

Cross-tolerance reduced pharmacologic effect when taking sedative-hypnotic drugs developed by alcoholics.

Cryptorchidism condition in which one or both testes fails to descend into the scrotum.

Crystalloid solutions solutions that consist of water and uniformly dissolved crystals such as salt (sodium chloride), other electrolytes, and sugar (glucose, dextrose).

Cultural competence (1) an understanding both of the nurse's own worldview as well as the client's worldview; (2) process in which a nurse consistently tries to work within the cultural context of the client and his or her family and community.

Cultural history information obtained during a client interview about the client's religious affiliation, cultural background, and health beliefs.

Culture (1) person's way of perceiving, behaving, and evaluating the world that includes his or her knowledge, beliefs, art, morals, laws, and customs; (2) a test used to identify bacteria within a specimen taken from a person with symptoms of an infection.

Cushing's syndrome endocrine disorder that results from excessive secretion of hormones by the adrenal cortex.

Cushing's triad three signs associated with an increase in intracranial pressure: pulse increases initially but then decreases, systolic BP rises, and pulse pressure widens.

Cushingoid syndrome physical changes that accompany excess endogenous production of steroid hormones or long-term corticosteroid therapy.

Cutaneous triggering technique in which the client lightly massages or taps the skin above the pubic area to stimulate relaxation of the urinary sphincter.

Cyanide a solid salt or volatile liquid chemical that can cause death in minutes.

Cystectomy surgical removal of the bladder.

Cystic fibrosis multisystem disorder affecting infants, children, and young adults that results from a defective autosomal recessive gene; the genetic mutation causes dysfunction of the exocrine glands, involving the mucus-secreting and eccrine sweat glands.

Cystitis inflammation of the urinary bladder.

Cystocele bulging of the bladder into the vagina.

Cystogram study that evaluates abnormalities in bladder structure and filling through the instillation of contrast dye and radiography.

Cystometrogram study that evaluates bladder tone and capacity using a retention catheter that is inserted into the bladder after the client voids and slowly filled with sterile saline until the client indicates at what point the first urge to void is felt and when the bladder feels full.

Cystoscope instrument consisting of a lighted tube with a telescopic lens used to examine the inside of the bladder.

Cystoscopy visual examination of the inside of the bladder using an instrument called a cystoscope.

Cystostomy surgical procedure in which a catheter is inserted through the abdominal wall directly into the bladder.

Cytokines immunologic chemical messengers released by lymphocytes, monocytes, and macrophages.

Cytotoxic T cells lymphocytes that bind to invading cells and destroy them by altering their cellular membrane and intracellular environment and releasing chemicals called lymphokines.

D

Deaf inability to hear well enough to process information.

Debridement natural, mechanical, enzymatic, or surgical removal of necrotic tissue.

Decerebrate posturing position in which the extremities are stiff and rigid following neurologic trauma; also called decerebrate rigidity.

Decibel unit for measuring the intensity of sound.

Decompensation stage stage in shock that occurs as compensatory mechanisms fail and the client's condition spirals downward into cellular hypoxia, coagulation defects, and cardiovascular changes.

Decorticate posturing position in which the arms are flexed, the fists clenched, and the legs extended following neurologic trauma; also called decorticate rigidity.

Decortication surgical removal of the pericardium to allow more adequate filling and contraction of the heart chambers.

Deep brain stimulation invasive procedure used to help manage the tremor cause by Parkinsonism and other neurologic conditions; also used to alter brain circuitry to relieve depression.

Deep vein thrombosis inflammation of a vein deep in the lower extremities accompanied by clot or thrombus formation.

Defibrillation emergency procedure that uses electrical energy to stop a life-threatening ventricular dysrhythmia.

Degenerative joint disease type of arthritis that is characterized by a slow and steady progression of destructive changes in weight-bearing joints and those that are repeatedly used for work.

Dehiscence separation of surgical wound edges without the protrusion of organs.

Dehydration significant reduction of body fluid in both extracellular and intracellular compartments.

Delegation transferring to a competent individual the authority to perform a selected task in a selected situation while retaining accountability for the delegation.

Delegator person who assigns a task to someone.

Delirium sudden, transient state of confusion.

Delusions fixed false beliefs that cannot be changed by logical reasoning and are often persecutory in nature.

Demand (or synchronous) mode pacemaker pacemaker that self-activates when a client's heart rate falls below a certain level.

Dementia gradual, irreversible loss of intellectual abilities.

Democratic leadership style of leadership characterized by participation in decision-making by a work group.

Demyelinating disease disorder that causes permanent degeneration and destruction of myelin.

Dendrites threadlike projections or fibers on a neuron that conduct impulses to its cell body.

Denial psychological defense mechanism in which a client refuses to believe certain information; the first stage in Elisabeth Kübler-Ross' five stages of grief.

Deontology theory of ethics that proposes that the rightness of an action is determined entirely by whether or not it follows from an ethical duty.

Dependent edema accumulation of fluid in the body areas most affected by gravity (the feet, ankles, sacrum, or buttocks).

Depolarization stage in electrophysiology when positive ions move inside the myocardial cell membranes, and the negative ions move outside.

Depot injections deep intramuscular injections of drugs in an oil suspension that are gradually absorbed over 2 to 4 weeks.

Depression the fourth stage in Elisabeth Kübler-Ross' five stages of grief in which a client realizes the reality of impending death and mourns potential losses such as separation from loved ones, the inability to fulfill future goals, or loss of control.

Dermabrasion method of removing surface layers of scarred skin using sandpaper, a rotating wire brush, chemicals, or a diamond wheel.

Dermatitis general term that refers to an inflammation of the skin.

Dermatome skin area supplied by a nerve.

Dermatophytes parasitic fungi that invade the skin, scalp, and nails.

Dermatophytoses superficial fungal infections.

Dermis layer of skin that lies below the epidermis.

Desensitization (1) form of immunotherapy in which a client receives weekly or twice weekly injections of dilute but increasingly higher concentrations of an allergen; (2) technique for overcoming anxiety by gradually exposing a person to whatever it is that provokes his or her anxiety.

Detoxification process of stabilizing a client with a sedative drug while alcohol is metabolized from his or her system.

Deviated septum irregularity in the septum that results in nasal obstruction.

Dexamethasone (cortisol) suppression test blood test that theoretically detects major depression.

Diabetes insipidus endocrine disorder that develops when antidiuretic hormone from the posterior pituitary gland is insufficient.

Diabetes mellitus endocrine disorder of the pancreas that affects carbohydrate, fat, and protein metabolism.

Diabetic ketoacidosis type of metabolic acidosis that occurs when there is an acute insulin deficiency or an inability to use whatever insulin the pancreas secretes.

Diabetic nephropathy progressive decrease in renal function that occurs with diabetes mellitus.

Diabetic retinopathy pathologic changes in the retina experienced by persons with diabetes.

Diagnosis-related group (DRG) classification of diagnoses that is used for medical reimbursement.

Dialysate solution used during dialysis that has a composition similar to normal human plasma.

Dialysis procedure for cleaning and filtering the blood that substitutes for kidney function when the kidneys cannot remove nitrogenous waste products and maintain adequate fluid, electrolyte, and acid-base balances.

Dialyzer semipermeable membrane filter within a machine that contains many tiny hollow fibers; during dialysis, blood moves through the hollow fibers and water and wastes from the blood move into the dialysate fluid that flows around the fibers, but protein and RBCs do not.

Diaphragm muscle that separates the thoracic cavity from the abdominal cavity.

Diaphyses long shafts of bones in the arms and legs.

Diastolic blood pressure arterial pressure during ventricular relaxation.

Diethylenetriaminepentaacetate (DTPA) injectable salt or inhalant spray containing calcium (Ca-DTPA) or zinc (Zn-DTPA) used to treat internal contamination with radioactive substances such as plutonium.

Diffusion process of oxygen and CO_2 exchange through the alveolar-capillary membrane.

Digital rectal examination technique used to assess the prostate for size as well as evidence of tumor.

Digitalization method of giving large doses of a digitalis drug at the beginning of treatment to build up therapeutic blood levels of the drug.

Dilation and curettage surgical procedure in which the cervix is stretched open and the endometrium is scraped to diagnose or treat various gynecologic problems and to remove fetal and placental tissue.

Diplopia double vision.

Directed donor blood blood obtained from specified blood donors among a client's relatives and friends.

Dirty bomb conventional explosive device (e.g., dynamite) that spreads small amounts of radiation in the form of powder or pellets.

Disaster threatening event of such destructive magnitude and force as to dislocate people, separate family members, damage or destroy homes, and injure or kill people.

Disease pathologic condition that presents with clinical signs and symptoms.

Disequilibrium syndrome neurologic condition believed to be caused by cerebral edema; the shift in cerebral fluid volume occurs when the concentrations of solutes within the blood are lowered rapidly during dialysis.

Diskectomy surgical procedure in which a ruptured intervertebral disk is removed.

Dislocation injury in which the articular surfaces of a joint are no longer in contact.

Distal sensory polyneuropathy disorder characterized by abnormal sensations, such as burning and numbness, in the feet and later in the hands.

Distress excessive, ill-timed, or unrelieved stress.

Distributive shock shock that occurs when fluid in the circulatory system does not facilitate effective perfusion of the tissue; sometimes called normovolemic shock.

Diverticulitis inflammation of diverticula.

Diverticulosis asymptomatic diverticula.

Diverticulum (pl. diverticula) sac or pouch caused by herniation of the mucosa through a weakened portion of the muscular coat of the intestine or other structure.

Documentation written record of client care.

Dopamine monoamine neurotransmitter of the sympathetic nervous system and precursor of norepinephrine; excess is associated with distortion of thoughts and sensory perception.

Double-barrel colostomy an opening in the colon that contains both a proximal stoma for expelling fecal material and a distal stoma to the anus.

Drop factor ratio of drops to mL delivered by tubing in the administration of IV solution.

Drop size volume of IV fluid determined by the opening in the tubing.

Drug cross-resistance diminished drug response among similar drugs.

Drug resistance ineffective response to a prescribed drug because of the survival and duplication of exceptionally virulent mutations.

Dumping syndrome syndrome in which the rapid emptying of large amounts of hypertonic chyme into the jejunum draws fluid from the circulating blood into the intestine, causing hypovolemia, which can produce syncope. As the syndrome progresses, the sudden appearance of carbohydrates in the jejunum stimulates the pancreas to secrete excessive amounts of insulin, which in turn causes hypoglycemia.

Dura mater tough outermost membrane that protects the brain.

Durable power of attorney legal designation of a person to make decisions regarding finances or healthcare when a person becomes incompetent.

Duty expected action based on moral or legal obligations.

Dysmenorrhea painful menstruation.

Dyspareunia discomfort during intercourse.

Dyspepsia epigastric pain or discomfort.

Dysrhythmia conduction disorder that results in an abnormally slow or rapid heart rate or one that does not proceed through the conduction system in the usual manner.

E

Early detection use of screening diagnostic tests and procedures to identify a disease process earlier, so that treatment may be initiated earlier and be more effective.

Eating disorders disorders in which eating is outside the range of normal.

Ecchymosis bruising.

Eccrine glands sweat glands that release water and electrolytes, such as sodium and chloride, in the form of perspiration.

Echocardiography diagnostic procedure that uses ultrasound waves to determine the functioning of the left ventricle and to detect cardiac tumors, congenital defects, and changes in the tissue layers of the heart.

Ectopic site conductive tissue that initiates an electrical impulse independently of the SA node.

Educator person who provides information.

Effector T cells killer (cytotoxic) T-cell lymphocytes.

Effluent discharged fecal material or liquid feces.

Effusion accumulation of fluid within two layers of tissue.

Ejaculation discharge of semen.

Ejection fraction percentage of blood the left ventricle ejects when it contracts.

Elective electrical cardioversion nonemergency procedure to stop rapid atrial dysrhythmias in which a machine delivers an electrical stimulation that does not disrupt the heart during ventricular repolarization.

Electrocardiography graphic recording of the electrical currents generated by the heart muscle.

Electroconvulsive therapy application of an electric stimulus to one or both temporal regions of the head to produce a brief, generalized seizure; used to treat severe depression.

Electrolytes substances that carry an electrical charge when dissolved in fluid.

Electromagnetic therapy technique of healing using either electricity, magnets, or both.

Electron beam computed tomography radiologic test that produces x-rays of the coronary arteries using an electron beam.

Electronic infusion device machine that regulates and monitors the administration of IV solutions.

Electronystagmography method used to evaluate vestibular function, the mechanisms that facilitate maintaining balance, by measuring the duration and velocity of eye movements during caloric stimulation.

Electrophysiology study procedure that enables a physician to examine the electrical activity of the heart, produce actual dysrhythmias by stimulating structures within the conduction pathway, determine the best method for preventing further dysrhythmic episodes, and, in some cases, eradicate the precise location in the heart that is producing the dysrhythmia.

Embolectomy surgical removal of an embolus.

Embolus moving mass of particles, either solid or gas, within the bloodstream.

Emerging infectious disease disorder caused by microorganisms that are new or have had a resurgence in the last 2 decades.

Emission movement of sperm and their mixture with fluid from the seminal vesicles and prostate gland into the urethra, a process mediated via the sympathetic nervous system.

Emmetropia normal vision, in which light rays are bent to focus images precisely on the retina.

Empathy intuitive awareness of what a client is experiencing.

Emphysema chronic pulmonary disease characterized by abnormal distention of the alveoli.

Empyema collection of pus in the pleural cavity.

Emulsion mixture of two liquids, one of which is insoluble in the other; when combined, the two are distributed throughout the mixture as small, undissolved droplets.

Encopresis involuntary passage of liquid stool around an obstructive mass of stool.

Endarterectomy surgical removal of the atherosclerotic plaque lining an artery.

Endocannabinoids endogenous chemicals that have marijuana-like properties that activate the appetite center.

Endocardium innermost layer of the heart.

Endogenous opiates natural morphine-like substances that modulate pain transmission by blocking receptors for substance P.

Endometrial ablation detachment of the lining of the uterus.

Endometriosis condition in which tissue that histologically and functionally resembles that of the endometrium is found outside the uterus.

Endophthalmitis disorder in which all three layers of the eye and the vitreous are inflamed.

Endotoxins harmful chemicals released from within a bacterial cell; probably the major cause of toxic shock.

End-stage renal disease stage in chronic renal failure in which less than 10% of nephron function remains and the point at which a regular course of dialysis or kidney transplantation is necessary to maintain life.

Energy medicine field of alternative and complementary therapies that uses techniques to manipulate electromagnetic fields in the body and may involve the use of mechanical vibration, laser beams, and electromagnetic forces of measurable wavelengths and frequencies.

Energy therapies techniques that claim to manipulate electromagnetic fields within the body.

Engraftment establishment of bone marrow that has been harvested and reinfused.

Enhanced external counterpulsation noninvasive and nonsurgical therapy that helps relieve angina using a pressure suit that moves blood toward the heart.

Enteroclysis study to determine subtle small bowel disease in which two contrast media fill and pass through the intestinal loops and are observed continuously through fluoroscope and periodic x-rays of the various sections of the small intestine.

Enterostomal therapist nurse who collaborates with the surgeon regarding stomal placement and the ostomate's educational needs.

Entry inhibitors drugs that interfere with the HIV's ability to fuse with and enter the CD4 cell; also known as *fusion inhibitors*.

Enucleation surgical removal of an eye.

Environmental tobacco smoke smoke given off by the burning end of a cigarette, pipe, or cigar and the exhaled smoke from the lungs of a smoker.

Enzyme-linked immunosorbent assay initial HIV screening test that is positive when there are sufficient HIV antibodies.

Eosinophils granulocytes that destroy parasites and play a major role in allergic reactions.

Epicardium inner serous layer of the pericardium; also called the *visceral pericardium*.

Epicondylitis painful inflammation of the elbow.

Epidemic rapidly spreading infectious disease in a particular region.

Epidermis outermost layer of skin.

Epididymitis inflammation of the epididymis.

Epidural hematoma bleeding within the skull that stems from arterial bleeding, usually from the middle meningeal artery, with blood accumulation above the dura.

Epiglottis cartilaginous valve flap that covers the opening to the larynx during swallowing.

Epilepsy chronic recurrent pattern of seizures.

Epinephrine neurotransmitter of the sympathetic nervous system produced and secreted by the adrenal medulla.

Epiphyses rounded, irregular ends of long bones.

Epistaxis nosebleed.

Epithelialization regrowth of skin.

Epstein-Barr virus virus that causes infectious mononucleosis.

Equianalgesic dose oral dose that provides the same level of pain relief as when the drug is given by a parenteral route.

Erectile dysfunction the inability to (1) achieve an erection, (2) achieve or maintain an erection sufficiently rigid for sexual activity, or (3) sustain an erection for a satisfactory period.

Erection parasympathetic nerve activity or state in which the penis becomes elongated and rigid, facilitating its insertion into the vagina.

Erythema redness of the skin.

Erythrocytes red blood cells.

Erythrocytosis increase in circulating erythrocytes.

Erythropoietin hormone released by the kidneys that stimulates the bone marrow to produce erythrocytes.

Eschar hard leathery crust of dehydrated skin that forms in areas of full-thickness burns.

Escharotomy incision into eschar to relieve constricting pressure.

Esophageal varices dilated, bulging esophageal veins.

Esophagitis inflammation of the lining of the esophagus.

Esophagogastro-duodenoscopy examination of the esophagus, stomach, and duodenum through an endoscope to inspect, treat, or obtain specimens from any of the upper GI structures.

Essential hypertension sustained elevated blood pressure with no known cause.

Estrogen hormone produced by the ovaries.

Ethics moral principles and values that guide the behavior of honorable people.

Ethmoidal sinuses honeycomb of small spaces contained in the ethmoid bone, located between the eyes.

Ethnicity bond or kinship that people feel with their country of birth or place of ancestral origin, regardless of whether they have ever lived outside of the United States.

Ethnobotanicals plants used for food, clothing, shelter, and medicine that grow in a region where specific groups of people live.

Ethnocentrism belief that one's own ethnic heritage is superior to that of others.

Eustress healthy amount of stress that helps individuals to pursue goals, learn to solve problems, and manage life's predictable and unpredictable crises.

Euthymic state in which a person is capable of experiencing a variety of feelings, all of which are situationally appropriate.

Evaluation step in the nursing process that involves the assessment and review of the quality and suitability of care and the client's responses to that care.

Evisceration protrusion of organs through a separated surgical wound.

Exacerbation periods of acute flare-ups of the symptoms of a disorder.

Exercise electrocardiography diagnostic test that images the electrical activity of the heart while the client walks on a treadmill, pedals a stationary bicycle, or climbs up and down stairs; also known as a *stress test*.

Excitability ability of cardiac tissue to respond to electrical stimulation.

Excretory urogram radiologic study used to evaluate the structure and function of the kidneys, ureters, and bladder by examining a radiopaque dye as it passes through the urinary tract.

Exertional dyspnea effort at breathing when physically active.

Expected outcomes client goals derived from nursing diagnoses that are measurable, achievable, and developed with the client, family, and other healthcare providers.

Expressive aphasia neurologic impairment of a person's ability to speak.

External fixation procedure in which metal pins are inserted into a fractured bone or bones from outside the skin surface and then attached to a compression device.

External radiologic contamination exposure to fallout on the skin, hair, and clothing.

Extracellular fluid water in the body located outside cells.

Extracorporeal circulation technique in which blood is mechanically circulated and oxygenated outside the body.

Extracorporeal shock wave lithotripsy procedure that uses shock waves to dissolve large kidney stones.

Extramedullary outside the spinal cord.

Extrapyramidal motor tracts fibers that originate in the motor cortex and project to the cerebellum and basal ganglia.

Extrapyramidal symptoms movement disorders associated with certain prescribed drugs.

Extravasation leaking of an intravenously administered drug into surrounding tissues.

F

Facilitated diffusion process in which dissolved substances require the assistance of a carrier molecule to pass through a semipermeable membrane.

Fallout cooling, condensation, and dropping back to earth of vapor containing radioactive material.

Fasciculations involuntary twitching of muscles.

Fasciotomy surgical incision of fascia and separation of muscle.

Fasting blood glucose blood test performed to detect and monitor diabetes mellitus.

Fear feeling of terror in response to someone or something specific that a person perceives as dangerous or threatening.

Feedback loop mechanism that turns hormone production off and on; negative feedback stimulates a releasing gland in response to a decrease in levels while positive feedback keeps concentrations of hormones within a stable range.

Fertilization union of an ovum and a spermatozoon.

Fetor hepaticus sulfurous breath odor.

Fibroadenoma solid, benign breast mass composed of connective and glandular tissue.

Fibrocystic breast disease benign breast disorder that affects women primarily between the ages of 30 and 50.

Fibroid tumor common benign uterine growth.

Fibromyalgia pain in the fibrous tissues of the body such as muscles, ligaments, and tendons.

Filtration process that promotes the movement of fluid and some dissolved substances through a semipermeable membrane using pressure differences.

Fingerspelling alphabetical substitute for words that have no sign.

Fissure tear in tissue.

Fistula channel from an organ to the surface of the body or from one organ to another.

Fistulectomy surgical procedure in which a fistulous tract is excised.

Fistulotomy surgical procedure involving incision of a fistula.

Fixed-rate (asynchronous) mode pacemaker cardiac device that produces an electrical stimulus at a preset rate (usually 72 to 80 beats/min), despite the client's natural heart rate and rhythm.

Flaccidity lack of motor response to stimuli.

Flail chest disorder that occurs when two or more adjacent ribs fracture in multiple places and the fragments are free-floating; affects the stability of the chest wall and impairment of chest wall movement.

Flashbacks feelings of reliving a traumatic event.

Flexible sigmoidoscopy procedure in which a flexible fiberoptic endoscope is used to examine the sigmoid colon.

Focus assessment detailed information about one body system or problem.

Follicle-stimulating hormone (FSH) hormone that stimulates development of ovum in the ovaries and sperm in the testes.

Fomites nonliving environment in which an infectious agent can survive and reproduce.

Food binges rapid consumption of a large number of calories.

Foramen magnum opening in the lower part of the skull through which the upper part of the spinal cord connects with the brain and which provides the only extracranial exit for brain tissue.

Formal teaching planned, organized conveying of information. See also *informal teaching*.

Fracture break in the continuity of a bone.

Frontal sinuses bony cavities that lie within the frontal bone that extends above the orbital cavities.

Fulguration removal of small, superficial bladder tumors through coagulation with a transurethral resectoscope.

Fulminant colitis a progression of severity of ulcerations associated with ulcerative colitis with severe pain, copious diarrhea, and potential dehydration and shock.

Full-thickness graft skin graft in which the epidermis, dermis, and some subcutaneous tissue are harvested from the client's skin.

Functional assessment determination of how well a client can manage activities of daily living.

Functional nursing task-oriented system of nursing care that evolved in the 1930s in which distinct duties are assigned to specific personnel.

Fundoplication surgical procedure to treat gastroesophageal reflux disorder that tightens the lower esophageal sphincter by wrapping the gastric fundus around the lower esophagus and suturing it into place.

Furuncle skin infection commonly called a boil.

Furunculosis condition of having multiple furuncles, or boils.

Fusion inhibitor category of AIDS drugs that interfere with the ability of HIV to fuse with and enter the CD4 cell.

G

Gallbladder series test used to identify the presence of stones in the gallbladder or common bile duct and tumors or other obstructions, and to determine the ability of the gallbladder to concentrate and store an iodine-based, radiopaque contrast medium.

Gamma-aminobutyric acid inhibitory neurotransmitter.

Gamma-knife radiosurgery non-invasive alternative for treating brain tumors deep within the brain or for treating those tumors that conventional surgery can only partially remove.

Gamma radiation energy released from unstable atoms that can penetrate and damage body cells.

Ganglion cystic mass that develops near tendon sheaths and joints of the wrist.

Gastrectomy surgical removal of the stomach.

Gastric decompression removal of gas and fluids from the stomach.

Gastritis inflammation of the stomach lining.

Gastroesophageal reflux disorder in which there is an upward flow of gastric contents into the esophagus.

Gastrostomy placement of a tube into the stomach via a surgically created opening into the abdominal wall.

Gender role societal determination of behaviors as either feminine or masculine.

Gene therapy technique for fighting cancer that involves replacing altered genes with normal genes, inhibiting defective genes, or introducing substances that destroy defective genes or cancer cells.

General adaptation syndrome nonspecific physiologic cyclical response to stress involving alarm, resistance, and exhaustion.

Generalization acknowledging that common trends exist within a cultural group but understanding that those trends may or may not apply to a particular individual.

Generalized anxiety disorder psychobiologic disorder characterized by chronic worrying on a daily basis for 6 or more months, generally with more than one focus of worry and often with the worrying being out of proportion with reality.

Generalized edema accumulation of fluid in all the interstitial spaces.

Genital herpes sexually transmitted infection caused by herpes simplex virus type 2 that results in genital and perineal lesions.

Genitalia organs of reproduction.

Genotype testing blood test used to detect drug resistance in which genetic changes in circulating HIV particles are measured.

Gerogogy techniques that enhance learning among older adults

Gerontology study of aging, including its physiologic, psychological, and social aspects.

Glaucoma eye disorder caused by an imbalance between the production and drainage of aqueous fluid.

Glomerulonephritis inflammatory renal disorder that occurs most frequently in children and young adults that is preceded by an upper respiratory infection with group A beta-hemolytic streptococci, impetigo (skin infection), or viral infections such as mumps, hepatitis B, or HIV.

Glottis opening between the vocal cords in the larynx.

Glucagon hormone that increases blood sugar levels by stimulating the breakdown of glycogen into glucose in the liver.

Glutamate neurotoxic neurotransmitter that contributes to neuronal cell death.

Glycemic index measure of how fast a carbohydrate food is likely to raise blood sugar.

Glycogenolysis process in which glycogen is broken down into glucose in the liver.

Glycosuria glucose in the urine.

Glycosylated hemoglobin amount of glucose stored within a hemoglobin molecule during its lifespan of 120 days.

Goiter enlarged thyroid gland.

Gonorrhea sexually transmitted infection caused by a bacterium, *Neisseria gonorrhoeae,* which invades the urethra, vagina, rectum, or pharynx, depending on the nature of sexual contact.

Good Samaritan laws laws that provide legal immunity for rescuers who provide first aid in an emergency (outside of a hospital) to accident victims.

Gout painful metabolic disorder involving an inflammatory reaction within the joints that usually affects the feet (especially the great toe), hands, elbows, ankles, and knees.

Granulocytes leukocytes that contain cytoplasmic granules.

Granuloma inflammatory nodular lesion.

Granuloma inguinale sexually transmitted infection caused by a bacillus, *Calymmatobacterium granulomatis,* and characterized by painless nodules in the genital, inguinal, and anal areas.

Guardianship court-appointed responsibility for managing a client's care and assets when the client is incompetent.

Gynecologic examination inspection and palpation of pelvic reproductive structures.

H

Hallucinations sensory experiences that others do not perceive; can be auditory, visual, tactile, olfactory, or gustatory (involving taste).

Hallux valgus deformity of the great (large) toe at its metatarsophalangeal joint.

Halo sign blood stain surrounded by a yellowish stain; highly suggestive of a cerebrospinal fluid leak.

Hammer toe flexion deformity of the interphalangeal joint that may involve several toes.

Hardiness effective coping style that includes a sense of having control over sources of stress and the perception of life events as a challenge rather than a threat.

Hard of hearing having hearing that is limited but allows for communication.

Head-to-toe method technique used for carrying out an examination by beginning at the top of the body and progressing downward. See also *systems method*.

Health state of complete physical, mental, and social well-being; not merely the absence of disease and infirmity.

Health beliefs client's opinions regarding what causes illnesses, the role of the sick person and the healthcare professional, what must occur to restore health, and how one stays healthy, often shaped and perpetuated by the client's cultural affiliations.

Healthcare delivery system full range of services available to people seeking prevention, identification, treatment, or rehabilitation of health problems.

Healthcare team group of specially trained personnel who work together to help clients meet their healthcare needs.

Health maintenance protecting one's current level of health by preventing illness or deterioration.

Health maintenance organization group insurance plans in which each participant pays a preset, fixed fee in exchange for healthcare services.

Health practices actions that a client takes to restore health or stay healthy, often a product of and perpetuated by the client's cultural affiliations.

Health promotion engaging in strategies to enhance health.

Health promotion diagnosis reflects clinical judgment of a client's motivation to increase well-being and enhance health behaviors.

Hearing perceiving sounds.

Heart block disorders in the conduction pathway that interfere with the transmission of impulses from the sinoatrial node through the atrioventricular node to the ventricles.

Heart failure inability of the heart to pump sufficient blood to meet the body's metabolic needs.

Heberden's nodes bony enlargement of the distal interphalangeal joints.

Helper T cells cells that recognize antigens and form additional T-cell clones that stimulate B-cell lymphocytes to produce antibodies against foreign antigens.

Hematopoiesis manufacture and development of blood cells.

Hematuria blood in the urine.

Heme pigmented, iron-containing portion of hemoglobin.

Hemianopia disorder in which the client is only able to see half of the normal visual field.

Hemiplegia paralysis on one side of the body.

Hemoconcentration high ratio of blood components in relation to watery plasma.

Hemodialysis technique in which blood is transported from a client through a dialyzer, a semipermeable membrane filter within a machine that removes water and wastes from the blood.

Hemodilution reduced ratio of blood components in relation to watery plasma.

Hemodynamic monitoring procedure used to assess the volume and pressure of blood within the heart and vascular system by means of a peripherally inserted catheter.

Hemoglobin iron-containing protein attached to erythrocytes that carries oxygen to cells.

Hemoptysis expectoration of blood or bloody sputum.

Hemorrhoidectomy surgical removal of hemorrhoids.

Hemorrhoids dilated veins outside or inside the anal sphincter.

Hepatic encephalopathy central nervous system manifestation of liver failure related to an increased serum ammonia level that often leads to coma and death.

Hepatic lobectomy surgical procedure in which a primary malignant or benign tumor confined to a single lobe of the liver is removed.

Hepatitis inflammation of the liver.

Hepatorenal syndrome renal failure associated with liver disease that ultimately alters fluid distribution and interferes with fluid excretion.

Herbal therapy use of plants for treating disease and disorders.

Hernia protrusion of any organ from the cavity that normally confines it; most commonly used to describe the protrusion of the intestine through a defect in the abdominal wall.

Hernioplasty surgical procedure in which the weakened area of a hernia is reinforced with wire, fascia, or mesh to prevent recurrence.

Herniorrhaphy surgical repair of a hernia.

Herpes simplex virus infectious agent responsible for genital and perineal lesions and associated with cold sores around the nose and lips.

Herpes zoster skin disorder (shingles) that develops later after an infection with varicella (chickenpox) due to an acute reactivation of the varicella-zoster virus, which lies dormant in nerve roots.

Heterograft skin graft obtained from animals, principally pigs, to temporarily cover large areas of tissue until the client's own skin can be used for skin grafting.

Hiatal hernia (diaphragmatic hernia) protrusion of part of the stomach through the diaphragm.

High-density lipoprotein lipoprotein that has a higher ratio of protein than cholesterol.

Highly active antiretroviral therapy HIV treatment with a combination of drugs; sometimes referred to as a "drug cocktail."

Hilus entrance of the bronchi to the lungs.

Histocompatible cells cells whose antigens match an individual's own genetic code.

Hodgkin's disease malignancy that produces enlargement of lymphoid tissue, the spleen, and the liver, with invasion of other tissues such as the bone marrow and lungs.

Holism viewing a person's health as a balance of body, mind, and spirit; considering the client's psychological, sociocultural, developmental, and spiritual needs to restore optimal health.

Homans' sign calf pain that increases on dorsiflexion of the foot.

Home healthcare delivery of healthcare services, for both long-term and short-term health needs, in a client's home.

Homeopathy belief that the remedy for an illness should produce symptoms similar to the disease itself.

Homocysteine amino acid created during the metabolism of protein; elevated levels are believed to impair memory and contribute to above-normal cholesterol levels.

Hordeolum (sty) inflammation and infection of the Zeis or Moll gland, a type of oil gland at the edge of the eyelid.

Hormone replacement therapy administration of estrogen combined with progestin to reduce perimenopausal symptoms, prevent osteoporosis, and reduce the atherosclerotic process.

Hormones chemicals secreted by the endocrine glands that accelerate or slow physiologic processes.

Hospice facility for the care of terminally ill clients where they can live out their final days with comfort, dignity, and meaningfulness.

Host person on or in whom a microorganism resides.

Human immunodeficiency virus (HIV) pathogen that causes acquired immunodeficiency syndrome (AIDS).

Human papillomavirus infectious agent that causes venereal warts; transmitted by genital-genital, genital-anal, or genital-oral contact with an infected person and contagious as long as the warts are present.

Humor therapeutic use of laughter, which stimulates the immune system and causes the release of neuropeptides.

Humoral response formation of antibodies.

Hydronephrosis condition in which an obstruction of urine from the ureter distends the renal pelvis.

Hyperalgesia amplified pain experience.

Hyperbaric oxygen treatment administration of 100% oxygen at three times greater than atmospheric pressure in a specially designed chamber.

Hyperglycemia elevated blood glucose level.

Hyperlipidemia high levels of fat in blood.

Hypernatremia elevated serum sodium level.

Hyperopia farsightedness; people who are hyperopic see objects that are far away better than objects that are close.

Hyperosmolar hyperglycemic nonketotic syndrome acute complication of diabetes characterized by hyperglycemia without ketosis.

Hyperparathyroidism disorder of the parathyroid gland that affects calcium and phosphorus levels.

Hyperplasia increase in the number of cells.

Hypertension sustained elevation of systolic arterial blood pressure of 140 mm Hg or higher, a sustained diastolic arterial blood pressure of 90 mm Hg or higher, or both.

Hypertensive cardiovascular disease stage of hypertension when elevated blood pressure causes both cardiac abnormality and vascular damage.

Hypertensive crisis potentially fatal condition with symptoms such as extremely elevated blood pressure, headache, nausea, vomiting, sweating, palpitations, visual changes, neck stiffness, sensitivity to light, and tachycardia.

Hypertensive heart disease stage of hypertension when elevated blood pressure causes a cardiac abnormality.

Hypertensive vascular disease stage of hypertension when elevated blood pressure causes vascular damage without heart involvement.

Hyperthyroidism disorder associated with hypersecretion of thyroid hormones in which metabolic rate increases.

Hypertonic solution solution that is more concentrated than body fluid and draws fluid into the intravascular compartment from the more dilute areas within the cells and interstitial spaces.

Hypertrophied turbinates enlargements of the nasal concha that interfere with air passage and sinus drainage, and eventually lead to sinusitis.

Hyperuricemia accumulation of uric acid in the blood.

Hypervolemia high volume of water in the intravascular fluid compartment.

Hyphae threadlike filaments within the cells of most fungi.

Hypnosis therapeutic intervention that facilitates a physiologic change through the power of suggestion.

Hypochondriasis psychobiologic disorder in which a person is preoccupied with minor symptoms and develops an exaggerated belief that they signify a life-threatening illness.

Hypoglycemia low blood glucose level.

Hypoparathyroidism deficiency of parathormone that results in hypocalcemia.

Hypophysectomy surgical removal of the pituitary gland.

Hypophysis pituitary gland.

Hypothalamus portion of the brain between the cerebrum and the brain stem that stimulates and inhibits the pituitary gland.

Hypothyroidism disorder that occurs when the thyroid gland fails to secrete adequate thyroid hormones.

Hypotonic solution solution that contains fewer dissolved substances in comparison to plasma and is effective in rehydrating clients experiencing fluid deficits.

Hypovolemia low volume of extracellular fluid.

Hypovolemic shock condition that occurs when the volume of extracellular fluid is significantly diminished, primarily because of a loss or reduction in blood or plasma.

Hypoxia decrease in the amount of oxygen reaching the cells.

Hysterectomy surgical removal of the uterus.

I

Ileoanal reservoir (anastomosis) creation of an internal reservoir for the storage of GI effluent.

Ileostomy surgically created opening between the distal small intestine and the skin.

Illness state of being sick; may be viewed as catastrophic (sudden, traumatic), acute, chronic, or terminal.

Illness prevention identification of risk factors such as a family history of hypertension or diabetes and assisting of clients to reduce the effects of risk factors on their health.

Imagery psychobiologic technique that uses the mind to visualize a positive physiologic effect.

Immune response target-specific system of defense against infectious, foreign, or cancerous cells carried out primarily by lymphocytes.

Immunoglobulins proteins produced by B lymphocyte plasma cells that bind with antigens and promote the destruction of invading cells; also known as antibodies.

Immunopeptides chemical messengers that relay messages throughout the immune system and the brain.

Immunotherapy use of biologic response modifiers to stimulate the body's natural immune system to restrict and destroy cancer cells.

Impedance plethysmography test used for diagnosing clots within deep veins by recording blood volume in the arm or leg before and after inflating a BP cuff to stop venous blood flow.

Implantation process in which a fertilized ovum, or zygote, travels down the uterus and attaches itself within the endometrium.

Implanted pacemaker permanent electrical device used to manage a chronic bradydysrhythmia.

Implementation step in the nursing process that involves carrying out the written plan of care, performing the interventions, monitoring the client's status, and assessing and reassessing the client before, during, and after treatments.

Impotence inability to achieve or maintain an erection sufficient for sexual activity.

Incident report documentation made by healthcare workers when they make or discover errors, or when an event occurs that results in harm; it identifies the nature of the incident, witnesses, what actions were taken at the time, and the client's condition.

Incompetent legal term for the inability to understand the risks or benefits of decisions.

Incontinence inability to control urinary or bowel elimination.

Infarct area of tissue that dies from inadequate oxygenation.

Infectious mononucleosis viral disease that affects lymphoid tissues such as the tonsils and spleen and can involve other organs such as the brain, meninges, and liver as well.

Infectious process cycle cycle involving the transmission of an infectious disease from a human or animal to a susceptible host. The six components needed for it to occur are an infectious microorganism, reservoir, portal for exit, means of transmission, portal of entry, and susceptible host, also known as *chain of infection*.

Infective endocarditis inflammation of the inner layer of heart tissue as a result of an infectious microorganism.

Inferior vena cava large blood vessel that delivers unoxygenated blood from the lower body to the right atrium.

Inflammatory bowel disease group of chronic illnesses characterized by exacerbations and remissions of inflammation and ulceration of the bowel lining. See also *ulcerative colitis* and *Crohn's disease*.

Influenza acute viral respiratory disease of relatively short duration.

Informal teaching unplanned, spontaneous conveying of information, usually at the client's bedside or while caring for the client at home. See also *formal teaching*.

Informed consent voluntary permission granted by a knowledgable client, or the client's assigned *medical proxy* for an invasive procedure or surgery.

Infratentorial below the tentorium (an area between the cerebrum and cerebellum).

Infusion pump device that exerts positive pressure to infuse IV solutions and adjusts the pressure according to the resistance it meets.

Injection sclerotherapy procedure in which a physician passes an endoscope orally to locate an esophageal varix, then passes a thin needle through the endoscope and injects a sclerosing agent directly into the varix to stop circulation through it.

In-line filter device that removes air bubbles as well as undissolved drugs, bacteria, and large molecules from an infusing solution.

Insight-oriented therapy technique that helps clients understand the cause and relationship between their emotional distress and physical symptoms.

Inspection systematic and thorough observation of a client and specific areas of a client's body.

Insulin pancreatic hormone necessary for the metabolism of glucose.

Insulin independence ability of a client's own naturally produced insulin to regulate blood glucose levels within consistently normal ranges.

Insulin resistance decreased sensitivity to insulin at the tissue level.

Integrase viral enzyme that incorporates a viral code into a host cell's DNA.

Integrase inhibitors antiretroviral drugs that block integrase thus preventing the incorporation of HIV DNA into the T-cell's DNA.

Integrated delivery system network formed by hospitals and other healthcare facilities to reduce the redundancy of healthcare services and increase economic leverage.

Integrative medicine combination of conventional medicine with complementary or alternative therapy.

Integument structures that cover the body's exterior surface; the primary structure is the skin, but the integument also includes accessory structures such as the hair and nails.

Intentional tort deliberate and willful act that infringes on another person's rights or property.

Interferons chemicals that enable cells to resist viral infection and slow viral replication.

Interleukins chemicals that coordinate the immune response.

Intermittent claudication leg pain with exercise.

Internal fixation procedure in which metal screws, plates, rods, nails, or pins are used to stabilize a reduced bone fracture.

Internal radiologic contamination fallout, entering an open wound, inhaled via contaminated air, or consumed through contaminated food and water.

Interstitial cystitis chronic inflammation of the bladder mucosa.

Interstitial fluid water located between cells.

Interstitium structure that lies between the alveoli and contains the pulmonary capillaries and elastic connective tissue.

Interventions actions for achieving outcomes in a plan of care.

Intimate space physical closeness between two people, which is only appropriate for interactions of a very personal nature.

Intra-aortic balloon pump device that acts as a temporary, secondary pump to supplement ineffectual contraction of the heart's left ventricle.

Intracellular fluid water located within cells.

Intracerebral hematoma bleeding within the brain that results from an open or closed head injury or from a cerebrovascular condition such as a ruptured cerebral aneurysm.

Intractable pain pain that does not respond to analgesic medications, noninvasive measures, or nursing management.

Intramedullary within the spinal cord.

Intraocular lens implant artificial lens that is inserted in the eye to improve or restore vision.

Intraoperative phase of perioperative care that includes the entire surgical procedure until transfer of the client to the recovery area.

Intravascular fluid water located in the plasma (serum) portion of blood.

Intravenous pyelogram radiologic study used to evaluate the structure and function of the kidneys, ureters, and bladder by examining a radiopaque dye as it passes through the urinary tract.

Intravenous (IV) therapy parenteral administration of fluids and additives into a vein.

Introductory phase stage of the nurse–client relationship during which a nurse and a client get acquainted and the client identifies one or more health problems for which he or she is seeking care.

Intussusception telescoping of one part of the intestine into an adjacent part.

Involucrum new bone cells.

Ions positively and negatively charged substances.

Iridectomy surgical or laser procedure in which holes are made in the iris to increase drainage of aqueous fluid.

Irreversible stage stage in shock that occurs when significant numbers of cells and organ systems become damaged and the client no longer responds to medical interventions.

Irritable bowel syndrome paroxysmal motility syndrome primarily affecting the colon, in which the client experiences alternating periods of constipation and diarrhea.

Ischemia impaired oxygenation of cells and tissues.

Islets of Langerhans hormone-secreting cells of the pancreas that release insulin and glucagon.

Isoenzyme one of several forms of an enzyme that can be identified separately.

Isolation negative developmental outcome of the young adult stage characterized by an inability to form close relationships with others.

Isotonic solution solution containing the same concentration of dissolved substances normally found in plasma; used to maintain fluid balance when clients temporarily cannot eat or drink.

J

Janeway lesions small, painless, red-blue macular sores.

Jejunostomy GI intubation in which the tube enters the jejunum of the or small intestine via a surgically created opening into the abdominal wall.

Joint junction between two or more bones.

K

Kaposi's sarcoma type of connective tissue cancer common among those with AIDS.

Kegel exercises isometric exercises designed to assist with stress incontinence.

Keratin tough protective protein formed by the outer layer of dead skin cells.

Keratitis inflammation of the cornea.

Keratoplasty corneal transplantation.

Kernig's sign inability to extend the leg when the thigh is flexed on the abdomen.

Ketoacidosis form of metabolic acidosis resulting from an accumulation of ketones in the blood.

Ketonemia increased ketones in the blood.

Ketones metabolic by-products of fat metabolism.

Kinesics study of nonverbal techniques of communication such as facial expressions, postures, gestures, and body movements.

Kussmaul respirations fast, deep breathing.

L

Labyrinthitis inflammation of the labyrinth of the inner ear.

Lactation production of breast milk.

Laissez-faire leadership style of leadership characterized by allowing a work group to individually set goals, make decisions, and take responsibility for their own management.

Laminectomy surgical procedure in which the posterior arch of a vertebra is removed to expose the spinal cord and allow the removal of a herniated disk, tumor, blood clot, bone spur, or broken bone fragment.

Lanugo fine body hair grown in the absence of subcutaneous fat to help maintain body temperature by reducing heat loss.

Laryngitis inflammation and swelling of the mucous membrane that lines the larynx.

Laryngoscopy endoscopic examination of the larynx.

Laryngospasm spasm of the laryngeal muscles, resulting in narrowing of the larynx.

Larynx cartilaginous framework between the pharynx and the trachea whose primary function is to produce sound; it also protects the lower airway from foreign objects because of its ability to facilitate coughing.

Laser angioplasty use of short pulses of light to vaporize arterial plaque.

Laws written rules governing conduct and actions.

Leadership ability to guide and influence another person, group, or both to think in a certain way, achieve common goals, or provide inspiration for change.

Learning capacity person's intellectual ability to understand, remember, and apply new information.

Learning needs those skills and concepts that a client and family must acquire to restore, maintain, or promote health.

Learning readiness degree to which a person is in an optimal position to process new information.

Learning style that manner in which a person best comprehends new information.

Left ventricular end-diastolic pressure retrograde pressure from the fluid on the left side of the heart at the end of left ventricular diastole.

Left-sided heart failure condition that results from various conditions that impair the left ventricle's ability to eject blood into the aorta.

Leptin substance manufactured in human fat cells believed to suppress appetite-stimulating chemicals.

Leukocytes white blood cells.

Leukocytosis increased number of leukocytes above normal limits.

Leukopenia decreased white blood cell count.

Lewisite chemical developed, but never used, during World War I that can damage exposed skin and mucous membranes on contact or can damage respiratory tissues if inhaled.

Liability legal responsibility.

Libido interest in or desire for sex.

Ligament fibrous tissue that connects two adjacent freely movable bones and helps protect joints by stabilizing their surfaces and keeping them in proper alignment.

Limbic system ring of cranial structures that is a physiologic network for emotions, survival and behavioral responses, motivation, and learning.

Lipoatrophy breakdown of subcutaneous fat at the site of repeated injections.

Lipohypertrophy buildup of subcutaneous fat at the site of repeated injections.

Lipolysis breaking down of fat by the body.

Listening attending to and becoming fully involved in what a client says.

Litholapaxy surgical procedure in which small bladder stones are removed through the transurethral route, using a stone-crushing instrument (lithotrite).

Lithotripsy nonsurgical procedure that uses shock waves to break up some types of kidney or gallstones.

Living will document that states a client's wishes regarding healthcare if he or she is terminally ill.

Lobectomy surgical removal of a lobe of a lung.

Loop colostomy procedure in which a loop of bowel is lifted through the abdomen and is supported in place with a glass rod or plastic butterfly device.

Low-density lipoprotein protein in blood that has a higher ratio of cholesterol than protein.

Lower gastrointestinal series study used to identify polyps, tumors, strictures, and other abnormalities of the colon through the fluoroscopic observation of rectally instilled barium solution.

Lumpectomy surgical procedure in which only a tumor is removed from the breast.

Lung abscess localized area of pus formation within the lung parenchyma.

Lungs paired elastic structures enclosed by the thoracic cage that contain the alveoli.

Luteinizing hormone hormone that initiates ovulation and, in both sexes, secretion of sex hormones.

Lyme disease chronic inflammatory process and multisystem disease caused by a spirochetal bacterium that is transmitted to humans from deer ticks.

Lymph watery fluid derived from plasma that exits the walls of capillaries and enters interstitial spaces.

Lymphadenitis inflammation of the lymph nodes.

Lymphangitis inflammation of the lymphatic vessels.

Lymphatics vessels that transport lymph.

Lymphedema disorder in which obstructed lymph circulation causes an accumulation of lymph within soft tissue.

Lymph nodes clusters of bean-sized structures located primarily in the neck, axilla, chest, abdomen, pelvis, and groin that contain specialized immune defensive cells that trap, destroy, and remove infectious microorganisms, cellular debris, and cancer cells.

Lymphocytes white blood cells with immune functions.

Lymphogranuloma venereum sexually transmitted infection caused by a strain of *C. trachomatis* and characterized by a small erosion or papule and the enlargement of adjacent lymph nodes, which can become necrotic.

Lymphokines type of cytokines that attracts neutrophils and monocytes to remove debris, promotes the maturation of more T cells when they detect antigens, and directs B cell lymphocytes to multiply and mature.

Lymphoma group of cancers that affect the lymphatic system.

M

Macrodrip tubing intravenous tubing that releases large-sized drops of IV solution. See also *microdrop tubing*.

Macrophages large phagocytes present in tissues such as the lungs, liver, lymph nodes, spleen, and peritoneum.

Macular degeneration breakdown of or damage to the macula, the point on the retina where light rays converge for the most acute visual perception.

Magnetic resonance imaging (MRI) diagnostic tool used to identify disorders that affect many different structures in the body without performing surgery; a magnetic field excites hydrogen atoms within the body creating a radio signal that is converted to an image on a computer monitor.

Major (unipolar) depression mood disorder characterized by a feeling of sadness with no obvious relationship to situational events. See also *reactive (secondary) depression*.

Malignant type of tumor that is invasive and capable of spreading.

Malignant hypertension dangerously elevated blood pressure accompanied by papilledema.

Malignant hyperthermia disorder in which body temperature, muscle metabolism, and heat production increase rapidly, progressively, and uncontrollably in response to stress and some anesthetic agents.

Malpractice professional negligence resulting from a licensed person's action or lack of action.

Mammography radiographic technique used to detect cysts or tumors of the breast, some of which may be too small to palpate.

Mammoplasty collective term for several different cosmetic breast procedures.

Managed care organization insurer that carefully plans and closely supervises the distribution of healthcare services.

Management planning, organizing, directing and controlling resources and personnel to meet specific objectives within an organization.

Mania frenzied state of euphoria.

Manipulative and body-based practices healing methods that focus on body structures and systems, including bones and joints, soft tissues, and the circulatory and lymphatic systems.

Massage therapy technique of applying pressure and movement to stretch and knead soft body tissues to stimulate circulation, relieve physical and psychological tension, and improve mobility or functional use of affected parts of the body.

Mastalgia breast pain.

Mast cells constituents of connective tissue that contain granules of heparin, serotonin, bradykinin, and histamine; the release of granules causes various allergic and inflammatory manifestations.

Mastectomy excision of breast tissue.

Mastitis inflammation of breast tissue; most common in women who are breast-feeding.

Mastoidectomy surgical procedure performed to remove diseased tissue from the mastoid process.

Mastoiditis inflammation of any part of the mastoid process.

Mastopexy surgical procedure to correct ptosis, or drooping, of the breast(s).

Maxillary sinuses cavities on either side of the nose in the maxillary bones; they are the largest sinuses and the most accessible to treatment.

Maze procedure surgical procedure to treat atrial fibrillation in which a new conduction pathway is created that eliminates the rapid firing of ectopic pacemaker sites in the atria.

Means of transmission method by which a microorganism is transferred from its reservoir to a susceptible host; the five potential means of transmission are contact, droplet, airborne, vehicle, and vector.

Mediastinum wall that divides the thoracic cavity into two halves.

Medical durable power of attorney person with legal authority to make healthcare decisions for a client if he or she is no longer competent or able to make these decisions.

Medical systems healing practices that have evolved from other cultures.

Medication lock sealed chamber that allows intermittent access to a vein.

Medulla oblongata part of the brain below the pons that transmits motor impulses from the brain to the spinal cord and sensory impulses from peripheral sensory neurons to the brain; contains vital centers concerned with respiration, heart rate, and vasomotor activity.

Melanin pigment that is manufactured by melanocytes located in the epidermis and which determines the color of the skin.

Melanin-concentrating hormone endogenous chemical which in low levels causes weight loss and in high levels promotes obesity.

Melatonin hormone that aids in regulating sleep cycles and mood and is believed to play a role in hypothalamic-pituitary interaction.

Melena black, tarry stools.

Memory cells immunologic cells that convert to plasma cells on re-exposure to a specific antigen.

Menarche first menstruation.

Ménière's disease episodic symptoms created by fluctuations in the production or reabsorption of fluid in the inner ear.

Meninges membranes that protect the brain and spinal cord.

Meniscectomy damaged cartilage.

Menopause physiologic change in the female reproductive system in which ovulation becomes irregular and eventually ceases.

Menorrhagia excessive bleeding at the time of menstruation.

Menstrual diary daily written record of a client's premenstrual symptoms.

Menstruation process that occurs when an ovum is not fertilized, the production of progesterone decreases, and the endometrium degenerates and is shed.

Mental status examination array of observations and questions that elicit information about a person's cognitive and mental state.

Mentation mental activity.

Metabolic syndrome cluster of physiologic alterations that includes obesity (especially in the abdominal area), high blood pressure, elevated triglyceride and low-density lipoprotein, blood glucose levels, and low high-density lipoprotein level.

Metastasis spreading of cancer cells to adjacent tissues, from lymph vessels into the tissues adjacent to lymphatic vessels, by transport from blood or lymph systems, or by diffusion within a body cavity.

Methadone maintenance therapy technique that involves substituting a synthetic addicting drug for another addicting drug to forestall withdrawal, avoid a toxic overdose, or reduce the potential for blood-borne infections.

Metrorrhagia vaginal bleeding at a time other than a menstrual period.

Microdrip tubing intravenous tubing that releases small-sized drops of IV solution. See also *macrodrop tubing*.

Microorganisms potentially infectious agents that are so small they can be seen only with a microscope; commonly called "germs."

Microphages phagocytes present in blood that migrate to tissue as necessary to ingest small sized debris.

Midbrain forward part of the brain stem that connects the pons and cerebellum with the two cerebral hemispheres.

Midclavicular catheter peripherally inserted catheter which extends from a superficial vein to the proximal end of the axillary or subclavian vein.

Midline catheter peripherally inserted venous access device inserted from just above or below the antecubital area in the basilic, cephalic, or median cubital vein until the tip rests in the upper arm just short of the axilla; used for clients who have limited peripheral veins or who require an extended period of IV fluid therapy.

Mind-body medicine techniques that rely on the power of the brain, emotions, social interactions, and spiritual factors to alter body functions or symptoms.

Minority group of people who differ from the majority of people within a given society in terms of cultural characteristics (such as religion), physical characteristics (such as skin color), or both.

Mitral regurgitation backward flow of blood that occurs when the mitral valve does not close completely; sometimes referred to as mitral insufficiency.

Mitral stenosis disorder in which the mitral valve does not open sufficiently to facilitate filling of the left ventricle.

Mitral valve prolapse disorder in which the mitral valve cusps enlarge, become floppy, and bulge backward into the left atrium.

Mitral valve prolapse syndrome cluster of symptoms associated with autonomic nervous system dysfunction in which changes in mitral valve tissue layers cause its cusps to distend, stretching the papillary muscles and leading to valvular incompetence.

Modified radical mastectomy surgical procedure in which the breast, some lymph nodes, the lining over the chest muscles, and the pectoralis minor muscle are removed.

Modulation phase of pain impulse transmission during which the brain interacts with the spinal nerves to alter the pain experience by releasing pain-inhibiting neurochemicals.

Monoamine hypothesis theory that depression results from imbalances in one or more of the monoamine neurotransmitters, serotonin, norepinephrine, and dopamine.

Monocytes large phagocytes present in tissues such as the lungs, liver, lymph nodes, spleen, and peritoneum.

Mood person's overall feeling state; may be thought of as a continuum with extremes of emotion existing at both ends or poles.

Mood disorders conditions in which a person experiences an extreme persistent mood or severe mood swings that interfere with social relationships.

Morbidity the number of sick persons with a particular disease in a specific population.

Morbid obesity having a body mass index of 40 or higher or when one weighs 100 lbs more, or 20% or more than his or her ideal weight.

Mortality the death rate or the ratio of the number of deaths for a specific population.

Motivation desire to acquire new information or implement a new activity.

Multicratic leadership style of leadership in which the manager uses a variety of styles and adapts his or her approach to the situation at hand.

Multidrug resistance ability of some types of bacteria to remain unaffected by several antimicrobial drugs such as antibiotics.

Multifocal PVCs pattern of premature ventricular contractions originating from more than one ectopic location.

Multiple gated acquisition (MUGA) scan most accurate noninvasive test that can measure the left ventricle's ejection fraction during rest and activity; also called a *gated blood pool scan*.

Multiple organ dysfunction syndrome complication of overwhelming inflammation that results in massive cellular, tissue, and organ injury.

Murmur atypical heart sound.

Myelin fatty substance that covers and serves as an insulating substance for some axons in the central nervous and peripheral nervous systems.

Myelosuppression decreased bone marrow function.

Myocardial disarray alteration in the usual alignment of myofibrils, the contractile component of muscle tissue.

Myocardial infarction infarct of an area of the heart muscle that results from occlusion of coronary arterial blood flow; also known as *heart attack*.

Myocardial oxygen demand amount of oxygen the heart needs to perform its work.

Myocardial revascularization surgical procedure that improves the delivery of oxygenated blood to the myocardium by using one or more coronary artery bypass grafts.

Myocarditis inflammation of the myocardium (the muscle layer of the heart).

Myocardium muscle layer of the heart.

Myofibrils contractile component of muscle tissue.

Myopia nearsightedness; people who are myopic hold things close to their eyes to see them well.

Myringoplasty surgical repair of a perforated eardrum.

Myringotomy incisional opening of the eardrum to allow drainage, ease pressure, and relieve pain.

Myxedema hypothyroidism in an adult.

N

Nasal polyps grapelike growths of tissue that arise from the nasal mucous membranes.

Nasal septum wall that divides the internal nose into two cavities.

Nasoenteric intubation placement of a tube that passes through the nose, esophagus, and stomach to the small intestine.

Nasogastric intubation placement of a tube that passes through the nose and esophagus into the stomach.

Nasopharynx part of the pharynx that is near the nose and above the soft palate.

Natriuretic factor hormone produced by the heart, a deficiency of which causes arteries and arterioles to remain in a state of sustained vasoconstriction.

Natriuretic peptides hormone-like substances that act in opposition to the renin-angiotensin-aldosterone system.

Natural killer cells lymphocyte-like cells that circulate throughout the body looking for virus-infected cells and cancer cells and release potent chemicals that lethally alter the target cell's membrane, leading to its demise.

Naturally acquired active immunity immunity that occurs as a direct result of infection by a specific microorganism.

Naturopathy concept that considers disease as an aberration in natural healing.

Near death experience event in which a person almost dies but is resuscitated.

Near point closest point at which a person can clearly focus on an object.

Nearing death awareness phenomenon characterized by a dying client's premonition of the approximate time or date of death.

Negative symptoms impoverished speech and inability to enjoy relationships or express emotions that are characteristic of schizophrenia.

Negligence failure to act as a reasonable person would have acted in a similar situation.

Neoangiogenesis new growth of blood vessels.

Neoplasms new growths of abnormal tissue; also called tumors.

Nephrectomy surgical removal of a kidney.

Nephrolithiasis presence of a kidney stone, the size of which may range from microscopic to several centimeters.

Nephrostomy tube catheter inserted through the skin into the renal pelvis and used to relieve an obstruction to urine flow above the bladder.

Nerve agents potent organophosphate compounds that cause fatal consequences by inhibiting acetylcholinesterase.

Neuralgia nerve pain.

Neurally mediated hypotension disorder in which individuals experience hypotension accompanied by fatigue after standing for more than 10 minutes.

Neurilemma sheath that covers myelin.

Neuritic plaques deposits of beta amyloid in the brain.

Neurofibrillary tangles twisted bundles of microtubules in brain cells.

Neurogenic bladder urinary bladder that does not receive adequate nerve stimulation.

Neurogenic shock shock that results from an insult to the vasomotor center in the medulla of the brain or to the peripheral nerves that extend from the spinal cord to the blood vessels.

Neurohypophysis posterior lobe of the pituitary gland.

Neurologic deficit disorder in which one or more functions of the central and peripheral nervous systems are decreased, impaired, or absent.

Neuron nerve cell.

Neuropathic joint disease common finding in tertiary syphilis, also called Charcot's joints.

Neuropathic pain discomfort that is processed abnormally by the nervous system as a result of damage to either the pain pathways in peripheral nerves or pain processing centers in the brain.

Neuropeptides neurotransmitters that include chemicals such as substance P, which transmits the sensation of pain, endorphins and enkephalins that interrupt the transmission of substance P and promote a feeling of well-being, and neurohormones released by interactions between the hypothalamus, pituitary, and the endocrine glands they stimulate.

Neurotransmitters chemical messengers that communicate information that affects thinking, behavior, and bodily functions across the synaptic cleft between neurons.

Neutropenia decreased neutrophils.

Neutrophils granulocytes that protect the body through the ingestion and digestion of bacteria and foreign substances.

Nits eggs laid by adult female lice that are tightly cemented to the side of hair shafts.

Nociceptive pain discomfort that arises from noxious stimuli that are transmitted from the point of cellular injury to the cerebral cortex of the brain.

Nociceptors specialized pain receptors located in the free nerve endings of peripheral sensory nerves.

Nocturia urination during the night.

Nomogram chart that calculates body surface area based on height and weight.

Non-Hodgkin's lymphomas group of malignant diseases that originate in lymph glands and other lymphoid tissue.

Nonpathogens microorganisms that are generally harmless to healthy humans.

Nonprofit agencies facilities such as universities or religious organizations owned and operated by nonprofit groups.

Nonverbal communication exchange of information without using words.

Norepinephrine monoamine neurotransmitter produced and secreted by the adrenal medulla whose levels may be low or high among people affected by depression; low levels help to explain why some depressed people develop psychomotor retardation, and high levels help to explain why some depressed people experience psychomotor agitation.

Normal eating eating that occurs in response to hunger and ceases when a feeling of comfortable fullness occurs.

Nosocomial infections infections acquired while being cared for in a healthcare agency that were not active, incubatory, or chronic at the time of admission.

Nuchal rigidity pain and stiffness of the neck and an inability to place the chin on the chest.

Nuclear blast explosion that produces an intense wave of heat, light, air pressure, and radiation.

Nuclear scan study that uses special equipment and a radioactive substance, taken orally or injected intravenously, to visualize certain organs or determine their activities.

Nurse–client relationship affiliation that exists during the period when a nurse interacts with clients, sick or well, to promote or restore their health, help them to cope with their illness, or assist them to die with dignity.

Nurse practice acts legal statutes that define nursing practice and set standards for nurses in each state.

Nursing diagnosis step in the nursing process in which the nurse identifies and defines health-related problems.

Nursing orders specific nursing directions given so that all health-care team members understand exactly what to do for the client.

Nursing process problem-solving approach for planning and implementing client care to achieve desired outcomes; the five steps of the nursing process are assessment, diagnosis, planning, implementation, and evaluation.

Nystagmus uncontrolled oscillating movement of the eyeball.

O

Objective data facts obtained during a client's assessment through observation, physical examination, and diagnostic testing. See also *subjective data*.

Obsession disturbing, persistent thought.

Obsessive-compulsive disorder psychobiologic disorder manifested by the performance of an anxiety-relieving ritual to terminate a disturbing, persistent thought.

Obstructive shock shock that occurs when the heart or great vessels are compressed.

Odynophagia painful swallowing.

Oligomenorrhea infrequent menses, usually caused by endocrine imbalances resulting from pituitary disorders or hypothyroidism, the stress response, or severely lean body mass.

Oliguria low urine output of less than 500 mL/day.

Oncology nursing nursing specialty related to the care of clients with cancer.

Onychocryptosis ingrown toenail.

Onychomycosis fungal infection of the fingernails or toenails.

Oocytes developing egg cells.

Oophorectomy surgical removal of the ovary.

Open cholecystectomy surgical procedure in which a gallbladder is removed through an abdominal incision.

Open-ended questions questions asked during a client interview that require discussion. See also *closed questions*.

Open head injury trauma to the head in which the scalp, bony cranium, and dura mater (the outer meningeal layer) are exposed.

Open method burn wound management technique in which the wound is left uncovered.

Open reduction surgical procedure in which a fractured bone is exposed and realigned.

Ophthalmoscopy examination of the fundus or interior of the eye.

Opiate dependence addiction to central nervous system depressant drugs (narcotics) that are either derived from or chemically similar to opium.

Opisthotonos extreme hyperextension of the head and arching of the back.

Opportunistic infections condition in which nonpathogenic or remotely pathogenic microorganisms take advantage of a favorable situation and overwhelm the host; also called *superinfections*.

Oral glucose tolerance test blood test used to evaluate a client's metabolism of orally ingested glucose.

Orchiectomy surgical removal of the testis.

Orchiopexy surgical procedure in which an undescended testis is secured within the scrotum.

Orchitis inflammation of the testis.

Orexin A and B neurohormones believed to contribute to binge eating and obesity in humans.

Orogastric intubation placement of a tube G through the mouth into the stomach.

Oropharynx part of the pharynx that is near the mouth.

Orthopnea breathing that is eased by sitting upright.

Osler's nodes purplish, painful nodules in the pads of the fingers and toes and palms and soles of the feet; indicative of bacterial endocarditis.

Osmoreceptors specialized neurons that sense the concentration of substances in blood.

Osmosis movement of water through a semipermeable membrane from a lower to higher concentration of solutes.

Ossification process in which inorganic minerals, such as calcium salts, are deposited in bone matrix.

Osteoblasts cells that build bones.

Osteoclasts cells involved in the destruction, resorption, and remodeling of bone.

Osteocytes mature bone cells involved in maintaining bone tissue.

Osteodystrophy condition in which the bones become demineralized as a result of hypocalcemia and hyperphosphatemia.

Osteomalacia metabolic bone disease characterized by inadequate mineralization of bone, resulting from a calcium or phosphate deficiency.

Osteomyelitis infection of the bone.

Osteoporosis disorder in which bone density decreases, resulting in porous and fragile bones.

Osteotomy procedure involving the cutting and removal of a wedge of bone (most often the tibia or femur) to change the bone's alignment and, as a result, improve function and relieve pain.

Ostomate client with an ostomy.

Ostomy surgically created opening between an internal body structure and the skin.

Otalgia sense of fullness or pain in the ears.

Otitis externa inflammation of the tissue within the outer ear.

Otitis media inflammation or infection in the middle ear.

Otorrhea leakage of cerebrospinal fluid from the ear.

Otosclerosis disorder characterized by a bony overgrowth on the stapes that is a common cause of hearing impairment among adults.

Otoscope hand-held instrument used to inspect the external acoustic canal and tympanic membrane.

Ototoxicity detrimental effect of certain medications on the eighth cranial nerve or hearing structures.

Ovaries female endocrine glands important in the development of secondary sex characteristics, the manufacture of hormones, and the development of ova.

Ovulation cyclical release of an ovum.

Ovum (pl., ova) female reproductive cell.

Oxytocin hormone that stimulates contraction of pregnant uterus and release of breast milk after childbirth.

P

P24 antigen test blood test that measures the number of viral particles in the blood and is used to guide drug therapy and follow the progression of a disease.

Pacemaker device that provides an electrical stimulus to the heart muscle to treat an abnormally slow cardiac rhythm.

Packed cells blood solution that has most of the plasma (fluid) removed; used for clients who need cellular replacements but do not need and may be harmed by the administration of additional fluid.

Paget's disease chronic bone disorder characterized by abnormal bone remodeling.

Pain privately experienced, unpleasant sensation usually associated with disease or injury.

Pain management techniques used to prevent, reduce, or relieve discomfort.

Pain perception conscious experience of discomfort.

Pain threshold point at which pain-transmitting neurochemicals reach the brain, causing conscious awareness of discomfort.

Pain tolerance amount of discomfort a person endures once the pain threshold has been reached.

Palliative treatment management of symptoms that reduces physical discomfort but does not alter a disease's progression.

Palpation assessing the characteristics of an organ or body part by touching and feeling it with the hands or fingertips.

Palsy decreased sensation and movement.

Pancolitis ulcerative colitis that affects the client's entire colon.

Pancreas gland with both exocrine and endocrine functions; the exocrine portion secretes digestive enzymes that the common bile duct carries to the small intestine, while the endocrine cells of the pancreas release insulin and glucagon.

Pancreatectomy (partial, total) surgical procedure in which some or all of the pancreas is removed.

Pancreatitis inflammation of the pancreas.

Pancytopenia conditions such as aplastic anemia in which numbers of all marrow-produced blood cells are reduced.

Pandemic rapidly spreading disease infecting large numbers of people throughout the world.

Panendoscopy examination of both the upper and lower GI tracts.

Panhysterectomy removal of the uterus, both fallopian tubes, and ovaries.

Panic disorder psychobiologic disorder in which a person experiences an abrupt onset of physical symptoms and terror.

Pannus destructive vascular granulation tissue.

Papanicolaou test test in which a sample of exfoliated cells are obtained during a pelvic examination and used to detect early cancer of the cervix, determine estrogen activity as it relates to menopause, or detect endocrine abnormalities.

Papilledema swelling of the optic nerve.

Paralanguage vocal sounds that communicate a message but that are not words.

Paralytic ileus disorder in which the intestine becomes adynamic from an absence of normal nerve stimulation to intestinal muscle fibers.

Paranasal sinuses extensions of the nasal cavity located in the surrounding facial bones.

Paraplegia paralysis of both legs resulting from spinal injuries at the thoracic level.

Parasympathetic nervous system division of the autonomic nervous system that works to conserve body energy and is partly responsible for slowing heart rate, digesting food, and eliminating body wastes.

Parathormone hormone that regulates the metabolism of calcium and phosphorus.

Parathyroid glands four small bean-shaped bodies embedded in the lateral lobes of the thyroid that secrete parathormone.

Paresthesia sensation of numbness and tingling.

Parietal pericardium tough outer layer of the pericardium

Parietal pleura saclike serous membrane that is the outer layer of the lungs.

Parkinsonism cluster of Parkinson-like symptoms that develop from several etiologies.

Paroxysmal nocturnal dyspnea being awakened by breathlessness.

Partial (or segmental) mastectomy surgical procedure in which the breast, axillary lymph nodes, and pectoralis major and minor muscles are removed. In some instances, sternal lymph nodes also are removed.

Passive diffusion process in which dissolved substances such as electrolytes move from an area of high concentration of solutes to an area of lower concentration of solutes through a semipermeable membrane.

Passive immunity immediate but short-lived immunity that develops when ready-made antibodies are given to a susceptible individual.

Past health history information obtained during a client interview regarding a client's childhood diseases, previous injuries, major illnesses, prior hospitalizations, surgical procedures, and drug history.

Pathogens microorganisms that have a high potential to cause infectious diseases.

Patient-focused care system of nursing care in which an RN partnered with one or more assistive personnel cares for a group of clients.

Pedagogy teaching children or people with cognitive ability comparable to children.

Pediculosis infestation with lice.

Pelvic inflammatory disease infection of the pelvic organs such as the uterus, fallopian tubes, pelvic vascular system, and pelvic supporting structures.

Peptic ulcer disease circumscribed erosion of tissue in an area of the GI tract that is in contact with hydrochloric acid and pepsin.

Perception phase of pain impulse transmission during which the brain experiences pain at a conscious level, helps to discriminate the location of the pain, determines its intensity, attaches meaningfulness to the event, and provokes emotional responses.

Percussion tapping a portion of the body to determine if there is tenderness or to elicit sounds that vary according to the density of underlying structures.

Percutaneous endoscopic gastrostomy (PEG) procedure in which an endoscope is introduced orally and advanced into the stomach so that the physician can see the correct location for a gastronomy tube.

Percutaneous liver biopsy procedure in which a small core of liver tissue is obtained by placing a needle directly into the liver through the lateral abdominal wall.

Percutaneous transluminal coronary angioplasty procedure in which a balloon-tipped catheter is inserted into a diseased coronary artery, then inflated to compress atherosclerotic plaque.

Perfusion supplying blood to cells, tissues, or organs.

Pericardiectomy surgical removal of the pericardium to allow more adequate filling and contraction of the heart chambers.

Pericardiocentesis needle aspiration of fluid from between the visceral and parietal pericardium.

Pericardiostomy procedure in which a surgical opening is made in the pericardium to drain fluid.

Pericarditis inflammation of the pericardium.

Pericardium sac-like structure that surrounds and supports the heart.

Perioperative entire time span of surgery, including before and after the actual operation.

Periorbital ecchymosis condition in which both eyes are blackened; also called "raccoon eyes."

Periorbital edema puffiness around the eyes.

Periosteum outer layer of bones that is rich in blood and lymph vessels, and supplies the bone with nourishment.

Peripheral nervous system part of the nervous system consisting of all nerves outside the central nervous system.

Peripheral vascular disease disorders that affect blood vessels distant from the large central blood vessels supplying the myocardium or that circulate blood directly in and out of the heart.

Peripheral venous sites superficial veins of the arm and hand; the most common sites for infusing IV fluids.

Peristalsis coordinated wavelike muscular contractions.

Peritoneal dialysis technique that uses the peritoneum, the semi-permeable membrane lining of the abdomen, to filter fluid, wastes, and chemicals.

Peritonitis inflammation of the peritoneum, the serous sac lining the abdominal cavity.

Peritonsillar abscess infection that develops in the connective tissue between the capsule of the tonsil and the constrictor muscle of the pharynx.

Personal space distance between two people that is appropriate for one-on-one interactions like interviewing and physical assessment.

Pessary firm, doughnut-shaped or ring device that can be inserted into the upper vagina to reposition and give support to the uterus when surgery cannot be done or if the client declines surgery.

Petechiae tiny reddish hemorrhagic spots on the skin and mucous membranes.

Phagocytes white blood cells that engulf and digest bacteria and foreign material.

Phagocytosis process of engulfing and digesting bacteria and foreign material.

Pharyngitis inflammation of the throat.

Pharynx body structure that carries air from the nose to the larynx, and food from the mouth to the esophagus.

Phenotype testing blood test used to detect drug resistance in which a measured amount of antiviral drug is mixed with a virus until there is a quantity that prevents the virus from reproducing.

Pheochromocytoma tumor of the adrenal medulla that causes hyperfunction.

Pheromones hormone-like chemicals that communicate reproductive and social information among a species.

Phlebitis inflammation of the vein.

Phlebothrombosis clot formation with minimal or no venous inflammation.

Phobic disorder psychobiologic disorder in which a person develops an exaggerated fear.

Phonocardiography graphic representation of normal and abnormal heart sounds.

Phosgene liquid respiratory toxin that becomes a gas when released in the atmosphere.

Photochemotherapy combination of ultraviolet light therapy and a photosensitizing psoralen drug; used for severe, disabling psoriasis that does not respond to other methods of treatment.

Photoperiods daytime hours that are short because of fewer hours of sunlight.

Photophobia sensitivity to light.

Phototherapy technique for treating seasonal affective disorder with artificial light that simulates the intensity of sunlight.

Physical assessment examination of a client's body structures.

Physical dependence condition in which a person experiences physical discomfort when a drug that he or she has taken routinely is abruptly discontinued.

Physician hospital organization creation of a corporate structure between a hospital and a group of its physicians by contracting with a managed care organization to negotiate fees for services for their self-insured employees.

Phytoestrogens plant sources of estrogen.

Pia mater delicate inner membrane that adheres to the brain and spinal cord.

Pilonidal sinus infection in the hair follicles in the sacrococcygeal area above the anus.

Pineal gland gland attached to the thalamus that secretes melatonin, which aids in regulating sleep cycles and mood.

Pitting edema indentations in the skin following compression.

Pituitary gland gland that regulates the function of the other endocrine glands.

Placebo inert or inactive substance that by its very nature cannot alter physiology, but does in a significant number of people.

Placebo effect healing or improvement that takes place simply because an individual believes a treatment method will be effective.

Planning step of the nursing process that involves setting priorities, defining expected outcomes, determining specific nursing interventions, and recording the plan of care.

Plaque fatty deposits composed chiefly of cholesterol.

Plasma liquid, or serum, portion of blood.

Plasma cells B-cell lymphocytes that produce antibodies.

Plasma expanders nonblood solutions that pull fluid into the vascular space and are used as an economical and virus-free substitute for blood and blood products.

Platelets disk-like cell fragments in blood that help control bleeding by forming a loose blood clot.

Pleura saclike serous membrane located around the lungs.

Pleural effusion collection of fluid between the visceral and parietal pleurae.

Pleural space area containing serous fluid that separates and lubricates the visceral and parietal pleurae.

Pleurisy inflammation of the pleura.

Pluripotential stem cells undifferentiated precursors in the bone marrow from which all blood cells develop.

Pneumoconiosis fibrous inflammation or chronic induration of the lungs after prolonged exposure to dust or gases.

Pneumocystis pneumonia type of pneumonia rare among individuals with intact immune systems, but clients infected with HIV are at particular risk for acquiring.

Pneumonectomy surgical removal of an entire lung.

Pneumonia inflammatory process affecting the bronchioles and alveoli.

Pneumothorax air that enters the pleural space causing a lung to collapse.

Podiatrist practitioner who specializes in the care for feet.

Poikilothermia condition in which the temperature of the body varies with that of the environment.

Point of maximum impulse place on the chest wall where heart pulsations are most strongly felt.

Point of service (POS) plan network of providers in which clients select a primary care physician within the group who then serves as the gatekeeper for other healthcare services.

Polarization stage during diastole when positive ions predominate outside myocardial cell membranes and negative ions predominate inside.

Polyarthritis inflammation of more than one joint.

Polycystic ovarian syndrome condition that affects women 20 to 40 years of age, characterized by a cluster of signs and symptoms that include amenorrhea and oligomenorrhea.

Polydipsia excessive thirst.

Polydrug abuse abuse of more than one substance.

Polymerase chain reaction test measures the number of viral particles in the blood and is used to guide drug therapy and follow the progression of HIV infection.

Polyphagia excessive eating.

Polysomnography test that monitors a client's respiratory and cardiac status while he or she is asleep to determine the nature of sleep apnea.

Polyuria excessive urine production.

Pons part of the brain located between the midbrain and medulla.

Portal hypertension congestion and increased fluid pressure in the venous pathway through the liver.

Portal of entry route through which an infectious agent gains entrance into a susceptible host.

Portal of exit route through which an infectious agent exits from a reservoir.

Positive inotropic agents drugs with beta-adrenergic activity that increase the heart rate and improve the force of heart contraction.

Positive symptoms delusions, hallucinations, and fluent but disorganized speech that are characteristic of schizophrenia.

Possible diagnosis nursing diagnosis that identifies problems for which the data are undeveloped or incomplete. See also *actual diagnosis* and *risk diagnosis*.

Postoperative phase of perioperative care that begins with admission to the recovery area and continues until the client receives a follow-up evaluation at home or is discharged to a rehabilitation unit.

Postphlebitic syndrome vascular complication which occurs up to 5 years after treatment of thrombophlebitis.

Postprandial glucose blood test used to assess blood sugar following a meal.

Post-traumatic stress disorder condition that involves a delayed anxiety response 3 or more months after an emotionally traumatic experience.

Postvoid residual amount of urine left in the bladder after voiding.

Potassium iodide prophylaxis for protecting the thyroid gland from absorption of radiation.

Power ability to control, influence, or hold authority over an individual or group.

Prebiotics nondigestible food ingredients like dietary fiber that beneficially affect a host by stimulating or inhibiting bacteria in the colon.

Precordial pain pain in the anterior chest overlying the heart.

Pre-diabetes condition characterized by impaired fasting glucose (level of 100 to 125 mg/dL after an overnight fast), impaired glucose tolerance (level of 140 to 199 mg/dL after a glucose tolerance test lasting 2 hours), or both.

Preferred provider organization insurer that creates a community network of providers willing to discount their fees for service in exchange for a steady supply of referred customers.

Prehypertension systolic blood pressure of 120 to 139 mm Hg or diastolic blood pressure between 80 and 89 mm Hg.

Preictal phase time immediately before a tonic-clonic seizure consisting of vague emotional changes, such as depression, anxiety, and nervousness.

Preload degree of stretch of the cardiac muscle fibers at the end of diastole.

Premature atrial contraction early electrical impulse initiated by neural tissue in the atria.

Premature ovarian failure disorder characterized by irregular menses and symptoms that resemble natural menopause; occurs when the ovaries cease to function in women younger than 40 years.

Premature ventricular contraction ventricular contraction that occurs early and independently in the cardiac cycle before the sinoatrial node initiates an electrical impulse.

Premenstrual syndrome group of physical and emotional symptoms that occur in some women 7 to 10 days before menstruation.

Preoperative phase of perioperative care beginning with the decision to perform surgery and continuing until the client reaches the operating area.

Presbycusis hearing loss associated with aging.

Presbyopia condition in which visual accommodation, the ability to focus an image on the retina, gradually declines with aging, as a result of lens inelasticity.

Pressure infusion sleeve device wrapped around an IV solution bag that exerts a squeezing action to facilitate rapid infusion.

Pressure sores skin impairment that occurs when capillary blood flow to an area is reduced, as when the skin over a bony prominence is compressed between the weight of the body and a hard surface for a prolonged period.

Primary care initial resource, person, or agency that a client contacts about a health need.

Primary nursing system of nursing care in which an RN assumes 24-hour accountability for a client's care and has total responsibility for the nursing care of assigned clients during his or her shift.

Primary tubing long tubing used to administer a large volume of IV solution over an extended period or a small volume through a medication lock.

Prion protein that does not contain nucleic acid and that, after undergoing a mutant change, is capable of becoming an infectious agent.

Probiotics microorganisms that exert beneficial health effects, such as *Lactobacillus acidophilus* to lower the frequency or duration of diarrhea.

Procedural sedation (conscious sedation) state in which clients are free of pain, fear, and anxiety and can tolerate unpleasant procedures while maintaining independent cardiorespiratory function and the ability to respond to verbal commands and tactile stimulation.

Procreate to reproduce.

Proctosigmoidoscopy examination of the rectum and sigmoid colon using a rigid endoscope inserted anally.

Progesterone hormone produced by the ovaries.

Prolactin hormone that promotes production and secretion of milk after childbirth.

Proprietary agencies term that often refers to for-profit agencies.

Proptosis disorder in which an extended or protruded upper eyelid delays closing or remains partially open.

Prostatectomy surgical removal of the prostate.

Prostatic specific antigen tumor marker whose presence in blood sometimes indicates prostate cancer.

Prosthesis an artificial device to replace a body part such as a joint.

Protease viral enzyme that cuts long chains of replicated viral particles and releases them into the cytoplasm of a cell.

Protease inhibitor antiretroviral drug that inhibits the ability of HIV particles to leave the host cell.

Proxemics use of space when communicating.

Pruritus itching.

Prussian blue dye used to treat internal contamination with ingested radioactive cesium.

Psoriasis chronic, noninfectious inflammatory disorder of the skin in which the cells of the epidermis proliferate so quickly that the upper layer of cells cannot be shed fast enough to make room for the newly produced cells.

Psyche mind.

Psychic numbing technique for coping with a tragedy in which the affected person avoids dealing with the tragedy and detaches himself or herself from others.

Psychobiologic disorders those conditions in which evidence supports a link between biologic abnormalities in the brain and altered cognition, perception, emotion, behavior, and socialization.

Psychobiology study of the biochemical basis of thought, behavior, affect, and mood.

Psychomotor agitation state characterized by insomnia, pacing, and distractibility.

Psychomotor learner person who processes information best by doing.

Psychomotor retardation state characterized by a lack of energy, increased sleep, and little interest in daily events or responsibilities.

Psychoneuroendocrinology study of how fluctuations in pituitary, adrenal, thyroid, and reproductive hormones alter cognition, perception, behavior, and mood.

Psychoneuroimmunology study of the connections among the emotions, central nervous system, neuroendocrine system, and immunologic system.

Psychosocial history information obtained during a client interview about the client's age, occupation, religious affiliation, cultural background, marital status, and home and working environments.

Psychosomatic diseases medical conditions associated with or aggravated by stress.

Psychotherapy treatment in which a client talks with a psychiatrist, psychologist, or mental health counselor to cope with emotional problems, gain insight into behaviors, and learn techniques that can improve well-being.

Psychotic depression extreme form of depressive disorder.

Ptosis drooping of the eyelids.

Puberty stage marked by the onset of sexual maturation.

Public space distance between people that is appropriate for large group interactions such as speeches and meetings with strangers.

Pulmonary artery only artery that carries deoxygenated blood; branches to deliver venous blood to the right and left lung.

Pulmonary capillary wedge pressure retrograde pressure from the fluid on the left side of the heart at the end of left ventricular diastole.

Pulmonary contusion crushing bruise of the lung.

Pulmonary edema fluid accumulation in the interstitium and alveoli of the lungs which interferes with gas exchange in the alveoli.

Pulmonary embolus thrombus that migrates to the pulmonary circulation.

Pulmonary hypertension high pressure within pulmonary circulation.

Pulmonary vascular bed capillary network surrounding the alveoli.

Pulmonic valve opening between the right ventricle of the heart and the pulmonary artery.

Pulsus paradoxus assessment finding characterized by a difference of 10 mm Hg or more between the first Korotkoff sound heralding systolic blood pressure heard during expiration and the first that is heard during inspiration.

Purge elimination of consumed nutrients with self-induced vomiting, laxatives, enemas, or diuretics.

PY test test in which a client's breath is analyzed after consuming ^{14}C-urea capsules to detect *Helicobacter pylori,* the bacteria associated with peptic ulcer disease.

Pyelonephritis acute or chronic bacterial infection of the kidney and the lining of the collecting system (kidney pelvis).

Pyeloplasty surgical repair of the ureteropelvic junction.

Pyramidal (motor tracts) motor pathways that originate in the motor cortex of the cerebrum, cross over at the level of the medulla, and end in the brain stem and spinal cord.

Pyrosis burning sensation in the esophagus.

Pyuria pus (a combination of bacteria and leukocytes) in the urine.

R

R on T phenomenon premature ventricular contraction whose R wave falls on the T wave of the preceding complex.

Race biologic differences in physical features such as skin color, bone structure, and eye shape, as opposed to ethnic or cultural differences.

Radiation therapy technique that uses high-energy ionizing radiation, such as high-energy x-rays, gamma rays, and radioactive particles (alpha and beta particles, neutrons, and protons) to destroy cancer cells.

Radical pancreaticoduodenectomy (Whipple procedure) surgical procedure to resect a tumor at the head of the pancreas.

Radiofrequency catheter ablation procedure in which a heated catheter tip destroys dysrhythmia-producing tissue.

Radioimmunoassay study that determines the concentration of a radioactive substance in blood plasma.

Radiologic disasters events in which people, animals, and the environment are exposed to harmful levels of gamma radiation.

Radionuclide atom with an unstable nucleus that emits electromagnetic radiation.

Radionuclide imaging technique used to detect lesions in organs using a radioactive natural or synthetic element that is injected intravenously or ingested orally.

Random blood glucose diagnostic test in which a blood specimen is obtained after 8 hours of fasting to test its glucose level.

Rapid opiate detoxification procedure for accelerating opiate drug withdrawal within 4 to 8 hours while the client is under anesthesia.

Reactive (secondary) depression feeling of sadness that can be directly attributed to a situation or cause. See also *major (unipolar) depression.*

Receptive aphasia neurologic impairment of a person's ability to understand spoken and written language.

Receptor structures found on the surface of cells to which chemical messengers attach.

Recommended dietary allowance the level of an essential nutrient necessary to meet the needs of most healthy persons.

Rectocele herniation of the rectum into the vagina.

Red bone marrow substance that manufactures blood cells and hemoglobin.

Reduction mammoplasty surgical procedure in which glandular breast tissue, fat, and skin are removed to decrease the size of large pendulous breasts.

Reed-Sternberg cells malignant cells resulting from mutated lymphocytes that are indicative of Hodgkin's disease.

Reemerging infectious disease disorder caused by microorganisms that are new or have had a resurgence in the last 2 decades within and beyond a geographic range.

Referred pain discomfort that is perceived in a general area of the body, but not in the exact site where a diseased organ is anatomically located.

Reflex incontinence disorder in which a client lacks awareness of the urge to void.

Reflexology technique of applying manual pressure to reflex centers on the feet and hands to promote natural healing.

Refraction changing of direction and speed of a ray of light.

Refractory period time in diastole during which cells are resistant to electrical stimulation.

Regulator T cells T-cell lymphocytes made up of helper and suppressor cells.

Reiki Japanese technique of healing by transferring energy through the laying-on of hands.

Relapse (1) exacerbation of an illness; (2) return of a recovering alcoholic to drinking.

Remission asymptomatic periods of a disorder.

Renal arteriogram study of the arterial supply to the kidneys using radiopaque dye.

Renal threshold ability of the kidney to reabsorb glucose and return it to the bloodstream.

Renin-angiotensin-aldosterone system chain of chemicals that increases both blood pressure and blood volume.

Repolarization stage in cardiac electrophysiology when ions realign themselves in their original position and wait for an electrical impulse.

Reservoir human, animal, or nonliving environment in which an infectious agent can survive and reproduce.

Residual urine urine retained in the bladder after the client voids.

Resorption reduction of bone tissue.

Resource management method of using money, supplies, equipment, buildings, and personnel optimally.

Respiration exchange of oxygen and CO_2 between atmospheric air and the blood and between the blood and the cells.

Respiratory toxin chemical agent that primarily causes pulmonary edema when inhaled.

Respite care use of family and friends for brief relief from caregiving responsibilities.

Responsibility duty to perform a specific task.

Restraint alternatives protective or adaptive devices for fall protection and postural support that the client can release independently.

Restrictive lung disease decreased volume of the lungs with an inability to expand completely.

Retention inability to urinate or effectively empty the bladder.

Retinal detachment disorder in which the sensory layer becomes separated from the pigmented layer of the retina.

Retrograde ejaculation condition in which semen is deposited in the bladder rather than discharged through the urethra at the time of orgasm.

Retrograde pyelogram study that provides visualization of the complete ureter and renal pelvis using a radiopaque contrast medium instilled with a urethral catheter.

Reuptake reabsorption.

Reverse transcriptase enzyme that copies RNA into DNA.

Reverse transcriptase inhibitor antiretroviral drug that interferes with the human immunodeficiency virus' ability to make a genetic blueprint.

Reverse transcription process in which the enzyme reverse transcriptase copies RNA into DNA.

Rheumatic carditis inflammatory cardiac manifestations of rheumatic fever in either the acute or later stage.

Rheumatic disorders term for different types of recognized inflammatory disorders that involve inflammation and degeneration of connective tissue structures, especially joints.

Rheumatoid arthritis systemic inflammatory disorder of connective tissue/joints characterized by chronicity, remissions, and exacerbations.

Rh factor protein surface marker on red blood cells.

Rhinitis inflammation of the nasal mucous membranes; also referred to as coryza or the common cold.

Rhinophyma skin condition of inflamed tissue that causes the nose to become permanently enlarged, red, nodular, and bulbous.

Rhinorrhea (1) clear nasal discharge; (2) leakage of cerebrospinal fluid from the nose.

Rhythmicity ability of cardiac tissue to repeat its cycle with regularity.

Rights freedoms or actions to which individuals have a just moral or legal claim.

Right-sided heart failure condition that occurs when the right ventricle fails to completely eject its diastolic filling volume.

Rinne test assessment technique used to detect hearing loss by comparing bone conduction and air conduction of sound using a tuning fork.

Risk diagnosis nursing diagnosis that identifies potential problems. See also *actual diagnosis* and *possible diagnosis*.

Risk management process of reviewing the problems that occur at the workplace, identifying common elements, and then developing methods to reduce the potential for reoccurrence.

Romberg test assessment technique used to evaluate a person's ability to sustain balance.

Rosacea chronic skin disorder characterized by a "rosy" appearance; generally affects fair-skinned people 30 to 60 years old.

Rotator cuff shoulder joint where tears can develop from traumatic injury or chronic overuse.

Roth's spots white areas in the retina surrounded by areas of hemorrhage.

Rule of one hundreds cluster of signs indicating sedative (alcohol) withdrawal; evidenced by body temperature greater than or equal to 100°F, pulse rate greater than or equal to 100 beats/min, or diastolic blood pressure greater than or equal to 100 mm Hg.

S

Safe sex practices sexual activities in which body fluids are not exchanged.

Salpingo-oophorectomy surgical removal of the ovary and fallopian tube.

Salvaged blood blood collected and reinfused during surgery or shortly thereafter.

Salvage therapy treatment option for individuals who have developed significant HIV drug resistance with limited possibilities for effective drug management.

Sarin dangerous nerve agent.

Satiety feeling of comfortable fullness that signals to stop eating.

Scabies skin disorder caused by infestation with the itch mite.

Schizophrenia thought disorder characterized by deterioration in mental functioning, disturbances in sensory perception, and changes in affect.

Seasonal affective disorder mood disorder characterized by depressive feelings that develop during darker winter months and then disappear in months with more sunlight.

Sebaceous glands glands that are connected to each hair follicle and secrete an oily substance called sebum.

Sebum lubricant released from hair follicles that prevents drying and cracking of the skin and hair.

Secondary hypertension elevated blood pressure that results from some other disorder.

Secondary tubing short intravenous tubing used to administer smaller volumes of solution through a port in the primary tubing.

Segmental resection (1) surgical procedure in which the cancerous portion of a colon is removed and the remaining portions of the GI tract are rejoined to restore normal intestinal continuity; (2) surgical removal of a lobe segment of the lung.

Seizure brief episode of abnormal electrical activity in the brain.

Sensitivity studies performed to determine which antibiotic inhibits the growth of a nonviral microorganism and will be most effective in treating an infection.

Sensitization development of antibodies to an antigen.

Sensorineural hearing loss hearing loss that is the result of nerve impairment.

Sentinel lymph node mapping/biopsy technique for identifying the first (sentinel) lymph nodes through which breast cancer cells spread to regional lymph nodes in the axilla using a nuclear isotope and blue dye.

Sepsis systemic inflammatory response syndrome resulting from infection.

Septicemia condition resulting from microorganisms escaping the lymph nodes and reaching the bloodstream, which may lead to sepsis.

Septic shock shock associated with overwhelming bacterial infections; also called toxic shock.

Septum tissue that separates two cavities; for example, the tissue that separates the right side of the heart from the left side.

Sequela condition that follows a disease.

Sequestrum pocket of necrotic bone.

Serotonin monoamine neurotransmitter that is lower in depressed people.

Serotonin syndrome potentially life-threatening condition that results from elevated levels of serotonin in the blood.

Serum osmolality concentration of substances in blood.

Severe sepsis pre-septic shock condition that develops when sepsis is combined with organ hypoperfusion.

Shearing physical force that separates layers of tissue in opposite directions, for example, when a seated client slides downward.

Shiatsu application of pressure within various body meridians, or energy channels, to rebalance the body's energy and restore health.

Shingles skin disorder that develops years after an infection with varicella (chickenpox).

Shock life-threatening condition that occurs when arterial blood flow and oxygen delivery to tissues and cells are inadequate.

Short bowel syndrome loss of absorptive surface resulting from the surgical removal of a large amount of intestine.

Sickle cell anemia hereditary disease in which erythrocytes become sickle- or crescent-shaped when oxygen supply in the blood is inadequate.

Signing shortened term for American Sign Language communication.

Sign language method of communication that uses a hand-spelled alphabet and word symbols.

Signs abnormal objective data; see also *symptoms*.

Silicosis fibrous inflammation or chronic induration of the lungs caused by the inhalation of silica.

Simmonds' disease rare endocrine disorder caused by destruction of the pituitary gland.

Simple (or total) mastectomy surgical procedure in which all breast tissue is removed, but no lymph node dissection is performed.

Single-barrel colostomy opening to the colon that has a single stoma through which fecal matter is released.

Sinus bradycardia dysrhythmia that proceeds normally through the conduction pathway but at a slower than usual rate (≤ 60 beats/min).

Sinusitis inflammation of the sinuses.

Sinus tachycardia dysrhythmia that proceeds normally through the conduction pathway but at a faster than usual rate (100 to 150 beats/min).

Skeletal muscles voluntary muscles that promote movement of the bones of the skeleton.

Skin tear shallow break in the skin.

Skin tenting assessment finding in which skin remains elevated and is slow to return to underlying tissue when pinched.

Skip lesions randomly occurring inflamed areas of the bowel alternating with healthy tissue.

Sleep apnea syndrome phenomenon characterized by frequent, brief episodes of respiratory standstill during sleep.

Slit graft skin graft in which skin is removed from a client's donor site and passed through an instrument that perforates it in multiple places so that a smaller piece of skin can be stretched to cover a larger area.

Smallpox highly contagious disease caused by the variola virus appearing as raised bumps on the face and body.

Social phobia fear of being in situations in which one must perform in front of or may capture the attention of others.

Social space distance between people that is appropriate in small group interactions such as lecturing or non-private conversations.

Soma body.

Somatic pain pain that arises from mechanical, chemical, thermal, or electrical injuries or disorders affecting bones, joints, muscles, skin, or other structures composed of connective tissue.

Somatostatin hormone secreted by delta islet cells that helps to maintain a relatively constant level of blood glucose by inhibiting the release of insulin and glucagons.

Somatotropin hormone that stimulates bone and muscle growth and promotes protein synthesis and fat mobilization.

Spastic colon paroxysmal intestinal motility disorder characterized by alternating periods of constipation and diarrhea.

Speech reading perception of conversation by following the movements of a speaker's lips.

Spermatocytes immature spermatozoa.

Spermatozoon (pl., spermatozoa) male reproductive cell.

Sphenoidal sinuses bony cavities that lie behind the nasal cavity.

Spinal fusion surgical procedure in which two or more vertebrae are immobilized.

Spinal shock loss of sympathetic reflex activity below the level of injury within 30 to 60 minutes of a spinal injury.

Spiritual healing restoration of health through a higher power such as God or some other metaphysical force.

Splint thin piece of wood or strip that immobilizes and supports an injured body part in a functional position.

Splinter hemorrhages black longitudinal lines in the nails.

Split-thickness graft skin graft in which the epidermis and a thin layer of dermis are harvested from the client's skin.

Sprain injuries to the ligaments surrounding a joint.

Stage 1 hypertension systolic blood pressure of 140 to 150 mm Hg or diastolic blood pressure between 90 and 99 mm Hg.

Stage 2 hypertension systolic blood pressure that equals or exceeds 160 mm Hg or diastolic pressure that equals or exceeds 100 mm Hg.

Standards of practice guidelines established by the nursing profession for clinical decision-making that evolve as research and evidence change treatments and procedures.

Stapedectomy surgical procedure to improve hearing loss in which all or part of the stapes is removed and a prosthesis is inserted.

Starling's law principle of physiology in which the strength of ventricular contraction is related to the blood-filling stretch of the myocardium.

Status epilepticus condition marked by a series of tonic-clonic seizures in which the client does not regain consciousness between seizures.

Statute of limitations designated time in which a person can file a lawsuit.

Statutory law law that any local, state, or federal legislative body enacts.

Steatorrhea increased fat in the stool resulting from poor fat digestion.

Stem cells undifferentiated precursors to various types of cells including lymphocytes, neutrophils, and monocytes.

Stereotyping assumption that all people within a particular cultural, racial, or ethnic group share the same values and beliefs, behave similarly, and are basically alike.

Sterility an inability to conceive.

Stoma surgically created opening on the exterior abdominal surface.

Stomatitis inflammation of the mouth.

Strain injury to a muscle when it is stretched or pulled beyond its capacity.

Stratum corneum outer lay of dead skin cells in the epidermis.

Stress physiologic response to biologic stressors such as surgical trauma or infection, psychological stressors such as worry and fear, or sociologic stressors such as starting a new job or increased family responsibilities.

Stress management technique for minimizing the harmful effects of stress through relaxation techniques and effective coping strategies.

Stress-related disorder medical condition associated with or aggravated by stress.

Stricture narrowing.

Stridor high-pitched, harsh sound during respiration, indicative of airway obstruction.

Stroke volume amount of blood pumped per contraction of the heart.

Subarachnoid space area between the pia mater and the arachnoid membrane.

Subculture particular group which shares characteristics that identify it as a distinct entity.

Subcutaneous emphysema presence of air in subcutaneous tissues.

Subcutaneous mastectomy surgical procedure in which all breast tissue is removed, but the skin and nipple are left intact.

Subcutaneous tissue layer of skin attached to muscle and bone that is primarily composed of connective tissue and fat cells.

Subdural hematoma bleeding below the dura mater that results from venous bleeding.

Subendocardial infarction death of tissue that does not extend through the full thickness of the myocardial wall.

Subjective data information based on statements the client makes about what he or she feels (e.g., nausea, pain).

Subluxation partial dislocation.

Substance abuse use of a drug that is different from its accepted purpose.

Sulfur mustard chemical that damages exposed skin and mucous membranes on contact and can damage respiratory tissues if inhaled.

Superinfections conditions in which nonpathogenic or remotely pathogenic microorganisms overwhelm the host; also called *opportunistic infections.*

Superior vena cava large blood vessel that delivers unoxygenated blood from the upper body to the right atrium.

Supervision process of guiding, directing, evaluating, and following-up on tasks delegated to others.

Suppressor T cells cells that limit or turn off the immune response in the absence of continued antigenic stimulation.

Supratentorial above the tentorium.

Supraventricular tachycardia atrial dysrhythmia in which the heart rate is dangerously high ($\geq$150 beats/min).

Surgical asepsis sterile technique.

Susceptibility potential for infection or disease.

Sweat glands structures within the dermis that release water and electrolytes or secrete substances such as cerumen.

Sympathectomy procedure that interrupts or suppresses some portion of the sympathetic nerve pathway.

Sympathetic nervous system division of the autonomic nervous system that accelerates the expenditure of energy.

Symptoms physical experiences reported by a client. See also *signs.*

Synapses junctions between the axon of one neuron and the dendrite of another.

Syncope sudden loss of consciousness.

Syndrome diagnosis nursing diagnosis that is associated with a cluster of other diagnoses.

Syndrome of inappropriate antidiuretic hormone secretion phenomenon that alters fluid and electrolyte balance due to excessive release of ADH.

Synovitis inflammation of a synovial membrane of a joint.

Syphilis sexually transmitted infection caused by the spirochete *Treponema pallidum* that can be transmitted directly from an infected person or across the placenta to an unborn infant.

Systemic inflammatory response syndrome (SIRS) inflammatory state without a proven source of infection.

Systemic lupus erythematosus a diffuse connective tissue disease.

Systems method technique for carrying out an examination by assessing each body system separately. See also *head-to-toe method.*

Systolic blood pressure arterial pressure during ventricular contraction.

T

Tabes dorsalis degenerative condition of the central nervous system that results in the loss of peripheral reflexes and of vibratory and position senses.

Tachydysrhythmias abnormally fast cardiac rhythms.

Tachypnea increased rate of breathing.

Tai chi technique developed in China that combines mental and physical exercises for the purpose of integrating body and mind.

Task-oriented touch personal contact with a client that is required when performing nursing procedures. See also *affective touch.*

Tattoo pigmentation of the dermal layer of skin with injection of needles containing dye.

Tau abnormal protein that causes microtubules within neurons of the brain to clump together forming neurofibrillary tangles.

Teaching plan organized arrangement of information to be conveyed in a specific time frame.

Team nursing system of nursing care in which teams made up of an RN team leader, other RNs, LP/LVNs, and nursing assistants provide care to a group of clients.

Telemetry process of sending ECG information over radio waves to a monitor that is distant from the client.

Telephonic interpreting over-the phone translation of foreign language.

Tendon cordlike structures that attach muscles to the periosteum of the bone.

Tendonitis inflammation of a tendon caused by overuse.

Tenesmus urgent desire to evacuate the bowel.

Tentorium double fold of dura mater in the brain that separates the cerebrum from the cerebellum.

Terminating phase stage of the nurse-client relationship reached when the nurse and client mutually agree that the client's immediate health problems have improved and the nurse's services are no longer necessary.

Terrorists people whose objective is to manipulate the politics and policies of a country by frightening and maiming its civilian population.

Tertiary care treatment management for clients in facilities where specialists and complex technology are available.

Testes male sex glands, important in the development of secondary sex characteristics, the manufacture of hormones, and the development of sperm.

Testicular self-examination technique for examining one's own testicles to detect any abnormal mass within the scrotum.

Testosterone hormone produced by the testes for the development and maintenance of male secondary sex characteristics, such as facial hair and a deep voice.

Tetany group of signs and symptoms associated with hypocalcemia.

Tetraiodothyronine hormone synthesized by the thyroid gland that regulates the body's metabolic rate; also known as T_4.

Tetraplegia paralysis of all extremities due to a high cervical spine injury.

Therapeutic communication using words and gestures to promote a person's physical and emotional well-being.

Third-spacing translocation of fluid from the intravascular or intercellular spaces to tissue compartments, where it becomes trapped and useless.

Thirst mechanism that promotes increased intake of oral fluid.

Thoracentesis aspiration of excess fluid or air from the pleural space.

Thoracotomy surgical opening of the thorax.

Thrill vibration.

Thrombectomy surgical removal of a thrombus (clot).

Thromboangiitis obliterans inflammation of blood vessels associated with clot formation and fibrosis of the blood vessel wall.

Thrombocytopenia decreased platelet count.

Thrombolytic agents drugs that dissolve blood clots.

Thrombophlebitis inflammation of a vein accompanied by clot or thrombus formation.

Thrombosis formation of a blood clot.

Thrombus stationary blood clot.

Thymopoietin hormone that aids in the proliferation and differentiation of T lymphocytes.

Thymosin hormone that aids in developing T lymphocytes, a type of white blood cell involved in immunity.

Thymus gland gland located in the upper part of the chest above or near the heart that secretes thymosin.

Thyroid gland structure located in the lower neck that concentrates iodine from food and uses it to synthesize tetraiodothyronine (thyroxine or T_4) and triiodothyronine (T_3).

Thyroiditis inflammation of the thyroid gland.

Thyroid-stimulating hormone (TSH) pituitary hormone that stimulates the production and secretion of thyroid hormones.

Thyrotoxic crisis abrupt and life-threatening form of hyperthyroidism, thought to be triggered by extreme stress, infection, diabetic ketoacidosis, trauma, toxemia of pregnancy, or manipulation of a hyperactive thyroid gland during surgery or physical examination.

Tilt-table test diagnostic test in which a client lays horizontally on a table that is elevated to approximately 70° for 45 minutes while blood pressure and pulse are monitored.

Time management organization and delegation of tasks to make optimal use of one's time.

Tinnitus disorder in which a client hears buzzing, whistling, or ringing noises in one or both ears.

Tolerance condition in which a client needs larger doses of a drug to achieve the same effect as when the drug was first administered.

Tonometry measurement of intraocular pressure.

Tonsillectomy surgical removal of the tonsils.

Tonsillitis inflammation of the tonsils.

Tonsils elliptically shaped lymphoid tissue located on either side of the upper oropharynx that protect the body from infection.

Tophi collections of urate crystals found in the cartilage of the outer ear (pinna), the great toe, hands, and other joints, ligaments, bursae, and tendons in clients with gout.

Topical hyperbaric oxygen therapy used to treat chronic, non-healing skin lesions by delivering oxygen above atmospheric pressure directly to the wound.

Tort physical, emotional, or financial injury that occurred because of another person's intentional or unintentional actions, or failure to act.

Tort law body of law that governs breaches of duty owed by one person to another.

Total parenteral nutrition hypertonic parenteral solution consisting of nutrients designed to meet nearly all the caloric and nutritional needs of clients who are severely malnourished or cannot consume food or liquids for a long time.

Toxic megacolon complication in which the colon dilates and becomes atonic and vulnerable to perforation.

Toxic shock syndrome life-threatening systemic reaction to the toxin produced by several kinds of bacteria.

Toxins pathologic substances produced by microorganisms.

Trabeculoplasty procedure in which a laser beam is directed at the trabecular network in the eye.

Trachea hollow tube composed of smooth muscle and supported by C-shaped cartilage that transports air from the laryngeal pharynx to the bronchi and lungs.

Tracheitis inflammation of the trachea.

Tracheobronchitis inflammation of the mucous membrane that lines the trachea.

Tracheostomy surgical opening into the trachea into which a tracheostomy or laryngectomy tube is inserted; may be temporary or permanent.

Tracheotomy surgical procedure that makes an opening into the trachea.

Traction method of pulling structures of the musculoskeletal system to relieve muscle spasm, align bones, and maintain immobilization.

Transcranial magnetic stimulation noninvasive method of stimulating the brain to treat depression by delivering short pulses of energy through an electromagnetic coil placed against the scalp near the forehead.

Transcultural nursing specialty in nursing that emphasizes providing nursing care within the context of another's culture.

Transcutaneous pacemaker external pacemaker used as a temporary, emergency measure for maintaining adequate heart rate.

Transduction phase of pain transmission involving the conversion of chemical information in the cellular environment to electrical impulses that move toward the spinal cord.

Transesophageal echocardiography ultrasound technique in which a tube with a small transducer is passed internally from the mouth to the esophagus to obtain images of the posterior heart and its internal structures.

Transient ischemic attack sudden, brief, fleeting attacks of neurologic impairment caused by a temporary interruption in cerebral blood flow.

Transillumination technique in which a light is shone through tissue.

Transmission phase of pain transmission during which peripheral nerve fibers form synapses with neurons within the spinal cord and the pain impulses move from the spinal cord to sequentially higher levels in the brain.

Transmission-based precautions actions that interfere with the manner in which a particular pathogen is spread.

Transmural infarction death of tissue that extends through the full thickness of the myocardial wall.

Transmyocardial revascularization laser procedure that improves oxygenation of myocardial tissue by creating channels into which oxygenated blood seeps and is absorbed by the ischemic myocardium.

Transvenous pacemaker temporary pulse-generating device that is used to manage transient bradydysrhythmias such as those that occur during acute MIs or after coronary artery bypass graft surgery, or to override tachydysrhythmias.

Triage evaluation of casualties.

Tricuspid valve opening between the right atrium and right ventricle of the heart.

Triiodothyronine hormone synthesized by the thyroid gland that regulates the body's metabolic rate; also called T_3.

Trousseau's sign assessment finding in which the hand spasms after placing a BP cuff on the client's upper arm and inflating it between the systolic and diastolic BP, for 3 minutes.

Trust positive developmental outcome of the infant stage in which a child has a sense of reliance on and confidence in others.

T-tube device used to drain bile while the surgical wound from an opening and exploration of the common bile duct heals.

Tuberculosis bacterial infectious disease caused by *Mycobacterium tuberculosis*.

Tumor markers substances synthesized by tumors that are released into the circulation in excessive amounts.

Tumor necrosis factor type of cytokine used to regulate various autoimmune and inflammatory disorders.

Tumor-specific antigen unique protein on cell surface of tumors; measurement helps to track the extent of cancer as malignant cells mature and become less differentiated.

Tuning fork instrument that produces sound in the same range as human speech; used to screen for conductive or sensorineural hearing loss.

Turbinates (conchae) bones that change the flow of inspired air to moisturize and warm it to a greater degree.

Tympanotomy incisional opening of the tympanic membrane.

U

Ulcerative colitis chronic inflammatory condition of the mucosal and submucosal layers of the colon.

Ulcerative proctitis chronic inflammation of the most distal area of the large intestine.

Ultrasonography technique that uses high frequency sound waves to show the size and location of organs and to outline structures and abnormalities.

Uncal herniation shifting of the brain to the lateral side.

Unintentional torts injuries caused by another person when the person responsible did not mean to cause any harm; negligence is the principal form of unintentional tort.

Unvented tubing type of intravenous tubing that does not draw air into a container of solution; used for solutions packaged in plastic bags. See also *vented tubing*.

Universal donor person with type O blood.

Universal recipient person with type AB blood.

Upper gastrointestinal series fluoroscopic observation of a client swallowing a flavored barium solution and its progress down the esophagus combined with radiographic observation of the barium moving into the stomach and the first part of the small intestine.

Uremia toxic state caused by the accumulation of nitrogen wastes in the blood.

Uremic frost precipitate that sometimes forms on the skin during chronic renal failure because it becomes the excretory organ for substances the kidney usually clears from the body.

Ureteral stent slender supportive device used to splint the ureter or divert urine past a possible tear in the ureteral wall.

Ureterolithiasis presence of a stone within the ureter.

Ureteroplasty removal of a narrowed section of ureter and reconnection of the patent portions.

Urethritis inflammation of the urethra.

Urethroplasty surgical repair of the urethra.

Urinalysis laboratory examination of the components and characteristics of urine.

Urinary diversion redirection of urine either to an external or an internal collecting system.

Urine osmolality measurement of the concentration of dissolved particles in urine expressed in osmoles of solute.

Urine protein test laboratory examination used to identify renal disease by detecting an increase in urine protein levels.

Urine specific gravity measurement of the kidney's ability to concentrate and excrete urine by comparing the density of urine with the density of distilled water.

Urodynamic studies tests that evaluate bladder and urethral function and are performed to assess causes of reduced urine flow, urinary retention, and urinary incontinence.

Uroflowmetry study performed to evaluate bladder and sphincter function by measuring the time and rate of voiding, the volume of urine voided, and the pattern of urination.

Urography radiologic study used to evaluate the structure and function of the kidneys, ureters, and bladder by examining a radiopaque dye as it passes through the urinary tract.

Urolithiasis condition of stones in the urinary tract.

Urosepsis serious systemic infection from microorganisms in the urinary tract that invade the bloodstream.

Urticaria hives.

Utilitarianism theory of ethics that determines the rightness of an action by its consequences; also referred to as teleologic theory.

Uveitis inflammation of the uveal tract.

V

Vaginitis condition in which the vagina is inflamed.

Vagus nerve stimulation treatment for depression in which a pulse generator sends intermittent electrical impulses directed toward the brain via the vagus nerve.

Values beliefs that individuals find most meaningful.

Valvular incompetence condition in which the aortic valve does not close tightly.

Valvular regurgitation leaking of blood backward through a valve that does not close tightly.

Valvuloplasty surgical procedure in which an incompetent cardiac valve is repaired.

Varicose veins dilated, tortuous veins.

Vasectomy surgical procedure involving the ligation of the vas deferens which results in permanent sterilization by interrupting the pathway that transports sperm.

Vasopressors drugs that increase peripheral vascular resistance and raise blood pressure.

Vegetations accumulation of inflammatory debris around the valve leaflets of the heart in rheumatic carditis.

Vein ligation surgical treatment for severe varicose veins in which the affected veins are tied off above and below the area of incompetent valves, but the dysfunctional vein remains.

Vein stripping surgical treatment for severe varicose veins in which the affected veins are severed and removed.

Vena caval filter surgically inserted umbrella-like sieve used to trap emboli before they reach the heart and lungs.

Vena caval plication surgical procedure that changes the lumen of the vena cava from a single channel to several small channels through the use of a suture or Teflon clip.

Venereal diseases diverse group of infections spread through sexual activity with an infected person.

Venereal warts (condylomas) sexually transmitted infection characterized as a; painless single lesion or cluster of soft, fleshy growths on the genitalia or cervix, within the vagina, or on the perineum, anus, throat, or mouth.

Venipuncture method for gaining access to the venous system by piercing a vein with one of various devices.

Venography procedure that uses radiopaque dye instilled into the venous system to identify a filling defect in the area of a clot.

Venous insufficiency peripheral vascular disorder in which the flow of venous blood is impaired through deep or superficial veins, or both.

Venous reflux retrograde flow of venous blood.

Venous stasis ulcer lesion that forms on the skin when the flow of venous blood is impaired.

Vented tubing intravenous tubing that draws air into a container of solution; used for administering solutions packaged in glass containers to facilitate their flow. See also *unvented tubing*.

Ventilation movement of air into and out of the respiratory tract.

Ventricles (1) hollow structures in the brain that manufacture and absorb cerebrospinal fluid; (2) lower chambers of the heart.

Ventricular assist device auxiliary heart pump that supplements the heart's ability to eject blood.

Ventricular fibrillation cardiac dysrhythmia in which the ventricles do not contract effectively and there is no cardiac output.

Ventricular tachycardia dysrhythmia in which a single, irritable focus in the ventricle causes the ventricles to beat very fast and cardiac output is decreased.

Ventriculomyomectomy procedure involving the removal of thickened myocardial muscle from the septum.

Venules smallest portion of veins.

Verbal communication communication that uses words (speaking, reading, and writing).

Vesicants intravenous medications that cause tissue necrosis if they infiltrate.

Viatical settlement arrangement in which a terminally ill individual agrees to name a person as beneficiary to his or her life insurance in exchange for immediate cash.

Video interpreting communication in which a person uses sign language in a remote location yet is visible to the health team member and client and visa versa.

Virchow's triad three factors that contribute to formation of thrombi; they include slowed circulation, altered blood coagulation, and trauma to the vein.

Virtual colonoscopy examination using a small catheter inserted in the rectum to instill air for dilating the colon and a CT scanner to visualize the colon.

Virulence power of a microorganism to produce disease.

Visceral pain discomfort that arises from diseased or injured internal organs.

Visceral pericardium inner serous layer of the pericardium; also called the *epicardium*.

Visceral pleura saclike serous membrane that covers the lung surface.

Visual acuity ability to see far images clearly.

Visual field examination test of peripheral vision and detection of gaps in the visual field.

Visually impaired condition in which visual acuity is between 20/70 and 20/200 in the better eye with the use of glasses.

Vocal cords folds of tissue within the larynx that vibrate and produce sound as air passes through.

Voice dismissal technique used to halt a hallucination by saying "stop" or "be gone."

Voiding cystourethrogram study that evaluates abnormalities in bladder function through the voiding of contrast dye and a rapid series of x-rays.

Volkmann's contracture claw-like deformity of the hand resulting from obstructed arterial blood flow to the forearm and hand.

Volumetric controller device that infuses IV solutions using gravity and compressing the tubing at a certain frequency to infuse the solution at a precise preset rate.

Volvulus kinking of a portion of the intestine.

Vulva collective term for external female genitalia.

W

Waiting for permission phenomenon situation in which some terminally ill clients forestall dying until their loved ones indicate they are prepared to deal with their death.

Water-hammer pulse assessment finding characterized as strong radial pulse with quick, sharp beats followed by a sudden collapse of force.

Water loading technique used by clients with anorexia nervosa to falsely demonstrate weight gain by consuming a large volume of water and avoiding urination before being weighed.

Webcam video camera that allows viewing via the internet.

Weber test assessment technique used to measure hearing loss by striking a tuning fork and placing its stem in the midline of the client's skull or center of the forehead; a person with normal hearing perceives the sound equally well in both ears.

Wedge resection surgical removal of a pie-shaped portion of diseased tissue from a lung.

Wellness state that involves good physical self-care, prevention of illness and injury, use of one's full intellectual potential, expression of emotions and appropriate management of stress, comfortable and congenial interpersonal relationships, and concern about one's environment and conditions throughout the world.

Wellness diagnosis category of nursing diagnoses that begins with the stem "potential for enhanced" and does not include related factors or supporting data.

Western blot test used to confirm an HIV diagnosis indicated by a positive enzyme-linked immunosorbent assay test.

White-coat hypertension elevated blood pressure that develops during evaluation by medical personnel as a result of anxiety.

Whole blood solution containing blood cells and plasma with preservative and anticoagulant added.

Whole medical systems alternative systems of healing theory and practice that evolved from non-Western cultures.

Withdrawal physical symptoms or craving for a drug that occur when a person abruptly stops using a drug that he or she has taken routinely for some time.

Withdrawal symptoms physical discomfort that follows when a person abruptly discontinues use of a drug taken routinely for some time.

Wood's light hand-held device that can identify fungal infections that fluoresce under long-wave ultraviolet light.

Working phase time during the nurse–client relationship when the nurse and client mutually plan the client's care and put the plan into action.

Worried well unaffected people in a disaster who believe they are at risk for physical consequences.

Wound, ostomy, and continent nurses (WOCNs) enterostomal therapy nurses who assist with marking placement of the stoma and collaborate with the surgeon on the client's educational needs.

X

Xerostomia dryness of the mouth.

Y

Y-administration tubing intravenous tubing used to administer whole blood or packed cells that contains two branches: one for blood and one for isotonic (normal) saline.

Yellow bone marrow bone marrow in long bones that consists primarily of fat cells and connective tissue.

Yoga technique developed in India that combines mental and physical exercises for the purpose of integrating body and mind.

Z

Zoonotic pathogens microorganisms that spread to animals and then to humans.

Zygote the fertilized ovum.

References and Suggested Readings

Chapter 1: Concepts and Trends in Healthcare

Agency for Healthcare Research and Quality Indicators (AHRQ) (2008). *AHRQuality Indicators*. (Online.) Available at www.qualityindicators.ahrq.gov/. Accessed October 2008.

Centers for Medicare and Medicaid Services (2008). *Medicare and You 2008*. Available at www.medicare.gov/publications. Accessed October 2008.

Cherry, B., & Jacob, S. R. (2008). *Contemporary nursing: Issues, trends, and management* (4th ed.). St. Louis, MO: Elsevier Mosby.

Chitty, K.K., & Black, B.P. (2007). *Professional nursing: Concepts and challenges* (5th ed.). St. Louis, MO: Elsevier Saunders.

Institute for Healthcare Improvement (2008). *Closing the quality gap*. Available at http://www.ihi.org. Accessed October 2008.

Safe Haven (2006). Safety first: What nurses are saying about patient safety. *LPN 2006, 2*(5), 16–21.

Hathaway, L. (2006). Saving 100,000 lives, one step at a time. *LPN 2006, 2*(2), 4–6.

Institute for Healthcare Improvement (2006). 5 Million lives campaign. Available at www.ihi.org. Accessed October 2008.

Office of Disease Prevention and Health Promotion, U.S. Department of health and Human Services (2008). *Healthy People 2020* Available at www.healthypeople.gov. Accessed October 2008.

Rafter, R.H., & Keown, S. (2006). Aim high: Achieving JCAHO's national patient safety goals. *LPN 2006, 2*(6), 18–20.

Safe Haven (2007). Saving 5 million lives, 1 patient at a time. *LPN 2007, 3*(5), 25–26.

The Joint Commission (2008). *2009 National Patient Safety Goals*. Available at http://www.jointcommission.org/PatientSafety/NationalPatientSafetyGoals/. Accessed October 2008.

U.S. Bureau of the Census (2000). *Profile of older Americans: 2000. Population projections of the United States by age, sex, race, and Hispanic origin: 1995–2050*. Washington, DC: Current Population Reports, pp. 25–1130.

U.S. Department of Health and Human Services. (2000). *Healthy people 2010: Understanding and improving health* (2nd ed.). Available at www.healthypeople.gov. Accessed October 2008.

Chapter 2: Settings and Models for Nursing Care

ANA (2003). *Nursing's social policy statement* (2nd ed.). Washington, DC: American Nurses Publishing.

Chitty, K. K., & Black, B. P. (2007). *Professional nursing: Concepts and challenges* (5th ed.). St. Louis, MO: Elsevier Saunders.

Ellis, J. R., & Hartley, C. L. (2008). *Nursing in today's world: Trends, issues, and management* (9th ed.). Philadelphia, PA: Lippincott Williams & Wilkins.

Seago, J. A., Spetz, J., Chapman, S., & Dyer, W. (2007). How can LPNs ease the nursing shortage? *LPN 2007, 3*(1), 16–19.

Chapter 3: The Nursing Process

Ackley, B.J., & Ladwig, G.B. (2008). *Nursing diagnosis handbook* (8th ed.). St. Louis, MO: Mosby Elsevier.

Alfaro-LeFevre, R. (2006). *Applying nursing process: A tool for critical thinking* (6th ed.). Philadelphia, PA: Lippincott Williams & Wilkins.

Carpenito-Moyet, L.J. (2008). *Nursing diagnosis: Application to clinical practice* (12th ed.). Philadelphia, PA: Lippincott Williams & Wilkins.

Carpenito-Moyet, L.J. (2007). *Understanding the nursing process: Concept mapping and care planning for students*. Philadelphia, PA: Lippincott Williams & Wilkins.

Maslow, A. H. (1968). *Toward a psychology of being*. New York, N.Y.: Van Nostrand Reinhold

NANDA International (2007). *Nursing diagnoses: Definitions & classification, 2007–2008*. Philadelphia, PA: Author.

Schuster, P. M. (2008). *Concept mapping: A critical thinking approach to care planning* (2nd ed.). Philadelphia, PA: F.A. Davis Company.

Smeltzer, S.C., Bare, B.G., Hinkle, J.L., et al. (2008). *Brunner & Suddarth's textbook of medical-surgical nursing* (11th ed.). Philadelphia, PA: Lippincott Williams & Wilkins.

Wilkinson, J.M (2007). *Nursing process and critical thinking* (4th ed.). Upper Saddle River, NJ: Pearson Prentice Hall.

Chapter 4: Interviewing and Physical Assessment

Chart Smart (2006). Getting the most from an admission interview. *Nursing 2006, 36*(12), 31.

Skill Building (2007). Now hear this: How to identify heart sounds. *LPN 2007, 3*(1), 4–7.

Weber, J. R. (2008). *Nurses' handbook of health assessment* (6th ed.). Philadelphia, PA: Lippincott Williams & Wilkins.

Chapter 5: Legal and Ethical Issues

Anderson, F. (2007). Finding HIPAA in your soup: Decoding the privacy rule. *American Journal of Nursing, 107*(2), 66–71.

Austin, S. (2006). Ladies and gentlemen of the jury, I present the nursing documentation. *Nursing 2006, 36*(1), 57–62.

Austin, S. (2006). Walk a fine line if your patient wants to leave AMA. *Nursing 2006, 36*(12), 48–49.

Brooke, P.S. (2005). Understanding HIPAA compliance. *LPN, 1*(4), 36–39.

Brooke, P.S. (2006). So you've been named in a lawsuit. What happens next? *Nursing 2006, 36*(7), 44–48.

Catalano, J.T. (2006). *Nursing now! Today's issues, tomorrow's trends,* (4th ed.). Philadelphia, PA: F.A. Davis.

Charting Checkup (2006). Making it clear with an incident report. *LPN 2006, 2*(3), 17–19.

Charting Checkup (2006). You're a witness: Know your role in obtaining informed consent. *LPN 2006, 2*(4), 15, 17.

Charting Checkup (2007). You're on trial: How to protect yourself. *LPN 2007, 3*(2), 16, 18.

Charting Checkup (2007). Your patient wants to see his medical record. *LPN 2007, 3*(5), 4–5.

Chitty, K.K., & Black, B. P. (2007). *Professional nursing: Concepts & challenges* (5th ed.). St. Louis, MO: Elsevier Saunders.

Croke, E.M. (2003). Nurses, negligence, and malpractice. *American Journal of Nursing, 103*(9), 54–62.

Dorloh, T. (2007). Document it! The importance of accurate charting. *LPN 2007, 3*(4), 25–26.

Ellis, J.R., & Hartley, C.L. (2008). *Nursing in today's world: Trends, issues, and management* (9th ed.). Philadelphia, PA: Lippincott Williams & Wilkins.

Gialanella, K.M. (2004). Documentation. *Advance for Nurses*, June 21, 22–24.

Helm, A., & Kihm, N.C. (2006). Liability insurance: Is it for you? *LPN 2006, 2*(3), 14–15.

Keefe, S. (2005). Ethical solutions. *Advance for Nurses*, March 14, 16–17.

LaDuke, S. (2003). Keeping up with standards. Your key to safe practice. *Nursing 2003, 33*(3), 45.

Leech, E.E. (2005). When your patient threatens to walk. *RN, 68*(9), 56–59.

Levine, C. (2006). HIPAA and talking with family caregivers. *American Journal of Nursing, 106*(8), 51–53.

Marquis, B.L., & Huston, C.J. (2008). *Leadership roles and management functions in nursing: Theory and application* (6th ed.). Philadelphia, PA: Lippincott Williams & Wilkins.

Martin, R.H. (2006, October 23). Incident reports. *Advance for Nurses*, 27–29.

Patient Education Series (2006a). Advance directives. *Nursing 2006, 36*(9), 43.

Patient Education Series (2006b). Protecting yourself against medical errors. *Nursing 2006, 36*(8), 49.

Quinn, C.A., & Smith, M.D. (1987). *The professional commitment: Issues and ethics in nursing.* Philadelphia, PA: W.B. Saunders.

Reising, D.L., & Allen, P.N. (2007, February). Protecting yourself from malpractice claims. *American Nurse Today*, 39–43.

Roman, L.M. (2007). 4 Nurse attorneys tell you how to stay out of legal hot water. *RN, 70*(1), 26–31.

Sullivan, G.H. (2004). Does your charting measure up? *RN, 67*(3), 61–65.

Taylor, C., Lillis, C., & LeMone, P. (2008). *Fundamentals of nursing: The art and science of nursing care* (6th ed.). Philadelphia, PA: Lippincott Williams & Wilkins.

Zerwekh, J., & Claborn J.C. (2006). *Nursing today: Transitions and trends* (5th ed.). St. Louis, MO: Elsevier Saunders.

Chapter 6: Leadership Roles and Management Functions

Anderson, P.S., Twibell, R.S., & Siela, D. (2006). Delegating without doubts. *American Nurse Today, 1*(11), 54–57.

Appold, K. (2007). Divvy up: Nurses have much to gain by delegating tasks. *Advance for LPNs.* Available at http://lpn.advanceweb.com. Accessed May 2008.

Corbo, S.A. (2006). Delegation defined. *Advance for Nurses*, July 17, 19–21.

Cox, S.S. (2006). How to delegate to UAPs. *Travel Nursing 2006, 36*(6), 10–11.

Ellis, J.R., & Hartley, C.L. (2004). *Managing and coordinating nursing care* (4th ed.) Philadelphia, PA: Lippincott Williams & Wilkins.

Ellis, J.R., & Hartley, C.L. (2008). *Nursing in today's world: Trends, issues, and management* (9th ed.). Philadelphia, PA: Lippincott Williams & Wilkins.

Hathaway, L.R. (2005). Safely delegating to unlicensed assistive personnel. *LPN 2005, 1*(5), 13–14.

Leiper, J. (2005). Nurse against nurse: How to stop horizontal violence. *Nursing 2005, 35*(3), 44–45.

Marquis, B.L., & Huston, C.J. (2008). *Leadership roles and management functions in nursing: Theory and application* (6th ed.). Philadelphia, PA: Lippincott Williams & Wilkins.

National Council of State Boards of Nursing (1995). *Delegation: Concepts and decision making process.* Chicago, IL: Author.

Orcajada, E., & Rao, L. (2005). The art and science of delegation. *Advance for Nurses*, August 29, 25–27.

Sherman, R.O., & Dyess, S. (2007). Be a coach for novice nurses. *American Nurse Today, 2*(5), 54–55.

Schroeder, S.J. (2007). Improving intershift handoff – and patient safety! *LPN 2007, 3*(2), 22–23.

Schroeder, S.J. (2006). Picking up the PACE: A new template for shift report. *Nursing 2006, 36*(10), 22–23.

Trossman, S. (2006). Issues up close: Getting a clearer picture on delegation. *American Nurse Today, 1*(10), 54–56.

Chapter 7: Nurse–Client Relationships

Brough, C. (2004). Developing and maintaining a therapeutic relationship: part 1. *Nursing Older People* 16(8): 26–27.

Brough, C. (2004). Developing and maintaining a therapeutic relationship. part 2—a case study. *Nursing Older People* 16(9): 26–28.

Brown, B. L. (1997). New learning strategies for generation X. Available at http://www.ericdigests.org/1998-1/x.htm. Accessed September 2007.

Feil, N. *Caring community: Wellness through life's end.* Available at http://caringcommunity.org/links/vfvalidation. Accessed May 2008.

Fursland, E. (2005). Finding the words: Nurses can learn how to communicate more effectively with patients who have aphasia. *Nursing Standard* 20(1): 24–25.

Gleeson, M., Timmins, F. (2005). A review of the use and clinical effectiveness of touch as a nursing intervention. *Clinical Effectiveness in Nursing* 9(1/2): 69–77.

Green-Hernandez, C., Quinn, A.A., Denman-Vitale, S., et al. (2004). Making nursing care culturally competent. *Holistic Nursing Practice* 18(4): 215–218.

Gruber, M., Hartman, R. (2007). Don't overlook "communication competence." *Nursing Management* 38(3): 12–13.

Hamilton, S. (2005). Clinical consultation. How do we assess the learning style of our patients? *Rehabilitation Nursing* 30(4): 129–131.

Holtschneider, M.E. (2007). Better communication, better care through high-fidelity simulation. *Nursing Management* 38(5): 55–57.

Joint Commission. (2008). National patient safety goals. Available at http://www.jointcommission.org/PatientSafety/National PatientSafetyGoals/08_npsg_facts. Accessed September 2007.

Manning, M.L. (2006). Improving clinical communication through structured conversation. *Nursing Economics* 24(5): 268–272.

Mauk, K.L. (2006). Healthier aging: reaching and teaching older adults. *Holistic Nursing Practice* 20(3): 158.

McAleer, M. (2006). Communicating effectively with deaf patients. Nursing Standard 20(19): 51–54.

National Council on Interpreting in Health Care. (2001). Terminology of health care interpreting: a glossary of terms. Available at http://www.ncihc.org/NCIHC_PDF/theterminologyofhealthcare interpreting.pdf. Accessed September 2007.

Roat, C. (2005) Addressing language access issues in your practice: A toolkit for physicians and their staff. Available at http://www.familydocs.org/assets/Multicultural_Health/Addressing%20Access Toolkit.pdf. Accessed September 2007.

Roberts, D. (2007). Clear communication—accept nothing less. *Med-Surg Nursing* 16(3): 142–143.

Skiba, D. J., & Barton, A. J. (2006). Adapting your teaching to accommodate the net generation of learners. *The Online Journal of Issues in Nursing*, 11(2): Manuscript 4. Available at http://nursingworld.org/MainMenuCategories/ANAMarketplace/ANAPeriodicals/OJIN/TableofContents/Volume112006/Number2May31/tpc30_416076.aspx. Accessed September 2007.

Stickley, T., Freshwater, D. (2006). The art of listening in the therapeutic relationship. *Mental Health Practice* 9(5): 12–18.

Tulgan, B., & Martin, C. A. (2001). Managing generation Y—Part 2. Available at http://www.businessweek.com/smallbiz/content/oct2001/sb2001105_229.htm. Accessed August 2007.

Williams, K., Kemper, S., & Hummert, L. (2004). Enhancing communication with older adults: overcoming elderspeak. *Journal of Gerontological Nursing* 30(10): 17–25.

Wilson-Sronks, A., & Galvex, E. (2007). Hospitals, language, and culture: a snapshot of the nation. Available at http://www.jointcommission.org/NR/rdonlyres/E64E5E89-5734-4D1D-BB4D-C4ACD4BF8BD3/0/hlc_paper.pdf. Accessed September 2007.

Zur, O., & Nordmarken, N. (2008). To touch or not to touch: Exploring the myth of prohibition on touch in psychotherapy and counseling. Available at http://www.zurinstitute.com/touchintherapy.html. Accessed September 2008.

Chapter 8: Cultural Care Considerations

Andrews, M. M., & Boyle, J. S. (2008). *Transcultural concepts in nursing care* (5th ed.). Philadelphia, PA: Lippincott Williams & Wilkins.

Carol, R. (2006). Culture is skin deep. *Minority Nurse*, Spring, 26–29.

Collins, S.D. (2006). Is cultural competency required in today's nursing care? *NSNA Imprint*, February/March, 52–54.

DeRosa, N., & Kochurka, K. (2006). Implement culturally competent healthcare in your workplace. *Nursing Management*, October, 18–26.

Diversity Rx (2003). Why language and culture are important. Available at www.diversityRx.org. Accessed April 2008.

ElGindy, G. (2005). Meeting Jewish and Muslim patients' dietary needs. *Minority Nurse*, Winter, 56–58.

ElGindy, G. (2005). Understanding Buddhist patients' dietary needs. *Minority Nurse*, Spring, 49–52.

Galanti, G. (2000). An introduction to cultural differences. *Western Journal of Medicine*. Available at http://www.ggalanti.com/articles/Intro.pdf. Accessed April 2008.

Giger, J.N., & Davidhizar, R.E. (2008). *Transcultural nursing: Assessment and intervention* (5th ed.). St Louis, MO: Elsevier Mosby.

Godshall, N., & Fenstermacher, K. (2006). *Advance for Nurses*, February 6, 64–65.

Jeffreys, M. (2006). Cultural competence in clinical practice. *NSNA Imprint*, February/March, 37–41.

Keefe, S. (2007). More than a melting pot. *Advance for Nurses*, March 26, 25–28.

Language Line Services; 1-877-886-3885. Available at http://www.languageline.com/. Accessed April 2008.

Leininger, M. (1977). Transcultural nursing and a proposed conceptual framework. In M. Leininger (ed.), *Transcultural nursing care of infants and children: Proceedings from the first transcultural conference*. Salt Lake City: University of Utah.

Leininger, M. (1991). Transcultural nursing. The study and practice field. *Imprint*, 38(2), 55–66.

Lipson, J.G., Minarik, P.A., & Dibble, S.L. (2005) *Culture and clinical care*. San Francisco, CA: UCSF Nursing Press.

McSweeney, J.C., Allan, J.D., & Mayo, K. (1997). Exploring the use of explanatory models in nursing research and practice. *IMAGE: Journal of Nursing Scholarship, 29*, 243–248.

Morris, A. H. (2007). *Factors influencing baccalareate of science in nursing students' perceptions of eldercare cultural self-efficacy*. Unpublished doctoral dissertation, Auburn University, Alabama.

Muñoz, C., & Hilgenberg, C. (2005). Ethnopharmacology. *American Journal of Nursing, 105*(8), 40–49.

Nardi, D.A. (2005). Cultural issues in home care. *Advance for Nurses*, May 23, 17–21.

Orlovsky, C. (2005). Transcultural nursing: Providing cultural care for all. *NurseZone, 3*(1), 6.

Purnell, L.D., & Paulanka, B.J. (2003). *Transcultural health care* (3rd ed.). Philadelphia, PA: F.A. Davis.

Sensor, C.S. (2006). Culturally competent care in the workplace. *NSNA Imprint*, February/March, 46–50.

Smeltzer, S.C., Bare, B.G., Hinkle, J.L., et al. (2008). *Brunner & Suddarth's textbook of medical-surgical nursing* (11th ed.). Philadelphia, PA: Lippincott Williams & Wilkins.

Waite, R.L. (2005). Beyond the color lines. *Advance for Nurses*, February 28, 31–32.

Wells, J.N., Cagle, C.S., & Bradley, P.J. (2006). Building on Mexican-American cultural values. *Nursing 2006, 36*(7), 20–21.

Chapter 9: Complementary and Alternative Therapies

Allyn, D.E. (2007). *Primum non nocere* (First, do no harm): prayer, culture, and evidence-based practice. Topics in Advanced Practice Nursing eJournal. Available at http://www.medscape.com/viewarticle/561760. Accessed October 2007.

Barrett, S. (2001). How the dietary supplement health and education act of 1994 weakened the FDA. Available at http://quackwatch.com/02ConsumerProtection/dshea.html. Accessed October 2007.

Cherniack, E. P., Ceron-Fuentes, J., Florenz H., et al. (2008). Influence of race and ethnicity on alternative medicine as a self-treatment preference for common medical conditions in a population of multi-ethnic urban elderly. *Complementary Therapies in Clinical Practice, 14*(2), 116–23.

Committee on the Use of Complementary and Alternative Medicine by the American Public (2005). Complementary and Alternative Medicine in the United States. Washington, DC: The National Academies Press. Available at http://www.nap.edu/catalog.php?record_id=11182. Accessed October 2007.

Gaydos, H.L.B. (2001). Complementary and alternative therapies in nursing education: Trends and issues. Available at http://www.nursingworld.org/MainMenuCategories/ANAMarketplace/ANA Periodicals/OJIN/TableofContents/Vol62001/Number2May31/Trendsandissues.aspx. Accessed October 2007.

Hospice and Palliative Nurses Association. (2000). Complementary and alternative medicine in the management of pain, dyspnea, and nausea and vomiting near the end of life: A symptomatic review. *Journal of Pain Symptom Management* 20(5): 374–387.

Jarvis, W.T. (2001). Why chiropractic is controversial. Available at http://www.chirobase.org.01General/controversy.html. Accessed October 2007.

Kuhn, M. (2002). Herbal remedies: Drug-herb interactions. *Critical care nurse, 22*(2), 22.

Mayo Clinic. (2007). *Mayo Clinic: Book of alternative medicine.* New York: Time Inc.

The National Academies. (2005). Complementary and alternative therapies and conventional medical therapies should be held to same standards; Revised regulation of dietary supplements is needed to ensure product quality and safety. Available at http://www8.nationalacademies.org/onpineews/newsitem.aspx?RecordID=1182. Accessed October 2007.

National Center for Complementary and Alternative Medicine. (2006). Herbal supplements: consider safety, too. Available at http://nccam.nih.gov/health/supplement-safety/. Accessed October 2007.

National Center for Complementary and Alternative Medicine. (2007a). Biologically-based practices: an overview. Available at http://www.nccam.nih.gov/health/backgrounds/mindbody.htm. Accessed October 2007.

National Center for Complementary and Alternative Medicine. (2007b). Consumer advisory. Available at http://www.nccam.nih.gov/health/alerts/vitamine/vitamine.htm. Accessed October 2007.

National Center for Complementary and Alternative Medicine. (2007c). Energy medicine: An overview. Available at http://www.nccam.nih.gov/health/backgrounds/energymed.htm. Accessed October 2007.

National Center for Complementary and Alternative Medicine. (2007d). Manipulative and body-based practices: An overview. Available at http://www.nccam.nih.gov/health/backgrounds/manipulative.htm. Accessed October 2007.

National Center for Complementary and Alternative Medicine. (2007e). Mind-body medicine: An overview. Available at http://www.nccam.nih.gov/health/backgrounds/energymed.htm. Accessed October 2007.

National Center for Complementary and Alternative Medicine. (2007f). Whole medical systems: An overview. Available at http://www.nccam.nih.gov/health/backgrounds/wholemed.htm. Accessed October 2007.

National Institute of Health Office of Dietary Supplements. (2006). Botanical dietary supplements: Background information. Available at http://ods.od.nih.gov/factsheets/BotanicalBackgroud.asp. Accessed November 2007.

Nutrition and Wellness Infocenter. (2007). Nutrition infocenter. Available at http://1stholistic.com/Nutrition/nutrition.htm. Accessed October 2007.

Ohio State University. (2004). About 70 percent of older adults use alternative medicine. Available at http://www.sciencedaily.com/releases/2005/04/050427134458.htm. Accessed October 2007.

Schrezenmeir, J., & deVrese, M. (2001). Probiotics, prebiotics, and symbiotics—Approaching a definition. *American Journal of Clinical Nutrition* 73(2): 361S–364S.

Silva, M.C., & Ludwick, R. (2001). Ethics: Ethical issues in complementary/alternative therapies. Available at http://www.nursingworld.org/MainMenuCategories/ANAMarketplace/ANAPeriodicals/OJIN/Columns/Ethics/EthicalIssues.aspx. Accessed October 2007.

Telepo, L.J. (2007). International Academy of Advanced Reflexology. Available at http://www.byregion.net/cgibin/users/profiles.pl?username=ranajean. Accessed October 2007.

United States Food and Drug Administration. (2004). FDA warns consumers that Actra-Rx "dietary supplements" promoted for sexual enhancement contains undeclared prescription drug ingredient. Available at http://www.fda.gov/bbs/topics/ANSWERS/2004/ans01322.HTML. Accessed October 2007.

Won, C., Hong, S., & Kim, C. (2007). Efficacy of Apitox (bee venom) for osteoarthritis. Available at http://www.apitherapy.org/efficacyarticle.htm. Accessed October 2007.

Chapter 10: End-of-Life Care

AJN Reports (2006). Understanding medical futility. *American Journal of Nursing, 106*(5), 25–26.

American Hospice Foundation. Available at http://www.american-hospice.org. Accessed April 2008.

Bensing, K. (2005). End-of-life care. *Advance for Nurses,* August 29, 38.

Corcoran, D. (2006). Near-death experiences. *Advance for Nurses,* May 8, 29–31.

DeSpelder, L.A., & Strickland, A.L. (2001). *The last dance: Encountering death and dying* (6th ed.). Mountain View, CA: Mayfield.

Department of Human Services, Office of Disease Prevention and Epidemiology (2006).

Tenth annual report on Oregon's Death with Dignity Act. Available at: http://www.oregon.gov/DHS/ph/pas/docs/year10.pdf. Accessed April 2008.

Dobbins, E.H. (2005). Helping your patient to a "good death." *Nursing 2005, 35*(2), 43–45.

Hascup, V.A. (2005). Nearing death awareness. *Advance for Nurses,* November 7, 27–28.

Kouch, M. (2006). Managing symptoms for a "good death." *Nursing 2006, 36*(11), 58–63.

Kübler-Ross, E. (1975). *Death: The final stage of growth.* Englewood Cliffs, NJ: Prentice-Hall.

Matzo, M. L., & Sherman, S. W. (2004). *Gerontologic palliative care.* St, Louis: Mosby.

Miller, C. A. (2009). *Nursing for wellness in older adults.* (5th ed.). Philadelphia, PA: Lippincott Williams & Wilkins.

Pomeranz, J., & Brustman, Sr. M.J. (2005). When's the time right to enter hospice care? *Nursing 2005, 35*(8), 43.

Puia, J., Bassett, C., & Dahnke, A. (2005). Palliative care in critical care settings. *Advance for Nurses*, January 3, 25–26.

Roman, L.M., & Metules, T.J. (2005). What we can learn from the Schiavo case. *RN, 68*(8), 53–57.

Rushton, C.H., Roshi, J.H., & Dossey, B. (2007). Being with dying. *American Nurse Today, 2*(9), 16–18.

Shellman, J. M. (2004). Nobody ever asked me before: Understanding life experiences of African American elders. *Journal of Transcultural Nursing, 15*(4), 308–316.

Smeltzer, S.C., Bare, B.G., Hinkle, J.L., et al. (2008). *Brunner & Suddarth's textbook of medical-surgical nursing* (11th ed.). Philadelphia, PA: Lippincott Williams & Wilkins.

Chapter 11: Pain Management

Acute and chronic pain: Assessment and management. (2004). Available at http://www.rn.com/main.php?uniq=57560&command=manage_courselist&data%5Bcourselist%5D%5Bid%5D=1375&da. Accessed October 2007.

American Geriatric Society Panel on Chronic Pain in Older Persons. *The management of chronic pain in older persons.* Available at www.americangeriatrics.org/products/chronic_pain.pdf. Accessed May 2009.

Barry, P. (2003). Many readers take drastic steps to get prescription medicine. American Association of Retired Persons Bulletin. Available at http://0-www.aarp.org.mill1.sjlibrary.org/bulletin/prescription/a2003-09-29-chasing_drugs.html. Accessed October 2007.

American Pain Society. (1999). New survey of people with chronic pain reveals out-of-control symptoms, impaired daily lives. Glenview, IL: American Pain Society.

Berkley, K. (1997). Sex differences in pain. *Behavioral and Brain Sciences* 20(3): 371–380.

Buckalew, N., Haut, M. W., Morrow, L., et al. (2008). Chronic pain is associated with brain volume loss in older adults: Preliminary evidence. *Pain Medicine, 9*(2), 240–248.

Bullock, B.L., & Henze, R. L. (2000). *Focus on pathophysiology*. Philadelphia, PA: Lippincott Williams & Wilkins.

Davis, G., Hiemenz, M., & White, T. (2002). Barriers to managing the chronic pain of older adults with arthritis. *Image: Journal of Nursing Scholarship* 34(2): 121–126.

DuPen, A, Shen, D., & Ersek, M. (2007). Mechanisms of opioid induced tolerance and hyperalgesia. *Pain Management Nursing* 8(3): 113–121.

Edwards, R.R., Haythornthwaite, J.A., Sullivan, M.J., et al. (2004). Catastrophizing as a mediator of sex differences in pain: differential effects for daily pain versus laboratory induced pain. *Pain* 111(3): 335–341.

Ferrell, B. A., & Gloth, M. A. (2005). Pain. In M. H. Beers (ed.). *The Merck manual of Geriatrics* (3rd ed.). Available at http://www.merck.com/mkgr/mmg/sec6/ch43/ch43a.jsp. Accessed May 2008.

Hsieh, R., Wee, W. (2002). One-shot percutaneous electrical nerve stimulation vs. transcutaneous electrical nerve stimulation for low back pain: Comparison of therapeutic effects. *American Journal of Physical Medicine & Rehabilitation* 8(11): 838–843.

Hospice and Palliative Nurses Association. (2004). HPNA position statement: Providing opioids at the end of life. Available at http://www.hpna.org/filemaintenance_view.aspx?ID=27. Accessed May 2009.

Jackson, T., Iezzi, T., Gunderson, J., et al. (2002). Gender differences in pain perception: The mediating role of self-efficacy beliefs. *Sex Roles* 47(11–12): 561–568.

Joint Commission. (2000a). *Pain assessment and management.* Oakbrook Terrace, IL: Joint Commission.

Joint Commission. (2000b). *Implementing the new pain management standards.* Oakbrook Terrace, IL: Joint Commission.

Joint Commission. (2007). Setting the Standard. The Joint Commission & Health Care Safety and Quality. Available at http://www.jointcommission.og/NR/rdonlyres/6C33FEDB-BB50-4CEE-9508-A6246DA4811E.0/setting_the-standard.pdf. Accessed October 2007.

Marcus, D. (2000). Treatment of nonmalignant chronic pain. *American Family Physician* 61, 1331–1338, 1345–1346.

McCaffery, M., & Beebe, A. (1989). *Clinical manual for nursing practice.* St. Louis, MO: Mosby.

McCaffery, M., & Ferrell, B.F. (1999). Opioids and pain management: What do nurses know? *Nursing* 29(3), 48–52.

Miguel, R. (2000). Interventional treatment of cancer pain. The fourth step in the World Health Organization analgesic ladder. *Cancer Control, 7,* 149–156.

National Institute of Neurological Disorders and Stroke (NINDS). (2007). Pain: Hope through research. Available at http://www.ninds.ni.gov/disorders/chronic_pain/detail_chronic_pain.htm. Accessed October 2007.

Pasero, C., & McCaffery, M. (1999). *Pain: clinical manual.* (2nd ed.). St. Louis, MO: Mosby.

Pasero, C., & McCaffery, M. (2005). No self-report means no pain-intensity rating: assessing pain in patients who cannot provide a report. *American Journal of Nursing* 105(10): 50–53.

Porth, C.M. (2006). *Essentials of pathophysiology: Concepts of altered states.* (2nd ed.). Philadelphia, PA: Lippincott Williams & Wilkins.

White, P.F. (2000). Percutaneous electrical nerve stimulation (PENS): A promising alternative approach to pain management. *American Pain Society Bulletin* 9(2): 1–8.

World Health Organization. (1996). *Cancer pain relief* (2nd ed.). Geneva, Switzerland: Author.

Chapter 12: Infection

Baseman, J.B., & Tully, J.G. (1997). Mycoplasmas: Sophisticated, reemerging, and burdened by their notoriety. *Emerging Infectious Diseases* 3(1): 1–14.

Centers for Disease Control and Prevention. (2007). BSE (Bovine spongiform encephalopathy, or mad cow disease). Available at http://www.cdc.gov/ncidod/dvrd/bse/. Accessed October 2007.

Centers for Disease Control and Prevention. (2001). Bovine spongiform encephalopathy and variant Cruetzfelt-Jakob disease: Background, evolution, and current concerns. Available at http://www.ninds.nih.gov/news_and_events/congressional_testimony_appendix.pdf. Accessed October 2007.

Durston, S. (2007). Uncompromising immunocompromised patient care. *Nursing Made Incredibly Easy*, 5(4): 52–56.

Eickhoff, T. C. (2005). *Immunization*. In M. H. Beers (ed.). *The Merck manual of geriatrics* (3rd ed.). Available at http://www.merck.com/mkgr/mmg/sec16/ch132/ch132a.jsp. Accessed June 23, 2008.

Eli Lilly and Company. (2007). Xigris (drotrecogin alfa) for severe sepsis: Efficiency. Available at http://www.xigris.com/320-efficacy.jsp. Accessed October 2007.

Gillis, J. (2001). FDA approves 1st drug for severe sepsis. Available at http://www.mercola.com/2001/dec/5/xigris.htm. Accessed October 2007.

Global patient safety challenge launched. (2006). *American Operating Room Nurses Journal* 83(1): 168.

Guideline for hand hygiene in healthcare settings. Recommendations of the Healthcare Infection Control Practices Advisory Committee and the HICPAC/SHEA/IDSA Hand Hygiene Task Force. (2002). *Morbidity and Mortality Weekly Report,* 51(RR16): 1–48.

Houghton, D. (2006). Healthcare acquired infection (HAI) prevention: The power is in your hands. *Nursing Management,* 37(5) Suppl: 1–7.

Meckler, L., & Ricks, C. (2001). Mad cow scare prompts Red Cross to tighten blood-donation rules. *Kalamazoo Gazette,* May 22, Section A, 2.

Now cardigans look set for a ban at work. (2007). *Nursing Standard,* 22(3): 6.

Prusiner, S.B. (1998). The prion diseases. *Brain Pathology,* 8: 499–513.

U.S. Food and Drug Administration. (2004). USDA and HHS strengthen safeguards against bovine spongiform encephalopathy. Available at http://www.fda.gov/bbs/topics/news/2004/NEW01084.html. Accessed October 2007.

Wilfinger, C. (2004). It's in your hands. *Nephrology Nursing Journal* 31(2): 250.

World Health Organization. (2006). Guidelines on hand hygiene in health care (advanced draft) Available at http://www.who.int/patientsafety/information_central/Last_April_versionHH_Guidelines%5b3%5d.pdf. Accessed October 2007.

Chapter 13: Intravenous Therapy

Beattie, S. (2007). Hemorrhage. *RN* 70(8): 30–34.

Cook, L.S. (2007). Choosing the right intravenous catheter. *Home Healthcare Nurse* 25(8): 523–531.

Gorski, L.A., & Czaokewski, L.M. (2004). Peripherally inserted central catheters and midline catheters for the homecare nurse. *Journal of Infusion Nursing* 27(6): 410–412.

Infusion Nurses Society. (2006). Infusion nursing standards of practice. *Journal of Infusion Nursing* 29(IS): S51.

Ingram, P., & Lavery, I. (2005). Peripheral intravenous therapy: Key risks and implications for practice. *Nursing Standard* 19(46): 55–65.

Joint Commission Resources. (2004). Special report! 2005 Joint Commission national patient safety goals: Practical strategies and helpful solutions for meeting these goals. Available at http://www.jcrinc.com/subscribers/printview.asp?durki=7916. Accessed May 2009.

Larouere, E. (2000a). Managing a midline catheter. *Nursing* 30(4): 17.

Larouere, E. (2000b). Placing a midline catheter. *Nursing* 30(3): 26.

Mitchell, D. (2004). Here's an easy way to make sense of IV fluid therapy. *RN* 67(10): 65.

Moureau, N. (2006). Focus on prevention of vascular access device complications. Available at http://www.piccexcellence.com/refrnc%20docs%20and20pdfs/P_revention%20article.pdf. Accessed November 2007.

Rh factor. (2007). Available at http://www.infoplease.com/ce6/sci/A0841716.html. Accessed November 2007.

Rosenthal, K. (2007). Bridging the IV access gap with midline catheters. *Nursing Made Incredibly Easy!* 5(3): 18–10.

The blood that you inherited. (2007). Available at http://www.bloodbook.com/type-facts.html. Accessed November 2007.

Ting, P. (2000a). Complications of blood transfusion—part 1 of 2. Immune complications hemolytic and non-hemolytic. Available at http://anesthesiology.info.com/articles/06232002.php. Accessed November 2007.

Ting, P. (2000b). Complications of blood transfusion—part 2 of 2. Complications of massive transfusion and infectious complications. Available at http://anesthesiologyinfo.com/articles/06232002.php. Accessed May 2009.

Chapter 14: Perioperative Care

Alonso, G.F. (2005). A wild reaction to a topical anesthetic. *RN,* 68(10), 57–60.

American Journal of Nursing (2004). *Medications associated with acute confusion in the elderly.* (Handout). Philadelphia, PA: Lippincott Williams & Wilkins.

Association of Perioperative Registered Nurses, Inc. Available at http://www.aorn.org. Accessed May 2008.

Baugh, N. (2007). Wounds in surgical patients who are obese. *American Journal of Nursing,* 107(6), 40–49.

Beattie, S. (2007). Bedside emergency: Wound dehiscence. *RN,* 70(6), 34–37.

Carpenito-Moyet, L. (2008). *Nursing care plans and documentation: Nursing diagnoses and collaborative problems* (5th ed.) Philadelphia, PA: Lippincott Williams & Wilkins.

Carter-Templeton, H. (2005). Malignant hyperthermia. *Nursing 2005, 35*(6), 8.

Cofer, M.J. (2005). Unwelcome companion to older patients: Postoperative delirium. *Nursing 2005, 35*(1), 32hn1–32hn3.

Crum, E., & Valenti, J. (2007). Can a bloodless surgery program work in the trauma setting? *Nursing 2007, 37*(3), 54–56.

Daniels, S.M. (2007). Improved care for surgical patients. *OR Nurse 2007, 1*(7), 18–22. Available at http://www.nursingcenter.com. Accessed December 2007.

D'Arcy, Y. (2005). What you need to know about fentanyl patches. *Nursing 2005, 35*(8), 73.

D'Arcy, Y. (2006a). How to care for a surgical patient with chronic pain. *Nursing 2006, 36*(3), 17.

D'Arcy, Y. (2006b). Managing postop pain in a patient who's delirious. *Nursing 2006, 36*(6), 17.

DeFazio-Quinn, D.M. (2006). How religion, language, and ethnicity impact perioperative nursing care. *Nursing Clinics of North America, 41*(2), 231–248.

Dixon, B.A., & O'Donnell, J.M. (2006). Is your patient susceptible to malignant hyperthermia? *Nursing 2006, 36*(12), 26–27.

Duchene, P. (2008). Perioperative concerns in older adults. *Advance for Nurses,* January 28, 28–29, 46.

Dunn, D. (2005). Preventing perioperative complications. *Nursing 2005, 35*(11), 36–43.

Griffin, F.A. (2005, November). Best practice protocols: Preventing surgical site infection. *Nursing Management,* 20–26.

Halliday, A.B. (2006). Shades of sedation. *Nursing 2006, 36*(4), 36–41.

Litwack, K. (2006). Adjusting postsurgical care for older patients. *Nursing 2006, 36*(1), 66–67.

Mamaril, M.E. (2006). Nursing considerations in the geriatric surgical patient: The perioperative continuum of care. *Nursing Clinics of North America, 41*(2), 313–328.

Millsaps, C.C.(2006). Pay attention to patient positioning. *RN,* *69*(1), 59–63.

Nettina, S. (2005). *The Lippincott manual of nursing practice* (8th ed.). Philadelphia, PA: Lippincott Williams & Wilkins.

Nursing News (2007). What's being done to make surgery safer. NurseZone.com. Available at http://www.nursezone.com. Accessed December 2007.

O'Connell, M.P. (2006). Positioning impact on the surgical patient. *Nursing Clinics of North America, 41*(2), 173–192.

Odom-Forren, J. (2006). Preventing surgical site infections. *Nursing 2006, 36*(6), 58–63.

O'Donnell, J. M., Bragg, K., & Sell, S. [2003]. Procedural sedation. *Nursing 2003,* 33[4], 38.

Sarvis, C. (2006). Postoperative wound care. *Nursing 2006, 36*(12), 56–57.

Schwartz, A.J. (2006). Learning the essentials of epidural anesthesia. *Nursing 2006, 36*(1), 44–49.

Smeltzer, S.C., Bare, B.G., Hinkle, J.L., et al. (2008). *Brunner & Suddarth's textbook of medical-surgical nursing* (11th ed.). Philadelphia, PA: Lippincott Williams & Wilkins.

Tabor, W. (2007). On the cutting edge of robotic surgery. *Nursing 2007, 37*(2), 48–50.

Up Front (2007). How herbal products increase surgical risks. *Nursing 2007, 37*(9), 24–25.

Wadlund, D.L. (2006). Prevention, recognition, and management of nursing complications in the intraoperative and postoperative surgical patient. *Nursing Clinics of North America, 41*(2), 151–171.

Chapter 15: Disaster Situations

Air Products and Chemicals, Inc. Cyanide: Health effects and treatments for medical professionals. Available at http://www.airproducts.com/NR/rdonlyres/F5FDBEE4-BB14-BA85-47A23036A3B5/0/CyanideMP.doc. Accessed February 2008.

Armanda, M., & Mendelson, M. (2002). Chemical terrorism update: Vesicants. *Emergency Medicine* 34(9): 51.

Boston Public Health Commission. (2005). Information on possible terrorist agents—radiological. Available at http://www.bphc.org/bphc/prepare_powerplant.asp. Accessed November 2007.

Centers for Disease Control and Prevention. (2005). Fact sheet, preparing for a terrorist bombing: A common sense approach. Available at http://www.bt.cdc.gov/masstrauma/pdf/preparing terroristbombing.pdf. Accessed November 2007.

Centers for Disease Control and Prevention. (1999). Bioterrorism readiness plan: A template for healthcare facilities. Available at http://www.cdc.gov/ncidod/dhqp/pdf/bt/13apr99APIC-CDCBioterrorism.PDF. Accessed November 2007.

Centers for Disease Control and Prevention. (2001). Abstract: Consensus statement: Smallpox as a biological weapon: Medical and public health management. Available at http://www.bt.cdc.gov/agent/smallpox/smallpox-biological-weapon.abstract.asp. Accessed November 2007.

Centers for Disease Control and Prevention. (2003a). Frequently asked questions about a nuclear blast. Available at http://www.bt.cdc.gov/radiation.nuclearfaq.asp. Accessed November 2007

Centers for Disease Control and Prevention. (2003b). Emergency preparedness & response. Available at http://www.bt.cdc.gov/agent/anthrax/. Accessed November 2007.

Centers for Disease Control and Prevention. (2004a). What you should know about a smallpox outbreak. Available at http://www.bt.cdc.gov/agent/smallpox/basics/outbreak.asp. Accessed November 2007.

Centers for Disease Control and Prevention. (2004b). Facts about cyanide. Available at http://emergency.cdc.gov/agent/cyanide/basics/facts.asp. Accessed November 2007.

Centers for Disease Control and Prevention. (2005). Fact sheet, preparing for a terrorist bombing: A common sense approach. Available at http://www.bt.cdc.gov/masstrauma/pdf/preparing terroristbombing.pdf. Accessed November 2007.

Chettle, C.C. (2002). Preparing for bioterrorism: Nurses on the front line. Available at http://www2.nursingspectrum.com/CESelf-Study_modules/tools/print.html?ID=375. Accessed November 2007.

Gebbie, K.M., & Qureshi, K. (2002). Emergency and disaster preparedness: Core competencies for nursings. *American Journal of Nursing* 102(1): 46–51.

Government Accounting Office. (2006). Nuclear power plants; efforts made to upgrade security, but the Nuclear Regulatory Commission's design basis threat process should be improved. Available at http://www.gao.gov/new.items/d06388.pdf. Accessed November 2007.

Hussar, D.A. (2005). New drugs '05, part 1. *Nursing* 35(2): 54–61.

Neel, J.V. (2002). The genetic effects of ionizing radiation on humans. Available at http://www.ibis-birthdefects.org/start.neelppr.htm. Accessed November 2007.

Sidell, F.R. (2002). Chemical agent terrorism. Available at http://www.totse.com/en/bad_ideas/guns_and_weapons/chemterr.html. Accessed November 2007.

Slepski, L. (2005). Weapons of mass destruction and emergency preparedness. Available at http://www.nursingspectrum.com/ce/Course45. Accessed November 2007.

Stilp, R. (2005). Biological weapons & emergency preparedness, part 1. Available at http://www.2.nursingspectrum.com/CE/Self-Study_modules/tools/print.html?ID=188. Accessed November 2007.

U.S. Environmental Protection Agency. (2007). Malathion for mosquito control. Available at http://www.epa.gov/pesticides/health/malathion4mosquitoes.htm. Accessed November 2007.

Willshire, L., Hassmiller, S.B., & Wodicka, K.A. (2004). Disaster preparedness and response for nurses. Available at http://www.nursingsociety.org/education/case_studies/SP0004.html. Accessed November 2007.

Chapter 16: Caring for Clients with Fluid, Electrolyte, and Acid-Bace Imbalances

Astle, S.M. (2005). Restoring electrolyte balance: A shift up, a shift down. Either way, an imbalance in electrolytes spells trouble for your patients. *RN* 68(5): 34–40.

Edwards, S. (2001). Regulation of water, sodium and potassium: Implications for practice. Available at http://www.nursing-standard.co.uk/archives/ns/vol15-22/pdfs/p3642v15w22.pdf. Accessed November 2007.

Garth, D. (2007). Hyperkalemia. Available at http://www.emedicine.com/emerg/topic261.htm. Accessed November 2007.

Goertz, S. (2006). Gauging fluid balance with osmolality. *Nursing* 36(10): 70–71.

Hill, J. (2002). Diagnostic and therapeutic uses of natriuretic peptides in patients with heart failure. Available at http://www.dcmsonline.org/jax-medicine/2002journals/Feb2002/peptides.htm. Accessed November 2007.

Holman, C., Martin, S., & Nicol, M. (2005). Promoting adequate hydration in older people. *Nursing Older People* 17(4): 31–32.

Kratz, A., Seigel, A.J., Verbalis, J.J., et al. (2005). Sodium status of collapsed marathon runners. *Archives of Pathology & Laboratory Medicine* 129(2): 227–230.

Mentes, J.C., (2004). Hydration management. Available at http://www.guideline.gov/summary/summary.aspx?doc_id=4832&nbr=003479&string=nurs Accessed November 2007.

National Heart, Lung, and Blood Institute. (2006). What is hypotension? Available at http://www.nhlbi.nih.gov/health/dci/Diseases/hyp/hyp_whatis.html. Accessed November 2007

Porth, C. (2007). *Essentials of pathophysiology: Concepts of altered health states* (2nd ed.). Philadelphia, PA: Lippincott Williams & Wilkins.

Rosenthal, K. (2006). Intravenous fluids: The why and wherefores. *Nursing* 36(7): 26–27.

Sherwood, L. (2007). *Human physiology: From cells to systems* (6th ed.). Florence, KY: Cengage Learning.

Shirreffs, S.M., & Sawka, M.N., Stone, M. (2006). Water and electrolyte needs for football training and match-play. *Journal of Sports Sciences* 24(7): 699-7-7.

Viejo, A., Nicolaus, M.J. (1999). Diabetes insipidus: A current perspective. *Critical Care Nurse* 19(6): 18–31.

Yaseen, S. (2007). Metabolic alkalosis. Available at http://www.emedicine.com/MED/topic1459.htm. Accessed November 2007.

Yucha, C. (2004). Renal regulation of acid-base balance. *Nephrology Nursing Journal* 31(2): 201–208.

Chapter 17: Caring for Clients in Shock

American National Red Cross. (2007). Practice guidelines for blood transfusion: A compilation from recent peer-reviewed literature (2nd ed). Available at https://www.prepare.org/services/biomed/profess/pgbtscreen.pdf. Accessed August 2008.

Chamberlain, N.R. (2004). From systemic inflammatory response syndrome to bacterial sepsis with shock. Available at http://www.kcom.edu/faculty/chamberlain/Website/lectures/lecture/sepsis.htm. Accessed November 2007.

Chavez, J.A., & Brewer, C. (2002). Stopping the shock slide. *Nursing* 65(9): 30–34.

Cheek, D. (2003). Stopping the shock slide. *RN* 65(9): 30–35.

Collins, T. (2000). Understanding shock. *Nursing Standard* 14(49): 35–39.

Cross, C. (2003). Consult stat: Causes and symptoms of neurogenic shock. *RN* 65(2): 76.

Diel-Oplinger, L., & Kaminski, M.F. (2004). Choosing the right fluid to counter hypovolemic shock. *Nursing* 34(3): 52–54.

Eli Lilly and Company. (2007). Xigris (drotrecogin alfa) for severe sepsis: Efficiency. Available at http://www.xigris.com/320-efficacty.jsp. Accessed October 2007.

Gessner, P. (2006). The effects of vasopressin on the renal system in vasodilatory shock. *Dimensions of Critical Care* 25(1): 1–8.

Hall, J.B., Schmidt, G.A., & Wood, L. (2005). *Principles of critical care* (3rd ed.). New York: McGraw-Hill.

Hanna, N.F. (2003). Sepsis and septic shock. *Topics in Emergency Medicine* 25(2): 158–165.

Holcomb, S.S. (2002). Cardiogenic shock: A success story. *Dimensions of Critical Care Nursing* 21(6): 232–235.

Kelly, D.M. (2005). Hypovolemic shock: An overview. *Critical Care Nursing Quarterly* 28(1): 2–19.

Kleinpell, R.M. (2007a). Recognizing and treating five shock states. Available at http://www.nurse.com/ce/orint.html?CCID=3723. Accessed November 2007.

Kleinpell, R.M. (2007b). Shock states: Knowing the similarities and differences is vital. Available at http://www.nurse.com/ce/print.html?CCID=3741. Accessed November 2007.

McAuley, D.F. (2005). What are the current recommendations regarding the use of vasopressin in the treatment of shock? Available at http://www.globalrph.com/vasopressin_shock.htm. Accessed November 2007.

Metules, T.J. (2003). IABP therapy: Getting patients treatment fast. *RN* 66(5): 56.

Muhlberg, A.H. (2004). Holistic care: Treatment and intervention for hypovolemic shock secondary to hemorrhage. *Dimension of Critical Care* 23(2): 55–59.

National Center for Emergency Medicine. (2004). APACHE II score. Available at http://ncemi.org/shared/etools_c/etools_c.pl?cmd=run&resource_fn=edecision_apache_ii_score_for_adults.xml. Accessed November 2007.

Peitzman, A.B., Rhodes, M., Schwab, C.W., et al. (2007). *The trauma manual: trauma and acute care surgery* (3rd ed). Philadelphia, PA: Lippincott Williams & Wilkins.

Powers, J., & Jacobi, J. (2003). Pharmacology consult: Treatment of severe sepsis with Xigris: Implications for the clinical nurse specialist. *Clinical Nurse Specialist: The Journal for Advanced Practice* 17(3): 128–130.

Smeltzer, S.C., Bare, B. G., Hinkle, J.L., et al. (2008). *Brunner & Suddarth's textbook of medical–surgical nursing* (11th ed.). Philadelphia, PA: Lippincott Williams & Wilkins.

Weil, M.H. (2007). Intravenous fluid resuscitation. Available at http://www.merck.com/mmpe/sec06/ch067/ch067c.html. Accessed August 2008.

Chapter 18: Caring for Clients with Cancer

American Cancer Society (2007). Cancer facts and figures. Available at http://www.cancer.org. Accessed June 2008.

American Cancer Society (2008). Information and resources. Available at http://www.cancer.org. Accessed June 2008.

Barton-Burke, M. (2006). Cancer-related fatigue and sleep disturbances. *American Journal of Nursing, 106*(3) supplement, 72–77.

Curtiss, C.P., Haylock, P.J., & Hawkins, R. (2006). Improving the care of cancer survivors. *American Journal of Nursing, 106*(3), 48–52.

Dawson, J.H., & Stewart, G.S. (2005). Taking control. *Advance for Nurses*, February 28, 29–30.

Dell, D.D. (2006). Caring for a client with lymphedema. *Nursing 2006, 36*(6), 49–51.

deNijs, E.J.M., Ros, W., & Grijpdonck, M.H. (2008). Nursing intervention for fatigue during the treatment of cancer. *Cancer Nursing, 31*(3), 191.

Dest, V. (2006). Cancer therapies. *RN, 69*(6), 31–36.

Held-Warmkessel, J. (2005). Managing critical cancer. *Nursing 2005, 35*(1), 58–63.

Hurter, B., & Bush, N.J. (2007). Cancer-related anemia: Clinical review and management update. *Clinical Journal of Oncology Nursing, 11*(3), 349–359.

Milligan, L. (2006). Epidemiology & cancer. *Advance for Nurses*, July 3, 19–21.

Nagel, T.J. (2004). Help patients cope with chemo. *RN, 67*(10), 25–30.

Nowlin, A. (2005). The promise of stem cells. *RN, 68*(4), 48–52.

Plaisance, L. (2005). Is your patient's cancer under control? *Nursing 2005, 35*(5), 52–55.

Polomano, R.C., & Farrar, J.T. (2006). Pain and neuropathy in camcer survivors. *American Journal of Nursing, 106*(3) supplement, 39–47.

Schwartz, A.L. (2007). Understanding and treating cancer-related fatigue. *Oncology, 21*(11), 30.

Smeltzer, S.C., Bare, B.G., Hinkle, J.L., et al. (2008). *Brunner & Suddarth's textbook of medical-surgical nursing* (11th ed.). Philadelphia, PA: Lippincott Williams & Wilkins.

Oncology nursing society and gerontology ontologic consortium (2007). Joint position on cancer care for older adults. Available at http://www.ons.org/publications/positions/Geriatric.shtml. Accessed September 2008.

Vachon, M. (2006). Psychosocial distress and coping after cancer treatment. *American Journal of Nursing, 106*(3) Supplement, 26–31.

Chapter 19: Introduction to the Respiratory System

DiNella, J.V. (2005). The ins and outs of pulmonary function testing. *Nursing 2005, 35*(12), 70–71.

Rushing, J. (2007). Obtaining a throat culture. *Nursing 2007, 37*(3), 20.

Smeltzer, S.C., Bare, B.G., Hinkle, J.L., et al. (2008). *Brunner & Suddarth's textbook of medical-surgical nursing* (11th ed.). Philadelphia, PA: Lippincott Williams & Wilkins.

Soetenga, D.J. (2007). Regional oxygen saturation: The new vital sign. *Nursing 2007, 37*(5), 56cc1–56cc2.

Chapter 20: Caring for Clients with Upper Respiratory Disorders

Andrews, P.L., & Habashi, N.M. (2006). Airway pressure release ventilation: A boost for spontaneous breathing. *American Nurse Today, 1*(10), 10–12.

Ballard, N., Holden-Huchton, P., & Pelter, M.M. (2006, December 4). Conquering VAP, *Advance for Nurses*, 25–27.

Belkner, L., & Craffey, A. (2005, May 24). Giving voice. *Advance for Nurses*, 15–17, 33.

Chulay, M. (2005). VAP prevention: The latest guidelines. *RN, 68*(3), 52–57.

Evans, B. (2005). Best-practice protocols: VAP prevention. *Nursing Management, 36*(12), 10–16.

Fitzgerald, M. (2007). Diagnosing and managing cough. *American Nurse Today, 2*(1), 44.

Gavaghan, S.R., & Jeffries, M. (2006). Your patient's receiving noninvasive positive-pressure ventilation. *Nursing 2006, 36*(5), 46–47.

International Association of Laryngectomees (IAL). Available at http://www.larynxlink.com. Accessed July 2008.

Keefe, S. (2005). Diabetes and sleep apnea. *Advance for Nurses*, August 1, 21–22.

Lindgren, V.A., & Ames, N.J. (2005). Caring for patients on mechanical ventilation. *American Journal of Nursing, 105*(5), 50–60.

Manno, M.S. (2005). Managing mechanical ventilation. *Nursing 2005, 35*(12), 36–41.

Mauk, K.L. (2005). Promoting sound sleep habits in older adults. *Nursing 2005, 35*(2), 22, 25.

Pagana, K.D. (2007). Sleeping in the danger zone. *American Nurse Today, 2*(9), 14–15.

Pruitt, B., & Jacobs, M. (2005). Clearing away pulmonary secretions. *Nursing 2005, 35*(7), 37–41.

Pruitt, B. (2005). Keeping respiratory syncytial virus at bay. *Nursing 2005, 35*(11), 62–64.

Pruitt, B., & Jacobs, M. (2006). Best-practice interventions: Ventilator-associated pneumonia? *Nursing 2006, 36*(2), 36–41.

Pruitt, B. (2006). Weaning patients from mechanical ventilation. *Nursing 2006, 36*(9), 36–41.

Schiech, L. (2007). Looking at laryngeal cancer. *Nursing 2007, 37*(5), 50–55.

Seckel, M.A. (2005, January 3). All about airways. *Advance for Nurses*, 27–28.

Smeltzer, S.C., Bare, B.G., Hinkle, J.L., et al. (2008). *Brunner & Suddarth's textbook of medical-surgical nursing* (11th ed.). Philadelphia, PA: Lippincott Williams & Wilkins.

Strohl, K., & Wylie, P. (2004). Automatic, continuous positive airway pressure delivered with expiratory pressure relief: an in-laboratory comparison with conventional continuous positive bivalve pressure therapy. Respironics. Available at http://cfler.respironics.com Accessed July 2008.

Willard, R.M., & Dreher, M. (2005). Wake-up call for sleep apnea. *Nursing 2005, 35*(3), 46–49.

Yantis, M.A., & Neatherlin, J. (2005). Obstructive sleep apnea in neurological patients. *Journal of Neuroscience Nursing, 37*(3), 150–155.

Chapter 21: Caring for Clients with Lower Respiratory Disorders

Adamow, S.M. (2005). Creating 'teachable moments'. *Advance for Nurses*, May 23, 30–32.

American Cancer Society (2007). Lung cancer. Available at http://www.cancer.org. Accessed July 2008.

Bademan, E.G. (2007). Act fast against pneumothorax. *American Nurse Today, 2*(5), 58.

Bullock, B.A., & Henze, R.L. (2000). *Focus on pathophysiology*. Philadelphia, PA: Lippincott Williams & Wilkins.

Carroll, P. (2005). Keeping up with mobile chest drains. *RN, 68*(10), 26–31.

Centers for Disease Control and Prevention (2008). Influenza. Available at cdcinfo@cdc.gov. Accessed July 2008.

Coughlin, A.M. (2007). Combating community-acquired pneumonia. *Nursing 2007, 37*(2), 64hn1–64hn3.

Coughlin, A.M., & Parchinsky, C. (2006). Go with the flow of chest tube therapy. *Nursing 2006, 36* (3), 36–41.

Cystic Fibrosis Foundation (2007). Living with cystic fibrosis. Available at http://www.cff.org. Accessed July 2008.

Day, M.W. (2005). Action stat: Pulmonary embolism. *Nursing 2005, 35*(9), 88.

deCastro, A.B., & Peterson, C. (2005). Preventing exposure to influenza. *American Journal of Nursing, 105*(1), 112.

Ebersole, P., Hess, P., Touhy, T.A., et al. (2008). *Toward healthy aging: Human needs and nursing response* (7th ed.). St. Louis, MO: Mosby/Elsevier.

Edmondson, D. (2008). Smoke out lung cancer. *LPN 2008, 4*(1), 38–49.

Gardner, J. (2007). What you ned to know about cystic fibrosis. *Nursing 2007, 37*(7), 52–55.

Goldrick, B.A. (2005). Update: Tuberculosis in the United States. *American Journal of Nursing, 105*(7), 85–86.

Holcomb, S.S. (2007). When your patient has pneumonia. *Nursing 2007, 37*(6), 48cc1–48cc3.

Jackson, M.M. (2006). Delayed diagnosis: The tuberculosis tragedy. *American Journal of Nursing, 106*(4), 13.

JAMA (2007). Trends in tuberculosis incidence – United States, 2006. *The JAMA 297*(16), 1765–1767.

McCarron, K. (2006). Take a deep breath: Assessing atelectasis. *LPN 2006, 2*(3), 20–25.

Pruitt, B. (2006). Help your patient combat postoperative atelectasis. *Nursing 2006, 36*(5), 64hn1–64hn6.

Pruitt, B. (2007). Clearing the air with chest tubes. *LPN 2007, 3*(5), 50–55.

Pruitt, B., & Jacobs, M. (2005). Caring for a patient with asthma. *Nursing 2005, 35*(2), 48–51.

Pruitt, B., & Jacobs, M. (2006). All clear. *LPN 2006, 2*(6), 46–55.

Pullen, R.L., & Hayes, D.D. (2007). Administering pneumococcal vaccine. *Nursing 2007, 37*(9), 59.

Roush, K. (2006). Helping patients quit smoking. *American Journal of Nursing, 106*(7), 71–72.

Rueling, S., & Adams, C. (2003). Close to the vest: A novel way to keep airways clear. *Nursing 2003, 33*(12), 56–57.

Sheff, B., & Hayes, D. (2005). Connecting the DOTS to treat pulmonary tuberculosis. *Nursing 2005, 35*(10), 24–25.

Smeltzer, S.C., Bare, B.G., Hinkle, J.L., et al. (2008). *Brunner & Suddarth's textbook of medical-surgical nursing* (11th ed.). Philadelphia, PA: Lippincott Williams & Wilkins.

Smith, S.K. (2006). Adult onset asthma. *Advance for Nurses*, September 11, 17–20.

Sniffing out pneumonia. The nose knows (2004). *Nursing 2004, 34*(7), 35.

Todd, B. (2007). Emerging infections: Extensively drug-resistant tuberculosis. *American Journal of Nursing, 107*(6), 29–31.

Warren, M.L., & Livesay, S. (2006). Taking action against acute COPD. *American Nurse Today, 2*(12), 12–15.

Weitzel, T., Robinson, S.B., & Holmes, J. (2006). Preventing nosocomial pneumonia. *American Journal of Nursing, 106*(9), 72A–72G.

White, M. (2005). Proning for ARDS makes a comeback. *Nursing 2005, 35*(4), 32cc1–32cc2.

World Health Organization (2007). Tuberculosis. Available at http://who.int. Accessed July 2008.

Chapter 22: Introduction to the Cardiovascular System

Bickley, L. (2007). *Bates guide to physical examination and history taking* (9th ed.). Philadelphia, PA: Lippincott Williams & Wilkins.

Cohen, B. J. (2006). *Memmler's structure and fuction of the human body* (8th ed.). Philadelphia, PA: Lippincott Williams & Wilkins.

Martini, F. H. (2006). *Fundamentals of anatomy and physiology.* San Francisco, CA: Benjamin Cummings.

Mehta, M. (2003). Assessing cardiovascular status. *Nursing, 33*(1): 56–58.

Springhouse. (2006a). *Health assessment made incredibly visual.* Philadelphia, PA: Lippincott Williams & Wilkins.

Springhouse. (2006b). *Straight As in anatomy and physiology.* Philadelphia, PA: Lippincott Williams & Wilkins.

Springhouse. (2008a). *Anatomy & physiology made incredibly easy* (3rd ed.). Philadelphia, PA: Lippincott Williams & Wilkins.

Springhouse. (2008b). *Anatomy & physiology made incredibly visual.* Philadelphia, PA: Lippincott Williams & Wilkins.

Springhouse. (2008c). *Assessment made incredibly easy* (4th ed.). Philadelphia, PA: Lippincott Williams & Wilkins.

Weber, J. R., Kelley, J. (2006). *Health assessment in nursing* (3rd ed). Philadelphia, PA: Lippincott Williams & Wilkins.

Chapter 23: Caring for Clients with Infectious and Inflammatory Disorders of the Heart and Blood Vessels

Aquila, A.M. (2001). Deep venous thrombosis. *Journal of Cardiovascular Nursing 15*(4): 25.

Brown, H. (2005). Action stat: cardiac tamponade. *Nursing 35*(3): 88.

Carter, T. (2005). Pericarditis: Inflammation or infarction? *Journal of Cardiovascular Nursing 20*(4): 239–244.

Cheitlin, M. (2006). Valvular heart disease. In M. H. Beers & T. V. Jones *The Merck manual of geriatrics* (3rd ed.). Available at http://www.merck.com/mkgr/mmg/sec11/ch89/ch89a.jsp. Accessed November 2008.

Chojnowski, D. (2004). Putting together the pieces of cardiomyopathy. *Nursing Made Incredibly Easy 2*(3): 18–28.

Church, V. (2000). Staying on guard for DVT & PE. *Nursing 30*(2): 34–44.

Cypher, S. (2006). Treament of heparin-induced thrombocytopenia: A practical argatroban dosing protocol for nurses. *Journal of Infusion Nursing 29*(6): 318–325.

Cook, H.C. (2004). Alternatives to heparin infusion. *Journal of Infusion Nursing 27*(6): 413–424.

Ennis, R.S. (2005). Deep venous thrombosis prophylaxis in orthopedic surgery. Available at http://www.emedicine.com/orthoped/topic600.htm. Accessed December 2007.

Fink, A.M. (2006). Endocarditis after valve replacement surgery. *American Journal of Nursing 106*(2): 40–51.

Goldrick, B.A. (2003). Emerging infections: Endocarditis associated with body piercings. *American Journal of Nursing 103*(1): 26–27.

Hawley, J., Dreher, H.M., & Vasso, M. (2003). Under pressure: Treating cardiac tamponade. *Nursing Management 34*(2): 44D–44H.

Holcomb, S.S. (2004). Critical care: Recognizing and managing endocarditis. *Nursing 34*(2): 32cc1–32cc2.

Holcomb, S.S. (2004). Critical care: Recognizing and managing pericarditis. *Nursing 34*(3): 32cc1–32cc5.

Holcomb, S.S. (2006). Carditis: Hearts afire. *Nursing Made Incredibly Easy.* 4(4): 14–24.

Jurynec, J. (2007). Hypertrophic cardiomyopathy: A review of etiology and treatment. *Journal of Cardiovascular Nursing 22*(1): 65–73.

Kehl-Pruett, W. (2006). Deep vein thrombosis in hospitalized patients: A review of evidence-based guidelines for prevention. *Dimensions of Critical Care Nursing 25*(2): 53–59.

Morgan, E. (2006). Action stat: Pericardial tamponade. *Nursing 36*(2):88.

Munson, B.L. (2005). Myths & facts…about infective endocarditis. *Nursing 35*(2): 71.

Nutescu, E.A., Helgason, & C.M., Briller, J., et al. (2004). New blood thinner offers first potential alternative in 50 years: Ximelagatran. *Journal of Cardiovascular Nursing* 19(6): 374–383.

Porth, C.A. (2006). *Essentials of pathophysiology: Concepts of altered states* (2nd ed). Philadelphia, PA: Lippincott Williams & Wilkins.

Understanding cardiomyopathies. (2004). *Nursing* 34(4): 62–63.

Wisniewski, A. (2003). Identifying infective endocarditis. *Nursing* 33(12): 30.

Wisniewski, A. (2004). Combating Infection: muscle up your knowledge of myocarditis. *Nursing* 34(10): 17.

Yee, C.A. (2005). Endocarditis: The infected heart. *Nursing Management* 36(2): 25–30.

Chapter 24: Caring for Clients with Valvular Disorders of the Heart

Baptiste, M.M. (2001). Aortic vavle replacement. *RN* 64(1): 58–64.

Bonow, R. O., Carabellow, B., Chatterjee, K., et al. (2006). ACC/AHA 2006 guidelines for the management of patients with valvular heart disease. *Journal of American College of Cardiology* 48 (3): 1–148.

Cheitlin, M. (2006). Valvular heart disease. In M.H. Beers & T.V. Jones. *The Merck Manual of Geriatrics* (3rd ed.). Available at http://www.merck.com/mkgr/mmg/sec11/ch89/ch89a.jsp Accessed November 2008.

Darty, S.N., Thomas, M.S., Neagle, C.M., et al. (2002). Cardiovascular magnetic imaging: As more patients undergoing examinations, will you know what to tell them about what to expect. *American Journal of Nursing* 102(12): 34–39.

Hayes, D.D. (2007). Patient education series: mitral valve prolapse. *Nursing* 37(1): 51.

Quillen, T.F. (2005). Myths & Facts…About mitral valve prolapsed *Nursing* 35(9): 71.

Sims, J.M., Miracle, V.A. (2007). An overview of mitral valve prolapsed. *Dimensions of Critical Care Nursing* 26(4): 145–149.

Skill Building: Now hear this: How to identify heart sounds. (2007) *LPN* 3(1): 5–7.

Todd, B. A., & Higgins, K. (2005). Recognizing aortic & mitral valve disease. *Nursing* 35(6): 58–63.

Yeo, K.K., & Low, R.I. (2007). Aortic stenosis: Assessment of the patient at risk. *Journal of Interventional Cardiology* 20(6): 509–516.

Ziegler, K., & Quillen, T.F. (2005). Action stat: Mitral valve regurgitation after myocardial infarction. *Nursing* 35(11):88.

Chapter 25: Caring for Clients with Disorders of Coronary and Peripheral Blood Vessels

Adam, F.M., Stone, M.A., Mendall, J.K., et al. (2002). Effect of treatment for *Chlamydia pneumonia* and *Helicobacter pylori* on markers of inflammation and cardiac events in patients with acute coronary syndromes. *Circulation*, 106(10): 1219–1223.

American College of Cardiology and American Heart Association. (2004). Guidelines for the management of patients with ST-elevation myocardial infarction—Executive summary. Available at http://www.acc.org/qualityandscience/clinical/guidelines/stemi/exec_summ/index.htm. Accessed December 2007.

American Heart Association. (2005). American Heart Association guidelines for cardiopulmonary resuscitation and emergency cardiovascular care. Part 7.5: Postresuscitation support. *Circulation*, 112(24_Supp.1):IV-84-IV-88.

Ashton, K.C. (2007). Nurses, women, and heart disease: Making the connection. Available at http://www.nurse.com/ce/print.html?CCID=4159. Accessed December 2007.

Braun, L.R. (2007). Risk factors lower age of heart attack onset in women. Available at http://www.healthcentral.com/newsdetail/408/8017478.html. Accessed December 2007.

Chu, J.J. (2004). Anxiety after AMI: the roles of sex and desires. *American Journal of Nursing*, 104(7): 72GG-72HH.

Cushman, M. (2005). Leukocyte count in vascular risk prediction. *Archives of Internal Medicine*, 165(5): 487–488.

Dudley-Brown, S. (2004). A shot of good cholesterol: Synthetic HDL, a new intervention for atherosclerosis. *Journal of Cardiovascular Nursing*, 19(6): 421–424.

Edston, E. (2006). The earlobe crease, coronary artery disease, and sudden cardiac death: An autopsy study of 520 individuals. *American Journal of Forensic Medicine & Pathology*, 27(2): 129–133.

Harrison, S. (2007). Guidelines to reduce mortality following MI. *Nursing Older People*, 19(5); 5.

King, K.B., & McGuire, M.A. (2007). Symptom presentation and time to seek care in women and men with acute myocardial infarction. *Heart and Lung*, 36(4): 235–243.

Lawson, W.E., & Hui, J.C.K. (2000). Enhanced external counterpulsation for chronic myocardial ischemia: How to use nonpharmacologic, noninvasive treatment for patients with angina. *Journal of Critical Illness*, 15: 629–636.

Mensah, G.A., Dunbar, S.B. (2006). A framework for addressing disparities in cardiovascular health. *Journal of Cardiovascular Nursing*, 21(6): 451–456.

Movius, M. (2006). What's causing that gut pain? Appendicitis? Diverticulitis?, Constipation?, MI? *RN*, 69(7): 25–30.

Mulestein, J.B., Anderson, J.L., Carlquist, J.F., et al. Randomized secondary prevention trial of azithromycin in patients with coronary artery disease: Primary clinical results of the ACADEMIC study. *Circulation*, 102(15): 1755–1760.

Mussi, L., DeMenezes, A.A., & Caramelli, B. (2007). Poor recognition of symptoms and access to medical care in women with myocardial infarction. *International Journal of Cardiology*, 116(1): 120.

Nissen, S.E., Tsunoda, T., Tuzcu, E.M., et al. (2003). Effect of recombinant ApoA-I Milano on coronary atherosclerosis in patients with acute coronary syndromes. *JAMA*, 290(17): 2292–2300.

O'Donnell, S., Condell, S., Begley, C., et al. (2006). Prehospital care pathway delays: gender and myocardial infarction. *Journal of Advanced Nursing*, 53(3): 268–276.

Reynolds risk score predicts risk for women. Available at http://www.redorbit.com/news/health/839691/reynolds_risk_score_predicts_risk_for_women/index.html. Accessed December 2007.

Ridker, P.M., Buring, J.E., & Rifai, N., et al. (2007). Development and validation of improved algorithms for the assessment of global cardiovascular risk for women: The Reynolds risk score. *JAMA*, 297(6): 611–619

Singh, V.N. (2005). Coronary artery atherosclerosis. Available at http://www.emedicine.com/med/topic446.htm Accessed December 2007.

Tarbutton, G.L., & Mitra, A.K. (2007). Is antibiotic treatment effective for coronary artery disease? *Journal of Applied Research* 7(1): 1–49.

Tindale, R. (2007). Myocardial infarction. *Emergency Nurse*, 14(9): 4–5.

You, T., Yang, R., Lyles, M.F., et al. (2005). Abdominal adipose tissue cytokine gene expression: Relationship to obesity and metabolic risk factors. *American Journal of Physiology, Endocrinology, and Metabolism* 288(4): E741–E747.

Chapter 26: Caring for Clients with Cardiac Dysrhythmias

American Heart Association. (2000). Early defibrillation. Available at http://www.americanheart.org/presenter.jhtml?identifier= 7252. Accessed December 2007.

Bonakdar, R.A., Guarneri, E. (2005). Coenzyme Q10. Available at http://www.aafp.org.afp/20050915/1065.html. Accessed December 2007.

Craig, K. (2005). Photo guide: How to provide transcutaneous pacing. *Nursing* 35(10): 52–53.

Crean, C.A. (2007). Eye on diagnostics: How can electrophysiology help your patients? *Nursing* 37(7): 60–61.

Dirks, J. (2007). Critical care: Supporting your patient through holiday heart syndrome: Excessive alcohol intake can cause dysrhythmias. Here's how to recognize trouble and respond appropriately. *Nursing* 37(2): 64cc1–64cc3.

Funk, M., Wood, K., Valderrama, A.L., et al. (2007). Supraventricular dysrhythmias: Nursing research to improve health outcomes. *Journal of Cardiovascular Nursing* 22(3): 196–217.

Geiter, H.B. (2004). Critical care: Getting back to basics with permanent pacemakers, part I. *Nursing* 34(10): 32cc1–32cc3.

Geiter, H.B. (2004). Critical care: Getting back to basics with permanent pacemakers, part II. *Nursing* 34(11): 32cc1–32cc2.

Gura, M.T. (2005). Implantable Cardioverter Defibrillator Therapy. *Journal of Cardiovascular Nursing* 20(4): 276–287.

Hayes, D.D. (2005). Action stat: Pacemaker malfunction. *Nursing* 35(7):88.

Horn, L, McCoin, M., Kris-Etherton, P., et al. (2008) The evidence for dietary prevention and treatment of cardiovascular disease. *Journal of the American Dietetic Association*, 108, 287–331.

Keeping pace with pacemakers. (2007). *LPN* 2(1): 18–24.

King, D.E., & Dickerson, L.M. (2002). Acute management of atrial fibrillation: Part II. Prevention of thromboembolic complications. Available at http://www.aafp.org/afp/20020715.261.html. Accessed December 2007.

Lazar, J., & Clark, A.D. (2007). Atrial fibrillation. Available at http://www.emedicine.com/emerg/topic47.htm. Accessed December 2007.

Mayo Clinic. (2006). Coenzyme Q10. Available at http://www.mayoclinic.com/health/coenzyme-q10/NS_patient-coenzymeq10. Accessed December 2007.

Reiffel, J.A., & Dizon, J. (2002). The implantable cardioverter-defibrillator; patient perspective. *Circulation* 105:1022–1024.

Taylor, B.A. (2006). Doing it better: Cutting surgical-site infection rate for pacemakers and ICDs. *Nursing* 36(3): 18–19.

Toth, P., & Knecht, J. (2004). Patient education series: Pacemakers. *Nursing* 34(1): 46.

Wolfe, D.A., Kosinski, D., & Gribb, B.P. (1998). Update on implantable cardiac defibrillators. *Postgraduate Medicine* 103: 115–116, 119–123, 129–130.

Woodruff, J., & Prudente, L.A. (2005). Update on implantable pacemakers. *Journal of Cardiovascular Nursing* 20(4). 261–268.

Zipes, D.P., Camm, A.J., Borgrefe, M., et al. (2006). ACC/AHA 2006 guidelines for the management of patients with ventricular arrhythmias and the prevention of sudden cardiac death: a report of the American College of Cardiology/American Heart Association Task Force and the European Society of Cardiology Committee for Practice Guidelines. *Journal of the American College of Cardiology* 48:e247–346.

Chapter 27: Caring for Clients with Hypertension

Bengtson, A., & Drevenhorn, E. (2003). The nurse's role and skills in hypertension care. Available at http://www.medscape.com/viewarticle/463185. Accessed May 2009.

Department of Health and Human Services. Agency for Healthcare Research and Quality. Nursing management of hypertension. (2005). Available at http://www.guideline.gov/summary/summary.aspx?ss=15&doc_id=8342&nbr=4669. Accessed January 2008.

Kinglsey, M. (2007). When hypertension strikes the young. Available at http://include.nurse.com/apps/pbcs.dll/article?AID=/20071203/NJ02/712030314. Accessed January 2008.

Maddox, T., & Parker, D.M. (2006). Peak technique: Don't let hypertension sneak by you. *Nursing Made Incredibly Easy* 4(1):9–11.

Moore, J. (2005). Hypertension: Catching the silent killer. *The Nurse Practitioner* 30(10):16–35.

National Heart, Lung and Blood Institute. (2003) Seventh Report of the Joint National Committee on Prevention, Detection, Evaluation, and Treatment of High Blood Pressure. Available at http://www.nhlbi.nih/gov/guidelines/hypertension/phycard.pdf. Accessed January 2008.

Pickering, T.G., Hall, J.E., Appel, L.J., et al. (2005). Recommendations for blood pressure measurement in humans and experimental animals. *Circulation* 111:697–716.

Woods, A. (2004). Loosening the grip of hypertension. *Nursing* 34(12): 36–43.

Woods, A. (2005). Lowering the risks of diabetes, hypertension, and heart disease. *Nursing* 35(2): 4–8.

Woods, A. (2004). Managing the silent killer. *Nursing Made Incredibly Easy* 2(2): 12–25.

Chapter 28: Caring for Clients with Heart Failure

Ancheta, I.B. (2007). B-type natriuretic peptide rapid assay: A diagnostic test for heart failure. *Dimensions of Critical Care Nursing* 25(4): 149–154.

Angerstein, R.L., Thronson, F., & Rasmusson, M.J. (2006). Enhancing care for cardiac resynchronization therapy patients, device, diagnostics, and clinical application. *Journal of Cardiovascular Nursing* 21(5): 397–404.

Brookes, L. (2004). Incorrect classification of patients by the AHA/ACC stages of heart failure. Available at http://www.medscape.com/viewarticle/490041. Accessed February 2008.

Chojnowski, D. (2006). Managing systolic heart failure. *Nursing* 36(7): 36–42

Chojnowski, D. (2007). Protecting patients from harm: Taking aim at heart failure. *Nursing* 37(11): 50–55.

Chojnowski, D. (2007). Treatment for the troubled heart. *Nursing Made Incredibly Easy* 5(4): 38–49.

Food and Drug Administration. (2006). FDA approves first totally implanted permanent artificial heart for humanitarian uses. Available at http://www.fda.gov/bbs/topics/NEWS/2006/NEW01443.html. Accessed October 2008.

Gray, N.A., & Selzman, C.H. (2006). Current status of the total artificial heart. *American Heart Journal* 152(1): 4–10.

Heart Failure Society of America. (2006). The stages of heart failure—New York Heart Association (NYHA) classification. Available at http://www.abouthf.org/questions_stages.htm. Accessed February 2008.

Moz, T. (2008). Cardiovascular disease: The heart of the matter. *LPN* 3(2): 34–44.

Rasmusson, K, Hall, J.A., & Renlund, D.G. (2007). The intricacies of heart failure. *Nursing Management* 38(5): 33–40.

Richards, N.M., & Stahl, M.A. (2007). Ventricular assist device in the adult. *Critical Care Quarterly* 30(2): 104–118.

Riggs, J.M. (2006). Manage heart failure. *Men in Nursing* 1(2): 18–26,

Riggs, J.M. (2006). Too pooped to pump: Managing chronic heart failure. *Nursing Made Incredibly Easy* 4(1): 28–39.

SAVER heart failure surgery (2004) Available at http://www.chfpatients.com/saver.htm. Accessed February 2008.

Schrock, D., & Ambler, M. (2008). Keeping heart failure patients on the right path. *LPB* 1(5): 18–28.

The Cleveland Clinic. (2005). Heart transplant. Available at http://www.medscape.com/viewarticle/465008. Accessed February 2008.

Wingate, S. (2007). Caring for persons with advanced heart failure. *Home Healthcare Nurse* 25(8): 511–520.

Chapter 29: Caring for Clients Undergoing Cardiovascular Surgery

American College of Cardiology/American Heart Association Task Force. (2004). ACC/AHA 2004 Guideline Update for Coronary Artery Bypass Graft Surgery.

Beattie, S. (2005). Cardiac tamponade. Available at http://www.rnweb.com/rnweb/article/articleDetauk.jsp?id=153932. Accessed February 2008.

CABG drug may increase likelihood of death. (2007). Available at http://wwww.rnweb.com/rnweb/Cardiovascular+Disease/CABG-drug-may-increase-likelihood-of death/ArticleStandard/Article/detail/425310. Accessed February 2008.

Cleveland Clinic Heart Center. (2005). Heart transplant. Available at http://www.medscape.com/viewarticle/465008. Accessed February 2008.

Croce, H.D. (2007). Aortic dissection. Available at http://rnweb.com/rnweb/CE+Library/Aortic-dissection/ArticleStandard/Article/detail/409198. Accessed February 2007.

Edwards Lifesciences. (2005). Edwards previews new minimally invasive heart monitor at SCCM. Available at http://www.edwards.com/newsroom/nr20050117.htm. Accessed February 2008.

Farley, T. (2004). Putting cardiac surgery patients on the "fast track." *Nursing* 34(3): 19.

George, E.L., & Shatzer, M. (2006). When the patient's history includes a transplant. Available at http://www.rnweb.com/rnweb/article/articleDetail.jsp?id=362473. Accessed February 2008.

Holcomb, S.S. (2004). Managing a sternal wound infection after cardiac surgery. *Nursing* 34(9): 68–69.

Hyett, J.M. (2004). Caring for a patient after CABG surgery. *Nursing* 34(7): 48–52.

Innovations in practice: A unique way to reduce patients' preop anxiety. (2006). Available at http://www.rnweb.com/rnweb/Clinical+Highlights/Innovations-in-practice-A-unique-way-to-reduce-pat/ArticleStandard/Article/detail/409198. Accessed February 2008.

Mayo Clinic. (2006). Heart transplant: A treatment for end-stage heart failure. Available at http://www.mayoclinic.com/health/heart-transplant/HB00045. Accessed February 2008.

National Kidney Foundation. (2006). Getting a heart transplant. Available at http://www.kidney.org/atoz/atozItem.cfm?id=158. Accessed February 2008.

Parks, R. (2006). Heart transplant. Available at http://www.webmd.com/heart-disease/heart-transplant-15646. Accessed February 2008.

Rosborough, D. (2006). Cardiac surgery in elderly patients: strategies to optimize outcomes. *Critical Care Nurse* 26(5): 24–31.

Smartt, S. (2004). Minimally invasive cardiac surgery: In search of the wizard. *Journal of PeriAnesthesia Nursing* 19(4):268.

Veronesi, J.F. (2004). Trauma nursing: Blunt chest injuries. Available at http://www.rnweb.com/rnweb/artical/articleDetail.jsp?id=110082. Accessed February 2008.

Whitman, G.R. (2004). Nursing-sensitive outcomes in cardiac surgery patients. *Journal of Cardiovascular Nursing* 19(5): 293–300.

Wright, J. (2006). Drug watch 2006: Cardiovascular meds. *RN* 69(5): 33–38.

Chapter 30: Introduction to the Hematopoietic and Lymphatic Systems

Beattie, S. (2007). Hands-on help: bone marrow aspiration and biopsy; perfect your skills before you assist with a bone marrow exam. *RN* 70(2): 41–43.

Campbell, K. (2005). Blood cells: part one—bone marrow. *Nursing Times* 101(40): 28–29.

Cohen, B. J., & Taylor, J. J. (2009). *Memmler's structure and function of the human body* [9th ed.]. Philadelphia, PA: Lippincott Williams & Wilkins

Cohen, B. J. (2009). *Memmler's the human body in health and disease* [11th ed.]. Philadelphia, Lippincott Williams & Wilkins.

Freedman, M. L. (2006). Aging and the Blood; Anemias; Hematologic Malignancies; Lymphomas. In *The Merck manual of geriatrics,* (3rd ed., updated online). Available at http://www.merck.com/mkgr/mmg/sec9/ch68/ch68d.jsp. Accessed September 2008.

Rogers, B. (2005). Looking at lymphoma and leukemia. *Nursing* 35(7): 56–63.

Springhouse. (2008). *Anatomy and physiology made incredibly easy* [3rd ed.]. Philadelphia, PA: Lippincott Williams & Wilkins. start

Weber, J., & Kelley, J. (2007). *Health assessment in nursing* (3rd ed.). Philadelphia, PA: Lippincott Williams & Wilkins.

Chapter 31: Caring for Clients with Disorders of the Hematopoietic System

Anderson, N. (2006). Hydroxyurea therapy: improving the lives of patients with sickle cell disease. *Pediatric Nursing* 32(6): 541–543, 550–551.

Ballas, S.K., Files, B., Luchtman-Jones, L., et al. (2004). Safety of purified poloxamer 188 in sickle cell disease: phase 1 study of a non-ionic surfactant in the management of acute chest syndrome. Available at http://www.ncbi.nlm.nih/pubmed/15182051. Accessed March 2007.

Bauer, J. (2006). Clinical highlights. Detecting a dangerous complication in sickle cell patients. *RN* 69(9): 24.

Bennett, L. (2005). Understanding sickle cell disorders. *Nursing Standard* 19(32): 52–62.

Bishop, L., & Pearce, H. (2007). Chronic lymphocytic leukaemia: a common but overlooked cancer. *Cancer Nursing Practice* 6(9): 29–35.

Burruss, N., & Holz, S. (2005). Managing the risks of thrombocytopenia. *Nursing* 35(6): 32hn1–32hn-4.

Cooney, M.F. (2006). Heparin-induced thrombocytopenia: advances in diagnosis and treatment. *Critical Care Nurse* 26(6). 30–37.

Dorman, K., & Roman, L.M. (2005). Sickle cell crisis! Managing the pain. *RN* 68(12): 33–7, 33–8.

Faiman, B. (2007). Clinical updates and nursing considerations for patients with multiple myeloma. *Clinical Journal of Oncology Nursing* 11(6): 831–840.

Freedman, M. L. (2006). Hematologic maliginancies. In *The Merck manual of geriatrics,* (3rd ed., updated online). Available at http://www.merck.com/mkgr/mmg/sec9/ch73/ch73a.jsp. Accessed September 2008.

Gibbs, W.J., & Hagemann, T.M. (2003). Purified poloxamer 188 for sickle cell vaso-occlusive crisis. Available at http://www.theannals.com/cgi/content/abstract/38/2/320. Accessed March 2007

Holcomb, S.S. (2005). Recognizing and managing anemia. *Nurse Practitioner* 30(12): 16–18, 23–24, 27–28+.

Huiras, R. (2007). Study focuses on sickle cell's painful reality. *Nursing Spectrum – Florida Edition* 17(11): 26–27.

International Myeloma Foundation. (2005). Bank on a Cure® understanding multiple myeloma. Available at http://myeloma.org/main.jsp?type=article&id=1560. Accessed March 2008.

Johnson, L. E. (2006). Vitamin and trace mineral disorders. In *The Merck manual of geriatrics,* (3rd ed., updated online). Available at http://www.merck.com/mkgr/mmg/sec8/ch60/ch60b.jsp. Accessed September 2008.

Jones, A.P., Davies, S.C., & Olujohungbe, A. (2007). Hydroxyurea for sickle cell disease. Cochrane Database of Systematic Reviews. CINAHL Accession Number: 2009716010.

Leukemia and Lymphoma Society (2008). *Leukemia.* Available at http://www.leukemia-lymphoma.org/all_page?item_id=7026#acute. Accessed September 2008.

Linton, A. D., & Lach, H. W. (2007). *Matteson and McConnell's gerontological nursing: Concepts and practices* (3rd ed.). Philadelphia, PA: Saunders/Elsevier.

Lynn, S.J. (2007). A product is approved for use in von Willebrand disease. *American Journal of Nursing* 107(6): 37.

Miller, C. A. (2009). *Nursing for wellness in older adults.* (5th ed.). Philadelphia, PA: Lippincott Williams & Wilkins.

National Heart, Lung, and Blood Institute. (2007). Nitric oxide inhalation to treat sickle cell pain crises. Available at http://clinicaltrials.gov/ct/show/NCTOO94887?ORDER=39. Accessed March 2007.

Perry, V. (2005). Myths & facts…About sickle cell disease. *Nursing* 35(12): 27.

Platt, A., & Beasley, J. (2005). Patho puzzler. Puzzled about sickle-cell disease? *Nursing Made Incredibly Easy* 3(6): 60–64.

Porth, C.M. (2008). *Pathophysiology: Concepts of altered health states* (8th ed). Philadelphia, PA: Lippincott Williams & Wilkins.

Rogers, B. (2005). Looking at lymphoma & leukemia. *Nursing* 35(7): 56–63.

Smith, P.J., Cox, C.L., & Kelly, D. (2007). Multiple myeloma: Understanding the impact of the disease. *Cancer Nursing Practice* 6(1): 25–28.

Spader, C. (2006). Shedding light on sickle cell anemia. *Nursing Spectrum – DC, Maryland & Virginia Edition* 16(5): 16–17.

University of Arkansas for Medical Sciences. (2007). UAMS performs record 7,000th myeloma stem-cell transplant. Available at http://www.uams.edu/update/absolutenm/templates/news2003v2.asp?articleid=7005&zoneid=18 Accessed March 2008

Walters-Fischer, P. (2005). Cord blood transplantation: May be option in treatment of acute leukemia. *American Journal of Nursing* 105(8): 72D.

Chapter 32: Caring for Clients with Disorders of the Lymphatic System

Ansell, S.M., & Armitage, J.O. (2006). Management of Hodgkin lymphoma. *Mayo Clinic Proceedings* 81(3): 419–426.

Ansell, S.M., Armitage, J.O. (2006). Non-Hodgkin lymphoma: diagnosis and treatment. *Mayo Clinic Proceedings* 80(8): 1087–1097.

Dell, D.D., & Doll, C. (2006). Caring for a patient with lymphedema. *Nursing* 36(6): 49–51.

Freedman, M. L. (2006). Lymphomas. In *The Merck manual of geriatrics,* (3rd ed., updated online). Available at http://www.merck.com/mkgr/mmg/sec9/ch74/ch74b.jsp. Accessed September 2008.

Holcomb, S.S. (2006). Putting the squeeze on lymphedema. *Nursing Made Incredibly Easy* 4(2): 36–34.

Horning, K.M., & Guhde, J. (2007). Lymphedema: An undertreated problem. *MEDSURG Nursing* 16(4): 221–228.

Hussar, D.A. (2004). New drugs04, Part III. *Nursing* 34(9): 56–62.

King, J.E., & Jenkins, T.J. (2006). Clinical queries. Can mononucleosis damage the liver? *Nursing* 36(4): 31.

Lacovara, J.E., & Yoder, L.H. (2006). Cancer: caring and conquering. Secondary lymphedema in the cancer patient. *MEDSURG Nursing* 15(5): 302–307.

Marrs, J. (2007). Oncology nursing 101. Lymphedema and implications for oncology nursing practice. *Clinical Journal of Oncology Nursing* 11(1): 19–21.

Mullen, E., & Zhong, Y. (2007). Hodgkin lymphoma: An update. *Journal for Nurse Practitioners* 3(6): 393–403.

Rogers, B. (2005). Looking at lymphoma and leukemia. *Nursing* 37(7): 56–63.

Winter, G. (2006). Epstein-Barr virus and the kissing disease. *Practice Nursing* 17(9): 453–455.

Zhong, Y. (2006). Non-Hodgkin lymphoma: What primary care professionals need to know. *Journal for Nurse Practitioners* 2(5): 309–315.

Chapter 33: Introduction to the Immune System

Ah, D.V., Kang, D.H., & Carpenter, J.S. (2007). Stress decreases immune function for breast cancer patients. *Research in Nursing & Health* 30:72–83.

Cohen, B. (2006). *Memmler's the structure and function of the human body* (8th ed.). Philadelphia, PA: Lippincott Williams & Wilkins.

Donaldson, T. (2007). Immune responses to infection. *Critical Care Nursing Clinics of North America* 19(1): 1–8.

Harrold-Wild, K. (2006). Nutrition, immunity and the infant and young child. *Journal of Family Health Care* 16(3): 66.

In defense of the body: How the immune system protects us from harm. (2004). *Nursing Made Incredibly Easy!* 2(3): 40–41.

Martini, F.H., & Bartholomew, E.F. (2007). *Essentials of Anatomy and Physiology* (4th ed.). San Francisco, CA: Benjamin Cummings.

Quinn, E. (2007). Yo-yo dieting may weaken immune system. Available at http://sportsmedicine.about.com/od/sportsnutrition/a/060304.htm Accessed April 2008

Springhouse. (2008). *Anatomy and physiology made incredibly easy* (3rd ed.). Philadelphia, PA: Lippincott Williams & Wilkins.

Starkwether, A.R., Witek-Janusek, L., & Mathews, H.L. (2005). Applying the psychoneuroimmunology framework to nursing research. Available at http://www.goliath.ecnext.com/coms2/gi_0199-4811716/Applying-the-psychoneuroimmunology-framework-to.html. Accessed April 2008.

Weber, R. (2005). The immunity challenge. I'm my own cytokine. *Dermatology Nursing* 17(5): 384.

Weber, R. (2005). The immunity challenge. The primary and secondary B-cell response. *Dermatology Nursing* 17(1): 71.

Chapter 34: Caring for Clients with Immune-Mediated Disorders

Benedict, M., & Jackson, R. (2006). Food allergies: New labeling guidelines issued by FDA. *Health Care Food & Nutrition Focus* 23(8): 7.

Bollinger, M.B. (2006). The safety of sublingual-swallow immunotherapy: An analysis of published studies. *Pediatrics* 118 (Supplement August 2006): S22-S23.

Cappellano, K.L. (2008). Food allergy and intolerances: The nuts and bolts of detection and management. *Nutrition Today* 43(1): 11–14.

Carpenito-Moyet, L.J. (2007). *Nursing diagnosis, application to clinical practice* (12th ed.). Philadelphia, PA: Lippincott Williams & Wilkins.

Centers for Disease Control and Prevention. (2004). Public health genomics at CDC, Accomplishments and priorities 2004. Available at http://www.cdc.gov/genomics/activities/ogdop/2004/cocid.htm Accessed May 2008

Centers for Disease Control and Prevention. (2007). Chronic fatigue syndrome; fact sheets for healthcare professionals. Available at http://www.cdc.gov/cfs/toolkit.htm Accessed May 2008

Charron, M., Kramer, J., & Crocetti, S. (2006). Allergy immunotherapy in the primary care setting: Integrating national practice standards to promote safe delivery. *Journal of Nursing Care Quality* 21(2): 187–193.

Conboy-Ellis, K., & Braker-Shaver, S. (2007). Intranasal steroids and allergic rhinitis. *The Nurse Practitioner: The American Journal of Primary Health Care* 32(4): 44–49.

Dellwo, A. (2008). RNase L. Available at http://chronicfatigue.about.com/od/cfsglossary/g/RNaseL.htm. Accessed May 2008.

Drug news: Parents fear using EpiPen on their kids. *Nursing* 35(10): 30.

Geddie, P.I. (2008). Nononcologic use of chemotherapy. *Journal of Infusion Nursing* 31(1): 28–38.

Gelfand, E.W. (2005). Critical decisions in selecting an intravenous immunoglobulin product. *Journal of Infusion Nursing* 28(6): 366–374.

Glenn, Y. (2008). Wound watch: Tape sensitivity: Avoiding a sticky situation. *LPN* 2(6): 10–11.

Hathaway, L.R. (2005). Patient education series: Anaphylaxis. *LPN* 1(3): 38–39.

Hayden, M.L. (2005). Ask the expert: The itchy 'runny' sneezy misery of allergic rhinitis. *Nursing Made Incredibly Easy* 3(2): 64.

National Center for Infectious Diseases. (2006). Chronic fatigue syndrome, information. Available at http://www.cdc.gov/ncidod/diseases/cfs/info.htm Accessed May 2008

Riser, N., & Murphy, M. (2005). Literature review. Insect sting allergy. *The Nurse Practitioner: The American Journal of Primary Health Care* 30(2): 62.

Smith, K., Wallace, A., & Smith-Campbell, B. (2004). What you should know about latex allergy. *The Nurse Practitioner: The American Journal of Primary Health Care* 29(12): 24.

Valente, S. Murray, L., & Fisher, D. (2007). Nurses improve medication safety with medication allergy and adverse drug reports. *Journal of Nursing Care Quality* 22(4): 322–327.

What is CFIDS? (2008). *Journal of Christian Nursing* 25(1): 43.

Wysocki, L. (2007). Red flags: Anaphylaxis doesn't have to be a shock. *Nursing Made Incredibly Easy!* 5(6): 9–13.

Chapter 35: Caring for Clients with HIV/AIDS

Bentley, D. W. (2006). *Human immunodeficiency virus infection.* In M. H. Beers & T. V. Jones *The Merck Manual of Geriatrics* (3rd ed.). Available at http://www.merck.com/mkgr/CVMHighLight?file=/mkgr/mmg/sec16/ch134/ch134a.jsp%3Fregion%3Dmerckcom&word=HIV&domain=www.merck.com#hl_anchor. Accessed November 2008.

Body Health Resources. (2004). Drug delivery strategies. Available at http://www.thebody.com/content/treat/art5571.html. Accessed June 2008.

Body Health Resources. (2003). Fuzeon—A review of the first entry inhibitor. Available at http://img.thebody.com/fuzeon/fuzeon.pdf. Accessed June 2008.

Capili, B., & Anastasi, J.K. (2006). HIV and hyperlipidemia: Current recommendations and treatment. MedSurg Nursing 15(1):14–21.

Centers for Disease Control and Prevention. (2008). HIV and AIDS in the United States: A picture of today's epidemic. Available at http://www.cdc.gov/hiv/topics/surveillance/united_states.htm. Accessed June 2008.

Centers for Disease Control and Prevention. (2003). Surveillance of healthcare personnel with HIV/AIDS as of December 2002. Available at http://www.cdc.gov/ncidod/dhqp/bp_hiv_hp_with.html. Accessed June 2008.

Childrens' AIDS Fund. (2005). The current status of HIV vaccines. Available at http://www.childrensaidsfund.org/showarticle.asp?id=61. Accessed June 2008.

Cichocki, M. (2007). HIV and the older adult – A growing population. Available at http://aids.about.com/cs/aidsfactsheets/a/seniors.htm. Accessed June 2008.

Cohen, B. (2007). Caring for a patient with HIV/AIDS. *MedSurg Nursing* 16(1): 53–54.

Coleman, C.L. (2006). Revisiting HIV/AIDS. *Men in Nursing* 1(6): 20–27.

Ehlers, V.J. (2006). Challenges nurses face in coping with the HIV/ AIDS pandemic in Africa. *International Journal of Nursing Studies* 43(6): 657–662.

Henry J. Kaiser Foundation. (2008). Kaiser daily HIV/AIDS report. Available at http://www.kaisernetwork.org/Daily_reports/rep_ index.cfm?DR_ID=52542. Accessed June 2008.

HIV and Hepatitis Treatment Advocates. (2007). Roche and Trimeris to discontinue "Biojector 2000" device for enfuvirtide (Fuzeon). Available at http://www.hivandhepatitis.com/recent/ 2007/100507_c.html. Accessed June 2008.

Hudson, K. (2006). Human immunodeficiency virus (HIV) and autoimmune deficiency syndrome. Available at http://www. dynamicnursingeducation.com/class.php?class_id=95&oid=20 Accessed June 2008.

Joint United Nations Programme on HIV/AIDS (UNAIDS). 2007. Sub-Saharan Africa. Available at http://www.unaids.org/en/ CountryResponses/Regions/SubSaharanAfrica.asp. Accessed June 2008.

Jones, S.G. (2006). A step-by-step approach to HIV/AIDS. *The Nursing Practitioner: The American Journal of Primary Care* 31(6): 26–39.

Medical News Today. 2005. Resistant strain of rapidly progressive HIV diagnosed in New York City. Available at http://www. medicalnewstoday.com/articles/19966.php. Accessed June 2008.

National Institute of Allergy and Infectious Diseases. (2004). The current status of HIV-1 vaccine development, 2004: Recommendations for the future. Available at http://www3.niaid.nih. gov/research/topics/HIV/vaccines/advisory/avis/PDF/AVRWG_ 2 11 04.pdf. Accessed June 2008.

National Institute of Allergy and Infectious Diseases. 2004. How HIV causes AIDS. Available at http://www.niaid.nih.gov/ factsheets/howhiv.htm. Accessed June 2008.

National Institute of Allergy and Infectious Diseases. (2005). International trial of two microbicides begins. Available at http:// www2.niaid.nih.gov/news/newsreleases/2005/microbicides.htm. Accessed June 2008.

Panel on Antiretroviral Guidelines for Adults and Adolescents. (2008). Guidelines for the use of antiretroviral agents in HIV-1-infected adults and adolescents. Department of Health and Human Services. Available at http://www.aidsinfo.nih.gov/ ContentFiles/AdultsandAdolescentGL.pdf. Accessed June 2008.

Scondras, D. (2004). Search for a cure. The latest news. Available at http://www.thebody.com/content/treat/art2747.html. Accessed June 2008.

Spooner, L.M., & Olin, J.L. (2007). New therapies for HIV infection. Available at http://www.uspharmacist.com/econnect/ Default.aspx?tabid=53&page=publish/content/8_2139.htm. Accessed June 2008.

Vaccines and Related Biological Products Advisory Committee. (2004) HIV-1 recombinant canarypox-vectored vaccine with recombinant gp120 B/E. Available at http://www.fda.gov/ ohrms/dockets/ac/04/briefing/4072B2_1.htm. Accessed June 2008.

Woods, M., Potts, E., & Connors, J. (2008). Building a high quality diet. Available at www.tufts.edu/med/nutrition-infection/hiv/ health_high_quality_diet.html. Accessed August 2008.

World Health Organization. (2007). AIDS epidemic update. Joint United Nations Programme on HIV/AIDS. Available at http://www.unaids.org/en/HIV_data/2007EpiUpdate/default.asp. Accessed June 2008.

Chapter 36: Introduction to the Nervous System

Assessing the cranial nerves. (2006). *Nursing* 36(11): 47–49.

Be creative teaching nurses to do neuro assessments. (2005). *ED Nursing* 8(5): 53–54.

Bolek, B. (2006). Strictly clinical. Facing cranial nerve assessment. *American Nurse Today* 1(2): 21–22.

Huntley, A. (2008). Chart smart. Documenting level of consciousness. *Nursing* 38(8): 63–64.

Iankova, A. (2006). The Glasgow Coma Scale. *Emergency Nurse* 14(8): 30–35.

Joynt, R. J. (2006). Aging and the nervous system. In M. H. Beers & T. V. Jones *The Merck manual of geriatrics* (3rd ed.). Available at http://www.merck.com/mkgr/mmg/sec6/ch42/ch42a.jsp. Accessed December 2008.

Katz, M.J., & Bauer, J. (2006). Save time! Do a 5-minute initial assessment. *RN* 69(3): 43–46, 50, 52.

McNett, M. (2007). A review of the predictive ability of Glasgow Coma Scale scores in head-injured patients. *Journal of Neuroscience Nursing* 39(2): 68–75.

Meyers, S. (2006). Clinical clips. Coma measurement system increases evaluation accuracy. *Nursing Spectrum (Midwest)* 7(4): 18–19.

New tool is coming for neuro assessments. (2006). *ED Nursing* 9(8): 87–88.

Rutenberg, C. (2008). How to recognize life-threatening emergencies over the phone. *Nursing* 38(2): 56hn1–56hn2, 56hn4.

Tips to teach nurses to do neuro assessments. (2005). *ED Nursing* 8(5): 54–55.

Waterhouse, C. (2005). The Glasgow Coma Scale and other neurological observations. *Nursing Standard* 19(33): 56–64, 66–67.

Wellington, B. (2005). Development of a guide for neurological observations. *Nursing Times* 101(39): 32–34.

White, A. (2006). Neurologic assessment: vital in prioritizing emergency department interventions. *American Journal for Nurse Practitioners* 10(9): 57–58, 60–67.

Chapter 37: Caring for Clients with Central and Peripheral Nervous System Disorders

Bole, K. (2007). Research teams uncover risk genes for multiple sclerosis. Available at http://pub.ucsf.edu/newsservices/ releases/200707301. Accessed July 2008.

Bonifazi, W. (2006). A question of balance. *Nursing Spectrum— Florida edition* 16(13): 20–21.

Centers for Disease Control and Prevention. (2008). West Nile virus: Background information for clinicians. Available at http:// www.cdc.gov/nciod/dvbid/westnile/clinicians/background.htm. Accessed July 2008.

Bourne, C., Clayton, C., Murch, A., et al. (2006). Cognitive impairment and behavioural difficulties in patients with Huntington's disease. *Nursing Standard* 20(35): 41–44.

Costello, F. (2006). Myasthenia gravis and multiple sclerosis: a review of the ocular manifestations. *The Journal of the American Society of Ophthalmic Registered Nurses* 31(3): 19–24.

Florea, N.R., Maglio, D., & Nicolau, D.P. (2003). Pleconaril, a novel antipiconaviral agent. Available at http://www.medscape.com/viewarticle/451846_5. Accessed July 2008.

Gangloff, J.M. (2004). Compassionate use offers access to unapproved drugs. Available at http://www.curetoday.com/backissues/v3n3/departments/specialreport/. Accessed July 2008.

Harms, S.L., Eberly, L.E., Garrard, J.M., et al. (2005). Prevalence of appropriate and problematic antiepileptic combination therapy in older people in the nursing home. *Journal of the American Geriatrics Society* 53(6): 1023–1028.

Heisters, D. (2007). Care planning for Parkinson's disease. *Nursing & Residential Care* 9(4): 164–166.

Hunka, K., Suchowersky, O., Wood, S., et al. (2005). Nursing time to program and assess deep brain stimulators in movement disorder patients. *Journal of Neuroscience Nursing* 37(4): 204–210.

Koski, C.L., & Patterson, J.V. (2006). Intravenous immunoglobulin use for neurologic diseases. *Journal of Infusion Nursing* 29(Supplement 3S): S21–28, S45–48.

Lettieri, C.J. (2006). Neurotrauma: Management of acute head injuries. Available at http:www.medscape.com/viewarticle/542508_4. Accessed July 2008.

Mathews, C., Miller, L., & Mott, M. (2007). Getting ahead of acute meningitis & encephalitis: learn how to distinguish between these common central nervous system infections and respond appropriately. *Nursing* 37(11): 36–41.

Miller, A. (2007). Guillain-Barre' Syndrome. Available at http://www.emedicine.com/EMERG/topic222.htm. Accessed July 2008.

Myers, F. (2000). Meningitis, the fears, the facts. *RN* 63(11): 52–58.

National Multiple Sclerosis Society. (2008). Nervous system repair & protection team. Available at http://nationalmssociety.org/research/research-we-fund/targeted-research/nervous-system-repair/french-constant-repair-team/index.aspx Accessed July 2008.

O'Maley, K., O'Sullivan, J., Woolin, J., et al. (2005). Teaching people with Parkinson's disease about their medication. *Journal of Nursing Older People* 17(1): 14–16, 18, 20.

Palese, A., & Infanti, S. (2006). The experiences of nurses who participate in awake craniotomy procedures. *American Operating Room Nurses Journal* 84(5): 811–812, 814, 816–819+.

Palmieri, R.L. (2005). Is it myasthenia gravis or Guillain-Barré syndrome? *Nursing* 35(12): 32hn1–32hn2, 32hn4.

Palmieri, R.L. (2005). Take aim at amyotrophic lateral sclerosis. *Nursing* 34(11): *Hospital Nursing*: 32hn1–32hn2.

Pountney, D. (2007). Parkinson's: not easy to detect. *Nursing Older People* 19(6): 12–13.

Rangel-Castillo, L., Gopinath, S., & Robertson, C.S. (2008). Management of intracranial hypertension. *Clinical Neurology* 26(2): 521–541.

Raymond, R. (2006). Providing quality care for residents with Parkinson's disease. *Nursing & Residential Care* 8(6): 275–277.

Schumacher, L., & Chernecky, C.C. (2005). *Critical care and emergency nursing*. St. Louis, MO: WB Saunders.

Skirton, H. (2005). Huntington's disease: a nursing perspective. *MEDSURG Nursing* 14(3): 167–173.

Sole, M.L., Moseley, M.J., & Klein, D.G. (2005). *Introduction to critical care nursing* (4th ed.). St. Louis, MO: WB Saunders.

Stover, N.P., Bakay, R.A., Subramanian, T., et al. (2005). Intrastriatal implantation of human retinal pigment epithelial cells attached to microcarriers in advanced Parkinson's disease. *Archives of Neurology* 62(12): 1833–1837.

Swann, J. (2005). Moving with a purpose in Parkinson's disease. *Nursing & Residential Care* 7(7): 316–318.

Thomure, A. (2006). Helping your patient manage Parkinson's disease. *Nursing* 36(8): 20–21.

Van den Berg, J.P., Kalmijn, S., Lindeman, E., et al. (2005). Multidisciplinary ALS care improves quality of life in patients with ALS. *Neurology* 65(8): 1264–1267.

Waterhouse, C. (2005). The Glasgow Coma Scale and other neurological observations. *Nursing Standard* 19(33): 56–64, 66–67.

Wisniewski, A. (2003). Closing in on clues to encephalitis. *Nursing* 33(4): 70–71.

Zink, E.K., & McQuillan, K. (2005). Managing traumatic brain injury. *Nursing* 35(9): 36–44.

Chapter 38: Caring for Clients with Cerebrovascular Disorders

Allen, G. (2007). Evidence for practice. Mild hypothermia during intracranial aneurysm surgery. *American Operating Room Nurses Journal* 86(1): 114, 116.

Alverzo, J.P., Brigante, M.A., & McNish, M.D. (2007). Hospital Extra. Improving stroke outcomes: rehabilitation strategies that work. *American Journal of Nursing* 107(11): Supplement: 72B-72D, 72F, 72H.

American Heart Association/American Stroke Association. (2008). Heart disease and stroke statistics – 2008 update at-a-glance. Available at http://www.www.americanheart.org/downloadable/heart/1200078608862HS_Stats%202008.final.pdf. Accessed July 2008.

Byrns, C., & Lynch, P.A. (2005). Hi-tech meets rehab nursing. *Nursing Spectrum – Florida Edition* 15(9): 12–13.

Caplan, L. R. (2006). Cerebrovascular disease. In M. H. Beers & T. V. Jones, *The Merck manual of geriatrics* (3rd ed.). Available at http://www.merck.com/mkgr/mmg/sec6/ch44/ch44a.jsp. Accessed December 2008.

Corcoran, L. (2005). Nutrition and hydration tips for stroke patients with dysphagia. *Nursing Times* 101(48): 24–27.

Daly, M.L., & Powers, J. (2007). Strictly clinical. Rapid response: Speeding to save a stroke victim. *American Nurse Today* 2(12): 20.

Hinkle, J.L., & Guanci, M.M. (2007). Acute ischemic stroke review. Journal of *Neuroscience Nursing* 39(5): 285–293, 310.

King, J.E., & Ezell, J. (2006). Clinical queries. How do I manage ischemic stroke in a menstruating woman. *Nursing* 36(1): 22.

Liechty, J.A., & Heinzekehr, J.B. (2007). Reflections. Caring for those without words: a perspective on aphasia. *Journal of Neuroscience Nursing* 39(5): 316–318.

Miller, J., Elmore, S. (2005). Call a stroke code. *Nursing* 35 (3): 58–64.

Morris, H. (2007). The impact and management of swallowing difficulties. *Nursing & Residential Care* 9(12): 562, 564, 566.

Morrison, K. (2007). Improving the care of stroke patients: Using an evidence-based quality improvement initiative enhances outcomes for stroke patients. *American Nurse Today* 2(4): 38–44.

National Institute of Neurological Disorders and Stroke. (2008). Headache—hope through research. Available at http://www.ninds.nih.gov/disorders/headache/detail_headache.htm Accessed July 2008.

National Institute of Neurological Disorders and Stroke. (2008). Stroke: Hope through research. Available at http://www.ninds.

nih.gov/disorders/stroke/detail_stroke.htm. Accessed July 2008.

Peters, M., Vydelingum, V., & Abu-Saad, H.H. (2007). Migraine and chronic daily headache management: implications for primary care practitioners. *Journal of Clinical Nursing* 16(7b): Supplement: 159–167.

Quinn, C.M. (2006). Quick! My patient is having an ischemic stroke. *Nursing* 36(7): *Critical Care*: 56cc1–56cc-2, 56cc4.

Smallwood, A., & Humphreys, M. (2007). Nurses' perceptions and experiences of initiating thrombolysis: a qualitative study. *Nursing in Critical Care* 12(3): 132–140.

Vacca, V.M., Jr. (2006). Action stat. Acute ischemic stroke. *Nursing* 36(9): 80.

Welch, E. (2005). Headache. *Nursing Standard* 19(24). 45–53.

Chapter 39: Caring for Clients with Head and Spinal Cord Trauma

Ash, D. (2005). Sustaining safe and acceptable bowel care in spinal cord injured patients. *Nursing Standard* 20(8): 55–64, 66, 68.

Brain Trauma Foundation, American Association of Neurological Surgeons, Congress of Neurological Surgeons. (2007). Guidelines for the management of severe traumatic brain injury. Steroids. Journal of Neurotrauma 24(Suppl1): S91-S95. Available at http://www.guideline.gov/summary/summary.aspx?doc_id=11003. Accessed July 2008.

Dworkin, R.H., O'Connor, A.B., Backonja, M., et al. (2007). Pharmacologic management of neuropathic pain: evidence based recommendations. Available at http://www.guideline.gov/summary/summary.aspx?doc_id=11724. Accessed July 2008.

Emory physician uses Botox injections to treat spasticity following stroke, spinal cord injury, and brain injury. (2003). Available at http://whsc.emory.edu/_releases/2003january.botox.html. Accessed July 2008.

Hansen, R.B., Sorensen, F.B., & Kristensen, J.K. (2007). Urinary calculi following traumatic spinal cord injury. Available at http://www.informaworld.com/smpp/content~content=a777126547db=allorder=page. Accessed July 2008.

Hill, C.E., Moon, L., & Wood, P.M. (2005). Labeled Schwann cell transplantation: cell loss, host Schwann cell replacement, and strategies to enhance survival. Glia 53(3): 338–343. Available at http://www3.interscience.wiley.com/journal/112139046/abstract. Accessed July 2008.

Jeffrey, S. (2006). Pregabalin effective for neuropathic pain after spinal cord injury. Available at http://www.medscape.com/viewarticle/548374. Accessed July 2008.

Lima, C., Pratas-Vital, J., Escada, P., et al. (2005). Olfactory mucosa autografts in human spinal cord injury: A pilot clinical study. Journal of Spinal Cord Medicine 29(3): 191–203. Available at http://www.pubmedcentral.nih.gov/articlerender.fcgi?artid=1864811. Accessed July 2008.

Matsas, R., Lavdas, A., Papastefanaki, F., et al. (2008). Schwann cell transplantation for CNS repair. *Current Medicinal Therapy* 15(2): 151–160.

Oudega, M., & Xu, X.M. (2006). *Journal of Neurotrauma* 23 (3–4): 453–467. Available at http://www.ncbi.nlm.nih.gov/pubmed/16629629. Accessed July 2008.

Parsa, C. (2008). Spinal cord injury nursing: An extraordinary specialty. *Imprint* 55(1): 49–51.

Raia, L., & Carlineo, G. (2006). *SCI Nursing* 23(4): 1.

Raisman, G. (2005). Repair of spinal cord injury by transplantation of olfactory ensheathing cells. Available at http://ist.inserm.fr/BASIS.elgis/fqmat/atelier/DDD/2334.doc. Accessed July 2008.

Regan, M., Teasell, R.W., & Mortenson, W.B. (2006). Pressure ulcers following spinal cord injury. Available at http://www.icord.org/scire/pdf/SCORE_CHAP20.pdf. Accessed July 2008.

Rehabilitation Institute of Chicago. (2008). Spinal cord injury: Tendon transfer surgery. Available at http://lifecenter.ric.org/content/2149/index.html?topic=1&subtopic=304. Accessed July 2008.

Spinal Cord InfoSheet. (2007). Sexuality for women with spinal cord injury. Available at http://www.spinalcord.uab.edu/show.asp?durki=1021&return=21479. Accessed July 2008.

Starkweather, A. (2006). Posterior lumbar interbody fusion: An old concept with new techniques. *Journal of Neuroscience Nursing* 38(1): 13–20, 30.

University of Washington. (2002). Common musculoskeletal problems after SCI: contractures, osteoporosis, fractures, and shoulder pain. Available at http://sci.washington.edu/info/forums/reports/musculoskeletal.asp. Accessed July 2008.

Chapter 40: Caring for Clients with Neurologic Deficits

Arias, M., & Smith, L.N. (2007). Early mobilization of acute stroke patients. *Journal of Clinical Nursing* 16(2): 282–288.

Bisanz, A. (2007). Chronic constipation. *American Journal of Nursing* 107(4): Hospital Extra: 72B-72D, 72F-72H.

Fletcher, K. (2005). Elimination: geriatric self-learning module. *MEDSURG Nursing* 14(2): 127–131.

Gray, M. (2007). Context for WOC (wound, ostomy, continence) practice: bowel and bladder management. *Journal of Wound, Ostomy & Continence Nursing* 34(6): 592–594

Myers, J.S. (2008). Factors associated with changing cognitive function in older adults: implications for nursing rehabilitation. *Rehabilitation Nursing* 33(3): 117–23.

Sturdy, D. (2008). Dependence and dignity. *Nursing Older People* 20(3). 10.

Wilson, L.A. (2005). Continuing professional development. Understanding bowel problems in older people: part 1. *Nursing Older People* 17(8): 25–29.

Chapter 41: Introduction to the Sensory System

American Academy of Ophthalmology (2008). Get your eyes screened at 40. Available at http://www.geteyesmart.org. Accessed August 2008.

ASHA (2008). Hearing assessment. Available at http://www.asha.org. Accessed August 2008.

Smeltzer, S.C., Bare, B.G., Hinkle, J.L., et al. (2008). *Brunner & Suddarth's textbook of medical-surgical nursing* (11th ed.). Philadelphia, PA: Lippincott Williams & Wilkins.

Chapter 42: Caring for Clients with Eye Disorders

Boyd-Monk, H. (2006). Glaucoma and macular degeneration. *LPN 2006, 3*(1), 46–53.

Covell, C.A., Graziano, J., Rich, D., et al. (2007). New outlook for age-related macular degeneration. *Nursing 2007, 37*(3), 22–24.

Infection Prevention (2007). All eyes on conjunctivitis. *LPN 2007, 3*(6), 23, 25.

International Society of Refractive Surgery of the American Academy of Ophthalmology (ISRS/AAO) (2008). Refractive Surgery Procedures. Available at http://www.aao.org/isrs. Accessed August 2008.

Monk, H.B. (2005). Bringing common eye emergencies into focus. *Nursing 2005, 35*(12), 46–51. National Eye Institute (2006). Age-related macular degeneration. Available at http://www.nei.nih.gov/health/macular degen. Accessed August 2008.

Rushing, J. (2007). Administering eyedrops. *Nursing 2007, 37*(5), 18.

Skill Building (2006). Understanding ocular drug delivery. *LPN 2006, 2*(6), 12–14.

Smeltzer, S.C., Bare, B.G., Hinkle, J.L., et al. (2008). *Brunner & Suddarth's textbook of medical-surgical nursing* (11th ed.). Philadelphia, PA: Lippincott Williams & Wilkins.

Spires, R. (2006). How you can help when older eyes fail. *RN, 69*(2), 38–43.

Whiteside, M.M., Wallhagen, M.I., & Pettengill, E. (2006). Sensory impairment in older adults: Part 2: Vision loss. *American Journal of Nursing, 106*(11), 52–61.

Chapter 43: Caring for Clients with Ear Disorders

Carpenito-Moyer, L.J. (2008). *Nursing diagnosis: Application to nursing practice* (12th ed.). Philadelphia, PA: Lippincott Williams & Wilkins.

Keefe, S. (2005). Cochlear implants: A culture issue. *Advance for Nurses*, June 20, 25–26.

Pullen, R.L. (2006). Spin control: Caring for a patient with inner ear disease. *Nursing 2006, 36*(5), 48–51.

Safe Haven (2006). Do you hear what I hear? *LPN 2006, 2*(3), 6–10.

Smeltzer, S.C., Bare, B.G., Hinkle, J.L., et al. (2008). *Brunner & Suddarth's textbook of medical-surgical nursing* (11th ed.). Philadelphia, PA: Lippincott Williams & Wilkins.

Wallhagen, M.I., Pettengill, E., & Whiteside, M. (2006). Sensory impairment in older adults: Part I: Hearing loss. *American Journal of Nursing, 106*(10), 40–47.

Chapter 44: Introduction to the Gastrointestinal System and Accessory Structures

Madsen, D., Sebolt, T., Cullen, L., et al. (2005). Listening to bowel sounds: An evidence-based practice project. *American Journal of Nursing, 105*(12), 40–49.

Mayo Clinic (2008). Early warning for liver disease: From MRI to MRE. *Discovery's Edge: Mayo Clinic's Online Research Magazine*. Available at http://discoverysedge.mayo.edu/de07-1-biotech-ehman/. Accessed November 2008.

Molle, E. (2005). Getting down to the lower GI tract. *Nursing 2005, 35*(11), 20–21.

Pagana, K.D. (2006). Virtual colonoscopy: A noninvasive look at the colon. *American Nurse Today, 1*(12), 20–21.

Porth, C.M. (2007). *Essentials of pathophysiology: Concepts of altered health states* (2nd ed.). Philadelphia, PA: Lippincott Williams & Wilkins.

Pullen, R.L. (2005). Tips for safe, accurate occult blood testing. *Nursing 2005, 35*(3), 28.

Smeltzer, S.C., Bare, B.G., Hinkle, J.L., et al. (2008). *Brunner & Suddarth's textbook of medical-surgical nursing* (11th ed.). Philadelphia, PA: Lippincott Williams & Wilkins.

Chapter 45: Caring for Clients with Disorders of the Upper Gastrointestinal Tract

Barba, K., Fitzgerald, P., & Wood, S. (2007). Managing peptic ulcer disease. *Nursing 2007, 37*(7), 56hn1–56hn4.

Beauchamp-Johnson, B.M. (2006). Scale down bariatric surgery's risk. *Nursing Management, 37*(9), 27–32.

Center for Disease Control and Prevention (CDC) (2008). Defining overweight and obesity. Available at http://www.cdc.gov/nccdphp/dnpa/obesity/defining.htm. Accessed September 2008.

Condon, M. (2007). Handling with care: The bariatric patient. *American Nurse Today, 2*(4), 50.

Fry, D.A. (2007). Exposing the source of peptic ulcer disease. *LPN 2007, 3*(3), 6–10.

Hathaway, L. (2005). A guide to GERD. *LPN 2005, 1*(6), 26–31.

Holmes, S.L. (2006). Gastroesophageal reflux disease. *Advance for Nurses*, December 18, 37–39.

Lawrence, B.L., & Taylor, D. Esophageal pH monitoring goes wireless. *Nursing 2007, 37*(10), 26–27.

Mayo Clinic Staff (2007). Gastric bypass surgery: What can you expect? *Mayo Clinic.com*. Available at http://wwww.mayoclinic.com/health/gastric-bypass/HQ01465. Accessed December 2008.

McGohan, L.D. (2005). Bariatric surgery: Helping your obese patients take control. *LPN 2005, 1*(5), 30–37.

Merrel, P., & Fisher, C. (2007). Fine-tuning your feeding-tube insertion skills. *American Nurse Today, 2*(8), 33–35.

Miller, S.K. (2007). Getting a grip on GERD. *American Nurse Today, 2*(6), 12–14.

Molle, E. (2005). Keep the GI tract from going downhill. *Nursing 2005, 35*(10), 28–29.

Nowlin, A. (2006). The dysphagia dilemma: How you can help. *RN, 69*(6), 44–48.

Peters, V.L. (2006a). Feeding patients with swallowing disorders. *LPN 2006, 2*(2), 13–17.

Peters, V.L. (2006b). Tube feeding: What you need to know. *LPN 2006, 2*(1), 4–7.

Reising, D.L., & Neal, R.S. (2005). Enteral tube flushing: What you think are best practices may not be. *American Journal of Nursing, 105*(3), 58–63.

Skill Building (2008). Caring for a client with a gastrostomy feeding tube. *LPN 2008, 4*(4).

Skill Building (2008). Hard to swallow: Understanding dysphagia. *LPN 2008, 4*(5), 22–23.

Smeltzer, S.C., Bare, B.G., Hinkle, J.L., et al. (2008). *Brunner & Suddarth's textbook of medical-surgical nursing* (11th ed.). Philadelphia, PA: Lippincott Williams & Wilkins.

Smith, B.L. (2005). Bariatric surgery: It's no easy fix. *RN, 68*(6), 58–63.

Smith, R-M., & Myers, S.A. (2005). 2 Devices that unclog feeding tubes. *RN, 68*(1), 36–41.

Chapter 46: Caring for Clients with Disorders of the Lower Gastrointestinal Tract

Amerine, E. (2007). Preventing and managing acute diverticulitis. *Nursing 2007, 37*(9), 56hn1–56hn6.

Amerine, E., & Keirsey, M. (2006a). Managing acute diarrhea. *Nursing 2006, 36*(9), 64hn1–64hn2.

Amerine, E., & Keirsey, M. (2006b). How should you respond to constipation? *Nursing 2006, 36*(10), 64hn1–64hn2.

Bauman, T. (2006, October 9). Hereditary colon cancer. *Advance for Nurses*, 33–35.

Bisanz, A. (2007). Chronic constipation. *American Journal of Nursing, 107*(4), 72B-72H.

Freeman, L.C. (2007). Responding to small-bowel obstruction. *Nursing 2007, 37*(5), 56hn1–56hn6.

Hill, R. (2007). Conquering constipation. *LPN 2007, 3*(4), 48–53.

Kather, T.A. (2005). Colorectal cancer: Guidelines for prevention, screening and treatment. *Advance for Nurses*, March 28, 15–17.

Kent, V.P. (2007). Caring for a patient with a bowel obstruction. *Nursing 2007, 3*(5), 30–33.

Mauk, K.L. (2005). Preventing constipation in older adults. *Nursing 2005, 35*(6), 22–23.

Mayo Clinic (2008). Irritable Bowel Syndrome. Available at http://www.mayoclinic.com/health/irritable-bowel-syndrome. Accessed September 2008.

Movius, M. (2006). What's causing that gut pain? *RN, 69*(7), 25–29.

Oriola, S. (2006). C. difficile: A menace in hospitals and homes alike. *Nursing 2006, 36*(8), 14–15.

Rocca, J.D. (2007). Minimizing the perils of appendicitis. *Nursing 2007, 37*(1), 64hn1–64hn3.

Skill Building (2007). Easy does it: Administering rectal suppositories and ointments. *LPN 2007, 3*(4), 4–5.

Smeltzer, S.C., Bare, B.G., Hinkle, J.L., et al. (2008). *Brunner & Suddarth's textbook of medical surgical nursing* (11th ed.). Philadelphia, PA: Lippincott Williams & Wilkins.

Todd, B. (2006). Emerging infections: Clostridium difficile: Familiar pathogen, changing epidemiology. *American Journal of Nursing, 106*(5), 33–36.

Chapter 47: Caring for Clients with Disorders of the Liver, Gallbladder, and Pancreas

Baltimore, J.J., & Davidson, J. (2007). Caring for a patient with acute cholecystitis. *Nursing 2007, 37*(3), 64hn1–64hn4.

Burruss, N., & Holz, S. (2005). Understanding acute pancreatitis. *Nursing 2005, 35*(3), 32hn1–32hn4.

Despins, L.A., Kivlahan, C., & Cox, K.R. (2005). Acute pancreatitis. *American Journal of Nursing, 105*(11), 54–57.

Durston, S. (2005). What you need to know about viral hepatitis. *Nursing 2005, 35*(8), 36–41.

Holcomb, S.S. (2005). Gallstones. *Nursing 2005, 35*(9), 45.

Holcomb, S.S. (2007). Stopping the destruction of acute pancreatitis. *Nursing 2007, 37*(6),

Hospital Nursing (2007). What are the options for managing ascites? *Nursing 2007, 37*(3), 64hn6.

Pellegrino, A. (2006). Looking at liver cancer. *Nursing 2006, 36*(10), 52–55.

Riehl, M. (2007). Help your patient cope with pancreatic cancer. *Nursing 2007, 37*(4), 54–57.

Shea, M.C. (2004). Radiofrequency ablation: Putting the heat on liver cancer. *Nursing 2004, 34*(12), 32hn1, 32hn4.

Smeltzer, S.C., Bare, B.G., Hinkle, J.L., et al. (2008). *Brunner & Suddarth's textbook of medical-surgical nursing* (11th ed.). Philadelphia, PA: Lippincott Williams & Wilkins.

Whiteman, K., & McCormack, C. (2005). When your patient is in liver failure. *Nursing 2005, 35*(4), 58–63.

Chapter 48: Caring for Clients with Ostomies

Pullen, R.L. (2006). Teaching your patient to irrigate a colostomy. *Nursing 2006, 36*(4), 22.

Skill Building (2007). How to apply and change an ostomy pouch. *LPN 2007, 3*(3), 20–22.

Chapter 49: Introduction to the Endocrine System

CCRN Review: endocrine and immunologic systems. (2006). *Nursing 36*(3): Critical care 64cc5–64cc-6.

Kimball, J. (2006). Hormones of the hypothalamus. Available at http://users.rcn.com/jkimball.ma.ultranet/BiologyPages/H/Hypothalamus.html. Accessed August 2008.

Marieb, E.N., & Hoehn, K. (2007). *Human anatomy & physiology* (7th ed.). Upper Saddle River, NJ: Pearson Benjamin Cummings.

Tomagno, G., Mioni, R., De Carlo, E., et al. (2004). Effects of a somatostatin analogue in occult gastrointestinal bleeding: a case report. *Digestive and Liver Disease 26*(12): 843–846.

Chapter 50: Caring for Clients with Disorders of the Endocrine System

Eason, H.H. (2006). Saved from the storm: one nurse's SOS for RRT (rapid response team) is another nurse's lifesaver. *Nursing Spectrum – DC, Maryland & Virginia edition 16*(13): 22–23.

Hanberg, A. (2005). Common disorders of the pituitary gland: hyposecretion versus hypersecretion. *Journal of Infusion Nursing 28*(1): 36–44, 68–71.

Marieb, E.N., & Hoehn, K. (2007). *Human anatomy & physiology* (7th ed.). Upper Saddle River, NJ: Pearson Benjamin Cummings.

Mathur, R. (2008). Hyperthyroidism. Available at http://www.medicinenet.com. Accessed August 2008.

Mauk, K.L. (2005). Healthier aging: caring for older adults. Rooting out hypothyroidism in the elderly. *Nursing 35*(12): 65–66.

National Institute of Diabetes and Digestive & Kidney Diseases. (2008). Acromegaly. Available at http://www.niddk.nih.gov/health/endo/pubs/acro/acro.htm Accessed August 2008.

Neal-Boylan, L. (2007). Health assessment of the very old person at home. *Home Healthcare Nurse 25*(6): 388–400.

Noble, K.A. (2006). Patho corner. Thyroid storm. *Journal of Peri Anesthesia Nursing 21*(2): 119–125.

Pfadt, E., & Carslon, D.S. (2006). Action stat. Acute adrenal crisis. *Nursing 36*(8):80.

Robertson, G.L. (2006). What is diabetes insipidus? Available at http://www.diabetesinsipidus.org/whatisdi.htm. Accessed August 2008.

Solan, J., McKiernan, J. (2007). Thyroidectomy: the ambulatory nurse's role in preventing long-term sequelae. *Oncology Nursing Forum 34*(2): 515.

Thyroid operations. (2005). Available at http://www.endocrineweb.com/surthyroid.html. Accessed August 2008.

Understanding goiter. (2001). *Nursing 31*(8): 78.

Vacca, V.M., Jr. (2005). Action stat. Cerebral salt wasting syndrome. *Nursing 35*(10): 88.

van der Lely, A.J., & Kopchick, J.J. (2006). Growth hormone receptor antagonists. *Neuroendocrinology 83*(3–4): 264–268.

Wilden, R.S. (2006). What is NDI (nephrogenic diabetes insipidus). Available at http://www.diabetesinsipidus.org/4_types_nephrogenic_di.htm. Accessed August 2008.

Chapter 51: Caring for Clients with Diabetes Mellitus

American Diabetes Association. (2002). Position statement: Insulin administration. Available at http://care.diabetesjournals.org/cgi/content/full/25/suppl_1/s112. Accessed August 2008

American Diabetes Association. (2007). Prevalence of diabetes rose 5% annually since 1990. Available at http://www.diabetes.org/doabetesmewsarticle.jsp?storyID=15351710&filename=20070623/ADA200706231182625856641EDIT.xml. Accessed August 2008.

American Diabetes Association (2008). Diagnosis and classification of diabetes mellitus. Diabetes Care 31: Supplement S55-S60.

Barzilai, N. (2006). Disorders of carbohydrate metabolism. In M. H. Beers & T. V. Jones, *The Merck manual of geriatrics* (3rd ed.). Available at http://www.merck.com/mkgr/mmg/sec8/ch64/ch64b.jsp. Accessed January 2009.

Becton, Dickinson and Company. (2009). Blood glucose testing on fingertip, palm, forearm and thigh. Available at http://www.bddiabetes.com/us/main.aspx?cat=1&id=236. Accessed January 2009.

Behr, M. (2007). Diabetes. *MEDSURG Nursing* 16(2): 122–123.

Brand-Miller, J., Foster-Powell, K., Colaqiuri, S., et al. (2007). *The new glucose revolution for diabetes: The definitive guide to managing diabetes and prediabetes using the glycemic index*. Cambridge, MA: Da Capo Press.

Bril, V., & Buchanan, R.A. (2006). Long-term effects of ranirestat (AS-3201) on peripheral nerve function in patients with diabetic sensorimotor polyneuropathy. Available at http://care.diabetes-journals.org/cgi/content/abstract/29/1/68. Accessed August 2008.

Centers for Disease Control and Prevention. (2008). National diabetes fact sheet:general information and national estimates on diabetes in the United States, 2007. Available at http://www.cdc.gov/diabetes/pubs/pdf/ndfs_2007.pdf. Accessed August 2008.

Children with Diabetes. (2008). Research into a cure – Dr. Faustman. Available at http://www.childrenwithdiabetes.com/faustman.htm. Accessed August 2008.

Danis, S.J. (2007). From lizards and laboratories: New diabetes options. Available at http://www.nurse.com/ce/CE378-60/CoursePage./ Accessed August 2008.

Dongsheng, C., Minsheng, Y., Frantz, D., et al. (2005). Local and systemic insulin resistance from hepatic activation of IKK-β and NF-κB. Available at http://www.pubmedcentral.nih.gov/articlerender.fcgi?artid=1440292. Accessed August 2008.

Dudek, S. G. (2010). *Nutrition essentials for nursing practice* (6th ed.). Philadelphia, PA: Lippincott Williams & Wilkins.

Fletcher, C. (2007). New type 2 drugs, Januvia and Byetta offer big benefits. Available at http://www.diabeteshealth.com/read/2007/05/02/5165.html. Accessed August 2008.

Friedman, E.A. (2007). Aminoguanidine in the prevention of diabetic complications. Available at http://www.uptodate.com/patients/content/topic.do?topicKey=BxZ9xAWqzJcrE42. Accessed August 2008.

Kimball, J. (2008). Hormones of the pancreas. Available at http://users.rcn.com/jkimball.ma.ultranet/BiologyPages/P/Pamcreas.html. Accessed August 2008.

Kordella, T. (2004). Research profile. Carbs and fats. How much of each? Diabetes Forecast 57(9): 90, 92–93.

Massachusetts General Hospital. (2005). Type 1 research – the search for a cure. Available at http://www.massgeneral.org/diabetes/laboratory_type1.htm. Accessed August 2008.

Matsumoto, T., Ono, Y., Kuromiya, A., et al. (2008). Long-term treatment with ranirestat (AS-3201), a potent aldose reductase inhibitor, suppresses diabetic neuropathy and cataract formation in rats. Available at http://www.ncbi.nlm.nih.gov/pubmed/18612195. Accessed August 2008.

McGill University Health Centre. (2008). McGill University Health Centre announces important support for advancing INGAP as a therapy for type 1 diabetes. Available at http://www.muhc.ca/media/news/item/?item_id=29493. Accessed August 2008.

National Center for Health Statistics. (2005). Diabetes. Available at http://www.cdc.gov/nchs/FASTATS/diabetes.htm. Accessed August 2008.

National Institute of Diabetes and Digestive and Kidney Diseases. (2008). National diabetes statistics, 2007. Available at http://diabetes.niddk.nih.gov/dm/pubs/statistics/. Accessed August 2008.

National Institute of Diabetes and Digestive and Kidney Diseases. (2007). Pancreatic islet transplantation. Available at http://diabetes.niddk.nih.gov/dm/pubs/pancreaticislet/. Accessed August 2008.

Pavlovich-Danis, S.J. (2007). New horizons in diabetes treatment. *Nursing Spectrum – DC, Maryland & Virginia Edition* 17(12): 12–15.

Peebles, M., & Seley, J.J. (2007). Diabetes care: The need for change. *American Journal of Nursing* 107(6): Supplement: 13–9.

Porth, C.M. (2008). *Pathophysiology: Concepts of altered health states*. (8th ed.). Philadelphia, PA: Lippincott Williams & Wilkins.

Reuters World News. (2008). Kinexum Metabolics, Inc. announces abstracts on INGAP peptide will be presented at Keystone Symposia. Available at http://www.reuters.com/article/pressRelease/idUS174267+04-Apr-2008+MW20080404. Accessed August 2008.

Ridge, R.A. (2007). Patient safety. Boosting insulin safety. *Nursing* 37(2): 14–15.

Seelandt, K.K., & Twedell, D. (2007). Clinical updates. Diabetes mellitus update. *Journal of Continuing Education in Nursing* 38(2): 54–55.

Seley, J.J., Weinger, K., & Mason, D.J. (2007). Diabetes self-care: a challenge to nursing. *American Journal of Nursing* 107(6): Supplement 4–5.

Seley, J.J., & Weinger, K. (2007). The state of the science on nursing best practices for diabetes self-management. *Diabetes Educator* 33(4): 616–618.

World Health Organization. (2004). The diabetes programme. Available at http://www.who.int/diabetes/facts/en/. Accessed August 2008.

Chapter 52: Introduction to the Reproductive System

American Cancer Soceity. (2008). Can prostate cancer be found early? Available at http://www.cancer.org/docroot/CRI/content/

CRI_2_4_3X_Can_prostate_cancer_be_found_early_36.asp. Accessed August 2008.

American Cancer Society. (2004). Guidelines for the early dectection of cancer, 2004. Available at http://canonline.amcancersoc.org/cgi/content/full/54/1/41. Accessed August 2008.

American Cancer Society. (2003). Updated breast cancer screening guidelines released. Available at http://www.cancer.org/docroot/NWS/content/NWS_1_1x_Updated_Breast_Cancer_Screeing_Guidelines_Released.asp. Accessed August 2008.

Herlihy, B., & Maebius, N.K. (2007). *The human body in health and disease*. Philadelphia, PA: W.B. Saunders.

Marieb, E.N., & Hoehn, K. (2007). *Human anatomy & physiology* (7th ed.). Upper Saddle River, NJ: Pearson Benjamin Cummings

National Cancer Institute. (2008). Human papillomaviruses and cancer: Questions and answers. Available at http://www.cancer.gov/cancertopics/factsheets/risk/HPV. Accessed August 2008.

Smeltzer, S.C., Bare, B.G., Hinkle, J.L., et al. (2008). *Brunner & Suddarth's textbook of medical-surgical nursing* (11th ed.). Philadelphia, PA: Lippincott Williams & Wilkins.

Chapter 53: Caring for Clients with Disorders of the Female Reproductive System

Ahlberg, K., Ekman, T., Gaston-Johansson, F. (2005). Fatigue, psychological distress, coping resources, and functional status during radiotherapy for uterine cancer. *Oncology Nursing Forum* 32(3): 633–640.

American Academy of Family Physicians. (2008). PMS. Available at http://familydoctor.org/141.xml. Accessed September 2008.

American Cancer Society. (2008). Cancer Facts & Figures 2008. Available at http://www.cancer.org/downloads/STT/2008CAFFfinalsecured.pdf. Accessed September 2008.

Bukovic, D., Sliovski, H., Sliovski, T., et al. (2008). Sexual functioning and body image of patients treated for ovarian cancer. *Sexuality & Disability* 26(2): 63–73.

Consult stat. How long do you keep "an eye on" this patient? (2005). RN 68(7): 58–60.

Dyer, K. (2005). Myths & facts...about endometriosis. *Nursing* 35(4): 68.

Fibroids: weighing the options. (2008). *Consumer Reports on Health* 20(4): 6.

Gallagher, K. (2006). Premenstrual syndrome (PMS) – other treatment. Available at http://health.yahoo.com/reproductive-treatment/premenstrual-syndrome-pms-other-treatment/healthwise-hw139700.html. Accessed September 2008.

Garcia, A.A. (2007). Ovarian cancer. Available at http://www.emedicine.com/med/TOPIC1698.htm. Accessed September 2008.

Heiss, G., Wallace, R., Anderson, G.L., et al. (2008). Health risks of long-term combination hormone therapy outweigh benefits for postmenopausal women. *JAMA* 299(9): 1036–1045.

National Cancer Institute. (2007a). NCI researchers uncover unusual association between cell survival proteins and ovarian cancer aggressiveness. Available at http://www.cancer.gov/newscenter/pressreleases/OvarianBAG4. Accessed September 2008.

National Cancer Institute. (2008). Recurrent or persistent ovarian epithelial cancer. Available at http://www.cancer.gov/cancertopics/pdq/treatment/ovarianepithelial/HealthProfessional/page7. Accessed September 2008.

National Institute of Child Health and Human Development. (2007). Premature ovarian failure. Available at http://www.nichd.nih.gov/health/topics/Premature_Ovarian_Failure.cfm. Accessed September 2008.

Porth, C. M. (2008). *Pathophysiology: Concepts of altered health states.* (8th ed.). Philadelphia, PA: Lippincott Williams & Wilkins.

Potera, C. (2007). Staying alert for signs of ovarian cancer. *American Journal of Nursing* 107(9): 21.

Screening tool: symptoms predict ovarian cancer. (2007). *Nursing* 37(3): 35.

The New York Times Health Guide. (2008). Ovarian cancer. Available at http://health.nytimes.com/health/guides/disease/ovarian-cancer/prognosis.html. Accessed September 2008.

University of Maryland Medical Center. (2006). Vaginitis. Available at http://www.umm.edu/altmed/articles/vaginitis-000172.htm. Accessed September 2008.

Vaughn, D. (2006). Knowing their odds. *Nursing Spectrum – Florida edition* 16(2): 22–24.

Chapter 54: Caring for Clients with Breast Disorders

American Cancer Society. (2008a). Cancer statistics 2008 presentation. Available at http://www.cancer.org/docroot/PRO/content/PRO_1_1_Cancer_Statistics_2008_Presentation.asp. Accessed September 2008.

American Cancer Society. (2008b). What is breast cancer? Available at http://www.cancer.org/docroot/CRI/content/CRI_2_4_1X_What_is_breast_cancer_5.asp. Accessed September 2008.

American Cancer Society. (2007). ACS advises MRIs for some at high risk of breast cancer. Available at http://www.cancer.org/docroot/NWS/content/NWS_1_1x_Society_Advises_MRIs_for_Some_Women_at_High_Risk_of_Breast_Cancer.asp. Accessed September 2008.

Barclay, L., & Murata, P. (2007). Breast cancer risk may decrease with increasing duration of NSAID use. Available at http://www.medscape.com/viewarticle/563580. Accessed September 2008.

Bevers, T.B. (2007). The STAR trial: evidence for raloxifene as a breast cancer risk reduction agent for postmenopausal women. *Journal of National Comprehensive Cancer Network* 5(8): 817–822.

Breast cancer vaccine heads for trial. (2005). Available at http://www.cancerline.com/cancerlinehcp/6096_15167_2_0_0.aspx. Accessed September 2008.

American Cancer Society News Center. (2003). Common painkillers to prevent breast cancer? Available at http://www.cancer.org/docroot/NWS/content/NWS_2_1x_Common_Painkillers_To_Prevent_Breast_Cancer.asp. Accessed September 2008.

Gardner, A. (2008). Breast cancer vaccine works against deadlier form of disease. Available at http://www.washingtonpost.com/wp-dyn/content/article/2008/04/13/AR2008041301616.html. Accessed September 2008.

Harris, R.E., Chlebowski, R.T., Jackson, R.D., et al. (2003). Inverse association of breast cancer and NSAIDs: Results from the women's health initiative (WHI). American Association for Cancer Research. Available at http://www.aspirin.org/studies/20030416.pdf. Accessed September 2008.

Karmanos Cancer Institute. (2008). DNA vaccine developed at the Karmanos Cancer Institute fights HER2-positive cancers. Available at http://www.karmanos.org/view_news.asp?id=521. Accessed September 2008.

Mayo Clinic. (2007a). Breast cancer. Available at http://www. mayoclinic.com/health/breast-cancer/DS00328/DSECTION=risk-factors. Accessed September 2008.

McCloskey, S.A., Botnick, L.E., Rose, C.M., et al. (2006). Long-term outcomes after breast conservation therapy for early stage breast cancer in a community setting. *The Breast Journal* 12(2): 138–144.

Narayanan, K., Jaramillo, A., Benshoff, N.D., et al. (2004). Response of established human breast tumors to vaccination with mammaglobin-A cDNA. *Journal of the National Cancer Institute* 96(18): 1399–1396.

National Cancer Institute. (2006). Estimating breast cancer risk: questions and answers. Available at http://www.cancer.gov/cancertopics/factsheet/estimating-breast-cancer risk Accessed September 2008.

National Institutes of Health. (2008). Vaccine therapy in treating patients with breast cancer. Available at http://clinicaltrials.gov/ct2/show/NCT00524277. Accessed September 2008.

National Cancer Institute. (2008). SEER (Surveillance Epidemiology and End Results) stat fact sheets – cancer of the breast. Available at http://seer.cancer.gov/statfacts/html/breast.html. Accessed September 2008.

National Cancer Institute. (2008). Tamoxifen: questions and answers. Available at http://www.cancer.gov/cancertopics/factsheet/therapy/tamoxifen. Accessed September 2008.

National Cancer Institute. (2007). Aromatase inhibitors come of age. Available at http://www.cancer.gov/cancertopics/treatment/breast/aromatase-inhibitors0307. Accessed September 2008.

National Cancer Institute. (2006). Advanced breast cancer patients benefit more from aromatase inhibitors than tamoxifen. Available at http://www.cancer.gov/clinicaltrials/results/aromatase-inhibitors1006. Accessed September 2008.

Oncology nursing society position: breast cancer screening. (2006). *Oncology Nursing Forum* 33(4): 685–686.

Peptide vaccine fights off breast tumors with aid of bacteria-mimicking agents. (2007). Available at http://www.sciencedaily.com/releases/2007/02/070201082202.htm. Accessed September 2008.

Quaglino, E. (2004). Breast cancer vaccine may halt tumor growth. *The Journal of Clinical Investigation* 113(3): 709–717.

Science Daily. (2007). Peptide vaccine fights off breast tumors with aid of bacteria mimicking (sic) agents. http://www.sciencedaily.com/releases/2007/02/070201082202.htm. Accessed April 2009.

Solin, L.J., Fourquet, A., Vicini, F.A., et al. (2005). Long term outcome after breast-conservation treatment with radiation for mammographically detected ductal carcinoma in situ of the breast. *Cancer* 103(6): 1137–1146.

Stermer, C. (2008). Helping your patient after breast reconstruction. *Nursing* 38(8): 28–32.

United States Food and Drug Administration. (2006). Breast implant questions and answers. Available at http://www.fda.gov/cdrh/breastimplants/qa2006.html. Accessed September 2008.

United States Food and Drug Administration. (2006). FDA approves silicone gel-filled breast implants after in-depth evaluation. Available at http://www.fda.gov/bbs/topics/NEWS/2006/NEW01512.html. Accessed September 2008.

Vivani, G.A., Stefano, E.J., Alfonso, S.L., et al. (2007). Breast-conserving surgery with or without radiotherapy in women with ductal carcinoma in situ: a meta-analysis of randomized trials. Available at http://www.pubmedcentral.nih.gov/articlerender.fcgi?artid=1952067. Accessed September 2008.

Wyatt, J.P. (2005). Patient education. Preparing for breast augmentation: informed consent. *Plastic Surgical Nursing* 25(4): 196–198.

Chapter 55: Caring for Clients with Disorders of the Male Reproductive System

American Cancer Society. (2006). Procedure for prostate treatment questioned. Available at http://www.cancer.org/docroot/NWS/content/NWS_1_1x_Procedure_for_Prostate_Cancer_Treatment_Questioned.asp. Accessed September 2008.

American Cancer Society. (2008). Cancer statistics 2008 presentation. Available at http://www.cancer.org/docroot/PRO/content/PRO_1_1_Cancer_Statistics_2008_Presentation.asp. Accessed September 2008.

American Cancer Society. (2008). Detailed guide: Prostate cancer. Can prostate cancer be found early? Available at http://www.cancer.org/docroot/CRI/content/CRI_2_4_3X_Can_prostate_cancer_be_ found_early_36.asp?rnav=cri. Accessed September 2008.

American Cancer Society. (2007). How is testicular cancer found? Available at http://www.cancer.org/docroot/CRI/content/CRI_2_2_3x_How_Is_Testicular_Cancer_Found_41.asp. Accessed October 2008.

American Cancer Society. (2006). Procedure for prostate treatment questioned. Available at http://www.cancer.org/docroot/NWS/content/NWS_1_1x_Procedure_for_Prostate_Cancer_Treatment_Questioned.asp. Accessed September 2008.

American Cancer Society. (2008). Prostate cancer. Available at http://www.cancer.org/downloads/PRO/ProstateCancer.pdf. Accessed September 2008.

American Cancer Society. (2002). PSA "bounce" no reason for concern. Available at http://www.cancer.org/docroot/NWS/content/NWS_1_1x_PSA_Bounce_No_Reason_For_Concern.asp. Accessed September 2008.

American Cancer Society. (2008). What are the key statistics about prostate cancer. Available at http://www.cancer.org/docroot/CRI/content/CRI_2_4_1X_What_are_the_key_statistics_for_prostate_cancer_36.asp. Accessed September 2008.

Center for Holistic Urology, Columbia University Medical Center. (2006). Prostate – BPH. Available at http://www.holisticurology.columbia.edu/_conditions/prostate_bph.html. Accessed September 2008.

Darst, E.H. (2007). Sexuality and prostatectomy: nursing assessment and intervention. *Urologic Nursing* 27(6): 534–541.

Edwards, J.L. (2008). Diagnosis and management of benign prostatic hyperplasia. *American Family Physician* 77(10): 1403–1410.

Erectile Dysfunction Guideline Update Panel (2005). *The management of erectile dysfunction: an update.* Baltimore, MD: American Urological Association Education and Research, Inc.

Mayo Clinic. (2007). Prostate cancer; grading and Gleason scores. Available at http://www.mayoclinic.com/health/prostate-cancer/PC99999/PAGE=PC00006. Accessed September 2008.

Mayo Clinic. (2006). Undescended testicle (cryptorchidism). Available at http://www.mayoclinic.com/health/undescended-testicle/DS00845. Accessed May 2009.

Montague, D.K., Jarow, J.P., Broderick, G.A., et al. (2006). *Erectile dysfunction guideline update panel. The management of erectile dysfunction: an update.* Linthicum, MD: American Urologic Association Education and Research, Inc.

Nichols, C. (2008). The testicular cancer resource center's expert Q & A page. Available at http://www.acor.org/TCRC/iu.html. Accessed October 2008.

Saper, R.B., Fletcher, S.W., & Rind, D.M. (2008). Clinical use of saw palmetto. Available at http://www.uptodate.com/patients/content/topic.do?topicKey=~MncdT5COgOVon. Accessed September 2008.

United States Preventive Services Task Force. (2008). Screening for prostate cancer; recommendation statement. Available at http://www.ahrq.gov/clinic/uspstf08/prostate/prostaters.htm. Accessed September 2008.

WCRF/AICR (2007). *Food, nutrition, physical activity, and the prevention of cancer: A global perspective.* Washington, DC: American Institute of Cancer Research.

Chapter 56: Caring for Clients with Sexually Transmitted Infections

American Social Health Association. (2006). STD/STI statistics. Available at http://www.ashastd.org/lcarn/lcarn_statistics.cfm. Accessed October 2008.

Centers for Disease Control and Prevention. (2008). Estimates of new HIV infections in the United States. Available at http://www.cdc.gov/hiv/topics/surveillance/resources/factsheets/incidence.htm. Accessed October 2008.

Centers for Disease Control and Prevention. (2006). Sexually transmitted diseases treatment guidelines, 2006. *Morbidity & Mortality Weekly Report* 55(RR11): 1–94.

Centers for Disease Control and Prevention. (2007). STD surveillance 2006, National Profile. Available at http://www.cdc.gov/std/stats/toc2006.htm. Accessed October 2008.

Centers for Disease Control and Prevention. (2007). Trends in reportable sexually transmitted diseases in the United States, 2007. Available at http://www.cdc.gov/STD/stats07/trends.htm. Accessed February 2009.

Centers for Disease Control and Prevention. (2007). *Update to CDC's Sexuallly Transmitted Diseases Treatment Guidelines, 2006:* Fluoroquinolones no longer recommended for treatment of gonococcal infections. *Morbidity & Mortality Weekly Report* 56(14): 332–336.

Duffin, C. (2008). Taking the risky our of frisky. *Nursing Older People* 20(5): 6–7.

Haddad, A. (2008). Ethics in action. Would you tell the parents? *RN* 71(3): 15.

Jemmott, L.S., Jemmott, J.B., Hutchinson, M.K., et al. (2008). Sexually transmitted infection/HIV risk reduction interventions in clinical practice settings. *Journal of Obstetric, Gynecologic, & Neonatal Nursing* 37(2): 137–145.

Leung-Chen, P. (2008). Syphilis makes another comeback: nurses can help in containing transmission, above all through education. *American Journal of Nursing* 108(2): 28–31.

National Institute of Allergy and Infectious Diseases. (2007). Human papillomavirus and genital warts. Available at http://www3.niaid.nih.gov/topics/genitalWarts/default.htm. Accessed October 2008.

O'Rourke, E., & Schween, S. (2007). Syphilis. Still a public health danger. *RN* 70(7): 26–32.

Porth, C.M. (2006). *Essentials of pathophysiology; Concepts of altered states.* Philadelphia, PA: Lippincott Williams & Wilkins.

Young, F. (2007). Sexually transmitted infections in men. *Journal of Family Health Care* 17(5): 175–178.

Chapter 57: Introduction to the Urinary System

American Nursing Student (November/December, 2005). Understanding the renal system. Author, p. 6–7.

Hathaway, L. (2006). Inserting an indwelling urinary catheter, step by step. *LPN 2006, 2*(5), 9–11.

Porth, C.M. (2007). *Essentials of pathophysiology: Concepts of altered health states* (2nd ed.). Philadelphia, PA: Lippincott Williams & Wilkins.

Smeltzer, S.C., Bare, B.G., Hinkle, J.L., et al. (2008). *Brunner & Suddarth's textbook of medical-surgical nursing* (11th ed.). Philadelphia, PA: Lippincott Williams & Wilkins.

Chapter 58: Caring for Clients with Disorders of the Kidneys and Ureters

Burrows-Hudson, S. (2005). Chronic kidney disease: An overview. *American Journal of Nursing, 105*(2), 40–49.

Campoy, S., & Elwell, R. (2005). Pharmacology & CKD. *American Journal of Nursing, 105*(9), 60–71.

Castner, D. (2007). Failed dialysis access. *Nursing 2007, 37*(8), 72.

Castner, D., & Douglas, C. (2005). Now onstage: Chronic kidney disease. *Nursing 2005, 35*(12), 58–63.

Coleman, T., Culkin, C., & Sierka, D. (2006). Kidney transplants in HIV clients? *RN, 69*(1), 33–38.

Dinwiddie, L.C., Burrows-Hudson, S., & Peacock, E.J. (2006). Stage 4 Chronic kidney disease. *American Journal of Nursing, 106*(9), 40–51.

Kear, T.M. (2006, July 5). Chronic kidney disease. *Advance for Nurses, 19*–21.

Kring, D. (2006). Sneak attack: Tracking down kidney stones. *LPN 2007, 2*(6), 36–43.

Legg, V. (2005). Complications of chronic kidney disease. *American Journal of Nursing, 105*(6), 40–49.

Leydig, E.J. (2005). Are you endangering your patients? *RN, 68*(2), 29–31.

Mahoney, C. (2007). Should patients eat during dialysis? *Nursing 2007, 37*(10), 57–58.

McCarley, P.B., & Salai, P.B. (2005). Cardiovascular disease in chronic kidney disease. *American Journal of Nursing, 105*(4), 40–53.

Porth, C.M. (2007). *Essentials of pathophysiology: Concepts of altered health states* (2nd ed.). Philadelphia, PA: Lippincott Williams & Wilkins.

Smeltzer, S.C., Bare, B.G., Hinkle, J.L., et al. (2008). *Brunner & Suddarth's textbook of medical-surgical nursing* (11th ed.). Philadelphia, PA: Lippincott Williams & Wilkins.

Thomas-Hawkins, C., & Zazworsky, D. (2005). Self-management of chronic kidney disease. *American Journal of Nursing, 105*(10), 40–49.

Wetherbee, S.L. (2006). New weapons to snuff out kidney cancer. *Nursing 2006, 36*(12), 58–63.

Ziegler, S.A. (2007). Prevent dangerous hemodialysis catheter disconnections. *Nursing 2007, 37*(3), 70.

Chapter 59: Caring for Clients with Disorders of the Bladder and Urethra

Bray, B., Van Sell, S.L., & Miller-Anderson, M. (2007). Stress continence: It's no laughing matter. *RN, 70*(4), 25–29.

Burrows-Hudson, S. (2005). Chronic kidney disease: An overview: Early and aggressive treatment is vital. *American Journal of Nursing, 105*(2), 40–50.

Campbell, B.D. (2006). Bladder cancer. *Nursing 2006, 36*(4), 54–57.

Cohen, N. (2005). Beating bladder cancer. *Advance for Nurses*, October 24, 29–30.

Mauk, K.L. (2005). Conservative therapy for urinary incontinence can help older adults. *Nursing 2005, 35*(8), 20–21.

Mennick, F. (2005). Urinary incontinence worsens with menopausal hormone therapy. *American Journal of Nursing, 105*(7), 22.

Polt, C.A. (2006). Taking the pressure off for women with stress incontinence. *Nursing 2006, 36*(2), 49–51.

Pullen, R.L. (2007). Clinical do's & don'ts: Replacing a urostomy drainage pouch. *Nursing 2007, 37*(6), 14.

Specht, J. (2005). Nine myths of incontinence in older adults. *American Journal of Nursing, 105*(6), 58 70.

Toughill, E. (2005). Indwelling catheters: Common mechanical and pathogenic problems. *American Journal of Nursing, 105*(5), 35–37.

Woods, A. (2005). Managing UTIs in older adults. *Nursing 2005, 35*(3), 12.

Chapter 60: Introduction to the Musculoskeletal System

Maintaining Mobility (2006). Bend and stretch: Performing range-of-motion exercises. *LPN 2006, 2*(3), 11–13.

Chapter 61: Caring for Clients Requiring Orthopedic Treatment

Best, J. (2005). Revision total hip and total knee arthroplasty. *Orthopaedic Nursing, 24*(3), 174–181.

D'Arcy, Y. (2005). Managing phantom limb pain. *Nursing 2005, 35*(11), 17.

D'Arcy, Y. (2006a). Easing the pain after total joint replacement. *LPN 2006, 2*(5), 7–8.

D'Arcy, Y. (2006b). Phantom limb pain: What it is, how to treat it. *LPN 2006, 2*(6), 15–17.

D'Arcy, Y. (2006c). Treating pain after a total joint replacement. *Nursing 2006, 36*(5), 26–28.

Day, M.W. (2006). Traumatic amputation. *Nursing 2006, 36*(10), 88.

Hohler, S.E. (2005). Looking into minimally invasive total hip arthroplasty. *Nursing 2005, 35*(6), 54–57.

Holmes, S.B., & Brown, S.J. (2005). Skeletal pin care: National Association or Orthopaedic Nurses guidelines for orthopaedic nursing. *Orthopaedic Nursing, 24*(2), 99–107.

Howell, B. (2007). Joint surgery: paving the way to a smooth recovery. *RN, 70*(1), 32–37.

Laskowski-Jones, L. (2006). First aid for amputation. *Nursing 2006, 36*(4), 50–51.

Maintaining Mobility (2005). Getting patients back on their feet. *LPN 2005, 1*(5), 15–16.

Maintaining Mobility (2006). One foot in front of the other. *LPN 2006, 2*(2), 43–44.

Chapter 62: Caring for Clients with Traumatic Musculoskeletal Injuries

Gore, T. (2005). Bone up on fat embolism syndrome. *Nursing 2005, 35*(8), 32hn1–32hn2.

Gross, K.A. (2006). Solid advice on managing vertebral compression fractures. *Nursing 2006, 36*(12), 64hn1–64hn4.

Hall, D. (2007). Detect compartment syndrome in time. *American Nurse Today, 2*(7), 42.

Laskowski-Jones, L. (2006). First aid for sprains. *Nursing 2006, 36*(8), 48–49.

Metules, T.J. (2007). Hands on help: Hot and cold packs. *RN, 70*(1), 45–48.

Porth, C.M. (2007). *Essentials of pathophysiology* (2nd ed.) Philadelphia, PA: Lippincott Williams & Wilkins.

Pullen, R.L. (2007). Using slings without errors. *Nursing 2007, 37*(7), 24.

Schoen, D.C. (2005). The mystery of ankle problems. *Orthopaedic Nursing, 24*(2), 166–169.

Smith, B.L. (2005). How to manage that pelvic fracture. *RN, 68*(8), 30–34.

Smeltzer, S.C., Bare, B.G., Hinkle, J.L., et al. (2008). *Brunner & Suddarth's textbook of medical-surgical nursing* (11th ed.) Philadelphia, PA: Lippincott Williams & Wilkins.

Veronesi, J.F. (2005). After the crash: Treating whiplash. *RN, 68*(9), 40–44.

Chapter 63: Caring for Clients with Orthopedic and Connective Tissue Disorders

American College of Rheumatology. (2008a). The 1982 Revised Criteria for Classification of Systemic Lupus Erythematosus. Available at http://www.rheumatology.org. Accessed October 2008.

American College of Rheumatology. (2008b). 1990 Criteria for classification of fibromyalgia. Available at http://www.rheumatology.org. Accessed October 2008.

American College of Rheumatology. (2008c). 2008 Recommendations for the Use of Nonbiologic and Biologic Disease-Modifying Antirheumatic Drugs in Rheumatoid Arthritis. Available at http://www.rheumatology.org. Accessed October 2008.

Arthritis Foundation (2008). Arthritis today: Drug guide. Available at http://www.arthritis.org. Accessed October 2008.

Bullock, B.A., & Henze, R.L. (2000). *Focus on pathophysiology*. Philadelphia, PA: Lippincott Williams & Wilkins.

Clinical Queries. (2006). Are NSAIDs safe for arthritis pain? *Nursing 2006, 36*(12), 24.

FitzGibbons, J. (2007). Be a myth-buster: Stop the misconceptions about fibromyalgia. *American Nurse Today, 2*(9), 40–44.

Hathaway, L.R. (2005). Lyme disease. *Nursing 2005, 35*(4), 44–45.

Hawkins, R. (2006). Osteoporosis. *American Journal of Nursing Supplement, 106*(3), 78–81.

Hetzell, C.B. (2005). New help for old bones. *Nursing 2005, 35*(5), 20–21.

Holcomb, S.S. (2006). Osteoporosis. *Nursing 2006, 36*(4), 48–49.

Keefe, S. (2006, June 5). Down to the bone. *Advance for Nurses*, 27–28.

Kelly, A.M. (2006). Managing osteoarthritis pain. *Nursing 2006, 36*(11), 20–21.

National Fibromyalgia Association (2009). Prevalence of fibromyalgia. Available at http://www.fmaware.org. Accessed March 2009.

Porth, C.M. (2007). *Essentials of pathophysiology* (2nd ed.) Philadelphia, PA: Lippincott Williams & Wilkins.

Rooney, J. (2005). Systemic lupus erythematosus. *Nursing 2005*, 35(11), 54–60.

Tencer, A.F. (2005). Biomechanics of falling. *Mayo Clinic Proceedings*, 80(7), 847–848.

Chapter 64: Introduction to the Integumentary System

Butta, M.F. (2007). Sex and the nose: Human pheromonal responses. *Journal of Social Medicine* 100(6): 268–274.

Hess, C.T. (2008). Practice points. Performing a skin assessment. *Advances in Skin & Wound Care* 21(8): 392.

Marieb, E., Mallatt, J., Wilhelm, P. (2007). *Human anatomy* (5th ed.). San Francisco, CA: Benjamin Cummings.

Peters, J. (2007). Examining and describing skin conditions. *Practice Nurse* 34(8): 39–40, 43, 45.

Stechmiller, J.K., Cowan, L., Whitney, J.D. (2008). Guidelines for the prevention of pressure ulcers. *Wound Repair & Regeneration* 16(2): 151–168.

van de Kerkof, P.C, Pasch, M.C., Scher, R.K., et al. (2005). Brittle nail syndrome: A pathogenesis-based approach with a proposed grading system. *Journal of the American Academy of Dermatology* 53(4): 644–651.

Werkman, H., Simodejka, P., & DeFilippis, J. (2008). Partnering for prevention: a pressure ulcer prevention collaborative project. *Home Healthcare Nurse* 26(1): 17–22.

Chapter 65: Caring for Clients with Skin, Hair, and Nail Disorders

American Dental Association. (2005). ADA statement on intraoral/perioral piercing and tongue splitting. Available at http://www.ada.org/prof/resources/positions/statements/piercing.asp Accessed October 2008.

Armstrong, M.L. (2004). Caring for the patient with piercings. *RN* 67(6): 46–52.

Armstrong, M.L. (2005). Tattooing, body piercing, and permanent cosmetics: a historical and current view of state regulations, with continuing concerns. *Journal of Environmental Health* 67(8): 38–43.

Bowles, D. (2005). Hope for the 'heartbreak of psoriasis'. *Nursing Spectrum* (DC, Maryland, Virginia edition) 15(13): 15–17.

Edmunds, K. (2006). Practice makes perfect; the removal of body piercings. *Emergency Nurse* 14(1): 21.

Ferringer, T., Pride, H., & Tyler, W. (2008). Body piercing complicated by atypical mycobacterial infections. *Pediatric Dermatology* 25(2): 219–222.

Freyenberger, B. (1998). Peer reviewed: Eland, J. (2004) Tattooing and body piercing: decision making for teens. Children's Hospital of Iowa. Available at http://lib.cpums.edu.cn/jiepou/tupu/atlas/www.vh.org/pediatric/patient/dermatology/tattoo/index.htm. Accessed October 2008.

Gorgos, D. (2003). Using lasers to remove tattoos. *Dermatology Nursing* 15(5): 486.

Hanson, D., Thompson, P.A., Langemo, D., et al. (2008). What you should know about psoriasis. *Nursing* 38(6): 58–59.

Hickin, L. (2008). Managing skin and nail infections. *Practice Nurse* 35(10): 19–21.

If you are thinking about body art. (2005). Patient Care for the Nurse Practitioner 8(4): 13.

Lasers safe and effective in removing tattoos. *Dermatology Nursing* 16(6): 538–539.

Loescger, L.J., Harris, R.B., Lim, K.H., et al. (2006). Thorough skin self-examination in patients with melanoma. *Oncology Nursing Forum* 33(3): 633–637.

Mascai, M.S., Mannis, M.J., & Huntley, A.C. (1996). Acne rosacea. *Eye and Skin Disease*. Philadelphia, PA: Lippincott-Raven.

Mayo Clinic. (2008). Piercings: Proper care can help prevent complications. Available at http://www.mayoclinic.com/health/piercings/SN00049. Accessed October 2008.

Mayo Clinic. (2008). Tattoos: Risks and precautions to know first. Available at http://www.mayoclinic.com/health/tattoos-an-piercings/MC00020. Accessed October 2008.

Melton, L.P. (2005). Psoriasis in the war zone. *American Journal of Nursing* 105(3): 52–54, 56.

Meltzer, D.I. (2005). Complications of body piercing. Available at http://www.aafp.org/afp/20051115/2029.html. Accessed October 2008.

Meyers, S. (2006). Clinical clips. It's that time of year: time to take on head lice. *Nursing Spectrum* (DC, Maryland, Virginia edition) 16(23): 6.

Mills, M. (2008). Practice makes perfect: scabies. *Emergency Nurse* 16(2): 18–19.

National Cancer Institute. (2005). What you need to know about skin cancer. Available at http://www.cancer.gov/cancertopics/wyntk/skin. Accessed October 2008.

National Institute of Arthritis and Musculoskeletal and Skin Diseases. (2005). What is rosacea? Fast facts: An easy-to-read series of publications for the public. Available at http://www.niams.nih.gov/Health_Info/Rosacea/default.asp. Accessed October 2008.

National Rosacea Society. (2008). All about rosacea. Available at http://www.rosacea.org/patients/allaboutrosacea.php. Accessed October 2008.

Porth, C.M. (2006). *Essentials of pathophysiology. concepts of altered states* (2nd ed.). Philadelphia, PA: Lippincott Williams & Wilkins.

Rosacea Treatment Clinic. (2008). Rosacea & inflammation: Demodex skin mites. Available at http://members.ozemail.com.au/~rosacea/rosacea-inflammation.htm. Accessed October 2008.

Rushing, J. (2008). Clinical do's & don'ts. Assessing a patient for lice infestation. *Nursing* 38(7): 20.

Sarabi, K., & Khachemoune, A. (2007). Tinea capitis: a review. *Dermatology Nursing* 19(6): 525–530.

Smith, J.P. (2007). Tattoos, body piercing, and nursing: A photo essay. *American Journal of Nursing* 107(4): 55–55.

Thomas, L. (2004). It might be the latest fashion, but getting a tattoo is not without risk. Nursing, *Standard* 18(42): 26.

Tjioe, M., & Vissers, W.H.P. (2008). Scabies outbreaks in nursing homes for the elderly: recognition, treatment options and control of reinfestation. *Drugs & Aging* 25(4): 299–306.

United States Food and Drug Administration (FDA). (2008). Tattoos and permanent makeup. Available at http://vm.cfsan.fda.gov/~dms/cos-204.html. Accessed October 2008.

Chapter 66: Caring for Clients with Burns

American Burn Association. (2007). Burn incidence and treatment in the US: 2007 fact sheet. Available at http://www.ameriburn.org/resources_factsheet.php. Accessed October 2008.

Burn Survivor Resource Center. (2002). Medical care guide. Medications. Available at http://burnsurvivor.com/medications.html. Accessed October 2008.

Callanno, C., & Jakubek, P. (2006). Wound bed preparation: The key to success for chronic wounds, Part II. Nursing, 36(3): 76–77.

Edlich, R.F. (2008). Burns, thermal. Available at http://www.emedicine.com/plastic/topic518.htm. Accessed October 2008.

Mishra, A., Whitaker, T., Potokar, T., et al. The use of aquacel Ag in the treatment of partial thickness burns: A national study. *Burns* 33(5): 670–680.

Naradzay, J., & Alson, R. (2006). Burns, thermal. Available at http://www.emedicine.com/emerg/TOPIC72.HTM. Accessed October 2008.

National Fire Protection Association. (2008). News release: Young children and older adults at highest risk of death from home fires. Available at http://www.nfpa.org/newsReleaseDetails.asp?categoryid=488&itemID=39938&rss=NFPAnewsreleases. Accessed October 2008.

Petherick, A., Harder, B. (2005). Spray-on skin cells could help burns heal. Available at http://news.nationalgeographic.com/news/pf/98107980.html. Accessed October 2008.

Singer, E. (2007). A better artificial skin. Available at http://www.technologyreview.com/biotech/18059/. Accessed October 2008.

Van Houten, S. (2007). Burns. Healthwise, Inc. Available at http://www.aolhealth.com/symptom/burns. Accessed October 2008.

Chapter 67: Interaction of Body and Mind

American Psychiatric Association. (2000). Diagnostic and Statistical Manual of Mental Disorders (4th ed.). Arlington, VA.

Crossroads Institute. QEEG brain mapping. Available at http://www.crossroadsinstitute.org/brainmap.html. Accessed March 2009.

Kobasa, S. (1979). Stressful life events, personality and health: An inquiry into hardiness. *Journal of Personality and Social Psychology* 42(1): 1–11.

Pelletier, K.R. (1977). *Mind as healer, mind as slayer*. New York: Delacorte and Delta.

Pelletier, K.R. (1995). *Sound mind – sound body: A new model for lifelong health*. New York: Simon & Schuster.

Pert, C.B. (1997). *Molecules of emotion: The science behind mind-body medicine*. New York: Simon & Schuster.

Porth, C.M. (2006). *Essentials of pathophysiology. Concepts of altered health states* (2nd ed.) Philadelphia, PA: Lippincott Williams & Wilkins.

Sanofi Adventis. (2009). The only FDA approved treatment for ALS. Available at http://www.rilutek.com/About_Rilutek/About_Rilutek.aspx. Accessed May 2009.

Schmidt, W., & Reith. M.E.A., eds. (2005). *Dopamine and glutamate in psychiatric disorders*. Totowa, NJ.: Humana Press.

Selye, H. (1956). *The stress of life*. New York: McGraw-Hill.

Sheldon, A.L., & Robinson, M.B. (2007). The role of glutamate transporters in neurodegenerative diseases and potential opportunities for intervention. *Neurochemistry international* 51(6–7): 333–355.

Townsend, M.C. (2009). *Psychiatric mental health nursing: Concepts of care in evidence-based practice* (6th ed.). Philadelphia, PA: FA Davis.

Videbeck, S.L. (2007). *Psychiatric-mental health nursing* (4th ed.). Philadelphia, PA: Lippincott Williams & Wilkins.

Chapter 68: Caring for Clients with Anxiety Disorders

Antai-Otong, D. (2007). The art of prescribing. Pharmacotherapy of obsessive-compulsive disorder: an evidence-based approach. *Perspectives in Psychiatric Care* 43(4): 219–222.

Beck, J.G., Coffey, S.F., Foy, D.W., et al. (2009). Group cognitive behavior therapy for chronic posttraumatic stress disorder. *Behavior Therapy* 40(1): 82.

Byer, G., & Pavlovich-Danis, S.J. (2009). Anxiety disorders. Available at http://www.nurse.com/ce/CE175-60. Accessed March 2009.

Crowe, M., Carlyle, D., & Farmar, R. (2008). Clinical formulation for mental health nursing practice. *Journal of Psychiatric & Mental Health Nursing* 15(10): 800–807.

Cyr, N.R. (2007). Special needs populations. Obsessive compulsive disorder. *Association of periOperative Registered Nurses (AORN) Journal* 86(2): 277–280.

Flood, M., & Buckwalter, K.C. (2009). Recommendations for mental health care in older adults: part 1 – an overview of depression and anxiety. *Journal of Gerontological Nursing* 35(2): 26–34.

Gibson, J., & Sloan, G. (2008). Developing general principles of psychological skills in mental health nursing. *Nursing Older People* 20(1): 31.

Hart, B.G. (2007). Cutting: the mystery behind the marks. *American Association of Occupational Health Nurses (AAOHN) Journal* 55(4): 161–168.

Hyer, K., Brown, L.M. (2008). The Impact of Event Scale – revised: a quick measure of a patient's response to trauma. *American Journal of Nursing* 108(11): 60–69.

Katz, A. (2008). Postcombat sexual problems. *American Journal of Nursing* 108(10): 35–39.

McDonald, R. (2008). Everything you wanted to know about anxiety but were afraid to ask. *Journal of Health Services Research & Policy* 13(4): 249–250.

National Institute of Mental Health. (2009). Anxiety disorders. Available at http://nimh.nih.gov/health/topics/anxiety-disorders/index.shtmtl. Accessed March 2009.

Sheldon, L.K., Swanson, S., Dolce, A., et al. (2008). Putting evidence into PRACTICE Evidence-based interventions for anxiety. *Clinical Journal of Oncology Nursing* 12(5): 789–797.

Stress, Anxiety & Depression Center. (2006). Anxiety disorders research at the National Institute of Mental Health. Available at w?>http://www.stress-anxiety-depression.org/anxiety/anxiety-disorders-research-nimh.html. Accessed March 2009.

Thobaben, M. (2008). Client assessment: generalized anxiety disorder. *Home Health Care Management & Practice* 21(1): 67–69.

van der Watt, G., Janca, A. (2008). Aromatherapy in nursing and mental health care. *Contemporary Nurse* 30(1): 69.

Videbeck, S.L (2007). *Psychiatric mental health nursing* (4th ed.). Philadelphia, PA: Lippincott Williams & Wilkins.

Wheeler, K. (2007). Psychotherapeutic strategies for healing trauma. *Perspectives in Psychiatric Care* 43(3): 132–141.

Wood, D.A. (2008). Support our soldiers. *Nursing Spectrum – DC, Maryland & Virginia Edition* 18(18): 16–17.

Chapter 69: Caring for Clients with Mood Disorders

American Psychiatric Association. (2002). Practice guideline for the treatment of patients with bipolar disorder. *American Journal of Psychiatry* 159(4s): 1–50.

CBS News. (2008). Magnet device aims to treat depression. Available at http://www.cbsnews.com/stories/2008/10/21/health/printable4535599.shtml. Accessed November 2008.

Center for Disease Control and Prevention. (2007). Suicide trends among youths and young adults aged 10–24 years— United States, 1990–2004. Available at http://www.cdc.gov.mmrw/preview/mmwrhtml/mm5635a2.htm. Accessed November 2008.

Deep brain stimulation. (2007). Available at http://www.neurosurgerytoday.org/what/patient_e/deep%20brain%20stimulation.asp. Accessed November 2008.

Fortinash, K.M., & Holoday-Worret, P. (2007). *Psychiatric mental health nursing* (4th ed.) Philadelphia, PA: WB Saunders.

Holmberg, M. (2006). Depression: Identifying symptoms and appropriate treatment. Available at http://www.pharmacytimes.com/issues/articles/2006-05_3521.asp. Accessed November 2008.

Kelsoe, J.R. (2004). Mood disorders: Genetics. In Sadock, B.J., & Sadock, V.A. *Kaplan and Sadock's Comprehensive textbook of psychiatry* (8th ed.). Philadelphia, PA: Lippincott Williams & Wilkins.

Mayo Clinic. (2008). Serotonin and norepinephrine reuptake inhibitors. Available at http://www.mayoclinic.com/health/antidepressants/MH00067. Accessed March 2009.

National Institute of Mental Health. (2008). Antidepressant medications for children and adolescents: Information for parents and caregivers. Available at http://www.nimh.nih.gov/health/topics/child-and-adolescent-mental-health/antidepressant-medications-for-children-and-adolescents- information-for-parents-and-caregivers.shtml. Accessed November 2008

National Institute of Mental Health. (2008). Older adults: depression and suicide facts. Available at http://www.nimh.nih.gov/health/publications/older-adults-depression-and-suicide-factsheet/index.shtml. Accessed November 2008.

National Strategy for Suicide Prevention. (2005). At a glance – suicide among the elderly. Available at http://mentalhealth.samhsa.gov/suicideprevention/elderly.asp. Accessed November 2008.

Neurosurgerytoday. (2007). Deep brain stimulation. Available at http://www.neurosurgerytoday.org/what/patient_e/deep%20brain%20stimulation.asp. Accessed May 2009.

Schiller, J. (2008). ECT: a method to lift depression: controlled seizures refocus brain waves in severe depression. *RN* 71(11): 30–34.

Schlaepfer, T.E., Frick, C., Zobel, A., et al. (2008). Vagus nerve stimulation for depression: efficacy and safety in a European study. Available at http://www.ncbi.nlm.nih.gov/pubmed/18177525. Accessed November 2008.

Timby, B.K., & Smith, N.E. (2005). Seasonal affective disorder: shedding light on the wintertime blues. Nursing, 35(1): 18.

Types of bipolar disorder. (2008). Available at http://www.webmd.com/bipolar-disorder/guide/bipolar-disorder-forms. Accessed November 2008.

Videbeck, S.L. (2007). *Psychiatric-mental health nursing* (4th ed.). Philadelphia, PA: Lippincott Williams & Wilkins.

Chapter 70: Caring for Clients with Eating Disorders

Baranowska, B., Wolinska-Witort, E., Martynska. M., et al. (2005). Plasma orexin A, orexin B, leptin, neuropeptide Y (NPY), and insulin in obese women. Available at http://nel.edu/26-2005_4_pdf/NEL260405A01_Baranowska.pdf. Accessed December 2008.

Budd, G. (2007). Disordered eating: young women's search for control and connection. *Journal of Child and Adolescent Psychiatric Nursing* 20(2): 96–06.

Bulik, C.M., Lundt, M., van Furth, E., et al. The genetics of anorexia nervosa. Available at http://www.arjournals.annualreviews.org/doi/abs/10.1146/annurev.nutr.27.06146.093713. Accessed December 2008.

Breier-Mackie, S. (2007). Enforced refeeding treatment in severe anorexia nervosa: the pros and cons of an ethical-legal collision course. *Gastroenterology Nursing* 30(2):142.

Cassels, C. (2008). Atypical antipsychotic may be safe, effective treatment for anorexia nervosa. Available at http://www.medscape.com/viewarticle/577666. Accessed December 2008.

Crawford, D.T., Freeman, M.K., & Cates, M.E. Atypical antipsychotics in the treatment of anorexia nervosa. International Journal of Pharmacy Education and Practice. Available at http://www.samford.edu/schools/pharmacy/ijpe/208/208.html#atypicals. Accessed December 2008.

Di Marzo, V. (2005). The endocannabinoid system: a general view and latest editions. Available at http://esi-topics.com/fmf/2005-VincenzoDiMarzo.html Accessed December 2008

Godar, K. (2007). Starved for cash: when mental health benefits end long before bulimics can be successfully treated, it's a legitimate nursing issue. *Nursing Spectrum, Florida edition* 17(22): 18–19.

Hatmaker, G. (2005). Boys with eating disorders. *Journal of School Nursing* 21(6): 329–332.

Inui, A. (2001). Eating behavior in anorexia nervosa–an excess of both orexigenic and anorexigenic signalling? *Molecular Psychiatry* 6(6): 620–624.

Kaye, W. (2008). Neurobiology of anorexia and bulimia nervosa. *Physiological Behavior* 94(1): 121–135.

Kirkham, T. (2007). Endocannabinoids and the neurochemistry of gluttony. Available at http://www.neuroendo.org.uk/content/view/96/11. Accessed December 2008.

Murphy, K. (2007). The skinny on eating disorders. *Nursing Made Incredibly Easy!* 5(3): 40–48.

National Association of Anorexia Nervosa and Associated Disorders. (2008). Facts about eating disorders. Available at http://www.anad.org/22385/index.html. Accessed December 2008.

Olson, A.H. (2006). The role of serotonin and dopamine in anorexia nervosa. Available at http://www.fulllifeconsulting.com/Serotonin_Dopamine_AN.html Accessed December 2008.

Rolls, E.T. (2005). The brain control of eating and reward in *Emotion Explained*. New York: Oxford University Press.

Smy, J. (2005). Improving bulimia care. *Nursing Times* 101(47): 16–17.

Souers, A.J. (2007). Melanin-concentrating hormone (MCH). *Current Topics in Medicinal Chemistry* 7(15): 1424.

Walsh, L. (2007). Caring for patients who have eating disorders. *Nursing Times* 103(28): 28–29.

Chapter 71: Caring for Clients with Chemical Dependence

Alcohol and Drug Treatment. (2006). The disease concept. Available at http://www.alcohol-drug-treatment.net/disease_concept.html. Accessed December 2008

Bailey, K.P., (2004). Psychopharmacology grand rounds. The brain's rewarding system and addiction. *Journal of Psychosocial Nursing & Mental Health Services* 42(6): 14–18.

Centers for Disease Control and Prevention. (2007). Adult cigarette smoking in the United States: Current estimates. Available at http://www.cdc.gov/tobacco/data_statistics/fact_sheets/adult_data/adult_cig_smoking.htm. Accessed December 2008.

Centers for Disease Control and Prevention. (2005). Cigarette smoking among adults—United States, 2004. Available at http://www.cdc.gov/mmwr/preview/mmwrhtml5444a2.htm. Accessed 2008.

Centers for Disease Control and Prevention. (2008). Smoking and tobacco use. Fact sheet, health effects of cigarette smoking. Available at http://www.cdc.gov/tobacco/data_statistics/fact_sheets/health_effects.htm. Accessed December 2008.

Chong, J. (2007). Number of U.S. smokers stays steady. Available at http://articles.latimes.com/2007/nov/09/science-smoking9. Accessed December 2008.

Clark, J., & Moore, K.A. (2008). The danger next door: methamphetamine. *RN 71*(5): 22–28.

Dougherty, P.L. (2008). Varenicline: a new pharmaceutical approach to smoking cessation. *Nursing for Women's Health* 12(1): 66–69.

Edenberg, HJ, & Foroud, T. (2006). The genetics of alcoholism: identifying specific genes through family studies. *Addiction Biology* 11(3–4): 386–396.

Fitzpatrick, J.J. (2006). Alcohol awareness. *Archives of Psychiatric Nursing* 20(5): 203–204.

How to get an honest answer on cocaine use. *ED Nursing* 11(10): 116.

Lewis, P.C. (2008). Tobacco: what is it and why do people continue to use it? *MEDSURG Nursing* 14(4): 260–261.

Lewis, T. (2008). Assessing an older adult for alcohol use disorders. Nursing, *38*(6): 60–61.

McGuiness, T. (2006). Emergency. Methamphetamine abuse. *American Journal of Nursing* 106(12): 54–59.

Mirkin, B. (2008). Smoking and weight gain. Available at http://www.ahealthyme.com/topic/quitgain. Accessed December 2008.

National Cancer Institute. (2008). Tobacco statistics snapshot. Available at http://www.cancer.gov/cancertopcs/tobacco/statisticssnapshot. Accessed December 2008.

Olms, D. (1983). The disease concept of alcoholism. Belleville, IL: Gary Whiteaker Company.

Pittman, H.J. (2005). Action stat. Methamphetamine overdose. *Nursing,* 35(4): 88.

Rossie, K.M., Brunk, M.J., Mecklenberg, R., et al. (2004). Tobacco dependence. Available at http://www1.tobaccofreepatients.com/?id=3135. Accessed December 2008

Schofield, C. (2004). How do I care for a patient with alcohol withdrawal syndrome? *Nursing 34*(8): 25.

Sutherland, J., Pavlovich-Davis, S.J. (2006). Coming soon to your neighborhood: meth abuse. Available at https://www.nurse.com/ce/CE395-60/CoursePage/? Accessed May 2009.

The meth epidemic. (2006). Available at http://www.pbs.org/wgbh/pages/frontline/meth/. Accessed December 2008.

When should you ask about cocaine use? (2008). *ED Nursing* 11(10): 115–116.

Chapter 72: Caring for Clients with Dementia and Thought Disorders

Alzheimer's Organization. (2008). Alzheimer's facts and figures. Available at http://www.alz.org/. Accessed December 2008.

Alzheimer's Research Forum. (2008). Drugs in clinical trial. Available at http://www.alzforum.org.drg/drc/detail.asp?id=108. Accessed January 2009.

Beebe, L.H., Smith, K., Crye, C., et al. (2008). Telenursing intervention increases psychiatric medication adherence in schizophrenia outpatients. *Journal of the American Psychiatric Nurses Association 14*(3): 217–224.

Communication style matters with Alzheimer's patients. (2008). *RN 71*(9): 14.

England, M. (2008). Significance of cognitive intervention for voice hearers. *Perspectives in Psychiatric Care* 44(1): 40–47.

Fisher Center for Alzheimer's Research Foundation. (2008). Scientists identify new genes that may be involved in Alzheimer's. Available at http://www.alzinfo.org/newsarticle/templates/newstemplate.asp?articleide=321&zoneid=10. Accessed December 2008.

Garwood, P. (2007). Working with voices: nurse-led delivery of psychosocial interventions. *Mental Health Practice* 10(9): 16–18.

Hawley, K.S., Cherry, K.E. (2008). Memory interventions and quality of life for older adults with dementia. *Activities, Adaptation & Aging* 32(2): 89–102.

Hermanns, M.L.S., & Russell-Broaddus, C.A. (2006). "But I'm not a psych nurse!" *RN* 69(12): 28–32.

Kennedy, G.J., & Leon, L.A. (2008). Recent advances in dementia research. Available at http://wwwprimarypsychiatry.com/aspx/article_pf.aspx?articleid=1881. Accessed January 2009.

Levine, D.S. (2008). Food for thought. Available at http://www.tjols.com/article-509.html. Accessed January 2009.

Mannion, E. (2008). Alzheimer's disease: the psychological and physical effects of the caregiver's role. Part 1. *Nursing Older People* 20(4): 27–32, 39.

Mannion, E. (2008). Alzheimer's disease: the psychological and physical effects of the caregiver's role. Part 2. *Nursing Older People* 20(4): 33–38, 39.

Medical News Today. (2008). Encouraging results from phase 2 clinical trial of bapineuzumab at international conference on Alzheimer's disease. Available at http://www.medicalnewstoday.com/articles/116769.php. Accessed January 2009.

Medical University of South Carolina. (2008) Alzheimer's disease what's new? Available at http://www.muschealth.com/health yaging/alzheimnew.htm. Accessed December 2008.

National Center for Health Statistics. (2008). U.S. mortality drops sharply in 2006, latest data show. Available at http://www.cdc.gov/nchs/pressroom/08newsreleases/mortality2006.htm. Accessed December 2008.

National Institute on Aging. (2008). How does AD begin, and what causes it to progress? Available at http://www.nia.nih.gov/Alzheimer's/Publications/ADProgress2005_2006/Part2/adbegin.htm.htm. Accessed December 2008.

NIH Senior Health. (2007). Alzheimer's disease. Available at http://nihseniorhealth.gov/alzheimersdisease.html. Accessed December 2008.

Peterson, B.L., Fillenbaum, G.G., Pieper, C.F., et al. (2008). Home or nursing home: does place of residence affect longevity in patients with Alzheimer's disease? The experience of CERAD patients. *Public Health Nursing* 25(5): 490–497.

Price, L.M. (2007). Transition to community: a program to help clients with schizophrenia move from inpatient to community care; a pilot study. *Archives of Psychiatric Nursing* 21(6): 336–344.

Qing, H., He, Guiqiong, H., Ly, P., et al. (2008). Valproic acid inhibits $A\beta$ production, neuritic plaque formation, and behavior deficits in Alzheimer's disease mouse models. *Journal of Experimental Medicine* 205(12): 2781–2789.

Rentz, C.A. (2008). Alzheimer's disease: an elusive thief. *Nursing Management* 39(6): 33–39.

Sharer, J. (2008). Tackling sundowning in a patient with Alzheimer's disease. *MEDSURG Nursing* 17(1): 27–29.

Tay, S.C. (2007). Compliance therapy: an intervention to improve inpatients' attitudes toward treatment. *Journal of Psychosocial Nursing & Mental Health Services* 45(6): 29–37.

Usher, K., Foster, K., & Park, T. (2006). The metabolic syndrome and schizophrenia: the latest evidence and nursing guidelines for management. *Journal of Psychiatric & Mental Health Nursing* 13(6): 730–734.

Index

Page numbers followed by followed by "b" denote boxes; those followed by "f" denote figures; those followed by "t" denote tables.

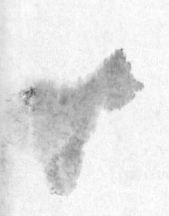

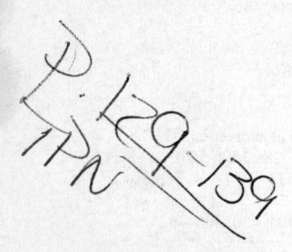